Community Health Nursing

Promoting and Protecting
the Public's Health

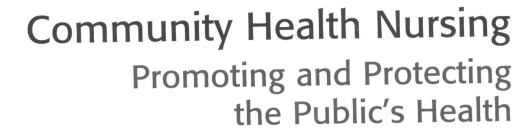

Community Health Nursing
Promoting and Protecting the Public's Health

7th Edition

Judith A. Allender, EdD, MSN, MEd, RN
Professor Emerita of Nursing
Department of Nursing, College of Health and Human Services
California State University, Fresno
Fresno, California

Cherie Rector, PhD, MSN, RN
Professor
Department of Nursing
California State University, Bakersfield
Bakersfield, California

Kristine D. Warner, PhD, MPH, RN
Associate Professor
School of Nursing
California State University, Chico
Chico, California

Wolters Kluwer | Lippincott Williams & Wilkins
Health
Philadelphia · Baltimore · New York · London
Buenos Aires · Hong Kong · Sydney · Tokyo

Senior Acquisitions Editor: Hilarie Surrena
Managing Editor: Katherine Burland
Production Project Manager: Cynthia Rudy
Director of Nursing Production: Helen Ewan
Senior Managing Editor / Production: Erika Kors
Design Coordinator: Joan Wendt
Manufacturing Coordinator: Karin Duffield
Production Services / Compositor: Aptara, Inc.

7th edition

9   8   7   6   5   4   3   2

Printed in China

Library of Congress Cataloging-in-Publication Data

Allender, Judith Ann.
    Community health nursing : promoting and protecting the public's health / Judith A. Allender, Cherie Rector, Kristine D. Warner. — 7th ed.
        p. ; cm.
    Includes bibliographical references and index.
    ISBN-13: 978-0-7817-6584-8
    ISBN-10: 0-7817-6584-6
  1.   Community health nursing. 2.   Public health nursing. I.   Rector, Cherie L. II.   Warner, Kristine D.
III.   Title.
    [DNLM: 1.   Community Health Nursing. 2.   Health Promotion. WY 106 A425c 2010]
    RT98S68 2010
    610.73'43—dc22

                                                                                            2008045578

LWW.com

To my husband Gil, with love and thanks.

Judy Allender

To my husband—my greatest supporter—and to my children and grandchildren, who make it all worthwhile.

Cherie Rector

To my son Sean and his wife Angela, my daughters Erin and Kathleen Whalen, and the best mom in the world, Dolores Warner—thank you for your unwavering love and support.

Kris Warner

About the Authors

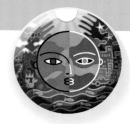

Dr. Judith A. Allender has been a nurse for more than 45 years. For 30 of those years, she taught nursing—first at Good Samaritan Hospital in Cincinnati, Ohio, and later at California State University, Fresno where she retired as a Professor Emerita. Her nursing practice experiences were varied. She worked with surgical patients, in intensive care units, as a school nurse, in-patient hospice, home care, and community health nursing. She has authored five nursing textbooks in addition to this one. During her long career, she received several awards. She was voted RN of the Year in Education for the Central Valley of California in 1998. The fourth edition of this textbook received a Robert Wood Johnson award in 2001 for the end-of-life care content. In 2005, she was inducted into the Central San Joaquin Valley, California Nursing Hall of Fame. Presently, Dr. Allender consults for a nonprofit immigrant and refugee center and writes a weekly health column for a local newspaper. She received her undergraduate nursing degree from the State University of New York in Plattsburgh; a master's degree in guidance and counseling from Xavier University in Cincinnati, Ohio; a master's in nursing from Wright State University in Dayton, Ohio; and a doctorate of education from the University of Southern California. When not busy at home, she can be found traveling around the world. She and her husband have a blended family with five children, 14 grandchildren, and two great-grandchildren.

Dr. Cherie Rector is a native Californian who is currently a Professor at California State University, Bakersfield Department of Nursing, where she teaches community health nursing. She served as director of the School Nurse Credential Program and the RN to BSN Program there and was formerly the coordinator of the School Nurse Credential Program at California State University, Fresno, where she also taught community health nursing. She has served as the director of Allied Health and the Disabled Students Program at College of the Sequoias. She has consulted with school districts and hospitals in the areas of child health, research, and evidence-based practice and has practiced community health and school nursing, as well as neonatal nursing in the acute care setting. She has taught undergraduate and graduate level courses in community health, vulnerable populations, research, and school nursing. Her grants, research, publications, and presentations have focused largely on child and adolescent health, school nursing, nursing education, and disadvantaged students. She earned an associate's degree in nursing from the College of the Sequoias more than 30 years ago, and a bachelor of science in nursing degree from the Consortium of the California State Universities, Long Beach. She has a master's degree in nursing (clinical specialist, community health) and a School Nurse Credential from California State University, Fresno. Her doctorate of philosophy in educational psychology is from the University of Southern California. Dr. Rector and her husband have three grown sons, five grandsons, and a granddaughter.

Dr. Kristine Warner, also a native Californian, is an associate professor at California State University, Chico with a specialization in public/community health nursing. With more than 3 decades of experience in the field of public/community health, she has taught in nursing programs in both Pennsylvania and California. Undergraduate and graduate courses she has taught include community health nursing, nursing research, program planning and development, and health policy. Her nursing career began in adult and pediatric acute care, and she has practiced home care and public health in rural and urban settings. Her current professional interests include evidence-based practice, nursing education, emergency preparedness, and health needs of vulnerable populations. Her grants, research, publications, and presentations have focused on emergency preparedness, poverty, chronic illness, and nutrition. Dr. Warner is a retired Navy Nurse Corps Captain, having ended a 29-year career of both active and reserve service in 2002. She was recalled to active duty and stationed in the Saudi Arabian desert during the first Gulf War as Assistant Charge Nurse of a 20-bed medical unit. She received her bachelor of science in nursing from Harris College of Nursing, Texas Christian University; master of public health (community health nursing) and master of science (community health nursing and nursing education) from the University of South Florida; and doctorate of philosophy in nursing from the University of Pennsylvania. Dr. Warner has three grown children and one daughter-in-law. She was a resident of Germany for 2 years in the early 1980s and has traveled extensively in Europe.

Contributors

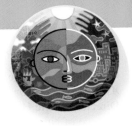

Elizabeth M. Andal, CNS, PhD, FAAN
Professor
Department of Nursing
California State University, Bakersfield
Bakersfield, California

Margaret Avila, MSN, MS, PHN, RN/NP
Assistant Professor
Mt. St. Mary's College
Los Angeles, California

Barbara J. Blake, RN, PhD, ACRN
Associate Professor
Kennesaw State University
WellStar School of Nursing
Kennesaw, Georgia

Lydia C. Bourne, BSN, RN, MA
Legislative Advocate
Bourne & Associates
Sacramento, California

Marie P. Farrell, EdD, MPH, RN, FAAN, ACC
Professor
Fielding Graduate University
Santa Barbara, California

Sheila Hoban, EdD, RN
Licensed Clinical Psychologist
Associate Professor
School of Nursing
California State University, Chico
Chico, California

Sheila M. Holcomb, EdD(c), RN, MSN
Clinical Faculty
Department of Nursing
Sacramento State University
Sacramento, California
School Nurse
Folsom Cordova Unified School District
Folsom, California

Mary Lashley, PhD, RN, APRN-BC
Professor
Community Health Nursing
Towson University
Towson, Maryland

Karin Lightfoot, MSN(c), RN-BC, PHN
Public Health Nurse II
Public Health Branch
Shasta County Department of Health & Human Services
Shasta County, California

Filomela A. Marshall, RN, EdD
Consultant
School of Nursing
Thomas Edison State College
Trenton, New Jersey

Erin D. Maughan, RN-BC, MS, PhD
Assistant Professor
College of Nursing
Brigham Young University
Provo, Utah

Debra Millar, MSN, RN
Senior Health Advisor
CHF International
Silver Spring, Maryland

Mary Ellen Miller, PhD, RN
Assistant Professor
Department of Nursing and Health
DeSales University
Center Valley, Pennsylvania

Cherie Rector, PhD, RN
Professor
Department of Nursing
California State University, Bakersfield
Bakersfield, California

Kathleen Riley-Lawless, RN, PhD, PNP-BC
Assistant Professor
School of Nursing
University of Delaware
Newark, Delaware
Pediatric Nurse Practitioner
Nemours/Alfred I. duPont Hospital for Children
Wilmington, Delaware

Phyllis G. Salopek, MSN, FNP
Assistant Professor
School of Nursing
California State University, Chico
Chico, California

Christine L. Savage, RN, PhD, CARN
Associate Professor
Director, Public Health Nursing Masters Program
College of Nursing
Associate Professor
Master of Public Health Program, College of Medicine
University of Cincinnati
Cincinnati, Ohio

Karen Smith-Sayer, RN, MSN
Immunization Coordinator and Communicable
Disease Control PHN
Nevada County Public Health Department
Nevada County, California

Mary E. Summers, PhD, MSN, RN, PHN
Professor Emeritus
Department of Nursing
Sacramento State University
Sacramento, California

Gloria Ann Jones Taylor, DSN, RNc
Professor
Kennesaw State University
WellStar School of Nursing
Kennesaw, Georgia

Rose Utley, PhD, RN, CNE
Associate Professor
Director, Nurse Educator Graduate Programs
Missouri State University
Springfield, Missouri

Kristine D. Warner, PhD, MPH, RN
Associate Professor
School of Nursing
California State University, Chico
Chico, California

Frances Wilson, RNC, MSN, OCN, PHN
Clinical Nurse Specialist
Acute Care Services/Telemetry
Kern Medical Center
Bakersfield, California

Joyce Zerwekh, EdD, RN
Director
Bachelor of Science Nursing Degree Program
College of Health & Human Services
Concordia University
Portland, Oregon

Reviewers

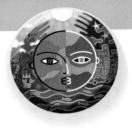

JoAnn Abegglen, APRN, MS, PNP
Brigham Young University
Provo, Utah

Joseph Adepoju, PhD, MA, BSN
Delaware State University
Dover, Delaware

Dolores Aguilar, RN, MS, APN
University of Texas, Arlington
Arlington, Texas

Jo Azzarello, PhD, RN
University of Oklahoma Health Science Center
Oklahoma City, Oklahoma

Margaret Bassett, MPH, MS, RN
Radford University
Radford, Virginia

Joyce Begley, BSN, MA, MSN
Eastern Kentucky University
Richmond, Kentucky

Carol Beltz, MSN, RN
Kent State University
Kent, Ohio

Anne Bongiorno, PhD, RN
SUNY Plattsburgh
Plattsburgh, New York

Cindy Bork, EdD, RN
Winona State University
Winona, Minnesota

Mary Bouchaud, RN, MSN
Thomas Jefferson University
Philadelphia, Pennsylvania

Kathleen Brewer, PhD, APRN, BC
Kansas State University Medical Center
Kansas City, Kansas

Alice Brnicky, MS, RN, BS
Texas Woman's University
Denton, Texas

Kathryn Burks, PhD, RN
University of Missouri, Columbia
Columbia, Missouri

Bonnie Callen, PhD, MA
University of Tennessee, Chattanooga
Chattanooga, Tennessee

Wilma Calvert, PhD, RN, BSN, MPE
University of Missouri, St. Louis
St. Louis, Missouri

JoAnne Carrick, RN, MSN
Penn State University
State College, Pennsylvania

Deborah Chaulk, MS, APRN, BC
University of Massachusetts, Lowell
Lowell, Massachusetts

Mary Clark, PhD, RN, BSN
University of Iowa
Iowa City, Iowa

Nancy Donovan
University of Pittsburgh School of Nursing
Pittsburgh, Pennsylvania

Mary Gallagher Gordon, MSN, RN, CNE
Drexel University
Philadelphia, Pennsylvania

Anita Hansberry
Southern University Baton Rouge
Baton Rouge, Louisiana

Sheila Hartung, PhD, RNC, BSN, MSN
Bloomsburg University of Pennsylvania
Bloomsburg, Pennsylvania

Margaret Kaiser, RN, PhD
University of Nebraska Medical Center
Omaha, Nebraska

Vicky Kent, PhD, RN
Towson University
Towson, Maryland

Judith Keswick
California State University Stanislaus
Turlock, California

Cheryl Krause-Parello, PhD, RN
Kean University
Union, New Jersey

Lynette Landry, PhD, MS, BSN
San Francisco State University
San Francisco, California

Mary Lashley, RN, PhD
Towson University
Towson, Maryland

Sandra Leh, MSN, BSN, DNS
Cedar Crest College
Allentown, Pennsylvania

Sherill Leifer, PhD, RN
Milwaukee School of Engineering
Milwaukee, Wisconsin

Shelly Luger, BSN, BA
Indiana State University
Terre Haute, Indiana

Beth Luthy, APRN, FNP-C
Brigham Young University
Provo, Utah

Carolyn Mason, MS, RN
Miami University of Ohio
Oxford, Ohio

Terran Mathers, RN, DNS
Spring Hill College
Mobile, Alabama

Erin D. Maughan, RN-BC, MS, PhD
College of Nursing
Brigham Young University
Provo, Utah

Susan McMarlin, RN, BSN, MSN, EdD
University of North Florida
Jacksonville, Florida

Phyllis More
Bloomfield College
Bloomfield, New Jersey

Nancy Mosca, PhD, RN, CS
Youngstown State University
Youngstown, Ohio

Ruth Mullins-Berg, PhD, RN, CPNP
California State University, Long Beach
Long Beach, California

Carol Ormond, MS
Georgia College & State University
Milledgeville, Georgia

DeAnne Parrott, BSN, MS
Oklahoma City University
Oklahoma City, Oklahoma

Cindy Parsons, BSN, MSN
University of Tampa
Tampa, Florida

Jenny Radsma, RN, MN
University of Maine at Fort Kent
Fort Kent, Maine

Rebecca Randall, MS, RN, BA
South Dakota State University
Brookings, South Dakota

Delbert Raymond, BSN, MSN, PhD
Wayne State University
Detroit, Michigan

Bobbie Reddick, EdD, MSN, PhD
Winston Salem State University
Winston Salem, North Carolina

Jerelyn Resnick, RN, PhD
University of Washington
Bothell, Washington

Will Anne Ricer
New Mexico State University, Las Cruces
Las Cruces, New Mexico

Carol Sapp, RN
Georgia College & State University
Milledgeville, Georgia

Charlotte Schober
Union College
Lincoln, Nebraska

Preface

The seventh edition of *Community Health Nursing: Promoting and Protecting the Public's Health* continues in the tradition of the previous editions of this text, beginning with Barbara Spradley's initial publication in 1981. The purpose of this textbook is to introduce undergraduate nursing students to the stimulating world of nursing outside the acute care setting—whether at a public health department, community health agency, school, or other setting. We hope to share our enthusiasm and devotion to this population-focused, community-oriented form of nursing. Compared with acute care nurses, those working in public or community health are often more autonomous and exert a greater influence on the overall health of their communities by being political advocates for their clients and aggregates.

This book is designed to give students a basic grounding in the principles of public health nursing and introduce them to key populations they may engage while working in the community setting. Entry-level public health nurses may also find it a helpful resource as they begin to familiarize themselves with their unique practice settings and target populations. The nexus of public health nursing lies in the utilization of public health principles along with nursing science and skills in order to promote health, prevent disease, and protect at-risk populations. We use the term *community health nurse* interchangeably with *public health nurse* to describe the practitioner who does not simply "work in the community" (physically located outside the hospital setting, in the community), but rather one who has a focus on nursing and public health science that informs their community-based, population-focused nursing practice.

ABOUT THE SEVENTH EDITION

This textbook has always strived to be a user-friendly resource for nursing students who are new to public health nursing, and this new edition is no exception. We have attempted to write in a style that is accessible to students, with a conversational quality and minimal use of unnecessary jargon and dry narrative. Throughout the book, we have made liberal use of case studies and highlighted student, practitioner, and instructor perspectives on pertinent issues. This is done to help students more readily grasp and apply necessary information to their real clients and better understand the common issues and problems they will face in this new area of nursing study. At the same time, our goal is to provide the most accurate, pertinent, and current information for students and faculty. We have sought out experts in various fields and specialty areas of public health nursing in order to provide a balanced and complete result. With the addition of more than 20 new contributors from across the country, the content reflects a broad spectrum of views and expertise.

ORGANIZATION OF THE TEXT

The seventh edition has five fewer chapters than the sixth edition, having been reorganized to combine some related topics while reducing duplication in other areas. We have chosen to continue the emphasis on *Healthy People 2010* goals and objectives throughout the text and to maintain a research emphasis by providing examples of evidence-based practice where applicable.

The book is now organized into eight units, with revised unit titles to better reflect content covered. In addition, some content has shifted to better align with the new units. The eighth unit was added to encompass the various settings for public health nursing practice or community-based nursing.

Unit 1, Foundations of Community Health Nursing, describes the core public health functions (Chapter 3), as well as the basic public health concepts of health, illness, wellness, community, aggregate, population, and levels of prevention (Chapter 1). Leading health indicators are introduced, along with *Healthy People 2010* goals and objectives (Chapter 1). The rich history of public health nursing is examined, along with social influences that have shaped our current practice (Chapter 2). Educational preparation is discussed, as well as the roles and functions of public health nurses (Chapters 2 and 3). Common settings for public health nursing are introduced (Chapter 3), and values, ethical principles, and decision making are also considered (Chapter 4). Evidence-based practice and research principles relating to community health nursing are discussed, along with the nurse's role in utilizing current research (Chapter 4). Cultural principles are defined and the importance of cultural diversity and sensitivity in public health nursing are highlighted, as well as cultural assessment and folk remedies (Chapter 5).

Unit 2, Public Health Essentials for Community Health Nursing, covers the structure of public health within the health system infrastructure, along with a basic overview of the economics of health care (Chapter 6). Epidemiology and communicable disease are examined, and principles of disease investigation and surveillance are explored from both an historical and practical perspective (Chapters 7 and 8). Chapter 9 focuses on issues of environmental health with particular attention to areas of concern to community health nursing practice. Emphasis is placed on prevention and using an ecological approach when addressing issues of environmental health and safety.

Unit 3, Community Health Nursing Toolbox, examines tools used by the public health nurse to ensure effectiveness in his or her practice. Communication and collaboration, as well as contracting with clients, are essential skills that must be mastered by all community health nurses (Chapter 10). Health promotion is examined in Chapter 11 with particular emphasis on achieving behavioral change through educational methodologies. Chapter 12 focuses on planning and developing community health programs with attention to the practical steps needed to achieve successful outcomes. Social marketing as an emerging tool in community health programs and grant funding are also explored. The community health nurse is an advocate for clients, and a basic knowledge of policy-making, political advocacy, and client empowerment strategies is needed (Chapter 13).

Unit 4, The Community as Client, examines the theoretical basis for public health nursing (Chapter 14). Moving the student's focus from the individual patient to the community as their client is emphasized in Chapter 15, as are community assessment strategies and resources. Chapter 16 describes the global community in which we now live, and provides examples of international health problems and practices. The timely topics of disaster and terrorism are covered in Chapter 17, with emphasis on the role of the community health nurse in emergency preparedness, both personally and professionally.

Unit 5, The Family as Client, introduces theoretical frameworks for promoting family health and better understanding and working with family dysfunctions (Chapter 18). Family assessment and application of the nursing process are included in Chapter 19. Chapter 20 examines family violence, spousal and child abuse, and effective measures that can be utilized by the community health nurse to provide resources and education.

Unit 6, Promoting and Protecting the Health of Aggregates with Developmental Needs, provides information about client groups as they are often delineated by public health departments—maternal–child and infants (Chapter 21), children and adolescents (Chapter 22), adult women's and men's health (Chapter 23), and the elderly (Chapter 24). These particular chapters can be very helpful in targeted health efforts for select population groups and build upon the content presented in Unit 5.

Unit 7, Promoting and Protecting the Health of Vulnerable Populations, examines theoretical frameworks, basic principles of vulnerability, and effective methods of working with vulnerable clients (Chapter 25). Clients with chronic illnesses and disabilities are also included (Chapter 26), as well as those with behavioral health problems, such as mental health and substance abuse (Chapter 27). The homeless client and the impact of poverty on these individuals and families are discussed in Chapter 28. Chapter 29 covers the unique challenges of rural and urban health care in terms of health care needs and types of service delivery options. The particular needs of migrant populations and issues of social justice are also explored.

Unit 8, Settings for Community Health Nursing, examines public (Chapter 30) and private (Chapter 31) settings in more depth. These chapters provide overviews of a number of practice options available to both new and experienced nurses. There is a vast array of opportunities for practice in public/community health, and this section is designed to enhance understanding of some of those options. Finally, the important roles of home health and hospice nursing are discussed in Chapter 32. With the aging of our population, many nurses are finding this practice area a challenging and satisfying option.

NEW AND REVISED CHAPTERS

Each of the chapters maintained from the sixth edition has been rigorously updated to provide clear and accurate information. Some content has been maintained, but reorganized into the new chapter format to keep the textbook to a manageable length and to enhance student learning. We are particularly pleased to present seven chapters that have been completely rewritten to reflect changes in nursing knowledge and to provide a fresh approach to valuable content. Chapter 12, on planning and developing community programs, now emphasizes the need for rigorous collaboration with community groups to both identify and solve health problems. Unit 7 contains three completely new chapters focusing on vulnerable populations, including how to work with vulnerable clients (Chapter 25), the unique aspects of behavioral health in the community (Chapter 27), and the homeless (Chapter 28). Chapter 26, dealing with disabilities and chronic illness, was new to the sixth edition, and has been updated and expanded here. Unit 8 is entirely new, with Chapters 30 and 31 focusing on practice settings in the public and private sector. Chapter 32 continues with the vital role of home care and hospice nursing in the aging of our population.

KEY FEATURES

The seventh edition of *Community Health Nursing: Promoting and Protecting the Public's Health* includes key features from previous editions as well as new ones. Features continued from previous editions include:

- An emphasis on aggregate-level nursing and the community health nurse's opportunity and responsibility not only to serve individuals and families, but also to promote and protect the health of communities and populations.
- An emphasis on health promotion, health protection, and illness prevention. This, in addition to the aggregate emphasis, reflects the view set forth in this text that community health nursing is the amalgamation of nursing science with public health science. Public health philosophy, values, knowledge, and skills are an essential part of all community health nursing practice.
- A balance of theory with application to nursing practice. The seventh edition continues the presentation of theoretical and conceptual knowledge to provide an understanding of human needs and a rationale for nursing actions. At the same time, the text presents practical information on the use of theory to undergird practice.
- A *Summary* of highlights at the end of each chapter provides an overview of material covered and serves as a review for study.
- *References* and *Selected Readings* at the end of each chapter provide you with classic sources, current research, and a broad base of authoritative information for furthering knowledge on each chapter's subject matter.
- A student-friendly writing style has been a hallmark of this text since the first edition. Topics are expressed and concepts explained to enhance understanding and capture interest. Writing style remains consistent throughout the

text (including contributed chapters) to promote an uninterrupted flow of ideas and enhance learning.

- *Internet Resources* have been improved and are included in nearly every chapter for quick and easy student reference.
- *Learning Objectives* and *Key Terms* sharpen the reader's focus and provide a quick guide for learning the chapter content.
- *Activities to Promote Critical Thinking* at the close of each chapter are designed to challenge students, promote critical-thinking skills, and encourage active involvement in solving community health problems. They include Internet activities, where appropriate.
- Recurring *displays, tables,* and *figures* throughout the text highlight important content and create points of interest for student learning.
- *Levels of Prevention Pyramid* boxes enhance understanding of the levels of prevention concept, basic to community health nursing. Each box addresses a chapter topic, describes nursing actions at each of the three levels of prevention, and is unique to this text in its complexity and comprehensiveness.
- Additional assessment tools can be found throughout the chapters. They are added to enhance assessment skills of aggregates, families, or individuals in unique situations.

FEATURES NEW TO THIS EDITION

Additional recurring displays new to this edition include:

- *Evidence-based Practice*—this feature incorporates current research examples and how they can be applied to public/community health nursing practice to achieve optimal client/aggregate outcomes.
- *From the Case Files*—presentation of a scenario/case study with student-centered, application-based questions. Emphasizing nursing process, students are challenged to reflect on assessment and intervention in typical yet challenging examples.
- *Perspectives*—this feature is included in most chapters and provides stories (viewpoints) from a variety of

sources. The perspective may be from a nursing student, a novice or experienced public health nurse, a faculty member, a policy maker, or a client. These short features are designed to promote critical thinking, reflect on commonly held misconceptions about public/community health nursing, or to recognize the link between skills learned in this specialty practice and other practice settings, especially acute care hospitals.

- New art has been added throughout the text to clarify important concepts and enhance interest in and understanding of material.

RESOURCES FOR INSTRUCTORS

A set of tools to assist you in teaching your course is available at http://thepoint.lww.com/allender7e. **thePoint*** is Lippincott Williams & Wilkins' web-based course and content management system that provides every resource instructors need in one easy-to-use site.

If, as an instructor, you want help structuring your lessons...
We've provided PowerPoint slides, which condense the material into bulleted lists, figures, and tables.

If you'd like your students to engage in further study of the material, beyond what's provided in the textbook...
We've provided journal articles and a listing of internet resources to facilitate research.

If you'd like your students to start applying what they've learned...
We've provided a set of case studies associated with units of the book to get students thinking about how their nursing knowledge works in real-world scenarios.

If you're concerned about preparing your students for the NCLEX exams...
We've provided a Test Generator that includes unique questions for each chapter. These questions are presented in traditional and in alternate-form NCLEX style, so students will become familiar with the format of the exams.

---

*thePoint is a trademark of Wolters Kluwer Health.

Acknowledgments

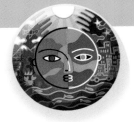

We are grateful to those who helped with the writing and publication of this text. To the contributors who brought their wealth of knowledge and experience to bear in writing their chapters, we acknowledge our debt and gratitude. We also thank former contributors whose work may remain, in part, in this edition. We appreciate the assistance of many other colleagues and friends who served as "sounding boards" and cheerleaders, and those who contributed ideas and suggestions, among them Linda Olsen Keller from the University of Minnesota; Dr. Linda Hewett from the University of California San Francisco and the Alzheimer's & Memory Center; Lieutenant Commander A. Karen Bryant from the U.S. Public Health Service; and Travis Hunter, RN, from the Utah State Prison.

To our managing editors, Katherine Burland and Betsy Gentzler, and acquisitions editor, Margaret Zuccarini, along with other staff at Lippincott Williams & Wilkins, we express our thanks.

We are in debt to our family and friends who "suffered" through this experience with us. We appreciate your flexibility and encouragement.

Contents

Chapter 9
Environmental Health and Safety 242

Kristine D. Warner

Unit 3
Community Health Nursing Toolbox

Chapter 10
Communication, Collaboration, and Contracting 276

Cherie Rector

Chapter 11
Health Promotion: Achieving Change Through Education 300

Kristine D. Warner, Debra Millar

Chapter 12
Planning and Developing Community Programs and Services 332

Mary E. Summers, Kristine D. Warner

Chapter 13
Policy Making and Community Health Advocacy 353

Lydia C. Bourne

UNIT 4
The Community as Client

Chapter 14
Theoretical Basis of Community Health Nursing 374

Kristine D. Warner, Karin Lightfoot

Chapter 15
Community as Client: Applying the Nursing Process 390

Filomela A. Marshall

Unit 7
Promoting and Protecting the Health of
Vulnerable Populations

Unit 8
Settings for Community Health Nursing

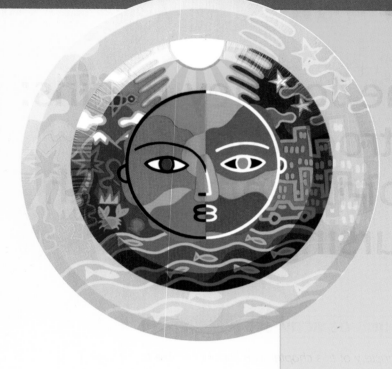

FOUNDATIONS OF COMMUNITY HEALTH NURSING

1

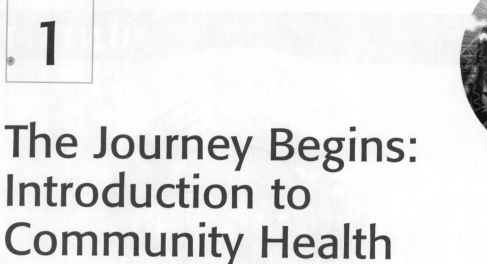

The Journey Begins: Introduction to Community Health Nursing

LEARNING OBJECTIVES

Upon mastery of this chapter, you should be able to:

◆ Define community health and distinguish it from public health.
◆ Explain the concept of community.
◆ Diagram the health continuum.
◆ Name three of the 10 leading health indicators.
◆ Discuss ways that public health nursing (PHN) practice is linked to acute care nursing practice.
◆ Discuss the two main components of community health practice (health promotion and disease prevention).
◆ Differentiate among the three levels of prevention.
◆ Describe the eight characteristics of community health nursing.

"A generation that acquires knowledge without ever understanding how that knowledge can benefit the community is a generation that is not learning what it means to be citizens in a democracy."

—Elizabeth L. Hollander, Author (1817–1885)

Opportunities and challenges in nursing are boundless and ever-changing. You have spent a lot of time and effort learning how to care for individual patients in medical-surgical and other acute-care oriented nursing specialties. Now you are entering a unique and exciting area of nursing—community/public health.

As one of the oldest specialty nursing practices, community health nursing offers unique challenges and opportunities. A nurse entering this field will encounter the complex challenge of working with populations rather than just individual clients, and the opportunity to carry on the heritage of early public health nursing efforts with the benefit of modern sensibilities. There is the challenge of expanding nursing's focus from the individual and family to encompass communities and the opportunity to affect the health status of populations. There also is the challenge of determining the needs of populations at risk and the opportunity to design interventions to address their needs. There is the challenge of learning the complexities of a constantly changing health care system and the opportunity to help shape service delivery. Community health nursing is community-based and, most importantly, it is population-focused. Operating within an environment of rapid change and increasingly complex challenges, this field of nursing holds the potential to shape the quality of community health services and improve the health of the general public.

You have provided nursing care in familiar acute care settings for the very ill, both young and old, but always with other professionals at your side. You have worked as part of a team, in close proximity, to welcome a new life, reestablish a client's health, or comfort someone toward a peaceful death. Now, you are being asked to leave the familiarity of the acute care setting and go out into the community—into homes, schools, recreational facilities, work settings, parishes, and even street corners that are familiar to your clients and unfamiliar to you. Here, you will find minimal or no monitoring devices, no charts full of laboratory data, nor professional and allied health workers at your side to assist you. You will be asked to use the nontangible skills of listening, assessing, planning, teaching, coordinating, evaluating, and referring. You will also draw on the skills you have learned through your acute care setting experiences (e.g., psychiatric mental health nursing, maternal child health nursing, medical surgical nursing), and begin to "think on your feet" in new and exciting situations. Often, your practice will be solo, and you will need to combine creativity, ingenuity, intuition, and resourcefulness along with these skills. You will be providing care not only to individuals but also to families and other groups in a variety of settings within the community. Talk about boundless opportunities and challenges! (See Perspectives: Student Voices.)

You may feel that this is too demanding. You may be anxious about how you will perform in this new setting. But perhaps, just perhaps, you might find that this new area is a rewarding kind of nursing—one that constantly challenges you, interests you, and allows you to work holistically with clients of all ages, at all stages of illness and wellness; one that absolutely demands the use of your critical-thinking skills. And you may decide, when you finish your community health nursing course, that you have found your career choice. Even if you are not drawn away from acute care nursing, your community health nursing experience will give you a deeper understanding of the people for whom you provide care—where and how they live, the family and cultural dynamics at play, and the problems they will face when discharged from your care. You will also discover myriad community agencies and resources to better assist you in providing a continuum of care for your clients. Finding out begins with understanding the concepts of community and health.

This chapter provides an overview of the basic concepts of community and health, the components of community health practice, and the salient characteristics of contemporary community health nursing practice, so that you can enter this field of nursing in concert with its intentions. The opportunities and challenges of community health nursing will become even more apparent as the chapter progresses. The discussion of the concepts and theories that make community health nursing an important specialty within nursing begins with the broader field of community health, which provides the context for community health nursing practice.

COMMUNITY HEALTH

Human beings are social creatures. All of us, with rare exception, live out our lives in the company of other people. An Eskimo lives in a small, tightly knit community of close relatives; a rural Mexican may live in a small village with hardly more than 200 members. In contrast, someone from New York City might be a member of many overlapping communities, such as professional societies, a political party, a religious group, a cultural society, a neighborhood, and the city itself. Even those who try to escape community membership always begin their lives in some type of group, and usually they continue to depend on groups for material and emotional support. Communities are an essential and permanent feature of the human experience.

The communities in which we live and work have a profound influence on our collective health and well-being (World Health Organization [WHO], 2006a). And, since the beginning, people have attempted to create healthier communities. Here are three recent examples:

- Asthma currently affects more than 31 million Americans—over three times the number reported in 1980. Worldwide, the number of asthma cases has increased 50% each decade, with over a quarter of a million people dying from asthma in 2005. Asthma-related costs are estimated to exceed those for tuberculosis and HIV/AIDS combined (Associated Press, 2006). Evidence of a connection between asthma attacks and community environments has been demonstrated both in the United States and abroad. In Harlem, 25% of the children were reported to have asthma—twice the expected rate. Public health officials note chronic environmental factors as a possible cause for increased asthma cases; pollution from high-traffic areas, secondhand smoke in homes, as well as poor living conditions characterized by dust mites, mold, industrial air pollution, mouse and cockroach droppings, and animal dander (Krisberg, 2006). In Atlanta, the 1996 Olympics brought an unexpected benefit; a 42% reduction in asthma-related

PERSPECTIVES
STUDENT VOICES

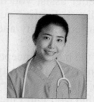

I was really terrified when I got to my community health rotation and found that I had to go to people's homes and knock on their doors! I was going to graduate in a few months, and I felt really comfortable in the hospital. . . . I knew the routines and the machines well. Now, I had to actually find houses and apartments in an area of the city I would normally never venture into! And, it wasn't clear to me what I was supposed to do! I didn't have much equipment—a baby scale, a blood pressure cuff, a stethoscope, a thermometer, and a paper tape measure—that was all! I was told to go visit this 16-year-old mother who had a 4-month-old baby, and to monitor the baby's progress. I don't even have children! What can I tell her? And, besides, she is a teenager who "knows it all." My clinical instructor told me to "build a relationship with her" and to "gain trust and rapport." That is hard to do when you are scared to death! I was afraid of her responses, of being out in that part of the city alone, and of trying to answer questions without anyone there to turn to. But, I wanted to get through nursing school, so I drove over there and knocked on her door. I was shocked to see the condition of the apartment building in which she lived. Peeling paint, loud music, trash everywhere, and strange characters at every turn. When she answered the door, she seemed uninterested—or maybe a little defensive. I told her who I was and why I was there, and she motioned me inside and pointed toward the baby, propped up on the tattered couch. I spent the next 15 weeks visiting Anna and her baby; weighing and measuring the baby, doing a Denver II and sharing the results with Anna, helping her schedule appointments for immunizations, listening to Anna's story of abuse and abandonment, and

realizing that what I was doing was actually exciting and rewarding. By the end of my rotation, I was truly going to miss Anna and little José! He always smiled at me, and I enjoyed "playing" with him as I instructed her about baby-proofing her apartment, finding resources for food and clothing, and getting birth control. We even talked about how she could finish high school. I thought about Anna and José occasionally, when young mothers would bring their babies into the emergency department, where I worked after graduation. I learned from my community health nursing rotation that I needed to look beyond the bravado of a teenage mother and try to "connect" with her in order to assure that she would follow through with the antibiotics and antipyretics we were prescribing for her baby's dangerously high fever and serious infection. A year and a half after I graduated, one day when it had been particularly hectic but was now calming down, I glanced up to see Anna and José. She looked so relieved to see me! She was frantic with worry about the serious burn José had on his right hand. The other nurses were mumbling about "child abuse" and how "irresponsible teen mothers always were." I learned that Anna had left José with a neighbor for an hour while she visited a nearby high school to see about getting her GED. The older neighbor was not used to dealing with a busy toddler, and she had left the handle of a pan of refried beans where José could reach it. The team treated José's burn, and I gave Anna instructions for follow-up care. The bond we had developed was still there. She trusted me, and I knew that she would follow through with the instructions. I also knew that the other nurses who were making comments about her did not know Anna's circumstances. I feel that I am a more effective ER nurse because of the things I learned in community health. Someday, when I get tired of the hospital, I may try working as a Public Health Nurse. You never know!

Courtney, Age 25

emergency room visits. With the Olympic congestion downtown, Atlanta restricted traffic and thus improved air quality. Internationally, Singapore also noticed a reduction in emergency room visits for asthma after it restricted automobile traffic in its central business district (*Milestones in Public Health*, 2006).

◆ Before the historic Surgeon General's *Report on Smoking and Health*, it was common to see people smoking on television, at work, in restaurants, and even in physician offices. Since that report linked tobacco to disease and death more than 40 years ago, much has changed in our living spaces. In most states, it is now uncommon to see smoking in public places, and smokers are often relegated to outdoor smoking areas. However, tobacco is still the leading cause of preventable disease and death in the United States (*Milestones in Public Health*, 2006). While U.S. consumption of tobacco

products has dropped by more than half, it is estimated that almost 5 million people die each year because of tobacco-related illnesses (*Morbidity and Mortality Weekly Report* [MMWR], 2006). With our present focus on bioterrorism, it is interesting to note the findings of a recent study showing that the worldwide mortality burden from tobacco averages 5,700 times that of international terrorism; in the United States, tobacco-related mortality is 1,700 times greater than terrorism-related mortality, and in Russia it is 12,900 greater (Thomson & Wilson, 2005). With the assistance of the Master Settlement Agreement negotiated by state attorneys general and the tobacco industry in 1999, $206 billion has been given to states to promote smoking cessation; create smoke-free environments in the workplace, restaurants, and bars; and develop antismoking public information campaigns (*Milestones in Public Health*, 2006). This is due to wide acceptance of the research showing deleterious effects of secondhand smoke for nonsmoking bystanders (*MMWR*, 2004).

♦ Exercise promotes health, and many people enjoy riding bicycles as a form of recreational exercise. However, risks for bicycle-related injury exist. State laws that require the use of helmets for bicyclists reduce the risk of head injuries (Macpherson, To, Macarthur, Chipman, Wright, & Parkin, 2002). Rodgers (2002, p. 42) found that state helmet laws significantly increased the use of bicycle helmets by children and adolescents. It is estimated that over 100,000 bicycle-related head injuries and over $81 million in direct health costs and $2.3 billion in indirect health costs could have been prevented if all bicycle riders wore helmets (Schulman, Sacks, & Provenzano, 2002). In many states, motorcyclists must also wear helmets, and research has found that helmet use decreases the severity of injuries and mortality rates (Hundley, Kilgo, Miller, Chang, Hensberry, Meredith, & Hoth, 2004). This study also showed that riders without helmets "monopolize hospital resources, incur higher hospital charges" and that the cost of caring for them is often borne by the larger community (p. 1091). In Florida, where the universal helmet law was amended to exclude those riders who were insured and over the age of 21, the death rate for motorcyclists increased significantly with a 25% greater likelihood of death (Kyrychenko & McCartt, 2006).

Just as systems theory reminds us that a whole is greater than the sum of its parts, the health of a community is more than the sum of the health of its individual citizens. A community that achieves a high level of wellness is composed of healthy citizens, functioning in an environment that protects and promotes health. Community health, as a field of practice, seeks to provide organizational structure, a broad set of resources, and the collaborative activities needed to accomplish the goal of an optimally healthy community.

When you worked in hospitals or other acute care settings, your primary focus was the individual patient. Patients' families were viewed as ancillary. Community health, however, broadens the view to focus on families, aggregates, populations, and the community at large. The community becomes the recipient of service, and health becomes the product. Viewed from another perspective, community health is concerned with the interchange between population groups and their total environment, and with the impact of that interchange on collective health. The narrow view of the solitary patient, so common in acute care nursing, is expanded to encompass a much wider vista.

Although many believe that health and illness are individual issues, evidence indicates that they are also community issues; and that the world is a community. The spread of the human immunodeficiency virus (HIV) pandemic, nationally and internationally, is a dramatic and tragic case in point, having spread to the "furthest corners of the world" (Coovadia & Hadingham, 2005, p. 1). Other community, national, and global concerns include the rising incidence and prevalence of tuberculosis (Zumla & Mullan, 2006), cardiovascular disease (WHO, 2006b), antibiotic resistance

(Zhang, Eggleston, Rotimi, & Zeckhauser, 2006), terrorism, and pollution-driven environmental hazards. While the United States fights rising rates of obesity, many countries in Africa battle malnutrition and starvation. Communities can influence the spread of disease, provide barriers to protect members from health hazards, organize ways to combat outbreaks of infectious disease, and promote practices that contribute to individual and collective health (Institute of Medicine [IOM], 1998; American Nurses Association [ANA], 2005).

Many different professionals work in community health to form a complex team. The city planner designing an urban renewal project necessarily becomes involved in community health. The social worker providing counseling about child abuse or working with adolescent substance abusers is involved in community health. A physician treating clients affected by a sudden outbreak of hepatitis and seeking to find the source is engaged in community health practice. Prenatal clinics, meals for the elderly, genetic counseling centers, and educational programs for the early detection of cancer all are part of the community health effort.

The professional nurse is an integral member of this team, a linch-pin and a liaison between physicians, social workers, government officials, and law enforcement officers. Community health nurses work in every conceivable kind of community agency, from a state public health department to a community-based advocacy group. Their duties range from examining infants in a well-baby clinic, to teaching elderly stroke victims in their homes, to carrying out epidemiologic research or engaging in health policy analysis and decision-making. Despite its breadth, however, community health nursing is a specialized practice. It combines all of the basic elements of professional clinical nursing with public health and community practice. Together, we will examine the unique contribution made by community health nursing to our health care system.

Community health and public health share many features. Both are organized community efforts aimed at the promotion, protection, and preservation of the public's health. Historically, as a field of practice, public health has been associated primarily with the efforts of official or government entities—for example, federal, state, or local tax-supported health agencies that target a wide range of health issues. In contrast, private health efforts or nongovernmental organizations (NGOs), such as those of the American Lung Association or the American Cancer Society, work toward solving selected health problems. The latter augments the former. Currently, public health practice encompasses both approaches and works collaboratively with all health agencies and efforts, public or private, which are concerned with the public's health. In this text, community health practice refers to a focus on specific, designated communities. It is a part of the larger public health effort and recognizes the fundamental concepts and principles of public health as its birthright and foundation for practice.

In the IOM's landmark publication, *The Future of the Public's Health* (1998), the mission of public health is defined simply as "fulfilling society's interest in assuring conditions in which people can be healthy" (p. 7). Winslow's classic 1920 definition of **public health** still holds true and forms the basis for our understanding of community health in this text:

Public health . . . is the science and art of preventing disease, prolonging life, and promoting health and efficiency through organized community efforts for the sanitation of the environment, the control of communicable infections, the education of the individual in personal hygiene, the organization of medical and nursing services for the early diagnosis and preventive treatment of disease, and the development of the social machinery to insure everyone a standard of living adequate for the maintenance of health. (Clinton County Health Department, 2006, p. 1)

More recent and concise definitions of public health include "an effort organized by society to protect, promote, and restore the people's health" (Trust for America's Health, 2006, p. 27) and "the health of the population as a whole rather than medical health care, which focuses on treatment of the individual ailment" (Public Health Data Standards Consortium, 2006, p. 120). The core public health functions have been delineated as assessment, policy development, and assurance. These will be discussed in more detail in Chapter 3.

Given this basic understanding of public health, the concept of community health can be defined. **Community health** is the identification of needs, along with the protection and improvement of collective health, within a geographically defined area.

One of the challenges community health practice faces is to remain responsive to the community's health needs. As a result, its structure is complex; numerous health services and programs are currently available or will be developed. Examples include health education, family planning, accident prevention, environmental protection, immunization, nutrition, early periodic screening and developmental testing, school programs, mental health services, occupational health programs, and the care of vulnerable populations. The Department of Homeland Security, for example, is a community health and safety agency developed in the aftermath of the terrorist attack on New York City and Washington, D.C., on September 11, 2001.

Community health practice, a part of public health, is sometimes misunderstood. Even many health professionals think of community health practice in limiting terms such as sanitation programs, health clinics in poverty areas, or massive public awareness campaigns to prevent communicable disease. Although these are a part of its ever-broadening focus, community health practice is much more. To understand the nature and significance of this field, it is necessary to more closely examine the concept of community and the concept of health.

THE CONCEPT OF COMMUNITY

The concepts of community and health together provide the foundation for understanding community health. Broadly defined, a community is a collection of people who share some important feature of their lives. In this text, the term **community** refers to a collection of people who interact with one another and whose common interests or characteristics form the basis for a sense of unity or belonging. It can be a society of people holding common rights and privileges (e.g., citizens of a town), sharing common interests (e.g., a community of farmers), or living under the same laws and

regulations (e.g., a prison community). The function of any community includes its members' collective sense of belonging and their shared identity, values, norms, communication, and common interests and concerns (Anderson & McFarlane, 2004). Some communities—for example, a tiny village in Appalachia—are composed of people who share almost everything. They live in the same location, work at a limited type and number of jobs, attend the same churches, and make use of the sole health clinic with its visiting physician and nurse. Other communities, such as members of Mothers Against Drunk Driving (MADD) or the community of professional nurses, are large, scattered, and composed of individuals who share only a common interest and involvement in a certain goal. Although most communities of people share many aspects of their experience, it is useful to identify three types of communities that have relevance to community health practice: geographic, common interest, and health problem or solution.

Geographic Community

A community often is defined by its geographic boundaries and thus is called a **geographic community**. A city, town, or neighborhood is a geographic community. Consider the community of Hayward, Wisconsin. Located in northwestern Wisconsin, it is set in the north woods environment, far removed from any urban center and in a climatic zone characterized by extremely harsh winters. With a population of approximately 2,200, it is considered a rural community. The population has certain identifiable characteristics, such as age and sex ratios, and its size fluctuates with the seasons: summers bring hundreds of tourists and seasonal residents. Hayward is a social system as well as a geographic location. The families, schools, hospital, churches, stores, and government institutions are linked in a complex network. This community, like others, has an informal power structure. It has a communication system that includes gossip, the newspaper, the "co-op" store bulletin board, and the radio station. In one sense, then, a community consists of a collection of people located in a specific place and is made up of institutions organized into a social system.

Local communities such as Hayward vary in size. A few miles south of Hayward lie several other communities, including Northwoods Beach and Round Lake; these three, along with other towns and isolated farms, form a larger community called Sawyer County. If a nurse worked for a health agency serving only Hayward, that community would be of primary concern; however, if the nurse worked for the Sawyer County Health Department, this larger community would be the focus. A community health nurse employed by the State Health Department in Madison, Wisconsin, would have an interest in Sawyer County and Hayward, but only as part of the larger community of Wisconsin.

Frequently, a single part of a city can be treated as a community. Cities are often broken down into *census tracts*, or neighborhoods. In Seattle, for example, the district near the waterfront forms a community of many transient and homeless people. In New York City, the neighborhood called Harlem is a community, as is the Haight-Ashbury district of San Francisco.

In community health, it is useful to identify a geographic area as a community. A community demarcated by geographic boundaries, such as a city or county, becomes a clear target for the analysis of health needs. Available data, such as morbidity and mortality figures, can augment assessment studies to form the basis for planning health programs. Media campaigns and other health education efforts can readily reach intended audiences. Examples include distributing educational information on safe sex, self-protection, the dangers of substance abuse, or where to seek shelter from abuse and violence. A geographic community is easily mobilized for action. Groups can be formed to carry out intervention and prevention efforts that address needs specific to that community. Such efforts might include more stringent policies on day care, shelters for battered women, work site safety programs in local hazardous industries, or improved sex education in the schools. Furthermore, health actions can be enhanced through the support of politically powerful individuals and resources present in a geographic community.

On a larger scale, the world can be considered as a global community. Indeed, it is very important to view the world this way. Borders of countries change with political revolution. Communicable diseases are not aware of arbitrary political boundaries. A person can travel around the world in less than 24 hours, and so can diseases. Children starving in Africa affect persons living in the United States. Political uprisings in the Middle East have an impact on people in Western countries. Floods or tsunamis in Southeast Asia have meaning for other national economies. The world is one large community that needs to work together to ensure a healthy today and a healthier and safer tomorrow. **Global health** has become a dominant phrase in international public health circles. Globalization raises an expectation of health for all, for if good health is possible in one part of the world, the forces of globalization should allow it elsewhere (Lopez, Mathers, Ezzati, Jamison, & Murray, 2006; Huynen, Martens, & Hilderink, 2005). Governments need to work together to develop a broader base for international relations and collaborative strategies that will place greater emphasis on global health security. We will learn more about global health issues and the global community in Chapter 16.

Common-interest Community

A community also can be identified by a common interest or goal. A collection of people, even if they are widely scattered geographically, can have an interest or goal that binds the members together. This is called a *common-interest community*. The members of a church in a large metropolitan area, the members of a national professional organization, and women who have had mastectomies are all common-interest communities. Sometimes, within a certain geographic area, a group of people develop a sense of community by promoting their common interest. Disabled individuals scattered throughout a large city may emerge as a community through a common interest in promoting adherence to federal guidelines for wheelchair access, parking spaces, toilet facilities, elevators, or other services for the disabled. The residents of an industrial community may develop a common interest in air or water pollution issues, whereas others who work but do not live in the area may not share that interest. Communities form to protect the rights of children, stop violence against women, clean up the environment, promote the arts, pre-

serve historical sites, protect endangered species, develop a smoke-free environment, or provide support after a crisis. The kinds of shared interests that lead to the formation of communities vary widely.

Common-interest communities whose focus is a health-related issue can join with community health agencies to promote their agendas. A group's single-minded commitment is a mobilizing force for action. Many successful prevention and health promotion efforts, including improved services and increased community awareness of specific problems, have resulted from the work of common-interest communities. Mothers Against Drunk Driving is one example. In 1980, after a repeat drunk-driving offender killed her 13-year-old daughter Cari, Candace Lightner gathered with a group of outraged mothers at a restaurant in Sacramento, California. Across the country, another mother was soon touched by a similar tragedy. Cindi Lamb's five-and-a-half month old infant daughter became a quadriplegic at the hands of a repeat drunk driver. Within a short time, the two women joined forces to form MADD and 2 years later, President Ronald Reagan organized a Presidential Task Force on drunk driving and invited MADD to participate. With media attention and perseverance, MADD quickly grew to over 100 chapters across the United States and Canada and worked to establish a federal legal minimum drinking age and standard blood alcohol levels of 0.08 percent, as well as to defend sobriety checkpoints before the Supreme Court. The National Highway Transportation and Safety Administration credited MADD when they released the 1994 figures showing a 30-year low in alcohol-related traffic deaths. Mothers Against Drunk Driving now claims more than 3 million members worldwide, and is one of the largest and most successful common-interest organizations (*Milestones in Public Health*, 2006).

Community of Solution

A type of community encountered frequently in community health practice is a group of people who come together to solve a problem that affects all of them. The shape of this community varies with the nature of the problem, the size of the geographic area affected, and the number of resources needed to address the problem. Such a community has been called a *community of solution*. For example, a water pollution problem may involve several counties whose agencies and personnel must work together to control upstream water supply, industrial waste disposal, and city water treatment. This group of counties forms a community of solution focusing on a health problem. In another instance, several schools may collaborate with law enforcement and health agencies, as well as legislators and policy makers, to study patterns of substance abuse among students and design possible preventive approaches. The boundaries of this community of solution form around the schools, agencies, and political figures involved. Figure 1.1 depicts some communities of solution related to a single city.

In recent years, communities of solution have formed in many cities to attack the spread of HIV/AIDS, and have worked with community members to assess public safety and security and create plans to make the community a safer place in which to live. Public health agencies, social service groups, schools, and media personnel have banded together

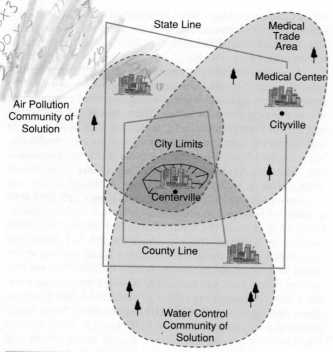

FIGURE 1.1 A city's communities of solution. State, county, and city boundaries (*solid lines*) may have little or no bearing on health solution boundaries (*dashed lines*).

to create public awareness of dangers that are present and to promote preventive behaviors (e.g., childhood obesity). Former President Bill Clinton organized the Alliance for a Healthier Generation in partnership with the American Heart Association, and they recently announced an agreement with beverage companies such as Coca-Cola and PepsiCo. Vending machines that once stocked calorie-laden sodas will now have supplies of low-calorie soft drinks and sports drinks, juices with no added sugar, tea, low or fat-free milk, and water (American Cancer Society, 2008). Although soft drinks are not the only culprit in the childhood obesity epidemic, this is an important step in helping kids make healthier choices. A community of solution is an important medium for change in community health.

Populations and Aggregates

The three types of communities just discussed underscore the meaning of the concept of community: in each instance, a collection of people chose to interact with one another because of common interests, characteristics, or goals. The concept of population has a different meaning. In this text, the term **population** refers to all of the people occupying an area, or to all of those who share one or more characteristics. In contrast to a community, a population is made up of people who do not necessarily interact with one another and do not necessarily share a sense of belonging to that group. A population may be defined geographically, such as the population of the United States or a city's population. This designation of a population is useful in community health for epidemiologic study and for collecting demographic data for purposes such as health planning. A population also may be defined by common qualities or characteristics,

such as the elderly population, the homeless population, or a particular racial or ethnic group. In community health, this meaning becomes useful when a specific group of people (e.g., homeless individuals) is targeted for intervention; the population's common characteristics (e.g., the health-related problems of homelessness) become a major focus of the intervention.

In this text, the term **aggregate** refers to a mass or grouping of distinct individuals who are considered as a whole, and who are loosely associated with one another. It is a broader term that encompasses many different-sized groups. Both communities and populations are types of aggregates. The aggregate focus, or a concern for groupings of people in contrast to individual health care, becomes a distinguishing feature of community health practice. Community health nurses may work with aggregates such as pregnant and parenting teens, elderly adults with diabetes, or gay men with HIV/AIDS.

The continuing shift away from acute care settings and toward community-based services as the focus of the health care system, along with a rising emphasis on the managed care of populations, underscores the importance of community health nursing's aggregate focus. In fact, some say it validates the focus of community health nursing as practiced over many decades (Porter-O'Grady, 2001). With the community as central to the health care model, it becomes essential for nurses to understand the meaning of community health and to assume leadership in aggregate-level health care (see What Do You Think?).

Community health workers, including community health nurses, need to define the community targeted for study and intervention: Who are the people who compose the community? Where are they located, and what are their characteristics? A clear delineation of the community or population must be established before the nurse can assess needs and design interventions. The complex nature of communities also must be understood. What are the characteristics of the people in terms of age, gender, race, socioeconomic level, and health status? How does the community interact with other communities? What is its history? What are its resources? Is the community undergoing rapid change, and, if so, what are the changes? These questions, as well as the tools needed to assess a community for health purposes, are discussed in detail in Chapter 15.

What Do You Think?

According to Porter-O'Grady (2001) during the past 20 to 30 years 70% of nurses worked in hospitals. That percentage has slowly diminished to 50% as we move through the early years of the 21st century. What do you think the continuing trend will be like as we get closer to 2050? Where do you think your career in nursing will take you over the next 25 years?

THE CONCEPT OF HEALTH

Health, in the abstract refers to a person's physical, mental, and spiritual state; it can be positive (as being in good health) or negative (as being in poor health). Health is extolled as a "dynamic state of well-being" (Bircher, 2005, p. 335) and, in a classic article from 1997, Sarrachi describes health as a "basic and universal human right" (p. 1,409). The World Health Organization (WHO) defines health positively as "a state of complete physical, mental, and social well-being and not merely the absence of disease or infirmity" (Ustin & Jakob, 2005). Our understanding of the concept of health builds on this classic definition. **Health**, in this text, refers to a holistic state of well-being, which includes soundness of mind, body, and spirit. Community health practitioners place a strong emphasis on **wellness**, which includes this definition of health, but also incorporates the capacity to develop a person's potential to lead a fulfilling and productive life—one that can be measured in terms of *quality of life*. Today, our health is greatly affected by the lifestyles we lead and the risk behaviors we engage in. An individual's behavioral risk factors, such as smoking, physical inactivity, or substance abuse, can be assessed through the use of various interview techniques and questionnaires or surveys (Glasgow, et al., 2005). The Behavioral Risk Factor Surveillance Survey, Jackson's Smoking Susceptibility Scale, and the Physical Activity and Nutrition Behaviors Monitoring Form are some examples.

There is increasing awareness of the strong relationship of health to environment. This is not a new concept. Almost 150 years ago, Florence Nightingale explored the health and illness connection with the environment. She believed that a person's health was greatly influenced by ventilation, noise, light, cleanliness, diet, and a restful bed. She laid down simple rules about maintaining and obtaining "health," which were written for lay women caring for family members to "put the constitution in such a state as that it will have no disease" (Nightingale, 1859, preface). The "built environment" is a concept under study by public health and other professionals, as the manmade structures and surroundings in a community (e.g., highways and bike paths, parks and open spaces, public buildings and housing developments) have an impact on the health of individuals and populations. Environment's relationship to health will be discussed in more detail in Chapter 9.

In some cultures, health is viewed differently. Some see it as the freedom from and absence of evil. Illness may be seen as punishment for being bad or doing evil (Lipson & Dibble, 2005). Many individuals come from families in which beliefs regarding health and illness are heavily influenced by religion, superstition, folk beliefs, or "old wives' tales." This is not unusual, and encountering such beliefs when working with various groups in the community is common. Chapter 5 explores these beliefs more thoroughly for a better understanding of how health beliefs influence every aspect of a person's life.

Although health is widely accepted as desirable, the nature of health often is ambiguous. Consumers and providers often define health and wellness in different ways. To clarify the concept for nurses who are considering community health practice, the distinguishing features of health are briefly characterized here; the implications of this concept for professionals in the field can then be examined more fully.

The Health Continuum: Wellness–Illness

Society suggests a polarized or "either/or" way of thinking about health: people either are well or they are ill. Yet wellness is a relative concept, not an absolute, and **illness** is a state of being *relatively* unhealthy. There are many levels and degrees of wellness and illness, from a robust 70-year-old woman who is fully active and functioning at an optimal level of wellness, to a 70-year-old man with end-stage renal disease whose health is characterized as frail. Someone recovering from pneumonia may be mildly ill, whereas a teenaged boy with functional limitations because of episodic depression may be described as mildly well.

The Human Genome Project, begun in 1990 and completed in 2000, and the genomic era of health care may skew the health continuum toward the healthy end (*Milestones in Public Health*, 2006). **Genomics**, the identification and plotting of human genes and the study of the interaction of genes with each other and the environment, will alter how we view and treat disease (Meadows, 2005). Primary and secondary preventive services will be individually designed based on genetic findings, and client lifestyle modifications will be recommended from birth. **Pharmacogenomics** will permit the design of drugs tailored to a person's genetic makeup or to a targeted disease. The capacity for this kind of health care will be a reality over the next decade, and we must guard against limiting access to this type of care and permitting further disenfranchisement of vulnerable populations (Eisenberg, 2005; Meadows, 2005).

Because health involves a range of degrees from optimal health at one end to total disability or death at the other (Fig. 1.2), it often is described as a continuum. This **health continuum** applies not only to individuals, but also to families and communities. A nurse might speak of a *dysfunctional family*, meaning one that is experiencing a relative degree of illness; or, a healthy family might be described as one that exhibits many wellness characteristics, such as effective communication and conflict resolution, as well as the ability to effectively work together and use resources appropriately. Likewise, a community, as a collection of people, may be described in terms of degrees of wellness or illness. The health of an individual, family, group, or community moves back and forth along this continuum throughout the lifespan. Healthy people make healthy communities and a healthy society. The Declaration of Alma Ata, which took place in 1978, noted that health is a "fundamental human right" and that the level of health must be raised for all countries in order for any society to improve their health (Bryant, 2003).

By thinking of health relatively, as a matter of degree, the scope of nursing practice can be broadened to focus on preventing illness or disability and promoting wellness. Traditionally, most health care has focused on treatment of acute and chronic conditions at the illness end of the continuum. Gradually, the emphasis is shifting to focus on the wellness end of the continuum, as outlined in the government document, *Healthy People 2010* (U.S. Department of Health and Human Services [USDHHS], 2000). The two main goals of Healthy People 2010 are: "1) to increase the quality and years of life, and 2) to eliminate health disparities" (¶ 3).

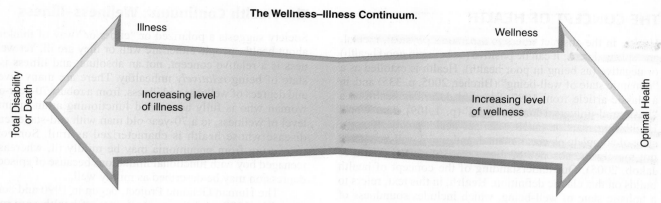

The Wellness–Illness Continuum.

The level (degree) of illness increases as one moves toward total disability or death; the level of wellness increases as one moves toward optimal health. This continuum shows the relative nature of health. At any given time a person can be placed at some point along the continuum.

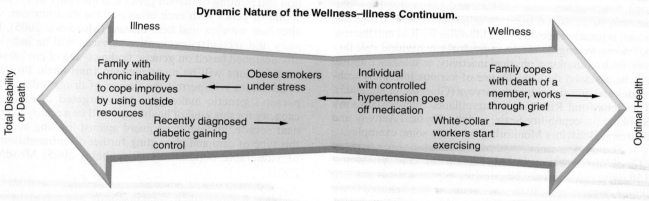

Dynamic Nature of the Wellness–Illness Continuum.

A person's relative health is usually in a state of flux, either improving or deteriorating. This diagram of the wellness-illness continuum shows several examples of people in changing states of health.

FIGURE 1.2   The health continuum.

These goals overarch the 28 focus areas (see Display 1.1) and the 467 objectives stated in measurable terms that specify targeted incidence and prevalence changes and address age, gender, and culturally vulnerable groups along with improvement in public health systems. Ten major health concerns were also identified as the **leading health indicators** (*Healthy People 2010,* 2006) and these are used in measuring the health of the U.S. population (see Display 1.2 for a list of resources pertaining to each of these health indicators):

◆ Physical activity
◆ Overweight and obesity
◆ Tobacco use
◆ Substance use
◆ Responsible sexual behavior
◆ Mental health
◆ Injury and violence
◆ Environmental quality
◆ Immunization
◆ Access to health care

Community health practice ranges across the entire health continuum; it always works to improve the degree of health in individuals, families, groups, and communities. In particular, community health practice emphasizes the promotion and preservation of wellness and the prevention of illness or disability.

Community characteristics of health have been described by the Centers for Disease Control as health-related quality of life indicators. These include such things as rates of poverty and unemployment, levels of high school education and severe work disability, mortality rates, and the proportion of adolescent births (*MMWR,* 2000). Canada has included such factors as life expectancy at birth, infant mortality, self-rated health, cancer incidence, body mass index (BMI) and dietary practices, life stress, smoking and alcohol use, unemployment rate, leisure-time physical activity, number of health professionals, as well as the total health expenditures in their list of health indicators (Canadian Institute for Health Information, 2006). How does the United States compare to other developed countries on population health indicators? See Chapter 6 for details. Healthy People in Healthy Communities is an outgrowth of the Healthy People 2010 movement (*Healthy People 2010,* 2001). A healthy community is defined as one that:

◆ Is characterized by a safe and healthy environment
◆ Offers access to health care services, focusing on both treatment and prevention for all members of the community

---

DISPLAY 1.1   ISSUES IN COMMUNITY HEALTH NURSING

Priority Areas for National Health Promotion and Disease Prevention

The context in which the document *Healthy People 2010* was developed differs from that in which Healthy People 2000 was framed—and will continue to evolve through the decade. Advances in preventive therapies, vaccines and pharmaceuticals, assistive technologies, and computerized systems will all change the face of medicine and how it is practiced. New relationships will be defined between public health departments and health care delivery organizations. Meanwhile, demographic changes in the United States—reflecting an older and more radically diverse population—will create new demands on public health and the overall health care system. Global forces—including food supplies, emerging infectious diseases, and environmental interdependence—will present new public health challenges (U.S. Department of Health and Human Services, 2000).

Its report, *Healthy People 2010,* states two broad goals: to (1) increase the quality and years of healthy life, and (2) eliminate health disparities. To accomplish these goals, measurable objectives were established under each of the following 28 priority areas:

Healthy People 2010 Focus Areas
1. Access to Quality Health Services
2. Arthritis, Osteoporosis, and Chronic Back Conditions
3. Cancer
4. Chronic Kidney Disease
5. Diabetes
6. Disability and Secondary Conditions
7. Educational and Community-Based Programs
8. Environmental Health
9. Family Planning
10. Food Safety
11. Health Communication
12. Heart Disease and Stroke
13. HIV
14. Immunization and Infectious Diseases
15. Injury and Violence Prevention
16. Maternal, Infant, and Child Health
17. Medical Product Safety
18. Mental Health and Mental Disorders
19. Nutrition and Overweight
20. Occupational Safety and Health
21. Oral Health
22. Physical Activity and Fitness
23. Public Health Infrastructure
24. Respiratory Diseases
25. Sexually Transmitted Diseases
26. Substance Abuse
27. Tobacco Use
28. Vision and Hearing

This national listing is a guide to policy makers and health planners at all levels. It provides a framework for prioritizing and addressing specific health needs in designated communities.

◆ Has roads, playgrounds, schools and other services to meet the needs of the population

Another description of a healthy community, first described by Cottrell (1976) as a *competent community*, is one in which the various organizations, groups, and aggregates of people making up the community do at least four things:

1. They collaborate effectively in identifying the problems and needs of the community.
2. They achieve a working consensus on goals and priorities.
3. They agree on ways and means to implement the agreed-on goals.
4. They collaborate effectively in the required actions.

Healthy communities and healthy cities impact the health of their populations and vice versa. In the 1980s, the WHO initiated the Healthy Cities movement to improve the health status of urban populations. A healthy city is defined as "one that is continually creating and improving those physical and social environments and expanding those community resources that enable people to mutually support each other in performing all functions of life and in developing their maximum potential" (WHO, 2004, ¶ 8). The eleven key components of a healthy city are listed in Display 1.3. How many of these are found in your city or community?

Health as a State of Being

Health refers to a state of being, including many different qualities and characteristics. An individual might be described in terms such as energetic, outgoing, enthusiastic, beautiful, caring, loving, and intense. Together, these qualities become the essence of a person's existence; they describe a state of being. Similarly, a specific geographic community, such as a neighborhood, has many characteristics. It might be characterized by the terms congested, deteriorating, unattractive, dirty, and disorganized. These characteristics suggest diminishing degrees of vitality. A third example might be a population, such as workers involved in a massive layoff, who band together to provide support and share resources to effectively seek new employment. This community shows signs of healthy adaptation and positive coping.

Health involves the total person or community. All of the dimensions of life affecting everyday functioning determine an individual's or a community's health, including physical, psychological, spiritual, economic, and sociocultural experiences. All of these factors must be considered when dealing with the health of an individual or community. The approach should be holistic. A client's placement on the health continuum can be known only if the nurse considers all facets of the client's life, including not only physical and emotional status, but also the status of home, family, and work.

DISPLAY 1.2 RESOURCES FOR THE LEADING HEALTH INDICATORS

The Leading Health Indicators will be used to measure the health of the nation over the next 10 years. Each of the 10 Leading Health Indicators has one or more objectives from *Healthy People 2010* associated with it. As a group, the Leading Health Indicators reflect the major health concerns in the United States at the beginning of the 21st century. The Leading Health Indicators were selected on the basis of their ability to motivate action, the availability of data to measure progress, and their importance as public health issues. Corresponding sample resources from the Federal government are listed here. The Federal consumer health information Web site, www.healthfinder.gov, is also a good starting point for more information on these topics.

Physical Activity
- President's Council on Physical Fitness and Sports 202-690-9000 http://www.fitness.gov
- Centers for Disease Control and Prevention (CDC) 888-232-3228 http://www.cdc.gov/nccdphp/dnpa

Overweight and Obesity
- Obesity Education Initiative, National Heart, Lung, and Blood Institute Information Center 301-592-8573 http://www.nhlbi.nih.gov/about/oei/index.htm
- The Weight-Control Information Network, National Institutes of Health (NIH) 877-946-4627 http://win.niddk.nih.gov/index.htm

Tobacco Use
- Office on Smoking and Health, National Center for Chronic Disease Prevention and Health Promotion, CDC 800-CDC-1311 http://www.cdc.gov/tobacco
- Cancer Information Service, NIH 800-4-CANCER http://cis.nci.nih.gov

Substance Abuse
- National Clearinghouse for Alcohol and Drug Information Substance Abuse and Mental Health Services Administration (SAMHSA) 800-729-6686; 800-487-4889 (TDD) http://www.health.org
- National Institute on Drug Abuse, NIH 301-443-1124 http://www.nida.nih.gov
- National Institute on Alcohol Abuse and Alcoholism, NIH 301-443-3860 http://www.niaaa.nih.gov

Responsible Sexual Behavior
- CDC National AIDS Hotline 800-342-AIDS (800-342-2437) http://www.cdc.gov/hiv/hivinfo/nah.htm
- CDC National Sexually Transmitted Diseases (STD) Hotline 800-227-8922 http://www.cdc.gov/std
- CDC National Prevention Information Network 800-458-5231 http://www.cdcnpin.org
- Office of Population Affairs 301-654-6190 http://opa.osophs.dhhs.gov

Mental Health
- Center for Mental Health Services, SAMHSA http://www.mentalhealth.samhsa.gov/cmhs/

- National Mental Health Information Center, SAMHSA 800-789-2647 http://www.mentalhealth.samhsa.gov
- National Institute of Mental Health Information Line, NIH 800-421-4211 http://www.nimh.nih.gov/healthinformation/depressionmenu.cfm

Injury and Violence
- National Center for Injury Prevention and Control, CDC 770-488-1506 http://www.cdc.gov/ncipc/ncipchm.htm
- Office of Justice Programs, U.S. Department of Justice 202-307-0703 http://www.ojp.usdoj.gov/home.htm
- National Highway Traffic Safety Administration U.S. Department of Transportation Auto Safety Hotline 888-DASH-2-DOT (888-327-4236) http://www.nhtsa.dot.gov/hotline

Environmental Quality
- Indoor Air Quality Information Clearinghouse U.S. Environmental Protection Agency 800-438-4318 (IAQ hotline) 800-SALUD-12; (725-8312) Spanish http://www.epa.gov/iaq/iaqinfo.html
- Information Resources Center (IRC) U.S. Environmental Protection Agency 202-260-5922 http://www.epa.gov/natlibra/hqirc/about.htm
- Agency for Toxic Substances and Disease Registry, CDC 888-442-8737 http://www.atsdr.cdc.gov

Immunization
- National Immunization Program/CDC 800-232-2522 (English); 800-232-0233 (Spanish) 888-CDC-FAXX (Fax-back) http://www.cdc.gov/nip

Access to Health Care
- Agency for Healthcare Research and Quality Office of Healthcare Information 301-594-1364 http://www.ahrq.gov/consumer/index.html#plans
- "Insure Kids Now" Initiative Health Resources and Services Administration 877-KIDS NOW (877-543-7669) http://www.insurekidsnow.gov
- Maternal and Child Health Bureau Health Resources and Services Administration 1-888-ASK-HRSA (HRSA Information Center) http://www.mchb.hrsa.gov
- Office of Beneficiary Relations, Centers for Medicare & Medicaid Services 800-444-4606 (customer service center) 800-MED-ICARE (Info Line) http://www.medicare.gov

For more health promotion and disease prevention information—Search online for thousands of free Federal health documents using healthfinder® at http://www.healthfinder.gov/.

For health promotion and disease prevention information in Spanish—Visit http://www.healthfinder.gov/espanol/.

For more information about *Healthy People 2010*, visit http://www.healthypeople.gov or call 800-367-4725. (Retrieved July 5, 2008 from: www.healthypeople.gov/LHI/EnglishFactSheet.htm)

DISPLAY 1.3   **WHAT ARE THE QUALITIES OF A HEALTHY CITY?**

- A clean, safe physical environment of a high quality (including housing quality)
- An ecosystem that is stable now and sustainable in the long term
- A strong mutually supportive and nonexploitative community
- A high degree of participation in and control by the citizens over the decisions affecting their lives, health, and well-being
- The meeting of basic needs (food, water, shelter, income, safety, and work) for all the city's people
- Access by the people to a wide variety of experiences and resources, with the chance for a wide variety of contact, interaction, and communication

- A diverse, vital, and innovative economy
- The encouragement of connectedness with the past, with the cultural and biologic heritage of city dwellers, and with other groups and individuals
- A form that is compatible with and enhances the preceding characteristics
- An optimum level of appropriate public health and sickness care services, accessible to all, and high health status (high levels of positive health and low levels of disease)

(Retrieved from www.euro.who.int/healthy-cities/introducing/20050202_4.)

When considering an aggregate or group of people in terms of health, it becomes useful for intervention purposes to speak of the "health of a community." With aggregates as well as individuals, health as a state of being does not merely involve that group's physical state but also includes psychological, spiritual, and socioeconomic factors. The health of the Gulf Coast region after hurricane Katrina made landfall in August 2005 is one example. Widespread damage occurred after the deadliest hurricane since the 1920s, and then, only 26 days later, hurricane Rita (the fourth most intense Atlantic hurricane on record) hit near the Texas–Louisiana border. The Centers for Disease Control (CDC) estimated that more than 200,000 people converged on evacuation centers, and the country watched in anguish as the Federal Emergency Management Agency (FEMA) struggled to meet the emergency needs of the survivors. At the same time, over 1,000 deaths have been attributed to Katrina, and the survivors are left with many physical, emotional, and social difficulties. The CDC estimated that almost 2 months after Katrina made landfall, more than 20% of houses did not have water, almost 56% of households had at least one member with a chronic health condition, and almost half of the adults had a level of emotional distress indicating a need for mental health services (*MMWR*, March 10, 2005; *MMWR*, January 19, 2006). Prior to that, on September 11, 2001, thousands of lives were lost in New York City's World Trade Center towers, in the Pentagon in Washington, DC, and in an airliner that crashed in Somerset County, Pennsylvania. The trauma of these events left our nation shaken. The health of many communities was dangerously poor. Communities needed to be restored, and the entire country needed to heal.

Subjective and Objective Dimensions of Health

Health involves both *subjective* and *objective* dimensions; that is, it involves both how people feel (subjective) and how well they can function in their environment (objective). Subjectively, a healthy person is one who feels well, who experiences the sensation of a vital, positive state. Healthy people are full of life and vigor, capable of physical and mental productivity. They feel minimal discomfort and displeasure with the world around them. Again, people experience varying degrees of vitality and well-being. The state of feeling well fluctuates. Some mornings we wake up feeling more energetic and enthusiastic than we do on other mornings. How people feel varies day by day, even hour by hour; nonetheless, how they feel overall is a strong indicator of their overall state of health.

Health also involves the objective dimension of ability to function. A healthy individual or community carries out necessary activities and achieves enriching goals. Unhealthy people not only feel ill, but are limited, to some degree, in their ability to carry out daily activities. Indeed, levels of illness or wellness are measured largely in terms of ability to function (Roach, 2000). A person confined to bed is labeled sicker than an ill person managing self-care. A family that meets its members' needs is healthier than one that has poor communication patterns and is unable to provide adequate physical and emotional resources. A community actively engaged in crime prevention or policing of industrial wastes shows signs of healthy functioning. The degree of functioning is directly related to the state of health (see Perspectives: Voices from the Community).

The ability to function can be observed. A man dresses and feeds himself and goes to work. Despite financial exigencies, a family nourishes its members through a supportive emotional climate. A community provides adequate resources and services for its members. These performances, to some degree, can be regarded as indicators of health status.

The actions of an individual, family, or community are motivated by their values. Some activities, such as walking and taking care of personal needs, are functions valued by most people. Other actions, such as bird watching, volunteering to help a charity, or running, have more limited appeal. In assessing the health of individuals and communities, the community health nurse can observe people's ability to function, but also must know their values, which may contrast sharply with those of the professional. The influence of values on health is examined more closely in Chapter 4.

The subjective dimension (feeling well or ill) and the objective dimension (functioning) together provide a clearer picture of people's health. When they feel well and demonstrate functional ability, they are close to the wellness end of the health continuum. Even those with a disease, such as arthritis or diabetes, may feel well and perform well within their capacity. These people can be considered healthy or closer to the wellness end of the continuum. Figure 1.3 depicts the relationships between the subjective and objective views of health.

Continuous and Episodic Health Care Needs

Community health practice encompasses populations in all age groups with birth to death developmental health care needs. These **continuous needs** may include, for example, assistance with providing a toddler-proof home or establishing positive toilet-training techniques, help in effectively dealing with the progressive emancipation of preteens and teenagers, anticipatory guidance for reducing and managing the stress associated with retirement, or help coping with the death of an aged parent. These are developmental events experienced by most people, and they represent typical life occurrences. The community health nurse has the skills to work at the individual, family, and group level to meet these needs. On an individual and family level, a home visit may be the appropriate place for intervention. If the nurse sees that the community has many young and growing families, and several families have similar developmental issues, a class for mothers and babies, parents and teenagers, or preretirement adults may be formed to meet weekly at the library or health clinic waiting room. In these instances, the nurse works with groups ranging from small to large.

In addition, populations may have a one-time, specific, negative health event, such as an illness or injury, that is not an expected part of life. These **episodic needs** might derive from the birth of an infant with Down syndrome, a head injury incurred from an automobile crash, or a diagnosis of HIV/AIDS.

In a given day, the community health nurse may interact with clients having either continuous or episodic health care needs, or both. For example, when can parents expect a child with Down syndrome to begin toilet training? How do middle-aged adults, planning their retirement and preparing for the death of an aged parent, deal with their adult child's AIDS diagnosis? Complex situations such as these may be positively influenced by the interaction with and services of the community health nurse.

COMPONENTS OF COMMUNITY HEALTH PRACTICE

Community health practice can best be understood by examining two basic components—promotion of health and prevention of health problems. The levels of prevention are a key to community health practice.

Promotion of Health

Promotion of health is recognized as one of the most important components of public health and community health practice (USDHHS, 2000). **Health promotion** includes all efforts that seek to move people closer to optimal well-being or higher levels of wellness. Nursing, in particular, has a social mandate for engaging in health promotion (Pender, Murdaugh & Parsons, 2006). Health promotion programs and activities include many forms of health education—for

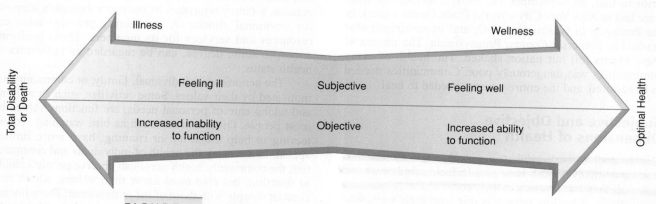

FIGURE 1.3 Subjective and objective views of the wellness–illness continuum.

example, teaching the dangers of drug use, demonstrating healthful practices such as regular exercise, and providing more health-promoting options such as heart-healthy menu selections. Community health promotion, then, encompasses the development and management of preventive health care services that are responsive to community health needs. Wellness programs in schools and industry are examples. Demonstration of such healthful practices as eating nutritious foods and exercising more regularly often is performed and promoted by individual health workers. In addition, groups and health agencies that support a smoke-free environment, encourage physical fitness programs for all ages, or demand that food products be properly labeled underscore the importance of these practices and create public awareness.

The goal of health promotion is to raise levels of wellness for individuals, families, populations, and communities. Community health efforts accomplish this goal through a three-pronged effort to:

1. Increase the span of healthy life for all citizens
2. Reduce health disparities among population groups
3. Achieve access to preventive services for everyone

Specifically, in the 1980s, the U.S. Public Health Service published the Surgeon General's report, *Healthy People,* and continued with *Promoting Health, Preventing Disease: 1990 Health Objectives for the Nation* and *Healthy People 2000.* The third set of health objectives for the nation, *Healthy People 2010* (USDHHS, 2000), built on the previous two decades of success in Healthy People initiatives. These documents provide guidance for promoting health as a nation.

The Surgeon General's report provided vision and an agenda for significantly reducing preventable death and disability nationwide, enhancing quality of life, and greatly reducing disparities in the health status of populations. It emphasized the need for individuals to assume personal responsibility for controlling and improving their own health destiny. It challenged society to find ways to make good health available to vulnerable populations whose disadvantaged state placed them at greater risk for health problems. Finally, it called for an intensified shift in focus from treating preventable illness and functional impairment to concentrating resources and targeting efforts that promote health and prevent disease and disability. The Institute of Medicine's 2001 report, *The Future of the Public's Health in the 21st Century*, notes that the majority of health care spending, "as much as 95%," focuses on "medical care and biomedical research," whereas evidence suggests that "behavior and environment are responsible for over 70% of avoidable mortality" and that health care is only one of many "determinants of health" (p. 2).

The implications of this national agenda for health have far-reaching consequences for persons engaged in health care. For centuries, health care has focused on the illness end of the health continuum, but health professionals can no longer justify concentrating most of their efforts exclusively on treating the sick and injured. We now live in an age when it is not only possible to promote health and prevent disease and disability, but it is our mandate and responsibility to do so (USDHHS, 2000).

Prevention of Health Problems

Prevention of health problems constitutes a major part of community health practice. Prevention means anticipating and averting problems or discovering them as early as possible in order to minimize potential disability and impairment. It is practiced on three levels in community health: primary prevention, secondary prevention, and tertiary prevention (Neuman, 2001). These concepts recur throughout the chapters of this text, in narrative format and in the Levels of Prevention Pyramids, because they are basic to community health nursing. Once the differences among the levels of prevention are recognized, a sound foundation on which to build additional community health principles can be developed.

Primary prevention obviates the occurrence of a health problem; it includes measures taken to keep illness or injuries from occurring. It is applied to a generally healthy population and precedes disease or dysfunction. Examples of primary prevention activities by a community health nurse include encouraging elderly people to install and use safety devices (e.g., grab bars by bathtubs, hand rails on steps) to prevent injuries from falls; teaching young adults healthy lifestyle behaviors, so that they can make them habitual behaviors for themselves and their children; or working through a local health department to help control and prevent communicable diseases such as rubeola, poliomyelitis, or varicella by providing regular immunization programs.

Primary prevention involves anticipatory planning and action on the part of community health professionals, who must project themselves into the future, envision potential needs and problems, and then design programs to counteract them, so that they never occur. A community health nurse who instructs a group of overweight individuals on how to follow a well-balanced diet while losing weight is preventing the possibility of nutritional deficiency (see Levels of Prevention Pyramid). Educational programs that teach safe-sex practices or the dangers of smoking and substance abuse are other examples of primary prevention. In addition, when the community health nurse serves on a fact-finding committee exploring the effects of a proposed toxic waste dump on the outskirts of town, the nurse is concerned about primary prevention. The concepts of primary prevention and planning for the future are foreign to many social groups, who may resist on the basis of conflicting values. The Parable of the Dangerous Cliff (Display 1.4) illustrates such a value conflict. How often does our nation put an ambulance at the bottom of the cliff?

Secondary prevention involves efforts to detect and treat existing health problems at the earliest possible stage, when disease or impairment is already present. Hypertension and cholesterol screening programs in many communities help to identify high-risk individuals and encourage early treatment to prevent heart attacks or stroke. Other examples are encouraging breast and testicular self-examination, regular mammograms and Pap smears for early detection of possible cancer, and providing skin testing for tuberculosis (in infants at 1 year of age and periodically throughout life, with increasing frequency for high-risk groups). Secondary prevention attempts to discover a health problem at a point when intervention may lead to its control or eradication.

LEVELS OF PREVENTION PYRAMID

SITUATION: Promotion of community nutritional status through healthy dietary practices.
GOAL: Using the three levels of prevention, negative health conditions are avoided, or promptly diagnosed and treated, and the fullest possible potential is restored.

Tertiary Prevention

Rehabilitation

- Encourage long-term follow-up for diagnosed eating disorders
- Reassess client dietary practices as necessary

Primary Prevention

Health Promotion & Education
- Encourage healthy meal preparation and consumption

Health Protection
- Use vitamin and mineral supplements as needed

Secondary Prevention

Early Diagnosis

- Provide dietary screening programs for high-risk groups: infants, adolescents, young female adults, elderly individuals
- Refer clients with eating disorders (underweight/overweight, anorexia, bulimia, compulsive eating) to nutritionist or primary care provider

Prompt Treatment

- Initiate educational and incentive programs to improve dietary practices
- Teach clients (individuals or families) on a one-to-one basis to modify dietary practices

Primary Prevention

Health Promotion & Education

- Provide nutrition educational programs to promote awareness at schools, work sites, food stores, etc.
- Encourage restaurants to offer healthy menu items
- Complete a kitchen cupboard survey in collaboration with client
- Recommend nutrition classes offered at neighborhood centers or health care facilities

Health Protection

- Supplement diet with vitamins and minerals that offer health protection (e.g., vitamins A, B, C, E)

This is the goal behind testing of water and soil samples for contaminants and hazardous chemicals in the field of community environmental health. It also prompts community health nurses to watch for early signs of child abuse in a family, emotional disturbances among widows, or alcohol and drug abuse among adolescents.

Tertiary prevention attempts to reduce the extent and severity of a health problem to its lowest possible level, so as to minimize disability and restore or preserve function. Examples include treatment and rehabilitation of persons after a stroke to reduce impairment, postmastectomy exercise programs to restore functioning, and early treatment and management of diabetes to reduce problems or slow their progress. The individuals involved have an existing illness or disability whose impact on their lives is lessened through tertiary prevention. In community health, the need to reduce disability and restore function applies equally to families,

groups, communities, and individuals. Many groups form for rehabilitation and offer support and guidance for those recuperating from some physical or mental disability. Examples include Alcoholics Anonymous, halfway houses for psychiatric patients discharged from acute care settings, ostomy clubs, and drug rehabilitation programs. In broader community health practice, tertiary prevention is used to minimize the effects of an existing unhealthy community condition. Examples of such prevention are insisting that businesses provide wheelchair access, warning urban residents about the dangers of a chemical spill, and recalling a contaminated food or drug product. When a community experiences a disaster such as an earthquake, a fire, a hurricane, or even a terrorist attack, preventing injuries among the survivors and volunteers during rescue is another example of tertiary prevention—eliminating additional injury to those already experiencing a tragedy.

DISPLAY 1.4 **PARABLE OF THE DANGEROUS CLIFF**

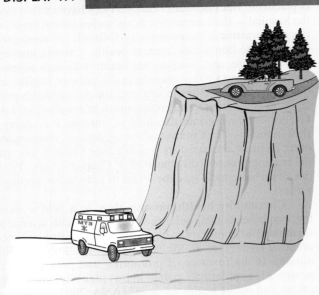

Twas a dangerous cliff, as they freely confessed,
  Though to walk near its crest was so pleasant;
But over its terrible edge there has slipped
  A duke, and full many a peasant.
The people said something would have to be done
  But their projects did not at all tally.
Some said, "Put a fence around the edge of the cliff";
  Some, "an ambulance down in the valley."
The lament of the crowd was profound and was loud,
  As their hearts overflowed with their pity;
But the cry of the ambulance carried the day
  As it spread through the neighboring city.
A collection was made to accumulate aid
  And the dwellers in highway and alley
Gave dollars or cents not to furnish a fence
  But "an ambulance down in the valley."

"For the cliff is all right if you're careful," they said.
  "And if folks ever slip and are dropping,
It isn't the slipping that hurts them so much
  As the shock down below when they're stopping."
So for years (we have heard), as these mishaps
    occurred,
  Quick forth the rescuers sally,
To pick up the victims who fell from the cliff,
  With the ambulance down in the valley.
Said one in his plea, "It's a marvel to me
  That you'd give so much greater attention
To repairing results than to curing the cause;
  You had much better aim at prevention.
For the mischief, of course, should be stopped at its
    source,
  Come neighbors and friends, let us rally.
It is far better sense to rely on a fence
  Than an ambulance down in the valley."
"He is wrong in his head," the majority said;
  "He would end all our earnest endeavor.
He's a man who would shirk this responsible work,
  But we will support it forever.
Aren't we picking up all, just as fast as they fall,
  and giving them care liberally?
A superfluous fence is of no consequence,
  If the ambulance works in the valley."
The story looks queer as we've written it here,
  But things oft occur that are stranger.
More humane, we assert, than to care for the hurt,
  Is a plan for removing the danger.
The very best plan is to safeguard the man,
  And attend to the thing rationally;
To build up the fence and try to dispense
  With the ambulance down in the valley.
Better still! Cut down the hill!

—*Author Unknown*

Health assessment of individuals, families, and communities is an important part of all three levels of preventive practice. Health status must be determined to anticipate problems and select appropriate preventive measures. Community health nurses working with young parents who themselves have been victims of child abuse can institute early treatment for the parents to prevent abuse and foster adequate parenting of their children. If the assessment of a community reveals inadequate facilities and activities to meet the future needs of its growing senior population, agencies and groups can collaborate to develop the needed resources.

Health problems are most effectively prevented by maintenance of healthy lifestyles and healthy environments. To these ends, community health practice directs many of its efforts to providing safe and satisfying living and working conditions, nutritious food, and clean air and water. This area of practice includes the field of preventive medicine, which is a population-focused, or community-oriented, branch of medical practice that incorporates public health sciences and principles (Kriebel & Tickner, 2001).

CHARACTERISTICS OF COMMUNITY HEALTH NURSING

As a specialty field of nursing, community health nursing adds public health knowledge and skills that address the needs and problems of communities and aggregates and focuses care on communities and vulnerable populations. Community health nursing is grounded in both public health science and nursing science, which makes its philosophical orientation and the nature of its practice unique. It has been recognized as a subspecialty of both fields. Recognition of this specialty field continues with a greater awareness of the important contributions made by community health nursing to improve the health of the public.

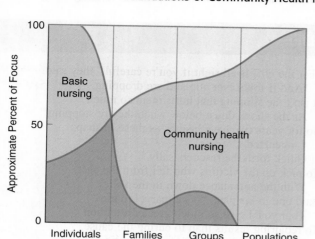

FIGURE 1.4 Difference in client focus between basic nursing and community health nursing.

Knowledge of the following elements of public health is essential to community health nursing (ANA, 2005; Quad Council, 2003; Williams, 1977):

◆ Priority of preventive, protective, and health-promoting strategies over curative strategies
◆ Means for measurement and analysis of community health problems, including epidemiologic concepts and biostatistics
◆ Influence of environmental factors on aggregate health
◆ Principles underlying management and organization for community health, because the goal of public health is accomplished through organized community efforts
◆ Public policy analysis and development, along with health advocacy and an understanding of the political process

Confusion over the meaning of "community health nursing" arises when it is defined only in terms of where it is practiced. Because health care services have shifted from the hospital to the community, many nurses in other specialties now practice in the community. Examples of these practices include home care, mental health, geriatric nursing, long-term care, and occupational health. Although community health nurses today practice in the same or similar settings, the difference lies in applying the public health principles to large groups and communities of people (Fig. 1.4). For nurses moving into this field of nursing, it requires a shift in focus— from individuals to aggregates. Nursing and other theories undergird its practice (see Chapter 14), and the nursing process (incorporated in Chapter 15 and 19) is one of its basic tools (see the levels of prevention discussed earlier).

Community health nursing, then, as a field of nursing, combines nursing science with public health science to formulate a community-based and population-focused practice (Anderson & McFarlane, 2004). "Public health nursing is the practice of promoting and protecting the health of populations using knowledge from nursing, social, and public health sciences" (ANA, 2005, p. 10) (see Display 1.5). For instance, community health nurses are nursing when their concern for homeless individuals sleeping in a park leads to development of a program providing food and shelter for this population. Community health nurses are nursing when they collaborate to institute an AIDS education curriculum in the local school system. When they assess the needs of elderly people in retirement homes to ensure necessary services and provide health instruction and support, they are, again, nursing.

During the first 70 years of the 20th century, community health nursing was known as **public health nursing**. The PHN section of the American Public Health Association's definition of a public health nurse is a "nursing professional with educational, preparation in public health and nursing science with a primary focus on population-level outcomes" and notes the primary focus for public health nursing is to "promote health and protect disease for entire population

---

DISPLAY 1.5   THE ROLE OF PUBLIC HEALTH NURSES

Public health nurses integrate community involvement and knowledge about the entire population with personal, clinical understandings of the health and illness experiences of individuals and families within the population. They translate and articulate the health and illness experiences of diverse, often vulnerable individuals and families in the population to health planners and policy makers, and assist members of the community to voice their problems and aspirations. Public health nurses are knowledgeable about multiple strategies for intervention, from those applicable to the entire population, to those for the family, and the individual. Public health nurses translate knowledge from the health and social sciences to individuals and population groups through targeted interventions, programs, and advocacy. Public health nursing may be practiced by one public

health nurse or by a group of public health nurses working collaboratively. In both instances, public health nurses are directly engaged in the interdisciplinary activities of the core public health functions of assessment, assurance, and policy development. Interventions or strategies may be targeted to multiple levels, depending on where the most effective outcomes are possible. They include strategies aimed at entire population groups, families, or individuals. In any setting, the role of public health nurses focuses on the prevention of illness, injury, or disability; the promotion of health; and the maintenance of the health of populations.

(Public Health Nursing Section, American Public Health Association [1996]. The definition and role of public health nursing. Washington, DC: APHA.)

groups" (1996, p. 2). The later title of community health nursing was adopted to better describe where the nurse practices. As used in this text, the terms are interchangeable.

Eight characteristics of community health nursing are particularly salient to the practice of this specialty:

1. The client or "unit of care" is the population.
2. The primary obligation is to achieve the greatest good for the greatest number of people or the population as a whole.
3. The processes used by public health nurses include working with the client(s) as an equal partner.
4. Primary prevention is the priority in selecting appropriate activities.
5. Selecting strategies that create healthy environmental, social, and economic conditions in which populations may thrive is the focus.
6. There is an obligation to actively reach out to all who might benefit from a specific activity or service.
7. Optimal use of available resources to assure the best overall improvement in the health of the population is a key element of the practice.
8. Collaboration with a variety of other professions, organizations, and entities is the most effective way to promote and protect the health of people. (ANA, 2005, pp. 12–14)

Population-focused

The central mission of public health practice is to improve the health of population groups. Community health nursing shares this essential feature: it is **population-focused**, meaning that it is concerned for the health status of population groups and their environment. A population may consist of the elderly living throughout the community or of Southeast Asian refugees clustered in one section of a city. It may be a scattered group with common characteristics, such as people at high risk of developing heart disease or battered women living throughout a county. It may include all people living in a neighborhood, district, census tract, city, state, or province. Community health nursing's specialty practice serves populations and aggregates of people.

Working with individuals and families as aggregates has been common for community health nursing; however, such work must expand to incorporate a population-oriented focus, a feature that distinguishes it from other nursing specialties. Basic nursing focuses on individuals, and community health nursing focuses on aggregates, but the many variations in community needs and nursing roles inevitably cause some overlap.

A population-oriented focus requires the assessment of relationships. When working with groups and communities, the nurse does not consider them separately but rather in context—that is, in relationship to the rest of the community. When an outbreak of hepatitis occurs, for example, the community health nurse does more than work with others to treat it. The nurse tries to stop the spread of the infection, locate possible sources, and prevent its recurrence in the community. As a result of their population-oriented focus, community health nurses seek to discover possible groups with a common health need, such as expectant mothers or groups at high risk for development of a common health problem (e.g., obese children at risk for type 2 diabetes, victims of child abuse).

Community health nurses continually look for problems in the environment that influence community health and seek ways to increase environmental quality. They work to prevent health problems, such as promoting school-based education about nutrition and physical activity or exercise programs for groups of seniors.

The Greatest Good for the Greatest Number of People

A population-oriented focus involves a new outlook and set of attitudes. Individualized care is important, but prevention of aggregate problems in community health nursing practice reflects more accurately its philosophy and benefits more people. The community or population at risk is the client (see Display 1.6). Furthermore, because community health nurses are concerned about several aggregates at the same time, service will, of necessity, be provided to multiple and overlapping groups. The ethical theory of *utilitarianism* promotes the greatest good for the greatest number. Further discussion of ethical principles in community health nursing can be found in Chapter 4.

Clients as Equal Partners

The goal of public health, "to increase quality and years of healthy life and eliminate health disparities" (USDHHS, 2000, ¶ 3), requires a partnership effort. Just as learning cannot take place in schools without student participation, the goals of public health cannot be realized without consumer participation. Community health nursing's efforts toward health improvement go only so far. Clients' health status and health behavior will not change unless people accept and apply the proposals (developed in collaboration with clients) presented by the community health nurse.

Community health nurses can encourage individuals' participation by promoting their autonomy rather than permitting a dependency. For example, elderly persons attending a series of nutrition or fitness classes can be encouraged to take the initiative and develop health or social programs on their own. Independence and feelings of self-worth are closely related. By treating people as independent adults, with trust and respect, community health nurses help promote self-reliance and the ability to function independently.

Frequently, consumers are intimidated by health professionals and are uninformed about health and health care. They do not know what information to seek and are hesitant to act assertively. For example, a migrant worker brought her 2-year-old son, who had symptoms resembling those of scurvy, to a clinic. Recognizing a vitamin C deficiency, the physician told her to feed the boy large quantities of orange juice but gave no explanation. Several weeks later, she returned to the clinic, but the child was much worse. After questioning her, the nurse discovered that the mother had been feeding the child large amounts of an orange soft drink, not knowing the difference between that beverage and orange juice. Obviously, the quality of care is affected when the consumer does not understand and cannot participate in the health care process. **Health literacy**, or the ability to "obtain, process, and understand basic health information and services needed to make appropriate health decisions," is an important concept that will be discussed more fully in Chapter 10 (Parker & Gazmararian, 2003, p. 116).

DISPLAY 1.6   PARABLE OF THE TREES: POPULATION-FOCUSED PRACTICE

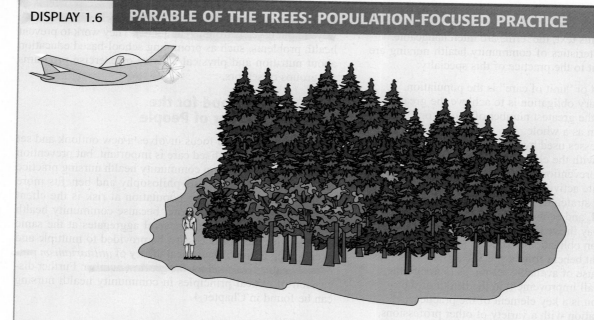

There were once two sisters who inherited a large tract of heavily forested land from their grandmother. In her will, the grandmother stipulated that they must preserve the health of the trees. One sister studied tree surgery and became an expert in recognizing and treating diseased trees. She also was able to spot conditions that might lead to problems and prevent them. Her work was invaluable in keeping single or small clusters of trees healthy. The other sister became a forest ranger. In addition to learning how to care for individual trees, she studied the environmental conditions that affected the well-being of the forest. She learned the importance of proper ecologic balance between flora and fauna and the impact of climate, geog-

raphy, soil conditions, and weather. Her work was to oversee the health and growth of the whole forest. Although she spent time walking through the forest assessing conditions, her aerial view from their small plane was equally important for spotting fires, signs of disease, or other potential problems. Together, the sisters preserved a healthy forest.

Nursing also has tree surgeons and forest rangers. Various nursing specialties, like the tree surgeons, serve the health needs of individuals and families. Community health nurses, like the forest rangers, study and address the needs of populations. Both are needed and must work together to ensure healthy communities.

When people believe that their health, and that of the community, is their own responsibility, not just that of health professionals, they will take a more active interest in promoting it. The process of taking responsibility for developing one's own health potential is called **self-care**. As people maintain their own lives, health, and well-being, they are engaging in self-care. Some examples of self-care activities at the aggregate level include building safe playgrounds, developing teen employment opportunities, and providing senior exercise programs.

When people's ability to continue self-care activities drops below their need, they experience a **self-care deficit**. At this point, nursing may appropriately intervene. However, nursing's goal is to assist clients to return to or reach a level of functioning at which they can attain optimal health and assume responsibility for maintaining it (Orem, 2001). To this end, community health nurses foster their clients' sense of responsibility by treating them as adults capable of managing their own affairs. Nurses can encourage people to negotiate health care goals and practices, develop their own programs, contact their own resources (e.g., support groups, transportation services), identify and implement lifestyle changes that promote wellness, and learn ways to monitor their own health.

When planning for the health of communities, for example, partnerships must be established and the values and priorities of the community incorporated into program planning, data collection and interpretation, and policy making.

Prioritizing Primary Prevention

In community health nursing, the promotion of health and prevention of illness are a first-order priority. Less emphasis is placed on curative care. Some corrective actions always are needed, such as cleanup of a toxic waste dump site, stricter enforcement of day care standards, or home care of the disabled; however, community health best serves its constituents through preventive and health-promoting actions (USDHHS, 2000). These include services to mothers and infants, prevention of environmental pollution, school health programs, senior citizens' fitness classes, and "workers' right-to-know" legislation that warns against hazards in the workplace.

Another distinguishing characteristic of community health nursing is its emphasis on positive health, or wellness (Anderson & McFarlane, 2004; Porter-O'Grady, 2001). Medicine and acute care nursing have dealt primarily with the illness end of the health continuum. With the potential of genomics just around the corner, the wellness end of the continuum will come into greater focus. In contrast, community health nursing always has had a primary charge to prevent health problems from occurring and to promote a higher level of health. For example, although a community health nurse may assist a population of new mothers in the community with postpartum fatigue and depression, the nurse also works to prevent such problems among women of child-bearing age by developing health education programs, establishing prenatal classes, and encouraging proper rest and nutrition, adequate help, and stress reduction.

Community health nurses concentrate on the wellness end of the health continuum in a variety of ways. They teach proper nutrition or family planning, promote immunizations among preschool children, encourage regular physical and dental checkups, assist with starting exercise classes or physical fitness programs, and promote healthy interpersonal relationships. Their goal is to help the community reach its optimal level of wellness.

This emphasis on wellness changes the role of community health nursing from a reactive to a proactive stance. It places a greater responsibility on community health nurses to find opportunities for intervention. In clinical nursing and medicine, the patients seek out professional assistance because they have health problems. As Williams put it decades ago, "patients select themselves into the care system, and the providers' role is to deal with what the patients bring to them" (1977, p. 251). Community health nurses, in contrast, seek out potential health problems. They identify high-risk groups and institute preventive programs. They watch for early signs of child neglect or abuse and intervene when any occur, often long before a request for help is made. They look for possible environmental hazards in the community, such as smoking in public places or lead-based paint in older housing units, and work with appropriate authorities to correct them. A wellness emphasis requires taking initiative and making sound judgments, which are characteristics of effective community health nursing.

Selecting Strategies That Create Healthy Conditions in Which Populations May Thrive

With our population focus, it is prudent for community health nurses to design interventions for "education, community development, social engineering, policy development, and enforcement" that "result in laws and rules, policies and budget priorities" (ANA, 2005, p. 13). Advocacy for our clients, whether they be individuals, families, aggregates, communities, or populations, is an essential function of public health nursing. We want to create healthy environments for our clients, so that they can thrive and not simply survive.

Actively Reaching Out

We know that some clients are more prone to develop disability or disease because of their vulnerable status (e.g., poverty, no access to health care, homeless). Outreach efforts are needed to promote the health of these clients and to prevent disease. In acute care and primary health care settings, like emergency rooms or physician offices, clients come to you for service. However, in community

health, nurses must "focus on the whole population and not just those who present for services" and seek out clients wherever they may be (ANA, 2005, p. 13). Like Lillian Wald and her Henry Street Settlement, community health nurses must learn about the populations they serve and be willing to search out the most at-risk. You will learn more about the rich history of community/public health nursing in Chapter 2. Chapter 25 will cover vulnerable populations.

Optimal Use of Available Resources

It is our duty to wisely use the resources we are given. For many public health agencies, budgets have been stretched to the limits. Tertiary health care uses up the greatest percentage of our health care dollar, leaving decreased funds for primary and secondary services. Decisions for programs or services are often made on the basis of the "cost-benefit or cost-effectiveness of potential strategies" (ANA, 2005, p. 13). It is vital that community health nurses ground their practice in research, and use that information to educate policy makers about best practices. Utilizing personnel and resources effectively and prudently will pay off in the long run.

Interprofessional Collaboration

Community health nurses must work in cooperation with other team members, coordinating services and addressing the needs of population groups. This interprofessional collaboration among health care workers, other professionals and organizations, and clients is essential for establishing effective services and programs. Individualized efforts and specialized programs, when planned in isolation, can lead to fragmentation and gaps in health services. For example, without collaboration, a well-child clinic may be started in a community that already has a strong Early and Periodic Screening and Developmental Testing (EPSDT) program, yet community prenatal services may be nonexistent. Interprofessional collaboration is important in individualized practice, because nurses need to plan with the client, family, physician, social worker, physical therapist, teacher, or counselor, and must keep them informed of the client's health status; however, it is a greater necessity when working with population groups, especially those from vulnerable or at-risk segments.

Effective collaboration requires team members who are strong individuals, with various areas of expertise and who can make a commitment to team goals. Community health nurses who think and act interdependently make a great contribution to the team effort. In appropriate situations, community health nurses also function autonomously, making independent judgments. Collaboration involves working with members of other professions on community advisory boards and health planning committees to develop needs assessment surveys and to contribute toward policy development efforts.

Interprofessional collaboration requires clarification of each team member's role, a primary reason for community health nurses to understand the nature of their practice. When planning a city-wide immunization program with a community group, for example, community health nurses need to explain the ways in which they might contribute to the program's objectives. They can offer to contact key community leaders, with whom they have established relationships, to build community acceptance of the program. They can share their knowledge of the public's preference about times and locations for the program. They can meet with various local agencies and organizations (e.g., health insurance companies, local hospitals) to gain financial support. They can help to organize and give the immunizations, and they can influence planning for follow-up programs. Another component includes development of policies to promote and protect the health of clients. This can be accomplished by meeting with local legislators and providing testimony to local, state, and national bodies in an effort to promote legislation to mandate helmets for cyclists, ban sugar-laden beverages in school vending machines, or provide funding for specific community-based programs. Collaboration is discussed further in Chapter 10.

Client participation is promoted when people serve as partners on the health care team. An aim of community health nursing is to collaborate with people, rather than do things for them. As consumers of health services are treated with respect and trust and, as a result, gain confidence and skill in self-care—promoting their own health and that of their community—their contribution to health programs becomes increasingly valuable. The consumer perspective in planning and delivering health services makes those services relevant to consumer needs. Community health nurses encourage the involvement of health care consumers by soliciting their ideas and opinions, by inviting them to participate on health boards and committees, and by finding ways to promote their participation in decisions affecting their collective health.

Summary

Community health nursing has opportunities and challenges to keep the nurse interested and involved in a community-focused career for a lifetime. Community health is more than environmental programs and large-scale efforts to control communicable disease. It is defined as the identification of needs and the protection and improvement of collective health within a geographically defined area. To comprehend the nature and significance of community health and to clarify it's meaning for the specialty practice of community health nursing, it is important to understand the concepts of community and of health.

A *community*, broadly defined, is a collection of people who share some common interest or goal. Three types were discussed in this chapter: geographic, common-interest, and health problem-solving communities. Sometimes, a community such as a neighborhood, city, or county is formed by geographic boundaries. At other times, a community may be identified by its common interest; examples are a religious community, a group of migrant workers, or citizens concerned about air pollution. A community also is defined by a pooling of efforts by people and agencies toward solving a health-related problem.

Health is an abstract concept that can be understood more clearly by examining its distinguishing features. First, people are neither sick nor well in an absolute sense but have levels of illness or wellness. These levels may be plotted along a continuum ranging from optimal health to total

disability or death. This is known as the *health continuum*. A person's state of health is dynamic, varying from day to day and even hour to hour.

Second, health is a state of being that includes all of the many characteristics of a person, family, or community, whether physical, psychological, social, or spiritual. These characteristics often indicate the degree of wellness or illness of an individual or community and suggest the presence or absence of vitality and well-being.

Third, health has both subjective and objective dimensions: the subjective involves how well people feel; the objective refers to how well they are able to function. Most often, functional performance diminishes dramatically toward the illness end of the health continuum.

Fourth, health care needs can be either continuing, as in developmental concerns that occur over a person's lifetime, or episodic, occurring unexpectedly once or twice in a lifetime. Community health nursing deals with continuing needs, whereas episodic needs are more often managed in acute care settings.

Community health practice incorporates the elements of promotion of health and prevention of health problems.

The eight important characteristics of community health practice are the client is the population, the greatest good for the greatest number of people, working with clients as equal partners, primary prevention is the priority, select strategies that create healthy environmental, social and economic conditions, reach out to all who might benefit, make optimal use of available resources, and collaborate with a variety of professions, organizations, and entities. ■

ACTIVITIES TO PROMOTE CRITICAL THINKING

1. Identify a community of people about whom you have some knowledge. What makes it a community? What characteristics do this group of people share? Work on this activity in a group of peers or family members. Do they think as you do? Is there a difference between the views of family members and those of nursing student peers?

2. Select three populations for whom you have some concern, and place each group on the health continuum. What factors influenced your decision?

3. Describe three preventive actions (one primary, one secondary, and one tertiary) that might be taken to move each of your selected populations closer to optimal wellness.

4. Select a current health problem and identify the three levels of prevention and corresponding activities in which you as a community health nurse would engage at each level.

5. Discuss how you might implement one health-promotion effort with each of your selected populations.

6. Browse the Internet for community health nursing research articles that focus on levels of prevention. Find one focusing on each level. For those involved

in the articles focusing on secondary and tertiary prevention, what could you as a community health nurse have done to keep the clients at the primary level of prevention?

7. Place yourself on the health continuum. What factors influenced your decision?

8. Using the eight characteristics of community health nursing outlined in this chapter, give examples of how a community health nurse might demonstrate meeting each characteristic.

References

American Cancer Society. (2008). Schools move to limit 'junk' foods. Retrieved August 2, 2008 from http://www.cancer.org/docroot/SPC/content/SPC_1_Schools_Move_to_Expel_Junk_Foods.asp.

American Nurses Association. (2005). *Public health nursing: Scope and standards of practice (draft document)*. Retrieved August 23, 2005 from I:\stathome\webpage\practice\publichealthnursing.doc.

American Public Health Association (APHA) Public Health Nursing Section. (1996). *The definition and role of public health nursing*. Washington, DC: APHA.

Anderson, E.T., & McFarlane, J. (2004). *Community as partner: Theory and practice in nursing*. Philadelphia, PA: Lippincott, Williams & Wilkins.

Associated Press, The. (June 15, 2006). Many asthma-related deaths involve children with mild cases. *Visalia Times-Delta*.

Bircher, J. (2005). Towards a dynamic definition of health and disease. *Medicine, Health Care & Philosophy, 8*, 335–341.

Bryant, J.H. (2003). Reflections on primary health care: 25 years after Alma Ata. Retrieved June 27, 2008 from www.who.int/chronic_conditions/primary_health_care/en/closing_jbryant.pdf.

Canadian Institute for Health Information. (2006). *Health indicators: 2006*. Ottawa, Ontario: Author.

Clinton County Health Department. (2006). A definition of public health. Retrieved June 27, 2008 from www.co.clinton.ny.us/Departments/Health/print_page/aboutus.pdf.

Coovadia, H.M., & Hadingham, J. (2005). HIV/AIDS: Global trends, global funds and delivery bottlenecks. *Globalization and Health, 1*(13), 1–10.

Cottrell, L.S. (1076). The competent community. In B.H. Kaplan, R.N. Wilson & A.H. Leighton (Eds.), *Further explanations in social psychiatry* (pp.195–209). New York: Basic Books.

Eisenberg, L. (2005). Are genes destiny? Have adenine, cytosine, guanine and thymine replaced Lachesis, Clotho and Atropos as the weavers of our fate? *World Psychiatry, 4*(1), 3–8.

Glasgow, R.E., Ory, M.G., Klesges, L.M., Cifuentes, M., Fernald, D., & Green, L.A. (2005). Practical and relevant self-report measures of patient health behaviors for primary care research. *Annals of Family Medicine, 3*, 73–81.

Healthy People 2010. (2006). What are the leading health indicators? Retrieved June 27, 2008 from www.healthypeople.gov/LHI/lhiwhat.htm.

Healthy People 2010. (2001). Healthy People in Healthy Communities: A community planning guide using Healthy People 2010. Retrieved June 27, 2008 from www.healthypeople.gov/Publications/HealthyCommunities2001/Chapter_1.htm.

Hundley, J., Kilgo, P., Miller, P., Chang, M., Hensberry, R., Meredith, J., & Hoth, J. (2004). Non-helmeted motorcyclists: A burden to society? A study using the National Trauma Data Bank. *Journal of Trauma, 57*(5), 944–949.

Huynen, M., Martens, P., & Hilderink, H. (2005). The health impacts of globalization: A conceptual framework. *Globalization and Health, 1*(14), 1–19.

Institute of Medicine. (2001). *The future of the public's health in the 21st century*. Washington, DC: National Academy Press.

Institute of Medicine. (1998). *The future of public health*. Washington, DC: National Academy Press.

Kriebel, D., & Tickner, J. (2001). Reenergizing public health through precaution. *American Journal of Public Health, 91*(9), 1351–1354.

Krisberg, K. (April, 2006). Safer housing conditions mean healthier lives for children. *The Nation's Health, 1*, 22–23.

Kyrychenko, S.Y., & McCartt, A.T. (2006). Florida's weakened motorcycle helmet law: Effects on death rates in motorcycle crashes. *Traffic Injury Prevention, 7*(1), 55–60.

Lipson, J., & Dibble, S. (2005). *Culture and clinical care*. San Francisco, CA: UCSF Nursing Press.

Lopez, A., Mathers, C., Ezzati, M., Jamison, D., & Murray, C. (2006). Global and regional burden of disease and risk factors, 2001: Systematic analysis of population health data. *Lancet, 367*(9524), 1747–1757.

Macpherson, A.K., To, T.M., Macarthur, C., Chipman, M.L., Wright, J.G., & Parkin, P.C. (2002). *Pediatrics, 110*(5), E60.

Meadows, M. (2005). Genomics and personalized medicine. *FDA Consumer.* Retrieved May 1, 2006 from www.fda.gov/fdac/features/2005/605_genomics.html.

Milestones in Public Health: Accomplishments in public health over the last 100 years. (2006). Pfizer, Inc.: New York, NY.

Morbidity and Mortality Weekly Report. (May 26, 2006). Use of cigarettes and other tobacco products among students aged 13–15 years: Worldwide, 1999–2005.

Morbidity and Mortality Weekly Report. (March 10, 2006). Public health response to hurricanes Katrina and Rita: United States, 2005.

Morbidity and Mortality Weekly Report. (January 19, 2006). Assessment of health-related needs after hurricane Katrina: Orleans and Jefferson Parishes, New Orleans area, Louisiana, October 17–22, 2005.

Morbidity and Mortality Weekly Report. (January 30, 2004). 40th anniversary of the First Surgeon General's Report on Smoking and Health/Prevalence of cigarette use among 14 racial/ethnic populations: United States, 1999–2001.

Morbidity and Mortality Weekly Report. (April 7, 2000). Community indicators of health-related quality of life: United States, 1993–1997.

Neuman, B. (2001). The Neuman systems model. In B. Neuman (Ed.), *The Neuman systems model* (4th ed.). Norwalk, CT: Appleton & Lange.

Nightingale, F. (1859/1992). Notes on nursing: What it is, and what it is not [Commemorative edition]. Philadelphia: Lippincott.

Orem, D. (2001). *Nursing concepts of practice* (6th ed.). St. Louis: Mosby-Year Book.

Parker, R., & Gazmararian, J. (2003). Health literacy: Essential for health communication. *Journal of Health Communication, 8*(Suppl 1), 116–118.

Pender, N.J., Murdaugh, C., & Parsons, M.A. (2006). *Health promotion in nursing practice* (5th ed.). Upper Saddle River, NJ: Prentice-Hall Health, Inc.

Porter-O'Grady, T. (2001). Profound change: 21st century nursing. *Nursing Outlook, 49*(4), 182–186.

Public Health Data Standards Consortium. (2006). Public Health Data Standards tutorial: Glossary of terms. Retrieved June 27, 2008 from www.phdatastandards.info/knowresources/tutorials/glossary.htm.

Quad Council. (2003). Public health nursing competencies. Retrieved June 27, 2008 from www.astdn.org/downloadablefiles/PHB%20competencies%20final%20comb.pdf.

Roach, S.S. (2000). *Introductory gerontological nursing*. Philadelphia: Lippincott Williams & Wilkins.

Rodgers, G.B. (2002). Effects of state helmet laws on bicycle helmet use by children and adolescents. *Injury Prevention, 8*(1), 42–46.

Sarrachi, R. (1997). The World Health Organization needs to reconsider its definition of Health. *British Medical Journal, 314*, 1409–1410.

Schulman, J., Sacks, J., & Provenzano, G. (2002). State-level estimates of the incidence and economic burden of head injuries stemming from non-universal use of bicycle helmets. *Injury Prevention, 8*(1), 47–52.

Thomson, G., & Wilson, N. (2005). Policy lessons from comparing mortality from two global forces: International terrorism and tobacco. *Global Health, 15*(1), 18.

Trust for America's Health. (2006). Ask the epidemiologist: Glossary of terms. Retrieved June 27, 2008 from http://healthyamericans.org/docs/?DocID=96.

U.S. Department of Health and Human Services (USDHHS). (2000). *Healthy People 2010* (Conference ed., in two volumes). Washington, DC: U.S. Government Printing Office.

Ustin, B., & Jakob, R. (2005). Calling a spade a spade: Meaningful definitions of health conditions. *Bulletin of the World Health Organization, 83*, 802.

Williams, C. (1977). Community health nursing: What is it? *Nursing Outlook, 25*(4), 250–254.

World Health Organization. (2006a). The world health report: 1998. Message from the Director-General. Retrieved January 20, 2006 from www.who.int/whr/1998/media_centre/dgmessage/ en/index.html.

World Health Organization. (2006b). Healthy cities: Reducing poverty through healthy cities programme. Retrieved January 20, 2006 from www.afro.who.int/des.

World Health Organization. (2004). WHO award for healthy cities. Retrieved June 27, 2008 from www.wpro.who.int/NR/rdonlyres/F23E3F1E-74F2-4894-8BAA-9F2ACC51E045/0/whoawardsforhealthycities2004.pdf.

Zhang, R., Eggleston, K., Rotimi, V., & Zeckhauser, R.J. (2006). Antibiotic resistance as a global threat: evidence from China, Kuwait and the United States [Electronic version]. *Global Health, 2*(1), article 6.

Zumla, A., & Mullan, Z. (2006). Turning the tide against tuberculosis. *Lancet, 367*(9514), 877–888.

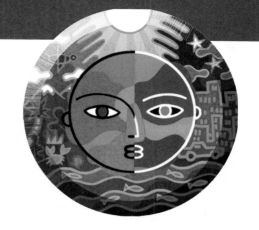

2

History and Evolution of Community Health Nursing

LEARNING OBJECTIVES

Upon mastery of this chapter, you should be able to:

◆ Describe the four stages of community health nursing's development.
◆ Recognize the contributions of selected nursing leaders throughout history to the advancement of community health nursing.
◆ Analyze the impact of societal influences on the development and practice of community health nursing.
◆ Explore the academic and advanced professional preparation of community health nurses.

❝*Our basic idea was that the nurse's peculiar introduction to the patient and her organic relationship with the neighborhood should constitute the starting point for a universal service to the region. . . . we considered ourselves best described by the term 'public health nurses.'*❞
—Lillian Wald (1867–1940), pioneer of public health nursing

You just left the home of a long-time client who is concerned about a new family who just moved into the building where she lives. The family of six lives in an apartment with barely enough room for two. After years in this neighborhood, you are well aware of the high rents charged for apartments with peeling paint, rodents, and garbage all around the buildings. Your client is concerned that the young mother looks "worn out" and coughs all the time. She said she tried to help, but the family doesn't speak much English. She describes four young children all under the age of about 5. She's never seen the husband, but you know that most of the men in this neighborhood leave early in the morning to try to get some day work, so you are not surprised. You assure your client that you will do what you can to help her new neighbors and thank her for being such a kind person. Thinking about how you will prepare for the visit to the family who doesn't even expect you, your thoughts are racing. At the top of your list is trying to find someone who speaks their language; you only know a few words. You suspect without even seeing the mother what the cough means, although you hope you are wrong. Then you think about the four young children living so close together and creating so much work for a woman who isn't well. The husband may want to help his wife more, but if he doesn't work, they can't get by. You wonder if he has the cough too.

As you read this scenario, what picture did you have in your mind? What language did this family speak? What disease did this young mother likely have? Now, think about when this event might have occurred. If you thought it was now, it certainly could be, but this scenario was actually set in the early 1900s. This family emigrated from Greece and hadn't yet mastered the English language. The mother likely had consumption (the old name for tuberculosis). Because birth control information was not available to most women, she had no idea how to space out her pregnancies. The filthy and overcrowded housing, often called *tenement housing*, was typical of the time. The husband found work as he could. Few social services were available; no work, no food for the family, and no money to pay the rent. The family came to America with the hope of a new start, but what they found was in many ways worse than what they had left. At least at home in Greece, they had family and friends to count on; here, they were alone. There were others from Greece who lived nearby, but it wasn't the same. Life was hard, and they worried most about their children, wondering what the future could hold for them.

Community health nurses in the early 20th century had to deal with many of the same issues we face today. We thought for a long time that tuberculosis was a disease of the past; now clients with multidrug-resistant strains are becoming alarmingly more common. Poverty, communicable diseases, poor housing, lack of social services, and limited access to family planning information remain as challenges to improving the health of our populations. As a community health nurse, you will be facing similar challenges to those faced by nurses of the past. History is not always exciting, but without it we often fail to see where we need to go next. The often misquoted saying by George Santayana (1863–1952), "Those who cannot remember the past are condemned to repeat it," serves to caution us not to "forget" our heritage (Kaplin, 1992, p. 588). As you read through this chapter, think about how your practice has been shaped by the hard work of the nurses who went before.

This chapter examines the international roots of community health nursing as a specialty, exploring the historical and philosophical foundations that undergird the dynamic nature of its practice. The chapter traces community health nursing's historical development, highlighting the contributions of several nursing leaders, and examining the global societal influences that shaped early and evolving community health nursing practice. The final section of the chapter describes the academic and advanced professional preparation required of community health nurses today. Nursing's past influences its present, and both guide the future of community health nursing in the 21st century.

HISTORICAL DEVELOPMENT OF COMMUNITY HEALTH NURSING

Before the nature of community health nursing can be fully grasped or its practice defined, it is necessary to understand its roots and the factors that shaped its growth over time. Community health nursing is the product of centuries of responsiveness and growth. Its practice has adapted to accommodate the needs of a changing society, yet it has always maintained its initial goal of improved community health. Community health nursing's development, which has been influenced by changes in nursing, public health, and society, can be traced through several stages. This section examines these stages.

The history of public health nursing, since its recognized inception in Europe, and more recently in America, encompasses continuing change and adaptation (Hein, 2001). The historical record reveals a professional nursing specialty that has been on the cutting edge of innovations in public health practice and has provided leadership to public health efforts. A summary of public health nursing made in the early 1900s still holds true:

> It is precisely in the field of the application of knowledge that the public health nurse has found her great opportunity and her greatest usefulness. In the nationwide campaigns for the early detection of cancer and mental disorders, for the elimination of venereal disease, for the training of new mothers, and the teaching of the principles of hygiene to young and old; in short, in all measures for the prevention of disease and the raising of health standards, no agency is more valuable than the public health nurse. (Central Hanover Bank and Trust Company, 1938, p. 8)

In tracing the development of public health nursing and, later, community health nursing, the leadership role has been clearly evident throughout its history. Nurses in this specialty have provided leadership in planning and developing programs, in shaping policy, in administration, and in the application of research to community health.

Four general stages mark the development of community health/public health nursing: (1) the early home care nursing stage, (2) the district nursing stage, (3) the public health nursing stage, and (4) the community health nursing stage. It is well worth referring to the Chapter 1 discussion of the interchangeable terms *public health nurse* and *community health nurse*. In the course of the historical evolution of this specialty, there was a definite shift in thinking about the focus of practice, resulting in the broader use of the term *community health nurse*. However, the discussion that follows is about the practice emphasis, not the title. There are still nurses in practice who use the title public health nurse, in addition to those called community health nurses; some even use the title community/public health nurse. Whether by custom, preference, or established employment title, nurses call themselves by many professional titles. It is important to recognize that the work of the nurse is, as it always has been, to improve the health of the community.

Early Home Care Nursing (Before Mid-1800s)

The prototype of **community-based nursing** can be seen within the historical development of home-care nursing. For many centuries, the sick were tended at home by female family members and friends. In fact, in 1837, Farrar (p. 57) reminded women, "You may be called upon at any moment to attend upon your parents, your brothers, your sisters, or your companions." The focus of this care was to reduce suffering and promote healing.

The Origins of Early Nursing

The early roots of home-care nursing began with religious and charitable groups. Even emergency care was provided. In 1244, a group of monks in Florence, Italy, known as the Misericordia provided first-aid care for accident victims on a 24-hour basis. Another example is the Knights Hospitalers, who were warrior monks in Western Europe. They protected and cared for pilgrims on their way to Jerusalem ("Men, monasteries, wars, and wards," 2001). These and other men's contributions to the early practice of nursing have been long overlooked. Further, the lack of attention to these early works "perpetuates the notion of men nurses as anomalies" (Evans, 2004, p. 321).

Medieval times saw the development of various institutions devoted to the sick, including hospitals and nursing orders. In England, the Elizabethan Poor Law, written in 1601, provided medical and nursing care to the poor and disabled. St. Frances De Sales organized the Friendly Visitor Volunteers in the early 1600s in France. This association was directed by Madame de Chantel and assisted by wealthy women who cared for the sick poor in their homes (Dolan, 1978). In Paris in 1617, St. Vincent de Paul started the Sisters of Charity, an organization composed of nuns and lay women dedicated to serving the poor and needy. The ladies and sisters, under the supervision of Mademoiselle Le Gras in 1634, promoted the goal of teaching people to help themselves as they visited the sick in their homes. In their emphasis on preparing nurses and supervising nursing care, as well as determining causes and solutions for clients' problems, the Sisters of Charity laid a foundation for modern community health nursing (Bullough & Bullough, 1978).

Unfortunately, the years that followed these accomplishments marked a serious setback in the status of nursing and care of the sick. From the late 1600s to the mid-1800s, the social upheaval after the Reformation caused a decline in the number of religious orders, with subsequent curtailing of nursing care for the sick poor. Babies continued to be delivered at home by self-declared midwives, most of whom had little or no training. Concern over high maternal mortality rates prompted efforts to better prepare midwives and medical students. One midwifery program was begun in Paris in 1720, and another in London by Dr. William Smellie in 1741 (Bullough & Bullough, 1978).

The Industrial Revolution created additional problems; among them were epidemics, high infant mortality, occupational diseases and injuries, and increasing mental illness in both Europe and America. Hospitals were built in larger cities, and dispensaries were developed to provide greater access to physicians. However, disease was rampant; mortality rates were high; and institutional conditions, especially in prisons, hospitals, and "asylums" for the insane, were deplorable. The sick and afflicted were kept in filthy rooms without adequate food, water, cover, or care for their physical and emotional needs (Bullough & Bullough, 1978). Reformers such as John Howard, an Englishman who investigated the spread of disease in hospitals in 1789 (Kalisch & Kalisch, 2004), revealed serious needs that would not be addressed until much later (Bullough & Bullough, 1978).

Both Catholic and Anglican religious nursing orders, although few in number, continued the work of caring for the sick poor in their homes. For example, in 1812, the Sisters of Mercy organized in Dublin to provide care for the sick at home. With the status of women at an all-time low, often only the least respectable women pursued nursing. In 1844, in his novel *Martin Chuzzlewit,* Charles Dickens (1910) portrayed the nurse Sairy Gamp as an unschooled and slovenly drunkard, reflecting society's view of nursing at the time. It was in the midst of these deplorable conditions and in response to them that Florence Nightingale began her work.

The Early Nightingale Years

Much of the foundation for modern community health nursing practice was laid through Florence Nightingale's remarkable accomplishments (Figure 2.1). She has been referred to as a reformer, a reactionary, and a researcher (Palmer, 2001). Born in 1820 into a wealthy English family, her extensive travel, excellent education—including training at the first school for nurses in Kaiserwerth, Germany—and determination to serve the needy resulted in major reforms and improved status for nursing. Her work during the Crimean War (1854–1856) with the wounded in Scutari is well documented (Florence Nightingale Museum Trust, 1997; Woodham-Smith, 1951). Conditions in the military hospitals during the war were unspeakable. Thousands of sick and wounded men lay in filth, without beds, clean coverings, food, water, or laundry facilities. Florence Nightingale organized competent nursing care and established kitchens and laundries that resulted in hundreds of lives being saved. Her work further demonstrated that capable nursing intervention could prevent illness and improve the health of a population at risk—precursors to modern community health nursing practice. Her subsequent work for health reform in the military was supported by implementing another public health strategy: the use of biostatistics. Through meticulously gathered data and statistical comparisons, Miss Nightingale demonstrated that military mortality rates, even in peacetime, were double those of the civilian population because of the terrible living conditions in the barracks. This work led to important military reforms.

Miss Nightingale's concern for populations at risk included a continuing interest in the population of the sick at

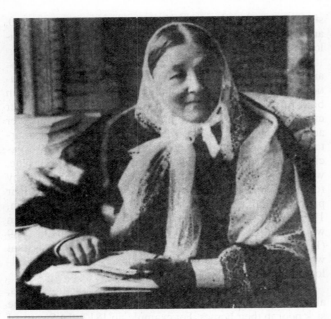

FIGURE 2.1 Florence Nightingale's concern for populations at risk, as well as her vision and successful efforts at health reform, provided a model for community health nursing today.

home. Her book, *Notes on Nursing: What It Is, and What It Is Not,* published in England in 1859, was written to improve nursing care in the home. It was also during this period that Nightingale clarified nursing as a woman's occupation (Evans, 2004). This gender distinction in nursing was due more to the culture of the times than as a direct exclusion of men from the practice; it was consistent with social norms of that period.

Florence Nightingale also became a skillful lobbyist for health care reform. Her exemplary influence on English politics and policy improved the quality of existing health care and set standards for future practice. Furthermore, she demonstrated how population-focused nursing works.

In her work to help establish the first nonreligious school for nurses in 1860 at St. Thomas Hospital in London, she promoted a standard for proper education and supervision of nurses in practice, known as the Nightingale Model. Principles she wrote about in *Notes on Nursing* relate directly to her early education and the notions held by Hippocrates in ancient Greece, which she had studied for years. Specifically, her concern with the environment of patients, the need for keen observation, the focus on the whole patient rather than the disease, and the importance of assisting nature to bring about a cure all reflect Hippocrates' teachings (Nightingale, 1859/1969; Palmer, 2001).

Another great nurse and healer in her own right was Mary Seacole (1805–1881), who has been called the "Black Nightingale." She was the daughter of a well-respected "doctress" who practiced Creole or Afro-Caribbean medicine in Jamaica, and began helping her mother at an early age. Spending many years developing her skills, she helped populations who experienced tropical diseases, especially cholera, in Central America, Panama, and the Caribbean. She attempted, through many formal channels, to join Florence Nightingale in Scutari, but was rejected again and again. Undaunted, she went to the Crimea on her own to open a hotel for sick and convalescing soldiers,

where she met Miss Nightingale and many of the troops she had cared for in Jamaica. Many of the military commanders sought her out for her knowledge of healing, and she was affectionately known by the troops as "Mother Seacole." After the war and into her old age, she continued to provide nursing care in London and when visiting Jamaica. She focused her caregiving among high-risk clients of the day and did so in an innovative, entrepreneurial manner unique for women, especially for women of color in the 1800s (Florence Nightingale Museum Trust, 1997).

District Nursing (Mid-1800s to 1900)

Nightingale's Continued Influence

The next stage in the development of community health nursing was the formal organization of visiting nursing, or **district nursing.** In 1859, William Rathbone, an English philanthropist, became convinced of the value of home nursing as a result of private care given to his wife. He employed Mary Robinson, the nurse who had cared for his wife, to visit the sick poor in their homes and teach them proper hygiene to prevent illness. The need was so great that it soon became evident that more nurses were needed. In 1861, with Florence Nightingale's help and advice, Rathbone opened a training school for nurses connected with the Royal Liverpool Infirmary and established a visiting nurse service for the sick poor in Liverpool. Florence Lees, a graduate of the Nightingale School, was appointed first Superintendent-General of the District Nursing System (Mowbray, 1997). As the service grew, visiting nurses were assigned to districts in the city—hence the name, district nursing. Subsequently, other British cities also developed district nursing training and services. An example is the Nurse Training Institution for district nurses, founded in Manchester in 1864. Privately financed, the nurses were trained and then "dispensed food and medicine" to the sick poor in their homes; they were "closely supervised by various middle and upper class women who collected the necessary supplies" (Bullough & Bullough, 1978, p. 143).

Although Florence Nightingale is best remembered for her professionalization of nursing, she had a full understanding of the need for community health nursing. This was documented in her writings and recorded conversations:

> Hospitals are but an intermediate stage of civilisation. At present hospitals are the only place where the sick poor can be nursed, or, indeed often the sick rich. But the ultimate object is to nurse all sick at home. (Nightingale, 1876)
>
> The aim of the district nurse is to give first-rate nursing to the sick poor at home. (Nightingale, 1876 [cited in Mowbray, 1997, p. 24])
>
> The health visitor must create a new profession for women. (conversation with Frederick Verney, 1891 [cited in Mowbray, 1997, p. 25])

For years, Miss Nightingale studied the social and economic conditions of India (Nightingale, 1864). The plight of the poor and ill in India led her to become involved with Frederick Verney in a pioneering "health at home" project in England in 1892. She wrote a series of papers on the need for "home missioners" and "health visitors," endorsing the view that prevention was better than cure (Mowbray, 1997).

DISPLAY 2.1	TWENTY YEARS IN HISTORY: 1873–1893

1873	First Nightingale-model nursing school established in the U.S. at Bellevue Hospital
1877	Francis Root—First Public Health Nurse hired by the Women's Branch of the New York Mission
1885	Visiting Nurse Association established in Buffalo, New York
1886	Visiting Nurse Associations established in Philadelphia and Boston
1893	Lillian Wald and Mary Brewster organize a visiting nurses service for the poor in New York, which would be named the Henry Street Settlement in 1906

Home Visiting Takes Root

In the United States, the first community health nurse, Frances Root, hired by the Women's Branch of the New York Mission in 1877, pioneered home visits to the poor in New York City. District nursing associations were founded in Buffalo in 1885, and in Boston and Philadelphia in 1886 (Display 2.1). These district associations served the sick poor exclusively, because patients with enough money had private home nursing care. However, the English model with its standards for visiting nurses' education and practice, established in 1889 under Queen Victoria, was not followed in the United States. Instead, visiting nursing organizations sprang up in many cities without common standards or administration. Twenty-one such services existed in the United States in 1890 (Bullough & Bullough, 1978; Kalisch & Kalisch, 2004).

Although district nurses primarily cared for the sick, they also taught cleanliness and wholesome living to their patients, even during that early period. For example, the Boston program, founded by the Women's Educational Association, "emphasized the teaching of hygiene and cleanliness, giving impetus to what was called instructive district nursing" (Bullough & Bullough, 1978, p. 144). This early emphasis on prevention and "health" nursing became one of the distinguishing features of district nursing and, later, of public health nursing as a specialty.

The work of district nurses in the United States focused mostly on the care of individuals. District nurses recorded temperatures and pulse rates and gave simple treatments to the sick poor under the immediate direction of a physician. They also instructed family members in personal hygiene, diet and healthful living habits, and the care of the sick. The problems of early home care patients in the United States were numerous and complex. Thousands of European and eastern European immigrants filled tenement housing in the poorest and most crowded slums of the large coastal cities during the late 1800s. Inadequate sanitation, unsafe and unhealthy working conditions, and language and cultural barriers added to poverty and disease. Nursing educational programs at that time did not prepare district nurses to cope with their patients' multiple health and social problems.

The sponsorship of district nursing changed over time. Early district nursing services in both England and the United States were founded by religious organizations. Later, sponsorship shifted to private philanthropy. Funding came from contributions and, in a few instances, from fees charged to patients on an ability-to-pay basis. Finally, visiting nursing began to be supported by public money. An early example occurred in Los Angeles where, in 1897, a nurse was hired as a city employee. Although one form of funding dominated, all three types of financing continued to exist, as they still do. Although the government was beginning to assume more responsibility for the public's health, most district nursing services during this time remained private.

In England, the establishment of "health visitors" in poor areas of London began early in the 19th century. These health care providers enhanced the English model of health visitor/district nurse/midwife as the backbone of the primary health care system in the second half of the 1800s. "The impact of early health visiting was clearly shown by the halving of infant mortality in the areas within two years" (Beine, 1996, p. 59). The main focus of the health visitor's work was giving advice to poor mothers and teaching hygiene to prevent infant diarrhea (Beine, 1996).

Public Health Nursing (1900 to 1970)

By the beginning of the 20th century, district nursing had broadened its focus to include the health and welfare of the general public, not just the poor. This new emphasis was part of a broader consciousness about public health. Robert Koch's demonstration that tuberculosis was communicable led the Johns Hopkins Hospital to hire a nurse, Reba Thelin, in 1903, to visit the homes of tuberculosis patients. Her job was to ensure that patients followed prescribed regimens of rest, fresh air, and proper diet and to prevent possible infection (Sachs, 1908). A growing sense of urgency about the interrelatedness of health conditions and the need to improve the health of all people led to an increased number of private health agencies. These agencies supplemented the often-limited work of government health departments. By 1910, new federal laws made states and communities accountable for the health of their citizens.

Nurses Making a Difference

Three years before Reba Thelin began her work with Johns Hopkins Hospital, Jessie Sleet was hired by the Charity Organization Society's (COS) tuberculosis committee as a temporary district nurse in New York City (Mosley, 2007). Her position called for her to visit the city's black community, which was ravaged by the disease. Jessie Sleet had been trained at the Provident Hospital in Chicago (a hospital for black patients), which had a nurse's training program for black women. Credited as the first black public health nurse, Ms. Sleet was not eagerly accepted by the COS membership, but they agreed in hope that she would be accepted by the black community. She was so successful in her efforts that, one year later, the society

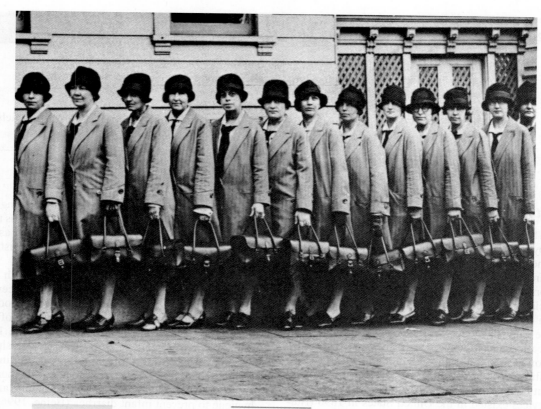

FIGURE 2.2 Public health nurses—uniforms and symbols. (Photograph courtesy of Visiting Nurses and Hospice of San Francisco.)

hired her as a permanent employee (Mosley, 2007). Jessie Sleet was a pioneer in early community health nursing practice and forged the way for many.

As specialized programs such as infant welfare, tuberculosis clinics, and venereal disease control were developed, there was an increased demand for nurses to work in these areas (Figure 2.2). As Bullough and Bullough commented, "Although the hospital nursing school movement emphasized the care of the sick, a small but growing number of nurses were finding employment in preventive health care" (1978, p. 143). In 1900, there were an estimated 200 public health nurses. By 1912, that number had grown to 3,000 (Gardner, 1936). "This development was important: it brought health care and health teaching to the public, gave nurses an opportunity for more independent work, and helped to improve nursing education" (Bullough & Bullough, 1978, p. 143).

The role of the district nurse expanded during this stage. Lillian D. Wald (1867–1940), a leading figure in this expansion, first used the term *public health nursing* to describe this specialty (Bullough & Bullough, 1978). District nurses, while caring for the sick, had pioneered in health teaching, disease prevention, and promotion of good health practices. Now, with a growing recognition of familial and environmental influences on health, public health nurses broadened their practice even more. Nurses working outside of the hospital increased their knowledge and skills in specialized areas such as tuberculosis, maternal and child health, school health, and mental disorders.

Lillian Wald's contributions to public health nursing were enormous. A graduate of the New York Hospital Training School, she started teaching home nursing but quickly changed to a career of social reform and nursing activism (Christy, 1970). Appalled by the conditions of an immigrant neighborhood in New York's Lower East Side, she and a nurse-friend, Mary Brewster, started the Henry Street Settlement in 1893 to provide nursing and welfare services. Her books, *The House on Henry Street* (1915) and *Windows of Henry Street* (1934), portray her work and views on public health nursing. Nursing visits conducted through her organization were supervised by nurses, in contrast to earlier models, in which nursing services were administered by lay boards and actual care was supervised by lay persons. It was during these early years that Wald asked Jessie Sleet to recommend another black nurse for service at the settlement (Mosley, 2007). Miss Sleet recommended her schoolmate Miss Elizabeth Tyler, a graduate of the Freedmen's Hospital Training School for Nurses (Washington, D.C.). In 1906, Miss Tyler became the first black nurse hired at the Henry Street Settlement; she would not be the last. This was no small event in the progress of public health nursing and was a clear demonstration of Miss Wald's commitment to social change.

Wald's Growing Influence

The work done at the Henry Street Settlement showed clearly that nursing could reduce illness-caused employee absenteeism. She demonstrated this in her early work with the city of New York. She would use this success to address the issue of childhood illness and school absenteeism (Bullough & Bullough, 1978). In the early 1900s, approximately 15 to 20 children per day were sent home from each school in New York City for health-related reasons. Wald suggested that

DISPLAY 2.2	TWENTY YEARS IN HISTORY: 1909–1929

1909	Metropolitan Life Insurance Company provided first insurance reimbursement for visiting nursing care
1910	Public Health Nursing program instituted at Teacher's College, Columbia University
1912	National Organization for Public Health Nursing formed, with Lillian Wald as first President
1917	U.S. entry into World War I
	18th Amendment passed by Congress (Prohibition)
1918	U.S. Public Health Service establishes Division of Public Health Nursing to aid the war effort
	World War I Armistice
	World-wide influenza epidemic begins
1919	19th Amendment passed by Congress (Vote)
1920	Women vote for the first time in a presidential election
1921	Margaret Sanger founds the American Birth Control League to distribute birth control information
	Bureau of Indian Affairs Health Division created (later to become the Indian Health Service)
1925	Frontier Nursing Service established
1929	Stock Market Crash

placing nurses in the schools would allow for follow-up on recurring cases and home visits during the periods of exclusion. She argued that the nurses could supplement the work done by local physicians, who occasionally examined the children. Offering the services of one nurse for 1 month, Wald hoped to demonstrate how effective a school nurse could be. The work done by this first school nurse, Lina Rogers, was a resounding success (Kalisch & Kalisch, 2004). One year after this initial experiment, the number of children sent home from the New York City schools had dropped dramatically. By September 1903, only 1,101 children needed to be excluded (compared with 10,567 one year earlier); a nearly 10-fold reduction. As a result, the New York Board of Health hired dozens of nurses to work at the schools.

Just 6 years after her efforts with the New York City schools, Wald embarked on another visionary path. In 1909,

she convinced the Metropolitan Life Insurance Company that nurse intervention could reduce death rates (Hamilton, 2007). In collaboration with the Henry Street Settlement, the company organized the Visiting Nurse Department and provided services to policy holders in a section of Manhattan (Display 2.2). The success of this program resulted in expansion to other parts of the city and to 12 other eastern cities within 1 year. By 1912, the company had organized 589 Metropolitan nursing centers and, when possible, contracted with local Visiting Nurses Associations, although they also hired their own nurses (Kalisch & Kalisch, 2004).

The legendary accomplishments of Lillian Wald reflect her driving commitment to serve needy populations. Through her efforts, the New York City Bureau of Child Hygiene was formed in 1908, and the Children's Bureau at the federal level in 1912 (Figure 2.3). Wald's emphasis on illness prevention

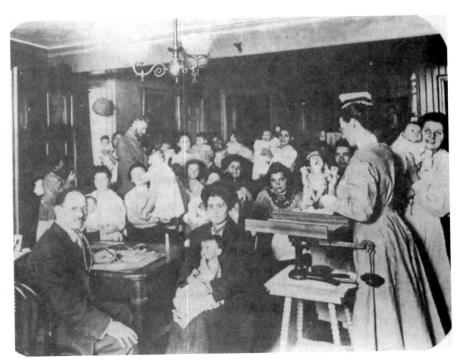

FIGURE 2.3   Examination of infants was part of early health department programs in which district nurses played a major role.

and health promotion through health teaching and nursing intervention, as well as her use of epidemiologic methodology, established these actions as hallmarks of public health nursing practice. She promoted rural nursing and family-focused nursing, and encouraged improved coursework at the Teachers College of Columbia University (New York) to prepare public health nurses for practice. Through her work and influence with the legislature to establish health and social policies, improvements were made in child labor and pure food laws, tenement housing, parks, city recreation centers, immigrant handling, and teaching of mentally handicapped children. In 1912, she helped to found and was first president of the National Organization for Public Health Nursing (NOPHN), an organization that set standards and guided public health nursing's further development and impact on public health (Christy, 1970). Her exemplary accomplishments truly reflect a concern for populations at risk. They further demonstrate how nursing leadership, involvement in policy formation, and use of epidemiology led to improved health for the public.

Another Nurse—Another Problem

During the same period that Lillian Wald and her contemporaries were working to alleviate the suffering caused by disease and poverty, another nurse, Margaret Sanger, began a different battle. Sanger, who was born in 1879, had seen her own mother die at the age of 48 after a long struggle with tuberculosis. Her 18 pregnancies undoubtedly contributed to her both contracting the disease and eventually succumbing to it. After her mother's death, she was accepted at White Plains Hospital as a nursing probationer (Ruffing-Rahal, 1986). Later, as a visiting nurse Sanger was prevented by the Comstock Act of 1873 from providing any information on contraception to the women she cared for (Draper, 2006). She knew, as did many at the time, that the affluent and educated in American society were the only ones to have reliable contraception. Even discussing the topic was prohibited, placing increased pressure on the poor and uneducated women who were most in need of this basic information. In 1912, Sanger watched helplessly as a 28-year-old mother of three died from abortion-induced septicemia. "A few months earlier, during a similar crisis, this woman had begged Sanger for the 'secret' of preventing future pregnancy" (Ruffing–Rahal, 1986, pp. 247–248). In 1916, Sanger openly offered birth control information in the Brownsville section of Brooklyn. Ten days after opening the first birth control clinic in America, Sanger was arrested and the clinic was closed. This was not the first nor would it be her last encounter with the legal system. Her open defiance of a law that she saw as unjust eventually resulted in the formation of the International Planned Parenthood Federation.

The Profession Evolves

By the 1920s, public health nursing was acquiring a more professional stature, in contrast to its earlier association with charity. Nursing as a whole was gaining professional status as a science, in addition to being an art. National nursing organizations began to form during this stage and contributed to nursing's professional growth. The first of these emphasized establishing educational standards for nursing. Called the American Society of Superintendents of Training Schools for Nurses in the United States and Canada, it was started by Isabel Hampton Robb in 1893, and later became known as the National League of Nursing Education in 1912. This was the forerunner of the National League for Nursing (NLN), which was established in 1952 (Ellis & Hartley, 2000). In 1890, a meeting of nursing leaders at the World's Fair in Chicago initiated an alumnae organization of 10 schools of nursing to form the National Associated Alumnae of the United States and Canada in 1896, which was created to promote nursing education and practice standards. In 1899, the group was renamed the Nurses' Associated Alumnae of the United States and Canada. Canada was excluded from the title in 1901, because New York, where the organization was incorporated, did not allow representation from two countries. In 1911, the organization went through a final name change to the American Nurses' Association (ANA), while Canadian nurses formed their own nursing organization (Ellis & Hartley, 2000). The previously mentioned NOPHN, founded by Lillian Wald and Mary Gardner, merged with the NLN in 1952. These three organizations, in particular, strengthened ties between nursing groups and improved nursing education and practice.

As nursing education became increasingly rigorous, collegiate programs began to include public health as essential content in basic nursing curricula. The first collegiate program with public health content to be accredited by the NLN began in 1944 (National Organization for Public Health Nursing, 1944) (Display 2.3). Previously, only postgraduate courses in public health nursing had been offered for nurses

DISPLAY 2.3	TWENTY YEARS IN HISTORY: 1933–1953
1933	18th Amendment repealed (Prohibition)
1935	Passage of Social Security Act
1937	Birth control information legal in all but two states (Massachusetts and Connecticut)
1941	U.S. entry into World War II
1943	Division of Nursing established at Public Health Service
1944	First basic program in nursing accredited as including sufficient public health content
1945	World War II ends
1946	Hill-Burton Act approved
	Communicable Disease Center established; forerunner of the Centers for Disease Control and Prevention
1950	U.S. involvement in Korean Conflict
1953	U.S. withdrawal from Korea

choosing this specialty. The first such course had been developed by Adelaide Nutting in 1912, at Teachers College in New York, in affiliation with the Henry Street Settlement. A group of agencies met in 1946 to establish guidelines for public health nursing, and by 1963, public health content was required for NLN accreditation in all baccalaureate nursing programs. The nurse practitioner (NP) movement, starting in 1965 at the University of Colorado, was initially a part of public health nursing and emphasized primary health care to rural and underserved populations. The number of educational programs to prepare NPs increased, with some NPs continuing in public health and others moving into different clinical areas.

During this period, as a result of the influence of Lillian Wald and other nursing leaders, the family began to emerge as a unit of service (Figure 2.4). The multiple problems faced by many families impelled a trend toward nursing care generalized enough to meet diverse needs and provide holistic services. Public health nurses gradually gained more autonomy in such areas as home care and instruction of good health practices to families and community groups. Their collaborative relationships with other community health providers grew as the need to avoid gaps and duplication of services became apparent. Public health nurses also began keeping better records of their services.

Industrial nursing, another form of public health nursing, also expanded during this period. The first known industrial nurse, Philippa Flowerday Reid, was hired in Norwich, England, by J. and J. Colmans in 1878. Her job was to assist the company physician and to visit sick employees and their families in their homes. In the United States, the Vermont Marble Company was first to begin a nursing service in 1895; other companies followed soon after. By 1910, 66 firms in the United States employed nurses. During World War I, the number of industrial nurses greatly increased with the recognition that nursing service reduced worker absenteeism (Bullough & Bullough, 1978). Early industrial nursing was the forerunner of modern occupational and environmental health nursing.

During this stage, the institutional base for much of public health nursing shifted to the government. By 1955, 72% of the counties in the continental United States had local health departments. Public health nursing constituted the major portion of these local health services and emphasized health promotion, as well as care for the ill at home (Scutchfield & Keck, 2003). Some of the district nursing services, known as *visiting nurse associations* (VNAs), remained privately funded and administered, offering their own home nursing care. In some places, city or county health departments joined administratively and financially with VNAs to provide a combination of services, such as home care of the sick and health promotion to families.

Rural public health nursing, which had already been organized around 1900 in Great Britain, Germany, and Canada, also expanded in the United States (see Chapter 29). Initially, starting in 1912, rural nursing was privately financed and largely administered through the Red Cross and the Metropolitan Life Insurance Company, but responsibility had shifted to the government by the 1940s (Bullough & Bullough, 1978). An innovative example of rural nursing was the Frontier Nursing Service, which was started by Mary Breckenridge (1881–1965) in 1925, to serve mountain families in Kentucky. From six outposts, nurses on horseback visited remote families to deliver babies and provide food and nursing services. Over the years, the service has expanded to provide medical, dental, and nursing care. The Frontier Nursing Service continues today, with its remarkable accomplishments of reducing mortality rates and promoting health among this disadvantaged population, as the parent holding company for the Frontier School of Midwifery and Family Nursing. It is the largest nurse-midwifery program in the United States. In addition, Mary Breckinridge Healthcare, Inc. consists of a home health agency, two outpost clinics,

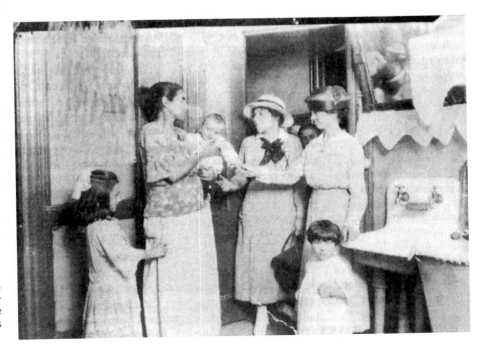

FIGURE 2.4 The public health nurse, carrying her bag of equipment and supplies, makes regular home visits to provide physical and psychological care, as well as health lessons to families.

one primary care clinic, and the Kate Ireland Women's Healthcare Clinic (Simpson, 2000).

The public health nursing stage was characterized by service to the public, with the family targeted as a primary unit of care. Official health agencies, which placed greater emphasis on disease prevention and health promotion, provided the chief institutional base.

Community Health Nursing (1970 to the Present)

The emergence of the term *community health nursing* heralded a new era. By the late 1960s and early 1970s, while public health nurses continued their work, many other nurses who were not necessarily practicing public health were based in the community. Their practice settings included community-based clinics, doctors' offices, work sites, and schools. To provide a label that encompassed all nurses in the community, the ANA and others called them community health nurses.

This term was not universally accepted, however, and many people—including nurses and the general public—had difficulty distinguishing community health nursing from public health nursing. For example, nursing education, recognizing the importance of public health content, required course work in public health for all baccalaureate students. This meant that graduates were expected to incorporate public health principles such as health promotion and disease prevention into nursing practice, regardless of their sphere of service. Consequently, some questioned whether public health nursing retained any unique content. Although leaders such as Carolyn Williams clearly stated that community health nursing's specialized contribution lay in its focus on populations (Williams, 1977), this concept did not appear to be widely understood or practiced.

To distinguish the domains of community and public health nursing, in 1984, the U.S. Department of Health and Human Services, Bureau of Health Professionals, Division of Nursing, convened a Consensus Conference on the Essentials of Public Health Nursing Practice and Education in Washington, D.C. (U.S. Department of Health and Human Services [USDHHS], Division of Nursing, 1984). This group concluded that *community health nursing* was the broader term, referring to all nurses practicing in the community, regardless of their educational preparation. *Public health nursing,* viewed as a part of community health nursing, was described as a generalist practice for nurses prepared with basic public health content at the baccalaureate level and a specialized practice for nurses prepared in public health at the masters level or beyond.

Confusion also arose regarding the question of whether community health nursing is a generalized or a specialized practice. Graduates from baccalaureate nursing programs were inadequately prepared to practice in public health; their education had emphasized individualized and direct clinical care and provided little understanding of applications to populations and communities. By the mid-1970s, various community health nursing leaders had identified knowledge and skills needed for more effective community health nursing practice (Roberts & Freeman, 1973). These leaders valued promoting the health of the community, but both education and practice continued to emphasize direct clinical care to individuals, families, and groups in the community (de Tornyay, 1980). Reflecting this view, the ANA's Division of Community Health Nursing developed *A Conceptual Model of Community Health*

Nursing in 1980. This document distinguished generalized community health nursing preparation at the baccalaureate level and specialized community health nursing preparation at the masters or postgraduate level. The generalist was described as one who provides nursing service to individuals and groups of clients while keeping "the community perspective in mind" (American Nurses Association, 1980, p. 9).

Finally, confusion also arose regarding the changing roles and functions of community health nurses. Accelerated changes in health care organization and financing, technology, and social issues made increasing demands on community health nurses to adapt to new patterns of practice. Many new kinds of community health services appeared. Hospital-based programs reached into the community. Private agencies proliferated, offering home care and other community-based services. Other community health professionals assumed responsibilities that traditionally had been the domain of public health nursing. For example, some school counselors in Oregon began coordinating home visits previously done by school nurses, and health educators (who were part of a more recently developed discipline) took over large segments of client education. Social workers, too, provided services that overlapped with community health nursing roles. Health educators, counselors, social workers, epidemiologists, and nutritionists working in community health came prepared with different backgrounds and emphases in their practice. Their contributions were and still are important. Their presence, however, forced community health nurses to reexamine their own contribution to the public's health and incorporate stronger interdisciplinary and collaborative approaches into their practice (see Levels of Prevention Pyramid).

The debate over these areas of confusion continued through the 1980s, and some issues are yet unresolved. Still, the direction in which public health and community health nursing must move remains clear: to care *for,* not simply *in,* the community. Public health nursing continues to mean the synthesis of nursing and the public health sciences applied to promoting and protecting the health of populations. Community health nursing, for some, refers more broadly to nursing in the community. In this text, the term *community health nursing* is used synonymously with *public health nursing* and refers to specialized, population-focused nursing practice, which applies public health science and nursing science. A possible distinction between the two terms might be to view community health nursing as a beginning level of specialization and public health nursing as an advanced level. Clarification and consensus on the meaning of these terms help to avoid misconceptions and misuse, and are explored more fully in Chapter 3. Whichever term is used to describe this specialty, the fundamental issues and defining criteria remain the same: (1) Are populations and communities the target of practice? and (2) Are the nurses prepared in public health and engaging in public health practice?

As community health nursing continues to evolve, many signs of positive growth are evident. Community health nurses are carving out new roles for themselves in primary health care. Collaboration and interdisciplinary teamwork are recognized as crucial to effective community nursing. Practitioners work through many kinds of agencies and institutions, such as senior citizen centers, ambulatory services, mental health clinics, and family planning programs. Community needs assessment, documentation of nursing outcomes, program evaluation, quality improvement, public

LEVELS OF PREVENTION PYRAMID

GOAL: Clarify and enhance the community health nurse's role to promote impact.

Tertiary Prevention

- Promote increasing influence of the nurse through an expanded role in service delivery
- Minimize the impact of community misunderstandings of the nurse's role through education

Secondary Prevention

- Promote aggregate-level interventions
- Foster nurse involvement on community boards and other political groups

Primary Prevention

- Participate in policy formation
- Be politically active
- Assist in acquiring funding for community health programs
- Conduct research on health and nursing outcomes to enhance evidenced-based practice
- Collaborate with the news media to publicize current public health issues

policy formulation, and community nursing research are high priorities. This field of nursing is assuming responsibility as a full professional partner in community health.

Internationally, community nursing services are well established in England, Scandinavia, the Netherlands, and Australia. Services, however, are relatively underdeveloped in France and Ireland. Furthermore, relatively few professional nurses are working in the community in central and eastern Europe and in the former Union of Soviet Socialist Republics (USSR). Ivanov and Paganpegara (2003) note that changes have occurred in nursing education subsequent to the collapse of the Soviet Union, but they have not included content in public health nursing. Moreover, the concepts of health promotion and health education are not well understood, with the vast majority of health care provided at the tertiary level. It is concerning that modernization in many countries has not included expansion of public health services in general and community health nursing more specifically. In many of the most populated regions of the world—such as China, Africa, and India—volunteers, lay providers, and paraprofessionals provide the bulk of community health services.

In 1978, a joint World Health Organization (WHO) and the United Nations Childrens' Fund International Conference in Alma-Ata, in the Soviet Union, adopted a declaration on primary health care as the key to attaining the goal of health for all by the year 2000. At this conference, delegations from 134 governments agreed to incorporate the concepts and principles of primary health care in their health care systems to reach this goal (WHO, 1978, 1998). This was adopted by the World Health Assembly and endorsed by the United Nations General Assembly in 1981. On paper, at least, everyone acknowledged the crucial need for nurses to be involved in reaching this goal. In practice, support has not been forthcoming in many countries. Policy makers and the public still need to be educated to realize that nursing's most effective contributions to the overall health of the population are based in the community.

Table 2.1 summarizes the most important changes that have occurred during community health nursing's four stages

TABLE 2.1   Development of Community Health Nursing

Stages	Focus	Nursing Orientation	Service Emphasis	Institutional Base (Agencies)
Early home care (Before mid-1800s)	Sick poor	Individuals	Curative	Lay and religious orders
District nursing (1860–1900)	Sick poor	Individuals	Curative; beginning of preventive	Voluntary; some government
Public health nursing (1900–1970)	Needy public	Families	Curative; preventive	Government; some voluntary
Emergence of community health nursing (1970–present)	Total community	Populations	Health promotion; illness prevention	Many kinds; some independent practice

of development. It shows these changes in terms of focus, nursing orientation, service emphasis, and institutional base.

SOCIETAL INFLUENCES ON THE DEVELOPMENT OF COMMUNITY HEALTH NURSING

Many factors have influenced the growth of community health nursing. To better understand the nature of this field, the forces that began and continue to shape its development must be recognized. Six are particularly significant: advanced technology, progress in causal thinking, changes in education, demographic changes and the role of women, the consumer movement, and economic factors.

Advanced Technology

Advanced technology has contributed in many ways to shaping the practice of community health nursing. For example, technologic innovation has greatly improved health care, nutrition, and lifestyle and has caused a concomitant increase in life expectancy. Consequently, community health nurses direct an increasing share of their effort toward meeting the needs of the elderly population and addressing chronic conditions. The advances in technology in the home can be life-altering. For example, homebound elders, disabled persons, and their caregivers found a new sense of camaraderie and friendship through use of a grant-sponsored website with discussion groups and a listserv (Bradley & Poppen, 2003). After 1 year, these individuals expressed increased satisfaction with the amount of contact with others, thus supporting the use of online access for isolated persons.

Online access to health information can provide a critical link to information for all elderly persons, but it is important to recognize that not all websites are reputable. An increasing number of online websites catering to the elderly provide inaccurate information and, in some cases, are designed to defraud (Moore, 2005) or possibly harm those who access the website. It is critical for the community health nurse to check carefully any websites that are recommended for clients. It is important for clients to access only reputable sites and participate in discussion groups that utilize a facilitator or moderator (Moore, 2005).

Advanced technology has been a strong force behind industrialization, large-scale employment, and urbanization. We are now primarily an urban society, with approximately 75% of the world's population living in urban or suburban areas. Population density leads to many health-related problems, particularly the spread of disease and increased stress. Community health nurses are learning how to combat these urban health problems. In addition, changes in transportation and high job mobility have affected the health scene. As people travel and relocate, they are separated from families and traditional support systems; community health nurses design programs to help urban populations cope with the accompanying stress. New products, equipment, methods, and energy sources in industry have also increased environmental pollution and industrial hazards. Community health nurses have become involved in related research, occupational health, and preventive education. Technologic innovation has promoted complex medical diagnostic and treatment procedures, making illness-oriented care more dramatic and desirable, as well

as more costly. Community health nurses face a challenge to demonstrate the physical and economic value of technology for wellness-oriented care.

Finally, innovations in communications and computer technology have shifted America from an industrial society to an "information economy." Our economy is built on information—the production and marketing of knowledge—making it global and active around-the-clock. Community health nurses now are in the business of information distribution, and they use computer technologies to enhance the efficiency and effectiveness of their services. Geographic Information Systems (GIS) is an example of emerging computer technology that the community health nurse can use to design and evaluate population-focused programs (Caley, 2004). GIS technology can be a valuable tool for many purposes, including examining health disparities and outbreaks of disease and for determining health priorities within a community (Riner, Cunningham, & Johnson, 2004). Telenursing, telehealth, and nursing informatics are part of our professional activities as community health nurses. We communicate by e-mail, use computer-based applications to enhance education among peers and with clients, and comfortably use the computers that are found in all areas where nurses function (Saba, 2001). As we move deeper into the 21st century, we move to "mobile care," using handheld, wireless technology tools that are nurse-friendly and compatible with the nurse's role. We have the ability to "tele-visit" our clients, and we regularly use smaller and smaller laptop computers for video conferencing (Saba, 2001). We even have the ability to take a "bird's-eye" view of the distribution of service providers and chronic disease clusters in a community through the use of GIS technology. Access to information is increasing, and the use of the information is limitless. The emerging difficulty is how to manage the sheer volume of information and still meet the needs of our communities.

Progress in Causal Thinking

Relating disease or illness to its cause is known as **causal thinking** in the health sciences. Progress in the study of causality, particularly in epidemiology, has significantly affected the nature of community health nursing (Fos & Fine, 2000; Thomas & Weber, 2001). The *germ theory* of disease causation, established in the late 1800s, was the first real breakthrough in control of communicable disease. At that time, it was established that disease could be spread or transmitted from patient to patient or from nurse to patient by contaminated hands or equipment. Nurses incorporated the teaching of cleanliness and personal hygiene into basic nursing care.

A second advance in causal thinking was initiated by the tripartite view that called attention to the interactions among a causative agent, a susceptible host, and the environment. This information offered community health nurses new ways to control and prevent health disorders. For example, nurses could decrease the vulnerability of individuals (hosts) by teaching them healthier lifestyles. They could instigate measles vaccination programs as a means of preventing the organism (agent) from infecting children. They could promote proper disinfection of a neighborhood swimming pool (environment) to prevent disease.

Further progress in causal thinking led to the recognition that not just one single agent, but many factors—a multiple causation approach—contribute to a disease or health disorder. A food poisoning outbreak that is associated with a restaurant might be caused not only by the *Salmonella* organism but also by improper food handling and storage, lack of adherence to minimum food preparation standards, and lack of adequate health department supervision and enforcement (see Chapter 7). A chronic condition such as coronary heart disease can be related to other kinds of multicausal factors, such as heredity, diet, lack of exercise, smoking, and personal and work stress.

Community health nurses can control health problems by examining all possible causes and then attacking strategic causal points. Efforts to prevent acquired immunodeficiency syndrome (AIDS) provide a dramatic case in point. Contact reporting, condom use, protection of health workers serving patients infected with the human immunodeficiency virus (HIV), screening for HIV infection, and public education about AIDS are examples of a multifaceted approach.

Current causal thinking has led to a broader awareness of unhealthy conditions; in addition to disease, problems such as accidents and environmental pollution are major targets of concern. Work-related stress, environmental hazards, chemical food additives, and alcohol and nicotine consumption during pregnancy are all examples of concerns in community health nursing practice.

Nursing's contribution to public health adds a further application to causal thinking. That is, nursing seeks to identify and implement the causes, or contributing factors, of wellness. Community health nurses do more than prevent illness; they seek to promote health. By conducting research and applying research findings, community health nurses promote health-enhancing behaviors. Nurses promote healthier lifestyle practices such as eating low-fat diets, exercising, and maintaining social support systems; promote healthy conditions in schools and work sites; and design meaningful activities for adolescents and the elderly.

Changes in Education

Changes in education, especially those in nursing education, have had an important influence on community health nursing practice. Education, once an opportunity for a privileged few, has become widely available; it is now considered a basic right and a necessity for a vital society. When people's understanding of their environment grows, an increased understanding of health usually is involved. For the community health nurse, health teaching has steadily assumed greater importance in practice. For the learner, education has led to more responsibility. As a result, people believe that they have a right to know and question the reasons behind the care they receive. Community health nurses have shifted from planning for clients to collaborating with clients.

Education has had other effects. Scientific inquiry, considered basic to progress, has created a dramatic increase in knowledge. The wealth of information relevant to community health nursing practice means that nursing students have more content to assimilate, and practicing community health nurses have to make greater efforts to keep abreast of knowledge in their field. In contrast to earlier times, when nurses were trained to work as apprentices in hospitals or health

agencies and to follow orders perfunctorily, today's educational programs, including continuing education, prepare nurses to think for themselves in the application of theory to practice. Community health nursing has always required a fair measure of independent thinking and self-reliance; now, community health nurses need skills in such areas as population assessment, policy making, political advocacy, research, management, collaborative functioning, and critical thinking. As the result of expanding education, community health nurses have had to reexamine their practice, sharpen their knowledge and skills, and clarify their roles.

Demographic Changes and the Role of Women

The changing demographics in the United States and the changing role of women have profoundly affected community health nursing. In the 20th century, the Women's Rights movement made considerable progress; women achieved the right to vote and gained greater economic independence by moving into the labor force. Today, 145 million people are employed in the United States, 46.6% of whom are female. In the decade between 1998 and 2008, the number of women in the labor force will likely increase by 15%, compared with 10% for men. In the same decade, the percentage of workers aged 45 years or older will increase from 33% to 40% of the workforce (USDHHS, 2004).

Women nurses are aging in a predominantly female profession. In 1996, the average age of a registered nurse was 42.3 years. By 2004, the average age had increased to 46.8 years. Looking back just 25 years, a dramatic shift has occurred in the ratio of younger to older registered nurses. In 1980, 40.5% of registered nurses were under the age of 35. By 2004, only 16.6% of registered nurses fit into that demographic age group (USDHHS, 2004). Although most nursing schools remain full and many have a waiting list, the number of nurses staying active in their profession is dwindling. Those remaining in the profession are "graying" and retiring. Added to this is the aging population of nursing faculty, which raises concern over meeting the increased demand for nurses in the coming decade.

Salaries for nurses compare favorably with those for other workers who have four years of education in fields other than health care, such as education, human services (social work), and business. When compared with other workers in the health care field, however, nurses make a lower salary. For example, among the 2,368,070 practicing registered nurses in the United States in 2005, the average salary was $56,880. In comparison, the average salary for physical therapists was $65,350; for dental hygienists, it was $60,620, and for occupational therapists, it was $59,100 (U.S. Department of Labor, 2006).

Changing demographics, such as shifting patterns in immigration, varying numbers of births and deaths, and a rapidly increasing population of elderly persons, affect community health nursing planning and programming efforts. Monitoring these changes is essential for relevant and effective nursing services. Equally important is a diverse and representative workforce in nursing. The 2004 findings of the National Sample Survey of Registered Nurses indicated that the vast majority of nurses (81.8%) specifying a racial background selected White (non-Hispanic). With 7.5% of nurses not specifying a racial background, that left 10.6% in one or more of the groups identified in the survey. Because of a change in the form of questioning, these figures are difficult to compare with earlier surveys. It is concerning, however, that in 2000, 12.3% of the registered nurses identified themselves as being non-White, whereas the 2004 estimate was only 10.6%; clearly, this is a move in the wrong direction if the 2004 estimate is correct. The 2004 data also showed the racial background of the nurses surveyed to be 4.6% Black/African American; 3.3% Asian/Pacific Islander; 1.8% Hispanic; 0.4% American Indian/Alaskan Native; and a further 1.5% indicated two or more racial backgrounds (USD-HHS, 2004). Increased racial and ethnic representation in community health nursing is essential and remains one of the major challenges facing the profession in the coming years.

Although the diversity of career options and employment opportunities for women has been a positive social factor, these gains have decreased the number of women entering nursing. As a profession, nursing's contributions and status have improved, but its ability to compete with careers offering higher pay and status remains problematic. Changes resulting from the women's movement continue. Nurses still struggle for equality—equality of recognition, respect, and autonomy, as well as job selection, equal pay for equal work, and equal opportunity for advancement in the health field. If community health nurses are to influence the field of community health, they need status and authority equal to that of their colleagues. This step requires nurses to demonstrate their competence and learn to be assertive in assuming roles as full professional partners. It is worth noting that, in 2002, men held more than one-third of the nursing administrative positions (U.S. Department of Labor, 2002). This is significant because, in that same year, men represented only 5.4% of the total registered nurse population. Despite efforts to recruit more men into nursing, the 2004 data suggest only minimal improvement to 5.7% of registered nurses (RNs) (USDHHS, 2004). The high proportion of leadership positions held by the men may in part reflect a larger proportion of women in nursing who have less than full-time careers. The women's movement has contributed to community health nursing's gains in assuming leadership roles, but a need for greater influence and involvement remains for all nurses.

Consumer Movement

The consumer movement also has affected the nature of community health nursing. Consumers have become more aggressive in demanding quality services and goods; they assert their right to be informed about goods and services and to participate in decisions that affect them regardless of sex, race, or socioeconomic level. This movement has stimulated some basic changes in the philosophy of community health nursing. Health care consumers are viewed as active members of the health team rather than as passive recipients of care. They may contract with the community health nurse for family care or group services, represent the community on the local health board, or act as ombudsmen by serving as representatives or advocates for their community constituents (e.g., to investigate complaints and report findings to protect the quality of care in a local nursing home). This assumption of consumers' responsibility for their own health means that the community health nurse often supplements clients' services, rather than primarily supervising them.

The consumer movement has also contributed to increased concern for the quality of health services, including a demand for more humane, personalized health care. Dissatisfied with fragmented services offered by an array of health workers, consumers seek more comprehensive, coordinated care. For example, senior citizens in a high-rise apartment building need more than a series of social workers, nutritionists, recreational therapists, nurses, and other callers ascertaining a variety of specific needs and starting a variety of separate programs. Community health nurses seek to provide holistic care by collaborating with others to offer more coordinated, comprehensive, and personalized services—a case-management approach. One example of the current attention given to the opinions of consumers is exemplified by the 2005 Gallup Poll discussed in Display 2.4. In this poll, nurses are the most highly rated profession with respect to honesty and ethics; not a bad position to be in.

Economic Forces

Myriad economic forces have affected the practice of community health nursing. Unemployment and the rising cost of living, combined with mounting health care costs, have resulted in numerous people carrying little or no health insurance. With limited or no access to needed health services, these populations are especially vulnerable to health problems and further economic stress. Other economic forces affecting community health nursing are changing health care financing patterns (including prospective payment and diagnosis-related groups); decreased federal, state, and local subsidies of public health programs; pressures for health care cost containment through managed care; and increased competition and managed competition among providers of health services (see Chapter 6).

Global economic forces also influence community health nursing practice. As the United States experiences

---

DISPLAY 2.4	NURSES RANK HIGH IN HONESTY AND ETHICAL STANDARDS

Nurses are again at the top of the list, according to a Gallup Poll taken in 2005. When asked how they would rate the honesty and ethical standards of members of various professions, Americans rated nurses highest. Each year, a random sample of Americans are asked to rate select professions on a five-point scale ranging from "very high" to "very low." Since being added to the list in 1999, nurses have been at the top of the list each year except 2001, when firefighters took the #1 spot ("Nurses Top List," 2006). Here are the results for the top scoring professions:

- Nurses   82%
- Pharmacists   67%
- Medical Doctors   65%
- High School Teachers   64%
- Policemen   61%
- Clergy   54%

increasing interdependence with foreign countries for trade, investment, and production of goods, the population has experienced a growing mobility and increased immigration, particularly among Hispanic and Asian groups. Under these conditions, the spread of communicable diseases poses a serious threat, as do problems associated with unemployment and poverty. Furthermore, the fastest-growing sector of the job market is in technical fields, which require new or retrained workers, and these jobs frequently are accompanied by health problems related to the stresses of ever-changing technology and financial and competitive pressures to produce.

Community health nursing has responded to these economic forces in several ways. One is by assuming new roles, such as health educators in industry or case managers for government and privately sponsored programs for the elderly. Another is by directly competing with other community health service providers, particularly in such areas as ambulatory care or home care. Still another is by developing new programs and service emphases. Elder day care, respite care, senior fall-prevention programs, teen pregnancy and drug prevention projects, and programs for the homeless are a few examples of the response by community health nursing to the changing community needs created by demographic and economic forces. Yet another community health nursing response has been to develop new revenue-generating services, such as workplace wellness or health screening programs, to augment depleted budgets.

Economic factors continue to play a significant role in shaping community health nursing practice. Limited dollars for health promotion services and a continued need for home care have drawn some public health agencies into more illness-oriented rather than wellness-oriented services. Yet, community health nurses continue to be resourceful in finding ways to foster the community's optimal health while adapting to changing economic conditions.

PREPARATION FOR COMMUNITY HEALTH NURSING

The demands of community health nursing practice are significant, as described in Chapter 1, and are elaborated elsewhere in this textbook. The daily routine of the community health nurse may include organizing a flu clinic for seniors in the community, making home visits, giving a presentation on playground safety at a parent–teacher meeting, participating in a team meeting in the health department office, answering telephone calls, and charting. All of the skills learned in a basic baccalaureate nursing program are needed to effectively manage this type of day. Furthermore, this day may not represent the bigger picture of the community health nurse's role in community advisory panels, grant writing for new programs, or participation in or presentation of in-service programs. Academic preparation for this role is necessary, as is continuous professional development, and this training must meet the requirements of both employers and, in many instances, state regulations.

Academic Preparation

The minimum preparation for community health nurses in many states has been graduation from a baccalaureate-level nursing program, a nursing major built on 2 years of liberal arts and sciences courses (Ellis & Hartley, 2000). This can be achieved in a variety of ways. Some students enter a baccalaureate program as their initial higher educational experience after high school or later. Others complete an associate degree program in nursing and continue on to a university to receive the baccalaureate degree. This requires additional courses in liberal arts and sciences, along with selected nursing courses, usually one or more courses in public health nursing, nursing research, and leadership-management courses. In some programs designed to extend an RN to a Bachelor of Science in Nursing (BSN), nurses with years of experience in acute care nursing can "challenge" the previously mentioned courses by taking a test to demonstrate clinical expertise or by presenting a portfolio of experience, or a combination of these. Nevertheless, whatever the initial entry into practice, a comprehensive nursing education that is rich in leadership, management, research, health maintenance and promotion, disease prevention, and community health nursing experience is needed to meet the demands of this specialty.

In some states, meeting criteria for entry into practice as a public health nurse is required by some employers. In California, the State Board of Registered Nursing (BRN) has established specific criteria, including completion of specific coursework (e.g., child abuse and prevention information), which must be documented in undergraduate classes. On graduation, a school transcript, application, and fee are sent to the BRN to receive the public health nursing certificate. After they pass the RN license examination (NCLEX), these nurses can sign "RN, PHN" after their names. Only those who have completed a baccalaureate nursing program can apply for this certificate, and only people with the certificate can take jobs as public health nurses. In California, this means that employment as an RN in settings such as health departments, schools, and Native American health services requires a PHN certificate.

Professional Development

Completion of a baccalaureate education may not be sufficient educational preparation for the more demanding community health nursing settings. Furthermore, to maintain licensure in most states, it is mandated that nurses participate in continuing education programs and receive continuing education units (Ellis & Hartley, 2000). In the United States, courses on specific topics are offered by employers, nursing associations, nursing journals, and private programs that travel to various cities. These help nurses to remain current on topics covered by the courses; however, a community health nurse may consider more lengthy and formal professional development opportunities such as advanced nursing practice (NP) programs or certification opportunities.

To someone who is just finishing an undergraduate nursing program, the thought of continuing in school may be overwhelming. However, within a few months or years after graduation, continuing in higher education may seem right. It can take time and experience to find a particular focus in nursing and to decide on specializing at an advanced level. When that time comes, a variety of course work and degree options are available. For example, short-term certificate programs specialize in a narrow focus of health care, such as early recognition and prevention of child abuse, research, grant writing, or team management. These may or may not be offered for university credit, but the content enhances a nurse's role in an agency.

Matriculation in an NP program or a master's degree program in nursing is a longer commitment and gives the nurse greater marketability. In some health departments, NPs run well-child clinics, and a school nurse with an NP license can direct a school-based clinic. Advanced practice in community health nursing can open doors into leadership positions in community health agencies. A master's degree in business, public health, education, or epidemiology can lead to management positions, private community health agency ownership, agency teaching, or research positions. A doctoral program may be the next educational step for those wanting tenure-track university teaching, research, or upper-level administrative positions.

The American Nurses Credentialing Center (ANCC) provides other opportunities by offering nurses certification in more than 36 specialty areas (2008). Currently, only one specialty is available in community health nursing: Advanced Public Health Nurse (APHN–BC). A generalist certificate in public/community health nursing had been available but was suspended in 2006, pending an ongoing review. Related certifications as an NP or in nursing administration also exist. Each certificate is awarded after completion of a certain number of years of practice in the specialty, payment of a fee, and passage of an ANCC Certification Examination. Many employers reward the initiative required for certification with promotion or a higher salary, accompanied by additional responsibilities and opportunities.

Summary

The specialty of community health nursing developed historically through four stages. The early home-care stage (before the mid-1800s) emphasized care to the sick poor in their homes by various lay and religious orders. The district nursing stage (mid-1800s) included voluntary home nursing care for the poor by specialists or "health nurses" who treated the sick and taught wholesome living to patients. The public health nursing stage (1900 to 1970) was characterized by an increased concern for the health of the general public. The community health nursing stage (1970 to the present) includes increased recognition of community health nursing as a specialty field, with focus on communities and populations.

Six major societal influences have shaped the development of community health nursing. They are advanced technology, progress in causal thinking, changes in education, the changing demographics and role of women, the consumer movement, and economic factors such as health care costs, access, limited funds for public health, and increased competition among health service providers.

Academic preparation for community health nursing begins at the baccalaureate level. However, students beginning at the diploma or associate degree level can advance to a BSN completion program and then are prepared to enter this challenging specialty in nursing. The demands of community health nursing require additional courses in liberal arts and science, along with courses in community health nursing practice at the student level. Once students achieve an undergraduate degree, completion of additional educational programs is required to keep current and, in most states, to maintain licensure, advance in practice opportunities, or branch out into administration, teaching, or research. ■

ACTIVITIES TO PROMOTE CRITICAL THINKING

1. Select one societal influence on the development of community health nursing and explore its continuing impact. What other events are occurring today that shape community health nursing practice? Support your arguments with documentation. Use the Internet to find your documentation.
2. Using the Internet, seek out information about a historical public health nursing leader. Using this information, determine how this practitioner might deal with current population-based issues such as AIDS, sexually transmitted diseases, or child neglect and abuse.
3. Assume that you have been asked to make a home visit to a 75-year-old man, living alone, whose wife recently died. Besides assessing his individual needs, what additional factors should you consider for assessment and intervention that would indicate an aggregate or population-focused approach? What self-care practices might you encourage or teach?
4. Interview a community health nursing director to determine what population-based programs are offered in your locality. Explore nursing's role in the assessment, development, implementation, and evaluation of these programs. Discuss with the director how community health nurses might expand their population-focused interventions.
5. Go to your university, nursing college, or school and locate brochures for advanced degrees in nursing and related areas. Peruse them and see whether any of the programs appeal to you. Request more information from at least one of these programs through the mail or the Internet.

References

American Nurses Association, Community Health Nursing Division. (1980). *A conceptual model of community health nursing* (Publication No. CH-10 2M 5/80). Kansas City, MO: Author.

American Nurses Credentialing Center. (2008). *Certification.* Retrieved August 9, 2008 from http://www.nursecredentialing.org/certification.aspx.

Beine, J. (1996). Changing with the times. *Nursing Times, 92*(48), 59–62.

Bradley, N., & Poppen, W. (2003). Assistive technology, computers and Internet may decrease sense of isolation for homebound elderly and disabled persons. *Technology and Disability, 15,* 19–25.

Bullough, V., & Bullough, B. (1978). *The care of the sick: The emergence of modern nursing.* New York: Neale, Watson.

Caley, L.M. (2004). Using geographic information systems to design population-based interventions. *Public Health Nursing, 21,* 547–554.

Central Hanover Bank and Trust Company, Department of Philanthropic Information. (1938). *The public health nurse.* New York: National Organization for Public Health Nursing.

Christy, T.W. (1970). Portrait of a leader: Lillian D. Wald. *Nursing Outlook, 18*(3), 50–54.

de Tornyay, R. (1980). Public health nursing: The nurse's role in community-based practice. *Annual Review of Public Health, 1*, 83.

Dickens, C. (1910). *Martin Chuzzlewit.* New York: Macmillan.

Dolan, J.A. (1978). *Nursing in society: A historical perspective.* Philadelphia: W.B. Saunders.

Draper, L. (2006). Working women and contraception: History, health, and choices. *AAOHN Journal, 54*, 317–324.

Ellis, J.R., & Hartley, C.L. (2000). *Nursing in today's world: Challenges, issues, and trends* (7th ed.). Philadelphia: Lippincott Williams & Wilkins.

Evans, J. (2004). Men nurses: A historical and feminist perspective. *Journal of Advanced Nursing, 47*, 321–328.

Farrar, E.W. (1837). *The young lady's friend—By a lady* (p. 57). Boston: American Stationer's Co.

Florence Nightingale Museum Trust. (1997). *The Florence Nightingale Museum's School Visit Pack.* London: Author.

Fos, P.J., & Fine, D.J. (2000). *Designing health care for populations: Applied epidemiology in health care administration.* San Francisco: Jossey-Bass.

Gardner, M.S. (1936). *Public health nursing* (3rd ed.). New York: Macmillan.

Hamilton, D. (2007). The cost of caring: The Metropolitan Life Insurance Company's Visiting Nurse Service, 1909–1953. *In* P. D'Antonio, E.D. Baer, S.D. Rinker, & J.E. Lynaugh (Eds.), *Nurses' work: Issues across time and place* (pp. 141–164). New York: Springer Publishing Company.

Hein, E.C. (2001). *Nursing issues in the 21st century: Perspectives from the literature.* Philadelphia: Lippincott Williams & Wilkins.

Ivanov, L.L., & Paganpegara, G. (2003). Public health nursing education in Russia. *Journal of Nursing Education, 42*, 292–295.

Kalisch, P.A., & Kalisch, B.J. (2004). *American nursing: A history* (4th ed.). Philadelphia: Lippincott Williams & Wilkins.

Kaplin, J. (Ed.). (1855/1992). *Bartlett's familiar quotations* (16th ed.). New York: Little, Brown and Company.

Men, monasteries, wars, and wards. (2001). *Nursing Times, 97*(44), 25–26.

Moore, G.A. (2005). On-line communities: Helping "senior surfers" find health information on the web. *Journal of Gerontological Nursing, 31*(11), 42–48.

Mosley, M.O.P. (2007). Satisfied to carry the bag: Three black community health nurses' contributions to health care reform, 1900–1937. *In* P. D'Antonio, E.D. Baer, S.D. Rinker, & J.E. Lynaugh (Eds.), *Nurses' work: Issues across time and place* (pp. 65–78). New York: Springer Publishing Company.

Mowbray, P. (1997). *Florence Nightingale museum guidebook.* London: The Florence Nightingale Museum Trust.

National Organization for Public Health Nursing. (1944). Approval of Skidmore College of Nursing as preparing students for public health nursing. *Public Health Nursing, 36*, 371.

Nightingale, F. (1859/1969). *Notes on nursing: What it is, and what it is not.* London: Harrison.

Nightingale, F. (1864). *How people may live and not die in India.* London: Longman, Green, Longman, Roberts, & Green.

Nightingale, F. (1876, April 14). [Letter to the editor]. *The Times* (London).

Nurses top list in honesty and ethics again in Gallup Poll. (2006, January/March). *New Mexico Nurse, 51*(1), 13.

Palmer, I.S. (2001). Florence Nightingale: Reformer, reactionary, researcher. *In* E.C. Hein, *Nursing issues in the 21st century: Perspectives from the literature* (pp. 26–38). Philadelphia: Lippincott Williams & Wilkins.

Riner, M.E., Cunningham, C., & Johnson, A. (2004). Public health education and practice using geographic information system technology. *Public Health Nursing, 21*, 57–65.

Roberts, D., & Freeman, R. (Eds.). (1973). *Redesigning nursing education for public health: Report of the conference* (Publication No. HRA 75–75). Bethesda, MD: U.S. Department of Health, Education, and Welfare.

Ruffing-Rahal, M. (1986). Margaret Sanger: Nurse and feminist. *Nursing Outlook, 34*, 246–249.

Saba, V.K. (2001). Nursing informatics: Yesterday, today, and tomorrow. *International Nursing Review, 48*, 177–187.

Sachs, T.B. (1908). The tuberculosis nurse. *American Journal of Nursing, 8*, 597.

Scutchfield, F.D., & Keck, C.W. (2003). *Principles of public health practice.* Albany, NY: Delmar.

Simpson, M.S. (2000). Nurses and models of practice: Then and now. *American Journal of Nursing, 100*(2), 82–83.

Thomas, J.C., & Weber, D.J. (2001). *Epidemiologic methods for the study of infectious diseases.* Oxford: Oxford University Press.

U.S. Department of Health and Human Services, Division of Nursing. (1984). *Consensus conference on the essentials of public health nursing practice and education: Report of the conference.* Rockville, MD: Author.

U.S. Department of Health and Human Services, Health Resources Service Administration. *Preliminary findings 2004 National Sample Survey of Registered Nurses.* Retrieved June 21, 2008 from http://www.bhpr.hrsa.gov.

U.S. Department of Health and Human Services, National Center for Health Statistics. (2002). *Health, United States, 2002 with chartbook on trends in the health of America* (DHHS Publication No. 1232). Washington, DC: Author.

U.S. Department of Health and Human Services, National Institute for Occupational Safety and Health. (2004). *Worker Health Chartbook, 2004.* Washington, DC: Author.

U.S. Department of Labor, Bureau of Labor Statistics. (2002). Retrieved June 21, 2008 from http://www.dol.gov.

U.S. Department of Labor, Bureau of Labor Statistics. (2006). Retrieved June 21, 2008 from http://www.dol.gov.

Wald, L.D. (1915). *The house on Henry Street.* New York: Holt.

Wald, L.D. (1934). *Windows of Henry Street.* Boston: Little Brown.

Williams, C.A. (1977). Community health nursing: What is it? *Nursing Outlook, 25*, 250–254.

Woodham-Smith, C. (1951). *Florence Nightingale.* New York: McGraw-Hill.

World Health Organization. (1978). *Primary health care: Report of the International Conference on Primary Health Care, Alma-Ata, USSR.* Geneva: Author.

World Health Organization. (1998). *The world health report: 1998.* Geneva: Author.

Selected Readings

100 years in pictures. (2000). *American Journal of Nursing, 100*(10), 40–45.

Baer, E.D., D'Antonio, P., Rinker, S., & Lynaugh, J.E. (2001). *Enduring issues in American nursing.* New York: Springer.

Bullough, V.L., & Sentz, L. (2000). *American nursing: A biographical dictionary* (Vol. 3). New York: Springer.

Chaska, N.L. (2001). *The nursing profession: Tomorrow and beyond.* Thousand Oaks, CA: Sage.

D'Antonio, P., Baer, E.D., Rinker, S.D., & Lynaugh, J.E. (Eds.). (2007). *Nurses' work: Issues across time and place.* New York: Springer Publishing Company.

Davis, A.T. (1999). *Early Black American leaders in nursing: Architects for integration and equality.* Sudbury, MA: Jones & Bartlett Publishers International.

Duffus, R.L. (1938). *Lillian Wald: Neighbor and crusader.* New York: Macmillan.

Fitzpatrick, M.L. (1975). Nursing and the Great Depression. *American Journal of Nursing, 75*(12), 2188–2190.

Hawkins, J.W., & Bellig, L.L. (2000). The evolution of advanced practice nursing in the United States: Caring for women and newborns. *Journal of Obstetric, Gynecologic, and Neonatal Nursing, 29*(1), 83–89.

Heistand, W.C. (2000). Think different: Inventions and innovations by nurses, 1850–1950. *American Journal of Nursing, 100*(10), 72–77.

Henderson, V. (1969/2000). Excellence in nursing: An AJN classic, October 1969. *American Journal of Nursing, 100*(10), 96I, 96K, 96M–96R.

Libster, M. (2001). *Demonstrating care: The art of integrative nursing.* Albany, NY: Delmar.

Lynaugh, J.E. (2002). *Nursing History Review: Official journal of the American Association for the History of Nursing.* New York: Springer.

Macrae, J.A. (2001). *Nursing as a spiritual practice: A contemporary application of Florence Nightingale's views.* New York: Springer.

Nichols, F.H. (2000). History of the women's health movement in the 20th century. *Journal of Obstetric, Gynecologic, and Neonatal Nursing, 29*(1), 56–64.

Sandelowski, M. (2000). Thermometers and telephones: A century of nursing and technology. *American Journal of Nursing, 100*(10), 82–86.

Sarnecky, M.T. (2001). Army nurses in "The Forgotten War." *American Journal of Nursing, 101*(11), 45–49.

U.S. Department of Health and Human Services. (2000). *Healthy people 2010* (Conference ed., Vols. 1 & 2). Washington, DC: Author.

Internet Resources

American Academy of Nursing: *http://www.aannet.org/*

American Assembly for Men in Nursing: *http://www.aamn.org*

American Nurses Association: *http://www.ana.org*

American Nurses Credentialing Center: *http://www.nursingworld.org/ancc/index.html*

American Nursing Informatics Association: *http://www.ania.org*

American Public Health Association: *http://www.apha.org*

Association of Community Health Nursing Educators: *http://www.achne.org/*

Frontier Nursing Service, Inc.: *http://www.frontiernursing.org/*

National Association of Hispanic Nurses: *http://thehispanicnurses.org/index.php*

National Black Nurses Association, Inc.: *http://nbna.org*

National Center for Health Statistics: *http://www.cdc.gov/nchs/*

National League for Nursing: *http://www.nln.org*

Sigma Theta Tau International Honor Society of Nursing: *http://www.nursingsociety.org*

U.S. Department of Labor. Bureau of Labor Statistics: *http://www.bls.gov*

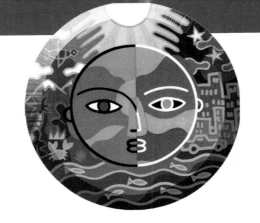

3

Setting the Stage for Community Health Nursing

LEARNING OBJECTIVES

Upon mastery of this chapter, you should be able to:

◆ Identify the three core public health functions basic to community health nursing.
◆ Describe and differentiate among seven different roles of the community health nurse.
◆ Discuss the seven roles within the framework of public health nursing functions.
◆ Explain the importance of each role for influencing people's health.
◆ Identify and discuss factors that affect a nurse's selection and practice of each role.
◆ Describe seven settings in which community health nurses practice.
◆ Discuss the nature of community health nursing, and the common threads basic to its practice, woven throughout all roles and settings.
◆ Identify principles of sound nursing practice in the community.

"One good community nurse will save a dozen policemen."

—Herbert Hoover

Historically, community health nurses have engaged in many professional roles. Nurses in this professional specialty have provided care to the sick, taught positive health habits and self-care, advocated on behalf of needy populations, developed and managed health programs, provided leadership, and collaborated with other professionals and consumers to implement changes in health services. Although the practice settings may have differed, the essential goal of the community health nurse has always been a healthier community. The home certainly has been one site for practice, but so too have public health clinics, schools, factories, and other community-based locations. Today, the roles and settings of community health nursing practice have expanded even further, offering a wide range of professional opportunities.

This chapter examines how the conceptual foundations and core functions of community health practice are integrated into the various roles and settings of community health nursing. It provides an opportunity to gain greater understanding about how and where community health nursing is practiced. Moreover, it will expand awareness of the many existing and future possibilities for community health nurses to improve the public's health. As you read through this chapter, think about client populations that you may have encountered in the acute care setting and consider your role with these same populations in a community setting. Perhaps you may discover a community health nursing specialty area that you never even considered.

CORE PUBLIC HEALTH FUNCTIONS

Community health nurses work as partners within a team of professionals (in public health and other disciplines), nonprofessionals, and consumers to improve the health of populations. The various roles and settings for practice hinge on three primary functions of public health: assessment, policy development, and assurance (Institute of Medicine [IOM], 1988). These functions are foundational to all roles assumed by the community health nurse and are applied at three levels of service: to individuals, to families, and to communities (Display 3.1). Regardless of the role or setting of choice, these three essential responsibilities direct the work of all community health nurses.

Assessment

An essential first function in public health, **assessment**, means that the community health nurse must gather and analyze information that will affect the health of the people to be served. As described in Display 3.1, assessment is *the systematic collection, assembly, analysis, and dissemination of information about the health of a community* (U.S. Department of Health & Human Services [USDHHS], Centers for Disease Control & Prevention [CDC], 2006). The nurse and others on the health team need to determine health needs, health risks, environmental conditions, political agendas, and financial and other resources, depending on the individuals, community, or population targeted for intervention. Data may be gathered in many ways; typical methods include interviewing people in the community, conducting surveys, gathering information from public records (many of which are available online), and using research findings.

The community health nurse is typically both trusted and valued by clients, agencies, and private providers. Trust placed in the community health nurse can often be attributed to consistency, honesty, dependability, and an ongoing presence in the community. Although securing and maintaining the trust of others is pivotal to all nursing practice, it is even more critical when working in the community. Trust can afford a nurse access to client populations that are difficult to engage, to agencies, and to health care providers. In the capacity of trusted professional, community health nurses gather relevant client data that enable them to identify strengths, weaknesses, and needs. It is important to recognize that as difficult as it may be for the nurse to gain the trust and respect of the community, if ever lost, these attributes can be difficult if not impossible to regain.

| DISPLAY 3.1 | PUBLIC HEALTH NURSING WITHIN THE CORE PUBLIC HEALTH FUNCTIONS MODEL |

The model includes assessment, policy development, and assurance surrounding the individual, family, and community. *Assessment* is "the systematic collection, assembly, analysis, and dissemination of information about the health of a community." *Policy development* uses the scientific information gathered during assessment to create comprehensive public health policies. *Assurance* is the "pledge to constituents that services necessary to achieve agreed-upon goals are provided by encouraging actions of others (private or public), requiring action through regulation, or providing service directly."

(From U.S. Department of Health and Human Services, Centers for Disease Control & Prevention, retrieved October 31, 2006 from *http://www.cdc.gov/epo/dphsi/AI/what_new.htm*.)

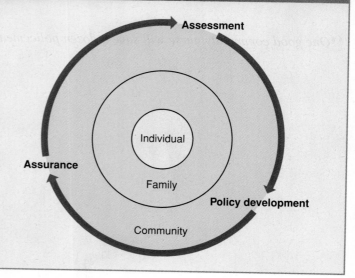

At the community level, assessment is done both formally and informally as nurses identify and interact with key community leaders. With families, the nurse can evaluate family strengths and areas of concern in the immediate living environment and in the neighborhood. At the individual level, people are identified within the family who are in need of services, and the nurse evaluates the functional capacity of these individuals through the use of specific assessment measures and a variety of tools. Assessment of communities and families as the initial step in the nursing process is discussed more fully in Chapters 15 and 19.

Policy Development

Policy development (defined in Display 3.1) is enhanced by the synthesis and analysis of information obtained during assessment. At the community level, the nurse provides leadership in convening and facilitating community groups to evaluate health concerns and develop a plan to address those concerns. Typically, the nurse recommends specific training and programs to meet identified health needs of target populations. This is accompanied by raising the awareness of key policy makers about factors such as health regulations and budget decisions that negatively affect the health of the community (see Chapter 13). With families, the nurse recommends new programs or increased services based on identified needs. Additional data may be needed to identify trends in groups or clusters of families, so that effective intervention strategies can be used with these families. At the individual level, the nurse assists in the development of standards for individual client care, recommends or adopts risk-classification systems to assist with prioritizing individual client care, and participates in establishing criteria for opening, closing, or referring individual cases.

Assurance

Assurance activities—activities that make certain that services are provided—often consume most of the community health nurse's time. With the shift in emphasis to programmatic funding and direct state reimbursement through Medicaid programs, community health nurses in many settings have been required to focus on direct service to individuals rather than on population-based services. Nonetheless, community health nurses perform the assurance function at the community level when they provide service to target populations, improve quality assurance activities, maintain safe levels of communicable disease surveillance and outbreak control, and collaborate with community leaders in the preparation of a community disaster plan. In addition, they participate in outcome research, provide expert consultation, promote evidence-based practice, and provide services within the community based on standards of care.

Essential Services

To more clearly articulate the services that are linked to the core functions of assessment, policy development and assurance, a list of 10 essential services was developed in 1994 by the Public Health Functions Steering Committee (USDHHS, 1997) (see Display 3.2). This initial effort to define the service components of the core functions provided an organized service delivery plan for public health providers across the country. A model depicting the relationships between the core functions and the essential services was eventually developed (USDHHS, 1999). The model (Fig. 3.1) shows the types of services necessary to achieve the core functions of assessment, policy development, and assurance. It also emphasizes the circular or ongoing nature of the process. The placement of research at the center of the model is a clear indication of the high priority placed on providing scientific evidence in all areas of service delivery. Research is essential to evidence-based practice and is vital to achieving healthy communities. As you review this model, think about what types of services might be provided in each category, depending on whether you are focusing on an individual, a family, or a community. It is not necessary that the community health nurse provide each of the listed services. Working in collaboration with an interdisciplinary team, the community nurse can support the efforts of others to achieve improved health in the community. What is important is that the team members all recognize their respective roles and are working toward the same goal.

DISPLAY 3.2 TEN ESSENTIAL SERVICES OF PUBLIC HEALTH

1. Monitor health status to identify community health problems.
2. Diagnose and investigate health problems and health hazards in the community.
3. Inform, educate, and empower people about health issues.
4. Mobilize community partnerships to identify and solve health problems.
5. Develop policies and plans that support individual and community health efforts.
6. Enforce laws and regulations that protect health and ensure safety.
7. Link people to needed personal health services and assure the provision of health care when otherwise unavailable.
8. Assure a competent public health and personal health care workforce.
9. Evaluate effectiveness, accessibility, and quality of personal and population-based health services.
10. Research for new insights and innovative solutions to health problems.

(From U.S. Department of Health and Human Services, Public Health Functions Project, 1997.)

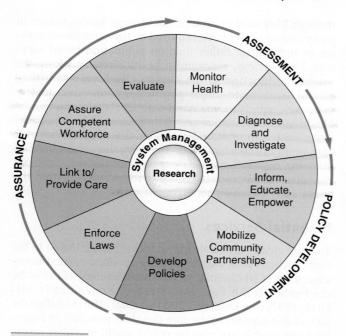

FIGURE 3.1 The Core Functions & Ten Essential Services of Public Health. From U.S. Department of Health and Human Services, Office of Disease Prevention & Health Promotion (1999), retrieved July 4, 2008 from *http://www.health.gov/phfunctions/public.htm.*

STANDARDS OF PRACTICE

In 1998, the American Association of Colleges of Nursing published the document *The Essentials of Baccalaureate Education for Professional Nursing Practice.* This document was a major step in providing clear guidelines as to what constituted professional nursing education. Roles of beginning professional nursing practice were grouped into three broad areas: provider of direct and indirect care to individuals, families, groups, communities, and populations; designer, manager, and coordinator of care; and member of a profession. Although this document describes educational preparation in all areas of nursing practice, the link to community health nursing is quite evident. The document lists seven areas of core knowledge seen as vital to the education of the nurse. Content typically associated with community health nursing is emphasized: health promotion, risk reduction, and disease prevention; global health care; and health care systems and policy. This document clearly articulates the growing need to prepare nurses to assume a variety of roles in the community (both domestic and international).

Community health nursing practice is further defined by specific standards developed under the auspices of the American Nurses Association (ANA) in collaboration with the Quad Council of Public Health Nursing Organizations (ANA, 2007c). The Quad Council is comprised of representatives from the American Nurses Association, Council on Nursing Practice and Economics; the American Public Health Association, Public Health Nursing Section; the Association of Community Health Nursing Educators; and the Association of State and Territorial Directors of Nursing. These four organizations represent academics and professional practitioners, providing a broad spectrum of views regarding professional practice in the field of community health nursing. Public Health Nursing: Scope and Standards of Practice provides guidance as to what constitutes public health nursing and how it can be differentiated from other nursing specialties. Standards of care are consistent with the nursing process and include assessment, diagnosis, outcomes identification, planning, assurance, and evaluation. This document is an important reference for all those practicing in the community. It provides the basis for evaluating an individual's performance in this field, and is used by many employers to assess job performance.

In addition to their work on the practice standards, the council completed work in 2003 on the *Quad Council Public Health Nursing Competencies,* which is designed as a tool to evaluate community health nursing practice. This guide was developed in conjunction with the more broadly focused *Core Competencies for Public Health Professionals,* with attention to areas specific to public health nursing practice. The list of competencies is applicable to two levels of practice; the staff nurse/generalist role and the manager/specialist/consultant role. Use of the competencies is seen as an appropriate assessment tool for practicing community health nurses and as a guide for agencies and academic programs as they plan educational experiences for both novice and experienced nurses (Association of Community Health Nursing Educators [ACHNE], 2003). General areas covered in the list of competencies include analytic assessment skills, policy development and program planning skills, communication skills, cultural competency skills, community dimensions of practice skills, basic public health sciences skills, financial planning and management skills, and leadership and systems thinking skills. It is also important to recognize that a specific objective in *Healthy People 2010* (23-8) stresses the need for public health agencies to utilize a competency-based assessment of their personnel (Display 3.3). The Quad Council competencies provide the basis for addressing that national objective.

DISPLAY 3.3	HEALTHY PEOPLE 2010—OBJECTIVE 23 PUBLIC HEALTH INFRASTRUCTURE

Ensure that federal, tribal, state, and local health agencies have the infrastructure to provide essential public health services effectively

Workforce

23-8 Competencies for public health workers
23-9 Training in essential public health services

23-10 Continuing education and training by public health agencies

Prevention Research

23-17 Population-based prevention research

The community health nurse provides nursing services based on other standards developed by the American Nurses Association (ANA), such as the *Code of Ethics for Nurses with Interpretive Statements* (2001), *Nursing's Social Policy Statement* (2003), and *Nursing: Scope and Standards of Practice* (2004). These three documents provide essential information regarding sound general nursing practice. When combined with Public Health Nursing: Scope and Standards of Practice (2007c), they provide the community health nurse with a clear understanding of accepted practice in this nursing specialty. With specific standards of practice and clear competencies to achieve, the community health nurse can integrate the core functions of assessment, policy development, and assurance throughout all of the various roles and community settings of practice.

ROLES OF COMMUNITY HEALTH NURSES

Just as the health care system is continually evolving, community health nursing practice evolves to remain effective with the clients it serves. Over time, the role of the community health nurse has broadened. This breadth is reflected in the description of public health nursing from the American Public Health Association, Public Health Nursing Section (1996):

> Public health nurses integrate community involvement and knowledge about the entire population with personal, clinical understandings of the health and illness experiences of individuals and families within the population. They translate and articulate the health and illness experiences of diverse, often vulnerable individuals and families in the population to health planners and policy makers, and assist members of the community to voice their problems and aspirations. Public health nurses are knowledgeable about multiple strategies for intervention, from those applicable to the entire population, to those for the family, and the individual. Public health nurses translate knowledge from the health and social sciences to individuals and population groups through targeted interventions, programs, and advocacy.

Public health nursing may be practiced by one public health nurse or by a group of public health nurses working collaboratively. In both instances, public health nurses are directly engaged in the interdisciplinary activities of the core public health functions of assessment, assurance, and policy development. Interventions or strategies may be targeted to multiple levels depending on where the most effective outcomes are possible. They include strategies aimed at entire population groups, families, or individuals. In any setting, the role of public health nurses focuses on the prevention of illness, injury or disability, the promotion of health, and maintenance of the health of populations.

Community health nurses wear many hats while conducting day-to-day practice. At any given time, however, one role is primary. This is especially true for specialized roles, such as that of full-time manager. This chapter examines seven major roles: clinician, educator, advocate, manager, collaborator, leader, and researcher. It also describes the factors that influence the selection and performance of those roles.

Clinician Role

The most familiar role of the community health nurse is that of clinician or care provider. The provision of nursing care, however, takes on new meaning in the context of community health practice. The **clinician** role in community health means that the nurse ensures health services are provided not just to individuals and families, but also to groups and populations. Nursing service is still designed for the special needs of clients, however, when those clients comprise a group or population, clinical practice takes different forms. It requires different skills to assess collective needs and tailor service accordingly. For instance, one community health nurse might visit elderly residents in a seniors' high-rise apartment building. Another might serve as the clinic nurse in a rural prenatal clinic that serves migrant farm workers. These are opportunities to assess the needs of entire aggregates and design appropriate services.

For community health nurses, the clinician role involves certain emphases that are different from those of basic nursing. Three clinician emphases, in particular, are useful to consider here: holism, health promotion, and skill expansion.

Holistic Practice

Most clinical nursing seeks to be broad and holistic. In community health, however, a holistic approach means considering the broad range of interacting needs that affect the collective health of the "client" as a larger system (Dossey, Keegan, & Guzzetta, 2005). Holistic nursing care encompasses the comprehensive and total care of the client in all areas, such as physical, emotional, social, spiritual, and economic. All are considered and cared for when the client is a large system, just as they should be with individual clients. The client is a composite of people whose relationships and interactions with each other must be considered in totality. Holistic practice must emerge from this systems perspective.

For example, when working with a group of pregnant teenagers living in a juvenile detention center, the nurse would consider the girls' relationships with one another, their parents, the fathers of their unborn children, and the detention center staff. The nurse would evaluate their ages, developmental needs, and peer influence, as well as their knowledge of pregnancy, delivery, and issues related to the choice of keeping or giving up their babies. The girls' reentry into the community and their future plans for school or employment would also be considered. Holistic service would go far beyond the physical condition of pregnancy and childbirth. It would incorporate consideration of pregnant adolescents in this community as a population at risk. What factors contributed to these girls' situations, and what preventive efforts could be instituted to protect other teenagers or these teens from future pregnancies? The clinician role of the community health nurse involves holistic practice from an aggregate perspective.

Focus on Wellness

The clinician role in community health also is characterized by its focus on promoting wellness. As discussed in Chapter 1, the community health nurse provides service along the entire range of the health continuum, but especially emphasizes promotion of health and prevention of illness. Effective services include seeking out clients who are at risk for poor health and offering preventive and health-promoting services, rather than waiting for them to come for help after problems arise. The community health nurse identifies people, programs, and agencies interested in achieving a higher level of health, and works with them to accomplish that goal and to sustain the expected changed behavior (Pender, Murdaugh, & Parsons, 2005). The nurse may help employees of a business learn how to live healthier lives or work with a group of people who want to quit smoking. The community health nurse may hold seminars with a men's group on enhancing fathering skills or assist a corporation with the implementation of a health promotion program. Groups and populations are identified that may be vulnerable to certain health threats, and preventive and health-promoting programs can be designed in collaboration with the community (Pender et al., 2005). Examples include immunization of preschoolers, family planning programs, cholesterol screening, and prevention of behavioral problems in adolescents. Protecting and promoting the health of vulnerable populations is an important component of the clinician role and is addressed extensively in the chapters in Unit VII on vulnerable aggregates.

Expanded Skills

Many different skills are used in the role of the community health clinician. In the early years of community health nursing, emphasis was placed on physical care skills. With time, skills in observation, listening, communication, and counseling became integral to the clinician role as it grew to encompass psychological and sociocultural factors. Recently, environmental and community-wide considerations—such as problems caused by pollution, violence and crime, drug abuse, unemployment, poverty, homelessness, and limited funding for health programs—have created a need for stronger skills in assessing the needs of groups and populations and intervening at the community level. The clinician role in population-based nursing also requires skills in collaboration with consumers and other professionals, use of epidemiology and biostatistics, community organization and development, research, program evaluation, administration, leadership, and effecting change (ANA, 2000; ANA, 2006). These skills are addressed in greater detail in later chapters.

Educator Role

A second important role of the community health nurse is that of **educator** or health teacher. Health teaching, a widely recognized part of nursing practice, is legislated through nurse practice acts in a number of states and is one of the major functions of the community health nurse (ANA, 2004; ANA, 2007c).

The educator role is especially useful in promoting the public's health for at least two reasons. First, community clients usually are not acutely ill and can absorb and act on health information. For example, a class of expectant parents, unhampered by significant health problems, can grasp the relationship of diet to fetal development. They understand the value of specific exercises to the childbirth process, are motivated to learn, and are more likely to perform those exercises. Thus, the educator role has the potential for finding greater receptivity and providing higher-yield results.

Second, the educator role in community health nursing is significant because a wider audience can be reached. With an emphasis on populations and aggregates, the educational efforts of community health nursing are appropriately targeted to reach many people. Instead of limiting teaching to one-on-one or small groups, the nurse has the opportunity and mandate to develop educational programs based on community needs that seek a community-wide impact. Community-wide antidrug campaigns, dietary improvement programs, and improved handwashing efforts among children provide useful models for implementation of the educator role at the population level and demonstrate its effectiveness in reaching a wide audience (Redman, 2007).

One factor that enhances the educator role is the public's higher level of health consciousness. Through plans ranging from the President's Council on Physical Fitness and Sports to local antismoking campaigns, people are recognizing the value of health and are increasingly motivated to achieve higher levels of wellness. When a middle-aged man, for example, is discharged from the hospital after a heart attack, he is likely to be more interested than before the attack in learning how to prevent another. He can learn how to reduce stress, develop an appropriate and gradual exercise program, and alter his eating habits. Families with young children often are interested in learning about children's growth and development; most parents are committed to raising happy, healthy children. Health education can affect the health status of people of all ages (Bastable, 2006; Pender et al., 2005). Today, in more businesses and industries, nurses promote the health of employees through active wellness-education and injury-prevention programs. The companies recognize that improving the health of their workers, which includes earning a living wage, means less absenteeism and higher production levels, in addition to other benefits (Halls & Rhodes, 2004). Some companies even provide exercise areas and equipment for employees to use and pay for the cost of their participation or allow paid time off for exercise.

Whereas nurses in acute care teach patients with a one-on-one focus about issues related to their hospitalization, community health nurses go beyond these topics to educate people in many areas. Community-living clients need and want to know about a wide variety of issues, such as family planning, weight control, smoking cessation, and stress reduction. Aggregate-level concerns also include such topics as environmental safety, sexual discrimination and harassment at school or work, violence, and drugs. What foods and additives are safe to eat? How can people organize the community to work for reduction of violence on television? What are health consumers' rights? Topics taught by community health nurses extend from personal and family health to environmental health and community organization.

As educators, community health nurses seek to facilitate client learning. Information is shared with clients both formally and informally. Nurses act as consultants to individuals or groups. Formal classes may be held to increase people's understanding of health and health care. Established community groups may be used in the nurse's teaching practice. For example, a nurse may teach parents and teachers at a parent–teacher meeting about signs of mood-modifying drug and alcohol abuse, discuss safety practices with a group of industrial workers, or give a presentation on the importance of early detection of child abuse to a health planning committee considering funding a new program. At times, the community health nurse facilitates client learning through referrals to more knowledgeable sources or through use of experts on special topics. Client self-education is facilitated by the nurse; in keeping with the concept of self-care, clients are encouraged and helped to use appropriate health resources and to seek out health information for themselves. The emphasis throughout the health teaching process continues to be placed on illness prevention and health promotion. Health teaching as a tool for community health nursing practice is discussed in detail in Chapter 11.

Advocate Role

The issue of clients' rights is important in health care. Every patient or client has the right to receive just, equal, and humane treatment. The role of the nurse includes client advocacy, which is highlighted in the ANA *Code of Ethics for Nurses with Interpretive Statements* (2001) and *Nursing's Social Policy Statement* (2003). Our current health care system is often characterized by fragmented and depersonalized services, and many clients—especially the poor, the disadvantaged, those without health insurance, and people with language barriers—frequently are denied their rights. They become frustrated, confused, degraded, and unable to cope with the system on their own. The community health nurse often acts as an **advocate** for clients, pleading their cause or acting on their behalf. Clients may need someone to explain which services to expect and which services they ought to receive, to make referrals as needed, and to write letters to agencies or health care providers for them. They need someone to guide them through the complexities of the system, and assure the satisfaction of their needs. This is particularly true for minorities and disadvantaged groups (Sequist, Cullen, & Ayanian, 2005; Traeger, Thompson, Dickson, & Provencio, 2006).

Advocacy Goals

Client advocacy has two underlying goals. One is to help clients gain greater independence or self-determination. Until they can research the needed information and access health and social services for themselves, the community health nurse acts as an advocate for the clients by showing them what services are available, those to which they are entitled, and how to obtain them. A second goal is to make the system more responsive and relevant to the needs of clients. By calling attention to inadequate, inaccessible, or unjust care, community health nurses can influence change.

Consider the experience of the Merrill family. Gloria Merrill has three small children. Early one Tuesday morning, the baby, Tony, suddenly started to cry. Nothing would comfort him. Gloria went to a neighbor's apartment, called the local clinic, and was told to come in the next day. The clinic did not take appointments and was too busy to see any more patients that day. Gloria's neighbor reassured her that "sometimes babies just cry." For the rest of the day and night, Tony cried almost incessantly. On Wednesday, Gloria and her children made the 45-minute bus ride to the clinic, and waited 3.5 hours in the crowded reception room; the wait was punctuated by interrogations from clinic workers. Gloria's other children were restless, and the baby was crying. Finally, they saw the physician. Tony had an inguinal hernia

that could have strangulated and become gangrenous. The doctor admonished Gloria for waiting so long to bring in the baby. Immediate surgery was necessary. Someone at the clinic told Gloria that Medicaid would pay for it. Someone else told her that she was ineligible because she was not a registered clinic patient. At this point, all of her children were crying. Gloria had been up most of the night. She was frantic, confused, and felt that no one cared. This family needed an advocate.

Advocacy Actions

The advocate role incorporates four characteristic actions: being assertive, taking risks, communicating and negotiating well, and identifying resources and obtaining results.

First, advocates must be assertive. Fortunately, in the Merrills' dilemma, the clinic had a working relationship with the City Health Department and contacted Tracy Lee, a community health nurse liaison with the clinic, when Gloria broke down and cried. Tracy took the initiative to identify the Merrills' needs and find appropriate solutions. She contacted the Department of Social Services and helped the Merrills to establish eligibility for coverage of surgery and hospitalization costs. She helped Gloria to make arrangements for the baby's hospitalization and the other children's care.

Second, advocates must take risks—go "out on a limb" if need be—for the client. The community health nurse was outraged by the kind of treatment received by the Merrills: the delays in service, the impersonal care, and the surgery that could have been planned as elective rather than as an emergency. She wrote a letter describing the details of the Merrills' experience to the clinic director, the chairman of the clinic board, and the nursing director. This action resulted in better care for the Merrills and a series of meetings aimed at changing clinic procedures and providing better telephone screening.

Third, advocates must communicate and negotiate well by bargaining thoroughly and convincingly. The community health nurse helping the Merrill family stated the problem clearly and argued for its solution.

Finally, advocates must identify and obtain resources for the client's benefit. By contacting the most influential people in the clinic and appealing to their desire for quality service, the nurse caring for the Merrill family was able to facilitate change.

Advocacy at the population level incorporates the same goals and actions. Whether the population is homeless people, battered women, or migrant workers, the community health nurse in the advocate role speaks and acts on their behalf. The goals remain the same: to promote clients' self-determination and to shape a more responsive system. Advocacy for large aggregates, such as the millions with inadequate health care coverage, means changing national policies and laws (see Chapter 13). Advocacy may take the form of presenting public health nursing data to ensure that providers deliver quality services. It may mean conducting a needs assessment to demonstrate the necessity for a shelter and multiservice program for the homeless. It may mean testifying before the legislature to create awareness of the problems of battered women and the need for more protective laws. It may mean organizing a lobbying effort to require employers of migrant workers to provide proper housing and working conditions. In each case, the community health nurse works with representatives of the population to gain their understanding of the situation and to ensure their input.

Manager Role

Community health nurses, like all nurses, engage in the role of managing health services. As a **manager**, the nurse exercises administrative direction toward the accomplishment of specified goals by assessing clients' needs, planning and organizing to meet those needs, directing and leading to achieve results, and controlling and evaluating the progress to ensure that goals are met. The nurse serves as a manager when overseeing client care as a case manager, supervising ancillary staff, managing caseloads, running clinics, or conducting community health needs assessment projects. In each instance, the nurse engages in four basic functions that make up the management process. The management process, like the nursing process, incorporates a series of problem-solving activities or functions: planning, organizing, leading, and controlling and evaluating. These activities are sequential, yet also occur simultaneously for managing service objectives (Cherry & Jacob, 2005). While performing these functions, community health nurses most often are participative managers; that is, they participate with clients, other professionals, or both to plan and implement services.

Nurse as Planner

The first function in the management process is planning. A planner sets the goals and direction for the organization or project and determines the means to achieve them. Specifically, planning includes defining goals and objectives, determining the strategy for reaching them, and designing a coordinated set of activities for implementing and evaluating them. Planning may be strategic, which tends to include broader, more long-range goals (Cherry & Jacob, 2005; USDHHS, 2000). An example of *strategic planning* is setting 2-year agency goals to reduce teenage pregnancies in the county by 50%. Planning may be operational, which focuses more on short-term planning needs. An example of *operational planning* is setting 6-month objectives to implement a new computer system for client record keeping.

The community health nurse engages in planning as a part of the manager role when supervising a group of home health aides working with home care clients. Plans of care must be designed to include setting short-term and long-term objectives, describe actions to carry out the objectives, and design a plan for evaluating the care given. With larger groups, such as a program for a homeless mentally ill population, the planning function is used in collaboration with other professionals in the community to determine appropriate goals for shelter and treatment, and to develop an action plan to carry out and evaluate the program (Burke, 2005). The concepts of planning with communities and families are discussed further in Chapters 15 and 19, respectively.

Nurse as Organizer

The second function of the manager role is that of organizer. This involves designing a structure within which people and tasks function to reach the desired objectives. A manager must arrange matters so that the job can be done. People, activities, and relationships have to be assembled to put the plan into effect. Organizing includes deciding on the tasks to be done, who will do them, how to group the tasks, who reports to whom, and where decisions will be made (Cherry & Jacob, 2005). In the process of organizing, the nurse manager provides a framework for the various aspects of service, so that each runs smoothly and accomplishes its purpose. The framework is a part of service preparation. When a community health nurse manages a well-child clinic, for instance, the organizing function involves making certain that all equipment and supplies are present, required staff are hired and are on duty, and that staff responsibilities are clearly designated. The final responsibility as an organizer is to evaluate the effectiveness of the clinic. Is it providing the needed services? Are the clients satisfied? Do the services remain cost-effective? All of these questions must be addressed by the organizer.

Nurse as Leader

In the manager role, the community health nurse also must act as a **leader**. As a leader, the nurse directs, influences, or persuades others to effect change that will positively impact people's health and move them toward a goal. The leading function includes persuading and motivating people, directing activities, ensuring effective two-way communication, resolving conflicts, and coordinating the plan. Coordination means bringing people and activities together, so that they function in harmony while pursuing desired objectives.

Community health nurses act as leaders when they direct and coordinate the functioning of a hypertension screening clinic, a weight control group, or a three-county mobile health assessment unit. In each case, the leading function requires motivating the people involved, keeping open clear channels of communication, negotiating conflicts, and directing and coordinating the activities established during planning, so that the desired objectives can be accomplished.

Nurse as Controller and Evaluator

The fourth management function is to control and evaluate projects or programs. A controller monitors the plan and ensures that it stays on course. In this function, the community health nurse must realize that plans may not proceed as intended and may need adjustments or corrections to reach the desired results or goals. Monitoring, comparing, and adjusting make up the controlling part of this function. At the same time, the nurse must compare and judge performance and outcomes against previously set goals and standards—a process that forms the evaluator aspect of this management function.

An example of the controlling and evaluating function was evident in a program started in several preschool day care centers in a city in the Midwest. The goal of the project was to reduce the incidence of illness among the children through intensive physical and emotional preventive health education with staff, parents, and children. The two community health nurses managing the project were pleased with the progress of the classes and monitored the application of the prevention principles in day-to-day care. However, staff became busy after several weeks, and some plans were not being followed carefully. Preventive activities, such as ensuring that the children coughed into their shirt sleeve and washed their hands after using the bathroom and before eating, were not being closely monitored. Several children who were clearly sick had not been kept at home. Including the quiet or reserved children in activities sometimes was overlooked. The nurses worked with staff and parents to motivate them and get the project back on course. They held monthly meetings with the staff, observed the classes periodically, and offered one-on-one instruction to staff, parents, and children. One activity was to establish competition between the centers for the best health record, with the promise of a photograph of the winning center's children and an article in the local newspaper. Their efforts were successful.

Management Behaviors

As managers, community health nurses engage in many different types of behaviors. These behaviors or parts of the manager role were first described by Mintzberg (1973). He grouped them into three sets of behaviors: decision-making, transferring of information, and engaging in interpersonal relationships.

Decision-Making Behaviors

Mintzberg identified four types of decisional roles or behaviors: entrepreneur, disturbance handler, resource allocator, and negotiator. A manager serves in the entrepreneur role when initiating new projects. Starting a nurse-managed center to serve a homeless population is an example. Community health nurses play the disturbance-handler role when they manage disturbances and crises—particularly interpersonal conflicts among staff, between staff and clients, or among clients (especially when being served in an agency). The resource-allocator role is demonstrated by determining the distribution and use of human, physical, and financial resources. Nurses play the negotiator role when negotiating, perhaps with higher levels of administration or a funding agency, for new health policy or budget increases to support expanded services for clients.

Transfer of Information Behaviors

Mintzberg described three informational roles or behaviors: monitor, information disseminator, and spokesperson. The monitor role requires collecting and processing information, such as gathering ongoing evaluation data to determine whether a program is meeting its goals. In the disseminator role, nurses transmit the collected information to people involved in the project or organization. In the spokesperson role, nurses share information on behalf of the project or agency with outsiders.

Interpersonal Behaviors

While engaging in various interpersonal roles, the community health nurse may function as a figurehead, a leader, and a liaison. In the figurehead role, the nurse acts in a ceremonial or symbolic capacity, such as participating in a ribbon-cutting ceremony to mark the opening of a new clinic or representing the project or agency for news media coverage. In the leader role, the nurse motivates and directs people involved in the project. In the liaison role, a network is maintained with people outside the organization or project for information exchange and project enhancement.

Management Skills

What types of skills and competencies does the community health nurse need in the manager role? Three basic management skills are needed for successful achievement of goals: human, conceptual, and technical. *Human skills* refer to the ability to understand, communicate, motivate, delegate, and work well with people (Cherry & Jacob, 2005). An example is a nursing supervisor's or team leader's ability to gain the trust and respect of staff and promote a productive and satisfying work environment. A manager can accomplish goals only with the cooperation of others. Therefore, human skills are essential to successful performance of the manager role. *Conceptual skills* refer to the mental ability to analyze and interpret abstract ideas for the purpose of understanding and diagnosing situations and formulating solutions. Examples are analyzing demographic data for program planning and developing a conceptual model to describe and improve organizational function. Finally, *technical skills* refer to the ability to apply special management-related knowledge and expertise to a particular situation or problem. Such skills performed by a community health nurse might include implementing a staff development program or developing a computerized management information system.

Case Management

Case management has become the standard method of managing health care in the delivery systems in the United States, and managed care organizations have become an integral part of community-oriented care. **Case management** is a systematic process by which a nurse assesses clients' needs, plans for and coordinates services, refers to other appropriate providers, and monitors and evaluates progress to ensure that clients' multiple service needs are met in a cost-effective manner. Managed care, the broader umbrella under which case management exists, is a cost-containing system of health care administration (Cohen & Cesta, 2005). Managed care, as an approach to delivering health care, is discussed in detail in Chapter 6. As clients leave hospitals earlier, as families struggle with multiple and complex health problems, as more elderly persons need alternatives to nursing home care, as competition and scarce resources contribute to fragmentation of services, and as the cost of health care continues to increase, there is a growing need for someone to oversee and coordinate all facets of needed service (Cohen & Cesta, 2005; Simpson, 2005). Through case management, the nurse addresses this need in the community.

The activity of case management often follows discharge planning as a part of continuity of care. When applied to individual clients, it means overseeing their transition from the hospital back into the community and monitoring them to ensure that all of their service needs are met. Case management also applies to aggregates. In this context, it involves overseeing and ensuring that a group's or population's health-related needs are met, particularly for those who are at high risk of illness or injury. For example, the community health nurse may work with battered women who come to a shelter. First, the nurse must ensure that their immediate needs for safety, security, food, finances, and child care are met. Then, the nurse must work with other professionals to provide more permanent housing, employment, ongoing counseling, and financial and legal resources for this group of women. Whether applied to families or aggregates, case management, like other applications of the manager role, uses the three sets of management behaviors and engages the community health nurse as planner, organizer, leader, controller, and evaluator.

Collaborator Role

Community health nurses seldom practice in isolation. They must work with many people, including clients, other nurses, physicians, teachers, health educators, social workers, physical therapists, nutritionists, occupational therapists, psychologists, epidemiologists, biostatisticians, attorneys, secretaries, environmentalists, city planners, and legislators. As members of the health team, community health nurses assume the role of **collaborator**, which means working jointly with others in a common endeavor, cooperating as partners. Successful community health practice depends on this multidisciplinary collegiality and leadership (Klinedinst, 2005; Umble et al., 2005). Everyone on the team has an important and unique contribution to make to the health care effort. As on a championship ball team, the better all members play their individual positions and cooperate with other members, the more likely the health team is to win.

The community health nurse's collaborator role requires skills in communicating, in interpreting the nurse's unique contribution to the team, and in acting assertively as an equal partner. The collaborator role also may involve functioning as a consultant.

The following examples show a community health nurse functioning as collaborator. Three families needed to find good nursing homes for their elderly grandparents. The community health nurse met with the families, including the elderly members; made a list of desired features, such as a shower and access to walking trails; and then worked with a social worker to locate and visit several homes. The grandparents' respective physicians were contacted for medical consultation, and in each case, the elderly member made the final selection. In another situation, the community health nurse collaborated with the city council, police department, neighborhood residents, and the manager of a senior citizens' high-rise apartment building to help a group of elderly people organize and lobby for safer streets. In a third example, a school nurse noticed a rise in the incidence of drug use in her schools. She initiated a counseling program after joint planning with students, parents, teachers, the school psychologist, and a local drug rehabilitation center.

Leadership Role

Community health nurses are becoming increasingly active in the leadership role, separate from leading within the manager role mentioned earlier. The leadership role focuses on effecting change (see Chapter 11); thus, the nurse becomes an agent of change. As leaders, community health nurses seek to initiate changes that positively affect people's health. They also seek to influence people to think and behave differently about their health and the factors contributing to it.

At the community level, the leadership role may involve working with a team of professionals to direct and coordinate such projects as a campaign to eliminate smoking in public areas or to lobby legislators for improved child day care facilities. When nurses guide community health decision-making, stimulate an industry's interest in health promotion, initiate group therapy, direct a preventive program, or influence health policy, they assume the leadership role. For example, a community health nurse started a rehabilitation program that included self-esteem building, career counseling, and job placement to help women in a halfway house who had recently been released from prison.

The community health nurse also exerts influence through health planning. The need for coordinated, accessible, cost-effective health care services creates a challenge and an opportunity for the nurse to become more involved in health planning at all levels: organizational, local, state, national, and international. A community health nurse needs to exercise leadership responsibility and assert the right to share in health decisions (Cherry & Jacob, 2005). One community health nurse determined that there was a need for a mental health program in his district. He planned to implement it through the agency for which he worked, but certain individuals on the health board were opposed to adding new programs because of the cost. The nurse's approach was to gather considerable data to demonstrate the need for the program and its cost-effectiveness. He invited individual, key board members to lunch to convince them of the need. He prepared written summaries, graphs, and charts, and at a strategic time, he presented his case at a board meeting. The mental health program was approved and implemented.

A broader attribute of the leadership role is that of visionary. A leader with *vision* develops the ability to see what can be and leads people on a path toward that goal. A leader's vision may include long- and short-term goals. In one instance, it began as articulating the need for stronger community nursing services to an underserved population in an inner-city neighborhood served by a community health nurse. In this densely populated, tenant-occupied neighborhood, drugs, crime, and violence were commonplace. One summer, an 8-year-old boy was shot and killed. The enraged immigrant families in the neighborhood felt helpless and hopeless. Several families were visited by the nurse, and they shared their concerns with her. The nurse felt strongly about this blighted community and offered to work with the community to effect change. She gathered volunteers from neighborhood churches, and together they began to discuss the community's concerns. Together they prioritized their needs and began planning to make theirs a healthy community. The nurse organized her work week to provide health screening and education to families in the basement of a church on one morning each week. Initially, only a few families accessed this new service. In a matter of months, it became recognized as a valuable community service, and it expanded to a full day; the expanding volunteer group soon outgrew the space. The community health nurse worked closely with influential community members and the families being served. They determined that many more services were needed in this neighborhood, and they began to broaden their outreach and think of ways to get the needed services.

Within a year, the group had written several grants to the city and to a private corporation in an effort to expand the voluntary services. The funding that they obtained allowed them to rent vacant storefront space, hire a part-time nurse practitioner, contract with the health department for additional community health nursing services, and negotiate with the local university to have medical, nursing, and social work students placed on a regular basis. The group, under the visionary leadership of the community health nurse, planned to add a one-on-one reading program for children, a class in English as a second language for immigrant families, a mentoring program for teenagers, and dental services. Even the police department had opened a substation in the neighborhood, making their presence more visible. This community health nurse's vision filled an immediate, critical need in the short term and developed into a comprehensive community center in the long term. Violence and crime diminished, and the neighborhood became a place where children could play safely.

Researcher Role

In the **researcher** role, community health nurses engage in the systematic investigation, collection, and analysis of data for solving problems and enhancing community health practice. But how can research be combined with practice? Although research technically involves a complex set of activities conducted by persons with highly developed and specialized skills, research also means applying that technical study to real-practice situations. Community health nurses base their practice on the evidence found in the literature to enhance and change practice as needed. For example, the work of several researchers over 15 years supports the value of intensive home visiting to high-risk families (Olds, 2006). The outcomes of this research are changing practice protocol to high-risk families in many health departments today.

Research is an investigative process in which all community health nurses can become involved in asking questions and looking for solutions. Collaborative practice models between academics and practitioners combine research methodology expertise with practitioners' knowledge of problems to make community health nursing research both valid and relevant. The ongoing need for evidence-based practice is supported by Healthy People 2010, which stresses the importance of population-based prevention research to our national health goals (Display 3.3).

The Research Process

Community health nurses practice the researcher role at several levels. In addition to everyday inquiries, community health nurses often participate in agency and organizational studies to determine such matters as practice activities, priorities, and education of public health nurses (Grumbach, Miller, Mertz, & Finocchio, 2004). Some community health nurses participate in more complex research on their own or in collaboration with other health professionals (Elliott, Crombie, Irvine, Cantrell, & Taylor, 2004). The researcher role, at all levels, helps to determine needs, evaluate effectiveness of care, and develop a theoretic basis for community health nursing practice. Chapters 4 and 12 will explain community health research in greater detail.

Research literally means to *search again*—to investigate, discover, and interpret facts. All research in community health, from the simplest inquiry to the most complex epidemiologic study, uses the same fundamental process. Simply put, the research process involves the following steps: (1) identify an area of interest, (2) specify the research question or statement, (3) review the literature, (4) identify a conceptual framework, (5) select a research design, (6) collect and analyze data, (7) interpret the results, and (8) communicate the findings (see Chapter 4).

Investigation builds on the nursing process, that essential dynamic of community health nursing practice, using it as a problem-solving process (Burns & Grove, 2007). In using the nursing process, the nurse identifies a problem or question, investigates by collecting and analyzing data, suggests and evaluates possible solutions, and either selects a solution or rejects them all and starts the investigative process over again. In a sense, the nurse is gathering data for health planning—investigating health problems to design wellness-promoting and disease-preventing interventions for community populations.

Attributes of the Researcher Role

A questioning attitude is a basic prerequisite for good nursing practice. A nurse may have revisited a patient many times and noticed some change in her condition, such as restlessness or pallor; consequently, the nurse wonders what is causing this change and what can be done about it. In everyday practice, numerous situations challenge the nurse to ask questions. Consider the following examples:

- A newspaper reports that another group of children has been arrested for using illegal drugs. Is there an increase in the incidence of illegal drug use in the community?
- Children attending a day care center appear to have excessive bruises on their arms and legs. What is the incidence of reported child abuse in this community? What could be done to promote earlier detection and improved reporting?
- Elderly persons are living alone and without assistance in a neighborhood. How prevalent is this situation, and what are this population's needs?
- Driving through a particular neighborhood, the nurse notices not a single playground. Where do the kids play?

Each of these questions places the nurse in the role of investigator. They demonstrate the fundamental attitude of every researcher: a spirit of inquiry.

A second attribute, careful observation, also is evident in the examples just given. The nurse needs to develop a sharpened ability to notice things as they are, including deviations from the norm and subtle changes suggesting the need for nursing action. Coupled with observation is open-mindedness, another attribute of the researcher role. In the case of the bruises seen on day care children, a community health nurse's observations suggest child abuse as a possible cause. However, open-mindedness requires consideration of other alternatives, and, as a good investigator, the nurse explores these possibilities as well.

Analytic skills also are used in this role. In the example of illegal drug use, the nurse already has started to analyze the situation by trying to determine its cause-and-effect relationships. Successful analysis depends on how well the data have been collected. Insufficient information can lead to false interpretations, so it is important to seek out the needed data. Analysis, like a jigsaw puzzle, involves studying the pieces and fitting them together until the meaning of the whole picture can be described.

Finally, the researcher role involves tenacity. The community health nurse persists in an investigation until facts are uncovered and a satisfactory answer is found. Noticing an absence of playgrounds and wondering where the children play is only a beginning. Being concerned about the children's safety and need for recreational outlets, the nurse gathers data about the location and accessibility of play areas, as well as expressed needs of community residents. A fully documented research report may result. If the data support a need for additional play space, the report can be brought before the proper authorities.

SETTINGS FOR COMMUNITY HEALTH NURSING PRACTICE

The previous section examined community health nursing from the perspective of its major roles. The roles can now be placed in context by viewing the settings in which they are practiced. The types of places in which community health nurses practice are increasingly varied and include a growing number of nontraditional settings and partnerships with non-health groups. Employers of community health nurses range from state and local health departments and home health agencies to managed care organizations, businesses and industries, and nonprofit organizations. For this discussion, these settings are grouped into seven categories: homes, ambulatory service settings, schools, occupational health settings, residential institutions, faith communities, and the community at large (domestic and international). This section of the chapter provides a brief overview of the various settings. Chapters 30 and 31 will provide much more detail on specific roles and settings, including both public and private practice settings.

Homes

Since Lillian Wald and the nurses at the Henry Street Settlement first started their practice at the beginning of the last century, the most frequently used setting for community health nursing practice was the home. In the home, all of the community health nursing roles are performed to varying degrees. Clients who are discharged from acute care institutions, such as hospitals or mental health facilities, are regularly referred to community health nurses for continued care and follow-up. Here, the community health nurse can see clients in a family and environmental context, and service can be tailored to the clients' unique needs.

For example, Mr. White, 67 years of age, was discharged from the hospital with a colostomy. Doreen Levitz, the community health nurse from the county public health nursing agency, immediately started home visits. She met with Mr.

White and his wife to discuss their needs as a family and to plan for Mr. White's care and adjustment to living with a colostomy. Practicing the clinician and educator roles, she reinforced and expanded on the teaching started in the hospital for colostomy care, including bowel training, diet, exercise, and proper use of equipment. As part of a total family care plan, Doreen provided some forms of physical care for Mr. White as well as counseling, teaching, and emotional support for both Mr. White and his wife. In addition to consulting with the physician and social service worker, she arranged and supervised visits from the home health aide, who gave personal care and homemaker services. She thus performed the manager, leader, and collaborator roles.

The home is also a setting for health promotion. Many community health nursing visits focus on assisting families to understand and practice healthier living behaviors. Nurses may, for example, instruct clients on parenting, infant care, child discipline, diet, exercise, coping with stress, or managing grief and loss.

The character of the home setting is as varied as the clients served by the community health nurse. In one day, the nurse may visit a well-to-do widow in her luxurious home, a middle-income family in their modest bungalow, an elderly transient man in his one-room fifth-story walk-up apartment, and a teen mother and her infant living in a group foster home. In each situation, the nurse can view the clients in perspective and, therefore, better understand their limitations, capitalize on their resources, and tailor health services to meet their needs. In the home, unlike in most other health care settings, clients are on their own "turf." They feel comfortable and secure in familiar surroundings and often are better able to understand and apply health information. Client self-respect can be promoted, because the client is host and the nurse is a guest.

Sometimes, the thought of visiting in clients' homes can cause anxiety for the nurse. This may be the nurse's first experience outside the acute care, long-term care, or clinic setting. Visiting clients in their own environment can make the nurse feel uncomfortable. The nurse may be asked to visit families in unfamiliar neighborhoods, and she must walk through those neighborhoods to locate the clients' homes. Frequently, fear of the unknown is the real fear—a fear that often has been enhanced by stories from previous nurses. This may be the same feeling as that experienced when caring for your first client, first entering the operating room, or first having a client in the intensive care unit. However, in the community, more variables exist, and basic safety measures should be used by all people when out in public. General guidelines for safety and making home visits are covered in detail in Chapter 19. Nevertheless, the specific instructions given during the clinical experience should be followed, and everyday, common-sense safety precautions should be used.

Changes in the health care delivery system, along with shifting health economics and service delivery (discussed in Chapter 6), are changing community health nursing's use of the home as a primary setting for practice. Many local health departments are finding it increasingly difficult to provide widespread home visiting by their public health nurses. Instead, many agencies are targeting populations that are most in need of direct intervention. Examples include families of children with elevated blood lead levels, low-birth-weight babies, clients requiring directly observed administration of tuberculosis medications, and families requiring ongoing monitoring due to identified child abuse or neglect. With limited staff and limited financial resources, the highest-priority clients or groups are targeted.

With skills in population-based practice, community health nurses serve the public's health best by focusing on sites where they can have the greatest impact. At the same time, they can collaborate with various types of home care providers, including hospitals, other nurses, physicians, rehabilitation therapists, and durable medical equipment companies, to ensure continuous and holistic service. The nurse continues to supervise home care services and engage in case management. The increased demand for highly technical acute care in the home requires specialized skills that are best delivered by nurses with this expertise. Chapter 32 further examines the nurse's role in the home health and hospice settings. The ANA documents *Home Health Nursing Scope and Standards of Practice* (2007a) and *Hospice and Palliative Nursing: Scope and Standards of Practice* (2007b) offer additional insight on these specialty areas.

Ambulatory Service Settings

Ambulatory service settings include a variety of venues for community health nursing practice in which clients come for day or evening services that do not include overnight stays. A community health center is an example of an ambulatory setting. Sometimes, multiple clinics offering comprehensive services are community based or are located in outpatient departments of hospitals or medical centers. They also may be based in comprehensive neighborhood health centers. A single clinic, such as a family planning clinic or a well-child clinic, may be found in a location that is more convenient for clients, perhaps a church basement or empty storefront. Some kinds of day care centers, such as those for physically disabled or adults with behavioral health issues, use community health nursing services. Additional ambulatory care settings include health departments (city, county, or state) and community health nursing agencies, where clients may come for assessment and referral or counseling. An increasing number of nurse-managed health centers have also been formed over the past decade, often as a community service component of schools of nursing. The mission of these centers varies, but they are typically used to enhance student clinical experiences while providing identified community needs in the areas of primary health care and health promotion (see Chapter 31).

Offices are another type of ambulatory care setting. Some community health nurses provide service in conjunction with a medical practice; for example, a community health nurse associated with a health maintenance organization sees clients in the office and undertakes screening, referrals, counseling, health education, and group work. Others establish independent practices by seeing clients in community nursing centers, as well as making home visits.

Another type of ambulatory service setting includes places where services are offered to selected groups. For example, community health nurses practice in migrant camps, on Tribal lands, at correctional facilities, in children's day care centers, through faith communities, and in remote mountain and coal-mining communities. In each ambulatory setting, all of the community health nursing roles are used to varying degrees (see Student Voices).

PERSPECTIVES
STUDENT VOICES

A Graduating Student Viewpoint on Postgraduation Employment

Before entering nursing school, I spent 6 years on active duty as a corpsman in the Navy. I remembered seeing some nurses who visited our hospital wearing what looked like Navy uniforms, but was told that they worked for the federal government and weren't in the Navy. I didn't think much of it until I was looking up information on the U.S. Public Health Service and the Surgeon General. Only then did it dawn on me that those nurses were part of the Commissioned Corps of the Public Health Service. I didn't even know they existed, much less what they did, so I looked around the section of the website dealing with nursing. It turns out that they do quite a bit—respond to disasters, provide health services to Native Americans, and even work with the federal prisons. It surprised me to find out that they hire new graduates for many of their positions. I still haven't decided what I want to do after I graduate, but I may seriously consider this option. They even have an extern program available while I'm still in school—who knows, I may be in uniform again.

Matt, Age 24

Schools

Schools of all levels make up a major group of settings for community health nursing practice. Nurses from community health nursing agencies frequently serve private schools at elementary and intermediate levels. Public schools are served by the same agencies or by community health nurses hired through the public school system. The community health nurse may work with groups of students in preschool settings, such as Montessori schools, as well as in vocational or technical schools, junior colleges, and college and university settings. Specialized schools, such as those for the developmentally disabled, are another setting for community health nursing practice.

Community health nurses' roles in school settings are changing. School nurses, whose primary role initially was that of clinician, are widening their practice to include more health education, interprofessional collaboration, and client advocacy. For example, one school had been accustomed to using the nurse as a first-aid provider and record keeper. Her duties were handling minor problems, such as headaches and cuts, and keeping track of such events as immunizations. This nurse sought to expand her practice and, after consultation and preparation, collaborated with a health educator and some of the teachers to offer a series of classes on personal hygiene, diet, and sexuality. She started a drop-in health counseling center in the school and established a network of professional contacts for consultation and referral.

Community health nurses in school settings also are beginning to assume managerial and leadership roles and to recognize that the researcher role should be an integral part of their practice. The nurse's role with school-age and adolescent populations is discussed in detail in Chapter 22. The ANA *School Nursing: Scope and Standards of Practice* (2005a) provides additional information on this important specialty.

Occupational Health Settings

Business and industry provide another group of settings for community health nursing practice. Employee health has long been recognized as making a vital contribution to individual lives, the productivity of business, and the well-being of the entire nation. Organizations are expected to provide a safe and healthy work environment, in addition to offering insurance for health care. More companies, recognizing the value of healthy employees, are going beyond offering traditional health benefits to supporting health promotional efforts. Some businesses, for example, offer healthy snacks, such as fruit at breaks, and promote jogging during the noon hour. A few larger corporations have built exercise facilities for their employees, provide health education programs, and offer financial incentives for losing weight or staying well.

Community health nurses in occupational health settings practice a variety of roles. The clinician role was primary for many years, as nurses continued to care for sick or injured employees at work. However, recognition of the need to protect employees' safety and, later, to prevent their illness led to the inclusion of health education in the occupational health nurse role. Occupational health nurses also act as employee advocates, assuring appropriate job assignments for workers and adequate treatment for job-related illness or injury. They collaborate with other health care providers and company management to offer better services to their clients. They act as leaders and managers in developing new health services in the work setting, endorsing programs such as hypertension screening and weight control. Occupational health settings range from industries and factories, such as an automobile assembly plant, to business corporations and even large retail sales systems. The field of occupational health offers a challenging opportunity, particularly in smaller businesses, where nursing coverage usually is not provided. Chapter 31 more fully describes the role of the nurse serving the working adult population.

Residential Institutions

Any facility where clients reside can be a setting in which community health nursing is practiced. Residential institutions can include a halfway house in which clients live temporarily while recovering from drug addiction or an inpatient hospice program in which terminally ill clients live. Some residential settings, such as hospitals, exist solely to provide health care; others provide a variety of services and support. Community health nurses based in a community agency maintain continuity of care for their clients by collaborating with hospital personnel, visiting clients in the hospital, and planning care during and after hospitalization.

Some community health nurses serve one or more hospitals on a regular basis by providing a liaison with the community, consultation for discharge planning, and periodic in-service programs to keep hospital staff updated on community services for their clients. Other community health nurses with similar functions are based in the hospital and serve the hospital community.

A continuing care center is another example of a residential site providing health care that may use community health nursing services. In this setting, residents usually are elderly; some live quite independently, whereas others become increasingly dependent and have many chronic health problems. The community health nurse functions as advocate and collaborator to improve services. The nurse may, for example, coordinate available resources to meet the needs of residents and their families and help safeguard the maintenance of quality operating standards. Chapter 24 discusses the community health nurse's role with elders aging in place. Chapter 32 discusses nursing services needed by clients after hospitalization through home care services or by families and clients in hospice programs. Sheltered workshops and group homes for mentally ill or developmentally disabled children and adults are other examples of residential institutions that serve clients who share specific needs.

Community health nurses also practice in settings where residents are gathered for purposes other than receiving care, where health care is offered as an adjunct to the primary goals of the institution. For example, many nurses work with camping programs for children and adults offered by religious organizations and other community agencies, such as the Boy Scouts, Girl Scouts, or the YMCA. Other camp nurses work with children and adults who have chronic or terminal illnesses, through disease-related community agencies such as the American Lung Association, American Diabetes Association, and American Cancer Society. Camp nurses practice all available roles, often under interesting and challenging conditions.

Residential institutions provide unique settings for the community health nurse to practice health promotion. Clients are a "captive audience" whose needs can be readily assessed and whose interests can be stimulated. These settings offer the opportunity to generate an environment of caring and optimal-quality health care provided by community health nursing services.

Faith Communities

Faith community nursing finds its beginnings in an ancient tradition. The beginnings of community health nursing can be traced to religious orders (see Chapter 2), and for centuries, religious and spiritual communities were important sources of health care. In faith community nursing today, the practice focal point remains the faith community and the religious belief system provided by the philosophical framework. Faith community nursing may take different names, such as church-based health promotion (CBHP), parish nursing, or primary care parish nursing practice (PCPNP). Whatever the service is called, it involves a large-scale effort by the church community to improve the health of its members through education, screening, referral, treatment, and group support.

In some geopolitical communities, faith community nurses are the most acceptable primary care providers. The role of the nurse can be broad, being defined by the needs of the members and the philosophy of the religious community. However, the goal is to enhance and extend services available in the larger community, not to duplicate them.

The ANA has written standards of care for faith community nursing practice in collaboration with Health Ministries Association, Inc. (ANA, 2005b). The standards act as guidelines for faith communities that plan to offer or are offering faith community nursing services. This specialty area of practice is guided by a variety of standards set up by several groups. Together, these standards provide guidance and direction for caregiving within the faith community.

When community health nurses work as faith community nurses, they enhance accessibility to available health services in the community while meeting the unique needs of the members of that religious community, practicing within the framework of the tenets of that religion. A nurse working within a faith community must be cognizant of the basic principles and practices of the religious group served. In most situations, the nurse is a practitioner of the same religious belief system. Chapter 31 provides more detailed information about this specialty area of practice.

Community at Large

Unlike the six settings already discussed, the seventh setting for community health nursing practice is not confined to a specific philosophy, location, or building. When working with groups, populations, or the total community, the nurse may practice in many different places (Display 3.4). For example, a community health nurse, as clinician and health educator, may work with a parenting group in a church or town hall. Another nurse, as client advocate, leader, and researcher, may study the health needs of a neighborhood's elderly population by collecting data throughout the area and meeting with resource people in many places. Also, a nurse may work with community-based organizations such as an AIDS organization or a support group for parents experiencing the violent death of a child. Again, the community at large becomes the setting for practice for a nurse who serves on health care planning committees, lobbies for health legislation at the state capital, runs for a school board

---

DISPLAY 3.4   INNOVATIVE COMMUNITY HEALTH NURSING PRACTICE

In some community health nursing courses, students do not have access to an established agency such as a health department or community center from which to establish a client base. Student nurses and practicing community health nurses can provide outreach services and do case-finding in innovative settings such as these:

Settings	Clients	Roles of the Community Health Nurse
1. Senior centers when flu shots are given or commodities are distributed	Older adults	Educator, Clinician, Advocate
2. Outside of grocery stores, department stores, movie theaters, large pharmacies	People of all ages and families	Educator, Clinician, Advocate
3. At PTA meetings, sporting events, dances, and school registration (in collaboration with school nurses)	Young adults, children, and teenagers	Educator, Clinician, Advocate
4. Outside of concerts, plays, the circus, etc.	People of all ages	Educator, Clinician, Advocate
5. Other public gatherings: farmers markets, neighborhood yard sales, etc.	People of all ages	Educator, Clinician, Advocate
6. Conferences or seminars	People of all ages	Leader, Educator, Clinician
7. "On the street"	Homeless persons, passersby, transients, low-income urban dwellers	Educator, Clinician, Advocate
8. Truck stops	Predominently employed men	Educator, Clinician, Advocate

Leader Role—initiate, plan, strategize, collaborate, and cooperate with community groups to present programs that are focused on specific population's needs.

Educator Role—teach nutrition, stress management, safety, exercise, prevention of sexually transmitted diseases, and other mens' and womens' health issues, child home/school/play and stranger safety, and child growth and development, and provide anticipatory guidance. Have pamphlets available to support verbal information on health and safety topics, specific diseases, Social Security, Medicare, and Medicaid.

Clinician Role—perform blood pressure screening, height, weight, blood testing for diabetes and cholesterol, occult blood test, hearing and vision tests, scoliosis measurements, and administration of immunizations.

Advocate Role—provide information regarding community resources as needed, cut "red tape" for those who need it, answer questions, and guide people to additional resources, such as Internet Web sites and "800" phone numbers.

position, or assists with flood relief in another state or another country.

Although the term "setting" implies a place, remember that community health nursing practice is not limited to a specific site. Community health nursing is a specialty of nursing that is defined by the nature of its practice, not its location, and it can be practiced anywhere. As you read through this chapter, perhaps an area of practice or a particular population captured your attention. If you are interested in Tribal health, you might consider working as a Public Health Service nurse, or if you find that you are more interested in providing comprehensive health promotion programs to rural individuals, a nurse-managed health center may be of interest. Opportunities for community health nursing include the American Red Cross, state and local health departments, the Peace Corps, and various international aide groups. Both private and public health agencies are actively seeking nurses with an interest in improving the health of their communities. Take some time to read over Chapters 30 and 31; perhaps you will find an opportunity that supports your professional goals.

Summary

Community health nurses play many roles, including that of clinician, educator, advocate, manager, collaborator, leader, and researcher. Each role entails special types of skills and expertise. The type and number of roles that are practiced vary with each set of clients and each specific situation, but the nurse should be able to successfully function in each of these roles as the particular situation demands. The role of manager is one that the nurse must play in every situation, because it involves assessing clients' needs, planning and organizing to meet those needs, directing and leading clients to achieve results, and controlling and evaluating the progress to ensure that the goals and clients' needs are met. A type of comprehensive management of clients that has become known as *case management* is an integral part of community health nursing practice.

As a part of the manager role, the nurse must engage in three crucial management behaviors: decision-making, transferring information, and relationship building. Nurses must also use a comprehensive set of management skills: human skills that allow them to understand, communicate, motivate, and work with people; conceptual skills that allow them to interpret abstract ideas and apply them to real situations to formulate solutions; and technical skills that allow them to apply special management-related knowledge and expertise to a particular situation or problem.

There also are many types of settings in which the community health nurse may practice and in which these roles are enacted. "Setting" does not necessarily refer to a specific location or site, but rather to a particular situation. These situations can be grouped into seven major categories: homes; ambulatory service settings, where clients come for care but do not stay overnight; schools; occupational health settings, which serve employees in business and industry; residential institutions such as hospitals, continuing care facilities, halfway houses, or other institutions in which people live and sleep; faith communities, where care is based on the philosophy of the religious organization; and the community at large, which encompasses a variety of expected and innovative locations. ■

ACTIVITIES TO PROMOTE CRITICAL THINKING

1. Discuss ways for a community health nurse to make service holistic and focused on wellness with
   a. preschool-age children in a day care setting.
   b. a group of chemically dependent adolescents.
   c. a group of elders living in a senior high-rise building.
2. Select one community health nursing role and describe its application in meeting the needs of your friend or next-door neighbor.
3. Describe a hypothetical or real situation in which you, as a community health nurse, would combine the roles of leader, collaborator, and researcher (investigator). Discuss how each of these roles might be played.
4. If your community health nursing practice setting is the community at large, will your practice roles be any different from those of the nurse whose practice setting is the home? Why? What determines the roles played by the community health nurse?
5. Interview a practicing community health nurse and determine which roles are part of the nurse's practice during 1 month of caregiving. Describe the ways in which each role is enacted. How many instances of this nurse's practice were aggregate focused? In which of the settings does the nurse mostly practice? If you were a public health consultant, what suggestions might you make to expand this nurse's role into aggregate-level practice?
6. Search the Internet or go to the library and find two sources of health-related information for consumers. Was the information accurate?
7. Search the Internet or go to the library and find two research articles on community health nursing. In what settings did the research take place? Did the nursing authors collaborate with interdisciplinary team members on this research? If so, how do you think this collaboration helped the research? If you were to conduct research in the community, would you conduct it with only nurses on the team, or would your team be interdisciplinary? Why? What would be the benefits or limits of each approach?

References

American Association of Colleges of Nursing. (1998). *The essentials of baccalaureate education for professional nursing practice.* Washington, DC: Author.

American Nurses Association. (2007a). *Home health nursing scope and standards of practice.* Silver Spring, MD: Nursesbooks.org.

American Nurses Association. (2000). *Public health nursing: A partner for healthy populations.* Washington, DC: American Nurses Publishing.

American Nurses Association. (2001). *Code for nurses with interpretive statements.* Kansas City, MO: American Nurses Publishing.

American Nurses Association/Hospice and Palliative Nurses Association. (2007b). *Hospice and palliative nursing: Scope and standards of practice.* Washington, DC: American Nurses Foundation.

American Nurses Association. (2003). *Nursing's social policy statement*. Washington, DC: American Nurses Publishing.

American Nurses Association. (2004). *Nursing: Scope and standards of practice*. Washington, DC: American Nurses Publishing.

American Nurses Association. (2005a). *School nursing: Scope and standards of practice*. Washington, DC: American Nurses Publishing.

American Nurses Association. (2005b). *Faith community nursing: Scope and standards of practice*. Washington, DC: American Nurses Publishing.

American Nurses Association. (2007c). *Public health nursing: Scope and standards of practice*. Silver Spring, MD: Nursesbooks.org.

American Public Health Association. (1996). *A Statement of APHA Public Health Nursing Section*. Retrieved October 31, 2006 from American Public Health Association Web site: http://www.apha.org/extranet/phn/default.htm.

Association of Community Health Nursing Educators. (2003). *Quad Council PHN Competencies*. Retrieved October 31, 2006 from http://www.achne.org/achne%20documents/Final_ PHN_Competencies.pdf.

Bastable, S.B. (2006). *Essentials of patient education*. Boston: Jones & Bartlett Publishers.

Burke, J. (2005). Educating the staff at a homeless shelter about mental illness and anger management. *Journal of Community Health Nursing, 22,* 65–76.

Burns, N., & Grove, S.K. (2007). Understanding nursing research: Building an evidence-based practice (4th ed.). St. Louis: Saunders.

Cherry, B., & Jacob, S.R. (2005). *Contemporary nursing: Issues, trends, and management* (3rd ed.). St. Louis: Mosby.

Cohen, E.L., & Cesta, T.G. (2005). *Nursing case management: From essential to advanced practice applications* (4th ed.). Philadelphia: Mosby.

Dossey, B.M., Keegan L., & Guzzetta, C.E. (2005). *Holistic nursing: A handbook for practice* (4th ed.). Sudbury, MA: Jones & Bartlett Publishers.

Elliott, L., Crombie, I.K., Irvine, L., Cantrell, J., & Taylor, J. (2004). The effectiveness of public health nursing: The problems and solutions in carrying out a review of systematic reviews. *Journal of Advanced Nursing, 45,* 117–125.

Grumbach, K., Miller, J., Mertz, E., & Finocchio, L. (2004). How much public health in public health nursing practice? *Public Health Nursing, 21,* 266–276.

Halls, C., & Rhodes, J. (2004). Employee wellness and beyond. *Occupational Health & Safety, 73,* 46–49.

Institute of Medicine. (1988). *The future of public health*. Washington, DC: National Academy Press.

Klinedinst, N.J. (2005). Effects of a nutrition education program for urban, low-income, older adults: A collaborative program among nurses and nursing students. *Journal of Community Health Nursing, 22,* 93–104.

Mintzberg, H. (1973). *The nature of managerial work*. New York: Harper & Row.

Olds, D. (2006). Progress in improving the development of low birth weight newborns. *Pediatrics, 117,* 940–941.

Pender, N.J., Murdaugh, C.L., & Parsons, M.A. (2005). *Health promotion in nursing practice* (5th ed.). Upper Saddle River, NJ: Prentice Hall.

Redman, B.K. (2007). *The practice of patient education* (10th ed.). St. Louis: Mosby.

Sequist, T.D., Cullen, T., & Ayanian, J.Z. (2005). Information technology as a tool to improve the quality of American Indian health care. *American Journal of Public Health, 95,* 2173–2179.

Simpson, A. (2005). Community psychiatric nurses and the care co-ordinator role: Squeezed to provide 'limited nursing'. *Journal of Advanced Nursing, 52,* 689–699.

Traeger, M., Thompson, A., Dickson, E., & Provencio, A. (2006). Bridging disparity: A multidisciplinary approach for influenza vaccination in an American Indian community. *American Journal of Public Health, 96,* 921–925.

Umble, K., Steffen, D., Porter, J., Miller, D., Hummer-McLaughlin, K., Lowman, A., et al. (2005). The National Public Health Leadership Institute: Evaluation of a team-based approach to developing collaborative public health leaders. *American Journal of Public Health, 95,* 641–644.

U.S. Department of Health and Human Services. (1997). *The public health workforce: An agenda for the 21st century*. Washington, DC: U.S. Government Printing Office.

U.S. Department of Health and Human Services, Office of Disease Prevention & Health Promotion. (1999). *Public Health Functions Project*. Retrieved October 31, 2006 from http://www.health.gov/phfunctions/public.htm.

U.S. Department of Health and Human Services. (2000). *Healthy people 2010*. (Conference ed., Vols. 1 & 2). Washington, DC: U.S. Government Printing Office.

U.S. Department of Health and Human Services, Centers for Disease Control and Prevention. (n.d.). *Assessment in public health*. Retrieved October 31, 2006 from http://www.cdc.gov/epo/dphsi/AI/what_new.htm.

Selected Readings

American Public Health Association. (2005). *APHA legislative advocacy handbook*. Washington, DC: Author.

Anderson, E.T., & McFarlane, J. (2004). *Community as partner: Theory and practice in nursing*. Philadelphia: Lippincott Williams & Wilkins.

Bastable, S. (2003). *Nurse as educator: Principles of teaching nursing practice* (2nd ed.). Boston: Jones & Bartlett Publishers.

Kotch, J.B. (Ed.) (2005). *Maternal and child health: Programs, problems, and policy in public health* (2nd ed.). Boston: Jones & Bartlett Publishers.

Leddy, S.K. (2006). *Integrative health promotion: Conceptual bases for nursing practice* (2nd ed.). Boston: Jones & Bartlett Publishers.

Norwood, S. L. (2002). *Nursing consultation: A framework for working with communities* (2nd ed.). Upper Saddle River, NJ: Prentice Hall.

Rice, R. (2006). *Home care nursing practice* (4th ed.). St. Louis: Mosby.

Solari-Twadell, P.A., & McDermott, M.A. (2006). *Parish nursing: Development, education, and administration*. St. Louis: Mosby.

Internet Resources

American Association of Colleges of Nursing: *http://aacn.campusrn.com/students/jobsearch.asp*

American Association of Occupational Health Nurses: *http://www.aaohn.org/*

American Nurses Association: *http://www.nursingworld.org/*

American Red Cross: *http://www.redcross.org/*

Association of Community Health Nursing Educators: *http://www.achne.org/*

Health Ministries Association, Inc.: *http://www.hmassoc.org/*

National Association of School Nurses: *http://www.nasn.org/*

National Nursing Centers Consortium: *http://www.nncc.us/*

Peace Corps: *http://www.peacecorps.gov/*

President's Council on Physical Fitness and Sports: *http://www.fitness.gov/*

U.S. Department of Health and Human Services: *http://www.hhs.gov/*

U.S. Public Health Service Commissioned Corps: *http://www.usphs.gov/*

4

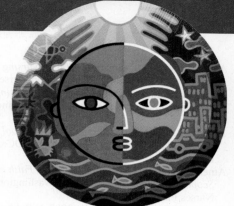

Evidence-based Practice and Ethics in Community Health Nursing

Upon mastery of this chapter, you should be able to:

◆ Discuss the concept of evidence-based practice (EBP).

◆ List the necessary steps in the process of EBP.

◆ Explain the difference between quantitative research and qualitative research.

◆ List the nine steps of the research process.

◆ Analyze the potential impact of research on community health nursing practice.

◆ Identify the community health nurse's role in conducting research and using research findings to improve his or her practice.

◆ Describe the nature of values and value systems and their influence on community health nursing.

◆ Articulate the impact of key values on professional decision-making.

◆ Discuss the application of ethical principles to community health nursing decision-making.

◆ Use a decision-making process with and for community health clients that incorporates values and ethical principles.

❝*Doing good to others is not a duty. It is a joy, for it increases your own health and happiness.*❞

—Zoroaster

KEY TERMS

Autonomy
Beneficence
Bioethics
Conceptual model
Control group
Descriptive statistics
Distributive justice
Egalitarian justice
Equity
Ethical decision-making
Ethical dilemma
Ethics
Evidence-based practice
Experimental design
Experimental group
Fidelity
Generalizability
Health policy evaluation
Inferential statistics
Instrument
Instrumental values
Integrative review
Justice
Meta-analysis
Moral
Moral evaluations
Nonexperimental design
Nonmaleficence
Qualitative research
Quantitative research
Quasi-experiment
Randomization
Randomized control trial (RCT)
Reliability
Research
Respect
Restorative justice
Self-determination
Self-interest
Systematic review
Terminal values
True experiment
Validity
Value
Value systems
Values clarification
Veracity
Well-being

As a new student in community health nursing, you may ask, "Can I really do something to make a difference in the lives of my clients?" You may often feel shocked and discouraged by the crushing poverty and overwhelming sense of helplessness many of your clients experience, and by the continual recurrence of substance abuse, domestic violence, job failure, and criminal activity. For the first time, you may truly confront the inequalities and injustices of our health care system. You will face many ethical dilemmas in community health nursing. You may ask, "Why should I bother to make home visits to pregnant teens? Why should I offer smoking cessation classes at the local homeless shelter? Why should I teach clients about the importance of taking their antituberculosis medications? Will it really matter?"

This chapter discusses current research as it relates to and impacts community health nursing practice. The steps of the research process are identified and discussed, and evidence-based practice (EBP) is emphasized. The chapter includes information on constructing a clinical question and incorporating client considerations and clinical guidelines, and helpful resources for finding and analyzing research studies. Ethics and values are also examined, as they relate to both research and community health nursing practice. This chapter explores the nature and function of values and value systems, the role of values and value systems in ethical decision-making, the central values related to health care choices and their potential conflicts, and the implications of values and ethics for community health nursing decision-making and practice.

Recent community health nursing research validates that nursing care *does* matter and that you really *can* make a difference in the lives of your clients. For example, nurse–family partnership programs, based on research conducted by David Olds and his colleagues, are reaping results in many communities across the United States (Nurse–Family Partnership, 2008). In a classic longitudinal study by Olds and his research team (1997), conducted with a primarily White sample in a semi-rural setting over a 15-year period, regular visits by public health nurses (PHNs) to poor, unmarried women and their first-born children resulted in dramatic differences when compared with similar mothers and children in a control group. Many of the women in the study were younger than 19 years of age, and nurses made an average of nine prenatal visits and 23 child-related visits (up to age 2 years). Statistically significant differences were noted in the following outcomes:

◆ Fewer subsequent pregnancies and increased percentage of live births
◆ Longer intervals between first and second births
◆ Fewer incidences of reported child abuse and neglect
◆ Fewer months on public assistance and food stamps
◆ Fewer arrests and convictions
◆ Less reported impairment by alcohol or other drug use

The effects of the intervention continued for up to 15 years after the birth of the first child. This is powerful evidence for the effectiveness of a program of regular community/PHN visits to this vulnerable group. The costs of community health nurse visits are more than offset by the large savings in both dollars and human suffering. The Rand Corporation estimates that programs of this type "generate a return to society ranging from $1.80 to $17.07 for each dollar spent" (2005, p. 1). Rand also noted that "stronger impacts" occurred when a nurse provided home visits "as opposed to a paraprofessional or lay professional home visitor" (2005, p. 2). So, community/PHNs really *do* make a difference!

The nurse–family partnership model was based on theory and research. Numerous other studies of public nursing practice have been done, across different locales and with different populations. For instance, David Olds and his colleagues (Kitzman et al., 2000) examined the enduring effects of a nurse home visitation program on a different population—a group of primarily Black urban women—and found that 3 years after visits ended, when compared with the women in the control group, the participants had:

◆ Fewer subsequent pregnancies
◆ Longer intervals between the births of their first and second children
◆ Fewer closely spaced subsequent pregnancies
◆ Fewer months of using welfare and food stamps

Women in the home visitation program had an average of only seven visits during their pregnancies and approximately one visit per month during the first 2 years of their children's lives—a relatively small investment of time and resources with potentially priceless returns.

In a follow-up study, the effects of this nurse visitation program were found to continue 4 years after the program ended (Olds et al., 2004). Mothers had fewer subsequent pregnancies and births, longer intervals between the births of first and second children, longer relationships with current partners, and fewer months of using food stamps and welfare. In addition, the children who were visited by community health nurses had fewer behavior problems and higher math achievement test scores, and they demonstrated less incoherence and aggression.

Child maltreatment and the early onset of problem behaviors were outcomes also examined by Olds, Eckenrode, and colleagues (1997). They reexamined the group of low-income unmarried women and their first-born children as the children were turning 15 years old; these researchers concluded that a 2-year program of nurse home visitation had moderated the risk of child maltreatment.

Do community health nurses really make the difference, or can other health care workers also get results? Olds and colleagues (2004) have examined differences between nurse and paraprofessional visitation in a large study of mostly Mexican American low-income first-time mothers. Initially, no statistical differences were noted between control and paraprofessional subjects. Two years after the end of the program, participants visited by paraprofessionals had fewer low-birth-weight babies and had better results than control subjects on measures of mastery and mental health, and home environments conducive to early learning—these benefits were only noticeable 2 years after the visits ended. However, mothers visited by nurses showed immediate as well as long-term benefits. They had longer intervals between first and second births, less domestic violence, and home environments conducive to early learning. Children of those mothers had better behavioral adaptation during testing, more advanced language scores, and better executive functioning. Olds and his fellow researchers are convinced that public/community health nurses are the key to success.

Other researchers have noted benefits of community health nurse visitation in nurse–family partnerships in California for Hispanic adolescent mothers and babies (Nguyen, Carson, Parris, & Place, 2003). Even using different protocols than the tightly controlled Olds' model, intense PHN visitation for Latina and African American adolescent mothers and infants was found to be more effective than traditional PHN care (Koniak-Griffin et al., 2003).

This evidence about the effectiveness of public health nursing visits can be gleaned only through conducting formal nursing research. **Research** is the systematic collection and analysis of data related to a particular problem or phenomenon. Research that is properly conducted and analyzed has the potential to yield valuable information that can affect the health of large groups of people. Indeed, it should guide our practice of community health nursing, and it often serves as the basis for changes in health care policies and programs. In the current national atmosphere of managed care and obstinately rising health care costs, the importance of valid research on how health care dollars can be spent to benefit the greatest number of people is vitally important.

❂ EVIDENCE-BASED PRACTICE

Dr. Archie Cochrane, a British epidemiologist, is widely regarded as the force behind evidence-based clinical practice in medicine (The Cochrane Collaboration, 2008). We certainly have ample evidence of the need for a shift to **evidence-based practice** (EBP) in health care: the Institute of Medicine has been studying the issues of health care quality and effectiveness over the past decade and has called for widespread and systematic changes through their reports—*To Err Is Human: Building a Safer Health System* (2000), *Crossing the Quality Chasm: A New Health System for the 21st Century* (2001), and *Priority Areas for National Action: Transforming Health Care Quality* (2003). These reports draw attention to the fact that we spend "billions in research to find appropriate treatments," and more than a trillion dollars are spent annually on health care, but "we repeatedly fail to translate that knowledge and capacity into clinical practice" (2003, p. 2). In response, the federal Agency for Healthcare Research and Quality (AHRQ) has established EBP centers across the United States and Canada. Schools of nursing, such as Arizona State University, University of Texas Health Science Center at San Antonio, Case Western Reserve, and the University of Rochester, also have established centers for EBP.

According to Melnyk and Fineout-Overholt (2005), EBP in nursing means just that—using evidence (or research findings), along with clinical judgment and patients' wishes, in making decisions about how to care for patients. Clinical reasoning is an important component. Higgs, Burn, and Jones (2001) reiterate that the practice knowledge of expert clinical nurses is vital to the process. For Porter-O'Grady (2006), EBP is the "integration of the best possible research" evidence with clinical knowledge and expertise, along with patient preferences and needs (p. 1). Thinking critically about practice problems is an important component of EBP. Reflecting on why we do things a particular way, and critically thinking through a problem in a purposeful, systematic way are vital steps in the process. For instance,

Porter O'Grady (2006) finds commonalities between EBP and critical thinking:

- ◆ Exploring a problem
- ◆ Addressing a purpose or goal
- ◆ Making assumptions about the problem derived from an assessment of the problem and its elements
- ◆ Clarifying the problem around central concepts or indicators
- ◆ Accessing data, evidence, information, and sources to better explain the problem
- ◆ Interpreting accumulated evidence about the specific situation or problem
- ◆ Using reasoning, processing, defining, planning, and documenting to guide subsequent actions in addressing the issue
- ◆ Acting on the problem, consistent with protocols and parameters, and "assessing process, impact, and effect" (p. 6)
- ◆ Evaluating, adjusting, generalizing, and applying to a broader problem set (indicative of a successful problem-solving process)

The effective practitioner utilizes his clinical judgment and expertise to reflect on the practice of community health nursing and determine if safe, effective, quality, and cost-efficient care is being delivered. Problems or situations that need clarification can then be identified, and current research can be reviewed to guide needed changes in practice. Although acknowledged barriers exist, they can be overcome utilizing available resources (Ciliska, Pinelli, DiCenso, & Cullum, 2001; Morris, Scott-Findlay, & Estabrooks, 2001). Melnyk and Fineout-Overholt (2005) stress the importance of systematically searching for all relevant research on a clinical question of interest and critically analyzing the evidence (Fig. 4.1). They argue that this is not merely research utilization, in which new interventions may be tried based on the results of one or two good studies, but "systematic reviews of randomized clinical trials (RCTs)" and critical reviews of both quantitative and qualitative studies pertinent to a particular question of interest (p. 7). While doing this, the nurse must keep in mind the unique needs and wants of the clients served, as well as current practice standards, guidelines, and ethical considerations. Sanares and Heliker (2006, p. 33) note that "nationally recognized clinical

---

Five Steps of Evidence-based Practice
1. Ask the burning clinical question.
2. Collect the most relevant and best evidence.
3. Critically appraise the evidence.
4. Integrate all evidence with one's clinical expertise, patient preferences, and values in making a practice decision or change.
5. Evaluate the practice decision or change.

FIGURE 4.1 Five steps of evidence-based practice. From Melnyk, B., & Fineout-Overholt, E. (2005). *Evidence-based practice in nursing and healthcare*, p. 9, with permission.

practice guidelines" should be reviewed (e.g., National Guideline Clearinghouse at www.guideline.gov), and expert clinicians could be interviewed for their opinions on the problem at hand. In fact, Thompson and colleagues (2004) note that nurses rely on colleagues as "experiential sources of information"; well-seasoned nurses and clinical nurse specialists can be "the most useful (and accessible) information sources" (p. 7).

Although expert nurses are a good starting point in collecting evidence, clinically relevant research that is both medically sound and patient-centered must be reviewed. Good places to begin are **integrative** or **systematic reviews** that compile all recent studies and summarize what is known about the problem or situation. The Cochrane Collaboration (www.cochrane.org) lists systematic reviews on various topics of interest to both physicians and nurses. For instance, a community health nurse working with a group of adults who have diabetes might be interested in the systematic review on the importance of exercise for type 2 diabetes clients. This review is based on 14 RCTs that compared the use of exercise in a group of 377 participants over periods of between 8 weeks to 12 months. When compared with those who got no exercise intervention, the results indicated decreased body fat and triglyceride levels and improved blood sugar control for those exercising (even for those who did not lose any weight). Although a community health nurse may certainly have a "hunch" that exercise is good for his or her clients, this systematic review of current studies provides solid evidence on which to base recommendations (Thomas, Elliott, & Naughton, 2006). A review on promoting adherence to antiretroviral therapy for human immunodeficiency virus (HIV)/acquired immune deficiency syndrome (AIDS) clients might be helpful to a PHN supervisor in designing an AIDS case management program utilizing community health nurses. Over 2,159 participants in 19 RCTs were part of this review, which found that interventions such as "practical medication management skills . . . administered to individuals vs. groups and . . . delivered over 12 weeks or more" had improved medication adherence (Rueda et al., 2006, ¶ 6). From this evidence, a community health nurse case manager can conclude that medication compliance can be effectively assured through development of a nurse–client relationship based on the nurse's consistent availability to the client—through home visits or individual appointments at clinics—and a focus on teaching medication management skills.

The AHRQ EBP centers also provide evidence reports that are easily accessible online (www.ahrq.gov-clinic/epcindex.htm). These can be searched by topical index, clinical area, or health care services (e.g., bioterrorism) and technical areas (e.g., community-based participatory research). Other sources for systematic or integrative reviews include:

- *Worldviews on Evidence-Based Nursing* from Sigma Theta Tau International (www.nursingsociety.org)
- *Evidence-Based Nursing*, a British online journal (www.ebn.bmjjournals.com)
- RAND Corporation research briefs (www.rand.org)

ASKING THE QUESTION

Melnyk and others suggest that the first step to solving the problem is "asking the burning clinical question" (2005, p. 8). This question may be about client care or effective interventions, such as:

- What methods are most effective in assuring client medication compliance with antiretroviral therapy for HIV/AIDS?
- What is the best information I can give new mothers about preventing sudden infant death syndrome (SIDS)?

It could also be about systems approaches to population health:

- What is the most effective method of immunizing toddlers?
- How can PHNs better collaborate with families, physicians, and hospitals in preventing complications of high levels of bilirubin in newborns coming home within 24 to 48 hours after birth?

There are some specific methods of phrasing or structuring questions (Fig. 4.2). The Association of Women's Health, Obstetric, and Neonatal Nurses (AWHONN) asked a "burning clinical question" when they wanted to find a scientific basis for the development of standards of practice for their members regarding counseling pregnant women on smoking cessation. The project, *Setting Universal Cessation Counseling, Education, and Screening Standards* (SUCCESS), was an attempt to integrate best practices in primary care settings where women of childbearing age receive care. They did extensive searches in the Cumulative Index on Nursing and Allied Health Literature (CINAHL) and MEDLINE for research studies relating to low-birth-weight infants, effects of prenatal smoking on infants, and effects of smoking cessation intervention on premature labor and birth weight with both pregnant women and those seeking care prior to conception (Albrecht, Maloni, Thomas, Jones, Halleran, & Osborne, 2004). They critically analyzed 98 articles, and found evidence of a higher incidence of many complications, including preterm labor, premature rupture of membranes, lower birth weight and length, spontaneous abortion, and placenta previa or abruption in women using tobacco. Infants and children exposed to secondhand smoke had a higher risk for ear infections, asthma and other respiratory problems, SIDS, and learning disorders. Significant evidence suggested that this was a problem that needed to be addressed. They also concluded "office-based assessment, client-specific tobacco counseling, skill development, and support programs serve as an effective practice guideline" for their members, so they developed protocols and began piloting them in 13 states (p. 298). They are currently continuing to collect evaluation research to determine the effectiveness of the protocols.

Critical analysis of the literature is a necessary step in EBP. Systematic reviews should be carefully examined to determine validity by asking these questions (University of Alberta Medical School, 2006):

- Did the review concentrate on a "focused clinical question" (¶ 1)?
- Were there appropriate inclusion criteria for articles?

PICO		
Patient population/disease	The patient population or disease of interest, for example: • Age • Gender • Ethnicity • With certain disorder (e.g., hepatitis)	(e.g., adolescent females ages 12–20)
Intervention	The intervention or range of interventions of interest, for example: • Exposure to disease • Prognostic factor A • Risk behavior (e.g., smoking)	(e.g., sexuality education program)
Comparison	What you want to compare the intervention against, for example: • No disease • Placebo or no intervention/therapy • Prognostic factor B • Absence of risk factor (e.g., nonsmoking)	(e.g., no intervention)
Outcome	Outcome of interest, for example: • Risk of disease • Accuracy of diagnosis • Rate of occurrence of adverse outcome (e.g., death)	(e.g., fewer unplanned pregnancies)

FIGURE 4.2 PICO: Components of an answerable, searchable question. Adapted from Melnyk, B., & Fineout-Overholt, E. (2005). *Evidence-based practice in nursing and healthcare*, p. 30.

◆ Were any important, relevant studies overlooked?
◆ Was the validity of all included studies taken into consideration?
◆ Were there similar results found in all studies?
◆ How reliable are the results?
  • Were sample sizes large enough?
  • Were results statistically significant?
  • Were there confounding factors (outside influences that make you doubt the results)?

Next, it is important to decide if incorporating this information into your practice will be helpful by asking:

◆ How can I apply these results to my community health nursing practice?
  • Will it benefit my clients?
  • Are my clients similar to the population studied?
  • Do I have the necessary resources?

To effectively practice evidence-based research, community health nurses must know how to correctly compose a clinical question, find an appropriate database to search for systematic reviews, critically review the evidence, consult practice guidelines and expert practitioners, and work with their clients to develop an appropriate plan of action. A clear understanding of basic research principles is needed to systematically review and incorporate research into community health nursing practice.

QUANTITATIVE AND QUALITATIVE RESEARCH

Scientific inquiry through research is generally pursued by means of two different approaches: quantitative research and qualitative research. **Quantitative research** concerns data that can be quantified or measured objectively. This could be as simple as counting the number of children receiving vaccination for varicella in immunization clinics during the past month and noting the number of reported cases of postvaccination complications. Another example of a rather simple quantitative study uses telephone survey methods to determine older rural adults' use of complementary health care (e.g., acupuncture, herbal remedies). Shreffler-Grant and colleagues (2005) picked a random sample of 325 older adults from rural communities in two states and found that, whereas only 17.5% had used complementary providers, over 45% had used some form of complementary health care—many of them finding out about these methods by word-of-mouth. They noted that this figure was similar to findings in larger national studies. This has implications for nurses working with rural older adults, who may think that this population doesn't have access to alternative forms of health care, thus risking the potential for possible drug interactions or side effects of these treatments in their clients.

Another study by Valente (2005) examined staff nurses' perceptions of improved knowledge with the use of research-based fact sheets. Concise, well-researched fact sheets on common topics (e.g., hypertension, heart failure, pressure ulcers, depression) were developed at a Veterans Administration hospital in an effort to improve nursing care. Over 93% of nurses felt that the use of the fact sheets improved their knowledge level. This led to other questions, such as the perceived quality of the fact sheets and the perceived areas needing improvement. The majority of nurses rated them as "excellent" and noted that they used them to improve patient "education, assessment, intervention, and follow-up care" (p. 171).

More variables can be added to quantitative studies. An example is a study by Remington (2002) that was also reported in an integrative review on the use of preferred music to decrease agitated behavior in elderly clients with dementia (Sung & Chang, 2005). The review concluded that music has "positive effects on decreasing agitated behaviours in older people with dementia" (p. 1,133), but the Remington study employed 10-minute periods of either calming music, hand massage, combined music and massage, or no treatment (control) to determine whether all of the three treatment groups had demonstrated benefits. By adding the variable of hand massage, another effective method of calming agitated clients with dementia was discovered—one that may be more appropriate for hearing-impaired elders.

Quantitative research is helpful in identifying a problem or a relationship between two or more variables, such as type of treatment (e.g., calming music) and an outcome (agitated behaviors in nursing home residents with dementia). In so doing, quantitative studies tend to examine isolated parts of problems or phenomena and do not generally pay attention to the larger context or overall health of individuals. Quantitative research involves a reductionistic tendency (focusing on the parts rather than the whole) and, if used exclusively, can limit nursing knowledge, because many of the important aspects of client services (e.g., quality of life, grieving, spirituality) cannot be measured objectively.

A more subjective or qualitative approach is needed to study those areas that need a broader focus or that do not lend themselves to objective measurement. **Qualitative research** emphasizes subjectivity and the meaning of experiences to individuals. An example of this type of research is a study examining the experiences of individuals who were quarantined because of severe acute respiratory syndrome (SARS) in Toronto (Cava, Fay, Beanlands, McCay, & Wignall, 2005). Quantitative research can tell us the number of people who were quarantined, but qualitative research is needed to understand the feelings and experiences of those affected. Interviews conducted with a sample of quarantined adults revealed that a variety of responses to the initial quarantine order ranged from "acceptance to fear, shock, disbelief, and anger" (p. 401). While in quarantine, many felt isolated and noted a sense of rejection, stigmatization, and scrutiny. A universal response of "relief" was noted when quarantine ended, and suggestions were made to prompt public health officials to improve communication in future episodes. "Timely and trustworthy information about SARS and quarantine" were recommended to decrease levels of confusion and frustration (p. 403).

It is not uncommon to find research studies in which both quantitative and qualitative approaches are used. A study examining the experiences of Hurricane Katrina evacuees in Houston shelters combined both survey and interview techniques to gather information about the demographics of the evacuees, their experiences during evacuation and emergency response to the storm, and their current well-being and future plans (Brodie, Weltzein, Blendon, & Benson, 2005). The results of the study indicated that those hardest hit by the storm were poor, working, uninsured, long-term residents of New Orleans, mostly African American, and reliant on safety-net providers for medical care. They were unlikely to have their own car or funds to pay for transportation, and were unlikely to have sources of alternative shelter once evacuated. Implications for policy makers, disaster planners, and health care providers were noted in an attempt to learn from past mistakes and deficiencies.

Another method of analyzing research in community health uses a statistical procedure known as **meta-analysis** to evaluate the results of many similar quantitative research studies in an attempt to integrate the findings and combine the sample sizes of many small studies to obtain a "single-effect measure" (Melnyk & Fineout-Overholt, 2005, p. 115). By combining the results of many similar studies, meta-analysis affords greater statistical power and can give the researcher a more complete general perspective, especially when research on a certain issue may seem inconclusive. An example of this type of research is highlighted in *Nursing Research* by Wewers, Sarna, and Rice (2006). In addition to discussing barriers to nursing research related to tobacco cessation and future directions to be taken, the authors cited a meta-analysis done by Rice and Stead (2004), in which 29 RCTs examining the effectiveness of nurses as cessation interventionists were analyzed. Both low- and high-intensity interventions were included (i.e., advice given at a single visit lasting less than about 10 minutes and a longer initial visit with follow-up visits that included additional strategies or materials). Through complex statistical measurements, the authors found that "nurse-delivered interventions were more effective than usual care in achieving abstinence at 6 months or longer" (p. 513). The statistical effect was found consistently in both high- and low-intensity nurse interventions. The moral of this meta-analysis is that even short discussions with your clients about smoking cessation, along with information on accessing support groups or other resources, may prove beneficial.

STEPS IN THE RESEARCH PROCESS

All effective research follows a series of predetermined, highly specific steps. Each step builds on the previous one and provides the foundation for the eventual discussion of findings. It is important to understand basic research principles in order to effectively implement EBP. Alone or in collaboration with others, community health nurses use the following nine steps to complete a research project:

1. Identify an area of interest.
2. Formulate a research question or statement.
3. Review the literature.
4. Select a conceptual model.
5. Choose a research design.
6. Obtain Institutional Review Board or Human Subjects Committee approval.

7. Collect and analyze data.
8. Interpret results.
9. Communicate findings.

Clear research questions, thorough review of the literature, human subjects protection, and a sound research design are factors to consider when evaluating the results of studies for incorporation into your practice.

Identify an Area of Interest

Identifying the problem or area of interest is frequently one of the most difficult tasks in the research process. The problem needs *specificity* (i.e., it must be specific enough to direct the formulation of a research question). For example, concern about child safety is too broad a problem; instead, the focus could be on a narrower subject, such as the use of child restraints and car seat availability and use in a particular community.

The problem must also be *feasible*. Feasibility concerns whether the area of interest can be examined, given available resources. For example, a statewide study of the needs of pregnant adolescents might not be practical if time or funding is limited, but a study of the same group in a given school district could be more easily accomplished.

The *meaning* of the project and its *relevance* to nursing must also be considered, such as exploring the implications for nursing practice in the study of pregnant adolescents. Areas for study often evolve from personal interests, clinical experience, or philosophical beliefs. The nurse's specialty influences the selection of a problem for study and also the particular perspective or approaches used. The community health nurse functions within a context that emphasizes disease prevention, wellness, and the active involvement of clients in the services they receive. Clients' physical and social environments, as well as their biopsychosocial and spiritual domains, are of major concern. Community health nurses think in terms of the broader community; their research efforts are developed with the needs of the community or specific populations in mind.

Problems recently identified and studied within community health nursing include:

◆ Cardiovascular health promotion in aging women: validating a population health approach (Sawatzky & Naimark, 2005)
◆ Childhood immunization refusal: provider and parent perceptions (Fredrickson, Davis, Arnould, Kennen, Hurniston, Cross, & Bocchini, 2004)
◆ Process evaluation of a nurse-delivered smoking relapse prevention program for new mothers (Groner, French, Ahijevych, & Wewers, 2005)
◆ The impact of just-in-time e-mail "reminders" on patient outcomes in home health care (Feldman, Murtaugh, Pezzin, McDonald, & Peng, 2005)
◆ Mothers' ranking of clinical intervention strategies used to promote infant health (Gaffney & Altieri, 2001)
◆ Racial differences in parenting dimensions and adolescent condom use at sexual debut (Cox, 2006)
◆ The volunteer potential of inactive nurses for disaster preparedness (Fothergill, Palumbo, Rambur, Reinier, & McIntosh, 2005)

◆ Public health nursing practice change and recommendations for improvement (Zahner & Gredig, 2005)

Each of these problem areas provides direction for the formulation of related research questions.

Formulate a Research Question or Statement

The research question or statement reflects the kind of information desired and provides a foundation for the remainder of the project. The manner in which the question or statement is phrased suggests the research design for the project. For example, the question "What are nurses' attitudes toward pregnant women who use methamphetamine?" determines that the design will be simple, nonexperimental, and exploratory (see later discussion). In contrast, the question "What is the effect of an educational program on nurses' attitudes toward drug-abusing pregnant women?" suggests an experiment that will evaluate changes in nurses' attitudes toward pregnant women who abuse drugs after receiving an educational intervention. The first research question suggests a broad, open-ended conversation with nurse participants, asking them to discuss their attitudes toward pregnant women who abuse drugs, such as methamphetamine. From the data obtained, general themes and patterns will emerge, leading the researcher to some overall conclusions. The second question examines the effects that an educational program may have on nurses' attitudes about pregnant women who abuse crack cocaine, for instance. This is most likely a quantitative, evaluative study that may involve pretesting to determine the nurses' attitudes, conducting one or more classes, and then posttesting to determine whether any change occurred in attitude or beliefs.

Well-formulated research questions identify the population of interest, the variable or variables to be measured, and the interventions (if any). It is very important when formulating research questions that specific terms be used to clearly represent the variables being studied. For example, if "stress" is identified as the variable measured in the research question, then it is important to note how stress is being defined. The researcher who wants to measure stress experienced by clients waiting for HIV test results must be careful not to measure other related variables, such as trait anxiety (a general personality trait) or depression. Consistency of terms used is crucial to the success of a project, so investigators must formulate the research question carefully. One must be clear about the variable and what is being measured to ensure validity of the results.

Formulation of a PICO question (*p*atient problem, *i*ntervention, *c*omparison, *o*utcome), related to EBP, is a similar process, especially in its specificity. Good examples of research questions addressed recently by community health nurses include:

◆ Are there differences in how rural and urban families [*population of interest*] view death and end-of-life care [*variables*] for their elderly family members with dementia residing in nursing homes (Gessert, Elliott, & McAlpine, 2006)?
◆ What is the effect of rural residence [*variable*] on unmet dental care [*variable*] for children with special

health care needs [*population of interest*] (Skinner, Slifkin, & Mayer, 2006)?

♦ What is the lived experience [*variable*] of adults being diagnosed with Lyme disease [*population of interest*] (Drew & Hewitt, 2006)?

♦ Are parents of low-income Ohio toddlers [*population of interest*] receiving information on lead poisoning prevention [*variable*], and how would they prefer to receive this information [*variable*] (Polivka, 2006)?

♦ Can father's clubs [*intervention variable*] improve the health of rural Haitian children [*population of interest*] (Sloand & Gebrian, 2006)?

Review the Literature

A review of the literature consists of two phases. The first phase consists of a cursory examination of available publications related to the area of interest. Although several nursing research journals publish studies reflecting all areas of nursing practice, most specialty areas have dedicated journals. *Public Health Nursing, Family and Community Health, Journal of Community Health Nursing, American Journal of Public Health, Journal of School Health, Nursing and Health Sciences*, and *Journal of School Nursing* are some of the journals that publish studies of particular interest to community health nurses. In this phase, the investigator develops knowledge about the area of interest that is somewhat superficial but sufficient to make a decision about the value of pursuing a given topic. If considerable research has already been conducted in the area, the investigator may decide to ask a different question or to pursue another area of interest.

The second phase of the literature review involves an in-depth, critically evaluated search of all publications relevant to the topic of interest. The goal of this phase is to narrow the focus and increase depth of knowledge. Journal articles describing research conducted on the topic of interest provide the most important kind of information, followed by clinical opinion articles (information on the topic described by experts in the field) and books. Journal articles provide more up-to-date information than do books, and systematic investigations provide a foundation for other studies. Prior research that has already been done on the topic of interest provides a solid foundation for later replication studies.

Criteria for compiling a good review of the literature include (a) using articles that closely relate to the topic of interest (relevancy); (b) using current articles that provide up-to-date and recent information—usually within the past 5 years (although earlier articles may be included based on their importance to the area of interest); and (c) using both primary and secondary sources. A *primary source* is a publication that appears in its original form. A *secondary source* is an article in which one author writes about another author's work; reviews fall into this category. Primary sources historically were preferred over secondary sources because they afford the investigator a more accurate and first-hand account of the study from which personal conclusions can be drawn. Secondary sources, however, are now seen as more helpful in guiding practice decisions, as integrative reviews of current research are a critical element of EBP.

A major component of a review of literature is the investigator's critical evaluation of the information collected. The conceptual base and research methods of studies must be critically assessed regarding the appropriateness of the methods used and the conclusions drawn, as well as how carefully the research was conducted.

After a careful, critical, and comprehensive review of the literature, the investigator writes a clear description of the information related to the area of interest, including conflicting findings and referencing each study or article. This review provides the basis for the proposed study or the clinical decision to be made. The conclusions from the literature review become the basis for the new study's assumptions and methodology. Rather than making a "leap of knowledge," the hypothesis or research question must be created by basing assumptions on previous research studies.

Select a Conceptual Model

In relation to research, a **conceptual model** is a framework of ideas for explaining and studying a phenomenon of interest. A conceptual model conveys a particular perception of the world; it organizes the researcher's thinking and provides structure and direction for research activities. Models are like a framework on which to "hang" concepts or variables, and they should be used to guide the design and methods for collecting research data.

All fields of study identify their major areas of concerns or boundaries. Nursing, since the early work of Florence Nightingale, is concerned with the interaction between humans and the environment in relation to health (Blais, Hayes, Kozier, & Erb, 2006). Widely used classic nursing conceptual models such as Orem's (1985) self-care model or King's (1989) open systems model reflect the boundaries and major concerns of nursing as a profession. Although nurse investigators frequently and successfully use conceptual models developed within other fields, the advantage of using nursing models is that they provide an understanding of the world in terms of nursing's major concerns (see Chapter 14).

The investigator can become familiar with various conceptual models by reviewing the literature in the area of interest and by reading any of the many texts available on conceptual models. A thorough understanding of the major concepts of a potential model and their relationships is necessary before one attempts to use a model as a framework for a study.

Choose a Research Design

The design of a research project represents the overall plan for carrying out the study. This overall plan guides the conduct of the study and, depending on its effectiveness, can influence investigators' confidence in their results. A major consideration in selecting a particular design is to try to control as much as possible those factors that are not included in the study but can influence the results. For example, in a classic study by Douglas and co-workers (1999), researchers wanted to discover the percentage of homes with functioning smoke alarms. They initially conducted a telephone survey, a commonly used method of survey research in community health, and found that 71% of households reported functioning smoke alarms. Concerned that this might be an inflated number, they conducted an on-site survey to confirm the results.

After face-to-face interviews, they found that only 66% of householders reported having functioning alarms. However, when researchers actually tested the smoke alarms in those homes, only 49% were fully functioning. By having researchers actually test the smoke alarms, this design controlled for inflated results of the more commonly conducted, convenient, and economical telephone survey. Is self-report always unreliable? A small study of working middle-aged women revealed that self-reported weekly physical activity was strongly associated with pedometer data, indicating that, in this case, self-report yielded reasonably reliable data (Speck & Looney, 2006). This is evidence that the community health nurse must determine the most efficacious method of obtaining necessary data.

In another example, researchers themselves controlled the variables to ensure true results. Kerr and colleagues (2001) knew from their review of the literature that posters encouraging exercise at the point of choice between stairs and escalators in public shopping areas could be effective in promoting greater use of stairs. They incorporated this fact into the design of their study. They used a control site and a study site (both shopping malls) and collected baseline data and a first observation 2 weeks after placing posters. Then, they followed up with stair-riser banners containing multiple messages placed on alternate stairs. Both sites were equal at baseline and the first observation; however, at the second observation time (at 4 weeks), there was a 6.7% increase in use of the stairs at the site with stair-riser banners. This simple yet novel approach motivated more people to use the stairs.

Complete descriptions of various research designs and specific methodologies are available in basic nursing research texts. For the purposes of this chapter, a few important considerations underlying design selection are described. First, quantitative approaches use two major categories of research design: experimental and nonexperimental (or descriptive).

Experimental design requires that the investigators institute an intervention and then measure its consequences. Investigators hypothesize that a change will occur as a result of their intervention, and then they attempt to test whether their hypothesis was accurate. Experimental design requires investigators to randomly assign subjects to an **experimental group** (those receiving the intervention) and a **control group** (those not receiving the intervention). This process, called **randomization**, is the systematic selection of research subjects, so that each one has an equal probability of selection.

Another important distinction made within the experimental category of research is between true experiments and quasi-experiments. **True experiments** are characterized by instituting an intervention or change, assigning subjects to groups in a specific manner (randomization), and comparing the group of subjects who experience the manipulation to the control group (those not receiving the intervention). **Randomized control trials (RCTs)** are generally considered the gold standard of experimental research—they are commonly used to determine the safety and efficacy of new medications or to test the effectiveness of one intervention over another, and they are a foundation of EBP (Melnyk & Fineout-Overholt, 2005). **Quasi-experiments** lack one of these elements, such as the randomization of subjects. Community health nurses conduct quasi-experiments more often than true experiments because it is often difficult (and some-

times impossible) to use randomization. For instance, a nurse may conduct a nutrition education intervention with fifth grade students at a particular school. Although the nurse can have one classroom participate in the intervention and another remain the control group, he or she cannot randomly assign the children to classrooms (i.e., intervention or control). Therefore, this research would be characterized as quasi-experimental in nature.

Nonexperimental designs (also called *descriptive designs*) are used in research to describe and explain phenomena or examine relationships among phenomena. Examples of this approach include examining the relationship between gender and smoking behaviors among adolescents, describing the emotional needs of families of clients with Alzheimer disease, and determining the attitudes of parents in a given community toward sex education in the schools. In each of these instances, the focus of the research is on the relationships observed or the description of what exists. Such nonexperimental designs are often the precursors of experiments. Once such an intervention is developed, further research can evaluate its appropriateness and, ultimately, its effectiveness. Other lines of clinically based research can also be designed. The choice of research design influences the ability to generalize the results, and the attention given to the details of the study affects the value of the knowledge derived. Research done with larger numbers of participants drawn from a geographically diverse area is more complete than small scale, exploratory studies done in an isolated area with a small, homogeneous sample. Valid tools or instruments and appropriately applied statistical methods lead to greater confidence in the results of the study.

Obtain Institutional Review Board or Human Subjects Committee Approval

Whenever research is to be conducted that involves human subjects, prior approval must be gained from either an Institutional Review Board or a Human Subjects Committee. The reason for this approval is to safeguard the rights of prospective study participants. Each health department should have a committee or a gatekeeper, such as the health officer, who understands the federal guidelines for protecting subjects involved in research studies.

One of the most egregious examples of exploitation of human subjects was a study carried out by the U. S. Public Health Service. The Tuskegee study, begun in 1932 and ended in 1972, sought to learn more about syphilis and to justify treatment services for Blacks in Alabama (Centers for Disease Control and Prevention [CDC], 2008). The 399 men with syphilis who participated in the study had agreed to be examined and treated. However, they were misled about the exact purpose of the study and were not given all of the facts; therefore, they were unable to give truly informed consent. Even after penicillin became the drug of choice for treatment of syphilis in 1947, the researchers failed to offer this treatment to the infected participants. Because of this experiment and earlier Nazi atrocities, the Nuremberg Code and the Declaration of Helsinki were adopted by the world scientific community, then revised in 1975, as a means of assuring ethical research practices (Blais, Hayes, Kozier, & Erb, 2006; CDC, 2003) (see Evidence-Based Practice: Ethics in Action).

EVIDENCE-BASED PRACTICE

Ethics in Action

Today, safeguards are in place to ensure that studies are stopped when either potential harm or insufficient benefit are noted. In January 2006, a major international study of a drug-conserving protocol for AIDS medication was stopped because those who were in the on-again, off-again group got sicker than those taking continuous medication therapy (Associated Press, 2006). More than 5,000 HIV patients in 33 countries participated in this study, which was halted by the National Institutes of Health. This large-scale study was initiated after several smaller studies had suggested a possible benefit from the on-and-off medication strategy. It was hoped that this strategy of only taking medications when immune cell levels dropped would not only cut costs, it would decrease medication side effects for patients. What researchers found was that this episodic strategy actually increased side effects related to the heart, liver, and kidney. Researchers say that the results are difficult to explain, but because of patient safety, it was best to stop the clinical trial. What ethical principles are involved here? Is there an ethical dilemma here? Consider the rights of a few versus the rights of many. Apply Iserson's (1999) three tests (see p. 80 of this text).

The following ethical principles are widely viewed as basic protections for research participants (U.S. Department of Health & Human Services, 2006a). Freedom from harm or exploitation encompasses several aspects. First, no research can be done that may inflict permanent or serious harm. Second, the research study must be stopped if it becomes evident that harm may come to participants. Debriefing, or allowing participants to ask questions of the researcher at the conclusion of the study, as a means of protecting them from any unseen psychological harm, is also a component. There should be some identified benefits from participation in the research study, and any costs or risks should be clearly enumerated, so that participants can more easily determine the cost–benefit ratio (referred to as *full disclosure*). Subjects should also be told that they may withdraw from the study at any time without prejudice or penalty (known as *self-determination*). Consent forms should include full disclosure of the nature of the study, the time and commitment required of subjects, the researcher's contact information, and a pledge of confidentiality (assurance of privacy).

Vulnerable subjects, determined by federal guidelines, include children, mentally or emotionally disabled people, physically disabled people, institutionalized people, pregnant women, and the terminally ill. Special care must be taken to ensure protection of vulnerable subjects. Once approval has been obtained from the proper entities, data collection can begin (U.S. Department of Health & Human Services, 2006b).

Collect and Analyze Data

The value of the data collected in any research project depends largely on the care taken when measuring the concepts of concern or variables. The specific tool used to measure the variables in a study, often a questionnaire or interview guide, is called an **instrument**. The accuracy of the instrument used and the appropriateness of the choice of instruments can clearly influence the results. For instance, Spielberger's State-Trait Anxiety Inventory is a well-researched questionnaire used in studying anxiety levels in adults. It has been shown to accurately measure state anxiety and the more stable tendency toward anxious personality—*trait anxiety*. One could infer that more accurate measurements of anxiety could be found using this instrument than a researcher-developed questionnaire that has never been tested for validity and reliability.

Validity and Reliability

Two tests are used to evaluate instrument accuracy: validity and reliability. **Validity** is the assurance that an instrument measures the variables it is supposed to measure. If a written questionnaire is being used in the study, the questions included would be evaluated to make certain that they are appropriate to the subject (content validity) and that the variable of interest is actually being measured (construct validity).

Reliability refers to how consistently an instrument measures a given research variable within a particular population. Test–retest reliability ensures that similar results are obtained using the same instrument with the same population at two separate testing times. If similar results are obtained on two separate occasions, the test can be considered reliable.

Statistical tests and measurements are often used to analyze subjects' responses to questionnaires to evaluate internal consistency. A questionnaire is internally consistent to the extent that all of its subparts measure the same characteristic. Cronbach's alpha (α) is often cited as a measure of internal consistency and is reported as a correlation coefficient, so that the closer the value is to $+1.0$, the greater the degree of internal consistency. Results higher than .7 are generally regarded as desirable.

Within the area of community health nursing research, instruments appropriate to the measurement of nursing concepts (e.g., caring) are often not available. Researchers may use questionnaires that have been designed and tested by other investigators, or they may begin the tedious task of developing their own. Both approaches to measuring the variables of interest are acceptable; however, using available instruments of known reliability and validity saves considerable time.

Methods of Collecting Data

A variety of methods can be used to collect data, including self-report (subjects report their own experience verbally or in written form), observation (investigators observe subjects and document their observations), physiologic assessment (investigators use measures of physical evidence, such as blood pressure or impaired mobility), and document analysis (investigators review and analyze written materials, such as health records). For example, using these four methods, investigators examining the stress level of the caregiver when a family member chooses to die at home might do the following:

1. Design or use an existing written questionnaire or interview schedule (self-report).
2. Outline a schema, such as a list of potential stress-induced behaviors, for observing caregivers as they function in the home (observation).
3. Measure various physiologic indicators of stress, such as hypertension, insomnia, or poor diet (physiologic assessment).
4. Ask caregivers to keep a diary of their activities and feelings for 2 weeks, and analyze the diaries for evidence of stress (document analysis).

In most instances, the nature of the data to be collected dictates the best method of collection. One or more methods may be appropriate, given the topic of concern. In the example mentioned, a combination of the first three methods would probably be appropriate, or the diary could be substituted for the questionnaire.

Methods of Analyzing Data

Once collected, data must be analyzed so that a meaningful interpretation can be made. Statistical procedures reduce great amounts of information to smaller chunks that can be easily interpreted. When deciding on an appropriate statistical procedure, it is helpful to consider the two major categories of statistical analysis: descriptive and inferential statistics.

Descriptive statistics portray the data collected in quantitative or mathematical terms. Commonly used descriptive statistical methods include calculating the average number (or *mean*) of a particular set of occurrences and calculating *standard deviations* (how much each score on the average deviates from the mean) and percentages. For example, an investigator analyzing data collected from 50 clients with chronic pain might find their mean pain score to be 4.96 (on a scale from 0 [no pain] to 10 [worst pain]), with a standard deviation of 0.83. These descriptive statistics suggest that clients are grouped around the middle of the pain scale and differ very little in the amount of pain they experience. The investigator may also report that more than 95% of the female clients experience pain rated between 4 and 6 on the 10-point pain scale. These descriptive statistics can be reported graphically (using graphs or charts) or in written form as shown in Table 4.1.

Inferential statistics involve making assumptions about features of a population based on observations of a sample. For example, the Gallup Poll, which surveys a sample of the population to determine what opinion they hold on a particular topic (e.g., favorite presidential candidate), uses inferential statistics to estimate the proportion of the total population that favors a particular candidate (McKenzie & Smeltzer, 2001). The potential for **generalizability**, the ability to apply the research results to other similar populations, has great value to health professionals. It allows researchers to test their hypotheses on smaller groups before instituting widespread changes in methods, programs, and even national health policies.

Inferential statistics are also used to test hypotheses in research; they provide information about the likelihood that an observed difference between two or more groups could have happened just by chance or might be the result of some intervention or manipulation. These statistical procedures provide a determination of the extent to which changes or differences between sets of data are attributable to chance fluctuations and estimate the confidence with which one can make generalizations about the data.

It is appropriate to use both descriptive and inferential statistics to analyze the data from a study. For example, in a study designed to examine the effects of prenatal education on the health status of pregnant women, investigators might use inferential statistics to find a significant difference in health status between the group who experienced the educational program (experimental group) and the group who did not (control group). The investigators might also use descriptive statistics to report the percentage of women from the experimental group who attended all classes and the means and standard deviations for the women's health status scores.

Interpret Results

The explanation of the findings of a study flows from the previously formulated research plan. The findings need to be a logical conclusion, based upon the building blocks of the literature review, conceptual framework, research question, and methodology. You can't jump to a conclusion for which you have not laid a foundation. Findings need to make sense, to be reasonable and logical. When findings support the directions developed in the research plan, their interpretation is relatively straightforward. For example, a group of community health nurse investigators might design a study to determine the effect of parenting classes on the self-esteem of single welfare mothers between 21 and 35 years of age. They could use Coopersmith's (1967) ideas on self-esteem as their conceptual model, hypothesize that self-esteem will improve

TABLE 4.1	Pain Ratings	
Value	Frequency	Percent (%)
3.00	1	2.0
4.00	11	22.0
5.00	30	60.0
6.00	6	12.0
7.00	1	2.0
8.00	1	2.0
MEAN 4.96	STANDARD DEVIATION 0.83	

as a result of the classes, and design an experiment to test their idea. If self-esteem does, in fact, increase, their finding flows logically from their framework.

If the findings do not support the hypothesis of the study, investigators question various aspects of the research to develop an explanation. In this instance, a number of questions could be posed. Coopersmith posited that self-esteem would relate to feelings of success in a given endeavor. Can that position be inaccurate? Could the parenting classes have been ineffective? Perhaps they did not enhance feelings of success. Could the intervention have been too weak to show a statistical difference (not enough sessions)? Were there problems with the methodology used: were there too few subjects, or intervening, confounding factors that affected the results? All of these questions and more should be considered in an attempt to explain the results.

If the study is descriptive in nature (i.e., one that was designed to describe particular characteristics of a population), the direction of the findings is not a concern. A detailed, accurate report of the results and their implications alone is appropriate. Given either an experimental or a descriptive design, the importance of accuracy cannot be overemphasized. Leaps of faith when reporting the results of a study are not appropriate unless labeled as such. For example, one could not conclude from the study on parenting classes that these classes develop expert parenting skills, given that parenting skills were not assessed.

A valuable contribution can be made to the advancement of nursing knowledge when investigators use their results to make suggestions for future research. The investigators' knowledge of a particular area and their experience in conducting a specific study give them an excellent background for identifying future research possibilities.

Communicate Findings

The findings of nursing research projects need to be shared with other nurses, regardless of the studies' outcomes. Negative as well as positive findings can make a valuable contribution to nursing knowledge and influence nursing practice. Whether or not the hypothesis was verified is not the most important part of research; it is equally important to know about results that are inconclusive or not statistically significant, because this information is also necessary to build the science of nursing. For instance, in the study by Eckenrode and colleagues (2000) cited at the beginning of this chapter, researchers found that participants who received nurse home visitation during pregnancy and through the child's second birthday had significantly fewer child maltreatment reports with the mother as perpetrator or the study child as subject than did participants not receiving nurse home visitation. However, for mothers reporting more than 28 incidents of domestic violence, no significant reductions were noted. This is important information, because ongoing domestic violence may limit the effectiveness of these types of programs. In the future, researchers may want to elicit more information about domestic violence when trying to evaluate the effectiveness of this type of intervention.

The research report should include the key elements of the research process. The research problem, methodology used, results of the study, and the investigators' conclusions and recommendations are presented. Whether investigators are presenting their findings verbally or writing for publication, they need to discuss the implications of their findings for nursing practice.

IMPACT OF RESEARCH ON COMMUNITY HEALTH AND NURSING PRACTICE

Research has the potential to have a significant impact on community health nursing in three ways, by affecting public policy and the community's health, the effectiveness of community health nursing practice, and the status and influence of nursing as a profession. Community health nurses have been involved in research addressing all three of these dimensions.

Public Policy and Community Health

Research, with policy implications for addressing the health needs of aggregates, has been conducted on numerous topics. Many studies done by nurses and others have examined issues related to prevention, lifestyle change, quality of life, and health needs of specific at-risk populations (see Evidence-Based Practice: A Change of Position).

Often both quantitative and qualitative methods are useful when conducting **health policy evaluation** studies to determine whether existing health services are appropriate and accessible, as well as effective. Remler and Glied (2003) wanted a better understanding of why many Americans who qualify for health insurance programs do not participate in them. They examined more than 100 articles about health insurance and other health policy–driven programs and found similar patterns and themes across all areas. The most consistent predictor of client participation was the size of the benefit measured over time, and they suggested that longer periods of coverage might promote greater participation. They noted that Medicare, Part A, had the highest percentage of participation (99%), whereas participation in Medicaid for eligible uninsured children ranged between 50% and 70%.

The results of health policy studies can influence public policy, the quality of services, and, in turn, the public's health. As an example, several studies conducted by a researcher at the University of Miami could lead to further policy changes regarding cigarette smoking. One study examined the projected health benefits and cost savings of raising the legal age for smoking in the United States to 21 (Ahmad, 2005a). Using a computer simulation model, the researcher concluded that changing the policy would net total savings of $212 billion in the United States and reduce the prevalence of cigarette smoking substantially. A similar study, looking only at the state of California, found that raising the legal smoking age to 21 would yield an 82% drop in prevalence in teen smoking and would save $24 billion over 50 years' time (Ahmad, 2005b). Taxes are another disincentive for smokers. California raised excise taxes on cigarettes in 1999, but Ahmad (2005c) used another computer simulation to reveal that an additional "20% tax-induced cigarette price increase would reduce smoking prevalence from 17% to 11.6% . . . and reduce smoking-related medical costs by $188 billion" (p. 276). Raising cigarette taxes again would both decrease the number of smokers and increase the tax revenue that could be used to further reduce smoking in California. But, other effective methods of reducing cigarette smoking may exist. Levy, Nikolayev, and Mumford (2005) noted that smoking prevalence declined between 1997 and 2003, and, although most of the change could be explained by price increases, researchers also found that clean air laws, widespread media campaigns, and more easily accessible smoking cessation interventions also played a part. They encouraged lawmakers to continue with tax increases and to strengthen clean air laws that ban smoking in public places. In a Minnesota study, smoke-free workplaces were found to be more effective than free nicotine replacement therapy (Ong & Glantz, 2005). Other researchers have found that antismoking advertising focusing on the addictive nature of cigarettes and the dangers of environmental tobacco smoke to children increased the chances of quitting among adult smokers who have children living in their homes (Netermeyer, Andrews, & Burton, 2005). Consistent and wide-ranging antismoking media campaigns that emphasize social unacceptability and easier access to smoking cessation classes were also emphasized to policy makers (Alamar & Glantz, 2006).

Community Health Nursing Practice

A primary purpose for conducting community health research is to gain new knowledge that will improve health services and promote the public's health. Consequently, most nursing research has implications for nursing practice. Many studies focus on a specific health need or at-risk population, then suggest nursing actions to be taken based on study findings. An example is a study examining effective approaches to take in promoting cardiovascular health in aging women (Sawatzky & Naimark, 2005). Historically, most care has focused on individual-level prevention and the treatment of risk factors such as hypertension and obesity. However, these nurse researchers found that a survey questionnaire, the Cardiovascular Health Promotion Profile, measured population-level determinants of health (i.e., income, social status, social support networks, employment and working conditions, level of education, utilization of health services, and biology and genetic factors) and could be a valuable method of promoting cardiovascular health in women. Individual-level measures are not thought to be as effective as population-based approaches in improving the health of a nation (Edelman & Mandle, 2006).

Nursing's Professional Status and Influence

The third way in which research has a significant impact on community health nursing is in its potential to enhance

EVIDENCE-BASED PRACTICE

A Change of Position

A good number of mothers today place their infants in a supine position—on their backs—to sleep. However, for most of us writing this textbook, the opposite was true— we were placed as sleeping infants in the prone position, on our stomachs. For generations, mothers were told that babies would be at risk of aspiration if they were put to sleep on their backs. Why did this change? In the late 1980s, research indicated that prone positioning of infants was related to greater incidences of sudden infant death syndrome (SIDS), according to a group at the National Institute of Child Health and Human Development (NIH) who conducted an epidemiologic study examining SIDS risk factors (Hoffman, Damus, Hillman, & Krongrad, 1988). In the early 1990s, an expert panel from the same institute and the American Academy of Pediatrics concluded that infant sleeping positioning was an important factor in prevention of SIDS and a recommendation was made for parents to place their infants on their backs when sleeping. The *Back to Sleep* campaign began in 1994 (First Candle, 2006). Since then, the incidence of SIDS has continued to drop steadily in the U.S. (Malloy & Freeman, 2000) and in other countries (Mitchell, Tuohy, et al., 1997)—as much as 50%. Despite this, SIDS is still the leading cause of death in infants between the ages of 1 month and 1 year (American Academy of Pediatrics, 2005). More recent research has focused on the use of side sleeping positions (considered to be as risky as prone positions), bed-sharing (not recommended), prenatal maternal smoking (a major risk factor), and genetic factors as additional variables to consider with SIDS

(Li, Petitti, Willinger, et al., 2003; Thogmartin, Siebert, & Pelian, 2001; Opdal & Rognum, 2004). Current recommendations from the American Academy of Pediatrics (2005) include continuing the *Back to Sleep* campaign and advising parents to:

- Place their sleeping infants in a supine position (not on side or stomach)
- Use a firm sleeping surface (no pillows or quilts under the baby)
- Keeping soft objects (e.g., stuffed animals) and loose bedding (e.g., extra quilts or loose bedding) out of baby's crib
- Not smoke during pregnancy and avoid baby's exposure to secondhand smoke
- Not share the bed with baby—put baby in a separate crib or bassinet with parents in the same room
- Offer a pacifier at sleep time throughout the first year of life (it has been shown to reduce the risk of SIDS)
- Avoid overheating (keep room temperature comfortable for lightly clothed adults—do not overbundle babies)
- Encourage "tummy time" to avoid development of positional plagiocephaly (uneven head)
- Avoid the use of apnea monitors (not shown to be effective) and other commercial devices marketed as effective in reducing SIDS cases (not sufficient proof of efficacy)

Do your community health clients put their babies to sleep on their backs? If not, how can you convince them that it is beneficial?

nursing's status and influence. As community health nursing research sheds light on the critical health needs of at-risk populations, exposes deficiencies in the health care system, demonstrates more efficient and cost-effective methods for delivering services, and documents the effectiveness of nursing interventions, the profession will gain a stronger voice and have a greater impact on health policy and programs. After all, PHNs have always been advocates for their clients and promoted policies that improved health.

An example of community-oriented research was conducted by Rothman and associates (2002). Community-developed strategies were used in a program to reduce lead poisoning in a poor area of Philadelphia. Four census tracts were selected for intervention, on the basis of pre-1950 built housing, poverty level, and percentage of Black citizens. Matching control census tracts were also studied. Adult block parties (using educational and motivational strategies) and interactive educational sessions for children (e.g., puppet shows) were used over the 3 years of study. Approximately 1,200 children and 900 adults participated. Initially, overall lead poisoning awareness was low. Testing of homes revealed that more than 90% were positive for lead. After the first intervention year, a 27% increase occurred in the number of children tested for lead in the intervention census tracts, and only a 10% increase in the control census tracts. An 11% reduction occurred in the percentage of children with excess blood lead levels in the intervention group, and only a 3% reduction in the control group. Participants readily accepted this community-developed and community-based intervention by nurses and a physician from Temple University. This research enhanced nursing's role in the community by engaging with community members on their turf and demonstrating nurses' roles in research.

Strong documentation supports the effectiveness of community health nursing interventions. Nurses in the community setting must provide empiric proof of their worth as professionals, as well as serve the needs of their clients. This kind of information must be made visible if it is to influence legislators, planners, administrators, and other decision-makers in health care. As visibility increases, nursing's status and influence will increase.

THE COMMUNITY HEALTH NURSE'S ROLE IN RESEARCH

The advantages of community health nursing include a focus on health promotion and disease prevention; provision of services across the lifespan where people live, work, and learn; development of community capacity building for health; and working with partnerships, coalitions, and policy makers to promote a healthier environment. Community health nurses have two important responsibilities with respect to research in community health: to apply research findings to practice (EBP) and to conduct or participate in nursing research. Because research results provide essential information for improving health policy and the delivery of health services, community health nurses must be knowledgeable consumers of research. That is, they need to be able to critically examine research reports and apply study findings to improve the public's health.

Many research textbooks describe the steps one can take to thoroughly assess a research study. Begin by looking carefully at the title and the journal in which the article is found. Abstracts afford an opportunity to quickly preview the article. The quality of the journal (based on its history, circulation, and caliber of editorial board, among other factors) is another consideration. Authors' educational and affiliative credentials give clues to their credibility and could reveal any financial interest they may have in relation to their research outcomes. For instance, authors whose research studies are funded by drug companies may have a conflict of interest, and the results of those studies could be questioned. Examine the currency of references and the extensiveness of the authors' literature review. When reading the article, keep in mind the steps in the research process and note how carefully the authors followed each one. Ask the following questions:

- ◆ Was the research question clearly stated?
- ◆ Was the literature review complete and current?
- ◆ Was an appropriate conceptual framework in place?
- ◆ How was the sample selected?
- ◆ Did the methodology follow logically from the research question and the conceptual framework?
- ◆ Were the instruments used valid and reliable and described in sufficient detail?
- ◆ Were the methods of data collection and data analysis clearly identified?
- ◆ Did the authors give ideas for future nursing research based on this study?

Review the findings and discussion sections of the research article carefully to determine what implications this study might have for nursing practice. Talk with colleagues and peers about the implications of the study and ways in which it might be replicated or its line of research extended.

Community health nurses have many opportunities to apply the results of other investigators' research, but a necessary prerequisite is to be informed about research findings. As an essential part of their role, community health nurses must read the journals focusing on public health and community health nursing. Subscribing to some of these journals enables nurses to make a regular review of research an ongoing part of their professional practice. Nursing agencies and employment sites in community health can encourage nurses to become more knowledgeable about research findings by subscribing to journals and circulating them among staff, by holding seminars to discuss recent research results, and by promoting nurses' application of research findings in their practice.

Second, although the amount of health nursing research is expanding, and its quality improving, many more community health nurses need to conduct research themselves. An increasing number of nurses have developed skill in research through advanced preparation, and they are conducting investigations related to aggregate health needs. Other community health nurses work collaboratively with trained investigators on a variety of research projects affecting community health. Whether initiated by the nurse or involving the nurse as a team member, these projects are an opportunity to influence the types of research questions that are addressed and the ways in which the research is carried out, factors that ultimately affect the community's health.

☼ VALUES AND ETHICS IN COMMUNITY HEALTH NURSING

Health care is replete with ethical questions, and the field of bioethics continues to expand as new discoveries are made (Beauchamp & Childress, 2001). Community health nurses face an expanding number of ethical dilemmas every day. Imagine, for example, that you are providing health care to a population of migrant farm workers whose housing lacks adequate toilets, bathing facilities, heating, and equipment for cooking and refrigerating food. You recognize that this is a valid health and safety issue. However, when you report the situation to your supervisor, you are told to ignore the conditions because the wineries that employ the workers contribute heavily to a high-profile clinic for all low-income children in your area. What would you do?

What if you were working in a homeless shelter and were told to evict someone who would not agree to take a tuberculin skin test. You agree that residents should comply with this demand, but would you hesitate to implement the eviction if the resident were elderly or the teenage mother of a newborn?

Within the United States, many marginalized people are failed by the public health care system or go without any health care at all. At the same time, affluent individuals enjoy a plethora of health care options, including preventive screenings and health promotion classes. Community health nurses often are confronted by this disparity when making ethical decisions about client care.

In addition to these dilemmas within U.S. borders, progress in the United States often is linked to the exploitation of people in less-developed countries, and this contributes to widening disparities in health, wealth, and human rights. Failure to respond to such global challenges only leads to greater poverty and deprivation, continuing conflict, escalating migration, and the spread of infectious disease, all further adding to our ethical dilemmas.

Advances in technology also contribute to ethical dilemmas. For example, electronic health records make client information readily accessible, thus raising issues of confidentiality, clients' rights, and informed consent (Ries & Moysa, 2005). Technology also forces nurses to confront the issues of genetic testing and stem cell research, as well as assisted suicide and euthanasia (Buroughs, 2005; Yoshimura, 2006; Hurst & Mauron, 2006). Further ethical questions arise regarding organ, tissue, and limb transplants and the decisions about who is to receive them (Delmonico, 2006). Underlying every issue and influencing every ethical and professional decision are *values*. Ethics and values are inextricably intertwined in professional decision-making, because values are the criteria by which decisions are made.

Values

What are values? A **value** is something that is perceived as desirable or a personally held abstract belief "about the truth and worth of thoughts, objects, or behavior" (Guido, 2006, p. 2). A value motivates people to behave in certain ways that are personally or socially preferable. Values are usually derived from societal norms, as well as from family and/or religious beliefs. We develop our value system as a result of our experiences with others (e.g., family, peers, schools, churches, jobs). As seen in Chapter 5, a group's culture often is defined by its members' common or shared values.

Standards for Behavior

In general, values function as standards that guide actions and behavior in daily situations or act as a code of conduct for living one's life. Once internalized by an individual, a value, such as honesty, becomes a criterion for that individual's personal conduct. Values may function as criteria for developing and maintaining attitudes toward objects and situations or for justifying a person's own actions and attitudes. Values also may be the standard by which people pass moral judgments on themselves and others.

Values have a long-term function in giving expression to human needs. Values motivate people in their work setting, in their personal lives, and in dealing with their health, as well as with the larger society. In addition, values are used as standards to guide presentation of the self to others, to ascertain personal morality and competency, and to persuade and influence others by indicating which beliefs, attitudes, and actions of others are worth trying to reinforce or change. As a practitioner, values act as a compass to direct the nurse when working with clients.

Qualities of Values

The nature of values can be described according to five qualities: endurance, hierarchical arrangement, prescriptive-proscriptive belief, reference, and preference.

Endurance

Values remain relatively stable over time, persisting to provide continuity to personal and social existence. Enduring religious beliefs, for example, offer stability to many people. This is not to say that values are completely stable over time; values do change throughout a person's life. Certainly, the values of children are different from adults. Moral development generally follows a prescribed path, according to Lawrence Kohlberg (Colby & Kohlberg, 1987) and Carol Gilligan (1982), researchers studying changes in moral behavior and judgment from childhood to adulthood. Yet social existence in the community requires standards within the individual as well as an agreement about standards among groups of individuals. As Kluckhohn (1951, p. 400) once pointed out, without values, "the functioning of the social system could not continue to achieve group goals; individuals . . . could not feel within themselves a requisite measure of order and unified purpose." A group's culture provides such a set of enduring values. By adding an element of collective purpose in social life, values most often guarantee endurance and stability in social existence.

Hierarchical System

Isolated values usually are organized into a hierarchical system in which certain values have more weight or importance than others. For instance, in a team sport such as baseball, values regarding individual performance, batting and running records, speed, and throwing and catching all fall into a hierarchy, with the values of team and winning being at the top. As an individual confronts social situations throughout life, isolated values learned in early childhood come into competition with other values, requiring a weighing of one value against another. Concern for others' welfare, for instance, competes with self-interest. Through experience and maturation, the individual integrates values learned in different contexts into systems in which each value is ordered relative to other values (Glasser, 1998).

Prescriptive–Proscriptive Beliefs

Rokeach (1973) described values as a subcategory of beliefs. He argues that some beliefs are *descriptive* or capable of being true or false (e.g., the chair on which I am sitting will hold me up). Other beliefs are *evaluative*, involving judgments of good and bad (e.g., that was an excellent lecture). Still other beliefs are *prescriptive–proscriptive*, determining whether an action is desirable or undesirable (e.g., this music is too loud, those baseball fans shouldn't yell when the pitcher is winding up). Values, Rokeach says, are prescriptive–proscriptive beliefs. They are concerned with desirable behavior or "what ought to be." For example, parents' values about child behavior determine how they choose to discipline their children, using either corporal punishment or a time-out. Some parents believe that their 2-year-old child has the capacity to control his bladder, and when the child wets his pants they are being "rebellious" and should be punished. Values have cognitive, affective, and behavioral components. According to Rokeach, to have a value, it is important to know the correct way to behave or the correct end state for which to strive (cognitive component); to feel emotional about it—to be affectively for or against it (affective component); and to take action based on it (behavioral component).

Reference

Values also have a reference quality. That is, they may refer to end states of existence called **terminal values**, such as spiritual salvation, peace of mind, or world peace, or they may refer to modes of conduct called **instrumental values**, such as confidentiality, keeping promises, and honesty. The latter can have a moral focus or a nonmoral focus, and these values may conflict. For example, a nurse may experience a conflict between two moral values, such as whether to act honestly (tell a client about a fatal diagnosis) or to act respectfully (honor the family's request not to tell the client). Similarly, the nurse may experience conflict between two nonmoral values, such as whether to plan logically (design a traditional group intervention for mental health clients) or to plan creatively (design an innovative field experience). The nurse also may experience conflict between a nonmoral value and a moral value, such as whether to act efficiently or to act fairly when establishing priorities for funding among community health programs.

Adults generally possess only a few—perhaps no more than 20—terminal values, such as peace of mind or achievement. These are influenced by complex physiologic and social factors. The needs for security, love, self-esteem, and self-actualization, proposed by Maslow (1969), are believed to be the greatest influences on terminal values. Although an individual may have only a few terminal values, the same person may possess as many as 50 to 75 instrumental values. Any single instrumental value, or several instrumental values combined, also may help to determine terminal values. For example, the instrumental values of acceptance, taking it easy, living one day at a time, and not being concerned about the future can shape the terminal value of peace of mind; whereas the instrumental values of hard work, driving oneself to compete, and not letting anyone get in the way can influence the terminal value of achievement. Figure 4.3 illustrates the influence of instrumental values and human needs on the development of terminal values.

Preference

A value may show preference for one mode of behavior over another, such as exercise over inactivity, or it may show a

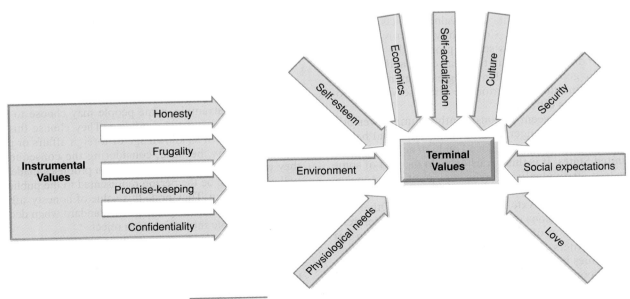

FIGURE 4.3 Factors influencing personal values.

preference for one end state over another, such as physical fitness and leanness over sedentary lifestyle and obesity. The preferred end state, or mode of behavior, is located higher in the personal value hierarchy.

Value Systems

Value systems generally are considered organizations of beliefs that are of relative importance in guiding individual behavior (Rokeach, 1973). Instead of being guided by single or isolated values, however, behavior at any point in time (or over a period of time) is influenced by multiple or changing clusters of values. Therefore, it is important to understand how values are integrated into a person's total belief system, how values assume a place in a hierarchy of values, and how this hierarchical system changes over time.

Hierarchical System of Values

Learned values are integrated into an organized system of values, and each value has an ordered priority with respect to other values (Rokeach, 1973). For example, a person may place a higher value on physical comfort than on exercising. This system of ordered priority is stable enough to reflect the continuity of someone's personality and behavior within culture and society, yet it is sufficiently flexible to allow a reordering of value priorities in response to changes in the environment or social setting (e.g., society's emphasis on physical fitness and youth) or changes based on personal experiences (e.g., diagnosis of type 2 diabetes). Behavioral change would be regarded as the visible response to a reordering of values within an individual's hierarchical value system.

Conflict Between Values in a System

When an individual encounters a social situation, several values within the person's value system are activated, rather than just a single value. Because not all of the activated values are compatible with one another, conflict between values occurs. This conflict between values is a part of the decision-making process, and resolving these value conflicts is crucial to making good decisions. Community health nurses face conflicting values when they seek to promote the well being of certain individuals, a result that may come at the expense of the public good. Even within a single community agency, nurses may find that they prioritize client service or programming values differently.

Some values seem to consistently triumph over others, persisting as stronger directives for individual behavior; an example is the value placed on high achievement in the United States. It is this persistence on the part of some values (e.g., individualism versus community) that makes universal coverage and other issues so controversial in health care reform (Axtell-Thompson, 2005). Other values lose their positions of importance in a value hierarchy (e.g., resuscitation of all hospital patients versus do not resuscitate orders [DNRs]). It is this changing arrangement of values in a hierarchical system that determines, in part, how conflicts are resolved and how decisions are made. In this way, people's value systems function as a learned organization of principles and rules that help them

to choose among alternative courses of action to reach decisions.

Values Clarification

One way to understand the influence and priority of values in your own behavior, as well as in that of community health clients, is to use various values clarification techniques in decision-making. **Values clarification** is a process that helps to identify the personal and professional values that guide your actions, by prompting you to examine what you believe about the worth, truth, or beauty of any object, thought, or behavior and where this belief ranks compared with your other values (Feldman-Stewart, Brennenstuhl, Brundage, & Roques, 2006). Because individuals are largely unaware of the motives underlying their choices, values clarification is important for understanding and shaping the kind of decisions people make. Only by understanding your values and their hierarchy can you ascertain whether your choices are the result of rational thinking or of external influences, such as cultural or social conditioning. Values clarification by itself does not yield a set of rules for future decision-making and does not indicate the rightness or wrongness of alternative actions. It does, however, help to guarantee that any course of action chosen by people is consistent and in accordance with their beliefs and values (Redman, 2001; Guido, 2006).

Process of Valuing

Before values clarification can take place, it must be understood how the process of valuing occurs in individuals. In 1977, Uustal listed the following seven steps, which remain useful today:

1. Choose the value freely and individually.
2. Choose the value from among alternatives.
3. Carefully consider the consequences of the choice.
4. Cherish or prize the value—feel good about the choice.
5. Publicly affirm the chosen value.
6. Incorporate the value into behavior, so that it becomes a standard or a pattern of behavior.
7. Consciously use the value in decision-making.

These steps provide specific actions for the discovery and identification of people's values. They also assist the decision-making process by explicating the process of valuing itself. For example, some people may choose to value honesty in a presidential candidate. They choose this over other values, such as knowledge of foreign affairs or public speaking ability, because, considering the consequences, they want a leader who will deliver on promises made, who will continue to be the person represented to the public during the campaign. They prize this value of honesty, affirm it publicly, and consciously use it as a standard when deciding on whom to vote into office or to reject.

Values Clarification Strategies

In 1978, Uustal offered several values clarification strategies that are ultimately useful to the decision-making process in community health nursing practice today. Strategy 1 is a way

---

Name Tag

Take a piece of paper and write your name in the middle of it. In each of the four corners, write your responses to these four questions:

1. What two things would you like your colleagues to say about you?
2. What single most important thing do you do (or would you like to do) to make your nurse–client relationships positive ones?
3. What do you do on a daily basis that indicates you value your health?
4. What are the three values you believe in most strongly?

In the space around your name, write at least six adjectives that you feel best describe who you are.

Take a closer look at your responses to the questions and to the ways in which you described yourself. What values are reflected in your answers?

FIGURE 4.4 Values clarification strategy 1.

for nurses to come to know themselves and their values better (Fig. 4.4). Strategy 2 assists in discovering value clusters and the priority of values within personal value systems (Fig. 4.5). Strategy 3 can be used to examine personal responses to selected issues in nursing practice. Each response helps to establish priorities of values by asking the nurse to choose among the alternatives presented or to indicate degree of agreement or disagreement (Fig. 4.6). Other values clarification strategies are included in the critical thinking activities at the end of this chapter to assist in understanding personal ordering of values and when considering directions for change. These strategies also help the nurse to assist community health clients to become clearer about their own values.

All of these strategies can be used to analyze and understand how values are meaningful to people and ultimately influence their choices and behavior. Clarification of a person's values is the first step in the decision-making process, and it affects the ability of people to make ethical decisions. Values clarification also promotes understanding and respect for values held by others, such as community health clients and other health care providers. As pointed out by Uustal (1977, p. 10), "Nurses cannot hope to give optimal, sensitive care to any patient without first understanding their own opinions, attitudes, and values." This values clarification process provides a backdrop for next exploring the role of values in ethical decision-making.

ETHICS

Values are central to any consideration of ethics or ethical decision-making. Yet, it is not always obvious at first what constitutes an ethical problem in health care or in the practice of community health nursing. Most nurses easily recognize the moral crisis in some kinds of decisions—for example, whether to let seriously deformed newborn infants die, whether to terminate pregnancies resulting from rape, or whether to provide universal health care coverage. However, other, less obvious moral dilemmas often found in the routine practice

---

Patterns

Which of the following words describe you? Draw a circle around the seven words that best describe you as an individual. Underline the seven words that most accurately describe you as a professional person. (You may circle and underline the same word.)

ambitious	reserved	assertive	opinionated
concerned	generous	independent	
easily hurt	outgoing	reliable	indifferent
capable	self-controlled	fun-loving	
suspicious	solitary	likable	dependent
intellectual	argumentative	dynamic	unpredictable
compromising	thoughtful	affectionate	obedient
logical	imaginative	self-disciplined	
moody	easily led	helpful	slow to relate

Reflect on the following questions:

1. What values are reflected in the patterns you have chosen?
2. What is the relationship between these patterns and your personal values?
3. What patterns indicate inconsistencies in attitudes or behavior?
4. What patterns do you think a nurse should cultivate?

FIGURE 4.5 Values clarification strategy 2.

Forced Choice Ranking

How do you order the following alternatives by priority? (There is no correct set of priorities.) What values emerge in response to each question?

1. With whom on a nursing team would you become most angry? The nurse who
   _____ never completes assignments.
   _____ rarely helps other team members.
   _____ projects his or her feelings on clients.

2. If you had a serious health problem, you would rather
   _____ not be told.
   _____ be told directly.
   _____ find out by accident.

3. You are made happiest in your work when you use
   _____ your technical skills in caring for adults with complex needs.
   _____ your ability to compile data and arrive at a nursing diagnosis.
   _____ your ability to communicate easily and skillfully with clients.

4. It would be most difficult for you to
   _____ listen to and counsel a dying person.
   _____ advise a pregnant adolescent.
   _____ handle a situation of obvious child abuse.

FIGURE 4.6 Values clarification strategy 3.

of community health nursing are not always considered to be ethical in nature.

What is *ethics* and what is *ethical*? The *Merriam Webster Online Dictionary* (2006) defines **ethics** as "a set of moral principles; a theory or system of moral values; the principles of conduct governing a group; a guiding philosophy; a consciousness of moral importance" (¶ 1). Ethics are often idealized as "what ought to be." **Ethical decision-making**, then, means making a choice that is consistent with a moral code or that can be justified from an ethical perspective. Of necessity, the decision-maker must exercise moral judgment. Remember that the term **moral** refers to conforming to a standard that is right and good. Community health nurses become "moral agents" by making decisions that have direct and indirect consequences for the welfare of themselves and others. **Bioethics** refers to using ethical principles and methods of decision-making in questions involving biologic, medical, or health care issues. The next section examines how a nurse makes these moral decisions.

Identifying Ethical Situations

Ethics involves making evaluative judgments. To be ethically responsible in the practice of community health nursing, it is important to develop the ability to recognize evaluative judgments as they are made and implemented in nursing practice. Nurses must be able to distinguish between evaluative and nonevaluative judgments. Evaluative statements involve judgments of value, rights, duties, and responsibilities. Examples are, "Parents should never strike their children," and "It is the duty of every citizen to vote." Among the words to watch for are verbs such as *want, desire, refer, should,* or *ought* and nouns such as *benefit, harm, duty, responsibility, right,* or *obligation.*

Sometimes, the evaluations are expressed in terms that are not direct expressions of evaluations but clearly are

functioning as value judgments. For example, the American Nurses Association (ANA) *Code for Nurses with Interpretive Statements* (2001), in its nine statements, has several that actually refer to "the nurse's obligation" or "owing the same duties to self as to others" and "nursing values" (see Code of Ethics for Nurses—Provisions).

Another important step is to distinguish between moral and nonmoral evaluations. **Moral evaluations** refer to judgments that conform to standards of what is right and good. Moral evaluations assess human actions, institutions, or character traits rather than inanimate objects, such as parks or architectural structures. They are prescriptive–proscriptive beliefs having certain characteristics separating them from other evaluations such as aesthetic judgments, personal preferences, or matters of taste. Moral evaluations also have distinctive characteristics (Thompson, Melia, & Boyd, 2000):

- *The evaluations are ultimate.* They have a preemptive quality, meaning that other values or human ends cannot, as a rule, override them.
- *They possess universality or reflect a standpoint that applies to everyone.* They are evaluations that everyone in principle ought to be able to make and understand, even if some individuals, in fact, do not.
- *Moral evaluations avoid giving a special place to a person's own welfare.* They have a focus that keeps others in view, or at least considers one's own welfare on a par with that of others.

Resolving Moral Conflicts and Ethical Dilemmas

When judgments involve moral values, conflicts are inevitable. In clinical practice, the nurse may be faced with moral conflicts, such as the choice between preserving the welfare of one set of clients over that of others. For example, the nurse may

---

CODE OF ETHICS FOR NURSES   PROVIDIONS, APPROVED AS OF JUNE 30, 2001

1. The nurse, in all professional relationships, practices with compassion and respect for the inherent dignity, worth, and uniqueness of every individual, unrestricted by considerations of social or economic status, personal attributes, or the nature of health problems.
2. The nurse's primary commitment is to the patient, whether an individual, family, group, or community.
3. The nurse promotes, advocates for, and strives to protect the health, safety, and rights of the patient.
4. The nurse is responsible and accountable for individual nursing practice and determines the appropriate delegation of tasks consistent with the nurse's obligation to provide optimum patient care.
5. The nurse owes the same duties to self as to others, including the responsibility to preserve integrity and safety, to maintain competence, and to continue personal and professional growth.

6. The nurse participates in establishing, maintaining, and improving health care environments and conditions of employment conducive to the provision of quality health care and consistent with the values of the profession through individual and collective action.
7. The nurse participates in the advancement of the profession through contributions to practice, education, administration, and knowledge development.
8. The nurse collaborates with other health professionals and the public in promoting community, national, and international efforts to meet health needs.
9. The profession of nursing, as represented by associations and their members, is responsible for articulating nursing values, for maintaining the integrity of the profession and its practice, and for shaping social policy.

Reprinted with permission from American Nurses Association, *Code of ethics for nurses with interpretive statements,* © 2001 Nursesbooks.org, Silver Spring, MD.

have to choose whether to keep a promise of confidentiality to persons who are infected by HIV when these individuals continue to have unprotected sex with unknowing partners. Nurses may have to choose between protecting the interests of colleagues or the interests of the employing institution by reporting a nurse who makes phone visits rather than home visits, so that she can spend more time shopping online from work. They may have to decide whether to serve future clients by striking for better conditions or to serve present clients by refusing to strike. Often, nurses' values are at odds with their employers' values and procedures. The moral values of a nurse may conflict with the policies and practices of a particular bureaucracy. Each decision involves a potential conflict between moral values and is called an **ethical dilemma**. An ethical dilemma occurs when morals conflict with one another, causing the nurse to face a choice with equally attractive or equally undesirable alternatives (Kelly, 2006; Thompson, Melia, & Boyd, 2000). When "two or more seemingly equivalent principles or values seem to compel different actions," you are faced with an ethical dilemma (Iserson, 1999, p. 298). It can create a decision-making problem, even in ordinary nursing situations.

Decision-making Frameworks

To resolve ethical dilemmas or the conflict between moral values in community health nursing practice, and to provide morally accountable nursing service, several frameworks for ethical decision-making have been proposed. Among these frameworks, three key steps are considered as fundamental to choosing alternative courses of action that reflect moral reasoning: separate questions of fact from questions of value, identify both clients' and nurse's value systems, and consider ethical principles and concepts.

The identification of clients' values and those of other persons involved in conflict situations is an important part of ethical decision-making. In the example given in From the Case Files I, what are Mr. Bell's values? What are the values of neighbors who are concerned about him, but feel that they can no longer care for him? What are the nurse's values? What are the values of the nurse's employing agency? What are society's values?

An ethical decision-making framework referred to as the DECIDE model is a practical method of making prudent value judgments and ethical decisions (Thompson, Melia, & Boyd, 2000). It includes the following steps:

D—*Define the problem (or problems).* What are the key facts of the situation? Who is involved? What are their rights and duties and your rights and duties?

E—*Ethical review.* What ethical principles have a bearing on the situation, and which principle or principles should be given priority in making a decision?

C—*Consider the options.* What options do you have in the situation? What alternative courses of action exist? What help, means, and methods do you need to use?

I—*Investigate outcomes.* Given each available option, what consequences are likely to follow from each course of action open to you? Which is the most ethical thing to do?

D—*Decide on action.* Having chosen the best available option, determine a specific action plan, set clear objectives, and then act decisively and effectively.

E—*Evaluate results.* Having initiated a course of action, assess how things progress, and when concluded, evaluate carefully whether or not you achieved your goals.

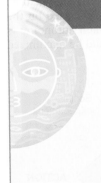

From the Case Files I

Mr. Bell

Community health nurses encounter value differences every day, and value differences, in turn, create ethical problems. Consider, for example, the dilemma faced by one nurse in Seattle on her first home visit to an elderly man, Mr. Bell, referred by concerned neighbors, this 82-year-old gentleman was homebound and living alone with severe arthritis under steadily deteriorating conditions. Overgrown shrubs and vines covered the yard and house, making access impossible except through the back door. A wood-burning stove in the kitchen was the sole source of heat, and that room, plus a corner of the dining room, were Mr. Bell's living quarters. The remainder of the once-lovely three-bedroom home, including the bathroom, was layered with dust, unused. His bed was a cot in the dining room; his toilet, a two-pound coffee can placed under the cot. Unbathed, unshaven, and existing on food and firewood brought by neighbors, Mr. Bell seemed to be living in deplorable conditions. Yet he prized his independence so highly that he adamantly refused to leave.

The conflict of values between Mr. Bell's choice to live independently and the nurse's value of having him in a safer living situation raises several ethical questions. When do health practitioners or family members have the right or duty to override an individual's preferences? When do neighbors' rights (Mr. Bell's home was an eyesore and his care was a source of anxiety for his neighbors) supersede one homeowner's rights? Should the nurse be responsible when family members can help but won't take action? Mr. Bell had one son living in a neighboring state.

In this case, the nurse entering Mr. Bell's home applied her values of respect for the individual and his right to autonomy even at the risk of public safety. Not until he fell and broke a hip did he reluctantly agree to be moved into a nursing home.

DISPLAY 4.1 A FRAMEWORK FOR ETHICAL DECISION-MAKING

1. *Clarify the ethical dilemma:* Whose problem is it? Who should make the decision? Who is affected by the decision? What ethical principles are related to the problem?
2. *Gather additional data:* Have as much information about the situation as possible. Be up to date on any legal cases related to the ethical question.
3. *Identify options:* Brainstorm with others to identify as many alternatives as possible. The more options identified, the more likely it is that an acceptable solution will be found.

4. *Make a decision:* Choose from the options identified and determine the most acceptable option, the one more feasible than others.
5. *Act:* Carry out the decision. It may be necessary to collaborate with others to implement the decision and identify options.
6. *Evaluate:* After acting on a decision, evaluate its impact. Was the best course of action chosen? Would an alternative have been better? Why? What went right and what went wrong? Why?

Other frameworks can be used. The framework for ethical decision-making shown in Display 4.1 helps to organize thoughts and acts as a guide through the decision-making process. The steps help to determine a course of action, with heavy responsibility at the evaluation level: here the outcomes need to be judged and decisions repeated or rejected in future situations. Figure 4.7 summarizes several views in the field on ethical decision-making. This framework advocates keeping multiple values in tension before resolution of conflict and action on the part of the nurse. It suggests that value conflict is not capable of resolution until all possible alternative actions have been explored. Iserson (1999) advocates the use of three tests: the impartiality test (e.g., Would you be willing to have this done to you?—the "golden rule"), the universalizablity test (e.g., If every nurse in similar circumstances did the same as you, would you be comfortable with that "universal rule"?), and the interpersonal justifiability test (e.g., Can you state a reason for your choice and justify your actions to your peers, supervisors, and society?). Final resolution of the ethical conflict occurs through a conscious choice of action, even though some values would be overridden by other stronger, presumably moral values.

The triumphant values would be those located higher in the decision-maker's hierarchy of values.

Basic Values That Guide Decision-making

When applying a decision-making framework, certain values influence community health nursing decisions. Three basic human values are considered key to guiding decision-making in the provider–client relationship: self-determination, well-being, and equity.

Self-determination

The value of **self-determination** or individual autonomy is a person's exercise of the capacity to shape and pursue personal plans for life (Guido, 2006). Self-determination is instrumentally valued because self-judgment about a person's goals and choices is conducive to an individual's sense of well-being. Informed consent derives from self-determination. When one respects self-determination, it is based on the belief that better outcomes will result when autonomy is held in high regard. The outcomes that could be maximized

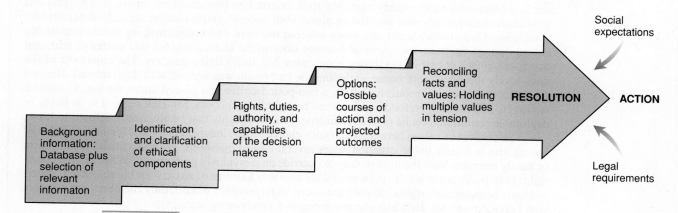

FIGURE 4.7 An ethical decision-making framework. Although legal requirements or social expectations may sway a decision one way or another, they are extrinsic to the ethical analysis and should not be confused with right and wrong. What is legal and what is expected are not necessarily right and wrong.

by respecting self-determination or autonomy include enhanced self-concept, enhanced health-promoting behaviors, and enhanced quality of care. Self-determination is a major value in the United States, but does not receive the same emphasis in all societies or ethnic groups.

In health care contexts, the desire for self-determination has been of such high ethical importance in U.S. society that it overrides practitioner determinations in many situations. Client empowerment is an approach that differs from the paternalistic approach to health care in which decisions are made for, rather than with, the client; instead, it enables patients and professionals to work in partnerships (Gagnon, Hibert, Dube, & Dubois, 2006; Aston, Meagher-Stewart, Sheppard-Lemoine, Vukic, & Chircop, 2006). Many physicians and other health providers, including community health nurses, fail to recognize the high value attributed to self-determination by many consumers or the differences in views of self-determination among ethnic groups.

The conflict between provider and consumer may be broader. When self-determination deteriorates into self-interest, it poses a major roadblock to equitable health care. **Self-interest** is the fulfillment of one's own desires, without regard for the greater good. Consumers mostly have to fend for themselves when they encounter the world of for-profit health care, just as they do in other commercial markets, where "buyer beware" is the standard (Darke & Chaiken, 2005).

When providing health care, self-determination and taking personal responsibility for health care decisions should be nurtured. This includes informing clients of options and the reasoning behind all recommendations. Yet self-determination and personal autonomy at times are impermissible or even impossible. For example, society must impose restrictions on unacceptable client choices, such as child abuse and other abusive behaviors, or situations in which clients are not competent to exercise self-determination, as is true for certain levels of mental illness or dementia. There are two situations in which self-determination should be restricted: when some objectives of individuals are contrary to the public interest or the interests of others in society (e.g., endangering others with a communicable disease), and when a person's decision-making is so defective or mistaken that the decision fails to promote the person's own values or goals. When a person cannot fully comprehend the options, the consequences of actions related to the options, and the true costs and benefits, he may not have adequate capacity for making health care decisions. In these situations, self-determination is justifiably overridden on the basis of the promotion of one's own well-being or the well-being of others—another important value in health care decision-making (Guido, 2006; Kelly, 2006).

Well-being

Well-being is a state of positive health. Although all therapeutic interventions by health care professionals are intended to improve clients' health and promote well-being, well-intended interventions sometimes fall short if they are in conflict with clients' preferences and needs. Determining what constitutes health for people and how their well-being can be promoted often requires knowledge of clients' subjective preferences. It is generally recognized that clients may be inclined to pursue different directions in treatment procedures based on individual goals, values, and interests. Community health nurses, who are committed not only to helping clients but also to respecting their wishes and avoiding harming them, must understand each client group's needs and develop reasonable alternatives for service from which clients may choose (see From the Case Files II). In addition, when individuals are not capable of making a choice, the nurse or other surrogate decision-maker is obliged to make health care decisions that promote the value of well-being. This may mean that the alternatives presented

---

From the Case Files II

Andrea Vargas, PHN—A Family Living in Poverty

Contrasting value systems may be seen in many community health practice settings. Andrea Vargas, a community health nurse, experienced such a contrast on her first home visit to a family living in poverty. Referred by a school nurse for the children's recurring problems with head lice and staphylococcal infections, the family was living in the worst conditions that Andrea had ever seen. Papers, moldy food, soiled clothing, and empty beer cans covered the floor. Andrea recoiled in dismay. The children, home from school, were clustered around the television. Their mother, a divorced, single parent—unkempt and obese—sat smoking a cigarette and drinking a soda. Although she worked part-time as a waitress, she had been unable to earn enough money to support her family, so they were now temporarily receiving state aid. The mother's main pleasure in life was watching soap operas on television. The nurse interpreted the situation through the framework of her own value system, in which health and cleanliness were priorities. Yet the mother, who might have shared those values in the past, appeared to prize pleasurable diversion, perhaps as a way to cope with her situation. In this instance, it is possible that environmental influences reordered the family's value system priorities. Rather than imposing her own values, Andrea chose to determine the priorities of the family, assess their needs, and begin where they were. Will she have a greater chance at success by doing this?

LEVELS OF PREVENTION PYRAMID

SITUATION: Provide distributive justice for battered women and children by changing a proposed state law that would eliminate funding for shelters for battered women and children to a law that preserves resources for this population.

GOAL: Using the three levels of prevention, negative health conditions are avoided, or promptly diagnosed and treated, and the fullest possible potential is restored.

Tertiary Prevention

Rehabilitation

If unable to stop the proposed law:
- Seek volunteer services to fill the gaps in funding paid employees
- Seek donations to support existing shelter buildings

Primary Prevention

Health Promotion & Education
- Educate the public regarding the need for lost/limited services using various forms of media and/or venues

Health Protection
- Seek private resources to fund shelters
- Propose a new bill to match private funding for shelters at the next legislative session

Secondary Prevention

Early Diagnosis
- Recognition that the proposed bill is going to pass

Prompt Treatment
- Advocate for amendments to the proposed bill to preserve limited funding for shelters

Primary Prevention

Health Promotion & Education
- Advocacy
- Active lobbying against the bill
- Garnering community support in favor of the revised bill

Health Protection

---

by the nurse for choice are only the alternatives that will promote well-being. With shared decision-making, the nurse not only seeks to understand clients' needs and develop reasonable alternatives to meet those needs, but also to present the alternatives in a way that enables clients to choose those they prefer. Well-being and self-determination are two values that are intricately related when providing community health nursing services.

Equity

The third value that is important to decision-making in health care contexts is the value of **equity** or justice, which means being treated equally or fairly. The principle of equity implies that it is unjust (or inequitable) to treat people the same if they are, in significant respects, unalike. In other words, different people have different needs in health care, but all must be served equally and adequately. Equity generally means that all individuals should have the same access to health care according to benefit or needs (see Levels of Prevention Pyramid).

The major problem with this definition of equity is, of course, that it assumes that an adequate level of health care can be economically available to all citizens. In times of limited technical, human, and financial resources, however, it may be impossible to fully respect the value of equity (Smith, Oveku, Homer, & Zuckerman, 2006; Franco, 2005). Choices must be made and resources allotted, while the value obligations of professional practice create conflicts of values that seem impossible to resolve.

Many of these conflicts are reflected in current health care reform efforts that focus on access to services, quality of services, and ways to control rising costs. However, the following list represents some of the most pressing aggregate health problems related to inequities in the distribution of and access to health and illness care facing our nation:

◆ *Too many women go without preventive care.* The overall rate of infant mortality (all infant deaths before 1 year of age) is 7 per 1,000 in the United States; it remains among the highest in the industrialized world (Centers for Disease Control [CDC], 2006). The rates for some people of color—African Americans (13.9), Native Hawaiian and other Pacific Islanders (9.6), and Native Americans (8.6) specifically—are higher than those for White, non-Hispanic (5.8) or Mexican Americans (5.4) (CDC, 2006). Forty-nine percent of pregnancies in the United States during 2001 were unintended—among White and Hispanic females 40% and 54%, respectively, were reported as unintended. But, among African American females, 69% report unintended pregnancies. Poverty is strongly related to difficulty in accessing family planning services (Finer & Henshaw, 2006).

◆ *Immunization rates for some diseases are at dangerously low levels.* For example, in 2004, about 82% of all children between 19 and 35 months of age had received full doses of childhood vaccines—below the 90% Healthy People 2010 objective. By ethnicity, though, only 76% of Black children, 81% of Hispanic children, and 74% of American Indian/Alaska Native children received those immunizations. When poverty level was factored in, the total dropped to 78% for those living below the poverty level, with only 73% of Black children immunized (CDC, 2006). Vast disparities in immunization rates also exist for adults along racial and ethnic lines, as well as poverty level (Office of Minority Health, 2006).

◆ *The uninsured are likely to go without physician care.* Differences in access to expensive, discretionary procedures emerge according to health insurance status, race, and ethnicity, as well as other sociodemographic factors. In 2003, 17% of Americans below the age of 65 reported having no health insurance, with Black and Hispanic Americans being more likely than White non-Hispanic Americans to lack health insurance coverage. Interestingly, only 30% of those without health insurance live below the poverty level (National Center for Health Statistics, 2005).

◆ *Environmental hazards threaten global health.* Global trade, travel, and changing social and cultural patterns make the population vulnerable to diseases that are endemic to other parts of the world, as well as to previously unknown diseases. Pollution of air, water, and soil to support industry contributes to pathogen mutations and threatens public health.

(See Display 4.2)

DISPLAY 4.2　SOCIETY AND INDIVIDUAL RESPONSIBILITY IN HEALTH CARE

To promote the achievement of equity, self-determination, and clients' well-being, certain conclusions drawn from the literature can enhance community health nursing practice (Des Jardin, 2001):

1. *Society has an ethical obligation to ensure equitable access to health care for all.* This obligation is centered on the special importance of health care and is derived from its role in relieving suffering, preventing premature death, restoring functioning, increasing opportunity, providing information about an individual's condition, and giving evidence of mutual empathy and compassion.

2. *The societal obligation is balanced by individual obligations.* Individuals ought to pay a fair share of the cost of their own health care and take reasonable steps to provide for such care when they can do so without excessive burdens.

3. *Equitable access to health care requires that all citizens can secure an adequate level of care without excessive burdens.* Equitable access also means that the burdens borne by individuals in obtaining adequate care ought not to be excessive or to fall disproportionately on particular individuals. Communities need to be empowered to address distribution problems.

4. *When equity occurs through the operation of private forces, there is no need for government involvement.* However, the ultimate responsibility for ensuring that society's obligation is met—through a combination of public and private sector arrangements—rests with the federal government.

5. *The cost of achieving equitable access to health care ought to be shared fairly.* The cost of securing health care for those who are unable to pay ought to be spread equitably at the national level and should not fall more heavily on the shoulders of particular practitioners, institutions, or residents of different localities.

6. *Efforts to contain rising health care costs are important but should not focus on limiting the attainment of equitable access for the least-served portion of the public.* Measures designed to contain health care costs that exacerbate existing inequities or impede the achievement of equity are unacceptable from a moral standpoint. Aggregates in the community should be involved in planning and problem-solving to increase the distribution of resources where those resources are most needed.

Ethical Decision-making in Community Health Nursing

The key values of self-determination, well-being, and equity influence nursing practice in many ways. The value of self-determination has implications for how community health nurses regard:

- the choices of clients,
- privacy,
- informed consent, and
- diminished capacity for self-determination.

The value of well-being has implications for how community health nurses seek to:

- prevent harm and provide benefits to client populations,
- determine effectiveness of nursing services, and
- weigh costs of services against real client benefits.

The value of equity has implications for community health nursing in terms of its priorities for:

- distributing health goods (macroallocation issues), and
- deciding which populations will obtain available health goods and services (microallocation issues).

Decisions based on one value mean that this value often will conflict with other values. For example, deciding primarily on the basis of client well-being may conflict with deciding on the basis of self-determination or equity. How community health nurses balance these values may even conflict with their own personal values or the professional values of nursing as a whole. In these situations, values clarification techniques used with an ethical decision-making process may assist in producing decisions that promote the greatest well-being for clients without substantially reducing their self-determination or ignoring equity.

Ethical Principles

Seven fundamental ethical principles provide guidance in making decisions regarding clients' care: respect, autonomy, beneficence, nonmaleficence, justice, veracity, and fidelity (Guido, 2006; Thompson, Melia, & Boyd, 2000).

Respect

The principle of **respect** refers to treating people as unique, equal, and responsible moral agents. This principle emphasizes one's importance as a member of the community and of the health services team. To apply this principle in decision-making is to acknowledge community clients as valued participants in shaping their own and the community's health outcomes. It includes treating them as equals on the health team and holding them, as well as their views, in high regard.

Autonomy

The principle of **autonomy** means freedom of choice and the exercise of people's rights. Individualism and self-determination are dominant values underlying this principle. As nurses apply this principle in community health, they promote individuals' and groups' rights to and involvement in decision-making. This is true, however, only so long as those decisions enhance these individuals' and groups' well-being and do not harm the well-being of others (Franco, 2005). When applying this principle, nurses should make certain that clients are fully informed and that the decisions are made deliberately, with careful consideration of the consequences (see From the Case Files III).

Beneficence

The ethical principle of **beneficence** means doing good or benefiting others. It is the promotion of good or taking action to ensure positive outcomes on behalf of clients. In community health, the nurse applies the principle of benef-

---

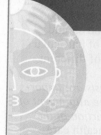

From the Case Files III

Tom Hardy, PHN—An Elderly Client Gives Up

Tom Hardy, PHN, has been assigned to monitor Mr. Jack, an elderly man who was diagnosed with tuberculosis (TB) (positive skin test, positive sputum and x-ray). Mr. Jack's wife unexpectedly died recently, and he is depressed and wants to "join her." He is not eating or sleeping much. He refuses to take his TB medications, nor his eight other medications for heart disease, thyroid insufficiency, type 2 diabetes, glaucoma, high cholesterol and triglycerides, and hypertension. He has consistently refused any of Tom's suggestions or assistance. He does not want to see a mental health counselor, and Tom wonders if he should continue to make home visits. He has a busy caseload and needs to focus on the most pressing cases. Mr. Jack's children feel that his depression and refusal of medications is a "temporary condition" in response to his wife's death, and ask for Tom's assistance in keeping him healthy. Why is this an ethical dilemma? What are the ethical principles involved? What does Mr. Jack value? What are his children's values? Prioritize your values. What are the possible actions you could take?

icence by making decisions that actively promote community clients' best interests and well-being. Examples might encompass the development of a seniors' health program that ensures equal access to all in the community who are in need, and the support of programs to encourage preschool immunizations.

Nonmaleficence

The principle of **nonmaleficence** means avoiding or preventing harm to others as a consequence of a person's own choices and actions. This involves taking steps to avoid negative consequences. Community health nurses can apply this ethical principle in decision-making by actions such as encouraging physicians to prescribe drugs with the fewest side effects, promoting legislation to protect the environment from pollutants emitted from gasoline even if it raises prices, and lobbying for lower speed limits or gun controls to save lives.

Justice

The principle of **justice** refers to treating people fairly. It means the fair distribution of both benefits and costs among society's members. Examples might include: equal access to health care, equitable distribution of services to rural as well as urban populations, not limiting the amount or quality of services because of income level, and fair distribution of resources—all of these draw on the principle of justice.

Within this principle are three different views on allocation, or what constitutes the meaning of "fair" distribution. One, **distributive justice**, says that benefits should be given first to the disadvantaged or those who need them most (see Levels of Prevention Pyramid). Decisions based on this view particularly help the needy, although it may mean withholding goods from others who also are also deserving but less in need (e.g., food stamps). The second view, **egalitarian justice**, promotes decisions based on equal distribution of benefits to everyone, regardless of need (e.g., Medicare). The third, **restorative justice**, determines that benefits should go primarily to those who have been wronged by prior injustice, such as victims of crime or racial discrimination. Programs are in place to compensate victims for their injury or families for their loss—a beginning step to "restore justice." Another example includes the funds that were set up by several agencies, corporations, and groups to assist the families of the victims of the September 11, 2001 terrorist attacks. The principle of justice seeks to promote equity, a value that was discussed in the previous section.

Veracity

The principle of **veracity** refers to telling the truth. Community clients deserve to be given accurate information in a timely manner. To withhold information or not tell the truth can be self-serving to the nurse or other health care providers and hurtful, as well as disrespectful, to clients. Truth-telling involves treating clients as equals, and it expands the opportunity for greater client involvement, as well as provides needed information for decision-making (Arries, 2006).

Fidelity

The final ethical principle, **fidelity**, means keeping promises. People deserve to count on commitments being met. This principle involves the issues of trust and trustworthiness. Nurses who follow through on what they have said earn their clients' respect and trust. In turn, this influences the quality of the nurse's relationship with clients, who then are more likely to share information, which leads to improved decisions and better health. Conversely, when a promise (e.g., a commitment to institute child care during health classes) is not kept, community members may lose faith and interest in participation.

Ethical Standards and Guidelines

As the number and complexity of ethical decisions in community health increase, so too does the need for ethical standards and guidelines to help nurses make the best choices possible. The ANA's *Code for Nurses with Interpretive Statements* (2001) provides a helpful guide. Some health care organizations and community agencies, using the ANA code or a similar document, have developed their own specific standards and guidelines.

More health care organizations are using ethics committees or ethics rounds to deal with ethical aspects of client services (Guido, 2006). These committees are common in the acute care setting and in senior and long-term care settings, and they may focus on such issues as caregiving dilemmas that may involve practitioner negligence or poor client outcomes and the related health care decisions. However, these committees also function in a variety of community health care settings. In long-term care and home care settings, such a committee may consider conflicts in client care issues that involve family members. In public health agencies, cases of clients with complicated communicable disease diagnoses and health care provider concerns are discussed as they relate to policy, protocols, and the health and safety of the broader population.

Summary

Involvement in community health nursing research can be an exciting opportunity to contribute to the body of nursing knowledge and influence changes in nursing practice and in community health programs and policies. Research findings also enable community health nurses to promote health and prevent illness among at-risk populations and to design and evaluate community-based interventions. Evidence-based practice is essential to ensuring cost-efficient and effective interventions for our clients. Systematic reviews can provide direction for those who have developed a "burning clinical question." Finding accurate, complete information and critically appraising it is vital (see Evidence-Based Practice: Handwashing).

Research is defined as the systematic collection and analysis of data related to a particular problem or phenomenon. *Quantitative research* concerns data that can be measured objectively. It is helpful in identifying a problem or a

EVIDENCE-BASED PRACTICE

Handwashing

As nurses, we are taught the importance of handwashing. In nursing school, we are educated to wash our hands before and after patient care—it is often drilled into us. But, when you work in the community, you do not always have ready access to soap and water. Many PHNs choose to carry small bottles of hand sanitizer as a practical alternative to handwashing. But, is this effective? A small study of health care workers in France found that handrubbing with an alcohol-based mixture was better than handwashing with antiseptic soap when it came to reducing hand bacterial contamination for workers in

intensive care settings (Girou, Loyeau, Legrand, et al., 2002). A larger French study found that handrubbing with an alcohol solution was as effective as handscrubbing with antiseptic soap in preventing infections of surgical sites. They noted no statistical differences in development of nosocomial infections of patients' surgical sites between the two groups (Parienti, Thibon, Heller, et al., 2002). Where would you go to find a systematic or integrative review of this subject? How would you go about presenting this information at a staff meeting to stimulate changes in policies and procedures?

---

relationship between two or more variables; however, because it requires the researcher to focus on a part instead of the whole, if used exclusively it can limit nursing knowledge. *Qualitative research* emphasizes subjectivity and the meaning of experiences to individuals.

The research process includes nine steps:

1. Identify an area of interest.
2. Formulate a research question or statement.
3. Review the literature.
4. Select a conceptual model.
5. Choose a research design.
6. Obtain Institutional Review Board or Human Subjects Committee approval.
7. Collect and analyze data.
8. Interpret results.
9. Communicate findings.

Although the process is the same regardless of nursing specialty, community health nurses have a unique opportunity to expand nursing knowledge in relation to community health issues and the health needs of aggregates and families.

Research has a significant impact on community health and nursing practice in three ways. It provides new knowledge that helps to shape health policy, improve service delivery, and promote the public's health. It contributes to nursing knowledge and the improvement of nursing practice. And it offers the potential to enhance nursing's status and influence through documentation of the effectiveness of nursing interventions and broader recognition of nursing's contributions to health services.

Nurses must become responsible users of research, keeping abreast of new knowledge and applying it in practice. Nurses must learn to evaluate nursing research articles critically, assessing their validity and applicability to their own practice. Nurses should subscribe to and read nursing research journals and discuss research studies with colleagues and supervisors. More community health nurses must also conduct research studies of their own or in collaboration with other

community health professionals. A commitment to the use and conduct of research will move the nursing profession forward and enhance its influence on the health of at-risk populations.

Values and ethical principles strongly influence community health nursing practice and ethical decision-making. Values are lasting beliefs that are important to individuals, groups, and cultures. A value system organizes these beliefs into a hierarchy of relative importance that motivates and guides human behavior. Values function as standards for behavior, as criteria for attitudes, and as standards for moral judgments, and they give expression to human needs. The nature of values can be understood by examining their qualities of endurance, their hierarchical arrangement, and their function as prescriptive–proscriptive beliefs, and by examining them in terms of reference and preference.

The nurse often is faced with decisions that affect client's values and involve conflicting moral values and ethical dilemmas. Understanding what personal values are and how they affect behavior assists the nurse in making ethical evaluations and addressing ethical conflicts in practice. Various strategies can guide the nurse in making these decisions; one example is values clarification, which clarifies what values are important. Several frameworks for ethical decision-making that include the identification and clarification of values impinging on the making of ethical decisions were discussed in this chapter.

Three key human values influence client health and nurse decision-making: the right to make decisions regarding a person's health (self-determination), the right to health and well-being, and the right to equal access and quality of health care. At times, these values are affected by the value of self-interest on the part of another person or a system. Seven fundamental principles guide community health nurses in making ethical decisions: respect, autonomy, beneficence, nonmaleficence, justice, veracity, and fidelity. ■

ACTIVITIES TO PROMOTE CRITICAL THINKING

1. As a community health nurse working in a large city, you notice a group of small children playing in a vacant, unfenced lot bordered by a busy street. List three research questions you might consider using to study the situation.
2. You want to determine whether a group of sexually active teenagers who are at risk for acquired immunodeficiency syndrome (AIDS) would be receptive to an educational program on HIV/AIDS. Formulate a research question, describe a conceptual framework you might use in your study, and defend your choice.
3. Select a community health nursing research article from the references listed in this chapter (or choose one of your own) and analyze its potential impact on health policy and on community health nursing practice.
4. You have just completed a study on the effectiveness of a series of birth control classes in three high schools, and the results show a reduction in the number of pregnancies over the last year. Describe three ways in which you could disseminate this information to your nursing colleagues and other community health professionals.
5. You are alarmed to note that the new area to which you have been assigned has high rates of tuberculosis. Using the Internet and your college library databases to research this topic, determine the most effective forms of treatment and discuss the feasibility of implementing some new approaches with your specific target population.
6. Describe where you stand on the following issues. For each statement, decide whether you strongly agree, agree, disagree, strongly disagree, or are undecided.
   a. Clients have the right to participate in all decisions related to their health care.
   b. Nurses need a system designed to credit self-study.
   c. Continuing education should not be mandatory to maintain licensure.
   d. Clients always should be told the truth.
   e. Standards of nursing practice should be enforced by state examining boards.
   f. Nurses should be required to take relicensure examinations every 5 years.
   g. Clients should be allowed to read their health record on request.
   h. Abortion on demand should be an option available to every woman.
   i. Critically ill newborns should be allowed to die.
   j. Laws should guarantee desired health care for each person in this country.
   k. Organ donorship should be automatic unless a waiver to refuse has been signed.
7. In a grid similar to the one shown, write a statement of belief in the space provided and examine it in relation to the seven steps of the process of valuing. Areas of confusion and conflict in nursing practice that should be examined are peer review, accountability, confidentiality, euthanasia, licensure, clients' rights, organ donation, abortion, informed consent, and terminating treatment. To the right of your statements, check the appropriate boxes to indicate when your beliefs reflect one or more of the seven steps in the valuing process. Is your belief a value according to the valuing process?

Statement	Freely chosen	Alternatives	Consequences	Cherished	Affirmed	Incorporated	Employed
	1	2	3	4	5	6	7

8. Rank in order the following 12 potential nursing actions, using "1" to indicate the most important choice in a client–community health nurse relationship and "12" to indicate the least important choice.
   _____ Touching clients
   _____ Empathetically listening to clients
   _____ Disclosing yourself to clients
   _____ Becoming emotionally involved with clients
   _____ Teaching clients
   _____ Being honest in answering clients' questions
   _____ Seeing that clients conform to professionals' advice
   _____ Helping to decrease clients' anxiety
   _____ Making sure that clients are involved in decision-making
   _____ Following legal mandates regarding health practices
   _____ Remaining "professional" with clients
   _____ (Add an alternative of your own)

(continued on next page)

Examine your ordering of these options. What values can be identified based on your responses in this exercise? How do these values emerge in your behavior?

9. Request to attend two or three sessions of an ethics committee meeting of a community health agency.

Observe and make notes on (a) what values are evident in the discussion, (b) what ethical principles are used, (c) what decision-making framework is used, and (d) what you would have liked to contribute if you had been a member of the committee.

References

Ahmad, S. (2005a). Closing the youth access gap: The projected health benefits and cost savings of a national policy to raise the legal smoking age to 21 in the United States. *Health Policy, 75*(1), 74–84.

Ahmad, S. (2005b). The cost-effectiveness of raising the legal smoking age in California. *Medical Decision Making, 25*(3), 330–340.

Ahmad, S. (2005c). Increasing excise taxes on cigarettes in California: A dynamic simulation of health and economic impacts. *Preventive Medicine, 41*(1), 276–283.

Alamar, B., & Glantz, S.A. (2006). Effect of increased social unacceptability of cigarette smoking on reduction in cigarette consumption. *American Journal of Public Health, 96*(8), 1359–1363.

Albrecht, S., Maloni, J., Thomas, K., Jones, R., Halleran, J., & Osborne, J. (2004). Smoking cessation counseling for pregnant women who smoke: Scientific basis for practice for WWHONN's SUCCESS project. *Journal of Obstetric, Gynecological and Neonatal Nursing, 33*(3), 298–304.

American Academy of Pediatrics. (2005). Policy statement: Task force on sudden infant death syndrome. *Pediatrics, 116*(5), 1245–1255.

American Nurses Association. (2001). *Code for nurses with interpretive statements.* Washington, DC: Author.

Arries, E. (2006). Virtue ethics: An approach to moral dilemmas in nursing. *Kidney International, 69*(6), 954–955.

Associated Press. (2006). U.S. halts enrollment in major AIDS drug study. Retrieved January 18, 2006 from http//www.msnbc.msn.com/id/10907973/print/1/displaymode/1098/.

Aston, M., Meagher-Stewart, D., Sheppard-Lemoine, D., Vukic, A., & Chircop, A. (2006). Family health nursing and empowering relationships. *Pediatric Nursing, 32*(1), 61–67.

Axtell-Thompson, L.M. (2005). Consumer directed health care: Ethical limits to choice and responsibility. *Journal of Medical Philosophy, 39*(2), 207–226.

Beauchamp, T., & Childress, J. (2001). *Principles of biomedical ethics* (5th ed.). Oxford, UK: Oxford University Press.

Blais, K.K., Hayes, J.S., Kozier, B., & Erb, G. (2006). *Professional nursing practice: Concepts and perspectives.* Upper Saddle River, NJ: Pearson Prentice Hall.

Burroughs, A.M. (2005). The medical examination in United States immigration applications: The potential use of genetic testing leads to heightened privacy concerns. *The Journal of Biolaw & Business, 8*(4), 22–32.

Cava, M., Fay, K., Beanlands, H., McCay, E., & Wignall, R. (2005). The experience of quarantine for individuals affected by SARS in Toronto. *Public Health Nursing, 22*(5), 398–406.

Centers for Disease Control & Prevention (CDC). (2008). *The Tuskegee timeline:* Retrieved August 2, 2008 from http://www.cdc.gov/tuskgee/timeline.htm.

Centers for Disease Control and Prevention (CDC). (2006). *Quickstats: Infant mortality rates by selected racial/ethnic populations, United States, 2002.* Retrieved July 4, 2008 from http://ww.cdc.gov/mmwr/preview/mmwrhtml/mm5405a5.htm.

Ciliska, D., Pinelli, J., DiCenso, A., & Cullum, N. (2001). Resources to enhance evidence-based nursing practice. *AACN Clinical Issues, 12*(2), 520–528.

Colby, A., & Kohlberg, L. (1987). *The measurement of moral judgment: Theoretical foundations and research validation* (Vol. 1). New York: Cambridge University Press.

Coopersmith, S. (1967). *The antecedents of self-esteem.* San Francisco: Freeman & Company.

Cox, M.F. (2006). Racial differences in parenting dimensions and adolescent condom use at sexual debut. *Public Health Nursing, 23*(1), 2–10.

Darke, P., & Chaiken, S. (2005). The pursuit of self-interest: Self-interest bias in attitude judgment and persuasion. *Journal of Personality & Social Psychology, 89*(6), 864–883.

Delmonico, F.L. (2006). What is the system failure? *Kidney International, 69*(6), 957–959.

Des Jardin, K. (2001). Political involvement in nursing: Politics, ethics, and strategic action. *AORN Journal, 74*(5), 614–626.

Douglas, M.R., Mallonee, S., & Istre, G.R. (1999). Estimating the proportion of homes with functioning smoke alarms: A comparison of telephone survey and household survey results. *American Journal of Public Health, 89*(7), 1112–1114.

Drew, D., & Hewitt, H. (2006). A qualitative approach to understanding patients' diagnosis of Lyme disease. *Public Health Nursing, 23*(1), 20–26.

Eckenrode, J., Ganzel, B., Henderson, C., Smith, E., Olds, D.L., Powers, J., et al. (2000). Preventing child abuse and neglect with a program of nurse home visitation: The limiting effects of domestic violence. *JAMA, 284*(11), 1385–1391.

Eckenrode, J., Zielinski, D., Smith, E., Marcynyszyn, L., Henderson, C., Kitzman, H., et al. (2001). Child maltreatment and the early onset of problem behaviors: Can a program of nurse home visitation break the link? *Developmental Psychopathology, 13*(4), 873–890.

Edelman, C., & Mandle, C. (2006). *Health promotion throughout the life span* (6th ed.). St. Louis: Elsevier-Mosby.

Feldman, P., Murtaugh, C., Pezzin, L., McDonald, M., & Peng, T. (2005). Just-in-time evidence-based e-mail "reminders" in home health care: Impact on patient outcomes. *Health Services Research, 40*(3), 865–885.

Feldman-Stewart, D., Brennenstuhl, S., Brundage, M., & Roques, T. (2006). An explicit values clarification task: Development and validation. *Patient Education and Counseling* (in press).

Finer, L.B., & Henshaw, S.K. (2006). Disparities in rates of unintended pregnancy in the United States, 1994 and 2001. *Perspectives on Sexual and Reproductive Health, 88*(2), 90–96.

First Candle. (2006). Back to Sleep Campaign. Retrieved July 4, 2008 from http://www.firstcandle.org/health/health_backto.html.

Fothergill, A., Palumbo, M., Rambur, B., Reinier, K., & McIntosh, B. (2005). The volunteer potential of inactive nurses for disaster preparedness. *Public Health Nursing, 22*(5), 414–421.

Franco, G. (2005). Ethical analysis of the decision-making process in occupational health practice. *Medical Law, 96*(5), 375–382.

Fredrickson, D., Davis, T., Arnould, C., Kennen, E., Hurniston, S., Cross, J., & Bocchini, J. (2004). Childhood immunization refusal: Provider and parent perceptions. *Family Medicine, 36*(6), 431–439.

Gaffney, K.F., & Altieri, L.B. (2001). Mothers' ranking of clinical intervention strategies used to promote infant health. *Pediatric Nursing, 27*(5), 510–515.

Gagnon, M., Hibert, R., Dube, M., & Dubois, M. (2006). Development and validation of an instrument measuring individual empowerment in relation to personal health care: The Health Care Empowerment Questionnaire (HCEQ). *American Journal of Health Promotion, 20*(6), 429–435.

Gessert, C., Elliott, B., & McAlpine, C. (2006). Family decision-making for nursing home residents with dementia: Rural-urban differences. *The Journal of Rural Health, 22*(1), 1–8.

Gilligan, C. (1982). *In a different voice.* Cambridge, MA: Harvard University Press.

Girou, E.M., Loyeau, S., Legrand, P., Oppein, F., & Brun-Buisson, C. (2002). Efficacy of handrubbing with alcohol based solution versus standard handwashing with antiseptic soap: Randomized clinical trial. *British Medical Journal, 325*, 362–365.

Glasser, W. (1998). *Choice theory: A new psychology of personal freedom.* New York: Harper Collins Publishers.

Groner, J., French, G., Ahijevych, K., & Wewers, M. (2005). Process evaluation of a nurse-delivered smoking relapse prevention program for new mothers. *Journal of Community Health Nursing, 22*(3), 157–167.

Guido, G.W. (2006). *Legal and ethical issues in nursing* (4th ed.). Upper Saddle River, NJ: Pearson-Prentice Hall.

Hoffman, H., Damus, K., Hillman, L., & Krongrad, E. (1988). Risk factors for SIDS. Results of the National Institute of Child Health and Human Development SIDS Cooperative Epidemiological Study. *Annals of the New York Academy of Sciences, 533*, 13–30.

Hurst, S., & Mauron, A. (2006). The ethics of palliative care and eiuthanasia: Exploring common values. *Palliative Medicine, 20*(2), 107–112.

Institute of Medicine. (2000). *To err is human: Building a safer health care system.* Washington, DC: National Academy Press.

Institute of Medicine. (2001). *Crossing the quality chasm: A new health system for the 21st century.* Washington, DC: National Academy Press.

Institute of Medicine. (2003). *Priority areas for national action: Transforming health care quality.* Washington, DC: National Academy Press.

Iserson, K.V. (1999). Ethical issues in emergency medicine. *Emergency Medicine Clinics of North America, 17*(2), 283–306.

Kelly, C. (2006). *Nurses' moral practice: Investing and discounting self.* Indianapolis, IN: Sigma Theta Tau International.

Kerr, J., Eves, F., & Carroll, D. (2001). Encouraging stair use: Stair-riser banners are better than posters. *American Journal of Public Health, 91*(8), 1192–1193.

Kitzman, H., Olds, D., Sidora, K., Henderson, C., Hanks, C., Cole, R., et al. (2000). Enduring effects of nurse home visitation on maternal life course: A 3-year follow-up of a randomized trial. *Journal of the American Medical Association, 283*(15), 1983–1989.

Kluckhohn, C. (1951). Values and value-orientations in the theory of action: An exploration in definition and classification. In Parsons, T., & Shils, E.A. (Eds.), *Toward a general theory of action* (pp. 388–433). Cambridge, MA: Harvard University Press.

Koniak-Griffin, D., Verzemnieks, I., Anderson, N., Brecht, M., Lesser, J., Kim, S., & Turner-Pluta, C. (2003). Nurse visitation for adolescent mothers: Two-year infant health and maternal outcomes. *Nursing Research, 52*(2), 127–136.

Levy, D., Nikolayev, I., & Mumford, E. (2005). Recent trends in smoking and the role of public policies: Results from the SimSmoke tobacco control policy simulation model. *Addiction, 100*(10), 1526–1536.

Li, D.K., Petitti, D., Willinger, M., McMahon, R., Odouli, R., Vu, H., & Hoffman, H. (2003). Infant sleeping position and the risk of sudden infant death syndrome in California, 1997–2000. *American Journal of Epidemiology, 157*, 446–455.

Malloy, M., & Freeman, D. (2000). Birth weight- and gestational age-specific sudden infant death syndrome mortality: United States, 1991 versus 1995. *Pediatrics, 105*(6), 1227–1231.

Maslow, A. (1969). *Toward a psychology of being* (2nd ed.). New York: Van Nostrand.

McKenzie, J.F., & Smeltzer, J.L. (2001). *Planning, implementing and evaluating health promotion programs: A primer* (3rd ed.). Needham Heights, MA: Allyn & Bacon.

Merriam Webster Online Dictionary. (2006). *Ethics.* Retrieved July 4, 2008 from http://www.m-w.com/dictionary/ethics.

Mitchell, E., Tuohy, P., Brunt, J., Thompson, J., Clements, M., Stewart, W., Ford, R., & Taylor, B. (1997). Risk factors for sudden infant death syndrome following the prevention campaign in New Zealand: A prospective study. *Pediatrics, 100*(5), 835–840.

Morris, M., Scott-Findlay, S., & Estabrooks, C. (2001). Evidence-based nursing Websites: Finding the best resources. *AACN Clinical Issues, 12*(4), 578–587.

Netermeyer, R., Andrews, J.C., & Burton, S. (2005). Effects of antismoking advertising-based beliefs on adult smokers' consideration of quitting. *American Journal of Public Health, 95*(6), 1062–1066.

Nguyen, J., Carson, M., Parris, K., & Place, P. (2003). A comparison pilot study of public health nursing home visitation program interventions for pregnant Hispanic adolescents. *Public Health Nursing, 20*(5), 412–418.

Nurse-Family Partnership. (2008). *Research evidence.* Retrieved August 2, 2008 from http://www.nursefamilypartnership.org/content/index.cfm?fuseaction=showContent&conentID=4&navID=4.

Olds, D., Eckenrode, J., Henderson, C., Kitzman, H., Powers, J., Cole, R., et al. (1997). Long-term effects of home visitation on maternal life course and child abuse and neglect: Fifteen-year follow-up of a randomized trial. *Journal of the American Medical Association, 278*(8), 637–643.

Olds, D., Kitzman, H., Cole, R., Robinson J., Sidora, K., Luckey, D., Henderson, C., Hanks, C., Bondy, J., & Holmberg, J. (2004). Effects of nurse home-visiting on maternal life course and child development: Age 6 follow-up results of a randomized trial. *Pediatrics, 114*(6), 1550–1559.

Olds, D., Robinson, J., Pettitt, L., Luckey, D., Holmberg, J., Ng, R.K., Isacks, K., Sheff, K., & Henderson, C.R. (2004). Effects of home visits by paraprofessionals and by nurses: Age 4 follow-up results of a randomized trial. *Pediatrics, 114*(6), 1560–1568.

Ong, M., & Glantz, S.A. (2005). Free nicotine replacement therapy programs vs. implementing smoke-free workplaces: A cost-effectiveness comparison. *American Journal of Public Health, 95*(1), 969–975.

Opdal, S., & Rognum, T. (2004). The sudden infant death syndrome gene: Does it exist? *Pediatrics, 114*(4), 506–512.

Parienti, J., Thibon, P., Heller, R., Le Roux, Y., von Theobald, P., Bensadoun, H., Bouvet, A., Lemarchand, F., & Coutour, X. (2002). Hand-rubbing with an aqueous alcoholic solution vs. traditional surgical hand-scrubbing and 30-day surgical site infection rates. *The Journal of the American Medical Association (JAMA), 288*(6), 722–727.

Polivka, B. (2006). Needs assessment and intervention strategies to reduce lead-poisoning risk among low-income Ohio toddlers. *Public Health Nursing, 23*(1), 52–58.

Porter-O'Grady, T. (2006). A new age for practice: Creating the framework for evidence. In Malloch, K., & Porter-O'Grady, T.

(Eds.), *Introduction to evidence-based practice in nursing and health care*, pp. 1–29. Sudbury, MA: Jones & Bartlett Publishers.

Rand Corporation. (2005). *Research brief: Proven benefits of early childhood interventions.* Santa Monica, CA: Author.

Redman, B.K. (2001). *Measurement tools in clinical ethics.* Thousand Oaks, CA: Sage.

Remington, R. (2002). Calming music and hand massage with agitated elderly. *Nursing Research, 51*(5), 317–323.

Remler, D., & Glied, S. (2003). What other programs can teach us: Increasing participation in health insurance programs. *American Journal of Public Health, 93*(1), 67–74.

Ries, H.N.M., & Moysa, G. (2005). Legal protections of electronic health records: Issues of consent and security. *Health Law Review, 14*(1), 18–25.

Rokeach, M. (1973). *The nature of human values.* New York: Free Press.

Rothman, N., Lourie, R., & Gaughan, J. (2002). Lead awareness: North Philly style. *American Journal of Public Health, 92*(5), 739–741.

Rueda, S., Park-Wyllie, L., Bayoumi, A., Tynan, A., Anoniou, T., Rourke, S., & Glazier, R. (2006). Patient support and education for promoting adherence to highly active antiretroviral therapy for HIV/AIDS. Cochrane Database of Systematic Reviews 2006, 3(CD001442). Retrieved July 4, 2008 from http://www.mrw.interscience.wiley.com/cochrane/clsysrev/-article/CD001442/frame.html.

Sanares, D., & Heliker, D. (2006). A framework for nursing clinical inquiry: Pathway toward evidence-based nursing practice. In Malloch, K., & Porter-O'Grady, T. (Eds.), *Introduction to evidence-based practice in nursing and health care*, pp. 31–64. Sudbury, MA: Jones & Bartlett Publishers.

Sawatzky, J., & Naimark, B. (2005). Cardiovascular health promotion in aging women: Validating a population health approach. *Public Health Nursing, 22*(5), 379–388.

Shreffler-Grant, J., Weinert, C., Nichols, E., & Ide, B. (2005). Complementary therapy use among older rural adults. *Public Health Nursing, 22*(4), 323–331.

Skinner, A., Slifkin, R., & Mayer, M. (2006). The effect of rural residence on dental unmet need for children with special health care needs. *The Journal of Rural Health, 22*(1), 36–42.

Sloand, E., & Gebrian, B. (2006). Fathers clubs to improve child health in rural Haiti. *Public Health Nursing, 23*(1), 46–51.

Smith, L., Oveku, S., Homer, C., & Zuckerman, B. (2006). Sickle cell disease: A question of equity and quality. *Pediatrics, 117*(5), 1763–1770.

Speck, B., & Looney, S. (2006). Self-reported physical activity validated by pedometer: A pilot study. *Public Health Nursing, 23*(1), 88–94.

Sung, H.C., & Chang, A.M. (2005). Use of preferred music to decrease agitated behaviours in older people with dementia: A review of the literature. *Journal of Clinical Nursing, 14*(9), 1133–1140.

The Cochrane Collaboration. (2008). *An introduction to Cochrane reviews and the Cochrane Library.* Retrieved August 2, 2008 from http://www.cochrane.org/reviews/clibintro.htm.

Thogmartin, J., Siebert, C., & Pellan, W. (2001). Sleep position and bed-sharing in sudden infant deaths: An examination of autopsy findings. *Journal of Pediatrics, 138*(2), 212–217.

Thomas, E., Elliott, E., & Naughton, G. (2006). Exercise for type 2 diabetes mellitus. *Cochrane Database of Systematic Reviews 2006, 3*(CD002968). Retrieved July 4, 2008 from http://www.mrw.interscience.wiley.com/cochrane/clsysrev/articles/CD002968/frame.html.

Thompson, C., Cullum, N., McCaughan, D., Sheldon, T., & Raynor, P. (2004). Nurses, information use, and clinical decision making—The real world potential for evidence-based decisions in nursing. *Evidence-Based Nursing, 7,* 68–72.

Thompson, I.E., Melia, K.M., & Boyd, K.M. (2000). *Nursing ethics* (4th ed.). Edinburgh: Churchill Livingstone.

University of Alberta Medical School. (2006). Finding and using articles about therapy. Retrieved July 4, 2008 from http://www.med.ualbrta.ca/ebm/therapy.htm.

U.S. Department of Health & Human Services (USDHHS). (2006a). *Informed consent checklist—basic & additional elements.* Retrieved from http://www.hhs.gov/ohrp/humansubjects/assurance.consentckls.htm.

U.S. Department of Health & Human Services. (2006b). Special requirements. Retrieved July 4, 2008 from http://www.hhs.gov/ohrp/humansubjects/guidance/basics.htm.

Uustal, D.B. (1977). The use of values clarification in nursing practice. *Journal of Continuing Education in Nursing, 8,* 8–13.

Uustal, D.B. (1978). Values clarification in nursing. *American Journal of Nursing, 78,* 2058–2063.

Valente, S.M. (2005). Evaluation of innovative research-based fact sheets. *Journal of Nurses Staff Development, 21*(4), 171–176.

Wewers, M.E., Sarna, L., & Rice, V.H. (2006). Nursing research and treatment of tobacco dependence: State of the science. *Nursing Research, 55*(4S), 511–515.

Willinger, M., James, L., & Catz, C. (1991). Defining the sudden infant death syndrome (SIDS): Deliberations of an expert panel convened by the National Institute of Child Health and Human Development. *Pediatric Pathology, 11*(5), 677–684.

Yoshimura, Y. (2006). Bioethical aspects of regenerative and reproductive medicine. *Human Cell: Official Journal of Human Cell Research Society, 19*(2), 83–86.

Zahner, S.J., & Gredig, Q.B. (2005). Public health nursing practice change and recommendations for improvement. *Public Health Nursing, 22*(5), 420–429.

Internet Resources

American Nurses Association: *http://www.ana.org*
American Nurses Foundation: *http://www.nursingworld.org/anf/*
Bioethics News: *http://www.bioethics.net*
Current Clinical Trials: *http://www.clinicaltrials.gov*
Eastern Nursing Research Society: *http://www.enrs.org*
Healthy People 2010: *http://www.health.gov/healthypeople*
International Council of Nurses: *http://www.icn.ch/index.html*
Midwest Nursing Research Society: *http://www.mnrs.org*
National Institute of Nursing Research: *http://www.nih.gov/ninr*
Sigma Theta Tau International Registry of Nursing Research: *http://www.stti.iupui.edu/VirginiaHendersonLibrary/RegistryofNursingResearch.aspx*
Southern Nursing Research Society: *http://www.snrs.org*
Triservice Nursing Research Program/Military Nursing: *http://www.usuhs.mil/tsnrp*
Western Institute of Nursing: *http://www.winuring.org*

5

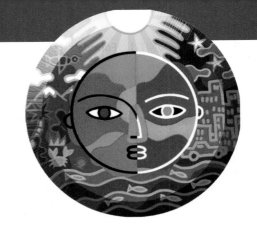

Transcultural Nursing in the Community

LEARNING OBJECTIVES

Upon mastery of this chapter, you should be able to:

◆ Define and explain the concept of culture.
◆ Discuss the meaning of cultural diversity and its significance for community health nursing.
◆ Describe the meaning and effects of ethnocentrism on community health nursing practice.
◆ Identify five characteristics shared by all cultures.
◆ Contrast the health-related values, beliefs, and practices of selected culturally diverse populations with those of the dominant U.S. culture.
◆ Conduct a cultural assessment.
◆ Apply transcultural nursing principles in community health nursing practice.

"People everywhere share common biological and psychological needs, and the function of all cultures is to fulfill such needs; the nature of the culture is determined by its function."

—Bronislaw Malinowski (1884–1942), Cultural Anthropologist

KEY TERMS

Complementary therapies
Cultural assessment
Cultural diversity
Cultural relativism
Cultural self-awareness
Cultural sensitivity
Culture
Culture shock
Dominant values
Enculturation
Ethnic group
Ethnicity
Ethnocentrism
Ethnorelativism
Folk medicine
Home remedies
Integrated health care
Microculture
Minority group
Norms
Race
Subcultures
Tacit
Transcultural nursing
Value

American society values individuality, and we are a country of immigrants. Many different cultural groups and races built this nation. For example, pilgrims came here hundreds of years ago, to seek freedom to practice their religious beliefs. It took powerful independence to pioneer the West in the 1800s. Partly because of this pioneer spirit, people from all nations have sought to live in America. Some came of their own free will for adventure and opportunity. Others saw this land as a refuge from political, religious, or economic strife. Still others were brought here against their will. Consequently, we have not become the ideal *melting pot* once described, but rather, an amalgamation of people who have different values, ideals, and behaviors.

Americans have many differences, but we also have much in common. In the Western culture, there is joy in seeing children grow and develop in unique ways. An individual's creative achievements are applauded. There is also respect for one another's personal preferences about food, dress, or personal beliefs. The right to be oneself—and thereby to be different from others—is even protected by state and federal laws.

Although individuality is a cherished American value, there are limits to the range of differences most Americans find acceptable. People whose behavior falls outside the acceptable range may be labeled as misfits. For example, the U.S. culture approves moderate social drinking, but not alcoholism. The beliefs and sanctions of the dominant or majority culture are called **dominant values**. In the United States, the majority culture is made up largely of European Americans whose dominant values include the work ethic, thrift, success, independence, initiative, privacy, cleanliness, youthfulness, attractive appearance, and a focus on the future. However, in some regions and states, European Americans are not the majority. For example, in California, 53% of the population are "people of color," and the dominant culture is no longer European American (California Pan-Ethnic Health Network, 2007, ¶ 3); the proportion of the population identified as White is projected to continue to fall below other ethnicities (Legislative Analyst's Office, 2000).

Dominant values are important to consider in the practice of community health nursing because they can shape people's thoughts and behaviors. Why are some client behaviors acceptable to health professionals and others not? Why do nurses have such difficulty persuading certain clients to accept new ways of thinking and acting? Explanations can be found by examining the concept of culture, especially its influence on health and on community health nursing practice. For example, an emphasis on the need for milk in the diet may reflect cultural blindness, considering the number of people in diverse ethnic groups who are lactose intolerant (Swagerty, Walling, & Klein, 2002). Regardless of their own cultural backgrounds, nurses are socialized throughout the educational process; the biomedical model is frequently the framework, and dominant social values are often involuntarily reinforced.

THE MEANING OF CULTURE

Culture refers to the beliefs, values, and behavior that are shared by members of a society and provide a design or "roadmap" for living. Culture tells people what is acceptable or unacceptable in a given situation. Culture dictates what to do, say, or believe. Culture is learned. As children grow up, they learn from their parents and others around them how to interpret the world. In turn, these assimilated beliefs and values prescribe desired behavior.

Anthropologists describe culture as the acquired knowledge that people use to generate behavior and interpret experience (Spradley & McCurdy, 2005). This knowledge is more than simply custom or ritual; it is a way of organizing and thinking about life. It gives people a sense of security about their behavior; without having to consciously think about it, they know how to act. Culture also provides the underlying values and beliefs on which people's behavior is based. For example, culture determines the value placed on achievement, independence, work, and leisure. It forms the basis for the definitions of male and female roles. It influences a person's response to authority figures, dictates religious beliefs and practices, and shapes childrearing. According to Giger and Davidhizar (2002, p. 80), "culture is a patterned behavioral response that develops over time as a result of imprinting the mind through social and religious structures and intellectual and artistic manifestations."

Every community and social or ethnic group has its own culture. Furthermore, all of the individual members believe and act based on what they have learned within that specific culture. As anthropologist Edward Hall (1959) said a half-century ago, culture controls our lives. Even the smallest elements of everyday living are influenced by culture. For instance, culture determines the proper distance to stand from another person while talking. A comfortable talking distance for Americans is at least 2.5 feet, whereas Latin Americans prefer a shorter distance, often only 18 inches, for dialogue. Culture also influences one's perception of time. In European American culture, when someone makes an appointment, it is expected that the other person will be on time or not more than a few minutes late; to keep a person waiting (or to be kept waiting) for 45 minutes or more is considered insulting. Yet other cultural groups, including Native Americans and Hispanics, have a much more flexible response to time; their members feel that time is much more elastic, and if someone is kept waiting, it is not considered a thoughtless act. So, as you can see, culture is the knowledge people use to design their own actions and, in turn, to interpret others' behavior (Spradley & McCurdy, 2005).

Cultural Diversity

Race refers to biologically designated groups of people whose distinguishing features, such as skin color, are inherited; examples include Asian, Black, and White. An **ethnic group** is a collection of people who have common origins and a shared culture and identity; they may share a common geographic origin, race, language, religion, traditions, values, and food preferences (Spector, 2004). A person's **ethnicity** is that group of qualities that mark her association with a particular ethnic group, or "who share cultural and/or physical characteristics including one or more of the following: history, political system, religion, language, geographical origin, traditions, myths, behaviours, foods, genetic similarities, and physical features" (Ethnicity Online, 2007, ¶ 1). When a variety of racial or ethnic groups join a common, larger group, cultural diversity becomes apparent. **Cultural diver-**

sity, also called *cultural plurality*, means that a variety of cultural patterns coexist within a designated geographic area. Cultural diversity occurs not only between countries or continents, but also within many countries, including the United States (Spector, 2009). However, the term *culture,* used alone, has no single definition. We have defined it for use in this book at the beginning of this section. Others have described culture as meaning the total, socially inherited characteristics of a group, comprising everything that one generation can tell, convey, or hand down to the next. Culture has also been described as "the luggage that each of us carries around for a lifetime" (Spector, 2004, p. 9).

Immigration patterns over the years have contributed to significant cultural diversity in the United States. Early settlers came primarily from European countries through the 1800s, peaking in numbers just after the turn of the 20th century, with almost 9 million immigrants admitted in the first decade. During much of that time, especially during the late 1600s through the early 1800s, African slaves were brought to the United States against their will, mostly to southern states, where they were sold to plantation owners as laborers. This "forced immigration" has had profound effects for many generations (Berlin, 2005). Immigration stayed high during the early 1900s, and then dropped sharply from 1930 to 1950. Immigration from non-European regions such as Asia and South America then steadily increased. The total number of immigrants from all countries in the 1990s almost equaled the number who arrived during the 1910s, when immigration was at a peak (Table 5.1).

As shown in Table 5.2, immigrants come from all regions of the world, in greater numbers from some areas than others. According to the U.S. Committee for Refugees and Immigrants (USCRI, 2006), in 2005, the United States hosted 176,700 refugees and asylum seekers, down by over half from 2001. The largest numbers of refugees are listed as coming from Haiti, Cuba, and China.

TABLE 5.2	Immigrants and Region of Birth (2006)
Origin	No. of Immigrants
All Countries	41,150
Africa	18,185
Asia	9,245
Europe	10,456
North America	3,145
Oceania	—
South America	119

From U. S. Department of Homeland Security, Yearbook of Immigration Statistics: 2006.

Although the numbers of legal immigrants have dropped, illegal immigration continues to be a *hot button topic* in this country, especially after 9/11. Proposals to end the flow of illegal immigrants from Mexico include building a 700-mile fence along the border, and legislation that would penalize employers of undocumented workers more stiffly. In 1994, Operation Gatekeeper sought to close the most commonly traversed border crossings with more guards and fences. That year, deaths along the border numbered 30. The numbers of migrants losing their lives while crossing illegally into this country continue to rise, from 147 in 1998 to 387 in 2001; in 2005, the number climbed to 451 (Hing, 2006). What is often not considered in the debate over this issue is the economic desperation that drives people to put themselves in such jeopardy.

The population of this country continues to increase. Five years after the 2000 census, the population grew by over 14 million; and Whites and Hispanic/Latinos showed the greatest increases (Table 5.3). Such numbers can be

TABLE 5.1	Immigrants Admitted to the United States in the 20th Century
Decade	Number of Immigrants
1901–1910	8,795,386
1911–1920	5,735,611
1921–1930	4,107,209
1931–1940	528,431
1941–1950	1,035,039
1951–1960	2,515,479
1961–1970	3,322,677
1971–1980	4,493,314
1981–1990	7,338,062
1991–2000	9,095,417

From U. S. Department of Commerce. (2001). *Statistical abstract of the United States, 2001* (121st ed.). Washington, DC: Government Printing Office.

TABLE 5.3	U.S. Population by Race and Hispanic/Latino Origin, Census 2000 and July 1, 2005	
Origin	Census 2000 (%)	July 1, 2005 (%)
White	75.1	80.2
Black	12.3	12.8
American Indian/ Alaska Native	.9	1
Asian	3.6	4.3
Two or More Races	2.4	1.5
Some Other Race	5.5	n/a*
Hispanic or Latino	12.5	14.4

*Those answering "Other" have been allocated to one of the recognized race categories.

From Population of the United States by Race and Hispanic/Latino Origin, Census 2000 and July 1, 2005. Retrieved January 5, 2007 from http://www.infoplease.com/ipa/A0762156.html; © 2000–2006 Pearson Education, publishing as Infoplease.

deceiving, however, because the 2000 census was the first one in which individuals were able to indicate two or more races or ethnic groups. Over 6 million people indicated multiple races or ethnic groups, with the number dropping to over 4 million in 2005. Approximately 50% of these people indicated Hispanic along with a second or third race or ethnic group (U.S. Department of Commerce, 2001).

People representing more than 100 different ethnic groups—more than half of them significant in size—live in the United States. Significant minorities include Hispanic Americans, numbering more than 35 million in 2000 and over 42 million in 2005 and currently representing over 14% of the population; African Americans, numbering over 37 million, or approximately 12.8% of the population; Asian Americans, numbering more than 12 million, or approximately 4.3% of the population; and American Indians and Alaska Natives, numbering 2.8 million, or 1% of the population. In 2000, Hispanics surpassed the African American population as the largest race/ethnic group in the United States (U.S. Department of Commerce, 2001; Infoplease, 2007). By 2050, the total number of Hispanic Americans is projected to double, making up 24.5% of the population; Asian–Pacific Islanders are expected to more than double their numbers, to 8.2% of the U.S. population; and the number of African Americans will increase to 15.4% of the population. The American Indian and Alaska Native population will probably stay at or near 1%. These changes, primarily resulting from immigration, are projected to result in 49.8% of the U.S. population in 2050 belonging to "minority" groups, and European Americans/Whites may no longer be the majority. In some states, especially those bordering Mexico and some industrialized states in the eastern part of the country, the most current information reveals that this change already has occurred or will occur much sooner than 2050 (U.S. Bureau of the Census, 1992) (see Display 5.1).

Immigration patterns are strongly influenced by immigration laws established since the 1800s. The Immigration Reform and Control Act of 1986 (Public Law 99–603) and the Immigration Act of 1990 (Public Law 101–649) set new limits on the number of immigrants admitted. These laws set annual numerical ceilings on certain immigrant groups while authorizing increases for highly skilled workers or family members of aliens who have recently achieved legal status. After the terrorist attacks on September 11, 2001, President Bush suspended all immigration for 2 months. Suspicion about people from Middle Eastern countries permeated the nation—worsening the social climate for immigrants.

This social climate is characterized by ambivalence about whether immigrants should be accepted and ambiguity about their status. The newcomers find an environment that is both welcoming and hostile. On one hand, they may find tolerance of diversity in the United States—demonstrated by interest in ethnic food, cultural celebrations, and sensitivity to employees from different backgrounds. On the other hand, a backlash is demonstrated by a rise in hate crimes, national and local policies that limit services to undocumented immigrants, restriction in English as a Second Language (ESL) and bilingual education, and limits to potential class action suits challenging practices of the Immigration and Nationalization Service.

Although broad cultural values are shared by most large national societies, those societies contain smaller cultural groups—called subcultures. **Subcultures** are relatively large aggregates of people within a society who share separate distinguishing characteristics, such as ethnicity (e.g., African American, Hispanic American), occupation (e.g., farmers, physicians), religion (e.g., Catholics, Muslims), geographic area (e.g., New Englanders, Southerners), age (e.g., the elderly, school-age children), gender (e.g., women), or sexual preference (e.g., gay, lesbian).

Within these subcultures are even smaller groups that anthropologists call **microcultures**. "Microcultures are systems of cultural knowledge characteristic of subgroups within larger societies. Members of a microculture usually share much of what they know with everyone in the greater society but possess a special cultural knowledge that is unique to the subgroup" (Spradley & McCurdy, 2005, p. 15). Examples of microcultures can range from a group of Hmong immigrants from Southeast Asia adopting selected aspects of the United States culture to a third-generation Norwegian American community whose members share unique foods, dress, and values.

The members of each subculture and microculture retain some of the characteristics of the society from which they came or in which their ancestors lived (Mead, 1960). Some of their beliefs and practices—such as the food they eat, the language they speak at home, the way they celebrate holidays, or their ideas about sickness and healing—remain an important part of their everyday life. American Indian groups have retained some aspects of their traditional cultures. Mexican Americans, Irish Americans, Swedish Americans, Italian Americans, African Americans, Puerto Rican Americans, Chinese Americans, Japanese Americans, Vietnamese Americans, and many other ethnic groups have their own microcultures.

Furthermore, certain customs, values, and ideas are unique to the poor, the rich, the middle class, women, men,

---

DISPLAY 5.1   HISPANIC POPULATION TREND IN THE UNITED STATES

A report conducted by the Pew Hispanic Center and the Brookings Institution Center on Urban and Metropolitan Policy and released in July 2002 indicated that the Hispanic population has spread out across the nation faster and farther than any previous wave of immigrants. Hispanics are moving from immigrant gateways into the heartland and suburbs at a rate possibly exceeding that of European immigrants in the early 20th century and of African Americans moving away from the Deep South in the years before World War II.

Although large metropolitan areas such as New York, Los Angeles, and Miami accounted for the largest increases in number of Hispanics between 1980 and 2000, smaller communities charted a faster rate of growth in their Hispanic populations.

More than half of Hispanics now live in suburbs, and many migrants are skipping metropolitan areas and heading straight to jobs and housing in outlying areas. Researchers indicate that this is not one trend replacing another, but several trends expanding at once.

Hispanic population spreads out. (2002, August 1). *The Fresno Bee,* p. A4.

youth, or the elderly. Many deviant groups, such as narcotics abusers, transient alcoholics, gangs, criminals, and terrorist groups, have developed their own microcultures. Regional microcultures, such as that of the White Appalachian people living in the hills and hollows of Kentucky or West Virginia, also have distinctive ways of defining the world and coping with life. Other microcultures, such as those of rural migrant farm workers or urban homeless families, acquire their own sets of beliefs and patterns for dealing with their environments. Many religious groups have their own microcultures. Even occupational and professional groups, such as nurses or attorneys, develop their own special languages, beliefs, and perspectives.

Ethnocentrism

There is a difference between a healthy cultural or ethnic identification and ethnocentrism. Anthropologists note "**ethnocentrism** is the belief and feeling that one's own culture is best. It reflects our tendency to judge other people's beliefs and behavior using values of our own native culture" (Spradley & McCurdy, 2005, p. 16). It causes people to believe that their way of doing things is right and to judge others' methods as inferior, ignorant, or irrational. Ethnocentrism blocks effective communication by creating biases and misconceptions about human behavior. In turn, this can cause serious damage to interpersonal relationships and interfere with the effectiveness of nursing interventions (Leininger, 2006).

People can experience a developmental progression along a continuum from ethnocentrism, feeling one's own culture is best, to **ethnorelativism**—seeing all behavior in a cultural context (Narayanasamy & White, 2005). Some people may stop progressing and remain stagnated at one step, and others may move backward on the continuum. The left side of the continuum represents the most extreme reaction to intercultural differences: refusal or denial. On the right side is the characterization of people who show the most sensitivity to intercultural differences: incorporation (Fig. 5.1).

CHARACTERISTICS OF CULTURE

In their study of culture, anthropologists and sociologists have made significant contributions to the field of community health. Their findings shed light on why and how culture influences behavior. Five characteristics shared by all cultures are especially pertinent to nursing's efforts to improve community health: culture is learned, it is integrated, it is shared, it is tacit, and it is dynamic.

Culture Is Learned

Patterns of cultural behavior are acquired, not inherited. Rather than being genetically determined, the way people dress, what they eat, and how they talk are all learned.

Spradley and McCurdy (2005, p. 14) offered the following explanation:

> At the moment of birth, we lack a culture. We don't yet have a system of beliefs, knowledge, and patterns of customary behavior. But from that moment until we die, each of us participates in a kind of universal schooling that teaches us our native culture. Laughing and smiling are genetic responses, but as infants we soon learn when to smile, when to laugh, and even how to laugh. We also inherit the potential to cry, but we must learn our cultural rules for when crying is appropriate.

Each person learns about culture through socialization with the family or significant group, a process called **enculturation**. As a child grows up in a given society, he or she acquires certain attitudes, beliefs, and values and learns how to behave in ways appropriate to that group's definition of the female or male role; by doing so, children are learning about their culture (Spradley & McCurdy, 2005; Spector, 2009).

Although culture is learned, the process and results of that learning are different for each person. Each individual has a unique personality and experiences life in a singular way; these factors influence the acquisition of culture. Families, social classes, and other groups within a society differ from one another, and this sociocultural variation has important implications (Wang, 2004). Because culture is learned, parts of it can be relearned. People might change certain cultural elements or adopt new behaviors or values. Some individuals and groups are more willing and able than others to try new ways and thereby influence change.

Culture Is Integrated

Rather than being merely an assortment of various customs and traits, a culture is a functional, integrated whole. As in any system, all parts of a culture are interrelated and interdependent. The various components of a culture, such as its social mores or religious beliefs, perform separate functions but come into relative harmony with each other to form an operating and cohesive whole. In other words, to understand culture, single traits should not be described independently. Each part must be viewed in terms of its relationship to other parts and to the whole.

A person's culture is an integrated web of ideas and practices. For example, a nurse may promote the need for consuming three balanced meals a day, a practice tied to the beliefs that good nutrition leads to good health and that prevention is better than cure. These cultural beliefs, in turn, are related to the nurse's values about health. Health, the nurse believes, is essential for maximum energy output and productivity at work. Productivity is important because it enables people to reach goals. These values are linked to

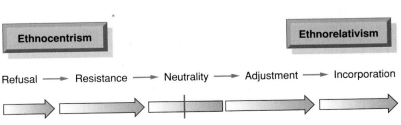

FIGURE 5.1 Cross-cultural sensitivity continuum. Being extremely ethnocentric (left of midpoint) and totally ethnorelative (far right) are reflected in the diagram. The steps toward ethnorelativism begin at the most ethnocentric view, with refusal and resistance. Neutrality is midpoint, and adjustment and incorporation bring the person to an ethnorelative perspective.

social or religious beliefs about hard work and taboos against laziness. Through such connections, these ideas and beliefs about nutrition, health, economics, religion, and family are all interrelated and work to motivate behavior.

For example, parents who are Jehovah's Witnesses may refuse a blood transfusion for their child. Their actions might seem irrational or ignorant to those who do not understand the parents' religious beliefs. However, the couple's choice represents behavior consistent with their cultural values and standards. The single behavior of refusing blood transfusions, when viewed in context, is seen to be part of a larger religious belief system and a basic component of the parents' culture. Even mothers' expectations for their children's development can vary between cultures, as evidenced by various research studies (Bornstein & Cote, 2004; Bradley & Corwyn, 2005; Pachter & Dworkin, 1997)—something to keep in mind when we use developmental screening tools.

In some cultural groups (e.g., Muslims), modesty for women may make it uncomfortable and perhaps traumatic to be examined by a person of the opposite sex. Asking certain Native American groups to comply with rigid appointment scheduling requires them to reframe their concept of time. It also violates their values of patience and pride (Spector, 2009). Before nurses attempt to change a person's or group's behavior, they need to ask how that change will affect the people involved through its influence on other parts of their culture. Extra time and patience or different strategies may be needed if change still is indicated. Nurses often may find, however, that their own practice system can be modified to preserve clients' cultural values.

Culture Is Shared

Culture is the product of aggregate behavior, not individual habit. Certainly, individuals practice a culture, but customs are phenomena shared by all members of the group. Over thirty years ago, anthropologist G. Murdock explained (1972, p. 258):

> Culture does not depend on individuals. An ordinary habit dies with its possessor, but a group habit lives on in the survivors and is transmitted from generation to generation. Moreover, the individual is not a free agent with respect to culture. He is born and reared in a certain cultural environment, which impinges on him at every moment of his life. From earliest childhood his behavior is conditioned by the habits of those around him. He has no choice but to conform to the folkways current in his group.

A culture's values are among its most important elements (see Chapter 4). A **value** is a notion or idea designating relative worth or desirability. For example, some cultures place value on honesty, loyalty, and faithfulness more than other traits. Also, there may be strong values against lying, stealing, and cheating—behaviors to avoid. Each culture classifies phenomena into good and bad, desirable and undesirable, right and wrong. When people respond in favor of or against some practice, they are reflecting their culture's values about that practice. One person may eagerly anticipate eating a steak for dinner. Another, who believes that eating meat is sacrilegious or unhealthful, experiences revulsion at the idea of steak for a meal. Some American

subcultures think that loud, vocal expressions are a necessary way to deal with pain; others value silence and stoicism. Some have high regard for speed and efficiency, whereas others prefer patience and thoughtfulness. Either way, values serve a purpose. Shared values give people in a specific culture stability and security and provide a standard for behavior. From these values, members know what to believe and how to act (Lockwood, Marshall, & Sadler, 2005). The normative criteria by which people justify their decisions are based on values that are more deeply rooted than behaviors and, consequently, more difficult to change.

Knowing that culture is shared helps us to better understand human behavior. For example, a community health nurse tried unsuccessfully to persuade a mother to limit the amount of catnip tea she fed her infant. The infant was pacified with the tea and was not consuming a sufficient amount of infant formula, thus putting him at risk for nutritional deficiencies and developmental problems. The nurse discovered that the mother was acting in the tradition of her rural subculture, which held that catnip promoted good health (it acts as an antispasmodic, perhaps causing relaxation and resulting in a more contented infant with fewer symptoms of colic [Spector, 2009]). The fact that all of the other mothers in her small rural community also used catnip with their babies proved a powerful deterrent to the change suggested by the nurse. Other members of the same culture frequently influence health behaviors. It is difficult for one person to eliminate a cultural practice, especially when that practice is reinforced by so many other members of the group. Group acceptance and a sense of membership usually depend on conforming to shared cultural practices (Spradley & McCurdy, 2005).

Community health nurses may need to focus on an entire group's health behavior to affect individual practices. In the example described, the pattern of consuming large amounts of catnip tea was modified after the nurse worked with the entire rural community. She began with a well-recognized cultural strategy: working through formal or informal leaders. She contacted the oldest woman in the community and discussed the cultural practice. The elder shared the group's beliefs that catnip tea is vital to the well-being of infants for the first 6 months. When the nurse explained her concerns about low formula intake and low weight gain, the community leader clarified that only 1 or 2 ounces of the tea a day was needed. The nurse and the community leader shared this information among the women, and as a result, the mothers gradually reduced the amount of tea they gave their infants. Consequently, the clients' infants drank more formula and gained weight appropriately. A cultural tradition was retained while the health of the infants was improved. The community health nurse could then use this new information and other supportive information from the community leader to improve the health of more infants.

Culture Is Mostly Tacit

Culture provides a guide for human interaction that is **tacit**—that is, mostly unexpressed and at the unconscious level. Members of a cultural group, without the need for discussion, know how to act and what to expect from one another. Culture provides an implicit set of cues for behavior, not a written set of rules. Spradley and McCurdy explained that culture often is "so regular and routine that it lies below a conscious level" (2005, p. 16). It is like a memory bank in which knowledge is stored for recall when the situation requires it, but this recall process is mostly unconscious. Culture teaches the proper tone of voice to use for each occasion. It prescribes how close to stand when talking with someone and how one should appropriately respond to elders. Individuals learn to make responses that are appropriate to their sex, role, and status. They know what is right and wrong. As an example, a recent study showed that cultural factors influence the desired affective state of children through their exposure to different types of storybooks (Tsai, Louie, Chen, & Uchida, 2007). All of these attitudes and behaviors become so ingrained—so tacit—that they are seldom, if ever, discussed.

Because culture is mostly tacit, realizing which of one's own behaviors may be offensive to people from other groups is difficult. It also is difficult to know the meaning and significance of other cultural practices. In some groups, such as American Indians or Islamic women, silence is valued and expected, but may make others uncomfortable. Offering food to a guest in many cultures is not merely a social gesture but an important symbol of hospitality and acceptance; to refuse it, for any reason, may be an insult and a rejection. Touching or calling someone by their first name may be viewed as a demonstration of caring by some groups, but is seen as disrespectful and offensive by others. Even how one trusts others in a group context is affected by cultural influences (Yuki, Maddux, Brewer, & Takemura, 2005). Consequently, community health nurses have a twofold task in developing cultural sensitivity: not only must we try to learn clients' cultures, but we also must try to make our own culture less tacit and more explicit. We must be more aware of our own biases and preconceived values and beliefs. Nurses bring both their professional and personal cultural history to the workplace, often developing unique values not shared with others who are not in the profession (Blais, Hayes, & Kozier, 2005). Cross-cultural tension can be resolved through conscious efforts to develop awareness, patience, and acceptance of cultural differences (Display 5.2).

Culture Is Dynamic

Every culture undergoes change; none is entirely static. Within every cultural group, some individuals generate innovations. More important, some members see advantages in doing things differently and are willing to adopt new practices. Each culture is an amalgamation of ideas, values, and practices from a variety of sources. This process depends on the extent of exposure to other groups. Nonetheless, every culture is in a dynamic state of adding or deleting components. Functional aspects are retained; less functional ones are eliminated.

When this adaptation does not occur, the cultural group may face serious difficulty. For example, Hmong teenagers from Southeast Asian refugee families in the United States are among the first generation to be raised in America. Their parents had high hopes for them to restore honor and pride to a displaced people, but the teens struggle to balance their American lifestyle with Hmong traditions. The stresses they feel as a result of the generational and cultural gaps between

---

DISPLAY 5.2   CULTURE SHOCK

An increasing number of immigrants and refugees from many different countries have been assimilated into American culture in recent years. Although they quickly adapt in many respects, such as learning the language and seeking housing and employment, they continue to operate within the framework of their own cultural beliefs and behaviors. The conflict between their culture and American culture often causes **culture shock**, "a state of anxiety that results from crosscultural misunderstanding . . . and an inability to interact appropriately in the new context" (Spradley & McCurdy, 2000, p. 16). Immigrants and refugees find themselves in a strange setting with people who act in unfamiliar ways. Speaking their own language in their homes and retaining values and familiar practices all help to promote some sense of security in the new environment.

The same is true for nurses and others working in unfamiliar countries. No longer are the small but important cues available that orient a stranger to appropriate behavior. Instead, a person in a different culture may feel isolated and anxious and even become dysfunctional or ill. Immersion in the culture over time and learning the new culture are the major remedies. As adjustment occurs, old beliefs and practices that are still functional in the new setting can be retained, but others that are not functional must be replaced.

---

themselves and their parents are often overwhelming. Many have not been successful in balancing these stresses and have chosen gang membership or suicide as a way to relieve their frustration and depression (Ellis, 2002). Hmong community leaders, community health workers, school districts, law enforcement, and Hmong families have joined together to develop interventions to address these issues (see Perspectives).

Another example of problematic cultural adaptation is the case of the "one child rule" in China. In an effort to contain population growth, in 1979, China began limiting married couples to having only one child. The government strictly enforces this policy, with few exceptions. Because male offspring are more highly valued than female in the Chinese culture, there is now a significant increase in the ratio of male to female births. Couples who have a female infant may choose to place the baby in an orphanage and make her available for adoption, but, although they are considered illegal, it is thought that a large number of sex-selective abortions occur. The goal of the government's policy was to change the Chinese culture from large- to small-family preference, and recent surveys indicate that this appears to be taking place; however, there are other untoward consequences of this cultural shift (Hesketh, Lu, & Xing, 2005). "Only-children" are now caring for their elderly parents, along with their "one child," as a widespread pension system does not yet exist in China. This strain, along with the shortage of women that leads to "kidnapping and trafficking of women for marriage, and increased numbers of commercial sex workers" are issues that must still be resolved (p. 1173).

Community health nurses must remember the dynamic nature of culture for several reasons. First, cultures and subcultures do change over time. Patience and persistence are key attributes to cultivate when working toward improving health behaviors. Second, cultures change as their members see greater advantages in adopting "new ways." Discussions of these advantages need to be conducted in a language understood by members and in the context of their own cultural value system. This is an important reason for nurses to develop an understanding of their clients' culture and to deliver culturally competent care (Callister, 2001; Giger & Davidhizar, 2002; Leininger, 2006). Third, it is important to remember that, within a culture, change is usually brought about by certain key individuals who are receptive to new ideas and are able to influence their peers. These key persons can adapt the change process, so that "new" practices are culturally consistent and fit with group values. Tapping into this resource becomes imperative for successful change. Finally, the health care culture is dynamic, too. Westerners are just beginning to appreciate the validity of many non-Western health care practices such as acupuncture, meditation, and the use of various therapeutic herbs and spices (e.g., turmeric, fenugreek). We can learn much from our clients and their cultures (Spector, 2009) (see Perspectives: Voices from the Community).

ETHNOCULTURAL HEALTH CARE PRACTICES

Throughout history, people have relied on natural elements to treat various maladies that family, clan, tribe, or community members experience. Knowledge of culturally recognized practices or substances, such as berries, plants, barks, or rituals and incantations usually becomes the responsibility of one person in the community. This revered community leader is known as a medicine man/woman, healer, or shaman (Spector, 2009). As time passes, this person teaches the skills of recognizing and treating ailments or performing rituals to an apprentice, thereby continuing the healing knowledge and traditions.

In the following sections, we discuss how various geographic or ethnocultural groups view health care, including the biomedical, magicoreligious, and holistic views. You may encounter many distinctive ways that your clients manage their health and illness, so we will discuss selected folk medicines and home remedies, such as herbs, over-the-counter (OTC) drugs, and patent medications. In addition to these forms of treatments, there are complementary or alternative therapies (e.g., folk remedies) and various self-care practices. This section concludes with the community health nurse's role and responsibilities to provide culturally competent care in relation to caring for, respecting, teaching, and treating clients from different cultures.

The World Community

Beliefs about the causes and effects of illness, health practices, and health-seeking behaviors are all influenced by a person's, a group's, or a community's perception of what causes illness and injury and what actions can best treat or cure the health problem. The three major views in the world community are biomedical, magicoreligious, and holistic health beliefs (Spector, 2009).

Biomedical View

Western societies in general have a biomedical view of health and illness. The biomedical view relies on scientific principles and sees diseases and injuries as life events controlled by physical and biochemical processes that can be manipulated through medication, surgery, and other treatments. Examples of this view include the following beliefs:

◆ Elements, such as bacteria, fungi, or viruses, are causes of illness.
◆ Lack of certain elements, such as an adequate diet, calcium, or iron, causes other health problems, such as malnutrition, osteoporosis, or anemia.
◆ An accepted treatment for many physical ailments is to remove diseased organs, or to treat injuries from falls or accidents.

People living in countries where Western medicine is practiced believe that theirs is the best and, perhaps the only way, to deal with illness or injury. The dominant values presume that science is value-free and not constructed by the social norms of the cultural group. The same is true, however, where Western medicine is not practiced and the social norms of the cultural group support the healing practices of that group (Leininger, 2006; Spector, 2009). Many people, including community health nurses, are not open to other ways of looking at a person's wellness capabilities. As a result, clients may not receive culturally competent care from their caregivers. To be effective with clients, community health nurses must be knowledgeable and accepting of others' cultural practices.

PERSPECTIVES
VOICES FROM THE COMMUNITY

"You are talking about parents who are medieval, coming to a country that is hundreds of years ahead of theirs. They're trying to catch up, but it's hard."— Mymee (college instructor)

"There is much research that shows people who stand in the middle of two cultures are really at risk of depression and anxiety."—Valerie (psychologist)

"The kids are constantly living between two cultures. At some point, they may give up."—Leng (psychologist. Southeast Asian adult services center)

"I think it's a topic that nobody wants to talk about. It's hard for me to say if the Hmong community is ready to deal with it."—Xong (social worker, Hmong suicide task force)

"We parents think we know only one way to raise our kids. We ignore that these children are living in America and are espousing everything that is American, good and bad."—Andy (Hmong parent)

Ellis, A.D. (2002, August 11). Hmong Teens: Lost in America [Special report]. The Fresno Bee, pp. 1–12.

Magicoreligious View

Magicoreligious themes of health and illness, which focus on the control of health and illness by supernatural forces, are prominent in some cultural groups. Diseases occur as a result of "committing sins" or "going against God's will." Good health is a gift from God, and illness is a form of punishment that affords an opportunity to be forgiven and to realign oneself with God. Prayer to God or other religious figures is used to cope with illness, seek intervention for healing, and ask for forgiveness and entrance into heaven, if death be God's will.

Some cultures mix traditional folk beliefs with organized religious practices and participate in forms of magic or voodoo. In cultures that have such beliefs, a hex or spell can be placed on another person through the use of incantations, elixirs, or an object resembling the person. For some, illness results from a look or a touch from another person considered to have special powers or intent to harm (Leininger, 2006; Spector, 2009). Later in this chapter, we discuss some specific health beliefs and practices common to cultural groups in North America.

Religious beliefs, an individual's spirituality, and how these factors interface with feelings of wellness and specific healing practices are personal and important to clients and cannot be separated from their culture. This makes it imperative for community health nurses to be familiar with folk beliefs commonly seen in their practice. Only then can culturally competent nursing care be provided.

Holistic View

Holistic health believers come from many different cultural groups and generally view the world as being in harmonious balance. If the principles guiding natural laws to maintain order are disturbed, an imbalance in the forces of nature is created, resulting in chaos and disease. For an individual to be healthy, all facets of the individual's nature—physical, mental, emotional, and spiritual—must be in balance.

Some cultural groups believe that all things in creation or the universe have a spirit and therefore are considered equal in value, purpose, and contribution (Lowe, 2002). Individuals have universal connectedness and are viewed as holistic beings. Persons are extensions of and integrated with family, community, tribe, and the universe. For example, "mother and fetus are viewed as interrelated and as affecting each other: They are one, but also they are two. In the circle of life, each individual is believed to be on a journey experiencing a process of being and becoming" (Lowe & Struthers, 2001, p. 6).

Folk Medicine and Home Remedies

Many of us remember our mothers giving us hot herbal tea with lemon, or slathering on ointments and piling on blankets to lessen the effects of a mild illness. Many folk medicines and home remedies came about as a means of providing health care to family members when no medical care was available or deemed affordable.

Folk medicine is a body of preserved treatment practices that has been handed down verbally from generation to generation. It exists today as the first line of treatment for many individuals. Some clients may never plan to seek Western medical treatment but may share with you, the community health nurse, a practice they are using to treat a family member. Your response and actions may mean the difference between health and illness or injury. Some maternal–child health practices from the U.S. rural Midwest or South that may be encountered in community health nursing practice include the following (Giger & Davidhizar, 2004; Spector, 2009):

- Not reaching above your head if you are pregnant, because doing so will cause the umbilical cord to strangle the baby
- Pregnant women eating handfuls of clay, dirt, or cornstarch
- Taping coins over a newborn's umbilical area to prevent hernias
- Giving catnip tea to infants because it saves their lives
- Holding a baby upside down by her heel to "wake up her liver"
- Not letting a cat in a room with a sleeping baby, because the cat will "suck the life" out of the baby

Home remedies are individualized caregiving practices that are passed down within families. Even individuals who routinely seek the guidance of a health care practitioner for diagnosis and treatment may try home remedies before seeking professional advice. Each of us has a set of home remedies our parents used on us that we are likely to use on our own children before or instead of calling the pediatrician. Examples include using baking soda paste on a bee sting, ice on a "cold sore," or cranberry juice to prevent a urinary tract infection.

Herbalism

Textbooks have been written on the many uses of medicinal herbs (Gruenwald, 2004). The use of some herbs has waxed and waned in favor. Some continue to be much touted, whereas others have been designated as dangerous and to be avoided (Medline Plus, 2007). Increasingly, the public is using herbal preparations in the form of self-selected over-the-counter (OTC) products for therapeutic or preventive purposes.

In an increasingly multicultural society, the source, form, and identity of many herbs, roots, barks, and liquid preparations become impossible for most community health nurses to distinguish. The most astute among us may be familiar with herbs used by one cultural group, whereas herbs used by another escape us. A book with pictures and descriptions, botanical form, purported indications and uses, and implications for nursing management is an important tool to keep handy when interacting with clients. *Nursing Herbal Medicine Handbook* (Lippincott, Williams, & Wilkins, 2005) is also available in software version for PDAs (Handango, 2007)—an even more efficient method of retrieving information quickly. Basic safety questions that community health nurses should answer about an herb when teaching or interacting with families include the following:

- Is the herb contraindicated with prescription medications the client is taking?
- Is the herb harmful? Does it have negative side effects?
- Is the client relying on the herb, without positive health changes, while neglecting to get effective treatment from a health care practitioner?

Herbs are not regulated as drugs and are not risk free. Dosages are not standardized and are left to the individual. Quality of the product may be suspect. For these reasons, herbs must be used only in moderation and with caution, preferably with guidance by a health care practitioner.

Prescription and Over-the-Counter (OTC) Drugs

The cautions mentioned about herbs can also apply to prescription and OTC medications. First, they are not risk free. In this country, prescription drugs are reviewed and tested by the U.S. Food and Drug Administration (FDA)'s Center for Drug Evaluation and Research (CDER), and OTC drugs go through a somewhat less-rigorous process through the CDER's Division of OTC Drug Products. Over-the-counter drugs comprise six out of every 10 medications bought in the United States (U.S. FDA, 2007). However, many OTC drugs were once available only by prescription, and remain powerful medicines. All drugs can have major side effects, may be contraindicated in people with certain conditions, and may not be safe to use in combination with certain other drugs. Medication instruction and review is an important part of the community health nurse's role on home visits, especially with elderly clients (see Chapter 24).

Second, some new prescription medications are so expensive that clients cannot afford to take them as prescribed. Often, older, less expensive, and more frequently used drugs work as well as the newer, more expensive ones, which are heavily marketed by drug companies to health care practitioners and consumers. If you encounter clients who are unable to pay for drugs, you may need to advocate for them with health care providers to prescribe a less expensive medication or change to the generic form of the same drug, usually sold at a fraction of the cost. Some health care practitioners have samples of drugs available and may be able to use them for medically indigent clients. Many pharmaceutical companies now have low-cost prescription assistance programs for those in need (NeedyMeds.com, 2007).

Third, the efficacy of medications must be assessed. At times, the use of a new drug or an additional drug does not have the intended effect. As someone who sees the client managing at home over time, the community health nurse may be able to give the best information to the health care provider about the effectiveness of new medications for a particular client.

Complementary Therapies and Self-care Practices

Complementary therapies (also called alternative medicine or alternative therapies) are practices used to complement contemporary Western medical and nursing care and are designed to promote comfort, health, and well-being (Snyder, 2001). The range of complementary therapies is broad and includes:

- Therapies (cancer diets, juice diets, fasting)
- Treatments (coffee enemas, high colonic enemas)
- Exercise activities (t'ai-chi, yoga)
- Exposure (aromatherapy, music therapy, light therapy)
- Manipulation (acupuncture, acupressure, reflexology)

Most cultural groups engage in some form of complementary therapy, either alone or in conjunction with Western medicine. **Integrated health care** is defined as the combination of complementary therapies with biomedical or Western health care (Snyder, 2001). Complementary therapies have become so commonplace today that many states are developing policies and guidelines for their use.

Consumers need to be well informed regarding the efficacy and safety of complementary therapies and how they can be true complements to other treatment modalities. The community health nurse should be aware of the variety of therapies available and how to get information for clients while remaining objective and supportive of the client's choices. At times, if a therapy contradicts the recommendations of the client's health care practitioner, the nurse may be in a position to provide the pros and cons of continuing the complementary therapy. On the other hand, the nurse may be able to suggest therapy forms that would complement Western medicine for the client, such as music therapy to promote relaxation and reduce stress or biofeedback for chronic pain management.

Self-care activities include complementary therapies, medications, and spiritual and cultural practices. They are uniquely individual for each person, as well as among different cultural groups. Chapter 19 includes a Self-Care Assessment Guide that may be helpful in assessing the self-care practices of families.

Role of the Community Health Nurse

When working with different cultural groups in the area of health care practices, the community health nurse can be an effective advocate for the client. First, however, the nurse must be prepared to speak knowledgeably about health care practices and choices. The nurse also must be able to assess the client or family adequately, so as to know what belief system motivates their choices. Finally, the nurse must be prepared to teach clients about the limits and benefits of cultural health care practices. The community health nurse should always individualize assessment and caregiving for the client within her culture and should not generalize about the client based on cultural group norms.

Preparation of the Community Health Nurse

To be effective when working with clients in the area of cultural health care and spirituality, the nurse must be prepared. Many ways exist for you to increase your cultural awareness and promote sensitivity to the differences among people from ethnocultural groups different from your own. You can acquire information from peers who are from the same cultural group as your clients; attend workshops or conferences on chosen cultural topics; read books on ethnocultural health care practices, herbalism, or complementary therapies; talk with clients about their views and practices and learn from them; keep an open mind and be curious about various practices; or attend community cultural events such as Native American powwows, ethnic food events held in some cities, or Cinco de Mayo celebrations. There are textbooks, novels, and articles about cultures in the community in which one practices. For example, the book *The Spirit Catches You and You Fall Down* (Fadiman, 1997) describes a Hmong child, her American doctors, and the collision of two cultures.

From the Case Files I

Learning About Other Cultures

I was always interested in learning about other countries and cultures, but I didn't realize that an overseas assignment would teach me so much about myself, in addition to other cultures and ways of living. The lessons were sometimes difficult, but always rewarding. I knew that my expectations would not always be met, yet it did surprise me how different the experience was from what I had imagined. My job assignment, location, and team members changed frequently. Flexibility, comfort with ambiguity, a sense of humor, a deeper reliance upon my faith, patience when results were not forthcoming, trust in others, and the ability to cross multiple cultures with some degree of ease were all skills that I developed over time. Most important to being successful at my job was to maintain the attitude of a "learner," not a "solver of problems" or the person "with all the answers." I made friends with people from all over the world who graciously accepted me into their lives, thus enriching mine. I learned that we all are different, but that every behavior has a reasonable explanation when you take the time to listen with your heart as well as with your ears. I found that I actually preferred other ways of doing and being while still maintaining those parts of my identity that were valuable to me. When I returned home, I found that my newly developed skills were still necessary—I had changed and had to adjust to re-entry back into my home culture!

Karin Urso, PHN

Universities offer courses in transcultural nursing, ethnic studies courses or programs, and cultural events that can be valuable. The experience of Karin Urso, who worked with people from many different countries and cultures, illustrates the benefits of being open-minded (see From the Case Files I).

Assessment

When beginning to work with a group or family, it is important for you to become as familiar with them as possible. In addition to a family assessment or an individual health assessment, you can enhance your aggregate care by doing an ethnocultural or self-care assessment. Such an assessment reveals information about day-to-day living, cultural/spiritual influences, traditional/cultural health care choices and practices, and cultural taboos. Often this type of information is most useful as you work with clients on a regular basis. Useful tools include the two cultural assessment reviews at the end of this chapter (see Tables 5.7 and 5.8) and the self-care assessment tool in Chapter 19.

Teaching

As you are aware from your studies and preparation, teaching is a most important role in nursing, both in acute care settings and in the home. When working with families as a community health nurse, teaching takes a good deal of your time, because health care education is vitally important to communities, groups, and families. However, teaching that is undertaken in ways that are incomplete, culturally inappropriate, or inadequate may be frustrating and even harmful to your clients. Becoming ethnoculturally focused and prepared to teach from the client's view of the world will start you in the right direction. The suggestions in Display 5.3 offer ideas for providing culturally competent care. Chapter 11 on Health Promotion and Education will help prepare you as well.

SELECTED CULTURAL COMMUNITIES

An examination of the meaning and nature of culture clearly underscores the need to recognize cultural differences and to understand clients in the context of their cultural backgrounds. Practically speaking, how can knowledge of cultural diversity be integrated into everyday community health nursing practice? What are the diverse cultural communities served by community health nurses? What are their differences? Do they share some features?

To provide insights and answers to these questions, this section describes five cultural communities, out of the more than 100 different ethnic groups living in the United States. Three are dominant in the United States; the other two represent populations native to North America and people from a Middle Eastern culture, an expanding group in the United States. These brief descriptions should not to be considered as a stand-alone guide to cultural competence; each culture is complex and unique, deserving of a more comprehensive study than is possible within the scope of this chapter. Many good references are available for nurses on cultural diversity (see References and Selected Readings).

Four of the groups highlighted represent those identified in *Healthy People 2010* (U.S. Department of Health and Human Services [USDHHS], 2000). The fifth group, Saudi Arabians, is presented because of the significant media attention people of the Middle East have received in recent years.

Healthy People 2010 (USDHHS, 2000) described significant disparities among members of some of the five groups highlighted here. Several of the disparities are displayed in Table 5.4.

Native American Indians, Aleut, and Eskimo Communities

Native American Indians and Alaska Natives (Eskimo communities residing in Alaska), the first known settlers of this continent, form a large cluster of tribal groups whose members are descendants of the original Native Americans who

DISPLAY 5.3	DEVELOPING CULTURAL COMPETENCE

First: Know that culture is dynamic.
It is a continuous and cumulative process.
It is learned and shared by people.
Cultural behaviors and values are exhibited by people.
Culture is creative and meaningful to our lives.
It is symbolically represented through language and interaction.
Culture guides us in our thinking, feeling, and acting.

Second: Become aware of culture in yourself.
Thought processes that occur within you also occur within others but may take on a different shape or meaning.
Cultural values and biases are interpreted internally.
Cultural values are not always obvious since they are shared socially with those you meet on a daily basis and are perceived through your senses.

Third: Become aware of culture in others, especially among client groups you serve.
This is best represented by the belief that there are many cultural ways that are correct, each in its own location and context.
It is essential to build respect for cultural differences and appreciation for cultural similarities.
Develop the ability to work within others' cultural context, free from ethnocentric judgments.

inhabited this country before White Europeans settled here. The earliest European explorers were the Vikings (circa 1010 AD); they were followed by various other Europeans in the 16th century (Spector, 2009). Native Americans, Aleuts, and Eskimos have adopted many European American values and practices, yet they preserve many aspects of their own culture.

Population Characteristics and Culture

Native Americans and Alaska Natives are a diverse group made up of different tribes and 561 federally recognized nations that speak approximately 250 languages. Eskimos, Aleuts, and Native Americans living in Alaska are known as Alaska Natives; those living in other states are known as Native Americans or

TABLE 5.4   *Healthy People 2010* and Disparities

Goal of Healthy People 2010	Baseline Values				
	White	Native American	Hispanic	Black	Asian
Health insurance: 79% of population	89%	79%	70%	84%	83%
Cancer deaths/100,000: 158.7	202.2	131.8	125.5	262.1	127.2
End-stage renal disease/1 million: 217	218	586	N/A	873	344
Diabetes deaths/100,000: 45	68	107	86	130	62
CHD deaths/100,000: 166	214	134	151	257	125
Stroke deaths/100,000: 48	60	39	40	82	55
HIV/AIDS deaths/100,000: 0.8	2.8	2.5	8.9	26.6	0.9
Deaths from firearms/100,000: 4.9	10.4	11.4	10.7	22.9	5.0
Motor vehicle deaths/100,000: 9.0	15.8	31.5	15.2	17.0	10.6
Unintentional injury deaths/100,000: 20.8	34.3	62.7	30.1	40.9	20.9
Residential fire deaths/100,000: 0.6	1.1	2.2	0.8	3.4	0.8
Homicides/100,000: 3.2	4.3	10.4	9.9	25.2	4.1
Low-birth-weight babies: 7.6% of births	6.5	6.8	6.4	13.0	7.2
Suicides/100,000: 6.0	12.8	12.4	6.4	6.3	7.0
Drug induced deaths/100,000:1.0	5.7	6.6	6.0	9.0	1.6
Smokers: 12% of population	25%	34%	20%	26%	16%

CHD, (coronary heart disease); HIV/AIDS, (human immunodeficiency virus/acquired immunodeficiency syndrome); N/A, (not available).
From U. S. Department of Health and Human Services. (2000). *Healthy people 2010* (Conference edition, Vols. 1 and 2). Washington, DC: Author.

American Indians. In this chapter, the term *Native American* is used to encompass all facets of this diverse group of people. These people make up just 1% of the U.S. population, or about 2.8 million people (Infoplease, 2007). In the 2000 Census, 4.1 million people said they were at least "part" Native American, and 2.5 million identified themselves only as Native American. These people proudly identify themselves as being Native American, unlike in the past, when to claim Native American blood carried a social stigma. In addition to societal changes in the acceptance of Native Americans, financial incentives exist for many Americans who are recognized tribal members. More than 300 of the Indian Nations receive revenue from gambling casinos—roughly half of all tribes have casinos (Walton, 2005). In 1988, when Congress passed the Indian Gaming Regulatory Act, casinos owned by Native Americans made $212 million; by 2000, they grossed $10 billion (U.S. Department of Commerce, 2001). By 2002, the 290 Native American casinos generated $12.7 billion, but only a small number of casinos (about 13%) generated the majority of the revenues (66%), and the amounts given to tribe members varied widely (e.g., less than $400 to over $200,000) (Barlett & Steele, 2002). To put this in perspective, 11 states have commercial (non-Indian) casinos that generated almost $29 billion in gross revenues in 2004 (Walton, 2005). Taylor and Kalt (2005) reported that real per capita income for gaming tribes increased by 36% between 1990 and 2000, while the total U.S. increase was 11%. However, even though the poverty rate fell for Native Americans overall, it is still three times the U.S. average. Although gaming and other ventures have improved access to health, education, and employment for most Native Americans, they still fall behind many other U.S. citizens.

The population of Native Americans and Alaska Natives is primarily concentrated in 26 states in the United States, including Alaska and the Aleutian Islands (Spector, 2009). Many live on reservations and in rural areas; however, more than half live in urban counties and have greater difficulty accessing the health care available to them through Indian Health Service (a federal program providing comprehensive health care to Native Americans) (Brenneman, Rhoades, & Chilton, 2006). The largest numbers live in Oklahoma, Arizona, California, New Mexico, North Carolina, and Alaska, as a result of forced westward migration (Spector, 2009). By 2050, the U.S. Census Bureau estimates about 4.5 million Native Americans will live in the United States, nearly double the number in 2000 (U.S. Department of Commerce, 2001). Some of this increase can be attributed to official recognition of persons who can provide information linking them to a tribe or nation; if they are accepted, they can then declare themselves as Native Americans.

Each tribe or nation has its own distinct language, beliefs, customs, and rituals. The community health nurse cannot assume that knowledge of one group can be generalized to others. Knowledge of certain similarities among the various Native American cultures (Display 5.4) can assist nurses working with members of a specific tribe. For many Native American groups, large, extended family networks reinforce cultural standards and expectations and provide emotional support and practical assistance.

Health Problems

Health problems among Native Americans tend to be both chronic and socially related. One third of Native Americans

DISPLAY 5.4 · SIMILARITIES AMONG NATIVE AMERICAN CULTURES

All of creation/universe has Spirit and is considered equal in value.
Everything is considered alive with energy and importance.
People have universal connectedness.
Harmony is a way of life based on cooperation and sharing.
Dignity of the individual, family, and community is valued.
Respect for advancing age is valued; elders are leaders.
There is present-time orientation, grounded in what is happening at the moment.
Symbolic arts and crafts are valued.
Life is lived in the present, with little concern for the distant future.
Generosity, harmony, and sharing are valued.
Religion is integrated into everyday life.
Herbal medicines and traditional healing practices are used.
Rituals and ceremonies are valued.
Silence is used as a way to practice presence and strength.
Thoughtful speech is valued.
Patience is valued.

Adapted from Lowe, 2002; Lowe and Struthers, 2001; and Spector, 2009.

live in abject poverty and experience the afflictions associated with poor living conditions, including malnutrition, tuberculosis (TB), and high maternal and infant death rates (Spector, 2009). The highest-ranking health problems in children include a postneonatal mortality rate double that of White infants (due largely to sudden infant death syndrome [SIDS], injuries, and congenital anomalies); overweight, obesity, and type 2 diabetes; and morbidity and mortality as a result of unintentional and intentional injuries (often motor vehicle injuries) (Brenneman, Rhoades, & Chilton, 2006). For adults, diabetes, TB, and obesity all rank higher among Native Americans than in the general population. Deaths from TB (seven times higher), alcoholism (six times higher), motor vehicle crashes (three times higher), diabetes (almost three times higher), unintentional injuries, and suicide and homicide (both 1.6 times higher) are higher for Native Americans than other Americans (Indian Health Service, 2006). Poor sanitation, crowded housing, and low immunization levels contribute to the prevalence of a variety of communicable diseases. On the other hand, the prevalence of heart disease is slightly lower in this population than among the population as a whole (236.2 versus 247.8 per 100,000) (Indian Health Services, 2006).

Alcoholism is the major health problem of Native Americans. Both traditional/cultural and medical explanations exist for the disproportionate number of alcohol-related health problems in Native Americans. Tribal medicine men have attributed the problems of alcoholism to losing "the opportunity to make choices," stating that until "people return to a sense of identification within themselves they will not rid themselves of this problem of alcoholism"

(Spector, 2004, p. 199). Medically, it appears that Native Americans have a much lower tolerance for alcohol and therefore demonstrate the effects of alcohol with lower amounts consumed. When individuals are under the influence of alcohol, other health and safety problems occur. Instances of domestic violence, child abuse and neglect, traffic injuries and deaths, and homicides are more frequent because of the abuse of alcohol. Along with these high rates of injuries and deaths, alcohol's destructive effects on the unborn lead to a high incidence of fetal alcohol syndrome (FAS) and fetal alcohol effects (FAE). Substance abuse is also prevalent among those living on reservations, and increasingly among youth using alcohol, tobacco, and other drugs (Substance Abuse & Mental Health Services Administration [SAMHSA], 2004).

Health Beliefs and Practices

Native Americans as a group prefer traditional healing practices and folk medicine to Western medicine. Most Native Americans today still seek out a medicine man or rely on traditional remedies before going to a health clinic. Many of their beliefs about health and illness have common traditional roots, regardless of tribe or location. Health and dietary practices are closely tied to cultural and religious beliefs. Beliefs about health reflect living in total harmony with nature. The Earth is considered a living organism that should be treated with respect, as should the body (Spector, 2009). Native Americans practice purification rituals such as immersion in water and the use of sweat lodges to maintain their harmony with nature and to cleanse the body and spirit. The basis of therapy lies in nature, with herbal teas, charms, and fetishes used as preventive and curative measures (Kavasch & Baar, 1999).

Because of decades of racism and government paternalism, many Native Americans feel oppressed and dehumanized and carry considerable resentment and lack of trust toward Whites. As a result, many maintain a degree of separateness from overall American culture. Nurses must overcome these barriers through patience, acceptance, and respect for their clients' culture, as illustrated in the case study of the community health nurse, Sandra Josten, and her new client from a Native American community (see From the Case Files II).

Blacks or African Americans

Some of the ancestors of Black Americans, or African Americans, originally came to this continent as free settlers as early as 1619, but most of the approximately 4 million who followed came as slaves in the 17th and 18th centuries, mostly from the west coast of Africa (Byrd & Clayton, 2002). Most African Americans living today were born in the United States; some, however, have recently emigrated from African countries. Other Black Americans come from the West Indies, the Dominican Republic, Haiti, and Jamaica, often to escape poverty or political persecution. These people do not self-identify as African Americans but as Hispanics, a fact that may cause some difficulty for others trying to identify and accommodate to their culture. (Similarly, some people from the Philippines have Hispanic surnames and skin tones similar to those of Mexicans or other Latinos; when Filipinos—a culturally distinct group—settle in areas with large Hispanic populations, they can be similarly misidentified and misunderstood [Spector, 2009].)

Population Characteristics and Culture

In 2004, African Americans numbered 38.6 million and constituted approximately 13% of the U.S. population; projections show an increase to 15.4% by the year 2050 (National Center for Health Statistics, 2007a; U.S. Census Bureau, 1992; U.S. Department of Commerce Bureau 2001). One-third of the African American population is younger than 18 years of age. Slightly more than 8% of African Americans are older than 65 years, and most of them are women; in comparison, 13% of the total population is older than 65 years of age. Fifty-eight percent of Black children live with their mothers only, compared with 21% of White children.

Despite improvements in the legal and social climate for African Americans, great disparities exist between them and White Americans (Byrd & Clayton, 2002). Average family income for African Americans is 62% of the income earned by White families. More than 26% of African Americans live in poverty, compared with 8.9% of Whites. Although African Americans make up only 13% of the population, more than 50% of prison inmates are Black. A greater percentage of Blacks use illicit drugs (7.7%), compared with Whites (6.6%) or Hispanics (6.8%) (Antai-Otong, 2002). Approximately 36% of African American families in households headed by women live below the poverty level. Unemployment among African Americans is 8.9%, compared with 3.9% for Whites (U.S. Department of Commerce, 2001).

Educational disparities also exist. Among people age 25 years and older, 76% of Blacks and 83.7% of Whites have a high school education. More than half of those African Americans with less than a high school education are not in the workforce, compared with 36% of Whites with a similar education. However, 89% of both Blacks and Whites with a college degree are employed; 14.7% of Blacks and 25% of Whites are college graduates (Williams & Collins, 2001). African American women acquire more educational training than their Black male counterparts do, but their earnings are lower than those of the men, as is also the case with White and Hispanic women compared with men in those groups.

Like Native Americans and Asian Americans, African Americans do not comprise a single culture; rather, this group forms a heterogeneous community. As with other large ethnic and racial groups, many factors influence their culture, resulting in much diversity within the African American population. Among the variables determining specific microcultures within the African American community are economic level, religious background, education, occupation, social class identity, geographic origin, and residence in an integrated or segregated neighborhood. For community health nurses, this means that specific groups of African Americans have their own unique values, character, lifestyle, and health needs.

The primary language of most African Americans is English. Recent Black immigrants from Caribbean or other countries may retain the language of their country of origin, but usually learn to use English as well. Many African Americans speak nonstandard dialects of English, also called Black English, Ebonics, or African American Vernacular English. These dialects evolved from pidgin English spoken during the era of slavery, and they have become a dynamic and meaningful language of their own. For some African Americans, Ebonics symbolizes racial pride and identity—it can also be used to differentiate them from the mainstream culture (Novak, 2000; Spector, 2009).

From the Case Files II

Sandra's New Clients

As she drove up the dirt road and parked her car next to the community hall, Sandra Josten felt apprehensive. She had been alerted by the previous community health nurse about the difficulty of working with these Native American people: "This tribe is lazy and unappreciative. You can't get anywhere with them." Only through the urging of Mrs. Brown, an Indian community aide, had a group of the women reluctantly agreed to meet with the new nurse. They would see what she had to say.

Sandra's steps echoed hollowly as she walked across the wooden floor of the large room to the far corner where a group of women sat silently in a circle. Only their eyes turned; their faces remained impassive. Mrs. Brown rose slowly, greeted the nurse, and introduced her to the group. Swallowing her fear, Sandra smiled. She told them of her background and explained that she had not worked with Indian people before. There was a long silence. No one spoke. Sandra continued, "I'd like to help you if I can, maybe with problems about care of your children when they are sick or questions about how to keep them healthy, but I don't know what you need or want." Silence fell again. She would like to learn from them, she repeated. Would they help her? Again Sandra felt an uncomfortable silence.

Then one woman began to speak. Quietly, but with deep feeling, she described several bad experiences with the previous nurse and the county social worker. Then others spoke up: "They tell us what we should do. They don't listen. They say our way is not good." Seeing Sandra's interest and concern, the women continued. One of their main concerns was their children's health. Another was the high incidence of accidents and injuries on the reservation. They wanted to learn how to give first aid. Other concerns were expressed. The group agreed that Sandra could help them by teaching a first-aid class.

In the weeks that followed, Sandra taught several classes on first aid and emergency care. She then began a series of sessions on child health. Each time, she asked the women to choose a topic or problem for discussion and then elicited from them their accustomed ways of dealing with each problem; for example, how they handled toilet training or taught their children to eat solid foods. Her goal was to learn as much as she could about their culture and incorporate that information into her teaching, which preserved as many of their practices as possible. Sandra also visited informally with the women in their homes and at community gatherings.

She learned about their way of life, their history, and their values. For example, patience was highly valued. It was important to be able to wait patiently, even if a scheduled meeting was delayed as much as 2 hours. It also was important for others to speak, which explained the Indian women's comfort with silences during a conversation. Other values influenced their way of life. Courage, pride, generosity, and honesty all were important determinants of behavior. These also were values by which they judged Sandra and other professionals. Sandra's honesty in keeping her promises enabled the women to trust her. Her generosity in giving her time, helping them occasionally with some household task and arranging for child care during classes won their respect.

The women came to accept her, and Sandra was invited to eat with them and share in tribal get-togethers. The women criticized and advised her on acceptable ways to speak and act. Her openness and patience to learn and her respect for them as a people had paved the way to improving their health. At first, Sandra felt that her progress was slow, but this slowness was an advantage. She had built a solid foundation of cross-cultural trust, and in the months that followed she saw many changes in her clients' health practices.

Health Problems

African Americans have much higher mortality rates than White Americans, with a life expectancy of 71.1 years (U.S. Department of Commerce, 2001). This number is the same as the life expectancy of Whites in 1966, revealing a 35-year lag for the Black population compared with the White population. This demonstrates the inequality in mortality and life expectancy, an outcome of health care, economic, and educational disparity (Levine et al., 2001). Life expectancy for Whites in 2000 was 76.8 years (U.S. Department of Commerce, 2001). The gap for Blacks is 6.3 years for males and 4.5 years for females (Harper, Lynch, Burris & Smith, 2007). The major health problems for Blacks include cardiovascular disease and stroke, cancer, diabetes mellitus, cirrhosis, a high infant mortality rate

(twice that of whites), homicide, accidents, and malnutrition (Display 5.5).

Stress and discrimination, poverty, lack of education, high rates of teen pregnancy, inadequate housing, and inadequate insurance for health care are among the risk factors influencing the health of this population. In the last three decades, a dramatic increase in Black households headed by women, single-parent births (most frequently among teenagers), and a limited presence of male role models has further exacerbated family vulnerability (Lewis, Gutierrez, & Sakamoto, 2001).

Leading causes of death for African Americans are heart disease, cancer, and stroke. As noted, infant death rates are higher in Blacks than in other groups (13.6 per 1,000 live births), leading many health departments to provide Black Infant Health programs (National Center for Health Statistics, 2007a). Mortality rates for communicable diseases,

DISPLAY 5.5	EXAMPLES OF CULTURAL PHENOMENA AFFECTING HEALTH CARE AMONG BLACK OR AFRICAN AMERICANS
Nations of Origin	• Many West African countries (as slaves) • West Indian Islands • Dominican Republic, Haiti, Jamaica
Environmental Control	• Traditional health and illness beliefs may continue to be observed by "traditional" people
Common Biological Variations	• Sickle-cell anemia • Hypertension • Cancer of the esophagus • Stomach cancer • Coccidioidomycosis • Lactose intolerance
Social Organization	• Family: many single-parent households headed by females • Large, extended family networks • Strong church affiliations within the community • Community social organizations
Communication	• National languages • Dialect: Pidgin • French, Spanish, Creole
Spatial Distancing	• Close personal space
Time Orientation	• Present over future

Adapted from Spector, R.E. (2004). *Cultural diversity in health and illness* (6th ed.). Upper Saddle River, NJ: Pearson Education, Inc.

including the acquired immunodeficiency syndrome (AIDS), also are higher for Blacks than for Whites. The incidence of TB in this population is rising, with many cases being diagnosed in conjunction with AIDS (see Chapters 8 and 26). Other infectious and parasitic diseases are three to six times more prevalent among African Americans than among Whites (U.S. Department of Health and Human Services, 2000). Hypertension is a real concern in this population (37% of men and 41% of women over the age of 20 report having hypertension). In the same age group, 66% of men and 79% of women are reported as overweight (National Center for Health Statistics, 2007a). In two health-related areas, Blacks demonstrate a lower incidence than Whites: suicide is 50% less prevalent among Blacks, and the rate of chronic obstructive pulmonary disease (COPD) is 20% to 30% less. All other leading causes of death are higher for Black populations, much of which can be attributed to lifestyle and poverty (Hong et al., 2006). However, some genetic studies have shown significant differences between African Americans and Whites in those genes associated with hypertension and cardiovascular disease (Lange et al., 2006; Wang et al., 2006).

Blacks may have specific skin problems (e.g., keloids, melasma). In addition, sickle cell anemia occurs in Blacks, an inherited genetic trait thought to have originated in Africa as a defense against malaria (Spector, 2009).

Health Beliefs and Practices

Although African Americans have assimilated into the more dominant European American culture in the United States,

some retain aspects of their ancestors' traditional values and practices. Some, for example, hold traditional African beliefs about health being a sign of harmony with nature and illness being evidence of disharmony. Evil spirits, the punishment of God, or a hex placed on the person might account for this disharmony. Healers treat body, mind, and spirit. Prayer, laying on of hands, magic or other rituals, special diets, wearing of preventive charms or copper bracelets, ointments, and other folk remedies sometimes are practiced (Spector, 2009). A recent study by Aaron, Levine, and Burstin (2003) found that, for African Americans, church attendance is significantly associated with positive health care practices (e.g., blood pressure measurements, Pap smears, mammograms, dental visits). This was even stronger for the chronically ill and uninsured subgroups. This is an important consideration when public health nurses plan programs targeting this population. Each African American community has its own set of health beliefs and practices that must be determined by the community health nurse before any interventions are planned.

Asian Americans

A third cultural cluster is composed of immigrants and refugees from various Pacific Rim countries, such as China, Korea, Japan, Thailand, Laos, the Philippines, Vietnam, and Cambodia (Display 5.6). Some Asian Americans have been transplanted fairly recently from their native countries and cultures to an entirely different culture, whereas others may have lived here many years or were born in America.

DISPLAY 5.6	ASIAN-PACIFIC POPULATIONS

Asian refers to:	Pacific Islander refers to:
Chinese	Polynesian
Filipino	Hawaiian
Japanese	Samoan
Asian Indian	Tongan
Korean	Micronesian
Vietnamese	Guamanian
Laotian	Melanesian
Thai	Fijian
Cambodian	Tahitian
Pakistan	Marshallese
Indonesian	Trilese
Hmong	
Mien	

Population Characteristics and Culture

In 2004, more than 14 million Asians and Pacific Islanders were living in the United States, representing 4.3% of the total population (National Center for Health Statistics, 2006; Infoplease, 2007; U.S. Department of Commerce, 2001).

The largest groups were Chinese and Filipinos, with more than 1.5 million persons from each country; Vietnamese numbered a close second. Other fairly large groups came from Korea, India, Laos, and Cambodia. Each group represents a distinct culture with its own unique challenges for community health nurses, as illustrated in the case study of the Kim family (see From the Case Files III).

Whereas each Asian culture is distinct in language, values, and customs, many Asians share some general traits. Traditional Asian families tend to be patriarchal (the father is the head of the household) and patrilineal (the genealogy is carried through the male line). Male members are valued over female members. Elders are respected. The male role generally is that of provider, whereas the female role is that of homemaker. Traditional Asians value achievement because it brings honor to the family name. Saving face or preserving dignity and family pride is important. Cooperation is valued over competition (Leininger, 2006; Spector, 2009).

Health Problems

Leading causes of death among Asians include cancer, heart disease, and stroke (National Center for Health Statistics, 2006). Smoking is lower in this group (18% of males and 6% of females over age 18 smoke). Health problems for Asian Americans include malnutrition, TB, mental illness, cancer, respiratory infections, arthritis, parasitic infestations, and chronic

From the Case Files III

The Kim Family

Armed with enthusiasm and pamphlets on pregnancy and prenatal diet, Paula Morrow, the community health nurse, began home visits to the Kim family. Paula's initial plan was to discuss pregnancy and fetal development, teach diet, and prepare the mother for delivery. Mr. Kim, a graduate student, was present to interpret, because Mrs. Kim spoke little English. Their two boys, ages 1½ and 3 years, played happily on the kitchen floor. The family offered tea to the nurse and listened politely as she explained her reasons for coming and asked, "How can I be most helpful to you? What would you like from my visits?"

The Kims were grateful for this approach. Hesitant at first, they hinted at Mrs. Kim's fears of American doctors and hospitals; her first two children had been born in Korea. None of the family had any experience with Western medicine. They shared some concents about adjustment to living in the United States. It was difficult to shop in American food stores with their overwhelming variety of foods, many of which the Kims found unfamiliar. Mrs. Kim, who had come from a family whose servants prepared the food, was an inexperienced cook. Servants also had cared for the children, and her role had been that of an aristocrat in hand-tailored silk gowns.

Listening carefully, Paula began to realize the striking differences between her own culture and that of her clients. Her care plans changed. In subsequent visits, she was determined to learn about Korean culture and base her nursing intervention on that knowledge. She learned about their traditional ways of raising children, the traditional male and female roles, and practices related to pregnancy and lactation. She respected their value of "saving face" and attempted never to offend their pride or dignity. As time went on, her interest and respect for their way of life won their trust. She inquired about their cultural practices before attempting any intervention. As a result, the Kims were receptive to her suggestions. Whenever possible, Paula adapted her teaching and suggestions to comply with the Kim's culture. For example, appropriate changes were made in Mrs. Kim's diet that were compatible with her food preferences and cultural eating patterns. Because she was not accustomed to drinking milk, she increased her calcium intake by learning to prepare custards (which disguised the milk flavor) and by eating more green, leafy vegetables. After 5 months, a strong, positive relationship had been established between this family and the nurse. Mrs. Kim delivered a healthy baby girl and looked forward to continued supportive visits from the community health nurse.

diseases associated with aging. Suicide rates and stress-related illness are particularly high among Asian refugee groups who have had to flee their countries under stressful conditions and among teens born in the United States to Asian immigrants; many of these children have difficulty living between two cultures (Mui & Kang, 2006). However, Asians can view mental illness as shameful, and the stigma attached to it prompts them to express the mental illness as a disturbed bodily function or to hide it as long as possible (Mui & Kang, 2006; Spector, 2009).

Health Beliefs and Practices

Asian health beliefs vary among subcultures. Many Asians believe in the Chinese concepts of *yin* (cold) and *yang* (hot), which do not refer to temperature but to the opposing forces of the universe regulating normal flow of energy. A balance of yin and yang results in *qi* (pronounced *chee*), which is the desired state of harmony. Illness results when an imbalance occurs in these forces. If the imbalance is an excess of yin, then "cold" foods, such as vegetables and fruits, are avoided, and "hot" foods, such as rice, chicken, eggs, and pork, are offered. Some Asians view Western medicines as "hot" and Eastern folk medicines and herbal treatments as "cold," which explains why some groups practice both for balance. The Vietnamese have a similar hot-and-cold belief, but call it *am* and *dong*. Other Asian groups, such as the Filipinos, view illness as an act of God and pray for healing, reflecting their strong religious beliefs as Catholics or Muslims. The Khmer of Cambodia believe that illness reflects a deviation from moral standards, and the Hmong consider illness to be a visitation by spirits (Her & Culhane-Pera, 2004; Spector, 2009).

Many Asian groups have traditional healers, who, depending on the culture, may include acupuncturists, herbalists, herb pharmacists, spirit and magic experts, or a shaman. Most Asian cultures also exercise traditional self-care practices, including herbal medicines and poultices, types of acupuncture, and massage (Davis, 2001; Kim et al., 2002; Plotnikoff et al., 2002; Ryan, 2003; Spector, 2009). Southeast Asians also practice dermabrasive techniques of coining, cupping, pinching, rubbing, and burning. These methods are used to relieve symptoms such as headache, sore throat, cough, fever, and diarrhea by bringing toxins to the skin surface or compensating for heat lost. Cupping was a common medical practice in colonial America (Cash, Christianson, & Estes, 1981). Because these techniques leave a bruise-like lesion on the skin, they can be mistaken for physical abuse. Each client requires a careful **cultural assessment** (a detailed data-gathering about the client's cultural practices) before nursing action is implemented (Leonard, 2001).

Hispanic Americans

A fourth cultural cluster comprises groups who are of Hispanic or Latino origin and have immigrated to the United States, some many generations ago. More than half come from Mexico, followed by Puerto Rico, Cuba, Central and South America, and Spain (Spector, 2009). Those with Mexican and Central American backgrounds generally are referred to as Latinos. Depending on the region of the country, socioeconomic status, immigration or citizenship status, or age, members of this large minority group refer to themselves as Mexican American, Spanish American, Chicano, Latin American, Latin, Latino, or

Mexican (Eggenberger, Grassley, & Restrepo, 2006; Spector, 2009). In this chapter, for convenience, the term *Hispanic* is used to encompass this entire diverse population.

The subgroups of Hispanics vary by their patterns of geographic distribution in the United States. Those from Mexico tend to live predominantly in the west (56.7%) and south (32.6%), Puerto Ricans are most likely to live in the northeast (63.9%), and Cubans are highly concentrated in the South (80.1%). Central and South Americans are concentrated in the northeast (32.3%), the south (34.6%), and the west (28.2%) (U.S. Census Bureau, 2001).

Population Characteristics and Culture

Hispanics are the fastest growing and largest ethnic group in the United States, and people of Hispanic origin are predicted to number more than 58 million, or 17.5% of the population, by 2025 (U.S. Department of Commerce, 2001). In 2004, this group comprised more than 42.6 million people and accounted for over 14% of the U.S. population (Infoplease, 2007; National Center for Health Statistics, 2007b).

The Hispanic population uses Spanish as its common and primary language; nonetheless, its diverse cultural and linguistic backgrounds account for diversity in dialects. Hispanic people value extended, cohesive families. Families have been patriarchal, with male members perceived as superior and female members seen as a family-bonding life force. These traditional family structures are changing because of migration, urbanization, women in the work force, and social movements. Spousal roles are becoming more egalitarian (Giger & Davidhizar, 2004; Eggenberger, Grassley, & Restrepo, 2006; Spector, 2009). However, vestiges of the *macho* man and the self-sacrificing woman still are evident in the Hispanic culture and continue to shape behavior (see From the Case Files IV).

Health Problems

Leading causes of death for the Hispanic population include heart disease, cancer, and accidents (unintentional injuries). A large number of this population is uninsured (34%) and do not have a usual source of health care (31% for adults, almost 10% for children) (National Center for Health Statistics, 2007b). Health problems among the Hispanic population are complicated by experiences in their countries of origin, as well as by socioeconomic and lifestyle factors in this country. Tuberculosis is high in this group, especially among those younger than 35 years of age. Hypertension, diabetes, and obesity are major concerns. Other problems include infectious diseases, particularly AIDS and pneumonia, parasitic infections, malnutrition, gastroenteritis, alcohol and drug abuse, accidents, and violence. Frequently, the most important health issues for Hispanics are related to the fact that the population is young and has a high birth rate (97.7 per 1,000 births) (National Center for Health Statistics, 2007b). Posttraumatic stress disorder is a major problem among refugees from Central and South America who have experienced war and physical and emotional torture.

Health Beliefs and Practices

Religion plays an important part in Hispanic culture. For most Hispanics, Catholicism is the dominant religion (95%

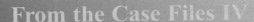

From the Case Files IV

Maria Juarez

Maria Juarez, a 53-year-old Mexican American widow, was referred to a community health nursing agency by a clinic. Her married daughter reported that Mrs. Juarez was having severe and prolonged vaginal bleeding and needed medical attention. The daughter had made several appointments for her mother at the clinic, but Mrs. Juarez had refused at the last minute to keep any of them.

After two broken home visit appointments, the community health nurse made a drop-in call and found Mrs. Juarez at home. The nurse was greeted courteously and invited to have a seat. After introductions, the nurse explained that she and the others were only trying to help. Mrs. Juarez had caused a lot of unnecessary concern to everyone by not cooperating, she scolded in a friendly tone. Mrs. Juarez quickly apologized and explained that she had felt fine on the days of her broken appointments and saw no need "to bother" anyone. Questioned about her vaginal bleeding, Mrs. Juarez was evasive. "It's nothing," she said. "It comes and goes like always, only maybe a little more." She listened politely, nodding in agreement as the nurse explained the need for her to see a physician. Her promise to come to the clinic the next day, however, was not kept. The staff labeled Mrs. Juarez as unreliable and uncooperative.

Mrs. Juarez had been brought up in traditional Mexican American culture that taught her to be submissive and interested primarily in the welfare of her husband and children. She had learned long ago to ignore her own needs and found it difficult to identify any personal wants. Her major concern was to avoid causing trouble for others. To have a medical problem, then, was a difficult adjustment. The pain and bleeding had caused her great apprehension. Many Mexican Americans have a particular dread of sickness and especially hospitalization. Furthermore, Mrs. Juarez's culture had taught her the value of modesty. "Female problems" were not discussed openly. This cultural orientation meant that the sickness threatened her modesty and created intense embarrassment. Conforming to Mexican American cultural values, she had first turned to her family for support. Often, only under dire circumstances do members of this cultural group seek help from others; to do so means sacrificing pride and dignity. Mrs. Juarez agreed to go to the clinic because refusal would have been disrespectful, but her fear of physicians and her reluctance to discuss such a sensitive problem kept her from going. Mrs. Juarez was being asked to take action that violated several deeply felt cultural values. Her behavior was far from unreliable and uncooperative. With no opportunity to discuss and resolve the conflicts, she had no other choice. Knowing this, how would you approach Mrs. Juarez?

of Mexican Americans, for example, are Catholic), but religious beliefs often consist of a blend of Catholicism and pre-Columbian Indian beliefs and ideology, along with magicoreligious practices. Hispanics believe in submission to the will of God and that illness may be a form of *castigo*, or punishment for sins. They cope with illness through prayers and faith that God will heal them. Their religion also determines the rituals used in healing. For example, *solito*, a condition of depression in women similar to a midlife crisis in American culture, is treated by having the patient lie on the floor while her body is stroked by the *curandero* (native healer) until the depression passes. Latino culture includes beliefs that witchcraft (*brujeria*) and the evil eye (*mal de ojo*) are supernatural causes of illness that cannot be treated by "Anglo" or Western medicine. *Empacho*, a stomachache in children that occurs after a traumatic event, is treated by the *curandero* with herbal mixtures made into teas. After tender loving care and a bowel movement, the child is considered healed (Table 5.5). As with Asians, Hispanics use "hot" and "cold" categories of foods to influence their diet during illness. Many Hispanics tend to be present-oriented, and consequently are not as concerned as the mainstream culture about keeping to time schedules or preparing for the future (Giger & Davidhizar, 2004; Leininger, 2006; Eggenberger, Grassley, & Restrep, 2006; Spector, 2009).

Arab Populations and Muslims

The final cultural community selected for this discussion is made up of groups of people who come from Arabic countries, especially those who espouse the Muslim religion. By comparison with the groups previously mentioned, the number of people from Arabic countries in the United States is small, but because of the terrorist attacks of September 11, 2001 and the wars in the Middle East, increasing racial and religious animosity has been directed toward people from this part of the world and against those who bear physical resemblance to members of these groups. This unwarranted ostracism has led to mental anguish and distress in Arab and Muslim communities (Giger & Davidhizar, 2002; Goodman, 2002). Hopefully, factual information about these groups of people will dispel myths and alleviate fear.

About 4 million people of Arab descent live in the United States. For purposes of the U.S. Census, Arabs are characterized as White (Electronic Resource Center, 2007a). Los Angeles County (California), Wayne County (Michigan), and Cook County (Illinois) have the largest populations of Arab Americans, with Detroit, Los Angeles, and New York metropolitan areas reporting the largest numbers (Samhan, 2006). Arab Americans have generally done very well economically: 41% are college graduates, over 50% own their

TABLE 5.5   Hispanic Health Beliefs and Folk Diseases

Belief Name	Explanation/Treatment
Ataque	Severe expression of shock, anxiety, or sadness characterized by screaming, falling to the ground, thrashing about, hyperventilation, violence, mutism, and uncommunicative behavior. Is a culturally appropriate reaction to shocking or unexpected news, which ends spontaneously.
Bilis	Vomiting, diarrhea, headaches, dizziness, nightmares, loss of appetite, and the inability to urinate brought on by livid rage and revenge fantasies. Believed to come from bile pouring into the bloodstream in response to strong emotions and the person "boiling over."
Bilong (hex)	Any illness may be caused by this; proper diagnosis and treatment requires consulting with a santero or santera (priest or priestess).
Caide de mollera	A condition thought to cause a fallen or sunken anterior fontanel, crying, failure to nurse, sunken eyes, and vomiting in infants. Popular home remedies include holding the child upside down over a pan of water, applying a poultice to the depressed area of the head, or inserting a finger in the child's mouth and pushing up on the palate. (Note: According to Western medicine, these symptoms are indicative of dehydration and can be life-threatening. The community health nurse's role is imperative—to promoting hydration and definitive health care.)
Empacho	Lack of appetite, stomach ache, diarrhea, and vomiting caused by poorly digested food. Food forms into a ball and clings to the stomach, causing pain and cramping. Treated by strongly massaging the stomach, gently pinching and rubbing the spine, drinking a purgative tea (estafiate), or by administering azarcon or greta, medicines that have been implicated, in some cases, in lead poisoning. (Note: The community health nurse must assess family for the use of these "medicines" and initiate appropriate follow-up).
Fatigue	Asthma-like symptoms treated with Western health care practices, including oxygen and medications.
Mal de ojo	A sudden and unexplained illness including vomiting, fever, crying, and restlessness in a usually well child (most vulnerable) or adult. Brought on by an admiring or covetous look from a person with an "evil eye." It can be prevented if the person with the "evil eye" touches the child when admiring him or her if the child wears a special charm. Treated by a spiritualistic sweeping of the body with eggs, lemons, and bay leaves accompanied by prayer.
Pasmo	Paralysis-like symptoms in the face and limbs treated by massage.
Susto	Anorexia, insomnia, weakness, hallucinations, and various painful sensations brought on by traumatic situations such as witnessing a death. Treatment includes relaxation, herb tea, and prayer.

Adapted from Spector, R. E. (2004). *Cultural diversity in health and illness* (6th ed.). Upper Saddle River, NJ: Pearson Education, Inc.

own home, 42% work as professionals or managers, and the median income for Arab American families is 4.6% higher than other Americans (Naim, 2005). Many Arab immigrants have only arrived since the 1990s, fleeing war-torn countries or repressive regimes (Goodman, 2002; Naim, 2005).

A common language (Arabic) and background unite them, yet only 18% of Muslims (followers of Islam) reside in Middle Eastern countries. Arabs are largely Christian or Muslim, although some Arabs may be Jews or Druze (Electronic Resource Center, 2007b). Christian Arabs first began emigrating to the U.S. in the late 19th and early 20th centuries (mostly from Syria and Lebanon), but during the middle of the 20th century, Muslim Arabs began to emigrate in greater numbers (commonly from Palestine, Egypt, Iraq, and Yemen). Islam is the fastest-growing global religion, with more than 1 billion followers worldwide. Most Muslims live in Indonesia, the southern Philippines, and the United States (Electronic Resource Center, 2007c). The Council on American–Islamic Relations (2008) reports that, in the U.S., 25% of Muslims are of Southeast Asian ancestry, while only 23% are of Arab descent. Approximately 8 million Americans are Muslim. In Britain, it is estimated that Muslim worshippers will outnumber Anglicans within a few years, and the Christian Research Organization in England projected that, if current

trends continue, by 2039 Muslims will surpass all British Christians in worship attendance (Baqi-Aziz, 2001). The tenets of Islam are interpreted more liberally in some nations and more strictly in others, but all practicing Muslims adhere to the five tenets of Islam in some fashion (Table 5.6).

Population Characteristics and Culture

An Arab is defined as "an individual who was born in an Arab country, speaks the Arabic language, and shares the values and beliefs of an Arab culture" (Kridli, 2002, p. 178). Arab Americans can trace their ancestry to the North African countries of Morocco, Tunisia, Algeria, Libya, Sudan, and Egypt, as well as the western Asian countries of Lebanon, Palestine, Syria, Jordan, Bahrain, Qatar, Oman, Saudi Arabia, Kuwait, United Arab Emirates, and Yemen. Iran is sometimes listed in this group, although Iraqis generally consider themselves to be Persian, not Arab (Arab American Institute Foundation, 2002). Assyrian/Chaldean/Syriac and Sub-Saharan (Somalian and Sudanese) groups are also noted as Arab. In general, the beliefs and practices of people from such disparate and distant countries cannot be encompassed into one culture. Despite the fact that some of these countries are highly Westernized, enjoy natural resources such as crude

TABLE 5.6   The Five Pillars (Tenets) of Islam

1. Faith	Declaration of faith (*shahada*) that there is no God but Allah and that Mohammad is the messenger of Allah.
2. Prayer	Obligatory prayers five times a day at dawn, noon, mid-afternoon, sunset, and when night falls (called *salat*) link the worshipper to God. Prayers are led by a learned man who knows the Quran, as there is no hierarchical authority in Islam (such as a minister or priest).
3. Almsgiving	This is like tithing and is a very important principle, as all wealth is thought to belong to God. It is called *zakat*, and each Muslim is expected to pay 2.5% of his or her wealth annually for the benefit of others in need.
4. Fast	To abstain from food, drink, and sexual intercourse during daytime (from dawn to sunset) throughout the ninth lunar month (Ramadan). It is a means of self-purification and spirituality. The sick, elderly, or pregnant/nursing women may be permitted to break the fast.
5. Pilgrimage	The pilgrimage to Makkah (the Hajj) once in a lifetime for those who are physically and financially able to do so. About 2 million people go to Makkah every year (located in Saudi Arabia).

Adapted from *The Five Pillars of Islam*. Retrieved from: http://www.islamicity.com/mosque/pillars.shtml.

oil and the riches that may follow, and are more liberal in following traditional cultural practices, others do not. It must also be noted that the Middle East has one of the slowest growing levels of personal income in the world and the highest unemployment rates among developing nations (Naim, 2005).

Arabs are mostly divided into two distinct religious groups: Muslims and Christians. Arabs value Western medicine, trust American health care workers, and do not generally postpone seeking medical care (Electronic Resource Center, 2007d). Several practices, however, are unfamiliar to most Americans. Many Arabic women stay at home and are not in the workforce. Families impose stricter rules for girls than for boys. After menarche, teenage girls may not socialize with boys. The adolescent female also begins to cover her head and perhaps wears a *hajab*, which takes the form of a modest dress and veil designed to diminish attractiveness and appeal to the opposite sex. Some Arab groups take this mode of dress to extremes, not even allowing a woman's eyes to show out of the hajab. Modesty is one of the core values for Arabs; it is expressed by both genders, although more evidently by females (Al-Shahri, 2002; Goodman, 2002).

Within the Arabic population, strict sexual taboos and social practices exist. All sexual contacts outside the marital bond are considered illegal. Those known to have been involved in such activities can be socially rejected, or in some countries even put to death. The stigma of lost honor can continue with their families for generations to come. Another social practice, at times mistakenly related to the Islamic religion, is the practice of female genital mutilation. This is practiced in a few of the Arabic countries on the African continent and has spread to southern Egypt, but it is rare or nonexistent in other Arabic countries. This horrific practice may include the removal of a young woman's labia, clitoris, or both, and it sometimes includes closing the vaginal opening by suturing (Kridli, 2002).

Health Problems

Health problems among Middle Easterners are most frequently lifestyle related. These include poor nutritional practices, resulting in obesity, especially among women; smoking among men; and lack of physical exercise (Al-Shahri, 2002). In some rural areas, especially in Saudi Arabia, men and women chew tobacco, and an increase of oral cancers is seen. Major public health concerns for most Arabs are related to motor vehicle accidents, maternal–child health, TB, malaria, trachoma, typhus, hepatitis, typhoid fever, dysentery, and parasitic infections (Giger & Davidhizar, 2002).

Most social restrictions are directed toward women and can affect their health. Pregnancy can be complicated by genital mutilation, which results in infections and difficult deliveries. Childbearing continues up until menopause, and 30% of marriages in some Arabic countries are between first cousins; both factors can contribute to the prevalence of genetically determined diseases (Giger & Davidhizar, 2002). The desire to have more sons than daughters often results in very large families and closely spaced pregnancies—often without the benefit of family planning. It is often debated whether birth control methods are sanctioned by Islam or not, but Akbar (2007) states that Muslims can reason for themselves, and notes that family planning is not forbidden by the beliefs of Islam. Abortion and infanticide are not accepted, however.

Health Beliefs and Practices

Traditional medicine is practiced in spite of the growth of Western medical services in some of the richer Arab nations. Traditional health care practices are much more common in the poorer Middle Eastern countries and in rural areas of all Arabic countries.

Muslims believe in predestination—that life is determined beforehand—and they attribute the occurrence of disease to the will of Allah. However, this does not prevent people from seeking medical treatment. Islamic law prohibits the use of illicit drugs, which include alcohol. Users of such substances are liable to trial, and those convicted of smuggling substances into an Arab country can be sentenced to death in some cases. *Sharaf*, or honor, is an important concept in Arab American beliefs, and drug addiction, mental illness, or unwed pregnancy of a family member brings shame to the entire family (Electronic Resource Center, 2007e). Conversely, when a member does something good or is recognized for an achievement, that honor is reflected on the family as a whole.

Cleanliness is paramount and ritualistic, especially before prayers and after sexual intercourse. The bodies of both genders are kept free of axillary and pubic hair. The left hand is used for cleaning the genitals and the right one is reserved for eating, hand shaking, and other hygienic activities. Muslims fast during Ramadan from sunrise to sunset, and this can include abstinence from all things (including medications or intravenous fluids). Illness can be an exception to this rule, but public health nurses should consult with a family elder or Muslim leader to encourage the client to continue with any necessary treatments. Also, Muslims pray several times daily, facing toward Mecca. Home visits should be planned so that prayers are not interrupted (Electronic Resource Center, 2007e).

When caring for Arabs in clinics or at home, a nurse of the same sex as the client should be assigned. Many topics (e.g., menstruation, family planning, pregnancy, and childbirth) must be discussed only with and by women; men are not included in these discussions.

Additional guidelines for nurses working with all immigrant groups include the following:

♦ Do not make assumptions about a client's understanding of health care issues.
♦ Permit more time for interviewing; allow time to evaluate beliefs and provide appropriate interventions.
♦ Provide educational programs to correct any misconceptions about health issues; this can occur in clinics, mosques, schools, or homes.
♦ Provide an appropriate interpreter to improve communication with immigrants who do not speak English well.

TRANSCULTURAL COMMUNITY HEALTH NURSING PRINCIPLES

Culture profoundly influences thinking and behavior and has an enormous impact on the effectiveness of health care. Just as physical and psychological factors determine clients' needs and attitudes toward health and illness, so too can culture. Kark emphasized over 30 years ago "culture is perhaps the most relevant social determinant of community health" (1974, p. 149). Culture determines how people rear their children, react to pain, cope with stress, deal with death, respond to health practitioners, and value the past, present, and future. Culture also influences diet and eating practices. Partly because of culturally derived preferences, dietary practices can be very difficult to change (Leininger, 2006; Spector, 2009).

Despite its importance, the client's culture often is misunderstood or ignored in the delivery of health care (Leininger, 2006). With the growth in non-White populations, "health care providers must be prepared for interactions with increasingly diverse health care team members and clients" (Giger & Davidhizar, 2002, p. 80). Especially in public health, the nurse must avoid ethnocentric attitudes and must attempt to understand and bridge cultural differences when working with others. It is important to develop knowledge and skill in serving multicultural clients and an ability to place clients' responses to experiences within the context of their lives, or else risk ineffectiveness in the face of a limited understanding and interpretation of client experience.

Overcoming ethnocentrism requires a concerted effort on the nurse's part to see the world through the eyes of clients. It means being willing to examine one's own culture carefully and to become aware that alternative viewpoints are possible. It means attempting to understand the meaning other people derive from their culture and appreciating their culture as important and useful to them (Campinha-Bacote, 2003). Ignoring consideration of clients' different cultural origins often has negative results, as illustrated in From the Case Files IV discussion about Maria Juarez.

Culture is a universal experience. Each person is part of some group, and that group helps to shape the values, beliefs, and behaviors that make up their culture. In addition, every cultural group is different from all others. Even within fairly homogeneous cultural groups, subcultures and microcultures have their own distinctive characteristics. Further differences, based on such factors as socioeconomic status, social class, age, or degree of acculturation, can be found within microcultures. These latter differences, called *intraethnic variations*, only underscore the range of culturally diverse clients served by community health nurses.

Given such diversity, community health nurses face a considerable challenge in providing service to cross-cultural groups. This kind of practice, known as **transcultural nursing**, means providing culturally sensitive nursing service to people of an ethnic or racial background different from the nurse's (Leonard, 2001; Leininger, 2006). Community health nurses in transcultural practice with client groups can be guided by several principles: develop cultural self-awareness, cultivate cultural sensitivity, assess the client group's culture, show respect and patience while learning about other cultures, and examine culturally derived health practices.

Develop Cultural Self-Awareness

The first principle of transcultural nursing focuses on the nurse's own culture. Self-awareness is crucial for the nurse working with people from other cultures (Leininger, 2006). Nurses must remember that their culture often is sharply different from the culture of their clients. **Cultural self-awareness** means recognizing the values, beliefs, and practices that make up one's own culture. It also means becoming sensitive to the impact of one's culturally based responses. The community health nurse who assisted Mrs. Juarez in the fourth Case File discussion probably thought that she was being friendly, efficient, and helpful. In terms of her own culture, this nurse's behavior was intended to reassure clients and meet their needs. Unaware of the negative consequences of her behavior, the nurse caused damage rather than meeting needs.

To gain skill in understanding their own culturally based behavior, nurses can complete a cultural self-assessment by analyzing their own:

♦ Racial background influences
♦ Verbal and nonverbal communication patterns
♦ Values and **norms,** or expected cultural practices or behaviors
♦ Beliefs and practices

Start with a detailed list of values, beliefs, and practices relative to each point. Next, enlist one or more close friends to call attention to selected behaviors, to bring them to a more conscious level. Videotaping practice interviews with colleagues and actual interviews with selected clients creates further awareness of the nurse's unconscious, culturally based responses. Finally, ask selected clients to critique nursing actions in light of the clients' own culture. Feedback from clients' perspectives can reveal many of the nurse's own cultural responses.

Because culture is mostly tacit, as discussed earlier, it takes conscious effort and hard work to bring the nurse's own cultural biases or influence to the surface. Doing so, however, rewards the nurse with a more effective understanding of self and enhanced ability to provide culturally relevant service to clients (Leonard, 2001; Narayanasamy, 2003).

Cultivate Cultural Sensitivity

The second transcultural nursing principle seeks to expand the nurse's awareness of the significance of culture on behavior. Nurses' beliefs and ways of doing things frequently conflict with those of their clients. A first step toward bridging cultural barriers is to recognize those differences and develop cultural sensitivity. **Cultural sensitivity** requires recognizing that culturally based values, beliefs, and practices influence people's health and lifestyles and need to be considered in plans for service (Campinha-Bacote, 2003; Leininger, 2006). Mrs. Juarez's values and health practices sharply contrasted with those of the clinic's staff. Failure to recognize these differences led to a breakdown in communication and ineffective care. Once differences in culture are recognized, it is important to accept and appreciate them. A nurse's ways are valid for the nurse; clients' ways work for them. The nurse visiting the Kim family in the third case file discussion avoided the dangerous ethnocentric trap of assuming that her way was best, and she consequently developed a fruitful relationship with her clients.

As a part of developing cultural sensitivity, nurses need to try to understand clients' points of view. They need to stand in their clients' shoes and try to see the world through their eyes. By listening, observing, and gradually learning other cultures, the nurse must add a further step of choosing to avoid ethnocentrism. Otherwise, the nurse's view of a different culture will remain distorted and perhaps prejudiced (Leonard, 2001; Leininger, 2006). The ability to show interest, concern, and compassion enabled one nurse to win the trust and respect of the Native American women in the second case file example and told the Kims that their nurse cared about them. These nurses attempted to understand the feelings and ideas of their clients; in this way, they established a trusting relationship and opened the door to the possibility of their clients' adopting healthier behaviors.

Assess the Client Group's Culture

A third transcultural nursing principle emphasizes the need to learn clients' cultures. All clients' actions, like one's own, are based on underlying culturally learned beliefs, values, and ideas (Ludwick & Silva, 2000; Spector, 2009). Mrs. Kim did not like milk because her culture had taught her that it was distasteful and many Asians are lactose intolerant. The Native American women's response to waiting or keeping someone else waiting was influenced by their valuing patience. There usually is some culturally based reason that causes clients to engage in (or avoid) certain actions. Instead of making assumptions or judging clients' behavior, the

nurse first must learn about the culture that guides that behavior (Giger & Davidhizar, 2002). During a cultural assessment, the nurse obtains health-related information about the values, beliefs, and practices of a designated cultural group. Learning the culture of the client first is critical to effective nursing practice. The Giger and Davidhizar Transcultural Assessment Model (2002) denotes six interrelated factors for assessing differences between people in cultural groups (Figure 5.2). Understanding these phenomena is a first step toward appreciating the diversity that exists among people from different cultural backgrounds. Interviewing members of a subcultural group can provide valuable data to enhance understanding (Eggenberger, Grassley, & Restrepo, 2006).

To fully understand a group's culture, it should be studied in depth, as Bernal maintains (1993, p. 231):

> Although a general knowledge base and skills are applicable transculturally, immersion in a given culture is necessary to understand fully the patterns that shape the behavior of individuals within that group. Experience with one group can be helpful in understanding the concept of diversity, but each group must be understood within its own ecologic niche and for its own historical and cultural reality.

Practically speaking, however, it is not possible to study in depth all of the cultural groups that the nurse encounters. Instead, the nurse can conduct a cultural assessment by questioning key informants, observing the cultural group,

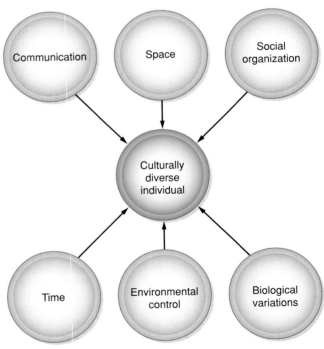

F I G U R E 5.2 Components of the Giger and Davidhizar Transcultural Assessment Model, showing the culturally diverse individual through communication, space, social organization, time, environmental control, and biologic variations. Adapted from Giger, J.N., & Davidhizar, R. (2002). Culturally competent care: Emphasis on understanding the people of Afghanistan, Afghan Americans, and Islamic culture and religion. *International Nursing Review, 49*(2), 79–86, with permission.

and reading additional information in the literature. The data can be grouped into six categories:

1. *Ethnic or racial background:* Where did the client group originate, and how does that influence their status and identity?
2. *Language and communication patterns:* What is the preferred language spoken, and what are the group's culturally based communication patterns?
3. *Cultural values and norms:* What are the client group's values, beliefs, and standards regarding such things as family roles and functions, education, child rearing, work and leisure, aging, death and dying, and rites of passage?

4. *Biocultural factors:* Are there physical or genetic traits unique to this cultural group that predispose them to certain conditions or illnesses?
5. *Religious beliefs and practices:* What are the group's religious beliefs, and how do they influence life events, roles, health, and illness?
6. *Health beliefs and practices:* What are the group's beliefs and practices regarding prevention, causes, and treatment of illnesses?

The cultural assessment guide presented in Table 5.7 gives suggestions for more detailed data collection.

Many cultural assessment guides can be found throughout the nursing literature. Nonetheless, a thorough cultural assessment may be too time-consuming and costly.

TABLE 5.7　Cultural Assessment Guide

Category	Sample Data
Ethnic/racial background	Countries of origin Mostly native-born or U.S. born? Reasons for emigrating if applicable Racial/ethnic identity Experience with racism or racial discrimination?
Language and communication patterns	Languages of origin Languages spoken in the home Preferred language for communication How verbal communication patterns affected by age, sex, other? Preferences for use of interpreters Nonverbal communication patterns (e.g., eye contact, touching)
Cultural values and norms	Group beliefs and standards for male and female roles and functions Standards for modesty and sexuality Family/extended family structures and functions Values re: work, leisure, success, time Values re: education and occupation Norms for child-rearing and socialization Norms for social networks and supports Values re: aging and treatment of elders Values re: authority Norms for dress and appearance
Biocultural factors	Group genetic predisposition to health conditions (e.g., hypertension, anemia) Socioculturally associated illnesses (e.g., AIDS, alcoholism) Group attitudes toward body parts and functions Group vulnerability or resistance to health threats? Folk illnesses common to group? Group physical/genetic differences (e.g., bone mass, height, weight, longevity)
Religious beliefs and practices	Religious beliefs affecting roles, childbearing and child-rearing, health and illness? Recognized religious healers? Religious beliefs and practices for promoting health, preventing illness, or treatment of illness Beliefs and rituals re: conception and birth Beliefs and rituals re: death, dying, grief
Health beliefs and practices	Beliefs re: causes of illness Beliefs re: treatment of illness Beliefs re: use of healers (traditional and Western) Health promotion and illness prevention practices Folk medicine practices Beliefs re: mental health and illness Dietary, herbal, and other folk cures Food beliefs, preparation, consumption Experience with Western medicine

TABLE 5.8   Two-Phased Cultural Assessment Process

Phase I—Data Collection

Stage 1	Assess values, beliefs, and customs (e.g., ethnic affiliations, religion, decision-making patterns).
Stage 2	Collect problem-specific cultural data (e.g., cultural beliefs and practices related to diet and nutrition). Make nursing diagnoses.
Stage 3	Determine cultural factors influencing nursing intervention (e.g., child-rearing beliefs and practices that might affect nurse teaching toilet training or child discipline).

Phase II—Data Organization

Step 1	Compare cultural data with Standards of client's own culture (e.g., client's diet compared with cultural norms) Standards of the nurse's culture Standards of the health facility providing service.
Step 2	Determine incongruities in above standards.
Step 3	Seek to modify one or more systems (client's, nurse's, or the facility's) to achieve maximum congruity.

Instead, the two-phase assessment process is proposed, as outlined in Table 5.8. Categories to explore in the assessment include values, beliefs, customs, and social structure components. Two methods that have proved highly effective for in-depth study of cultural groups are ethnographic interviewing and participant observation. Classic models of these methods have been published by Spradley (1979, 1980).

Show Respect and Patience While Learning About Other Cultures

The fourth transcultural nursing principle emphasizes key behaviors for the nurse to practice during the cultural learning process. Respect is the first behavior, and it is shown in many ways. When Sandra Josten involved the Native American women in decisions and gave them choices, she was showing respect. When the nurse gave positive recognition to the importance of the Kims' culture, she was showing respect. Attentive listening is a way to show respect and to learn about a client's culture. Within the United States, people of minority groups particularly need respect (Cowan & Norman, 2006). At times, for groups with limited English skills and a community health nurse who is not bilingual, an interpreter who can assist with communication becomes a necessity (Display 5.7).

A **minority group** is part of a population that differs from the majority and often receives different and unequal treatment. Their ways contrast with those of the dominant culture. It is difficult for them to retain pride in their lifestyles, or in themselves, when the majority culture suggests that they are inferior (Leininger, 2006; Spector, 2009). This message may be only implied or even unintentional, as was the case for Mrs. Juarez in From the Case Files IV. The clinic's routine and the manner of the staff were not intended to show disrespect. They did, nevertheless, and Mrs. Juarez was intimidated and was unable to receive the help that she needed. Everyone needs respect to enhance pride, dignity, and self-esteem; it is an important contributor to good mental health. Showing respect also is an important means for breaking down barriers in cross-cultural communication. For community health nurses, culturally relevant care means practicing cultural relativism. **Cultural relativism** is recognizing and respecting alternative viewpoints and understanding values, beliefs, and practices within their cultural context.

In addition to respect, patience is essential. It takes time to build trust and effect cultural change. It can be difficult to

establish the nurse–client relationship when it involves two different cultures. Trust must be won, and winning it may take weeks, months, or years. Time must be allowed for both nurse and clients to learn how to communicate with one another, to test one another's trustworthiness, and to learn about one another. Change in behavior (learned aspects of the culture) occurs gradually. Some aspects of both the nurse's and the clients' cultures can, and probably will, change. The Kims' nurse, Paula Morrow, for example, modified

DISPLAY 5.7   INTERPRETER GUIDELINES

1. Unless the community health nurse is thoroughly effective and fluent in the client's language, an interpreter should be used.
2. Speak at a normal to slow pace and make eye contact with the client.
3. Confidentiality must be maintained by the interpreter, who divulges nothing without the full approval of the client and community health nurse.
4. Evaluate the interpreter's style, approach to clients, and ability to develop a relationship of trust and respect. Try to match the interpreter to the client.
5. Be patient. Careful interpretation often requires that the interpreter use long, explanatory phrases.
6. Interpreters must interpret everything that is said by all of the people in the interaction but should inform the community health nurse if the content might be perceived as offensive, insensitive, or harmful to the dignity and well-being of the client.
7. When appropriate, encourage interpreters to explain cultural differences to the client and to yourself.
8. Interpretation conveys the content and spirit of what is said, with nothing omitted or added.
9. Volunteer interpreters receive no fee. Employed interpreters receive their fee or salary from the hiring agency. They should not accept money or favors from clients or the community health nurse. A sincere "thank you" is most appropriate (Kaufert & Putsch, 1997; Putsch, 1985. University of Washington Medical Center, 2008).

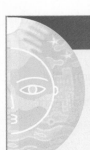

From the Case Files V

The Importance of Cultural Sensitivity

In Australia, well-intentioned government officials, including representatives of the health ministry, identified problems related to substandard housing among a particular aggregate of aboriginal people. To assist this community, the officials spent a great deal of time, energy, and finances planning and building homes for the Aborigines. The homes were small but modern and offered many of the conveniences that officials believed would improve the quality of life for the community.

The Aborigines were appreciative of the group's efforts and moved into their new homes. Before long, however, officials realized that one by one the community members were moving back to their "substandard" housing. When asked about their lack of appreciation for the improved lifestyle, the group informed the officials that their watering hole was their life-line and that the houses were not only uncomfortable to them but were too far from their watering hole. Soon, all of the aboriginal families had returned to living on the land, and the homes were part of a veritable ghost town in the middle of nowhere.

QUESTIONS
- Was the aboriginal community truly "poor," as the officials seemed to think?
- Discuss your perception of the following issues:
  - Cultural imposition
  - Cultural poverty
  - Dignity and spirit
- If you were part of an international health team assigned to return to the community to try again to improve their quality of life, what steps would you take to ensure that previous mistakes are not repeated?

---

some of her usual practices and adapted them to the Kims' culture and needs. They, in turn, began to assume some American practices and values. However, the process took several months. Time, respect, and patience help to break down cultural barriers (Campinha-Bacote, 2003).

Examine Culturally Derived Health Practices

The final transcultural nursing principle involves scrutiny of the client group's cultural practices, as they affect the group's health status. Once the community health nurse has assessed the culture of the client group, cultural practices affecting the health of the client group need to be examined. Are these behaviors preserving and enhancing the group's health, or are they harmful to their health? Some traditional practices, such as customary diet, birth rituals, and certain folk remedies, may promote both physical and psychological health. These can be considered healthful. Other practices may be neither harmful nor particularly health-promoting but are useful in preserving the culture, security, and sense of identity of a particular ethnic group. And some traditional practices may be directly harmful to health. Examples include using herbal poultices to treat an infected wound or "burning" the abdomen to compensate for heat loss associated with diarrhea (Leininger, 2006).

Cultural assessment and aggregate health assessment must go hand in hand. If the group is experiencing a high incidence of low-birth-weight babies, pregnancy complications, skin infections, mental illness, or other evidence of health problems, these can be clues to prompt an examination of cultural health practices. Those that are clearly damaging to health can be discussed with group leaders and healers. In this situation, knowing the group's cultural norms for authority and decision-making can be helpful. Often, a cultural practice can be continued or modified while combined with Western medicine,

so that respect for the culture is maintained while full treatment efficacy is accomplished (see From the Case Files V).

Summary

Community health clients belong to a variety of cultural groups. A culture is a design for living; it provides a set of norms and values that offer stability and security for members of a society and plays a major role in motivating behaviors. The increase in and great variety of cultural groups reinforce the need for community health nurses to understand and appreciate cultural diversity. Ethnocentrism is the bias that a person's own culture is best and others are wrong or inferior. It can create serious barriers to effective nursing care. Understanding cultural diversity and being sensitive to the values and behaviors of cultural groups often is the key to effective community health intervention.

Culture has five characteristics: it is learned from others; it is an integrated system of customs and traits; it is shared; it is tacit; and it is dynamic. Every culture preserves its integrity by deleting nonfunctional practices and acquiring new components that better serve the group. To gain acceptance, nurses must strive to introduce improved health practices that are presented in a manner consistent with clients' cultural values.

Five transcultural nursing principles, drawn from an understanding of the concept of culture, can guide community health nursing practice:

1. Develop cultural self-awareness.
2. Cultivate cultural sensitivity.
3. Assess the client group's culture.
4. Show respect and patience while learning other cultures.
5. Examine culturally derived health practices. ■

ACTIVITIES TO PROMOTE CRITICAL THINKING

1. Based on your own cultural background, how would you feel and what behaviors would you exhibit if you were:
   a. A client sitting in a clinic waiting room in a foreign country whose language you did not know?
   b. Part of a nutrition class being told to eat foods you had never heard of before?
   c. Visited in your home by a nurse who told you to discipline your child in a way that contradicted everything you had been raised to believe about parenting?
2. Describe three tacit cultural rules that govern your own behavior. How might these affect your interactions with clients from another culture?
3. What does the term *ethnocentrism* mean to you? Have you ever experienced someone else's being ethnocentric in their attitude toward you? If so, describe that experience. Using the Cross-Cultural Sensitivity Continuum (see Fig. 5.1), explore where your own attitudes are on the continuum toward several of the cultural groups with which you regularly come in contact or from which you know people well.
4. Imagine that you are assigned to work with a Mexican American migrant population. What steps would you take to gather the appropriate information to provide culturally relevant nursing service? What sources might provide that information?
5. A Hmong father who severely beat his 12-year-old son with a belt, leaving cuts and bruises, is charged with child abuse. "If I can't discipline my son, how can he be a good child?" said the father. What nursing responses would show respect for this cultural group's norms and values, yet be constructive in resolving the cultural conflict?
6. Find websites that elaborate on transcultural nursing and cross-cultural health care concerns. Print materials of interest and develop a resource file for your professional use.
7. Interprofessional communication techniques among diverse health care disciplines are imperative to effective caregiving. How comfortable are you with knowing the linguistic style, practice, and research backgrounds of social workers, pharmacists, physical therapists, educators, psychologists, and others? Seek out a colleague from a different interprofessional discipline and discuss developing a "shared language."

References

Aaron, K.F., Levine, D., & Burstin, H.R. (2003). African American church participation and health care practices. *Journal of General Internal Medicine, 18*(18), 908–913.

Akbar, K.F. (2007). *Family planning and Islam: A review*. Retrieved July 5, 2008 from http://muslim-canada.org/family.htm.

Al-Shahri, M. (2002). Culturally sensitive caring for Saudi patients. *Journal of Transcultural Nursing, 13*(2), 133–138.

Antai-Otong, D. (2002). Culturally sensitive treatment of African-Americans with substance-related disorders. *Journal of Psychosocial Nursing, 40*(7), 14–21.

Baqi-Aziz, M. (2001). Where does she think she is? *American Journal of Nursing, 101*(11), 11.

Bartlett, D.J., & Steele, J.B. (2002, December 8). *Wheel of misfortune*. Retrieved August 9, 2008 from http://www.time.com/time/magazine/article/0,9171,397526-1,00.html.

Berlin, I. (2005). African immigration to Colonial America. *History Now: American History Online, 3*. Retrieved March 1, 2008 from http://www.historynow.org/03_2005/historian3.html.

Bernal, H. (1993). A model for delivering culture-relevant care in the community. *Public Health Nursing, 10*(4), 226–232.

Blais, K.K., Hayes, J.S., & Kozier, B. (2005). *Professional nursing practice: Concepts and perspectives* (5th ed.). Upper Saddle River, NJ: Prentice Hall.

Bornstein, E., & Cote, J. (2004). "Who is sitting across from me?": Immigrant mother's knowledge of parenting and children's development. *Pediatrics, 114*, 557–564.

Bradley, M., & Corwyn, A. (2005). Caring for children around the world: A view from HOME. *International Journal of Behavioral Development, 29*, 468–478.

Brenneman, G., Rhoades, E., & Chilton, L. (2006). Forty years in partnership: The American Academy of Pediatrics and the Indian Health Service. *Pediatrics, 118*, 1257–1263.

Byrd, W.M., & Clayton, L.A. (2002). *An American health dilemma: Race, medicine, and health care in the United States 1900-2000*, Vol. II. New York: Routledge.

California Pan-Ethnic Health Network. (2007). *Racial/ethnic makeup (California, 2000)*. Retrieved July 5, 2008 from http://www.cpehn.org/demochartdetail.php?btn_viewchart=1&view_1.x=52&view_1.y=17&view_1=Get+Statistics%21.

Callister, L.C. (2001). Culturally competent care of women and newborns: Knowledge, attitude, and skills. *Journal of Obstetric, Gynecologic, and Neonatal Nursing, 30*(2), 209–215.

Campinha-Bacote, J. (2003). Many faces: Addressing diversity in health care. *Online Journal of Issues in Nursing, 8*(1). Retrieved July 5, 2008 from http://www.nursingworld.org/ojin/topic20/tpc20_2.htm.

Cash, P., Christianson, E., & Estes, J.W. (1981). Medicine in Colonial Massachusetts, 1620–1820. *The New England Quarterly, 54*(4), 583–585.

Council on American-Islamic Relations. (2008). *About Islam & American Muslims*. Retrieved August 8, 2008 from http://www.cair.com/AboutIslam/IslamBasics.aspx.

Cowan, D.T., & Norman, I. (2006). Cultural competence in nursing: New meanings. *Journal of Transcultural Nursing, 17*, 82–88.

Davis, R.E. (2001). The postpartum experience for Southeast Asian women in the United States. *The American Journal of Maternal Child Nursing, 26*(4), 208–213.

Eggenberger, S.K., Grassley, J., & Restrepo, E. (2006). Culturally competent nursing care: listening to the voices of Mexican American women. *Online Journal of Issues in Nursing, 11*(3), Article 7.

Electronic Resource Center. Management Sciences for Health. (2007a). *Challenges to health and well-being of Arab-Americans families & communities*. Retrieved July 5, 2008 from http://erc.msh.org/mainpage.cfm?file=5.4.2k.htm&module=providers&language=English.

Electronic Resource Center. Management Sciences for Health. (2007b). *Arab-Americans*. Retrieved July 5, 2008 from http://erc.msh.org/mainpage.cfm?file=5.4.2h.htm&module=providers&language=English.

Electronic Resource Center. Management Sciences for Health. (2007c). *What is Islam, and who are Muslims?* Retrieved July 5, 2008 from http://erc.msh.org/mainpage.cfm?file=5.4.6a.htm&module=providers&language=English.

Electronic Resource Center. Management Sciences for Health. (2007d). *Strengths and protective factors in Arab-American families and communities.* Retrieved July 5, 2008 from http://erc.msh.org/mainpage.cfm?file=5.4.2j.htm&module=providers&language=English.

Electronic Resource Center. Management Sciences for Health. (2007e). *Principles for culturally competent health care for Muslim families and communities.* Retrieved July 5, 2008 from http://erc.msh.org/mainpage.cfm?file=5.4.6g.htm&module=providers&language=English.

Ellis, A.D. (2002, August 11). Hmong teens: Lost in America [Special report]. *The Fresno Bee*, 1–12.

Ethnicity Online. (2007). *Cultural awareness in health care: Ethnicity is....* Retrieved July 5, 2008 from http://www.ethnicityonline.net/ethnicity_is.htm.

Fadiman, A. (1997). *The spirit catches you and you fall down.* New York: Noonday Press.

Giger, J.N. (2002). The Giger and Davidhizar transcultural assessment model. *Journal of Transcultural Nursing, 13*(3), 185–188.

Giger, J.N., & Davidhizar, R.E. (2004). *Transcultural nursing* (4th ed.). St. Louis, MO: Elsevier.

Giger, J.N., & Davidhizar, R. (2002). Culturally competent care: Emphasis on understanding the people of Afghanistan, Afghanistan Americans, and Islamic culture and religion. *International Nursing Review, 49*, 79–86.

Goodman, D. (2002). Arab American and American Muslims express mental health needs. *SAMSHA News, X*(1). Retrieved July 5, 2008 from http://www.samhsa.gov/SAMHSA_News/VolumeX_1/article1.htm.

Gruenwald, J. (2004). *Physicians desk reference for herbal medicines* (3rd ed.). Montvale, NJ: Thompson Health Care.

Hall, E.T. (1959). *The silent language.* Garden City, NY: Doubleday.

Handango. (2007). *Nursing herbal medicine handbook* (3rd ed.). Retrieved July 7, 2008 from http://www.handango.com/PlatformProductDetail.jsp?&siteId=1&productType=2&platformId=1&catalog=1&productId=52567.

Her, C., & Culhane-Pera, K. (2004). Culturally responsive care for Hmong patients: Collaboration is a key treatment component. *Postgraduate Medicine, 116*(6), 39–42.

Hesketh, T., Lu, L., & Xing, Z.W. (2005). The effect of China's one-child family policy after 25 years. *New England Journal of Medicine, 353*(11), 1171–1176.

Hing, B.O. (2006). Immigration death trap. *San Francisco Chronicle.* Retrieved July 7, 2008 from http://www.sfgate.com/cgi-bin/article.cgi?file=/chronicle/archive/2006/01/02/EDG5TG18EB1.DTL&type=printable.

Hispanic population spreads out. (2002, August 1). *The Fresno Bee*, A4.

Hong, S., Nelesen, R., Krohn, P., et al. (2006). The association of social status and blood pressure with markers of vascular inflammation. *Psychosomatic Medicine, 68*(4), 517–523.

Infoplease. (2007). *Population of the United States by race and Hispanic/Latino origin, census 2000 and July 1, 2005.* Infoplease.com (Pearson Education). Retrieved July 7, 2008 from http://www.infoplease.com/ipa/A0762156.html.

Indian Health Services (IHS). (2006). *Facts on Indian health disparities.* Retrieved July 7, 2008 from http://infoihs.gov/Files/DisparitiesFacts-Jan2006.pdf.

Kark, S.L. (1974). *Epidemiology and community medicine.* New York: Appleton-Century-Crofts.

Kavasch, E.B., & Baar, K. (1999). *American Indian healing arts: Herbs, rituals, and remedies for every season of life.* New York: Bantam Books.

Kim, M.J., Cho, H., Cheon-Klessig, Y.S., et al. (2002). Primary health care for Korean immigrants: Sustaining a culturally sensitive model. *Public Health Nursing, 19*(3), 191–200.

Kridli, S.A. (2002). Health beliefs and practices among Arab women. *The American Journal of Maternal Child Nursing, 27*(3), 178–182.

Lange, L.A., et al. (2006). Association of polymorphisms in the CRP gene with circulating C-reactive protein levels and cardiovascular events. *Journal of the American Medical Association, 296*(22), 2703–2711.

Leininger, M. (2006). *Culture, care, diversity, and universality: A theory of nursing* (2nd ed.). Boston, MA: Jones & Bartlett Publishers.

Legislative Analyst's Office. (2000). *No single ethnicity to dominate California's population: California's ethnic mix in 2000.* Retrieved July 7, 2008 from http://www.lao.ca.gov/2000/calfacts/2000_calfacts_demographics.html.

Leonard, B.J. (2001). Quality nursing care celebrates diversity. *Online Journal of Issues in Nursing, 6*(2). Retrieved July 7, 2008 from http://www.nursingworld.org/ojin/topic15/tpc15_3.htm.

Levine, R.S., Foster, J.E., Fullilove, R.E., et al. (2001). Black-White inequalities in mortality and life expectancy, 1933–1999: Implications for *Healthy People 2010. Public Health Reports, 116*(5), 474–483.

Lewis, E., Gutierrez, L., & Sakamoto, I. (2001). Women of color. In A. Gitterman (Ed.). *Handbook of social work practice with vulnerable and resilient populations*, 2nd ed. (pp. 820–840). New York: Columbia University Press.

Lippincott, Williams, & Wilkins. (2005). *Nursing herbal medicine handbook* (3rd ed.). Philadelphia: Author.

Lockwood, P., Marshall, T., & Sadler, P. (2005). Promoting success or preventing failure: Cultural differences in motivation by positive and negative role models. *Personality and Social Psychology Bulletin, 31*(3), 379–392.

Lowe, J. (2002). Balance and harmony through connectedness: The intentionality of Native American nurses. *Holistic Nursing Practice, 6*(4), 4–11.

Lowe, J., & Struthers, R. (2001). A conceptual framework of nursing in the Native American culture. *Journal of Nursing Scholarship, 33*(3), 279–283.

Ludwick, R., & Silva, M.C. (2000). Nursing around the world: Cultural values and ethical conflicts. *Online Journal of Issues in Nursing.* Retrieved July 7, 2008 from http://www.nursingworld.org/ojin/ethicol/ethics_4.htm.

Mead, M. (1960). Cultural contexts of nursing problems. In F.C. MacGregor (Ed.). *Social science in nursing.* New York: Wiley.

Medline Plus. (2007). *Herbal medicine.* Retrieved July 7, 2008 from http://www.nlm.nih.gov/medlineplus/herbalmedicine.html.

Mui, A., & Kang, S. (2006). Acculturation stress and depression among Asian immigrant elders. *Social Work, 51*(3), 243–255.

Murdock, G. (1972). The science of culture. In M. Freilich (Ed.). *The meaning of culture: A reader in cultural anthropology.* (pp. 252–266). Lexington, MA: Xerox College Publishing.

Naim, M. (2005). *Arabs in foreign lands: What the success of Arab Americans tells us about Europe, the Middle East, and the power of culture. Foreign Policy.* Retrieved July 7, 2008 from http://www.foreignpolicy.com/story/cms.php?story_id=2781&print=1.

Narayanasamy, A. (2003). Transcultural nursing: How do nurses respond to cultural needs? *British Journal of Nursing, 12*(3), 185–194.

Narayanasamy, A., & White, E. (2005). A review of transcultural nursing. *Nurse Educator Today, 25*(2), 102–111.

National Center for Health Statistics. (2007a). *Health of Black or African American population.* Retrieved July 7, 2008 from http://www.cdc.gov/nchs/fastats/black_health.htm.

National Center for Health Statistics. (2007b). *Health of Hispanic/Latino population.* Retrieved July 7, 2008 from http://www.cdc.gov/nchs/fastats/hispanic_health.htm.

National Center for Health Statistics. (2006). *Health of Asian or Pacific Islander population.* Retrieved July 7, 2008 from http://www.cdc.gov/nchs/fastats/asian_health.htm.

NeedyMeds.com. (2007). *Information you need to get your medicine*. Retrieved July 7, 2008 from http://www.needymeds.com/.

Novak, S.M. (2000). *American shibboleth: Ebonics*. Retrieved July 7, 2008 from http://www.csa.com/discoveryguides/ebonics/overview.php.

Pachter, L.M., & Dworkin, P.H. (1997). Maternal expectations about normal child development in four cultural groups. *Archives of Pediatrics and Adolescent Medicine, 151*(13), 1144–1156.

Plotnikoff, G., Numrich, C., Wu, C., et al. (2002). Hmong shamanism. Animist spiritual healing in Minnesota. *Minnesota Medicine, 85*(6), 29–34.

Ryan, T.J. (2003). Use of herbal medicines in wound healing: A perspective paper. *International Journal of Lower Extremity Wounds, 2*(1), 22–24.

Samhan, H. (2006). Arab Americans. *Grolier's multimedia encyclopedia*. Retrieved from http://www.aaiusa.org/foundation/358/arab-americans.

Snyder, M. (2001). Overview and summary of complementary therapies: Are these really nursing? *Online Journal of Issues in Nursing, 6*(2). Retrieved July 7, 2008 from http://www.nursingworld.org/ojin.topic145/tpc15ntr.htm.

Spector, R.E. (2009). Cultural diversity in health and illness (7th ed.). Upper Saddle River, NJ: Prentice-Hall Allied Health.

Spector, R.E. (2004). Cultural diversity in health and illness (6th ed.). Upper Saddle River, NJ: Pearson Education, Inc.

Spradley, J.P. (1979). *The ethnographic interview*. New York: Holt.

Spradley, J.P. (1980). *Participant observation*. New York: Holt.

Spradley, J.P., & McCurdy, D.W. (2005). *Conformity and conflict: Readings in cultural anthropology*, 12th ed. Boston, MA: Allyn & Bacon Publishing.

Substance Abuse & Mental Health Services Administration (SAMHSA). (2004). *National survey on drug use and health. Risk and protective factors for substance use among American Indian or Alaska Native youths*. Retrieved July 7, 2008 from http://oas.samhsa.gov/2k4/AmindianYouthRF/AmindianYouthRF.htm.

Swagerty, S.L., Walling, A.D., & Klein, R.M. (2002). Lactose intolerance. *American Family Physician, 65*(9). Retrieved July 7, 2008 from http://www.aafp.org/afp/20020501/1845.html.

Taylor, J.B., & Kalt, J.P. (2005). *American Indians on reservations: A databook of socioeconomic change between the 1990 and 2000 censuses*. Cambridge, MA: Harvard University.

Tsai, J., Louie, J., Chen, E.E., & Uchida, Y. (2007). Learning what feelings to desire: Socialization of ideal affect through children's storybooks. *Personality and Social Psychology Bulletin, 33*(1), 17–30.

U.S. Census Bureau. (1992). *Population projections of the US, 1992-2050*. Retrieved July 7, 2008 from http://www.wonder.cdc.gov/wonder/sci_data/census/post/type_txt/proj2050.asp.

U.S. Census Bureau. (2001). *Hispanic population of the United States*. Retrived August 4, 2008 from http://www.census.gov/population//www/socdemo/hispanic/ho01.html.

U.S. Committee for Refugees and Immigrants (USCRI). (2006). *World Refugee Survey 2005: The Americas and the Caribbean*. Retrieved February 20, 2007 from http://www.refugees.org/data/wrs/06/docs/refugee_and_asylum_seekers_worldwide.pdf.

U.S. Department of Commerce. (2001). *Statistical abstract of the United States, 2001*, 121st ed. Washington, DC: Government Printing Office.

U.S. Department of Health and Human Services. (2000). *Healthy People 2010*, Conference ed., Vols. 1 & 2. Washington, DC: Author.

U.S. Food & Drug Administration. (2007). *Over-the-counter drug review process*. Retrieved July 7, 2008 from http://www.fda.gov/cder/handbook/otcpage.htm.

Walton, M. (2005 July 6). *The business of gambling*. CNN. Retrieved July 7, 2008 from http:// cnn.worldnews.printthis.clickability.com/pt/cpt?action=cpt&titl...2Fcnn25.top25.gambling%2Findex.html&partnerID=2006&showBibliography=Y.

Wang, Q. (2004). The emergence of cultural self-constructs: Autobiographical memory and self-description in European American and Chinese children. *Developmental Psychology, 40*(1), 3–15.

Wang, X., Zhu, H., Dong, Y., et al. (2006). Effects of angiotensinogen and angiotensin II type I receptor genes on blood pressure and left ventricular mass trajectories in multiethnic youth. *Twin Research in Human Genetics, 9*(3), 393–402.

Williams, D.R., & Collins, C. (2001). Racial residential segregation: A fundamental cause of racial disparities in health. *Public Health Reports, 116*(5), 404–416.

Yuki, M., Maddux, W., Brewer, M., & Takemura, K. (2005). Cross-cultural differences in relationship- and group-based trust. *Personality and Social Psychology Bulletin, 31*(48). Retrieved July 7, 2008 from http://www.psp.sagepub.com/cgi/congtent/abstract/31/1/48.

Selected Readings

Adams, P., Dey, A., & Vickerie, J. (2007). Summary health statistics for the U.S. population: National Health Interview Survey, 2005. *Vital Health Statistics, 10*(233), 1–104.

Andrews, M.M., & Boyle, J.S. (2007). *Transcultural concepts in nursing care* (5th ed.). Philadelphia: Lippincott Williams & Wilkins.

Arorian, K., Katz, A., & Kulwicki, A. (2006). Recruiting and retaining Arab Muslim mothers and children for research. *Journal of Nursing Scholarship, 38*(3), 255–261.

Azaiza, F., & Cohen, M. (2006). Health beliefs and rates of breast cancer screening among Arab women. *Journal of Women's Health, 15*(5), 520–530.

Baker, L., Afendulis, C., Chandra, A., et al. (2007). Differences in neonatal mortality among Whites and Asian American subgroups: Evidence from California. *Archives of Pediatric & Adolescent Medicine, 161*(1), 69–76.

Brown, S.A., Garcia, A.A., Kouzekanani, K., & Hanis, C.L. (2002). Culturally competent diabetes self-management education for Mexican Americans. *Diabetes Care, 25*(2), 259–268.

Couzin, J. (2007). Cancer research: Probing the roots of race and cancer. *Science, 315*(5812), 592–594.

Devlin, H., Roberts, M., Okaya, A., & Xiong, Y. (2006). Our lives were healthier before: Focus groups with African American, American Indian, Hispanic/Latino, and Hmong people with diabetes. *Health Promotion Practice, 7*(1), 47–55.

Edinburgh, L., Saewyc, E., Thao, T., & Levitt, C. (2006). Sexual exploitation of very young Hmong girls. *Journal of Adolescent Health, 39*(1), 111–118.

Engebretson, J. (2001). Alternative and complementary healing: Implications for nursing. In E.C. Hein (Ed.). *Nursing issues in the 21st century: Perspectives from the literature.* (pp. 150–167). Philadelphia: Lippincott Williams & Wilkins.

Fitzpatrick, L., Sutton, M., & Greenberg, A. (2006). Toward eliminating health disparities in HIV/AIDS: The importance of the minority investigator in addressing scientific gaps in Black and Latino communities. *Journal of the National Medical Association, 98*(12), 1906–1911.

Jonas, W.B. (2001). Alternative medicine: Value and risks. In E.C. Hein (Ed.). *Nursing issues in the 21st century: Perspectives from the literature.* (pp.145–149). Philadelphia: Lippincott Williams & Wilkins.

Jones, M.E., Bercier, O., Hayes, A.L., et al. (2002). Family planning patterns and acculturation level of high-risk, pregnant Hispanic women. *Journal of Nursing Care Quality, 16*(4), 46–55.

Kandula, N., Lauderdale, D., & Baker, D. (2007). Differences in self-reported health among Asians, Latinos, and non-Hispanic Whites: The role of language and nativity. *Annals of Epidemiology, 17*(3), 191–198.

Keswick, R., & McNeil, L. (2006). Reaching out to the Arabic community. *Behavioral Healthcare, 26*(11), 32.

Kogan, S., Brody, G., Crawley, C., et al. (2007). Correlates of elevated depressive symptoms among rural African American adults with type 2 diabetes. *Ethnicity & Disease, 17*(1), 106–112.

Leininger, M. (2002). Culture care theory: A major contribution to advance transcultural nursing knowledge and practice. *Journal of Transcultural Nursing, 13*(3), 189–192.

Malepede, C., Greene, L., Fitzpatrik, S., et al. (2007). Racial influences associated with weight-related beliefs in African American and Caucasian women. *Ethnicity & Disease,17*(1), 1–5.

McLaughlin, D.K., & Stokes, S. (2002). Income inequality and mortality in U.S. counties: Does minority racial concentration matter? *American Journal of Public Health, 92*(1), 99–104.

National Center for Cultural Competence. (2007). *Cultural competence health practitioner assessment (CCHPA).* Retrieved July 7, 2008 from http://www.11.georgetown.edu/research/gucchd/nccc/features/CCHPA.html.

Oppenheimer, G.M. (2001). Paradigm lost: Race, ethnicity, and the search for a new population taxonomy. *American Journal of Public Health, 91*(7), 1049–1055.

Pappas, G., Aktar, T., Gergen, P.J., et al. (2001). Health status of the Pakistani population: A health profile and comparison with the United States. *American Journal of Public Health, 91*(1), 93–98.

Parker, M.W., Bellis, J.M., Bishop, P., et al. (2002). A multidisciplinary model of health promotion incorporating spirituality into a successful aging intervention with African American and White elderly groups. *The Gerontologist, 42*(3), 406–415.

Satcher, D. (2000). Eliminating racial and ethnic disparities in health: The role of the ten leading health indicators. *Journal of the National Medical Association, 92*(6), 315–318.

Yang, R., Mills, P., & Dodge, J. (2006). Cancer screening, reproductive history, socioeconomic status, and anticipated cancer-related behavior among Hmong adults. *Asian Pacific Journal of Cancer Prevention, 7*(1), 79–85.

Ypinazar, V., & Margolis, S. (2006). Delivering culturally sensitive care: The perceptions of older Arabian Gulf Arabs concerning religion, health, and disease. *Qualitative Health Research, 16*(6), 773–787.

Internet Resources

AltaVista's Translator—translates any web page to one of eight languages: *http://abelfish.altavista.com*

American Academy of Child and Adolescent Psychiatry (AACAP), Facts for Families (available in four languages): *http://www.aacap.org/publications/factsfam/index.htm*

American Diabetes Association, Facts and Figures: *http://www.diabetes.org*

American Immigration Resources on the Internet—general references for immigrants: *http://theodora.com*

Association of Asian Pacific Community Health Organizations (AAPCHO). Health education information to improve the health status of Asians and Pacific Islanders in the United States. Available in 12 languages. *http://www.aapcho.org*

Cultural Competence Compendium: *http://www.ama-assn.org*

Cultural Competence Health Practitioner Assessment: *http://www11.georgetown.edu/research/gucchd/nccc/CCHPA.html*

Culture and Diversity: *http://www.amsa.org*

Ensuring Linguistic Access in Health Care Settings: Legal Rights and Responsibilities: *http://www.kff.org*

Indian Health Service—an agency within the U.S. Department of Health and Human Services that provides health services and information about American Indians and Alaska Natives: *http://www.ihs.gov*

Milstead, J.A. (2003). Interweaving policy and diversity. *Online Journal of Issues in Nursing, 8*(1), manuscript 4. Retrieved from http://www.nursingworld.org/MainMenuCategories/ANAMarketplace/ANAPeriodicals/OJIN/TableofContents/Volume82003/Num1Jan31_2003/InterweavingPolicyandDiversity.aspx.

Multicultural Health Communication Service. The goal of this Australian site is to provide quality health care information to people of non–English-speaking backgrounds. Information is offered in 36 languages, including Arabic, Chinese, Russian, and Vietnamese: *http://www.mhcs.health.nsw.gov.au/*

Office of Minority Health: *http://www.omhrc.gov/*

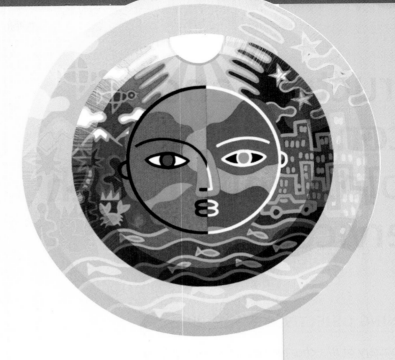

PUBLIC HEALTH ESSENTIALS FOR COMMUNITY HEALTH NURSING

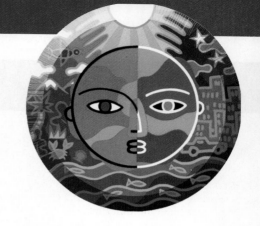

6

Structure and Economics of Community Health Services

Upon mastery of this chapter, you should be able to:

◆ Trace historic events and philosophical developments leading to today's health services delivery systems.

◆ Outline the current organizational structure of the public health care system.

◆ Examine the three core functions of public health as they apply to health services delivery.

◆ Differentiate between the functions of public versus private sector health care agencies.

◆ Examine the public health services provided by selected international health organizations.

◆ Explain the influence of selected legislative acts in the United States on shaping current health services policy and practice.

◆ Explore how the structure and functions of community health services affect community health nursing practice.

◆ Define the concept of health care economics.

◆ Describe three sources of health care financing.

◆ Compare and contrast retrospective and prospective health care payment systems.

◆ Analyze the trends and issues influencing health care economics and community health services delivery.

◆ Explain the causes and effects of health care rationing.

◆ List the pros and cons of managed competition as opposed to a single-payer system.

◆ Explain the philosophical implications of health care financing patterns on community health nursing's mission and values.

❝There are 10^{11} stars in the galaxy. That used to be a huge number. But it's only a hundred billion. It's less than the national deficit! We used to call them astronomical numbers. Now we should call them economical numbers.❞

—Richard Feynman (1918–1988)

Adverse selection
Assessment
Assurance
Capitation rates
Competition
Consumer-driven health plan (CDHP)
Core public health functions
Cost sharing
Cost shifting
Demand
Diagnosis-related groups (DRGs)
Economics
Fee-for-service
Gross domestic product (GDP)
Health care economics
Health maintenance organization (HMO)
Health savings account (HSA)
Macroeconomic theory
Managed care
Managed competition
Medicaid
Medical home
Medically indigent
Medicare
Microeconomic theory
Nongovernmental organizations (NGOs)
Official health agencies
Point of service plan (POS)
Policy development
Preferred provider organization (PPO)
Proprietary health services
Prospective payment
Public Health Service
Quarantine
Rationing
Regulation
Retrospective payment
Sanitation
Shattuck Report
Single-payer system
Supply
Third-party payments
Universal coverage
Voluntary health agencies

Nurses preparing for population-based practice need to be familiar with how the health care delivery system is organized and operates, because it is through this system that we are able to offer community health services (see Chapter 3). This system forms an organizing framework for the design and implementation of programs aimed at improving the health of communities and vulnerable groups. It is within this system or framework that community health nurses labor, realize the opportunity to shape future health services, and develop innovative and more effective means of improving community health.

Nurses concerned with the delivery of needed community health services also must understand how those services are financed. In an era when health care costs are rising while resources are limited and providers are competing for scarce dollars, nurses must be well-informed about the issues related to health care financing and about ways to obtain funding to address identified health needs in the community. The structure and economics of community health care are intertwined. **Health care economics** is a specialized field of economics that describes and analyzes the production, distribution, and consumption of goods and services, as well as a variety of related problems such as finance, labor, and taxation (Aday, 2005). The goal of health care economics, much like public health, is to overcome scarcity by making good choices and providing essential services.

Service delivery systems directed at restoring or promoting the public's health have evolved over centuries. The structure, function, and financing of health care systems have changed dramatically during that time in response to evolving societal needs and demands, scientific advancements, more effective methods of service delivery, new technologies, and varying approaches to resource acquisition and allocation (Barton, 2003). Although progress has been made toward a healthier global society, many problems remain, particularly those of controlling health care costs, assuring equitable distribution and effectiveness of health services, and assuring the quality of and access to those services (Pan American Health Organization, 2001; U.S. Department of Health and Human Services [USDHHS], 2000).

This chapter examines the current structure and functions of community health services in the United States and reviews historical and legislative events that influenced the planning for and the delivery of those services. It also provides an overview of health care economics and the ever-changing landscape of financial incentives and disincentives for enhancing the public's health.

HISTORICAL INFLUENCES ON HEALTH CARE

Despite centuries of change, some personal and community hygiene and health care practices have gone on from the beginning of time. Many primitive tribes engaged in sanitary practices such as burial of excreta, removal of the dead, and isolation of members with certain illnesses. Treatment of the sick has always included using a variety of therapeutic agents administered by a "healer."

Whether health care practices were based on superstition, derived from survival needs, or primarily tied to religious beliefs is unknown. Nonetheless, records show that in Egypt and the Middle East, as early as 3000 BC, people were building drainage systems, using toilets and systems for water flushing, and practicing personal cleanliness (Scutchfield & Keck, 2003). The Hebrew hygienic code, described in the Bible in Leviticus circa 1500 BCE, probably was the first written code in the world and was the prototype for personal and community sanitation. It emphasized bodily cleanliness, protection against the spread of contagious diseases, isolation of lepers, disinfection of dwellings after illness, sanitation of campsites, disposal of excreta and refuse, protection of water and food supplies, and maternal hygiene (Scutchfield & Keck, 2003). Even more advanced were the Athenians, circa 1000 to 400 BCE, who emphasized personal hygiene, diet, and exercise in addition to a sanitary environment, albeit for the benefit of the wealthy. Their successors, the Romans, added more community health measures, such as laws regulating environmental sanitation and nuisances and construction of paved streets, aqueducts, and a subsurface drainage system.

The Middle Ages (from about 500 to 1500 AD) were distinguished by a distinct change in health beliefs and practices in Europe, based on the philosophy that to pamper the body was evil. During this regressive period in history, health care was scarce, private, and reserved for the wealthy few, whereas public health problems were rampant, and only minimally and ineffectively addressed.

Neglected personal hygiene (e.g., infrequent bathing), improper diets, and accumulation of refuse and body wastes led to widespread epidemics and pandemics of disease, including cholera, plague, and leprosy (Hecker, 1839). Increased trade between Europe and Asia, military conquests, and Christian crusades to the Middle East furthered the spread of disease. Bubonic plague, known as the Black Death, was the most devastating of pandemics, reportedly killing more than 60 million people in the mid-1300s (Hecker, 1839). Fear of Black Death caused Venice to ban entry of infected ships and travelers—a form of quarantine.

Quarantine is a period of enforced isolation of persons exposed to a communicable disease during the incubation period of the disease, to prevent its spread should infection occur. The first known official quarantine measure was instituted in 1377, at the port of Ragusa (now Dubrovnik in Croatia, formerly Yugoslavia), where travelers from plague areas were required to wait 2 months and to be free of disease before entry.

By the 1700s, more enlightened Europeans began to challenge the prevailing beliefs and conditions (e.g., disease as a punishment for sin). Even in the 1800s, many people in the United States thought that disease and poverty were visited upon the ignorant and the dirty. We now know the cause of disease; however, stigma regarding such conditions as leprosy and tuberculosis (TB) still exists today, and some regard sexually transmitted diseases and acquired immune deficiency syndrome (AIDS) as punishment for immoral conduct. During the late 18th century, new efforts at reform were influenced by a growing emphasis on human dignity, human rights, and the search for scientific truth. These efforts continued through the 19th and 20th centuries (Scutchfield & Keck, 2003).

Despite improvement during the 17th and 18th centuries, serious problems persisted and new ones developed. Industrialization, masses of people moving to cities, and low regard for human life all contributed to deplorable living and working conditions. Hundreds of poor children died in England's abusive but socially approved workhouses and apprentice slavery system. Most European communities were characterized by unspeakable misery and filth. Householders dumped their refuse from windows or doors into the streets. Rivers and water supplies were seriously contaminated. Diseases, including cholera, typhus, typhoid, smallpox, and TB, took a tremendous toll on human life (Greene, 2001).

In the 16th and 17th century, London was one of the largest cities in the world, with the population tripling by the end of the 17th century (Cockayne, 2007, p. 9). By the mid 18th century, noise from carriages and carts, animals, and vendors created a "hideous din" (Cockayne, p. 107). Air pollution from burning coal and wood for fuel caused Londoners to cough and spit. People "rarely washed their bodies and lived in the constant sight and smell of human feces and human urine" (Cockayne, p. 60).

Around the turn of the 19th century, England's leaders became increasingly concerned about social and sanitary reform. The term **sanitation** refers to the promotion of hygiene and prevention of disease by maintenance of health-enhancing (sanitary) conditions. The first sanitary legislation, passed in 1837, established vaccination stations in London. One of the most notable reformers, Edwin Chadwick, the father of modern public health, published his *Report on an Inquiry into the Sanitary Conditions of the Laboring Population of Great Britain* in 1842 (Richardson, 1887). His efforts resulted in passage of the English Public Health Act and establishment of a General Board of Health for England in 1848, as reported by Lewis more than a century later (1952).

An epidemiologist and anesthetist, John Snow (1813–1858) worked on the cholera outbreak in London in 1854. His investigations of cholera outbreaks and conclusions led to changes in the practice of sewage dumping into the Thames River, thus improving London's morbidity and mortality from cholera (see Chapter 7). His 1855 work, *On the Mode of Communication of Cholera* (2nd ed.), was a landmark public health contribution. Conditions improved, and scientific study advanced in England and, concurrently, in France, Germany, Scandinavia, and other European countries. England, however, set the pace for application of research, particularly with reference to public health measures, through steadily improved legislation. British laws subsequently became the pattern for American sanitary ordinances (Greene, 2001).

PUBLIC HEALTH CARE SYSTEM DEVELOPMENT IN THE UNITED STATES

The current U.S. public health care system was long in developing. Most health-related services in the United States were initially reactive, responding to the pressure of immediate needs and uncoordinated from one locality to another. Over time, events and insights contributed to a gradually improving system of programs and services, along with recognition that the health of individuals was affected by the health of the wider community (Table 6.1 highlights some of these changes). Our current public health system is not really a "single entity, but rather a loosely affiliated network of approximately 3,000 federal, state, and local

governmental health agencies often working closely with private sector voluntary and professional health associations" (Trust for America's Health, 2005, p. 8).

Precursors to a Health Care System

Early health care in the American colonies consisted of private practice, with occasional (but infrequent) governmental action for the public good. Action usually was in the form of isolated local responses to specific dangers or nuisances, such as the 1647 regulation to prevent pollution of Boston Harbor or the 1701 Massachusetts law requiring ship quarantine and isolation of smallpox patients. New York City, in the late 1700s, formed a public health committee to monitor water quality, sewer construction, marsh drainage, and burial of the dead. Physicians in the early 19th century had few tools at their disposal and could do little to change the course of illness. They made house calls, as most quality care was given in the home, not in hospitals (Cutler, 2004). The U.S. Constitution, adopted in 1789, made no direct reference to public health, nor did the federal government take an active stance on health matters. It was the responsibility of each sovereign state to manage its own health affairs. The first federal intervention for health problems was the Marine Hospital Service Act of 1798. It subsidized medical and hospital care for sick and injured merchant seamen, with the first marine hospital being located in Boston.

During the early years, a scourge of epidemics, especially smallpox, cholera, typhoid, and typhus, caused deaths throughout the colonies and decimated the Native American population (Woodward, 1932). Slave trade further threatened the lives of colonists by introducing diseases, such as yaws (an infectious nonvenereal disease caused by a spirochete), yellow fever, and malaria (Marr, 1982). Local control of quarantine efforts proved ineffective. In 1837, Congress finally instituted the national port quarantine system, which was regulated and enforced by the Marine Hospital Service. Epidemics were quickly checked, causing society to recognize the benefits of uniform central government policy. However, improvements in public health and sanitation on a state and local level competed with other needs, such as police and fire protection (Greene, 2001) (see Table 6.2).

Calls for Sanitary Reforms

The **Shattuck Report**, a landmark document, made a tremendous impact on sanitary progress. Lemuel Shattuck, a physician and legislator, chaired a legislative committee that studied health and sanitary problems in the Commonwealth of Massachusetts. In 1850, he produced the *Report of the Sanitary Commission of Massachusetts* (Shattuck et al., 1850) describing the public health concepts and methods that form the basis for current public health practice. Shattuck advocated the establishment of state and local boards of health, environmental sanitation, collection and use of vital statistics, systematic study of diseases, control of food and drugs, urban planning, establishment of nurses' training schools (there were none before this time), and preventive medicine.

A similar report by John Griscom on conditions of the working poor in New York City, published in 1845, concluded that illness, premature death, and poverty were directly related and were not the result of immoral or intemperate

TABLE 6.1 Changes in Health Status and Health Care Services

Turn of the 20th Century	Turn of the 21st Century
MORBIDITY AND MORTALITY	
Then	**Now**
High communicable disease and mortality	High chronic disease morbidity and mortality
Little prevention	Old and new sexually transmitted diseases
Infrequent cure	Resurgence of tuberculosis
Life span of 47 yr	Life span of 76 yr
High infant mortality	Significant infant mortality
High maternal mortality	High teenage pregnancy
Alcohol abuse	Multiple substance abuse
Many undiagnosed and untreated conditions	New strains of multidrug-resistant diseases, long-term chronicity, and disability
ACCESS TO HEALTH CARE	
Then	**Now**
Access primarily for those who could pay a fee	Access for those with health insurance
No health insurance	Insurance with copayments shifting to managed care
Public health clinics for poor and underserved	Free health clinics for medically indigent (especially children)
Limited treatments available	Multitude of treatments with regular new advances
HEALTH CARE DELIVERY SYSTEM	
Then	**Now**
Extended hospital stays	Short-term, acute-care hospitalizations
Discharge on recovery	Recovery occurs at home or in a transitional setting
Extended maternal and newborn hospitalization	Short-stay maternal and newborn care
Many home deliveries with lay assistance	Few home deliveries with skilled assistance
Home care through not-for-profit agencies	Home care through not-for-profit and proprietary agencies
PHN begun in health departments	Shifting PHN role in health departments
Health departments provide personal care services for poor and underserved	Health department's personal care services a part of managed care systems

Adapted from Erickson, G.P. (1996). To pauperize or empower: Public health nursing at the turn of the 20th and 21st centuries. *Public Health Nursing, 13*(3), 163–169.

behaviors, as many public health officials advocated. He recommended sanitary reform as did others, such as Barton, Jarvis, and Martin Snow (Duffy, 1990). Almost 25 years passed before these recommendations were fully appreciated and implemented.

Recent Calls to Action

In 1988, the Institute of Medicine published *The Future of Public Health*, highlighting the state of disarray in our current public health system and calling for improvements in the public health infrastructure—largely focusing on governmental responsibilities. In 2002, the Institute issued a new publication, *The Future of the Public's Health in the 21st Century*. This report called for expanding the responsibilities of the public health system beyond governmental agencies to include private and nongovernmental entities. The report outlined how partnerships could be formed with communities, businesses, the media, universities, and other components of the health care delivery system to expand the reach of public health and achieve the Healthy People 2010 goals (Institute of Medicine, 2002). Other needed changes included a spotlight on multiple determinants of health along with a population focus, transdisciplinary utilization of evidence-based practice, and better communication and systems of accountability.

Official Health Agencies

The beginnings of an organized health care system in the United States came in the form of **official health agencies**, later called public health agencies. These were publicly funded and operated by state or local governments with a goal of providing population-based health services. Development occurred initially at the local level. Many cities established local boards of health in the late 1700s and early to middle 1800s. Among the earliest were those in Baltimore, Maryland (1798); Charleston, South Carolina (1815); and Philadelphia, Pennsylvania (1818). As their efforts expanded from handling public "nuisances" to dealing with epidemics and complex public health problems, local health boards recognized that full-time staffs were needed, and thus health departments were formed. Louisiana was first in 1855; Massachusetts followed in 1869.

Again at the national level, the Marine Hospital Service, now with a broader function, became the Public Health and Marine Hospital Service in 1902. Congress gave it a more clearly defined organizational structure and specific functions

TABLE 6.2 Societal Events and Situations Affecting Health Care Needs

Turn of the 20th Century	Turn of the 21st Century
SOCIETAL AND POPULATION SHIFTS	
Then	**Now**
Industrial society focusing on production	Postindustrial, service and information oriented
Rural to urban	Urban to suburban
Limited violence	Rampant violence and terrorism
Wide gaps between rich and poor	Widening gaps between rich and poor
Growing philanthropy	Declining support for charitable health care
Intense immigration from eastern Europe	Moderate immigration—Africa, Europe, Asia
ENVIRONMENT	
Then	**Now**
Overcrowded, unsanitary housing	Deteriorating inner-city neighborhoods
Unsafe workplaces, lack of worker safeguards	Environmental hazards in some workplaces
Rampant child labor	Homelessness
Poor public sanitation	Good public sanitation
Multiple health risks	Increasing environmental and behavioral risks
SKILL CHANGES AND EMPLOYMENT	
Then	**Now**
Farm to factory	Factory to service and information
Low wages	Improving wages, limited benefits
Dramatic disparity in wages between men and women	Slowly resolving disparity in male/female wage differences
Not enough jobs	Downsizing, layoffs, corporate streamlining, failing companies
PEOPLE LIVING IN POVERTY	
Then	**Now**
Women and children	Women, children, the aged
Immigrants—European	Immigrants—Hispanic, Caribbean, Middle Eastern, and Asian
Migration—south to north	Seasonal migration of farm workers

Adapted from Erickson, G.P. (1996). To pauperize or empower: Public health nursing at the turn of the 20th and 21st centuries. *Public Health Nursing, 13*(3), 163–169.

for its director, the Surgeon General. In 1912, it was renamed the United States Public Health Service (PHS) (Melosi, 2000; Turnock, 2004; USDHHS, 2007; Ward & Warren, 2007).

Rapidly expanding through World War I and the Great Depression, the PHS strengthened its research activity through the National Institutes of Health (NIH, founded in 1912), added demonstration projects, and initiated greater cooperation with the states. Responding to increasingly complex needs, the NIH added programs significant to public health, such as the Children's Bureau (1912); the National Leprosarium at Carville, Louisiana (1917); examination of arriving aliens (1917); the Division of Venereal Diseases (1918); the Food and Drug Administration [FDA] (1927); and the Narcotics Division (1929), which later became the Division of Mental Hygiene. Title VI of the 1935 Social Security Act promoted stronger federal support of state and local public health services, including health workforce training (USDHHS, 2007; Ward & Warren, 2007).

As health, welfare, and educational services proliferated, the need for consolidation prompted the creation of the Federal Security Agency in 1939. In 1953, the agency was enlarged and renamed the Department of Health, Education,

and Welfare (DHEW), under President Eisenhower. In 1979, education was made a separate cabinet-level department, and the DHEW was renamed the Department of Health and Human Services (DHHS). Other significant events include the establishment during World War II of the Communicable Disease Center in Atlanta, currently known as the Centers for Disease Control and Prevention (CDC), and the development after World War II of the National Office of Vital Statistics, now called the National Center for Health Statistics (NCHS) (Centers for Disease Control & Prevention, 2006).

Voluntary Health Agencies

The private sector responded first to America's health problems and continues to complement and supplement the government's role in providing health services. By the late 1800s, **voluntary health agencies** (sometimes called private agencies or **nongovernmental organizations [NGOs]**) began to emerge. They were privately funded and operated to address specific health needs. The first of these was the Anti-Tuberculosis Society of Philadelphia, which was formed in 1892 to educate the public and the government about TB, then causing 10% of all deaths. Other agencies followed: the National Society to Prevent Blindness was formed in 1908, the Mental Health Association in 1909, the American Cancer Society in 1913, the National Easter Seal Society for Crippled Children and Adults in 1921, and the Planned Parenthood Federation of America, also in 1921. In the late 1800s, organized charities such as the Red Cross, previously denounced for promoting dependent poverty, began to be recognized for their contributions to health and welfare. Philanthropy, too, became prominent with the establishment of the Rockefeller Foundation in 1913, followed by the Carnegie-Mellon, Kellogg, and Robert Wood Johnson Foundations (Public Health Encyclopedia, 2007).

Health-related Professional Associations

Many health-related professional associations have influenced the quality and type of community health services delivery. Among these, the National Organization for Public Health Nursing, from 1912 to 1952, significantly influenced early preparation for and the quality of public health nursing services (Abrams, 2004). The American Public Health Association (APHA), founded in 1872, maintains a prominent role in the dissemination of public health information, influence on health policy, and advocacy for the nation's health. Other nursing and community health organizations that have promoted quality efforts in community health include the Association of State and Territorial Directors of Nursing (ASTDN), the Association of State and Territorial Health Officers (ASTHO), the National League for Nursing (NLN), the American Nurses Association (ANA), and the Association for Community Health Nursing Educators (ACHNE).

HEALTH ORGANIZATIONS IN THE UNITED STATES

Over the years, responsibility for meeting community health needs has shifted between private groups and governing institutions, each offering different viewpoints and benefits. Only within the last century have they gradually begun to work together to create a loosely structured system of health care.

Barton spoke of the growing interdependence of the public and private sectors (2003), and this partnership was encouraged by the Institute of Medicine (2002). How does that system work today? What are its strengths and weaknesses? To answer these questions, its structure must first be examined. Structure is important because it becomes the operational base for assessment, diagnosis, planning, implementation, and evaluation of services—and it provides a framework for intersystem and intrasystem communication and coordination.

Health services occur at four levels: local, state, national, and international. Like ever-widening concentric circles, these levels encompass broader populations. The organization of health services at each level can generally be classified as one of two types: public or private sector.

Public Sector Health Services

Government health agencies, the tax-supported arm of the public health effort, perform a vital function in community health practice. With their jurisdiction and types of service dictated by law, they coordinate and administer activities that often can be carried out only by group or community-wide action (e.g., proper sewage disposal, provision of sanitary water systems, or regulation of toxic wastes). Many community health activities require an authoritative legal backing to ensure enforcement—another useful function of public health agencies—in areas such as environmental pollution, highway safety practices, communicable disease control, and proper, safe handling of food. Official or public health agencies provide important record-keeping services, including the collection and monitoring of vital statistics. They also conduct research, provide consultation, and sometimes financially support other community health efforts.

Core Public Health Functions

Public health services encompass a wide variety of activities, but all can be grouped under one of three **core public health functions** (Institute of Medicine, 1988). They are assessment, policy development, and assurance (Figure 3.1). As discussed in Chapter 3, public health nurses practice as partners with other public health professionals within these core functions.

Assessment refers to measuring and monitoring the health status and needs of a designated community or population. As a core function, it is a continuous process of collecting data and disseminating information about health, diseases, injuries, air and water quality, food safety, and available resources. This function helps to identify trends in morbidity, mortality, and causative factors. It identifies available health resources, unmet needs, and community perceptions about health issues.

Policy development is the formation of a guide for action that determines present and future decisions affecting the public's health. As a core public health function, good public policy development builds on data from the assessment function and incorporates community values and citizen input. It provides leadership and administration for the development of sound health policy and planning.

Assurance is the process of translating established policies into services. This function ensures that population-based services are provided, whether by public health agencies or private sources. It also monitors the quality of and access to those services. The specific functions of assessment, policy development, and assurance are described in Table 6.3.

The roles of public health agencies vary by level, with each level carrying out the core functions in different ways to form a partnership in protecting the public's health (Turnock, 2004; Williams & Torrens, 2002). International health agencies focus on issues of global concern, setting policy, developing standards, and monitoring health conditions and programs. At the national level, government health agencies engage in similar functions aimed at regional or nationwide concerns.

The federal level provides funds (e.g., through the Medicaid program, block grants, categorical grants) and develops policy (e.g., air pollution policy, occupational safety) but depends on the states to implement them. Agencies at the federal level also develop facilities and programs for special groups, such as Native Americans, migrant workers, inmates of federal prisons, and military personnel and veterans, whose health care is not the direct responsibility of any one state or locality (CDC, 2002).

TABLE 6.3 Core Public Health Functions Applied to Populations and People at Risk

Population-Wide Services

Assessment
- Health status monitoring and disease surveillance

Public Policy
- Leadership, policy, planning, and administration

Assurance
- Investigation and control of diseases and injuries
- Protection of environment, workplaces, housing, food, and water
- Laboratory services to support disease control and environmental protection
- Health education and information
- Community mobilization for health-related issues
- Targeted outreach and linkage to personal services
- Health services quality assurance and accountability
- Training and education of public health professionals

Personal Services and Home Visits for People at Risk

- Primary care for unserved and underserved people
- Treatment services for targeted conditions
- Clinical preventive services
- Payments for personal services delivered by others

State government health agencies function fairly autonomously while working within federal guidelines. They assess, develop, and monitor statewide health needs and services. Historically, they have been responsible for communicable disease control, vital statistics, laboratory services, environmental sanitation and hygiene, health education and maternal–child health, with the addition of categorical programs (e.g., heart disease, migrant health) in the 1950s (Scutchfield & Keck, 2003). In the 1980s, block grants were instituted to give more flexibility to states in how funds are targeted.

At the local level, one may find a city government health agency, a county agency, or a combination of both to assess, plan, and serve the health needs of that locality. Most local health departments are under county jurisdiction, with only a small percentage of cities (usually large cities) having local health departments. Some are city–county agencies or special districts, and most local health departments report to either local government councils or boards of health (Scutchfield & Keck, 2003). In some states, local health departments also report to state public health agencies. In about 30% of the states, local health departments are operated by the state health agency, which provides services locally, without city or county oversight (Turnock, 2004).

Unlike private organizations that tend to have a specific focus, government health agencies exist to accomplish a broad goal of protecting and promoting the health of the total population under their jurisdiction. Such a task requires a wide range of services and the combined talents of many types of professional disciplines. Among them are nurses, physicians, health educators, sanitarians, epidemiologists, statisticians, engineers, administrators, accountants, computer programmers, planners, sociologists, nutritionists, laboratory technicians, chemists, physicists, veterinarians, dentists, pharmacists, demographers,

and meteorologists. Furthermore, public health agencies must function not only on an interdisciplinary basis but also on an interorganizational basis. Other government services (e.g., education) can meet their goals fairly autonomously, but public health cannot accomplish its important objectives without the collaboration of many agencies and organizations, both public and private (Barton, 2003; Williams & Torrens, 2002). To manage the AIDS epidemic, for example, public health agencies, educational institutions, welfare agencies, mental health programs, home care services, Medicaid, and private groups, among others, may be called upon to collaborate.

Many different government agencies contribute to the health of a community. Most obvious are the local and state health departments, which provide a variety of direct and indirect health services, including community health nursing. Other tax-supported agencies that sponsor health care or health-related services include welfare departments, departments of public works, public schools and hospitals, police departments, county agricultural services, and local housing authorities.

Local Public Health Agencies

At the grassroots level, government health agencies vary considerably in structure and function from one locality to the next. This partly results from variations in local needs and the size and resources of the community. For example, a rural community served by a county or state health department may have needs and services that differ widely from those of a densely populated urban community (see Chapter 29). Differing health care standards and regulations, as well as the type and stipulations of funding sources, also contribute to variations in the structure and function of health agencies. Nonetheless, each local governmental health agency shares some commonly held responsibilities, functions, and structural features.

The primary responsibilities of the local health department are to assess the population's health status and needs, determine how well those needs are being met, and take action toward satisfying unmet needs (Scutchfield & Keck, 2003). Specifically, local government health agencies should fulfill these core functions as follows:

- Monitor local health needs and the resources for addressing them.
- Develop policy and provide leadership in advocating equitable distribution of resources and services, both public and private.
- Evaluate availability, accessibility, and quality of health services for all members of the community.
- Keep the community informed about how to access public health services.

The local health agency represents a critical level of health services' provision because of its closeness to the ultimate recipients—health care consumers. The most recent survey of local health departments revealed the top three expenditure categories as enforcing laws and regulations; informing, educating, and empowering people; and ensuring the provision of care (Barry et al., 1998).

The structure of the local health department varies in complexity with the setting. Rural and small urban agencies need only a simple organization, whereas large metropolitan agencies require more complex organizational structures to support the greater diversity and quantity of work.

Where a board of health exists, it holds the legal responsibility for the health of its citizens. About 80% of local public health departments work with a board of health, and they are more commonly found with smaller populations (Turnock, 2004). Health board members may be appointed by the mayor if the board of health serves a city, by a board of supervisors if the board of health serves a county, or by voters if they are publicly elected. In turn, the board of health usually appoints a health officer (about 80%)—often a physician (about 50%) with public health training (about 15%)—who directs the remaining staff of the health department, including public health nurses, environmental health workers, health educators, and office personnel (Turnock, 2004). Others, such as nutritionists, statisticians, epidemiologists, social workers, physical therapists, veterinarians, or public health dentists, may be added as needs and as resources dictate. The number of staff at local health departments can range from five to over 100, depending upon the size of the agency and population served (Scutchfield & Keck, 2003).

Revenues to support local health departments come from various sources. Local and county general appropriations make up the largest share of the local health department's budget—around 44%. State revenues account for about 30% of the total local budget—with additional funds provided through special levies and programs such as school health, Head Start, air pollution, toxic substance control, primary care, immunizations, fees, and private foundation grants. Federal funds provide another source of revenue (about 3%) targeted at specific efforts, such as AIDS research and services, family planning, child health, environmental protection, and hypertension and nutrition programs. According to Turnock (2004), fees, reimbursements, and additional miscellaneous sources, such as state laboratory revenues and food supply supplements, make up the remaining portion of the budget (about 23%). A good number of health departments bill Medicaid for personal health services rendered (e.g., prenatal care, TB treatment, well-baby care), but an increasing number of states are offering Medicaid managed care, and moving personal health care out of local health departments (Scutchfield & Keck, 2003). Figure 6.1 depicts the organization of one local health department serving a population of approximately 300,000.

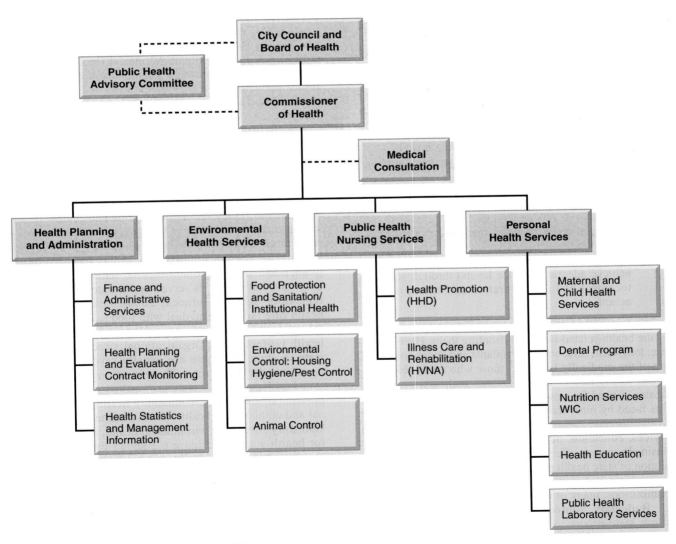

FIGURE 6.1   Organizational chart of a city public health department.

State Public Health Agencies

State-level government health agencies also vary in structure and in how they carry out the core functions. Each state, as a sovereign government, establishes its own health department, which in turn determines its goals, actions, and administrative structure. The state health department is responsible for providing leadership in and monitoring of comprehensive public health needs and services in the state. It establishes statewide health policy standards, assists local communities, allocates funds, promotes state-level health planning, conducts and evaluates state-level health programs, promotes cooperation with voluntary (private) health agencies or NGOs, and collaborates with the federal government for health planning and policy development (Scutchfield & Keck, 2003). Of the various levels of government health agencies, the states recently have played the most pivotal role in health policy formation.

General functions of state health departments include (Scutchfield & Keck, 2003):

◆ Statewide health planning
◆ Intergovernmental and other agency relations
◆ Intrastate agency relations
◆ Certain statewide policy determinations
◆ Standards setting
◆ Health regulatory functions

Specifically, the Institute of Medicine (1988) described the role of state government related to health. Summarized, it includes:

◆ A statewide method of collecting and analyzing data to assess health needs
◆ Adequate statutory base for state health activities
◆ Statewide health objectives (holding localities accountable where power for implementation has been delegated)
◆ Statewide development and maintenance of essential personal, educational, and environmental health services
◆ Identification of problems that threaten the health of the state
◆ Support for local health services (when needed to achieve adequate service levels) through subsidies, technical and administrative assistance, or direct action

State public health agencies face a challenge in addressing the health-related issues confronting them. Health insurance, long-term care, organ transplants and donations, AIDS, care of the **medically indigent** (those who are unable to pay for and totally lack medical services), malpractice, and certificates of need for new health services are among the problems faced by most states. Clearly, state health departments must collaborate closely with other agencies, such as social services, education, public works, the legislature, and the housing bureau, to effectively solve such problems. Thus, the solution of state health problems and delivery of health services requires the functioning of an interdependent network of organizations, many of which are not health agencies per se.

Budgetary sources for a state health department include state-generated funds, federal grants and contracts, and fees and reimbursements. A large source of federal monies to the states comes through the Department of Agriculture, which supports the Women, Infants, and Children (WIC) Program, a supplemental nutrition program. State health agencies often provide grant opportunities for local health departments (often through federal grant monies awarded to states). Fragmentation of public health roles and functions among different state agencies poses problems for coordinating the core public health functions at this level (Turnock, 2004). Funding for state public health agencies comes largely from state coffers, with less than 40% coming from federal contracts and grants, and a smaller percentage generated from fees and third-party reimbursements, local taxes and funds, as well as other sources (Scutchfield & Keck, 2003). The Department of Agriculture, the Centers for Disease Control and Prevention, and Health Resources and Services Administration (HRSA) all provide substantial funding at the state level. Less than 6% of all state health care expenditures go toward population health (e.g., health promotion, chronic disease control), even with the addition of new federal bioterrorism monies (Milbank Memorial Fund et al., 2003). In many states, these new funds have been accompanied by state and local funding cuts that actually leave agencies in worse financial shape (Elliott, 2002).

State-level population health expenditures in 2001 accounted for 6.3% of all health care expenditures. Most expenditures were for promotion of chronic disease control and healthy behaviors, along with environmental hazards control programs (Milbank Memorial Fund et al., 2003). Prevention of epidemics and communicable disease control, injury prevention, disaster preparation and response, and health infrastructure were also included under this spending category.

Each of the 50 state health departments in the United States has developed its own unique structure. Some are strongly centralized organizations, whereas others are decentralized. In most states, the appointed director or executive of the agency reports to a state board of health or directly to the governor. Some states have advisory boards that make health policy recommendations and review departmental activities. Significant variation occurs in the types of programs managed by state health agencies—in 2002, about 90% reported administrative responsibility for the WIC program, public health laboratories, vital statistics, and tobacco programs, but only 25% served as the state's environmental regulatory agency (Turnock, 2004). Over 70% regulate health care facilities and deal with food safety and environmental health issues, while over 30% regulate licensing of health professionals. Organizational structures vary from state to state, but there are usually several divisions or bureaus under the director. Those most commonly found in state health department organizational structures are disease prevention and control, community health services, maternal and child health, health systems and technical services, laboratory services, environmental health, and a state center for health statistics. Figure 6.2 shows the organizational chart of a state health department.

National Public Health Agencies

The national level of public health organization consists of many government agencies. They can be clustered into four groups. First and most directly focused on health is the

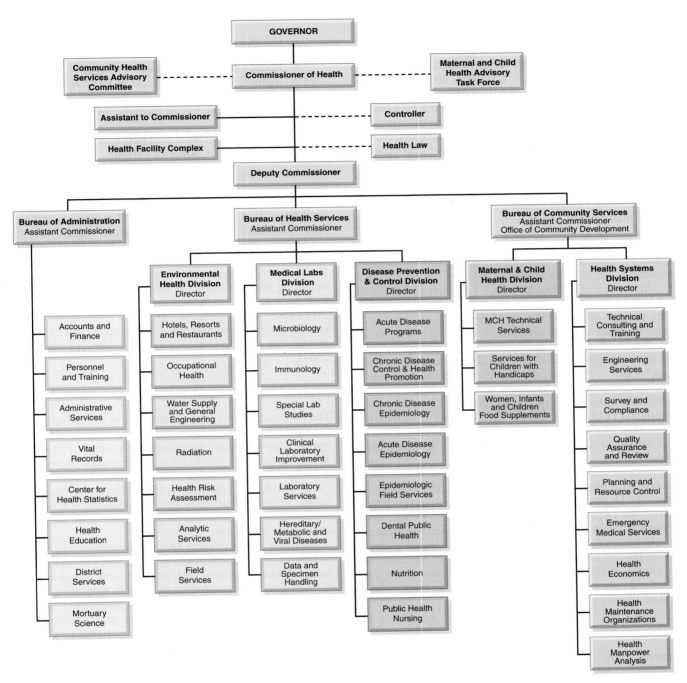

FIGURE **6.2** Organizational chart of a state public health department.

Public Health Service (PHS). It is concerned with the broad health interests of the country and is a functional (not organizational) unit of DHHS (see Chapter 30 for more on the PHS Commissioned Corps).

The Secretary of Health and Human Services (a cabinet-level position) has ultimate responsibility for the PHS. The PHS consists of the Office of Public Health and Science (headed by the Assistant Secretary for Health), and comprises the Commissioned Core (over 6,000 uniformed health professionals), the Office of the Surgeon General, and 12 public health offices (e.g., Office of Women's Health, National Vaccine Program Office, Office of HIV/AIDS Policy, Office of Minority Health). The PHS is made up of eight functional branches: the CDC, the FDA, the NIH, the Substance Abuse and Mental Health Services Administration (SAMHSA), the HRSA, the Agency for Healthcare Research & Quality (AHRQ), the Indian Health Service, and the Agency for Toxic Substances and Disease Registry (ATSDR). One of its major functions through these eight branches is the administration of grants and contracts with other government agencies, private organizations, and individuals. In some instances, the PHS provides hospital, clinical, and other types of health services, for example, for Native Americans and Eskimos through the Indian Health Service. Through the CDC and the

NIH, it provides epidemiologic surveillance and numerous research programs. The FDA of the PHS monitors the safety and usefulness of various food and drug products, as well as cosmetics, toys, and flammable fabrics (Office of the Public Health Service Historian, 2004; USDHHS, 2006, 2007).

Through its staff offices, the PHS offers other services. It has responsibility for the formation, planning, and evaluation of health policy; health promotion; health services management; health research and statistics; intergovernmental affairs; legislation; population affairs; and international health. It provides financial assistance to the states through grants-in-aid—monies raised by Congress through taxes for specific purposes. It also offers consultation through national advisory health councils and special advisory committees made up of lay experts. The PHS maintains 10 regional offices to make its services more readily available to the states. These offices are located in New York City, Boston, Philadelphia, Atlanta, Chicago, Kansas City, Dallas, Denver, Seattle, and San Francisco.

At the federal level, the primary agencies concerned with health are organized under the DHHS. Assistant secretaries manage offices for Health, Administration and Management, Resources and Technology, Planning and Evaluation, Public Health Emergency Preparedness, Legislation, and Public Affairs. Within the DHHS, clusters of federal agencies deal with the needs of special population groups, such as the elderly (Administration on Aging), children (Administration for Children and Families), and Native Americans (Bureau of Indian Affairs), and government health insurance programs (Centers for Medicare and Medicaid Services) (USDHHS, 2006). Figure 6.3 is the organizational chart for USDHHS.

Another cluster of service departments addresses special programs or problems. Examples are the Department of Labor, the Department of Education, the Department of the Interior, the Department of Agriculture, and the Department of Transportation. A final cluster of federal agencies focuses on international health concerns of interest to the nation. Two important ones are the U.S. Agency for International Development (USAID), an independent agency, and the Office of International Health Affairs, under the Department of State (Turnock, 2004).

Budgets and Funding for Public Health

Annually, only 8% of health spending goes toward health promotion and improvement, while 92% is spent for medical care (Trust for America's Health, 2005). Actual government spending for public health is estimated at only 3% of total U.S. health spending (Sensenig, 2007). In 2000, the state and local levels contributed about 70% of spending for public health service. Federal funds for public health are more often directed toward research, health status monitoring, program evaluation, and workforce training (Turnock, 2004). In 2004, the CDC spent just under $15 per capita, with individual state spending ranging between just above $9 to almost $46 per person (Trust for America's Health, 2005). The sum is paltry considering that total current per capita annual health expenditure well exceeds $6,100 (Colliver, 2007). This disproportionate funding for health continues despite estimations that more "robust" public health funding would provide the following benefits:

◆ Prevent 43,000 amputations, 165,000 kidney failures, and over 10,000 cases of eye disease among diabetics every year
◆ Reduce annual traffic deaths by 9,000
◆ Reduce, by 50%, new cases of HIV (40,000 annually)
◆ Reduce the number of alcohol-exposed fetuses by two-thirds
◆ Eliminate childhood lead poisoning by the year 2010 (Trust for America's Health, 2005, p. 7)

Most of the Healthy People 2010 goals remain unmet, and strategies for wide scale change and capturing of sufficient funding have not materialized. The Public Health Foundation (n.d., ¶1) estimates that "2 million deaths may occur this decade . . . as a result of not meeting only nine of the Healthy People 2010" objectives. But, in addition to health promotion, public health services must be ready for disasters, bioterrorism, and pandemics, and evidence is mounting that the system is structurally weak and suffers from poor access and inconsistent preparation (CDC, 2002, 2008; Institute of Medicine, 2002). To meet the necessary standards and immediate needs, an estimated $10 billion plus in new funding is required (Public Health Foundation, 2007).

Private Sector Health Services

The nongovernmental and voluntary arm of the health care delivery system includes many types of services. Privately owned, nonprofit health agencies (most hospitals and welfare agencies) make up one large group. Privately owned (proprietary), for-profit agencies are another. Private professional health care practice, composed largely of physicians in solo or group practice, forms a third group. These make up the non–tax-supported, nongovernmental dimension of community health care.

Private health services are complementary and supplementary to government health agencies. They often meet the needs of special groups, such as those with cancer or heart disease; they offer an avenue for private enterprise or philanthropy; they are less constrained than government agencies in developing innovations in health care; and they have been spurred to development, in part, by impatience or dissatisfaction with government programs. Their financial support comes from voluntary contributions, bequests, or fees (Scutchfield & Keck, 2003).

For-Profit and Not-for-Profit Health Agencies

Proprietary health services are privately owned and managed. They may be nonprofit or for-profit. Many hospitals and nursing homes offer nonprofit services, but must generate sufficient revenues to keep ahead of operating costs. Often, one or more special services offered by a hospital generate enough income to cover the drain from more expensive programs or uncompensated care. As more hospitals have merged or been integrated into larger health conglomerates, the practice in many cases has been to establish a separate, for-profit corporation that generates revenues so that the basic organization can retain its nonprofit, tax-exempt status.

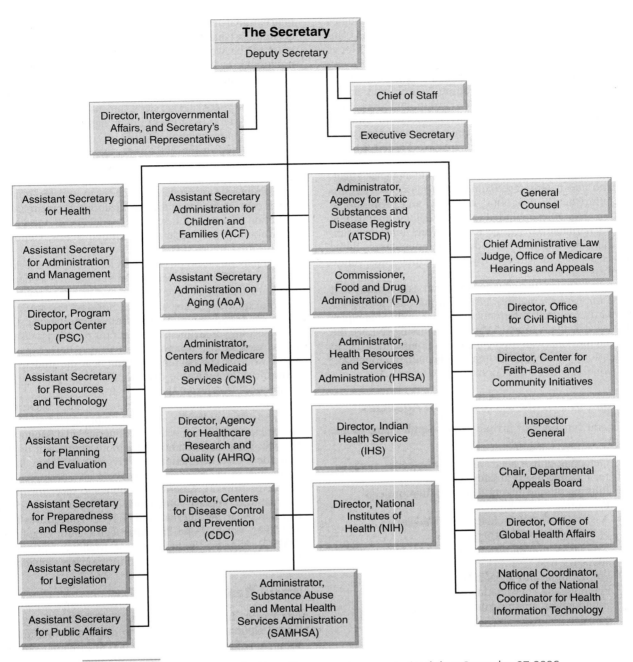

FIGURE 6.3   Department of health and human services organizational chart, September 27, 2006.

Examples of for-profit health services include a wide range of private practices by physicians, nurses, social workers, psychologists, and laboratory and radiology technologists. With the greater demand for home care services since the 1980s, the number of new, for-profit services (e.g., home care agencies, nursing personnel pools, and durable medical equipment supply companies) increased dramatically. Medicare's annual costs for home care services per enrollee went from $4 in 1969 to more than $300 by the late 1990s (Tyson, 2001). Partially in response to these escalating home care costs to Medicare, the Balanced Budget Act of 1997 was passed, and payments for home health care services to the elderly dropped by 12.5% annually through

the year 2000 (Meara, White, & Cutler, 2004). Even with these budget adjustments, average total Medicare expenditures grew from $5,080 per person in 1991 to $7,310 in 2001 (Congressional Budget Office, 2005).

Not-for-profit private health agencies are organizations that are established and administered by private citizens for a specific health-related purpose. Often, this purpose is seen as a special need either not addressed or served inadequately by government. An example is visiting nurse associations, which were formed to provide care for the sick in their homes. The contribution of the private, not-for-profit health agency then becomes complementary to public health services.

Three types of private, not-for-profit health agencies have specialized interests. Some, such as the American Cancer Society and the American Diabetes Association, focus on specific diseases. Others, such as the National Society for Autistic Children, Planned Parenthood Federation of America, and the National Council on Aging, focus on the needs of special populations. A third group, including agencies such as the American Heart Association and the National Kidney Foundation, are concerned with diseases of specific organs. All of these agencies are funded through private contributions.

Another group of private, not-for-profit agencies affecting health and health care includes the many foundations that support health programs, research, and professional education. Examples include the W.K. Kellogg Foundation, the Pew Charitable Trusts, the Robert Wood Johnson Foundation, and the Bill and Melinda Gates Foundation. Some agencies, such as the United Way, exist to fund other voluntary efforts.

Another group includes professional associations that work to improve the public's health through the promotion of standards, research, information, and programs. Examples are the APHA, the National League for Nursing (NLN), the ANA, and the American Medical Association (AMA). These organizations are funded primarily through membership dues, bequests, and contributions.

Functions of Private-sector Health Agencies

The general functions of private-sector health agencies are as follows:

◆ Detecting unmet needs or exploring better methods for meeting needs already identified
◆ Piloting or subsidizing demonstration projects
◆ Promoting public knowledge
◆ Assisting official agencies with innovative programs not otherwise possible
◆ Evaluating official programs and assuming a public advocacy role
◆ Promoting health legislation
◆ Planning and coordinating to promote collaboration among voluntary services and between voluntary and official agencies
◆ Developing well-balanced community health programs that seek to make services relevant and comprehensive

Both public and private agencies are needed to maintain a viable public health system (Porche, 2004). Future functions of both private and public sectors most likely will remain much the same. However, the structure of the organizations within both sectors is changing dramatically and will continue to do so as managed care organizations blur the lines between private and public sectors. The blurring of the private and public health care sectors has opened the doors to emerging creative health care services.

INTERNATIONAL HEALTH ORGANIZATIONS

The health of countries around the world cannot be ignored. Besides important humanitarian and moral concerns, there are pragmatic reasons for addressing health issues at the international level. Today, health—along with politics and economics—has become a global issue. Health care among most of the world's population continues to be based on traditional medicine. At the same time, technology is revolutionizing health practices via distance education, training, and telemedicine. The nations of the world depend on one another for goods and services, and, as in any set of interdependent systems, a problem in one nation has repercussions on others (Jamison et al., 2006).

As stated in the 2002 executive summary of the Pan American Health Organization (PAHO), *Health in the Americas,* "new information technologies have played an invaluable role in improving access to and the quality of health care, as well as in the organization, administration, and operation of new health services models being introduced in the Region [the Americas, the United States, Central and South America]" (p. 14).

It may not seem possible that the health of a resident of a country 9,000 miles away can affect that of a student from the United States or vice versa; however, when boarding an international flight for a school holiday, the student will likely be seated among people from many nations. Despite close scrutiny of airline passengers for passports, visas, customs regulations, weapons, and drugs, how can anyone know whether any passenger sitting near the student has an airborne communicable disease that is resistant to known antibiotics? (See From the Case Files I.)

International cooperation in health dates back to early concerns for epidemics. In 1851, representatives from 12 countries met in Paris for the First International Sanitary Conference. They later established a more permanent organization, the Office Internationale d'Hygiene Publique, in 1907. Epidemics in the Western Hemisphere also prompted representatives from 21 American republics to meet for the First International Sanitary Conference in Mexico City in 1902. In that same year, the International Sanitary Bureau was formed and, later, renamed the Pan American Health Organization (PAHO) (Geneva Foundation for Medical Education & Research, 2007). (See Chapter 16 for more on global health.)

World Health Organization

The World Health Organization (WHO), an agency of the United Nations, was developed to direct and coordinate the promotion of health worldwide. It was formed after World War II, in 1948, and assumed the functions of the League of Nation's health organization. The PAHO remained separate but became the WHO regional office for the Americas. The WHO began with 61 member nations, one of which was the United States. By 1998, membership had expanded to 193 nations and two associate members (WHO, 2007a). The mission of the WHO is to serve as the one directing and coordinating authority on international health. From its inception, the WHO has influenced international thinking with its classic definition of health as "a state of complete physical, mental, and social well-being and not merely the absence of disease or infirmity" (Grad, 2002, p. 984). The primary function of the WHO is to help countries improve their health status and services by assisting them to help themselves and each other. To accomplish this, it provides member countries with technical services, information from epidemiology and statistics reports, advisory and consulting services, and demonstration teams.

From the Case Files I

Medication-Resistant Tuberculosis

In 2007, the Centers for Disease Control and Prevention (CDC) ordered federal isolation (or quarantine)—something it hadn't done since 1963—for a 31-year-old Atlanta lawyer diagnosed with tuberculosis (TB). In his initial examination, Andrew Speaker says he was told he had TB but was "not contagious or a danger to anyone" and was not forbidden to fly to Greece and Europe for his wedding and honeymoon, but rather told by county health officials that they preferred that he didn't fly (*Toronto Star*, 2007, p. 5). While he and his new wife were honeymooning, lab test results revealed that he had an extensively drug resistant (XDR) strain of tuberculosis, and the CDC warned him not to take another long flight home. However, he and his wife disregarded this admonition, flying back to Canada on Czech Air and then "sneaking" across the border to the United States. He was quarantined a day later and sent to National Jewish Medical and Research Center in Denver, Colorado—a hospital with a long history of TB research and treatment. Several months later, new tests showed that his sputum samples were positive for multi-drug resistant (MDR) TB, with no signs of the XDR TB first noted on bronchoscopy samples. MDR TB is less resistant to antituberculosis medications and requires less intensive treatment than XDR TB (although it sometimes requires surgical removal of diseased sections of the lung). The CDC recommended that fellow travelers on Mr. Speaker's transatlantic flights have TB tests to determine if they contracted the disease. Although a number of lawsuits have been filed, no TB cases have been reported (Hitti, 2007). This incident brought TB to the forefront and reinforced the concept of the world as a global community.

For 20 years, the WHO had a realistic expectation that by the year 2000, no individual citizen in any country would have a level of health below an acceptable minimum, and that the global community would later adopt a new strategy to take people further toward the goal of health for all in the future (WHO, 1998). The target date of the year 2000 was intended as a challenge to the member nations. Although the goal has not been met entirely, WHO continues to focus on environmental health, control of infectious and diarrheal diseases, maternal and child health care, poverty and hunger, and education (WHO, 2007b). These emphases point to a change in focus from primarily reactive programs (e.g., stopping epidemics, instituting quarantines) to the more proactive promotion of health for the world community.

Headquartered in Geneva, Switzerland, WHO has six regional offices. The Regional Office for the Americas is located in Washington, D.C. (WHO, 2007c). The other regional offices are in Copenhagen, Denmark (Europe), Alexandria, Egypt (Eastern Mediterranean), Brazzaville, Congo (Africa), New Delhi, India (Southeast Asia), and Manila, Philippines (Western Pacific). Funding comes from member countries and from the United Nations. The WHO holds an annual World Health Assembly to discuss international health policies and programs. The organization publishes several periodicals of interest to the global community, which are available by subscription for a fee and in partial text through WHO's various websites www.who.int/publications/en/.

Bulletin of the World Health Organization—monthly
WHO Drug Information—quarterly
Weekly Epidemiological Record—weekly
Pan American Journal of Public Health—monthly.

Pan American Health Organization

The PAHO, the central coordinating organization for public health in the Western Hemisphere, is the oldest continuously functioning international health organization in the world. Its budget comes from assessments contributed by member states, augmented by funds from WHO, the United Nations, and other sources, including private donations (PAHO, 2007a).

As WHO's regional office for the Americas, PAHO disseminates epidemiologic information, provides technical assistance, finances fellowships, and promotes cooperative research and professional education. Conferences convened by PAHO provide an opportunity for delegates from member nations to discuss issues of concern and plan strategies for addressing health needs. The most widely read journal published by PAHO is the *Pan American Journal of Public Health,* published monthly (PAHO, 2007b).

United Nations International Children's Emergency Fund

Organized in 1946, the United Nations Children's Fund, now called the United Nations International Children's Emergency Fund (UNICEF), was established initially as a temporary emergency program to assist the children of war-torn countries. That focus has broadened, and UNICEF is now a permanent agency for promoting child and maternal health and welfare globally, through a variety of programs and activities, including provision of food and supplies to underdeveloped countries, immunization programs in cooperation with the WHO, disease control, prevention demonstrations, and, in particular, promotion of family planning in developing countries (UNICEF, 2007).

United States Agency for International Development

Existing for more than 30 years, the U.S. Agency for International Development (USAID) lists goals of improving the health, education, and well-being of the populations of developing countries. It is "an independent agency that provides economic, development and humanitarian assistance around the world in support of the foreign policy goals of the United States" (USAID, 2006, ¶1).

Other International Health Organizations

Many other organizations deal with health concerns at the international level. The United Nations Educational, Scientific, and Cultural Organization (UNESCO) promotes "cooperation . . . . in the fields of education, science, culture and communication" (UNESCO, 2007, ¶2). The World Bank addresses health problems through funding and technical assistance. The Food and Agriculture Organization (FAO) works to "defeat hunger" by providing information and technical assistance (FAO, 2007, ¶1). In addition to these international organizations, most developed countries have agencies that provide assistance, some in major proportions, to underdeveloped countries.

SIGNIFICANT LEGISLATION

During the past century in the United States, an ever-widening sense of responsibility for health in the public sector led to passage of an increasing amount of health-related legislation. Some acts are of particular significance to the financing and delivery of community health services (see Display 6.1). Only after World War I and the Great Depression did the U.S. government enact significant legislation that affected the health and well-being of a wider range of citizens. Before that, legislation dealt with specific sectors of society (e.g., merchant seamen, mothers and infants).

In 1935, the Social Security Act ensured greater public health services and programs and provided retirement income to participating workers age 65 years and older. The act also included aid to dependent children and unemployment insurance (Social Security Administration, 2003). Later legislation provided federal support for expansion of hospitals; care for the mentally retarded; and research and support for heart disease, cancer, and stroke, as well as the training of health care personnel.

The landmark Medicare and Medicaid legislation moved the federal government deeper into the role of providing health care, especially for many elderly and poor people who, prior to this time, either could not get services or had to rely on charity care. More recent legislation, especially during President Reagan's term, sought to contain health care spending, assure the quality of health care, promote national health objectives, and facilitate data collection and research (see Display 6.2). More recent laws have protected the confidentiality of health records and made it easier for workers to continue insurance coverage after being laid off.

President Clinton made an attempt at universal health care during his first term in office and supported legislation to reform the welfare system. In 1997, the State Children's Health Insurance Program (SCHIP) was created to expand coverage to uninsured children at no or low cost (USDHHS, 2007). President George W. Bush added prescription drug benefits to Medicare and promoted Health Savings Accounts (HSAs).

Development of the Current Health Care System

In 1900, a total of 20% of infants died before they reached the age of 10, and life expectancy was about 47 years. Infectious diseases and poor sanitation and nutrition contributed to the poor outcomes. Physicians were not well trained, and the AMA had only 8,000 members (PBS, 2007). Hospital infection rates were high, and most care was given in the home—and then only to those who could afford to pay for it or those who received charity care. (See From the Case Files II.)

As the public health system acted to improve water supplies, sanitation, and personal hygiene, the incidence of infectious disease began to diminish. Antibiotics, first widely available during World War II, and better-trained physicians began to change the health care system in the 1950s—although medical and surgical care was not at all sophisticated by today's standards. (See From the Case Files III.)

Since 1950, Americans have come to expect longer lives made possible by medications and treatments that can cure or control a wide variety of diseases and by expanding technology and services that provide a dizzying array of choices to health care consumers. These advances have come at a price, however. Health spending in 2006 represented 16% of the U.S. **gross domestic product (GDP)**—the total amount of goods and services produced within a year; whereas health spending in 1950 represented 4.5%. Viewed as a separate economy, U.S. health care today would be the fourth largest economy in the world and, by 2016, U.S. health spending is projected to exceed $4 trillion (Gardner, 2007; Rice & Rhodes, 2002). Clearly, to gain a deeper understanding of this phenomenon, some basic concepts must be examined. For instance, what are the economic principles behind this rapid growth in health care costs?

THE ECONOMICS OF HEALTH CARE

Economics is defined as the science of making decisions regarding scarce resources. Economics permeates our social structure—it affects and is affected by policies. Consequently, health is closely tied to economic growth and development, in that a healthy population is necessary for adequate national productivity. Ample evidence exists for a "health–income gradient," as personal income (specifically poverty) is linked to health status (Aday, 2005, p. 191).

Health economics can be better understood by examining the two basic theories underlying the science of economics: microeconomics and macroeconomics. In addition, concepts of health care payment must be understood.

Microeconomics

Microeconomic theory is concerned with supply and demand. **Supply** is the quantity of goods or services that providers are willing to sell at a particular price. **Demand** denotes the consumer's willingness to purchase goods or services at a specified price (Chang, Price, & Pfoutz, 2001). In our free market–driven economy, supply-and-demand is a key concept. Economists using microeconomic theory study the supply of goods and services as these relate to how we, as consumers, allocate and distribute our resources—as well as how markets compete. They further study how allocation and

DISPLAY 6.1	LANDMARK HEALTH CARE LEGISLATION

The Shepard-Towner Act of 1921

The Shepard-Towner Act of 1921 provided federal grant-in-aid funds to the states for administration of programs to promote the health and welfare of mothers and infants. The act expired in 1929, but it set a pattern for maternal and child health programs that later was revived and strengthened through the successful and far-reaching efforts of the Children's Bureau (now known as the Maternal and Child Health Bureau), housed in the Department of Labor. Through the leadership of this bureau, many programs were instituted that enhanced children's health. Among them were services targeting prematurity, perinatal mortality, nutrition, mental retardation, audiology, rheumatic fever, cerebral palsy, epilepsy, dentistry, juvenile delinquency, and the problems of migrant workers' children (Scutchfield & Keck, 2003). The Children's Bureau maintained its impact through several administrative changes (it was moved to the Federal Security Agency in 1946 and to the Department of Health, Education, and Welfare in 1953), but was phased out in 1972, when it became the Office of Maternal and Child Health. Now under the Department of Health and Human Services, it is known as the Maternal and Child Health Bureau (Ruhl, 2007).

The Social Security Act of 1935

The Social Security Act of 1935 had tremendous consequences for public health. In addition to its revolutionary welfare insurance and assistance programs, which particularly benefited high-risk mothers and children, Title VI of the act financially assisted states and localities in providing public health services. These funds were and still are allocated on the basis of population public health problems, economic need, and need for training of public health personnel. Many of the grants had to be matched by the states or localities. This served to increase their knowledge of and commitment to health programs. The act strengthened local health departments and health programs in most states (Scutchfield & Keck, 2003; Social Security Online, 2007). Most commonly, this act is known for retirement benefits for those over age 65, but it also provides aid for dependent children and unemployment insurance (Social Security Administration, 2003). In 2007, over 50 million Americans will receive more than $602 billion in benefits; the vast majority of recipients are retired workers (Social Security Administration, 2007a; 2007b).

The Hill-Burton Act (Hospital Survey and Construction Act) of 1946

The Hill-Burton Act of 1946 was an important breakthrough in nationwide health facilities planning. It marked the first real effort to link health planning with population needs on a comprehensive basis. The act provided federal funds to states for hospital construction (about one-third of the total cost). It helped to provide access, especially in rural areas, to acute care services, but did not address public health or preventive care. It also required participating hospitals to provide services to residents, such as "community services," regardless of "race, color, national origin, or creed" (USDHHS, 2006, ¶2).

Emergency services were to be provided "without regard to the person's ability to pay" (¶1). A 1961 medical facilities bill expanded grant money to states for public health services, nursing homes, and planning for hospitals, as well as for outpatient services for elderly and chronically ill. Expenditures for this act ended in 1975, but it has provided close to 500,000 hospital beds, and has had a lasting effect on the U.S. health care system. Few people remember that this bill was sponsored by the American Hospital Association in response to a proposal by President Harry Truman to add a comprehensive medical insurance program to Social Security—an effort to provide universal health coverage (Brookings Institution, 2007; Perlstadt, 1995).

The Maternal and Child Health and Mental Retardation Planning Amendments of 1963

Although the Social Security Act of 1935 provided for some services for "crippled children," the Maternal and Child Health and Mental Retardation Planning Amendments of 1963 opened the door for improved services to selected mothers and children. Recognizing the nation's high infant mortality rate and the accompanying problems of premature births, handicapping conditions, and mental retardation, Congress—through this law—authorized grants to fund projects offering comprehensive care to high-risk, low-income mothers and children. It also provided grants to states to design comprehensive programs addressing mental retardation (National Center for Education in Maternal & Child Health, 2007).

The Heart Disease, Cancer, and Stroke Amendments of 1965 (PL 89–239)

The Heart Disease, Cancer, and Stroke Amendments of 1965 are noteworthy for their establishment of regional medical programs, one of the first real efforts at comprehensive health planning. Fifty-six regions in the United States were designated, and each was charged with the responsibility to evaluate the overall health needs of its region and cooperate with other regions for program development. Although the amendments initially were categorical (limited to heart disease, cancer, and stroke), amendments in 1970 expanded the legislation's focus. The act was important for two additional reasons: it encouraged local participation in health planning, which was previously done at federal and state levels, and it funded program operations and planning (National Library of Medicine, 2003).

The Social Security Act Amendments of 1965 (PL 89–97)

The Social Security Act Amendments of 1965 addressed a concern for some version of national health insurance. Title XVIII, Medicare, provided federally funded health insurance for the elderly (65 years and older) and for disabled persons. Title XIX, Medicaid, is a joint federal–state welfare assistance program that serves the blind, certain families with dependent children, the disabled, and eligible elderly. These two pieces of legislation have enabled many of the poor, disabled, and elderly to receive quality

(text continues on page 140)

health care that otherwise would not be available to them (Scutchfield & Keck, 2003; Williams & Torrens, 2002).

The Comprehensive Health Planning and Public Health Service Amendments Act (Partnership for Health Act) of 1966 (PL 89–749)

The Partnership for Health Act of 1966 promoted further advances in comprehensive health planning. It established comprehensive health planning agencies and coordinated the many categorical health and research efforts into an integrated system. It emphasized comprehensive health planning and cost containment at local, state, and regional levels. Its goals were improved efficiency and effectiveness of health care, and it also provided for some public health services and training (Brookings Institution, 2007).

The Health Manpower Act of 1968 (PL 90–490)

The Health Manpower Act of 1968 increased the supply of health personnel by providing federal money to educational institutions for construction, training, special projects, student loans, and scholarships. This act replaced several previous acts that had similar goals but resulted in only fragmentary efforts to address the problem. Among them were the Health Amendment Acts of 1956, the Nurse Training Act (1966), and the Allied Health Professions Personnel Training Act (1966). In 1976, Congress passed the Health Professions Education Assistance Act (Pub. L. No. 94–484) to effect a better balance between the country's health needs and the supply of available health professionals. One of its major emphases was to address the problem of physician misdistribution between underserved (rural) and overserved (urban) areas through educational incentive programs (National Institutes of Health, 2007). The Health Professions Education Extension Amendments (1992) also provided educational assistance to many in the health professions (Duffy, Chen, & Sampson, 1998).

The Occupational Safety and Health Act of 1970 (PL 91–956)

The Occupational Safety and Health Act of 1970 provided protection to workers against personal injury or illness resulting from hazardous working conditions. It established the National Institute for Occupational Safety and Health (NIOSH) and OSHA—the Occupational Safety and Health Administration (U.S. Environmental Protection Agency, 2007).

The Professional Standards Review Organization Amendment to the Social Security Act of 1972 (PL 92–603)

The Professional Standards Review Organization (PSRO) Amendment to the Social Security Act of 1972 had two goals: cost containment and improved quality of care. The PSRO legislation created autonomous organizations, external to hospitals and ambulatory health care agencies, to monitor and review objectively the quality of care delivered to Medicare and Medicaid patients. The PSRO review boards, composed mostly of physicians, examined such things as need for care, length of stay, and quality of care against predetermined standards developed locally. Failure to meet standards could mean

denial of federal funding. In 1983, Professional Review Organizations replaced PSROs. These private organizations, employed by government agencies to review medical records and avoid excessive and inappropriate costs to taxpayers, strive to identify "best practices" (Dranove, 2000).

The Health Maintenance Organization Act of 1973 (PL 93–222)

In a cost-controlling move, the Health Maintenance Organization Act of 1973 added federal support to the concept of prepayment for medical care. President Nixon, a proponent of wage controls, was concerned about the rising costs of health care for employers and citizens. Congress authorized funding for feasibility studies, planning, grants, and loans to stimulate growth among qualifying health maintenance organizations (HMOs). In addition, this act required a business employing 25 people or more to offer an HMO health insurance option, if available locally. A subsequent law, the Employee Retirement Income Security Act (ERISA), passed in 1974, served to protect HMOs from many malpractice lawsuits, even though the intent of the law was to standardize employee benefit laws among the states (Wood, 2001).

The National Health Planning and Resource Development Act of 1974 (PL 93–641)

The National Health Planning and Resource Development Act of 1974 was a major breakthrough in comprehensive health planning. Replacing the Partnership for Health Act, it combined Hill-Burton, comprehensive health planning agencies, and regional medical programs into a single, new program. It fostered not only comprehensive health planning, but also regulation and evaluation, and it promoted collaborative efforts among regional, state, and federal governments. An important contribution of this act was its emphasis on consumer involvement in health planning. The act was divided into two titles. Title XV, National Health Planning and Development, established national health priorities and assisted the development of area-wide and state planning through Health Systems Agencies (HSAs) and state health planning and development agencies. Title XVI, Health Resources Development, coordinated health facilities planning with health planning, replacing the Hill-Burton Act. The HSAs set targets and limited services, reviewing certificates of need (CON) for all health care facilities seeking to expand. If a facility expanded without HSA approval, its Medicaid and Medicare reimbursements could be denied. Because many providers were members of the HSA and supported each other's projects, and others learned to "work the system," these cost-control systems failed to produce the desired results and were ended during the Reagan era (Dranove, 2000).

The National Center for Health Statistics of 1974 (PL 93–353)

The National Center for Health Statistics (NCHS), established in 1974, arose from the earlier National Office of Vital Statistics and became part of the Centers for Disease Control (CDC) under the Public Health Service in 1987. The NCHS operates data collection systems that provide vital information for public health planning and service delivery (National Committee on Vital and Health Statistics, 2000).

The Omnibus Budget Reconciliation Act of 1981 (PL 97–35)

The Omnibus Budget Reconciliation Act (OBRA) of 1981 had a profound effect on public health. In this act, Congress halted the progress made in most of the public health laws of the previous 45 years, substantially reducing their funding authorization. To shift more power to the states and reduce the budget, the Reagan administration consolidated categorical grants into four block grants (Centers for Medicare and Medicaid Services, 1981). The first block grant targeted general preventive health services; the second addressed alcohol, drug abuse, and mental health; the third focused on maternal and child health; and the fourth addressed primary care, which covered federal support for community health centers. Although block grants provide some advantages, these came with limiting restrictions on the amount and use of the funds. The result was a significant reduction in funding for state and local health programs, but states worked to better coordinate health promotion and disease prevention (Scutchfield & Keck, 2003).

The Social Security Amendments of 1983 (PL 98–21)

The Social Security Amendments of 1983 became law in response to accelerating health care costs. The act represented a major reform in health care financing from retrospective to prospective payment. It introduced a billing classification system consisting of 467 diagnosis-related groups (DRGs), with Medicare payments provided to hospitals based on a fixed rate set in advance (Social Security Online, 2007). The fixed payment could not be increased if hospital costs for care exceeded that amount. Conversely, if costs were less than the paid amount, the hospital could keep the difference. Thus, a positive incentive was introduced to reduce hospital costs and promote timely patient discharge (Institute of Medicine, 2001).

The Consolidated Omnibus Budget Reconciliation Act of 1985 (PL 99–272)

The Consolidated Omnibus Budget Reconciliation Act (COBRA) of 1985 extended the Medicare prospective payment system. The act also expanded Medicaid services and permitted states to offer hospice services to terminally ill recipients (CMMS, 1985). It also authorized demonstration projects to determine the effectiveness of health promotion and disease prevention services for Medicare recipients. The 1990 extension of this act mandated longer-term evaluation of the demonstration projects. Results of the experimental design showed a 12% improvement in self-reported health status and better results in the areas of exercise, seat belt use, recent mammograms, and alcohol consumption (Gale Group, 2004).

Omnibus Budget Reconciliation Act Expansion of 1986 (PL 99–509)

The OBRA Expansion of 1986 extended the prospective payment system for hospital outpatient services, and required certain employers to provide extended (eventually up to 36 months) group-rate insurance coverage for laid-off workers and their dependents. This expense is paid by the former employee, but cannot exceed 102% of the cost for other employees (U.S. Department of Labor, 2007). In 1989, a further OBRA expansion regulated fee schedules for physicians and mandated other measures to attempt to slow the growth in both Medicare and Medicaid (Kaiser Family Foundation, 2007b). Also under OBRA 1989, nursing home reforms were instituted, and the Agency for Health Care Policy and Research was established to study the effectiveness of health care services.

The Medicare Catastrophic Coverage Act of 1988 (PL 100–360)

The Medicare Catastrophic Coverage Act (MCCA) of 1988 expanded Medicare benefits significantly. Coverage was extended to include a portion of outpatient prescription drug costs and greater post-hospital extended care facility and home health benefits. Also, the MCCA set limits on beneficiary liability and provided increased inpatient hospital benefits, as well as set up a commission to examine the possibility of providing long-term care benefits through Medicare (Kaiser Family Foundation, 2007b). In 1989, a second MCCA rescinded the drug benefit and the limits on out-of-pocket spending, among other things.

The Family Support Act of 1988 (PL 100–485)

The Family Support Act of 1988 reformed the federal welfare system to emphasize work and child support. It established child support programs, work opportunities, and basic skill and training programs. It included a requirement that recipients seek employment and that states establish an education, training, and work program, along with the child care support. It established the Commission on Interstate Child Support to aid in locating absent parents and assure payment of child support. It also provided for paternity testing and withholding of wages in cases in which child support was in arrears (Office of Inspector General, 1989).

The Health Objectives Planning Act of 1990 (PL 101–582)

The Health Objectives Planning Act of 1990 was significant for its support of the report by the Institute of Medicine, *Healthy People 2000,* with funding to improve the health status of the nation. Funding for health promotion and disease prevention was added in the 1991 legislative session (Centers for Disease Control & Prevention [CDC], 1991). Ten years later, *Healthy People 2010* followed.

Preventive Health Amendments of 1992 (PL 102–531)

The Preventive Health Amendments of 1992 placed a focus by the federal government on preventive health and primary prevention initiatives. It added *prevention* to the CDC (now the Centers for Disease Control and Prevention). It enhanced services to Migrant Health Centers, especially in maternal and child health and community education, as well as lead poisoning prevention. It promoted international exchange programs for public health officials from around the world who have an interest in working in another country (Woolley & Peters, 2007).

Personal Responsibility and Work Opportunity Reconciliation Act of 1996 (PL 104–193)

The Personal Responsibility and Work Opportunity Reconciliation Act of 1996 is commonly known as the "Welfare Reform Bill." It amended the Social Security Act to reform the federal welfare system, imposing a 5-year lifetime limit on welfare benefits. It ended Aid to Families with Dependent Children (AFDC) and enacted Temporary Assistance to Needy Families (TANF). It provided child care to working parents or those receiving training or education, and required unmarried minor parents to live with their parents or another responsible adult and attend school or training programs in order to receive government assistance. Finally, it restricted benefits to legal immigrants (Administration for Children & Families, 2008). As aid to children and families is usually tied to Medicaid benefits, this legislation affected health by moving people off welfare rolls and onto payrolls—but often at minimum-wage jobs without insurance benefits.

Health Insurance Portability & Accountability Act (HIPAA) of 1996 (PL 104–191)

This landmark piece of legislation has two major components: one that provides protection for workers in group health insurance plans and another that protects the privacy of health records. It first became effective in 2001, with compliance dates set for 2003 and 2004 (for smaller health plans). It set national standards for protecting individually identifiable health information (including electronic health data), and limited exclusions for workers with preexisting conditions as well as prohibited discrimination based upon health status (Office of Civil Rights, 2003; U.S. Department of Labor, 2004). This legislation made it easier for people to obtain or keep health insurance.

Nurse Reinvestment Act of 2002 (PL 107–205)

The Nurse Reinvestment Act of 2002 addresses the nation's critical shortage of nurses. Developed with support and input from female legislators, the bill is well designed to address several issues contributing to the nursing shortage. It emphasizes a media campaign to promote the nursing profession, offers scholarships for nursing students who agree to work upon graduation in an agency facing a critical shortage of nurses, cancels student loans, provides grants to hospitals and other medical facilities that are willing to offer career incentives to nurses to advance in their field and to take on larger responsibilities for organizing and directing patient care, and includes strategies to attack the burn-out and frustration that are driving many people out of nursing. It also promotes career ladders, recruitment of minority students into nursing, increased interprofessional collaboration, encouragement of nurses to focus on community-based practices and to address the needs of vulnerable populations. It provides forgivable loans for new nursing faculty as well (Donley et al., 2002).

Medicare Prescription Drug, Improvement, and Modernization Act of 2003 (PL 108–173)

Commonly known as Medicare Part D, this voluntary program was added to Medicare Part A and Part B in 2003, and extended and improved coverage for beneficiaries beginning in January 2006 (Medicare Advocacy, 2007). Participants can enroll in one of over 100 private plans to be covered, unlike the original Medicare program that is administered through the federal government. The plans must offer the standard benefit package, or a comparable one. The 2007 deductible was $265. Beneficiaries pay 25% of the cost of covered medications up to $2,400, at which point they reach the *coverage gap* (or "donut hole") and must pay for all covered medications above the set limit. After spending $3,850 out-of-pocket in one calendar year, they reach *catastrophic coverage* and then pay only $2.15 for covered generic medications (Medicare Advocacy, 2007). The annual enrollment period for Medicare Part D is from November 15 to December 31. Senior citizens can change plans or begin coverage during that time period.

distribution affect consumer demand for these goods and services. The concepts of supply and demand are influenced by each other and, in turn, affect prices. In a simplified example, an increase in, or oversupply of, certain products usually leads to less overall consumption (decreased demand) and, usually, lowered prices. The opposite also is true. Limited availability of desired products means that supply does not meet demand, and prices usually increase. An example is the price of a gallon of gasoline. When demand for oil is high and supply begins to dwindle, the prices go up. When demand drops and supplies become more plentiful, prices go down to attract more purchasers. This occurs as long as there are no monopolies to artificially control prices, or only a few choices for goods and services that inhibit competition.

In health care, demand-side policies are enacted to reduce demand for health care (e.g., raising insurance deductibles and co-payments), and supply-side policies restrict the supply of resources (e.g., preadmission screening to reduce the likelihood of insuring someone with a serious health condition, denial of coverage for specific services, utilization of preferred providers who practice within boundaries set by insurance companies) (Nyman, 2003).

Microeconomic theory is useful for understanding price determination, resource allocation, consumer income, and spending distribution at the level of individuals and organizations (Aday, 2005). Microeconomic theory comes into play when health care competition increases, because the success of the supply-and-demand concept depends upon a competitive market. Issues such as cost containment, competition between providers, accessibility of services, quality, and need for accountability continue as targets of major concern in the 21st century.

Macroeconomics

Macroeconomic theory is concerned with the broad variables that affect the status of the economy as a whole. Economists using macroeconomics study factors influencing

DISPLAY 6.2	DATA COLLECTION SYSTEMS

The National Center for Health Statistics Data Collection Systems

Some collection systems of the National Center for Health Statistics (NCHS) are ongoing annual systems, and others are conducted periodically. There are two major types of data systems: those based on populations (these data are collected by personal interview and examination) and those based on records, with data collected from vital and medical records.

National Health Interview Survey

The National Health Interview Survey (NHIS) is a continuous nationwide survey of illness and disability. It is the main source of data on the health of the U.S. population (nonmilitary, noninstitutionalized). This survey, which monitors the health of the nation, has been conducted since 1957.

National Health and Nutrition Examination Survey

The National Health and Nutrition Examination Survey (NHANES) provides physical, physiologic, and biochemical data related to nutrition of national population samples. Conducted for over 40 years, NHANES provided data that led to the development of pediatric growth charts, vitamin fortification of grains and cereals, and phasing out of lead-based gasoline. It also provided information about the link between cholesterol and heart disease and information on smoking, bone density, obesity, and changes in diet over time.

National Health Care Survey

The National Health Care Survey (NHCS) is a series of surveys of providers that yields clear information about health care services, patients, organizations, and providers.

Ambulatory Health Care Data (NAMCS/NHAMCS): Gathers data from physicians on ambulatory services by specialty and target population

Hospital Discharge and Ambulatory Survey Data: Provides annual data on such things as length of stay, diagnosis, procedures performed, and patient use patterns

National Home and Hospice Care Survey: Administrators and staff are personally interviewed to retrieve information about patients and discharges

National Nursing Home Survey: Collects data about nursing home services, staff, and residents regarding need, level of care, costs, and use patterns

National Employer Health Insurance Survey: Provides estimates on employer-sponsored health insurance, the types of plans provided, and detailed information about the plans

National Vital Statistics System

The National Vital Statistics System is the oldest survey and best example of public health intergovernmental data sharing. Vital statistics registries around the country provide uniform data to the national system on the following categories: births, marriages, divorces, deaths, and fetal deaths. Specific data are available through the following systems:

- Birth data
- Mortality data
- Fetal death data
- Linked birth/infant deaths
- National Mortality Followback Survey
- National Maternal and Infant Health Survey

National Survey of Family Growth

The National Survey of Family Growth (NSFG) assembles information on marriage and divorce, pregnancy, use of contraception, family life, infertility, and women's and men's health. The data is used to plan health programs and services.

National Immunization Survey

The National Immunization Survey is a list-assisted random-digit-dialing survey employed to gather information on vaccination coverage rates for children between the ages of 19 and 35 months. A mailed survey follows the telephone call, and this produces timely estimates of the rates of recommended vaccine doses.

The Longitudinal Studies of Aging

The Longitudinal Studies of Aging (LSOAs) are done as a collaboration between the National Center for Health Statistics (NCHS) and the National Institute on Aging (NIA). These studies measure changes in functional status, living arrangements, health, and the utilization of health services for persons age 70 and above. They involves two cohorts of Americans moving into old age and on to the oldest ages.

State and Local Area Integrated Telephone Survey

The State and Local Area Integrated Telephone Survey (SLAITS) collects in-depth data needed at state and local levels to meet the needs of program planners, policy makers, and government agencies. Some of the topics researched include access to care, utilization of services, health insurance coverage, perceived health status, and measurement of child well-being. The same random-digit-dialing method employed by NIS is utilized on a regional basis.

From National Center for Health Statistics. Surveys and Data Collection Systems. Retrieved July 7, 2008 from http://www.cdc.gov/nchs/express.htm.

"aggregate consumption, production, investment and international trade, as well as inflation and unemployment" (Aday, 2005, p. 186). The focus is on the larger view of economic stability and growth. Macroeconomic theory is useful for providing a global or aggregate perspective of the variables affecting the total economic picture (Aday, 2005).

Macroeconomic theory has been useful in providing a large-scale perspective on health care financing, ultimately resulting in various proposals for national health plans, health care rationing, competition, and managed care. For instance, when the United States compares overall health spending with countries across the world, it becomes clear

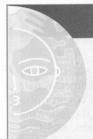

From the Case Files II

20th and 21st Century Hospital Care

At the turn of the 20th century, riots occurred in Milwaukee when a child suspected of having smallpox was to be taken to a local hospital by ambulance. One of the child's siblings had already died of smallpox in the same hospital, and his family did not want the second child to risk death at the same institution. A crowd of 3,000 or more people, carrying clubs, kept the ambulance attendants at bay. Why was there such concern about hospitalizing a sick child? In the 1890s, when this occurred, hospitals were rife with infection, and doctors could do little to halt its spread (Cutler, 2004).

In the early 21st century, are hospitals any safer? The Centers for Disease Control and Prevention (CDC) reports that over 1.7 million health care-related infections occur annually, resulting in almost 100,000 deaths (2007). Can you be assured of good care when you or your loved one enters a hospital emergency room (ER)? In the case of a busy trauma center located in South Los Angeles, you might have reason for concern. Martin Luther King/Drew Medical Center was created after the 1965 Watts Riot, and has a history of providing stellar neonatal care—95% of babies under 2 pounds survive—and excellent training for trauma surgeons—one-fourth of U.S. military surgeons have trained there (The Associated Press, 2004). But, numerous incidents of patients in the ER going untreated and unnoticed have been reported. In 2004, a 20-year-old art student entered the ER writhing in pain and vomiting. He was left alone in the crowded ER for 18 hours, whiled his heart rate climbed and his blood pressure fell. He was later found dead, having dropped to the floor covered in his own vomit—he died of gangrene of the bowel (The Associated Press, 2004). Another patient died in the ER after waiting 22 hours to be treated. The patient had a gangrenous leg, a pneumothorax, and was in kidney failure. In 2003, two patients died while on cardiac monitors, and the hospital blamed the lapse in care on the nursing shortage. Inpatient care was often no better, though, as a 46-year-old man admitted for meningitis was given chemotherapy medication for 4 days. Even after the pharmacy error was noted, nurses continued to give medications in error (at least 40 incidents). The patient subsequently lost vision in one eye. In 2007, a 43-year-old woman was admitted to the now-named Martin Luther King/Harbor Medical Center three times in 3 days complaining of intense stomach pain. Her diagnosis was listed as gallstones and she was prescribed pain medication and released each time. After the third discharge, she remained on the hospital grounds and was eventually taken to the ER by police, who were notified of a woman screaming for help. According to the police officers, the ER triage nurse refused to help the woman, and she lay on the floor in severe pain for almost an hour. She "spit up a dark-colored substance, which her boyfriend said was blood" and security cameras showed a janitor mopping around her as she lay in agony on the floor (Ornstein, 2007, p. 11). By fall 2007, after the federal government withdrew $200 million in annual funding, the hospital closed its doors (Ornstein, Weber, & Leonard, 2007).

What is different about these two scenarios is the reaction of the public. In the last century, it was an angry mob trying to keep a child out of harm's way by not allowing ambulance personnel to take him to the hospital. In this century, it was the federal and local government who moved to close what was deemed an unsafe facility. Some in the community are happy to see the closure, especially those who lost loved ones to what they feel was substandard care. Others are sad to see a much-needed neighborhood medical center close—its ER saw almost 50,000 patients in 2006—and wonder where they can go now for care (Ornstein, Weber, & Leonard, 2007).

that we spend a large percentage of our GDP on health care—more than any other country, and we often have worse indicators of health (e.g., life expectancy, infant mortality) (University of Maine, 2001). See Figure 6.4 for a comparison of health care expenditure per capita among 10 industrialized countries.

The economics of health care encompasses both microeconomics and macroeconomics, and an intricate and complex set of interacting variables. Health care economics is concerned with supply and demand: Are available resources sufficient to meet the demand for use by consumers? Are the resources expended achieving the desired outcomes? When health care resources are scarce or insufficient to address all needs (for example for programs and services for at-risk populations), how should they be applied?

Supply and Demand in Health Care Economics

When you purchase textbooks, for instance, you as the purchaser are able to determine the best value for your money (generally based on price, availability, and condition of the book). As a health care consumer, however, can you truly be an efficient and effective purchaser of health care goods and services? How does a patient determine what services are needed, where to buy them, and how to evaluate the quality of the goods and services—much less how to coordinate all necessary services? Does health care truly represent a competitive free market, then? For instance, when purchasing a new LCD flat-screen television, consumers often rely on word-of-mouth from friends and relatives, advice from experts, past experiences with brands, and

From the Case Files III

Care for Cardiovascular Patients

In 1950, the role that hypertension and high cholesterol levels played in heart disease was unclear. Only when someone presented with chest pain were they then monitored for blood pressure and cholesterol control. Doctors frequently recommended that their patients cut down on salt consumption and lose weight. They were also counseled to "slow down" and "rest around midday," as there were essentially no effective medications to treat these two problems (Cutler, 2004, p. 50). It was not until the 1960s that the Framingham Heart Study confirmed that hypertension leads to cardiovascular disease, and oral antidiuretic medications were used to control it. In the 1950s and 1960s, epidemiologist Ancel Keys' research revealed that high cholesterol intake was associated with cardiovascular disease. In the 1950s, cardiac patients were treated with absolute bed rest for a minimum of 6 weeks, morphine for pain, and oxygen. That was the state-of-the-art regimen prescribed for President Eisenhower after his heart attack in 1955 (Cutler, 2004).

Today, bed rest is known to promote blood clots, and is ineffective in treating myocardial infarctions (MIs)—or heart attacks. Quick, intensive therapy is the standard. Aspirin, heparin, beta (β)-blockers, and thrombolytic medications help to prevent and reduce blood clots, reduce the workload on the heart, and dissolve tiny clots in cardiac vessels (Cutler, 2004). Cardiac catheterization permits physicians to visualize arterial blockages. Percutaneous angioplasty to open the blocked arteries or coronary artery bypass graft (CABG) surgery is now routine. Well-trained emergency medical service personnel and specialized cardiac intensive care units with highly expert nurses are found in most communities. CPR is promoted and automated external defibrillators (AEDs), which are now placed in schools, shopping malls, government buildings, and other common spaces, have saved the lives of many victims of heart disease (AED.com, 2006; Cutler, 2004). Because of all of these advances in the last 50 years, post-MI death rates have dropped by 75%. Antihypertensive and cholesterol-lowering medications, along with healthier lifestyles that include no smoking, regular exercise, and diets low in sodium and saturated fats, have also reduced the rates of hypertension and hyperlipidemia. About 25% fewer people develop serious cardiovascular disease today than in 1950 (Cutler, 2004).

With all of these advances over the past half-century, it is reasonable to expect increased health care costs. In return, more lives have been saved and extended. But, how much can we afford to pay in the future? How many more new advances lie ahead? And, what will we receive in return for our investment?

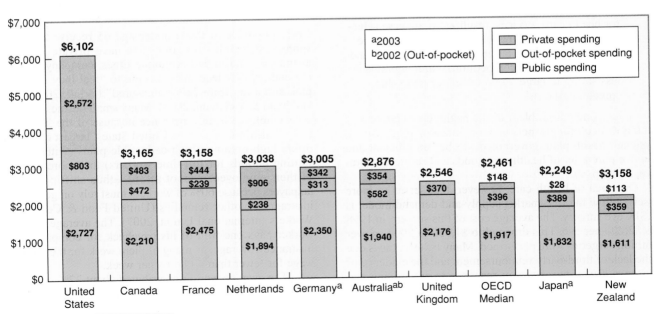

F I G U R E 6.4 Health care expenditure per capita by source of funding in 2004: adjusted for differences in cost of living. (From Shea, Holmgren, Osborn & Schoen. [2007, May]. *Health system performance in selected nations: a chartpack.* As cited originally in Cylus & Anderson. [2007, April]. *Multinational Comparisons of Health Systems Data, 2006.* New York: The Commonwealth Fund, used with permission.)

rating services like *Consumer Reports*. Also, we most often plan for large purchases, like newer and bigger televisions, in advance.

With health care, this is seldom the case; health care is typically unpredictable and difficult to research. Even with the growth of health information (and sometimes misinformation) available on the Internet, physicians are still the system's main gatekeepers, and patients must trust that these care providers have the competence to appropriately diagnose and treat them, and coordinate necessary resources to provide quality health care. Further, they trust that physicians will put the patients' interests before their own (e.g., give them accurate information about risks and benefits and not induce them to have expensive procedures to enrich the provider) (Dranove, 2000; Newhouse, 2002). Now, enter health insurance companies and managed care into the mix, and you can see why health care purchases are not straightforward and easily understood. In a free-market system, competition is an important factor, but is competition truly possible with employer-based health insurance that limits the choice of plans and providers?

In 1963, economist Kenneth Arrow wrote an influential article about health care economics detailing the lack of information in the medical marketplace (cited in Newhouse, 2002). The main points of the article noted that consumers:

◆ Do not know when or if they will become ill—but they know they will need and want medical treatment, thus the demand for health insurance
◆ Do not know what services will be needed and what works best for their condition—thus the need for physicians
◆ Do not know about the quality of health care good and services—thus the need for government regulation (e.g., licensing, certification) and malpractice lawsuits
◆ Have an asymmetric level of information, compared to the insurer, about the likely demand for health care services, resulting in **adverse selection** (e.g., high-risk patients are denied insurance or care) and market failure (e.g., inefficiencies and lack of appropriate competition)—although this is less severe in large group insurance plans that spread out the risk

A fundamental problem of the health care economy is that it is difficult for any person or organization (e.g., patient, physician, health plan, government) to be "an efficient and effective purchaser of health care goods and services" (Dranove, 2000, p. 9).

One area of health care, however, that seems to more closely follow the free-market supply-and-demand model is LASIK eye surgery. The average cost of this surgery in 1998 was $2,200 per eye. This dropped to $1,350 in 2004 as over 3 million surgeries were performed. Many believe this is due to the lack of third-party reimbursement and the evidence of *consumer driven purchases* in response to advertising and competition (Tabarrok, 2004).

Health Insurance Concepts

Conventional theories posit that people pay small premiums monthly to offset the risk of large medical bills should they become seriously ill. This represents an *indemnity policy*, much like car or homeowners' insurance, and this is the type of health insurance first offered in the United States. In the past, patients could choose any doctor or hospital and submit the providers' bills to the insurance company for payment. "Moral hazard" is the term used by economists to explain how health insurance changes the behavior of people, resulting in more risk-taking and wasteful behaviors. They liken it to fire insurance without a deductible, noting that a person may be less careful about clearing brush from a house if it costs the owner nothing to have the home replaced. If a person has health insurance, many economists posit, they are less likely to take good care of themselves, and if they don't pay for their health care (through premiums, co-payments, deductibles), they are more likely to misuse it or overuse it (Gladwell, 2005). In other words, insurance has a paradoxical effect and often leads to wasteful and risk-taking behaviors. In this scenario, patients will demand expensive health care, even if it provides only the smallest benefit (Dranove, 2000). The concept of moral hazard is the reason behind larger deductibles and co-payments—it is an effort to control wasteful and excessive use of health care resources.

A newer theory states that consumers purchase health insurance not to avoid risk, but to earn a "claim for additional income (i.e., insurance paying for medical care) if they become ill" and that co-payments and managed care actually work against the system by reducing the amount of income transferred to ill persons or limiting their access to needed services (Nyman, 2003). Some economists argue that moral hazard doesn't accurately apply to health insurance, as even those with unlimited insurance coverage don't just "check into the hospital because it's free" (Gladwell, 2005, ¶11). Most people do not seek infinite numbers of colonoscopies or surgeries, for instance.

Employer-sponsored Health Insurance

Currently, 63% of those under age 65 receive employer-sponsored health care (only 5% have private nongroup insurance), and in bad economic times, company downsizing and lay-offs lead many people to "feel they are only a pink slip away from being uninsured" (Brink, 2002, p. 63; Goldman & McGlynn, 2005). Many small businesses do not offer employee health insurance because of the high costs. Even Wal-Mart, one of the United States' largest employers, offers high-premium/high-deductible plans (with 6-month waiting periods for full-time workers) that more than half of their employees cannot afford—thus shifting costs to taxpayers because 60% of workers must rely on government insurance or other remedies (United Food & Commercial Workers International Union, 2007). The average Wal-Mart worker pays one-fifth of his paycheck for company health insurance coverage, as many of them work for the minimum wage for fewer than 40 hours per week.

The average worker contributed about 27% of the total cost of group insurance in 2004 (around $10,000 for a family of four). Few people (between 5% and 7%) purchase individual insurance, and these small numbers have fallen even more over the past 15 years. Cost keeps many people from purchasing insurance; one study found that premiums for individual insurance rose 25% in a 7-year period (Goldman & McGlynn, 2005; 2006). The Kaiser Family Foundation

(2006a), in its 2006 Employer Health Benefits Survey, reported an 87% increase in premiums since 2000, and noted an increase to $11,480 for the average family group policy, with the cost to workers at just under $3,000 annually. However, the Foundation also noted that the increase in premiums for 2006 (7.7%) was down from the past 2 years (9.2% and 13.9%, respectively). See Figure 6.5 for trends in health insurance premium costs as compared to wages and overall inflation.

The most chilling fact is that a minimum-wage worker in 2005 earned an average of $10,712, but the cost of an annual premium for a family of four averaged $10,880—helping to explain the large number of uninsured Americans (Colliver, 2005). Employers are either not offering health insurance or are passing along the higher costs to employees in the form of higher employee premiums, deductibles, co-payments, and stricter enrollment requirements. According to a study by the Agency for Healthcare Research and Quality (Stanton & Rutherford, 2004), even though offers of workplace health insurance increased from 1996 to 2002, eligibility and enrollment rates dropped—mostly because of rising employee costs (e.g., over 65% increases in employee premium contributions). In 2003, about 5 million fewer jobs provided health insurance, even though employers shopped around for the best value and about one-third either changed insurance carriers or changed the type of insurance plan offered to employees (Gabel et al., 2004). The number of small companies offering health plans continues to decline, and state efforts to reform small-group health insurance have been relatively unsuccessful in increasing the numbers of employers offering coverage (Gabel et al., 2004; RAND Health, 2005).

About 25% of Americans who are insured are under-insured, and 33% report problems accessing medical care, as well as paying for it. They often exhaust their savings, run up credit card debt, or else delay necessary medical care to avoid going into debt (RAND Health, 2006; Forbes, 2007).

SOURCES OF HEALTH CARE FINANCING: PUBLIC AND PRIVATE

Financing of health care significantly affects community health and community health nursing practice. It influences the type and quality of services offered, as well as the ways in which those services are used. Sources of payment may be grouped into three categories: third-party payments, direct consumer payment, and private or philanthropic support.

Third-Party Payments

Third-party payments are monetary reimbursements made to providers of health care by someone other than the consumer who received the care. The organizations that administer these funds are called *third-party payers* because they are a third party, or external, to the consumer–provider relationship. Included in this category are four types of payment sources: private insurance companies, independent or self-insured health plans, government health programs, and claims payment agents (Harrington & Estes, 2004).

Private Insurance Companies

Private insurance companies currently pay the majority of U.S. health care expenditures for those under age 65. They market and underwrite policies aimed at decreasing consumer risk of economic loss because of a need to use health services. Traditional indemnity health insurers have been experiencing decelerating growth for more than a decade as the result of a shift to lower-cost managed-care plans offered through employers. In 2006, only 3% of those under age 65 who were insured had this type of plan (Kaiser Family Foundation, 2006a).

There are three types of private insurers. First are commercial stock companies that sell health insurance, usually as a sideline. They are private, stockholder-owned corporations that sell insurance nationally; examples are Aetna,

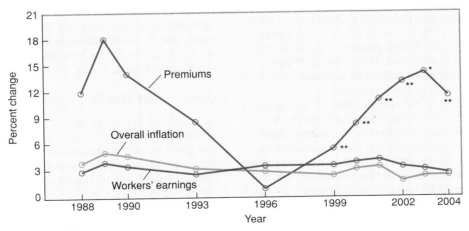

FIGURE 6.5 Increases in employer health insurance premiums compared with other indicators, selected years 1988–2004. Data on premium increases reflect the cost of health insurance premiums for a family of four. Statistical significance indicators denote that premium estimates are statistically from the previous year shown (*$p < .10$, ** $p < .05$). (From Gabel et al. [2004]. Health benefits in 2004: Four years of double-digit premium increases take their toll on coverage. *Health Affairs, 23*(5), 200–209, used with permission.)

Travelers, and Connecticut General (CIGNA). A second type of insurer operates in the national marketplace and is owned by policyholders—a *mutual company*. Examples are Mutual of Omaha, Prudential, and Metropolitan Life. The third type, *nonprofit insurance* plans, includes companies such as Blue Cross, Blue Shield, and Delta Dental. These operate under special state-enabling laws that give them an exclusive franchise to the whole state (or a part of it) and to a specific type of insurance. For example, traditionally, Blue Cross sold only hospital coverage; Blue Shield, only medical insurance; and Delta Dental, only dental insurance. Because they are nonprofit, they are tax exempt and, at the same time, subject to tighter state regulation than are the commercial health insurance companies. Combined, the nonprofit and commercial carriers have sold most of the private health insurance in the United States over the last decade (Lee, Estes, & Rodriguez, 2003).

A recent trend in private insurance is the move to consumer-directed or **consumer-driven health plans (CDHP)** and **health savings accounts (HSAs)**. Beginning in 2004, legislation provided for tax-exempt HSAs tied to high-deductible health insurance plans that can be rolled over yearly and move with the employee (Gabel, Pickreign & Whitmore, 2006). The high deductibles (e.g., over $1,100 for an individual and over $2,200 for a family) allow for lower premiums, but the attendant HSAs can only be used on medical expenses—nothing else—or tax-exempt status is lost and a penalty is also incurred (Mayo Clinic, 2007). Most plans require employees to pay a percentage of their total health costs (coinsurance, e.g., 20%)—not just a small co-payment per office visit or prescription as in many other plans. Some think that this improves **cost sharing**—whereby the insured assumes a greater share of health care costs, without a third-party payer intervening. Others think that this trend will not result in expanded coverage for the uninsured, and may lead to more employees forgoing health insurance offered by their employers (Glied & Remier, 2005).

Employers may or may not contribute to HSAs, and when they do, the cost savings in premiums are nullified and the accounts usually cannot be moved to a new employer. Only about 4% of workers are enrolled in these types of plans, and 39% of those who did enroll in 2006 had no other choice of health plan. When given a choice, few workers have chosen CDHPs, even though premiums are lower than for any other type of plan (Gabel, Pickreign, & Whitmore, 2006). See Table 6.4 for a comparison of premium costs for CDHP and other forms of health insurance.

A large-scale study of the effect of cost on compliance with antihyperlipidemic (cholesterol-lowering) therapy found that for every $10 increase in prescription co-payment, patient compliance levels fell by 5%. Researchers concluded that lowered patient compliance with medication regimens was inversely related to utilization of expensive medical services (e.g., emergency room [ER] visits, hospitalizations); in other words, when people didn't properly take their medications (or stopped taking them), they were more likely to need hospitalization, thereby increasing health care costs. These researchers also provided projections showing that requiring no prescription drug co-payments for high-risk patients would result in fewer hospitalizations and ER visits, for savings of more than $1 billion (Goldman, Joyce, & Karaca-Mandic, 2006).

TABLE 6.4	Comparison of Consumer-Directed Health Plans with Other Health Plans When Enrollees Have a Choice of Plans, 2006			
	CDHP	**HMO**	**PPO**	**POS**
Monthly premium, single	$299	$339	$364	$363
Monthly employer contribution*	$243	$288	$303	$307
Monthly employee contribution	$56	$51	$61	$56
Average single deductible, in-network	$1,459	$30	$261	$94
% Employees with office visit co-payments	15%	95%	79%	98%

*Average monthly employer contribution to CDHP savings account $54 in addition to premium.
Adapted from Gabel, J.R., Pickreign, J.D., & Whitmore, H. (2006). Behind the slow growth of employer-based consumer-driven health plans. *Center for Studying Health System Change*, Issue Brief No. 107, ¶14.

Independent or Self-insured Health Plans

Independent or self-insured health plans underwrite the remaining private health insurance in the United States. These plans have been offered through a limited number of organizations, such as large businesses, unions, school districts, consumer cooperatives, and medical groups. Employers with self-insured plans take on all or a major part of the risk for health care costs of their employees. These plans may be self-administered or utilize third-party claims administrators. Minimum premium plans are another form of self-insurance for which employers pay medical costs up to an agreed-upon limit, and insurers assume responsibility for the excess claims (Bureau of Labor Statistics, 2002). Self-insurance plans are not subject to regulation by the states, and it is estimated that 54% of employees receiving work-related insurance benefits are part of self-insurance plans (Dow, Harris, & Liu, 2006; Lawlor & Hall, 2005).

Government Health Programs

Government health programs make up the next largest source of third-party reimbursement in the United States. The government's four major health insurance programs are Medicare, Medicaid, the Federal Employees Health Benefits Plan, and the Civilian Health and Medical Program of the Uniformed Services (CHAMPUS). As a whole, the proportion of government funding of health care in the United States is less than that of many other countries. Of the government's health insurance programs, Medicare and Medicaid are the largest. Medicare pays the majority of health care costs (56%) for citizens age 65 and older, while private insurance pays for 54% of health care costs for those under age 65 (Goldman & McGlynn, 2005). In 2005, Medicare covered 42.5 million people at a cost of $330 billion for health care costs (Centers for Medicare & Medicaid Services [CMMS], 2006). Spending for Medicaid in 2006 was $180.6 billion (Center on Budget & Policy Priorities, 2006). Less than half of the total health care expenditure per person is paid by public sources in the United States, compared with the United Kingdom (England) at close to 90% and Canada at 71% (Cylus & Anderson, 2006; Lemieux, 2006; Organization for Economic Cooperation & Development, 2007).

Medicare and Social Security Disability Insurance

Medicare, known as Title XVIII of the Social Security Act Amendments of 1965, has provided mandatory federal health insurance since July 1, 1966, for adults age 65 years and older who have paid into the Social Security system. It also covers certain disabled persons. Medicare is the largest health insurer in the United States, covering about 16% of the population. Of the approximately 42 million beneficiaries, over 7 million qualify for Social Security Disability Insurance (SSDI); these recipients are younger than age 65 and permanently disabled or chronically ill (CMMS, 2007; Kaiser Family Foundation, 2006b). The Medicare population is projected to grow to 44.5 million by 2008, and to more than 63 million by 2027, and their share of GDP is expected to grow from just under 3% in 2005 to over 9% in 2050 (Van de Water & Lavery, 2006) (see Figs 6.6 and 6.7).

Medicare is administered by the Centers for Medicare and Medicaid Services (formerly the Health Care Financing Administration—HCFA) of the U.S. Department of Health and Human Services.

Part A of Medicare, the hospital insurance program, covers inpatient hospitals, limited-skilled nursing facilities, home health, and hospice services to participants eligible for Social Security. It is financed through trust funds derived from employment payroll taxes. A total tax of 2.8% of employee wages is split between the employer and employee. These payroll taxes, along with interest earned on trust fund investments, provide the income for this program (Van de Water & Lavery, 2006).

Part B, the supplementary and voluntary medical insurance program, primarily covers physician services, but also covers home health care for beneficiaries not covered under

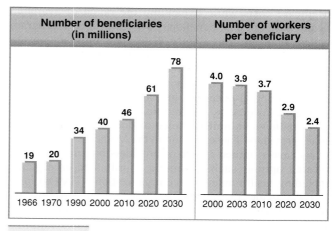

FIGURE 6.7 Historical and projected number of Medicare beneficiaries and number of workers per beneficiary. (From *Fact sheet: Medicare spending & financing*. [2005, April]. Kaiser Family Foundation, Publication No. 7305. This information was reprinted with permission from the Henry J. Kaiser Family Foundation. The Kaiser Family Foundation, based in Menlo Park, California, is a nonprofit, private operating foundation focusing on the major health care issues facing the nation and is not associated with Kaiser Permanente or Kaiser Industries.)

part A. It is funded through enrollee monthly premiums ($88.50 in 2006) (Van de Water & Lavery, 2006).

Part D, the prescription benefit plan added through the Medicare Prescription Drug, Improvement and Modernization Act of 2003 cost just over $27 monthly in 2007—although premiums can vary across regions, with plans from $9.50 for a basic prescription drug plan (PDP) to $135 for a PDP with enhanced benefits (Van de Water & Lavery, 2006; Kaiser Family Foundation, 2007a).

Medicare was managed in the same manner for more than 30 years until August 1997, when President Clinton signed the Balanced Budget Act (PL No. 105–33). This act, which took effect in 1998, provided Medicare beneficiaries with markedly different options. Among the most significant alterations brought about by the Balanced Budget Act are those to the fast-growing managed-care side of Medicare (Kaiser Family Foundation, 2001). To control

FIGURE 6.6 Measures of Medicare spending, 2005–2014. (From *Fact sheet: Medicare spending & financing*. [2005, April]. Kaiser Family Foundation, Publication No. 7305. This information was reprinted with permission from the Henry J. Kaiser Family Foundation. The Kaiser Family Foundation, based in Menlo Park, California, is a nonprofit, private operating foundation focusing on the major health care issues facing the nation and is not associated with Kaiser Permanente or Kaiser Industries.)

	2005	2006	2010	2012	2014
Spending as % of Gross Domestic Product	2.7%	3.3%	3.5%	3.7%	4.0%
Spending as % of National Health Expenditures	17.2%	20.4%	20.2%	20.3%	20.8%
Years to HI Trust Fund Depletion (2005 projections)	15 years	14 years	10 years	8 years	6 years
General Revenue as a Share of Total Medicare Spending	36.8%	42.8%	44.5%	45.6%	47.9%

Medicare costs while expanding the range of available health care options, beneficiaries were offered a program called Medicare Plus Choice Plans. This program was an effort to accelerate the migration of patients away from Medicare's traditional and more expensive fee-for-service (FFS) program into various managed care options. Enrollees opting to remain in traditional Medicare continued to be covered by the traditional FFS program, which gives patients unlimited choice of doctors, hospitals, and other providers. Those moving to the Medicare Plus Choice plans have a limited choice of providers but, in return, are offered options such as joining coordinated care plans, including health maintenance organizations (HMOs), preferred provider organizations (PPOs), provider-sponsored organizations, private FFS plans, and on a limited basis, medical savings account plans. As benefit coverage for these managed care plans was cut and premiums increased, along with cost sharing for physician and hospital visits, a good number of seniors chose to return to the traditional Medicare coverage (Gold & Achman, 2002). For more information on Medicare trends and concerns about its solvency, see Chapter 24.

Medicaid

Medicaid, known as Title XIX of the Social Security Act Amendments of 1965, provides medical assistance for children; for those who are aged, blind, or disabled; and for people who are eligible to receive federally assisted income maintenance payments (CMMS, 2005). In 2001, almost 44 million Americans received Medicaid-sponsored health and long-term care (Kaiser Family Foundation, 2001). It is jointly funded between federal and state governments to assist the states in providing adequate medical care to eligible needy persons. The states have some discretion in determining which groups their Medicaid programs will cover and the financial criteria for Medicaid eligibility, as well as the scope of services, rate of payment, and how the program will be administered (CMMS, 2005). To be eligible for federal funds, however, states are required to provide Medicaid coverage for most individuals who receive federally assisted income maintenance payments (welfare), as well as for related groups not receiving cash payments (especially the elderly). The states determine the type, amount, duration, and scope of services. According to the Centers for Medicare and Medicaid Services (2005), the following are examples of mandatory Medicaid eligibility groups:

◆ Citizens on federally assisted income maintenance, including Supplemental Security Income recipients
◆ Offspring of Medicaid-eligible pregnant women
◆ Children younger than 6 years and pregnant women who meet the state's assisted income maintenance requirements or whose family income is at or below 133% of the federal poverty level (FPL)
◆ Children on adoption assistance and foster care under Title IV of the Social Security Act
◆ Medicare beneficiaries (qualified disabled workers and certain poor Medicare recipients)
◆ Protected groups who lose cash assistance because of the cash programs' rules (e.g., earnings from

work or increases in Social Security benefits—may keep Medicaid for a period of time)
◆ Minors born after September 30, 1983, who are under age 19, from families at or below the FPL

Optional "categorically related" groups also exist, which states may or may not choose to cover (¶ 7). These include infants and pregnant women with a family income at or below 185% of the FPL, people under age 21 who meet more liberal criteria than those listed above, individuals who are institutionalized or are receiving care under waivers for home and community-based services, some working disabled persons, some TB-infected persons, women with low incomes who need breast and cervical cancer screenings, and "medically needy" persons (often elderly who must spend down their resources in order to be covered for long-term care) (¶ 9).

Coverage includes preventive, acute, and long-term care services. Potential Medicaid recipients must apply for coverage and prove their eligibility in terms of category and limited income. About 65% of Medicaid funds are spent on the elderly and disabled, with 25% going to children and adults with low incomes (Kaiser Family Foundation, 2001).

Medicaid has historically reimbursed providers at a lower rate than Medicare and other insurances, and this has caused problems with access to care. Even with lower reimbursement rates, costs continue to rise. As with Medicare, Medicaid programs moved to a managed care concept, following mandates within the Balanced Budget Act of 1997. In 2006, over 29 million Medicaid enrollees participated in a managed care plan (Kaiser Family Foundation, 2006c).

The move has not been without its problems for those receiving Medicaid. Medicaid beneficiaries are economically disadvantaged, frequently reside in medically underserved areas, and often have more complex health and social needs than do Americans with higher incomes. Early evidence on the implementation of Medicaid managed care showed "some improvement in access to a regular provider but more difficulties in obtaining care and dissatisfaction with care" compared with those in Medicaid FFS (Kaiser Family Foundation, 2001, ¶12). In recent years, many people who were never before eligible for Medicaid benefits have become eligible as a result of downward national economic trends, company downsizing, and corporate scandals. Subsequent to these economic issues, families have lost employer-subsidized health care benefits, and some now find themselves among those eligible for Medicaid managed care programs.

Medicaid's use of managed care has grown dramatically. The percentage of Medicaid recipients enrolled in a broad array of managed care arrangements increased from just below 10% in 1991 to almost 56% in 2000. However, during that same time, the number of commercial plans withdrawing from the Medicaid market increased, and new plans entering the market decreased (Kaiser Family Foundation, 2001). The future success of Medicaid managed care depends on the adequacy of the **capitation rates** (fixed amounts of money paid per person by the health plan to the provider for covered services) and the ability of state and federal governments to monitor access and quality. Quality performance standards are evolving. Ensuring access and quality of care in a managed care environment will require fiscally solvent plans, established provider networks, education of providers and beneficiaries about managed care, and awareness of the unique needs of the Medicaid population.

State Children's Health Insurance Plan

In 1997, as another part of the Balanced Budget Amendment, the State Children's Health Insurance Plan (SCHIP) provided health coverage to uninsured children under age 19 for families caught in the gap between Medicaid and affordable health insurance (Congresspedia, 2007; FirstGov, 2007). All 50 states participate, and for little or no cost, provide insurance for hospitalization, physician visits, prescription drugs, and in some cases dental and vision services (FirstGov, 2007). There are variations among the states, but SCHIP is geared to working families who may earn up to $34,100 yearly for a family of four (FirstGov, 2007). In 2007, SCHIP coverage was expanded by imposing an excise tax on tobacco products (Congresspedia, 2007).

Other Government Programs

In addition to third-party reimbursement, the government offers some direct health services to selected populations, including Native Americans, military personnel, veterans, merchant marines, and federal employees. Government support, largely through grants administered through the CDC, provides immunizations and well-child care, as well as prenatal care and other programs at the state and local level.

Payment Concepts in Health Care

Reimbursement for health care services generally has been accomplished through one of two approaches: retrospective or prospective payment. Conceptually, these approaches are polar opposites. It is helpful to understand their differences and their meaning for the financing and delivery of health services, past and present.

Retrospective Payment

A traditional form of reimbursement for any kind of service, including health care, is **retrospective payment**, which is reimbursement for a service after it has been rendered. A fee may be established in advance. However, payment of that fee occurs after the fact, or retrospectively. This is known as the **fee-for-service** (FFS) approach (Cutler, 2004; Newhouse, 2002).

In health care, limited accountability in the use of retrospective payment has created several problems. With third-party payers (e.g., insurance companies, the government) serving as intermediaries, neither consumers nor providers of health services were accountable for containing costs. Patients and providers alike often insisted on expensive or unnecessary tests and treatments. Because reimbursement was made retrospectively by the insuring agency, there was no incentive to keep a lid on this spending. Third-party reimbursement increased, along with other factors, to create an inflationary spiral of escalating costs. Abuse of the FFS system made it more difficult to develop retrospective payment for other health care providers, including nurses (Chang, Price, & Pfoutz, 2001).

A further problem associated with the FFS concept was its tendency to encourage sickness care rather than wellness services. Physicians and other providers were rewarded financially for treating illness and for providing additional tests and services. There were few incentives for prevention or health promotion in an industry that reaped its revenues from keeping hospital beds full and caring for the sick and injured. Although retrospective payment worked well in other industries, from a cost-containment as well as a public health perspective, it was problematic in health care.

Prospective Payment

Prospective reimbursement, although not a new concept, was implemented for inpatient Medicare services in 1983, in response to the health care system's desperate need for cost containment (Newhouse, 2002). It has since influenced the Medicaid program, as well as private health insurers. The prospective payment form of reimbursement has virtually eliminated the retrospective payment system (Chang, Price, & Pfoutz, 2001; Newhouse, 2002). **Prospective payment** is a payment method based on rates derived from predictions of annual service costs that are set in advance of service delivery. Providers receive payment for services according to these fixed rates, set in advance. Payments may be in the form of premiums paid before receipt of service or in response to fixed-rate (not cost) charges. To correct unlimited reimbursement patterns and counteract disincentives to contain costs, prospective payment involves four classic steps (Dowling, 1979):

1. An external authority is empowered (by statute, market power, or voluntary compliance by providers) to set provider charges, third-party payment rates, or both.
2. Rates are set in advance of the prospective year during which they will apply and are considered fixed for the year (except for major, uncontrollable occurrences).
3. Patients, third-party payers, or both pay the prospective rates rather than the costs incurred by providers during the year (or charges adjusted to cover these costs).
4. Providers are at risk for losses or surpluses.

The concept of prepayment, or consumers paying in advance of health care, has existed for many years. As far back as 1933, prepaid medical groups were advocated to reduce costs and make services more accessible (Premera, 2007). Examples of early plans were the Health Insurance Program of Greater New York City and the Kaiser Plan (Chang, Price, & Pfoutz, 2001). The success of these two plans helped to influence the growth of the HMO, a type of managed care discussed later in this chapter.

Prospective payment imposes constraints on spending and provides incentives for cutting costs. The federal government, as mentioned earlier, enacted a prospective payment plan (Social Security Amendments Act 1983; see Landmark Health Care Legislation). The plan is a billing classification system known as **diagnosis-related groups (DRGs)**. The system is based on about 500 diagnosis and procedure groups. It provides fixed Medicare reimbursement to hospitals based on weighted formulas (Newhouse, 2002). Flat rates of payment are based on average national costs for a specific group, adjusted annually, with some regional variations accounting for higher wages and other costs (Chang, Price, & Pfoutz, 2001). This system was enacted to curb Medicare spending in hospitals and to extend the program's solvency period. The regulatory approach of DRGs changed Medicare hospital reimbursement from a cost-based retrospective payment system, in which a hospital was paid its costs, to a fixed-price prospective payment system. It was designed to create incentives for hospitals to be more efficient in delivering services.

Indeed, the prospective payment system has reduced Medicare's rate of increase in inpatient hospital spending and increased hospital productivity (Institute of Medicine, 2001). Thought to reduce hospital stays and unnecessary admissions, the system led to "DRG creep" (e.g., classifying patients into more lucrative categories) and "patient dumping" (e.g., transferring patients whose reimbursement is expected to be lower than actual costs of services) in an effort to counteract the losses in revenue to hospitals that spend more on Medicare patients than they are reimbursed (Dranove, 2000, p. 52). It also led to fierce competition among providers and mounting concern about quality of care—in hospitals, ambulatory settings, and home care.

A more vigorous version of prospective payment is *capitation*. As noted before, capitation refers to a fixed fee per person that is paid to a managed care organization for a specified package of services. Fees remain in effect until renegotiated, regardless of the number of services provided. Because profit margins are very tight, utilization, quality, and costs are carefully monitored (Chang, Price, & Pfoutz, 2001).

The prospective payment concept has proved useful from a public health perspective. Prepaid services create incentives for providers to keep their enrollees healthy, thus reducing provider costs. A potential, indirect benefit from fixed rates and reduced costs is that more of the health care dollar is available to spend on prevention programs.

Claims Payment Agents

Claims payment agents administer the process for government third-party payments. That is, the government contracts with private fiscal agents to handle the claims payment process and function as an intermediary between them and the health care provider. More than 80% of the government's third-party payments have been handled by these private contractors, who sometimes are known as fiscal intermediaries (when processing Medicare hospital claims), carriers (when dealing with insurance under Medicare), or fiscal agents (as applied to Medicaid programs). As an example, Blue Cross, in addition to being a private insurance company, also is a claims payment agent for Medicare (Virginia Commonwealth University, 2007).

Direct Consumer Reimbursement or Out-of-Pocket Payment

Another source of health care financing comes from direct fees paid by consumers. This refers to individual out-of-pocket payments made for several different reasons, such as payments made by individuals who have no insurance coverage (fees must be paid directly for health and medical services) or payments for limited coverage, insurance caps, and exclusions (services for which the consumer must bear the entire expense).

For example, some individuals carry only major medical insurance and must pay directly for physician office visits, prescriptions, eyeglasses, and dental care. In other instances, the insurance contract may include a deductible amount that must be paid by the insured before reimbursement begins (e.g., $500 for individuals, $1,500 for a family). The contract may be established on a coinsurance basis, which determines a percentage to be paid by the insurer and the rest by the individual (e.g., 80/20 plans for which individuals pay 20% of costs after deductibles). Or, the individual may pay the remainder of a health service bill after the insurer has paid a previously agreed-on fixed amount, such as a fixed fee (known as a coverage cap) for labor and delivery, for example. About 21% of people under age 65 pay out-of-pocket for health care costs; about 16% of people age 65 and more pay health care costs directly (Goldman & McGlynn, 2005).

Another important factor for those paying directly for their health care expenses is **cost shifting**. This practice of charging different prices to different consumers most often affects those without health insurance who are paying out-of-pocket for care (Morrissey, 2003). As health insurance plans or large companies contract with hospitals and physicians for services, they purchase these services at a reduced cost. Those without this "buying power" pay full price. For example, a $500 radiology procedure may be discounted to $225 for an insurance plan, but an individual paying out-of-pocket will pay the full price.

Private and Philanthropic Support

Private or philanthropic support, a third funding source, contributes both directly and indirectly to health care financing. Many private agencies fund programs, underwrite research, and provide benefits for people who otherwise would go without services. In addition, volunteerism, the efforts of numerous individuals and organizations that donate their time and services (e.g., hospital guild members), provides tremendous cost savings to health care institutions. It also enables many individuals to receive services, such as home-delivered meals or transportation to health care facilities, at no charge.

Philanthropic financing of health care has significantly decreased in the last two decades. One study tracking physicians noted that over 76% offered charity care in 1996–1997, but that number decreased to just over 68% in 2004–2005, and that the charity care hours per 100 people decreased by 18% in the same time period (Cunningham & May, 2006). Surgeons were most often noted to provide free care to patients without insurance, and hospitals are required to provide emergency care to everyone. Uncompensated care costs for hospitals, though, have remained steady, and their payments from private insurance have risen faster than their costs (Cunningham & May, 2006). Even though some providers offer charity care, continued private support is essential, particularly when federal and state monies for health and social programs have been severely restricted (Harrington & Estes, 2004).

Further understanding of health economics and its impact on community health and community health nursing can be obtained by examining methods of health care finance, trends and issues influencing health care economics, and the effects of finance patterns on community health practice.

TRENDS AND ISSUES INFLUENCING HEALTH CARE ECONOMICS

The High Cost of Health in America

America paid over $6,100 per person for health care in 2004 (Davis et al., 2007) through a combination of public tax money, individual and corporate contributions to insurance plans, and other sources. Not only do we pay almost twice the per capita expenditure of Canada and Germany and almost three times that of New Zealand and the United Kingdom, but we have had "one of the highest growth rates in per capita health care spending since 1980 among higher income countries"(Davis et al., 2007; Kaiser Family Foundation, 2007c, ¶2).

Many Americans believe that we have the best health care system in the world. But what actually constitutes a good health care system? Are we truly getting our money's worth? The WHO's groundbreaking report of member countries outlined a *good health system* as one that provides good health for the whole population over the entire life cycle, responds to client's expectations for respectful treatment and a client-oriented system of health care providers, and ensures that costs are distributed according to ability to pay and provides financial protection for all (2000). A "good and fair" health care system exhibits (p. 2):

◆ Overall good health (e.g., low infant mortality)
◆ Fair distribution of good health (e.g., long life expectancy distributed evenly across population groups)
◆ High level and fair distribution (across population groups) of overall responsiveness
◆ Fair distribution of health care financing (e.g., based on ability to pay, distributed fairly, so that everyone has equal protection from financial risks incurred by illness)

What researchers found was that the U.S. health care system was the "most expensive . . . in the world" largely because of high administrative costs (estimated then to range between 19.3% and 24.1%), the system of complex multiple payers, and the rising costs of prescription medications and advanced medical technology (p. 2). They also noted the shift from nonprofit to for-profit hospitals and the aging population as causative factors, along with the high proportion of uninsured people (and the attendant high cost of untreated illness). Access was a significant problem, as the United States was found to be "the only country in the developed world, except for South Africa, that does not provide health care for all of its citizens" (p. 3). In the United States, the patchwork quilt of private and public insurance—mostly tied to either employment or low-income status—makes it difficult for many people to get the care they need. The researchers noted that those without health insurance are "sicker and die younger than people with health insurance" (p. 4).

Americans believe that we have a quality health care system, and that this can make up for other deficits. The United States did rank first among all WHO countries on *responsiveness*—a construct relating to how respectfully clients are treated. However, as noted in Chapter 25, for many racial and ethnic minorities, this is not the case.

Disability-adjusted life expectancy (DALE, or the average number of healthy years expected in a population) was very low, and the United States was ranked 24th, with an unequal distribution, especially among males. The United States was ranked lowest among 14 industrialized nations and placed 54th among WHO countries on the measure of *fairness in financing* (Anderson & Hussey, 2001; WHO, 2000). This inequality disproportionately affects the poor, underinsured, and the uninsured, as many public health nurses (PHNs) can corroborate.

Compared to the other 190 countries studied by the WHO, the United States ranked 15th for attainment of the criteria listed above, and 37th for *performance* (a comparison of how well it *could* perform based on available resource levels). Also, only 40% of those in the United States reported that they were *satisfied* with the health care system. Many factors contribute to this, and shrinking patient choices, increased influence of managed care, and nursing shortages, along with quality of care, were noted as important (University of Maine, 2001; WHO, 2000).

The Commonwealth Fund created a *National Scorecard on U.S. Health System Performance*, and defined several dimensions of a "high performance health system" (Schoen, Davis, How, & Schoenbaum, 2006, p. 457) as:

◆ Long, healthy, and productive lives
◆ Quality
◆ Access
◆ Efficiency
◆ Equity

On a total possible score of 100, the United States scored 66 overall, and only 51 on the dimension of *efficiency*. The researchers also found that less than half of U.S. adults receive preventive care and all recommended screening tests (using national standards), and that 30-day hospital readmission rates varied greatly. They were over 50% greater in regions with the highest rates when compared with those with the lowest rates—highlighting a wide disparity in quality care across the country.

Increasing influenza and pneumonia vaccinations would cost between $200 and $400 million annually, but could save between 20,000 and 40,000 deaths. Other inefficiencies could be corrected by the widespread implementation of *health information technology* (HIT)—including computerized physician order entry and electronic medical records (Hillestad et al., 2005). Over $77 billion per year could be saved if hospitals and outpatient clinics adopted widespread use of these technologies. Over 200,000 adverse drug events could be avoided annually, with a savings exceeding $1 billion and many lives spared. Earlier research found a "fragmented system fraught with waste and inefficiency"—indicating what could be termed an "*un-system*" of health care. It was also noted that the United States spends more than two times the per capita average for health care among industrialized nations (Gauthier & Serber, 2005, ¶1).

Why does health care cost so much? Explanations include the following:

◆ Medical malpractice costs and the need to practice *defensive medicine* by ordering excessive tests and x-rays (Sage & Kersch, 2006; RAND Institute for Civil Justice, 2004)

◆ An aging population (Cutler, 2004)
◆ Advances in and the spread of medical technology; for instance, in the last decade 12 of 19 Nobel prizes in medicine have been awarded to U.S. scientists—and this comes at a price (Cowan, 2006; Morris, 2005)
◆ Rapidly rising prescription drug and hospital costs (Goldman & McGlynn, 2005; Rice & Rhodes, 2006)
◆ The failure of market forces, in that health care doesn't respond to supply and demand as in other areas of the economy (Nyman, 2003; Rice & Rhodes, 2006; Sharma, 2006)
◆ High costs of insurance administration—in some cases, three times that of the cost in other nations (Commonwealth Fund Commission on a High Performance Health System, 2006; Nyman, 2003)
◆ Ineffective, inappropriate, and inadequate health care leading to increased morbidity and mortality and costs (Institute of Medicine, 2001)
◆ High proportion of uninsured—it has been estimated that the U.S. economy would benefit by $130 billion a year if all citizens were provided health insurance (Commonwealth Fund Commission on a High Performance Health System, 2006)
◆ Americans' demand for high-tech health care and preference for freedom of choice among providers and services (Jones, 2005)
◆ The higher U.S. cost of living and level of income—things just cost more in the USA. Some argue that the high proportion of GDP spent on health care actually benefits the U.S. economy (Gaynor & Gudipati, 2006)

A study by Anderson, Hussey, Frogner, and Waters (2005) examined two commonly held views regarding U.S. health care and rejected these arguments:

◆ Restriction of the supply of health care in many countries leads to decreased spending but also long waiting lists.
◆ U.S. malpractice litigation results in higher malpractice insurance costs and defensive medicine practices to protect physicians from lawsuits.

They noted that, despite high per capita expenditures, the United States was in the bottom 25% of countries in the Organization for Economic and Co-operative Development (OECD) for per capita hospital beds, and the average malpractice payment was 36% below the United Kingdom and 14% below Canada. While generally more malpractice claims are filed in the United States than in other countries, payments for claims were lower on average and the total costs of malpractice only encompassed less than .5% of the total expenditures for health care.

A striking example of cost differences found in different countries involves prescription drugs. For example, the cancer drug Campath (alemtuzumab) costs $2,400 in the United States, but only $760 in France, $660 in Sweden, $570 in the United Kingdom, and only $500 in Italy (McKenzie, 2007). Canada has enacted price controls that limit costs of new classes of medications to the median price paid by other countries, making the price for Campath in Canada $600. The United States is the only industrialized country without some form of price control on patented drugs. Drug companies say that limiting prices on new medications will reduce innovation and research for new drugs; however, for instance, in Canada only a handful of U.S. medications are not readily available (McKenzie, 2007).

Controlling Costs

As noted earlier, cost-control measures utilizing both supply-side and demand-side strategies have been attempted. Utilization review techniques have further enhanced utilization and cost control (Sultz & Young, 2006). Yet, despite various public and private cost-control strategies, health care costs continue to rise (Cutler, 2004). Although expenditures in the 1990s decelerated slightly from the escalation experienced during the 1970s and 1980s, in the early 2000s costs rose and continue to rise. Many factors influenced this increase. Between 1965 and 2001, the price per day of hospitalization rose tenfold from under $200 to over $1,300 (Kaiser Family Foundation, 2007c). As medical care became more complex, insurance costs rose dramatically, as did costs of public health care financing through Medicare and Medicaid (Cutler, 2004). More than half of the health care dollar goes to hospital and physician costs (31% and 22%, respectively) (Goldman & McGlynn, 2005). The explosion of medical technology has been characterized as a "medical arms race" by some (Dranove, 2000, p. 46), and a youth-oriented culture and unwillingness to accept illness and death has helped fuel this and the growth of elective procedures, such as plastic surgery.

A focus on primary prevention demands a paradigm shift in thinking about the practice and delivery of health care (see Chapter 1). It is one that fits more closely with the mission of public health. It expects that citizens are involved in their health care, are knowledgeable about their health status, can manage self-care practices, and can modify lifestyle behaviors to promote wellness. This creates a rich environment for community health nurses to collaborate with primary care practitioners and other health care professionals to control health care costs while providing quality care focusing on primary prevention.

Access to Health Services: The Uninsured and Underinsured

A growing segment of the U.S. populace (estimated at between 16% and 33%) is uninsured, resulting in limited or no access to health care (Aday, 2005; Forbes, 2007). More than 45 million Americans are currently without any form of health insurance coverage (Collins et al., 2006). There is wide variation between states—from 11% in Minnesota to over 30% in Texas—contributing to great inconsistencies in health care quality and access (Collins, 2007). By 2015, the number of uninsured is expected to reach 54 million (Broder, 2005).

As noted earlier, about 25% of Americans who have health insurance are underinsured (Forbes, 2007), and they often must chose between paying insurance and health-related expenses or foregoing needed care. The underinsured are more likely to "go without care because of costs" at a rate similar to those without health insurance, and 46% of underinsured were contacted by debt collectors, while 35% reported changing their usual way of life to pay medical expenses (Himmelstein, Warren, Thorne, & Woolhandler, 2005, p. 6). As an example of this, one large-scale study found that those with private health insurance paid close to $13,500 in out-of-pocket expenses for medical costs in 2001—while those who were uninsured paid close to $11,000 (Himmelstein et al., 2005). In addition, many underinsured have no dental or vision coverage, and have higher deductibles.

A particularly ominous study indicates that adults in the 50- to 64-year age range—baby boomers—have unstable health insurance coverage (Collins et al., 2006). More than half of these working older adults with annual incomes below $25,000 report that they have times without insurance coverage, and one-third of those with incomes between $25,000 and $39,999 also experience insurance instability. People in this age group have higher rates of chronic illness (62% had at least one chronic condition, such as diabetes or hypertension) and higher medical expenses. One-third of those in the study reported that they had problems paying medical bills or that they were paying off medical debt. Two-thirds were concerned that they would be unable to afford medical care in the future.

Medical Bankruptcies

Bankruptcy filings have been rising over the last decade—as much as 360%. In a 2001 study conducted by Harvard and Ohio University researchers, almost half of participants cited illness—sometimes with loss of work—and medical expenses as the chief cause for their bankruptcy (Himmelstein, Warren, Thorne & Woolhandler, 2005). The average study participant who filed for bankruptcy was a "42-year-old woman with children and at least some college education" (¶ 22). Most owned a home, and more than 75% of them had insurance coverage at the start of the illness that led to their bankruptcy. The reasons that those without insurance lacked coverage included unaffordable premiums, pre-existing conditions, lack of employer insurance coverage, gaps in coverage, and loss of employment. Of those filing medical bankruptcies, over 20% had gone without food, over 40% had their phone service disconnected, and around 30% lost electricity or water in the 2 years before filing. About 60% reported going without a needed doctor or dentist visit during that same time (Himmelstein, Warren, Thorne, & Woolhandler, 2005).

The consequences of not getting needed medical care are not trivial and can result in unnecessary hospitalization and serious health problems—along with increased costs. Death rates for the uninsured are 25% higher each year than for those with health insurance (Gladwell, 2005). It is estimated that not having health insurance leads to 18,000 deaths annually, making it the sixth leading cause of death for adults between age 25 and 64 (Davis, 2003). One of the largest groups among the uninsured are young adults between ages 19 and 29 (Collins et al., 2007), as well as workers and their families with low incomes. Most of these families have one member working full time; some have two or more full-time workers.

Access to health care is a prime concern for the uninsured. Many have no **medical home**—defined as seeing the same health care provider for regular care. Because there is a lack of care coordination, duplicative and wasteful services are often the case (Collins, 2007). And without a reliable care provider, the uninsured tend to use ERs for non-emergency care. Recent research noted that 33% of ER visits could have been handled in a primary physician's office (Davis, 2003). Other consumers utilize public clinics and other charity care services. Cost estimates for uncompensated care in 2001 reached $34.5 billion.

Government costs to reimburse "safety net" hospitals and other entities involved in care of the uninsured exceed $30 billion yearly—exemplifying just some of the costs to taxpayers. Because of the instability of the system, about half of the uninsured lose their health insurance coverage in a year—racking up higher administrative costs as they move between private and public insurers and change their usual sources of medical care. Interruptions in care, duplication in medical records, and verification of eligibility all lead to higher costs for everyone (Davis, 2003).

In the private sector, numerous firms do not offer health insurance to their employees; almost 80% of the uninsured are employees of these firms or are their dependents (Hellander, 2002). Self-employed individuals also find it difficult to pay the higher costs of insurance premiums without the benefit of group rates. Consequently, many of the self-employed can access health services only by purchasing expensive individual insurance policies with high-deductibles and coinsurance or by making expensive out-of-pocket payments.

Managed Care

The term **managed care** became popular in the late 1980s. It refers to systems that coordinate medical care for specific groups to promote provider efficiency and control costs. Although the term *managed care* is relatively new, the concept has been practiced for many years through various models of alternative health care delivery. Managed care is a cost-control strategy used in both public and private sectors of health care. Care is *managed* by regulating the use of services and levels of provider payment. This approach includes using HMOs and PPOs. In contrast to FFS models, managed care plans operate on a prospective payment basis and control costs by managing utilization and provider payments. The managed care model encourages the provision of services within fixed budgets, thus avoiding cost escalation. Because costs are tight, preventive services are generally encouraged, so that more expensive tertiary care costs can be avoided, if possible.

Health Maintenance Organizations

The HMOs and various companies' self-insured plans also are included in this category. Usually, they sell only health insurance; in some cases, they also may provide actual health services. They focus on a localized population. As a group, they generate a large amount of premium revenues; HMOs represent 20% of employer-sponsored group insurance (Kaiser Family Foundation, 2006a). Consumers have often resisted the strenuous cost-containment policies of many HMOs, and prefer to have their physicians make decisions about their care—not insurance company employees. However, employers are often drawn to alternatives as a cost-saving method. HMO premiums are usually lower than other types of insurance premiums, and out-of-pocket costs to consumers are generally lower (Gabel, Pickreign, & Whitmore, 2006).

A **health maintenance organization (HMO)** is a system in which participants prepay a fixed monthly premium to receive comprehensive health services delivered by a defined network of providers. The HMOs are the oldest model of coordinated or managed care. Several HMOs have existed for decades, but many have developed more recently. HMO enrollees benefit from a lower premium, reduced cost sharing, and fewer administrative costs.

From 1930 to 1965, the HMO movement, supported initially by the private sector, gradually gained federal backing. Group plans were included as a part of Medicare and Medicaid legislation. The HMO Act of 1973 demonstrated stronger federal support and assistance for growth of this industry (Chang, Price, & Pfoutz, 2001). Amendments to this act in 1976 lifted restrictions and further encouraged HMO growth. The skyrocketing employer health insurance costs of the 1980s and 1990s encouraged many companies to move from traditional insurance and FFS to HMOs. Currently, there are numerous HMOs with a variety of configurations. The unique set of properties of HMOs include:

◆ A contract between the HMO and the beneficiaries (or their representative), the enrolled population
◆ Absorption of prospective risk by the HMO
◆ A regular (usually monthly) premium to cover specified (typically comprehensive) benefits paid by each enrollee of the HMO; few additional charges are levied, because the payment mechanism is not FFS
◆ An integrated delivery system with provider incentives for efficiency; the HMO contracts with professional providers to deliver the services due the enrollees, and the basis for reimbursing those providers varies among HMOs (Harrington & Estes, 2004)

Official encouragement, government subsidies, and the pressures for cost control spurred the growth of HMOs. Some HMOs follow the traditional model, employing health professionals (e.g., physicians, nurses), building their own hospital and clinic facilities, and serving only their own enrollees. Other HMOs provide some services while contracting for the rest. Variations of the HMO model include solo practice physicians (some also continuing FFS medicine) who affiliate with hospitals (Chang, Price, & Pfoutz, 2001; Cutler, 2004). Enrollment in HMOs through employer-based programs numbered more than 77.7 million in 2006 (Managed Care Online [MCOL], 2007).

HMOs have been viewed as a positive alternative delivery system because of their potential for conserving costs, which results from their emphasis on prevention, health promotion, and ambulatory care, with a concomitant reduction in hospital and medical care utilization. However, there are questions as to whether the cost savings result partly from favorable selection of enrollees. Quality concerns also have been raised about the dangers of underserving enrollees in order to stay within payment limits (Baker et al., 2004; Sultz & Young, 2006). Scanlon, Swaminathan, Chernew, and Lee (2006) examined longitudinal data, and found that HMO competition was related to consumer satisfaction surveys, but not necessarily to better quality of care for chronic

conditions. Greater penetration of HMOs in some regions of the United States was associated with better outcomes for six common medical conditions (e.g., hip fracture, heart attack), but in other areas, the outcomes were worse—indicating no solid evidence of either higher or lower quality of care (Escarce, Jain, & Rogowski, 2006).

These concerns about HMOs and managed care in general have not gone unattended. The Health Insurance Portability and Accountability Act (HIPAA) and the Newborns' and Mothers' Health Protection Act are both significant pieces of legislation, addressing health care concerns among the nation's citizens and official organizations, such as the APHA. HIPAA reassured people that they would not lose health care coverage if they changed jobs. In addition, for a while in the United States, insurance for labor and delivery hospitalization covered only 24 or fewer hours after birth. Infants and mothers were being sent home in unstable post-delivery conditions. Newborns would go home when younger than 1 day of age, in some cases so soon after birth that body temperature was not stabilized and the ability to suck and take breast milk or formula was not established. The Newborns' and Mothers' Health Protection Act eliminated these "drive through deliveries," ensuring that mothers and newborns would have the right to remain in the acute care setting for at least 48 hours, covered by their insurance plan (see Landmark Health Care Legislation).

In response to concerns from managed care clients, recommendations from the Advisory Commission on Consumer Protection and Quality (1998) stipulated that health plans should subscribe to *The Patient's Bill of Rights*:

◆ *Information disclosure*: This is the right to accurate and easily understood information about the health plan, health care professionals, and facilities. This includes information in the patient's primary language.
◆ *Choice of providers and plans:* This is the right to a sufficient choice of providers to ensure access to appropriate, quality health care.
◆ *Access to emergency services:* This is the right to receive timely screening and stabilization emergency services whenever and wherever needed, without prior authorization or financial penalty, under certain circumstances (e.g., severe pain, injury).
◆ *Participation in treatment decisions:* Patient's have the right to know treatment options and to participate in care decisions.
◆ *Respect and nondiscrimination:* This is the right to considerate, respectful, and nondiscriminatory care from providers and others associated with the health care plan.
◆ *Confidentiality of health information:* Patient's have a right to talk confidentially with their health care provider and to have health information protected. This also includes the right to review and copy the patient's own medical records and the ability to request changes when indicated.
◆ *Complaints and appeals:* This is the right to a fast, fair, and objective review of any complaints against the health plan, providers, or other personnel, including waiting times, hours of operation,

conduct of personnel, and adequacy of health care system facilities.

These principles have been adopted by many health plans, on a voluntary basis. Legislation requiring these and more stringent rules (e.g., liability for medical malpractice, external appeals processes, discontinuation of provider financial incentives to reduce service utilization) have failed to be enacted by Congress (House of Representatives, 1998).

Preferred Provider Organizations

A **preferred provider organization (PPO)** is another model of managed or coordinated care that developed earlier than the HMO. A PPO is a network of physicians, hospitals, and other health-related services that contracts with a third-party payer organization to provide comprehensive health services to subscribers on a fixed FFS basis. Because of contractual fixed costs, employing organizations that subscribe can offer medical services to their employees at discounted rates. In PPOs, consumer choice exists. Enrollees have a choice among providers within the plan and contracted providers out of the plan. The PPOs practice utilization review and use formal standards for selecting providers (Chang, Price, & Pfoutz, 2001).

PPOs did not exist in their present form until after 1980. Enrollment in PPOs grew from about 10 plans in 1981 to more than 700 plans in the 1990s. The number of people enrolled in PPOs also increased, from an estimated 10.4% of individuals with private insurance in 1988 to 40% by the late 1990s, with the numbers leveling off as the decade came to a close (Dranove, 2000; Sultz & Young, 2006). As consumers became more frustrated with limits imposed by HMOs, they began to move toward PPOs that provide more choices. In 2006, 81.3 million

Americans were enrolled in a PPO, more than the number in HMOs (MCOL, 2007). Early use of PPOs appeared to promote cost savings, but the long-range cost effectiveness of this model has yet to be proved (Hurley, Strunk, & White, 2004). PPOs have been criticized for their lack of vigorous case management—more often found in HMOs—and some have begun to move toward this model, especially in the case of chronic diseases (e.g., hypertension, diabetes) (Porter & Teisberg, 2006).

Point of Service Plans

A variation on the just-mentioned plans is the **point-of-service (POS) plan**, which permits more freedom of choice than a standard HMO or PPO. At an extra cost, enrollees can go outside the HMO or PPO network of contracted providers unless their primary physician has made a specific referral (California Healthcare Foundation, 2007). This type of plan covers a small percentage of the market, estimated at around 10 million people (Dranove, 2000). For a look at the trend in types of health plan coverage among those employees who are covered by their employers, see Figure 6.8.

Health Care Rationing

The concept of **rationing** in health care refers to limiting the provision of health care services to save costs. Sometimes, this may jeopardize the well-being of groups of individuals. Rationing implies that resources are fixed or limited and therefore must be used sparingly. Rationing may occur by restricting people's choices, denying access to services, or by limiting the supply of services or personnel. It may be overt, as in the oft-cited case of Britain, or more covert, as

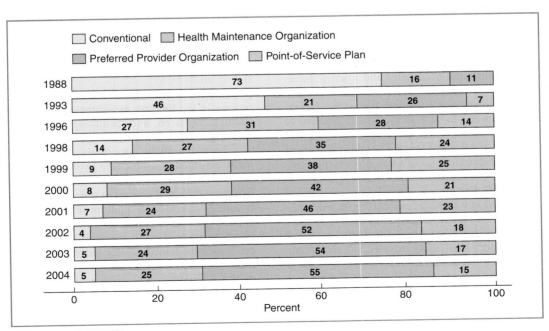

FIGURE **6.8** Health plan enrollment among covered workers, by type of plan, selected years 1988–2004. For 1998, 1999, 2000, 2001, and 2003, the distribution is significantly different from the previous year shown, at the 0.05 level. (From Gabel et al. [2004]. Health benefits in 2004: Four years of double-digit premium increases take their toll on coverage. *Health Affairs, 23*(5), 200–209, used with permisson.)

practiced by many managed care organizations or health plans. Often, insurers and providers of health care services make rationing decisions to contain costs. With rationing, there is a danger of compromising quality and effectiveness (Aaron, 2005).

Rationing in health care has been practiced for many years. With limited resources for health services delivery, government programs have had to establish strict eligibility levels and monitor the use of these resources to ensure the most equitable distribution. To maintain viability and some kind of profit margin, private insurers have engaged in rationing by excluding enrollees who are at greatest risk for health problems—and, thus, higher expenditures (Dranove, 2000; Porter & Teisberg, 2006; Sultz & Young, 2006).

Advances in knowledge and technical capabilities through research and technology compound rationing decisions. When several individuals need an organ transplant and only one organ is available, what criteria should be used to select the recipient? Now that it is known that certain lifestyle behaviors, such as smoking and alcohol consumption, or driving without restraints, create health risks, should people who engage in these activities pay a higher price for health care or be excluded from certain services? Should a younger person needing specialized surgery take priority over an elderly person needing similar care? There are no easy answers. Providers and insurers have struggled with these difficult policy issues for years.

With today's health care costs, the problems are even more complex. As health care spending rises, calls for rationing may intensify. The spending for Medicare and Medicaid in 2040 could be as great as our current combined income and payroll taxes (Aaron, 2005). Technological advances have added years to life and improved national welfare, but as spending continues to consume more and more of the GDP, many will ask if the costs outweigh the benefits and may seek to limit high-cost, low-benefit health procedures, such as expensive MRIs for rare conditions or conditions with no effective treatments or cures.

Oregon began a system of rationing in 1994. The state approached the problem pragmatically and openly. In an effort to reach universal coverage, Medicaid was expanded to cover all state residents with incomes below the federal poverty level, and then health care services were planned to be rationed to pay for the increase public coverage. A list of 709 medical services was decided upon. The state envisioned a plan for legislative determination of a cutoff point, depending on yearly budget allocations (Dranove, 2003; Loewy & Loewy, 2001). In 1999, Oregon's Medicaid program covered 574 of 743 conditions; however, the current Medicaid benefit package is still considered more generous than the state's previous plan (there is better coverage for dental care and mental health) and better than many private insurance plans (Oberlander, Marmor, & Jacobs, 2001). Although Oregon has not seen substantial savings with this plan and has not been able to achieve true universal coverage, it did reduce the number of uninsured residents to 11% (below the national average of around 16%). Some feel that the failure to reach universal coverage was partly due to the breakdown of legislation requiring business to provide insurance for all employees. Oregon made very public decisions about rationing health care, but more subtle means of rationing—budgetary caps, limits to the spread of technology—may

actually be more effective in achieving lower costs (Oberlander et al., 2001).

Competition and Regulation

Often, competition and regulation in health economics have been viewed as antagonistic and incompatible concepts. **Competition** means a contest between rival health care organizations for resources and clients. **Regulation** refers to mandated procedures and practices affecting health services delivery that are enforced by law. In a society in which long-held values of freedom of choice and individualism reign supreme, competition provides opportunities for entrepreneurial endeavor, free enterprise, and scientific advancement. Yet, to promote the public good, oversee equitable distribution of health services, and foster community-wide participation, regulation also serves an important role.

Health care incorporates four major kinds of regulation (Sultz & Young, 2006):

◆ Laws
◆ Regulations
◆ Programs
◆ Policies

Laws that regulate health care include any legislation that governs financing or delivery of health services, such as legislation regulating Medicare reimbursement to hospitals. Regulations guide and clarify implementation; they are issued under the authority of law and are part of most federal health care programs. Examples include regulations governing project grants such as HMO development; formula grants, such as those provided under the Hill-Burton Act; and entitlements, such as Medicare and Medicaid. Regulatory programs are created from legislative enactments and are designed to accomplish specific goals, such as accreditation and licensing rules for hospitals, public health agencies, and other health service providers. Regulatory policies have a broader focus and involve decisions that shape the health care system by channeling the flow of resources into it and setting limits on key players' actions. Examples of regulatory policies are found by reviewing state or federal budget proposals for funding programs, such as health manpower training, research, and technology development (Porter & Teisberg, 2006).

From the 1950s through the 1970s, the federal government assumed a strong role in regulating health services. First, federal subsidy of health care costs increased, and there was greater federal control of state programs. Health services became regionalized and more comprehensive. Federal appropriations supported operational as well as capital and planning costs. Health research and the training of health professionals gained greater federal support. Group medical practice multiplied as a cost-saving measure. More than 60% of the population was covered by some form of prepaid health insurance, largely because of the effects of Medicare and Medicaid. Interagency health planning cooperation increased, and health program evaluation improved. Neighborhood health centers, community mental health centers, and other programs were developed to improve health care access for everyone. Although costs rose, the period was one of relative economic stability that emphasized quality of care, with the federal government assuming a major role in regulating the planning, use, and reimbursement of health care services (Dranove, 2000; Sultz & Young, 2006).

In the early 1980s, government cost control measures were greatly diminished as the Reagan era ushered in deregulation in many areas. The passage of the Omnibus Budget Reconciliation Act caused dramatic changes affecting health care. The federal government, having failed to contain rising health care costs, shifted responsibility for the public's health and welfare back to state and local governments. Large amounts of federal funding for health research, health manpower training, and public health programs were withdrawn. Continued escalation of health care costs prompted a concentrated effort among public and private providers alike to find cost-containment measures. From all this grew the competition-versus-regulation debate (Dranove, 2000; Sultz & Young, 2006).

The 1990s were marked by "merger mania" and the move from nonprofit to for-profit hospitals (Dranove, 2000, p. 115). The Clinton health plan failed to gain support, and many hospitals downsized, laying off nurses. Managed care became more popular as a means of reducing employer premiums in the early 1990s, but by the late 1990s, as they restricted benefits, fears were raised about managed care organizations withholding necessary care and a consumer "backlash" resulted (Marquis, Rogowski, & Escarce, 2004/2005, p. 1). Many states and the federal government enacted benefit laws between 1990 and 2002, in response to these concerns (Laugesen et al., 2006, p. 1,081). During this time, many smaller managed care plans merged to gain a larger market share and provide more "efficiencies, avoid duplication, and improve services" (p. 121). We are still feeling the results of these changes, and one of the most obvious consequences deals with competition in health care.

Competition, its proponents say, offers wider consumer choice and positive incentives for cost containment and enhanced efficiency (Porter & Teisberg, 2006; Sultz & Young, 2001); that is, consumers are free to select among various health plans on the basis of cost, quality, and range of services. Competing providers must develop efficient production and distribution methods to stay in business, and consumers are more likely to use only necessary services, because of the required cost sharing that is part of the competition model.

Examples of competition are increasingly evident as more health plans, including HMOs and PPOs, vie with traditional insurance companies for subscribers. Many hospitals, too, compete aggressively for patients. Some hospitals now advertise maternity care depicting a new mother and father having a candlelight dinner in the hospital with their newborn infant in the bassinet beside them. Some surgical centers advance the "hotel guest" concept, with beautifully appointed rooms, including meals and lodging for a guest.

Although it appears that competition offers the best service for the least cost, regulation advocates have for almost 20 years argued that there are at least four problems associated with the competition model: (1) consumers often do not make proper health care choices because of limited knowledge of health services; (2) competition may discriminate against enrolling certain consumers, especially high-risk, high-cost patients, thus excluding those who may need services the most; (3) the competition model may not encourage enough teaching and research—expensive

elements of our present system; and (4) quality may be sacrificed to keep costs down.

Regulation advocates conclude that standardization and controls are needed to guarantee quality and equal access. Leaders in the field have concluded that both competition and regulation are needed (Kongstvedt, 2004; Sultz & Young, 2006). With foresight, McNerney wrote in 1980, "It is rapidly becoming apparent that what we need is a proper balance between competition and regulation with more effective links [and] regulation [should be] used as a force to keep the market honest" (p. 1,091).

HEALTH CARE REFORM POSSIBILITIES

HMOs and PPOs have become accepted methods of delivering health care in the United States in the past 30 years. During recent decades, other methods have been considered, yet not passed by legislation and adopted as law. Two plans worth further review are managed competition and universal coverage, with and without a single-payer system. The benefits and drawbacks of each are important to discuss here.

Managed Competition

The idea of managed competition, as a health care delivery method, was born from the controversy regarding competition versus regulation and was driven by the need for health care reform. **Managed competition**, it was hoped, would combine with market competition to achieve cost savings with government regulation to achieve expanded coverage. This idea, whose origin is credited to economist Alain C. Enthoven of Stanford University, has played a major part in debates on health care reform. It sought to address the two fundamental issues driving reform: cost containment and universal access to health care (Enthoven & Talbott, 2004).

Managed competition has been viewed as a market-based solution that places accountability for resolving the health care crisis with the insurance industry and with consumers. Insurers would be required to accept all applicants, without excluding those at poorer risk. At the same time, the insurers must control costs. Consumers would choose among competing health insurance plans, paying above fixed amounts paid by their employers to receive the best value. But for true competition, employers must offer real choices and a wide variety of plans. To do this, employers may form "regional exchanges" that select health plans, manage risk selection, and establish equity rules (those plans with sicker participants would be subsidized by plans with younger, healthier participants) (Sipkoff, 2003, ¶6).

Another concept of managed competition is consumer choice, and consumers must be able to access information, so that they can make responsible choices and feel that they have purchased something of value for their money. Other common features of managed competition proposals include regulations that prevent screening-out of high-risk enrollees, penalties for companies that try to achieve better risk pools, community ratings to prevent companies from setting rates by risk pool, and guaranteed coverage for all who apply. Another critical component involves management; some standardization must be established among benefit packages and an effort must be made to dismantle health care monopolies that endeavor to gain uneven market power—in other words, a more level playing field (Enthoven, 2004).

Proponents of managed competition cite many advantages. Managed competition would encourage insurance companies to compete on price and quality of services to attract enrollees. It would also offer consumers tax incentives to purchase the lowest-cost plans that meet minimum benefit requirements. Managed competition, although market driven, would be highly regulated to ensure quality and access. Cost-effectiveness and quality/outcomes information must be made available to consumers, although currently this information is not always easy to find or to decipher. Providers have not widely accepted systems of ranking on measures of quality. According to its proponents, managed competition, as a reform concept, would have the potential for reducing expenditures and improving access to health care coverage (Enthoven, 2004).

Managed competition may not be beneficial for physicians, however. A study commissioned by the AMA found that, in many regions of the United States, only a few health insurance companies dominate the market, and they exert significant market power. Because physicians are often unable to exert bargaining power against these large insurers—in 64% of areas studied, one health plan had a 50% or greater market share—they have called for antitrust action by the federal government to stem the further consolidation of health plans (AMA, 2007).

This example highlights some of the problems with the managed competition concept. Can market forces really work in the health care market? It remains fully untested anywhere in the world, and many believe that it would fail to achieve the needed cuts in the growth of health care spending. Similar models, such as HMOs and the Federal Employee Health Benefits Program, have failed to slow increasing health care costs (Sultz & Young, 2006).

Some argue that managed care networks, which enhance managed competition and enable health insurance plans to control cost and quality, also would limit consumers' choices in selecting their own providers and hospitals. Consumers would have to pay out of pocket if they chose services from outside the network. Cost-saving incentives built into managed competition networks still have the potential for reducing quality of services and denying care to enrollees. Other countries, such as New Zealand, have initiated health care reforms based on principles of managed competition, and these plans have not been well received by voters (Laugesen, 2005). Recent research found that health plan competition did not measurably improve quality (Encinosa & Hagan, 2006).

Another major criticism of managed competition is its potential failure to provide equitable and universal coverage. This was one of the key provisions of the Clinton Health Security Act (Budetti, 2004). It is possible that large employers would benefit financially under managed competition, but small businesses would find the cost burden heavy, and many individuals, such as the self-employed, would remain uninsured. A basic benefits package, critics argue, must address the special concerns affecting groups such as women and elderly adults, including coverage for long-term care, home care, mental health, dental care, and prescribed drugs. Competition among providers would be inefficient in rural areas, where there are fewer provider choices, such as county nursing agencies and isolated small-town hospitals scattered over great distances.

Although the private insurance industry and many physicians have endorsed the managed competition concept, a number of respectable groups in the United States strongly oppose it. Among the organizations that oppose managed competition and support some kind of single-payer plan are the ANA, the National League for Nursing, the APHA, Physicians for a National Health Program, and the American Association for Retired Persons (AARP). Dissatisfaction with managed competition as a reform solution has spurred a host of different proposals, all addressing cost savings and access issues.

Universal Coverage and a Single-payer System

A different approach to health care reform emphasizes universal health insurance coverage, often through a stronger role played by government. Some proponents of this system of health care promote a **single-payer system** that would replace the health insurance companies in the United States with a single, public-sector insurer that would entitle all citizens to **universal coverage** (everyone would have health insurance of some type, assuring better access to care). Efforts to accomplish this approach have been evident for many years.

Since the time of Teddy Roosevelt in 1912, national health insurance (NHI) has been debated while its proponents have sought comprehensive health care protection, in particular, for the aged, children, and the needy. Presidents Roosevelt (both Theodore and Franklin), Truman, Nixon, Carter, and Clinton have all lobbied for some form of NHI or universal health coverage (Cutler, 2004). Growing concern over the cost and accessibility of health services in the 1960s and again in the mid 1970s led to a renewed focus on NHI as a solution by which health insurance coverage could be provided for all citizens through a single-payer system or a mix of public and private insurers. Numerous attempts to pass some form of NHI resulted in piecemeal legislation that added various benefits for Social Security recipients. The Kerr-Mills bill (1960) set a precedent of public financing for elderly persons who were medically needy but not receiving public assistance. Medicare (1965) was the first compulsory NHI program in the United States. By 2001, it reached some 40 million people—only 16% of the total U.S. population (CMMS, 2007).

Most other developed countries offer some type of NHI or attempt to provide universal health coverage to their citizens. Other countries believe that health care is a fundamental right, and provide it as a social service, unlike the United States, which tends to view it as a commodity that is only available based on one's ability to pay (Woolhandler et al., 2003). The APHA has long been an advocate of universal health care, initially endorsing a single-payer system. The APHA is now endorsing more incremental extensions of current forms of health coverage along with health care delivery system reforms (Akhter, 2003).

Although many agree that insuring all Americans will improve overall national health and performance, the concept of a government-sponsored, single-payer system is controversial (Himmelstein & Woolhandler, 2003). Even though polls reveal that Americans are dissatisfied with the current health care system, they usually report being satisfied with their own arrangements for health care—and they are uncomfortable with the idea of a government-controlled health plan (Blendon et al., 2006). Single-payer plans could provide cost savings from reduced overhead and administrative costs. Compelling evidence suggests that between $320 billion to $1.1 trillion could be saved through universal health care coverage over the first decade, and the quality of the health care system would substantially improve (Broder, 2005). Once everyone has access to health care, attention can focus more on primary interventions and less on expensive tertiary care because people will either remain healthier or be treated earlier at lower costs (Broder, 2005).

What is the best way to provide universal coverage? Should health insurance still be linked to employment? How can the expense be funded? Should citizens become more responsible for their health outcomes? How can quality be ensured and costs managed? These are important questions, and many policy makers and health care economists are working on potential solutions (Heskett, 2007).

In testimony to Congress, experts from the Commonwealth Fund encouraged the design of a universal health care system that meets four criteria: improves access to care, has the potential to slow cost increases and improve efficiency, improves equity in the system, and has the potential to improve health care quality (Collins, 2007).

Some politicians propose expanding Medicare, Medicaid, and the SCHIP programs, or focusing more on prevention and individual responsibility. Other groups support a system of tax credits, employer and individual taxes, and more "transparent information about costs and quality" (International Foundation for Education, Benefits & Compensation [IFEBC], 2007, ¶10). Some states have begun to initiate legislation to extend coverage to uninsured residents. Illinois extended coverage to all children through a program called *All Kids*, and ways to extend coverage to uninsured adults are being examined. Washington extended insurance coverage for unmarried dependents to age 25 and organized a "state purchasing pool" to help small businesses find health insurance for employees (¶ 27). Maryland attempted to tax large, for-profit employers (the "Wal-Mart bill") in an effort to provide health coverage for the large uninsured population, but the attempt was overturned in the courts. Massachusetts initiated universal health coverage in 2006, and created a state agency to provide information on health insurance plans to consumers and employers. At the same time, Massachusetts requires all residents above a set income level to get insurance coverage from their employer or purchase it individually (IFEBC, 2007). Some people think that universal coverage will not be attained because of the partiality toward private insurers and the plan's lack of cost control measures and lack of adequate provisions for low-income families (Himmelstein & Woolhandler, 2007). Setting potential inadequacies aside, some states have at least begun to incrementally approach the problem of universal coverage.

Proposals to build upon the current mix of public and private insurance may be most acceptable (Tooker, 2003). This could be accomplished by expanding Medicare, Medicaid, and SCHIP coverage, along with a new group insurance program with a variety of options similar to the Federal Employees Health Benefits Program (FEHBP) and requirements for insurance coverage for all with income-related subsidies, as needed (Broder, 2005; Collins, 2007; Tooker,

2003). Currently, the federal government provides health insurance through FEHBP to over 9 million employees (e.g., members of congress, park rangers, postal workers) by contracting with a variety of insurers who must agree to provide coverage to everyone at the same premium rate (Cutler, 2004). Most agree that a combination of higher taxes and employer/employee fees could subsidize a public–private plan that could cover all Americans (Cutler, 2004; Kahn & Pollack, 2001).

How much will universal coverage cost? It depends upon which type of plan is chosen, but most agree it will not come cheaply. One economist projected costs of coverage for the current uninsured population to run about $75 billion annually. However, by the end of 10 years, net savings would be between $125 billion and $182 billion annually (Broder, 2005). Others have projected $200 billion cost savings annually by providing universal health coverage and "eliminating the high overhead and profits of the private, investor-owned insurance industry and reducing spending for marketing and other satellite services" (Woolhandler, et al., 2003, p. 798).

Even if everyone receives health insurance, how can quality be assured? Some believe that the overall performance of the health care system will improve as everyone gains access to care. However, others propose "quality-based bonus payments" as an incentive (Cutler, 2004, p. 115). Still others think that a system providing incentives to *both* providers and patients to use services efficiently and effectively will produce the best results (Collins, 2007). Providing information to consumers is another component of quality assurance, and this is sorely lacking. But, information is becoming more readily available. For instance, the Leapfrog Group (2007) promotes *transparency* through surveys of standard measurements and practices to enable comparisons, and reimbursement incentives to encourage quality and efficiency. Scores for local hospitals can be reviewed at the Leapfrog website (see Internet Resources at the end of this chapter). The quality of insurance plans, measured by the Health Plan Employer Data and Information Set (HEDIS), includes information on patient satisfaction, data on risk factor control, and procedures such as prescribing beta (β)-blockers after heart attacks, and is monitored by the National Committee for Quality Assurance (NCQA). Other systems of quality measurement, like health outcomes, the process of care, and adherence to standardized guidelines, among other things, are still needed (Cutler, 2004).

Health Care Reform: Making the Change

The cry for health care reform is not new. Perkins examined the work of the 1927 to 1932 Committee on the Costs of Medical Care. More than 75 years ago, the committee defined *costs* as the major problem and *business models of organization* as the major solution (Perkins, 1998). Today, consumers and professionals agree that health care reform is needed in the United States. The disagreement lies in the form that it should take and the speed at which it should be completed. At issue is a fundamental conflict in values between advocates of the managed competition model and advocates of the universal coverage or single-payer plan. On the one hand are those who strongly value the competition model, which ensures a free market, individualism, and the right to choose the type of health care desired. On the other hand are those who propose a more regulated, statutory model.

Proponents of universal coverage argue that more comprehensive benefits are needed to include the unemployed and those who are physically or economically disadvantaged and cannot afford individual health care coverage. Furthermore, they argue that universal coverage emphasizes prevention and primary health care as key factors in reducing long-range health care costs and, more importantly, in ensuring improved levels of health for the public (Collins, 2007). *Nursing's Agenda for Health Care Reform* (American Nurses Association [ANA], 2002) supports this emphasis by promoting nurses as primary providers of health care. The ANA's nursing's agenda proposes a *core of care* that involves restructuring of the health care system, a federally defined standard package of essential health care services, planned change to anticipate the needs of a population with changing demographics, steps to decrease costs, insurance reform, case management, assured access to health care for all, and establishment of public/private sector review. This plan is enthusiastically endorsed by more than 60 nursing organizations and four non-nursing organizations.

Designers of health reform have faced a difficult challenge in reconciling these conflicting views. As a result, elements of both models have been used to shape an improved system. Reform proposals include an incremental plan that allows for a flexible transition and opportunities for states to experiment with both approaches. Sultz and Young (2006) and Collins (2007) point out the importance of separating the task of financing (how insurance funds are collected) from that of disbursement (how providers receive payment) and implementation (how to put a plan in place). Financing might be tried through an income-based premium that would go into a publicly administered health insurance fund. The methods of collection and administration can then be decided. Japan and Germany have used a payroll-collection method for years to successfully finance their health care systems. Supplemental financing (to adjust for low-income or no-income households) might come from an extra tax on those with moderate to high incomes or from a tax on products that are known to contribute directly to health care costs, such as alcohol and tobacco. Some have even proposed a tax on fat in foods as a means of raising revenues while impacting the problem of obesity (Chouinard, Davis, LaFrance, & Perloff, 2007).

Disbursement of health insurance funds could occur in at least two ways. First, a strictly federal program could enroll all Americans who are not privately insured and disburse funds through a program similar to Medicare or the Federal Employees Health Benefits Plan, as noted earlier. A second option could be to disburse capitation funds from the federal government to the states for payment to providers. In some cases, state funds could supplement federal disbursement. Forms of either the single-payer or the managed competition models could be tried to accomplish disbursement, allowing states to adjust for local preferences and existing delivery systems (Cutler, 2004; Sultz & Young, 2006).

Another aspect of health care reform that has been considered is a global budget. In this system, a single, nationwide health budget would help to control certain aspects of national health spending. Much like the Oregon Health Plan (mentioned earlier), funding might come from income-based premiums plus supplemental sources (Loewy & Loewy, 2001). The amount of money in this budget would help to determine the size of disbursements to federal programs (e.g., Medicare) and to the states. States could choose to spend more on health care out of their own resources, or to limit the provision of services.

A standard set of benefits, set by law and enjoyed by the entire population, regardless of age, health, income, and employment status, is an important health care reform element. Many countries have successfully implemented such a package under a plan called a *statutory model*. Various versions of this model have worked well in Austria, France, Belgium, Japan, Germany, Israel, Poland, the Netherlands, and Switzerland. In this model, health insurance falls under the rubric of social security, and is funded through government-mandated payroll premiums or taxes. Payment is made to private-sector health insurers, from a fund called a *sickness fund* in some countries (Loewy & Loewy, 2001). Individuals select among nationwide plans and choose their doctor and hospital, and can switch plans when desired. This element of consumer choice is thought to encourage the sickness funds to respond to consumer preferences and improve efficiency in the health care system (van de Ven et al., 2007). Reimbursement for services is made directly by insurers to providers. In Germany, a disease management program was added to the statutory health insurance plan in the 1990s; its purpose is to both promote competition and increase the quality of care (Stock, Redaelli, & Lauterbach, 2007). This statutory model eliminates the need for separate programs such as Medicaid and Medicare. It also provides uniform and comprehensive benefits (Harrington & Estes, 2004; Loewy & Loewy, 2001). See Display 6.3 for a comparison of health systems in four developed countries.

Other issues to be addressed in health reform include making the system more accountable, eliminating adverse risk-selection, and providing informed choices to consumers. Although reform is under way, the need continues for strong advocates of universal access and cost containment. Furthermore, health reform proposals must be encouraged to focus on the central question: Do they fund the promotion of health and prevention of illness or simply pay for the diagnosis and treatment of those who are already ill? World Bank evaluations show that public health interventions have been found to be consistently more cost-effective than medical services, yet health reform proposals have often paid minimal attention to this critical issue. In addition, "the current emphasis on managing medical care for cost containment disregards the social and environmental genesis of many health problems" (McIntosh, 2002, p. 85). Community health nurses can play an influential role in emphasizing health promotion services as being central to future health reform efforts through political involvement and policy development.

EFFECTS OF HEALTH ECONOMICS ON COMMUNITY HEALTH PRACTICE

Health economics has significantly affected community health and community health practice by advancing disincentives for efficient use of resources, incentives for illness care, and conflicts with public health values.

DISPLAY 6.3   HOW FOUR OTHER COUNTRIES APPROACH UNIVERSAL HEALTH CARE

Canada

- Publicly financed, provincially run insurance plans that cover *all* residents (70% from national and provincial funds)
  - Covers all "medically necessary" physician and hospital care
  - Nonprofit administration of health plans
  - Comprehensive coverage, portability between provinces, not dependent on employment, addresses universality and accessibility
- Has intermittent problems and some complaints of long wait times, but access, quality, and satisfaction is generally high

France (ranked first by the WHO in 2000 when the French reached 100% coverage)

- Public and private mix (funding from general revenues for social insurance and patient cost sharing)
  - Covers ambulatory and hospital care, medications, dental and vision, nursing home, thermal spa cures, and some other alternative therapies
  - Compulsory universal coverage
- Higher health status indicators, consumer satisfaction, more health care resources

Germany

- German Statutory Health Insurance since 1883 (93% covered by national health insurance, remainder by private insurance; between 7% and 10% have both)
  - Mandatory contributions by employers and employees (work-based social insurance and patient cost sharing)
  - Choice of physician, hospital, long-term care facility; medication and dental
- Portability of coverage, legally set caps or fixed budgets, modest co-payments and no deductibles

Great Britain (United Kingdom)

- National Health Service since World War II (funded from general revenues)
  - Well-designed system, but chronically underfunded

- Tax-based, free at point of service (covers ambulatory care, hospital, medications, long-term care, vision)
- Choice of physician, generally short wait times for appointments, but longer waiting lists for elective referrals to specialists (average of 46 days)
- Private care is available (11.5% have this), and patients with this are seen more quickly and have more luxurious accommodations; new additions include registered nurse call-in service, web-based information, and integrated services (social/community-based)

All Four Nations

- Spend substantially lower percentage than the United States for health expenditures
- Pay physicians less and have fewer specialized and high-tech services
- Try to cap health spending (budget caps, spending targets, linking health cost increases to wage increases, utilize waiting lists, offer less widely diffused technology)
- Are working to improve integration of care (networks of care, comprehensive integrated community-based care, better managed care)
- Have interest in analytic tools (evidence-based medicine, report cards, cost-effectiveness analysis)
- Report high levels of satisfaction with their systems (but they are not without some criticism)
- Have strong central government leadership (states, provinces, and regional bodies consult on policy making and administrative decisions)

Adapted from Brown, L.D. (2003). Comparing health systems in four countries: Lessons for the United States. *American Journal of Public Health, 93*(1), 52–56.

Disincentives for Efficient Use of Resources

All of the system structures that directly or indirectly promote cost escalation and prevent cost containment contribute to disincentives for efficient use of resources. For example, retrospective financial reimbursement, with its lack of setting limits, encourages spending on nonessential tests and treatments and drives up costs. Tax-deductible employer contributions for health care coverage and nontaxable employee health benefits encourage unnecessary use of services and result in cost increases. Lack of cost sharing by consumers and of financial risk for decisions made by providers may create further disincentives to keep costs down (Cutler, 2004; Dranove, 2000).

Community health has been affected in several ways. Abuse of resources in some parts of the system leads to depletion in other areas. The trend of diminished federal and state allocations has had profound effects on community and public health programs, and severe budget cuts have affected even basic community health services. Competition from the private sector in home care and other community services, such as health education programs, has forced traditional public health agencies to reexamine their traditional programs and seek new avenues for the provision of services, along with new revenue sources (Institute of Medicine, 2002). Costs indirectly affect even appropriate use of nursing personnel in community health. Failing to recognize the differences in skill levels of community health nurses and their less-prepared counterparts, public health departments and agencies often have hired persons who are underqualified to give the high-caliber and comprehensive care required. Finally, the advent of prospective payment and limits on lengths of stay have encouraged early hospital discharge, resulting in more acutely ill people needing home care services. The immediate effect was an increase in the demand for highly skilled and more expensive home care services, which required changes in provision patterns of community health care. As acute care nursing shortages have intensified and salaries have increased, the number of open, unfilled PHN positions has mounted (Chiha & Link, 2003). The long-range effects of this phenomenon on family stress and caregiver health, on community health care reimbursement, and on the nature and structure of community health services, including the role of the community health nurse, have yet to be determined.

Incentives for Illness Care

The traditional American health care system tends to promote illness, because health care providers have primarily been rewarded for treating problems, not for preventing them. Hospitals derive more income when their beds are full of sick or injured people. Health insurance plans compete, not by lowering costs or increasing quality, but by "avoiding the sick"—leaving many without access to necessary health care (Woolhandler et al., 2003, p. 798).

The bulk of most reimbursable health services centers on treating illness or disability in hospitals, nursing homes, and ambulatory care facilities, using physicians or skilled nursing care in the home (home health services)—situations in which the individual must play the role of patient. Our disease-focused system of health care is thought by many to be the basic problem (Adams, 2006). It rewards disease by paying doctors who diagnose, treat, and refer ill patients. It does not pay them for keeping their patients healthy. Most preventive care is woefully inadequate and largely overlooked by both practitioners and patients alike: Remember, fewer than half of all U.S. adults receive recommended health screening tests annually (Schoen et al., 2006). Health promotion nursing activities, such as comprehensive prenatal, maternal, and infant care; health education; childhood immunizations; and home services to enable the elderly to live independently have not always been consistently covered by most insurers.

A system that financially supports illness care affects community health practice in several ways. The number and severity of health problems in a community increase when individuals postpone care because they cannot afford visits to the doctor or clinic. It has been more difficult to encourage community clients to assume responsibility for their own health and to engage in self-care, prevention, and active health promotion. Furthermore, such illness-oriented incentives create a basic societal valuing of illness care that, conversely, devalues wellness care. Health promotion and disease prevention efforts become second-ranked priorities in the competition for scarce resources. In communities where a greater proportion of community health practice is spent in the treatment of disorders and rehabilitation, resources are more limited for prevention and health promotion.

Prepayment methods and the growth of managed care have been positive moves in the direction of a more wellness-oriented financial incentive structure. An HMO has the incentive to offer preventive and health-promoting services, such as early detection and treatment of symptoms, regular physical examinations, and health teaching, because the HMO loses money when it must pay out for expensive tertiary care. Health care reform proposals show promise of greater recognition of the cost-saving value of prevention efforts. In the Michael Moore documentary, *Sicko*, British physicians reveal that they are awarded "bonuses" for encouraging healthy behaviors (e.g., getting patients to stop smoking) and for successful management of diseases (e.g., hypertensive patients who remain on medications to control blood pressure and cholesterol levels). Some in the United States have proposed a paradigm shift to "health consultants" or "healers" who "only get paid when you stay healthy, not when you are sick," and a change from managed care to *life maintenance organizations* (LMOs) that provide life insurance and advise on needed health care—thus, having a true incentive to keep you in good health because they will be paying your life insurance claim if your life is shortened by an avoidable illness (Adams, 2006, ¶4; Hanson, 1994). The focus of the system would be on proper nutrition, exercise, health education, and prescription drugs to keep people healthy, not just treating disease.

Managed care has evolved but remains a "system of business strategies employed to make health care services efficient and cost-effective," with the highest priority to maximize market principles (Drevdahl, 2002, p. 163). This makes individual rights significant, whereas societal obligations are pushed to the background. "Freedom of choice and action take precedence over issues of equality and equity" (p. 163). The managed care organizations (MCOs) have business-focused goals that are given more consideration than is the issue of equal access to health care.

Managed Care and Public Health Values

Initially, MCOs focused on event-driven cost avoidance. Strategies included decreasing inpatient days, decreasing specialty physician use, using physician extenders, and implementing provider discounting. This evolved into a second stage, in which the principal objective was to control resource intensity and improve the delivery process. Strategies used to meet this objective included capitation of specialist costs, controls on units of service, patient-focused redesign, clinical pathways, and total quality management.

> The emphasis, however, is now shifting to a focus on community-based health status improvement that goes beyond just measuring utilization of care or mortality outcomes. This focus calls for new strategies, such as community health assessments, identification of high-risk individuals, targeted interventions, case management, and management of illness episodes across the continuum. (Weiss, 1997, p. 28)

Some believe that community health assessments could become standard quality tools for MCOs (Porche, 2004; Weiss, 1997). Community assessments establish the baseline health status of a community and measure changes in the health of the community over time. Community health assessments must include source information that is both primary (health status assessment surveys, focus groups, and satisfaction surveys) and secondary (data collected by public health agencies and state agencies, such as birth rates, mortality rates, and incidence of communicable diseases in the community) (see Chapter 15).

Improving the health status of a community mandates that the MCO—the organization providing health care services through managed care agencies, such as an HMO or PPO—be actively involved in accurately assessing the community's health status and the major issues facing the community. This involves "informing health care consumers of how to care for themselves, and empowering them to do so, and developing a community action plan that fosters collaboration among organizations and focuses on preventive service strategies" (Weiss, 1997, p. 29). Are these not the proposals that public health advocates have been making for more than a century?

In 2002, Drevdahl expressed concerns regarding the paradoxical missions of public health and managed care. One relies on partnerships for fostering health care equity and creating healthy communities and populations as it embraces a social justice mission, whereas the other "falls more along the line of market justice" (p. 163). Perhaps the incentive to keep costs down will be the motivation needed to work with clients at the primary prevention level of care. Although public health proponents have advocated preventive care as the best care for the individual, family, and community as long as the goal of community health is reached, the motivating factor becomes insignificant. If the community health approach is embraced by MCOs, the conflict with public health can be minimized and perhaps eliminated.

Competition in health care is a reality with which community health practice must cope. Although competition offers several benefits, it poses some dilemmas for community health that may be difficult to resolve. Values underlying the competition model can be in direct conflict with several basic public health values (Drevdahl, 2002; Scutchfield & Keck, 2003). Competition for the healthier and younger enrollee, for example, encourages MCOs to develop market strategies that entice the client to choose one plan over another. This is a win–lose situation for the MCO: one MCO wins while another loses. Public health, however, operates on the basis of collaboration and cooperation.

Competition among MCOs serves a selected market partly determined by those who are able to purchase products or services. Public health is committed to serving all persons in need, regardless of ability to pay. Traditionally, the competition model has focused on individuals and has been oriented to the present. Public health is concerned with aggregates and is future oriented, emphasizing prevention. Competition establishes relatively fixed limits for service, whereas public health must remain flexible if it is to respond to the health needs of the entire population. These dramatic differences between MCOs and public health are beginning to blur and, out of necessity, will continue to be less adversarial and more collegial. By shifting their focus to community health as a systems outcome, MCOs can create several positive changes, including a safe environment, wholesome nutrition, healthy lifestyle, adequate education, sufficient income, meaningful spirituality, challenging work, recreation, and functional families (Meador & Linnan, 2006; Weiss, 1997).

If enrollees in health insurance programs like Medicare, Medicaid, or other MCOs become empowered to assume responsibility for their own self-care and well-being, a cooperative and collaborative relationship can be achieved between MCOs and public health. A nurse-directed diabetes management program at a county public health clinic in Los Angeles County reflects the potential benefits of public health services for clients of MCOs and other private health care plans. PHNs were able to significantly reduce the numbers of urgent care and ER visits, along with hospitalizations, for diabetic patients from a minority population (Davidson, Ansari, & Karlan, 2007). Working together, better health can be achieved for large numbers of patients.

Along with philosophical differences, other constraints exist, such as civil service restrictions and political influences, under which most public health agencies must operate and that make it difficult for them to compete. Likewise, MCOs have stockholders, boards of directors, employees, and state and federal regulations that they must satisfy. Public health agencies must remain committed to providing the health promotion and disease prevention services that are their public trust. This may become the commitment of MCOs as they see the cost savings and health benefits of disease prevention. Yet, some aspects of competition seem necessary if both forms of health care delivery are to stay in business. Exclusion from health care competition, freedom from unreasonable constraints, and dependable financial support are needed to maintain the organizational viability of many public health agencies. Public health systems can incorporate marketing principles common to MCOs as a means of improving utilization and visibility (Lega, 2006). Competition also may stimulate new and innovative community health services and the introduction of new roles and revenue sources for traditional public health agencies. The evolution of the reform of health care implementation may see developing public and private health care partnerships, with MCOs contracting with public health agencies for certain services and MCOs more effectively expanding the reach of public health agencies into the suburbs or rural areas. Reform will need to continue to address issues affecting the delivery of public health services.

IMPLICATIONS FOR COMMUNITY HEALTH NURSING

The structure and functions of the health care delivery system, as well as particular legislative acts, have had a significant impact on community health nursing. Community health nurses have had to adapt to a constantly changing system. They have developed innovative modes of service delivery, such as community-based nursing centers for health education, counseling, and screening of low-income populations. They have learned to practice in a variety of settings extending beyond homes, worksites, schools, churches, clinics, and voluntary agencies. They have acquired skills in teamwork, leadership, and political activism. They have recognized the importance of outcomes research to document the value of nursing interventions with at-risk populations.

At the national, state, and local level, community health nursing has important ties to both private and public health agencies. Either type of organization may employ community and public health nurses. When serving in the public sector, they often provide consultation, serve on boards, volunteer their services, or collaborate with private-sector health organizations to ensure quality and access of care to the broader community. Examples include joint efforts to promote certain types of health legislation and collaboration to produce and disseminate health education materials targeting specific populations (Porche, 2004). Sometimes, community health nursing services operate within a single organization that combines public- and private-sector organization and funding. An example is the Metropolitan Visiting Nurse Association of Minneapolis, Minnesota, which is a combined public–private agency supported by taxes and voluntary funds.

Community health nurses also have many opportunities to serve in international health. Some work with the WHO, PAHO, or other agencies to assist in direct care projects such as famine relief, immunization efforts, or nutritional screening and education programs (see Chapter 16). Other nurses serve as health planners, assist with policy development, conduct collaborative needs assessment projects and research efforts, or engage in program development.

Summary

Many factors and events have influenced the current structure, function, and financing of community health services. Understanding this background gives the community health nurse a stronger base for planning for the health of the population under her care.

Historically, health care has progressed unevenly, marked by numerous influences. Primitive practices of early centuries were replaced with more advanced sanitary measures by the Greeks and Romans. The Middle Ages saw a serious health decline in Europe, with raging epidemics leading to extensive 19th-century reform efforts in England and, later, in the United States.

Organized health care in the United States developed slowly. Public health problems, such as the need for isolation of persons with communicable diseases and control of environmental pollution, prompted the gradual development of official interventions. For example, quarantines to control the spread of communicable disease were imposed in the late 1700s. Sanitary reform was pursued more vigorously during the 1800s. Local and then state health departments were formed starting in the late 1700s. By the early 1900s, the federal government had assumed a more active role in public health, with a proliferation of health, education, and welfare services.

For years, efforts to address community health needs have been made by public agencies and private individuals. These two arms of service were not well coordinated in the past. Only gradually and recently have they begun to work together to form an emerging health care system.

The public arm of health services includes all government, tax-supported health agencies and occurs at four levels: local, state, national, and international. Each level deals with the health needs of the population encompassed within its boundaries. Each level has a different structure and set of functions. Public health services include three core public health functions: assessment, policy development, and assurance.

Private health services are the unofficial arm of the community health system. They include voluntary nonprofit agencies as well as privately owned (proprietary) and for-profit agencies. Their financial support comes from voluntary contributions, bequests, or fees. Private health organizations often supplement and complement the work of official agencies.

The delivery and financing of community health services has been significantly affected by various legislative acts. These acts have prompted such innovations as health insurance and assistance for the poor, the elderly, and the disabled; money to train health personnel and conduct health research; standards for health planning and delivery; health protection for workers on the job; and the financing of health services.

Health care economics studies the production, distribution, and consumption of health care goods and services to maximize the use of scarce resources to benefit the most people. This science underlies the financing of the health care system. It is influenced by microeconomics as well as macroeconomics.

Health care is funded through public and private sources, which fall into three categories: third-party payers, direct consumer payment, and private support. Health care services have been reimbursed either retrospectively, typical of FFS plans, or prospectively, typical of most HMOs.

Several trends and issues have influenced community health care financing and delivery and are important in understanding health care economics and helping to improve community health. They include cost control, financial access, managed care, health care rationing, competition and regulation, managed competition, universal coverage, a single-payer system, and health care reform.

The changing nature of health care financing has adversely affected community health and its practice in three important ways: (1) retrospective payment without limiting costs, tax-deductible employer contributions for health care coverage and nontaxable employee health benefits, together with a lack of consumer involvement in cost sharing, have created disincentives for efficient use of resources; (2) because the health care system traditionally has reimbursed only for treatment of the ill or disabled, with no reward for health promotion and prevention efforts, it has promoted incentives to focus only on illness care; and (3) the competition model, which has long driven up health care costs and eliminated many from being able to afford health care services, has generated a conflict with the basic public health values of health promotion and disease prevention for all persons. Health care reforms have been proposed, but the United States remains the only industrialized nation without some type of universal health coverage. We also rank significantly lower than most other developed countries on health indicators, such as infant mortality and life expectancy.

Public health nurses can lead the effort in making health care more accessible to all citizens and encourage policies and practices that promote health, rather than reward illness. ∎

ACTIVITIES TO PROMOTE CRITICAL THINKING

1. Interview someone at your local health department. How do the services offered compare with those listed in this chapter? How do PHNs in this agency incorporate the core public health functions?

2. Make an onsite visit to your state health department or visit its website. Compare its functions with the core public health functions described in this chapter. Identify areas where improvement may be needed.

3. Conduct an interview onsite with someone at a private health agency, voluntary agency, or community-based

non-governmental organization (or NGO). Compare the agency's functions with those listed in this chapter for private health agencies. Describe how this agency works collaboratively with public health agencies and other community organizations. What is the role of the nurse in this agency? How does the role compare to PHNs in the local public health agency?

4. Look up various international health agencies online. Explore websites that discuss current international health care issues. What topics are of current concern? For example, are new epidemics or emerging strains of a virus being highlighted? What could (or should) a community health nurse in your local community do with this information?

5. With your classmates, debate the pros and cons of a strong federal role in health care provision, as opposed to decentralized (state and local) control.

6. Interview two consumers about their perception of the problems and strengths of our health care system. Select people who represent distinctly different age groups and life situations, such as a single 25-year-old mother of three children making minimum wage and a 75-year-old widower.

7. Form two teams and debate the advantages and disadvantages of managed competition as opposed to mandatory universal coverage. What are the advantages and disadvantages of a single-payer system? Is some form of national health insurance feasible in the United States? What would be the most efficient way of assuring universal coverage?

8. Locate recent articles and legislation on health care reform, strengths and weakness of the public health system, and the uninsured population. What are the most common themes on each issue? What most surprised you about your results?

9. Talk with your classmates and other students at your college or university about their access to health care and if they have some type of health insurance. Does your campus have a student health center? What services are offered there? What are the average costs to students?

References

Aaron, H.J. (2005). *Healthcare rationing: what it means.* Brookings Policy Brief Series, No. 148. Retrieved August 11, 2008 from http://www.brookings.edu/papers/2005/12useconomics_aaron.aspx?rssid=aaronh.

Abrams, S.E. (2004). From function to competency in public health nursing, 1931 to 2003. *Public Health Nursing, 21*(5), 507–510.

Adams, M. (2006). Health care economics: Diseases are too profitable to prevent or cure. *News Target.* Retrieved July 7, 2008 from http://www.newstarget.com/z019475.html.

Aday, L.A. (Ed.). (2005). *Reinventing public health: Policies and practices for a healthy nation.* San Francisco, CA: Jossey-Bass.

Administration for Children & Families. U.S. Department of Health & Human Services. (2008). *Office of Family Assistance (OFA): What is the Temporary Assistance for Needy Families (TANF) program?* Retrieved August 9, 2008 from http://www.acf.hhs.gov/opa/fact_sheets/tanf_factsheet.html.

AED.com. (2006). *Layperson-operated automatic defibrillators shown to save lives.* Retrieved July 7, 2008 from http://www.aed.com/survivor/story_detail.cfm?key=196.

Akhter, M. (2003). APHA policies on universal health care: Health for a few or health for all? *American Journal of Public Health, 93*(1), 99–101.

American Medical Association (AMA). (2007). *Competition in health insurance: A comprehensive study of U.S. markets: 2007 update.* Retrieved July 7, 2008 from http://www.ama-assn.org/ama1/pub/upload/mm/368/compstudy_52006.pdf.

American Nurses Association. (2002). *Nursing's agenda for health care reform.* Retrieved July 7, 2008 from http://nursingworld.org/readingroom/magenda.htm.

Anderson, G., & Hussey, P.S. (2001). Comparing health system performance in OECD countries. *Health Affairs, 20*(3), 219–232.

Anderson, G., Hussey, P.S., Frogner, B., & Waters, H. (2005). Health pending in the United States and the rest of the industrialized world. *Health Affairs, 24*(4), 903–914.

Associated Press, The. (April 23 2004). Crisis threatens landmark medical center: Five top administrators have been fired for ignoring problems. *MSNBC.com.* Retrieved July 7, 2008 from http://www.msnbc.msn.com/id/4780341/.

Baker, L.C., Phillips, K., Haas, J., et al. (2004). The effect of area HMO market share on cancer screening. *Health Services Research, 39*(6 Pt. 1), 1751–1772.

Barry, M.A., Centra, L., Pratt, Ed., et al. (1998). *Where do the dollars go? Measuring local public health expenditures.* Retrieved July 7, 2008 from http://www.phf.org/Reports/Expend1/exec_summ.htm.

Barton, P.L. (2003). *Understanding the U.S. health service system,* 2nd ed. Chicago: Health Administration Press.

Blendon, R., Brodie, M., Benson, J., et al. (2006). Americans' views of health care costs, access, and quality. *Millbank Quarterly, 84*(4), 623–657.

Brink, S. (2002). Living on the edge. *U.S. News & World Report, 133*(14), 58–64.

Broder, D. (2005). An urgent case for fixing health care. *The Washington Post,* B07.

Brookings Institution. (2007). *Government's 50 greatest endeavors.* Retrieved July 7, 2008 from http://www.brookings.edu/gs/cps/research/projects/50ge/endeavors/healthcare.htm.

Brown, L. (2003). Comparing health systems in four countries: Lessons for the United States. *American Journal of Public Health, 93*(1), 52–56.

Budetti, P.P. (2004). Ten years after the Health Security Act failure: Subsequent developments and persistent problems. *Journal of the American Medical Association, 292*(16), 2000–2006.

Bureau of Labor Statistics. (2007). *Definitions of health insurance terms.* Retrieved July 7, 2008 from http://www.bls.gov/ncs/ebs/sp/healthterms.pdf.

California Healthcare Foundation. (2007). *Reference guide, coverage types: Point-of-service plan (POS).* Retrieved July 7, 2008 from http://www.healthcoverageguide.org/referenceguide/index.cfm?itemID=21391.

Center on Budget & Policy Priorities. (2006). *Medicaid costs are growing more slowly than costs for Medicare or private insurance.* Retrieved July 7, 2008 from http://www.cbpp.org/11-13-06health.htm.

Centers for Disease Control & Prevention (CDC). (1991). Health objectives for the nation consensus set of health status indicators for the general assessment of community health status: United States. *Morbidity & Mortality Weekly Report, 40*(27), 449–451.

Centers for Disease Control & Prevention (CDC). (2002). *Fact sheet: Public health infrastructure.* Retrieved July 7, 2008 from http://www.cdc.gov/od/oc/media/pressrel/fs020514.htm.

Centers for Disease Control & Prevention (CDC). (2006). *CDC timeline.* Retrieved July 7, 2008 from http://www.cdc.gov/od/oc/media/timeline.htm.

Centers for Disease Control & Prevention (CDC). (2007). *Estimates of health care-related infections.* Retrieved August 12, 2008 from http://www.cdc.gov/ncidod/dhqp/hai.html.

Centers for Disease Control & Prevention (CDC). (2008). *Public health preparedness: mobilizing state by state. Executive summary.* Retrieved August 13, 2008 from http://emergency.cdc.gov/publications/feb08phprep/executivesummary.asp.

Centers for Medicare & Medicaid Services. (1985). *Legislative summaries: Consolidated Omnibus Budget Reconciliation Act of 1985.* Retrieved July 7, 2008 from http://www.cms.hhs.gov/RelevantLaws/LS/ItemDetail.asp?ItemID=CMS029310.

Centers for Medicare & Medicaid Services. (2005). *Medicaid program: General information.* Retrieved July 7, 2008 from http://www.cms.hhs.gov/MedicaidGenInfo/03_Technical Summary.asp#TopOfPage.

Centers for Medicare & Medicaid Services. (2006). *Medicare trustees report.* Retrieved July 7, 2008 from http://www.cms.hhs.gov/apps/media/press/release.asp?Counter=1846.

Centers for Medicare & Medicaid Services. (2007). *Medicare enrollment: All beneficiaries: As of July 2005.* Retrieved July 7, 2008 from http://www.cms.hhs.gov/MedicareEnRpts/Downloads/05All.pdf.

Chang, C.F., Price, S.A., & Pfoutz, S.K. (2001). *Economics and nursing: Critical professional issues.* Philadelphia, PA: F.A. Davis Co.

Chiha, Y., & Link, C. (2003). The shortage of registered nurses and some new estimates of the effects of wages on registered nurses labor supply: A look at the past and a preview of the 21st century. *Health Policy, 64*(3), 349–375.

Chouinard, H., Davis, D., LaFrance, J., & Perloff, J. (2007). Fat taxes: Big money for small change. *Forum for Health Economics & Policy, 10*(2), Article 2. Retrieved July 7, 2008 from http://www.bepress.com/fhep/10/2/2/.

Cockayne, E. (2007). *Hubbub, filth, noise & stench in England 1600-1770.* New Haven, CT: Yale University Press.

Collins, S. (2007). Congressional testimony: Universal health insurance: Why it is essential to a high performing health system and why design matters. *The Commonwealth Fund.* Retrieved July 7, 2008 from http://www.commonwealthfund.org/publications/publications_show.htm?doc_id=506778#areaCitation.

Collins, S., Davis, K., Schoen, C., et al. (2006). Health coverage for aging baby boomers: Findings from the Commonwealth Fund survey of older adults. *The Commonwealth Fund,* Pub. No. 884.

Collins, S., Schoen, C., Kriss, J., et al. (August 8 2007). Rite of passage? Why young adults become uninsured and how new policies can help. *The Commonwealth Fund.* Retrieved July 7, 2008 from http://www.commonwealthfund.org/publications/publications_show.htm?doc_id-=514761.

Colliver, V. (September 15 2005). Health plans dwindle in U.S.: Number of firms offering insurance drops as costs rise. *San Francisco Chronicle.* Retrieved July 7, 2008 from http://sfgate.com/cgi-bin/article.cgi?file=/c/a/2005/09/15/BUG8OENLE61.DTL&type=printable.

Colliver, V. (July 10 2007). We spend far more, but our health care is falling behind. *San Francisco Chronicle.* Retrieved July 7, 2008 from http://sfgate.com/cgi-bin/article.cgi?file=/c/a/2007/07/10/MNGNUQTQJB1.DTL&type=printable.

Commonwealth Fund Commission on a High Performance Health System. (2006). *Why not the best? Results from a national scorecard on U.S. health system performance.* Retrieved July 7, 2008 from http://www.commonwealthfund.org/publications/publications_show.htm?doc_id=401577.

Congressional Budget Office. (2005). *High-cost Medicare beneficiaries.* Retrieved July 7, 2008 from http://www.cbo.gov/ftpdoc.cfm?index=6332&type=0.

Congresspedia. (2007). *State Children's Health Insurance Plan (SCHIP) U.S.* Retrieved July 7, 2008 from http://www.source-watch.org/index.php?title=State_Children's_Health_Insurance_Plan#Background.

Cowan, T. (October 5 2006). Poor U.S. scores in heath care don't measure Nobels and innovation. *The New York Times.* Retrieved July 7, 2008 from http://www.nytimes.com/2006/10/05/business/05scene.html?ex=1317700800&en=5889b4819eaf787a&ei=5090&partner=rssuserland&emc=rss.

Cunningham, P.J., & May, J.H. (March 2006). A growing hole in the safety net: Physician charity care declines again. *Center for Studying Health System Change.* Tracking Report, No. 13.

Cutler, D.M. (2004). *Your money or your life: Strong medicine for America's health care system.* New York: Oxford University Press.

Cylus, J., & Anderson, G. (2006). *Multinational comparisons of health systems data, 2006.* The Commonwealth Fund. Retrieved July 7, 2008 from http://www.commonwealthfund.org/usr_doc/Shea_hltsysperformanceselectednations_chartpack.pdf?section=4039.

Davidson, M., Ansari, A., & Karlan, V. (2007). Effect of a nurse-directed diabetes disease management program on urgent care/emergency room visits and hospitalizations in a minority population. *Diabetes Care, 30*(2), 224–227.

Davis, K. (2003). The costs and consequences of being uninsured. *Medical Care Research and Review, 60*(2), S89–S99.

Davis, K., Schoen, C., Schoenbaum, S., et al. (May 15, 2007). Mirror, mirror on the wall: An international update on the comparative performance of American health care. *The Commonwealth Fund,* Vol. 59. Retrieved July 7, 2008 from http://www.commonwealthfund.org/publications/publications_show_htm?doc_id=482678#areaCitation.

Donley, R., Flaherty, M.J., Sarsfield, E., et al. (2002). What does the Nurse Reinvestment Act mean to you? *Online Journal of Issues in Nursing, 8*(1) [manuscript 5]. Retrieved July 7, 2008 from http://www.nursingworld.org/ojin/topic14/tpc14_5.htm.

Dow, W.H., Harris, D.M., & Liu, Z. (2006). Differential effectiveness in patient protection laws: What are the causes? An example from the drive-through delivery laws. *Journal of Health Politics, Policy & Law, 31*(6), 1107–1127.

Dowling, W.L. (1979). Prospective rate setting: Concept and practice. *Topics in Health Care Financing, 3*(2), 35–42.

Dranove, D. (2000). *The economic evolution of American health care: From Marcus Welby to managed care.* Princeton, NJ: Princeton University Press.

Dranove, D. (2003). *What's your life worth? Health care rationing: Who lives, who dies, who decides.* Upper Saddle River, NJ: Financial Times Prentice-Hall.

Drevdahl, D. (2002). Social justice or market justice? The paradoxes of public health partnerships with managed care. *Public Health Nursing, 19*(3), 161–169.

Duffy, J. (1990). *The sanitarians: A history of American public health.* Urbana, IL: University of Illinois Press.

Duffy, R., Chen, D., & Sampson, N. (1998). History of federal legislation in health professions educational assistance in dental public health, 1956–1997. *Journal of Public Health Dentistry, 58*(S1), 84–89.

Elliott, V.S. (October 28 2002). Public health funding: Feds giveth but the states taketh away. *American Medical News.* Retrieved July 7, 2008 from http://www.ama-assn.org/amednews/2002/10/28/hll21028.htm.

Enthoven, A.C., & Talbott, B. (2004). Stanford University's experience with managed care. *Health Affairs, 23*(6), 136–140.

Escarce, J., Jain, A., & Rogowski, J. (2006). Hospital competition, managed care, and mortality after hospitalization for medical conditions: Evidence from three states. *Medical Care Research & Review, 63*(6 Suppl.), 112–140.

FirstGov. (2007). *Your child may be eligible for free or low-cost health insurance!* U.S. Department of Health & Human

Services. Health Resources & Services Administration. Retrieved July 7, 2008 from http://www.insurekidsnow.gov.

Food and Agriculture Organization (FAO). (2007). *About us: The Food and Agriculture Organization of the United Nations.* Retrieved July 7, 2008 from http://www.fao.org/UNFAO/about/index_en.html.

Forbes. (August 7 2007). *Underinsured risking debt to pay health bills.* Retrieved July 7, 2008 from http://www.forbes.com/forbeslife/health/feeds/hscout/2007/08/07/hscout607092.html.

Gabel, J.R., Pickreign, J.D., & Whitmore, H.H. (December 2006). *Behind the slow growth of employer-based consumer-driven health plans.* [Issue brief No. 107]. Retrieved July 7, 2008 from http://www.hschange.org/CONTENT/900/?PRINT=1.

Gale Group. (2004). *COBRA Medicare prevention demonstration: Consolidated Omnibus Budget Reconciliation Act of 1985.* Retrieved July 7, 2008 from http://findarticles.com/p/articles/mi_m0795/is_n1_v15/ai_15268447/print.

Gardner, A. (February 21 2007). US health care costs to top $4 trillion by 2016. *Health On the Net News.* Retrieved July 7, 2008 from http://www.hon.ch/News/HSN/602078.html.

Gauthier, A., & Serber, M. (2005). *US health care system: Improving access, quality, and efficiency.* The Commonwealth Fund. Retrieved July 7, 2008 from http://www.cmwf.org/publications/publications_show.htm?doc_id=302833.

Gaynor, M., & Gudipati, D. (2006). *Health care costs: Do we need a cure? The Heinz School Review.* Carnegie Mellon University. Retrieved July 7, 2008 from http://journal.heinz.cmu.edu/articles/health-care-costs-do-we-need-cure/.

Geneva Foundation for Medical Education & Research. (2007). *World Health Organization: The mandate of a specialized agency of the United Nations. Chronology.* Retrieved July 7, 2008 from http://www.gfmer.ch/TMCAM/WHO_Minelli/A3.htm.

Gladwell, M. (August 29 2005). The moral-hazard myth. *The New Yorker.* Retrieved July 7, 2008 from http://www.newyorker.com/archive/2005/08/29/050829fa_fact?printable=true.

Glied, S.A., & Remier, D.K. (April 2005). The effect of health savings accounts on health insurance coverage. *Issue Brief: The Commonwealth Fund, 811,* 1–8.

Gold, M., & Achman, L. (2002). *Average out-of-pocket health care costs for Medicare Choice enrollees increase substantially in 2002.* NY: The Commonwealth Fund.

Goldman, D.P., Joyce, G.F., & Karaca-Mandic, P. (2006). Varying pharmacy benefits with clinical status: The case of cholesterol-lowering therapy. *The American Journal of Managed Care, 12*(1), 21–28.

Goldman, D.P., & McGlynn, E.A. (2005). *U.S. health care: Facts about cost, access, and quality.* Santa Monica, CA: RAND Health.

Grad, F.P. (2002). The preamble of the constitution of the World Health Organization. *Bulletin of the World Health Organization, 80*(12), 981–984.

Greene, V.W. (2001). Personal hygiene and life expectancy improvements since 1850: Historic and epidemiologic associations. *American Journal of Infection Control, 29*(4), 203–206.

Hanson, R. (1994). Buy health, not health care. *Cato Journal, 14*(1). Retrieved July 7, 2008 from http://hanson.gmu.edu/buyhealth.html.

Harrington, C., & Estes, C.L. (2004). *Health policy and nursing: Crisis and reform in the U.S. health care delivery system,* 4th ed. Sudbury, MA: Jones & Bartlett.

Hecker, J.F.C. (1839). *The epidemics of the Middle Ages.* London: Trubner and Company.

Hellander, I. (2002). A review of data on the health sector of the United States, January 2002. *International Journal of Health Services, 32*(3), 579–599.

Heskett, J. (March 2 2007). What is the government's role in US healthcare? *Harvard Business School (HBS) Working Knowledge for Business Leaders.* Retrieved July 7, 2008 from http://hbswk.hbs.edu/cgi-bin/print.

Hillestad, R., Bigelow, J., Bower, A., et al. (2005). Can electronic medical record systems transform healthcare? An assessment of potential health benefits, savings, and costs. *Health Affairs, 24*(5), 1103–1111.

Himmelstein, D., Warren, E., Thorne, D., & Woolhandler, S. (February 2 2005). Market Watch: Illness and injury as contributors to bankruptcy. *Health Affairs,* DOI: 10.1377/hlthaff.w5.63.

Himmelstein, D., & Woolhandler, S. (2003). National health insurance or incremental reform: Aim high, or at our feet? *American Journal of Public Health, 93*(1), 102–105.

Himmelstein, D., & Woolhandler, S. (2007). Massachusetts' approach to universal coverage: High hopes and faulty economic logic. *International Journal of Health Services, 37*(2), 251–257.

Hitti, M. (July 3 2007). Andrew Speaker's TB reclassified. *WebMD Medical News.* Retrieved July 7, 2008 from http://www.webmd.com/news//20070703/andrew-speakers-tb-reclassified?print=true.

House of Representatives (HR). (1998). *H.R. 3605 Patient's Bill of Rights Act of 1998: Summary.* Retrieved July 7, 2008 from http://energycommerce.house.gov/comdem/pbor/summ.htm.

Hurley, R., Strunk, B., & White, J. (2004). The puzzling popularity of the PPO. *Health Affairs, 23*(2), 56–68.

Institute of Medicine. (1988). *The future of public health.* Washington, DC: National Academy Press.

Institute of Medicine. (2001). *Crossing the quality chasm: A new health system for the 21st century.* Washington, DC: New Academy Press.

Institute of Medicine. (2002). *The future of the public's health in the 21st century.* Retrieved July 7, 2008 from http://www.iom.edu/Object.File/Master/4/165/AssuringFINAL.pdf.

International Foundation for Education, Benefits & Compensation. (2007). *The US health care dilemma: Who has the answer?* Retrieved July 7, 2008 from http://www.febp.org/Rsources/News/Health+Care+Reform+Discussion/.

Jamison, D.T., Breman, J.G., Measham, A.R., et al., (Eds.). (2006). *Disease control priorities in developing countries,* 2nd ed. New York, NY: Oxford University Press.

Jones, C.I. (May 27 2005). More life vs. more goods: Explaining rising health expenditures. *Federal Reserve Bank of San Francisco (FRSBF) Economic Letter, 2005*(10), 1–4.

Kahn, C., & Pollack, R. (2001). Building a consensus for expanding health coverage. *Health Affairs, 20*(1), 40–48.

Kaiser Family Foundation. (2001). Medicaid and managed care. *Kaiser Commission on Key Facts: Medicaid and the uninsured.* Fact Sheet #2068-03.

Kaiser Family Foundation. (2006a). *Health insurance premium growth moderates slightly in 2006, but still increases twice as fast as wages and inflation.* Retrieved July 7, 2008 from http://www.kff.org/insurance/ehbs092606nr.cfm.

Kaiser Family Foundation. (2006b). *Total Social Security Disability Insurance (SSDI) beneficiaries ages 18–64; December, 2005.* Retrieved July 7, 2008 from http://www.statehealthfacts.org/comparemaptable.jsp?ind=344&cat=6&yr=16&typ=1&o=a&sort=n.

Kaiser Family Foundation. (2006c). *Medicaid managed care enrollees, as of June 30, 2006.* Retrieved from http://www.statehealthfacts.org/comparemaptable.jsp?cat=4&ind=216.

Kaiser Family Foundation. (2007a). The Medicare prescription drug benefit. *Medicare Fact Sheet.* Publication #7044-06.

Kaiser Family Foundation. (2007b). *Medicare: A timeline of key developments.* Retrieved July 7, 2008 from http://www.kff.org/medicare/timeline/pf_85.htm.

Kaiser Family Foundation. (2007c). *Health care spending in the United States and OECD countries.* Retrieved July 7, 2008 from http://www.kff.org/insurance/snapshot/chcm010307oth.cfm.

Kongstvedt, P.R. (2004). *Managed care: What it is and how it works,* 2nd ed. Boston: Jones & Bartlett.

Laugesen, M. (2005). Why some market reforms lack legitimacy in health care. *Journal of Health Politics, Policy & Law, 30*(6), 1065–1100.

Laugesen, M., Paul, R., Luft, H., et al. (2006). A comparative analysis of mandated benefit laws, 1949–2002. *Health Services Research, 41*(3 Pt. 2), 1081–1103.

Lawlor, J.S., & Hall, M.A. (2005). Do employers voluntarily include patient protections in self-insured managed care plans? *Managed Care Interface, 18*(1), 76–80.

Leapfrog Group, The. (2007). *Leapfrog accomplishments.* Retrieved July 7, 2008 from http://www.leapfroggroup.org/media/file/Leapfrog_Accomplishments_3-07.pdf.

Lee, P.R., Estes, C.L., & Rodriguez, F.M. (Eds.). (2003). *The nation's health,* 7th ed. Boston: Jones & Bartlett.

Lega, F. (2006). Developing a marketing function in public healthcare systems: A framework for action. *Health Policy, 78*(2–3), 340–352.

Lemieux, P. (April 23 2006). Canada's 'free' health care has hidden costs. *The Wall Street Journal.* Retrieved July 7, 2008 from http://www.independent.org/newsroom/article.asp?id=1292.

Lewis, R.A. (1952). *Edwin Chadwick and the public health movement, 1832–1854.* New York: Longman's.

Loewy, E.H., & Loewy, R.S. (2001). *Changing health care systems from ethical, economic, and crosscultural perspectives.* Norwell, MA: Kluwer Plenum.

Managed Care Online (MCOL). (2007). *National managed care enrollment, 2006.* Retrieved July 7, 2008 from http://www.mcareol.com/factshts/mcolfact.htm.

Marr, J. (1982, Winter). Merchants of death: The role of the slave trade in the transmission of disease from Africa to the Americas. *Pharos,* 31.

Marquis, S., Rogowski, J., & Escarce, J. (2004/2005). The managed care backlash: Did consumers vote with their feet? *Inquiry, 41,* 376–390.

Mayo Clinic. (2007). *Health savings accounts: Is an HSA right for you?* Retrieved July 7, 2008 from http://www.mayoclinic.com/print/health-savings-accounts/GA00053/GA00053/METHOD=print.

McIntosh, M.A.E. (2002). The cost of healthcare to Americans. *JONA's Healthcare Law, Ethics, and Regulation, 4*(3), 78–89.

McKenzie, J. (2007). Critical condition: Cheaper in Canada. Why do drugs cost less outside the United States? *ABC News.* Retrieved July 7, 2008 from http://abcnews.go.com/WNT/print?id=129359.

McNerney, W.J. (1980). Control of health care costs in the 1980s. *The New England Journal of Medicine, 303,* 1088–1095.

Meador, M.G., & Linnan, L.A. (2006). Using the PRECEDE model to plan men's health programs in a managed care setting. *Health Promotion in Practice, 7*(2), 186–196.

Meara, E., White, C., & Cutler, D. (2004). Trends in medical spending by age, 1963–2000. *Health Affairs, 23*(4), 176–183.

Medicare Advocacy. (2007). *Medicare prescription drug coverage 2007.* Retrieved July 7, 2008 from http://www.medicareadvocacy.org/FAQ_PartD_Info.htm#_ftn1.

Melosi, M. (2000). *The sanitary city: Urban infrastructure in America from colonial times to the present.* Baltimore: Johns Hopkins University Press.

Milbank Memorial Fund, the National Association of State Budget Officers & the Reforming States Group. (2003). *2000–2001 state health care expenditure report.* Retrieved July 7, 2008 from http://www.milbank.org/reports/2000shcer/index.html#direct11.

Morris, C.R. (April 8 2005). The economics of health care: It's going to cost a lot more. *The Commonwealth Magazine, CXXXII*(7). Retrieved July 7, 2008 from http://www.commonwealmagazine.org/article.php3?id_article=1181.

Morrissey, M.A. (October 8 2003). Cost shifting: New myths, old confusion, and enduring reality. *Health Affairs.* Retrieved July 7, 2008 from http://content.healthaffairs.org/cgi/content/full/hltaf.w3.489v/DC1.

National Center for Education in Maternal and Child Health. (2007). *Landmark federal MCH legislation.* Retrieved July 7, 2008 from http://images.main.uab.edu/isoph/MCH/Tech_Reports/MCHLegislation.pdf.

National Committee on Vital and Health Statistics (NCVHS). (2000). *NCVHS 1949-1999: A history.* Retrieved July 7, 2008 from http://www.ncvhs.hhs.gov/50history.htm.

National Institutes of Health. (2007). *Health manpower act. NIH historical data: Legislative chronology.* Retrieved July 7, 2008 from http://www.nih.gov/about/almanac/historical/legislative_chronology.htm#19.

National Library of Medicine. (2003). *Profiles in science: Regional medical programs collection.* Retrieved July 7, 2008 from http://profiles.nlm.nih.gov/RM/A/A/U/C/.

Newhouse, J.P. (2002). *Pricing the priceless: A health care conundrum.* Cambridge, MA: The MIT Press.

Nyman, J.A. (2003). *The theory of demand for health insurance.* Menlo Park, CA: Stanford University Press.

Oberlander, J., Marmor, T., & Jacobs, L. (2001). Rationing medical care: Rhetoric and reality in the Oregon Health Plan. *Canadian Medical Association Journal, 164*(11), 1583–1587.

Office of Civil Rights. (2003). *General overview of standards for privacy of individually identifiable health information.* U.S. Department of Health & Human Services. Retrieved July 7, 2008 from http://www.hhs.gov/ocr/hipaa/guidelines/overview.pdf.

Office of Inspector General. (1989). *The Family Support Act of 1988: What do frontline workers know? What do they think?* Department of Health & Human Services. Retrieved July 7, 2008 from http://www.oig.hhs.gov/oei/reports/oei-05-89-01220.pdf.

Office of Public Health Service Historian. (2004). *FAQs.* Retrieved August 10, 2008 from http://www.lhncbc.nlm.nih.gov/apdb/phsHistory/faqs.html.

Organization for Economic Cooperation & Development (OECD). (2007). *OECD health data 2007: How does the United States compare?* Retrieved July 7, 2008 from http://www.oecd.org/dataoecd/46/2/38980580.pdf.

Ornstein, C. (July 17 2007). Police won't be charged in death at hospital: Prosecutors say L.A. County officers did more than the King-Harbor staff to help woman get medical care. *Los Angeles Times.* Retrieved July 7, 2008 from http://www.calendarlive.com/services/site/la-me-kingcops17jul17,1.2667620.story.

Ornstein, C., Weber, T., & Leonard, J. (August 11 2007). King-Harbor fails final check, will close soon. *Los Angeles Times.* Retrieved July 7, 2008 from http://www.latimes.com/news/local/la-me-king11aug11,0,4847476,print.story?coll=la-home-center.

Pan American Health Organization. (2001). *Equity & Health: Views from the Pan American Sanitary Bureau.* Washington, DC: Author.

Pan American Health Organization. (2002). *Executive Summary: Health in the Americas.* Washington, D.C.: Author.

Pan American Health Organization (PAHO). (2007a). *About PAHO.* Retrieved July 7, 2008 from http://www.paho.org/English/PAHO/about_paho.htm.

Pan American Health Organization (PAHO). (2007b). *PAHO publishing.* Retrieved July 7, 2008 from http://www.paho.org/English/DD/PUB/pubHome.asp.

PBS. (2007). *Healthcare crisis: Healthcare timeline.* Retrieved July 7, 2008 from http://www.pbs.org/healthcarecrisis/history.htm.

Perkins, B.B. (1998). Economic organization of medicine and the Committee on the Costs of Medical Care. *American Journal of Public Health, 88*(11), 1721–1726.

Perlstadt, H. (1995). The development of the Hill-Burton legislation: Interests, issues and compromises. *Journal of Health & Social Policy, 6*(3), 77–96.

Porche, D.J. (2004). *Public & community health nursing practice: A population-based approach.* Thousand Oaks, CA: Sage Publications.

Porter, M., & Teisberg, E. (2006). *Redefining health care: Creating value-based competition on results.* Cambridge, MA: Harvard Business School Press.

Premera. (2007). *History: The Premera Blue Cross story.* Retrieved July 7, 2008 from https://www.premera.com/stellent/groups/public/documents/xcpproject/CompanyHistory.asp.

Public Health Encyclopedia. (2008). *Non-governmental organization.* Retrieved July 7, 2008 from http://www.answers.com/topic/non-governmental-organization.

Public Health Foundation. (n.d.). *A strong public health infrastructure can help save lives.* Retrieved July 7, 2008 from http://www.phf.org/infrastructure/resources/PHFactSheet.pdf.

Public Health Foundation. (2007). Understanding public health infrastructure. *Public Health Infrastructure Resource Center.* Retrieved July 7, 2008 from http://www.phf.org/infrastructure/.

RAND Health. (2005). *State efforts to insure the uninsured: An unfinished story.* Retrieved July 7, 2008 from http://www.rand.org/pubs/research_briefs/2005/RAND_RB4558-1.pdf.

RAND Health. (2006). *Consumer decision making in the insurance market.* Santa Monica, CA: Author.

RAND Institute for Civil Justice. (2004). *Changing the medical malpractice dispute process.* Retrieved July 7, 2008 from http://www.rand.org/pubs/research_briefs/RB9071/index1.html.

Rice, C.L., & Rhodes, R.S. (2002). Health care economics: The larger context: Introduction. *ACS Surgery Online.* Retrieved July 7, 2008 from http://www.medscape.com/viewarticle/535641_print.

Richardson, B.W. (1887). *The health of nations: A review of the works of Edwin Chadwick,* Vol. 2. London: Longmans, Green.

Ruhl, T. (2007). *Children's Bureau name and hierarchy: Roots and history.* Retrieved July 7, 2008 from http://www.mchlibrary.info/history/names.html.

Sage, W. & Kersch, R. (Eds.). (2006). *Medical malpractice and the U.S. healthcare system.* New York: Cambridge University Press.

Scanlon, D., Swaminathan, S., Chernew, M., & Lee, W. (2006). Market and plan characteristics related to HMO quality and improvement. *Medical Care Research & Review, 63*(6 Suppl.), 56–89.

Schoen, C., Davis, K., How, S., & Schoenbaum, S. (September 20 2006). US health system performance: A national scorecard. *Health Affairs, 56,* W457–W475.

Schoen, C., Doty, M., Collins, S., & Holmgren, A. (June 13 2005). Insured but not protected: How many adults are underinsured? *Health Affairs,* Web Exclusive, W5–289–W5–302.

Scutchfield, F.D., & Keck, C.W. (Eds.). (2003). *Principles of public health practice,* 2nd ed. Albany, NY: Delmar Thomson Learning.

Sensenig, A.L. (2007). Refining estimates of public health spending as measured in national health expenditures accounts: The United States experience. *Journal of Public Health Management & Practice, 13*(2), 103–104.

Sharma, A.K. (2006). Redesigning the US healthcare model. *The Heinz School Review.* Carnegie Mellon University. Retrieved July 7, 2008 from http://journal.heinz.cmu.edu/articles/redesigning-us-healthcare-model/.

Shattuck, L., et al. (1850). *Report of the Sanitary Commission of Massachusetts.* Cambridge, MA: Harvard University Press (Original work published by Dutton & Wentworth in 1850).

Sipkoff, M. (August 2003). Managed competition: The future, not the past. *Managed Care Magazine.* Retrieved July 7, 2008 from http://www.managedcaremag.com/archives/0308/0308.enthoven.html.

Snow, J. (1855). *On the mode of communication of cholera,* 2nd ed. London: John Churchill.

Social Security Administration (SSA). (2003). *Historical background and development of Social Security.* Retrieved July 7, 2008 from http://www.ssa.gov/history/briefhistory3.html.

Social Security Administration (SSA). (2007a). *SSA History.* Retrieved July 7, 2008 from http://www.ssa.gov/history/35actinx.html.

Social Security Administration. (2007b). *Fact sheet: Social Security.* Retrieved July 7, 2008 from http://www.ssa.gov/pressoffice/factsheets/basicfact-alt.pdf.

Social Security Online. (2007). *Legislative history: 1935 Social Security Act.* Retrieved July 7, 2008 from http://www.ssa.gov/history/35actinx.html.

Stanton, N.W., & Rutherford, M.K. (September 2004). Employer-sponsored health insurance: Trends in cost and access. Rockville, MD: Agency for Healthcare Research & Quality (AHRQ). *Research in Action* Issue #17. AHRQ Pub. No. 04-0085.

Stock, S., Redaelli, M., & Lauterbach, K. (2007). Disease management and health care reforms in Germany: Does more competition lead to less solidarity? *Health Policy, 80*(1), 86–96.

Sultz, H.A., & Young, K.A. (2006). *Health care USA: Understanding its organization and delivery,* 5th ed. Boston: Jones & Bartlett.

Tabarrok, A. (November 23 2004). *Seeing is believing (in the free market).* Retrieved July 7, 2008 from http://www.marginalrevolution.com/marginalrevolution/2004/11/seeing_is_belie.html.

Tooker, J. (2003). Affordable health insurance for all is possible by means of a pragmatic approach. *American Journal of Public Health, 93*(1), 106–109.

Toronto Star. (2007, June 3). Doctors monitor TB flyer. *Associated Press.* Retrieved July 7, 2008 from http://www.thestar.com/printArticle/220973.

Trust for America's Health. (2005). *Shortchanging America's health: A state-by-state look at how federal public health dollars are spent.* Washington, DC: Author.

Turnock, B.J. (2004). *Public health: What it is and how it works,* 3rd ed. Boston: Jones & Bartlett Publishers.

Tyson, L.D. (2001). Healing Medicare. In E.C. Hein (Ed.). *Nursing issues in the 21st century: Perspectives from the literature.* (pp. 459–468). Philadelphia: Lippincott Williams & Wilkins.

United Food & Commercial Workers International Union. (2007). *Wal-Martization of health care.* Retrieved July 7, 2008 from http://www.ufcw.org/pres_room/fact_sheets_and_backgrounder/walmart/benefits.cfm.

United Nations Educational Scientific & Cultural Organization (UNESCO). (2007). *What is it? What does it do?* Retrieved July 7, 2008 from http://portal.unesco.org/en/ev.php-URL_ID=3328&URL_DO=DO_PRINTPAGE&URL_SECTION=201.html.

United Nations International Children's Emergency Fund (UNICEF). (2007). *What we do.* Retrieved July 7, 2008 from http://www.unicef.org/whatwedo/index.html.

University of Maine. (2001). *The US health care system: Best in the world, or just the most expensive?* Retrieved July 7, 2008 from http://dll.umaine.edu/ble/U.S.%20HCweb.pdf.

U.S. Agency for International Development (USAID). (2006). *Frequently asked questions.* Retrieved July 7, 2008 from http://www.usaid.gov/faws.html.

U.S. Department of Health and Human Services. (2000). *Healthy people 2010,* Conference ed., Vols. 1 & 2. Washington, DC: Author.

U.S. Department of Health and Human Services. (2006). *Fact sheet: Your rights under the community service assurance provision of the Hill-Burton act.* Retrieved July 7, 2008 from http://www.hhs.gov/ocr/hburton.html.

U.S. Department of Health & Human Services. (2007). *Historical highlights.* Retrieved July 7, 2008 from http://www.hhs.gov/about/hhshist.html.

U.S. Department of Health and Human Services. U.S. Public Health Service Commissioned Corps. (2007). *About the Commissioned Corps: History.* Retrieved July 7, 2008 from http://commcorps.shs.net/AboutUs/history.aspx.

U.S. Department of Labor. (2004). *The Health Insurance Portability and Accountability Act (HIPAA): Fact sheet.* Retrieved July 7, 2008 from http://www.dol.gov/ebsa/pdf/fshipaa.pdf.

U.S. Department of Labor. (2007). *FAQs about COBRA continuation health coverage.* Employee Benefits Security Administration. Retrieved July 7, 2008 from http://www.dol.gov/ebsa/faqs/faq_consumer_cobra.html.

U.S. Environmental Protection Agency. (2007). *Occupational safety and health act: 29 U.S.C., 651 et seq. (1970).* Retrieved July 7, 2008 from http://www.epa.gov/Region5/defs/html/osha.htm.

Van de Ven, W., Beck, K., Van de Voorde, C., et al. (2007). Risk adjustment and risk selection in Europe: 6 years later. *Health Policy, 83*(2–3), 162–179.

Van de Water, P.N., & Lavery, J. (2006). Medicare finances: Findings of the 2006 trustees report. *National Academy of Social Insurance, Medicare Brief, No. 13.* Retrieved July 7, 2008 from http://www.nasi.org/usr_doc/medicare_brief_013.pdf.

Virginia Commonwealth University. (2007, August 9). Medicare claims processing. *Work World.* Retrieved July 7, 2008 from http://www.workworld.org/wwwebhelp/medicare_claims_processing.htm.

Ward, J., & Warren, C. (Eds.). (2007). *Silent victories: The history and practice of public health in twentieth-century America.* New York: Oxford University Press.

Weiss, M. (1997). The quality evolution in managed care organizations. *Journal of Nursing Care Quality, 11*(4), 27–31.

Williams, S.J., & Torrens, P.R. (2002). *Introduction to health services,* 6th ed. Albany, NY: Delmar Thomson Learning.

Wood, D. (2001). *The rise of the HMO.* CNN Interactive. Retrieved July 7, 2008 from http://www.cnn.com/SPECIALS/2000/democracy/doctors.under.the.knife/stories/hmo.history/index.html.

Woodward, S.B. (1932). The story of smallpox in Massachusetts. *New England Journal of Medicine, 206,* 1181.

Woolhandler, S., Himmelstein, D., Angell, M., et al. (2003). Proposal of the Physicians' Working Group for Single-Payer National Health Insurance. *Journal of the American Medical Association, 290*(6), 798–805.

Woolley, J., & Peters, G. (2007). *George Bush: Statement on signing the Preventive Health Amendments of 1992. The American Presidency Project.* Retrieved July 7, 2008 from http://www.presidency.ucsb.edu/ws/index.php?pid=21681.

World Health Organization (WHO). (1998). *Health for all policy for the twenty-first century* (Resolution WHA51.7). Geneva: Author.

World Health Organization. (2000). *The world health report 2000. Health systems: Improving performance.* Retrieved July 7, 2008 from http://www.who,.int/whr/2000/en/.

World Health Organization (WHO). (2007a). *Countries.* Retrieved July 7, 2008 from http://www.who.int/countries/en/.

World Health Organization (WHO). (2007b). *Health in the millennium development goals.* Retrieved July 7, 2008 from http://www.who.int/mdg/goals/en/print.html.

World Health Organization (WHO). (2007c). *WHO regional offices.* Retrieved July 7, 2008 from http://www.who.int/about/regions/en/.

Selected Readings

Blevins, S.A. (2001). *Medicare's midlife crisis.* Washington, DC: CATO Institute.

Cunningham, P.J., & Trude, S. (2001). Does managed care enable more low income persons to identify a usual source of care? Implications for access to care. *Medical Care, 39*(7),716–726.

Drummond, M.F., & McGuire, A. (2001). *Economic evaluation in health care: Merging theory with practice.* New York: Oxford University Press.

Emanuel, E.J. (2000). Justice and managed care: Four principles for the just allocation of health care. *Hastings Center Report, 30*(2), 8–16.

Erickson, G.P. (1996). To pauperize or empower: Public health nursing at the turn of the 20th and 21st centuries. *Public Health Nursing, 13*(3), 163–169.

Goody, B., Mentnech, R., & Riley, G. (2002). Changing nature of public and private health insurance. *Health Care Financing Review, 23*(3), 1–7.

Hurley, R., & Zuckerman, S. (2002). *Medicaid managed care: State flexibility in action.* Washington, DC: Urban Institute.

Institute of Medicine. (2001). *Coverage matters: Insurance and health care.* Washington, DC: National Academy Press.

Institute of Medicine. (2002). *Unequal treatment: What healthcare providers need to know about racial and ethnic disparities in healthcare.* (pp. 1–8). Washington, DC: National Academy of Sciences.

Jacobs, J.R. (2002). *The economics of health and medical care,* 5th ed. Gaithersburg MD: Aspen Publishers.

Jonas, S., & Kovner, A.R. (2005). *Health care delivery in the United States,* 8th ed. New York: Springer.

Kleinke, J.D. (2001). *Oxymorons: The myth of the US health care system.* San Francisco, CA: Jossey-Bass.

Langner, B.E. (2001). The uninsured: A chronic American problem: Finding the elusive solution. *Journal of Professional Nursing 17*(6), 277.

Leavitt, J.K., & Beacham, T.B. (2002). Policy perspectives: The effects of September 11 on health policy. *American Journal of Nursing, 102*(9), 99–102.

Lopez, A.D., Ahmad, O.B., Gulliot, M., et al. (2002). *World mortality in 2000.* Geneva: World Health Organization.

Mays, G.P., Halverson, P.K., & Stevens, R. (2001). The contributions of managed care plans to public health practice: Evidence from the nation's largest local health departments. *Public Health Reports, 116*(1 Suppl. 2001), 50–67.

Mays, G.P., Miller, C.A., & Halverson, P.K. (2000). *Local public health practice: Trends and models.* Washington, DC: American Public Health Association.

McCarthy, M. (2002). What's going on at the World Health Organization? *The Lancet, 360,* 1108–1112.

McDonald, R. (2002). *Using health economics in health services: Rationing rationally?* Philadelphia: Open University Press.

Millenson, M.L. (2002). Demanding medical excellence: Doctors and accountability in the information age. Chicago, IL: University of Chicago Press.

Moon, M., & Storeygard, M. (2002). *Solvency or affordability? Ways to measure Medicare's financial health.* Menlo Park, CA: Henry J. Kaiser Family Foundation.

Nunn, P., Harries, A., Godfrey-Faussett, P., et al. (2002). The research agenda for improving health policy, systems performance, and service delivery for tuberculosis control: A WHO perspective. *Bulletin of the World Health Organization, 80,* 471–476.

Pan American Health Organization. (2002). *Health in the Americas,* Vols. I & II. Washington, DC: Author.

Phelps, C.E. (2003). *Health economics,* 3rd ed. Reading, MA: Addison-Wesley.

Scott, C. (2001). *Public and private roles in health care systems: Reform experience in seven OECD countries.* Philadelphia, PA: Open University Press.

Stone, P.W., Curran, C.R., & Bakken, S. (2002). Economic evidence for evidence-based practice. *Journal of Nursing Scholarship, 34*(3), 277–282.

Tulchinsky, T., & Varavikova, E. (2000). *The new public health: An introduction for the 21st century.* San Diego, CA: Academic Press.

Walshe, K. (2002). *Regulating healthcare: A prescription for improvement?* Philadelphia: Open University Press.

Warren, M. (2000). *A chronology of state medicine, public health, welfare and related services, 1066–1999.* London: Faculty of Public Health Medicine of the Royal Colleges of Physicians of the United Kingdom.

Zwanziger, J., & Khan, N. (2006). Safety-net activities and hospital contracting with managed care organizations. *Medical Care Research & Review, 63*(6 Suppl.), 90–111.

Internet Resources

Center for Medicare and Medicaid Services: *http://www.cms.hhs.gov*

Department of Health and Human Services, Health Resources and Services Administration: *http://www.hrsa.gov*

Joint Commission on Accreditation of Healthcare Organizations: *http://www.jointcommission.org*

Kaiser Family Foundation: *http://www.kff.org*

The Leapfrog Group: *http://www.leapfroggroup.org*

National Center for Health Statistics: *http://www.cdc.gov/nchs/*

National Committee for Quality Assurance: *http://www.ncqa.org*

Pan American Health Organization: *http://www.paho.org*

Population Reference Bureau: *http://www.prb.org*

Rollins School of Public Health InfoLinks: Reference Resources—The History of Public Health: *http://www.sph.emory.edu/PHIL/history.html*

U.S. Agency for International Development: *http://www.usaid.gov*

World Health Organization: *http://www.who.org*

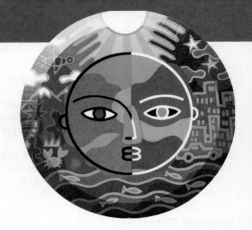

7

Epidemiology in Community Health Care

LEARNING OBJECTIVES

Upon mastery of this chapter, you should be able to:

◆ Explore the historical roots of epidemiology.
◆ Explain the host, agent, and environment model.
◆ Describe theories of causality in health and illness.
◆ Explain a *web of causation* matrix that assists you with recognizing multi-causal factors in disease or injury occurrences.
◆ Define immunity and compare passive immunity, active immunity, cross-immunity, and herd immunity.
◆ Explain how epidemiologists determine populations at risk.
◆ Identify the four stages of a disease or health condition.
◆ List the major sources of epidemiologic information.
◆ Distinguish between incidence and prevalence in health and illness states.
◆ Use epidemiologic methods to describe an aggregate's health.
◆ Discuss the types of epidemiologic studies that are useful for researching aggregate health.
◆ Use the seven-step research process when conducting an epidemiologic study.

"Investigation may be likened to the long months of pregnancy, and solving a problem to the day of birth. To investigate a problem is, indeed, to solve it."
—Mao Tse-Tung

KEY TERMS

Agent
Analytic epidemiology
Case-control study
Causality
Cohort
Cross-sectional study
Descriptive epidemiology
Endemic
Environment
Epidemic
Epidemiology
Experimental epidemiology
Experimental study
Global health patterns
Host
Immunity
Incidence
Morbidity rate
Mortality rate
Natural history
Pandemic
Prevalence
Prevalence study
Prospective study
Rates
Retrospective study
Risk

Epidemiology is "concerned with the distribution and determinants of health and diseases, morbidity, injuries, disability, and mortality in populations" (Friis & Sellers, 2004, p. 5). It is a specialized form of scientific research that can provide health care workers, including community health nurses, with a body of knowledge on which to base their practice and methods for studying new and existing problems. The term is derived from the Greek words *epi* (upon), *demos* (the people), and *logos* (knowledge): the knowledge or study of what happens to people. Epidemiologists ask such questions as the following:

◆ What is the occurrence of health and disease in a population?
◆ Has there been an increase or decrease in a health state over the years?
◆ Does one geographic area have a higher frequency of disease than another?
◆ What characteristics of people with a particular condition distinguish them from those without the condition?
◆ What factors need to be present to cause disease or injury?
◆ Is one treatment or program more effective than another in changing the health of affected people?
◆ Why do some people recover from a disease and others do not?

The ultimate goals of epidemiology are to "determine the extent of disease in a population, identify patterns and trends in disease occurrence, identify the causes of disease, and evaluate the effectiveness of prevention and treatment options" (Aschengrau & Seage, 2008, p. 33). With knowledge regarding the scale and nature of human health problems, solutions to prevent disease can be sought, thereby contributing to the improved health of the entire population.

Epidemiology offers community health nurses a specific methodology for assessing the health of aggregates. Furthermore, it provides a frame of reference for investigating and improving clinical practice in any setting. For example, if a community health nursing goal is to lower the incidence of sexually transmitted diseases (STDs) in a given community, such a prevention plan requires information about population groups. How many STD cases have been reported in this community in the past year? What is the expected number of STD cases (the morbidity rate)? Which members of the community are at highest risk of contracting STDs? To be effective, any program of screening, treatment, or health promotion regarding STDs must be based on this kind of information about population groups. Whether the community health nurse's goals are to improve a population's nutrition, control the spread of human immunodeficiency virus (HIV), deal with health problems created by a flood, protect and promote the health of battered women, or reduce the number of automobile crash injuries and fatalities at a specific intersection, epidemiologic data are essential.

HISTORICAL ROOTS OF EPIDEMIOLOGY

The roots of epidemiology can be traced to Hippocrates, a Greek physician who lived from about 460 to 375 BCE and who is sometimes referred to as the first epidemiologist.

Hippocrates and other members of the Hippocratic School believed that disease not only affects individuals but also affects the masses. This was one of the earliest associations of the occurrence of disease with lifestyle and environmental factors, specifically geographic location (Lawson & Williams, 2001). Not until the late 19th century however, did modern epidemiology come into existence.

An **epidemic** refers to a disease occurrence that clearly exceeds the normal or expected frequency in a community or region. In past centuries, epidemics of cholera, bubonic plague, and smallpox swept through community after community, killing thousands of people, changing the community structure, and altering the lifestyle of masses of people. When an epidemic, such as the bubonic plague (also called pneumonic plague or the Black Death) or acquired immunodeficiency syndrome (AIDS), is worldwide in distribution, it is called a **pandemic**.

Epidemic and pandemic diseases clearly prompted the development of epidemiology as a science. Epidemiology became a distinct branch of medical science through its concern with massive waves of infectious diseases. In 1348 and 1349, the Black Death (likely caused by the bacillus *Yersinia pestis*) swept through continental Europe and England, killing millions of people. In England alone, the epidemic resulted in the deaths of 30% to 60% of the population (Theilmann & Cate, 2007).

The plague continued in Europe, but with less force, for three centuries and then waned, only to reappear in an epidemic in Hong Kong in 1894. Discovery of the plague bacillus was first attributed to Shibasaburo Kitasato (1852–1931), a Japanese bacteriologist (Solomon, 1997). Procedural issues with Kitasato's work however, eventually resulted in the attribution to Alexandre Yersin (1863–1943), who worked in Hong Kong at the same time (Solomon, 1997). The name of the bacillus, *Yersinia pestis* reflects his acknowledged discovery. Within 4 years, another scientist, Paul-Louis Simond, had traced the bacillus life cycle from rats to fleas to humans; he postulated that the bite of a *Yersinia*-infected flea caused plague in humans. Although viewed with skepticism, by 1906 the scientific community finally accepted the route of disease transmission described by Simond and others (Simond, Godley, & Mouriquand, 1998). With this combined knowledge, intervention was now possible, and public health officials declared war on rats, seeking to make ships and wharf buildings rat-proof.

One early example of a community-wide campaign against rats occurred after the outbreak of plague in California in 1900 (Evans, 1939). The campaign proved successful, and bolstered confidence in efforts to control disease outbreaks by attacking the likely source. Understanding the role that rats played in the transmission of the disease led to an effective approach for disease control. Unfortunately, plague has not been eradicated, and wild rodents, especially ground squirrels, as well as rabbits and domestic cats, remain a natural reservoir of the plague bacillus (Heymann, 2004). Cases still occur occasionally in the western half of the United States, and there are sporadic outbreaks in South America. The disease is an ongoing threat in major areas of Asia and Africa, especially in rural regions. In Europe, the area near the Caspian Sea continues to harbor wild rodent plague (Heymann, 2004). The continuing presence of a disease or infectious agent in a given geographic area, such as plague in Vietnam or malaria in the tropics of Brazil and Indonesia, means that the disease is **endemic** to that area.

As the threat of the great epidemic diseases declined, epidemiologists began to focus on other infectious diseases, such as diphtheria, infant diarrhea, typhoid, tuberculosis, and syphilis. They also studied diseases linked to occupations, such as scurvy among sailors and scrotal cancer among chimney sweeps. In recent years, epidemiologists turned to the study of major causes of death and disability, such as cancer, cardiovascular disorders, AIDS, violence, mental illness, accidents, arthritis, and congenital defects.

Florence Nightingale: Nurse Epidemiologist

Nursing's epidemiologic roots can be traced to Florence Nightingale (1820–1910). Her detailed records, morbidity (sickness) statistics, and careful description of the health conditions among the soldiers in the Crimean War represent one of the first systematic descriptive studies of the distribution and patterns of disease in a population. She used wedge-shaped graphs that were shaded and colored to illustrate preventable deaths of the hospitalized Crimean soldiers, compared with hospitalized soldiers in England at the time. The sophisticated level of detail in her studies heralded her as the first nurse researcher. Changes made according to her suggestions, which are common knowledge now—establishing a clean environment, providing edible foods, cleaning wounds and using new bandages, and separating infectious soldiers from injured soldiers—brought dramatic proof of the authenticity of her observations and knowledge. Forty-four of every 100 British troops were dying in the Crimea before Nightingale instituted environmental and nutritional changes in the hospital and field. When her work was finished, the mortality (death) rate was only 2% (Gabriel & Metz, 1992).

William Farr

Nightingale's epidemiologic approach grew from her decades-long collaboration with friend and colleague William Farr (Kudzma, 2006). Farr, a physician and self-taught mathematician, is considered one of the founders of modern epidemiology (Aschengrau & Seage, 2008). As head of the Office of the Registrar General for England and Wales (Kudzma, 2006), he developed a "more sophisticated system for coding medical conditions than was previously in use" (Friis & Sellers, 2004, p. 31). Arguments for the health care reforms Nightingale sought were bolstered by her collaboration with Farr. With Nightingale's data on the frequency of mortality among groups and Farr's broader population statistics, it was now possible to make "comparisons to the population at risk as a whole" (Kudzma, 2006, p. 63). The professional liaison between Nightingale and Farr is a wonderful example of collaborative practice in addressing public health; the merging of expertise from these two disciplines resulted in much more than either could accomplish individually.

Nightingale's use of statistical data, along with her commitment to environmental reform, strongly influenced nursing's evolution into a profession whose service addressed public health problems as well as hospital care (Kopf, 1978). As nursing has evolved, public health nurses have been increasingly challenged to intervene at the aggregate level, using epidemiologic approaches to address the needs of high-risk groups and populations.

Eras in the Evolution of Modern Epidemiology

Modern epidemiology can be described as having four distinct eras, each based on causal thinking, sanitary statistics, infectious-disease epidemiology, and chronic-disease epidemiology. In light of new research, the eco-epidemiology era is currently emerging.

Early causal thinking was dominated by the *miasma theory,* which had its origins in the work of the Hippocratic School and was formally developed in the early 1700s. This theory held that a substance called *miasma* was composed of malodorous and poisonous particles generated by the decomposition of organic matter and was the cause of disease. Prevention based on this theory attempted to eliminate the sources of the miasma or polluted vapors. Despite its base on faulty reasoning, this type of prevention had positive consequences because it made people aware that decaying organic matter can be a source of infectious diseases. This theory dominated until the first half of the 19th century. Nightingale herself never accepted the link between microorganisms and disease (Kudzma, 2006) and based her practice on this same approach. Her work in the Crimea, with its emphasis on sanitation, had positive results nonetheless.

Similarly, the pioneering work of John Snow in identifying the source of cholera in England in the mid 1800s was based on a faulty assumption that the climate was involved. Even so, he was able to trace the source of the infectious agent to the water supply and brought public attention to the link between sanitary conditions and disease. We owe much to these individuals; that they didn't understand the exact mechanisms in disease causation does not diminish their pioneering work in applied epidemiology.

The era of infectious-disease epidemiology was dominated by the *contagion theory* of disease, which developed by the mid 18th century. Prompted by the development of increasingly sophisticated microscopes, this theory attempted to identify the microorganisms that cause diseases as a first step in prevention. It inspired various theories of immunity, and even prompted some initial attempts at vaccination against smallpox. Additionally, once an agent had been identified, measures were taken to contain its spread. Fumigating ships to kill rats, protecting wharf buildings and human habitations from rats, and removing rat food supplies from easy access were all measures taken to protect the public by further preventing the spread of plague bacilli. Based on the work of Louis Pasteur, Jakob Henle, and Robert Koch, the contagion theory was refined and became best known as the *germ theory of disease* (Aschengrau & Seage, 2008), which was predominant from the late 19th century through the first half of the 20th century (Lawson & Williams, 2001).

In the era of infectious-disease epidemiology, scientists viewed disease in terms of a simple cause-and-effect relationship. Finding a single cause (plague bacilli) and attacking it (eliminating rats) seemed to be the solution for preventing many diseases. In the case of bubonic plague, this approach appeared to be quite effective. However, scientific research eventually revealed that disease causation was much more complex than first suspected. For example, although most members of a group might be exposed to the plague, many did not contract it.

With bubonic plague, as with many other infectious diseases, the characteristics of the host can determine both the spread of the disease and its individual impact. Not everyone in a population is at equal risk; it is now known that untreated bubonic plague has a case-fatality rate of 50% to 60%; meaning that about half of those who contract the disease and are not treated will eventually die (Heymann, 2004). Furthermore, the agent and course of transmission can be quite complex. Although a flea carries the bacilli from rats to humans in bubonic plague, many infectious diseases spread directly from one human being to another. Finally, the environment must be considered as part of the cause of disease. Evidence suggests that the plague originated in the high plains of Asia and spread to other parts of the world. However, questions remain as to whether the bacillus spread from rats to ground squirrels or had always been part of the squirrels' ecology.

After World War II, the causative agents of major infectious diseases were identified, methods of prevention were recognized, and antibiotics and chemotherapy were added to the arsenal to fight communicable diseases. The focus then became understanding and controlling the new chronic disease epidemics. Researchers completed case-control and cohort studies (discussed later) that linked the causative factors of cholesterol levels and smoking with coronary heart disease and associated smoking with lung cancer. Today, the major causes of mortality in the United States are noninfectious diseases. Chronic diseases of the heart, cancer, and stroke alone account for nearly 60% of deaths; accidents (including road traffic injuries), suicide, and homicide account for another 6.5% (Miniño, Heron, & Smith, 2006). These major health problems are not caused by infectious agents.

We are entering a new era of *eco-epidemiology*, distinguished by transforming global health patterns and technological advances. **Global health patterns**, the route, form, and virulence in which diseases appear in countries around the world, with consideration of environmental, ecologic, human, technologic, and political factors, are in transformation. The West Nile virus, severe acute respiratory syndrome (SARS), and the HIV epidemic illustrate this transformation. In most cases, causative organisms and critical risk factors are known, yet diseases occur, spread, and suddenly appear in countries or regions previously free of them. We

know which social behaviors need to change, but we are at a loss about how to create a climate of permanent change, even when entire populations are at stake. For example, we know how to prevent the transmission of HIV, yet thousands of new cases are reported each year. How can preventive practices be promoted in populations at risk for communicable diseases? The same is true for many current chronic diseases. How many nurses smoke? Do you exercise as you know you should? Do you know your cholesterol level, and eat appropriate foods accordingly? What are we missing to effectively change social behaviors?

Developments in technology drive research, primarily in biology and biomedical techniques and in information system capabilities. For example, the possibility now exists through DNA studies to recognize both viral and genetic components in insulin-dependent diabetes. HIV, tuberculosis, and other infections can be tracked from person to person through identifying the molecular specificity of the organisms, and a gene to track and mark one form of breast cancer has been identified. On a broader scale, using new technology, we are now able to track the geographic distribution of disease and correlate that data with other important health risks. For instance, using these geocoding systems, overweight and obesity in children can be correlated with other factors, such as after-school recreation opportunities, distribution of fast food restaurants, farmer's markets, or socioeconomic status. Recognizing the power of such capability, one of the goals of Healthy People 2010 (U.S. Department of Health and Human Services [USDHHS], 2000) was to use geocoding at all levels (national, state, and local). In the Healthy People 2010 Midcourse Review, this goal was revised to: "increase the proportion of major national health data systems that use geocoding to promote nationwide use of geographic information systems (GIS)" (USDHHS, 2006, p. 23.13). Even with the removal of the state and local emphasis, with a baseline of 50% in 2000, the national target of this goal is 100% by 2010. The possibilities of learning through technology have just begun in this current epidemiologic era. Table 7.1 summarizes the four eras in the evolution of modern epidemiology.

TABLE 7.1   Eras in the Evolution of Modern Epidemiology

Era	Paradigm	Analytic Approach	Prevention Approach
Sanitary statistics (1800–1850)	Miasma: poisoning from foul emanations	Clustering of morbidity and mortality	Drainage, sewage, sanitation
Infectious disease epidemiology (1850–1950)	Germ theory: single agent related to specific disease	Laboratory isolation and culture from disease sites and reproduce lesions	Interrupt transmission (vaccines, isolation, and antibiotics)
Chronic disease epidemiology (1950–2000)	Exposure related to outcome	Risk ratio of exposure to outcome at individual level in populations	Control risk factors by modifying lifestyle (diet), agent (guns), or environment (pollution)
Eco-epidemiology (emerging)	Relations within and between localized structures organized in a hierarchy of levels	Analysis of determinants and outcomes at different levels of organization using new information systems and biomedical techniques	Apply both information and biomedical technology to find leverage at efficacious levels

Adapted from Susser, M., & Susser, E. (1996a). Choosing a future for epidemiology: I. Eras and paradigms. *American Journal of Public Health, 86*(5), 668–673; and Susser, M., & Susser, E. (1996b). Choosing a future for epidemiology: II. From black box to Chinese boxes and eco-epidemiology. *American Journal of Public Health, 86*(5), 674–677.

CONCEPTS BASIC TO EPIDEMIOLOGY

The science of epidemiology draws on certain basic concepts and principles to analyze and understand patterns of occurrence among aggregate health conditions.

Host, Agent, and Environment Model

Through their early study of infectious diseases, epidemiologists began to consider disease states generally in terms of the *epidemiologic triad*, or the *host, agent, and environment model*. Interactions among these three elements explained infectious and other disease patterns.

Host

The **host** is a susceptible human or animal who harbors and nourishes a disease-causing agent. Many physical, psychological, and lifestyle factors influence the host's susceptibility and response to an agent. Physical factors include age, sex, race, and genetic influences on the host's vulnerability or resistance. Psychological factors, such as outlook and response to stress, can strongly influence host susceptibility. Lifestyle factors also play a major role. Diet, exercise, sleep patterns, and healthy or unhealthy habits all contribute to either increased or decreased vulnerability to the disease-causing agent.

The concept of resistance is important for public health nursing practice. People sometimes have an ability to resist pathogens. This is called *inherent resistance*. Typically, these people have inherited or acquired characteristics, such as the various factors mentioned earlier, that make them less vulnerable. People who maintain a healthful lifestyle may not contract influenza even if exposed to the flu virus. Resistance can be promoted through preventive interventions that support a healthful lifestyle. For example, one study found that regular use of a multivitamin in the periconceptual period reduced the risk of preeclampsia by 45% ($n = 1,835$); but only in those women who were not overweight (Bodnar, Tang, Ness, et al., 2006). If confirmed by additional studies, multivitamin use could be recommended as a preventive measure for those women planning pregnancies. These findings can also be viewed as supporting efforts to reduce overweight and obesity in women of child-bearing age.

Agent

An **agent** is a factor that causes or contributes to a health problem or condition. Causative agents can be factors that are present (e.g., bacteria that cause tuberculosis, rocks on a mountain road that contribute to an automobile crash) or factors that are lacking (e.g., a low serum iron level that causes anemia or the lack of seat belt use that contributes to the extent of injury during an automobile crash).

Agents vary considerably and include five types: biologic, chemical, nutrient, physical, and psychological. Biologic agents include bacteria, viruses, fungi, protozoa, worms, and insects. Some biologic agents are infectious, such as influenza virus or HIV. Chemical agents may be in the form of liquids, solids, gases, dusts, or fumes. Examples are poisonous sprays used on garden pests and industrial chemical wastes. The degree of toxicity of the chemical agent influences its impact on health. Nutrient agents include essential dietary components that can produce illness conditions if they are deficient or are taken in excess. For example, a deficiency of niacin can cause pellagra, and too much vitamin A can be toxic. Physical agents include anything mechanical (e.g., chainsaw, automobile), material (rock slide), atmospheric (ultraviolet radiation), geologic (earthquake), or genetically transmitted that causes injury to humans. The shape, size, and force of physical agents influence the degree of harm to the host. Psychological agents are events that produce stress leading to health problems.

Agents may also be classified as infectious or noninfectious. Infectious agents cause communicable diseases, such as AIDS or tuberculosis—that is, the disease can be spread from one person to another. Certain characteristics of infectious agents are important for community health nurses to understand. Extent of *exposure* to the agent, the agent's *pathogenicity* (capacity to cause disease in the host), its *infectivity* (capacity to enter the host and multiply), its virulence (severity of disease), *toxigenicity* (capacity to produce a toxin or poison), *resistance* (ability of the agent to survive environmental conditions), *antigenicity* (ability to induce an antibody response in the host) (Friis & Sellers, 2004), and its structure and chemical composition all influence the effect of the agent on the host. (Chapter 8 examines the subject of communicable disease in greater depth.) Noninfectious agents have similar characteristics in that their relative abilities to harm the host vary with type of agent and intensity and duration of exposure.

Environment

The **environment** refers to all the external factors surrounding the host that might influence vulnerability or resistance. The physical environment includes factors such as geography, climate and weather, safety of buildings, water and food supply, and presence of animals, plants, insects, and microorganisms that have the capacity to serve as reservoirs (storage sites for disease-causing agents) or vectors (carriers) for transmitting disease. The psychosocial environment refers to social, cultural, economic, and psychological influences and conditions that affect health, such as access to health care, cultural health practices, poverty, and work stressors, which can all contribute to disease or health.

Host, agent, and environment interact to cause a disease or health condition. For example, the agent responsible for Lyme disease is the spirochete *Borrelia burgdorferi*; humans of all ages are susceptible hosts, along with dogs, cattle, and horses. Ticks that feed on wild rodents and deer transfer the spirochete to human hosts after feeding on them for several hours. Environmental factors, such as working or playing in tick-infested areas, influence host vulnerability. The host, agent, and environment model, shown in Figure 7.1, offered the epidemiologists who first studied Lyme disease in 1982 a plan for intervention. As soon as the agent was identified, measures could be taken to keep the spirochete from infecting human hosts, such as wearing protective clothing or tick repellent in tick-infested areas and promptly removing the attached ticks (Heymann, 2004).

In another example, the West Nile virus, which was widespread in Africa and the Middle East, arrived in the United States in 1999 and began to spread (Heymann,

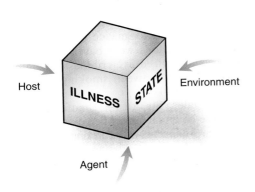

FIGURE 7.1 Epidemiologic triad. Epidemiologists study the causal agent, the susceptible host, and environmental factors that contribute to an illness, an injury, or a wellness state. Intervention may focus on any of these three to prevent the spread of illness or to improve health in a population.

2004). The first reported cases were in New York, where 45 people were infected. In that year, the region experienced a total of 59 hospitalized cases of West Nile disease, resulting in seven deaths. By 2006, West Nile virus had been reported in 43 states and the District of Columbia, with a total of 4,269 cases and 177 deaths (Centers for Disease Control and Prevention [CDC], 2007b). As of mid-2007, only Alaska and Hawaii had no confirmed presence of the virus in humans, birds, animals, or mosquitoes.

The encephalitis-causing disease is transmitted by a mosquito bite. The virus survives winter in the body of the adult *Culex* mosquito (Heymann, 2004). The infected mosquito bites a bird and infects it. Other mosquitoes bite the bird and in turn become infected. The infected mosquitoes pass the virus on to birds, humans, or horses. Many dead birds in an area may mean that the virus is circulating between the bird and mosquito populations and should be reported. In humans and animals with intact immune systems, the virus is usually destroyed in the bloodstream. If the virus survives in the body, it can infect membranes around the spinal cord and brain and cause encephalitis. Those at highest risk are the elderly, children, and people with impaired immune systems.

Prevention includes avoiding mosquito bites by applying insect repellent containing N,N-diethyl-meta-toluamide (DEET) when outdoors; wearing long-sleeved clothing and long pants treated with DEET-containing repellents; staying indoors at dawn, dusk, and in the early evening; eliminating standing water sources where mosquitoes lay their eggs; reporting dead birds; and ensuring that an organized mosquito control program exists in the area (CDC, 2004a). Using the model in Figure 7.1, can you categorize each of these six recommendations by their target (host, agent, or environment)?

Causality

Causality refers to the relationship between a cause and its effect. A purpose of epidemiologic study has been to discover causal relationships to understand why conditions develop and offer effective prevention and protection. As scientific knowledge of health and disease has expanded, epidemiology has changed its view of causality. The following section discusses some of those changes in thinking that began in the 1960s and are continually refined to this day.

Chain of Causation

As the scientific community's thinking about disease causation and the tripartite model (host-agent-environment) grew more complex, epidemiologists began to use the idea of a chain of causation (Fig. 7.2). The chain begins by identifying the reservoir (i.e., where the causal agent can live and multiply). With plague, that reservoir may be other humans, rats, squirrels, and a few other animals. With malaria, infected humans are the major reservoir for the parasitic

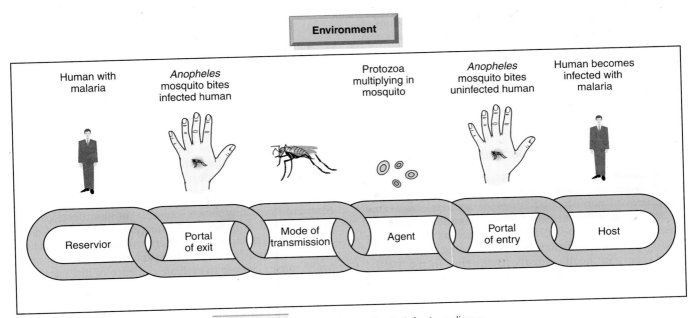

FIGURE 7.2 Chain of causation in infectious disease.

agents, although certain nonhuman primates also act as reservoirs (Heymann, 2004). Next, the agent must have a portal of exit from the reservoir, as well as some mode of transmission. For example, the bite of an *Anopheles* mosquito provides a portal of exit for the malaria parasites, which spend part of their life cycle in the mosquito's body; the mosquito in this case is the mode of transmission. The next link in the chain of causation is the agent itself. Malaria, for example, actually consists of four distinct diseases caused by four kinds of microscopic protozoa (Heymann, 2004). The next link is the portal of entry. In the case of malaria, the mosquito bite provides a portal of exit as well as a portal of entry into the human host.

The box surrounding the chain of causation in Figure 7.2 represents the environment, which can have a profound influence at almost any point along the chain. Consider the impact of environmental factors on the 1934–1935 malaria epidemic in Ceylon (an island country in the Indian Ocean off southern India). Historically, malaria occurred frequently in the dry northern area, where sparse vegetation allowed pools of water to be exposed to the sun, providing excellent breeding grounds for the *Anopheles* mosquito. In contrast, the more populous southwestern area usually had heavy monsoon rains and was relatively free from malaria. In 1934, however, a severe drought changed this environment drastically; throughout Ceylon, rivers almost dried up, leaving stagnant pools of water for mosquito breeding. Widespread crop failure caused the population to become badly undernourished, which added to conditions that would foster a malaria epidemic. The epidemic occurred in October 1934, affecting 2 to 3 million people and causing 80,000 deaths. The environment must certainly be seen as a major part of this causal chain (Burnet, 1962).

Another tragic example of the influence of environment on the causal chain occurred in the African country of Rwanda in July of 1994. Civil war caused a large percentage of the population to flee in the face of mass genocide of "unprecedented swiftness" that left up to 800,000 dead (U.S. Department of State, 2007). Hundreds of thousands of people filled refugee camps to overflowing, with over 50,000 deaths in the first month alone (Connolly et al., 2004). Conditions of squalor and poor sanitation led to contaminated water and resulted in a large-scale epidemic of cholera, a severe form of bacterial dysentery. Relief workers had limited supplies of intravenous or oral rehydration solutions and could do little to help. Thousands lost their lives. The unstable political environment, unsanitary conditions, scarcity of clean water, and malnourishment were all part of the causal chain.

Causation in Noninfectious Disease

With the availability of vaccines and antibiotics in the United States and the developed world, attention shifted to the causes of noninfectious diseases such as cancer and diabetes. A new causal paradigm was clearly needed. The linear thinking embodied in models such as the *chain of causation* were insufficient in understanding the causes of these emerging health threats. Beginning in the 1950s, there was a growing interest in the role smoking played in the development of lung cancer. In 1964, the publication of *Smoking and Health: Report of the Advisory Committee to the Surgeon General of the Public Health Service* con-

cluded that smoking caused lung and laryngeal cancer in men (U.S. Public Health Service [USPHS], 1964). The Committee's conclusions were based on review of over 7,000 articles and utilized five criteria for judging the significance of the link between smoking and lung cancer (Friis & Sellers, 2004).

One year later, Sir Austin Bradford Hill proposed expanding those criteria to nine when evaluating the relationship between environmental exposure and potential health outcomes. Although these guidelines are often viewed as necessary for causal attribution, Hill stressed that they were a tool, not strict criteria (Legator & Morris, 2003). The elements added by Hill included biologic gradient, plausibility, experiment, and analogy. The criteria can be used with infectious disease, yet their significance lies with attributing cause in noninfectious disease. Each of the nine elements is summarized below (Aschengrau & Seage, 2008; Friis & Sellers, 2004):

1. *Strength of association:* This refers to the ratio of disease rates in those with and without the suspected causal factor. A strong association would be noted if disease rates are much higher in the group with the factor than in the group without it.
2. *Consistency:* An association is demonstrated in varying types of studies among diverse study groups (i.e., replication).
3. *Specificity:* A cause leads to one effect (not always the case in noninfectious diseases).
4. *Temporality:* Exposure to the suspected factor must precede the onset of disease (i.e., time order or time sequence).
5. *Biological gradient:* This relationship is demonstrated if, with increasing levels of exposure to the factor, there is a corresponding increase in occurrence of the disease (i.e., dose–response relationship).
6. *Plausibility:* The hypothesized cause makes sense based on current biologic or social models (i.e., it is possible).
7. *Coherence of explanation:* The hypothesized cause makes sense based on current knowledge about the natural history or biology of the disease (i.e., scientific knowledge).
8. *Experiment:* Experimental and nonexperimental studies support the association (e.g., reduced tobacco use in a population should lead to reduced lung cancer rates).
9. *Analogy:* Similarities between the association of interest and others (e.g., potential links to birth defects from new drugs is a concern since we already recognize this potential from the use of the drug thalidomide).

Based on the work of Hill and others, a basis was formed to critically assess causality in noninfectious diseases, as well as in new and emerging infectious diseases. The elements described by Hill are still utilized by epidemiologists and provide the fundamental principles community health nurses can use to evaluate evidence of disease causation in all types of published reports, both scientific and lay. In health education, these principles can be utilized to teach disease causation risk, especially when the evidence is not yet complete. For instance, a pregnant teen asks a nurse if

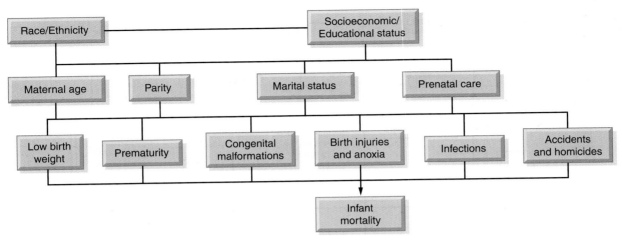

FIGURE 7.3   Web of causation for infant mortality, based on information available from birth and death certificates. From Anderson, E.T., & McFarlane, J. (2003). *Community as partner,* 4th ed. Philadelphia: Lippincott Williams & Wilkins, with permission.

she should drink diet soda while she is pregnant. The nurse can share with her that the evidence to date supports the safety of artificial sweeteners for most adults (experiment), but that it is probably not wise to drink diet soda while pregnant. When she asks why (since there isn't any reported risk), the nurse can respond that any chemical has the potential to cause harm (plausibility and analogy), and the effects on a growing fetus (biologic gradient) are often unknown until decades later (temporality and experiment).

Multiple Causation

As health care professionals began to understand the complexity of many of the infectious and noninfectious disease threats, they came to realize that causation was never completely straightforward. Even with long-recognized contagious diseases like cholera, the organism was only part of the equation. Factors such as availability of clean water, the number of trained nurses and doctors, the overall nutrition of the population, and even political upheaval could influence the spread of disease and the number who ultimately died. Causation was beginning to be viewed as multifactorial. Fortunately, with recognition of the complexity of each health threat, came multiple opportunities to find solutions. The following section discusses the complexity of causal factors on health outcomes and implications for reduced morbidity and mortality.

Web of Causation

In the 1960s, the concept of multiple causation emerged to explain the existence of health and illness states and to provide guiding principles for epidemiologic practice. A causal paradigm that gained attention was referred to as the *web of causation.* The implication was that intervention (or breaking of the web at any point nearest to the disease) could profoundly impact the development of that disease (Aschengrau & Seage, 2008). This was a significant shift in thinking about disease and health, positing that the combination of multiple factors was the deciding factor in the

development of poor outcomes. This refinement in causal thinking also provided opportunities for health care interventions at a variety of levels. Another common term used for this approach is *causal matrix.*

Utilizing the multicausal approach, Figure 7.3 depicts a causal matrix for infant mortality. Data from birth and death certificates were used to identify the complex interactions among multiple causal factors that produce a negative health condition leading to infant mortality. Another example (Fig. 7.4) shows a web of causation for automobile crashes. All of the numerous factors involved must be considered when diagramming a web of causation. Speed, faulty equipment, heavy traffic, confusing traffic patterns, road construction, poor visibility, weather conditions, driver inexperience, and drinking or drug use, in any combination, can cause an automobile crash.

All health conditions can be diagramed to depict a matrix of causation. A communicable disease with one clearly identified organism as the agent has the ability to be diagramed based on factors such as availability of emergency services (treatment), diagnostic skill of health professionals (early diagnosis), availability of medications and vaccines to treat the disease (reduced morbidity), and community communication networks (public awareness). Any of these factors could greatly influence the progression of disease within the community.

Association is a concept that is helpful in determining multiple causality. Events are said to be associated if they appear together more often than would be the case by chance alone (see Perspectives). Such events may include risk factors or other characteristics affecting disease or health states. Examples are the frequent association of cigarette smoking with lung cancer, obesity with heart disease, and severe prematurity with infant mortality. The study of associated factors suggests possible causality and points for intervention. Contemporary epidemiologists continue to explore new and more comprehensive ways of viewing health and illness. The associations among lifestyle, behavior, environment, and stress of all kinds and the ways in which they affect health states are gaining importance in epidemiology.

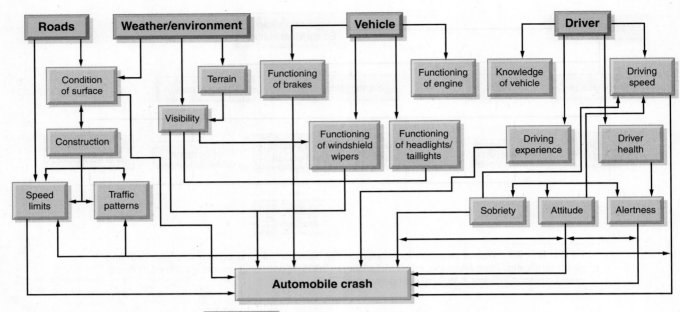

FIGURE 7.4 Web of causation for automobile crashes.

In the host, agent, and environment model, a shifting emphasis of investigation over time may be noted. Early epidemiologists worked to identify and manage the causative agent; the focus of concern was the disease state. The emphasis then shifted to the host: Who was susceptible? What characteristics led to susceptibility? Through immunization and health promotion, efforts were made to improve host resistance. Increasingly, however, public health workers came to realize the limitations imposed on individual control of health. Even individuals who are in the best of health cannot withstand toxic agents in the workplace—for example, nuclear wastes in the atmosphere from power plant accidents—or other debilitating conditions created by modern society. More and more, public health professionals are studying the environment and looking for methods to change conditions that contribute to illness.

Immunity

Immunity refers to a host's ability to resist a particular infectious disease–causing agent. This occurs when the body forms antibodies and lymphocytes that react with the foreign antigenic molecules and render them harmless. For public health nursing, this concept has significance in determining which individuals and groups are protected against disease and which may be vulnerable. Four types of immunity are important in community health: passive immunity, active immunity, cross-immunity, and herd immunity.

Passive Immunity

Passive immunity refers to short-term resistance that is acquired either naturally or artificially. Newborns, through maternal antibody transfer, have natural passive immunity that lasts up to 1 year for certain diseases (CDC, 2007a). This maternally provided protection seems to work best with measles, rubella, and tetanus, and less well with other

diseases (e.g., polio and pertussis). Artificial passive immunity is attained through inoculation with antibody products to provide temporary resistance. Examples of such products include immune globulin (hepatitis A and measles), hyperimmune globulins (hepatitis B, rabies, tetanus, and varicella), and hyperimmune serum (equine antitoxin for use with botulism and diphtheria). These products are used to boost a susceptible person's immunity, and administration must be repeated periodically to maintain immunity levels (CDC, 2007a).

Active Immunity

Active immunity is long-term and sometimes lifelong resistance that is acquired either naturally or artificially. Naturally acquired active immunity comes through host infection. That is, a person who contracts a disease often develops long-lasting antibodies that provide immunity against future exposures. Artificially acquired active immunity is attained through vaccine inoculation. Such vaccines are prepared from killed (inactivated) or live attenuated (weakened) organisms administered to artificially produce or increase immunity to a particular disease (CDC, 2007a). The concept of active immunity underlies public health immunization programs that have successfully kept polio, diphtheria, smallpox, and other major diseases under control worldwide.

Cross-immunity

Cross-immunity refers to a situation in which a person's immunity to one agent provides immunity to a related agent as well. The immunity can be either passive or active. Sometimes, infection with one disease, such as cowpox, gives immunity to a related disease, such as smallpox. The concept of cross-immunity has also been useful in the development and administration of vaccines. Inoculation with a vaccine

PERSPECTIVES
STUDENT VOICES

Vaccine Adverse Event Reporting System— Example of Epidemiological Surveillance

I graduated in 2006 and started working in the emergency department (ED) of our local hospital. All through school I knew the ED was exactly where I wanted to work. Just about every course I took brought me that much closer to my dream . . . with one exception—Public Health Nursing. It just didn't interest me—and it didn't seem to have much relevance to working as an ED nurse. Six months after I graduated, my view changed.

My community is pretty rural—we have a great hospital, but it's small and we don't have all the specialty areas available, such as pediatric surgeons. At about 0300, we had a 4-month-old come in a great deal of distress; vomiting and crying inconsolably. While I was interviewing the mother, she said he had been a very healthy baby up until about 8 hours ago and had even been seen by his pediatrician a few days earlier for his regular check-up. She handed me his immunization record as proof. We ended up airlifting the baby to the nearest children's hospital when it seemed likely that he had intussusception, which is a folding of the bowel on itself and pretty serious. After the child and the mother were gone, I realized that I still had the child's immunization record and hadn't yet looked at it either. I called the other hospital to tell them I had the immunization record and that I could fax over a copy. The nurse I spoke with asked me which immunizations the child had recently received. Thinking he just wanted to see if the child was up-to-date, I told him he just had a well-child visit a few days ago. He persisted and told me he needed to know the exact dates and which vaccines were given. As I read through the list, I realized I wasn't familiar with one of the vaccines and asked him what it was. He explained that it was the rotavirus vaccine and had been licensed about 10 months ago—adding that an earlier vaccine had been pulled off the market in 1999 due to an association with

intussusception. He had my attention! The nurse wanted to know if the lot numbers for the vaccines were on the record—and they were. I asked if he thought the child's condition was due to the vaccine—he didn't believe so, but that he would be making a VAERS report on the case once the physician confirmed the diagnosis and the lab's findings were back. I didn't know what this VAERS report was but thanked him and went to fax the immunization copy. I had a break coming up, so I went online to see what this report was. Turns out that VAERS stands for the *Vaccine Adverse Event Reporting System* and anyone (even parents) can make a report, if they think that a health condition might be the result of an immunization. The report can be made by phone or online at www.vaers.hhs.gov. The system monitors reports from all over the country to determine if there might be a problem with a particular vaccine. As I read more, I found out that the system is designed so that epidemiologists can look at the information and determine if there is a real association; they don't want to leave a vaccine on the market if it's potentially dangerous or pull vaccines off unnecessarily. The old vaccine for the rotavirus was pulled off the market after reports came in from VAERS and other sources. While I was sitting there taking this all in, I started recognizing that I had encountered two public health situations with just this one patient, and I had missed both of them. The first was assuming that because the child had a well-child check-up that he was up-to-date with his immunizations (I should have checked the record). The second was disease surveillance—if I had paid attention to the current recommendations for the rotavirus vaccine, I might have been alert to the possible connection with intussusception with the old vaccine and been aware of the VAERS system. Since that night, I have been following the reports on the vaccine's safety, and so far it looks like the association with intussusception is no more than would be expected in unvaccinated children—but I'll keep checking. I'm now the nurse that everyone comes to for information on vaccines, the need to make sure all the children we treat are up-to-date, and how to provide data to help monitor potential problems with vaccines. Who knew you could use public health nursing skills in an ED?

—Minerva G., RN/BSN (a.k.a. PHN)

made from one disease-causing organism can provide immunity to a related disease-causing organism. Field trials in Uganda and Papua, New Guinea and a study in India in the 1990s examined the administration of bacille Calmette-Guérin (BCG) vaccine, which is used to prevent tuberculosis, to people who had been exposed to Hansen disease (leprosy). The vaccine against *Mycobacterium tuberculosis* appeared to provide these individuals with a degree of cross-immunity to the related infectious agent, *Mycobacterium leprae,* and prevented their contracting disease (Heymann, 2004).

Herd Immunity

Herd immunity describes the immunity level that is present in a population group. A population with low herd immunity is one with few immune members; consequently, it is more susceptible to a particular disease. Nonimmune people are more likely to contract the disease and spread it throughout the group, placing the entire population at greater risk. Conversely, a population with high herd immunity is one in which the immune people in the group outnumber the susceptible people; consequently, the incidence of a particular disease is reduced (Friis & Sellers, 2004). The level of herd immunity may vary with diseases. For instance, a level of community immunity of between 85% and 90% may be necessary for rubella, but for diphtheria a level of 70% may be effective (Friis & Sellers, 2004). Mandatory preschool immunizations and required travel vaccinations are applications of the herd immunity concept.

Risk

To determine the chances that a disease or health problem will occur, epidemiologists are concerned with **risk**, or the probability that a disease or other unfavorable health condition will develop. For any given group of people, the risk of developing a health problem is directly influenced by their biology, environment, lifestyle, and system of health care (Dever, 1984; Lalonde, 1974). A person's inherited health capacity, the environment lived in, the person's lifestyle choices, and the quality and accessibility of the health care system either negatively or positively affect health, thereby increasing or decreasing the likelihood that a health problem will occur. Negative influences are called *risk factors*. For example, low-birth-weight babies (biology, environment, and system of health care) tend to be at greater risk for health problems, as are people who smoke cigarettes, have diets high in cholesterol, and are sedentary (lifestyle). The degree of risk is directly linked to susceptibility or vulnerability to a given health problem.

Epidemiologists study populations at risk. A *population at risk* is a collection of people among whom a health problem has the possibility of developing because certain influencing factors are present (e.g., exposure to HIV) or absent (e.g., lack of childhood immunizations, lack of specific vitamins in the diet), or because there are modifiable risk factors present (e.g., cardiovascular disease). A population at risk has a greater probability of developing a given health problem than other groups do. Epidemiologists measure this difference using the *relative risk ratio,* which statistically compares the disease occurrence in the population at risk with the occurrence of the same disease in people without that risk factor.

$$\text{Relative risk ratio} = \frac{\text{Incidence rate in exposed group}}{\text{Incidence rate in unexposed group}}$$

If the risk of acquiring the disease is the same regardless of exposure to the risk factor studied, the ratio will be 1:1, and the relative risk will be 1.0. A relative risk greater than 1.0 indicates that those with the risk factor have a greater likelihood of acquiring the disease than do those without it; for instance, a relative risk of 2.54 means that the exposed group is 2.54 times more likely to acquire the disease than the unexposed group. This statistic may be used, for example, to compare the incidence of heart disease among smokers (smoking is a risk factor) with the incidence among nonsmokers, assuming that all other factors are the same. The relative risk ratio assists in determining the most effective points for community health intervention in regard to particular health problems. It also provides a more easily understood method for explaining the risk of certain behaviors in the development of illness or injury to the public.

Natural History of a Disease or Health Condition

Any disease or health condition follows a progression known as its **natural history**; this refers to events that occur before its development, during its course, and during its conclusion. This process involves the interactions among a susceptible host, the causative agent, and the environment. The natural progression of a disease occurs in four stages as they affect a population—susceptibility, preclinical (subclinical) disease, clinical disease, and resolution (Fig. 7.5). The last stage, resolution, includes recovery, disability, or death (Gerstman, 2003).

Susceptibility Stage

The first stage is *susceptibility.* During this state, the disease is not present and individuals have not been exposed. However,

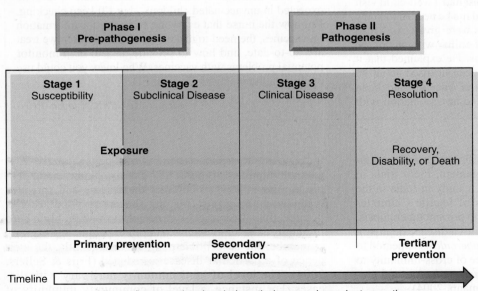

FIGURE 7.5 Natural history stages of a disease or health condition. Adapted From: Gerstman, B.B. (2003). *Epidemiology kept simple: An introduction to traditional and modern epidemiology,* 2nd ed. Hoboken, NJ: Wiley-Liss, Inc.

host and environmental factors could very likely influence people's susceptibility to a causative agent and lead to development of the disease. For example, college students with poor eating habits and fatigue from lack of sleep during final examinations present risk factors that promote the occurrence of the common cold. "If exposure to an agent occurs at this time, a response will take place. Initial responses reflect the normal adaptation response of the cell or functional system (e.g., the immune system). If these adaptation responses are successful, then no disease occurs and the process is arrested" (Valanis, 1999, p. 22). In 1994, the overcrowded conditions and poor sanitation of Rwandan refugee camps in Africa, described earlier, as well as refugees' stress, fatigue, and malnutrition, made them extremely vulnerable to contracting cholera and other diseases. However, in a later tragedy in Kosovo in 1999, the thousands of refugees fleeing for their lives from Yugoslavian Serbs were housed in refugee border camps with adequate supplies and services, and many found temporary or permanent refuge in other countries, including the United States. They endured a shorter period of stress and fatigue with better nutrition than the refugees in Rwanda; as a result, malnutrition was not as rampant. Because improved conditions in refugee camps eliminated major outbreaks of cholera and other diseases, susceptibility to disease in the group as a whole was reduced. Nevertheless, the psychological trauma from the attempts at "ethnic cleansing" of the people in Kosovo remained an existing health problem for years.

Subclinical Disease Stage

The stage of *subclinical disease* begins when individuals have been exposed to a disease but are as yet asymptomatic. It is followed by an *incubation period*, during which the organism multiplies to sufficient numbers to produce a host reaction and clinical symptoms. Vulnerable children who have been exposed to chickenpox (varicella) but do not yet display signs of fever or lesions are in this stage. For diseases caused by infectious agents, the incubation period is relatively short, hours to months. One noteworthy exception to this is infection with HIV, which has an incubation period of 1–3 months, with progression to AIDS (Acquired Immunodeficiency Syndrome) from 1 year to 15 years or longer (Heymann, 2004). In other conditions caused by noninfectious agents, the time from exposure to onset of symptoms, known as the *induction period* or *latency period*, is often years to decades. For example, children exposed to radiation may have a 5-year latency period for leukemia. Lung cancer caused by exposure to asbestos may have a latency period of 40 years between exposure and detection of the disease.

Clinical Disease Stage

During the *clinical disease stage*, signs and symptoms of the disease or condition develop. In the early phase of this period, the signs may be evident only through laboratory test findings, such as tubercular lesions on radiographs or premalignant cervical changes evident on Papanicolaou (Pap) smears. Later in this stage, acute symptoms are clearly visible, as in the case of widespread enterocolitis in a salmonellosis (food poisoning) outbreak. In this early clinical stage or early discernible lesions stage, evidence of the disease or condition is present and diagnosis occurs.

Resolution Stage

In the *resolution stage*, the disease or health condition causes sufficient anatomic or functional changes to produce recognizable signs and symptoms. Disease severity may vary from mild to severe. The disease may conclude with a return to health, a residual or chronic form of the disease with some disabling limitations, or death. This can also be called the *advanced disease stage*, because the disease or condition has completed its course.

Community health nurses can intervene at any point during these four stages to delay, arrest, or prevent the progression of the disease or condition. Primary, secondary, and tertiary prevention can be applied to each of the stages (see Levels of Prevention Pyramid).

Epidemiology of Wellness

The public health science of epidemiology has traditionally studied the occurrence of disease and health problems. Because of their devastating effect on the health of populations, infectious diseases such as plague, cholera, and AIDS, as well as chronic illnesses such as heart disease or cancer, and fatal or debilitating injuries all require a continued epidemiologic focus. Nonetheless, the need to examine the epidemiology of wellness grows increasingly urgent, for if we continually examine and uncover new health promotion practices and encourage them, we can focus on wellness at the ideal primary level of prevention.

Epidemiology has moved from concentrating only on illness to examining how host, agent, and environment are involved in wellness at various levels. In response to an escalating need for improved methods of health planning and health policy analysis, epidemiology has developed more holistic models of health (Dever, 1984, 1991). These evolving epidemiologic models are organized around four attributes that influence health: (1) the physical, social, and psychological environment; (2) lifestyle with its self-created risks; (3) human biology and genetic influences; and (4) the system of health care organization. In the United States, *Healthy People 2010* (USDHHS, 2000) and greater recognition of the importance and cost-effectiveness of illness prevention and health promotion are driving new efforts to develop policy and research initiatives for public health (see Display 7.1).

Wellness models that at first focused on individual behavior now include approaches that encompass aggregates. A variety of wellness models can be found for groups of seniors (see Chapter 24), in occupational health settings (see Chapter 31), at innovative schools where wellness programs for children and teens are initiated (see Chapter 22), and throughout the services provided for beginning and growing families (see Chapter 21). Programs designed for aggregates focus on a wellness approach to growth and development. Examples include programs for pregnant teens and for infant and child development (e.g., Healthy Start, Head Start) that are funded by state and federal monies. Societal changes, such as the aging population, the communication revolution, the global economy, environmental threats, technology development, and the holism and wellness movements, are driving these new approaches.

The four stages of the natural history of disease can apply to an understanding of any health condition, including wellness states. In stage one, *susceptibility*, people can become amenable

LEVELS OF PREVENTION PYRAMID

SITUATION: Apply the levels of prevention during the four stages of the natural history of a disease to eradicate or reduce risk factors (examples of possible conditions provided).

GOAL: Using the three levels of prevention negative health conditions are avoided, or promptly diagnosed and treated, and the fullest possible potential is restored.

Tertiary Prevention

Rehabilitation	Primary Prevention	
	Health Promotion & Education	Health Protection
• Reduce the extent and severity of a health problem to minimize disability • Restore or preserve function	• Training for employment – homeless population • Group treatment and rehabilitation – adolescent drug users • Food, shelter, rest/sleep, exercise	• Health services • Immunizations as needed

Secondary Prevention

Early Diagnosis	Prompt Treatment
The third stage in the natural history of disease, the early pathogenesis or onset stage: • Screening programs – breast and testicular cancer, vision and hearing loss, hypertension, tuberculosis, diabetes	• Initiate prompt treatment • Arrest progression • Prevent associated disability

Primary Prevention

Health Promotion & Education	Health Protection
May include • Nutrition counseling – diabetes • Sex education – pregnancy• • Smoking cessation – lung cancer	May include • Improved housing and sanitation – waterborne diseases • Immunizations – communicable diseases • Removal of environmental hazards – accidents

to healthier practices and improved health system organization. In stage two, *subclinical*, a community can learn about these health-promoting behaviors. Stage three, *clinical disease stage*, could be a period of trying out the beneficial policies and activities, and stage four, *resolution*, could encompass full adoption and a higher level of well-being for the community. This approach has important implications for preventive and health-promotion practices in community health nursing.

Community health nursing can play a primary role in the investigation and identification of factors that not only prevent illness but also promote health. This means sharpening skills in epidemiologic research to uncover the factors

that contribute to a full measure of healthful living. The time for an epidemiology of wellness has come.

Causal Relationships

One of the main challenges to epidemiology is to identify causal relationships in disease and health conditions in populations. As was previously suggested, the assessment of causality in human health is difficult at best; no single study is adequate to establish causality. Causal inference is based on consistent results obtained from many studies. Frequently, the accumulation of evidence begins with a clinical

---

DISPLAY 7.1 **HEALTHY PEOPLE 2010 & MIDCOURSE REVIEW—EPIDEMIOLOGICAL FOCUS (OBJECTIVE SHORT TITLES AND OBJECTIVES)**

Data & Information Systems

23-2. *Public Access to Information and Surveillance Data*
(Developmental) Increase the proportion of Federal, Tribal, State, and local health agencies that have made information available for internal or external public use in the past year based on health indicators related to *Healthy People 2010* objectives.

23-3. *Use of Geocoding in Health Data Systems*
Increase the proportion of major national health data systems that use geocoding to promote nationwide use of geographic information systems (GIS).

23-4. *Data for All Population Groups*
Increase the proportion of population-based Healthy People 2010 objectives for which national data are available for all population groups identified for the objective.

23-6. *National Tracking of Healthy People 2010 Objectives*
Increase the proportion of Healthy People 2010 objectives that are tracked regularly at the national level.

23-7. *Timely Release of Data on Objectives*
Increase the proportion of Healthy People 2010 objectives for which national data are released within 1 year of the end of data collection.

Public Health Organizations

23-14. *Access to Epidemiology Services*
Increase the proportion of Tribal, State, and local public health agencies that provide or assure comprehensive epidemiology services to support essential public health services.

Prevention Research

23-17. *Population-based Prevention Research*
(Developmental) Increase the proportion of Federal, Tribal, State, and local health agencies that conduct or collaborate on population-based prevention research.

Sources:
U.S. Department of Health and Human Services. (2000). *Healthy People 2010: Understanding and improving health* (2nd ed.) Washington, DC: U.S. Government Printing Office.
 U.S. Department of Health and Human Services. (2006). *Healthy People 2010: Midcourse review.* Washington, DC: U.S. Government Printing Office.
 Note: Objectives 23-1; 23-5; & 23-16 were removed at midcourse and were not included in this list.

---

observation or an educated guess that a certain factor may be causally related to a health problem.

A **cross-sectional study** (which explores a health condition's relation to other variables in a specified population at a specific point in time) can show that the factor and the problem coexist. For example, one study compared the incidence of gonorrhea in a 55-block area in urban New Orleans with a "broken window index," which measured housing quality, abandoned cars, graffiti, trash, and public school deterioration (Cohen et al., 2000). The broken window index predicted the variance for gonorrhea rates more accurately than did a poverty index measuring income, unemployment, and low education.

A **retrospective study** (which looks backward in time to find a causal relationship) allows a fairly quick assessment of whether an association exists. Looking back at the use of lead in interior paint in the United States, history shows that even though the particular dangers to children were documented in English-language literature as early as 1904, the U.S. lead industry did nothing to discourage the use of lead paint on interior walls and woodwork. In fact, some paint companies (e.g., Dutch Boy Paint) used children in their advertising through the 1920s (Markowitz & Rosner, 2000). Not until the 1950s did the industry adopt a voluntary standard limiting the amount of lead in interior paints, and then only under increasing pressure. Not until 1978 was interior lead paint prohibited.

A **prospective study** (which looks forward in time to find a causal relationship) is crucial to ensure that the presumed causal factor actually precedes the onset of the health problem. The prospective approach is concerned with current information and provides a direct measure of the variables in

question. For example, the U.S. Nurses Health Study provided an opportunity for a prospective analysis of the association between night shift work and sleep deprivation and the risk of developing Parkinson disease. In a sample of nearly 85,000 registered nurses, those with 15 or more years of night shift work had a 50% lower risk of developing the disease than those nurses who never worked the night shift. Increased sleep duration was positively associated with disease risk. The data suggest one of two options: that night shift work is protective against the development of Parkinson disease or that low tolerance for night shift work is an indicator of the disease (Chen, Schernhammer, Schwarzschild, & Ascherio, 2006). Studies such as these provide a mechanism to evaluate a variety of factors that precede the development of disease and then assess issues of association and ultimately causation.

Finally, if ethically possible, an **experimental study** (in which the investigator controls or changes factors suspected of causing the condition and observes results) is used to confirm the associations obtained from observational studies (in which the investigator merely observes data or people without controlling or changing any factors). It often requires many years to accumulate enough evidence to suggest a causal relationship.

Epidemiologically, a causal relationship may be said to exist if two major conditions are met: the factor of interest (causal agent) is shown to increase the probability of occurrence of the disease or condition as observed in many studies in different populations, and evidence suggests that a reduction in the factor decreases the frequency of the given disease. The synthesis of data begins by selecting as many of the various types of epidemiologic studies of the problem as possible. After those studies that are not methodologically sound are discarded, the studies are reviewed. The better the data meet the criteria outlined by Hill (discussed earlier), the more likely it is that the factor of interest is one of several causes of the disease (strength of association, consistency, specificity, time sequence, biologic gradient, plausibility, coherence, experiment, and analogy).

The goal of any epidemiologic investigation is to identify causal mechanisms that meet these nine criteria and to develop measures for preventing illness and promoting health. The community health nurse may need to gather new data for this type of investigation, but pertinent existing data should be thoroughly examined first. This type of information can be obtained by the community health nurse from a variety of sources, which are discussed in the next section.

SOURCES OF INFORMATION FOR EPIDEMIOLOGIC STUDY

Epidemiologic investigators may draw data from any of three major sources: existing data, informal investigations, and scientific studies. The public health nurse will find all three sources useful in efforts to improve the health of aggregates.

Existing Data

A variety of information is available nationally, by state, and by section, such as county, region, or urbanized area. This information includes vital statistics, census data, and morbidity statistics on certain communicable or infectious diseases. Local health departments often can provide these data on request. Public health nurses seeking information on communities may find local health system agencies helpful. These agencies collect health information for groups of counties within states and interact with health planning authorities at the state level. They have access to many types of information and can give advice on specific problems.

Vital Statistics

Vital statistics refers to the information gathered from ongoing registration of births, deaths, adoptions, divorces, and marriages. Certification of births, deaths, and fetal deaths are the most useful vital statistics in epidemiologic studies. The community health nurse can obtain blank copies of a state's birth and death certificates to become familiar with the information contained in each (Displays 7.2 and 7.3). Much more information is recorded than the fact and cause of death on the death certificate. Birth certificates also can provide helpful information (e.g., weight of the infant, amount of prenatal care received by the mother), which can be used to identify high-risk mothers and infants.

Sources for vital statistical information include state websites on the Internet, local and state health departments, city halls, and county halls of records (see list of Internet resources at the end of this chapter). Statistics regarding general morbidity and mortality for specific states are located in the aggregate from the Centers for Disease Control and Prevention (CDC) at the national level (National Center for Health Statistics). State statistics are obtained from state health departments, and county information (spe-

cific cities or census tracts) can be obtained from either the state or the county health department.

Census Data

Data from population censuses taken every 10 years in many countries are the main source of population statistics. This information can be a valuable assessment tool for the community health nurse who is taking part in health planning for aggregates. Population statistics can be analyzed by age, sex, race, ethnic background, type of occupation, income gradient, marital status, educational level, or other standards, such as housing quality. Analysis of population statistics can provide the community health nurse with a better understanding of the community and help identify specific areas that may warrant further epidemiologic investigation. Data from the U.S. Census Bureau is found on its website (see the Internet section at the end of this chapter) and is an easily accessed source of population-level data.

Reportable Diseases

Each state has developed laws or regulations that require health organizations and practitioners to report to their local health authority cases of certain communicable and infectious diseases that can be spread through the community (Heymann, 2004). This reporting enables the health department to take the most appropriate and efficient action. All states require that diseases subject to international quarantine regulations be reported immediately. However, many of these diseases (e.g. plague, cholera, yellow fever, and polio) are virtually unknown now in developed countries (World Health Organization [WHO], 2007). Health care professionals have not had experience identifying another reportable disease, smallpox, because no cases have been reported since 1977 (CDC, 2004b). In 1980, the World Health Organization (WHO) declared the global eradication of smallpox after more than 10 years of international effort. (Chapter 17 discusses the concern over the use of smallpox as a bioterrorism threat.) Numerous other diseases under surveillance by WHO (e.g., tuberculosis, malaria, viral influenza, and severe acute respiratory syndrome [SARS]) must also be reported (WHO, 2007). Other reportable diseases (numbering between 20 and 40 in each state) are usually classified according to the speed with which the health department should be notified. Some should be reported by phone or e-mail, others weekly by regular mail. They vary in potential severity from varicella (chickenpox) to rabies and include AIDS, encephalitis, meningitis, syphilis, and toxic shock syndrome. Community health nurses should obtain the list of reportable diseases from their local or state health department office. Following-up on occurrences of these diseases is a task frequently assigned to public health nurses working for local health departments. Chapter 8 includes an example of a Confidential Morbidity Report (CMR) used to report and track communicable diseases at the local, regional, and national level.

Disease Registries

Some areas or states have disease registries or rosters for conditions with major public health impact. Tuberculosis and rheumatic fever registries were more common when these

DISPLAY 7.2 **STANDARD BIRTH CERTIFICATE**

U.S. STANDARD CERTIFICATE OF LIVE BIRTH

LOCAL FILE NO.

BIRTH NUMBER:

CHILD

1. CHILD'S NAME (First, Middle, Last, Suffix)	2. TIME OF BIRTH (24 hr)	3. SEX	4. DATE OF BIRTH (Mo/Day/Yr)

5. FACILITY NAME (If not institution, give street and number)	6. CITY, TOWN, OR LOCATION OF BIRTH	7. COUNTY OF BIRTH

MOTHER

8a. MOTHER'S CURRENT LEGAL NAME (First, Middle, Last, Suffix)	8b. DATE OF BIRTH (Mo/Day/Yr)

8c. MOTHER'S NAME PRIOR TO FIRST MARRIAGE (First, Middle, Last, Suffix)	8d. BIRTHPLACE (State, Territory, or Foreign Country)

9a. RESIDENCE OF MOTHER-STATE	9b. COUNTY	9c. CITY, TOWN, OR LOCATION

9d. STREET AND NUMBER	9e. APT. NO.	9f. ZIP CODE	9g. INSIDE CITY LIMITS? ☐ Yes ☐ No

FATHER

10a. FATHER'S CURRENT LEGAL NAME (First, Middle, Last, Suffix)	10b. DATE OF BIRTH (Mo/Day/Yr)	10c. BIRTHPLACE (State, Territory, or Foreign Country)

CERTIFIER

11. CERTIFIER'S NAME: _____

TITLE: ☐ MD ☐ DO ☐ HOSPITAL ADMIN. ☐ CNM/CM ☐ OTHER MIDWIFE

☐ OTHER (Specify)_____

12. DATE CERTIFIED ____/____/____ MM DD YYYY	13. DATE FILED BY REGISTRAR ____/____/____ MM DD YYYY

INFORMATION FOR ADMINISTRATIVE USE

MOTHER

14. MOTHER'S MAILING ADDRESS: ☐ Same as residence, or: State: _____ City, Town, or Location: _____

Street & Number: _____   Apartment No.: _____   Zip Code: _____

15. MOTHER MARRIED? (At birth, conception, or any time between) ☐ Yes ☐ No
IF NO, HAS PATERNITY ACKNOWLEDGEMENT BEEN SIGNED IN THE HOSPITAL? ☐ Yes ☐ No

16. SOCIAL SECURITY NUMBER REQUESTED FOR CHILD? ☐ Yes ☐ No

17. FACILITY ID. (NPI)

18. MOTHER'S SOCIAL SECURITY NUMBER:

19. FATHER'S SOCIAL SECURITY NUMBER:

INFORMATION FOR MEDICAL AND HEALTH PURPOSES ONLY

MOTHER

20. MOTHER'S EDUCATION (Check the box that best describes the highest degree or level of school completed at the time of delivery)

☐ 8th grade or less

☐ 9th - 12th grade, no diploma

☐ High school graduate or GED completed

☐ Some college credit but no degree

☐ Associate degree (e.g., AA, AS)

☐ Bachelor's degree (e.g., BA, AB, BS)

☐ Master's degree (e.g., MA, MS, MEng, MEd, MSW, MBA)

☐ Doctorate (e.g., PhD, EdD) or Professional degree (e.g., MD, DDS, DVM, LLB, JD)

21. MOTHER OF HISPANIC ORIGIN? (Check the box that best describes whether the mother is Spanish/Hispanic/Latina. Check the "No" box if mother is not Spanish/Hispanic/Latina)

☐ No, not Spanish/Hispanic/Latina

☐ Yes, Mexican, Mexican American, Chicana

☐ Yes, Puerto Rican

☐ Yes, Cuban

☐ Yes, other Spanish/Hispanic/Latina

(Specify)_____

22. MOTHER'S RACE (Check one or more races to indicate what the mother considers herself to be)

☐ White
☐ Black or African American
☐ American Indian or Alaska Native
   (Name of the enrolled or principal tribe)_____
☐ Asian Indian
☐ Chinese
☐ Filipino
☐ Japanese
☐ Korean
☐ Vietnamese
☐ Other Asian (Specify)_____
☐ Native Hawaiian
☐ Guamanian or Chamorro
☐ Samoan
☐ Other Pacific Islander (Specify)_____
☐ Other (Specify)_____

FATHER

23. FATHER'S EDUCATION (Check the box that best describes the highest degree or level of school completed at the time of delivery)

☐ 8th grade or less

☐ 9th - 12th grade, no diploma

☐ High school graduate or GED completed

☐ Some college credit but no degree

☐ Associate degree (e.g., AA, AS)

☐ Bachelor's degree (e.g., BA, AB, BS)

☐ Master's degree (e.g., MA, MS, MEng, MEd, MSW, MBA)

☐ Doctorate (e.g., PhD, EdD) or Professional degree (e.g., MD, DDS, DVM, LLB, JD)

24. FATHER OF HISPANIC ORIGIN? (Check the box that best describes whether the father is Spanish/Hispanic/Latino. Check the "No" box if father is not Spanish/Hispanic/Latino)

☐ No, not Spanish/Hispanic/Latino

☐ Yes, Mexican, Mexican American, Chicano

☐ Yes, Puerto Rican

☐ Yes, Cuban

☐ Yes, other Spanish/Hispanic/Latino

(Specify)_____

25. FATHER'S RACE (Check one or more races to indicate what the father considers himself to be)

☐ White
☐ Black or African American
☐ American Indian or Alaska Native
   (Name of the enrolled or principal tribe)_____
☐ Asian Indian
☐ Chinese
☐ Filipino
☐ Japanese
☐ Korean
☐ Vietnamese
☐ Other Asian (Specify)_____
☐ Native Hawaiian
☐ Guamanian or Chamorro
☐ Samoan
☐ Other Pacific Islander (Specify)_____
☐ Other (Specify)_____

Mother's Name

Mother's Medical Record No.

26. PLACE WHERE BIRTH OCCURRED (Check one)
☐ Hospital
☐ Freestanding birthing center
☐ Home Birth: Planned to deliver at home? ☐ Yes ☐ No
☐ Clinic/Doctor's office
☐ Other (Specify)_____

27. ATTENDANT'S NAME, TITLE, AND NPI

NAME: _____ NPI:_____

TITLE: ☐ MD ☐ DO ☐ CNM/CM ☐ OTHER MIDWIFE
☐ OTHER (Specify)_____

28. MOTHER TRANSFERRED FOR MATERNAL MEDICAL OR FETAL INDICATIONS FOR DELIVERY? ☐ Yes ☐ No
IF YES, ENTER NAME OF FACILITY MOTHER TRANSFERRED FROM:

_____

REV. 11/2003

MOTHER

29a. DATE OF FIRST PRENATAL CARE VISIT
____ / ____ / _____   □ No Prenatal Care
MM   DD   YYYY

29b. DATE OF LAST PRENATAL CARE VISIT
____ / ____ / _____
MM   DD   YYYY

30. TOTAL NUMBER OF PRENATAL VISITS FOR THIS PREGNANCY
_____ (If none, enter "0".)

31. MOTHER'S HEIGHT
_____ (feet/inches)

32. MOTHER'S PREPREGNANCY WEIGHT
_____ (pounds)

33. MOTHER'S WEIGHT AT DELIVERY
_____ (pounds)

34. DID MOTHER GET WIC FOOD FOR HERSELF DURING THIS PREGNANCY? □ Yes □ No

35. NUMBER OF PREVIOUS LIVE BIRTHS (Do not include this child)

35a. Now Living	35b. Now Dead
Number _____	Number _____
□ None	□ None

36. NUMBER OF OTHER PREGNANCY OUTCOMES (spontaneous or induced losses or ectopic pregnancies)

36a. Other Outcomes
Number _____
□ None

37. CIGARETTE SMOKING BEFORE AND DURING PREGNANCY
For each time period, enter either the number of cigarettes or the number of packs of cigarettes smoked. IF NONE, ENTER "0".

Average number of cigarettes or packs of cigarettes smoked per day.

	# of cigarettes		# of packs
Three Months Before Pregnancy	_____	OR	_____
First Three Months of Pregnancy	_____	OR	_____
Second Three Months of Pregnancy	_____	OR	_____
Third Trimester of Pregnancy	_____	OR	_____

38. PRINCIPAL SOURCE OF PAYMENT FOR THIS DELIVERY
□ Private Insurance
□ Medicaid
□ Self-pay
□ Other (Specify) _____

35c. DATE OF LAST LIVE BIRTH
____ / _____
MM   YYYY

36b. DATE OF LAST OTHER PREGNANCY OUTCOME
____ / _____
MM   YYYY

39. DATE LAST NORMAL MENSES BEGAN
____ / ____ / _____
MM   DD   YYYY

40. MOTHER'S MEDICAL RECORD NUMBER

MEDICAL AND HEALTH INFORMATION

41. RISK FACTORS IN THIS PREGNANCY (Check all that apply)

Diabetes
□ Prepregnancy (Diagnosis prior to this pregnancy)
□ Gestational (Diagnosis in this pregnancy)

Hypertension
□ Prepregnancy (Chronic)
□ Gestational (PIH, preeclampsia)
□ Eclampsia

□ Previous preterm birth

□ Other previous poor pregnancy outcome (Includes perinatal death, small-for-gestational age/intrauterine growth restricted birth)

□ Pregnancy resulted from infertility treatment-If yes, check all that apply:
  □ Fertility-enhancing drugs, Artificial insemination or Intrauterine insemination
  □ Assisted reproductive technology (e.g., in vitro fertilization (IVF), gamete intrafallopian transfer (GIFT))

□ Mother had a previous cesarean delivery
  If yes, how many _____

□ None of the above

42. INFECTIONS PRESENT AND/OR TREATED DURING THIS PREGNANCY (Check all that apply)

□ Gonorrhea
□ Syphilis
□ Chlamydia
□ Hepatitis B
□ Hepatitis C
□ None of the above

43. OBSTETRIC PROCEDURES (Check all that apply)

□ Cervical cerclage
□ Tocolysis

External cephalic version:
□ Successful
□ Failed

□ None of the above

44. ONSET OF LABOR (Check all that apply)

□ Premature Rupture of the Membranes (prolonged, ∃12 hrs.)
□ Precipitous Labor (<3 hrs.)
□ Prolonged Labor (∃ 20 hrs.)
□ None of the above

45. CHARACTERISTICS OF LABOR AND DELIVERY (Check all that apply)

□ Induction of labor
□ Augmentation of labor
□ Non-vertex presentation
□ Steroids (glucocorticoids) for fetal lung maturation received by the mother prior to delivery
□ Antibiotics received by the mother during labor
□ Clinical chorioamnionitis diagnosed during labor or maternal temperature ≥38°C (100.4°F)
□ Moderate/heavy meconium staining of the amniotic fluid
□ Fetal intolerance of labor such that one or more of the following actions was taken: in-utero resuscitative measures, further fetal assessment, or operative delivery
□ Epidural or spinal anesthesia during labor
□ None of the above

46. METHOD OF DELIVERY

A. Was delivery with forceps attempted but unsuccessful?
□ Yes □ No

B. Was delivery with vacuum extraction attempted but unsuccessful?
□ Yes □ No

C. Fetal presentation at birth
□ Cephalic
□ Breech
□ Other

D. Final route and method of delivery (Check one)
□ Vaginal/Spontaneous
□ Vaginal/Forceps
□ Vaginal/Vacuum
□ Cesarean
  If cesarean, was a trial of labor attempted?
  □ Yes
  □ No

47. MATERNAL MORBIDITY (Check all that apply) (Complications associated with labor and delivery)

□ Maternal transfusion
□ Third or fourth degree perineal laceration
□ Ruptured uterus
□ Unplanned hysterectomy
□ Admission to intensive care unit
□ Unplanned operating room procedure following delivery
□ None of the above

NEWBORN INFORMATION

NEWBORN

48. NEWBORN MEDICAL RECORD NUMBER

49. BIRTHWEIGHT (grams preferred, specify unit)
9 grams   9 lb/oz

50. OBSTETRIC ESTIMATE OF GESTATION:
_____ (completed weeks)

51. APGAR SCORE:
Score at 5 minutes: _____
If 5 minute score is less than 6,
Score at 10 minutes: _____

52. PLURALITY - Single, Twin, Triplet, etc.
(Specify) _____

53. IF NOT SINGLE BIRTH - Born First, Second, Third, etc. (Specify) _____

54. ABNORMAL CONDITIONS OF THE NEWBORN (Check all that apply)

□ Assisted ventilation required immediately following delivery
□ Assisted ventilation required for more than six hours
□ NICU admission
□ Newborn given surfactant replacement therapy
□ Antibiotics received by the newborn for suspected neonatal sepsis
□ Seizure or serious neurologic dysfunction
□ Significant birth injury (skeletal fracture(s), peripheral nerve injury, and/or soft tissue/solid organ hemorrhage which requires intervention)

9 None of the above

55. CONGENITAL ANOMALIES OF THE NEWBORN (Check all that apply)

□ Anencephaly
□ Meningomyelocele/Spina bifida
□ Cyanotic congenital heart disease
□ Congenital diaphragmatic hernia
□ Omphalocele
□ Gastroschisis
□ Limb reduction defect (excluding congenital amputation and dwarfing syndromes)
□ Cleft Lip with or without Cleft Palate
□ Cleft Palate alone
□ Down Syndrome
  □ Karyotype confirmed
  □ Karyotype pending
□ Suspected chromosomal disorder
  □ Karyotype confirmed
  □ Karyotype pending
□ Hypospadias
□ None of the anomalies listed above

56. WAS INFANT TRANSFERRED WITHIN 24 HOURS OF DELIVERY? 9 Yes 9 No
IF YES, NAME OF FACILITY INFANT TRANSFERRED TO: _____

57. IS INFANT LIVING AT TIME OF REPORT?
□ Yes □ No □ Infant transferred, status unknown

58. IS THE INFANT BEING BREASTFED AT DISCHARGE?
□ Yes □ No

Mother's Name

Mother's Medical Record No.

Rev. 11/2003

NOTE: This recommended standard birth certificate is the result of an extensive evaluation process. Information on the process and resulting recommendations as well as plans for future activities is available on the Internet at: http://www.cdc.gov/nchs/vital_certs_rev.htm.

DISPLAY 7.3 STANDARD DEATH CERTIFICATE

U.S. STANDARD CERTIFICATE OF DEATH

TYPE/PRINT IN PERMANENT BLACK INK FOR INSTRUCTIONS SEE OTHER SIDE AND HANDBOOK

LOCAL FILE NUMBER

STATE FILE NUMBER

DECEDENT

1. DECEDENT'S NAME (First, Middle, Last)

2. SEX

3. DATE OF DEATH (Month, Day, Year)

4. SOCIAL SECURITY NUMBER

5a. AGE—Last Birthday (Years)

5b. UNDER 1 YEAR — Months | Days

5c. UNDER 1 DAY — Hours | Minutes

6. DATE OF BIRTH (Month, Day, Year)

7. BIRTHPLACE (City and State or Foreign Country)

8. WAS DECEDENT EVER IN U.S. ARMED FORCES? (Yes or no)

9a. PLACE OF DEATH (Check only one; see instructions on other side)
HOSPITAL: ☐ Inpatient ☐ ER/Outpatient ☐ DOA
OTHER: ☐ Nursing Home ☐ Residence ☐ Other (Specify)

9b. FACILITY NAME (If not institution, give street and number)

9c. CITY, TOWN, OR LOCATION OF DEATH

9d. COUNTY OF DEATH

10. MARITAL STATUS—Married, Never Married, Widowed, Divorced (Specify)

11. SURVIVING SPOUSE (If wife, give maiden name)

12a. DECEDENT'S USUAL OCCUPATION (Give kind of work done during most of working life. Do not use retired.)

12b. KIND OF BUSINESS/INDUSTRY

13a. RESIDENCE—STATE

13b. COUNTY

13c. CITY, TOWN, OR LOCATION

13d. STREET AND NUMBER

13e. INSIDE CITY LIMITS? (Yes or no)

13f. ZIP CODE

14. WAS DECEDENT OF HISPANIC ORIGIN? (Specify No or Yes—If yes, specify Cuban, Mexican, Puerto Rican, etc.) ☐ No ☐ Yes Specify:

15. RACE—American Indian, Black, White, etc. (Specify)

16. DECEDENT'S EDUCATION (Specify only highest grade completed)
Elementary/Secondary (0-12) | College (1-4 or 5+)

PARENTS

17. FATHER'S NAME (First, Middle, Last)

18. MOTHER'S NAME (First, Middle, Maiden Surname)

INFORMANT

19a. INFORMANT'S NAME (Type/Print)

19b. MAILING ADDRESS (Street and Number or Rural Route Number, City or Town, State, Zip Code)

DISPOSITION

20a. METHOD OF DISPOSITION
☐ Burial ☐ Cremation ☐ Removal from State
☐ Donation ☐ Other (Specify) _____

20b. PLACE OF DISPOSITION (Name of cemetery, crematory, or other place)

20c. LOCATION—City or Town, State

21a. SIGNATURE OF FUNERAL SERVICE LICENSEE OR PERSON ACTING AS SUCH

21b. LICENSE NUMBER (of Licensee)

22. NAME AND ADDRESS OF FACILITY

PRONOUNCING PHYSICIAN ONLY

Complete items 23a-c only when certifying physician is not available at time of death to certify cause of death.

23a. To the best of my knowledge, death occurred at the time, date, and place stated.
Signature and Title ▶

23b. LICENSE NUMBER

23c. DATE SIGNED (Month, Day, Year)

ITEMS 24-26 MUST BE COMPLETED BY PERSON WHO PRONOUNCES DEATH

24. TIME OF DEATH — M

25. DATE PRONOUNCED DEAD (Month, Day, Year)

26. WAS CASE REFERRED TO MEDICAL EXAMINER/CORONER? (Yes or no)

CAUSE OF DEATH

27. PART I. Enter the diseases, injuries, or complications that caused the death. Do not enter the mode of dying, such as cardiac or respiratory arrest, shock, or heart failure. List only one cause on each line.

Approximate Interval Between Onset and Death

IMMEDIATE CAUSE (Final disease or condition resulting in death) ▶
a. _____
DUE TO (OR AS A CONSEQUENCE OF):

Sequentially list conditions, if any, leading to immediate cause. Enter UNDERLYING CAUSE (Disease or injury that initiated events resulting in death) LAST
b. _____
DUE TO (OR AS A CONSEQUENCE OF):
c. _____
DUE TO (OR AS A CONSEQUENCE OF):
d.

PART II. Other significant conditions contributing to death but not resulting in the underlying cause given in Part I.

28a. WAS AN AUTOPSY PERFORMED? (Yes or no)

28b. WERE AUTOPSY FINDINGS AVAILABLE PRIOR TO COMPLETION OF CAUSE OF DEATH? (Yes or no)

29. MANNER OF DEATH
☐ Natural ☐ Pending Investigation
☐ Accident
☐ Suicide ☐ Could not be Determined
☐ Homicide

30a. DATE OF INJURY (Month, Day, Year)

30b. TIME OF INJURY — M

30c. INJURY AT WORK? (Yes or no)

30d. DESCRIBE HOW INJURY OCCURRED

30e. PLACE OF INJURY—At home, farm, street, factory, office building, etc. (Specify)

30f. LOCATION (Street and Number or Rural Route Number, City or Town, State)

CERTIFIER

31a. CERTIFIER (Check only one)
☐ CERTIFYING PHYSICIAN (Physician certifying cause of death when another physician has pronounced death and completed Item 23)
To the best of my knowledge, death occurred due to the cause(s) and manner as stated.
☐ PRONOUNCING AND CERTIFYING PHYSICIAN (Physician both pronouncing death and certifying to cause of death)
To the best of my knowledge, death occurred at the time, date, and place, and due to the cause(s) and manner as stated.
☐ MEDICAL EXAMINER/CORONER
On the basis of examination and/or investigation, in my opinion, death occurred at the time, date, and place, and due to the cause(s) and manner as stated.

31b. SIGNATURE AND TITLE OF CERTIFIER ▶

31c. LICENSE NUMBER

31d. DATE SIGNED (Month, Day, Year)

32. NAME AND ADDRESS OF PERSON WHO COMPLETED CAUSE OF DEATH (ITEM 27) (Type/Print)

REGISTRAR

33. REGISTRAR'S SIGNATURE ▶

34. DATE FILED (Month, Day, Year)

NAME OF DECEDENT: For use by physician or institution

SEE INSTRUCTIONS ON OTHER SIDE

SEE DEFINITION ON OTHER SIDE

SEE INSTRUCTIONS ON OTHER SIDE

SEE DEFINITION ON OTHER SIDE

DEPARTMENT OF HEALTH AND HUMAN SERVICES – PUBLIC HEALTH SERVICE – NATIONAL CENTER FOR HEALTH STATISTICS – 1989 REVISION

PHS-T-003

diseases occurred more frequently. Cancer registries provide useful incidence, prevalence, and survival data, and assist the community health nurse in monitoring cancer patterns within a community. Community health nurses can access these registries through state health department websites. At the federal level, the Agency for Toxic Substances and Disease Registry (ATSDR, n.d.) maintains three registries of major public concern: the World Trade Center Health Registry (comprehensive and confidential health survey of those directly exposed to fallout and debris on Sept. 11, 2001), the Tremolite Asbestos Registry (asbestos exposure in Libby, Montana), and the National Exposure Registry (listing of persons exposed to certain hazardous substances).

Environmental Monitoring

State governments, through health departments or other agencies, now monitor health hazards found in the environment. Pesticides, industrial wastes, radioactive or nuclear materials, chemical additives in foods, and medicinal drugs have joined the list of pollutants (see Chapter 9 for a detailed discussion). Concerned community members and leaders view these as risk factors that affect health at both community and individual levels. Public health nurses can also obtain data from federal agencies such as the Food and Drug Administration (FDA), the Consumer Product Safety Commission, the Environmental Protection Agency (EPA), and, as previously mentioned, the ATSDR.

National Center for Health Statistics Health Surveys

The National Center for Health Statistics (NCHS) furnishes valuable health prevalence data from surveys of Americans. Published data are also frequently available for regions. The National Health Interview Survey (formerly known as National Health Survey) was established by Congress in 1956 and provides a continual source of information about the health status and needs of the entire nation (NCHS, 2007a). The National Health Interview Survey includes interviews from approximately 43,000 households each year and provides information about the health status and needs of the entire

country (NCHS, 2007a). The National Nursing Home Survey primarily samples institutional records of hospitals and nursing homes; it provides information on those who are using these services, along with diagnoses and other characteristics (NCHS, 2007b). The National Health and Nutrition Examination Survey (NHANES) reports physical measurements on smaller samples of the population and augments the information provided by interviews. It also provides prevalence information on injuries, diseases, and disabilities that appear frequently in the population. The National Survey of Family Growth (NSFG) focuses on fertility and family planning as well as other aspects of family health (NCHS, 2007b). Other studies investigate vital statistics events and characteristics of ambulatory patients in physicians' community practices.

Each of these nationally sponsored efforts suggest ways in which community health nurses can examine health problems or concerns affecting their communities (see From the Case Files). Interviews, physical examinations of subsets of community members, and surveillance of institutions, clinics, and private physicians' practices can be carried out locally after needs are identified and funds made available. Other sources may be found in data kept routinely but not centrally on the health problems of workers in local industries or the health problems of schoolchildren; a key issue for many community health nurses. Existing epidemiologic data can be used to plan parent education programs, health promotion among students, and almost any other type of service.

Another service of the CDC is its important publication, the *Mortality and Morbidity Weekly Report (MMWR)*. This publication presents weekly summaries of disease and death data trends for the nation. It includes reports on outbreaks or occurrences of diseases in specific regions of the country and international trends in disease occurrences that may affect the U.S. population. Most health departments subscribe to this publication, which provides important information both for epidemiologists and community health nurses.

Informal Observational Studies

A second information source in epidemiologic study is informal observation and description. Almost any client group encountered by the community health nurse can trigger such

From the Case Files

I am one of only four Public Health Nurses in our county—which is not many considering that our service area is very large, very rural, and very poor. Before I came, which was about 10 years ago, they had at least 10 nurses, and the population was maybe half of what it is now. We have growing numbers of residents with tuberculosis (TB), high teenage pregnancy, too many low-birth-weight babies, and to top it off, many of our residents lack health insurance. The county is in a budget crisis (again), and public health is high on the list for further reductions. I have been asked to speak at the next county supervisors meeting about what Public Health Nurses do and basically fight to keep us in the budget. I don't have much time to pull together information to give them, and will only have about 15 minutes for the presentation. They are all business owners, so I know they will appreciate data. I know other counties have all their morbidity and mortality figures online, but not here. Where to even start?

In preparing for this presentation, what specific types of data would you recommend to this nurse? What would be the sources of this data? Are those sources from local, state, or national resources? How could Healthy People 2010 and the Midcourse Review help frame this presentation?

a study. If, for example, the nurse encounters an abused child at a clinic, a study of the clinic's records to screen for additional possible instances of child abuse and neglect could lead to more case findings. If several cases of diabetes come to the attention of a nurse serving on a Navajo reservation, a widespread problem might come to light through informal inquiries about the incidence and age at onset of the disease among this Native American population. In a study of culture, sexuality, and women's agency in the prevention of HIV/AIDS, two researchers explored the awareness among women in southern Africa of the HIV epidemic and methods they might use to protect themselves from the virus. Interviews and informal field observations were carried out over a 7-year period at five sites "that were selected to reflect urban and rural experiences, various populations, and economic and political opportunities for women at different historical moments over the course of the HIV epidemic" (Susser & Stein, 2000, p. 1042). The findings indicated that most women saw themselves as active participants in the search for a way to protect themselves in sexual situations and were not helpless victims. At all sites over the 7 years, women desired to control their own bodies and felt they had the right to use the female condom. However, political and economic concerns, combined with historically powerful patterns of gender discrimination and neglect of women's sexuality, were considered to be the main barriers to the development and distribution of methods that women could control. Collecting such information and complementing it with existing data about a population served by a community health nurse could lead to improved women's health promotion practices to prevent HIV/AIDS in the United States. Informal observational study often raises questions and suggests hypotheses that form the basis for designing larger-scale epidemiologic investigations, such as this study in Africa.

Scientific Studies

The third source of information used in epidemiologic inquiry involves carefully designed scientific studies. The nursing profession has recognized the need to develop a systematic body of knowledge on which to base nursing practice. Already, systematic research is becoming an accepted part of the community health nurse's role. Findings from epidemiologic studies conducted by or involving nurses are appearing more frequently in the literature. For example, concern about testicular cancer and the patterns of testicular self-examination (TSE) among young adult men was the impetus for a nurse to conduct a study between 1999 and 2001 among 191 men attending occupational health fairs in the American Midwest (Wynd, 2002). The nurse learned that 64% rarely or never performed TSE and 36% practiced TSE monthly or every few months. Those who infrequently performed TSE more often were African American or Hispanic and had less than a college education. Factors associated with infrequent TSE practice included less satisfaction with job assignment and with life in general; greater worries interfering with daily life; more serious family problems involving spouse, children, or parents; and fewer people to turn to for support. In another study, concern regarding negative birth outcomes prompted exploration on the association between maternal chronic disease and preterm birth (PTB), low birth weight (LBW), and infant mortality (Graham, Zhang, & Schwalberg, 2007). Working in collaboration with other health professionals, the nurse researcher examined birth and death certificates between 1999 and 2003 in a cohort of over 200,000 singleton infants born to African American and White mothers. The research showed that, irrespective of maternal race, chronic hypertension and diabetes were significantly associated with at least one negative birth outcome. Concerning too was the finding that, for African American mothers, cardiac disease was strongly associated with LBW and PTB (Graham et al.). Systematic studies such as these, as well as informal studies and existing epidemiologic data, can provide the community health nurse with valuable information that can be used to positively affect aggregate health.

METHODS IN THE EPIDEMIOLOGIC INVESTIGATIVE PROCESS

The goals of epidemiologic investigation are to identify the causal mechanisms of health and illness states and to develop measures for preventing illness and promoting health. Epidemiologists employ an investigative process that involves a sequence of three approaches that build on one another: descriptive, analytic, and experimental studies. All three approaches have relevance for community health nursing (see Chapter 4 for a more detailed description).

Descriptive Epidemiology

Descriptive epidemiology includes investigations that seek to observe and describe patterns of health-related conditions that occur naturally in a population. For example, a community health nurse might seek to learn how many children in a school district have been immunized for measles, how many home births occur each year in the county, how many cases of STDs have occurred in the city in the past month, or how many automobile crashes have occurred near the community high school. At this stage in the epidemiologic investigation, the researcher seeks to establish the occurrence of a problem. Data from descriptive studies suggest hypotheses for further testing. Descriptive studies almost always involve some form of broad-based quantification and statistical analysis.

Counts

The simplest measure of description is a count. For example, an epidemiologic study to assess the impact of the varicella vaccine (licensed in 1995) on death due to the disease, examined data from the NCHS (1990–2001) Multiple Cause-of-Death Mortality Data (Nguyen, Jumaan, & Seward, 2005). Data from the period prior to and following vaccine availability showed that varicella-related deaths dropped by more than 45%, from an average 145 per year between 1990 and 1994 to 66 per year during 1999–2001. The findings also showed that varicella-related deaths declined among children and adults (20–49 years) alike and for all racial and ethnic groups. As positive as these results were, reported deaths occurred among those who were eligible to receive the vaccine and not among those with high-risk conditions such as HIV, as might be expected. The most current figures from the NCHS reflect an even more precipitous drop, with 19 reported varicella-related deaths during 2004 (NCHS, 2006).

Obtaining a count of this type always depends on the definition of what is being counted and when it was counted. This particular count, for example, utilizes a large database that takes time to be made public and therefore may not provide a current picture of actual deaths. Use of this type of data should always consider the time delay involved. If a community health nurse needs more current information within a specific community or state, hospital records or death certificates may be another source. However, before making use of any statistics, whether from official state offices, the Census Bureau, or a health agency, it is necessary to determine what the information represents.

Rates

Rates are statistical measures expressing the proportion of people with a given health problem among a population at risk. The total number of people in the group serves as the denominator for various types of rates. To express a count as a proportion, or rate, the population to be studied must first be identified. For instance, total West Nile virus fatalities in the United States for 2006 were 177 out of 4,269 confirmed infections (CDC, 2007b). If those deaths are considered in relation to the total number of cases in the country, there will be one rate; if, however, those fatalities are considered in relation to the total population, there will be a quite different rate. It is important when reviewing rates that you understand which measures are being compared.

In epidemiology, the population represents the universe of people defined as the objects of a study. Because it is often difficult, if not impossible, to study an entire population, most epidemiologic studies draw a sample to represent that group. Sometimes, it is important to seek a random sample (in which everyone in the population has an equal chance of selection for study and choice is made without bias). At other times, a sample of convenience (in which study subjects are selected because of their availability) is sufficient. In many small epidemiologic studies, it may be possible to study almost every person in the population, eliminating the need for a sample. Several rates have wide use in epidemiology. Those most important for the public health nurse to understand are the prevalence rate, the period prevalence rate, and the incidence rate.

Prevalence refers to all of the people with a particular health condition existing in a given population at a given point in time. The *prevalence rate* describes a situation at a specific point in time (Friis & Sellers, 2004). If a nurse discovers 50 cases of measles in an elementary school, that is a simple count. If that number is divided by the number of students in the school, the result is the prevalence of measles. For instance, if the school has 500 students, the prevalence of measles on that day would be 10% (50 measles/500 population).

$$\text{Prevalence rate} = \frac{\text{Number of persons with a characteristic}}{\text{Total number in population}}$$

In the study of varicella deaths, on the other hand, the investigators had a count for 1-year periods from 1991 to 2001 (Nguyen et al., 2005). Rather than portraying only 1 day, this number covered an extended period of time (1 year). The prevalence rate over a defined period of time is called a *period prevalence rate*:

$$\text{Period prevalence rate} = \frac{\text{Number of persons with a characteristic during a period of time}}{\text{Total number in population}}$$

Not everyone in a population is at risk for developing a disease, incurring an injury, or having some other health-related characteristic. The *incidence rate* recognizes this fact. **Incidence** refers to all new cases of a disease or health condition appearing during a given time. Incidence rate describes a proportion in which the numerator is all new cases appearing during a given period of time and the denominator is the population at risk during the same period. For example, some childhood diseases give lifelong immunity. The school children who have had such diseases would be removed from the total number of children at risk in the school population. Three weeks after the start of a measles epidemic in a school, the incidence rate describes the number of cases of measles appearing during that period in terms of the number of persons at risk:

$$\frac{200}{1,000} \quad \text{or} \quad \frac{200 \text{ new cases}}{1,000 \text{ persons at risk}}$$

The health literature is not always consistent in the use of the term *incidence;* sometimes, this word is used synonymously with *prevalence rates,* and the reader must take this into consideration.

$$\text{Incidence rate} = \frac{\text{Number of persons developing a disease}}{\text{Total number at risk per unit of time}}$$

Another rate that describes incidence is the attack rate. An *attack rate* describes the proportion of a group or population that develops a disease among all those exposed to a particular risk. This term is used frequently in investigations of outbreaks of infectious diseases such as influenza. If the attack rate changes, it may suggest an alteration in the population's immune status or that the disease-causing organism is present in a more or less virulent strain.

Computing Rates

To make comparisons between populations, epidemiologists often use a common base population in computing rates. For example, instead of merely saying that the rate of an illness is 13% in one city and 25% in another, the comparison is made per 100,000 people in the population. This population base can vary for different purposes from 100 to 100,000. To describe the **morbidity rate**, which is the relative incidence of disease in a population, the ratio of the number of sick individuals to the total population is determined. The **mortality rate** refers to the relative death rate, or the sum of deaths in a given population at a given time. Display 7.4 includes formulas for computing rates commonly used in community health.

The goal of descriptive studies is to identify the patterns of occurrence of any health-related condition. They can be *retrospective* (identify cases and controls, then go back to review existing data) or *prospective* (identify groups and exposure factors, and then follow them forward in time).

DISPLAY 7.4 COMMON EPIDEMIOLOGIC RATES

General Mortality Rates

Crude Mortality Rate =
$$\frac{\text{Number of Reported Deaths During 1 Year}}{\text{Estimated Population as of July 1 of Same Year}} \times 100,000$$

Cause-Specific Mortality Rate =
$$\frac{\text{Number of Deaths From a Stated Cause During 1 Year}}{\text{Estimated Population as of July 1 of Same Year}} \times 100,000$$

Case Fatality Rate =
$$\frac{\text{Number of Deaths From a Particular Disease}}{\text{Total Number With the Same Disease}} \times 100$$

Proportional Mortality Ratio =
$$\frac{\text{Number of Deaths From a Specific Cause Within a Given Time Period}}{\text{Total Deaths in the Same Time Period}} \times 100$$

Age-Specific Mortality Rate =
$$\frac{\text{Number of Persons in a Specific Age Group Dying During 1 Year}}{\text{Estimated Population of the Specific Age Group as of July 1 of Same Year}} \times 100,000$$

Specific Rates for Maternal and Infant Populations

Crude Birth Rate =
$$\frac{\text{Number of Live Births During 1 Year}}{\text{Estimated Population as of July 1 of Same Year}} \times 1,000$$

General Fertility Rate =
$$\frac{\text{Number of Live Births During 1 Year}}{\text{Number of Females Aged 15–44 as of July 1 of Same Year}} \times 1,000$$

Maternal Mortality Rate =
$$\frac{\text{Number of Deaths From Pueperal Causes During 1 Year}}{\text{Number of Live Births During Same Year}} \times 100,000$$

Infant Mortality Rate =
$$\frac{\text{Number of Deaths Under 1 Year of Age for Given Year}}{\text{Number of Live Births Reported for Same Year}} \times 1,000$$

Perinatal Mortality Rate =
$$\frac{\text{Number of Fetal Deaths Plus Infant Deaths Under 7 Days of Age During 1 Year}}{\text{Number of Live Births Plus Fetal Deaths During Same Year}} \times 1,000$$

In a descriptive study of child abuse, for example, the investigator would note the age, gender, race or ethnic group, and physical and emotional conditions of the children affected. In addition, data would be collected that described the economic status and occupation of parents, the location and setting of abusive behavior, and the time and season of the year when abuse occurred. In the retrospective study on reported varicella deaths, the investigators described the age, sex, ethnic background, and birthplace of victims and other information, such as whether varicella was an underlying or contributing cause of death (Nguyen et al., 2005). Describing facets of these deaths provides information for further study and suggests avenues for intervention or prevention.

Analytic Epidemiology

A second type of investigation, **analytic epidemiology**, goes beyond simple description or observation and seeks to identify associations between a particular human disease or health problem and its possible causes. Analytic studies tend to be more specific than descriptive studies in their focus.

They test hypotheses or seek to answer specific questions and can be retrospective or prospective in design. Analytic studies fall into three types: prevalence studies, case-control studies, and cohort studies.

Prevalence Studies

When examining prevalence, it is helpful to remember that the health condition may be new or may have affected some people for many years. A **prevalence study** describes patterns of occurrence, as in the study of varicella-related deaths. It may examine causal factors, but a prevalence study always looks at factors from the same point in time and in the same population. Hypothesized causal factors are based on inferences from a single examination and most likely need further testing for validation.

Case-control Studies

A **case-control study** compares people who have a health or illness condition (number of cases with the condition) with those who lack this condition (controls). These studies begin with the cases and look back over time (retrospectively) for presence or absence of the suspected causal factor in both cases and controls. In a case-control study to explore the risks of delivering a small-for-gestational-age (SGA) infant based on certain occupational patterns, women delivering single births between 1997 and 1999 were interviewed by telephone after delivery (Croteau, Marcoux, & Brisson, 2006). Comparisons between the cases and controls revealed that irregular and shift work increased the risk of a SGA birth, but that changing those occupational patterns before 24 weeks could reduce the risk substantially. In a case-control study, the two groups should share as many characteristics as possible, to isolate possible causes. In the study by Croteau and colleagues, the control group mothers were randomly selected from all singleton births during that same period and in the same region of the country. In this way, differences between the cases (SGA births) and those with a normal-weight infant are more easily identified.

Cohort Studies

A **cohort** is a group of people who share a common experience in a specific time period. Examples are a group of the elderly or the employees of an industry. In epidemiology, a cohort of people often becomes a focus of study. Cohort studies, rather than measuring the relationship of variables in existing conditions, study the development of a condition over time. A cohort study begins by selecting a group of people who display certain defined characteristics before the onset of the condition being investigated. In studying a disease, the cohort might include individuals who are initially free of the disease but are known to have been exposed to a particular factor. They would be observed over time to evaluate which variables were associated with the development or nondevelopment of the disease. These types of studies are often utilized with environmental hazard exposures, as with the World Trade Center Health Registry, the Tremolite Asbestos Registry, and the National Exposure Registry discussed earlier (ATSDR, n.d.). All of these registries provide the capability to conduct a cohort study on postexposure disease development and enable those affected to access the most current information on their exposure risks.

In 1993, the Women's Health Study, a 10-year national longitudinal, experimental, cohort study involving nearly 40,000 female health professionals was initiated (clinicaltrials.gov, 2007; Nabel, 2005). Sponsored by the National Heart, Lung, and Blood Institute and the National Cancer Institute, it consisted of a randomized trial evaluating the benefits and risks of low-dose aspirin and vitamin E in the prevention of cancer and cardiovascular disease. Depending on the random assignment of the women, participants took 100 mg of aspirin or placebo and 600 IU of vitamin E or placebo every other day. This was a double-blind study: neither the participants nor the researchers knew which subjects were taking the study drugs or placebos. The study has been funded through 2009 to provide observational follow-up of study participants. The only positive results to date show that women over age 65 may benefit from low-dose aspirin to prevent strokes. The aspirin regimen was not effective in preventing a first heart attack or death from cardiovascular causes. The research findings support adopting healthy lifestyle habits including "eating for heart health, getting regular physical activity, maintaining a healthy weight, not smoking, and controlling high cholesterol levels, high blood pressure, and diabetes" (Nabel, 2005). With respect to cardiovascular health and vitamin E, there was no demonstrated benefit or risk.

In practice, the various types of studies just discussed are frequently mixed. A case-control study may include description and analysis with a retrospective focus; a cohort study may be conducted prospectively or retrospectively. The Women's Health Study just discussed is an example of a case-control study, a cohort study, and an experimental study. Flexibility is essential to allow the investigator as much freedom as possible in choosing the most useful methodology.

Experimental Epidemiology

Experimental epidemiology follows and builds on information gathered from descriptive and analytic approaches. It is used to study epidemics, the etiology of human disease, the value of preventive and therapeutic measures, and the evaluation of health services (Valanis, 1999). In an experimental study, the investigator actually controls or changes the factors suspected of causing the health condition under study, then observes what happens to the health state. In human populations, experimental studies should focus on disease prevention or health promotion rather than testing the causes of disease, which is done primarily on animals.

Experimental studies are carried out under carefully controlled conditions. The investigator exposes an experimental group to some factor thought to cause disease, improve health, prevent disease, or influence health in some way (as in the Women's Health Study). Simultaneously, the investigator observes a control group that is similar in characteristics to the experimental group but without the exposure factor.

The public health nurse should be alert for opportunities to conduct experimental studies in the course of working with groups. A study need not be elaborate to provide important data for future nursing practice. For example, a community health nurse can provide focused instruction to 20 new mothers encouraging them to breast-feed and then compare the health of their infants with infants of 20 mothers in the same service area who use formula.

A nurse can look at the number of automobile crashes at an intersection where there is a traffic light compared with a similar intersection that has stop signs. Based on the results of the investigation, the nurse may bring the information to the city council and petition for a stop light at the intersection. Study results can be used to bring about change in the community and are not limited to communicable or chronic diseases. Improving community safety is also an essential outcome.

An expanding area of experimental epidemiology involves the use of computers to simulate epidemics. With mathematical models, it is possible to determine the probabilities of various aspects of disease occurrence. This approach is making an increased contribution to epidemiologists' knowledge of etiology and prevention.

Occasionally, an experiment occurs naturally, thus affording the researcher the chance to make important discoveries. John Snow discovered such a "natural experiment" in London in 1854 (as discussed earlier in the chapter). In his seminal study of an epidemic of cholera, he observed one group that contracted the disease and another that did not. Closer inspection revealed that the major difference between these groups was their water supply. Eventually, the spread of cholera was traced to the water supply of the group with the high morbidity rate (Valanis, 1999).

A *community trial* is a type of experimental study done at the community level. Geographic communities are assigned to intervention (experimental) or nonintervention (control) groups and compared to determine whether the intervention produces a positive change in the community. Community trials can be extremely expensive and are not undertaken unless there is substantial evidence that the intervention will make a difference at the aggregate level. There are times when these community trials occur spontaneously, and it is important for the community health nurse to recognize these opportunities. For instance, one community public health department institutes an aggressive campaign to educate health care workers on the signs of elder abuse. Selecting a similar community where that level of training is not available, the community health nurse can then compare the rates of elder abuse reporting between these two communities. If you were conducting this research, what outcome would you expect in the community with the enhanced training? Where could you obtain this information? Think about what other measures you might be interested in comparing between these two communities.

CONDUCTING EPIDEMIOLOGIC RESEARCH

The community health nurse who engages in an epidemiologic investigation becomes a kind of detective. First, there is a problem to solve, a puzzle to unravel, or a question to answer. The nurse begins to search for basic information, for clues that might help answer the question. Information is never self-explanatory, and, like a detective, the nurse must analyze and interpret every additional clue. Slowly, there is a narrowing of possible suspects until the causes of a disease, the consequences of a prevention plan, or the results of treatment are identified. On the basis of this investigation, the nurse can draw further conclusions and make new applications to improve health services.

As discussed previously, epidemiologic studies are a form of research. The steps outlined here are similar to those discussed in Chapter 4. Epidemiologic research involves seven steps. Everything from an informal study in the course of nursing practice to the most comprehensive epidemiologic research project can be undertaken with these steps:

1. Identify the problem.
2. Review the literature.
3. Design the study.
4. Collect the data.
5. Analyze the findings.
6. Develop conclusions and applications.
7. Disseminate the findings.

Each step is considered here in the context of a single nursing study that examined receipt of lead-poisoning prevention information by parents of children enrolled in one state's Medicaid program (Polivka, 2006). Although research as a community health nursing role is covered in a separate chapter, the analysis of one epidemiologic study reinforces the integration of research in the nurse's role.

Identify the Problem

Community health nurses are constantly confronted with threats to the health and well-being of the community. Almost daily, questions are raised, puzzles presented, and problems identified. Pregnant women who smoke or use cocaine threaten the health of their unborn children: What can be done to reduce this behavior? Rape is increasing: What can be done to prevent such violence or to bring aid to victims? Children are injured and die from bicycle accidents: Why do these occur and how can they be prevented? Many farm workers have been killed or injured in farm equipment accidents: What can be done to prevent them? Any threat to the health of a group offers fertile ground for epidemiologic investigation.

One nurse researcher was concerned with lead-poisoning prevention education among parents of young children. To explore this issue, the researcher sought to examine parental receipt of educational materials on lead-poisoning prevention, as well their preferred method of receiving that information (Polivka, 2006). Using a cross-sectional design, parents of 1- to 2-year-old children who were enrolled in the Medicaid program were mailed a survey developed by the researcher. From the nearly 90,000 children meeting the study criteria, a sample of 1,656 was selected, which allowed for a low but realistic 24% return rate. The response rate ($n = 532$) was actually higher than predicted, and the majority of the respondents reported receiving lead-poisoning prevention information. Of concern, however, was that only 28% reported receipt of some type of reminder to have their child's blood drawn for a lead level assessment. The findings also indicated that most respondents preferred to receive lead-poisoning prevention information from brochures/pamphlets (71%) or directly from health care providers (48%).

Review the Literature

All too often, after identifying a problem, health professionals rush to take immediate action without reviewing solutions that have been tried previously. Every epidemiologic investigation should begin with a review of the literature. Even discovering that little research has been done on the problem can be valuable information. Conversely, if many studies have already been conducted in the area, this information can help narrow the study to areas not previously investigated or allow researchers to replicate earlier studies to confirm findings in a different setting. One of the most valuable sources in the literature is the review article, which essentially summarizes all the research that has been conducted on a subject.

A review of the literature often suggests hypotheses from discoveries made in other studies. In the lead-poisoning prevention education survey, a review of the literature provided helpful background information (Polivka, 2006). The literature review also revealed that other studies have found varied levels of receipt of lead-poisoning prevention education among parents and caregivers, from as low as about 30% to as high as 60%.

Design the Study

The first step in designing a study is to formulate one or more specific questions to answer or hypotheses to test.

Sometimes, the question or hypothesis emerges from the review of the literature; it also may be developed through the researcher's own analysis and hunches. It is a good idea to write out one or more hypotheses to test or questions to answer. In the lead-poisoning education survey, the researcher did not explicitly state a hypothesis; however, in previous focus groups conducted by the researcher and a colleague, "parents revealed they had little knowledge regarding the sources of lead poisoning, and they preferred to receive information via videos and television ads" (Polivka & Gottesman, 2005). This piece of information helped inform the current study and the current research questions:

◆ Have parents received lead-poisoning prevention information or reminders about lead testing?
◆ With whom have parents talked about lead poisoning?
◆ How would parents prefer to receive lead-poisoning prevention education? (Polivka, 2006, p. 53)

The next step is to plan what study type (descriptive, analytic, or experimental) or combination of study types, best suits the goals of the research and how the study will be conducted. Will the data be collected retrospectively from existing records, or will new data be collected? Who will conduct interviews? What kinds of data will be needed to measure the outcomes of intervention? Polivka (2006) used a retrospective analytic approach in the design of this cross-sectional survey. A mailed survey was selected as an effective means to sample the population of interest.

Collect the Data

The survey tool used in the Polivka (2006) study was a researcher-developed instrument that was assessed for both face and content validity by a team of experts in the field. The next step was to pilot test the survey tool with individuals similar to the target population. In this case, the researcher used a small group of women who were enrolled in the WIC program (Special Supplemental Nutrition Program for Women, Infants, and Children, U.S. Department of Agriculture) and revised the survey based on their suggestions.

Following review by a human subjects committee, the survey was mailed to the identified parents along with a cover letter and stamped preaddressed envelope. To increase the return rate from the parents, a small incentive was included in the survey, and a thank-you card and reminder to return the survey (for nonrespondents) was mailed out 1 week later. For those not returning surveys after 3 to 7 weeks, another survey was sent out in hope of increasing the rate of return. For those who completed the survey, a small thank-you gift was mailed out. The steps taken by the researcher were all important to achieving a return rate of 32%, well over the expected rate of 24%.

As in the Polivka (2006) study, it is useful to perform a pilot study that pretests an interview guide, questionnaire, or treatment. If one wishes to interview women about battering during pregnancy, it might be useful to prepare a guide and interview one or two people, then revise the guide on the basis of the experience. If development of a questionnaire to assess the nutritional needs of elderly people living alone is

part of the study design, it would be helpful to test the survey on some volunteers to determine its clarity and relevance. And, if the study is to provide a specific treatment such as coaching, teaching, or demonstration, it is important to practice it on a small group of people with characteristics similar to those of the subjects. In community health nursing, data collection often can occur as part of ongoing practice. Unless the study has been carefully designed, however, data may be collected for months or years, only to discover that important questions have been omitted.

Analyze the Findings

In most epidemiologic studies, data analysis consists of summarizing the findings, computing rates and ratios, and displaying the findings in tables and graphs. At this stage, the data are used to address the original question or test the original hypothesis. Was the hypothesis supported or not supported by the data? Summarized data can also generate more questions or indicate areas that warrant further investigation. For example, in the Polivka (2006) study, 60% of the parents reporting receipt of some type of lead-poisoning prevention information tended to be over age 25, unmarried, and with more than a high school education. These results certainly suggest that younger parents and those with less education should be a target of educational interventions to address lead-poisoning prevention. Moreover, any educational materials developed should keep in mind the reading capability of those parents.

Develop Conclusions and Applications

Stating conclusions is an outcome of analysis and interpretation. The investigators summarize the results and their meaning for the purpose of making this information useful to other health services providers. Many times, research has direct practical application for improving health services, continuing or discontinuing services, or conducting future research. It is also important to describe mistakes made and lessons learned about study design and other aspects of the research, to assist future investigators.

In the Polivka study, the researcher suggests that "public health nurses need to collaborate with other health care providers in implementing individual, community, and system level lead-poisoning prevention educational interventions for parents of at-risk children" (2006, p. 55). Citing the continued need for efforts to reduce lead-poisoning and the Healthy People 2010 goal of eliminating lead poisoning in U.S. children (USDHHS, 2000), the author also states that "public health nurses can be pivotal in educational reminder efforts by determining specific targeted population segments and identifying appropriate educational methods for those segments at the individual, community, and system levels" (Polivka, p. 56). The author had clearly outlined the leadership role that community health nurses can and should take to reach this national goal.

Disseminate the Findings

Finally, research findings should be shared. Information gained from epidemiologic studies must be disseminated throughout the professional community to strengthen the knowledge base for improved practice and to promote future research. In the lead-poisoning prevention education study, the author selected a well-known nursing journal; one that specifically focuses on public health nursing practice. Careful selection of this specialty venue helps assure that those practicing in community and public health nursing are more likely to read the article. The author's use of the term *lead poisoning* in the title of the article was also very important for dissemination. Nurses interested in lead poisoning are very likely to have this article selected in a database reference search, such as the Cumulative Index to Nursing & Allied Health Literature (CINAHL), based on the use of that term alone.

Summary

Epidemiology is the study of the distribution and determinants of health, health conditions, and disease in human population groups. It shares with community health nursing the common focus of the health of populations. It is a specialized form of scientific research that can provide public health professionals with a body of knowledge on which to base their practice and methods for studying new and existing problems. To understand epidemiology, one must first understand some basic epidemiologic concepts: the host, agent, and environment model; causality; immunity; the natural history of disease or health conditions; risk; and prevention strategies.

Community health nurses can use three sources of information when conducting epidemiologic investigations: existing epidemiologic data, informal investigations, and carefully designed scientific studies.

Epidemiology employs three investigative approaches: descriptive studies, analytic studies, and experimental studies. Although studies can be either retrospective or prospective, some merely describe existing conditions (descriptive studies), whereas others seek to explain causes (analytic studies). Experimental studies seek to confirm causal relationships identified in descriptive and analytic studies. Analytic studies can be of three types: prevalence, case-control, or cohort. In practice, all these types of studies often become combined in various ways. They also make use of quantitative concepts such as count, prevalence rate, incidence rate, mortality rate, and various types of morbidity (sickness) rates.

Epidemiologic research includes seven steps:

1. Identify the problem, which is usually a threat to the population's health.
2. Review the literature to determine what other studies have found.
3. Carefully design the study.
4. Collect the data.
5. Analyze the findings.
6. Develop conclusions and applications.
7. Disseminate the findings.

Thinking epidemiologically can significantly enhance community health nursing practice. Epidemiology provides both the body of knowledge—information on the distribution and determinants of health conditions—and methods for investigating health problems and evaluating services. ∎

ACTIVITIES TO PROMOTE CRITICAL THINKING

1. Identify an aggregate-level health problem in your community. Using the host, agent, and environment model, explain who is the host, what are the causative agents, and what environmental factors have promoted or delayed the development of the problem.
2. Select an aggregate health (wellness) condition, such as preschoolers' normal growth and development or elders' healthy aging, and list all the causal factors that might contribute to this healthy state. Now, plot these schematically in a diagram to show the web of causation model for this condition.
3. Using the same health condition that you selected in the previous exercise, describe the natural history of this condition, outlining its four stages. Identify three preventive nursing interventions, one for each level of prevention that could apply to this condition.
4. Select an article that reports an epidemiologic study from a recent nursing or public health journal, and record your responses to the following questions:
   - What prompted the study, and what was its purpose?
   - Was it descriptive, analytic, or experimental research?
   - Was the study design retrospective or prospective?
   - Why did the investigators choose this design?
   - What existing sources of epidemiologic data did this study use? List all sources specifically, such as *Morbidity and Mortality Weekly Report* or incomes by household in census data.
   - What were the study findings? Identify the population group that will benefit from this research.
5. Interview one or more practicing public health nurses in your community, and identify an aggregate-level problem that needs epidemiologic investigation. Propose a rough draft study design to research this problem.

References

Agency for Toxic Substances and Disease Registry. U.S. Department of Health and Human Services. (n.d.). *Data resources.* Retrieved July 28, 2007 from http://www.atsdr.cdc.gov/2p-data-resources.html.

Aschengrau, A., & Seage, G.R. (2008). *Essentials of epidemiology in public health*, 2nd ed. Sudbury, MA: Jones and Bartlett Publishers.

Bodnar, L.M., Tang, G., Ness, R.B., et al. (2006). Periconceptual multivitamin use reduces the risk of preeclampsia. *American Journal of Epidemiology, 164*, 470–477.

Burnet, M. (1962). *Natural history of infectious diseases,* 3rd ed. Cambridge, England: Cambridge University Press.

Centers for Disease Control and Prevention, Division of Vectorborne Diseases. (2004a). *West Nile Virus Basics.* Retrieved July 22, 2007 from http://www.cdc.gov/ncidod/dvbid/westnile/prevention_info.htm.

Centers for Disease Control and Prevention. (2004b). *Smallpox fact sheet: Smallpox disease overview.* Retrieved July 28, 2007 from http://www.bt.cdc.gov/agent/smallpox/overview/disease-facts.asp.

Centers for Disease Control and Prevention. (2007a). *Epidemiology and prevention of vaccine preventable diseases,* 10th ed. Retrieved July 23, 2007 from http://www.cdc.gov/vaccines/pubs/pinkbook/pink-chapters.htm.

Centers for Disease Control and Prevention, Division of Vectorborne Diseases. (2007b). *West Nile Virus: Statistics, surveillance, and control.* Retrieved July 22, 2007 from http://www.cdc.gov/ncidod/dvbid/westnile/surv&control.htm.

Chen, H., Schernhammer, E., Schwarzschild, M.A., & Ascherio, A. (2006). A prospective study of night shift work, sleep duration, and risk of Parkinson's Disease. *American Journal of Epidemiology, 163,* 726–730.

Clincaltrials.gov. (2007). *Women's Health Study (WHS).* Bethesda, MD: National Institutes of Health. Retrieved July 29, 2007 from http://clinicaltrials.gov/ct/show/NCT00000479.

Cohen, D., Spear, S., Scribner, R., et al. (2000). "Broken Windows" and the risk of gonorrhea. *American Journal of Public Health, 90,* 230–236.

Connolly, M.A., Gayer, M., Ryan, M.J., et al. (2004). Communicable diseases in complex emergencies: Impact and challenges. *Lancet, 364,* 1974–1983.

Croteau, A., Marcoux, S., & Brisson, C. (2006). Work activity in pregnancy, preventive measures, and the risk of delivering a small-for-gestational-age infant. *American Journal of Public Health, 96,* 846–855.

Dever, G.E.A. (1984). *Epidemiology in health services management.* Rockville, MD: Aspen Systems Corporation.

Dever, G.E.A. (1991). *Community health analysis: Global awareness at the local level,* 2nd ed. Gaithersburg, MD: Aspen Publishers, Inc.

Evans, G.H. (1939). Bubonic plague outbreak in San Francisco: Year 1900. *California West Medicine, 50*(2), 121–123. Retrieved July 21, 2007 from http://www.pubmedcentral.nih.gov/articlerender.fcgi?artid=1659815.

Friis, R.H., & Sellers, T.A. (2004). *Epidemiology for public health practice,* 3rd ed. Sudbury, MA: Jones and Bartlett Publishers.

Gabriel, R.A., & Metz, K.S. (1992). *A history of military medicine: From the Renaissance through modern times,* Vol. II. New York: Greenwood Press.

Gerstman, B.B. (2003). *Epidemiology kept simple: An introduction to traditional and modern epidemiology,* 2nd ed. Hoboken, NJ: Wiley-Liss, Inc.

Graham, J., Zhang, L., & Schwalberg, R. (2007). Association of maternal chronic disease and negative birth outcomes in a non-Hispanic Black-White Mississippi birth cohort. *Public Health Nursing, 24,* 311–317.

Heymann, D.L. (Ed.). (2004). *Control of communicable diseases manual,* 18th ed. Washington, DC: American Public Health Association.

Kopf, E.W. (1978). Florence Nightingale as statistician. *Research in Nursing and Health, 1*(3), 93–102.

Kudzma, E.C. (2006). Florence Nightingale and healthcare reform. *Nursing Science Quarterly, 19,* 61–64.

Lalonde, M. (1974). A new perspective on the health of Canadians. Ottawa, Canada: Office of the Canadian Minister of National Health and Welfare.

Lawson, A.B., & Williams, F.L.R. (2001). *An introductory guide to disease mapping.* Chichester, UK: John Wiley & Sons.

Legator, M.S., & Morris, D.L. (2003). What did Sir Bradford Hill really say? *Archives of Environmental Health, 58,* 718–720.

Markowitz, G., & Rosner, D. (2000). Public health then and now. "Cater to the children": The role of the lead industry in a public health tragedy, 1900–1955. *American Journal of Public Health, 90,* 36–46.

Miniño, A.M., Heron, M.P., & Smith, B.L. (2006). Deaths: Preliminary data for 2004. *National Vital Statistics Report, 54*(19), 1–52. Retrieved July 22, 2007 from http://www.cdc.gov/nchs/data/nvsr/nvsr54/nvsr54_19.pdf.

Nabel, E.G. (2005). *Statement from Elizabeth G. Nabel, M.D., Director of the National Heart, Lung, and Blood Institute of the National Institutes of Health on the Finding of the Women's Health Study. NIH News.* Retrieved July 29, 2007 from http://www.nih.gov/news/pr/mar2005/nhlbi-07.htm.

National Center for Health Statistics. (2006). *Worktable IV: Deaths from each cause, by month, race, and sex: United States 2004.* Retrieved July 29, 2007 from http://0-www.cdc.gov.mill1.sjlibrary.org/nchs/data/dvs/mortfinal2004_worktableIV_part1.pdf.

National Center for Health Statistics. (2007a). *National Health Interview Survey (NHIS). Celebrating the first 50 years: 1957–2007.* Retrieved July 28, 2007 from http://www.cdc.gov/nchs/about/major/nhis/hisdesc.htm.

National Center for Health Statistics. (2007b). *Surveys and data collection systems.* Retrieved July 28, 2007 from http://www.cdc.gov/nchs/express.htm.

Nguyen, H.Q., Jumaan, A.O., & Seward, J.F. (2005). Decline in mortality due to Varicella after implementation of varicella vaccination in the United States. *New England Journal of Medicine, 352,* 450–458.

Polivka, B.J. (2006). Needs assessment and intervention strategies to reduce lead-poisoning risk among low-income Ohio toddlers. *Public Health Nursing, 23,* 52–58.

Polivka, B.J., & Gottesman, M.M. (2005). Parental perceptions of barriers to blood lead testing. *Journal of Pediatric Health Care, 19*(5), 276–284.

Simond, M., Godley, M.L., & Mouriquand, P.D.E. (1998). Paul-Louis Simond and his discovery of plague transmission by rat fleas: A centenary. *Journal of the Royal Society of Medicine, 91,* 101–104

Solomon, T. (1997). Hong Kong, 1894: The role of James A. Lowson in the controversial discovery of the plague bacillus. *Lancet, 350,* 59–62.

Susser, I., & Stein, Z. (2000). Culture, sexuality, and women's agency in the prevention of HIV/AIDS in southern Africa. *American Journal of Public Health, 90,* 1042–1048.

Susser, M., & Susser, E. (1996a). Choosing a future for epidemiology: I. Eras and paradigms. *American Journal of Public Health, 86,* 668–673.

Susser, M., & Susser, E. (1996b). Choosing a future for epidemiology: II. From black box to Chinese boxes and eco-epidemiology. *American Journal of Public Health, 86,* 674–677.

Theilmann, J., & Cate, F. (2007). A plague of plagues: The problem of plague diagnosis in Medieval England. *Journal of Interdisciplinary History, 37,* 371–393.

U.S. Department of Health and Human Services. (2000). *Healthy People 2010: Understanding and improving health,* 2nd ed. Washington, DC: U.S. Government Printing Office.

U.S. Department of Health and Human Services. (2006). *Healthy People 2010: Midcourse review.* Washington, DC: U.S. Government Printing Office.

U.S. Department of Health and Human Services. (2007). *Vaccine Adverse Event Reporting System.* Retrieved August 2, 2007 from http://www.vaers.hhs.gov/.

U. S. Department of State – Bureau of African Affairs. (2007). *Background note: Rwanda.* Retrieved July 22, 2007 from http://www.state.gov/r/pa/ei/bgn/2861.htm.

U.S. Public Health Service. (1964). *Smoking and health: Report of the Advisory Committee to the Surgeon General of the Public Health Service.* Washington, DC: Author. Retrieved July 23, 2007 from http://www.cdc.gov/tobacco/data_statistics/sgr/history.htm.

Valanis, B. (1999). *Epidemiology in health care,* 3rd ed. Stamford, CT: Appleton & Lange.

World Health Organization. (2007). *International health regulations 2005.* Retrieved July 28, 2007 from http://www.who.int/csr/ihr/en/.

Wynd, C.A. (2002). Testicular self-examination in young adult men. *Journal of Nursing Scholarship, 34,* 251–255.

Selected Readings

American Academy of Pediatrics. (2007). *Red Book online: Status of licensure and recommendations for new vaccines.* Elk Grove Village, IL: Author. Retrieved August 2, 2007 from http://aapredbook.aappublications.org/news/vaccstatus.pdf.

Anderson, C.T., & McFarlane, J. (2006). *Community as partner: Theory and practice in nursing,* 5th ed. Philadelphia: Lippincott Williams & Wilkins.

Karon, J.M., Fleming, P.L., Steketee, R.W., & DeCock, K.M. (2001). HIV in the United States at the turn of the century: An epidemic in transition. *American Journal of Public Health, 91*(7), 1060–1068.

Kidder, T. (2004). *Mountains beyond mountains: The quest of Dr. Paul Farmer, a man who would cure the world.* New York: Random House, Inc.

Ott, M., Brown, G., Byrne, C., et al. (2006). Recreation for children on social assistance, 4–17 years old, pays for itself the same year. *Journal of Public Health, 28,* 203–208.

Rothman, K.J., & Greenland, S. (2005). Causation and causal inference in epidemiology. *American Journal of Public Health, 95*(Suppl. 1), 144–150.

Sawatzky, J.V., & Naimark, B.J. (2005). Cardiovascular health promotion in aging women: Validating a population health approach. *Public Health Nursing, 22,* 379–388.

Internet Resources

American Public Health Association—Epidemiology Section: *http://www.apha.org/membergroups/sections/aphasections/epidemiology/*

Association for Professionals in Infection Control and Epidemiology, Inc.: *http://www.apic.org*

Centers for Disease Control and Prevention: *http://www.cdc.gov*

Certification Board of Infection Control and Epidemiology, Inc.: *http://www.cbic.org*

Environmental Protection Agency: *http://www.epa.gov*

Immunization Action Coalition: *http://www.immunize.org*

March of Dimes (Perinatal Statistics): *http://www.marchofdimes.com/peristats/*

National Cancer Institute (Surveillance Epidemiology and End Results [SEER]–cancer statistics): *http://seer.cancer.gov/*

National Health Statistics: *http://www.health.gov*

Nurses Health Study: *http://www.NursesHealthStudy.org*

Safety and Health Statistics: *http://www.bls.gov/iif/*

UCLA Center for Health Policy Research (University of California, Los Angeles): *http://www.healthpolicy.ucla.edu/*

UIC School of Public Health (Public Health Games): *http://www.publichealthgames.com/*

United Nations International Children's Fund [UNICEF] (statistics): *http://www.unicef.org/infobycountry/index.html*

U. S. Bureau of Census: *http://www.census.gov/*

Women's Health Initiative—National Heart, Lung, and Blood Institute [NHLBI]: *http://www.nhlbi.nih.gov/whi/*

World Health Organization (statistics): *http://www.who.int/research/en/*

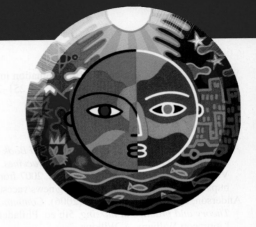

8

Communicable Disease Control

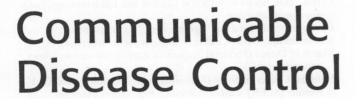

KEY TERMS

Acquired
    immunodeficiency
    syndrome (AIDS)
Active immunity
Communicable disease
Direct transmission
Fomites
Herd immunity
Human immunodeficiency
    virus (HIV)
Immunization
Incubation period
Index case
Indirect transmission
Infectious
Isolation
Passive immunity
Quarantine
Reservoir
Ring vaccination
Screening
Surveillance
Vaccine
Vector

LEARNING OBJECTIVES

Upon mastery of this chapter, you should be able to:

◆ Describe the nurse's role in communicable disease control.

◆ Describe the three modes of transmission for communicable diseases.

◆ Explain the strategies used for the three levels of prevention in communicable disease control.

◆ Explain the significance of immunization as a communicable disease control measure.

◆ Differentiate between human immunodeficiency virus (HIV) infection and acquired immunodeficiency syndrome (AIDS).

◆ Describe major issues that affect the control and elimination of tuberculosis (TB).

◆ Discuss specific ways to prevent sexually transmitted diseases, including HIV/AIDS.

◆ Identify six globally emerging communicable diseases.

◆ Discuss the global and national trends and issues in communicable disease control.

◆ Discuss the consequences of biologic terrorism with weapons such as anthrax and smallpox.

◆ Discuss ethical issues affecting communicable disease and infection control.

"*Illness is the doctor to whom we pay most heed; to kindness, to knowledge, we make promise only; pain we obey.*"

—Marcel Proust

Communicable diseases pose a major threat to public health and are of significant concern to community health nurses. A **communicable disease** is one that can be transmitted from one person to another, is caused by an agent that is **infectious** (capable of producing infection), and is transmitted from a source, or **reservoir**, to a susceptible host (Heymann, 2004). The majority of communicable diseases that the community health nurse will encounter and investigate are considered infectious; other diseases are not infectious, but are just as potentially problematic to a community. An example of a noninfectious disease is Lyme disease. The infections or diseases that are investigated are reportable through a process mandated by the individual state in which the nurse practices (Heymann, 2004).

Knowledge of communicable diseases is fundamental to the practice of community health nursing because these diseases typically spread through communities of people. Understanding the basic concepts of communicable disease control, as well as the numerous surrounding issues, helps a community health nurse work effectively to prevent and control communicable disease in populations and groups. It also helps nurses teach important and effective preventive measures to community members, advocate for those affected, and protect the well-being of uninfected persons (including nurses themselves).

In the last century, numerous changes occurred in the lives of people globally, as well as nationally, related to issues of public health. Achievements in health, safety, longevity, and disease control improved the lives of many populations in developed nations, and with the work of many global organizations, will continue to improve for developing nations as well. With progress, come challenges and concerns related to community health nursing services (Centers for Disease Control [CDC] 1999b; World Health Organization [WHO], 2003b), such as:

◆ Higher morbidity among various age and population groups related to communicable diseases, rather than death.
◆ Continuing disproportionate morbidity and mortality among lower socioeconomic populations.
◆ Emergent, newly identified, or reemerging diseases related to changing environments, global mobility, and need for space. Examples of these are hantavirus, severe acute respiratory syndrome (SARS), and West Nile virus.
◆ Development of multidrug resistant (MDR) strains of bacteria and viruses that pose significant occupational health challenges as well as practice issues for health workers.
◆ Rising fear of terrorist attacks utilizing biologic agents.
◆ Ongoing public empowerment through education regarding healthy life practices, and current health research associated with disease and cancer prevention through diet, immunization, and the environment.

This chapter provides you with valuable information to better understand the communicable disease burden in your community. It describes ways to plan and implement appropriate prevention interventions, including immunization of children and adults, environmental interventions, community education, screening programs, and disease case/source investigation and contact finding. Ethical issues of communicable disease control are also discussed. A list of communicable disease information sources useful to you, the public health nurse, is provided at the end of this chapter.

BASIC CONCEPTS REGARDING COMMUNICABLE DISEASES

Communicable diseases have challenged health care providers for centuries. They have led to the development of countless nursing and medical preventive measures, from simple procedures such as handwashing, sanitation, and proper ventilation to the research and development of vaccines and antibiotics (CDC, 1999b).

Evolution of Communicable Disease Control

Because preventive measures have greatly reduced the spread of communicable diseases, many people consider communicable diseases to be a threat of the past. Yet this is not the reality. Communicable diseases, particularly those of epidemic and pandemic probability, such as TB, influenza, or acquired immunodeficiency syndrome (AIDS), continue to cost millions of lives and billions of dollars to the global human society every year (WHO, 2003b).

As mentioned in Chapter 7, the first documented global threat from a communicable disease began in the 13th century in the form of bubonic plague. It was responsible for killing 25% of the population in some European countries over the years following the Crusades and during the years of exploration and trade by ship—in the 1400s to 1600s.

As commerce and industry continued to grow, people migrated from rural areas to towns and cities. However, health and hygiene practices that worked in remote areas did not transfer to the new urban settings. In tenements and overcrowded parts of towns, water for drinking easily became contaminated with human waste; mounting garbage and trash, unable to be composted or buried as was done in farming communities, created a rich habitat for rodents and other animals and insects, encouraging them to breed and become vectors for many communicable diseases.

Not until the 1700s and 1800s were the causative organisms for various infectious diseases recognized through the assistance of increasingly sophisticated microscopes. With these discoveries came early attempts to create ways to prevent the spread of such organisms, either by decreasing their power or by eliminating them. Pasteurization of milk was invented, and efforts to eliminate rats from ships and food storage areas began. These measures commenced a global effort to eliminate communicable diseases (Weatherall, Greenwood, Chee, & Wasi, 2005).

One disease, smallpox, is a classic example of a communicable disease control success story. For centuries, the infectious disease of smallpox killed millions of people and scarred survivors for life—in fact, it is thought that smallpox is responsible for more deaths than any other infectious disease (Children's Hospital of Philadelphia, 2007). Smallpox first responded to a crude vaccine that was developed in the 18th century, almost accidentally, when Dr. Edward Jenner noted that milkmaids seemed to be unaffected by the illness when it swept through the English countryside every few years. He posited that the mild infections they incurred while milking cows and coming in contact with the blisters on cow's udders gave them protection from the more serious smallpox infections. He injected fluid from the cows' blisters into volunteers, including his own young son (Children's Hospital of Philadelphia, 2007). Notable people of the time withstood the months-long after effects of the smallpox vaccine, including the family of our second president, John Adams (McCullough, 2001). The vaccine was studied and perfected and was used globally for decades. A major worldwide eradication campaign began in 1967. The last naturally acquired case of smallpox in the world occurred in October 1977; global eradication was certified 2 years later by the World Health Organization (WHO) and confirmed by the World Health Assembly in May 1980. Since then, no cases of smallpox have been identified in any country (Heymann, 2004).

However, the threat of biologic warfare using smallpox or other disease organisms raises concerns about how to prepare for the future. A smallpox immunization program began in 2002 with President George W. Bush being immunized. The plan was to follow with military personnel, health care providers, and then voluntary immunization among the general population. In 2002, the Centers for Disease Control and Prevention (CDC) issued guidelines for state and local health departments to develop smallpox response plans. The plans were to include a mass vaccination strategy in the event of an outbreak (CDC, 2002).

Community Health Nurse and Reporting Communicable Disease

Most health departments or districts have PHNs who work in disease control and prevention. Some agencies utilize a combination of nurses, epidemiologists, and communicable disease investigators. Each state has a state-level department of health services, which is either the primary or guiding agency for local disease control policies that are mandated through the health and safety codes of each state. States utilize the national reportable disease list as the guidance for state reportable diseases and may add to this list as they choose, reflecting the types of conditions that are unique to a state or region of the United States (CDC, 2006g). The CDC is the federal agency that provides guidance and recommendations for each state health department to utilize in developing individual state recommendations for the local agencies. The CDC is also available to each individual citizen via phone or the internet (www.cdc.gov).

The local health department/agency is the initial point of notification of a communicable disease investigation. The notifications may come from a laboratory, which is a mandated reporter of infectious reportable diseases and must report both to the ordering physician as well as to the health department. The physician is also a mandated reporter, and must complete the state's Confidential Morbidity Report (CMR) (see Fig. 8.1). Each local health department/agency will investigate the specific disease using a protocol set either by the state or local health officer (CDC, 2006g).

Global Trends—Achievements and Challenges

During the last several decades, substantial progress has been made in controlling some major infectious diseases around the world, although other diseases have not been as well managed. The following are some of the major accomplishments, as well as continuing dilemmas:

◆ WHO's Expanded Program on Immunization (EPI) was launched in 1974. As a result, by 2005, more than 78% of the world's children had been immunized against diphtheria, tetanus, whooping cough (pertussis), poliomyelitis, measles, and TB, compared with fewer than 5% in 1974 (WHO, 2005).

◆ Eradication of *smallpox* was achieved in 1980.

◆ The tropical disease *yaws* has virtually disappeared. The first yaws campaign was launched in Haiti in 1950, and by 1965, 46 million people in 49 countries had been successfully treated with penicillin. The disease is no longer a significant problem in most of the world.

◆ Improved sanitation and hygiene has decreased outbreaks of *relapsing fever*, transmitted by lice and fleas.

◆ The elimination of polio has been a goal since the 1988 Global Polio Eradication Initiative was developed by WHO (2006c). Achievement of this goal was earmarked for the year 2000, and it was looking like it might happen (WHO). As of 2003, only six of the original 125 countries were still experiencing polio—Nigeria, India, Pakistan, Niger, Afghanistan, and Egypt. By the end of 2003, India reported a reduction in cases from previous years to 225 cases—an all-time low. Unfortunately, in August of 2003, several northern states in Nigeria suspended their vaccination campaign, citing issues with what they believed to be problems with the vaccine. Because of this deferment of vaccinations, another outbreak occurred, which led to the disease being imported to once polio-free regions of Africa. Through the efforts and diplomacy of WHO, trust was regained, leading to a swift resurrection of the vaccination campaign (WHO, 2006c).

◆ The global threat of *plague* has declined in the last 40 years, largely as a result of the use of antibiotics and insecticides (Heymann, 2004).

◆ *Leprosy* (Hansen disease), once a major communicable disease, is almost eliminated. In 1966, there were 10.5 million reported cases worldwide. As of 2002, only 620,000 cases were diagnosed worldwide. The WHO will no longer consider leprosy a public health problem when fewer than one case per 10,000 population occurs—a goal that has been achieved in 110 of 122 endemic countries (Heymann, 2004).

Some major communicable diseases and areas of concern remain, including the following:

◆ *Malaria* remains a major threat, even though the mortality rate has improved in the last 25 years. In 1954, there were 2.5 million deaths annually and 250 million cases of malaria worldwide; in 2002, there were an estimated 1 million deaths and 300 to 500 million cases yearly (WHO, 2006d). Tropical Africa has 90% of the cases, and malaria is endemic in 92 countries (Heymann, 2004).

◆ *Cholera* was mainly confined to Asia in the early 20th century, but has been spread worldwide by

CONFIDENTIAL MORBIDITY REPORT

NOTE: For STD, Hepatitis, or TB, complete appropriate section below. Special reporting requirements and reportable diseases on back.

DISEASE BEING REPORTED: _____

Patient's Last Name

Social Security Number

Ethnicity (✓ one)
- ☐ Hispanic/Latino
- ☐ Non-Hispanic/Non-Latino

First Name/Middle Name (or initial)

Birth Date   Month   Day   Year

Age

Race (✓ one)
- ☐ African-American/Black
- ☐ Asian/Pacific Islander (✓ one):

Address: Number, Street

Apt./Unit Number

- ☐ Asian-Indian   ☐ Japanese
- ☐ Cambodian   ☐ Korean
- ☐ Chinese   ☐ Laotian

City/Town   **State**   **ZIP Code**

- ☐ Filipino   ☐ Samoan
- ☐ Guamanian   ☐ Vietnamese

Estimated Delivery Date   Month   Day   Year

- ☐ Hawaiian

Area Code   **Home Telephone**   **Gender** M F   **Pregnant?** Y N Unk

- ☐ Other: _____
- ☐ Native American/Alaskan Native
- ☐ White: _____

Area Code   **Work Telephone**   **Patient's Occupation/Setting**
- ☐ Food service ☐ Day care ☐ Correctional facility
- ☐ Health care ☐ School ☐ Other _____

- ☐ Other: _____

DATE OF ONSET   Month   Day   Year

Reporting Health Care Provider

REPORT TO

Reporting Health Care Facility

DATE DIAGNOSED   Month   Day   Year

Address

City   **State**   **ZIP Code**

DATE OF DEATH   Month   Day   Year

Telephone Number (   )   **Fax** (   )

Submitted by   **Date Submitted** (Month/Day/Year)

(Obtain additional forms from your local health department.)

SEXUALLY TRANSMITTED DISEASES (STD)

Syphilis
- ☐ Primary (lesion present)
- ☐ Secondary
- ☐ Early latent < 1 year
- ☐ Latent (unknown duration)
- ☐ Late latent > 1 year
- ☐ Late (tertiary)
- ☐ Congenital
- ☐ **Neurosyphilis**

Syphilis Test Results
- ☐ RPR   Titer: _____
- ☐ VDRL   Titer: _____
- ☐ FTA/MHA: ☐ Pos ☐ Neg
- ☐ CSF-VDRL: ☐ Pos ☐ Neg
- ☐ Other: _____

Gonorrhea
- ☐ Urethral/Cervical
- ☐ PID
- ☐ Other: _____

Chlamydia
- ☐ Urethral/Cervical
- ☐ PID
- ☐ Other: _____

- ☐ **PID (Unknown Etiology)**
- ☐ **Chancroid**
- ☐ **Non-Gonococcal Urethritis**

STD TREATMENT INFORMATION
- ☐ Treated (Drugs, Dosage, Route): _____
  Date Treatment Initiated   Month   Day   Year
- ☐ **Untreated**
  - ☐ Will treat
  - ☐ Unable to contact patient
  - ☐ Refused treatment
  - ☐ Referred to: _____

VIRAL HEPATITIS

		Pos	Neg	Pend	Not Done
☐ **Hep A**	anti-HAV IgM	☐	☐	☐	☐
☐ **Hep B**	HBsAg	☐	☐	☐	☐
☐ Acute	anti-HBc	☐	☐	☐	☐
☐ Chronic	anti-HBc IgM	☐	☐	☐	☐
	anti-HBs	☐	☐	☐	☐
☐ **Hep C**	anti-HCV	☐	☐	☐	☐
☐ Acute	PCR-HCV	☐	☐	☐	☐
☐ Chronic					
☐ **Hep D (Delta)**	anti-Delta	☐	☐	☐	☐
☐ Other: ___		☐	☐	☐	☐

Suspected Exposure Type
- ☐ Blood transfusion
- ☐ Other needle exposure
- ☐ Sexual contact
- ☐ Household contact
- ☐ Child care
- ☐ Other: _____

TUBERCULOSIS (TB)

Status
- ☐ **Active Disease**
  - ☐ Confirmed
  - ☐ Suspected
- ☐ **Infected, No Disease**
  - ☐ Convertor
  - ☐ Reactor

Site(s)
- ☐ Pulmonary
- ☐ Extra-Pulmonary
- ☐ Both

Mantoux TB Skin Test
Month   Day   Year
Date Performed
☐ Pending
Results: _____ mm ☐ Not Done

Chest X-Ray   Month   Day   Year
Date Performed
- ☐ Normal   ☐ Pending   ☐ Not done
- ☐ Cavitary   ☐ Abnormal/Noncavitary

Bacteriology   Month   Day   Year
Date Specimen Collected
Source _____
Smear: ☐ Pos ☐ Neg ☐ Pending ☐ Not done
Culture: ☐ Pos ☐ Neg ☐ Pending ☐ Not done
Other test(s) _____

TB TREATMENT INFORMATION
- ☐ **Current Treatment**
  - ☐ INH   ☐ RIF   ☐ PZA
  - ☐ EMB   ☐ Other: _____
  Month   Day   Year
  Date Treatment Initiated
- ☐ **Untreated**
  - ☐ Will treat
  - ☐ Unable to contact patient
  - ☐ Refused treatment
  - ☐ Referred to: _____

REMARKS

FIGURE 8.1 Confidential Morbidity Report.

global travel in the second half of the century. In countries where communities lack sanitary drinking water and sewage disposal, as well as safe food-handling practices, the rates can be very high. This disease can be lethal to the very young, elderly, and those with compromised health, as dehydration from the loss of fluids from diarrhea and vomiting can occur rapidly. Vaccine development, improved sanitation, and education regarding food handling are ongoing strategies being utilized in the cholera-endemic regions of the world (WHO, 2006a).

◆ *Tuberculosis* has made a powerful resurgence in the last three decades as many countries let their control programs become complacent. In 1993, WHO declared TB a global emergency. One-third of the incidence of TB in the last 5 years can be attributed to human immunodeficiency virus (HIV) infection. Drug-resistant strains of the TB bacillus have infected up to 50 million people worldwide. Each year, 8 million people develop TB, and 1.8 million die of the disease. The highest incidence rates are found in Africa and Southeast Asia (Borgdorff, Floyd, & Broekmans, 2002; CDC, 2006o).

◆ *Yellow fever* is endemic in tropical regions of South American and Africa. Integration of yellow fever vaccination into the regular childhood immunization schedule and mosquito abatement efforts are key to decreasing this disease (Heymann, 2004).

Global successes and failures in the control of communicable diseases are affected by many factors. First, the geopolitical nature of an area influences who can respond when a communicable disease occurs in a country. Second, the natural and manmade resources of an area influence the health status of the population before a disease strikes, contributing to both disease resistance and the ability to survive once a communicable disease is contracted. This is one reason that poorer nations have higher incidences and greater numbers of deaths from communicable diseases. Finally, weather and climate factors can influence health and illness. For example, both droughts and floods can lead to crop failure and subsequent famine, which directly affect an individual's ability to fight disease or recover (Weatherall et al., 2005).

National Trends

At the national level, for several decades in the late 20th century, medical research and funding focused on major chronic diseases such as arteriosclerosis and cancer. During those years, it seemed that the war against communicable disease was being won, and the nation became complacent about communicable diseases (CDC, 1999a).

New, Emerging, and Reemerging Diseases

In the early 1980s, HIV/AIDS had emerged as a new and devastating disease. But because of the political atmosphere of the time, valuable time was lost in recognizing the potentially deleterious effects that this disease would cost in human suffering and lives lost. Not only was this new epidemic ignored, but at the same time, it was also discovered that many children were not being immunized against communicable diseases—U.S. rates were as high as those in poorer nations. Tuberculosis was also coming back with a vengeance, and in many cases was resistant to the recognized treatment (Fauci, 2005).

Clearly, communicable diseases will always present challenges to health care. Pathogens that are considered to be under control because they respond well to current treatment can mutate and produce new, virulent, and resistant strains. Diseases that have been almost eliminated can emerge again if public health efforts slacken; and diseases that are eradicated in the United States can revisit this country on any one of the international flights arriving each day at our airports. As a result, present concerns focus on three types of communicable disease: new diseases, emerging diseases, and reemerging diseases (Fauci, 2005).

Some communicable diseases have been affecting us for centuries or millennia, but a major new disease, HIV/AIDS, which is discussed in this chapter and in more detail in Chapter 26, was first recognized only in 1981. Legionnaires' disease, which was first detected in Philadelphia in 1976, occurred sporadically in other countries since then. In 1999, West Nile virus was first diagnosed in the United States in New York City. In subsequent years, surveillance programs were developed to track West Nile virus activity as it crossed the country. In 2005, as more cases were confirmed, West Nile virus disease in humans became a reportable disease (CDC, 2006g). In 2006, West Nile virus activity reflected mild to severe symptoms in 4,052 human cases and resulted in 146 deaths nationally. These diseases are disturbing reminders that new threats to public health are always on the horizon (see Fig. 8.2).

Emerging diseases are diseases rarely or never before seen in the United States. These diseases may also be new to public health officials in other countries. Emerging diseases occurring in the United States include Hantavirus, seen in the southwestern region in 1993; and typhoid, seen in a native Nigerian in New York City in 1994. Typically, diseases that are uncommon in the United States, such as malaria, plague, Lassa fever, cholera, and yellow fever, accompany people as they travel from one country to another on airlines and cruise ships. Sudden acute respiratory syndrome (SARS) emerged in 2003, causing a worldwide panic and a crisis for health care systems. Global travel patterns enabled this infectious agent to spread quickly to other countries from its epicenter in China (Murphy, 2006). Dr. Mohammad Akhter, while serving as executive director of the American Public Health Association, said "the [CDC] is just like the Justice Department before 9/11. It only comes in to investigate once a crime has been committed" (Mullins, 2002).

Reemerging diseases are those communicable diseases that have been endemic in some parts of the world, but are now endemic in more countries and are increasing to epidemic proportions in others. Often, the resurgence is caused by the emergence of new, drug-resistant strains of a familiar organism, such as the MDR TB bacillus. *Staphylococcus aureus* infections now are characterized by some strains so powerful that they no longer respond to vancomycin. Fortunately, the infection still responds to two new antibiotics, but those could also lose effectiveness. This is a watershed

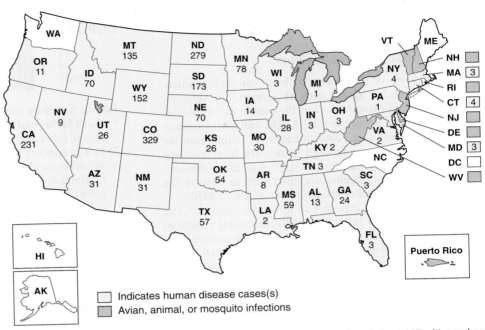

FIGURE 8.2 2007 West Nile Virus activity in the United States (reported to the CDC as of September 18, 2007).

Map shows the distribution of avian, animal, or mosquito infection occuring during 2007 with number of human cases if any, by state. If West Nile virus infection is reported to CDC from any area of a state, that entire state is shaded.

moment in the fight to stay ahead of communicable diseases. In addition to *S. aureus* and the TB bacillus, the list of antimicrobial-resistant organisms includes strains of *Haemophilus influenzae, Neisseria gonorrhoeae, Bordetella pertussis,* and *Streptococcus pneumoniae.* Tuberculosis is currently the communicable disease that affects the greatest number of people in the United States in regard to strains of drug-resistant microbes.

Healthy People: The Prevention Agenda for the Nation

The *Healthy People 2010* document (U.S. Department of Health and Human Services [USDHHS], 2000) groups the nation's health objectives somewhat differently from its predecessor, *Healthy People 2000* (USDHHS, 1991). Nevertheless, many objectives still focus on infectious diseases and immunizations, aiming to decrease morbidity and mortality from infectious diseases and to increase the number of immunized children and adults. In addition, the document attempts to guide the nation toward health with goals and objectives that include new focus areas such as arthritis, osteoporosis, chronic back conditions, chronic kidney diseases, respiratory diseases, vision and hearing, medical product safety, health communication, and public health infrastructure.

Healthy People 2010 objectives were formulated with input from more than 350 national and 250 state public health, medical, and environmental agencies, in addition to lay advisors from around the country. These collaborators began to meet in 1996 to design the structure and content of the document. During its development, the Office of Disease Prevention and Health Promotion accepted electronic comments at its website and in writing, making this truly a document of the people. With so many people involved, achievement of the document's goals is much more likely.

Modes of Transmission

As discussed in Chapter 7, the reservoir of infection can be a person, animal, insect, or inanimate material in which the infectious agent lives and multiplies and which serves as a source of infection to others. Transmission of a communicable disease can occur by direct, indirect, airborne, or vector methods.

Direct Transmission

Direct transmission occurs by immediate transfer of infectious agents from a reservoir to a new susceptible host. It requires direct contact with the source, through touching, biting, kissing, or sexual intercourse—that is, contact with oral secretions, blood, or other potentially infectious fluid, such as the drainage from a skin lesion. Coughing or sneezing secretions into the face of a susceptible individual can directly transmit respiratory infections, such as measles or pertussis. Close proximity is required—about 3 feet—to transmit an organism from one person to another (National Institutes of Health [NIH], 2006).

Indirect Transmission

Indirect transmission occurs when the infectious agent is transported within contaminated inanimate materials such as air, water, or food. It is also commonly referred to as *vehicle-borne transmission.* Chapter 9 describes both the government's role and the nurse's role in helping to prevent food and water contamination by infectious agents (NIH, 2006).

Food- and Water-related Illness

Reportable food- or water-related illness can include infections from bacterial agents such as *Salmonella, Shigella, E. coli* 0157, and *Camplyobacter*; the protozoan agent *Giardia*; and the viral agent hepatitis A. The contamination can occur at the source (e.g., contamination by animal into the food or water chain) or through unsanitary food handling practices, which are referred to as the *fecal–oral route*. Ingestion of the pathogenic organism sets in motion the events of a food- or water-related illness (CDC, 2005d).

Most commonly, exposure to infectious food or water results in symptoms related to gastrointestinal function, including diarrhea, nausea, vomiting, stomach cramps, and bloating. Fever accompanies these infections as well. Onset of symptoms may occur within a few hours after exposure or not until days or even weeks later, depending on the organism. This time interval between exposure and onset of symptoms is called the **incubation period**.

Bacterial contamination of food resulting in human illness occurs as a result of either infection or intoxication. Infection occurs through ingestion of food contaminated with adequate doses of *Salmonella, Shigella, E. coli,* or other pathogens. The cycle begins when the infectious agent multiplies and grows in the food medium. The agent subsequently invades the host after ingestion of the food. Infection then occurs—which is the entry and development or multiplication of an infectious agent in the body. Infection is usually accompanied by an immune response, such as the production of antibodies with or without clinical manifestation. The infectious organism produces illness by direct irritation of the normal gastrointestinal mucosa. By contrast, intoxication is caused by the production of toxins as a by-product of the normal bacterial life cycle. This commonly occurs when cooked food is left standing at room temperature. It is ingestion of the toxin, rather than the microbe itself, that produces the illness (CDC, 2005d).

The distinction between infection and intoxication is relevant for a number of reasons. Toxins may be difficult to isolate and identify, particularly in the absence of the bacteria; some suspected food-borne illnesses go unidentified for this reason. Although the bacteria may be killed after heating of foodstuffs before consumption, some bacteria-produced toxins are stable at normal cooking temperatures, so that food cannot be rendered safe. Bacteria established in the human gastrointestinal system may require medical treatment to be eradicated. In contrast, individuals with food intoxication typically require essentially supportive care while in the process of ridding themselves of the toxin (CDC, 2005d).

The most important aspects of food- or water-related diseases for nurses in community health may be, first of all, recognizing that outbreaks of illness affecting large numbers of people continue to occur fairly regularly, despite well-recognized standards for decontamination of water supplies and safe commercial food preparation. Second, such outbreaks may not be detectable by local surveillance means because of individuals' mobility or the routine transportation of foods from one

---

DISPLAY 8.1   CORRECT METHODS FOR PRESERVING THE SAFETY AND CLEANLINESS OF FOOD

Before handling food:
- Wash hands and all food preparation surfaces and utensils thoroughly with soap and water.

When preparing food:
- Wash foods that are to be eaten raw and uncooked thoroughly in clean water. This includes foods that are to be peeled that grow on the ground or come in contact with soil.
- Cook all meat products thoroughly.
- Do not allow cooked meats to come in contact with dishes, utensils, or containers used when the foods were raw and uncooked.

When storing leftover foods:
- Cool cooked foods quickly; store under refrigeration in clean, covered containers.

When reheating leftover foods:
- Heat foods thoroughly. Bacteria contaminating food grow and multiply in a temperature range between 39°F and 140°F.

---

state to the other (CDC, 2005d). For example, an outbreak of *E. coli* 0157 was associated with spinach grown in one state and sold nationally. This illness outbreak was detected through identification in multiple state laboratories and compared through sentinel disease detection centers. It was then traced back to the source—through local investigations of ill persons (CDC, 2006i). Third, such outbreaks can serve to remind all community health practitioners of the continuing need to teach and observe the most basic methods for preventing food and water contamination. Display 8.1 summarizes correct methods for maintaining the safety and cleanliness of food.

Vector Transmission

When transmission occurs through a **vector** (a nonhuman carrier such as an animal or insect), it is known as vector-borne transmission. Common vectors include bats, fleas, lice, mosquitoes, raccoons, rats, skunks, squirrels, and ticks. During vector-borne transmission, the infectious agent may be transported mechanically without multiplication or change, or the infectious agent may develop biologically before passage to a susceptible host.

Diseases transmitted through vectors prove challenging in communicable disease control, because individuals who become infected typically have no direct personal contact with other infected persons. Rather, isolated cases occur within areas inhabited by the vector. Nevertheless, vector-borne diseases have significantly affected human history. Louse-borne typhus and flea-borne plague together were responsible for a majority of the devastating epidemics that occurred over the last 600 years. Currently, mosquito-borne malaria and snail-borne schistosomiasis cause major human suffering for hundreds of millions of people in tropical settings every year (Heymann, 2004).

Control strategies directed toward vector-borne diseases typically involve community education and environmental measures to hinder the vector from reaching the host (see Chapter 9). Control strategies may include:

◆ Minimizing the population of insect vectors (e.g., by spraying insecticides to kill mosquitoes)
◆ Educating the public to the natural habitat of the vector to reduce the population density
◆ Exterminating rodents that carry diseases, such as rats
◆ Using barriers between the susceptible human and the vector, such as mosquito nets or screened windows to control malaria or protective clothing and sprays against tick-borne diseases
◆ Educating the public about preventive and protective measures, including actions to take when attacked by the vector to prevent disease from developing

In the United States, vector-borne illnesses have received renewed attention with accumulating information about Lyme disease, caused by a bacterium *Borrelia burgdorferi* that is transmitted to humans by a tick vector. Lyme disease results in symptoms of varying severity, including rash, joint pain, progressive weakness, vision changes, and other neuromuscular dysfunction. Other vector-borne diseases receiving attention in the 1990s included tick-borne fevers (e.g., Rocky Mountain spotted fever and relapsing fever) and rabies, whose vector usually is an infected domestic animal, bat, skunk, or raccoon. As mentioned earlier, West Nile virus was first seen in the United States in 1999. Occasionally, imported vector-borne tropical diseases, including malaria and dengue fever, are reported (Heymann, 2004).

Airborne Transmission

Airborne transmission occurs through droplet nuclei—the small residues that result from evaporation of fluid from droplets emitted by an infected host. Sneezing and coughing are common examples of airborne transmission. They may also be created purposely by atomizing devices or accidentally in microbiology laboratories. Because of their small size and weight, they can remain suspended in the air for long periods before they are inhaled into the respiratory system of a host. Airborne transmission can also occur in dust. Small particles of dust from soil containing fungus spores may cling to clothing, bedding, or floors. Alternatively, the spores may become separated from dry soil by the wind and then be inhaled by the host (CDC, 2006b).

PRIMARY PREVENTION

In the context of communicable disease control, two approaches are useful in achieving primary prevention: Education using mass media, and targeting health messages to aggregates and immunization.

Education

Health education in primary prevention is directed both at helping at-risk individuals understand their risk status and at promoting behaviors that decrease exposure or susceptibility.

Chapter 11 deals more extensively with the concepts of learning theory and the variety of health education approaches and materials available to community health nurses today.

Use of Mass Media for Health Education

All people need to be informed about the risks of communicable diseases. Often, use of health marketing techniques through mass media can be an effective way to reach the largest number of people (Rall & Meyer, 2006; Renaud et al., 2006). Additionally, many target groups, such as low-income and racially and ethnically diverse communities at high risk for communicable diseases, are very hard to reach one-on-one. Media can be an effective method to reach them. To disseminate public health information to large numbers of people, mass media plays four major roles:

1. *Use the media as a primary change agent:* Community education programs can successfully increase knowledge about communicable diseases and preventive measures.
2. *Use the media as a complement to other disease prevention efforts:* The media can effectively model preventive behaviors, such as condom use and drug abstinence.
3. *Use the media as a promoter of communicable disease control programs:* The media can help to increase participation of community members in primary prevention services.
4. *Use the media to promote disease prevention messages:* The media can contribute to the creation of a social environment that promotes health (e.g., increasing acceptance of regular condom use in the prevention of sexually transmitted diseases [STDs]).

The body of literature on mass communication for promoting health and preventing disease through the voluntary adoption of healthy behaviors is growing rapidly (Rall & Meyer, 2006; Renaud et al., 2006). Television, as a significant medium, reaches into most American homes, and public health campaigns are creatively designed to reach the target audiences.

The urgency to combat AIDS, as well as other life-threatening diseases, provides a strong rationale and impetus for developing effective disease prevention and control messages for dissemination through the media.

Messages need to be tailored to the specific characteristics of target audiences and the media channels to which the audiences are exposed. Disadvantaged or stigmatized groups, such as the poor, ethnic minorities, gay men, injection drug users, and prostitutes, are more vulnerable to infectious diseases and need mass media messages targeted to them. Those people who watch more television and listen to more radio respond to health promotion messages received through these media more often than groups who do not (CDC, 2006f).

Behavioral change is essential to control the spread of communicable diseases, and that change depends on successful communication between community health providers and target audiences, using the most appropriate media possible. Participation in media and education efforts depends on the awareness of target groups (e.g., injection drug users) about available programs and how to access them. Carefully and thoughtfully designed disease prevention messages disseminated through the media are a reliable and effective way of reaching hard-to-reach populations.

Targeting Meaningful Health Messages to Aggregates

To effectively deliver a communicable disease prevention message, the message must reach the target (at-risk) population. This requires correct identification of the characteristics of the target audience in terms of educational level, salience of the issue, involvement of the target audience with the issue, and access of the target audience to the media channels used. Cultural issues affect people's interpretation of messages and must be considered in the presentation of a disease-prevention message to ethnic and racial minority groups (Rall & Meyer, 2006; Renaud et al., 2006). Principles for adapting health messages to specific population subgroups include:

1. Develop educational materials from the community perspective, reflecting respect for community values and traditions, relevance to community needs and interests, and participation of the community in the preparation and use of the materials.
2. Ensure that materials are an integral part of a health education program, supported by other components of intervention—materials should not stand alone.
3. Materials must be related to the delivery of health services that are available, accessible, and acceptable to the target population.
4. All materials must be pretested and have demonstrated attractiveness, comprehension, acceptability, ownership, and persuasiveness.
5. Materials must be distributed with instructions for their use (i.e., how, when, and with whom they are to be used).

Immunization

Control of acute communicable diseases through immunization has been a common practice since the 19th century in the United States. **Immunization** is the process of introducing some form of disease-causing organism into a person's system to promote the development of antibodies that will resist that disease. In theory, this process makes the person immune to that particular infectious disease (i.e., able to resist a specific infectious disease–causing agent). That immunization requirements are acceptable in American society today is evidence that high levels of immunization in school children and aggressive enforcement of school immunization requirements, starting in the late 1970s, have not met widespread opposition. This continues to be true even during the last decade, when common immunizations have been changed and the number of immunizations has increased.

The schedule for administration of vaccines officially changes every January. In 2004, the CDC conducted the National Immunization Survey. Overall, 77.2% of children 18 to 35 months of age at the time of the survey had received all of the recommended immunizations (National Center for

Health Statistics, 2004). Adolescent vaccination, however, has lagged behind the rates achieved by younger children over the last decade. Barriers that must be overcome include lack of parental knowledge, inadequate access to medical care, and inadequate or no insurance coverage (National Foundation for Infectious Diseases, 2005). With adults, good progress has been made. Influenza vaccine coverage rates increased from 42% in 1991 to 65% in 2003, and pneumococcal vaccine coverage rates increased from 21% to 34% over the same period (CDC, 2005g).

The statutes that exist to ensure adequate immunization levels at the time of school entry place the school in the role of a controlling agency, whereas public health departments and private health care providers are authorized to administer the required vaccines (see Chapter 22). An emerging drawback of this mechanism is that many parents delay immunizations until the child's fifth year (Scutchfield & Keck, 2003). Preschool-age children represent a major proportion of all cases of vaccine-preventable diseases and are the group at highest risk for infection. A national objective stated in *Healthy People 2000* (USDHHS, 1991) was for 90% of American children to be vaccinated by their second birthday with four doses of DTaP, three doses of polio, and one dose of the combined measles, mumps, and rubella vaccine. *Healthy People 2010* (USDHHS, 2000) reinforced this goal by including an objective for reducing or eliminating all indigenous cases of vaccine-preventable disease (Table 8.1).

Although childhood immunization rates historically have been lower in minority populations compared with the White population, rates for minority preschool children have been increasing at a more rapid pace, and the gap has significantly

TABLE 8.1 *Healthy People 2010* Vaccine-preventable Disease Objectives

Disease	2003	2010 Target
Congenital rubella syndrome	0	0
Diphtheria	1	0
Haemophilus influenzae type b	2013	0
Hepatitis B	7526	0
Measles	56	0
Mumps	231	0
Pertussis	11,647	2000
Polio	0	0
Rubella	0	0
Tetanus	20	0
Varicella (chickenpox)	20,948	400,000

Sources:
Centers for Disease Control and Prevention (CDC). (2007a). *Epidemiology and prevention of vaccine-preventable diseases* (10th ed.). Atkinson, W., Hamborsky, J., McEntyre, L., & Wolfe, S. (Eds.), Washington, DC: Public Health Foundation.
 U.S. Department of Health and Human Services. (2000). *Healthy People 2010: Understanding and improving health* (2nd ed.). Washington, DC: U.S. Government Printing Office.

narrowed (CDC, 2005b; CDC, 2006h). The National Immunization Survey has documented substantial progress toward achieving 1996 Childhood Immunization Initiative coverage goals by racial and ethnic groups. However, efforts to increase vaccination coverage need to be intensified, particularly for children living in poverty (CDC, 2006h)

It is critical to discover the social and cultural characteristics affecting health status, attitudes about preventive measures, behaviors in seeking services, acceptability of interventions, and perceptions of health care providers that determine parental action in having a child immunized in a regular and timely fashion (see From the Case Files I, and Display 8.2). This is a unique area of health care delivery, one in which nurses must rely on parental initiative to obtain a form of care for the well child that may be perceived as producing pain and temporary illness for no observable benefit (CDC, 2006h).

Vaccine-preventable Diseases

Vaccine-preventable diseases (VPD), such as hepatitis B, *H. influenzae* type b, measles, polio, diphtheria, pertussis, and chickenpox, are diseases that can be prevented through immunization. Immunity may be either passive or active. **Passive immunity** is short-term resistance to a specific disease-causing organism; it may be acquired naturally (as with newborns through maternal antibody transfer) or artificially through inoculation with pooled human antibody (e.g., immune globulin) that gives temporary protection. **Active immunity** is long-term (sometimes lifelong) resistance to a

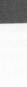

From the Case Files I

Personal Belief Exemption and Immunization

A whooping cough outbreak occurred in a small rural county last year. Whooping cough or pertussis is a vaccine-preventable disease. It is highly contagious, and most devastating to the very young and very old. In this community, the population is not very ethnically diverse, but it is philosophically diverse. Many community members are against vaccinating their children. The outbreak of pertussis occurred in a small charter school, with the majority of the children unvaccinated for reasons of personal belief. Personal belief exemption is an option for a family. Unfortunately, with a large unvaccinated population, as in this school, the spark of a contagious, vaccine-preventable infection can spread rapidly. This is what happened at this school, with 22 cases among children and family members. The school had to be closed a week early for winter break to help halt the spread. Three waves of illness occurred in this school from November to April.

One might think that the entire problem lies with the group of individuals who will not vaccinate their children, but this is not what was discovered upon investigation. The issue of personal belief exemption was discussed among public health nurses and school nurses in this community. We discussed the issue with parents and teachers at the charter school. The two highlights from our discussions were that parents either signed the exemption out of true conviction or out of frustration that the school was hounding them to get their child vaccinated. For whatever reason, some parents just cannot seem to make the time to get the necessary immunizations completed. These parents tend to be the high-risk families who keep a school nurse busy. It was discovered that in some of the schools with high-risk families, the personal belief exemption was signed in order to not be pestered any longer.

So, which group do you extend your efforts to as a public health nurse? The answer is both. The parents who will not vaccinate their children will not be convinced otherwise. Parents who chose the easy way out may need more assistance. Here was the solution that the county's immunization coordinator came up with. Utilizing the community's immunization coalition and the school nurses, it was determined that the school secretaries needed an inservice on how to properly offer the exemption to a family and what information parents would need to make an informed decision before signing the exemption.

The immunization coordinator developed an education tool that explained the parent responsibility to the community at large if their child were to become ill with a vaccine-preventable illness. The document covered points, such as the family having a medical plan with their physician, learning how to care for and isolate the child, working with a public health nurse, and so on (see Display 8.2). The school secretaries were asked to give this document to parents who were interested in exempting, along with community resource information as to where to send families who may not have access to affordable immunizations.

The parents at the charter school were very accepting of the information on what to do for an ill child, and the school secretaries expressed relief regarding dealing with parents who may want to exempt out for convenience rather than conviction. In time, we should be able to see if this approach has improved vaccination rates in the community.

Karen, RHN

DISPLAY 8.2	WHAT PARENTS SHOULD KNOW WHEN SIGNING A PERSONAL BELIEFS AFFIDAVIT EXEMPTION OF IMMUNIZATION

1. Measles, mumps, rubella, chicken pox, pertussis, diphtheria, polio, Haemophilus influenza type b, hepatitis A, and hepatitis B are infectious to others and are avoidable through immunization.
2. Please educate yourself to the symptoms and possible complications that can arise from a vaccine-preventable disease. Information for parents about these diseases may be found at the National Immunization Program site http://www.cdc.gov/nip/ or by calling the Nevada County Public Health Department (530) 265-1450.
3. These diseases have many symptoms that require close monitoring and care so that complications are minimized. It is essential to have a plan of care, coordinated with your health care provider, to act upon the mildest to most severe symptoms of the disease.
4. The school or school nurse is responsible for maintaining a list of the school children who have parent-signed exemption to immunization for medical, religious, or personal belief. This list allows the school nurse to quickly identify any child who is at risk of exposure to a vaccine-preventable disease.
5. An unimmunized child will be excluded from school by the County Health Officer when a vaccine-preventable disease is identified in the school. The ill child will also be excluded from school.
6. When a child is excluded from school, it is the responsibility of the parent or guardian to keep the

child isolated* from the public at large to prevent spread of infection to the community.
7. Vaccine-preventable diseases are considered **reportable communicable diseases** under the Health and Safety Codes of California. If your child contracts one of these diseases, a Public Health Nurse will contact you. Be prepared to provide information about the illness to the investigator. **This information is confidential.**
8. The parent or guardian is also at risk of contracting any of these diseases when exposed to an ill child. If unimmunized, the parent or guardian may also be considered exposed and incubating the disease, since this may continue the cycle of infection to others. This in turn requires that the parent or guardian remain in isolation from the community through the incubation period.
9. The child who is exposed to the disease may be offered preventive medication or immunization to prevent the disease from occurring—either may keep the child from being excluded from school.

———————————————   ——————————
Parent signature   Date

*The isolation time frame is determined by the county health officer. Isolation means that the exposed or ill child cannot leave home except for medical care. **No social gatherings!**

specific disease-causing organism; it also can be acquired naturally or artificially. Naturally acquired active immunity occurs when a person contracts a disease and develops long-lasting antibodies that provide immunity against future exposure. Artificially acquired active immunity occurs through inoculation with a vaccine, such as the diphtheria, pertussis, tetanus vaccination series given to children. A **vaccine** is a preparation made from a live organism or an inactivated form of the organism. Live attenuated vaccines are made from weakened wild virus organisms that are used to create an immune response in the recipient. It only takes a small amount to initiate an immune response, and the organisms must replicate to be effective. Inactivated vaccines are made from a viral organism that has been inactivated by heat or chemicals. These vaccines cannot replicate in the recipient (CDC, 2007a).

Because of the success of immunization strategies, few practicing nurses in the United States today have treated clients with tetanus or diphtheria, or even measles (although some have cared for clients with residual polio disabilities). However, VPDs still exist in force in the developing world, and outbreaks occur in the United States in groups of nonimmunized or susceptible populations. For example, certain people are medically exempt from immunization, and others decline immunization for religious or personal reasons. Even with global and national efforts at reducing and eliminating VPDs, some national goals have not been met. In fact, statistics for some diseases have gotten worse. Rates of

immunization coverage have declined in some areas, with subsequent increases in VPDs (e.g., pertussis). Pertussis has become endemic, with frequent outbreaks (Broder et al., 2006).

Schedule of Recommended Immunizations

A schedule for the administration of childhood vaccinations, based on recommendations by the Advisory Committee on Immunization Practices (ACIP), the American Academy of Pediatrics (AAP), the American Academy of Family Physicians (AAFP), and the CDC, is published annually (Table 8.2). The CDC also provides "catch-up" schedules for children not receiving their first immunizations at birth, according to the standard schedule. Current recommendations call for a child to receive 10 different vaccines or toxoids (many in combination form and all requiring more than one dose) in six or seven visits to a health care provider between birth and school entry, with boosters in the preteen to early teen years (CDC, 2007b).

Factors influencing the recommended age at which vaccines are administered include the age-specific risks of the disease, the age-specific risks of complications, the ability of persons of a given age to produce an adequate and lasting immune response, and the potential for interference with the immune response acquired from passively transferred maternal antibodies. In general, vaccines are recommended for the youngest age group at risk whose members are known to develop an acceptable antibody response to vaccination (CDC, 2007a).

TABLE 8.2   Vaccines for Infants and School Entry

DEPARTMENT OF HEALTH AND HUMAN SERVICES • CENTERS FOR DISEASE CONTROL AND PREVENTION

Recommended Immunization Schedule for Persons Aged 0–6 Years—UNITED STATES • 2007

Vaccine▼　　　　Age▶	Birth	1 month	2 months	4 months	6 months	12 months	15 months	18 months	19–23 months	2–3 years	4–6 years
Hepatitis B[1]	HepB	HepB		see footnote 1		HepB				HepB Series	
Rotavirus[2]			Rota	Rota	Rota						
Diphtheria, Tetanus, Pertussis[3]			DTaP	DTaP	DTaP		DTaP				DTaP
Haemophilus influenzae type b[4]			Hib	Hib	*Hib*[4]	Hib		Hib			
Pneumococcal[5]			PCV	PCV	PCV	PCV				PCV / PPV	
Inactivated Poliovirus			IPV	IPV		IPV					IPV
Influenza[6]						Influenza (Yearly)					
Measles, Mumps, Rubella[7]						MMR					MMR
Varicella[8]						Varicella					Varicella
Hepatitis A[9]						HepA (2 doses)				HepA Series	
Meningococcal[10]										MPSV4	

Range of recommended ages

Catch-up immunization

Certain high-risk groups

This schedule indicates the recommended ages for routine administration of currently licensed childhood vaccines, as of December 1, 2006, for children aged 0–6 years. Additional information is available at http://www.cdc.gov/nip/recs/child-schedule.htm. Any dose not administered at the recommended age should be administered at any subsequent visit, when indicated and feasible. Additional vaccines may be licensed and recommended during the year. Licensed combination vaccines may be used whenever any components of the combination are indicated and other components of the vaccine are not contraindicated and if approved by the Food and Drug Administration for that dose of the series. Providers should consult the respective Advisory Committee on Immunization Practices statement for detailed recommendations. Clinically significant adverse events that follow immunization should be reported to the Vaccine Adverse Event Reporting System (VAERS). Guidance about how to obtain and complete a VAERS form is available at http://www.vaers.hhs.gov or by telephone, 800-822-7967.

1. **Hepatitis B vaccine (HepB).** *(Minimum age: birth)*
   At birth:
   - Administer monovalent HepB to all newborns before hospital discharge.
   - If mother is hepatitis surface antigen (HBsAg)-positive, administer HepB and 0.5 mL of hepatitis B immune globulin (HBIG) within 12 hours of birth.
   - If mother's HBsAg status is unknown, administer HepB within 12 hours of birth. Determine the HBsAg status as soon as possible and if HBsAg-positive, administer HBIG (no later than age 1 week).
   - If mother is HBsAg-negative, the birth dose can only be delayed with physician's order and mother's negative HBsAg laboratory report documented in the infant's medical record.
   After the birth dose:
   - The HepB series should be completed with either monovalent HepB or a combination vaccine containing HepB. The second dose should be administered at age 1–2 months. The final dose should be administered at age ≥24 weeks. Infants born to HBsAg-positive mothers should be tested for HBsAg and antibody to HBsAg after completion of ≥3 doses of a licensed HepB series, at age 9–18 months (generally at the next well-child visit).
   4-month dose:
   - It is permissible to administer 4 doses of HepB when combination vaccines are administered after the birth dose. If monovalent HepB is used for doses after the birth dose, a dose at age 4 months is not needed.

2. **Rotavirus vaccine (Rota).** *(Minimum age: 6 weeks)*
   - Administer the first dose at age 6–12 weeks. Do not start the series later than age 12 weeks.
   - Administer the final dose in the series by age 32 weeks. Do not administer a dose later than age 32 weeks.
   - Data on safety and efficacy outside of these age ranges are insufficient.

3. **Diphtheria and tetanus toxoids and acellular pertussis vaccine (DTaP).** *(Minimum age: 6 weeks)*
   - The fourth dose of DTaP may be administered as early as age 12 months, provided 6 months have elapsed since the third dose.
   - Administer the final dose in the series at age 4–6 years.

4. ***Haemophilus influenzae* type b conjugate vaccine (Hib).**
   (Minimum age: 6 weeks)
   - If PRP-OMP (PedvaxHIB® or ComVax® [Merck]) is administered at ages 2 and 4 months, a dose at age 6 months is not required.
   - TriHiBit® (DTaP/Hib) combination products should not be used for primary immunization but can be used as boosters following any Hib vaccine in children aged ≥12 months.

5. **Pneumococcal vaccine.** *(Minimum age: 6 weeks for pneumococcal conjugate vaccine [PCV]; 2 years for pneumococcal polysaccharide vaccine [PPV])*
   - Administer PCV at ages 24–59 months in certain high-risk groups. Administer PPV to children aged ≥2 years in certain high-risk groups. See *MMWR* 2000;49(No. RR-9):1–35.

6. **Influenza vaccine.** *(Minimum age: 6 months for trivalent inactivated influenza vaccine [TIV]; 5 years for live, attenuated influenza vaccine [LAIV])*
   - All children aged 6–59 months and close contacts of all children aged 0–59 months are recommended to receive influenza vaccine.
   - Influenza vaccine is recommended annually for children aged ≥59 months with certain risk factors, health-care workers, and other persons (including household members) in close contact with persons in groups at high risk. See *MMWR* 2006;55(No. RR-10):1–41.
   - For healthy persons aged 5–49 years, LAIV may be used as an alternative to TIV.
   - Children receiving TIV should receive 0.25 mL if aged 6–35 months or 0.5 mL if aged ≥3 years.
   - Children aged <9 years who are receiving influenza vaccine for the first time should receive 2 doses (separated by ≥4 weeks for TIV and ≥6 weeks for LAIV).

7. **Measles, mumps, and rubella vaccine (MMR).** *(Minimum age: 12 months)*
   - Administer the second dose of MMR at age 4–6 years. MMR may be administered before age 4–6 years, provided ≥4 weeks have elapsed since the first dose and both doses are administered at age ≥12 months.

8. **Varicella vaccine.** *(Minimum age: 12 months)*
   - Administer the second dose of varicella vaccine at age 4–6 years. Varicella vaccine may be administered before age 4–6 years, provided that ≥3 months have elapsed since the first dose and both doses are administered at age ≥12 months. If second dose was administered ≥28 days following the first dose, the second dose does not need to be repeated.

9. **Hepatitis A vaccine (HepA).** *(Minimum age: 12 months)*
   - HepA is recommended for all children aged 1 year (i.e., aged 12–23 months). The 2 doses in the series should be administered at least 6 months apart.
   - Children not fully vaccinated by age 2 years can be vaccinated at subsequent visits.
   - HepA is recommended for certain other groups of children, including in areas where vaccination programs target older children. See *MMWR* 2006;55(No. RR-7):1–23.

10. **Meningococcal polysaccharide vaccine (MPSV4).** *(Minimum age: 2 years)*
    - Administer MPSV4 to children aged 2–10 years with terminal complement deficiencies or anatomic or functional asplenia and certain other high-risk groups. See *MMWR* 2005;54(No. RR-7):1–21.

The Recommended Immunization Schedules for Persons Aged 0–18 Years are approved by the Advisory Committee on Immunization Practices (http://www.cdc.gov/nip/acip), the American Academy of Pediatrics (http://www.aap.org), and the American Academy of Family Physicians (http://www.aafp.org).

SAFER • HEALTHIER • PEOPLE™

Recommendations for vaccine administration may be revised in light of specific circumstances. For example, it is now recommended that infants receive hepatitis B vaccine at birth, whether or not their mothers have a positive or negative response to the hepatitis B surface antigen. This approach will catch any infants born to mothers who lack prenatal testing, or who may live in households with individuals with unknown hepatitis B status (CDC, 2005a). Rotavirus—a diarrheal illness of infants—can safely be prevented by the use of a new vaccine RotaTeq, approved in February 2006 (CDC, 2007a). It has been reintroduced into the childhood immunization schedule recommendations.

Assessing Immunization Status of the Community

Determining the immunization status of children in a community can be a time-consuming but worthwhile task. Community health nurses may consider assessing groups of children with some common characteristics, such as children served by the Women, Infants, and Children program (WIC), those served by private medical providers, or those attending public schools in various neighborhoods. Because all children attending school in the United States must show proof of immunization upon school entry, review of immunization records at school can provide a means of retrospectively determining the proportion of these children whose immunizations were up to date at age 3 months or at age 2 years. It is strongly recommended that retrospective school vaccination record surveys be done as a means of estimating current levels of immunization status and monitoring trends over time. If no unusual immunization events occur in the intervening period, this retrospective record review gives a reasonable estimate of current immunization status of those age groups in the community. In addition, such a record review targeting children who were not up-to-date on their immunizations before school entry helps identify younger siblings who may also not be up-to-date (American Academy of Pediatrics [AAP], 2003).

With increasing numbers of children entering day care services in the preschool years, more states now require immunizations for preschool children, often including immunization against influenza, which is not presently required for older age groups. Preschool or day care center operators now obtain information about immunization status of this younger cohort, a group that previously often escaped surveillance and immunization initiatives (AAP, 2003).

Of interest to community health nurses, the ACIP and CDC in 2006 expanded the group of children eligible for influenza vaccine coverage under the Vaccines for Children (VFC) program. The resolution extends VFC coverage for influenza vaccine to all VFC-eligible children aged 6 to 59 months, as well as VFC-eligible children aged 2 to 18 years who are household contacts of children younger than 2 years of age. This resolution became effective in June 2006, so that flu vaccine could be administered during the 2006–2007 influenza vaccination season and subsequent seasons. These changes were expanded because of the increased risk for influenza-related hospitalizations among those younger than 59 months of age (CDC, 2006k).

Other community settings in which community health nurses may identify underimmunized children include homeless shelters and other public service settings or agencies used by families and children, including local religious centers. A family with one underimmunized child may have underimmunized children of other ages, as well as any number of other unmet preventive health care needs that the community health nurse can help address (AAP, 2003).

Herd Immunity

Herd immunity is central to understanding immunization as a means of protecting community health. As described in Chapter 7, herd immunity is the immunity level present in a particular population of people (Heymann, 2004). If few immune persons exist within a community, herd immunity is low, and the spread of disease is more likely. Vaccination of more individuals in the community, so that a high proportion has acquired resistance to the infectious agent, contributes to higher herd immunity. High herd immunity reduces the probability that the few unimmunized persons will come in contact with one another, making spread of the disease less likely. Outbreaks may occur if the immunization rate falls to less than 85% (Scutchfield & Keck, 2003) or if nonimmunized susceptible persons are grouped together rather than dispersed throughout the immunized community (see Evidence-Based Practice).

Barriers to Immunization Coverage

Improving immunization coverage requires examination of the reasons why children are not immunized. Many barriers exist. They include religious, financial, social, and cultural factors, as well as philosophical objections and provider limitations that form barriers to adequate immunization coverage.

Religious Barriers

The right to religious freedom gives some groups of individuals in the United States the constitutional right to exemption from immunization if they object to vaccination on religious grounds. Children from these families are identified at school entry. Such exemptions must be specifically enacted by law and, although it is not necessary to belong to a specific denomination, courts have required those seeking exemption to demonstrate that such belief against immunization is sincere and that no clear danger exists from the particular disease. Problems arise when members of exempted groups are found together in school or community settings, raising the risk of disease spread because of a lower herd immunity (Heymann, 2004).

Financial Barriers

Until recently, finances may have been a significant factor for immunization delays in families with limited incomes. Such families may have had more immediate priorities than vaccinations for an otherwise well child. In the late 1990s, two major initiatives significantly improved the financing of childhood immunizations. The VFC program and the Child Health Insurance Program (CHIP) cover children on Medicaid, uninsured children, and American Indian and Alaska Native children (USDHHS, 2006). In addition, underinsured children who receive immunizations at federally qualified health centers and rural health clinics are covered. These initiatives should eliminate low income as a barrier.

EVIDENCE-BASED PRACTICE

"Cocooning" to Protect Unvaccinated Infants

Over the past several years, a method known as *cocooning* has gained increased attention as a means to prevent communicable diseases, such as influenza and pertussis, in unvaccinated and incompletely vaccinated individuals. Children who are at high risk for infection, but not old enough to receive the current influenza vaccine, would be one of the target groups for this approach. Theoretically, by having all close family contacts immunized, the belief is that the risk of infection can be greatly reduced. This concept has been promoted in a variety of venues, including the Centers for Disease Control and Prevention (CDC) (2006) and the U.S. Food and Drug Administration (2006). Using the concept of herd immunity, this approach seems to hold great promise. The Cocooning Project at Renoun Regional Medical Center was the first in the nation to launch this innovative program in 2006 (CDC, 2006). The program provides immunizations for pertussis and influenza to all family contacts of babies born at the medical center.

The actual effectiveness of this program, however, has yet to be demonstrated. A literature search on this topic yielded only one discussion article regarding this type of intervention, and it cast some doubt on whether it can be an effective approach. De Serres and Duval (2005) note that less than half of the pertussis deaths in the United States had a traceable source of infection within their household contacts; meaning that other sources of infection are problematic. The 2006 proceedings of the Advisory Committee on Immunization Practices (CDC, 2006, p. 44) also noted that solid evidence has not yet been produced. Although the approach may have merit, the evidence is not yet apparent. In planning for an immunization program such as this, the public health nurse must approach this situation with cau-

tion. A number of questions must be addressed in considering whether cocooning is a viable option in a community: (a) Does this approach actually reduce infections in the target population and where is the evidence? (b) What is the risk to the household members being vaccinated? (c) What is the cost of this program? and (d) Are there unintended consequences from this approach, such as delayed immunizations in the target population?

Innovations are an important source of improved health-promoting practices and should not be discouraged, but as always, solid research evidence is vital. With limited health care dollars, efforts must target the most cost effective and proven methods possible. Only time and research will show whether cocooning can be an effective tool in the public health arsenal.

References and Selected Readings

Advisory Committee on Immunization Practices, CDC. (June 29–30, 2006). *Record of Proceedings.* Retrieved June 25, 2007 from http://www.cdc.gov/vaccines/recs/acip/downloads/min-jun06.pdf.

Centers for Disease Control and Prevention (CDC). (2006). *National Influenza Vaccine Summit Newsletter.* "Cocooning" Project. Retrieved June 25, 2007 from http://www.cdc.gov/flu/professionals/bulletin/pdf/2006-07/bulletin5_113006_si.pdf.

De Serres, G. & Duval, B. (2005). Pertussis vaccination beyond childhood. *Lancet,* 365, 1015–1016.

U.S. Food and Drug Administration. (2006). Influenza: Vaccination still the best protection. *FDA Consumer Magazine.* Retrieved June 25, 2007 from www.fda.gov/fdac/features/2006/506_influenza.html.

Social Barriers

Educational levels, transportation problems, as well as access to and overcrowding of facilities pose further barriers to adequate immunization coverage. The formidable quantities of paperwork involved in obtaining the informed consent of parents may be intellectually intimidating as well as time-consuming. Working parents may find it difficult, if not impossible, to reach an immunization clinic with their child during working hours. Requirements for appointments (instead of walk-in clinics) or for a physical examination before vaccination may present additional deterrents. Pockets of need continue to exist in areas of every major city where substantial numbers of underimmunized children live. These areas are of great concern because, particularly in large urban areas with traditionally underserved populations, a great potential exists for disease outbreaks (USDHHS, 2000).

Cultural Barriers

Meeting the immunization needs of minority groups may involve cultural barriers related to differing concepts of

health care and preventive measures among cultures. Language barriers may lead parents to feel confused, overwhelmed, and unable to access services. Depending on how long a family has resided in the United States and their level of active sponsorship, parents may not be familiar with expectations of the health care system in regard to their actions on behalf of the well child (Kennedy, Brown, & Gust, 2005).

Philosophical Objections

Many affluent, well-educated, caring parents have philosophical objections to immunization. They fear harm to their children, as has periodically been reported in the media. Parents may object to one or more of the vaccines, or prefer to delay or separate the vaccines; this puts the child "behind" on immunizations, according to the AAP schedule. Community health nurses should be aware that caring parents are talking about these issues, reading about them, and trying to make informed decisions about them (Kennedy et al., 2005). When possible, it may be helpful to offer information or websites that address the many myths surrounding childhood immunizations (see the Internet resources at the end of this chapter for more information).

Provider Limitations

Another barrier to immunization coverage is provider limitations. Health care providers may have contact with an eligible child, yet may fail to offer vaccination. This occurs when providers see children for different reasons and do not review their immunization records, thus missing the opportunity to provide vaccination services at what may be a very convenient time for parents. Sometimes, children come for immunization services and receive some vaccines but not others, although the safety and efficacy of administering multiple vaccines on the same occasion are well established and recommended by the CDC. Providers may erroneously defer administration of a vaccine based on a condition (e.g., symptom of illness) that is not a true contraindication to immunization. To address this particular issue, the CDC has developed guidelines for providers showing misconceptions concerning contraindications to vaccination (Table 8.3). Another provider limitation or barrier to timely immunization coverage is that few providers have the initiative and resources to establish a uniform system for recall and notification when the next immunization is due. In the United States, even clients of private providers often are not encouraged or assisted to maintain their own copies of personal written medical records (Margolis et al., 2001; Szilagyi et al., 2002).

Planning and Implementing Immunization Programs

Immunization programs targeting specific subgroups can be effective if they include the following: (a) community assessment parameters by race or other cultural groupings in the planning phase; (b) assessment of specific characteristics of the groups such as language, child care practices, preventive health behaviors, extreme poverty, or high illiteracy; and (c) appropriate planning decisions to deal with these potential barriers. Successful outreach efforts are motivated by the desire to reach the target population, even if specific or unusual accommodations must be made. Clinics can be scheduled and held at times and places specifically intended to make the service more accessible and convenient to the target group (Szilagyi et al., 2002). Materials should be designed and presented with the needs and abilities of target parents in mind. Interpreters must be provided as needed (Talking Quality.gov, 2006). Display 8.3 outlines the necessary steps and considerations for administering immunization clinics in community settings.

Adult Immunization

Many people erroneously assume that vaccinations are for children only. Well-advertised influenza vaccination campaigns in recent years have, to some extent, helped to correct this notion. However, media coverage about the adverse effects of such vaccination has done little to increase either community or provider enthusiasm about adult vaccination in general. Adults are at increased risk for many VPDs, and approximately 45,000 adult deaths each year are associated with complications from pneumococcal disease and influenza (CDC, 2006k). As the nation's population ages, increasing numbers of adults will be at risk for these major causes of death and illness.

Adults may require vaccination for a variety of reasons. Occupational exposure to blood, blood products, or other potentially contaminated body fluids provides the basis for Occupational Safety and Health Administration (OSHA) requirements for hepatitis B vaccine. All persons should receive tetanus vaccine every 10 years unless they experience major or contaminated wounds. If such a wound is sustained, the individual should receive a single booster of a tetanus toxoid on the day of the injury if more than 5 years has elapsed since the last tetanus toxoid dose.

In addition to the previously mentioned influenza and pneumonia vaccinations, the newly licensed version of the childhood diphtheria/tetanus/acellular pertussis (DTaP) vaccine—tetanus/diphtheria/acellular pertussis (Tdap)—is available for 11- to 64-year-olds and will now make an impact upon pertussis disease in the community (CDC, 2007b). Other reasons for promoting the necessity of adult vaccination include history of high-risk conditions, such as heart disease, diabetes, and chronic respiratory diseases; international travel; and suspected failure of earlier vaccines to produce lasting immunity. Table 8.4 displays the *Healthy People 2010* objective for influenza and pneumonia vaccines for people older than 18 years of age (USDHHS, 2000).

Substantial numbers of VPDs still occur among adults despite the availability of safe and effective vaccines (CDC, 2006h). At least six factors contribute to low vaccination levels among adults:

1. Limited comprehensive vaccine delivery systems are available in the public and private sectors.
2. Although statutory requirements exist for vaccination of children, no such requirements exist for all adults.
3. Vaccination schedules are complicated because of detailed recommendations that may vary by age, occupation, lifestyle, or health condition.
4. Health care providers frequently miss opportunities to vaccinate adults during contacts in offices, outpatient clinics, and hospitals.
5. Comprehensive vaccination programs have not been established in settings where healthy adults congregate (e.g., the workplace, senior centers).
6. Clients and providers may fear adverse effects after vaccination.

International Travelers, Immigrants, and Refugees

As Americans interact more and more with their neighbors in other parts of the world, the incidence of Americans with tropical or imported diseases also rises. Within 36 hours of beginning a trip, any destination in the world can be reached. That amount of time is within the incubation period of most infectious diseases, and microbial agents are rapidly spread around the globe.

Information necessary for a potential traveler to travel to new and exotic places, remain healthy, and return healthy is available from a number of sources. At a minimum, all

TABLE 8.3   Guide to Contraindications[a] and Precautions[b] to Commonly Used Vaccines —*Listed by Vaccine*

Vaccine	True Contraindications and Precautions[c]	Untrue (Vaccines Can Be Administered)
General for all vaccines, including diphtheria and tetanus toxoids & acellular pertussis vaccine (DTaP); pediatric diphtheria-tetanus toxoid (DT); adult tetanus-diphtheria toxoid (Td); inactivated poliovirus vaccine (IPV); measles-mumps-rubella vaccine (MMR); Haemophilus influenzae type b vaccine (Hib); hepatitis A vaccine, hepatitis B vaccine; varicella vaccine; pneumococcal conjugate vaccine (PCV); influenza vaccine; and pneumococcal polysaccharide vaccine (PPV)	**Contraindications** • Serious allergic reaction (e.g., anaphylaxis) after a previous vaccine dose • Serious allergic reaction (e.g., anaphylaxis) to a vaccine component **Precautions** • Moderate or severe acute illness with or without fever	• Mild acute illness with or without fever • Mild to moderate local reaction (i.e., swelling, redness, soreness); low-grade or moderate fever after previous dose • Lack of previous physical examination in well-appearing person • Current antimicrobial therapy • Convalescent phase of illness • Premature birth (hepatitis B vaccine is an exception in certain circumstances)[d] • Recent exposure to an infectious disease • History of penicillin allergy, other nonvaccine allergies, relative with allergies, receiving allergen extract immunotherapy
DTaP	**Contraindications** • Severe allergic reaction after a previous dose or to a vaccine component • Encephalopathy (e.g., coma, decreased level of consciousness; prolonged seizures) within 7 days of administration of previous dose of DTP or DTaP • Progressive neurologic disorder, including infantile spasms, uncontrolled epilepsy, progressive encephalopathy; defer DTaP until neurologic status clarified and stabilized. **Precautions** • Fever of >40.5°C ≤48 hours after vaccination with a previous dose of DTP or DTaP • Collapse or shock-like state (i.e., hypotonic hyporesponsive episode) ≤48 hours after receiving a previous dose of DTP or DTaP • Seizure ≤3 days of receiving a previous dose of DTP/DTaP[e] • Persistent, inconsolable crying lasting ≥3 hours ≤48 hours after receiving a previous dose of DTP or DTaP • Moderate or severe acute illness with or without fever	• Temperature of <40.5°C, fussiness or mild drowsiness after a previous dose of diphtheria toxoid-tetanus toxoid-pertussis vaccine DTP or DTaP • Family history of seizures[e] • Family history of sudden infant death syndrome • Family history of an adverse event after DTP or DTaP administration • Stable neurologic conditions (e.g., cerebral palsy, well controlled convulsions, developmental delay)
DT, Td	**Contraindications** • Severe allergic reaction after a previous dose or to a vaccine component **Precautions** • Guillain-Barré syndrome ≤6 weeks after previous dose of tetanus toxoid-containing vaccine • Moderate or severe acute illness with or without fever	

(continued)

TABLE 8.3 Guide to Contraindications[a] and Precautions[b] to Commonly Used Vaccines —Listed by Vaccine (Continued)

Vaccine	True Contraindications and Precautions[c]	Untrue (Vaccines Can Be Administered)
IPV	**Contraindications** • Severe allergic reaction to previous dose or vaccine component **Precautions** • Pregnancy • Moderate or severe acute illness with or without fever	
MMR[f]	**Contraindications** • Severe allergic reaction to previous dose or vaccine component • Pregnancy • Known severe immunodeficiency (e.g., hematologic and solid tumors; congenital immunodeficiency; long-term immunosuppressive therapy[h] or severely symptomatic human immunodeficiency virus [HIV] infection) **Precautions** • Recent (≤11 months) receipt of antibody-containing blood product (specific interval depends on product)[i] • History of thrombocytopenia or thrombocytopenic purpura • Moderate or severe acute illness with or without fever	• Positive tuberculin skin test • Simultaneous TB skin testing[g] • Breast-feeding • Pregnancy of recipient's mother or other close or household contact • Recipient is child-bearing-age female • Immunodeficient family member or household contact • Asymptomatic or mildly symptomatic HIV infection • Allergy to eggs
Hib	**Contraindications** • Severe allergic reaction to previous dose or vaccine component • Age <6 weeks **Precautions** • Moderate or severe acute illness with or without fever	
Hepatitis B	**Contraindications** • Severe allergic reaction to previous dose or vaccine component **Precautions** • Infant weighing <2,000 grams • Moderate or severe acute illness with or without fever	• Pregnancy • Autoimmune disease (e.g., systemic lupus erythematosis or rheumatoid arthritis)
Hepatitis A	**Contraindications** • Severe allergic reaction to previous dose or vaccine component **Precautions** • Pregnancy • Moderate or severe acute illness with or without fever	
Varicella[f]	**Contraindications** • Severe allergic reaction to previous dose or vaccine component • Substantial suppression of cellular immunity • Pregnancy	• Pregnancy of recipient's mother or other close or household contact • Immunodeficient family member or household contact[j] • Asymptomatic or mildly symptomatic HIV infection • Humoral immunodeficiency (e.g., agammaglobulinema)

(continued)

TABLE 8.3 **Guide to Contraindications[a] and Precautions[b] to Commonly Used Vaccines —*Listed by Vaccine* (*Continued*)**

Vaccine	True Contraindications and Precautions[c]	Untrue (Vaccines Can Be Administered)
	Precautions • Recent (≤11 months) receipt of antibody-containing blood product (specific interval depends on product)[i] • Moderate or severe acute illness with or without fever	
PCV	**Contraindications** • Severe allergic reaction to previous dose or vaccine component **Precautions** • Moderate or severe acute illness with or without fever	
Influenza	**Contraindications** • Severe allergic reaction to previous dose or vaccine component, including egg protein **Precautions** • Moderate or severe acute illness with or without fever	• Nonsevere (e.g., contact) allergy to latex or thimerosal • Concurrent administration of coumadin or aminophylline
PPV	**Contraindications** • Severe allergic reaction to previous dose or vaccine component **Precautions** • Moderate or severe acute illness with or without fever	

[a]**Contraindications.** A contraindication is a condition in a recipient that increases the risk for a serious adverse reaction. A vaccine will not be administered when a contraindication is present. Consult the MMWR article, "General Recommendations on Immunizations" for a full definition including examples.

[b]**Precautions.** A precaution is a condition in a recipient that might increase the risk for a serious adverse reaction or that might compromise the ability of the vaccine to produce immunity. Injury could result, or a person might experience a more severe reaction to the vaccine than would have otherwise been expected; however, the risk for this happening is less than expected with a contraindication. Under normal circumstances, vaccinations should be deferred when a precaution is present. However, a vaccination might be indicated in the presence of a precaution because the benefit of protection from the vaccine outweighs the risk for an adverse reaction. Consult the MMWR article, "General Recommendations on Immunizations" for a full definition including examples.

[c]Events or conditions listed as precautions should be reviewed carefully. Benefits and risks of administering a specific vaccine to a person under these circumstances should be considered. If the risk from the vaccine is believed to outweigh the benefit, the vaccine should not be administered. If the benefit of vaccination is believed to outweigh the risk, the vaccine should be administered. Whether and when to administer DTaP to children with proven or suspected underlying neurologic disorders should be decided on a case-by-case basis.

[d]Hepatitis B vaccination should be deferred for infants weighing <2,000 grams if the mother is documented to be hepatitis B surface antigen (HbsAg)-negative at the time of infant's birth. Vaccination can commence at chronological age 1 month. For infants born to HbsAg-positive women, hepatitis B immunoglobulin and hepatitis B vaccine should be administered at or soon after birth regardless of weight. See MMWR article, "General Recommendations on Immunizations" text for details.

[e]Acetaminophen or other appropriate antipyretic can be administered to children with a personal or family history of seizures at the time of DTaP vaccination and every 4–6 hours for 24 hours thereafter to reduce the possibility of post-vaccination fever (Source: American Academy of Pediatrics. Active immunization. In Pickering LK, ed. *2000 Red Book: Report of the Committee on Infectious Diseases,* 25th ed. Elk Grove Village, IL; American Academy of Pediatrics, 2000.)

[f]MMR and varicella vaccines can be administered on the same day. If not administered on the same day, these vaccines should be separated by ≥28 days.

[g]Substantially immunosuppressive steroid dose is considered to be >2 weeks of daily receipt of 20 mg or 2 mg/kg body weight of prednisone or equivalent.

[h]Measles vaccination can suppress tuberculin reactivity temporarily. Measles-containing vaccine can be administered on the same day as tuberculin skin testing. If testing cannot be performed until after the day of MMR vaccination, the test should be postponed for >4 weeks after the vaccination. If an urgent need exists to skin test, do so with the understanding that reactivity might be reduced by the vaccine.

[i]See text for details.

[j]If a vaccinee experiences a presumed vaccine-related rash 7–25 days after vaccination, avoid direct contact with immunocompromised persons for the duration of the rash.

Source: California Department of Public Health.

| DISPLAY 8.3 | ADMINISTRATIVE ASPECTS OF IMMUNIZATION PROGRAMS |

Study the Target Community
- Assess disease incidence and level of immunization coverage.
- Identify the target group.
- Assess conditions in the community: Is the target group scattered or localized?
- Assess level of community involvement and awareness of the problem.
- Identify means of communicating with target group: Through the media or through leaders or other.
- Consider political and social structure of the community. Identify important leaders.
- Identify sites for immunization clinics that are appropriate, accessible, and available.

Plan the Immunization Program
- Review budget for immunization services.
- Determine goals for clinic performance or outcome measures.
- Communicate with target group to notify them of need and promote involvement and participation.
- Estimate needs for vaccines and supplies and obtain them. Plan care of vaccines before, during, and after clinic.
- Develop team coordination among staff.
- Plan clinic logistics: Available supply of needed materials, medical waste disposal, anaphylaxis supplies, records and means of clinic registration, staffing, floor plan for traffic control and efficient management of crowds.
- Prepare staff with information regarding objectives for clinic, criteria for who shall not be immunized,

mechanisms for referral of clients with other health needs.

Publicity
- Inform target group of date, location, and times of immunization clinic.
- Provide information on reasons for and benefits of (and contraindications to) immunization.
- Encourage parents to bring existing immunization records to clinic.
- Provide contact information for those with questions or inquiries.

Immunization Clinic
- Registration system and records (for parent and clinic) ready.
- Registrar or assistant(s) ready to assist parents not familiar with language of paperwork.
- Parent education: informed consent, reporting of adverse reactions, date next vaccine due.
- System for call-back, follow-up.
- System for dealing with other health issues and/or adverse events.

Evaluation of Program
- Assess numbers of immunizations given in relation to goals.
- Assess suitability of approach in identification of target group, selection of sites, means of communication with group, availability of resources, and so forth.
- Invite parental as well as community and staff feedback.
- Evaluate results in relation to expenditures.

TABLE 8.4 *Healthy People 2010* **Target for Influenza and Pneumonia Immunization in Adults**

Objective: Increase to 90% the rate of immunization coverage among adults 65 years of age or older; 60% for high-risk adults 18 to 64 years of age.

Recommended Immunization	1998 (unless noted)	Target 2010
Noninstitutionalized adults 65 years of age or older		
Influenza vaccine	64%	90%
Pneumococcal vaccine	46%	90%
Noninstitutionalized high-risk adults 18 to 64 years of age		
Influenza vaccine	26%	60%
Pneumococcal vaccine	13%	60%
Institutionalized adults (persons in long-term or nursing homes)		
Influenza vaccine	59% (1997)	90%
Pneumococcal vaccine	25% (1997)	90%

Retrieved July 13, 2008 from http://www.healthpeople.gov/documents/html/volume1/14 immunization.htm
- Age-adjusted to the year 2000 standard population.
- National Nursing Home Survey estimates include a significant number of residents who have an unknown vaccination status.

international travelers must take steps to be adequately immunized as required by international health practices. These steps include being immunized with the recommended vaccines for the particular area of the world, having the necessary chemical prophylaxis on hand (i.e., antimalarial medications as prescribed), and being knowledgeable about food and water hygiene precautions as well as basic first aid for the care of simple injuries (CDC, 2005e). Every year, travelers who neglect to take the recommended travel vaccines or medications end up with generally preventable illnesses, which can cost them time, money, and their health. In many major cities of the United States, one finds tropical medicine or travelers' medicine specialists who can assist in adequate preparation for travel (CDC, 2005e).

Refugees and international travelers who arrive in the United States are often unfamiliar with U.S. health systems, health precautions, and practices. Refugees and immigrants must follow prescribed guidelines for their acculturation, including extensive health screening mandated by U.S. immigration laws. More than ever before, community health nurses have professional contact with these new Americans, whether close to their time of arrival or later, in schools, immunization clinics, or other locations. Visitors from other countries may also require the assistance of other community health professionals. For this reason, community health nurses are encouraged to develop and maintain a global perspective on communicable diseases

(CDC, 2006d). See Chapter 16 for more information on global health.

SECONDARY PREVENTION

Two approaches to secondary prevention of communicable disease are possible: screening, and disease case and contact investigation with partner notification.

Screening

The term **screening** is used in community health and disease prevention to describe programs that deliver a testing procedure to detect disease in groups of asymptomatic, apparently healthy individuals. Common screening measures can include: (a) prenatal hepatitis B, (b) urine chlamydia and gonorrhea, and (c) Mantoux tuberculin skin tests for TB infection. For HIV, several screening tests are available—including oral fluids testing, rapid finger stick, or the more sensitive screening enzyme immunoassay (EIA). All of these must be confirmed by a supplemental test such as the Western blot or an immunofluorescence assay (IFA) when positive results appear on screening tests (CDC, 2006j). All screening tests are discussed later in this chapter. Screening is a secondary prevention method because asymptomatic cases can be discovered and provided with prompt early treatment.

It is important to remember that the screening itself is not diagnostic, but rather seeks to identify those persons with positive or suspicious test findings who then require further medical evaluation or treatment. As a community health nurse working with clients in a screening setting, you must be prepared to clearly and correctly explain to individuals that screening tests are not definitive and that positive findings require subsequent investigation before diagnostic conclusions can be drawn.

Criteria for Screening Tests

Some important criteria are used in deciding whether to carry out a screening intervention in a community. They include validity and reliability, and predictive value and yield.

Validity and Reliability

The screening test must be valid and reliable. *Validity* refers to the test's ability to accurately identify those with the disease. *Reliability* refers to the test's ability to give consistent results when administered on different occasions by different technicians.

Predictive Value and Yield

The *predictive value* of a screening test is important for determining whether the screening intervention is justified. *Yield* refers to the number of positive results found per number tested. The predictive value and the yield of screening tests become important in planning screening programs for communicable disease detection and prevention because they can help planners locate screening efforts in areas or within population groups that are known to be at high risk for the disease. The predictive value of screening tests increases as the prevalence of the disease increases. For example, a screening test for syphilis targeted at the population associated with crack houses in a particular city would have greater predictive value and yield than a screening test for syphilis given to the city population at large.

Epidemiologic criteria for screening interventions for the detection of health problems include:

1. Is the disease an important public health problem?
2. Is there a valid and reliable test?
3. Is there an effective and tolerable treatment that favorably influences the early stages of the disease?
4. After a positive screening result, are facilities for diagnosis and treatment available and accessible?
5. Is there a recognizable early asymptomatic or latent stage in the disease?
6. Do clear guidelines for referral and treatment exist?
7. Is the total cost of the screening justifiable compared with the costs of treating the disease if left undiscovered?
8. Is the screening test itself acceptable?
9. Will screening be ongoing?

The ethics or values represented by these statements include a clear and unwavering respect for the dignity and worth of individuals across racial, gender, religious, sexual, tribal, ethnic, and geographic lines. They include a commitment to ensuring that resources are allocated to areas where they will have the most benefit in preventing disease and premature death. They speak to respect for the individual receiving the screening service, in that the person should take on the burden of diagnosis only if access to acceptable further intervention exists.

Socioeconomically disadvantaged persons are often at greatest risk for disease, yet they are the least likely to receive screening services because of financial barriers, including lack of health insurance coverage for preventive care (Coughlin, 2006).

Case and Contact Investigation, Partner Notification

Another secondary prevention approach is known as case and contact investigation with partner notification. In this approach, the community health nurse investigates a reported communicable disease case to discover and notify those who have had contact with the infected person, such as with TB reactors, and to notify partners in the case of STDs. The objective of a contact investigation and partner notification is specifically to reach contacts of the **index case** (diagnosed person) before the contacts, in turn, become infectious (CDC, 2006j). Therefore, the rapidity with which contact investigation can be accomplished is vital.

Healthy People 2010 (USDHHS, 2000) guidelines differentiate between two types of partner notification. *Patient referral* describes those clients who voluntarily advise their partners of the risk of disease and the need for contact with a health provider. *Provider referral* describes the community health workers who contact individuals exposed to the index case and either assist the individual in obtaining medical care or strongly encourage them to seek appropriate medical care. In both types of notification, clients need information and encouragement as well as assurance of confidentiality (Hogben et al., 2004).

Not all individuals who have a disease can accurately identify the persons with whom they have had close or intimate contact. This is particularly the case with STDs associated with drug use and the selling of sex for drugs. It is also true in situations involving highly mobile or transient people whose lifestyles preclude establishing relationships that can be traced or followed. These problems lead to the need for alternative approaches in finding contacts or new cases, including the provision of screening activities in locations where people with similar risky lifestyle behaviors are likely to congregate. It further points to the critical need for tests that provide reliable results very rapidly, because it may not be possible to locate the person for follow-up 24 hours or 2 weeks later (CDC, 2007b).

Contact investigation is most commonly practiced today in STD and TB control programs. The same interviewing and data collection techniques can transfer to use with food-borne illness or other disease outbreak control efforts. Understanding the disease being investigated, incubation period, various stages of infection (active or latent), and urgency of evaluation and treatment are important considerations in determining the timeline of the investigation (Dato, Wagner, & Fapohunda, 2004).

Tertiary Prevention

The approaches to tertiary prevention of communicable disease include isolation and quarantine of the infected person and safe handling and control of infectious wastes.

Isolation and Quarantine

Communicable disease control includes two methods for keeping infected persons and noninfected persons apart to prevent the spread of a disease. **Isolation** refers to separation of the infected persons (or animals) from others for the period of communicability to limit the transmission of the infectious agent to susceptible persons. **Quarantine** refers to restrictions placed on healthy contacts of an infectious case for the duration of the incubation period to prevent disease transmission if infection should develop (Heymann, 2004).

Safe Handling and Control of Infectious Wastes

Also important to the control of infection in community health is the proper disposition of contaminated wastes. The CDC has developed *universal precautions*, which encourage health care workers to think of all blood and body fluids, and materials that have come in contact with them, as potentially infectious. Although universal precaution observance is primarily considered while the nurse is giving hands-on treatment or care to a patient, keeping these principles in mind while making community health visits in the primary and secondary setting is paramount to the safety of both the client and the nurse (Heymann, 2004).

Universal precautions include the following:

◆ Hand-washing after contact with the client or with potentially contaminated articles and before care of other clients
◆ Discarding or bagging and labeling of articles contaminated with infectious material before it is sent for decontamination and reprocessing

◆ Isolation based on the mode of transmission of the specific disease, which may include strict isolation, contact isolation, respiratory isolation, TB isolation (acid-fast bacilli [AFB] isolation), enteric precautions, or drainage/secretion precautions

The Environmental Protection Agency (EPA, 2007) defines infectious waste as waste capable of producing an infectious disease. The agency notes that for waste to be infectious, it must contain pathogens with sufficient virulence and quantity so that exposure to the waste by a susceptible host could result in an infectious disease. EPA requirements for medical waste disposal are for waste to be segregated into categories of (a) used and unused sharps, (b) cultures and stocks of infectious agents, (c) human blood and blood products, and (d) human pathologic, isolation, and animal waste. Although incineration has long been recognized as an efficient method for disposing safely of sharps and other contaminated medical waste, fewer incinerators are available now because of increasing regulation of emissions, and particularly those regulations related to burning chemical wastes (Occupational Safety and Health Administration, 2006).

Four key elements of an infectious waste management program are applicable to community practice:

1. Health professionals must be able to correctly distinguish waste that poses a significant infection hazard from other biomedical waste that poses no greater risk than general municipal waste, and such infectious waste must be clearly defined.
2. The waste management program must have administrative support and authority to institute practice guidelines and provide the containers and other resources needed for safe disposal of infectious wastes.
3. Handling of the infectious wastes must be minimized. Containers should be rigid, leak resistant, and impervious to moisture; they should have sufficient strength to prevent rupture or tearing under normal conditions; and they should be sealed to prevent leakage. Containers for sharps must also be puncture resistant.
4. An enforcement or evaluation mechanism must be in place to ensure that the goal of reducing the potential for exposure to infectious waste in the community is met.

MAJOR COMMUNICABLE DISEASES IN THE UNITED STATES

Community health nurses encounter several communicable diseases in their practice. Many are reportable, but some are not—although they are just as transmittable to others as the reportable infections. As mentioned previously, each state department of health has the capacity to determine which diseases will be reportable based upon the federal reportable disease list. These diseases are frequently diagnosed and treated in the community care setting rather than the hospital. The most commonly reported diseases are the STDs: chlamydia, gonorrhea, and syphilis are reportable in all states; and genital herpes and human papillomavirus (HPV) genital warts are not reportable in all states. Hepatitis,

HIV/AIDS, influenza (seasonal and avian), pneumonia, and TB are mandated reportable diseases. The following sections discuss some of the more common communicable diseases, but the list is not inclusive of all that are reportable. Diseases are presented in groups by similarity, rather than by virulence or prevalence.

Chlamydia

Chlamydia trachomatis (CT) infections are the most commonly reported notifiable STD in the United States. Since 1994, CT has made up the largest proportion of all STDs reported to the CDC. In women, chlamydial infections, which are usually asymptomatic, may result in pelvic inflammatory disease (PID)—a major cause of infertility, ectopic pregnancy, and chronic pelvic pain (CDC, 2005h). Chlamydia is a sexually transmitted bacterial infection of great concern, with 436,350 cases reported to the CDC in 1997, 702,093 in 2000, and 976,445 in 2005. The number of cases has increased primarily because of an increase in recognition, testing, and mandatory reporting by the states in the past two decades (CDC, 2005h; Heymann, 2004).

Until recently, chlamydia was probably the least recognized of the STDs. Only since 2000 has reporting of chlamydia been required by all states, including the District of Columbia (CDC, 2005h). People with uncomplicated infection are quite often symptom free until late and serious complications occur. Women and children typically are the most adversely affected, particularly in terms of sequelae, including PID, ectopic pregnancy, infertility, infant conjunctivitis, and infant pneumonia (Heymann, 2004).

Screening programs have been extremely effective in reducing the chlamydia burden in groups that are screened regularly. One of the goals of *Healthy People 2010* is to reduce the prevalence of CT infections among young people (15 to 24 years of age) to no more than 3.0%, but as of 2004, the average was 6.3% (CDC, 2005h). In 2004, the reported rate of chlamydial infection among women in the United States (485 cases per 100,000) was nearly four times higher than the reported rate among men (147 cases per 100,000); however, this difference probably reflects a greater number of women being screened for this disease (CDC, 2005h). The lower rate among men suggests that many of the sex partners

of women with chlamydia are not diagnosed or reported. However, with the use of the highly sensitive nucleic acid amplification tests for testing urine, symptomatic and asymptomatic men are now regularly being diagnosed with chlamydial infection (CDC, 2005h). As a result of increased screening efforts in many settings outside of the medical office, reported rates of chlamydia continue to increase (Fig. 8.3).

Control of chlamydial infections of the cervix is considered key to effective reduction in the rates of PID, particularly among teenage women. A recent investigation of people in a health maintenance organization (HMO) demonstrated that screening and treatment of cervical infection reduces the likelihood of PID (CDC, 2005k). In one study of teen and young adult men who had their urine screened for chlamydia (Ku et al., 2002), 3.1% of the teenagers (age 15 to 19 years) and 4.5% of the young adults (age 22 to 26 years) had chlamydial infections. Also, the great majority of the participants were asymptomatic. The federal government reports that almost half of reported cases are 15- to 19-year-old girls, and an additional one-third of cases are women between the ages of 20 and 24 (Agency for Healthcare Research and Quality [AHRQ], 2001).

Barriers exist to successful prevention, diagnosis, and treatment of chlamydia. As noted, many people who are diagnosed with chlamydia are asymptomatic and often report their use of prophylactic protection during sexual intercourse as sporadic. In the study by Ku and colleagues (2002), the number of reported partners per year was about three for both age groups. Another major barrier to effective control is lack of compliance with the required 7-day treatment regimen of doxycycline (100 mg twice a day) or tetracycline four times a day. The use of azithromycin (1 g in a single dose) is also highly effective and leads to better compliance as on-the-spot treatment in the clinic setting is possible.

"Patient-delivered partner treatment" has been shown to be more effective than encouraging the patient to notify their partner(s) to seek testing and treatment. However, for men who have sex with men, this practice is not as customary, as there may be other co-infection issues that need evaluation and treatment as well (CDC, 2006m; Schillinger et al., 2003). To minimize the risk for reinfection, clients should be instructed to abstain from sexual intercourse until all of their sex partners have been treated. Clients do not need to be retested for chlamydia after completion of treatment with

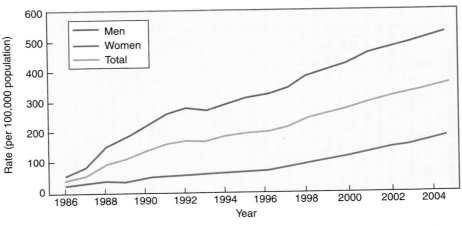

FIGURE 8.3 Chlamydia rates: Total and by sex: United States, 1986–2005.

NOTE: As of January 2000, all 50 states and the District of Columbia had regulations requiring the reporting of chlamydia cases.

doxycycline or azithromycin unless symptoms persist or reinfection is suspected. A test of cure may be considered 3 weeks after completion of treatment with erythromycin (CDC, 2006m). Condom use is important in decreasing the spread of chlamydia infection.

Prenatal screening of pregnant women can prevent chlamydial infection among neonates. Neonatal *C. trachomatil* infection may involve the mucous membranes of the eye, oropharynx, urogenital tract, and rectum. It is most often recognized by the presence of conjunctivitis, which develops 5 to 12 days after birth. Chlamydia is the most frequent identifiable infectious cause of opthalmia neonatorum. Chlamydia also is a common cause of subacute, afebrile pneumonia with onset at 1 to 3 months of age. Either of these conditions may be observed when you are making a home visit for post-delivery, family follow-up (CDC, 2005h).

Genital Herpes

Genital herpes is an STD caused by the herpes simplex viruses, type 1 (HSV-1) and type 2 (HSV-2). Most cases of genital herpes are caused by HSV-2. Most individuals have no or only minimal signs or symptoms from HSV-1 or HSV-2 infection. Primary and recurrent infections occur, with or without symptoms, and first occurrences may take up to 2 or 4 weeks to heal. In women, sites of primary disease are the cervix and the vulva. Recurrent disease generally involves the vulva, perineal skin, legs, and buttocks. In men, lesions appear on the penis, and in the anus and rectum of those engaging in anal sex. Typically, another outbreak can appear weeks or months after the first, but it almost always is less severe and briefer than the first outbreak. The infection can remain in the body indefinitely, and the number of outbreaks will decrease over a period of years (Heymann, 2004).

Nationwide, at least 45 million people ages 12 and older, or one of five adolescents and adults, have had genital HSV infection. Genital HSV-2 infection is more common in women (approximately one of four women) than in men (almost one of five). This may be due to male-to-female transmissions being more likely than female-to-male transmission. Generally, a person can only get HSV-2 infection during sexual contact with someone who has a genital HSV-2 infection. Transmission can occur from an infected partner who does not have a visible sore and may not know that he or she is infected (CDC, 2006m).

Most people infected with HSV-2 are not aware of their infection. However, if signs and symptoms occur during the first outbreak, they can be quite pronounced. The first outbreak usually occurs within 2 weeks after the virus is transmitted. Other signs and symptoms during the primary episode may include a second crop of sores, and flu-like symptoms, including fever and swollen glands. Most individuals with HSV-2 infection may never have sores, or they may have very mild signs that they do not even notice or that they mistake for insect bites or another skin condition (CDC, 2006m).

Health care providers can diagnose genital herpes by visual inspection if the outbreak is typical, and by taking a sample from the sore(s) and testing it in a laboratory. HSV infections can be difficult to diagnose between outbreaks. Blood tests, which detect HSV-1 or HSV-2 infection, may be helpful, although the results are not always clear (Heymann, 2004).

Three antiviral medications provide clinical benefit for genital herpes: acyclovir, valacyclovir, and famciclovir. Each is given orally for 7 to 10 days for a first clinical episode; for recurrent genital herpes, the recommended regimen is similar doses given twice daily. The drugs have been shown to reduce shedding of the virus, diminish pain, and accelerate healing. Intravenous acyclovir therapy is provided for clients who have severe disease or complications that necessitate hospitalization, such as disseminated infection, pneumonitis, hepatitis, or complications of the central nervous system (e.g., meningitis, encephalitis). These antiviral medications can shorten and prevent outbreaks during the period when the person takes the medication. In addition, daily suppressive therapy for symptomatic herpes can reduce transmission to partners (CDC, 2006m).

Gonorrhea

The overall rate of gonorrhea in the United States has decreased to 115.5 cases per 100,000 in 2005, compared with the 1997 case rate of 122.7 cases per 100,000. The causative agent is gonococcus bacteria—*Neisseria gonorrhoeae*. Consistently, the highest rates have been among women age 15 to 19 years (624.7 cases per 100,000) and 20- to 24-year-old men (436.8 cases per 100,000) (CDC, 2005i). Overall, we have yet to reach the *Healthy People 2010* target of 19 cases per 100,000 (Heymann, 2004; USDHHS, 2000) (see Fig. 8.4).

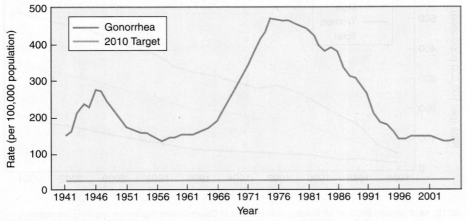

NOTE: The Healthy People 2010 target for gonorrhea is 19.0 cases per 100,000 population.

FIGURE 8.4 Gonorrhea rates: United States, 1941–2005 and the Healthy People 2010 target.

Antimicrobial resistance continues to be a concern in treating gonorrhea. Overall, 15.9% of isolates collected in the United States in 2004 from 28 Gonnococcal Isolate Surveillance Project (GISP) STD clinic sites were resistant to penicillin, tetracycline, or both. Resistance is more prevalent on the West Coast and in Hawaii (California Department of Health Services, STD Guidelines [CADHS], 2004). Globally, the prevalence of drug-resistant strains of gonococcal infections in developing countries are a cause for added concern (Indian Council of Medical Research, 2006).

Gonorrhea commonly manifests in men as a purulent drainage from the penis, accompanied by painful urination within 2 to 7 days after an infecting exposure. In women, the symptoms may be so mild as to go unnoticed. Progression of untreated gonorrhea in women can lead to serious reproductive system involvement causing PID and subsequent infertility. Treatment for gonorrhea will vary across the country due to the antibiotic resistance seen on the West Coast and among men who have sex with men. The recommended treatment regimen will need to reflect the surveillance data related to drug susceptibility. The practitioner must be vigilant in questioning recent travel or local acquisition of the infection and base treatment choice on this information (CDC, 2005i; Heymann, 2004). Because treatment failure with the combined ceftriaxone/doxycycline regimen is rare, a follow-up test of cure is not considered essential except for pregnant women, who should have a culture performed.

Syphilis

Syphilis, a genital ulcerative disease, manifests in several forms during the life cycle of the disease. Approximately 3 weeks after exposure, a primary lesion called a *chancre* characteristically appears as a painless ulcer at the site of initial invasion of the causative organism *Treponema pallidum,* a spirochete. This first stage is considered primary syphilis. After 4 to 6 weeks, the chancre heals without treatment, to be replaced by the development of a more generalized secondary skin eruption, classically appearing on the soles of the feet and palms of the hands, often accompanied by fatigue. This stage is secondary syphilis. These secondary manifestations resolve spontaneously, and a latent period follows, which may last from weeks to years. These stages are latent, late latent, and tertiary or neurosyphilis. Unpredictably, severe, systemic involvement with disability, or even death may occur. Transmission of untreated syphilis can occur in any stage (Heymann, 2004).

Syphilis is the first STD for which control measures were developed and tested. The incidence of primary syphilis cases in the United States decreased between 1990 and 2000, from 50,000 to 5,979 reported cases. But, an increase occurred between 2000 and 2004, mainly among men. An increase in primary syphilis cases reported in 2005 was 8,724. Between the years 2003 and 2004, the rate among women has remained the same, and the highest rate remains among men having sex with men. Syphilis contributes to HIV transmission in those parts of the country where rates of both infections are high. Only in the South do rates remain higher than the rest of the United States, with an average rate of 3.6 cases per 100,000 people. The target for 2010 is 0.2 cases per 100,000, and the opportunity exists to eliminate syphilis within the U.S. borders (CDC, 2005j).

Elimination of syphilis would have far-reaching public health implications because it would remove two devastating consequences of the disease—increased likelihood of HIV transmission and compromised ability to have healthy babies due to spontaneous abortions, stillbirths, and multisystem disorders caused by congenital syphilis acquired from mothers with syphilis. (USDHHS, 2000, Section 25, p. 18)

Treatment of early primary, secondary, and early latent syphilis is generally accomplished through antibiotic therapy. The specific treatment is a long-acting penicillin G (benzathine penicillin), 2.4 million units given in a single intramuscular dose on the day of diagnosis. Clients should be reexamined serologically at 3 and 6 months after treatment to ensure cure; however, the single-dose treatment is considered effective therapy even if the client fails to return (Heymann, 2004).

Viral Warts

Condyloma acuminata, verruca vulgaris, papilloma venereum, and the common wart are all forms of a viral disease manifested by a variety of mucous membrane and skin lesions (Heymann, 2004). All are transmitted by direct contact, but condyloma acuminata, or genital warts caused by HPV, are usually sexually transmitted.

Researchers have identified more than 100 types of papilloma viruses, and at least 30 of these types of the virus are sexually transmitted. Several of the subtypes of HPV are associated with cervical dysplasia and genital cancers, which can occur 5 to 30 years after the initial infection, accounting for more than 90% of cervical cancers (CDC, 2006c). The CDC estimates that about 6.2 million Americans get a new genital HPV infection each year.

Sexually active individuals are at risk for contracting any one or several of the types of genital warts that exist. Because few produce the actual bumpy, visual signs of warts, and some produce no notable symptoms, many cases go undiagnosed. This asymptomatic state leads to ongoing transmission between or among sexual partners (CDC, 2006m). Sexually active women can be diagnosed at the time of Papanicolaou smear (Pap) during the woman's health examination. This test can detect abnormal cytologic changes, and viral tests can be performed on the sample to determine the presence of HPV. Biopsy of the site may also be needed to examine the tissue more thoroughly (CDC, 2006m).

Treatment depends on the size and location of the warts. Even though the warts may be removed, the viral infection can't be cured, which is why the warts often return. Some of the medications used to treat genital warts cannot be used during pregnancy, so it is important for clients to tell their doctors if they could be pregnant. Small warts may be treated with medications applied to the skin. In some cases, applying liquid nitrogen (cryotherapy) to warts will freeze the tissue and make warts disappear. Some larger warts require laser treatment or surgical removal (CDC, 2006c; CDC, 2006m).

A vaccine released in 2006 has the potential to impact the rates of cervical cancer caused by HPV in women. The vaccine, Gardasil, protects against four HPV types (6, 11, 16, and 18), which together cause 70% of cervical cancers and 90% of genital warts. The vaccine is available to females between the ages of 9 and 26 years. The vaccine is not available to males at this time, although studies are under way

(CDC, 2006c). Some states now require this vaccine for girls enrolled in middle schools.

Hepatitis

Of five viral hepatitis infections that constitute serious liver disease, three commonly reported types are hepatitis A, B, and C. The number of people being infected with hepatitis is globally epidemic. Nationally, substantial progress is being made in the elimination of hepatitis viruses through the primary prevention practices of education and immunization for forms A and B.

Hepatitis A

Hepatitis A, caused by infection with the hepatitis A virus (HAV), occurs worldwide and is sporadic and epidemic, with cyclic recurrences affecting children and young adults most frequently. Case rates are high in Central and South America, the Caribbean, Mexico, Asia (except Japan), Africa, and southern and eastern Europe. Hepatitis A is identified by the presence of immunoglobulin M (IgM) antibodies against HAV in the serum of acutely or recently ill individuals (Heymann, 2004). The disease is transmitted from person to person by the fecal–oral route and is characterized by the abrupt onset of symptoms including fever, malaise, anorexia, nausea, and abdominal discomfort, followed by jaundice in more severe cases. Mild illnesses last 1 to 2 weeks, but more severe cases last 1 month or longer. It is generally a self-limited disease that does not result in chronic infection or chronic liver disease (Heymann, 2004).

Where environmental sanitation conditions are poor, infection is common and occurs at an early age. In the United States, most cases are transmitted in day care centers among diapered children, to household and sexual contacts of acute cases, and among travelers to countries where the disease is endemic. At times, common-source outbreaks are related to contaminated water, food contaminated by infected food handlers, raw or undercooked shellfish harvested from contaminated water, or contaminated produce, such as lettuce or strawberries (CDC, 2005e; Fiore, 2004).

Inactivated hepatitis A vaccines are prepared from formalin-inactivated, cell-culture–derived HAV and have been available in the United States since 1995 (CDC, 2007a). Administered in a two-dose series, these vaccines induce protective antibody levels in virtually all adults, providing the opportunity to eliminate this disease as a pubic health problem in the United States. The vaccine is recommended as a routine VFC vaccine and, as of 2005, is now available for children older than 12 months (CDC, 2007a). A combined hepatitis A and B vaccine has been developed for adults. Community health nurses play an important role in the prevention (pre-travel vaccination) and control of this disease, including case investigation, education, and identifying exposed contacts who need referral or assistance in obtaining postexposure prophylaxis and vaccination (CDC, 2006e).

Hepatitis B

Hepatitis B is a serious disease caused by a virus that attacks the liver. The virus, called hepatitis B virus (HBV), can cause lifelong infection, cirrhosis (scarring) of the liver, liver cancer, liver failure, and death. In very few cases, the infection will resolve, providing immunity (Heymann, 2004).

Hepatitis B is a global problem, with 66% of the world's population living in areas where high levels of infection by HBV occur. More than 2 billion people (one-third of the world's population) have evidence of resolved or current HBV infection, and 350 million people are chronic carriers of the virus. HBV causes 60% to 80% of all cases of primary liver cancer, which is one of the three top causes of cancer deaths in East Asia, Southeast Asia, the Pacific Basin, and sub-Saharan Africa (Heymann, 2004).

In the United States, cases of HBV are related to exposures common in certain high-risk groups, including injection drug users and homeless youth (Beech, Myers, & Beech, 2002), heterosexuals with multiple partners, homosexual men, incarcerated populations, and clients and staff in institutions for the developmentally disabled (Charuvastra et al., 2001).

The symptoms of HBV range from unnoticeable to fulminating, and include anorexia, vague abdominal discomfort, nausea and vomiting, and rash, often progressing to jaundice. The diagnosis is confirmed by the presence of specific antigens or antibodies (or both) to HBV in serum (Heymann, 2004).

Vaccination is the most effective way of preventing HBV transmission. Following WHO recommendations, 158 member states have integrated hepatitis B vaccine into their national immunization programs. The WHO and the United Nations Children's Fund (UNICEF) have sought means to help the poorest and neediest countries procure the vaccine. Effective implementation of this strategy could effectively eliminate transmission of hepatitis B by the year 2025 (WHO, 2005).

Community health nurses have an important role in the prevention and control of hepatitis B. Most importantly, this role includes teaching that encourages immunization compliance and consistent adherence to universal precautions (discussed earlier), especially for people in high-risk lifestyles or occupations (CDC, 2006a).

Hepatitis C

Hepatitis C was first identified in 1989 and has already become a major public health problem. It causes a complex infection of the liver and is one of the leading known causes of liver disease in the United States. It is a common cause of cirrhosis and hepatocellular carcinoma, as well as liver transplantation. It is believed that at least 4 million people in this country are infected with HCV. The incidence is not well known, but prevalence studies have led the WHO to estimate that 200 million people worldwide and 4 million people in the United States are infected with the hepatitis C virus (HCV) (NIH, 2002).

Hepatitis C is more widespread than AIDS, and many infected people are unaware that they are infected (Lauer & Walker, 2001). About 170 million people are chronic carriers, at risk for development of liver cirrhosis and liver cancer. In the United States, four times as many people have contracted HCV as have contracted HIV infection. Approximately 30,000 new acute infections and 8,000 to 10,000 deaths occur each year, and hepatitis C has become a leading reason for liver transplantation (Sarbah & Younossi, 2000).

Symptoms are similar to those of hepatitis A and B, and may be unrecognizably mild to fulminating. Diagnosis depends on the demonstration of antibody to HCV, and a screening test for blood donors was established in 1992 (Heymann, 2004). Before this test, HCV was the most common cause of posttransfusion hepatitis worldwide, accounting for approximately 90% of cases in the United States. The incidence of hepatitis C in the United States is highest in injection drug users (approximately 60%), hemophilia patients, and hemodialysis patients; it is also more frequently found among heterosexuals with multiple sexual partners, homosexual men, and health care workers than in the general public. Tattooing and body piercing provide an additional source of HCV transmission, and the exact role of tattooing is being studied. HCV testing is recommended for the following groups (Hench & Simpkins, 2002):

- People who inject nonprescribed drugs, including those who injected once or a few times in the past and do not consider themselves drug users
- Clients who received transfusions or organ transplants before 1992 and recipients of blood from a positive donor
- People with selected medical conditions, including recipients of clotting factors before 1987, people undergoing chronic hemodialysis, and those with persistently elevated alanine aminotransferase levels
- Those exposed to HCV-positive sources, such as needlesticks, sharps, or mucosal exposures
- Children born to HCV-positive women (after 12 months in order to make sure maternal antibodies have dissipated)

A community health nurse's role includes case-finding, encouraging testing for people who received blood transfusions before 1992, and reinforcing universal precautions (see earlier discussion), along with strong nursing assessment skills and compassion. There is no vaccine, and chronic hepatitis C is a life-altering event; clients need emotional support, and community health nurses can provide this support, as well as education for clients and families. New drugs and clinical trials are being continually introduced, and nurses can provide up-to-date information.

HIV/AIDS

The **human immunodeficiency virus (HIV)** is a retrovirus that attacks the body's immune system. Two types have been identified: type 1 (HIV-1) and type 2 (HIV-2). These viruses are relatively distinct serologically and geographically, but they have similar epidemiologic characteristics. The pathogenicity of HIV-2 appears to be less than that of HIV-1 (Heymann, 2004). Twenty-five years have passed since the identification of this infection, and it is viewed by many to be a chronic, manageable disease process; however, in most of the world, HIV continues to devastate populations of people who do not have access to life-extending medical care and medications. This section explores the acute nature of the infection, surveillance, investigation, and education. The chronic nature of this illness, along with treatment and disease management is discussed in Chapter 26.

Acquired immunodeficiency syndrome (AIDS) is a severe, life-threatening condition, representing the late clinical stage of infection with HIV, in which there is progressive damage to the immune and other organ systems—particularly the central nervous system. Most people infected with HIV remain symptom free for long periods, but viral replication is active during all stages of infection. AIDS eventually develops in almost all HIV-infected people who are not receiving antiretroviral therapy (ART) or highly active antiretroviral therapy (HAART), from months to 17 years after infection—with a median of 10 years (CDC, 2005f).

In recent years, the incidence of HIV infection among heterosexuals has grown. In the 1980s, most HIV infections occurred in men who had sex with men and in injection drug users. When HIV entered the country's blood supply, it affected transfusion patients, hemophiliacs, and other persons who received infected blood or blood products. As more women of childbearing age became infected, newborns were at increased risk for acquiring HIV infection. Today, almost all infections in infants and children are caused by transmission from the mother before or during birth. Today, most new cases of HIV/AIDS are transmitted through heterosexual or homosexual contact, the sharing of HIV-contaminated needles and syringes, or during the perinatal period from mother to child (CDC, 2006n).

HIV/AIDS was recognized as an emerging disease 25 years ago, and it has rapidly established itself throughout the world, creating a global pandemic. It is now prevalent in virtually all parts of the world (CDC, 2005f). An estimated 39.5 million adults and children worldwide were living with HIV/AIDS in 2006, with 1 million of them in the United States (CDC, 2006n).

Populations at Risk

AIDS was first recognized as a distinct syndrome in 1981. During the early years, it was seen as a disease of male homosexuals, intravenous drug abusers, and people with a history of multiple blood transfusions. The at-risk population for HIV/AIDS now includes people with a large number of sexual partners, adolescents, injection drug users and their sexual partners, homosexual men and their male or female partners, people who exchange sex for drugs or money, and people already infected with an STD (CDC, 2005f). Sexual transmission of HIV is closely associated with other STDs, particularly those that have an ulcerative phase, including syphilis. With belated but growing global awareness, the AIDS epidemic is recognized as a universal threat to the health and well-being of individuals and populations.

Adolescents and young adults are considered to be at particular risk for HIV infection because many of them engage in high-risk behaviors, believing they are invulnerable to infection. In addition to the considerable risks posed by potential HIV infection, other adverse outcomes related to early initiation of sexual activity include higher levels of all STDs (Quander, 2001).

Prevention Education

National HIV prevention and intervention efforts depend on two important factors: self-perception of risk, and adoption of risk-reducing behaviors in response to awareness of the risk. Consequently, education about HIV/AIDS, including safe sex and injection drug use behaviors, has become the key to prevention. Public health workers seek to identify and intervene with the at-risk population, providing counseling and prevention education as well as testing services. The primary purposes of counseling are to prevent further spread of HIV infection and, whenever possible, to slow the progression of HIV infection to AIDS. HIV counseling can help uninfected people initiate and sustain behaviors to reduce their risk of infection, help infected people adopt behaviors to reduce the risk of transmission to others, encourage spouses and partners of infected people to adopt safe behaviors, and help infected people take better care of themselves. Properly using condoms, reducing the number of sexual partners, and abstaining from injection drug use all decrease, but do not eliminate, the risk of HIV infection (CDC 2006j).

The role of a community health nurse may vary from state to state regarding surveillance, investigation, and contact notification. Only 33 states and territories have confidential name-based reporting systems, others have unique identifier reporting mechanisms. Both types of surveillance systems require physicians or medical practitioners to complete a reporting document with vital information regarding exposure risks, dates of testing, diagnosis, treatment, opportunistic illnesses, and patient identification (unique or named-based). From this information, the nurse may be able to facilitate ongoing community services, either through direct patient contact or the patient's medical provider. Partner notification is on a case-by-case basis, depending upon which system is in place in each state (CDC, 2006j).

Sexually Transmitted Disease Prevention and Control

Human history has been shaped by disease, and all historical events played a part in creating the preconditions for epidemics. Of all the communicable diseases, perhaps none are as closely interrelated with human activities and attitudes as STDs. Many have occurred in epidemic proportions; most have existed for centuries.

Sexually transmitted diseases are those infections that are spread by transfer of organisms from person to person during sexual contact. Sexually transmitted diseases are of critical importance in any discussion of communicable disease control because, as a single class of disease, gonorrhea, CT, syphilis, HIV, and hepatitis B are among the top ten diseases reported for 2004 (most current national data) (CDC, 2006n). The STDs discussed in this section included gonorrhea, syphilis, chlamydia, genital herpes, and HPV (genital warts). AIDS, of course, is an STD, as is hepatitis B, although transmission of these diseases can also occur through intravenous drug use, transfusion of blood products before 1986, or needle-stick injury (CDC, 2006n).

Of further concern to community health nurses is the fact that women and children suffer an inordinate STD burden. Aside from the risk of AIDS and subsequent death, the most serious complications of STDs are PID, sterility, ectopic pregnancy, blindness, cancer associated with HPV, fetal and infant death, birth defects, and mental retardation. The medically underserved, particularly the poor and marginalized, as well as ethnic and racial minorities, shoulder a disproportionate share of this problem—experiencing higher rates of disability and death than the population as a whole. Some notable disproportionately affected groups are sex workers, adolescents and adults in detention, and migrant workers (USDHHS, 2000). However, STDs can affect teen and young women who do not plan on becoming sexually active. Sexual

violence and sexual coercion are significant problems for America's young women. Studies show that not all sexually experienced young females enter a sexual relationship as a willing partner (Hanson, 2002) and that sexual assault or date rape is not uncommon on high school and college campuses.

Healthy People 2010 guidelines identify the availability and quality of public services for STD as key factors in reducing the spread of STDs and preventing complications (USDHHS, 2000). Effective health promotion approaches in the community must include STD prevention in the curricula of middle and secondary schools. Preventing the initiation of sexual activity early in life results in a decreased number of sexual partners over a person's lifetime, and education is needed to assist youth in cognitively establishing the behavioral link between sexual activity and STD exposure.

In addition to the need for more innovative and effective sexual health promotion approaches in school settings, a number of recommendations have been made for improvements in current delivery systems (USDHHS, 2000):

◆ The number of clinics offering STD screening, diagnosis, treatment, counseling, and referral services should increase substantially to improve access to comprehensive services.

◆ Increased allocation of resources must be directed to the quality-of-life issues that operate in young adults' lives and contribute to inappropriately early initiation of unprotected sexual activity.

◆ Improved collaboration is needed among health care providers, community health departments, and community health nurses in case management regarding medical treatment, follow-up strategies to confirm cure, and notification and treatment of sexual partners.

Changes in behavior require diverse and multidisciplinary interventions over an extended period. Such interventions must integrate the efforts of parents, families, schools, religious organizations, health departments, community agencies, and the media. The goals of educational programs should be to provide adolescents with the knowledge and skills they need to refrain from sexual intercourse, and to increase the use of condoms as well as other contraceptive measures among those unwilling to postpone onset of sexual activity. Parent–child conversations about sexual matters are associated with delays in the initiation of sexual activity and with increased use of contraceptives by adolescents who engage in sexual intercourse. Additional recommendations to promote sexual health in adolescent populations include: (a) innovations for early detection and treatment of STDs among teenagers, (b) specialized training for clinicians providing health services for adolescents, (c) school education combined with accessible clinical services, and (d) behavioral interventions to prevent exposure to and acquisition of STDs (CDC, 2006n; USDHHS, 2001).

Influenza (Seasonal, Avian) and Pandemic Preparedness

Influenza (flu) is identified as an acute communicable viral disease of the respiratory tract characterized by fever, headache, myalgia, prostration, coryza, sore throat, and cough. Influenza A virus causes the most severe and widespread disease (pandemics); influenza B causes milder disease outbreaks, and influenza C is connected with only sporadic cases of milder respiratory disease. Influenza is usually seasonal in nature, but may be found year round if testing is done. Seasonal flu preparedness is in the form of vaccine preparation, utilizing the previous year's flu strain information to calculate the next year's subtype through complex formulations done globally and nationally by public health authorities (CDC, 2006k; Kilbourne, 2006).

Influenza derives its importance from the rapidity with which epidemics evolve, the widespread morbidity, and the seriousness of complications, namely pneumonias (Heymann, 2004). Influenza, an Italian word that means *influence of the cold*, has been recognized since 412 BCE and was first described by Hippocrates. It existed throughout the early centuries, and about 30 possible pandemics have been documented in the past 400 years. Three have occurred in the 20th century—in 1918, 1957, and 1968. The 1918 "Spanish flu" pandemic was the most devastating, killing more than 20 million people worldwide from 1918 to 1920 (Kilbourne, 2006). This pandemic occurred because the new virus was easily transmitted from person to person, and the general population had not been previously exposed to this subtype of influenza.

Influenza infections occur primarily in the winter months, affecting individuals in all age groups and causing approximately 20,000 deaths and 110,000 hospitalizations annually in the United States (CDC, 2006k; Prisco, 2002). Children have the highest rates of infection, but individuals age 65 years and older and those with medical conditions who are at risk for complications have the highest rates of serious morbidity and mortality. Older adults account for more than 90% of the deaths attributed to influenza and pneumonia (CDC, 2006k; Prisco, 2002).

Influenza immunization is available every flu season; vaccines are closely matched to the circulating strains of the virus. Children younger than 2 years of age are at substantially increased risk for influenza-related hospitalizations. The key CDC (2006k) recommendations include providing vaccine to:

- Children 6 months to 59 months
- Women who will give birth or be pregnant during the influenza season
- Persons 50 years old or older
- Children and adolescents (aged 6 months–18 years) who are receiving long-term aspirin therapy and, therefore might be at risk for Reye syndrome after influenza infection
- Adults and children with medical conditions that put them at risk for poor outcomes if influenza is contracted
- Adults or children with any respiratory condition that would be compromised further by influenza infection
- Nursing home or other long-term care facility residents with chronic health conditions
- Health care workers

The injectable influenza vaccine is inactivated. The nasally inhaled version is a live attenuated vaccine (CDC, 2006k). In the elderly, immunization may be less effective in preventing illness, but may reduce the severity of disease. With vaccination, the incidence of complications among the elderly is reduced by 50% to 60%, and death by approximately 80% (Heymann, 2004). The vaccine should be given every year *before* influenza is expected in the community (i.e., November to March in the United States). For those living or traveling outside the United States, timing of the immunization should be based on the seasonal patterns of influenza in the area to which they are traveling (CDC, 2005e).

Community health nurses play a major role in primary prevention. Influenza vaccination clinics are frequently planned and organized by or with the local public health agency, with the injections usually administered by community health nurses. Health departments typically schedule vaccination clinics in line with the state recommendations and provide these services with minimal monetary charge to the at-risk community members. Private entities, such as pharmacies or home care agencies, often choose to provide vaccine for profit at venues around the community. Private physicians and HMOs provide immunization for their patients or members. The community influenza clinic is a primary prevention activity often occurring during the fall of each year (CDC, 2006k).

In 1997, a new influenza virus called A(H5N1) was identified in chickens in Hong Kong. This virus produces a strain of avian influenza, which is common in wild birds and domestic poultry. Although the Hong Kong avian strain caused numbers of human cases of avian flu, the transmission was from direct exposure to infected poultry, not through human-to-human transmission (Kilbourne, 2006). Infected poultry were exterminated before the avian flu could mutate into a human-to-human subtype. In 2003, this strain of avian flu reemerged worldwide, in both domestic chicken flocks and wild fowl, spread by bird-to-bird transmission following bird migration patterns (WHO, 2007). Although human illness has been documented, it has not occurred through person-to-person contact. It is feared, however, that a mutation could change the mode of transmission, and this situation is being closely watched worldwide.

Sources of influenza virus include swine, birds, and poultry, and many types of flu can pass from animals to humans. Influenza virus mutate readily; it is possible that the A (H5N1) subtype could mutate to jump species from bird to swine and then to man, considering that many types of swine flu are readily passed to humans (Kilbourne, 2006).

Pandemics occur when a flu subtype has not circulated previously (new strain) or has reemerged in a population that has never been exposed (Kilbourne, 2006). If the A (H5N1) subtype mutates, for example, it could then be available for human-to-human infection and thus spark a possible pandemic (Kilbourne, 2006).

The WHO Network for Global Influenza Surveillance, which involves 116 national influenza centers worldwide, maintains constant vigilance for new influenza viruses. FluNet is an Internet-based tool for worldwide influenza surveillance. This program allows for the electronic submission of influenza data from participating global laboratories. Only designated users can submit data, but the results—graphics, maps, and tables of influenza activity on a global scale—are available to the general public. As new data arrive and are verified, the maps and tables are revised to give users an up-to-date overview of the influenza situation. FluNet has expedited the sharing of information on influenza patterns and virus strains, and is becoming an essential tool in preparing for and preventing influenza pandemics. Collaborating Influenza Surveillance Centers have created a task force of influenza experts to develop a plan for the global management and control of such a pandemic, and world public health leaders work diligently to prevent another influenza pandemic similar to the devastating outbreak of 1918 (WHO, 2006b). It is unknown when or where the next flu epidemic or pandemic will occur, but the CDC has charged the individual states with the duty to develop statewide plans that can be used by individual counties as templates for countywide preparedness (Kilbourne, 2006).

Pneumonia

Pneumonia is a pulmonary infection that causes inflammation of the lobes of the lungs, bronchial tree, or interstitial space. The causative organism can be viral (50% of all cases), bacterial, or fungal (Schultz, 2002). Symptoms of pneumonia include sudden onset with a shaking chill, fever, pleural pain, dyspnea, a productive cough of "rusty" sputum, and tachypnea. The onset is less abrupt in elderly individuals, and the diagnosis may need to be confirmed by radiographic studies. In infants and young children, fever, vomiting, and convulsions may be the initial symptoms.

Community-acquired pneumonia is a significant cause of morbidity and mortality. It is the sixth leading cause of death and the first leading cause of infectious death in the United States. An increased incidence of pneumonia often accompanies epidemics of influenza. An estimated 3 million cases occur yearly, with approximately 20% requiring hospital admission, and 50,000 deaths occurring yearly from bacterial pneumonia (Schultz, 2002). Hospital admissions and mortality related to pneumonia are far more common among people older than age 65; the mortality rate is approximately 50%. This is not a reportable infectious disease, but, nevertheless, it can have a great impact upon the community (Heymann, 2004).

The incidence of pneumonia is highest in winter. Pneumonia is spread by droplets, by direct oral contact, and through **fomites**, which are any inanimate objects freshly soiled with respiratory discharges. People most susceptible to pneumonia are the elderly and people with a history of chronic diseases, a compromised immune system, or any condition affecting the anatomic or physiologic integrity of the lower respiratory tract.

Primary prevention is the best course of action, and includes a pneumococcal vaccine, especially for the high-risk groups, ages 2 years old and up. High-risk groups include those with chronic diseases, immune-suppressing health conditions, or those who are asplenic. Reimmunization is recommended only for high-risk children, or adults over 65 years who had their first vaccination before age 65. The vaccine is not effective in children younger than 2 years of age and is not recommended for the healthy population between the ages of 2 and 65 years. For these people, education about preventing pneumonia is a major part of the community health nurse's role (CDC, 2007a).

Secondary prevention includes the early diagnosis and prompt treatment of affected individuals. Antimicrobial agents such as penicillin and erythromycin are the drugs of first choice for treating pneumonia.

Tuberculosis

Tuberculosis is a disease primarily of the lungs and larynx, caused by the mycobacterium tuberculosis complex, *M. africanum*, *M. tuberculosis*, and *M. canettii*, all gram-positive bacillii. Tuberculosis can also infect other parts of the body, when it is referred to as *extrapulmonary TB* (outside of the lungs). Tuberculosis has two stages: latent infection, which is noninfectious to others, and active disease, which is highly infectious to others. Tuberculosis is airborne, and is spread by droplet nuclei, sprayed from the mouth by coughing, sneezing, laughing, yelling, singing, or any way in which air is expelled vigorously from the lungs through the mouth. Infection occurs after inhaling the bacilli exhaled by the person with active TB. The incubation time for TB is approximately 10 to 12 weeks. The Mantoux TB skin test is the acceptable screening test for this infection. A positive test result depends upon the situation and the state in which the test is performed (Heymann, 2004).

Exposure to TB does not lead to actual disease in all cases. A long latent period may persist for many years (even for a lifetime) before the infected person develops disease and becomes infectious. The probability of becoming infected depends primarily on the amount of exposure to air contaminated with *M. tuberculosis,* the proximity to the infectious person, and the degree of ventilation. Most individuals exposed to people with TB do not become infected. Of those who do, all but about 5% to 10% will remain disease free, perhaps for a lifetime. The remaining 90% harbor the organism; although they are not infectious, they represent a persistent pool of potential cases in a population. The likelihood of being among the 10% who develop clinical infectious disease is variable, depending on the initial dose of infection and certain other risk factors. Groups at increased risk include children younger than 3 years of age, adolescents, young adults, the aged, and the immunosuppressed (CDC, 2006l; Heymann, 2004).

Once almost eradicated, TB has reemerged as a serious public health problem. In 2005, the CDC reported that the number of cases had decreased by 44%. Between 1993 and 2003, there was a decrease in active TB cases from 25,108 to 14,840. As of 2005, the total number of active TB cases was listed as 14,097 (CDC, 2005c). Although this is good news, there is evidence of sharply disparate rates among minority populations—the number of active TB cases among African Americans was 3,954 (28%), Hispanic Americans had 4,043 cases (29%), and Asian Americans reported 3,209 cases (CDC, 2006i) (see Fig. 8.5). In addition, the worldwide TB situation has worsened over the past two decades, especially in Africa because of the HIV/AIDS epidemic (a fatal association exists between TB and HIV/AIDS). The rate of TB among children is increasing, and there has been a proliferation of MDR strains, especially in Eastern Europe, where the deterioration of the health infrastructure presents a significant threat not only to clients but also to their caregivers (Borgdorff et al., 2002).

Incidence and Prevalence

Roughly one-third of the world's population is infected with *M. tuberculosis.* These 2 billion people have the potential for developing active TB at some point in time. Each year,

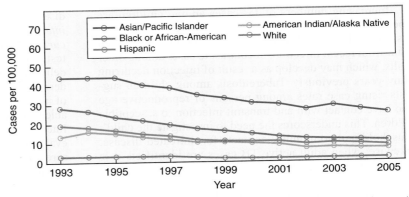

FIGURE 8.5 Tuberculosis case rates by race/ethnicity.

*All races are non-Hispanic. In 2003, Asian/Pacific Islander category includes persons who reported race as Asian only and/or Native Hawaiian or Other Pacific Islander only.
**Updated as of April 6, 2007, CDC.

8 million people worldwide develop active TB, and 1.8 million people die from it. Approximately 80% of TB cases are found in 23 countries; the highest incidence rates are in Africa and Southeast Asia (Borgdorff et al., 2002). In the United States, 10 to 15 million people are infected with *M. tuberculosis* without displaying symptoms (latent TB), and about 1 in 10 of these individuals will develop active TB at some time in their lives. This makes TB the leading infectious killer of adults, despite the fact that effective anti-TB treatment has existed since the 1940s. Tuberculosis is also a leading cause of death among people infected with HIV (Heymann, 2004; "WHO Reviews," 2002).

Surveillance

In the past, TB was called *consumption, wasting disease,* and the *white plague*. This disease has been one of the greatest scourges since times before recorded history. It was the leading cause of death in the United States through the 1930s because no cure was available. A diagnosis of TB was a slow death sentence, and the best chance of recovery was rest, sunshine, and plenty of food. Consequently, sanatoriums—rest homes where patients followed a prescribed routine every day—were built and were occupied for months until the patient recovered or died.

Surveillance of a disease refers to the continuous scrutiny of all aspects of occurrence and spread of the disease that are pertinent to effective control (Heymann, 2004). In 1953, when uniform national surveillance for TB was initiated, there were more than 84,000 TB cases in the United States. With the introduction of effective antibiotics in the 1940s to 1960s, there was a 73% decline in the number of TB cases, and it was thought that the problem of TB had been solved. From 1953 through 1984, the number of TB cases decreased by an average of 6% each year, and in 1985 they reached an all-time low of 22,201. The decrease in the number of TB cases contributed to medical and political complacency that resulted in a lack of progress in the development of new approaches and tools to control TB, and the disease is now resurging (Cowie, Field, & Enarson, 2002). In fact, TB dramatically increased in developing countries, prompting the WHO in 1993 to declare TB a "global emergency" at a time when many Western countries were anticipating the impending elimination of the disease (WHO, 2003a).

Populations at Risk

Minority populations tend to be at greater risk for TB. An increasing percentage of U.S. TB cases are occurring among people who were born in Asian, African, or Latin American countries, where TB rates are five to 30 times higher than in the United States. In the 1990s, TB cases among U.S.-born individuals declined 38%, whereas the number of TB cases among foreign-born persons in the United States increased by 6%. The TB case rate for foreign-born individuals has remained at least four to five times higher than for the U.S.-born, and the proportion of U.S. cases occurring in foreign-born persons has increased steadily since the mid-1980s, reaching 46% in 2000 (Saraiya et al., 2002). Tuberculosis disease cases occur predominantly among the following groups: foreign-born persons (46%), the elderly (23%), homeless people (5%), and individuals infected with HIV (8%). Higher incidences of TB are found among low-income people, persons with alcohol or drug abuse problems, the underserved, the malnourished, people in correctional facilities, people with other medical conditions, and individuals working where people at risk for TB are grouped together (e.g., homeless shelters, drug treatment centers, health care facilities). Tuberculosis rates are highest among refugees and immigrants, and noncompliance with treatment in all groups is a major factor in continued transmission of the disease, as well as in development of MDR organisms.

HIV infection is the strongest known risk factor for the development of TB. Immune-suppressed individuals, such as those with AIDS, can develop fulminant active TB within weeks after exposure to the mycobacterium, and the disease progresses much faster than in those with a normal, competent immune system. Consequently, a suspected case of TB in a person with AIDS is usually treated immediately, without waiting for the results of sputum tests or chest radiography.

During the last 20 years, the incidence of HIV infection has shifted from a predominantly homosexual, White, middle-class male population to a more impoverished, heterosexual, inner-city minority population with a high prevalence of *M. tuberculosis* infection. Consequently, the incidence of HIV-related TB mortality has risen. The risk of HIV-infected clients for TB infection is further complicated by the possible false-negative reactions of the tuberculin skin test resulting from the client's impaired immunity (Desvarieux, Hyppolite, Johnson, & Pape, 2001).

Increasing numbers of TB cases among children are especially worrisome because they point to escalated transmission in the United States. Cases in children most often result from recent infection, in contrast to cases among older adults, which may develop as a result of infection occurring many years previously. Tuberculosis among children suggests rising case rates among persons of reproductive age who have contact with and transmit infection to susceptible children. This underscores the need to investigate the child's household and community contacts for untreated disease. Likewise, when adult active TB cases are identified, it is essential to evaluate child contacts of the infected person (CDC, 2005c).

Among children with active TB, minority groups account for a vast majority of the cases. Girls have a much higher incidence during elementary and high school years than do boys of the same age. Susceptibility in children and adolescents peaks during infancy and again in puberty. Infants show decreased ability to localize infection and have limited stores of acquired antibodies. The occurrence of TB infection and disease in children provides important information about its spread in homes and communities. For example, if a child has TB infection or disease, it must have been transmitted relatively recently; therefore, the person who transmitted the TB may still be infectious. Other adults and children in the household or community have probably been exposed, and, if infected, others may develop TB disease in the future (CDC, 2005c).

Prevention and Intervention

Tuberculin testing, the standard method for evaluating TB infection, is a simple skin test that measures—by visible reaction—whether the body has had immunologic experience with *M. tuberculosis* (Table 8.5). From there, evaluation procedures determine the classification status of the disease, ranging from 0 to 5. The two most used terms are *infected without current disease* (classification 2) and *with current TB disease* (classification 3) (Table 8.6). The skin test itself is not diagnostic of disease. The Mantoux test delivers 0.1 mL of PPD (purified protein derivative) by intradermal injection. Because the dose is measured at the time of injection, the Mantoux test is considered to be more reliable than other methods, like the TB Tine test (CDC, 2005c). Interpretation of the tuberculin test is critical to subsequent evaluation of the client's status. The interpretation of this screening method must be as sensitive as possible while maintaining specificity for exposure.

The community health nurse may encounter an individual who, at the time of the TB skin test, discloses having had the bacillus Calmette-Guerin vaccine (BCG) in her home country. The BCG vaccine is an attenuated strain of *M. bovis* (bovine strain), which is not used in the United States. The efficacy of the BCG vaccine is questionable, as the protective value wanes over time and there is no consistency in how the vaccine is made. Because of these shortcomings, BCG is recommended in the United States *only* for infants and children with negative skin tests who (a) are at high risk for intimate and prolonged exposure to persistently untreated or ineffectively treated people with infectious pulmonary TB and cannot be removed from the source of exposure or placed on long-term preventive therapy, or (b) are continuously exposed to persons with TB who have bacilli resistant to both isoniazid and rifampin.

Successful interventions require TB control programs to focus resources on high-risk people, including contacts of people recently diagnosed as having TB disease. Also targeted for prevention efforts are members of racial and ethnic minorities and people born in countries where TB prevalence is high. People with TB infection who have conditions placing them at increased risk for active TB (e.g., HIV infection) also require special attention.

TABLE 8.5   Classification of the Tuberculin Skin Test Reaction

5 or more millimeters	10 or more millimeters	15 or more millimeters
An induration of **5 or more millimeters** is considered positive in • HIV-infected persons • A recent contact of a person with TB disease • Persons with fibrotic changes on chest radiograph consistent with prior TB • Patients with organ transplants • Persons who are immunosuppressed for other reasons (e.g., taking the equivalent of >15 mg/day of prednisone for 1 month or longer, taking TNF-alpha antagonists)	An induration of **10 or more millimeters** is considered positive in • Recent immigrants (<5 years) from high-prevalence countries • Injection drug users • Residents and employees of high-risk congregate settings • Mycobacteriology laboratory personnel • Persons with clinical conditions that place them at high risk • Children <4 years of age • Infants, children, and adolescents exposed to adults in high-risk categories	An induration of **15 or more millimeters** is considered positive in any person, including persons with no known risk factors for TB. However, targeted skin testing programs should only be conducted among high-risk groups

Retrieved April 15, 2008 from http://www.cdc.gov/tb.

TABLE 8.6 Classification System for Tuberculosis (TB)

Class	Type	Description
0	No TB exposure	Not infected: no history of exposure, negative reaction to tuberculin skin test (TST) or negative in vitro laboratory diagnostic tests.
1	TB exposure	No evidence of infection: history of exposure and negative reaction to TST or negative in vitro LTBI laboratory diagnostic tests.
2	Latent TB infection, no disease	Positive TST or positive in vitro LTBI laboratory diagnostic tests, negative bacteriologic studies (if done) and no clinical and/or radiographic evidence of active TB. Patients with isolated calcified granulomas (calcified solitary pulmonary nodules), calcified hilar lymph nodes, or pleural thickening are generally classified as TB 2.
3	TB, clinically active	Laboratory, clinical, bacteriological, and/or radiographic evidence of current disease.
4	Tuberculosis, not clinically active	History of previous episode(s) of TB, *or* Abnormal stable radiographic findings in a person with positive reaction to TST ($\geq$5 mm) or positive in vitro LTBI laboratory diagnostic tests and negative bacteriologic studies (if done) and no clinical and/or radiographic evidence of current disease.
5	TB suspect	Diagnosis pending. Diagnosis of TB being considered, whether or not treatment has been started, pending completion of diagnostic procedures. Persons should not be in this class more than 3 months. When diagnostic procedures have been completed, the person should be placed in one of the preceding classes.

From Centers for Disease Control & Prevention (CDC). (2002). *Core curriculum on tuberculosis.* *Chapter 2.* Retrieved August 13, 2008 from http://www.cdc.gov/TB/pubs/corecurr/ Chapter_2/Chapter_2_Classification_System.htm

According to the CDC Division of TB Elimination (DTBE) (2005c), a well-functioning TB control program is the best way to prevent TB and the emergence of drug resistance to TB. This program should ideally strive for:

◆ Standardized public health practices
◆ Prompt sputum conversion in people with active disease
◆ Identification of contacts of people with active TB to identify and treat other cases and people recently exposed
◆ A high completion-of-therapy rate within 1 year after diagnosis
◆ Assurance of adequate funding and a dedicated TB control infrastructure

One of the most effective ways to achieve a high completion-of-therapy rate is through directly observed treatment (DOT). In endemic countries, such as Africa, directly observed treatment short-course (DOTS) is used. This strategy assures treatment success because the client takes the medication in the presence of a health care worker. The American Thoracic Society and the CDC propose treating all patients with DOT because it reduces the sources of infection in the community (Jasmer et al., 2004; Potter, Rindfleish, & Kraus, 2005).

This labor-intensive approach has proved effective for the most difficult of TB cases in the United States. The more difficult clients are those who do not realize their personal or social responsibility for health and those who do not have the resources to focus on health when there are other stressors or diversions in their life. For these reasons, clients such as alcohol and drug abusers, transient homeless people, and low-income people may become the source for new cases of TB. DOT therapy ensures that clients take a daily or intermittent dose of prescribed medication, locating them wherever they may be—in neighborhood bars, sleeping on the sidewalk, in a homeless shelter, or in a drug rehabilitation center. Most health departments and TB control programs have a percentage of their clients receiving DOT therapy, with licensed staff or community health workers assigned to administer the TB drug regimen. These ancillary staff members are often former program participants, trained and supervised by professional health workers (Jasmer et al., 2004; Potter et al., 2005). A program like DOTS needs sustained political commitment, with the governments of nations recognizing the long-term benefits of providing the resources and staff necessary to ensure its proper implementation.

Commitment and flexibility on the part of health care providers and services can substantially enhance medication compliance. Significant improvement in compliance has been demonstrated with programs designed to provide DOT therapy for all clients, using community-based health workers who meet with clients in residences, at job sites, and at other local venues. In addition, new variations on the standard treatment regimens are being researched. Approaches include allowing individuals to take larger medication doses on a twice-weekly schedule, or providing an observed medication program for a limited period, followed by a course of self-administered medication with periodic reevaluation by health care providers (CDC, 2006p).

Multidrug-resistant Tuberculosis

Epidemiologists and communicable disease specialists cite a number of factors that contribute to the development and spread of TB strains resistant to one or more of the standard arsenal of TB drugs. Strains now exist that are resistant to as many as nine of 11 standard anti-TB drugs. In South Africa, an area that has been hard-hit with HIV/AIDS and TB, officials are now combating extremely drug-resistant tuberculosis (XDR-TB) that has killed close to 200 people in a few months, most of them with HIV (WHO, 2006e). Chief among the factors contributing to drug resistance seems to be the political and social response to declining rates of TB over past decades, which has resulted in funding cuts for surveillance, treatment, and research, and a premature sense that TB was defeated. On an individual case basis, the most common means by which resistant organisms are acquired is by noncompliance with therapy for the full, recommended period. Public health departments with limited resources have been unable to provide the intensive follow-up necessary to ensure that people who essentially feel well continue taking their medication (which may produce unpleasant although usually mild and manageable side effects) for the length of time considered necessary to achieve cure. Public health officials face a challenge and need to network effectively to provide continuous case management for highly mobile and often disenfranchised infected minority populations (Jasmer et al., 2004; Potter et al., 2005).

When candidates for drug therapy are identified, it is essential to provide program support to ensure that the maximum number of individuals comply with their medication regimen for the full duration of therapy. Isoniazid therapy for individuals who are infected with TB but have no evidence of active disease has been shown to be highly effective in preventing progression to infectiousness and clinical symptoms. Isoniazid is also a key component of the treatment for active disease (CDC, 2005c).

Clients with HIV and Tuberculosis

HIV infection is associated with an increased possibility of developing primary TB after exposure to a source. Someone with latent TB infection and HIV infection is up to 800 times more likely to develop active TB disease during her lifetime than someone without HIV (AVERT, 2007). The connection between TB and HIV/AIDS is dramatic, with one-third of the incidence of TB in the last 5 years attributed to HIV. In the United States, it is estimated that 26% of adult TB cases are attributable to HIV infection (CDC, 2005c).

People with HIV infection should be given high priority for preventive therapy, regardless of their age. For HIV-infected people, preventive therapy consists of isoniazid daily for up to 1 year (the usual regimen for preventive therapy is 6 months). These clients must be monitored closely for effectiveness of the preventive therapy and for tolerance to isoniazid. This drug has the capacity to develop adverse reactions or negative side effects. Isoniazid can cause hepatitis or damage the liver; close monitoring and regular follow-up are necessary to detect early symptoms such as nausea, vomiting, abdominal pain, fatigue, and dark urine signifying bleeding. Any combination of these symptoms is sufficient to initiate liver function tests (Springhouse, 2006).

As mentioned earlier, HIV-positive clients may not have the ability to react to a skin test for TB because of a weakened immune system. Therefore, other methods to determine TB status are employed. If it is determined that TB disease is present, HIV-infected clients should begin a regimen of drugs according to the schedule used by their physicians or clinics. The clients should be closely monitored for response to treatment; if they do not seem to be responding, they should be reevaluated.

Community health nurses have a responsibility to help HIV-infected clients experience a successful TB treatment regimen. Caregiving includes observing for adherence to treatment, administering medications (either directly through DOT or through DOT supervision by ancillary staff), observing for signs and symptoms of adverse reactions, monitoring for overall health and well-being, educating, and making referrals as needed.

Infectious Diseases of Bioterrorism

Information about anthrax and smallpox is presented here because of the threat that these diseases present to the community as weapons of terrorism (see Chapter 17 regarding disasters and terrorism). Because community health nurses work in the community, they are in a position of responsibility to allay fears, provide correct information, and to help people in the decision-making process regarding immunization in regard to possible terrorist attacks. Although other disease-causing organisms may be weaponizable, anthrax and smallpox have a history of use as terrorist weapons and will be discussed here (Secor-Turner & O'Boyle, 2006).

Anthrax

Shortly after the terrorist attacks of September 11, 2001, the U.S. population was further terrorized by anthrax. Several people who handled or delivered mail inhaled and touched anthrax spores concealed in envelopes. Many acquired anthrax, and deaths were reported. The pervasiveness of the fear this act created was felt nationwide. No person or country has yet claimed responsibility, or has been accused with spreading the causative organism.

In nature, anthrax is primarily a disease of herbivores, with humans and carnivores as incidental hosts. There are infrequent and sporadic human infections in most industrialized countries. It is an occupational hazard among workers who process animal hides, hair, bone and bone products, and wool in some countries. In fact, it has been called *woolsorter disease* and *ragpicker disease* (Heymann, 2004).

In humans, anthrax is an acute bacterial disease that affects mainly the skin or respiratory tract. The two main forms—cutaneous anthrax and inhalation anthrax—account for most human anthrax cases. The case-fatality rate for cutaneous anthrax is 5% to 20%. Skin becomes itchy where exposed, a lesion becomes papular and then vesicular, and in 2 to 6 days a depressed black eschar, surrounded by extensive edema, develops. The infection may spread to the lymph system and cause septicemia. With inhalation anthrax, the initial symptoms are mild and nonspecific but progress to respiratory distress. Fever and shock follow in 3 to 5 days, and death is the expected outcome (Heymann, 2004).

The causative organism, *Bacillus anthracis* is a gram-positive, encapsulated, spore-forming agent found in livestock and wildlife as the main reservoirs. The incubation period is short (hours to 1 week), and most cases occur within 48 hours after exposure. Transmission from person to person is rare, but articles and soil contaminated with spores may remain infective for decades (Heymann, 2004).

An anthrax vaccine exists, and all lots of this vaccine are owned by the Department of Defense. Troublesome side effects (fatigue, muscle or joint pains, and mental impairment) are experienced by 5% to 35% of recipients, and six doses are required over an 18-month period in addition to yearly booster doses. The vaccine was approved in 1970 for the treatment of cutaneous anthrax and has been administered primarily to members of the armed forces. However, it is not licensed for use with aerosol exposure, the form of anthrax that would be faced in a terrorist attack. Vaccination for anthrax remains voluntary (Nass, 2002).

Smallpox

Smallpox is a disease from our history books. In fact, the last case of smallpox was reported in 1978, and in 1980 WHO declared the disease eliminated worldwide. However, as recently as 1966, the disease was widespread in 31 countries. Some 10 to 15 million people were contracting smallpox annually, 2 million people died each year, and millions more were permanently disfigured or blinded (Sibley, 2002). By the late 1970s, just over one decade later, the global eradication campaign had pushed smallpox to the brink of extinction. The last known naturally occurring case of smallpox was in Somalia in 1977. Officially, the smallpox virus presently exists at only two places: the CDC in Atlanta and the State Research Centre of Virology and Biotechnology, Koltsovo, Novosibirsk Region, Russian Federation (Heymann, 2004; Sibley, 2002).

In the United States, routine vaccination against smallpox ended in 1972, and the smallpox vaccine has not been available for general distribution since May 1983. Few health care practitioners today have seen cases of smallpox or have administered the vaccine. In 2002, community health nurses in some communities became involved in the primary prevention of smallpox and learned the intricate techniques of smallpox vaccination and treatment of vaccine side effects in preparation for immunization of large portions of the population. That year, voluntary smallpox vaccinations were resumed for the first time in three decades (Spake, 2002). Initially, key military units were inoculated, beginning in 2002, followed by "first responders" such as emergency health care providers and health department personnel. The general public is not currently targeted for immunization (Veenema & Toke, 2006).

The plan for smallpox preparedness utilized the previously successful **ring vaccination** strategy—containing an outbreak by rapidly isolating and vaccinating people who have had close, face-to-face contact with the victim. This method refers to concentric rings, with those in the center ring being closest to the victim. Nonetheless, it is not clear whether any groups other than the United States and Russia possess the virus; furthermore, the rate of transmission of smallpox is complex and is contingent on many social and biological factors. "Therefore, it's difficult both to determine how real the threat is and to calculate a meaningful risk–benefit ratio in regard to compulsory mass vaccination" (Veenema, 2002, p. 35). However, one bright spot with smallpox prevention is that people who come in contact with a victim can receive protection if they are vaccinated within up to 7 days after exposure. This is unlike other VPDs and provides a window of time to reach exposed people (California Department of Health Services [CDHS], 2003).

Smallpox vaccination has risks. It is not a benign vaccine, and some experts allege that the morbidity associated with the vaccine has been understated (Veenema, 2002). One to 2 deaths per 1 million recipients of the vaccine can be expected, in addition to hundreds of cases of generalized vaccinia, eczema vaccinatum, and postvaccinal encephalitis (Heymann, 2004). Less severe but more common side effects include the formation of satellite lesions, regional lymphadenopathy, fever, headache, nausea, muscle aches, fatigue, and chills. In addition, the vaccine is contraindicated for the immunosuppressed, those with eczema, pregnant women, and infants younger than 1 year (Bicknell, 2002).

The variola virus causes smallpox and is transmitted from person to person. Initial infection begins with a febrile prodromal period that occurs 1 to 4 days before the onset of the rash. Fever is 101°F or higher, and victims experience at least one of the following: prostration, headache, backache, chills, vomiting, and severe abdominal pain. These physical symptoms are followed by the classic smallpox lesions—characterized as deep-seated, firm/hard, round, well-circumscribed vesicles or pustules. The lesions are in the same stage of development, anywhere on the body. Practitioners must prepare to recognize and differentiate smallpox from other diseases. The smallpox lesion can be confused with other conditions, such as varicella (chicken pox), disseminated herpes zoster, impetigo, drug eruptions, contact dermatitis, scabies, or disseminated HSV. Accurate diagnosis depends on the practitioner's skill to clearly recognize the classic smallpox lesion, identify that the lesions are in the same stage of development, and get an accurate history of prodromal symptoms (Heymann, 2004).

Community health nurses must raise their awareness and bioterrorism preparedness. As advocates for clients, families, groups, aggregates, and populations, community health nurses can do the following (Veenema, 2002):

- Become knowledgeable about the infectious agents that pose the most significant threats of being used in cases of bioterrorism (e.g., anthrax, botulism, plague, smallpox).
- Implement educational programs designed to inform the public of the potential consequences of the smallpox vaccine and of mass vaccination.
- Stay current on evolving vaccination policies, evaluating their potential impact on community health.
- Get involved in the national smallpox vaccination policy debate.
- Participate in designing bioterrorism disaster response plans within your professional organizations and at the state and local level; anticipate the challenges associated with the plans.
- Assist your facility in preparing for the responsibilities it would assume in the event of a change in national policy mandating universal smallpox vaccination.

◆ Be ready to participate in the design and implementation of large-scale immunization programs.
◆ Explore and educate yourself about voluntarily taking the vaccine if you work in a high-risk (first-response) clinical practice, such as an outpatient clinic or health department.

GLOBAL ISSUES IN COMMUNICABLE DISEASE CONTROL

Our planet has many common concerns, and communicable disease control is one of them. A new issue is the increasing number of emerging communicable diseases occurring globally. New diseases bring new challenges in case investigations, surveillance, and control. To conquer these challenges, community health nurses are assisted by the steps of the nursing process.

Globally Emerging Communicable Diseases

Emerging diseases are those that either have newly appeared or are rapidly increasing in incidence or geographic range. Most emerging diseases are not caused by genuinely new pathogens; rather, ecologic, environmental, and demographic factors place nonimmune people in increased contact with a pathogen or its host, or promote the pathogen's dissemination. As mentioned earlier in this chapter, the current volume, speed, and reach of international travel make the emergence of communicable diseases truly a global problem. The following is a brief profile of some old and new emerging infectious diseases. (See Chapter 16 for more on global health issues.)

Ebola hemorrhagic fever, a severe acute viral illness with sudden onset of fever, malaise, myalgia, headache, pharyngitis, vomiting, diarrhea, and a maculopapular rash, has been confined to countries in tropical Africa. It was first identified in 1976, in the Democratic Republic of the Congo, where the case-fatality rate has ranged from 50% to 90%. Person-to-person transmission occurs by direct contact with infected blood, secretions, organs, or semen. People of all ages are susceptible (Heymann, 2004).

Legionnaires' disease (legionellosis) is a form of a potentially fatal pneumonia caused by bacteria that contaminate the water in air-conditioning systems, faucets, and humidifiers. It was first identified at a convention of members of the American Legion, held in Philadelphia, Pennsylvania, in 1976. It is characterized by anorexia, malaise, myalgia, and headache; within 1 day, there is a rapidly rising fever associated with chills, a nonproductive cough, abdominal pain, and diarrhea. The case-fatality rate has been as high as 39% in hospitalized clients and higher among those with compromised immune systems. The disease occurs more frequently with increasing age, with most patients being older than 50 years of age (Heymann, 2004).

Hantavirus is an old virus with a newly recognized clinical illness. It first occurred in Manchuria before World War II. In 1951, it was recognized in Korea. It is considered a major, expanding public health problem in China, with 40,000 to 100,000 cases reported annually. It was first seen in the United States in 1993, in the area where Utah, Colorado, New Mexico, and Arizona meet; 28 people died from hantavirus infection. The severe form of the disease is endemic in Eurasia and Scandinavia. Deer mice appear to be the reservoir, and transmission is by way of aerosolization of infected droppings. It is an acute viral disease characterized by abrupt onset of fever, low back pain, varying degrees of hemorrhagic manifestations, renal involvement, hypotension, and shock. Prevention is focused on rodent control, and surveillance for the infection in wild rodents (Heymann, 2004).

E. coli O157:H7 was first identified as a pathogen in the United States in 1982. An outbreak of severe bloody diarrhea was traced to contaminated hamburgers. In January 1993, a large outbreak caused by this *E. coli* strain affected 700 people who ate undercooked hamburgers in the Puget Sound area of Washington. Other outbreaks have been caused by unpasteurized milk and by apple cider made from apples contaminated by cow manure. More recent outbreaks have included fresh spinach grown in California. Children younger than 5 years of age are most susceptible and are at greatest risk of developing hemolytic-uremic syndrome as a complication.

E.coli infections are recognized to be an important problem in Europe, South Africa, Japan, South America, and Australia. Humans may serve as a reservoir for person-to-person transmission. Primary prevention can be accomplished by following federal guidelines, which require commercially prepared meat to be cooked to an internal temperature of 140°F, and by safe and hygienic cooking practices at home. Raw meats should be kept separated from fruits, vegetables, and cooked meats during preparation; separate cutting boards should be used, and they should be cleaned with soap and hot water and rinsed using a bleach solution (Heymann, 2004).

Lyme disease was first discovered in the United States in the 1970s when an unusually high incidence of children developed rheumatoid arthritis in Lyme, Connecticut. It is an infection caused by a spirochete called *Borrelia burgdorferi* and is characterized by a distinctive skin lesion, systemic symptoms, and neurologic, rheumatologic, and cardiac involvement occurring over a period of months to years. A bite from a tick that can be carried by dogs and cats passes the disease to humans. All 48 contiguous states have reported cases, but it is most prevalent in the Northeast. It is the most common tick-borne disorder in the United States. Lyme disease is treatable and is not communicable from person to person. Primary prevention includes educating the public about the mode of transmission and being aware of high-risk areas. In wooded, brushy, and tall-grass areas, people should walk in the middle of trails, wear a long-sleeved shirt, wear a hat, spray tick repellent on clothes and shoes, and wear long pants tucked into high socks. They should check for ticks after an outing. Light-colored clothing makes it easier to see ticks. If a tick is found, it should be removed with forceps (tweezers), trying not to crush the tick's body, and pulling it straight out of the tissue it adheres to (Heymann, 2004).

Dengue fever, an acute febrile viral condition, is not transmitted from person to person but through the bite of an infected mosquito. Symptoms include sudden onset beginning with fever, severe headache, myalgia, arthralgia, retroorbital pain, anorexia, gastrointestinal disturbances, and rash. Children have milder symptoms than do adults. The prevalence has increased as a result of increasing worldwide urbanization during the last few decades. Dengue and dengue hemorrhagic fever (DHF) have been reported from more than 100 countries in the world, but not in Europe. These two diseases often occur in massive epidemics, most recently in 1996, when severe epidemics were reported in 27 countries in the Americas and in Southeast Asia. Outbreaks of DHF were recently reported in Brazil, Cuba, India, and Sri Lanka. The WHO strategy of control is based on prevention of transmission by controlling the vector mosquito. Such measures start with eliminating areas for breeding, such as small pools of stagnant water, even in empty flowerpots or abandoned tires (Heyman, 2004; WHO, 2002).

Other Diseases

In 1996, England reported the first cases of new-variant Creutzfeldt-Jakob disease (a fatal neurologic condition), probably related to eating contaminated beef. In 1997, cases of *S. aureus* with reduced susceptibility to vancomycin occurred in Japan and the United States, raising concern for a return to the preantibiotic era. In that same year, an outbreak of avian influenza in Hong Kong raised concerns about a potential pandemic; it was the first time an avian influenza virus had infected humans (Kilbourne, 2006). In 2002, SARS, an atypical pneumonia with a 10% fatality rate, was recorded in mainland China, Taiwan, and Hong Kong. By June of 2003, more than 8,400 cases and 772 deaths were reported in 13 countries (WHO, 2004).

Global Response to Communicable Diseases

Communicable diseases are not limited to specific regions of the world; they are the problem of all people. In 1996, WHO focused on completing the unfinished business of eradication and elimination of specific diseases; tackling "old" diseases, such as TB and malaria, and the problem of antimicrobial resistance, as well as combating newly emerging diseases. The WHO continues to focus on safeguarding the gains already achieved, which depends largely on sharing health and medical knowledge, expertise, and experience on a global scale. During the 50 years of its existence, WHO has taken a three-pronged approach to communicable diseases: case-finding, surveillance and control, and elimination and eradication (WHO, 2004).

Case-finding is an important beginning to communicable disease control and eventual eradication. Because of the changing nature of the world's demographics, use of space, and accelerating technology, old or once unknown diseases are reemerging, and others are being seen on our planet for the first time. Differentiation of one set of symptoms from those of another disease is an essential first step in case-finding. Once a disease has been identified, all cases need to be found through the traditional case-finding methods of contact investigation. Each contact leads to another piece of information and becomes part of communicable disease detective work.

Once a disease has been identified and is known to exist in a particular community, the steps of *surveillance and control* begin. Questions need to be answered and acted upon: How is the disease spread? What must be done to reduce the impact of the source? Do infected persons need to be isolated? Does the disease respond to antimicrobial therapy? Weekly, monthly, and yearly documentation of disease frequency and distribution is gathered and shared globally. Control measures then begin. Some developing countries may need more technical and financial support to achieve control. The cost of locating cases, eliminating vector pools, and providing immunizations and/or treatment can be a burden beyond the capabilities of poorer nations.

Effective surveillance and control can lead to the goal of *elimination and eradication* of a disease in many cases. We have been successful with smallpox and are closing in on polio. Within the next 25 years, other diseases, such as measles and TB, have the potential for elimination. Global collaboration, using the strengths from all nations, is needed to achieve these goals.

USING THE NURSING PROCESS FOR COMMUNICABLE DISEASE CONTROL

As mentioned in Chapters 4 and 7, the nursing process has steps similar to the research process and the epidemiologic process when approaching any health problem or condition. Therefore, using the nursing process to achieve communicable disease control should be an important and natural process for community health nurses.

Assessment

The first step of the nursing process, assessment, aligns itself with case-identification and case-finding in communicable disease control. The community health nurse must use all assessment skills and tools available during contact with clients, so as not to overlook the possibility of a communicable disease. Assessment must be comprehensive, producing physical, social, and environmental data. There is no place for assumption. At times, a nurse can become lulled into the usual patterns of inquiry, and this oversight may prove fatal to the client. An example follows:

> "Baby Josephine is irritable," says the mother. "Well, babies sometimes are," says the nurse. "How are you feeding her? Show me how you hold her. Does she sleep well? Try rocking her in the rocking chair before bedtime. And burp her more frequently. I'll check back with you in 2 weeks." Did the nurse record the baby's temperature, look at her for a rash, compare present weight with last weight, ask about bowel habits or vomiting, inquire about illnesses in the family, check on breast-feeding technique or watch while the mother demonstrated formula preparation, inspect the family's water source, ask about other foods the baby is eating, and so forth?

Broader inquiry into such a simple statement from the mother in this example may lead to the discovery of a life-threatening, undiagnosed communicable disease.

Assessment in the broader, community health nursing role may involve assessing a community's need for communicable disease surveillance and new or improved control programs. Nurses are in the community and can get a feel for the increasing or decreasing numbers of communicable diseases. They are often the first ones to know of a new outbreak of communicable disease in the community.

Planning

The planning step in the nursing process involves different activities, depending on whether the planning is for an individual, family, group, or entire community. At the individual level, the nurse may assist a client with a communicable disease to get immunizations or definitive treatment. Or, the nurse may assist the client in ways to care for the communicable disease symptoms that provide relief and comfort and reduce the chance of transmitting the disease to others in the family or community. When working with families, the nurse's actions are similar to those with individual clients and include assisting the family in getting available and needed immunizations, controlling the disease if present, limiting it to the people already exposed, and getting appropriate treatment and meaningful rehabilitation, if needed. With groups and communities, planning includes the collaboration of many different groups. Whether an immunization clinic is proposed or a flu shot day is planned for senior citizens, there are location, staff, and supplies to prepare, which may include writing grants, establishing contracts, and training and orienting staff, before implementation can begin.

Implementation

During the implementation step, the nurse actually takes the action that was identified as necessary during assessment and planned for with clients and others in collaboration. In the implementation step, the nurse may actually deliver the service or may supervise other staff or volunteers. On a large scale, such as with the implementation of a new immunization clinic, the fact that this will be an ongoing service has to be considered in an agency's budget. Staff turnover issues, relief when an absence occurs, and continuous formative (during the implementation process) evaluation of the services with minor changes to improve day-to-day operation can be introduced.

Implementing plans with small groups or families may involve arranging for transportation, so that several people can get to the immunization site or can be seen by a primary care provider. It may include gathering stool samples for laboratory analysis from a family recovering from a *Salmonella* infection. Education on primary prevention of future infections is an essential part of the implementation phase. Agency record keeping, state-required contact investigation, and reporting cases of communicable diseases are essential in this phase. Figure 8.1 is an example of a reporting form.

Evaluation

Evaluation is an essential step in the nursing process with all conditions, diseases, and services community health nurses provide. When dealing with communicable diseases, it is most important to determine whether actions have achieved the established goals. Have the outcomes been accomplished? Are all family members immunized? Are all family members free of the disease? Do families know how to prevent this and other diseases from occurring or recurring? Does the community have the communicable disease services it needs? Is the community free of the disease? What needs to be done now to keep the community safe from communicable diseases? Are there funding issues, programs nearing completion that need support, or growth of services needed that can be addressed before a critical need occurs? These are examples of questions that need answers during evaluation. The community health nurse who is concerned with the health and safety of the community follows the steps of the nursing process to achieve healthy community goals.

ETHICAL ISSUES IN COMMUNICABLE DISEASE CONTROL

When working to effectively control communicable diseases in communities and population groups, it is important to ensure that the activities undertaken are ethically sound and justified. It is important in communicable disease control to consider the ethical aspects of access to disease prevention and treatment services; enforced compliance with preventive measures; screening programs; privacy, confidentiality, and discrimination; and issues involving the health worker employee who is infected with or is a carrier of an infectious agent.

On a larger scale are ethical dimensions related to the cause and elimination of barriers to accessibility of drugs in developing countries. Making the inexpensive measles vaccine available to children in African villages, providing effective malaria treatment for people in South Asia, applying DOTS protocols for use in rural Brazil, and making ART and HAART drugs available to people with HIV/AIDS in developing countries (NIH, 2001) are examples of these issues (see Chapters 4 and 16 for further discussion).

Health Care Access in Communicable Disease Control

Access to health care means that people needing services find them available, acceptable, appropriate, and unrestricted by barriers to use. Such access has been advocated as an essential public health value, yet the global economy has been experiencing rising inequality, with income gaps between and within countries continuing to widen (Casas-Zamora & Ibrahim, 2004).

It would be misleading to say that rates of communicable diseases in population subgroups provide reliable indicators of health care access. The issue is significantly compounded when health care providers miss opportunities to vaccinate and when parents, who have the means, fail to seek out services to ensure that immunizations are up-to-date. It is clear that, in the absence of access to health care services, opportunities for people to receive the information and services necessary to prevent transmission and progression of infectious diseases are sharply curtailed (CDC, 2004).

Enforced Compliance

Legally, the responsibilities of public health officials in communicable disease control include the police power to enforce compliance with treatment or restrict the activity of infectious people to protect the welfare of others (Heymann, 2004). In disease prevention, completely voluntary measures to encourage healthier lifestyles tend to be ineffective.

Regulations that enforce compliance with disease prevention strategies are a justifiable restriction if the measures proposed are demonstrably effective and grounded in ethical principles. Coercion must be of the mildest sort compatible with achieving the goals of the regulation. Information must be provided to allow consumers to see the consequences of deleterious habits and the value choices that must be made. Inducements should be favored over disincentives. Regulation should be confined to actions with direct public impact and should be limited severely in matters that are personal and private (CDC, 2006d).

Confidentiality, Privacy, and Discrimination

To carry out communicable disease interventions, client needs for confidentiality and privacy must be ensured. Screening and other interventions must take place in a physical setting that does not allow overt differentiation between those clients with positive and negative results. As agency and national data systems and programs continue to evolve, it is essential to make confidentiality and data protection measures clear priorities. As many as 60 to 100 people are thought to have access to any average hospital record. Anonymity is frankly incompatible with early intervention. Two areas of current practice that may benefit from closer ethical scrutiny in regard to protection of privacy are contact investigation in STD programs and school-based screening for pediculosis (head lice).

Human society has a longstanding aversion to infectious diseases. Ostracism, which in the past included people with leprosy and other contagious conditions, has shifted to discrimination against people with TB, AIDS, head lice, and other current forms of communicable disease. Such discrimination should be of as much concern in the public health field as in the legal sector (CDC, 2006j).

Passage of the Americans with Disabilities Act in 1990 has resulted in legal protections for people diagnosed with communicable diseases who suffer discrimination, regardless of status of infectiousness. The issue of confidentiality has always been a major concern in contact investigation. It continues to be a source of debate in balancing the values of protection of the individual with protection of the public's health. The identity of the individual must be protected to the maximum extent possible, and any breaches of confidentiality must be clearly justified on the basis of a threat to the safety of an individual. That is, failure to provide essential information must jeopardize the well-being of the exposed person or contact. It is important to ensure that accessible services exist for the exposed partner or contact in the event that, as a result of screening intervention, they are burdened with the emotional, physical, and financial consequences of diagnosis (CDC, 2006j).

Summary

Communicable diseases pose a major threat to the public's health and have done so since the beginning of humankind. In today's world, such diseases are transmitted globally as the result of mobile populations, increased urbanization, and international travel. These diseases are transmitted through direct contact from one person to another or indirectly through contaminated objects (air, water, food) or a vector (animal or insect). Communicable diseases affect all types of people and have worldwide significance.

Ideally, prevention of communicable diseases is accomplished through primary prevention methods such as utilizing mass media education campaigns, one-on-one education, and immunization. Knowledge of VPDs, the schedule of vaccinations, a community's immunization status, herd immunity, barriers to immunization coverage, planning and implementing immunization programs, adult immunizations, and the immunization needs of international travelers, immigrants, and refugees have been discussed.

Secondary prevention activities of screening and contact investigation and casefinding are the steps to be taken when primary prevention activities have failed. Tertiary prevention is needed to ensure additional people are not infected. This is accomplished through isolation and quarantine, universal precaution practices among health care workers, and the safe handling and control of infectious wastes.

Becoming familiar with the major communicable diseases affecting our nation is essential baseline information for community health nurses. Tuberculosis, resurging since the 1980s, may be one of the biggest public health problems in the new millennium. Nurses must be aware of the populations at risk, how the disease is prevented, and the use of appropriate interventions during diagnosis and treatment. Issues compounding the control of TB are twofold: increasing infections with MDR strains, and the increasing number of people with TB and HIV/AIDS, making diagnosis and treatment more complicated.

A second major disease, HIV/AIDS, was first identified in the 1980s. In the last 25 years, 36 million people worldwide have become infected. With the success of antiviral drugs, HIV/AIDS is becoming a chronic disease for clients in industrialized nations, with an average life expectancy of 10 to 15 years after diagnosis. Africa is deeply affected by the massive numbers of women and children who are HIV positive, without access to the life-prolonging drugs available to people in developed nations.

Sexually transmitted diseases threaten the health and lives of millions of citizens. At risk are the sexually active, particularly adolescents and young adults, as well as minorities, women of childbearing age, and children born exposed to an STD. Control of STDs can be accomplished through effective screening, treatment, contact investigation, and aggressive public education. Several common STDs were discussed, including gonorrhea, syphilis, chlamydia, genital herpes, and anogenital viral warts.

Hepatitis is more common than HIV, and can lead to life-threatening events, such as cirrhosis and liver cancer. Yet, these diseases do not garner the attention they need. Most of the public is unaware of the types of hepatitis, prevention, transmission, and treatment. Vaccines for two of the forms (hepatitis A and hepatitis B) are now available, and hepatitis B vaccine is required in the routine childhood vaccine schedule.

Influenza and pneumonia are "old" diseases that are causing newly increased morbidity and mortality in the United States. These diseases cause the most morbidity and mortality in the frailest citizens—the very young and the very old—although vaccines are available to prevent them. A national objective for 2010 is to increase the immunized population, achieving a herd immunity to prevent such diseases.

Smallpox (an eradicated disease) and anthrax have been identified as potential bioterrorism weapons. The community health nurse has several areas of responsibility in regard to bioterrorism. First, the nurse must know the signs and symptoms of potential infectious diseases used as weapons. Also, the nurse has a responsibility to the community to allay fears about bioterrorism and to provide information about prevention. Finally, community health nurses and other nurses are becoming technically skilled in providing smallpox vaccine as the nation prepares for possible bioterrorism at home or during war.

Several emerging or new diseases are occurring globally. Such diseases as Ebola, hantavirus, *E. coli,* Legionnaires' disease, Lyme disease, dengue fever, Creutzfeldt-Jakob disease, antibiotic resistant *S. aureus,* SARS, and avian influenza are occurring in increasingly alarming numbers. It may not be unusual for community health nurses to come across these diseases in their practice.

Internationally, the WHO has been working for 50 years to make the world a healthier place in which to live. By providing all nations with the technical support, resources, and education they need, the WHO is aggressively tackling communicable diseases. Case-finding, surveillance, control, elimination, and eradication are steps toward meeting WHO's goals for communicable diseases.

Community health nurses use the nursing process in their important role with regard to all populations at risk for communicable diseases. Nurses concerned with communicable disease control must recognize who is at risk, where the potential reservoirs and sources of infectious disease agents are located, what environmental factors promote their spread, and what are the characteristics of vulnerability of community members and groups—particularly those subject to intervention. Community health nurses must work collaboratively with other public health professionals to establish immunization and education programs, improve community infection control policies, and develop a broad range of services to populations at risk.

Ethical issues in communicable disease and infection control include access to health care, enforced compliance, the justifiability of screening, preservation of confidentiality and privacy, and the avoidance of discrimination against infected people. ■

ACTIVITIES TO PROMOTE CRITICAL THINKING

1. Interview a professional in your local or state health department who works in communicable disease control. Determine (a) how she conducts communicable disease surveillance, (b) what diseases must be reported in your state, and (c) which communicable diseases are posing the greatest threat to the health of your state's citizens.

2. Compare a recent issue of *Mortality and Morbidity Weekly Report* with the same issue published a year earlier, in terms of cases of specific notifiable diseases in the United States. Which diseases appear to be increasing? Decreasing? Select one disease and read at least one recent publication on this subject to determine the reasons for its rise or decline.

3. Determine, through your local health department, what percentage of preschool children are immunized in your city or county. Is this a safe level of herd immunity? Propose some recommendations for preserving or raising this level.

4. Select one high-risk population discussed in this chapter and list the factors that make this group vulnerable to communicable disease. Use at least one other published source to enhance your understanding. Propose one nursing intervention (such as a specific screening or educational program) and outline how it might be accomplished.

5. Interview a professional who works in STD services or with the HIV-infected population. Determine what methods she uses for contact investigation. How does this health care worker preserve privacy and confidentiality? What measures have proved most effective in reaching contacts? What is your evaluation of their success?

6. Access the CDC through the Internet (*http://www.cdc.gov*) and browse the site to learn about its various services. Are there special travelers' warnings in certain countries at this time? What are some of the CDC's current concerns regarding communicable diseases? Select a communicable disease and identify the number of cases presently reported. Return to the same website 1 month later. Has the incidence of the disease increased or decreased?

References

Agency for Healthcare Research and Quality (AHRQ). (2001). *Screening for Chlamydial infection: What's new from the Third USPSTF.* Retrieved April 23, 2007 from http://www.ahrq.gov/clinic/prev/chlamwh.htm.

American Academy of Pediatrics. (2003). Standards for child and adolescent immunization practices. National Vaccine Advisory Committee. *Pediatrics, 112,* 958–963.

AVERT. (2007). *AIDS, HIV and Tuberculosis.* Retrieved April 23, 2007 from http://www.avert.org/tuberc.htm.

Beech, B.M., Myers, L., & Beech, D.J. (2002). Hepatitis B and C infections among homeless adolescents. *Family Community Health, 25*(2), 28–36.

Bicknell, W.J. (2002). The case for voluntary smallpox vaccine. *New England Journal of Medicine, 346,* 1323–1325.

Borgdorff, M.W., Floyd, K., & Broekmans, J.F. (2002). Interventions to reduce tuberculosis mortality and transmission in low- and middle-income countries. *Bulletin of the World Health Organization, 80*(3), 217–227.

Broder, K.R., Cortese, M.M., Iskander, J.K., et al. (2006). Preventing tetanus, diphtheria, and pertussis among adolescents: Use of tetanus toxoid, reduced diphtheria toxoid and acellular pertussis vaccines. *Morbidity and Mortality Weekly Report, 55*(RR-3), 1–22.

California Department of Health Services. (2003). California smallpox vaccination program. *Guide A, surveillance, contact tracing, and epidemiological investigations,* A1–A23.

California Department of Health Services. (2004). *STD/HIV prevention training center, STD treatment guidelines.* Retrieved November 25, 2006 from http://www.std/hivtraining.org.

Casas-Zamora, J.A., & Ibrahim, S.A. (2004). Confronting health inequity: The global dimension. *American Journal of Public Health, 94,* 2055–2058.

Centers for Disease Control and Prevention. (1999a). Achievements in public health, 1990–1999: Control of infectious diseases. *Morbidity and Mortality Weekly Report, 48*(29), 621–629.

Centers for Disease Control and Prevention. (1999b). Ten great public health achievements: United States 1900–1999. *Morbidity and Mortality Weekly Report, 48*(12), 241–243.

Centers for Disease Control and Prevention. (2002). *Supplemental guidance for planning and implementing the National Smallpox Vaccination Program (NSVP).* Retrieved January 2, 2007 from http://www.bt.cdc.gov/agent/smallpox/vaccination/supplemental-guidance-nsvp.asp.

Centers for Disease Control and Prevention. (2004). *Racial & Ethnic Adult Disparities in Immunization Initiative.* Retrieved April 23, 2007 from http://www.cdc.gov/nip/specint/readii/default.htm.

Centers for Disease Control and Prevention. (2005a). A comprehensive immunization strategy to eliminate transmission of hepatitis B virus infection in the United States. Recommendation of the ACIP. Part 1: Immunization of Infants, children, and adolescents. *Morbidity and Mortality Weekly Report 54*(RR-16), 1–33.

Centers for Disease Control and Prevention. (2005b). *Childhood immunization rates surpass Healthy People 2010 goal.* [Press release, July 26th.] Retrieved April 23, 2007 from http://www.cdc.gov/od/oc/media/pressrel/r050726.htm.

Centers for Disease Control and Prevention. (2005c). Controlling Tuberculosis in the United States. Recommendations for the American Thoracic Society, CSC, and the Infectious Diseases Society of America. *Mortality and Morbidity Weekly Report, 54*(RR-12), 1–81.

Centers for Disease Control and Prevention. (2005d). *Foodborne illness. Division of bacterial and mycotic diseases.* Retrieved January 2, 2007 from http://www.cdc.gov/ncidod/dbmd/diseaseinfo/foodborneinfections_g.htm.

Centers for Disease Control and Prevention. (2005e). *Health Information for International Travel 2005–2006.* Retrieved April 23, 2007 from http://www2.ncid.cdc.gov/travel/yb/utils/ybBrowseC.asp.

Centers for Disease Control and Prevention. (2005f). *HIV/AIDS Surveillance Report, 17,* 1–52.

Centers for Disease Control and Prevention. (2005g). *Influenza Vaccine Bulletin #1.* Retrieved April 23, 2007 from http://www.cdc.gov/flu/professionals/bulletin/2005-06/bulletin1_062905.htm.

Centers for Disease Control and Prevention. (2005h). *STD surveillance 2005: National profile chlamydia.* National STD Surveillance Report. Retrieved June 21, 2007 from http://www.cdc.gov/std/stats/chlamydia2004/.

Centers for Disease Control and Prevention. (2005i). *STD surveillance 2005: National profile gonorrhea.* National STD Surveillance Report. Retrieved June 21, 2007 from http://www.cdc.gov/std/stats/gonorrhea2004/.

Centers for Disease Control and Prevention. (2005j). *STD surveillance 2005: National profile syphilis.* National STD Surveillance Report. Retrieved June 21, 2007 from http://www.cdc.gov/std/stats/Syphilis2004/.

Centers for Disease Control and Prevention. (2005k). *Surveillance 2005: Special focus profiles STDs in women and infants.* Retrieved June 21, 2007 from http://www.cdc.gov/std/stats/2000sfwomen&inf.htm.

Centers for Disease Control and Prevention. (2006a). A comprehensive immunization strategy to eliminate transmission of hepatitis B virus infection in the United States. Recommendation of the ACIP. Part 2: Immunization of Adults. *Morbidity and Mortality Weekly Report 55*(RR-16), 1–25.

Centers for Disease Control and Prevention. (2006b). *Airborne precautions.* Retrieved April 23, 2007 from http://www.cdc.gov/ncidod/dhqp/gl_isolation_airborne.html.

Centers for Disease Control and Prevention. (2006c). *Genital HPV Infection: CDC Fact Sheet.* Retrieved April 23, 2007 from http://www.cdc.gov/std/HPV/STD Fact-HPV.htm.

Centers for Disease Control and Prevention. (2006d). *Global migration and quarantine.* Retrieved April 23, 2007 from http://www.cdc.gov/ncidod/dq/health.htm.

Centers for Disease Control and Prevention. (2006e). *Guidelines for viral hepatitis surveillance and case-management.* Retrieved April 23, 2007 from http://www.cdc.gov/ncidod/diseases/hepatitis/resource/surveillance.htm#hepa.

Centers for Disease Control and Prevention. (2006f). *National Center for Health Marketing. Health marketing basics.* Retrieved April 23, 2007 from http://www.cdc.gov/healthmarketing/basics.htm.

Centers for Disease Control and Prevention. (2006g). *Nationally notifiable infectious diseases, United States 2006.* Retrieved April 23, 2007 from http://www.cdc.gov/epo/dphsi/phs/infdis2006.htm.

Centers for Disease Control and Prevention, Office of Minority Health. (2006h). *Eliminate disparities in adult & child immunization rates.* Retrieved April 23, 2007 from http://www.cdc.gov/omh/AMH/factsheets/immunization.htm.

Centers for Disease Control and Prevention. (2006i). Ongoing multi-state outbreak of escherichia coli serotype 0157:H7 infections associated with the consumption of fresh spinach. *Morbidity and Mortality Weekly Report Dispatch, 55,* 1–2.

Centers for Disease Control and Prevention. (2006j). *Partners services.* Retrieved April 23, 2007 from http://www.cdc.gov/hiv/topics/prev_prog/AHP/resources/guidelines/Interim_partnercounsl.htm.

Centers for Disease Control and Prevention. (2006k). Prevention and control of influenza, Recommendations of the ACIP. *Morbidity and Mortality Weekly Report, 55*(RR-10).

Centers for Disease Control and Prevention. (2006l). *Reported TB rates in minorities. Division of TB elimination.* Retrieved January 2, 2007 from http://www.cdc.gov/nchstp/tb/worldtbday/2006/graph1htm.

Centers for Disease Control and Prevention. (2006m). Sexually transmitted diseases treatment guidelines. *Morbidity and Mortality Weekly Report, 55*(RR-11), 1–94.

Centers for Disease Control and Prevention. (2006n). Twenty-five years after HIV/AIDS-US 1981 to 2006. *Morbidity and Mortality Weekly Report, 55*(21), 585–592.

Centers for Disease Control and Prevention. (2006o). World TB day. *Morbidity and Mortality Weekly Report, 55*(11), 1.

Centers for Disease Control and Prevention. (2006p). *TB facts for health care workers.* Retrieved August 13, 2008 from http://www.cdc.gov/TB/pubs/Tbfacts_HealthWorkers/treatment.htm.

Centers for Disease Control and Prevention. (2007a). *Epidemiology and prevention of vaccine- preventable diseases,* 10th ed. In Atkinson W., Hamborsky J., McIntyre L., & Wolfe S., (Eds.). Washington, DC: Public Health Foundation.

Centers for Disease Control and Prevention. (2007b). Recommended childhood and adolescent immunization schedule: United Stated, 2007 harmonized childhood and adolescent immunization schedule. *Morbidity and Mortality Weekly Report, 55*(51), Q1–Q4.

Charuvastra, A., Stein, J., Schwartzapfel, B., et al. (2001). Hepatitis B vaccination practices in state and federal prisons. *Public Health Reports, 116*(3), 203–209.

Children's Hospital of Philadelphia. (2007). *Vaccine education center. A look at each vaccine: Smallpox vaccine.* Retrieved April 23, 2007 from http://www.chop.edu/consumer/jsp/division/generic.jsp?id=75742.

Coughlin, S. (2006). Ethical issues in epidemiologic research and public health practice. *Emerging Themes in Epidemiology, 3*(16), 1–10.

Cowie, R.L., Field, S.K., & Enarson, D.A. (2002). Tuberculosis in immigrants to Canada: A global problem which requires a global solution. *Canadian Journal of Public Health, 93*(2), 85–86.

Dato, V., Wagner, M.M, & Fapohunda, A. (2004). How outbreaks of infectious disease are detected: A review of surveillance systems and outbreaks. *Public Health Reports, 119*(5), 464–468.

Desvarieux, M., Hyppolite, P.R., Johnson, W.D., & Pape, J.W. (2001). A novel approach to directly observed therapy for tuberculosis in an HIV-endemic area. *American Journal of Public Health, 91*, 138–141.

Environmental Protection Agency (EPA). (2007). *Detailed definitions of waste types under federal incinerator regulations.* Retrieved April 23, 2007 from http://yosemite.epa.gov/R10/AIRPAGE.NSF/283d45bd5bb068e68825650f0064cdc2/23cb99ded687884588257060006faf83/$FILE/Detailed%20Definitions%20of%20Waste%20Types%20under%20Federal%20Incinerator%20Regulations%20%20.pdf.

Fauci, A.S. (2005). Emerging and reemerging infectious diseases: The perpetual challenge. *Academic Medicine, 80*, 1079–1085.

Fiore, A.E. (2004). Hepatitis A transmitted by food. *Clinical Infectious Diseases, 38*, 705–715.

Hanson, R.F. (2002). Adolescent dating violence: Prevalence and psychological outcomes. *Child Abuse & Neglect, 26*, 449–453.

Hench, C., & Simpkins, S. (2002). Continuing education. Hepatitis C: Risk factors, assessment and diagnosis (Part 1). *Nurseweek, 15*(13), 19–21.

Heymann, D.L. (Ed.) (2004). *Control of communicable diseases manual,* 18th ed. Washington, DC: American Public Health Association.

Hogben, M., St. Lawrence, J.S., Montaño, D.E., et al. (2004). Physicians' opinions about partner notification methods: Case reporting, patient referral, and provider referral. *Sexually Transmitted Infections, 80*, 30–34.

Indian Council of Medical Research. (2006). Emerging problem of antimicrobial resistance in developing countries: Intertwining socioeconomic issues. *Regional Health Forum WHO Southeast Asia Region, 7*(1). Retrieved April 23, 2007 from http://www.searo.who.int/EN/Section1243/Section1310/Section1343/Section1344/Section1357_5353.htm.

Jasmer, R.M., Seaman, C.B., Gonzalez, L.C., et al. (2004). Tuberculosis treatment outcomes. Directly observed therapy compared with self-administered therapy. *American Journal of Respiratory and Critical Care Medicine, 170*, 561–566.

Kennedy, A.M., Brown, C.J., & Gust, D.A. (2005). Vaccine beliefs of parents who oppose compulsory vaccination. *Public Health Reports, 120*(3), 252–258.

Kilbourne, E.D. (2006). Influenza pandemics of the 20th century. *Emerging Infectious Diseases, 12*(1), 9–14.

Ku, L., St. Louis, M., Farshy, C., et al. (2002). Risk behaviors, medical care, and chlamydial infection among young men in the United States. *American Journal of Public Health, 92*, 1140–1143.

Lauer, G., & Walker, B.D. (2001). Hepatitis C virus infection. *New England Journal of Medicine, 345*(1), 41–53.

Margolis, P.A., Stevens, R., Bordley, W.C., et al. (2001). From concept to application: The impact of a community-wide intervention to improve the delivery of preventive services to children. *Pediatrics, 108*(3), 42–67.

McCullough, D. (2001). *John Adams.* New York: Simon & Schuster.

Mullins, M.E. (September 24, 2002). West Nile's spread exposes health agency's weakness. *USA Today,* 11A.

Murphy, C. (2006). The 2003 SARS outbreak: Global challenges and innovative infection control measures. *Online Journal of Issues in Nursing, 11*(1), 1–15.

Nass, M. (2002). The anthrax vaccine program: An analysis of the CDC's recommendations for vaccine use. *American Journal of Public Health, 95*(5), 715–721.

National Center for Health Statistics. (2004). *The National Immunization Survey.* Retrieved April 23, 2007 from http://cdc.gov/nis.

National Foundation for Infectious Diseases. (2005). *Adolescent vaccination: Bridging from a strong childhood foundation to a healthy adulthood. Report on strategies to increase adolescent immunization rates.* Retrieved April 23, 2007 from http://www.nfid.org/pdf/publications/adolescentvacc.pdf.

National Institutes of Health Office of AIDS Research (OAR). (2001). *National Institutes of Health: HIV/AIDS research programs.* Bethesda, MD: Author.

National Institutes of Health. (2002). *Management of Hepatitis C: 2002.* National Institutes of Health Consensus Conference Statement. Retrieved April 23, 2007 from http://consensus.nih.gov/2002/2002HepatitisC2002116html.htm.

National Institutes of Health. (2006). *Understanding emerging and re-emerging infectious diseases.* Retrieved April 23, 2007 from http://www.niaid.nih.gov/publications/pdf/curriculum.pdf.

Occupational Safety and Health Administration. (2006). *Hazardous Materials Compliance guidelines – 1910.120 App C.*

Potter, B., Rindfleisch, K., & Kraus, C.K. (2005). Management of active tuberculosis. *American Family Physician, 72*(11), 2225–2232, 2235.

Prisco, M.K. (2002). Update your understanding of influenza. *The Nurse Practitioner, 27*(6), 32–39.

Quander, L. (2001, Spring). HIV/AIDS prevention programs: What's working with our youth? In *HIV Impact, A Closing the Gap Newsletter of the Office of Minority Health* (pp. 1–2, 4). Washington, DC: U. S. Department of Health & Human Services, Office of Minority Health.

Rall, M., & Meyer, S.M. (2006). The role of the registered nurse in the marketing of primary health care services, as part of health promotion. *Curationis, 29*(1), 10–24.

Renaud, L., Bouchard, C., Caron-Bouchard, M., et al. (2006). A model of mechanisms underlying the influence of media on health behaviour norms. *Canadian Journal of Public Health, 97*(2), 149–52.

Saraiya, M., Cookson, S.T., Tribble, P., et al. (2002). Tuberculosis screening among foreign-born persons applying for permanent US residence. *American Journal of Public Health, 92*, 826–829.

Sarbah, S.A., & Younossi, Z. (2000). Hepatitis C: An update on the silent epidemic. *Journal of Clinical Gastroenterology, 30*(2), 1–26.

Schillinger, J.A., Kissinger, P., Calvet, H., et al. (2003). Patient-delivered partner treatment with azithromycin to prevent repeated Chlamydia trachomatis infection among women: A randomized, controlled trial. *Sexually Transmitted Diseases, 30*(1), 49–56.

Schultz, T.R. (2002). Straight talk about community-acquired pneumonia. *Nursing, 32*(1), 46–49.

Scutchfield, F.D., & Keck, C.W. (2003). *Principles of public health practice,* 2nd ed. Albany, NY: Delmar.

Secor-Turner, M., & O'Boyle, C. (2006). Nurses and emergency disasters: What is known. *American Journal of Infection Control, 34*(7), 414–420.

Sibley, C.L. (2002). Smallpox vaccination revisited. *American Journal of Nursing, 102*(9), 26–32.

Spake, A. (2002). Small defense. *U.S. News & World Report, 133*(13), 64.

Springhouse. (2006). *Nursing 2007 drug handbook,* 27th ed. Philadelphia: Lippincott, Williams & Wilkins.

Szilagyi, P.G., Schaffer, S., Shone, L., et al. (2002). Reducing geographic, racial, and ethnic disparities in childhood immunization rates by using reminder/recall interventions in urban primary care practices. *Pediatrics, 110*(5), 58–74.

Talking Quality.com. (2006). *Testing your materials and dissemination strategy.* Retrieved January 2, 2007 from http://www.talkingquality.gov/docs/section5/5_1.htm.

U.S. Department of Health and Human Services. (1991). *Healthy People 2000: National health promotion and disease prevention objectives* S/N 017-001-00474-0. Washington, DC: U. S. Government Printing Office.

U.S. Department of Health and Human Services. (2000). *Healthy People 2010: Understanding and improving health*, 2nd ed. Washington, DC: U.S. Government Printing Office.

U.S. Department of Health and Human Services. (2001). *The Surgeon General's call to action to promote sexual health and responsible behavior.* Retrieved April 23, 2007 from http://www.surgeongeneral.gov/library/sexualhealth/call.htm.

U.S. Department of Health and Human Services. (2006). *The State Children's Health Insurance Program (SCHIP).* Retrieved April 23, 2007 from http://www.cms.hhs.gov/LowCost HealthInsFamChild.

Veenema, T.G. (2002). The smallpox vaccine debate. *American Journal of Nursing, 102*(9), 33–38.

Veenema, T.G., & Toke, J. (2006). Early detection and surveillance for biopreparedness and emerging infectious diseases. *Online Journal of Issues in Nursing, 11*(1) [Manuscript 2]. Retrieved April 1, 2007 from http://www.nursingworld.org/ojin/topic29/tpc29_2.htm.

Weatherall, D., Greenwood, B., Chee, H.L., & Wasi, P., (2005). Science and technology for disease control: Past, present, and future. In D.T. Jamison, et al. (Ed.). *Disease control priorities in developing countries,* 2nd ed. Disease Control Priorities Project. Washington, DC: World Bank. Retrieved from http://www.dcp2.org/pubs/DCP.

WHO reviews, approves acceptable HIV/AIDS drugs. (2002, May). *The Nation's Health, 14.*

World Health Organization. (2002). Dengue and Dengue haemorrhagic fever. Retrieved April 23, 2007 from http://www.who.int/mediacentre/factsheets/fs117/en/.

World Health Organization. (2003a). Media Centre. *Who reports 10 million TB patients successfully treated under "DOTS" 10 years after declaring TB a global emergency.* Retrieved April 23, 2007 from http://www.who.int/mediacentre/news/releases/2003/pr25/en/index.html.

World Health Organization. (2003b). *The world health report, 2003: Shaping the future.* Retrieved January 2, 2007 from http://www.who.int/whr/2003/en/index.html.

World Health Organization. (2004). *Communicable disease surveillance and response (CSR), SARS.* Retrieved June 21, 2007 from http://www.who.int/entity/CSR/SARS/country/2003_06_04/en.

World Health Organization. (2005). *Expanded program on immunization (EPI).* Retrieved June 21, 2007 from http://www.who.int/countries/eth/areas/immunization/en/.

World Health Organization. (2006a). *Cholera: Prevention and control 1–2.* Retrieved April 23, 2007 from http://www.who.int/topics/cholera/control/en/index.html.

World Health Organization. (2006b). *Core Terms of reference for WHO collaborating centres for reference and research on influenza.* Retrieved April 23, 2007 from http://www.who.int/csr/disease/influenza/whocccoretor2006.pdf.

World Health Organization. (2006c). *Global polio eradication initiative. 2005 annual report, 2–11.* Retrieved April 23, 2007 from http://www.polioeradication.org/content/publications/annualreport2005.asp.

World Health Organization. (2006d). *Malaria in Africa, roll back malaria.* Retrieved April 23, 2007 from http://www.rbm.who.int/cmc_upload/0/000/015/370/RBMInfosheet_3.htm.

World Health Organization. (2006e). Southern Africa is moving swiftly to combat the threat of XDR-TB. Retrieved June 21, 2007 from http://www.who.int/bulletin/volumes/84/12/06-011206/en/index.html.

World Health Organization. (2007). *Cumulative number of confirmed human cases of avian influenza A/(H521) reported to WHO.* Retrieved August 11, 2008 from http://www.who.int/csr/disease/avian_influenza/country/cases_table_2007_02_06/en/index.html.

Selected Readings

Bast, R., Brewer, M., Zou, C., et al. (2007). Prevention and early detection of ovarian cancer: Mission impossible? *Recent results in cancer research, 174,* 91–100.

Brown-Peterside, P., Rivera, E., Lucy, D., et al. (2001). Retaining hard-to-reach women in HIV prevention and vaccine trials: Project ACHIEVE. *American Journal of Public Health, 91*(9), 1377–1379.

Cullen, P.A. (2007). From genomes to protective antigens: Designing vaccines (GPADV 2006): Designing improved and novel vaccines in the future. *IDrugs, 10*(2), 109–111.

Essex, M., Mboup, S., Kanki, L., (2002). *AIDS in Africa,* 2nd ed. Norwell, MA: Kluwer Plenum.

Kolata, G. (1999). *Flu: The story of the great influenza pandemic of 1918 and the search for the virus that caused it.* New York: Farrar Straus & Giroux.

Mansoor, O.D., & Salama, P. (2007). Should hepatitis B vaccines be used for infants? *Expert Review of Vaccines, 6*(1), 29–33.

Paino, G.B. (2007). Sublingual immunotherapy: The optimism and the issues. *Journal of Clinical Immunology, 29*(2), 796–801.

Public Health, 91(8), 1187–1189.

Sander, C., & McShane, H. (2007). Translational mini-review series on vaccines: Development and evaluation of improved vaccines against tuberculosis. *Clinical & Experimental Immunology, 147*(3), 401–411.

Selke, M., Meens, J., & Springer, S. (2007). Immunization of pigs to prevent human disease: Construction and protective efficacy of a *Salmonella Typhimurium* live negative marker vaccine. *Infection & Immunity, 75*(2), 2476–2483.

St. Lawrence, J.S., Montano, D.E., Kasprzyk, D., et al. (2002). STD screening, testing, case reporting, and clinical and partner notification practices: A national survey of U.S. physicians. *American Journal of Public Health, 92*(11), 1784–1788.

Internet Resources

AIDS Info: U.S. Department of Health & Human Services: *http://aidsinfo.nih.gov/*

American Public Health Association: *http://www.apha.org/*

Center for International Health Information: *http://www.cihi.com*

Centers for Disease Control and Prevention: *http://www.cdc.gov*

CDC National Prevention Information Network: *http://www.cdcnpin.org*

Frances J. Curry National Tuberculosis Center: *http://www.nationaltbcenter.edu/*

HCV Advocate: *http://www.hcvadvocate.org*

Hepatitis Foundation International: *http://www.hepfi.org*

Immunization Action Coalition Immunization Web sites: *http://www.immunize.org/; http://www.immunizationinfo.org/; http://www.harlemtbcenter.org/*

National Immunization Program (NIP): *http://www.cdc.gov/nip*

National Institute of Allergy and Infectious Diseases: *http://www.niaid.nih.gov*

National Institutes of Health: *http://www.nih.gov*

Pandemicflu.Gov: *http://www.pandemicflu.gov/plan/states/index.html*

UNICEF: *http://www.unicef.org/*

Vaccine/vaccination information: *http://www.vaccineinformation.org; http://www.pediatricsnow.com; http://www.kidshealth.org*

WHO Epidemic & Pandemic Alert & Response: *http://www.who.int/csr/en/*

WHO Network for Global Influenza Surveillance: *http://www.who.int/csr/disease/influenza/surveillance/en/*

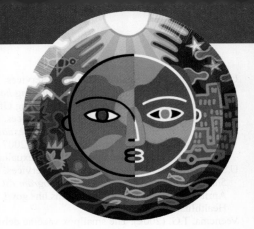

9

Environmental Health and Safety

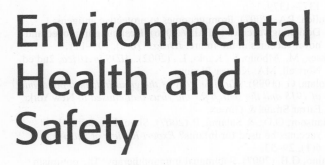

LEARNING OBJECTIVES

Upon mastery of this chapter, you should be able to:

◆ Discuss the importance of applying an ecologic perspective to any investigation of human–environment relationships.

◆ Explain the concepts of prevention and long-range environmental impact and their importance for environmental health.

◆ Identify at least five global environmental concerns and discuss hazards associated with each area.

◆ Relate the effect of the described hazards on people's health.

◆ Discuss appropriate interventions for addressing these health problems, including community health nursing's role.

◆ Describe how national health objectives for the year 2010 target environmental health.

◆ Describe strategies for nursing collaboration and participation in efforts to promote and protect environmental health.

> ❝*When we try to pick out anything by itself, we find it hitched to everything else in the Universe.*❞
>
> —John Muir, 1911

KEY TERMS

Built environment
Contaminant
Deforestation
Demographic entrapment
Desertification
Ecologic perspective
Ecosystem
Environmental health
Environmental impact
Environmental justice
Extinction
Global warming
Pollution
Toxic agent
Wetlands

Our environment—the conditions within which we live and work, including the quality of our air, water, food, and working conditions—strongly influences our health status. Consequently, the study of environmental health has tremendous meaning for community health nurses. Broadly defined, **environmental health** is concerned with assessing, controlling, and improving the impact people make on their environment and the impact of the environment on them. The field of environmental health is concerned with all elements of the environment that influence people's health and well-being. The conditions of workplaces, homes, or communities, including the many chemical, physical, and psychological forces present in the environment that affect human health, are important considerations.

Different environments pose different health problems and benefits. Consider the effects of climate change, soil erosion, and insect invasions on a rural community or the effects of industrial toxic wastes, auto emissions, and airport noise on urban residents. The health effects of a hot, dry climate are different from those of an arctic area, and the environmental conditions of an industrialized nation are dramatically different from those of a developing country.

This chapter describes conceptual and theoretic approaches to environmental health and examines historical perspectives, global environmental health issues, and the primary environmental areas of concern to community health nurses. Those primary environmental areas include air pollution, water pollution, contaminated food, waste disposal, insect and rodent control, and specific hazards in the home, worksite, and community. The role of the public health nurse in efforts to mitigate or remove environmental toxins and other hazards is stressed.

CONCEPTS AND THEORIES CENTRAL TO ENVIRONMENTAL HEALTH

Assessing environmental health means more than looking for illness or disease-causing agents; it also means examining the quality of the environment. Do the conditions of both the manmade and the natural environment combine to provide a health-enhancing milieu? Are people's surroundings safe and life-sustaining? Are they clean and aesthetically enriching? Is the environment not only physically but also psychologically health-enhancing? To answer these questions and gain greater understanding, the nurse needs to consider the conceptual and theoretic approaches that are essential to assessing and controlling environmental health.

Preventive Approach

The study of environmental health has become increasingly complex as people's influence on the environment has increased. With the unprecedented advances in science and technology that have taken place in the past few decades, society's ability to affect the environment has expanded, and the implications of these effects are not fully comprehended. New forms of energy, new synthetic chemical substances, and genetic engineering research bombard us with such rapidity that it is almost impossible to anticipate all the potential side effects on the environment and, in turn, on people's health. For each advance and presumed improvement, the toll to be paid is often unknown until years or even decades later. In many

cases, unfortunately, the risks have been known but ignored. For example, lead was recognized in the 19th century as a hazard, and white lead-based interior paint was banned in parts of Europe in the early 1900s. Despite this, it wasn't until 1978 that lead-based paint and lead-based paint products were finally banned in the United States (Wigle, 2003). The cost, just in terms of lost potential for those poisoned with lead can never be adequately measured. The impact of nearly 75 years of lead paint use is felt even to this day.

For these reasons, the concept of prevention is vital to environmental health. Scientists must use foresight as they design innovations; government agencies, business organizations, and citizens must play watchdog; and those concerned with human and environmental health must monitor new developments and intervene to prevent problems from occurring. Health practitioners need to determine causal links between people and their environment, with an eye to improving the health and well-being of both. Nurses must be particularly aware of environmental factors that have the potential to either promote or adversely affect the health of communities. All three levels of prevention (primary, secondary, and tertiary) must be employed, but most important is primary prevention. Prevention of a disease or *hazard* (a source of danger and risk particularly affecting human health) from occurring at all has the greatest benefit to the community.

Although small-scale preventive and health-promoting measures, such as safety education in the home or workplace, are important, the larger environmental problems ultimately place many, if not all, members of a given community at risk. Community health nurses can develop an understanding of these environmental threats, as well as the collaborative skills needed to work with other members of the public health team to prevent or alleviate them.

Ecologic Perspective

It is important to consider issues of environmental health from an **ecologic perspective**, keeping in mind the total relationship or pattern of relationships among people and their environment. Even when environmental health efforts focus on a specific health hazard or single environmental factor that poses a health threat, a broad view of human–environment relationships must be maintained. In most cases, a single causal factor cannot be isolated, because there may be many causal relationships. An example is childhood asthma; although the exact causes are not known, factors such as allergens (e.g., dust mites), irritants (e.g., tobacco smoke, air pollution), weather, exercise, and infections can induce symptoms (National Library of Medicine, 2007a). The risk of developing the disease is further increased with family history (genetics) and poverty (environment). These various causal mechanisms join to increase the risk for the development of asthma, with no single mechanism being sufficient. This relationship has been referred to as the *causal pie model* (Rothman & Greenland, 2005).

An **ecosystem** is a community of living organisms and their interrelated physical and chemical environment. Within an ecosystem, any manipulation of one element or organism may have hazardous effects on the rest of the system. Therefore, no one factor, whether organism or substance, can be viewed in isolation. For example, in produce processing, there are several points at which contamination can occur: at production and harvest (growing, picking, and bundling); during initial processing (washing, waxing, sorting, and boxing); during distribution (trucking); and during final processing (slicing, squeezing, shredding, and peeling). Several different pathogens are associated with a variety of food-borne diseases from produce and animals grown and raised in the United States, Mexico, and Central America (U.S. Department of Agriculture [USDA], 2006). Pathogens may have been introduced in the irrigation water, with the fertilizer, or from lack of field sanitation during production and harvest; from contaminated wash water and handling at initial processing; from contaminated ice and dirty trucks during distribution; or in the final processing from dirty wash water, improper handling, or cross-contamination. By taking an ecologic approach to the study of environmental health, the community health nurse acknowledges that people can affect their environment, and the environment can affect them. Preventive and health-promoting measures may be applied to all aspects of the environment, as well as to the people in it. Humans share this planet with millions of other living creatures, and we must consider the ecologic balance and anticipate the far-reaching consequences of our actions before introducing environmental change through contaminants or toxic agents. A **contaminant** is organic or inorganic matter that enters a medium, such as water or food, and renders it impure. A **toxic agent** is a poisonous substance in the environment that produces harmful effects on the health of humans, animals, or plants.

Using a model similar to the epidemiologic triad introduced in Chapter 7, a triangle of human disease ecology is created. This model stresses the links between habitat, population, and behavior (Fig. 9.1). *Habitat* includes aspects of the environment in which people live, including housing, workplaces, communication systems, flora, fauna, climate, topography, services, and economic and political structures of societies and local communities. *Population* factors include the characteristics of the population (age, gender, and genetic predisposition), which help to determine health status and disease susceptibility. *Behavioral* factors include health-related beliefs and behaviors, which are shaped by a range of social and economic factors. The triangular relationship among these factors suggests that no real boundaries exist between them and that the health of populations is a result of the interaction of all factors. It also indicates that action on one part of the system in isolation is unlikely to be effective without complementary action on other relevant factors.

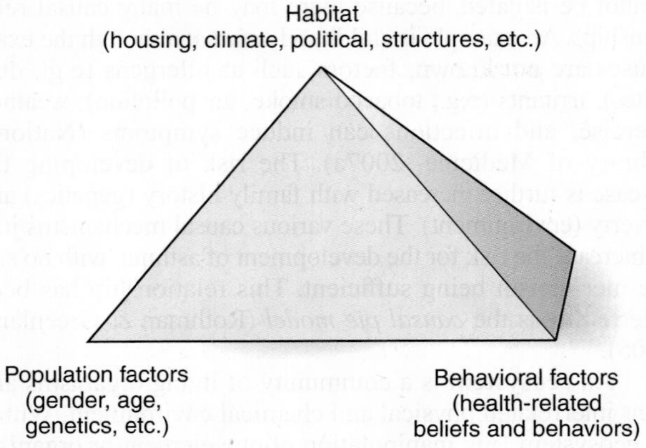

Environmental justice is a movement that has sought to ensure that no particular part of the population is disproportionately burdened by the negative effects of pollution. The U.S. Environmental Protection Agency (EPA) uses the following definition:

> Environmental Justice is the fair treatment and meaningful involvement of all people regardless of race, color, national origin, or income with respect to the development, implementation, and enforcement of environmental laws, regulations, and policies. . . . It will be achieved when everyone enjoys the same degree of protection from environmental and health hazards and equal access to the decision-making process to have a healthy environment in which to live, learn, and work. (2006b)

Industrial plants, waste facilities, and other potential polluters are more likely to be situated in poorer communities, and pollutants from these facilities can make the people who live there ill. The problem is even more pronounced with respect to the poor in developing countries; little global attention is rarely paid them until catastrophe strikes (Butler & McMichael, 2006). One of the world's worst industrial cataclysms occurred in Bhopal, India, in 1984, when methylisocyanate was uncontrollably released from a Union Carbide plant. The initial result was at least 3,800 people dead and over half a million people exposed. Well over 100,000 still suffer the after-effects of exposure (Bhopal Medical Appeal, n.d.; Butler & McMichael, 2006). It is very possible that, as poor countries industrialize and embrace Western development and consumerism, more disasters will occur. However, action can be taken in advance to prevent such incidents. Environmental legislation, preventive maintenance strategies, worker-training programs, environmental education programs, research on product safety, development of systematic hazard-evaluation models, and emergency planning are all examples of possible preventive activities.

In the United States, it is not unusual to identify communities that are exposed to higher levels of pollutants than others. Often, members of these communities are not well equipped to deal with pollution problems because of their limited involvement in the political process. In addition, they may not be aware of their exposure to pollutants and may be more vulnerable to health problems because of poor nutrition and inadequate health care.

Aesthetics is the appreciation of beauty that is culturally pleasing to the person observing the person, place, or thing. Even accounting for cultural differences, some things exist, such as a woodland path, a rocky beach, or a colorful sunset, that most people would find aesthetically pleasing. How does the aesthetics or beauty of our environment affect us? People themselves are the best sources for ideas regarding the things that they cherish as being beautiful. However, an environment that is well-landscaped and free of waste material, clutter, and foul smells can contribute to the inhabitants' well-being.

Habitat
(housing, climate, political, structures, etc.)

Population factors
(gender, age,
genetics, etc.)

Behavioral factors
(health-related
beliefs and behaviors)

FIGURE 9.1 The triangle of human disease ecology. Adapted from Curtis, S., & Tacket, A. (1996). *Health and Societies: Changing Perspectives*. London: Arnold.

PERSPECTIVES: STUDENT VOICES

I am definitely not an activist by any stretch of the imagination—at least I wasn't until a few months ago. One of my first public health nursing course assignments was to look into the smoke detector requirements in our community. I actually picked this project because it sounded easy—after all, doesn't everyone have a smoke detector in their home? Granted, I know that there is a problem with people removing batteries from them; but if they have a fire, that's their fault, right? Well, did I have a lot to learn! It turns out that smoke detectors are only good for about 8 years before they need to be replaced, and you need more than one in a house or apartment, especially inside each bedroom and right outside that area. To make matters worse, our city only requires multiple smoke detectors in housing built after 1992! So, if you live in older rental housing, like many of our elderly, poor, and even college students, the owners don't need more than one to be within code! This is scary and worse, it is perfectly legal. A few of the other students in the class took an interest in this, and we wrote a letter to our city council. It has taken some time, but it looks like they may be able to change the codes. You can be certain that I will be watching to make sure they do! Who would have guessed . . . I've become an activist! I guess I have what it takes to be a public health nurse after all.

Anna M., Nursing Student

The benefits of aesthetically pleasing surroundings are difficult to measure. Nevertheless, we know how good it makes us feel when we experience it, that we would like to linger there longer, and that we would not like to let it disappear. If people were able to feel this way about their home, their neighborhood, and their community, the world would be a more harmonious and healthier place.

A related issue concerns the **built environment**. The term refers "to urban areas and structures (e.g., roads, parks, and buildings) constructed by human beings, as opposed to undeveloped, rural areas" (Friis, 2007, p. 74). Increasingly, the built environment is thought to be a force of either positive or negative impact on the health of populations. For instance, the massive migration out of the cities that began in the 1950s and continues to the present has had a dramatic impact on both the environment and, inadvertently, the health of the population. As more and more land is developed and agricultural areas are converted to housing, the need for increased use of automobiles follows. With the automobile use comes the added impact of increased air pollution. Add to that the lack of services (schools, stores, recreation, and faith communi-

ties) within walking distance and normal daily physical activity is impeded, which can lead to overweight and obesity. This is a simplistic example, but it points out how unintended consequences can result from the environment we live in. Many communities are now looking for ways to discourage overdependence on automobiles and to encourage physical activity. They are planning new developments with major services that are easily accessible by walking, bicycling, or public transportation. One possible by-product of these efforts may be the strengthening of community ties. Although long thought to be unhealthy environments, cities actually encourage walking, and residents in poor neighborhoods tend to walk more than those in more affluent areas (Vlahov, Galea, & Freudenberg, 2005). With collaborative efforts by all stakeholders, our communities can become more health-promoting and life-enhancing to all residents.

Long-range Environmental Impact

When studying environmental health, it is important to consider the effect of positive or negative changes on the environment and on the people, animals, and plants living in it. This **environmental impact** must be viewed not only in terms of its consequences for people living now but also in terms of long-range impact on the human species. One must consider the health of future generations as well as present ones. Considerations should include food and fuel limitations of the natural environment, attendance to conservation through balancing of present and future needs, and prevention of the consequences of environmental abuse. This last point broadens the focus even more. Certainly, one should determine how current practices and toxins are hurting humans today, but it is also imperative to discover what threats they pose to the biosphere and thus to future generations—their long-range environmental impact. For example, carbon monoxide gas given off by factories and automobiles is toxic and can be lethal, causing dizziness, headaches, and lung diseases in humans who inhale it at certain concentrations. It has also been found to contribute to the formation of ground-level ozone, more commonly referred to as *smog* (EPA, 2007e), posing a serious ecologic threat both now and in the future. The National Institute of Environmental Health Sciences (NIEHS) 2006–2011 Strategic Plan calls for increased research and partnerships with industry to find effective means to better protect the health of the public (NIEHS, 2006). Efforts such as these will help policy makers weigh the possible environmental risks of any new industrial or business facility against its potential job and tax benefits for local citizens.

EVOLUTION OF ENVIRONMENTAL HEALTH

Environmental influences on health have been present throughout human history. Interactions with the environment, and the conditions of that environment, have shaped humans' mental, emotional, and physical health since the beginning of time. From ancient tribal practices of burial of excreta to modern-day sewage treatment, humans have been concerned with how the environment would provide for their needs and affect their well-being.

Global Perspective

In an effort to promote human health, people have taken steps to control, alter, and adapt to their environment. Demonstrations of this concern go back to Biblical times, when the Israelites observed strict rules governing food preparation, practiced sanitation, and quarantined people with infectious diseases (e.g., leprosy). For example, rules governing the proximity of tanneries, furnaces, animal slaughterhouses, and cemeteries served to protect the village water supply (Novick & Morrow, 2008).

As populations became more settled and urbanized, many different environmental health concerns developed. Community actions to deal with these developments have been recorded as far back as 2500 BCE. Archaeologists have discovered remnants of sophisticated water and waste systems in ancient cities of northern India and in the Middle Kingdom of Egypt. Early Roman engineers built aqueducts for supplying fresh water, and they developed management operations for overseeing water and sewage systems. (The use of lead pipes by the Romans in their water delivery systems likely resulted in chronic lead poisoning and may have contributed to the downfall of the empire [Friis, 2007]). Many of the innovations in sanitation brought to Europe by the Romans were lost for centuries. Ultimately, the decline in sanitary conditions would prove a breeding ground for major outbreaks of diseases such as plague and cholera.

A major environmental issue in the medieval world was the spread of infectious diseases brought about by the growth of cities, increased trade, and wars. The most severe infectious diseases were outbreaks of leprosy and bubonic plague during the 13th and 14th centuries (McGrew, 1985; Zgodzinski & Fallon, 2005). As leprosy spread and peaked in Europe in the early 13th century, people recognized a connection between the environment and spread of the disease. They instituted epidemic control by isolating people with signs of the disease and checking newcomers to the community (Novik & Morrow, 2008). Therefore, long before science had discovered the true causes of these diseases, people were instinctively changing or avoiding harmful environmental circumstances in an effort to promote health. Simple city ordinances restricted locals from washing their clothes or tanners from cleaning their skins in rivers that supplied drinking water. A law passed in London in 1309 governed the disposal of waste into the Thames River. Similarly, people passed rules governing the sale of old or spoiled meat to local residents, and "in Basel, leftover fish were displayed at a special inferior food stall and sold only to strangers" (McGrew, 1985, p. 139). This early concern for sanitary conditions became a major focus in public health, reaching its peak between 1840 and 1880.

The sanitary movement, which began about 1830, called for societal transformation to create a truly healthful environment that emphasized bathing, clean water, and controlled human waste disposal (Zgodzinski & Fallon, 2005). During the middle to late 1800s, Florence Nightingale in England and Dr. Ignaz Semmelweiss in Vienna pioneered the promotion of clean hospital and surgical conditions to prevent illness (Friis & Sellers, 2004; Nightingale, 1860/1969). Oliver Wendell Holmes made the connection between exposure to sepsis and maternal infection in Boston in 1843 (Holmes, 1843/1909–1914). John Snow first documented environmental spread of disease in London in 1849 when he linked the spread of cholera with contaminated drinking water (Aschengrau & Seage, 2008). The work of Pasteur and Koch demonstrated the role of bacteria in disease (Zgodzinski & Fallon, 2005). All of these, in addition to greater use of the microscope, shed further light on the relationship of the environment to health.

Awareness of the environmental impact on health was first documented in the *Report on the Sanitary Condition of the Labouring Population of Great Britain* by Edwin Chadwick in 1842 (Hanley, 2006; Library of Congress, 2007). This document addressed the necessity for a healthy environment. About the same time, a similar report called *Report of the Sanitary Commission of Massachusetts* was published in the United States (1850). This document, often referred to as the *Shattuck Report* after the chairman of the commission, Lemuel Shattuck, provided original insights into environmental health issues, including smoke prevention, urban planning, and sanitation programs (Gordon, 2002; Wilcox, 2005). These documents marked the first organized concern for public health and environmental health controls. Since that time, the focus has gradually expanded from sanitation to the problems generated by advances in technology, chemical production, and pollution, which are discussed in this chapter.

An important international agency, the World Health Organization (WHO), was created in 1948 and has helped to identify and address world health problems, including issues of environmental concern. Because many modern technological discoveries cause far-reaching health hazards that affect the environment and the health of the entire global population, this organization and others like it will play increasingly important roles in the future.

National Perspective

In the United States, all levels of government have worked diligently to assess, prevent, and correct environmental health hazards. The major environmental health efforts of the federal government have come primarily since the early 1970s. Local governments assume responsibility for proper waste disposal, pure water supply, and efficient sanitary and safety conditions within the community. State governments, represented by different agencies, handle broader issues that deal with the creation of state regulations, policies, and supervision of local health efforts. The federal government is charged with establishing and enforcing health standards and regulations (Mays, 2008). During the past several decades, the public concern for human health in relation to the environment, as well as concern for the environment itself, has stimulated increased government actions. The Environmental Protection Agency (EPA) was established in 1971 and was given extensive authority over all environmental concerns and protection of public health. The Food and Drug Administration (FDA) was established within the U.S. Public Health Service in 1968; the Occupational Safety and Health Administration (OSHA), for regulation, and the National Institute for Occupational Safety and Health

---

DISPLAY 9.1 HEALTHY PEOPLE 2010 OBJECTIVES RELATED TO ENVIRONMENTAL HEALTH

Goal: Promote health for all through a healthy environment.

Number   Objective Short Title

Outdoor Air Quality
8-1   Harmful air pollutants
8-2   Alternative modes of transportation
8-3   Cleaner alternative fuels
8-4   Airborne toxins

Water Quality
8-5   Safe drinking water
8-6   Waterborne disease outbreaks
8-7   Water conservation
8-8   Surface water health risks
8-9   Beach closings
8-10   Fish contamination

Toxics and Waste
8-11   Elevated blood lead levels in children
8-12   Risks posed by hazardous sites
8-13   Pesticide exposures
8-14   Toxic pollutants
8-15   Recycled municipal solid waste

Healthy Homes and Healthy Communities
8-16   Indoor allergens
8-17   Office building air quality

8-18   Homes tested for radon
8-19   Radon-resistant new home construction
8-20   School policies to protect against environmental hazards
8-21   Disaster preparedness plans and protocols
8-22   Lead-based paint testing
8-23   Substandard housing

Infrastructure and Surveillance
8-24   Exposure to pesticides
8-25   Exposure to heavy metals and other toxic chemicals
8-26   Information systems used for environmental health
8-27   Monitoring environmentally related diseases
8-28   Local agencies using surveillance data for vector control

Global Environmental Health
8-29   Global burden of disease
8-30   Water quality in the U.S.–Mexico border region

U.S. Department of Health and Human Services. (2000). *Healthy People 2010: Understanding and improving health* (2nd ed.). Washington, DC: U.S. Government Printing Office.

(NIOSH), for research, were both established in 1970. The Public Health Service, under the U.S. Department of Health and Human Services (USDHHS), has helped to focus environmental control efforts through development of objectives published in 1979 and again in 1991. Its 1991 document, *Healthy People 2000,* listed objectives in major target areas. In the 2000 follow-up document, *Healthy People 2010,* objectives for improvement in environmental health parameters continued (Display 9.1).

Private business has become more conscious of health and safety issues, following enhanced legislation such as the Products Liability Law and product monitoring by the U.S. Consumer Product Safety Commission (CPSC). Private business and industry have often been accused of having total disregard for the health of the environment and its effect on human health, but this image seems to be slowly changing. Many companies, when confronted by concerned environmentalists or consumer protection groups that have formed in recent years, have been forced to change their practices. Boycotts of products, listings of environmentally conscientious firms, and general public outrage have put a stop to many harmful practices. A number of companies have been concerned for some time with the environmental impact of their business operations; they have sought not only reduction of health hazards but also ways to promote environmental and public health. Timber companies, for example, have actively engaged in reforestation projects. Private business has been a major contributor to many non-profit, environmentally concerned projects and agencies, such as the Sierra Club.

Maintaining a healthy environment and balanced ecology and promoting the health of those living in it remain challenging. Past efforts to accomplish these goals have been only partially successful. However, increased public awareness and concern for future generations have exerted tremendous pressure to create new and more effective legislative acts and activities (Display 9.2).

MAJOR GLOBAL ENVIRONMENTAL CONCERNS

The global perspective, and specifically the national perspective, of environmental health provides a picture of humankind's attempts to protect populations. However, for much of our world's history, protecting people, other living beings, or the Earth itself has not been a priority or even a concern. Because of this history, major global environmental concerns now face the world, including overpopulation, ozone depletion, global warming, deforestation, wetlands destruction, desertification, energy depletion, inadequate housing, aesthetics, and environmental justice issues (Friis, 2007).

Overpopulation

Human population took hundreds of thousands of years to reach 1 billion in the 1800s and until 1960 to reach 3 billion. Less than 50 years later, it has more than doubled to 6.7 billion. Every 11 years, the world gains 1 billion people. Assuming that overall fertility rates continue to decline as

DISPLAY 9.2	SELECTED ENVIRONMENTAL HEALTH ACTS/AGENCIES/ACTIVITIES INFLUENCING HEALTH IN THE UNITED STATES

Date	Act/Agency/Activity
1850	The Shattuck Report
1872	The American Public Health Association was founded
1872	The American Forestry Association was established
1890	Yosemite National Park in California became the first national park in the United States
1936	The National Wildlife Federation was founded
1970	The Environmental Protection Agency was formed
1970	The Clean Air Act
1970	Poison Prevention Packaging Act
1970	Occupational Health and Safety Act (OSHA)
1970	National Institute of Occupational Safety and Health (NIOSH) formed
1970	Hazardous Materials Transportation Control
1970	National Environmental Policy Act
1970	First annual Earth Day was held
1971	Lead-Based Paint Poisoning Prevention Act
1972	Federal Water Pollution Control Act Amendments
1972	Noise Control Act
1974	Safe Drinking Water Act (amended in 1996)
1976	Resource Conservation and Recovery Act
1976	Toxic Substances Control Act
1977	Clean Water Act
1979	U.S. Department of Health and Human Services helped to focus environmental control efforts

Date	Act/Agency/Activity
1980	Low Level Radiation Waste Policy Act
1980	Comprehensive Environmental Response, Compensation, and Liability Act (Superfund)
1991	*Healthy People 2000* set environmental health objectives as a priority
1992	The United States, the European community, and 153 other nations signed the United Nations Framework Convention on Climate Change (UNFCCC), an agreement pledging to reduce greenhouse gases to the 1990 level by the year 2000
1995	*Healthy People 2000: Midcourse Review and 1995 Revisions* gave update on environmental health progress
1996	The Food Quality Protection Act
1996	The World Health Organization, scientists, and United Nations officials called for stronger efforts to combat global warming
2000	*Healthy People 2010* used the 1995 review and revisions and input from professionals from around the country to establish 2010 environmental health goals
2002	Homeland Security Act of 2002 authorized the formation of the Department of Homeland Security
2005	Kyoto Treaty ratified by 140 nations set emission reduction standards for 2012 (U.S. and Australia did not sign)
2006	*Healthy People 2010 Midcourse Review* update on environmental health progress

they have since the 1970s, by 2050 there may still be well in excess of 9.2 billion inhabitants of Earth. If however, the fertility rates remain constant, the population could reach 11.9 billion (Population Action International, 2007a, 2007b). The environmental impact of continued growth could translate into increasing food scarcity, water shortages, and depletion of other vital resources, ultimately threatening our very survival (Friis, 2007). Uncontrolled population growth is indisputably a public health issue.

The burden of population growth is being carried by the poorest developing countries, such as those in Sub-Saharan Africa, India, and Asia. According to the U.S. Census Bureau, the less-developed countries of Asia and Oceania (excluding India and China) will be more populous than any other region in the world by 2050 (Fig. 9.2). Long the most populated country in the world, at present growth rates, China will likely be eclipsed by India in 2037. Between one-third and one-half of the population in most developing countries is younger than 15 years of age, in part because advances in public health have lowered mortality among all age groups, but especially among infants and children. Globally, nearly one-third of the population is younger than 15 years (U.S. Census Bureau, 2007).

Until most recently, the elderly population (those 65 years and over) made up a relatively small percentage of the world's population. In 2002, this age group accounted for approximately 7% of the overall population. Compare that to projections for 2050, when the absolute number is expected to be tripled, bringing the percentage up to nearly 17% (U.S. Census Bureau, 2004). The growth in the population over 65 will increasingly strain existing health care, pension, and social service systems (Research Brief, 2005).

In some nations, the population is projected to shrink. If low fertility rates continue in Germany, Italy, Russia, and Spain for instance, their populations will decrease by anywhere from 2% to 10 % by the year 2025. In contrast, countries such as Nigeria, Zambia, and Jordan have high fertility rates, and it is likely that their populations will increase by 30% to 60% over the same period (U.S. Census Bureau, 2005).

What do these statistics and trends mean for the health of populations and the ecosystem? When a population exceeds the ability of its ecosystem to either support it or acquire the support needed, or when it exceeds its ability to migrate to other ecosystems in a manner that preserves its standard of living, the population is said to be experiencing **demographic entrapment**. Such a population faces the four tragedies of

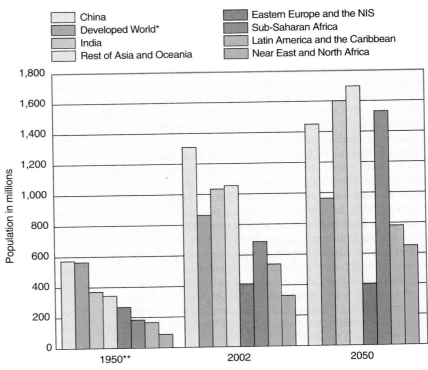

Legend:
- China
- Developed World*
- India
- Rest of Asia and Oceania
- Eastern Europe and the NIS
- Sub-Saharan Africa
- Latin America and the Caribbean
- Near East and North Africa

FIGURE 9.2   Regional Distribution of Global Population: 1950, 2002, and 2050. Population rankings of major world regions continue to shift in favor of developing regions. From U.S. Census Bureau. *International Population Reports WP/02. Global population profile: 2002*. Washington, DC: U.S. Government Printing Office.

* "Developed World" refers to North America (excluding Latin America and the Caribbean), Western Europe, Japan, Australia, and New Zealand. Rest of Asia and Oceania refers to Asia excluding Japan, China, and India plus Oceania excluding Australia and New Zealand. NIS indicates the New Independent States of the former Soviet Union.
** Current boundaries.

entrapment. Depending on cultural, political, and ecologic factors, it can starve, die from disease, slaughter itself or others, or be supported indefinitely by aid from others.

Government's Role

The government has a responsibility to prevent a population from exceeding the limits of the nation's resources and boundaries. The possible methods of preventing overpopulation, or solutions to it, are controversial, depending on one's culture, religious beliefs, and personal values and convictions. Ideally, the political system governing a country has a responsibility to provide a well-formed infrastructure of health and safety services for its population; economic development that provides employment, housing, and services; and political strength to provide stability to the nation. Many countries with unstable political systems are unable to deal effectively with overpopulation issues.

Where countries experience a decline in population, as is currently occurring in the European Union (EU), efforts have been undertaken to implement pronatalist policies. A growing aging population and a shrinking workforce are seen as threatening EU goals of full employment, economic growth, and social cohesion. Immigration may slow but not mitigate the problem and is not seen as a feasible long-term solution. Faced with one of the lowest birth rates in Europe, France instituted generous child-care subsidies and rewards for families having at least three children (Research Brief,

2005). Population stability clearly has an impact on developing and developed societies alike.

Nurse's Role

Public health professionals, including community health nurses, have a responsibility in the area of overpopulation, both globally and locally. Productive interventions include the following: (a) teaching families that birth spacing improves child and maternal survival and that a planned family is the best environment for a child's development; (b) preventing high-risk pregnancies, such as those among teens and adult women who are infected with the human immunodeficiency virus (HIV) or have the acquired immunodeficiency syndrome (AIDS); (c) preventing the growing epidemic of HIV/AIDS; (d) providing family planning education to prevent worldwide deaths from unsafe abortions; and (e) providing prenatal care—because healthy mothers equal healthy children. These are key areas in which public health efforts can reap major rewards for families.

Air Pollution

For many centuries, people have known that air quality affects human health. In Europe and America in the 1800s and early to middle 1900s, documented episodes of concentrated air pollution due to thermal atmospheric inversion caused many reported deaths. **Pollution** refers to the act of contaminating or defiling the environment to the extent that it negatively affects people's health. Air pollution is now recognized as one of the most hazardous sources of chemical contamination. It is especially prevalent in highly industrialized and urbanized areas where concentrations of motor vehicles and industry produce large volumes of gaseous pollutants.

Air pollution is a global problem. Recognizing the threat, the WHO published the first global standards for air quality in 2005 (WHO, 2006). Outdoor air pollution contributes to cardiovascular and respiratory diseases and is believed responsible for nearly 1 million lung cancer deaths yearly. With respect to children, infant mortality in the first year of life, bronchitis, asthma, and reduced lung development are additional health threats (Licari, Nemer, & Tamburlini, 2005). In Europe, outdoor air pollution and specifically particulate matter, is believed to cause 13,000 deaths per year among children younger than 4 years of age (WHO, 2006). U.S. children as well suffer disproportionately from the effects of both indoor and outdoor air pollution. One result of air pollution, asthma, accounts for 14 million lost school days each year and is the third leading cause of hospitalizations for children under 15 years; sadly, the number of U.S. children dying from asthma nearly tripled from 93 deaths in 1979 to 266 in 1996 (CDC, 2007a).

In the U.S., guidelines developed by the EPA serve to both regulate and monitor pollutants (EPA, 2006a). From 1980 to 2005, overall emissions of the six major pollutants measured by the federal government (carbon monoxide, nitrogen dioxide, ozone, particulate matter, sulfur dioxide, and lead) decreased substantially. However, the EPA also reported that in 2005 approximately 122 million people in the United States lived in counties where the air pollution levels exceeded the National Ambient Air Quality Standards (NAAQS) (EPA, 2006a). Airborne pollutants have adverse effects on many areas of human life; the costs to property, productivity, quality of life, and especially human health are enormous. The list of diseases and symptoms of ill health associated with specific air pollutants is lengthy, ranging from minor nose and throat irritations, respiratory infections, and bronchial asthma to emphysema, cardiovascular disease, lung cancer, and genetic mutations (Fig. 9.3).

As with other toxic chemicals, it is often difficult to establish a cause-and-effect relationship between air pollution and illness. A relatively short, high level of exposure is normally easier to identify. A number of poignant examples have occurred. One acute episode in Donora, Pennsylvania in 1948 caused 20 deaths, 400 hospitalizations, and nearly half of the town's 14,000 residents were sickened. Industrial contaminants

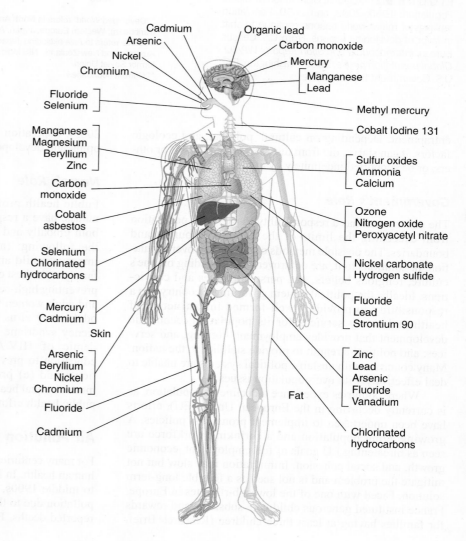

FIGURE 9.3 Body system targets of major air pollutants.

from iron and steel mills, coal-fired home stoves, and factory burning of coal combined with fog to create a deadly mix (Friis, 2007). Most affected by this disaster were residents over 55 years of age; those with existing heart or lung disease were most at risk for adverse outcomes (Friis). Another event occurred in London in 1952, when an atmospheric inversion trapped coal-burning smoke and fog over the city for almost a week. Between 4,000 and 8,000 people, mostly the elderly and those who were vulnerable because of respiratory and cardiac diseases, died as a result (Yassi et al., 2001). Although these disasters and others like them are dramatic and frightening, the effects of long-term exposure to low levels of pollution, such as environmental tobacco smoke exposure in the home (second-hand smoke), are perhaps even more threatening. Indoor air pollution is definitely more difficult to record, measure, understand, define, correlate, and control. It may be impossible to ever document the total effects.

Certain geographic areas are more susceptible to the ill effects of air pollution because of weather conditions or physical terrain. The episode in London occurred when a lack of wind combined with low temperatures to create a temperature inversion—a phenomenon in which air that normally rises is trapped under a layer of cold air, allowing air contaminants to build up to intolerable levels. Los Angeles, another city troubled by air pollution, is surrounded by mountains that prevent winds from clearing away smoke and fumes. A further condition occurs in urban areas: buildings create a "heat island effect," in which warm air traps pollution in the atmosphere around the city. In examining the effects of air pollution, it is necessary to take into account the climate conditions and topography of an area.

TABLE 9.1 The Air Quality Index (AQI)		
AQI Values	Levels of Health Concern	Colors
When the AQI is in this range. . .	. . .air quality conditions are. . .	. . .as symbolized by this color.
0–50	Good	Green
51–100	Moderate	Yellow
101–150	Unhealthy for Sensitive Groups	Orange
151–200	Unhealthy	Red
201–300	Very Unhealthy	Purple
301–500	Hazardous	Maroon

AIRNow. *Air Quality Index (AQI)—A Guide to Air Quality and Your Health.* http://www.airnow.gov/index.cfm?action=static.aqi

The EPA has developed a tool to provide the public with timely and easy-to-understand information on local air quality and whether air pollution levels pose a health concern. The Air Quality Index (AQI) lets the public know how clean the air is and whether they should be concerned for their health. The AQI is focused on health effects that can happen within a few hours or days after breathing polluted air (Table 9.1). Depending on the topography and general air flow patterns of the area, some communities use the index to inform the public as to

EVIDENCE-BASED PRACTICE

Helping Reach the HP 2010 Goal of Reduced Environmental Tobacco Exposure for Young Children—But How?

Environmental tobacco exposure (ETS), passive smoking, second-hand smoke—by any name, it is extremely harmful to young children. Their small size and lung capacity, coupled with rapid breathing rates as compared to adults, add to the risk of health problems, both short- and long-term. The problem is well known to public health nurses, but the question remains: How do you change adult behaviors so that fewer children are exposed? More and more public health nurses are looking to public policy change and community health education programs to address health problems such as this. A systematic review of literature regarding population-level options to support smoke-free homes found a correlation between comprehensive tobacco control programs and reduced prevalence of smoking in homes in Britain, the United States, Australia, and New Zealand (Thomson, Wilson, & Howden-Chapman, 2006). Most notably, efforts at reducing workplace smoking seemed to have a positive association with smoke-free homes. Chan and Lam (2006) implemented a simple health education program to reduce ETS in homes with sick children. Mothers were the target of this intervention, with reported

achievement of short-term motivation to reduce smoking exposure produced by fathers as well. Which approach, health education or policy change, do you think shows the most promise and why? Are there other sources of information to help guide you, such as systematic reviews? If you had 1 minute to present a case for a program to reduce ETS in homes to a politician, what would you say? What if you had that same short amount of time with a young mother who smokes? What would your 1-minute message be? How would you address privacy issues and right to self-determination?

References

Chan, S., Lam, T. H. (2006). Protecting sick children from exposure to passive smoking through mother's actions: A randomized controlled trial of a nursing intervention. *Journal of Advanced Nursing, 54,* 440–449.

Thomson, G., Wilson, N., & Howden-Chapman, P. (2006). Population level policy options for increasing the prevalence of smoke-free homes. *Journal of Epidemiology and Community Health, 60,* 298–304.

when use of wood-burning fireplaces or burning of trash piles or leaves is ill-advised or illegal. In the San Francisco area, residents may ride free on public transportation on those days when the air quality is poor. This program is designed for both short- and long-term behavioral change to reduce air pollution (Bay Area Air Quality Management District, 2007).

Dusts, Gases, and Naturally Occurring Elements

Dusts can contain numerous types of chemical irritants and poisons. Many hazardous dusts are associated with the workplace; for example, coal miners have developed black lung disease from inhaling coal dust, and a respiratory disease called silicosis is caused by exposure to silica dust (common in mining, sandblasting, and tunnel work). Dusts are also associated with farming and grain elevator work, as well as highway construction. Asbestos fibers, which are found in insulation and fireproofing materials, textiles, and many other products, have been associated with lung cancer. Although people who smoke are at 30 times greater risk of developing lung cancer than those who do not smoke, environmental tobacco smoke (ETS) is estimated to cause approximately 3,000 lung cancer deaths in nonsmokers each year, and 150,000 to 300,000 infants and children younger than 18 months of age experience lower respiratory tract infections annually because of exposure to second-hand smoke. In addition, asthma and other respiratory conditions are triggered or worsened by tobacco smoke (USDHHS, 2000).

Although much air pollution results from some type of human activity, naturally occurring elements, such as pollen from plants and flowers, ash from volcanic eruptions, and airborne microorganisms, can also have ill effects on health. A long list of gaseous pollutants, including sulfur oxides and nitrogen oxides produced by industrial emissions, pose additional problems for community health. Such gases cause respiratory disease, asphyxiation, and other problems in humans, and they can harm plant and animal life as well. Other gases, including chlorine, ozone, sulfur dioxide, and carbon monoxide, are all harmful to individual health, as well as to the broader environment and the ecosystem.

Radon is another gas that has been a topic of concern in recent years. This colorless, odorless, radioactive gas is formed by the breakdown of uranium in rock, groundwater, and soil in some geographic areas (Yassi et al., 2001). Radon is believed to be one of the leading causes of lung cancer, accounting for up to 20% of all lung cancers (Friis, 2007). Among nonsmokers, radon is the leading cause of lung cancer (EPA, 2007f), whereas lung cancer risk is increased 10-fold in smokers who are also exposed to radon in the home (EPA, 2007b). The link between radon exposure and lung cancer first came to light following studies of miners exposed to high levels of radon gas (Friis, 2007). Radon is a risk to all of us since it can seep into houses and public buildings through cracks in basement walls or through sewer openings, exposing people who inhabit, attend school, or work in the affected buildings. Furnaces and exhaust fans can help pull radon into a house, although the highest levels tend to be found in basements, where the gas enters. Home testing for radon was recommended by the EPA and the U.S. Public Health Service starting in 1988. Despite the health risks of radon exposure, a study to examine awareness of radon and its health consequences in low-income rural residents found very troubling results. In an area at high risk for radon exposure, only 21% accurately assessed their own risk, over 52% were unsure about the causal nature of health problems from radon, and 39% disagreed that the long-term health of their children could be improved with reduced radon exposure (Hill, Butterfield, & Larsson, 2006).

Healthy People 2010 (USDHHS, 2000) has two objectives focused on radon concerns. One goal is to increase the proportion of persons who live in homes tested for radon concentrations from 17% to 20%, and the other is to increase the number of new homes constructed to be radon-resistant from 1.4 million (in 1997) to 2.1 million by 2010. According to the EPA (2007h), radon-resistant construction techniques include installation of a gas-permeable layer beneath the slab or flooring system, plastic sheeting on top of the gas-permeable layer and under the slab, sealing and caulking of all openings in the concrete foundation, installation of a vent pipe from the gas-permeable layer to the outside of the house, and possibly the installation of a venting fan. Since 2001, 6% of new homes nationwide have been constructed with radon-reducing features. In areas with high radon risk (Zone 1), approximately 12% of new homes built incorporate the needed features (EPA, 2007h). Clearly, increased public awareness and action is needed (Fig. 9.4).

Acid Precipitation (Acid Rain)

The emission of hazardous chemicals into the Earth's atmosphere has a serious effect on the environment. Air pollutants such as sulfur dioxide from power plant emissions or nitrogen oxides from motor vehicle exhaust combine with rainwater, snow, and other forms of precipitation to produce sulfuric and nitric acid, commonly called "acid rain" (EPA, 2007a; Friis, 2007). The problem has been most severe and most heavily documented in Canada (from emissions arising in the U.S. Midwest) and Scandinavia (from emissions arising in Germany and Britain). Similar situations occur in Russia and Eastern Europe and probably in China, India, and Central Asia. Acid rain can extensively alter the biology of small bodies of water (Yassi et al., 2001). Although acid rain does not seem to pose any direct danger to humans, it kills small forms of life and endangers forest and freshwater ecologies.

Ozone Depletion and Global Warming

Two new and very threatening environmental hazards, stratospheric ozone layer depletion and global warming, are closely related. **Global warming** is the trapping of heat radiation from the Earth's surface that increases the overall temperature of the world, causing a "greenhouse effect." This warming is caused by carbon dioxide and other gases that enter the atmosphere through a depleted ozone layer and become trapped (Friis, 2007; Yassi et al., 2001). The direct health effects of ozone depletion include increased risks for skin cancer and cataracts. Greater indirect effects could result from global warming through damage to the food chain, an increase in the global population exposed to vector-borne diseases, raised ocean levels, and a variety of effects on crop production (Friis, 2007). Of additional concern, in 1995, at least 25 million people (sometimes called *environmental refugees*) could no longer support their families in their

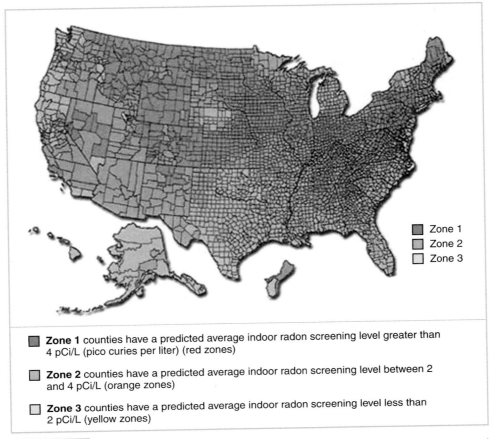

Zone 1

Zone 2

Zone 3

Zone 1 counties have a predicted average indoor radon screening level greater than 4 pCi/L (pico curies per liter) (red zones)

Zone 2 counties have a predicted average indoor radon screening level between 2 and 4 pCi/L (orange zones)

Zone 3 counties have a predicted average indoor radon screening level less than 2 pCi/L (yellow zones)

FIGURE 9.4 Environmental Protection Agency map of radon zones. From U.S. Environmental Protection Agency, http://www.epa.gov/radon/zonemap.html.

homelands because of drought, soil erosion, desertification, deforestation, and other environmental problems. By 2010, this number could well double, further stressing existing economic and environmental resources (Myers, 2005).

In the past, changes in the Earth's climate resulted from natural causes and enabled the evolution of species over hundreds of thousands of years. The accumulation of stratospheric ozone shields the Earth from damaging ultraviolet light, filtering and reducing the extent of radiation that reaches the Earth. Today, human activities are affecting our climate in serious and immediate ways. The ozone layer is being destroyed as a result of chemical interactions among air pollutants, primarily chlorofluorocarbons (CFCs). Most of these ozone-destroying chemicals and greenhouse gases are produced in the wealthier countries. Efforts to curb use of ozone-depleting gases in the U.S. and internationally is now having a measureable impact. Although the ozone is expected to continue to degrade over the next few years, gradual recovery is expected within 50 years (EPA, 2008); assuming continued worldwide efforts to phase out these chemicals are maintained.

Government's Role

Government regulation of air pollution has been relatively slow in developing. In 1963, the U.S. federal government passed the first series of Clean Air Acts. These set standards for air quality and industrial emissions and delegated funds to assist in pollution control programs. Although progress has been made, further public health efforts are needed to help identify pollution sources and related health hazards (see Display 9.2).

Even if the air is cleaner than it was 40 years ago, work remains to be done. In 2005, the EPA issued the Clean Air Interstate Rule (CAIR), designed to reduce power plant emissions by the largest amount in more than a decade. Currently, 28 states in the East, Southeast, and Midwest are covered by the rule. The health benefits are expected to exceed 25 times the cost of compliance, with results published in 2015 (EPA, 2005). This rule was enacted in conjunction with the Clean Air Mercury Rule, the first ever federally mandated requirements for reduced mercury emissions from coal-fired electric utilities. The automobile is a continued target of efforts to reduce pollutant production, and new steps will include reducing the sulfur content of gasoline, tightening emission standards, and removing loopholes that allow certain groups of vehicles to defy emission standards.

The EPA has identified ways in which people can help reduce greenhouse gases at home, work, school, and on the road. These are useful suggestions that the community health nurse can use and pass along to clients. Seven easy suggestions for the home include (EPA, 2007d):

1. Change five lights (e.g., replace five frequently used fixtures or bulbs with *Energy Star* options).

2. Look for *Energy Star* qualified products (e.g., lighting, home electronics, heating and cooling equipment, and appliances).
3. Heat and cool smartly (e.g., change filters regularly, install adequate insulation, have equipment serviced regularly).
4. Use green power (e.g., use electricity from renewable sources).
5. Reduce, reuse, and recycle (e.g., reduce waste generation and water consumption, participate in community recycling programs).
6. Be green in your yard (e.g., compost food and yard waste).
7. Calculate your household's *carbon footprint* (use EPA Personal Greenhouse Gas Emissions Calculator available at: http://www.epa.gov/climatechange/wycd/calculator/ind_calculator.html).

Nurse's Role

Community health nurses can influence air quality through detection, community education, and lobbying for appropriate legislation. People are exposed to numerous impurities in the air in their homes and workplaces. Nurses can promote health by helping to detect indoor pollutants and informing people of existing or potential dangers. Many household products and building materials emit vapors that can cause problems. Cigarette smoke and cigar smoke are common indoor pollutants that can have ill effects on non-smokers as well as smokers. Infants and other vulnerable persons are at risk from such exposure (Friis, 2007; Wigle, 2003). Carbon monoxide poisoning may result from stove and furnace emissions or from car exhaust accumulating in a garage. Radon gas trapped in basements or tightly insulated homes is also a major concern. Nurses can assist with the prevention or elimination of these health hazards by ensuring that the indoor environment is well ventilated (oxygenated) and heating equipment properly maintained, and by looking for possible sources of pollution. Installation and maintenance of residential carbon monoxide detectors outside the sleeping area in every home should also be encouraged (U.S. Consumer Product Safety Commission, n.d.).

Water Pollution

Water is such an essential element to human survival that the available quantity and quality of water within a community has become a prime environmental health issue. Water has many uses other than consumption by humans. It serves as a means of transportation. It cleans and cools the body or other objects. It is the basis for many forms of recreation and sports, such as swimming and boating, and it provides a vehicle for disposing of human and industrial wastes and controlling fires. Apart from serving human needs, water also acts as a medium for sustaining other living organisms, as a home to plant and animal life, and as a means of carrying and distributing necessary nutrients in the environment. Although nursing's environmental health role concerns the safe consumption of water by humans, it is important, taking an ecologic perspective, to keep in mind water's other uses and users.

Drinking water comes from two main sources: surface water (such as lakes and streams) and underground sources (called *groundwater*), which collects in areas known as *aquifers* and comes to the surface through wells and springs. In general, underground sources are thought to be less subject to contamination than surface sources, which are open to runoff from agricultural pesticides or industrial wastes. However, groundwater too may be contaminated if seepage occurs. It is important to recognize that public water supplies may originate from either surface or underground sources. Well water may refer to an individual residential well or to a large municipal facility. In the Middle Ages, disease epidemics spread as people drank water contaminated by human waste; this is still a problem today in developing countries and, at times, in other countries, if flooding occurs. Residential well water may contain fecal contaminants from improper septic tank drainage. Toxic agents that may affect groundwater include buried hazardous wastes, nitrate contamination of wells in rural areas, and arsenic in drinking water, which is linked to bladder, kidney, and liver cancers (Friis, 2007).

In most industrialized nations, lack of sufficient water for drinking has not been a serious issue. Areas with limited water supplies have devised facilities to store water during high-flow periods, so that it is available to satisfy the year-round needs of a given community. Adequate water supply to meet agricultural demands still has not been achieved, however.

The major concern with regard to water is purity. Every time you turn on the faucet in your home, workplace, or in the community, the expectation is that the water is clean, clear, and free of contamination. In the United States, we take it for granted that the water we drink is safe; this is not always the case. More concerning is that, in many parts of the world, access to safe sources does not exist. As much as 20% of the world's population may not have access to safe sources of drinking water (Friis, 2007). Water can be contaminated and made unsafe for drinking in many different ways. Three are discussed here.

1. Water may be infected with bacteria or parasites that cause disease. *Giardia lamblia* is a parasite that enters the water supply through contamination from human or wild animal feces. It can cause giardiasis, a gastrointestinal disease that results in diarrhea and malabsorption of nutrients. For example, beavers in the northern Cascade Mountains often contaminate water. Humans using the area for recreation must treat the water by boiling before drinking it. Water may also be contaminated with bacteria such as *Vibrio cholerae,* resulting in cholera, or with viruses leading to hepatitis A (Heymann, 2004).
2. Toxic substances, such as pesticides, are introduced by humans into water systems and constitute another form of water pollution. These substances may contaminate streams, lakes, and wells. Industrial pollutants may also enter drinking water through oil spills, careless dumping, or buried hazardous wastes that seep into underground water sources. Such wastes not only harm the quality of the water but also have been implicated in diseases such as leukemia. They can contaminate local fish and shellfish, making them unfit for consumption. One

such example is mercury, which, through bioaccumulation has reached levels in some seafood (shark, swordfish, king mackerel, and tilefish) that make them unsafe for consumption, especially by pregnant women, nursing mothers, and young children (U.S. Food and Drug Administration [FDA], 2004; Friis, 2007).

3. Pollutants may upset the ecosystem, affecting natural organisms that help purify water systems. Power plants or other industries dissipate excess heat into lakes and streams and cause water temperatures to rise. This *thermal pollution* kills off beneficial organisms in the water.

In response to the various potential water pollutants, most cities and local communities with public or semipublic water systems in operation have set up water testing and treatment purification centers to ensure safe drinking water. Unfortunately, testing for bacteria and toxins often does not occur until after illness has been reported. Another major problem arises in rural areas, where most water supplies are private and therefore not subject to systematic testing and treatment. Testing of water for coliforms as indicator organisms has proven useful (EPA, 2006c). Water frequently is treated with chlorine to disinfect it, but this has led to a small but potential risk of chloroform exposure, a by-product which is linked to small for gestational age (SGA) and preterm delivery (Wright, Schwartz, & Dockery, 2004).

Recreational uses of water, such as public swimming, have health implications. Lakes, oceans, rivers, and even hot tubs often carry infectious agents and result in a number of health problems including swimmers' itch; diarrheal diseases, such as cryptosporidiosis caused by a parasite; and the bacterial infection leptospirosis, which presents with fever and malaise and may progress to jaundice or meningitis (Heymann, 2004). Many disease outbreaks have been caused by polluted water systems serving campgrounds, parks, and other public areas. Between 2003 and 2004, the most commonly reported gastroenteritis outbreak associated with recreational water exposure was caused by cryptosporidium (Dziuban et al., 2006).

The marine ecosystem can be altered by any changes that affect the oceans, such as water temperatures at the surface, nutrient levels, winds, currents, and precipitation patterns. This can lead to possible increases in diseases transmitted from fish and shellfish, toxic "red tides" (Backer et al., 2005; Heymann, 2004), and a dormant form of cholera that develops when pH, temperature, salinity, and nutrient levels are insufficient (Hoskins, 2001). In addition, coming in contact with marine waters that are contaminated with domestic sewage can cause nonenteric illnesses among swimmers, including febrile respiratory illness from fecal streptococci and ear ailments from fecal coliform exposure.

Government's Role

Most of the responsibility for maintaining water quality rests with state and local governments. The federal government took a needed step in 1974 by passing the Safe Drinking Water Act, which gave the EPA authority to establish water standards and to ensure that these standards were upheld. The federal government also provided funds to assist state and local governments in this effort. In 2000, the EPA revised regulations on public notification to expedite sharing of vital information with the public. In fiscal year 1998 alone, 25% of the public water systems had violations requiring public notification. Of these 124,000 violations, the majority were for monitoring and testing violations, with 1.5% pertaining to real short-term health threats. In cases of acute health risks, water systems had 24 hours to notify affected populations (EPA, 2002). These long-awaited rules set the minimum requirements for healthy drinking water and helped to ensure the safety of drinking water supplies. However, policies related to groundwater quality protection need continued monitoring. Saltwater intrusion caused by excessive withdrawal of water from the aquifer can also threaten drinking water supplies in coastal areas (Friis, 2007). As in many communities across the country, almost half of all residential drinking water consumption in South Florida is used for landscape irrigation. With concern for continued viability of the water supply, many communities have implemented water use restrictions (South Florida Water Management District, 2007). With conservation, it is hoped that the progress of saltwater intrusion will be mitigated or reversed.

Globally, because of the enormous health problems in developing nations caused by unclean water, the WHO declared the 1980s as the International Clean Water Decade and established a goal to have safe drinking water for all by the year 1990. This goal was not met; only 50% of the world's population had a safe water supply in 1980, 55% in 1985, and 66% in 1990 (WHO, 2000). By 2002, the percentage had increased to 83%, yet slow progress in areas such as Sub-Saharan Africa tempered the achievement. In 2005, a new global initiative, the *International Decade for Action: Water for Life 2005–2015* was launched with the goal of increasing awareness of the basic need for safe drinking water and finding solutions to achieve global access (WHO, 2005). Efforts to address water purity globally continue to assume high priority, however the focus is shifting from drinking water quality alone toward overall improvement of the environment.

Nurse's Role

What role can community health nurses play in the effort to keep water safe? As nurses work in a community, they can help by examining household or city drinking water. Is there a strange odor or discoloration? Are particles or sediment visible in the water? Being aware of drinking water quality and possible contaminants in a given locality alerts the nurse to consider a possible causal relationship if a problem exists. Asking clients to observe and report changes in water quality further assists the nurse in the monitoring process. If such changes occur, the proper authorities, such as health department officials, should be notified and water samples tested. Community health nurses can also be alert to increased incidence of illnesses that might be water related. For example, if several children exhibit similar symptoms, the nurse might inquire as to whether all have been swimming in the same pool or drinking from the same water fountain. Although water quality monitoring is ultimately the responsibility of environmental health authorities, it is incumbent on the nurse, as a collaborating member of the health team, to observe and report any information that would further the goal of safe and healthy water for communities.

Deforestation, Wetlands Destruction, and Desertification

Deforestation is the clearing of tropical and temperate forests for cropland, cattle grazing, or urbanization. Elimination of these natural habitats is dooming some species of insects and animals to **extinction**, the loss of a species from the Earth forever. **Wetlands** are natural inland bodies of shallow water, such as marshes, ponds, river bottoms, and flood plains, which filter contaminated surface waters and support wildlife reproduction and growth. They can be as small as a neighborhood seasonal stream bed or as large as the Everglades in Florida. At one time, the Everglades covered the lower 20% of the state but, in 1948, the U.S. Army Corps of Engineers constructed an elaborate system of roads and water control structures that converted thousands of acres and ultimately led to urbanization and loss of much of the original habitat (National Park Service, 2000). Today, only 50% of the original wetlands still exist in South Florida. The destruction of this major U.S. wetland has caused numerous species of wildlife to disappear from the area or become extinct. There is discussion to reclaim some of the land and convert it back to much-needed wetlands. **Desertification** refers to the conversion of fertile land into desert, which is unable to support crop growth or wildlife.

Any natural or manmade process that changes life-supporting regions into land for other use or into barren wastelands upsets the ecosystem of the area. The destruction of forests and the upturning of Earth for urban sprawl uncovers organisms hidden for eons, to which humans and animals are then exposed. In addition, gases that were once absorbed by lost trees remain in the atmosphere and contribute to ozone depletion, which increases global warming. Deforestation, in turn, contributes to desertification, because forests provide protection for the surrounding topsoil by way of their roots, fallen leaves, and undergrowth. When this protection is lost, landslides and other geographic changes occur. Global temperature increases cause riverbeds to dry up and create desert areas that are unable to support the people who once inhabited them. Drought, famine, and starvation often follow in such areas. The loss of forests and wetlands, along with increasing desertification, affects millions of people each year, with a potential for catastrophic environmental damage in the future.

Government's Role

Our government (both state and federal) has the power to make decisions that save the wetlands and forests in the United States. The decision to save these lands is made when constituents express their concern loudly enough for their congressperson or senator to hear and respond positively. Often, developers of housing and industrial facilities are more influential, and their interests prevail. If the importance of the wetlands and forests is not recognized where decisions are made, then they will be lost.

Nurse's Role

Community health nurses can make a difference in this area. Perhaps no other person knows a community more intimately than the community health nurse. This role gives a valid voice of concern at the local level. By using leadership and collaborative skills, the nurse can initiate grassroots efforts to save wetlands and forests in the community. Chapters 12 and 13 provide information for bringing about change, beginning at the local level.

Energy Depletion

Most of the energy sources we use today are not renewable. Wood has been used for thousands of years and was our first fuel. It is still a primary source of home heating for most of the world's population (with resultant deforestation and air pollution). Natural gas for heat and fuel can be a highly efficient energy source, but pipelines must be built for hundreds or thousands of miles in some cases—a luxury that smaller and poorer countries cannot afford. Coal takes thousands of years to create, and although substantial reserves remain, not all coal extraction is environmentally or economically feasible (Energy Information Administration, 2007). Some countries do not have coal as a natural resource and have similar problems with natural gas.

Nuclear energy has been used for at least 50 years. This source of energy has been controversial since its first use, yet it has proved to be an effective power product. Nevertheless, there have been some near-disasters and real disasters caused by human error. In 1979, a nuclear power plant on Three Mile Island near Harrisburg, Pennsylvania, had a near-disaster in one of its cooling towers, with a partial meltdown of the core. Fortunately, the nuclear core was never exposed. This scare caused many people in the United States to lobby against nuclear power plants in their communities, and these protests have effectively stopped new construction (Friis, 2007). The largest radiation disaster occurred in April, 1986, at the Chernobyl nuclear power plant in Ukraine. Five million people in Ukraine, Belarus, and the Russian Federation were exposed to ionizing radiation. Twenty-eight of the 444 people at the plant who were directly exposed died within 3 months, and 300 were hospitalized. Psychological effects among people living in the surrounding areas resulted from the lack of information immediately after the accident, the stress and trauma of compulsory relocation, a break in social ties, and fear that radiation exposure could cause health damage in the future (Yassi et al., 2001). An increase in the incidence of childhood thyroid cancer has been noted, particularly in Belarus (Friis). The final impact in terms of increased cancer rates resulting from the breach may never be known. The area remains unsafe to enter today.

The building of nuclear power plants is only one community concern; the disposal of the nuclear waste products also raises environmental, safety, and ethical issues. The permanent disposal of all high-level radioactive waste falls under the regulations of the Nuclear Waste Policy Act of 1982. The act provides that all high-level waste will be disposed of underground and in a deep geologic repository, and that the Yucca Mountain, Nevada site is the current preferred site. The three federal agencies involved in the disposal are the Department of Energy, which develops permanent disposal capacity for spent fuel; the EPA, which develops environmental standards to evaluate the geologic repository; and the Nuclear Regulatory Commission, which develops regulations to implement the EPA safety standards and licensing of the repository (U.S. Nuclear Regulatory

Commission [NRC], 2007). The Yucca Mountain site was originally slated for licensing review in 2004, but legal challenges and financial complications have delayed that process (Yucca Mountain Information Office, 2007). With disposal issues and safety concerns at the forefront, the expansion of nuclear energy in the United States remains controversial.

Government's Role

Other renewable sources of energy need to be discovered, rediscovered, or tapped. Newer and more "environmentally friendly" energy sources are used experimentally in limited areas. They include landfill gas recovery, solar power, and wind power. These sources can make a difference:

- The National Wind Coordinating Collaborative (2007), established by utility companies, consumers groups, state and federal regulators, and the U.S. Department of Energy, serves as a forum for discussions about the use and expansion of wind power. The stated goal of the organization is "self-sustaining commercial markets for wind power that is environmentally, economically, and politically sustainable." Environmental impact issues, such as wildlife mortality and land use considerations are explored.
- The U.S. Department of Energy (DOE) is working closely with industry and universities to develop photovoltaic (PV) systems for harnessing the rays of the sun to generate power. As far back as the 1996 Olympics in Atlanta, the swimming competitions took place under lights powered by PV. Today, many emergency telephones along the nation's highways are powered by PV systems, and efforts are underway to expand this energy source for utility power production (DOE, 2006).
- The DOE is working to address the need for growing and harvesting crops that can be turned into biomass fuels and to reclaim waste products from agricultural crops and forestlands for generating electricity. The agency currently supports five regional organizations to advance the use of biomass. Since 2002, 60 awards for biomass research and development have been supported by the federal government. In 2007, $18 million was earmarked for these efforts (DOE, 2007a).
- The DOE also is involved in geothermal technology. One program *GeoPowering the West* is working with the western states, including Alaska and Hawaii, to dramatically increase the use of geothermal heat sources, including heat pump systems. The oldest and largest geothermal power complex in the United States is The Geysers. Located 100 miles north of San Francisco, it is a source of 725 megawatts of power, with plans to increase this amount by 80 megawatts by 2012 (DOE, 2007b).

It will take both a global effort to increase awareness and accompanying technology to use these energy sources in enough areas to make an environmental difference.

Nurse's Role

A community health nurse may not have a direct role in the creation of new energy sources or the use of a particular source. However, the nurse can educate people about energy conservation, discuss alternative energy sources presently available in the community, and encourage people to become interested in and knowledgeable about the importance of the potential for energy depletion in the future.

Conservative use of existing energy sources can be a part of the community health nurse's teaching with families in the community. In addition to saving precious energy resources, measures taken to cut energy use can save the family money on monthly utility bills. Conservation methods include ensuring that a home or apartment is well insulated and free from drafts; broken windows and improperly fitted windows or doors are repaired; caulking and weather stripping is used where needed; and heating and cooling of the home are modified by setting the thermostat at 68 degrees in the winter and no lower than 78 degrees in the summer. Families should be encouraged to wear warmer clothing or layers of clothing indoors in the winter and to dress in cool cotton garments in the summer. In the summer, encourage families to use indoor free-standing or ceiling fans, and to close blinds and curtains on the sunny sides of the house to help to keep it cooler.

In many communities, the utility company provides home energy inspections free of charge to help families recognize areas in their home where they are losing energy. Often, these programs provide funding to make the needed changes, especially among low-income families.

Unhealthy or Contaminated Food

The food supply, and particularly the quality of that food, is affected by the environment, and numerous health hazards are associated with food. The community health nurse needs to ask how the environment influences the safety of food for human consumption. Three types of hazardous foods must be considered when examining food as a possible health problem: inherently harmful foods, contaminated foods, and foods with toxic additives.

Inherently Harmful Foods

Poisonous foods, such as certain types of mushrooms or inedible berries, do not pose a serious threat to most people. The general public can identify and avoid harmful plants and substances, so poisonings are rare. There are, however, numerous household plants and outdoor flowers, shrubs, and trees that are poisonous if consumed. A searchable database of poisonous plants is available through Cornell University at: http://www.ansci.cornell.edu/plants/alphalist.html. Children in particular are at risk because some of these plants bear berries or colorful flowers that can capture a child's interest, including the following examples (Texas A&M University, n.d.):

House Plants
- Hyacinth
- Dieffenbachia
- Elephant ear

Flower Garden
- Larkspur
- Lily-of-the-valley
- Iris

Ornamental Plants
◆ Wisteria
◆ Azalea
◆ Yew
◆ Rhododendron

Trees and Shrubs
◆ Oaks
◆ Elderberry
◆ Black locust

Plants in Wooded Areas
◆ Jack-in-the-pulpit
◆ Mistletoe

Plants in Fields
◆ Nightshade
◆ Buttercups
◆ Poison hemlock

Contaminated Foods

Contaminated foods pose a more serious health problem. The Centers for Disease Control and Prevention (CDC) estimates that 76 million people in the United States experience food-borne illnesses each year, accounting for 325,000 hospitalizations and more than 5,000 deaths—an average of almost 100 deaths per week (National Institute of Allergy and Infectious Diseases [NIAID], 2007). Food may contain harmful bacteria that cause outbreaks of disease, such as *Salmonella enterica, Campylobacter jejuni, Clostridium botulinum, Shigella sonnei*, or *Escherichia coli 0157:H7*. These are the most common or serious of the more than 250 different known causes of food-borne diseases (Heymann, 2004; NIAID, 2007). Of these, salmonellosis is the most common (Friis, 2007).

There are other causes of foodborne illnesses. Parasitic transmission usually takes the form of trichinosis, which is caused by ingestion of *Trichinella spiralis* in undercooked pork and is rarely seen in the United States (Heymann, 2004). Various types of worm infestations have created serious health problems, particularly in developing countries. Viral food transmission is rare. Different types of chemical food contamination result from improper food handling or processing (e.g., dirty machines used in food processing factories), from use of pesticides and herbicides by farmers, and from polluted water (e.g., mercury in fish).

International trade and travel, together with changes in demographics, consumer lifestyles, food production, and microbial adaptation, have led to the emergence of new food-borne diseases. Globalization of the food supply means that people are exposed, through foods purchased locally, to pathogens native to remote parts of the world. As a result of international travel, people who are exposed to food-borne hazards in a foreign country may bring disease into their own country when they return, possibly exposing others in a location thousands of miles from the original source of the infection (Friis, 2007).

Foods with Toxic Additives

A third health hazard from food comes from the intentional introduction of additives to food products. Because present-day consumers demand convenience foods and time-saving devices—and businesses want to produce food items with long shelf-lives, enhanced flavor, and lasting, vibrant colors—many foreign chemicals and synthetic products have been added to foods. Animals that are raised for food, such as chickens, pigs, and beef cattle, are often fed or injected with substances to speed their growth. As consumers shift toward healthier eating, they do not know and are only starting to question the effects these additives may have over time. For example, red dye no. 2 once was added to improve the color of certain food products but has since been identified as carcinogenic. Preservatives and chemical flavorings such as saccharin have also proved hazardous in large doses. It is still questionable what small doses may do with prolonged use. More recently, questions have been raised about potential long-range effects of NutraSweet (aspartame), a sugar substitute. Furthermore, such natural flavor enhancers as salt and processed sugars appear in excessive quantities in some canned and packaged foods and are linked to unhealthy dietary consequences, such as hypertension or obesity. In small doses, these additives may not be harmful, but when additives are consumed in combination and over prolonged periods, they may create serious health consequences.

The most recently available sugar substitute *Splenda* (Sucralose) was first introduced in 1999 following FDA approval (McNeil Nutritionals, 2007). It is now found in a wide variety of foods, including snacks and treats for school-aged children, and is actively marketed to families with children. Although the substitute was tested in more than 100 scientific studies and approved by major organizations such as the Joint Food and Agriculture Organization/World Health Organization Expert Committee on Food Additives (JECFA), the Health Protection Branch of Health and Welfare Canada, and Australia's National Food Authority (McNeil Nutritionals), there are those who question the long-term safety of the additive and its effectiveness in reducing obesity. With respect to young children, a nutritionally sound and low-sugar diet would be far preferable to the use of artificial sweeteners.

Food Irradiation

One promising tool for global food safety not yet mentioned is food irradiation. It is a process of imparting ionizing energy to food to kill microorganisms. Sometimes it is referred to as *cold pasteurization* (Friis, 2007). Just as with traditional heat pasteurization of milk, food irradiation can enhance the safety of foods such as meat, chicken, seafood, and spices, which cannot be pasteurized by heat without changing their nature to a cooked rather than a raw form. Irradiation is not a substitute for safe food handling and good manufacturing practices by processors, retailers, and consumers, but it is a method of promoting food safety that has been approved by some 50 countries worldwide. It has been applied commercially in the United States, Japan, and several European countries such as Belgium, France, and the Netherlands for many years—in some for longer than two decades.

Only certain ionizing energy sources can be used for food irradiation. Permitted gamma (γ) sources are the isotopes cobalt 60 and cesium 137 (Friis, 2007). More recently, electron beams (e-beams) have become available as a source of ionizing energy in the United States and other countries. All of the previously mentioned organisms that cause food-borne diseases can be eradicated with the use of food irradiation. Although

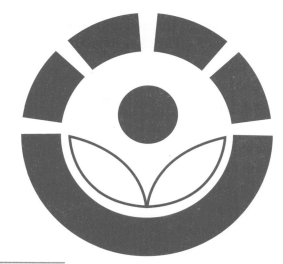

FIGURE 9.5 International symbol for irradiated food (Radura logo).

many questions have been raised about its safety and efficacy, food irradiation is an accepted practice globally (International Atomic Energy Agency [IAEA], 2005) and "after decades of research, development, public debate and consumer acceptance trials in many countries, irradiation has emerged as a safe and viable technology for ensuring the safety and quality of food and for combating food-borne diseases" (IAEA, n.d., p.2). The international symbol, the Radura logo, indicating that food has been irradiated can be seen in Figure 9.5.

Government's Role

It is the legal responsibility of food producers, processors, and manufacturers to guarantee the quality and safety of food products. However, conflicting motives, such as concern over loss of profit, often lead to careless or inadequate monitoring. Governmental regulatory agencies exist on the local, state, and federal levels to set standards and to control the quality of food sold to the public. Such public health authorities as the FDA, the U.S. Department of Agriculture, and the USDHHS are all necessary to help ensure the purity of commercial food products. Included in their jurisdiction is supervision of the food service industry. Licensing requirements, sanitation standards, and inspections serve as control measures.

Governmental agencies cannot cover all the bases, however. For example, inadequate inspection of the quality of commercial fish sold for food has led to numerous outbreaks of hepatitis A and other illnesses. With the wide variety of possible contaminants and potential dangers, consumers' best protection lies in supervising their own food quality (see Internet Resources at the end of this chapter).

Nurse's Role

Community health nurses can have a significant impact through health education. Most bacterial and viral food-borne diseases can be prevented if people know and practice proper cooking and storage of food as well as proper personal hygiene.

Nurses can teach the basics of keeping perishable products sufficiently refrigerated, discarding foods that may be old or spoiled, cooking foods thoroughly, and bringing water to a full boil when appropriate to be certain of eliminating microbes. A consumer education program that is sponsored by the Partnership for Food Safety Education is called Fight BAC! This is a public–private partnership of industry, government, and consumer groups created to educate the public about safe food handling to help reduce food-borne illness. Educational materials are available for use by teachers, health educators, and community health nurses when working with groups in the community (Partnership for Food Safety Education, 2006).

Nurses can emphasize washing and cleaning of produce and tools used in food processing, including the preparer's own hands. Finally, nurses can educate people to watch for signs of contamination. A dented can, for example, may signal the presence of living bacteria that are using the oxygen within the container and contaminating its contents. Nurses can raise public awareness regarding the conditions of supermarkets, restaurants, and other food handlers. They can also help promote community standards, enabling legislation, and policies for safer food supplies.

Waste Disposal

The United States generates more solid and hazardous waste per capita than any other industrialized nation. In 1990, each person in the United States produced, on average, 4.3 pounds per day of combustible or landfill-maintained waste. In 1995, this figure was 4.4 pounds per day, equivalent to 1,600 pounds of municipal solid waste each year. More frightening is the fact that U.S. industry produces the equivalent of more than 1 ton of *hazardous* waste per person each year. In addition, some 8.1 million tons of toxins were released into the air in 1993. The year 2010 target is 2.0 tons (USDHHS, 2000).

With the vast amounts of waste produced in the form of household garbage, human excreta, and agricultural and industrial byproducts, including hazardous chemical and radioactive substances, it is no wonder that waste management and disposal has become an important and pressing topic in recent decades. New technology has effectively addressed some of the problems, but there is still much need for improvement. Solid and hazardous wastes pose a wide range of public health concerns. Therefore, it is imperative that health officials, including community health nurses, become aware of the possible health hazards that these wastes present to individuals and to communities.

Disposal of Human Waste

One of the oldest environmental health hazards comes from improper disposal of human excreta. Although industrialized nations have successfully addressed the problem, it continues to be widespread in developing nations and in rural, poverty-stricken communities. Human wastes, particularly feces, provide a perfect environment in which bacteria and disease-causing parasites can live and reproduce.

Therefore, contaminated drinking water, food grown in contaminated soil, and, of course, direct contact with the contaminated water or soil can cause infections. For example, hookworm, a problem in the United States in the early part of the 20th century, usually enters the body through the skin of bare feet (Heymann, 2004; Rockefeller Archive Center, n.d.).

Disposal of Garbage

Dumping, burning, and burying are the most common solid-waste disposal methods. Dumping is problematic, because garbage dumps provide perfect conditions for the breeding of rats, flies, and other disease-carrying organisms and may potentially be a source of water contamination from runoff. Dumps are also eyesores that take up valuable land resources. Burning of waste reduces the volume of garbage, but it also produces noxious odors and pollutes the air. Sanitary landfills have generally replaced dumps as a more effective way to dispose of refuse by burying it. With proper handling, including covering and daily sealing (to prevent insect and rodent breeding), this method has proved satisfactory for solid waste.

Disposal of Hazardous Waste

Disposal of toxic chemical and radioactive wastes produced by industry is another grave concern. The threat is serious, because one cannot be certain of all of the effects of these wastes or whether present methods of disposal are foolproof. Furthermore, many of these wastes escape containment or accidentally leak into water systems and into the soil to contaminate drinking water and food.

In 1980, the federal government enacted the Comprehensive Environmental Response, Compensation, and Liability Act (CERCLA), commonly referred to as the Superfund. Under the act, uncontrolled or abandoned hazardous-waste sites are cleaned up. In addition, the act provides for accidents, spills, and other emergency releases (Friis, 2007). Another feature of the act is the identification and prioritization of the most hazardous substances by the Agency for Toxic Substances and Disease Registry (ATSDR), in cooperation with the EPA. The agencies prepare the National Priorities List (NPL), which is used to identify those sites eligible for Superfund action (Friis, 2007). The top 20 hazardous substances from the 2005 list can be reviewed in Table 9.2.

Primary methods of hazardous waste disposal include burial in double-lined cells in landfills, surface impoundments for special treatment and storage, waste-injected underground steel- and concrete-lined wells, solid waste piles, and land treatment facilities. Some hazardous wastes are incinerated before disposal. With the disposal of hazardous waste, it is always a concern that storage containers may not be leak proof, and interference with dump sites or storage facilities may expose the environment to these toxic substances. Examples of chemical contamination have been discovered in communities such as Elizabeth, New Jersey; Times Beach, Michigan; and Love Canal, New York, where residents developed cancer and other health problems because of exposures to toxic chemicals. There is also the continuing problem of securing disposal sites for the increasing volume of hazardous wastes. Communities seek

TABLE 9.2   Top 20 Hazardous Substances— 2005 CERCLA Priority List

1	Arsenic
2	Lead
3	Mercury
4	Vinyl chloride
5	Polychlorinated biphenyls
6	Benzene
7	Polycyclic aromatic hydrocarbons
8	Cadmium
9	Benzo(a)pyrene
10	Benzo(b)fluoromethane
11	Chloroform
12	DDT, p,p'-
13	Aroclor 1254
14	Aroclor 1260
15	Dibenzo(a,h)anthracene
16	Trichloroethylene
17	Dieldrin
18	Chromium, hexavalent
19	Phosphorus, white
20	DDE, p,p'-

Source: ATSDR. *2005 CERCLA Priority List of Hazardous Substances.* Retrieved July 16, 2007, from http://www.atsdr.cdc.gov/cercla/05list.html.

the advantages of new technology but do not wish to bury the resulting wastes in their backyards. In many instances, legislators and public officials have faced serious conflict in their efforts to locate acceptable toxic waste dump sites.

With burgeoning industry and new technology in the world today, society has developed more sophisticated means of energy production, more labor-saving devices, and more practical and innovative products. This massive new product development has created a problem for the environment—how to handle the vast amount of waste created from discarded goods, by-products of production, and the "throwaway mentality." For example, more than 3.5 million tons of disposable diapers, estimated to account for 1.4% of all municipal wastes, are dumped in landfills each year in the United States. Debate is ongoing as to whether reusable cloth diapers or one-time use diapers have a more negative environmental impact, but consensus is growing to support reusable diapers as the more environmentally friendly option (California Integrated Waste Management Board, 2007; National Geographic, 2006). With each child using between 5,000 and 8,000 diapers during the early years of life, the issue is of great importance. Additionally, the vast majority of disposable diapers are discarded directly into the trash instead of first flushing fecal material down the toilet.

Consequently, a large amount of raw, untreated sewage is ending up in landfills, with the potential for serious problems in the future. In the United States, modern landfills are designed to restrict leaching of contaminants directly into the groundwater, but this is not the case in all countries. Not only does the development of such products take an enormous toll on natural resources, but the quantity and nature of the resulting wastes also pose serious health hazards and environmental problems. Improper disposal of domestic products, such as toxic insect sprays, some household cleaners, partially used paint cans, used auto oil, and termite fumigation chemicals, causes health dangers (Calvert et al., 1998). The availability of toxic substances in the home is especially dangerous to young children. Estimates for 2001 are that nearly 40% of toxic agents most commonly ingested by children younger than 6 years of age included cosmetics, cleaning products, topical agents, pesticides, arts/crafts/office supplies, and hydrocarbons (Wilkerson, Northington, & Fisher, 2005).

Government's Role

The government's role is to establish standards for safe waste disposal and to monitor and enforce compliance. In most modernized urban areas, the public sewage system handles waste by treating raw sewage and disposing of it into a body of water. In most instances in the United States, state health departments oversee proper waste treatment and disposal. In rural areas, where people often have private septic systems, the supervision of proper waste handling is difficult and not as consistent. Health workers in rural settings should be alert to the potential dangers posed by inconsistent monitoring. Communities across the country are beginning to address the issue of household hazardous waste by developing both disposal and recycling programs. These programs must meet or exceed current EPA guidelines (EPA, 2006d).

More research is needed to determine the effects of various disposal methods and to improve disposal practices. It is imperative that people not only learn how to dispose of wastes safely—to protect humans, the environment, and future generations—but that they also look seriously at other options. More emphasis must be placed on transforming waste into usable products, increasing the amounts and kinds of recycling done, and reducing the amount of refuse produced in the first place.

Nurse's Role

Community health nurses can encourage the positive actions described by educating the public and lobbying for enabling legislation. Nurses can promote greater sensitivity among citizens to the problems of accumulating waste with its potential health hazards; encourage clients to buy products that can be recycled, and discourage use of aerosol spray containers, plastics, and other nonrecyclable items. Such information sharing occurs during home visits when conducting family and home assessments; during group educational opportunities that arise in apartment complexes or neighborhoods where several families are being served; with school children when the community health nurse is invited into the classroom by the teacher; or in conjunction with environmental health services when a community is blighted by waste management problems and the nurse speaks to groups of parents, teens, or children. The possibilities are limited only by the nurse's imagination, priorities, community connections, and time constraints.

Insect and Rodent Control

All human communities are affected by the insects and rodents living in their environment. On the least dangerous level, they can cause irritation (e.g., mosquito or flea bites) and discomfort (e.g., infestations of bedbugs or lice). They can also pose a direct threat to health through such things as attacks by diseased rats or squirrels. Insects and rodents can consume and, in turn, contaminate food. However, by far the most serious health hazard they impose is through their role as *vectors*—nonhuman carriers of disease organisms that can transmit these organisms directly to humans.

The most common vectors are mosquitoes, flies, ticks, roaches, fleas, rats, mice, and ground squirrels. All of these agents can serve as reservoirs for germs that they then transmit through physical contact with humans or by contaminating human foodstuffs or water. Cases of vector-spread diseases range from the 14th-century bubonic plague epidemic spread by rat fleas, which killed a quarter of the European population, to the mosquito-spread outbreaks of West Nile virus that began in New York in 1999.

Government's Role

Vector surveys, research, and control are usually left to local and state health departments. These agencies have also implemented community awareness and pest control programs. Once vectors have been found, health workers can attempt to control them through many methods. Approaches used in the past included trapping of rodents, poisoning, spraying with pesticides, and eliminating areas where vectors breed (e.g., draining or filling marshes to control mosquito populations). In planning any approach, it is essential to consider the possible health hazards to humans or other living organisms and the effect the method will have on the ecosystem—how it may upset the ecologic balance. In 1986, the WHO advocated that the most basic, yet effective, approach is to improve sanitary conditions and practices to the extent that the conditions encouraging the multiplication of insects and rodents no longer exist (WHO, 1986).

Nurse's Role

The community health nurse can contribute through awareness of the presence and possible health threat of rodents and insects. By remaining alert to the presence of rodents and insects in homes, schools, and communities, nurses can take measures to educate affected persons and notify proper authorities when corrective action is needed. They can assist this effort by surveying homes and neighborhoods for exposed rubbish or conditions that might attract insects and rodents. They can also promote preventive efforts through education and influencing policy makers.

Some of the simple changes families can make that will help to eliminate rodents and insects include the following:

◆ Ensure that screens are present on all open windows, and use screen doors.

- Wash dishes, pots, and pans after meals, and clean counter surfaces.
- Keep pet food off the floor; fill the pet dish when the pet eats, and do not leave it on the floor for extended periods.
- Keep foodstuffs that insects may infest, such as cereals, corn meal, and flour, in closed plastic containers.
- Ensure that doors and windows fit properly; use calking if the outside can be seen through gaps in doors or windows.
- Eliminate food supplies for rodents and insects by keeping floors swept and vacuumed in rooms where people eat; preferably, eat only in the kitchen or dining room.
- Remove trash bags that include food scraps and food packaging from the home daily and place in garbage containers that are kept outside and have tight-fitting lids.

Safety in the Home, Worksite, and Community

As we have seen, the environments of the home, workplace, and community at large significantly affect people's health. This section addresses six additional problems that affect people's safety: exposure to toxic chemicals, radiation exposure, injury hazards, noise pollution, and psychological hazards (Display 9.3).

Exposure to Toxic Chemicals

The number of natural and synthetic chemicals in the environment and the threats they pose to human and environmental health are overwhelming. Approximately 10 million chemical compounds were synthesized in laboratories in the 20th century (Yassi et al., 2001). Most chemicals are intermediates in the manufacture of end-products for human use. All chemicals are toxic to some degree, with the health risk being primarily a function of the severity of the toxicity and the extent of exposure. About 1,500 toxins constitute the greatest threat of hazardous exposures, but only some 450 have established threshold limit values and adequate toxicity testing. The *Household Products Database*, which is available to the public, links over 7,000 consumer brands to their health effects as described in the *Material Safety Data Sheets* (MSDS) provided by the manufacturers (NLM, 2007b). The number of new chemicals that come into use each year is of great concern, especially since many of them are essentially untested. Products originating from foreign sources, where consumer protection laws may be lax or nonexistent, are an ongoing threat. This section presents a general overview of the different categories of environmental chemicals, where they are found, the dangers they impose, and the community health nurse's role in forestalling or detecting those dangers.

Toxic chemicals include those that do not contain carbon, are not derived from living matter, are usually of mineral composition, and have an inherent capacity to cause injury to a living organism (Yassi et al., 2001). Inorganic toxic chemicals include halogens, corrosive materials, and metals. Substances such as zinc, iron, calcium, sodium, potassium, magnesium, and copper often play an important

| DISPLAY 9.3 | TOXIC SUBSTANCES SCAVENGER HUNT |

Do you know what toxic substances are in your community's air and water? You can find out by examining the Toxmap website. Other helpful sites may be found through the Centers for Disease Control & Prevention, the Environmental Protection Agency and local air resources boards or agencies. Go on a computer scavenger hunt and see what you can find:

- Look around your city or neighborhood. What are the most common environmental hazards? Find the ToxMap website and enter your zip code. For your city or area, which three companies have the highest amounts of emissions? Are there any VOCs (volatile organic compounds), metals, or polycyclic aromatic hydrocarbons listed for the top company?
- If you were an occupational health nurse, what safety measures would you want in place to respond to accidental exposures to these chemicals? What could you do for emergency first aid until assistance arrives?
- Search the web again to find the following information: What are the most deadly occupations? Which of the top three occupations are found in your area?
- Take another computer tour and learn more about air pollution. What is your estimated cancer risk from inhalation of air pollution? What other health problems arise from high levels of air pollution? Using the three Core Public Health Functions, state three things that a public health nurse can do to promote cleaner air and fewer health problems for clients.

U.S. National Library of Medicine—*Toxmap: Environmental Health e-Maps* http://toxmap.nlm.nih.gov/toxmap/main/index.jsp.

and healthful role in human physiology, but they become toxic if a person is exposed to large quantities. A toddler's accidental ingestion of several chewable vitamins with iron can cause mild gastrointestinal distress or, if many are ingested, devastating physiologic damage.

Lead is a toxic agent that is frequently found in occupational or industrial settings. Workers must be careful to avoid inhaling lead fumes or exposing their families to lead dust on their clothing. Lead, once widely used in paint and gasoline, can still be found in batteries and leaded gasoline sold in some parts of the world, mostly in developing countries. It is the top home environmental health hazard for children, with 310,000 children aged 1 to 5 years at risk for exposure (CDC, 2005). Although elevated blood lead levels (BLL) have been steadily and dramatically declining since the late 1970s, certain populations of children remain at high risk: minorities; children in low-income households; those exposed to lead-containing home remedies, cosmetics, and ceramics; children in contact with occupationally exposed adults; and those who live in older homes (EPA, 2007g). In 1997, there were 122,641 confirmed cases of elevated BLL (>10 μg/dL) in children under 6 years of age; by 2005, this number had dropped to 46,770 (CDC, 2007b).

Prenatal lead exposure is another concern. Even low-level exposure of pregnant women to lead has a dangerous cumulative effect leading to nerve damage, neurobehavioral problems, learning disabilities, and mental retardation in the child. It has also been linked to preterm birth, decreased gestational maturity, and reduced postnatal growth (CDC, 2007c). Display 9.4 shows some common sources of lead.

In occupational settings, workers have been exposed to lead since long before the Industrial Revolution, because lead was used for making pipes, pigments, and bullets. Workers in some occupations, such as smelters, have been exposed to high levels of lead, as have those exposed to leaded gasoline and lead-containing paints.

DISPLAY 9.4   WHERE LEAD IS FOUND

In general, the older your home, the more likely it has lead-based paint.

- **Paint.** Many homes built before 1978 have lead-based paint. The federal government banned lead-based paint from housing in 1978. Some states stopped its use even earlier. Lead can be found:
  - In homes in the city, country, or suburbs.
  - In apartments, single-family homes, and both private and public housing.
  - Inside and outside of the house.
- **In soil around a home.** Soil can pick up lead from exterior paint, or other sources such as past use of leaded gas in cars.
- **Household dust.** Dust can pick up lead from deteriorating lead-based paint or from soil tracked into a home.
- **Drinking water.** Your home might have plumbing with lead or lead solder. Call your local health department or water supplier to find out about testing your water. You cannot see, smell, or taste lead, and boiling your water will not get rid of lead. If you think your plumbing might have lead in it:
  - Use only cold water for drinking and cooking.
  - Run water for 15 to 30 seconds before drinking it, especially if you have not used your water for a few hours.
- **The job.** If you work with lead, you could bring it home on your hands or clothes. Shower and change clothes before coming home. Launder your work clothes separately from the rest of your family's clothes.
- **Old painted toys and furniture.**
- **Food and liquids** stored in lead crystal or lead-glazed pottery or porcelain.
- **Lead smelters** or other industries that release lead into the air.
- **Hobbies** that use lead, such as making pottery or stained glass, or refinishing furniture.
- **Folk remedies** that contain lead, such as *greta* and *azarcon* used to treat an upset stomach.

U.S. Environmental Protection Agency. Retrieved July 4, 2007, from http://www.epa.gov/lead/pubs/leadinfo.htm#where.

With new awareness of the dangers of lead exposure, most workplaces have instituted safeguards to protect workers from exposure. However, the accidental exposure of children to lead in the environment remains an important issue.

Community health nurses need to check with clients for possible exposure and to examine client homes for lead-based paint. Lead-based paint is now restricted in residential use, but any painted building that is more than 30 years old may still have lead paint. In particular, nurses can warn parents to keep their young children from eating paint chips from windowsills, walls, or furniture painted with lead-based paint; to keep them away from lead-infused dirt near roads; and to avoid dust and debris when older buildings are being torn down or renovated. The U.S. Department of Housing and Urban Development (HUD) *Lead-Safe Housing Rule,* enacted in 1999, has helped to reduce lead poisoning risk from paint in federally owned or subsidized housing (HUD, 2007).

Mercury is also highly toxic. It is used in many scientific instruments, electronic equipment, crop fungicides, and in the processing of dental fillings. Historically, mercury was used in goldsmithing, mirror-making, explosive detonators, and as an antiseptic and antifungal agent. Inorganic mercury can be changed through bacterial action in industrial processes to more toxic organic compounds, as in the bleach used for paper manufacturing. Toxic mercurials then escape into the environment and contaminate the food chain. In 1956, at Minamata Bay on the island of Kyushu, Japan, many people died and more were disabled with permanent neurologic impairment from eating mercury-contaminated seafood (Friis, 2007). In Iraq in 1971, hundreds of fatalities occurred among people who used methylmercury fungicide–treated seeds to make bread (Merson, Black, & Mills, 2004). The seeds had been supplied by USAID (U.S. Agency for International Development) for planting and were dyed red to indicate they shouldn't be eaten. Hungry farmers found that they could wash off the dye and make bread but not all the fungicide was removed. The end result was over 500 people dead and approximately 5,000 hospitalized.

Other harmful metals include aluminum, which recently was associated with certain mental disorders and has been found in high levels in the brain tissues of patients with Alzheimer disease. More research is needed to determine the role, if any, that aluminum exposure has in this debilitating disease. Chromium, nickel, and arsenic are other toxic compounds with severe health consequences from exposure (ATSDR, 2005).

Many toxic chemicals are by-products of the petroleum industry, including many alcohols, ethers, hydrocarbons (e.g., benzene), medicines, and plastics that contain carbon. Ingestion or exposure can cause cancer, liver and kidney disease, birth defects, and many other health problems. Pesticides for household and crop use have created major health hazards. Dichlorodiphenyltrichloroethane (DDT), a very dangerous chemical used for pest control, was banned in 1972 in the United States because of environmental and health concerns. However, it is still present in the environment and continues to be used in developing countries, thus posing a danger to their populations, but most especially to children (Friis, 2007).

Exposure to toxic chemicals can have far-reaching effects on humans. People may come in contact with these toxins in their homes through building materials, cleaning products, or airborne dust. Another source is the workplace, where many different compounds are created and used each day. Toxic substances also may be transferred home from the workplace in motor vehicles and on clothing or shoes. In the greater community, pollutants in the air and food chain create further hazards. Toxic chemicals can cause illness when they are inhaled, come into contact with the skin (as in industrial accidents where chemicals are spilled), or are ingested (as when a child drinks from a liquid cleaning solvent bottle). Table 9.3 lists some common workplace carcinogens. The Occupational Safety and Health Administration (OSHA, 2006) standards require that information on toxic substances be made available in all workplaces that utilize chemical products. The regulations are extensive, but the essential components are:

◆ Industrial chemical manufacturers and importers are required to evaluate the hazards of the chemicals they produce or import.

◆ Manufacturers and importers must prepare labels and material safety data sheets (MSDSs) to convey the hazard information to their downstream customers.
◆ All employers with hazardous chemicals in their workplaces must display labels and MSDSs for their exposed workers, and train them to handle the chemicals appropriately.

Recognizing the key role that nurses play in environmental health, the *Environmental Health Nursing Initiative* was begun by ATSDR, with the goal to "make environmental health an integral component of nursing practice, education, and research" (ATSDR, 2007). The ATSDR notes that, in addition to protecting the health of all people, nurses also have the "credibility and access that enables them to provide scientifically sound information about environmental issues and toxic exposure." A wide variety of educational tools and resources are available from the website at http://www.atsdr.cdc.gov/EHN/.

TABLE 9.3 Occupational Carcinogens

Carcinogen	Cancer Site	Examples of Exposed Occupations
4-Aminodiphenyl	Bladder	Dye manufacturing, rubber manufacturing
Auramine		
β-Napthylamine		
Magenta		
Benzidine		
Arsenic	Skin, lung, liver	Metal smelting, arsenic pesticide production, metal alloy workers
Asbestos	Lung, mesothelium, gastrointestinal tract	Asbestos miners, insulators, shipyard workers
Benzene	Leukemia (blood-forming organs)	Petrochemical workers, chemists
Bischloromethyl ether (BCME)	Lung	Organic chemical synthesizers
Cadmium	Prostate	Cadmium alloy workers, welders
Chromium/chromates	Lung, nasal sinuses	Chromate producers, metal workers
Coke oven emissions	Lung, kidney	Coke oven workers
Foundry emissions	Lung	Foundry workers
Leather dust	Nasal cavity, nasal sinuses, bladder	Shoe manufacturing
Nickel	Lung, nasal passages	Nickel smelting, metal workers
Radiation (x-rays)	Leukemia (blood-forming organs), skin, breast, thyroid, bone	Radiologists, industrial radiographers, atomic energy workers
Radon gas	Lung	Uranium and feldspar miners
Soots, tars, and oil	Skin, lung, bladder, scrotum	Roofers, chimney sweepers, shale oil workers
Petroleum (aromatic hydrocarbons)		
Ultraviolet light	Skin	Outdoor workers
Vinyl chloride	Liver, brain, lung	Polyvinyl chloride synthesizers, rubber workers
Welding fumes	Lung	Welders
Wood dust	Nasal passages	Hardwood workers, furniture makers

From Blumenthal, D., & Ruttenber, J. (1994). *Introduction to environmental health*, (2nd ed). New York: Springer.

LEVELS OF PREVENTION PYRAMID

SITUATION: Increase to at least 20% the proportion of homes in which homeowners/occupants have tested for radon concentrations (Baseline: 11% in 1994 from Healthy People 2010, USDHHS, 2000)

GOAL: Using the three levels of prevention, negative health conditions are avoided, promptly diagnosed and treated, and/or the fullest possible potential is restored.

Tertiary Prevention

Rehabilitation	Primary Prevention	
	Health Promotion & Education	*Health Protection*
• Seal cracks in basement floors and walls • Install subslab exhaust system below basement floors	• Educate the surrounding community members regarding their risk	• Require building modifications where radon concentrations are high

Secondary Prevention

Early Diagnosis	Prompt Treatment
• Periodic testing of radon levels	• Circulate air with fans in homes with low concentrations • Use fan and positive-ion generator to decrease inhaled concentrations

Primary Prevention

Health Promotion & Education	Health Protection
• Conduct community education regarding the nature and dangers of inhaling radon gas	• Require sealed basement construction to avoid release of radon into building from underlying soil

Exposure to Radiation

Radiation is technically defined as a process by which energy is propagated through space or matter. Natural radiation from the sun, soil, and minerals can be found in virtually all areas of the Earth's environment. The largest natural source of radiation exposure is airborne radon. Some radioactive substances produce particles, and others produce rays. Radiation in its manmade form has numerous beneficial uses in science and industry for lasers, radiographs (x-rays) that help in the diagnosis of disease, and the production of nuclear energy. It is found in many home electronic devices, such as television sets, smoke detectors, and microwave ovens (see Levels of Prevention Pyramid).

Regardless of its source, radiation is a threat to human health in the workplace and in the general environment. The extent of danger depends on the dose and type of radiation. For example, casualties among miners can be attributed to their prolonged and intense exposure to radioactive minerals such as uranium. Prolonged exposure can cause skin ulcers, damage to cells, cancer, premature aging, kidney dysfunction, and genetic disorders in the children of those whose cells have been damaged.

A certain amount of natural radiation exposure from the sun is important for the production of vitamin D. However, intentional exposure by sunbathing, still a popular activity in many areas, must be tempered with the use of lotions with sunscreen. The current recommendations are that sunscreen products used have a sun protection factor (SPF) of at least 15. Debate has been ongoing since 1999 as to the value of SPF factors above 30; until resolution, many products advertise a SPF greatly exceeding 30. What remains clear is that sunscreen products must be reapplied frequently for continued protection, especially during and after swimming or activities that promote sweating. They should be used by people of all ages when exposed to the sun for more than 10 to 15 minutes in winter or summer. Sunscreen is more important at higher elevations and when participating in outdoor snow activities, such as skiing, because the snow reflects the sun's rays. An

DISPLAY 9.5	UV INDEX SCALE

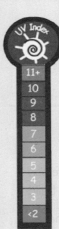

2 or less: Low

A UV Index reading of 2 or less means low danger from the sun's UV rays for the average person:

- Wear sunglasses on bright days. In winter, reflection off snow can nearly double UV strength.
- If you burn easily, cover up and use sunscreen.

3–5: Moderate

A UV Index reading of 3 to 5 means moderate risk of harm from unprotected sun exposure.

- Take precautions, such as covering up, if you will be outside.
- Stay in shade near midday when the sun is strongest.

6–7: High

A UV Index reading of 6 to 7 means high risk of harm from unprotected sun exposure. Apply a sunscreen with a SPF of at least 15. Wear a wide-brim hat and sunglasses to protect your eyes.

- Protection against sunburn is needed.
- Reduce time in the sun between 10 AM and 4 PM.
- Cover up, wear a hat and sunglasses, and use sunscreen.

8–10: Very High

A UV Index reading of 8 to 10 means very high risk of harm from unprotected sun exposure. Minimize sun exposure during midday hours, from 10 AM to 4 PM. Protect yourself by liberally applying a sunscreen with an SPF of at least 15. Wear protective clothing and sunglasses to protect the eyes.

- Take extra precautions. Unprotected skin will be damaged and can burn quickly.
- Minimize sun exposure between 10 AM and 4 PM. Otherwise, seek shade, cover up, wear a hat and sunglasses, and use sunscreen.

11+: Extreme

A UV Index reading of 11 or higher means extreme risk of harm from unprotected sun exposure. Try to avoid sun exposure during midday hours, from 10 AM to 4 PM. Apply sunscreen with an SPF of at least 15 liberally every 2 hours.

- Take all precautions. Unprotected skin can burn in minutes. Beachgoers should know that white sand and other bright surfaces reflect UV and will increase UV exposure.
- Try to avoid sun exposure between 10 AM to 4 PM.
- Seek shade, cover up, wear a hat and sunglasses, and use sunscreen.

Adapted from: U.S. Environmental Protection Agency. Retrieved July 4, 2007, from http://www.epa.gov/sunwise/uvindex2.html.

---

easily understood public health advisory system, the UV Index, shows the risk level for that day and the steps that should be taken to reduce exposure (see Display 9.5).

A major area of concern centers on the problems associated with nuclear energy and nuclear weapons. The production of radioactive wastes, the threat of accidental exposure from unsafe reactors, and possible fallout from weapons testing generate real fears. These fears were confirmed by the nuclear reactor accidents at Three Mile Island and Chernobyl, which were discussed earlier in this chapter. Accidents of this type are uncommon, however, and the safe operation of nuclear power plants exposes communities to much less radiation than other sources, such as medical or natural radiation.

Injury Hazards

When assessing a population's health risk, one environmental characteristic that must be considered is the community's level of physical safety. How likely is it that injuries will occur? This is a very important question when one considers that, in the United States, unintentional injuries kill more people during the first three decades of life than any other cause of death (National Center for Injury Prevention and Control [NCIPC], 2003). In 2003, a total of 109,277 Americans died from unintentional injuries (NCIPC, 2003). Groups at highest risk are the young, the elderly, the poor, minorities, and rural residents. Many of these deaths could have been prevented through community safety planning, which can enhance the built environment to reduce accidents and injuries.

Not surprisingly, motor vehicle accidents were the leading cause of death in 2003 for those aged 4 to 34 years (Subramanian, 2006). In all age groups, more than 43,000 deaths resulted from vehicular accidents, and approximately 40% of all motor vehicle deaths are alcohol-related. The second-ranked cause of injury death is falls, followed by poisoning, drowning, and residential fires. Alcohol plays a major role in many of these injuries and subsequent deaths, particularly with motor vehicle crashes and drowning (USD-HHS, 2000).

Community health nurses have a responsibility to assess situations for the threat of potential physical harm and to work with other professionals to design preventive measures. Safety education and primary prevention is a major role of the community health nurse. Because infants and children are particularly vulnerable to accidents, this teaching can begin one-on-one or in groups of pregnant women attending clinics or Women, Infants, and Children (WIC) appointments. The topics to be discussed are many but usually include anticipatory guidance to enhance infant safety, creating a child-proof home, and acquiring a car seat and using it properly. Topics and clients will change as the nurse branches out to preschools, schools, youth clubs, parent–teacher organizations, and other groups. The nurse may become a resource for others who do the teaching, and knowing where to find safety information, brochures, and other "handouts" is important in information dissemination.

Exposure to Noise Pollution

People in the United States are bombarded by noise from many sources. Noise has two definitions. One, related to its physical properties, defines noise as *a sound, generally random in nature, the spectrum of which does not exhibit clearly defined frequency components*. A simpler and more subjective definition is *any unwanted sound* (Behar, Chasin, & Cheesman, 2000). Household appliances, traffic, radios, machinery, and voices are typical noise sources. To a degree "noise" depends on the listener; a teen's loud music choice may be a source of noise to his parents. Noise is measured three ways. First, noise is measured by magnitude, or *decibels*. A whisper may measure 10 to 20 decibels, and a fire engine siren may measure 80 to 100 decibels. Another way to measure is by the high and low tones of the noise, referred to as *frequency*. A male voice usually has a lower frequency than a female voice does, and a tuba is lower than a flute. A third factor is the *time history*, or the length of time one has been exposed to the noise.

Noise has been cited as a major environmental health problem. Prolonged exposure (months to years) to extremely loud noises, such as pneumatic drills or rock music, can cause temporary or permanent hearing loss (Behar et al., 2000). Other noises, perhaps occasional machinery noises at the workplace or residential exposure to airport traffic, can lead to general annoyance; headaches; sleep, speech, and task interference; alterations in emotions; stress; lowered body resistance to disease; ulcers; and aggravation of existing physical disorders. The effects vary in severity depending on the intensity and duration of the noises and the disposition of the people concerned. Ototoxic "refers to agents that can produce hearing loss" and may result from a combination of noise and workplace chemical exposures (Friis, 2007, p. 331).

Noise control comprises four methods. First, the source of the noise can be relocated (e.g., having the teen band practice in the garage instead of the family room) or replaced (e.g., fixing or replacing a broken toy or appliance). Another method is to do something about the path of the noise. A barrier, enclosure, or muffler may be effective. This is often seen along highways, where 8- to 10-foot high walls have been built between the highway traffic noises and housing developments. An automobile muffler serves a similar purpose of *muffling* the engine's sound. A third method of control is to relocate the receiver. For instance, if parents are annoyed by the loudness and music choice of their teenager, they may want to go to another room in the house. Finally, the receiver can use hearing protectors such as ear plugs. For example, airline ground-crew members wear highly sophisticated hearing protectors.

Community responses to noise pollution take many forms. Community standards usually enforce noise abatement after 10 PM and before 8 AM, and police will respond if a neighbor complains about a loud neighborhood party. As highways creep into suburban neighborhoods, barriers are erected in the form of walls or noise-absorbing trees and shrubbery. Standards for the decibel levels of appliances and tools are set by manufacturers, following OSHA standards. Packaging instructions indicate whether hearing protectors should be used when the tool or piece of equipment is in use.

Community health nurses can inform families of the damage or annoyance noises can inflict and help people quiet their environment. If community-generated noise comes from industry, the nurse can collaborate with health team members from the offending company and work to bring about positive changes that improve the relationship between the company and the community. In one low-income community during the 1950s, an aluminum factory created a loud, repetitive booming noise all day long that made it impossible for people in nearby housing to speak to each other within their homes without raising their voices or shouting. It was impossible to sit on a porch and hear someone nearby speak. OSHA did not exist at the time, and community attempts at changing the situation did not make an impact. It was not until the company's manufacturing processes changed years later that the community felt relief. In the meantime, many families left the neighborhood as soon as they were able, leaving the housing choices near the factory for the uninformed.

Exposure to Biologic Pollutants

Biologic pollutants or hazards include all of the forms of life, as well as the nonliving products they produce, that can cause adverse health effects. Some common indoor biologic pollutants include animal dander (minute scales from hair, feathers, or skin), dust mite and cockroach parts, fungi, molds, infectious agents (bacteria and viruses), plants, pollen, and a wide variety of toxins and allergens (Wigle, 2003).

Breathing indoor air contaminated with biologic pollutants can cause health problems or make existing health problems worse, especially among infants, young children (Wigle, 2003), the elderly, and those with chronic illnesses. The effects range from allergic symptoms (conjunctival inflammation, rhinitis, sneezing, nasal congestion, itching, dyspnea, coughing, wheezing, chest tightness, headache, and malaise) to infections and toxicity.

Home conditions that promote this type of pollution include dampness, which encourages the growth and build-up of biologic pollutants. It is estimated that 30% to 50% of all structures, mostly in warm, moist climates, have damp conditions. One especially concerning fungus is *Stachybotrys chartarum*, commonly referred to as *toxic mold*. *S. chartarum* is a greenish-black fungus that is being investigated in the deaths of infants in Cleveland, Ohio, and as the cause of other serious health problems in other areas of the United States. It is known to produce toxigenic spores, and it grows on high-cellulose materials such as fiberboard and gypsum board, which are commonly used in home construction. The EPA does not currently have evaluation or remediation guidelines to address this potential threat (EPA, 2007c).

There are particular items and areas in homes and personal environments where biologic pollutants are commonly found and where proper cleaning or care is especially important. These include:

◆ Humidifiers and dehumidifiers
◆ Bathrooms without vents or windows

- Kitchens without vents or windows
- Refrigerator drip pans
- Laundry rooms with an unvented dryer
- Unventilated attics
- Damp basement floors with carpeting
- Bedding
- Closets on outside walls
- Heating/air conditioning systems
- Bookshelves, curio cabinets, and other areas that accumulate dust
- Dog and cat bedding, litter boxes, bird cages, fish tanks, and so forth
- Areas with water damage (around windows, the roof, or the basement)
- In automobile ventilation systems where moisture pools after use of the air conditioner

The most important role of the community health nurse is to assess clients' homes for possible biologic pollutants and then to provide them with the information they need to correct or improve the situation. If clients are renting a house or apartment, and the dampness is caused by structural conditions or owner negligence, the nurse may act as an advocate for the clients to remedy the potentially hazardous situation. Display 9.6 includes a list of assessment questions the nurse should apply during home visits when clients may have been exposed to biologic pollutants.

Psychological Hazards

A discussion of environmental health and safety would not be complete if it overlooked the psychological hazards that people must face in their environments. Environment plays a significant role in the mental health of a community. The psychological variables that affect people often lead to physiologic illnesses. Such elements as noise, overcrowding, traffic, inadequate housing, lack of privacy, unavailability of work, lack of natural beauty, and boredom can be detrimental to peoples' well-being.

Another psychological hazard is urban crowding. Early studies on crowding done by J. B. Calhoun demonstrated serious effects on behavior. When healthy, naturally clean laboratory mice were forced to live in overcrowded conditions, they experienced dramatic behavior changes. Gross unsanitary conditions led to aggressive behavior, attacks by strong mice on the weak, symptoms of regression and mental disturbance, mating decline, and neglect or cannibalization of weaker offspring. Although this is an extreme example, it perhaps provides some insight into the conditions of urban areas and the psychological stress that urban conditions can create (Nakamura, 1999).

The daily psychological stresses of the modern world are innumerable. Excessive stimulation comes from rapid societal changes created by new technology, an accelerated pace of living, increased work production demands, and other causes. All can create potential health hazards.

Government's Role

The government plays an active role in promoting public safety. Standards and regulations have been set at the federal level regarding toxic chemicals, radiation exposure,

---

| DISPLAY 9.6 | ASSESSMENT QUESTIONS TO DETECT BIOLOGIC POLLUTANTS IN HOMES |

- ❑ Does anyone in the family have frequent headaches, fevers, itchy watery eyes, a stuffy nose, dry throat, or a cough?
- ❑ Does anyone complain of feeling tired or dizzy all the time?
- ❑ Is anyone wheezing or having difficulties breathing on a regular basis?
- ❑ Did these symptoms appear after you moved to this home/apartment?
- ❑ Do the symptoms disappear when you go to school or work or go away on a trip, and return when you come back home?
- ❑ Have you (or your landlord or apartment manager) recently remodeled your home or done any energy conservation work, such as installing insulation, storm windows, or weather stripping?
- ❑ Does your home feel humid?
- ❑ Can you see moisture on the windows or on other surfaces, such as walls and ceilings?
- ❑ What is the usual temperature in your home? Is it very hot or cold?
- ❑ Have you recently had water damage?
- ❑ Do you have a basement? Is it wet or damp?
- ❑ Is there any obvious mold or mildew in the basement, closets, bathrooms?
- ❑ Does any part of your home have a musty or moldy odor?
- ❑ Is the air stale?
- ❑ Do you have pets? (Consider all—including fish, turtles, snakes.)
- ❑ Do you have house plants? Do they show signs of mold?
- ❑ Do you have air conditioners or humidifiers that have not been properly cared for or cleaned?
- ❑ Does your home have cockroaches or rodents?

Adapted from U.S. Consumer Product Safety Commission. (2007). *Biologic pollutants in your home* (CPSC Document #425). Bethesda, MD: Author. Retrieved July 5, 2007, from http://www.cpsc.gov/CPSCPUB/PUBS/425.html.

---

occupational safety practices, noise abatement, biologic hazards, and other safety issues. State and local governments seek to enforce business, industry, and community compliance with these standards. Health departments and other government agencies assist with monitoring of chemical use and production, as well as promotion of public education programs to alert people to the presence and potential dangers of toxic chemicals and exposure to radiation in the environment. Researchers are examining the biologic effects of chemicals and radiation. Those in medical and dental fields have developed simple safety procedures, such as having patients wear lead aprons during radiographs and having technicians stand behind metal walls.

Because the government holds companies liable for the safety of their products, industry now invests considerable resources into researching and designing safe goods. Many products have been modified to make them safer, such as childproof caps on medication bottles, flame-retardant children's clothing, and seat belts and airbags in automobiles. Industries must also warn consumers if one of their products is inherently dangerous (e.g., toys with sharp edges or parts small enough to be ingested by toddlers). Bright-orange, frowning faces on bottles that contain harmful substances have helped to warn consumers and reduce the number of poisonings. Children learn to avoid poisonous plants and other potential hazards through school and community education efforts.

Community safety organizations, government agencies, and public health officials all play their part in assessing community safety and taking measures to prevent accidents. Organizations such as *Health Care Without Harm*, the *Natural Resources Defense Council*, as well as consumer advocates such as Ralph Nader, continue to serve as watchdogs for environmental safety. Federal and state legislation to enforce speed limits has helped to reduce the number of automobile crashes, and supervision of recreational and occupational areas has led to discovery of health hazards and promoted the development of safety programs. State-established boating safety regulations and the assignment of adequate lifeguards to monitor busy swimming beaches are measures that help to reduce the number of recreational accidents. Community surveys of intersections where multiple traffic crashes have occurred have led to installation of traffic signals and a reduction of crashes.

Nurse's Role

It is difficult to monitor all the possible contacts a person or community may be experiencing with toxic chemicals, biologic agents, or radiation, but such monitoring is necessary in order to estimate health risks and establish correlations. Multiple exposures in small doses from many different sources may add up. Are clients' homes well ventilated? Is the burning of fossil fuels polluting the air with sulfur oxides? Does home, school, or worksite insulation contain asbestos? Are all household chemical agents stored in a childproof place? Is the home free of molds and other biologic hazards? Monitoring difficulties arise from the many opportunities for exposure to toxic chemicals, biological hazards, or radiation; cumulative exposure over time; and the fact that disease symptoms may not appear until years after exposure, when the agent may no longer be in the immediate environment. The best protection is to promote and monitor the safe use and disposal of chemical hazards, seek out and treat or remove biologic contaminants, and limit radiation exposure to prevent health problems from occurring.

Community health nurses can promote environmental safety and prevent injuries in many ways. Six target areas in which to concentrate preventive measures are highways, homes, worksites, schools, farms, and recreational sites. Working with the police, fire personnel, social services, schools, drug rehabilitation counselors, and many other community groups, the nurse can help to develop programs focused on failed smoke detectors, unsafe playground equipment, and much more. In homes, nurses can encourage safe storage of toxic materials and removal of biologic hazards. Railings can be installed on stairways and in bathrooms used by elderly individuals. Gates at the tops of stairways and window guards can prevent falls by small children. Nonskid decals can be used in bathtubs to prevent slipping.

Safety education offers one of the most vital preventive measures. When people are made aware of possible dangers and unsafe areas, they can avoid injuring themselves. Local community programs to educate people on the dangers of driving while intoxicated, to instruct them on the proper handling of home machinery such as chain saws, or to encourage viewing community sponsored and professionally conducted fireworks during holiday celebrations rather than attempting to use them at home, can also help to reduce injuries. In the event that an injury does occur, public education about appropriate responsive actions can help to reduce the potential impact. Promotion of first aid and cardiopulmonary resuscitation (CPR) classes can be beneficial.

Community health nurses need to be aware of the effects noise can have on hearing health and overall well-being. This knowledge will help the nurse identify specific health problems caused by increased noise. Teaching employers, employees, teachers, and children about the potential harm of repeated loud noises in their environment (even the noise from a headset that is turned to a high decibel level) is essential.

It is necessary for community health nurses to be aware of psychological hazards in the environment, to recognize the potential they have for affecting both psychological and physiologic health, and to encourage stress reduction wherever possible (see From the Case Files). Some specific ways in which community health nurses can promote a psychologically healthy environment include active lobbying for neighborhood crime prevention, reduction of workplace stressors, and the development of educational and support programs to reduce lifestyle stressors.

STRATEGIES FOR NURSING ACTION IN ENVIRONMENTAL HEALTH

Each of the preceding sections has discussed actions and given examples of ways in which the community health nurse can be involved in environmental health. To summarize, the nurse has a two-part challenge: to help protect the public's health from potential threats in the environment, and to help protect and promote the health of the environment itself, so that it can be life- and health-enhancing for its human inhabitants. The following strategies for collaboration and participation provide a summary of the nurse's role and can assist the nurse in addressing this two-part goal:

1. Learn about possible environmental health threats. The nurse has a responsibility to keep abreast of current environmental issues and to know the proper authorities to whom problems should be reported.

From the Case Files

Occupational Environmental Health and the Nurse's Role

Scenario

Metropolis Tool Company is a manufacturing plant that employs 1200 workers. Most of the employees work in assembly or data entry jobs. Recently, there have been increasing complaints of work-related stress, with employees citing pressure to perform and produce at higher levels as the root of the stress. You are an occupational health nurse working for the company.

It has come to your attention that there has been a significant increase in insurance claims for the following conditions:
- Stress-related migraine headaches
- Early pregnancy leave for women experiencing low maternal weight gain

Metropolis Tool Company has been in business for more than 29 years, Recently, competition in the manufacturing industry has increased, and the company's executives are looking for ways to cut expenses. Insurance premiums cost the company a considerable amount, and rates will increase if the number of claims continues to rise. Your employer recently became aware of the problems leading to increased utilization of disability benefits. He approached you and asked you to "fix" these problems in an expeditious manner.

Available assessment data that may be related to the problems include the following:
- The plant recently moved to rotating shifts and is now operating around the clock
- Staff layoffs are predicted within 6 months
- Increasing corporate completion has led to higher productivity standards and expectations

Questions

1. Discuss additional assessment data needed and how you will go about gathering these data.
2. Describe your role related to the issue of environmental health and safety.
3. Discuss interventions that your program may perform at the following levels of prevention:
   - Primary
   - Secondary
   - Tertiary
4. Your supervisor in your role of occupational health nurse is a company vice president. He is very knowledgeable about business but knows little about health issues. Where will you turn to obtain information to assist you in addressing the problems identified in this scenario?
5. How will you evaluate the effects of your interventions?
6. What issues does this scenario elicit regarding:
   Fears and anxiety in this role.
   Lack of immediate resources (supervisor)
   Social justice
   Building partnerships within your communities
   Globalization of public health

2. Assess clients' environment and detect health hazards. Careful observation and an environmental checklist can assist in this assessment.
3. Plan collaboratively with citizens and other professionals to devise protective and preventive strategies. Remember that environmental health work is generally a team effort.
4. Assist with the implementation of programs to prevent health threats to clients and the environment.
5. Take action to correct situations in which health hazards exist. Nurses can use direct intervention (e.g., in an unsafe home situation), notify proper authorities, or publicly protest if corrective measures are beyond their sphere.
6. Educate consumers and assist them to practice preventive measures. Examples of preventive

measures include radon testing in homes and well-water testing in rural communities.
7. Take action to promote the development of policies and legislation that enhance consumer protection and promote a healthier environment.
8. Assist with and promote program evaluation to determine the effectiveness of environmental health efforts.
9. Apply environmentally related research findings and participate in nursing research.

Summary

Environmental health is a discipline encompassing all of the elements of the environment that influence the health and well-being of its inhabitants. Public health workers, including community health nurses, need to monitor and determine causal links between people and their environment with a concern as to how they may promote the health and well-being of both.

An ecologic perspective of environmental health is important to understand the human–environment relationship and how the health of one affects the health of the other. Prevention and strategic or long-range concerns are also important in considering environmental health, because what is done today may affect the health of many generations in the future.

Major global environmental concerns exist, such as overpopulation, ozone depletion and global warming, deforestation, desertification and wetlands destruction, energy depletion, air pollution, water pollution, contaminated food, waste disposal, insect and rodent control, biologic pollutants, safety (in the home, worksite, and community). Each has its own set of problems, concerns, and solutions.

Both public and private sectors are involved in regulating, monitoring, and preventing environmental health problems, and have accomplished much during the past 35 years. Much, however, is still left to be done, and new problems continue to develop. The community health nurse is an important member of the team of health professionals who promote and protect the reciprocal relationship between the environment and the public's health. The nurse can follow several important strategies to accomplish the two-part goal of protecting the public's health from environmental threats and promoting a healthy and health-enhancing environment. ■

ACTIVITIES TO PROMOTE CRITICAL THINKING

1. You are planning a visit to a young family who live in an older home. You know that older homes may have radon, lead pipes and lead-based paint, asbestos insulation, and other safety, fire, and health threats, such as those from biologic pollutants. Using the nursing process, design a plan for (a) determining whether any of these threats are present, (b) deciding what actions should be taken if the dangers exist, (c) assisting the family in taking corrective action, and (d) evaluating successful removal of existing threats.

2. Data from the local health department show that, in the past year, five people from the same rural portion of the county died of cancer. What collaborative actions would be appropriate for you to take to determine whether an environmental relationship exists? What other members of the health team should be involved in the investigation? Write a letter to the mayor and the county commissioners to justify why nurses should be involved in this study.

3. Select an article from the mass media (e.g., newspaper, weekly news magazine) that deals with an "environmental health" problem. Analyze and critique the article by answering the following questions: What are the characteristics of the community involved? What appear to be the sources of the problem? What evidence is provided in the article to substantiate the cause? Does the news coverage describe health effects? What population is at risk? Does the coverage provide adequate information for consumers to understand the problem and seek any needed assistance? What suggestions do you have for improving the article?

4. Design a list of items to include in a checklist for assessing clients' home, school, or worksite environments. Consider each of the environmental areas of concern described in this chapter and what potential health threats might be present in each area. Review this list with an environmental health expert for accuracy and completeness. Use the list as a teaching tool with two different sets of clients, and evaluate its effectiveness for assessment and diagnosis of environmentally related health hazards.

5. Identify an environmental health problem in your community or state. Become informed about this problem by talking with experts in the area, reading recent literature and research reports, and searching the Internet for information about the problem. Meet with a senator or congressperson who has been involved in legislation related to the problem, and learn what he or she plans to do about it. Summarize what you have learned, and present it in writing as a letter to the editor of your city newspaper.

References

Agency for Toxic Substances & Disease Registry. (2005). *2005 CERCLA Priority List of Hazardous Substances.* Retrieved July 16, 2007 from http://www.atsdr.cdc.gov/cercla/05list.html.

Agency for Toxic Substances & Disease Registry. (2007). *The ATSDR Environmental Health Nursing Initiative.* Retrieved July 16, 2007 from http://www.atsdr.cdc.gov/EHN/.

Aschengrau, A., & Seage, G.R. (2008). *Essentials of epidemiology in public health*, 2nd ed. Sudbury, MA: Jones & Bartlett Publishers.

Backer, L.C., Kirkpatrick, B., Fleming, L.E., et al. (2005). Occupational exposure to aerosolized Brevetoxins during Florida Red Tide events: Effects on a healthy worker population. *Environmental Health Perspectives, 113*, 644–649.

Bay Area Air Quality Management District. (2007). *Spare the air program.* Retrieved July 13, 2007 from http://www.sparetheair.org/.

Behar, A., Chasin, M., & Cheesman, M.E. (2000). *Noise control: A primer.* San Diego, CA: Delmar.

Bhopal Medical Appeal & Sambhavna Trust. (n.d.). *What happened in Bhopal?* Retrieved July 4, 2007 from http://www.bhopal.org/whathappened.html.

Butler, C.D., & McMichael, A.J. (2006). Environmental health. In B.S. Levy, & V.W. Sidel (Eds.). *Social injustice and public health.* (pp. 318–336). New York: Oxford University Press, Inc.

California Integrated Waste Management Board. (2007). *Diapers.* Retrieved July 15, 2007 from http://www.ciwmb.ca.gov/WPIE/Healthcare/Diapers.htm.

Calvert, G.M., Mueller, C.A., Fajen, J.M., et al. (1998). Health effects associated with sulfuryl fluoride and methyl bromide exposure among structural fumigation workers. *American Journal of Public Health, 88*(12), 1774–1780.

Centers for Disease Control and Prevention. (2005). Blood lead levels: United States, 1999–2002. *Morbidity and Mortality Weekly Report, 54*(20), 513–516.

Centers for Disease Control and Prevention. (2007a). *Asthma's impact on children and adolescents.* Retrieved July 13, 2007 from http://www.cdc.gov/asthma/children.htm.

Centers for Disease Control and Prevention. (2007b). *CDC National Surveillance Data, 1997–2005.* Retrieved July 16, 2007 from http://www.cdc.gov/nceh/lead/surv/stats.htm.

Centers for Disease Control and Prevention. (2007c). Lead exposure among females of childbearing age: United States, 2004. *Morbidity and Mortality Weekly Report, 56*(16), 397–400.

Dziuban, E.J., Liang, J.L., Craun, G.F., et al. (2006). Surveillance for waterborne disease and outbreaks associated with recreational water: United States, 2003–2004. *Morbidity and Mortality Weekly Report, 55*(SS-12), 1–30.

Energy Information Administration (2007). *Coal reserves current and back issues.* Retrieved August 12, 2008 from http://www.eia.doe.gov/cneaf/coal/reserves/reserves.html.

Friis, R.H. (2007). *Essentials of environmental health.* Sudbury, MD: Jones & Barlett Publishers.

Friis, R.H., & Sellers, T.A. (2004). *Epidemiology for public health practice,* 3rd ed. Sudbury, MD: Jones & Barlett Publishers.

Gordon, L. (2002). *Introduction [Forward to Report of the Sanitary Commission of Massachusetts, 1850].* Dutton & Wentworth, State Printers: Boston. Retrieved July 3, 2007 from http://www.deltaomega.org/shattuck.pdf.

Hanley, J.G. (2006). Parliament, physicians, and nuisances: The demedicalization of nuisance law, 1831–1855. *Bulletin of the History of Medicine, 80,* 702–732.

Heymann, D.L. (Ed.). (2004). *Control of communicable diseases manual,* 18th ed. Washington, DC: American Public Health Association.

Hill, W.G., Butterfield, P., & Larsson, L.S. (2006). Rural parent's perceptions of risks associated with their children's exposure to radon. *Public Health Nursing, 23,* 392–399.

Holmes, O.W. (1843/1909–1914). The contagiousness of puerperal fever. In *Harvard Classics,* Vol. 38, Part 5. (Original work published 1843). Retrieved July 5, 2007 from http://www.bartleby.com/38/5/1.html.

Hoskins, R. (2001, Fall/Winter). *Climate change: Why public health practitioners should care.* Northwest Public Health. Retrieved July 14, 2007 from http://nwpublichealth.org/docs/nph/f2001/hoskins_f2001.pdf.

International Atomic Energy Agency. (2005). *Food and environmental protection newsletter. IAEA/RCA Final review meeting on the application of food irradiation for food, security, safety and trade* (RAS/5/042); Daejon, Republic of Korea; 21–25 February 2005. Retrieved July 15, 2007 from http://www.iaea.org/programmes/nafa/d5/public/fep-nl-8-1.pdf.

International Atomic Energy Agency. (n.d.). *Irradiation for food safety.* Retrieved July 15, 2007 from http://www-tc.iaea.org/tcweb/publications/factsheets/FoodIrradiation.pdf.

Library of Congress. (2007). *On-line catalog.* Retrieved July 3, 2007 from http://catalog.loc.gov/.

Licari, L., Nemer, L., & Tamburlini, G. (2005). *Children's health and environment: Developing action plans.* Copenhagen, Denmark: World Health Organization. Retrieved July 13, 2007 from http://www.euro.who.int/document/E86888.pdf.

Mays, G.P. (2008). Organization of the public health delivery system. In L.F. Novik, C.B. Morrow, & G.P. Mays (Eds.). *Public health administration: Principles for population-based management,* 2nd ed. (pp. 69–126). Sudbury, MA: Jones & Bartlett Publishers.

McGrew, R. (1985). *Encyclopedia of medical history.* (pp. 137–141). New York: McGraw-Hill.

McNeil Nutritionals, LLC. (2007). *Splenda brand timeline.* Retrieved July 15, 2007 from http://www.splenda.com/page.jhtml?id=splenda/newspromotions/press/timelines.inc.

Merson, M.H., Black, R.E., & Mills, A. (2004). *International public health: Diseases, programs, systems, and policies.* Boston: Jones & Bartlett Publishers.

Muir, J. (1911/1988). *My first summer in the Sierra.* Boston: Houghton Mifflin Sierra Club Books. (p. 110). Retrieved July 17, 2007 from http://www.sierraclub.org.

Myers, N. (2005, May). Environmental refugees: An emergent security issue. In *Session III – Environment and Migration, 13th Economic Forum.* Retrieved July 14, 2007 from http://www.osce.org/documents/eea/2005/05/14488_en.pdf.

Nakamura, R.M. (1999). *Health in America: A multicultural perspective.* Boston: Allyn & Bacon.

National Center for Injury Prevention and Control. (2003). *Ten leading causes of death by age group, United States: 2003.* Atlanta, GA: Centers for Disease Control and Prevention. Retrieved July 16, 2007 from http://www.cdc.gov/ncipc/osp/charts.htm.

National Geographic. (2006). *The green guide: Diapers.* Retrieved July 15, 2007 from http://www.thegreenguide.com/reports/product.mhtml?id=45.

National Institute of Allergy and Infectious Diseases. (2007). *Foodborne diseases.* Bethesda, MD: National Institutes of Health. Retrieved July 15, 2007 from http://www3.niaid.nih.gov/healthscience/healthtopics/foodborne/default.htm.

National Institute of Environmental Health Sciences. (2006). *New frontiers in environmental sciences and human health: The 2006–2011 NIEHS strategic plan.* Bethesda, MD: National Institutes of Health. Retrieved July 5, 2007 from http://www.niehs.nih.gov/external/plan2006/.

National Library of Medicine. (2007a). *Asthma in children.* Retrieved July 13, 2007 from http://www.nlm.nih.gov/medlineplus/asthmainchildren.html.

National Library of Medicine. (2007b). *Household products database.* Retrieved July 16, 2007 from http://householdproducts.nlm.nih.gov/about.html.

National Park Service. (2000). *Early development: Everglades National Park: The predrainage system and early development.* Retrieved July 14, 2007 from http://www.nps.gov/archive/ever/eco/develop.htm.

National Wind Coordinating Collaborative. (2007). *Collaborative objectives.* Retrieved July 15, 2007 from http://www.nationalwind.org/about/objectives.htm.

Nightingale, F. (1860/1969). *Notes on nursing: What it is and what it is not.* New York: Dover Publications, Inc.

Novick, L.F., & Morrow, C.B. (2008). Defining public health: Historical and contemporary developments. In L.F. Novik, C.B. Morrow, & G.P. Mays (Eds.). *Public health administration: Principles for population-based management,* 2nd ed. (pp. 1–34). Sudbury, MA: Jones & Bartlett Publishers.

Occupational Safety and Health Administration: U.S. Department of Labor. (2006). *Hazard communication: Foundation of workplace chemical safety programs.* Retrieved July 16, 2007 from http://www.osha.gov/SLTC/hazardcommunications/index.html.

Partnership for Food Safety Education. (2006). *Fight BAC.* Washington, DC: Author. Retrieved July 15, 2007 from http://www.fightbac.org/.

Population Action International. (2007a). *Population & environment.* Washington, DC: Author. Retrieved July 3, 2007 from http://www.populationaction.org/Issues/Population_and_Environment/Index.shtml.

Population Action International. (2007b). *Population: Facts and figures. Some population facts and figures.* Washington, DC: Author. Retrieved July 3, 2007 from http://www.populationaction.org.

Research Brief. (2005). *Population implosion? Low fertility and policy responses in the European Union.* Cambridge, UK: Rand Corporation. Retrieved July 5, 2007 from http://www.rand.org/pubs/research_briefs/2005/RAND_RB9126.pdf.

Rockefeller Archive Center. (n.d.). *Rockefeller Sanitary Commission for the Eradication of Hookworm Disease.* Retrieved July 15, 2007 from http://archive.rockefeller.edu/collections/rockorgs/hookwormadd.php?printer=1.

Rothman, K.J., & Greenland, S. (2005). Causation and causal inference in epidemiology. *American Journal of Public Health, 95,* (Suppl. 1), 144–150.

South Florida Water Management District. (2007). *Quick facts on residential/community water-use restrictions phase II.* Retrieved July 14, 2007 from http://www.sfwmd.gov/images/pdfs/splash/phase2_resident.pdf.

Subramanian, R. (2006). *Motor vehicle traffic crashes as a leading cause of death in the United States, 2003.* Washington, DC: National Highway Traffic Safety Administration. Retrieved July 16, 2007 from http://www-nrd.nhtsa.dot.gov/pdf/nrd-30/NCSA/RNotes/2006/810568.pdf.

Texas A&M University. (n.d.). *Poisonous plants and plant parts.* Retrieved July 15, 2007 from http://plantanswers.tamu.edu/publications/poison/poison.html.

U.S. Census Bureau. (2002). *International Population Reports WP/02. Global population profile: 2002.* Washington, DC: U.S. Government Printing Office. Retrieved July 5, 2007 from http://www.census.gov/ipc/prod/wp02/wp-02003.pdf.

U.S. Census Bureau. (2004). *Global Population at a Glance: 2002 and Beyond* (WP/02-1). Retrieved July 5, 2007 from http://www.census.gov/ipc/prod/wp02/wp02-1.pdf.

U.S. Census Bureau. (2005). *International Data Base: IDB summary demographic data.* Retrieved July 5, 2007 from http://www.census.gov/ipc/www/idbsum.html.

U.S. Census Bureau. (2007). *World population by age and sex. Table 094. Midyear population, by age and sex.* Retrieved July 15, 2007 from http://www.census.gov/cgi-bin/ipc/idbagg.

U.S. Consumer Product Safety Commission. (2007). *Biological pollutants in your home* [CPSC Document #425]. Washington, DC: Author. Retrieved July 5, 2007 from http://www.cpsc.gov/CPSCPUB/PUBS/425.html.

U.S. Consumer Product Safety Commission. (n.d.). *Carbon monoxide questions and answers* [CPSC Document #466]. Retrieved July 14, 2007 from http://www.cpsc.gov/CPSCPUB/PUBS/466.html.

U.S. Department of Agriculture. (2006). *Foodborne illness: What consumers need to know.* Washington, DC: Author. Retrieved July 5, 2007 from http://www.fsis.usda.gov/Fact_Sheets/Foodborne_Illness_What_Consumers_Need_to_Know/index.asp.

U.S. Department of Energy. (2006). *PV in use: Getting the job done with solar electricity.* Retrieved July 15, 2007 from http://www1.eere.energy.gov/solar/pv_use.html.

U.S. Department of Energy. (2007a). *Biomass research and development initiative.* Retrieved July 15, 2007 from http://www.brdisolutions.com/default.aspx.

U.S. Department of Energy. (2007b). *Geothermal technologies program: GeoPowering the West.* Retrieved July 15, 2007 from http://www1.eere.energy.gov/geothermal/gpw/index.html.

U.S. Department of Health and Human Services. (1991). *Healthy People 2000: National health promotion and disease prevention objectives* [Publication No. S/N 017-001-00474-0]. Washington, DC: U.S. Government Printing Office.

U.S. Department of Health and Human Services. (2000). *Healthy People 2010: Understanding and improving health,* 2nd ed. Washington, DC: U.S. Government Printing Office.

U.S. Department of Housing and Urban Development. (2007). *Healthy homes and lead hazard control: The Lead Safe Housing Rule.* Retrieved July 16, 2007 from http://www.hud.gov/offices/lead/leadsaferule/.

U.S. Environmental Protection Agency. (2002). *Fact sheet: Final drinking water public notification regulations.* Washington, DC: Author. Retrieved July 14, 2007 from http://www.epa.gov/safewater/publicnotification/regulations_rulefactsheet.html.

U.S. Environmental Protection Agency. (2005). *Clean Air Interstate Rule.* Washington, DC: Author. Retrieved July 14, 2007 from http://www.epa.gov/interstateairquality/.

U.S. Environmental Protection Agency. (2006a). *Air quality summary through 2005.* Washington, DC: Author. Retrieved July 13, 2007 from http://www.epa.gov/airtrends/2006/aq_summary_2005.html.

U.S. Environmental Protection Agency. (2006b). *Environmental justice.* Washington, DC: Author. Retrieved July 5, 2007 from http://www.epa.gov/compliance/environmentaljustice/index.html.

U.S. Environmental Protection Agency. (2006c). *Mid-Atlantic integrated assessment: Fecal coliform.* Washington, DC: Author. Retrieved July 14, 2007 from http://www.epa.gov/maia/html/fecal.html.

U.S. Environmental Protection Agency. (2006d). *Safe hazardous waste recycling.* Retrieved July 15, 2007 from http://www.epa.gov/epaoswer/general/manag-hw/e00-001d.pdf.

U.S. Environmental Protection Agency. (2007a). *Acid rain.* Washington, DC: Author. Retrieved July 13, 2007 from http://www.epa.gov/acidrain/index.html.

U.S. Environmental Protection Agency. (2007b). *Assessment of risks from radon in homes.* Washington, DC: Author. Retrieved July 13, 2007 from http://www.epa.gov/radon/risk_assessment.html.

U.S. Environmental Protection Agency. (2007c). *Children's health initiative: Toxic mold.* Retrieved July 16, 2007 from http://www.epa.gov/appcdwww/iemb/child.htm.

U.S. Environmental Protection Agency. (2007d). *Climate change & you: What you can do at home.* Washington, DC: Author. Retrieved July 14, 2007 from http://www.epa.gov/climatechange/wycd/downloads/wycd-home.pdf.

U.S. Environmental Protection Agency. (2007e). *Health and environmental impacts of CO.* Washington, DC: Author. Retrieved July 5, 2007 from http://www.epa.gov/air/urbanair/co/hlth1.html.

U.S. Environmental Protection Agency. (2007f). *Health risks: Exposure to radon causes lung cancer in non-smokers and smokers alike.* Washington, DC: Author. Retrieved July 5, 2007 from http://www.epa.gov/radon/healthrisks.html.

U.S. Environmental Protection Agency. (2007g). *Lead and lead paint.* Retrieved July 16, 2007 from http://www.epa.gov/Region2/health/leadpoisoning.htm.

U.S. Environmental Protection Agency. (2007h). *Radon-resistant new construction.* Washington, DC: Author. Retrieved July 13, 2007 from http://www.epa.gov/radon/construc.html.

U.S. Environmental Protection Agency. (2008). *Environmental indicators: Ozone depletion.* Retrieved August 12, 2008 from http://www.epa.gov/ozone/science/indicat/index.html.

U.S. Food and Drug Administration. (2004). *What you need to know about mercury in fish and shellfish: 2004 EPA and FDA Advice for: Women who might become pregnant, women who are pregnant, nursing mothers, young children* [EPA-823-R-04-005]. Washington, DC: Author. Retrieved July 14, 2007 from http://www.cfsan.fda.gov/~dms/admehg3.html.

U.S. Nuclear Regulatory Commission. (2007). *High-level waste disposal.* Washington, DC: Author. Retrieved July 14, 2007 from http://www.nrc.gov/waste/hlw-disposal.html.

Vlahov, D., Galea, S., & Freudenberg, N. (2005). Toward and urban health advantage. *Journal of Public Health Management & Practice, 11,* 256–258.

Wigle, D.T. (2003). *Child health and the environment.* New York: Oxford University Press, Inc.

Wilcox, L.S. (2005). Health education from 1775 to 2005. *Preventing Chronic Disease, 2* (Special issue), 1–3. Retrieved July 3, 2007 from http://www.cdc.gov/pcd/issues/2005/nov/05_0134.htm.

Wilkerson, R., Northington, L., & Fisher, W. (2005). Ingestion of toxic substances by infants and children: What we don't know can hurt us. *Critical Care Nurse, 25*(4), 35–44.

World Health Organization. (1986). *Health and the environment* (WHO Regional Publications, European Series, no. 19; pp. 12–16). Vienna: Author.

World Health Organization. (2000). *The world health report 2000*. Geneva, Switzerland: Author.

World Health Organization. (2005). *Celebrating water for life: The International Decade for Action 2005–2015. World Day for Water 2005*. Geneva, Switzerland: Author. Retrieved July 14, 2007 from http://www.who.int/water_sanitation_health/2005advocguide/en/print.html.

World Health Organization. (2006). *Air pollution*. Retrieved July 13, 2007 from http://www.euro.who.int/childhealthenv/Risks/AirTop.

Wright, J.M., Schwartz, J., & Dockery, D.W. (2004). The effect of disinfection by-products and mutagenic activity on birth weight and gestational duration. *Environmental Health Perspectives, 112*, 920–925.

Yassi, A., Kjellstrom, T., de Kok, T., & Guidotti, T.L. (2001). *Basic environmental health*. Oxford: Oxford University Press.

Yucca Mountain Information Office. (2007). Yucca Mountain licensing update. Retrieved July 14, 2007 from http://www.yuccamountain.org/license.htm.

Zgodzinski, E.J., & Fallon, L.F. (2005). The history of public health. In L.F. Fallon, & E.J. Zgodzinski (Eds.). *Essentials of public health management*. (pp. 7–17). Sudbury, MA: Jones & Bartlett Publishers.

Selected Readings

American Public Health Association, Public Health Nursing Section. (2005). *Environmental health principles & recommendations for public health nursing*. Washington, DC: Author.

Berke, E.M., Koepsell, T.D., Moudon, A.V., et al. (2007). Association of the built environment with physical activity and obesity in older persons. *American Journal of Public Health, 97*, 486–492.

Choi, M., Afzal, B., & Sattler, B. (2006). Geographic information systems: A new tool for environmental health assessments. *Public Health Nursing, 23*, 381–391.

Harnish, K.E., Butterfield, P., & Hill, W.G. (2006). Does Dixon's Integrative Environmental Health Model inform an understanding of rural parents' perceptions of local environmental health risks? *Public Health Nursing, 23*, 465–471.

National Center for Injury Prevention and Control. (2006). *Injury Fact Book 2006*. Atlanta, GA: Centers for Disease Control and Prevention. Retrieved July 16, 2007 from http://www.cdc.gov/ncipc/fact_book/factbook.htm.

Resnick, D.B., & Wing, S. (2007). Lessons learned from the Children's Environmental Exposure Research Study. *American Journal of Public Health, 97*, 414–418.

Ryan, M.A. (2006). The politics of risk: A human rights paradigm for children's environmental health research. *Environmental Health Perspectives, 114*, 1613–1616.

Schim, S.M., Benkert, R., Bell, S.E., et al. (2006). Social justice: Added metaparadigm concept for urban health nursing. *Public Health Nursing, 24*, 73–80.

Internet Resources

Agency for Toxic Substances and Disease Registry [ATSDR]: *http://www.atsdr.cdc.gov/default.htm*

ATSDR Environmental Health Nursing Initiative: *http://www.atsdr.cdc.gov/EHN*

American Public Health Association (Section on Environment): *http://depts.washington.edu/aphaenv/*

Centers for Disease Control and Prevention (Environmental Health): *http://www.cdc.gov/Environmental/*

Health Care Without Harm: *http://www.noharm.org*

Household Products Database: *http://householdproducts.nlm.nih.gov/*

Luminary Project: *http://www.TheLuminaryProject.org*

National Center for Health Housing: *http://www.healthyhomestraining.org/Nurse/PEHA.htm*

National Environmental Health Association: *http://www.neha.org/*

National Institute of Environmental Health Sciences: *http://www.niehs.nih.gov/*

National Library of Medicine (Tox Town): *http://toxtown.nlm.nih.gov/*

Natural Resources Defense Council: *http://www.nrdc.org*

Physicians for Social Responsibility: *http://www.envirohealthaction.org/*

Population Action International: *http://www.populationaction.org/*

U.S. Consumer Product Safety Commission: *http://www.cpsc.gov/*

U. S. Environmental Protection Agency (Climate Change): *http://www.epa.gov/climatechange/*

U. S. Environmental Protection Agency (UV Index Forecast Map): *http://www.epa.gov/sunwise/uvindex.html#map*

U. S. Food and Drug Administration: *http://www.fda.gov/*

U.S. Geological Survey (Toxic Substances Hydrology Program): *http://toxics.usgs.gov*

University of Maryland – School of Nursing: *http://envirn.umaryland.edu/*

World Health Organization: *http://www.who.int/topics/environmental_health/en/*

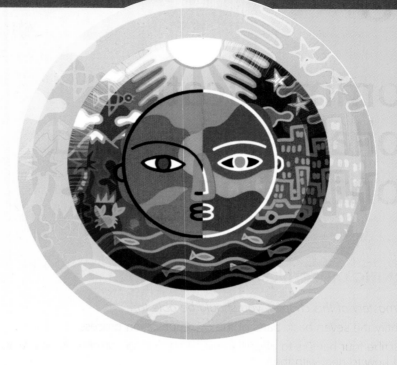

COMMUNITY
HEALTH NURSING
TOOLBOX

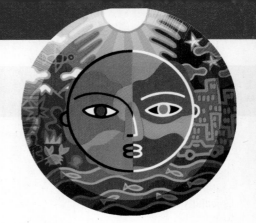

10

Communication, Collaboration, and Contracting

LEARNING OBJECTIVES

Upon mastery of this chapter, you should be able to:

◆ Identify the seven basic parts of the communication process.

◆ Describe four barriers to effective communication in community health nursing and how to deal with them.

◆ Explain three sets of skills necessary for effective communication in community health nursing.

◆ Summarize the key issues related to health literacy.

◆ Explain the stages of group process.

◆ Differentiate between task roles and maintenance roles.

◆ Describe five characteristics of collaboration in community health.

◆ Compare the three phases common to the collaboration process.

◆ Identify four features of contracting in community health nursing.

◆ Discuss the value of contracting to both clients and community health nurses.

◆ Design an aggregate-level contract useful in community health nursing.

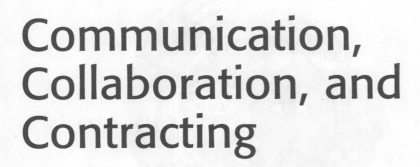

"Think like a wise man but communicate in the language of the people."
—William Butler Yeats (1865–1939)

KEY TERMS

Active listening
Brainstorming
Channel
Collaboration
Communication
Contracting
Critical pathway
Decoding
Delphi technique
Electronic meetings
Empathy
Encoding
Feedback loop
Formal contracting
Group process
Health literacy
Informal contracting
Message
Nominal group technique
Nonverbal messages
Nursing informatics
Paraphrasing
Receiver
Sender
Verbal messages

Communication, collaboration, and contracting are primary tools for community health nurses. They form the basis for effective relationships that contribute both to the prevention of illness and to the protection and promotion of aggregate health. To use these concepts skillfully in community health practice, it is important to understand their meaning and value. Because of its relationship to health promotion and disease prevention and management, health literacy is a concept that is becoming more important to health care providers, especially those in public settings. For the nurse accustomed to communicating one-on-one with clients, communication with aggregates, along with a wide range of professionals and lay community workers, requires new skills. Application of group process skills will facilitate work with both task and support groups. The computer, with its teleconferencing, telehealth, Internet and e-mail capabilities, as well as personal digital assistants, global positioning, and information systems, enriches communication and virtually brings the world into the home and work settings. Group work is a key component of community health nursing. Unlike ordinary social relationships, collaborative relationships are based on a team approach with shared responsibilities and mutual participation in establishing and carrying out goals. Clients and health care professionals enter into a working agreement, or contract, tailored to address specific client needs. The concept of contracting can further assist the collaborative process. This chapter examines these tools and discusses their integration into community health nursing practice.

COMMUNICATION IN COMMUNITY HEALTH NURSING

Groups cannot exist without communication, nor can nurses practice without communication. These facts often are taken for granted, since most people spend most of their waking hours communicating: speaking, listening, reading, or writing. Yet, the quality of people's communication has far-reaching effects. Lack of effective communication can lead to misunderstanding, poor performance, interpersonal conflict, ineffective programs, weak public policy, medical mistakes, and many other undesirable outcomes (Arora, Johnson, Lovinger, Humphrey, & Meltzer, 2005; Kurtz, Silverman, & Draper, 2005; McKnight, Stetson, Bakken, et al., 2002). Effective communication is vital to all areas of nursing, and techniques can be used to improve communication (Boyle & Kochinda, 2004). To communicate, people must have, construct, or create shared realities and meanings. In other words, they must engage in an exchange that is both understood and meaningful. **Communication** involves transferring meaning and enhancing understanding.

Communication is the lifeblood of effective community health nursing practice. A recent study identified public health nurses' (PHNs) use of communication as a "core concept of client supervision," and found that important components included "building a trusting relationship, . . . creating a partnership and equality, . . . and . . . trying to act in the clients' best interest" (Tveiten & Severinsson, 2006, p. 235).

Communication provides a two-way flow of information that nourishes professional–client and professional–professional relationships. It also establishes the base of information on which health planning decisions are made and programs developed. For communication to take place, clients and professionals need to send and receive messages.

As participants in the communication process, community health nurses play both roles: sender and receiver. The nurse working with a group of abused women must learn to "read" the messages these women send. Similarly, as a member of a health planning team, the nurse must be able to elicit ideas as well as contribute to the planning process by speaking and acting in ways that communicate effectively.

Communication serves several functions in community health nursing. It provides information for decision-making at all levels of community health. From the choice of goals for a small client support group to health policy affecting a population at risk, decisions are enhanced through effective communication. Communication functions as a motivator by clarifying information, so that consensus is reached and the people involved can move forward with commitment to shared goals. Effective communication facilitates the expression of feelings and promotes closer working relationships. It also controls behavior by providing clear expectations and boundaries for group-member actions.

The Communication Process

Communication occurs as a sequence of events or a process. The process consists of seven basic parts that work together to result in the transference and understanding of meaning. These parts are:

1. a message
2. a sender
3. a receiver
4. encoding
5. a channel
6. decoding
7. a feedback loop (Finkelman, 2006).

The first part of the communication process is a **message**, which is an expression of the purpose of communication. Without the message, there can be no communication. The next two parts include a sender and a receiver. The **sender** is the person (or persons) conveying a message, and the **receiver** is the person (or persons) to whom the message is directed and who is the intended recipient of the message. The fourth step is the act of **encoding**, which refers to the sender's conversion of the message into symbolic form. This involves how the sender translates the message to the receiver. It can be accomplished through verbal and/or nonverbal means. For example, a nurse teaching breathing techniques to a prenatal class may explain verbally while also demonstrating the correct procedures. The degree of the sender's success in encoding is influenced by the sender's communication skills, knowledge about the topic of the message, attitudes and feelings related to the message and the receiver, and the feelings, beliefs, and values held by the sender. The fifth part involves a **channel**, or the medium through which the sender conveys the message. The channel may be a written, spoken, or nonverbal expression. Examples include an e-mail stating a request, a report providing information, a written care plan, a verbal request for clarification, or a facial expression indicating confusion. Communication channels may be formal, such as a written grant proposal, or informal, such as a face-to-face verbal statement or an e-mail message.

Once the sender has conveyed a message through a channel, the receiver must translate the message into an understandable form, called **decoding**, which is the sixth

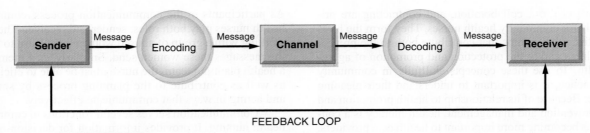

FEEDBACK LOOP

FIGURE 10.1 The communication process (feedback loop).

part of the communication process. The receiver's ability to decode the message is influenced by knowledge of the topic, skills in reading and listening, attitudes, and sociocultural values. All communication involves perception and expectation. We interpret messages based upon prior experiences; either with the sender/receiver or with others who have influenced our lives (e.g., families, peers, bosses) (Finkelman, 2006). The seventh and final part is a **feedback loop**, which refers to the receiver's indication that the message has been understood (decoded) in the way that the sender intended (encoded). It requires feedback from the receiver to the sender, serving as a check on the success of the transference of meaning (Finkelman, 2006). Figure 10.1 portrays the seven components of the communication process.

Communication Barriers

Community health nurses should be aware of the barriers that block effective communication. This section discusses four barriers that pose particular problems: selective perception, language barriers, filtering, and emotions (Robbins, 2003).

Selective Perception

Receivers in the communication process interpret a message through their own perceptions, which are influenced by their own experience, interests, values, motivations, and expectations. They project this perceptual screen onto the communication process as they decode a message. They might distort or misinterpret the meaning from the sender's original intent. For example, the nurse may propose a class session on nutrition to a group of elderly persons, and the clients may translate that message to mean a focus on dieting for weight loss, which is not the intended meaning. Nurses can overcome this barrier by using the feedback loop to ask clients or others involved to voice their understanding of the message. In this case, the nurse could ask the elderly clients what the term *nutrition* means to them. This provides an opportunity for clarification and correction of misunderstandings, which is an essential step in the communication process and helps to prevent miscommunication that can lead to mistakes (see Perspectives: Student Voices).

 PERSPECTIVES
STUDENT VOICES

The Case of the Misunderstood Directions

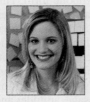 When I was in my junior year of nursing school, my grandfather began to have some intestinal problems. He thought at first it was just a little constipation, and he started drinking prune juice and added more fiber to his diet. The problem got worse, so he went to his family doctor and was told that he had a fecal impaction and needed to "take some enemas" before coming back to see the doctor who would then manually remove the fecal impaction. Because I had worked for this physician during the past two summers, he did not take a lot of time explaining the procedure to my grandfather. My grandfather is a very quiet man, a hard-working retired farmer who reads a lot and likes to listen to radio news and talk shows. The doctor told him to "take a couple of Fleets enemas, and then an oil retention enema" and to come back and see him in 2 days for removal of the fecal impaction. My grandfather had never before in his 79 years had an enema and didn't quite understand what he was supposed to do. Also, he was a bit embarrassed and didn't ask me about it either. He lives alone, and bought the enemas at a local chain drugstore—also not asking for directions from the clerk there. When he returned for his appointment, the doctor asked him how it went with the enemas. My grandfather replied, "Well the little ones weren't so bad, but that big oily one was really hard to swallow." You can imagine the doctor's reaction! My intelligent, confident grandfather had drunk the enemas! The doctor assumed that a man of his age, with a granddaughter in nursing school, would know what to do with enemas. He was sorely mistaken and very embarrassed! As was my grandfather, upon learning the correct administration of an enema. I was amazed that this could have happened and relieved that my grandfather didn't aspirate the oil retention enema. You always think that only poor, uneducated, or non-English speaking patients have problems like this, but that is not always the case. I learned that day how important it is to always have the patient explain their perception of your instructions back to you. It has come in handy in my community health nursing rotation, where many of my clients have real communication barriers. I always think about my grandfather, with all of his experience and knowledge, and remember that not everyone understands things the way you think you have explained them.

Rachel, age 34

Language Barriers

People interpret the meaning of words differently, depending on many variables, such as age, education, cultural background, and primary spoken language. An adolescent understands the terms *sweet* and *tight* to mean that something is fashionable or desirable, whereas an 80-year-old woman might understand the terms to mean sugary and confining, respectively. In community health, nurses work with a wide range of clients and professionals whose disparate ages, education levels, and cultural backgrounds lead to different communication patterns. The use of scientific terminology or jargon by some health professionals can be confusing, as in the case of the Hmong refugee woman who was asked whether her son had experienced enuresis—a term she had never heard before. If the nurse had not used medical jargon, or had explained the term, or even asked the question using an illustrative example, the woman would have been able to more accurately answer the question. Instead of just nodding her head "yes"—meaning "I hear you," the mother could have conveyed the correct message "no, my son does not wet the bed at night" (see From the Case Files). The use of unfamiliar terms can become a barrier to communication. Client differences in language and communication style must be taken into consideration during the communication process (Rubenfeld & Scheffer, 2006).

Filtering Information

A third barrier to communication is filtering, which means manipulation of information by the sender to influence the receiver's response. To gain favor with receivers, senders sometimes say what they believe receivers want to hear rather than the whole truth (Robbins, 2003). Clients sometimes use filtering during a needs assessment process, giving only partial or distorted information because they think this is what health professionals want to hear. Filtering can also affect PHNs. Cole (1990), in a classic work, notes that we have "filters" through which we view others—often influenced by culture and socioeconomic class or even gender—and these can lead to miscommunication. Cole's premise is that dissimilar people actually view the world differently, thus confounding communication and leading to prejudice and stereotyping. Another intent of filtering is to slant information. Prepared minutes from a meeting or a department's quarterly report can emphasize some points and omit or de-emphasize others, giving (sometimes unintentionally) false impressions that influence decision-making.

Emotional Influence

How a person feels at the time a message is sent or received influences its meaning. Senders can distort messages and

---

From the Case Files

Mr. Sanchez Needs an Interpreter

I am in community health nursing now, but I work as an extern at our small, local county hospital helping out in the ER. A man came in one Saturday a month or so ago with a bad cut to his right hand from a push lawnmower—you know, the kind without a motor. Mr. Sanchez was trying to clean the grass from the blades and cut himself pretty badly. The ER doc asked him if he had received a tetanus shot recently, and he quickly nodded "yes." He spoke a little English, but I could tell that he was having some trouble understanding some of our questions. His friend, who brought him to the ER, did not speak English at all. We couldn't find an interpreter—they are always stretched so thin. None of us spoke Spanish. Anyway, we didn't give him a tetanus booster—just cleaned his wound, closed it with stitches, bandaged it, and told him to keep it clean. He was given a prescription for an antibiotic medication. It was a busy night, and I didn't think about it much. A few weeks later, Mr. Sanchez was back in the hospital because his wound had gotten infected and he had used a needle to drain some pus from his hand (he hadn't gotten the prescription filled because he had no insurance and no money because he was off work now). Unfortunately, by poking around with the needle, he had provided a perfect, anaerobic place for tetanus to flourish. He now was in the ICU with full blown tetanus. I have never seen anything like this! He was on a ventilator and had to be "paralyzed," so that we could get air into him. I had only read about opisthotonos—in which the body arches with only feet and head touching the bed because of a tetanic spasm—but now I was seeing it firsthand. This poor man was completely rigid, and we were trying to give him meds to relax him and permit the ventilator to work, but at the same time we were working to keep his blood pressure from dropping too low from the meds. Mr. Sanchez spent 30 agonizing days in ICU—all because he nodded "yes" to the doc's question about the tetanus booster. In hindsight, he evidently just wanted to get out of the ER and didn't truly understand the question. A $5 tetanus booster could have prevented all of this misery and expense. (He had no insurance and was an illegal alien, so the county paid the bill.) We should have used an interpreter; should have insisted on it; should have waited until one was available. They are always in short supply—but I truly understand the importance of a translator now. I have some Spanish-speaking clients in my community health nursing rotation. I do my best to speak with them, but when I need to be sure that something is fully understood—I request that an interpreter accompany me on my home visits. I remember Mr. Sanchez and what happens when you don't use an interpreter.

Amy, age 24

receivers can interpret messages incorrectly when emotions cloud their perception. Emotions can interfere with rational and objective reasoning, thus blocking communication. Nurses need to be aware of their own emotions as they send messages. To avoid misunderstandings, they also need to ascertain the emotional status of clients or health professionals with whom they are communicating. For example, it is important for community health nurses to remain calm and unruffled when dealing with families in crisis. Family communication may be angry, blaming, and confrontational because of a serious health crisis with a child, for instance. A PHN who responds with frustration, defensiveness, or anger only heightens the family's emotional reactions. A calm, firm, reassuring presence can go far in diffusing the situation and promoting clearer and more constructive communication. It is always helpful to be aware of the receiver's emotional status and help the receiver to identify it. You may say, "I sense that you are feeling upset about Joey's diagnosis. Are there any questions I can answer for you? How can I be of assistance?"

Core Communication Skills

Overcoming the barriers to effective communication just described requires the development of sound communication skills. Community health nurses need to cultivate three sets of communication skills: sending skills, receiving skills, and interpersonal skills.

Sending Skills

Sending skills enable nurses to transmit messages effectively. Through these skills, nurses convey information to clients and other persons. Two important considerations influence the clarity and effectiveness of message sending. First, the extent of the nurse's self-awareness affects the communication. Does the nurse feel anxious, angry, tired, impatient, or concerned? Does the nurse find certain individuals irritating or offensive? What motives and interests prompt the communication? Second, the nurse's awareness of the receiver influences the sending of messages. What do clients or the professionals with whom the nurse is interacting want or need? Is the message suited to their cultural background and level of understanding? Does the message have significance for them? How are receivers responding as the nurse sends the message?

Two main channels are used to send messages: nonverbal and verbal. **Nonverbal messages**, those conveyed without words, constitute a large portion of the messages transmitted in normal communication. People send messages nonverbally in many ways. Personal appearance, dress, posture, facial expression, gestures, and physical distance between sender and receiver all communicate messages. These nonverbal statements may enhance or discredit what someone says verbally (Robbins, 2003; Finkelman, 2006). Body language often speaks louder than words. Facial expressions convey acceptance or rejection, interest or boredom, anger or patience, fear or confidence. Gestures and bodily movements, such as clenched hands, crossed arms, tapping fingers, hands on hips, or a turned shoulder, all communicate messages. Eye contact, or lack of it, carries additional meaning—and may be culturally mediated. Tone of voice and use of silence also send nonverbal messages. Accepting food in certain situations may communicate approval and the desire to be friendly. Nonverbal messages may have different cultural meanings or social interpretations (Spector, 2009). Nurse self-awareness and validation of meaning can save considerable misunderstanding.

Verbal messages are communicated ideas, attitudes, and feelings transmitted by speaking or writing. Nurses cannot assume that the intent of their words always is understood by clients or other professionals. Effective sending skills depend on asking for feedback to make certain that receivers have understood the verbal message's intent. Communication is more effective if speakers avoid using jargon that is unfamiliar to clients. Like all occupations, nursing has its own vocabulary, or jargon, that may not be understood by clients and that may make them feel ignorant or inferior. For example, the terms *critical pathways* or *case-management approach* may have little meaning to a community group. Nurses must make a special effort to avoid using jargon that is part of nursing's everyday speech. The basic rules for effective sending can be summarized in this manner:

1. Keep the message honest and uncomplicated.
2. Use as few words as possible to state it.
3. Ask for reactions (feedback) to make certain that the message is understood.

Receiving Skills

Receiving skills are as important to communication as sending skills. They involve not only listening to what people say but also observing their behavior and nonverbal cues. They enable nurses to receive accurate and complete messages. If members of a seniors' exercise class agree to certain exercises but do not participate in them, they are sending a message. What message is their behavior sending? Were the proposed exercises too difficult? Did they misunderstand the nurse's instructions about how to perform the exercises? Are they resisting in other areas of the program? Effective receiving skills require attending to nonverbal as well as verbal messages and seeking feedback to understand their meaning.

An essential skill needed for receiving messages is **active listening** or reflective listening, which is the skill of assuming responsibility for and striving to understand the feelings and thoughts in a sender's message. Instead of expecting clients or others to help the nurse understand, the nurse should actively work to discover what clients mean. Understanding the message from the sender's perspective demands careful attention, which arises from a genuine interest in what the speaker has to say. Active listeners demonstrate their interest, perhaps by sitting forward, sustaining eye contact, nodding the head, and asking occasional questions for clarification (Fowler, 2006; Kar, Arcalay, & Alex, 2001). At times, **paraphrasing**, or repeating back to the sender what the receiver heard, is helpful in clarifying the sender's meaning. Summarizing your perceptions at the end of a home visit, for instance, helps to assure that the client's communication has been accurately interpreted. Active listening keeps us engaged; behaviors, such as daydreaming or pretending to be listening, block communication. Because we can listen to over 600 words a minute, but we can speak fewer than 200 words a minute, it is important to focus and concentrate to stay engaged and keep your mind from wandering. Fowler (2006) suggests that you mentally repeat key words as your client speaks to you; this will help to reinforce your understanding and keep you from straying from the conversation. Also, the content and feeling of the sender's message may be overwhelming at times, and you can become preoccupied with formulating a response rather than listening actively. Nadig (2006) notes that we often listen to our own personal beliefs and values when clients are speaking, and make judgments about their messages. This interferes with effective communication; in these situations, paraphrasing can help you to stay focused. An example of the skill of paraphrasing follows:

Client: I don't think I can manage my elderly mother at home any longer. I know she never wanted to go to a nursing home, but with my job and the kids, caring for her is becoming impossible. My husband is so helpful, but I feel guilty burdening him. I'll be going against my mother's wishes if I place her somewhere, though.

Nurse: You sound like you are feeling frustrated caring for your mother and your family while maintaining a job, and you're not sure what is the best action to take.

Nurses also can listen actively by asking reflective questions that restate what clients or others have said to clarify the received meaning. Reflective questions have a twofold purpose: to show a sincere attempt to understand the senders' messages, and to make clear that the messages and the people who send them are important to the nurse. An example of a reflective question follows:

Class members state: Quitting smoking is impossible.
The nurse asks: Do you feel you can't quit smoking?

Active listening helps to communicate acceptance and increase trust, especially when the listener refrains from making any negative judgments of the message or the way it is delivered. Clients may simply need to be "heard and acknowledged" before they can accept suggestions (Nadig, 2006, p. 12). A critical response to the client's message by the nurse cuts off communication. Many nurses note that "a curtain drops"—a visible change of expression takes place—when the client *disengages* in response to a nurse's judgmental response. Active listening enables nurses to encourage clients to deliberate carefully and to exercise problem-solving skills; it avoids the pitfall of telling clients what to do. It is also a good initial response when your client seems hurt or angry, or is expressing dissatisfaction with you (Nadig, 2006). By asking reflective questions, the nurse continues to clarify the messages clients send. You can reflect back to clients their:

- Facts and information
- Thoughts and beliefs
- Feelings and emotions
- Wants, needs, motivations
- Hopes and expectations (Nadig, 2006).

Interpersonal Skills

Effective communication in community health nursing also requires interpersonal skills. Three types of interpersonal skills build on sending and receiving skills but go beyond the mere exchange of messages. They are showing respect, empathizing, and developing trust and rapport.

Showing Respect

Showing respect means conveying the attitude that clients and others have importance, dignity, and worth—a concept basic to nursing practice (Harper, 2006). Community health nurses can express respect by treating clients' ideas and comments as valuable and worthy of attention. You can demonstrate an interest in wanting to understand the situation from the other person's point of view. We show respect by the manner in which we address people—for instance, by using the courtesy titles of "Mr." or "Mrs." until it is determined how the client wants to be addressed. On a more subtle level, the tone of voice the nurse uses can show respect or make people feel inferior and insignificant. Nonverbal cues and active listening can indicate to clients that you are fully engaged and interested in their issues. Clients, community members, and other professionals need to feel respected if they are to enter fully into the mutual exchange necessary for effective communication (Display 10.1).

DISPLAY 10.1 **HEALTH COMMUNICATION—ONE DISPARITY: LOW-LITERACY CLIENTS**

Most poorly educated populations, those with the lowest literacy levels, have the highest mortality and morbidity. Changing demographics suggest that low literacy is an increasing problem among certain racial and ethnic groups, non–English-speaking populations, and persons older than 65 years of age, although the majority of people with low literacy are white native-born Americans (U. S. Department of Health and Human Services, 2000). Yet it has been well documented that most health information pamphlets, brochures, and other materials cannot be read or comprehended by low-literacy adults. Communication with these high-risk groups should be simplified and should include easy-to-read materials. At the same time, there is the danger of making the communication so simple that the reader feels insulted. Low literacy does not necessarily mean low intelligence. How does the nurse find the right balance?

The goal of communication is to achieve understanding. If clients are to understand health communication—whether the messages are spoken or written—they must be given ample opportunity to provide feedback. Pamphlets and other written health information should be reviewed by their intended audiences before final printing and distribution. Proposed users should comment on the readability and acceptability of both text and graphics. With spoken communication, nurses should regularly solicit feedback to make certain that messages are understood.

Empathizing

Empathizing is another important interpersonal skill. **Empathy** is the ability to communicate understanding and to vicariously experience the feelings and thoughts of others—a type of "emotional engagement" (Edelman & Mandle, 2006, p. 82). It is similar to the "moral value" of compassion (Von Dietze & Orb, 2000, p. 166) and involves "perspective-taking" (Lobchuk, 2006, p. 330). We show empathy by striving to put ourselves in our client's shoes—by reflecting their feelings and expressing that message in the receiver's language. The nurse should use the same terms and, if possible, the same tone of voice as the other person did. For example, you should assume a serious manner if the speaker seems serious. Empathy conveys the message, "This is the way it seems to me. Is that correct?" The nurse should keep validating the speaker's true feelings to be certain that the message is being interpreted correctly. Empathy focuses attention on receivers and their feelings, thus reducing clients' anxiety and defensiveness. It builds trust and a greater level of understanding, and shows that the nurse shares clients' concerns and makes them feel that their contributions are valued (Edelman & Mandle, 2006; Finkelman, 2006).

Developing Trust and Rapport

Developing trust is necessary for effective communication. Rapport—a warm, friendly, trusting relationship—develops when nurses are open, genuine, and demonstrate true concern for their clients. Building trust and rapport with clients is usually the first goal for community health nurses. Clients and others will not express their true feelings if they do not fully trust the nurse. Many times, clients say what they think the nurse wants to hear. They may agree to a plan of action simply because they do not want to displease the nurse, or they may hide their true feelings because they think that the nurse is eager for a decision. Agreeing with others, especially with people who are in powerful positions and from different cultures, is the polite and respectful thing to do in some cultures (Spector, 2009). The nurse who is unaware of this fact may interpret the client's agreement as understanding, thus a "teachable moment" is lost.

Nurses develop trust in the communication process by being trustworthy—doing as they have promised, being reliable. We can also do this by showing that we truly accept others, that we believe in them as people. In a qualitative study by Falk-Rafael, clients of PHNs noted that a trusting relationship is developed when the PHN shows respect and enhances their dignity while "creating a safe environment" by being nonjudgmental and showing empathy (2001, p. 5). Trust generates trust; as the nurse shows confidence in clients and the other professionals with whom the nurse is communicating, they will respond in kind. Treating people as fully participating partners in the communication process means demonstrating that they are trustworthy and responsible. Trust also is developed through an open, honest, and patient approach with others. Candid discussion in a flexible timeframe encourages people to share their real feelings and to move at their own pace. We can model behaviors we want our clients to adopt. Clients appreciate nurses who are "authentic" and honest with them, who are "down to earth"

and admit when they don't have all of the answers (Falk-Rafael, 2001, p. 5). We can promote trust by:

◆ Trusting our clients to do as they have committed.
◆ Clarifying expectations, anticipated behaviors, and boundaries of the nurse–client relationship.
◆ Demonstrating consistency.
◆ Being aware of attitudes and behaviors that do not promote trust (Gallant, Beaulieu, & Carnevale, 2002).

As trust develops, communication becomes more free-flowing and productive. When that occurs, you can become much more effective as a community health nurse and better able to assist your clients.

Factors Influencing Communication

In a helping relationship, it is important for the community health nurse to demonstrate effective communication. It is important to project:

◆ Openness, genuineness, and self-awareness (ability to reflect on one's strengths and weaknesses)
◆ Sensitivity, acceptance, concern, and respect for the client
◆ Knowledge, self-confidence, creativity, and empathy
◆ Ability to problem-solve and to confront when necessary (Edelman & Mandle, 2006, p. 87)

Effective communication, both sending and receiving, is strongly influenced by three factors: previous experiences, culture, and relationships.

Previous experiences of both sender and receiver influence their perceptions and the meanings they attach to messages. For example, adolescents who are having difficulty with parents' authority may hear the nurse's suggestion to "learn more about sexually transmitted diseases" as an authoritarian command or effort to exert control. Requests for clarification help to verify that messages are being received as intended.

The respective cultures of sender and receiver influence understanding and acceptance of messages. A nervous laugh, appropriate as an outlet in one culture, may appear rude and disrespectful to someone from another culture. Silence, which in Native American cultures indicates patience and thoughtfulness, may be interpreted as weakness or indifference to someone not familiar with these cultural practices. With many clients, the nurse must communicate cross-culturally, which requires patience and constant effort to ensure accurate and inoffensive messages (Williams, 2006; Spector, 2009).

Health Literacy and Health Outcomes

Health literacy has been defined as "the ability to read, understand, and act on health information" (Andrus & Roth, 2002, p. 282). Nutbeam (2000) delineates three different levels of health literacy and their outcomes (Table 10.1). Comprehension of health information, either verbal or written, is important for clients in maintaining their health and the health of their families (Nielsen-Bohlman, 2004)—in fact, poor health literacy has been associated with poorer health status and increased health costs (Andrus & Roth, 2002).

TABLE 10.1 Levels of Health Literacy

Health Literacy Level	Outcome
Functional health literacy	Communication of factual information on health risks, health services and screenings; better compliance with prescribed actions
Interactive health literacy	Improved ability to independently act on knowledge and develop skills; increased motivation
Critical health literacy	Empowerment of individuals and communities; better resilience to economic and social problems; community action on economic and social determinants of health

Adapted from Nutbeam, D. (2000). Health literacy as a public health goal: A challenge for contemporary health education and communication strategies into the 21st century. *Health Promotion International, 15*(3), p. 266.

A recent study found that lower scores on a measure of functional health literacy were statistically correlated with poorer glycemic control and retinopathy in a group of type 2 diabetic patients (Schillinger, Grumbach, Piette, et al., 2002). In a study of 653 Medicare enrollees with chronic diseases, almost one-quarter of the participants tested had inadequate health literacy, and over 10% had only marginal skills in that area (Gazmararian, Williams, Peel, & Baker, 2003). Those patients with health literacy difficulties demonstrated significantly less understanding of their disease than those without health literacy problems—a fact that could lead to greater complications and costs. Health literacy can also affect health promotion and disease prevention.

Another study found that low health literacy was a better predictor of cervical cancer knowledge than either education or ethnicity in a group of English-speaking ambulatory clinic patients (Lindau, Tomori, Lyons, et al., 2002). Over 40% of the women in this study were tested and found to have low health literacy. Understanding the purposes for receiving regular Papanicolaou (Pap) tests is a fundamental prerequisite to getting them—and the benefits of regular Pap testing are well documented.

Almost half of U.S. adults have been found to have deficits in regard to reading and math skills, and could be classified as having only basic literacy or a level below that—meaning that they can perform only simple everyday activities or have only the most simple and concrete skills (Andrus & Roth, 2002; National Assessment of Adult Literacy [NAAL], 2003). Health literacy goes beyond the basic definitions of literacy, however, and can include such things as cultural literacy and computer literacy, as well as scientific, media, and technological literacy (Kickbusch, 2001). *Healthy People 2010* defines health literacy as: "The capacity to obtain, interpret, and understand basic health information and services and the competence to use such information and services to enhance health" (USDHHS, Health Communication, 2006, ¶ 16).

Health literacy is characterized as critical to health promotion and disease prevention, and *Healthy People 2010* goals include improvement of health literacy and health communication for our population (Display 10.2). Health communication encompasses the concept of health literacy, but also incorporates health messages and campaigns, along with mass media and consumer health issues that are targeted to populations. Population health promotion is best achieved by health communication that uses "multiple communication channels . . . to reach specific audience segments with information that is

---

DISPLAY 10.2 *HEALTHY PEOPLE 2010:* HEALTH LITERACY AND HEALTH COMMUNICATION

These are only a portion of the *Healthy People 2010* objectives related to health literacy or health communication:

11-2. Improve the health literacy of persons with inadequate or marginal literacy skills.

11-3. Increase the proportion of health communication activities that include research and evaluation.

11-4. Increase the proportion of health-related World Wide Web sites that disclose information that can be used to assess the quality of the site.

11-5. Increase the number of centers for excellence that seek to advance the research and practice of health communication.

7-3. Increase the proportion of college and university students who receive information from their institution on each of the six priority health-risk behavior areas.

7-7. Increase the proportion of health care organizations that provide patient and family education.

7-8. Increase the proportion of patients who report that they are satisfied with the patient education they receive from their health care organization.

7-9. Increase the proportion of hospitals and managed care organizations that provide community disease prevention and health promotion activities that address the priority health needs identified by their community.

7-11. Increase the proportion of local health departments that have established culturally appropriate and linguistically competent community health promotion and disease prevention programs.

23-2. Increase the proportion of Federal, Tribe, State, and local health agencies that have made information available to the public in the past year on the Leading Health Indicators, Health Status Indicators, and Priority Data Needs.

From *www.healthypeople.gov/hpscripts/searchobjectives_FT.asp*

appropriate and relevant to them" (USDHHS, Health Communication, 2006, ¶ 5). More information on these topics can be found in Chapter 11.

Because much of community health nursing involves groups, the relationships among group members can significantly influence the effectiveness of communication. When many people are involved, group communication patterns can be complex, and interaction requires skill on the nurse's part to elicit feedback from all members and to generate a common understanding among the group's members.

Communicating with Groups

An important aspect of communication in community health nursing involves working with groups of people. Community health nurses are regularly involved in committees, task forces, and other work-related groups. Nurses also work with aggregates in small groups—often teaching, gathering community assessment and evaluation data, and facilitating support groups. We need to understand how to organize groups and how groups function and develop over time, as well as techniques for facilitating group support and decision-making.

Group Development

Think about the first time you walked into a nursing classroom—you didn't know the teacher or any of the other students in your group. What were your feelings? What did you expect or need the teacher to do? How did your feelings and expectations about the students and teacher change by the end of the term? Changes in group dynamics over time are termed **group process**.

Groups may consist of organized workgroups or they may simply come together because of a common need or task. When a group of people first comes together, group members are often hesitant, quiet, and depend very much on the group leader or facilitator to give them structure and guidance (George Mason University Center for Service and Leadership [CSL], 2006). Members may feel awkward and need to be reassured. Acceptance is foremost in each group member's mind. This first stage of group development is termed *forming* (see Display 10.3).

At this stage, the group leader's task is to help the members become oriented to each other and the work or purpose at hand. Ice-breaker activities, to introduce members to each and move past the awkwardness and hesitancy, are often used at the first group meeting. Conflict and sensitive topics, or too much self-disclosure by leaders or group members, are to be avoided at this stage. Rather, it is important to set ground rules (e.g., no sharing personal information outside of support group) and define the scope of work and timeline for completion. A component of group process involves how members address the work of the group (task role) and the personal or relationship issues (maintenance role) derived from membership in the group (USDHHS Substance Abuse and Mental Health Services Administration [SAMHSA], 2006). In the first stage, task roles are the major focus, with maintenance roles emerging in later stages (see Task, Maintenance and Nonfunctional Roles, Display 10.4).

The next stage is called *storming*,, because conflict and competition become more common as the group develops ideas about the task in a work group, or gets down to sharing more sensitive issues in a support group. Some conflict may not be readily apparent, as some members choose to be quiet and not express their feelings. It is important for the leader to make sure that all members have an opportunity to participate. Problem-solving is the goal of this stage, along with listening to others' opinions. Modeling maintenance roles, by encouraging group members, asking for a quiet member to contribute to the group, and summarizing group feelings, is helpful in moving group members along in maintenance as well as task roles.

By the time group members begin to show signs of cohesiveness, they have moved on to the *norming* stage, and work begins to progress. Trust and openness are much more apparent, and there is a shared sense of "belonging" to the group. Creativity and shared ideas and opinions characterize this stage. Until this time, most groups function at the task level, but by this stage, maintenance activities are more apparent as members draw others in and constructively share feelings. The leader should continue to role model good maintenance behaviors to move the group along in its work.

The *performing* stage may not occur with all groups; it is characterized by the ability to work as a total group, in subgroups, or independently. This is considered the "most

DISPLAY 10.3	STAGES OF GROUP DEVELOPMENT
Forming	Group dependent on facilitator; anxiety high, need safe environment, structure, and avoid too much self-disclosure; agree on guidelines for group work/behavior; orient to task or purpose of group
Storming	Competition and conflict; need for structure; problem-solving; need to draw out quiet members; continue to clarify group task or purpose
Norming	Group now more cohesive and creative; acknowledge others' contributions; shared leadership; trust increases; work moves along more quickly
Performing	Not reached by all groups; true interdependence—can work as group, or as individuals, and in subgroups; most productive; least reliant on facilitator
Adjourning	The termination phase; conclusion of activities and resolution of relationships; formal acknowledgement of group work

Adapted from Tuckman, D. (1965). Developmental sequence in small groups. *Psychological Bulletin, 63,* 384–399.

DISPLAY 10.4 TASK, MAINTENANCE, AND NONFUNCTIONAL ROLES IN GROUPS

Task Roles: Required in selecting and carrying out group tasks.

Maintenance Roles: Required in strengthening and maintaining group relationships and activities.

Nonfunctional Roles: Roles that harm the group and its work—often self-oriented behavior.

Task Role Behaviors

Initiating Activity: Proposing solutions; suggesting new ideas, new definitions of the problem, new approaches to the problem or new organization of material.

Seeking Information: Asking for clarification of suggestions; requesting additional information or facts.

Seeking Opinions: Looking for an expression of feeling about something from members; seeking clarification of values, suggestions or ideas.

Giving Information: Offering facts or generalizations; relating one's own experiences to the group problem to illustrate a point.

Giving Opinions: Stating an opinion or belief concerning a suggestion or suggestions; particularly concerning its value rather than its factual basis.

Elaborating: Clarifying, giving examples or developing meanings, trying to envision how a proposal might work if adopted.

Coordinating: Showing relationships among various ideas or suggestions, trying to pull ideas and suggestions together, trying to draw together activities of various subgroups or members.

Summarizing: Pulling together related ideas or suggestions; restating suggestions after the group has discussed them.

Maintenance Role Behaviors

Encouraging: Being friendly, warm, responsive to others, praising others and their ideas, agreeing with and accepting contributions of others.

Gatekeeping: Trying to make it possible for another member to make a contribution to the group by saying "We haven't heard anything from Jim yet," or suggesting limited talking time for everyone, so that all will have a chance to be heard.

Standard Setting: Expressing standards for the group to use in choosing its content or procedures or in evaluating its decisions; reminding the group to avoid decisions that conflict with group standards.

Following: Going along with decisions of the group; thoughtfully accepting ideas of others; serving as audience during group discussion.

Expressing Group Feelings: Summarizing what group feeling is sensed to be; describing reactions of the group to ideas or solutions.

Both Task and Maintenance Role Behaviors

Evaluating: Submitting group decisions or accomplishments to compare with group standards; measuring accomplishments against goals.

Diagnosing: Determining sources of difficulties; appropriate steps to take next; analyzing the main block to progress.

Testing for Consensus: Tentatively asking for group opinions in order to find out whether the group is nearing consensus on a decision; sending up trial balloons to test group opinions.

Mediating: Harmonizing, conciliating differences in points of view, suggesting compromise solutions.

Relieving Tension: Draining off negative feelings by jesting or pouring oil on troubled waters; putting a tense situation in a wider context.

Types of Nonfunctional Behaviors

Being Aggressive: Working for status by criticizing or blaming others; showing hostility toward the group or some individual; deflating egos or status of others.

Blocking: Interfering with the progress of the group by going off on a tangent; citing personal experiences unrelated to the problem; arguing too much on a point; rejecting ideas without consideration.

Self-confessing: Using the group as a sounding board; expressing personal, nongroup-oriented feelings or points of view.

Competing: Vying with others to produce the best idea, talk the most, play the most roles, gain favor with the leader.

Seeking Sympathy: Trying to induce other group members to be sympathetic to one's problems or misfortunes; deploring one's own situation, or disparaging one's own ideas to gain support.

Special Pleading: Introducing or supporting suggestions related to one's own pet concerns or philosophies, lobbying.

Horsing Around: Clowning, joking, mimicking, disrupting the work of the group.

Seeking Recognition: Attempting to call attention to one's self by loud or excessive talking, extreme ideas, unusual behavior.

Withdrawal: Acting indifferent or passive, using excessive formality, daydreaming, doodling, whispering to others, wandering off the subject.

From USDHHS Substance Abuse & Mental Health Services Administration (SAMHSA). (2006). *Training Tool #13: Roles in a Group.* Retrieved August 6, 2008 from http://preventiontraining.samhsa.gov/Cmhc02/01h-atod.t13.htm.

productive" stage, and a true balance is achieved between task and maintenance functions (George Mason University CSL, 2006, ¶ 7). Group leaders are less involved with moving along the work of the group. Members now work together more smoothly and do not need a lot of direction from the facilitator.

When either work or support groups end, the final stage of development is termed *adjourning*. This is a withdrawal from both task and relationship activities. Group leaders may plan a small party or ceremony—something to formally commemorate the group's time together and help members successfully disengage (George Mason University CSL, 2006).

Group Functions in Decision-Making

Groups, regardless of size, perform many functions. Four functions of particular relevance to group decision-making include:

1. *Group members share information.* In community health nursing, groups often include clients, health professionals, and community members who share their experience and expertise to arrive at solutions and decisions. Something one member says may spur others to think of more creative solutions or share similar problems (Nijstad & Stroebe, 2006).
2. *Groups are heterogeneous and present diverse views,* which enriches the number and types of alternatives in the problem-solving process. Group decisions are often better than individual ones because of the diversity of experiences and perspectives (Connery & Vohs, 2006).
3. *Groups influence their members' thinking* by broadening their perspectives and presenting new ways of thinking about the issues. This influencing function can improve the quality of group decision-making and reduce the likelihood of making serious mistakes in judgment (Nijstad & Stroebe, 2006).
4. *Groups progress toward consensus* or resolution by discussing a set of alternatives and arriving at solutions. Time pressures and the desire for completion help to move this process along. (Connery & Vohs, 2006).

Techniques for Enhancing Group Decision-Making

As a member of many decision-making groups in the community, the community health nurse can facilitate the process through certain techniques. Robbins (2003) describes four useful strategies commonly used in community health settings: brainstorming, nominal group technique, Delphi technique, and electronic meetings.

Brainstorming

Brainstorming is an idea-generating process that encourages group members to freely offer suggestions. When brainstorming, members sit around a table (if group size permits) and take turns presenting ideas. They are encouraged to be creative and "think out of the box"; no idea is too bizarre. Furthermore, no criticism or discussion is allowed until all ideas have been exhausted and recorded. This technique is helpful for generating creative possibilities and is most useful in the early stages of decision-making. Research has shown that brainstorming generates a large number of ideas, as well as a higher quality of ideas (Munoz, 2005).

Nominal Group Technique

Nominal group technique is a group decision-making method in which ideas are pooled and discussed face-to-face after members initially think and write down their ideas independently. In this approach, members generally meet together but first spend time silently writing down their ideas. Or, members may write down ideas and thoughts in advance of the meeting. Afterward, members take turns presenting one idea at a time to the group without discussion until all ideas have been recorded. Discussion then follows for clarifying and judging. Next, members independently and silently rank-order the ideas and read these rankings to the group. This allows the decisions to be narrowed down to the one with the highest aggregate ranking and facilitates earlier consensus. One example of the use of this technique led to the identification of health priorities among several rural districts in Tanzania, Africa. Input was gathered from lay people (e.g., religious leaders, community and youth leaders, elders). As was the case with health experts, the lay people identified malaria as the leading health concern, but noted that hunger, lack of water, and poverty were also issues that ranked high on the list of priorities needing to be addressed (Makundi, Manongi, Mushi, et al., 2005).

Delphi Technique

The **Delphi technique** is a method of arriving at group consensus through a systematic pooling of individuals' judgments by using a written questionnaire and suggestions. Members do not need to be physically present to participate. The technique follows a series of steps:

1. The researcher identifies a problem or topic and designs a questionnaire to elicit responses from members (often a predetermined expert panel).
2. Members respond independently and anonymously and return the questionnaire.
3. The researcher compiles the information from the original questionnaire, then sends a "feedback report" and a revised questionnaire to the members (Anderson & McFarlane, 2004, p. 300).
4. Members offer new responses or solutions, based on the feedback report and earlier results, and return the questionnaires.
5. Steps 3 and 4 are repeated either for a preset number of times or as needed until consensus is reached.

This process is useful for polling experts who may be geographically distant from one another (Irvine, 2006). It also provides a way to reach a decision without group members unduly influencing each other. Its disadvantages are that it is time-consuming and can be expensive. By using e-mail, instead of "snail mail," the Delphi technique provides practicality.

Electronic Meetings

Electronic meetings provide a fourth group decision-making method. This method is often used in business settings and by government and voluntary health organizations. It applies nominal group technique combined with computer technology. Using meeting-productivity software, group members can access meeting agendas and pertinent information in a central location. Decisions are recorded and minutes of meetings are kept. Past minutes can be easily accessed, and timers can even be added to keep group members on task (Effective Meetings, 2006). This method promotes greater honesty and speed. Experts claim that electronic meetings are significantly faster than face-to-face meetings, perhaps by as much as 50% (Robbins, 2003; Effective Meetings, 2006). Electronic meetings are becoming so common that resources about rules and parliamentary procedure have been specifically developed (National Association of Parliamentarians, 2006).

In community health, the availability of such technology may be limited in many settings. Nonetheless, computer-assisted decision-making is becoming increasingly useful and available. Computers are used with other group decision-making techniques for recording ideas and research findings, tabulating rankings, voting and election of officers in professional organizations, and conducting simulations.

Nursing Informatics

Nursing informatics is a term for the collective technological sciences currently available to nurses in the health care delivery system for the delivery of nursing care. The classic definition of nursing informatics comes from Graves and Corcoran (1989, p. 227):

> A combination of computer science, information science, and nursing science designed to assist in the management and processing of nursing data, information, and knowledge to support the practice of nursing and the delivery of nursing care.

Nursing informatics as a nursing specialty was approved in 1992 by the American Nurses Association. Specialty certification is awarded to nurses with a baccalaureate degree and either specialized education or practice in the field (Blais, Hayes, & Kozier, 2006). Graduate degrees in nursing informatics, including the Ph.D., can be found across the country. The computer is changing all aspects of health care. Educational efforts include online journals, workshops, courses, and conferences for professionals, and a vast amount of consumer-oriented health information can be found on the Web. The documentation process increasingly uses the computer, with paperless charting becoming commonplace. This technology is no longer used exclusively in acute care settings but in the community at clinics, with home health nurses, with advanced-practice nurses, and in PHN settings. Various practitioners use the computer to research diseases, treatment methodologies, and educational resources for clients, or to search for sites of clinical trials. Informatics can provide a framework for interdisciplinary study and research, thus enhancing individual and group decision-making.

In many community health settings, computer databases aid in tracking immunizations, and computerized charting and billing systems are commonly used. Community health nurses access computerized nursing information systems that assist with quality measurement and improvement (see Chapter 12), home visiting documentation according to protocols, documentation of all client contacts, time management, and work schedules. PHNs in four local health departments in Minnesota collaborated on a project to use "standardized nursing language" and create an "automated platform" for articulation of data and documentation of "client assessments, service delivery information, and client outcomes" (Monsen, Fitzsimmons,

Lescenski, Lytton, Schwichtenberg, & Martin, 2006, p. 152). Although there were barriers and frustrations when working across departments, the nurses felt that the project met its goals and improved the quality of nursing care. The technique of documenting everything on paper in handwriting is being replaced. Electronic health records make client information readily accessible (Ries & Moysa, 2005). The U.S. Department of Health and Human Services (USDHHS) is supporting the development of "prototypes for a Nationwide Health Information Network (NHIN)" (USDHHS, 2005, ¶ 1) that will standardize patient data and ensure ease of access by various providers while protecting privacy and security of patient records. Through its Consolidated Health Informatics initiative, the USDHHS Office of the National Coordinator for Health Information Technology (ONC) has begun to identify uniform standards among government agencies and a portfolio of 27 health domains (ONC, 2005). This work is in response to President George W. Bush's directive for development of personal electronic health records. We may soon be able to swipe a card and access a patient's health history and current health data (e.g., laboratory and x-ray results).

Computerized geographic information systems (GISs) are used to display, analyze, and manipulate spatial data. This allows community health and safety organizations to use three-dimensional graphics to locate and track diseases, toxic waste sites, ground water sources, and vehicle crashes on roads in a region, county, or census tract, and so on. With such information, community health and safety can be enhanced and traffic patterns can be altered to make roads safer; health care personnel resources can be redistributed based on disease distribution; and dumps and waste sites can be relocated to protect valuable ground water sources. In a survey, researchers from Pennsylvania and Tennessee found that GIS software is not often used to its full potential by public health professionals (Scotch, Parmanto, Gadd, & Sharma, 2006). Researchers used this advanced technology to map clusters of tuberculosis (TB) cases in Almora, India, and noted the potential for its use in TB surveillance (Tiwari, Adhikari, Tewari, & Kandpal, 2006).

Many of us are already familiar with personal digital assistants (PDAs) and enjoy the many features they provide. The use of PDAs is well established among physicians and medical students (Garrity & El Emam, 2006), and is growing among nursing students (Goldsworthy, Lawrence, & Goodman, 2006). Acute care nurses and nurse practitioners have found them to be helpful in managing complex patients, prescribing medications, and following complicated protocols (Taylor, 2005; Tilghman, Raley, & Comway, 2006).

However, PHNs may also benefit from the use of PDAs not only for calendaring appointments and keeping brief notes, but also for charting (Menachemi, Ettel, Brooks, & Simpson, 2006) and disease reporting. A case reporting system (RSVP) was developed jointly by University of Washington researchers and the Denver Public Health Department (Lober, Bliss, Dockrey, Davidson, & Karras, 2003). PDAs and wireless networks were used to collect data, notify the health department of reportable diseases (both routine and bioterrorism cases), and add cases to a reporting database, as well as access updated database files. A study in South Africa used PDAs and Bluetooth-linked global positioning system (GPS) receivers to assist in locating homes of

TB clients needing treatment followup (directly observed therapy [DOTS]). Because many people live in crowded areas with inadequate house numbering, and some live in "backyard shacks" or "informal settlements" without property numbers, it is often very difficult to locate clients for follow-up visits (Dwolatzky, Trengove, Struthers, McIntyre, & Martinson, 2006, ¶ 7). The researchers found that volunteers could locate homes more easily using the PDA/GPS systems versus aerial photographs.

The work of the community health nurse can be assisted as more technologies become available. Online chat rooms may be utilized for facilitating support groups; discussion boards can be used as a means of training for staff and students; and telehealth (the use of telecommunications and electronic information technologies to provide long-distance health care, professional and patient health education and public health administration) can be expanded to provide health care to medically underserved populations in remote areas (Copeland, 2002; Deering & Eichelberger, 2002; USDHHS Health Resources & Services Administration [HRSA], 2006).

COLLABORATION AND PARTNERSHIPS IN COMMUNITY HEALTH NURSING

Interprofessional and interdisciplinary collaboration is an "essential element of quality health care" (Coeling & Cukr, 2000, p. 63). **Collaboration**, for community health nurses, means a purposeful interaction between nurses, clients, other professionals, and community members based on shared values, mutual participation, and joint effort. It involves building trust and confidence and is "more often voluntary," with its roots "found in natural social skills developed by children through play" (Petersen, 2003, ¶ 1). These thoughts highlight two basic features of collaboration: it has a goal, and it involves several parties assisting one another to achieve that goal. The overriding purpose or goal of collaboration in community health practice is to benefit the public's health. To that end, many players must work together—agencies, professionals, clients, and lay health workers. There are key strategies for establishing partnerships and collaboration with interprofessional team members (Allender, Carey, Castanon, et al., 1997):

- ◆ Think "outside the box" when looking for partners or collaborators.
- ◆ Partners must be part of the planning.
- ◆ Plans are *guides* toward a goal; stay flexible.
- ◆ When adding new partners, be prepared to re-plan.
- ◆ Maintain different levels of collaboration (different team members have more resources, come in later to the project, or leave the project earlier).
- ◆ Use consensus-building techniques that are creative and visual.
- ◆ Establish a shared vision, then share the plans and the leadership.

Like group process, collaboration among agencies or groups of people may occur in stages:

- ◆ Competition. Competing backgrounds, ideas, and motivations, and a search to find shared values, goals, and ethical principles

- ◆ Networking/Communication. Sharing information promotes development of trust and role clarity, and reduces miscommunication caused by stereotypical views of other disciplines, professions, or entities
- ◆ Cooperation/Coordination. More sharing of resources, less duplication, and formal communication through structure and agreements; more mutual respect
- ◆ Coordination/Partnership. Becoming more invested in the success of all partners, better able to manage and share resources; full support of agencies involved
- ◆ Coalition. Shared leadership and decision-making; resources benefit all members; sufficient power and authority to work collectively
- ◆ Collaboration. Shared mission and vision, open and trusting communication, strong relationships, sense of belonging, and shared accomplishment and goals (Petersen, 2003; Lewandowski & GlenMaye, 2002)

Addressing the needs of aggregates requires a variety of team players. Community health nursing practice draws on the expertise and assistance of numerous individuals. The list includes health planners and policy makers, epidemiologists, biostatisticans, community citizens, demographers, environmentalists, educators, politicians, housing experts, safety professionals, and industrial hygienists in addition to physicians, social workers, psychologists, physical therapists, dentists, and most of the other professionals involved in health services. Depending on the need to be addressed, community health nurses may work with many of these people on a single project. Furthermore, perhaps the most important team players are community clients—those populations and groups who are the targets of community health services. Clients' cultural background, experience in collaboration and partnership building, perspectives, and expressions of need provide important information for the planning and delivery of services (Display 10.5). Their participation, either collectively or through representatives, ensures more comprehensive and accurate information as well as commitment to fully using the health programs designed for their benefit.

Characteristics of Collaboration and Partnerships

To explore the meaning of collaboration in the context of community health nursing, this section examines five characteristics that distinguish collaboration from other types of interaction: shared goals, mutual participation, maximized resources, clear responsibilities, and set boundaries.

Shared Goals

First, collaboration in community health nursing is goal directed. The nurse, clients, and others involved in the collaborative effort or partnership recognize specific reasons for entering into the relationship. For example, a lumber company with 150 employees seeks to develop a wellness program. The community health nurse, company employee representatives, a safety expert, an industrial hygienist, a health educator, an exercise therapist, a nutritionist, and a psychologist might work together to develop specific physical and

DISPLAY 10.5	CROSS-CULTURAL COLLABORATION GUIDELINES

1. Practice—we get better at cross-cultural collaboration when we practice it.
2. Do not use generalizations about other cultures to stereotype or oversimplify your ideas about another person or group.
3. Do not assume that there is only one right way (yours) to communicate. Keep questioning your assumptions about the "right way" to communicate.
4. Do not assume that breakdowns in communication occur because other people are on the wrong track. Search for ways to make communication work, rather than searching for who should receive the blame.

5. Listen actively and empathetically. Try to put yourself in the other person's shoes, especially when another person's ideas or perceptions are different from your own. Be willing to step outside your comfort zone.
6. Respect other opinions.
7. Stop, suspend judgment, and try to look at the situation as an outsider.
8. Be aware of power imbalances and the effects on communication.
9. Remember that cultural norms may not apply to the behavior of any particular individual. Start from where they are. Check your interpretations and ask for clarification.

From the National Institute for Dispute Resolution.

mental health goals. The team enters into the collaborative relationship with broad needs or purposes to be met and specific objectives to accomplish.

Mutual Participation

Second, in community health nursing, collaboration involves mutual participation; all team members contribute and are mutually benefited (Leonard, Graham, & Bonacum, 2004). Collaboration involves a reciprocal exchange in which individual team players discuss their intended involvement and contribution, and it is important for all members of a team to feel equally valued—no hierarchies should exist. The lumber company representatives may outline assessed areas of need, such as back-strengthening exercises to facilitate lifting and reduce strain. The professionals, including the nurse involved in the collaboration, will offer their own specific ideas and expertise to design the wellness program. In interdisciplinary teams, physicians, nurses, lay community health workers, clients, outside agency personnel, and others must be able to effectively share ideas and frustrations on an equal, reciprocal basis.

Maximized Use of Resources

A third characteristic of collaboration is that it maximizes the use of community resources. That is, the collaborative partnership is designed to draw on the expertise of those who are most knowledgeable and in the best positions to influence a favorable outcome. If the lumber company team has identified a need for health education materials, the nurse and other members of the collaborating team may explore health education resources through the local health department and within their own professions. In this age of dwindling resources, it is common for outside funding agencies to require proof of collaboration and coalitions in order to apply for grant or government funding.

Clear Responsibilities

Fourth, the collaborating team members work in partnership and assume clearly defined responsibilities. As in a football team, each member in the partnership plays a specific role with related tasks. The nurse may play a case-management or group leadership role, whereas others assume roles appropriate to their areas of expertise. Effective collaboration clearly designates what each member will do to accomplish the identified goals. The nurse, for example, might coordinate the planning effort for the lumber company wellness program and work with the health educator to develop classes on various topics. The psychologist might advise on a chemical dependency program, and the industrial hygienist would provide assistance with safety measures. Each member of the team develops an understanding of individual responsibilities based on realistic and honest expectations. This understanding comes through effective communication. The collaborating partners explore necessary resources, assess their capabilities, and determine their willingness to assume tasks.

Boundaries

Fifth, collaboration in community health practice has set boundaries, with a beginning and an end that fall within the goals of the communication. An important part of defining collaboration is determining the conditions under which it occurs and when it will be terminated. The temporal boundaries sometimes are determined by progress toward the goal, sometimes by the number of team member contacts, and often by setting a time limit. The collaborating group might target 6 months as a completion date for the lumber company wellness program and establish a timeline with designated activities to reach the goal. Once the purpose for the collaboration has been accomplished, the group as a formal entity can be terminated.

In some settings, the partnership may desire to continue to work on other, mutually agreed upon activities. If so, the process begins again with different goals. Some partnerships are ongoing. For example, a university with a department of nursing might use a neighborhood community center for clinical experiences for the students. The community center has needs that may include health assessments and in-home health teaching among community members, flu shots given at the center for elders without transportation, or health education classes for the adults in an English as a Second Language (ESL) class or for preschoolers in a Head Start program. The center and the university work in partnership so that, each semester, ongoing services are provided by the nursing students and coordinated by a faculty member or graduate nursing student in collaboration with the community center staff. Each partner wins. The students receive a rich educational experience, and the neighborhood center gets services they would otherwise do without. Within such a model, there are opportunities for students and volunteers. Students from other educational disciplines—social work, theater arts, physical therapy, early elementary education, and other areas—can be integrated into a center that serves people of all ages. Professionals (e.g., dentist, pediatrician) who are willing to volunteer (e.g., one-half or one day per week) enhance the services provided, as can lay volunteers, who can read to the children, answer the telephone, or participate in fund-raising. Any number of possibilities exist when people collaborate and work in partnership together.

Fostering Client Participation

This chapter has stressed that communication and collaboration are based on mutual participation. The extent of clients' involvement in that participation varies, however, depending on their readiness and ability to participate (Chatterjee & Leonard, 2001). The client's level of wellness at the time of the initial professional–client encounter directly influences participation. Some people are not physically or emotionally well enough to assume an active role in the relationship. Women recently discharged from the hospital after a mastectomy, for example, have many physical and emotional adjustments with which to cope. Their families, too, must expend additional energies to provide needed support and to cope with the temporary loss of the woman's usual role in the family. They may find it difficult to engage actively in identifying their needs and goals at the start of the collaborative process. The nurse may have to take a stronger initial leadership role; however, the goals of collaboration are not abandoned. Gradually, as the client's wellness level improves or the client's family becomes more involved, the nurse can encourage more active participation. Developmentally disabled clients, or others who are cognitively impaired, may not have the full capacity for true collaboration.

Sometimes a client's previous experiences with health personnel limit participation in collaboration. Clients from poverty-stricken areas, those from different cultural backgrounds, or those with little education may need extensive encouragement to participate actively. Also, clients who were not previously encouraged to participate in decision-making by physicians, nurses, or other professionals may follow the pattern of a passive role and not truly collaborate. Unless the nurse persists in efforts to reduce the dependence of clients, the relationship can fall short of the therapeutic goals.

The nurse's own view of collaboration also influences the degree of client participation. Nurses who are accustomed to relating to clients in an adult-to-child manner restrict client involvement. If nurses see their position as more informed, and the client's position as one of complete ignorance and

need, a paternalistic relationship may develop. All clients have resources on which to build, and the community health nurse helps clients to discover these resources and use them to enhance collaboration and attain health goals.

Clients who initiate or seek service frequently are best able to assume an active participant role; examples include abused women seeking protection and elderly widowed persons seeking support. These clients have already demonstrated a sense of responsibility for their health by identifying a need and asking for assistance. They also are experts regarding their situation. This intimate knowledge of the problem makes the client an expert partner and a colleague in problem-solving. The nurse still must work carefully to build mutual participation and respond with concern and caring to foster continued interest and participation by clients.

Structure of Collaborative Relationships

Effective collaboration occurs within a particular structure and sequence. During this process, the work of identifying and meeting the client's needs takes place. Because most collaborative and partner relationships are bound by time, the structure involves several phases: (1) a beginning phase when the team relationship is just being established; (2) a middle, working phase; and (3) a termination phase when the relationship ends.

The first phase is a period of establishing and defining the team relationship. All of the team members, including clients, are getting to know each other; they seek to establish communication patterns and develop trust. From these bases, they identify the clients' needs and determine the goals toward which they will work.

The second phase occurs when team members start working together to accomplish desired goals. Their work may include assessment and planning as well as implementation and evaluation. The cycle of the nursing process is repeated as needed during this working phase until goals are satisfactorily accomplished.

The third or termination phase occurs when the need for team members to work together has ended. When team members have grown close in the relationship, termination can be difficult. Termination should never occur abruptly or without participation. It often requires careful advance preparation to make certain that all parties understand when and why it is taking place. Termination helps to ensure a clear-cut end to the collaborative relationship. For example, a nurse, physician, social worker, psychologist, and nutritionist collaborated with a refugee group for almost 1 year. As the group's multiple needs declined, the professionals began to taper off their assistance. Two months before the relationship was ended, termination of the group was discussed. At first, client group members were frightened at the loss of group support, but slowly they took ownership and control, and with their newly acquired skills, they assumed more responsibility for their health needs.

Barriers to Effective Collaboration

Communication barriers and miscommunication can inhibit effective collaboration. This is sometimes caused by misconceptions on the part of team members regarding the professional knowledge and motives of other team members. Stereotypes and the perception of unequal power and authority granted to certain disciplines can sabotage the effectiveness of communication and true collaboration. Apprehension about sharing information with the team, inflexibility and uneasiness with the more fluid boundaries required in collaboration, and a failure to develop a common purpose and goals are all barriers for effective teamwork and collaboration. It is helpful for team members to share information about their respective disciplines and backgrounds, as well as personal expectations related to collaborative efforts. Structural factors, such as inadequate time, resources, and agency support, are also cited as barriers (Lewandowski & GlenMaye, 2002). Conflict is inevitable when dealing with groups of diverse individuals, but how that "dissent and disagreement" is handled is the key (Lewandowski & GlenMaye, 2002, p. 246). Open, honest communication must prevail. "Carefronting" has been described as a method of addressing and resolving conflict by confronting other professionals in a "caring, self-asserting, responsible manner" (Kupperschmidt, 2006, ¶ 4). It involves using "I" messages and "negotiating differences in clear, respectful, truthful ways" (¶ 2). It is more fruitful to focus on the issue or problem at hand in a safe environment where all members can voice their opinions openly, and not on personal determinations of who is right or wrong (Leonard, Graham, & Bonacum, 2004).

CONTRACTING IN COMMUNITY HEALTH NURSING

Contracting means negotiating a working agreement between two or more parties in which they come to a shared understanding and mutually consent to the purposes and terms of the transaction. Some kinds of contracts are familiar, such as when a buyer signs a contract agreeing to pay a certain amount over a certain period of time to purchase an automobile. Paying tuition for an education involves a form of contracting: although no formal document is signed, students agree with an educational institution on a purpose (to obtain a degree), with the terms of the contract being regular tuition payments and regular learning opportunities over a specified period of time. For students in individual university courses, their syllabus is a contract. It spells out what is offered, what is expected, and what the outcomes may include. Sometimes, learning contracts are utilized within a course to further clarify roles and responsibilities, and students may "contract" for a grade—agree to do a specific number of assignments in exchange for a predetermined grade.

In contrast to legal contracts, which are written and legally binding, contracts in a collaborative relationship or a nurse–client alliance are flexible and changing, and are based on mutual understanding and trust. They are working agreements that may be renegotiated continuously between clients and health professionals. The flexibility built into nurse–client contracting makes it a valuable tool for community health nurses.

The same format is followed with clients who are receiving home health care services. The contract that develops from the partnership between client and home health care nurse often is referred to as a **critical pathway**. It consists of the written plans for client care with a timetable. This represents a more formal type of contracting:

it is typically a fiscally driven and agency-required tool designed to document standards and quality of care while reducing costs (see Chapters 12 and 32).

Characteristics of Contracting

The concept of contracting, as used in the collaborative relationship, incorporates four distinctive characteristics: partnership and mutuality, commitment, format, and negotiation.

Partnership and Mutuality

All aspects of contracting involve shared participation and agreement between team members; they become partners in the relationship. There is also a mutuality to the nurse–client relationship: if we were to document nurse–client collaboration on a continuum, paternalism would be at one extreme and autonomy at the other. Mutuality becomes the midpoint, balance, or ideal of these two extreme positions. For example, a parenting group of 15 couples requested community health nursing involvement. The group entered into a mutual partnership with the nurse and came to an agreement on what they needed and what the nurse could provide. Together, they developed goals, outlined methods to meet those goals, explored resources to help achieve them, defined the time limits for the contract, and outlined their separate responsibilities. The contract involved reciprocal negotiation and shared evaluation. A partnership with mutuality means that all parties are responsible for setting up and carrying out the terms of the agreement within a dynamic balance. Display 10.6 shows an individual service plan, which includes a contract, that is used by one community health nursing program in a California county health department with clients in their Perinatal Outreach Education program.

Commitment

Second, every contract implies a commitment. The involved parties make a decision that binds them to fulfilling the purpose of the contract. In community health collaboration, contracting does not mean making a binding agreement in the legal sense; rather, it is a pledge of trust and dedication. Accompanying that sense of dedication is a strong motivation to see the contract through to completion. All parties feel responsible for keeping promises; all want to achieve the intended outcomes. When the nurse and the parenting group identified their separate tasks, they committed themselves: "Yes, we will do thus and so."

Format

Format, the third distinctive feature of contracting, involves outlining the specific terms of the relationship. Clients and professionals gain a clear idea of the purpose of the relationship, their respective responsibilities, and the specific limits within which they will work. Expectations are clarified for all parties involved. The format of contracting provides the framework for collaboration. Once the terms of the contract have been spelled out, there is no question about what has to be done, who is to do it, or within what timeframe it is to be accomplished. This format helps to avoid the difficulty of terminating long-term relationships and shifts health care responsibilities from the professionals to the individual or

DISPLAY 10.6	CLIENT SERVICE PLAN WITH CONTRACT

Madera County Public Health Department
Public Health Nursing: Client Individual Service Plan

Client Name: ___Angelica Luz-Smith___   Client Signature: ___Angelica Luz-Smith___

Case Manager: ___J. Allender, RN, PHN___   Start Date: ___6-02-10___

| Date: _6-02-10_

 Strengths Identified:

 Desires to have a healthy baby

 Problems/Risks/ Concerns Identified:

 Doesn't like vegetables

 Doesn't like many fruits | Client Goal:

 1. Eat 5 fruits + vegetables daily

 A. Start with 1—2 fruits + 1—2 vegetables/day

 B. Try new ones (use list provided) at least 1/week

 (May use cheese and/or ranch dressing) | Case Manager: Teaching/Counseling/ Referral

 –value of fruits + vegs
 –nutrients not available in any "vitamin"
 –reviewed vegs—client likes corn, canned green beans, V-8 juice
 –reviewed fruits—client likes apples, bananas + strawberries
 –Cl will try peas + carrots + pears | Follow-up/Reassessment Date: _6-30-10_

 Outcome/Evaluation
 –Client eating 4 vegs/day on 24 hr dietary recall
 –Client eating 1 fruit/day (banana)

 Teaching-
 –reviewed fruite in season
 –client will try a fresh peach or grapes each day | Follow-up/Reassessment Date: _____

 Outcome/Evaluation |
| Date: _____

 Strengths Identified:

 Problems/Risks/ Concerns Identified: | Client Goal: | Case Manager: Teaching/Counseling/ Referral | Follow-up/Reassessment Date: _____

 Outcome/Evaluation | Follow-up/Reassessment Date: _____

 Outcome/Evaluation |

group. At times, having something in writing helps the client 'legitimize' the nurse–client interaction. The goals and specific objectives are visualized and can be referred to and followed by all parties, as seen in Display 10.6.

Negotiation

Finally, contracting always involves negotiation. The nurse and other team members propose to accept certain responsibilities and then ask whether the clients agree. The nurse might ask, "What do you feel you can do to achieve this goal?" A period of give-and-take then occurs in which ideas are discussed and conclusions and consensus are reached— no coercion should be involved. Team members may find over time that terms or goals on which they had agreed need modification. Perhaps clients have assumed more responsibility than they can realistically handle at this time and need to redefine their specific responsibilities. Perhaps the nurse feels a need to involve another professional in the collaborative process. The importance of effective interpersonal communication between clients and professionals to keep contracts updated is emphasized. Negotiation during contracting allows for changes that facilitate the ultimate achievement of goals. It provides built-in flexibility and encourages ongoing communication among all team members. Negotiation gives contracting a dynamic quality. Also, we need to remember that, although we may be experts in community health nursing and feel that we know best what is needed for our clients, they know more about their life circumstances and how health and illness impact them (Mayor, 2006). Mutual respect and regard are necessary before effective contracting can take place.

Value of Contracting

The value of contracting has been demonstrated in many settings and disciplines. Contracts have been used for many years in psychiatric and other nursing settings to promote client self-respect, problem-solving skills, autonomy, and motivation. Other disciplines, such as social work, have long

LEVELS OF PREVENTION PYRAMID

SITUATION: A population of elderly clients, interacting with a community health nurse on a monthly basis at a senior center health clinic, will experience healthful living to the fullest extent of their ability.

GOAL: Using the three levels of prevention, negative health conditions are avoided, promptly diagnosed and treated, and/or the fullest possible potential is restored.

Tertiary Prevention

Rehabilitation	Primary Prevention	
	Health Promotion & Education	Health Protection
• In collaboration with elders, select appropriate activities to prevent recurrence of health problems or to restore the elders to a healthful level of functioning within their limitations	• Promote healthful lifestyle with adequate diet, rest/sleep, and exercise	• Maintain appropriate immunization schedule

Secondary Prevention

Early Diagnosis	Prompt Treatment
• Identify factors contributing to existing health limitations and functional status • Refer to appropriate professionals for diagnosis	• In collaboration with elders, select appropriate activities to achieve individual and group goals designed to resolve health limitations and functional status • Encourage client follow-up of treatment regimen designed by CHN or other health care practitioner

Primary Prevention

Health Promotion & Education	Health Protection
• Assess health status • Identify specific activities that will improve current health status and functional ability • Provide homework for elders to work on between meetings with the CHN	• Provide immunizations, e.g., flu, pneumonia, tetanus/diphtheria

used contracting as a tool in helping to enhance realistic planning and emphasize partnership (Madden, 2003). Educational contracts between students and instructors have proved valuable for facilitating learning (Chan & Chien, 2000; Donovan, 2001; Waddell & Stephens, 2000). In the Levels of Prevention Pyramid, the three levels of prevention are used to provide a framework of care for elderly clients in which contracting may be useful.

Community health nursing also has used the concept of contracting for many years. Without always labeling it as contracting, community health nurses have used these techniques with clients who, for example, want to lose weight. In this case, the contract involves mutual agreement on certain exercise and eating patterns for clients and teaching and support responsibilities for the nurse. Often, it has set a time limit,

such as 6 months, within which to achieve the intended weight loss. In each case, a partnership is developed, with agreement about the purpose of the relationship and the conditions under which it will be carried out. Nurses and clients are, in effect, contracting even though they may see it simply as setting goals with clients, and no written documentation is developed.

As more nurses seek to promote client autonomy and self-care, the wide applicability of contracting to nursing practice is being increasingly recognized (Buelow & Range, 2001). Community health nurses have provided case management for HIV/AIDS clients, care for infants receiving total parenteral nutrition, worked with outpatients receiving chemotherapy, and collaborated with prenatal groups, postpartum mothers, and home health clients using various forms of contracting with the clients.

The advantages of contracting in community health nursing are summarized as follows:

1. It involves clients in promoting their own health.
2. It motivates clients to perform necessary tasks.
3. It focuses on clients' unique needs, regardless of aggregate size.
4. It increases the possibility of achieving health goals identified by collaborating team members.
5. It enhances all team members' problem-solving skills.
6. It fosters client participation in the decision-making process.
7. It promotes clients' autonomy and self-esteem as they learn self-care.
8. It makes nursing service more efficient and cost-effective.

Potential Problems with Contracting

Emphasis on contracting as a method rather than a concept can create problems. If a client has experienced contracts only in a business setting, it is possible to carry the stereotype of a cold, formal arrangement into the nursing practice setting. Some nurses fear that asking clients to negotiate a contract will place clients under stress, impede the development of trust, and negatively influence the relationship. Others have found that some clients prefer to have the nurse make decisions for them and are not ready to enter into any kind of negotiation. These problems in contracting can be overcome by understanding the true concept of contracting. Contracting is not a panacea, however. Some clients cannot fully participate in a collaborative relationship. Developmentally delayed clients and those with serious mental or cognitive impairments (e.g., mental illness, dementia) may be unable to fully participate in the nurse–client contract.

Process of Contracting

Contracting applies the basic principles of adult education: self-direction, mutual negotiation, and mutual evaluation. It need not be a formal, written, or complex negotiation; it may be formal or informal, written or verbal, simple or detailed, and signed or unsigned by client and nurse. It should be adapted to the particular client's abilities to assess, plan, implement, and evaluate, which may vary greatly from situation to situation (Friedman, Bowden, & Jones, 2003). The tool shown in Display 10.6 seeks input from the client. The client's goals are mutually set, and the goals are spelled out. Initial interventions are dated, as are follow-up and reassessment visits. In addition, there is a place for a continuing assessment of outcomes and for evaluation on future dates. Like all nursing tools, contracting enhances client health only if it is adapted to each particular set of client needs and abilities.

Contracting follows a sequence of steps. As a working agreement, it depends on knowing what clients want, agreeing on goals, identifying methods to achieve these goals, knowing the resources that collaborating members bring to the relationship, using appropriate outside resources, setting limits, deciding on responsibilities, and providing for periodic reviews. Each of these tasks requires discussion among members of the contractual group. The tasks are incorporated into the contracting process and can be described in eight phases that follow the nursing process:

Assessment
1. *Explore needs:* Assess clients' health and needs: done by clients, nurse, and other relevant persons

Nursing Diagnosis/Goal Setting
2. *Establish goals:* Discussion followed by agreement among contracting members on goals and objectives

Plan/Intervention
3. *Explore resources:* Define what each member has to offer and can expect from the others; identify appropriate resources and agencies
4. *Develop a plan:* Identify methods, activities, and a timeline for achieving the stated goals
5. *Divide responsibilities:* Negotiate the activities for which each member will be responsible
6. *Agree on time frame:* Setting limits for the contract in terms of length of time or number of meetings

Evaluation
7. *Evaluation:* Formative and summative assessments of progress toward goals occur at agreed-on intervals
8. *Renegotiation or termination:* Agree to modify, renegotiate, or terminate the contract

As community health nurses use this process to negotiate a contract, they must adapt it to each situation. The sequence of phases may change, and some steps may overlap. Nevertheless, the basic elements remain important considerations for successful contracting (Fig. 10.2).

Levels of Contracting

Community health nurses use contracts at levels ranging from formal to informal. The degree of formality depends on the demands of the situation. To fund a community health program for preventing child abuse, for example, a formal contract in the form of a written grant proposal may be needed. To conduct a wide-scale needs assessment of a homeless population, the services of an epidemiologist and statistician may require a formal contract to clarify roles and expectations. **Formal contracting** involves all parties' negotiating a written contract by mutual agreement, signing the agreement, and sometimes having it witnessed or notarized. This level of contract has been used with mental health or substance-abusing clients, where the seriousness of the working agreement and the need to actively involve the client are important aspects of therapy.

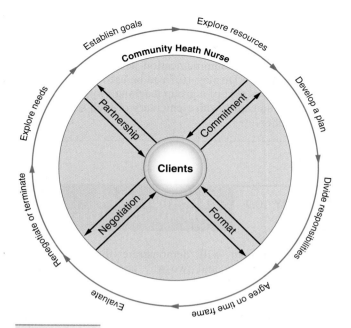

FIGURE 10.2 The concept and process of contracting. Contracting is based on four distinctive features, shown here as spokes that support a wheel. These features form the basis for a reciprocal relationship among clients, nurse, and other persons. This relationship is not static; it is a dynamic process that moves through phases, represented here as the outer rim of the wheel. The process moves forward, focused on meeting clients' needs, and enables the collaborating group to facilitate ultimate achievement of clients' goals.

Some situations best lend themselves to a modified and less formal use of contracting, in which the nursing plan becomes the written contract. For example, a school nurse forms a support group for pregnant adolescents. The nurse uses modified contracting by discussing with the girls the purpose of the group and the number of sessions needed and obtaining their agreement to attend all sessions.

Informal contracting involves some form of verbal agreement about relatively clear-cut purposes and tasks. A client group may agree to prioritize their list of needs, the nurse may agree to conduct health teaching sessions, the social worker may agree to obtain informational materials, and so on. Sometimes, nurses use contracting informally without realizing it. They conclude a session with clients by agreeing with them about the purpose and time of the next meeting. Conscious use of contracting, however, is a more effective way to provide structure for the relationship and foster client involvement, regardless of the level at which it is applied.

The level of contracting also may change during the development of communication and collaboration. Clients often need education about their options. Initially, they may have difficulty in identifying needs and making choices. The professional team can work to promote clients' self-confidence and help them to assume increasing responsibility for their own health. Through these efforts, contracting becomes a consciously recognized part

of the relationship, and clients become fully participating partners.

Summary

Communication and collaboration are important tools for community health nurses to promote aggregate health. Communication involves the transfer and understanding of meaning between individuals. The communication process comprises seven parts: a message, a sender, a receiver, encoding, a channel, decoding, and a feedback loop. Barriers to effective communication include selective perception, language barriers, clients filtering out parts of the message, and emotional influence. Core skills essential to effective communication in community health nursing include sending skills, which allow the nurse to transmit messages effectively; receiving skills, which allow the nurse to receive accurate and complete messages; and interpersonal skills, which allow the nurse to interact and respond to the messages from clients. These skills include special techniques of active listening, the ability to show respect regardless of the message (whether positive or negative), the ability to empathize with clients' thoughts and feelings, and the ability to develop trust. Many factors can influence the quality of communication, such as negative previous experience, cultural influence, and relationships among the people involved. The community health nurse must consider all of these factors when trying to foster good communication.

In community health, nurses frequently need to promote communication in groups and in-group decision-making. Decisions made by groups have many advantages, including sharing of members' experience and expertise, diversity of opinions, potential for broadening members' perspectives, and a focus on arriving at consensus solutions. Several methods of enhancing group decision-making are available, including brainstorming, nominal group technique, Delphi technique, and electronic meetings. Nursing informatics, encompassing all of the computer-generated tools created to enhance communication, is changing the form of communication in community health nursing, as it has in the acute care setting.

Collaboration and partnership building is a purposeful interaction among the nurse, clients, community members, and other professionals based on mutual participation and joint effort. It is characterized by shared goals, mutual participation, maximized use of resources, clear responsibilities, and set boundaries. Clients play an important role in the collaborative relationship.

Contracting is a helpful tool in promoting clients' participation, independence, and motivation. It is used at all levels in community health nursing to promote partnership in the collaborative process, to encourage commitment to health goals, and to ensure a format and a means for negotiation among the collaborating group. Contracts can be formal or informal, written or verbal, simple or complex. The nurse must know the needs and abilities of clients and must tailor the type of contracting to best suit the client's particular situation. ■

ACTIVITIES TO PROMOTE CRITICAL THINKING

1. Discuss how you would handle the communication barrier of selective perception with a group of clients.

2. Practice active listening with a colleague and analyze the factors that interfered with your total concentration. Identify three actions to take to improve your active listening and apply them during the next week, keeping a log of your progress. Think of a patient you have worked with who may have low health literacy. What kinds of things can you do to help them better communicate with their physician and other health professionals? Why is good health literacy important not only for the patient as an individual, but for the community and society as a whole?

3. Use nominal group technique with a group of classmates to arrive at a rank-ordering of barriers to cross-cultural communication. What did you learn about arriving at a quality decision in the process?

4. Attend an open meeting (e.g., student body council, school board, city council) and watch for task and maintenance roles among the members. Are any members displaying nonfunctional role behaviors? Can you recognize task, maintenance, and nonfunctional role behaviors in some of the student groups in which you participate?

5. Organize a group of classmates to represent a group of clients, professionals, and community members who are collaborating to address the needs of an inner-city homeless population. Analyze how well you integrated the five characteristics of collaboration into your activity.

6. Explain the concept of contracting as it applies to aggregates. Discuss its four distinctive characteristics and the advantages that contracting offers to the community health nurse.

7. Develop a hypothetical contract with a group of elderly widows who need support and outlets to alleviate their loneliness. What other community members and professionals might be helpful as part of a collaborative team to address the widows' needs?

8. Become a good listener. This exercise asks you to list your closest friends, relatives, school peers, and work associates. Rank them on a scale of 1 to 10, with 1 meaning always fascinating and 10 meaning boring. If you find that you've labeled most as boring, you probably have one of two problems: you are either socializing and working with the wrong people, or you are a poor listener. The likelihood is the latter. To improve listening skills, compliment people and encourage them; this increases the chance that they will continue conversing with you, and it is a valuable skill in both your personal and professional life.

9. Experiment in communication. The activity described in Display 10.7 can be used with your peers or as part of a group teaching project on communication with elementary or high school students.

DISPLAY 10.7 EXPERIMENT IN COMMUNICATION

Purpose
The experiment will demonstrate the differences between one-way and two-way communication and demonstrate the advantages of the latter.

Setting
The experiment can be conducted in the classroom with any size group. Each person will need paper and pencil.

Procedure
Have the group members select one person who everyone believes can communicate clearly and effectively to be the "sender." Place this person so that he or she is out of sight but can be clearly heard by the rest of the group (the "receivers"). The sender is to describe a diagram, and the receivers are to draw it. The sender should explain the diagram with the intention that the receivers will be able to recreate it exactly, without any further communication with the sender or with other group members. Time the exercise. When the receivers are finished, rank the accuracy of their drawings by placing them on a Likert scale (a 10-point scale, with 1 as Least Accurate to 10 as Most Accurate). Ask receivers how they felt and how the sender probably felt. Ask the sender how she or he felt.

Next, begin the two-way communication demonstration by allowing the sender to remain in sight of the group as he or she explains a second diagram and the receivers draw it. Allow the receivers to ask questions. The sender may reply, but may not use gestures. Record the time required and rank the drawings for accuracy. Discuss how the receivers felt and how the sender probably felt. Ask the sender how she or he felt this time.

Analysis
Compare your findings with the following statements:
1. Two-way communication takes longer.
2. Two-way communication results in greater accuracy among the drawings.
3. In one-way communication, the sender often feels relatively confident; the receiver, uncertain or frustrated.
4. In two-way communication, the sender may feel frustrated or angry; the receiver relatively confident.

References

Allender, J.A., Carey, K.T., Castanon, J.G., et al. (1997, April). *Interprofessional training project: California State University, Fresno. Serving children and families.* Monmouth, OR: Teaching Research Division.

Anderson, E.T., & McFarlane, J. (2004). *Community as partner: Theory and practice in nursing,* 4th ed. Philadelphia, PA: Lippincott Williams & Wilkins.

Andrus, M.R., & Roth, M.T. (2002). Health literacy: A review. *Pharmacotherapy, 22*(3), 282–302.

Arora, V., Johnson, J., Lovinger, D., et al. (2005). Communication failures in patient sign-out and suggestions for improvement: A critical incident analysis. *Quality and Safety in Health Care, 14*(6), 401–407.

Blais, K.K., Hayes, J.S., & Kozier, B. (2006). *Professional nursing practice: Concepts and perspectives,* 5th ed. Upper Saddle River, NJ: Prentice Hall.

Boyle, D.K., & Kochinda, C. (2004). Enhancing collaborative communication of nurse and physician leadership in two intensive care units. *Journal of Nursing Administration, 34*(2), 60–70.

Buelow, G., & Range, L. (2001). No-suicide contracts among college students. *Death Studies, 25*(7), 583–591.

Chan, S., & Chien, W. (2000). Implementing contract learning in a clinical context: Report on a study. *Journal of Advanced Nursing, 31*(2), 298–305.

Chatterjee, N., & Leonard, L. (2001). Partners-in-health: A new front line for disease prevention and health promotion in the community. *American Journal of Health Education, 32*(1), 52–55.

Coeling, H., & Cukr, P. (2000). Communication styles that promote perceptions of collaboration, quality, and nurse satisfaction. *Journal of Nursing Care Quality, 14*(20), 63–74.

Cole, J. (1990). *Filtering people: Understanding and confronting our prejudices.* Philadelphia, PA: New Society Publishers.

Connery, B.A., & Vohs, J.L. (2006). *Group work and collaborative writing.* University of California, Davis: Teaching Resource Center. Retrieved July 17, 2008 from http://trc.ucdavis.edu/TRC/papers/vohs/index.html.

Copeland, M. (2002). E-community health nursing. *Journal of Holistic Nursing, 20*(2), 152–165.

Deering, C.G., & Eichelberger, L. (2002). Mirror, mirror on the wall: Using online discussion groups to improve interpersonal skills. *CIN: Computers, Informatics, Nursing, 20*(4), 150–154.

Donovan, H. (2001). Learning contracts: Friend or foe? *The Practising Midwife, 3*(1), 42.

Dwolatky, B., Trengove, E., Struthers, H., et al. (2006). Linking the global positioning system (GPS) to a personal digital assistant (PDA) to support tuberculosis control in South Africa: A pilot study. *International Journal of Health Geographics, 5*:34 doi:10,1186/1476-072X-5-34.

Edelman, C.L., & Mandle, C.L. (2006). *Health promotion throughout the lifespan,* 6th ed. St. Louis, MO: Mosby, Inc.

Effective Meetings. (2006). *Electronic meetings.* Retrieved July 17, 2008 from http://www.effectivemeetings.com/technology/mrtools/electronic_meetings.asp.

Falk-Rafael, A. (2001). Empowerment as a process of evolving consciousness: A model of empowered caring. *Advances in Nursing Science, 24*(1), 1–16.

Finkelman, A. (2006). *Leadership and management in nursing.* Upper Saddle River, NJ: Pearson Education, Inc.

Fowler, K. (2006). Active listening: Hear what people are really saying. Mind Tools. Retrieved July 17, 2008 from http://www.mindtools.com/CommSkll/ActiveListening.htm.

Friedman, M., Bowden, V., & Jones, E. (2003). *Family nursing: Research, theory, and practice,* 5th ed. Upper Saddle River, NJ: Prentice Hall.

Gallant, M., Beaulieu, M., & Carnevale, F. (2002). Partnership: An analysis of the concept within the nurse-client relationship. *Journal of Advanced Nursing, 40,* 149–157.

Garrity, C., & El Emam, K. (2006). Who's using PDAs? Estimates of PDA use by health care providers: A systematic review of surveys. *Journal of Medical Internet Research, 8*(2), E7.

Gazmararian, J., Williams, M., Peel, J., & Baker, D. (2003). Health literacy and knowledge of chronic disease. *Patient Education and Counseling, 51*(3), 267–275.

George Mason University Center for Service and Leadership. (2006). *Leadership tips: 5 stages of group development.* Retrieved July 17, 2008 from http://www.gmu.edu/student/csl/5stages.html.

Goldsworthy, S., Lawrence, N., & Goodman, W. (2006). The use of personal digital assistants at the point of care in an undergraduate nursing program. *CIN: Computers, Informatics, Nursing, 24*(3), 138–143.

Graves, J., & Corcoran, D. (1989). The study of nursing informatics. *Image: Journal of Nursing Scholarship, 21*(3), 227–231.

Harper, M.G. (2006). Ethical multiculturalism: An evolutionary concept analysis. *Advances in Nursing Practice, 29*(2), 110–124.

Irvine, F. (2006). Exploring district nursing competencies in health promotion: The use of the Delphi technique. *Journal of Clinical Nursing, 14*(8), 965–975.

Kar, S.B., Arcalay, R., & Alex, S. (2001). *Health communication: A multicultural perspective.* Thousand Oaks, CA: Sage.

Kickbusch, I. (2001). Health literacy: Addressing the health and education divide. *Health Promotion International, 16*(3), 289–297.

Kupperschmidt, B.K. (2006). Addressing multigenerational conflict: Mutual respect and carefronting as strategy. *Online Journal of Issues in Nursing, 11*(2). Retrieved June 27, 2008 from http://www.medscape.com/viewarticle/536481_1.

Kurtz, S., Silverman, J., & Draper, J. (2005). *Teaching and learning communication skills in medicine.* Abingdon, UK: Radcliffe Publishing.

Leonard, M., Graham, S., & Bonacum, D. (2004). The human factor: The critical importance of effective teamwork and communication in providing safe care. *Quality and Safety in Health Care, 13,* 185–190.

Lewandowski, C., & GlenMaye, L. (2002). Teams in child welfare settings: Interprofessional and collaborative processes. *Families in Society, 83*(3), 245–256.

Lindau, S., Tomori, C., Lyons, T., et al. (2002). The association of health literacy with cervical cancer prevention knowledge and health behaviors in a multiethnic cohort of women. *American Journal of Obstetrics and Gynecology, 186*(5), 938–943.

Lobchuk, M.M. (2006). Concept analysis of perspective-taking: Meeting informal caregiver needs for communication competence and accurate perception. *Journal of Advanced Nursing, 54*(3), 330–341.

Lober, W., Bliss, D., Dockrey, M., et al. (2003). Communicable disease case entry using PDAs and public wireless networks. Association of Medical Informatics Association Annual Symposium Proceedings. Retrieved July 17, 2008 from http://www.pubmedcentral.nih.gov/articlerender.fcgi?tool=pubmed&pubmedid=14728422.

Madden, R.G. (2003). *Essential law for social workers.* New York, NY: Columbia University Press.

Makundi, E., Manongi, R., Mushi, A., et al. (2005). The use of nominal group technique in identifying community health priorities in Moshi rural district, northern Tanzania. *Tanzanian Health Research Bulletin, 7*(3), 133–141.

Mayor, V. (2006). Long-term conditions. 3: Being an expert patient. *British Journal of Community Nursing, 11*(2), 59–63.

McKnight, L., Stetson, P., Bakken, S., et al. (2002). Perceived information needs and communication difficulties of inpatient physicians and nurses. *Journal of the American Medical Informatics Association, 9,* S64–S69.

Menachemi, N., Ettel, D., Brooks, R., & Simpson, L. (2006). Charting the use of electronic health records and other information technologies among child health providers. *BMC Pediatrics, 6*, 21.

Monsen, K., Fitzsimmons, L., Lescenski, B., et al. (2006). A public health nursing informatics data-and-practice quality project. *CIN: Computers, Informatics, Nursing, 24*(3), 152–158.

Munoz, A.A. (2005). Does quantity generate quality? Testing the fundamental principle of brainstorming. *Spanish Journal of Psychology, 8*(2), 215–220.

Nadig, L.A. (2006). *Tips on effective listening.* Retrieved July 17, 2008 from http://www.drnadig.com/listening.htm.

National Assessment of Adult Literacy (NAAL). (2003). *National Center for Education Statistics.* Retrieved July 17, 2008 from http://www.nces.ed.gov/NAAL/index.asp?file=KeyFindings/Demographics/Overall.asp&Pageld=16.

National Association of Parliamentarians. (2006). *Meeting resources: 2005 report on e-meetings.* Retrieved July 17, 2008 from http://www.parliamentarians.org/store/itemdetail.php7id=400-SC.

Nielsen-Bohlman, L. (2004). *Health literacy: A prescription to end confusion.* Washington, DC: National Academies Press.

Nijstad, B.A., & Stroebe, W. (2006). How the group affects the mind: A cognitive model of idea generation in groups. *Personality & Social Psychology Review, 10*(3), 186–213.

Nutbeam, D. (2000). Health literacy as a public health goal: A challenge for contemporary health education and communication strategies into the 21st century. *Health Promotion International, 15*(3), 259–267.

Petersen, C.R. (2003). What does collaboration look like? In *Coming together: Building collaboration and consensus.* Retrieved July 17, 2008 from http://www.communitycollaboration.net.

Ries, H.M., & Moysa, G. (2005). Legal protections of electronic health records: Issues of consent and security. *Health Law Review, 14*(1), 18–25.

Robbins, S.P. (2003). *Essentials of organizational behavior,* 7th ed. Upper Saddle River, NJ: Prentice-Hall.

Rubenfeld, M.G., & Scheffer, B.K. (2006). *Critical thinking tactics for nurses.* Sudbury, MA: Jones & Bartlett Publishers.

Schillinger, D., Grumbach, K., Piette, J., et al. (2002). Association of health literacy with diabetes outcomes. *Journal of the American Medical Association, 288*(4), 475–482.

Scotch, M., Parmanto, B., Gadd, C., & Sharma, R. (2006). Exploring the role of GIS during community health assessment problem solving: Experiences of public health professionals. *International Journal of Health Geographics, 5*, 39. Retrieved July 17, 2008 from http://www.ij-healthgeographics.com/content/5/1/39.

Spector, R.E. (2009). *Cultural diversity in health and illness,* (7th ed.) Upper Saddle River, NJ: Prentice-Hall Allied Health.

Taylor, P.P. (2005). Use of handheld devices in critical care. *Critical Care Nursing Clinics of North America, 17*(1), 45–50.

Tilghman, J., Raley, D., & Conway, J. (2006). Family nurse practitioner students utilization of PDAs: Implications for practice. *ABNF Journal, 17*(3), 115–117.

Tiwari, N., Adhikari, C.M., Tewari, A., & Kandpal, V. (2006). Investigation of geo-spatial hotspots for the occurrence of tuberculosis in Almora district, India, using GIS and spatial scan statistic. *International Journal of Health Geographics, 10*(5), 33. Retrieved July 17, 2008 from http://www.pubmedcentral.nih.gov/articlerender.fcgi?tool=pubmed&pubmedid=16901341.

Tuckman, B.W. (1965). Developmental sequence in small groups. *Psychological Bulletin, 63*, 384–399.

Tveiten, S., & Severinsson, E. (2006). Communication: A core concept in client supervision by public health nurses. *Journal of Nursing Management, 14*(3), 235–243.

United States Department of Health and Human Services, Office of the National Coordinator for Health Information Technology (ONC). (2005). *Consolidated health informatics.* Retrieved July 17, 2008 from http://www.hhs.gov/healthit/chi.html.

United States Department of Health and Human Services. (Nov. 10, 2005). *News release: HHS awards contracts to develop nationwide health information network.* Retrieved July 17, 2008 from http://www.hhs.gov/news/press/2005pres/20051110.html.

United States Department of Health and Human Services, Health Resources and Services Administration (HRSA). (2006). *What is telehealth?* Retrieved July 17, 2008 from http://www.hrsa.gov/telehealth.

United States Department of Health and Human Services. (2006). *Healthy People 2010. 11—Health Communication.* Retrieved July 17, 2008 from http://www.healthypeople.gov/document/html/volume1/11healthcom.htm#_ednref30.

United States Department of Health and Human Services, Substance Abuse and Mental Health Services Administration (SAMHSA). (2006). *Training tool #13: Roles in a group.* Retrieved July 17, 2008 from http://preventiontraining.samhsa.gov/Cmhc02/01h-atol.t12.htm.

Von Dietz, E., & Orb, A. (2000). Compassionate care: A moral dimension of nursing. *Nursing Inquiry, 7,* 166–174.

Waddell, D., & Stephens, S. (2000). Use of learning contracts in a RN-to-BSN leadership course. *Journal of Continuing Education in Nursing, 31*(4), 79–84.

Williams, A. (2006). *Resolving conflict in a multicultural environment.* Conflict Research Consortium. Retrieved July 17, 2008 from http://www.colorado.edu/conflict/peace/example/will5746.htm.

Selected Readings

Alexander, C., & McKenna, S. (2001). A sound partnership for end-of-life care. *American Journal of Nursing, 101*(12), 75–77.

American Nurses Association. (2006). *Nursing informatics and technology.* ANA Nursing World. Retrieved July 17, 2008 from http://www.nursingworld.org/rnindex.nit.htm.

Arons, R.R. (2001). Using technology to advance the public's health. *American Journal of Public Health, 91*(8), 1178–1179.

Green, L., Daniel, M., & Novick, L. (2001). Partnerships and coalitions for community-based research. *Public Health Reports, 116*(Suppl. 1), 20–31.

Hardin, S., & Langford, D. (2001). Telehealth's impact on nursing and the development of the interstate compact. *Journal of Professional Nursing, 17*(5), 243–247.

Healey, A., Undre, S., & Vincent, C. (2006). Defining the technical skills of teamwork in surgery. *Quality and Safety in Health Care, 15*(4), 213–234.

Hojat, M., Nasca, T.J., Cohen, M.J.M., et al. (2001). Attitudes toward physician-nurse collaboration: A cross-cultural study of male and female physicians and nurses in the United States and Mexico. *Nursing Research, 50*(2), 123–128.

Jenkins, R.L., & White, P. (2001). Telehealth advancing nursing practice. *Nursing Outlook, 49*(2), 100–105.

Kim, J.J., Cho, H., Cheon-Klessig, Y.S., et al. (2002). Primary health care for Korean immigrants: Sustaining a culturally sensitive model. *Public Health Nursing 19*(3), 191–200.

Lingard, L., Espin, S., Rubin, B., et al. (2005). Getting teams to talk: Development and pilot implementation of a checklist to promote interprofessional communication in the OR. *Quality and Safety in Health Care, 14*(5), 340–346.

Malone, G., & Morath, J. (2001). Pro-patient partnerships. *Nursing Management, 32*(7), 46–47.

Maurana, C.A., & Rodney, M.M. (2000). Strategies for developing a successful community health advocate program. *Family and Community Health, 23*(1), 40–49.

Riegelman, R., & Persily, N.A. (2001). Health information systems and health communications: Narrowband and broadband technologies as core public health competencies. *American Journal of Public Health, 91*(8), 1179–1183.

Saba, V.K., & McCormick, K.A. (2005). *Essentials of nursing informatics,* 4th ed. New York, NY: McGraw-Hill Medical.

Saba, V.K. (2001). Nursing informatics: Yesterday, today and tomorrow. *International Nursing Review, 48,* 177–187.

Scholes, M. (2000). *International nursing informatics: A history of the first forty years, 1960–2000.* London: British Computer Society.

Sharpe, C.C. (2001). *Telenursing: Nursing practice in cyberspace.* Westport, CT: Auburn House.

Singh, H., Petersen, L., & Thomas. E. (2006). Understanding diagnostic errors in medicine: A lesson from aviation. *Quality and Safety in Health Care, 15(*3), 159–164.

Strader, T.N., Collins, D.A., & Noe, T.D. (2000). *Building healthy individuals, families, and communities: Creating lasting connections.* Norwell, MA: Kluwer Plenum.

Sullivan, M., & Kelly, J.G. (2001). *Collaborative research: University and community partnership.* Washington, DC: American Public Health Association.

Tan, J.K.H. (2001). *Health management information systems: Methods and practical applications,* 2nd ed. Gaithersburg, MD: Aspen.

United Nations Programme on HIV/AIDS (UNAIDS). (2001). *Effective prevention strategies in low HIV prevalence settings.* Washington, DC: Family Health International.

United States Department of Health and Human Services. (2000). *Healthy people 2010* [Conference ed., Vols. I & II]. Washington, DC: U.S. Government Printing Office.

Internet Resources

American Medical Informatics Association (AMIA): *http://www.amia.org*

American Nursing Informatics Association (ANIA): *http://www.ania.org*

Canada's Health Informatics Association: *http://www.coachorg.com*

Cumulative Index to Nursing and Allied Health Literature (CINAHL): *http://www.cinahl.com*

Groupwork: An Interdisciplinary Journal for Working with Groups. IngentaConnect: *http://www.ingentaconnect.com/content/wab/gijwg*

Health Literacy Project, American Medical Association Foundation: *http://www.ama-assn.org/ama/pub/category/8115.html*

Health Communication Activities, Office of Disease Prevention and Health Promotion: *http://www.health.gov/communication/literacy/default.htm*

Health Literacy Facts Sheets and Evaluation Tools, Center for Health Care Strategies, Inc.: *http://www.chcs.org/publications3960/publications_show.htm?doc_id=291711*

International HIV/AIDS Alliance. Information on working with groups: *http://www.aidsmap.com/en/docs/340F9B37-C484C-ACAA-D5FDB909748.asp*

Midwest Alliance for Nursing Informatics: *http://www.maninet.org*

North Central Regional Educational Laboratory. 21st Century Skills: Effective communication: *http://www.ncrel.org/engauge/skills/effcomm.htm*

Nursing-Informatics.com: *http://www.nursing-informatics.com*

Online Journal of Nursing Informatics: *http://www.eaa-knowledge.com/ojni/*

11

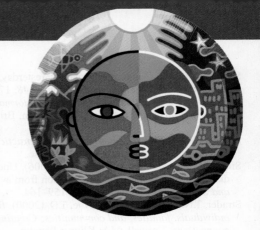

Health Promotion: Achieving Change Through Education

LEARNING OBJECTIVES

Upon mastery of this chapter, you should be able to:

◆ Explain the three stages of change.

◆ Identify three planned-change strategies.

◆ Summarize six principles for effecting change in community health.

◆ Describe the community health nurse's role as educator in promoting health and preventing or postponing morbidity.

◆ Identify educational activities for the nurse to use that are appropriate for each of the three domains of learning.

◆ Select learning theories that are applicable to an individual, family, or aggregate client.

◆ Identify health-teaching models for use when planning health education activities.

◆ Select teaching methods and materials that facilitate learning for clients at different developmental levels.

◆ Develop teaching plans focusing on primary, secondary, and tertiary levels of prevention for clients of all ages.

◆ Identify teaching strategies for the community health nurse to use when encountering clients with special learning needs.

KEY TERMS

Accommodation
Adaptation
Affective domain
Anticipatory guidance
Assimilation
Change
Cognitive domain
Empiric-rational change strategy
Evolutionary change
Force field theory
Gestalt-field
Health Promotion
Learning
Normative-reeducative change strategy
Operationalize
Planned change
Power-coercive change strategy
Psychomotor domain
Revolutionary change
Stages of change
Teaching

"As I see it, every day you do one of two things: build health or produce disease in yourself."

—Adelle Davis

300

Think of a time when you were so influenced by a teacher that you stopped an unhealthy habit, altered a long-held belief, or embarked on a new endeavor. What precisely was it that motivated the change? Was it simply the content of the teaching, or was it how the teacher presented the content? What is good teaching, and why is it so important to community health nursing?

Teaching has been a critical part of the community health nurse's role since the origins of the profession, and it frequently is the primary role or function. Community health nurses develop partnerships with clients to achieve behavior changes that promote, maintain, or restore health. This partnership focuses on self-care—the ability to effectively advocate and manage a person's own health. The rationale for health teaching is to equip people with the knowledge, attitudes, and practices that will allow them to live the fullest possible life for the greatest length of time. The goals of *Healthy People 2010* emphasize not only health status and longevity but also the quality of our lives, emphasizing that even the later years should be full of vigor (U.S. Department of Health and Human Services [USDHHS], 2000). Table 11.1 provides a list of *Healthy People 2010* objectives for educational, community-based programs.

When the community health nurse identifies a need that is best met through health education, the nurse is faced with a series of questions: How can I teach effectively? What content should I cover? What method of presentation will communicate most effectively? What resources can I use as teaching tools? How do I know when the client has grasped the information or mastered the skills? How do I help clients with special learning needs? The nurse must understand what makes teaching effective, how teaching skills are acquired, and how mastery is measured. The nurse might also need to consider why some individuals adopt new health practices and others do not. This chapter addresses these questions and discusses teaching as a basic intervention tool in community health nursing practice. For health education to be effective, awareness of the underlying principles of behavior change is

---

TABLE 11.1   *Healthy People 2010* Objectives for Educational and Community-Based Programs

	Objective	2010 Goals	Baseline
7.1	High school completion	Increase the high school completion rate to at least 90%.	85%
7.2	School health education	Increase to at least 70% the proportion of middle/junior high and senior high schools that require 1 school year of health education.	28%
7.3	Undergraduate health risk behavior information	Increase to at least 25% the proportion of undergraduate students attending postsecondary institutions who receive information from their college or university on all six priority health risk behavior areas—behaviors that cause unintentional and intentional injuries, tobacco use, alcohol and other drug use, sexual behavior, dietary patterns that cause disease, and inadequate physical activity.	6%
7.4	School nurse-to-student ratio	Increase to at least 50% the proportion of the middle/junior and senior high schools that have a nurse-to-student ratio of at least 1:750.	28%
7.5	Work site health-promotion programs	Increase to 75% the proportion of work sites (with more than 50 employees) that offer a comprehensive health-promotion program to their employees.	33–50%
7.6	Participation in employer-sponsored health-promotion activities	Increase to at least 75% the proportion of all employees (over age 18) who participate in employer-sponsored health-promotion activities.	61%
7.8	Patient satisfaction with health care provider communication	This objective is developmental: increase the proportion of patients who report that they are satisfied with the patient education they receive from their health care organization.	–
7.10	Community-based health promotion	This objective is developmental: increase the proportion of tribal and local health service areas or jurisdictions that have established a community health promotion program that addresses multiple *Healthy People 2010* focus areas.	–
7.11	Culturally appropriate community health-promotion programs	Increase the proportion of local health departments to at least 50% that have established culturally appropriate and linguistically competent community health-promotion and disease-prevention programs for racial and ethnic minority populations.	13-27%
7.12	Elderly participation in community health promotion	Increase to at least 90% the proportion of people age 65 and older who have participated during the preceding year in at least one organized health-promotion program.	12%

U.S. Department of Health and Human Services (USDHHS). (2000). *Healthy people 2010:* Understanding and Improving Health (2nd ed.). Washington, DC: U.S. Government Printing Office.

vital. The community health nurse should consider what motivates people to adopt new behaviors and what factors may inhibit or prevent that change. By understanding the principles of teaching and behavior change, the community health nurse can work toward the ultimate goal of health promotion for individuals, families, groups, and communities.

HEALTH PROMOTION THROUGH CHANGE

Health promotion has been defined as "behavior motivated by the desire to increase well-being and actualize human health potential" (Pender, Murdaugh, & Parsons, 2006, p.7). Another term often confused with health promotion is *disease prevention* (or *health protection*), which is "behavior motivated by a desire to actively avoid illness, detect it early, or maintain functioning within the constraints of illness" (Pender et al., p. 7). These two terms, so often used interchangeably, are clearly both important aspects of health education efforts, yet they imply a decidedly different motivation. For the community health nurse, both terms are aligned to practice at the primary level of prevention. The Levels of Prevention Pyramid at the end of this chapter describes educational activities within both of these approaches in relation to primary prevention. For instance, a community health nurse may plan an educational program for community-dwelling older adults to learn about the need for a balanced diet, rich in fruits and vegetables. This would be an example of a health promotion focus, since there is no clear disease or condition at issue. As the nurse continues to work with these individuals, he learns that several clients have had recent falls. Fortunately, none of the falls was serious, yet the nurse recognizes the need to discuss foods that will help reduce bone loss and promote healthy bone growth. To protect the clients' health, the nurse provides information on a variety of foods rich in calcium and explains the need for adequate vitamin D. This effort would be still primary prevention, but with the purpose of health protection.

For the community health nurse, teaching is the primary means to influence health at all levels, primary, secondary, and tertiary. But consider the community health nurse's educational program just described: He has provided a well-developed educational program that was well received by the participants. They listened attentively, took the nurse's well-prepared handouts home, and even promised to add more fruits, vegetables, and calcium-rich foods to their diet. A few weeks later, in another educational program, the nurse learns from the participants that they have not altered their dietary patterns in the slightest. This is an example of how understanding the principles of behavior change may have provided guidance to this nurse in planning a more effective program, with greater prospects for success.

The Nature of Change

To be a community health nurse is to be a health educator with the goal of effecting change in people's behaviors. When nurses suggest that families adopt healthier communication patterns, they are asking them to change. Teaching parenting skills to teenagers is introducing a change. Promoting a community's self-determination in choosing a safer environment requires that the individuals involved must change. Therefore, it becomes imperative for community health nurses to understand the nature of change, how

---

DISPLAY 11.1   CHANGING BEHAVIOR

- People decide to change for lots of different reasons.
- People try and fail several times before they successfully change habits.
- Working at some changes can be life-long.
- Most people change on their own; they don't need special programs.
- What works for one person may not help another.

Adapted from Center for the Advancement of Health. (2006). *What we know about changing behavior.* Retrieved June 13, 2008 from http://www.cfah.org/about/whatweknow.cfm.

---

people respond to it, and how to effect change for improved community health (see Display 11.1).

Definitions and Types of Change

Change is "any planned or unplanned alteration of the status quo in an organism, situation, or process" (Lippitt, 1973, p. 37). This classic definition explains that change may occur either by design or by default. Over the years, various theorists have contributed to understanding the nature of change. From a systems perspective, change means that things are out of balance or the system's equilibrium is upset (Roussel, Swansburg, & Swansburg, 2006; Rowitz, 2006). For instance, when a community is devastated by a flood, its normal functioning is thrown off balance. Adjustments are required; new patterns of behavior become necessary.

Other classic theorists have explained change as the process of adopting an innovation (Spradley & McCurdy, 1994). Something different, such as an organization-wide smoke-free policy, is introduced; change occurs when the innovation is accepted, tried, and integrated into daily practice. Some have explained change in terms of its effect on behavior—change requires adjustment in thinking and behavior, and people's responses to change vary according to their perceptions of it. Change threatens the security that people feel when following established and familiar patterns (Cherry & Jacob, 2005). It generally requires adopting new roles. Change is disruptive. The way people respond to change depends partly on the type of change. The change process can be described as sudden or drastic (revolutionary) or gradual over time (evolutionary).

Evolutionary change is change that is gradual and requires adjustment on an incremental basis. It modifies rather than replaces a current way of operating. Some examples of evolutionary change include becoming parents, gradually cutting back on the number of cigarettes smoked each day, and losing weight by eliminating desserts and snacks. Because it is gradual, this kind of change does not require radical shifts in goals or values. For the most part, people resist discarding their own ideas. Accepting another's idea can reduce their self-esteem and is resisted. Gradual change may "ease the pain" that change brings to some individuals. Sometimes this type of change may be viewed as *reform*.

Revolutionary change, in contrast, is a more rapid, drastic, and threatening type of change that may completely upset the balance of a system. It involves different goals and perhaps radically new patterns of behavior. Sudden unemployment, stopping smoking overnight, losing the town's football team in a plane accident, suddenly removing children from abusive parents, or suddenly replacing human workers with computers are examples of revolutionary changes. In each instance, the people affected have little or no advance warning and little or no time to prepare. High levels of emotional, mental, and sometimes physical energy and rapid behavior change are required to adapt to revolutionary change. If the demands are too great, some may experience defense mechanisms such as incapacitation, resistance, or denial of the new situation.

The impact of a proposed change on a system clearly depends on the degree of the change's evolutionary or revolutionary qualities, a factor to be considered in planning for change. Some situations lend themselves better to one kind of change than another. A community in need of improved facilities for the handicapped (e.g., ramps, wider doors) can introduce this change on an evolutionary, incremental basis, whereas a community that is involved in an unsafe, intolerable, or life-threatening situation, such as a flood or serious influenza epidemic, may require revolutionary change.

Stages of Change

The phrase **stages of change** refers to the three sequential steps leading to change: unfreezing (when desire for change develops), changing (when new ideas are accepted and tried out), and refreezing (when the change is integrated and stabilized in practice). These stages were first described by Kurt Lewin in the 1940s and early 1950s, and they have become a cornerstone for understanding the change process in more recent years (Lewin, 1947, 1951; Lippitt, Watson, & Westley, 1958).

Unfreezing

The first stage, unfreezing, occurs when a developing need for change causes disequilibrium in the system. A system in disequilibrium is more vulnerable to change. People are motivated to change either intrinsically or by some external force. People have a sense of dissatisfaction; they feel a void that they would like to fill. The unfreezing stage involves initiating the change.

Unfreezing may occur spontaneously: A family requests help in solving a problem with alcoholism, a group seeks assistance in adjusting to retirement, a community desires a solution to noise pollution. However, the nurse as change agent may need to initiate the unfreezing stage by attempting to motivate clients, through education or other strategies, to see the need for change.

Changing/Moving

The second stage of the change process, changing or moving, occurs when people examine, accept, and try the innovation. For instance, this is the period when participants in a prenatal class are learning exercises or when elderly clients in a senior citizens' center are discussing and trying ways to make their apartments safe from accidents. During the changing stage, people experience a series of attitude transformations, ranging from early questioning of the innovation's worth, to full acceptance and commitment, to accomplishing the change. The change agent's role during this moving stage is to help clients see the value of the change, encourage them to try it out, and assist them in adopting it (Cherry & Jacob, 2005).

Refreezing

The third and final stage in the change process, refreezing, occurs when change is established as an accepted and permanent part of the system. The rest of the system has adapted to it. Because it is no longer viewed as disruptive, threatening, or new, people no longer feel resistant to it. As the change is integrated, the system becomes refrozen and stabilized. It is evident that refreezing has occurred when weight-loss clients, for example, are routinely following their diets and losing weight, or when senior citizens are using grab bars in their bathrooms and have removed scatter rugs from their homes, or when a community has erected stop signs and established crosswalks at dangerous intersections.

Refreezing involves integrating or internalizing the change into the system and then maintaining it. Because a change has been accepted and tried does not guarantee that it will last. Often, there is a tendency for old patterns and habits to return. Consequently, the change agent must take special measures to ensure maintenance of the new behavior. A later section discusses ways to stabilize change.

Planned/Managed Change

Leaders in community health nursing have been change agents for decades. They have planned and managed change in a variety of systems. **Planned change** is a purposeful, designed effort to effect improvement in a system with the assistance of a change agent (Spradley, 1980). Planned change, also known as managed change (Roussel, et al. 2006), is crucial to the development of successful community health nursing programs. The following characteristics of planned change are key to its success:

The change is purposeful and intentional: There are specific reasons or goals prompting the change. These goals give the change effort a unifying focus and a specific target. Unplanned change occurs haphazardly, and its outcomes are unpredictable.

The change is by design, not by default: Thorough, systematic planning provides structure for the change process and a map to follow toward a planned destination.

Planned change in community health aims at improvement: That is, it seeks to better the current situation, to promote a higher level of efficiency, safety, or health enhancement. Planned change aims to facilitate growth and positive improvements. Plans to provide shelter and health care for a homeless population, for example, are designed to improve this group's well-being.

Planned change is accomplished through an influencing agent: The change agent is a catalyst in developing and carrying out the design; the change agent's role is a leadership role; often as an educator.

Planned Change Model

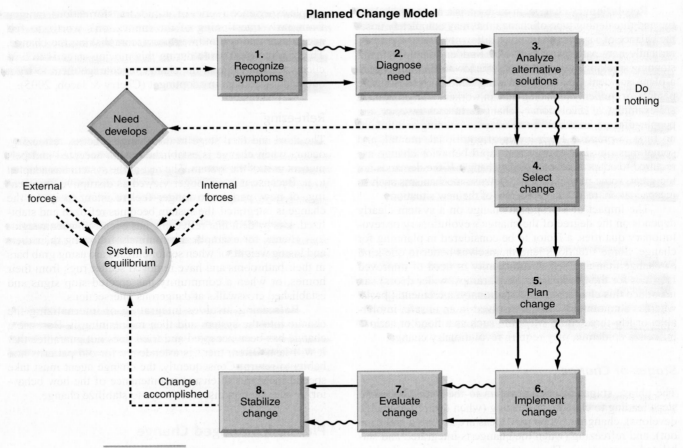

FIGURE 11.1 Planned change model. The planned change process begins when one recognizes a need. When the change agent fails to respond to a need for change, the need continues and may escalate. Client system (those involved and affected by the change) and change agent must work together throughout the entire planned change process. Their respective roles vary depending on the situation and the players' abilities, but no planned change is truly effective without utilization of this collaborative relationship. The client system (*wavy arrow*), which may be an entire community, will fluctuate in its involvement with the change process. The change agent (*straight arrow*), as a good leader, analyzes the situation thoroughly, plans carefully, and sets a steady course for effecting the change.

Planned Change Process

The planned change process involves a systematic sequence of activities that follows the nursing process. Following its eight basic steps leads to the successful management of change: (1) recognize symptoms, (2) diagnose need, (3) analyze alternative solutions, (4) select a change, (5) plan the change, (6) implement the change, (7) evaluate the change, and (8) stabilize the change (Spradley, 1980). Figure 11.1 shows how forces acting on a system create a need for change using the planned-change model.

Step 1: Recognize (Assess) Symptoms

The first step in managing change is to recognize and assess the symptoms that indicate a need for change. This step requires gathering and examining the presenting evidence, not diagnosing or jumping ahead to treatment. For instance, assume that a group of clients shows interest in receiving help with parenting skills. The nurse cannot assume that these clients feel inadequate in the parent role, nor can the nurse

assume that they lack information about parenting or are having difficulty with their children. The nurse must assess the specific needs to discover that some of the parents have trouble talking to their teenagers, others wonder whether their children's behavior is normal, a few question how strictly they should set limits, and still others are not certain about how to handle punishment. These symptoms are pieces of evidence that will assist diagnosis in the next step. This first step is an assessment phase. Before moving on, however, change agents need to ask themselves what their motives are for pursuing this change. Inappropriate motives on the change agent's part, such as wanting to feel needed, can cloud judgment and interfere with effective management of change.

Step 2: Diagnose Need

Diagnosis involves analyzing the symptoms and reaching a conclusion about what needs changing. First, describe the situation as it is now (the real) and compare it with the way it should be (the ideal). For example, loud arguing and conflict may be normal and functional behavior for an adolescent support group. There is no discrepancy between the real and the ideal and, therefore, no need for change within the group. If, however, a discrepancy exists between the real and the ideal, then a need exists and a change effort is justified (Hersey, Blanchard, & Johnson, 2008). For example, the community health nurse, in talking with a group of parents, hears the following comment: "I'm not sure how much freedom to allow Karen. She came in late twice last week and I'm not sure how to punish her." Clearly, the nurse notices a discrepancy between this family's present and ideal situations; hence, a need exists.

The next step is to determine the nature and cause of the need. Gathering data by questioning clients, checking the literature, or seeking consultation is important for making a more accurate diagnosis. The parents should be questioned in more detail about the difficulties that they are having with their children. The nurse asks questions such as the following: How do they feel about being parents? What are the most difficult aspects of parenting for them? Have they read any books or used any other resources to help them in their parenting activities? To whom do they talk about parenting problems? When they have a problem raising their children, how do they usually solve it? Secondary data should be obtained by checking the literature to determine the most effective approaches to solving parenting problems or by consulting an expert on family life to get ideas about what this group of parents might need. The parents also should be asked directly what information they desire or need. Conclusions should be drawn about the specific changes needed for these parents. Unless the diagnosis is made accurately, the entire change effort may address the wrong problem. Also, the client system should help the nurse to diagnose their problem; the nurse should ask the parents what it is that they want and need.

These findings should be formulated into a single, diagnostic statement that also includes the problem's cause. After data collection, the nurse discovers that the parents are insecure in their parenting roles, partially because of lack of knowledge about how to carry out parental responsibilities, but primarily because they lack a supportive reference group. Most of them live some distance from relatives or no longer maintain close ties with them. The diagnosis for these parents is insecurity in the parenting role resulting from a lack of support and knowledge.

Step 3: Analyze Alternative Solutions

Once the diagnosis and its cause are determined, it is time to identify solutions or alternative directions to follow. Brainstorming is helpful here, and the client system should be involved as much as possible in the process. Reviewing the literature is helpful at this point to suggest solutions tried by others. Make a list of all reasonable, broad alternatives and then analyze them thoroughly to determine the advantages, disadvantages, possible consequences, and risks involved in each. For the parents, general alternatives might be considered, such as family counseling, a support group, or education in family life. Each of these alternatives includes some advantages and disadvantages toward meeting the parents' need for confidence in their roles.

Next, each alternative should be analyzed. For example, the counseling solution could provide insight and awareness into family behavior. It would give family members opportunities to express feelings and gain understanding of how other family members feel. However, it would not provide a frame of reference that the clients could use to compare their own parenting behaviors with other acceptable ones, nor would it provide adult peer support for the parents. The consequences of this alternative most likely would be to promote parents' self-understanding and better family communication. Risks would include the possibility that children, especially teenagers, might not be willing to participate and that parents might not gain self-confidence in their roles. Each alternative should be examined to determine its usefulness and feasibility, again literature and other resources (e.g., consultants) can be used to learn the best ways to meet the parents' need for change.

Step 4: Select a Change

After all alternatives have been carefully analyzed, the best solution must be selected. The parents favor the idea that the best solution is a parenting support group. The risks involved in the choice of change should be reexamined, such as whether this action might be too costly in terms of time, money, or potential for failure. Ways to reduce these risks might be explored.

To know what the change is aiming to accomplish, a clearly stated goal should be formulated. For this parenting group, the mutually agreed-on goal is to provide a supportive, reinforcing climate while increasing members' parenting skills.

Step 5: Plan the Change

Step 5 is at the heart of planned change, because at this stage, the change agent and client system together prepare the design, or blueprint, that guides the change action. In steps 1 through 4, data are gathered, a diagnosis is made, resources are assessed, and a goal is established—all preparatory actions for planning the change. The plan tells the change agent and the client system how to meet that goal. Preferably, they develop the plan together.

The nurse talks with the parents about ways to meet their goal, considering such possibilities as weekly discussion groups on selected topics, monthly meetings with an informed speaker, or reading books and articles on parenting and holding regular sessions to discuss their application. After analysis and discussion, the group decides to meet one evening a month, rotating the location among members' homes. Group sessions will include a variety of approaches: a speaker will be invited every 4 months, a book or article discussion will be held quarterly, and the remaining meetings will be spent on topics of the group's choice. All sessions will provide opportunities for parents to discuss their concerns or problems. The nurse and the group design this plan around a set of objectives.

The most important activity in planning is to have clear, specific objectives. These should be measurable and, preferably, stated as outcomes. For example, the following objective is measurable and describes an outcome: "By the end of the second session, each parent in the group will have participated in the discussion at least once." It is helpful to prepare a list of activities to help accomplish each objective and to develop a time plan. It also is important to assess the potential costs in terms of time, money, materials, and the number of people needed and to determine the resources available. Then the evaluation plan is designed, and a list of ways to stabilize (refreeze) the change is made.

During planning, it is useful to perform a *force field analysis* (Hersey, Blanchard, & Johnson, 2008), a technique developed by Kurt Lewin for examining all positive (driving) and negative (restraining) forces that are influencing a change situation. **Force field theory** describes driving forces, which favor change, and restraining forces, which decrease or discourage change. Examples of driving forces include clients' desire to be healthier, to be more productive, or to have a safer environment. Examples of restraining forces include apathy, habits, fear of something new, perceived loss of power, low self-esteem, insecurity, and hostility (Roussel, Swansburg, & Swansburg, 2006). When the strength of the driving forces is equal to the strength of the restraining forces, equilibrium exists. To introduce a change and move the client system to a higher level of health, that balance must be altered. The change agent either increases the driving forces, decreases the restraining forces, or both. The change agent uses force field analysis to study both sets of forces and to develop strategies to influence the forces in favor of the change (Fig. 11.2).

The procedure for conducting a force field analysis follows a few simple steps. The change agent may perform the analysis alone but preferably consults with clients and a change-planning resource group such as community health colleagues. The steps for conducting force field analysis are as follows:

1. Brainstorm to produce a list of all driving and restraining forces. (For the parenting group, one driving force is the parents' desire to be more suc-

cessful parents; a restraining force might be lack of group agreement on discussion topics.)
2. Estimate the strength of each force.
3. Plot the forces on a chart such as the one shown in Figure 11.2.
4. Note the most important forces, then research and analyze them.
5. List and document possible responses or actions that might strengthen each important driving force or weaken each important restraining force.

Finally, as a consideration in planning the change and in analyzing the driving and restraining forces, the change agent studies the social network and interactions within the system involved in the change. The change agent needs to be aware of formal and informal leaders, cliques within larger groups, influential persons, and all other social network influences on the change process. For instance, one nurse attempting to improve the infant-feeding practices among a group of young southeast Asian mothers failed to consider the strong cultural influence of the infants' grandmothers living nearby. The older women had strong opinions based on long-held cultural traditions about what infants were to eat and how they were to be fed. To ignore their influence could cause the proposed change to fail; involving the grandmothers could be a way of turning their influence into a driving force for the change.

Step 6: Implement the Change

The implementation step involves enacting the change plan. Because the objectives and activities have been clearly defined in previous steps, the change agent and client system know what needs to be done and how to begin the process.

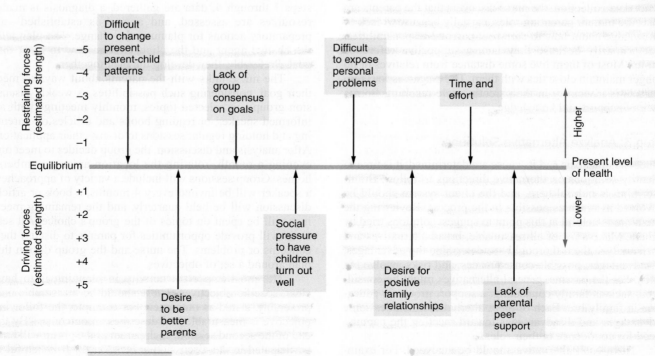

FIGURE 11.2 Analysis of restraining and driving forces.

For example, the parenting group and their nurse/change agent begin group discussions meeting every Tuesday evening at a local school.

At the start of implementation, be certain that all persons concerned clearly understand and are prepared for the change. When working with an aggregate, for example, the nurse may do most of the planning with a few key members. The nurse must be sure that each member who will be affected by the proposed change understands (a) what to expect, (b) the meaning of the change, and (c) what will be required of them in adapting to it. An unprepared client system, especially in a large group or organization, may bring disaster (Tiffany & Lutjens, 1998). No matter how well a change effort is planned, people who are unprepared for it may resist it strongly and render it useless.

When implementing change that will affect a large group of people, such as introduction of a mass screening or immunization program, it is helpful to do a *pilot study*. The pilot study is done to test the change on a small scale, iron out problems, and revise the change before implementing it in the larger system. One advantage of a pilot study is that it demonstrates the change to the client system on a small scale, which is less threatening, so that clients are more receptive. It gives people time to adjust their thinking and to discover that the change will not disrupt their lives too much or require drastic adaptations.

Step 7: Evaluate the Change

The success of step 7 depends on how well the change is planned. Well-written objectives with specific criteria for their measurement make the evaluation step simpler. However, evaluation does not end with saying whether the objectives were met. Each objective requires analysis: Was it met? What evidence (documentation) shows that it was met? Was it accomplished using the best means possible, or would another method have been better? The objective for the parenting group stated that each member should enter into the discussion by the end of the second session. Although this objective could easily be evaluated by the nurse leader, the objective could have been improved by more a specific description of how this participation would occur. A better method to achieve this objective would have been to suggest that more active group members could solicit ideas from those who did not have an opportunity to speak. This would facilitate more group participation, rather than having the nurse educator call on nontalkers to speak. Finally, considering the evaluation, the change agent makes needed modifications in the change before stabilization.

Step 8: Stabilize the Change

The final step in the planned change process requires taking measures to reinforce and maintain the change. A well-developed change plan includes a design for stabilization. The change agent actively encourages continued use of the innovation by establishing two-way communication. In this way, future resistance can be overcome, and the client's full commitment to the change can be maintained. Stabilization occurs by soliciting reactions from the client system. Do the clients perceive any potential problems? Do they have doubts? Reinforcing the desired behavior and following up on the change as long as necessary will help to ensure its permanence.

Alcoholics Anonymous, for example, stabilizes the change to nondrinking by providing a regular support group that reinforces the nondrinking pattern. The group rewards compliance with praise and replaces drinking with other satisfying experiences, such as social acceptance, to keep the alcoholic from returning to the old behavior. In the example of the parenting group, the nurse stabilizes changed behaviors by focusing on the group's increased confidence in their parenting roles and emphasizing the increased success in coping with their children. The group decides to reward successes by giving a "Parent of the Month" plaque to the member who demonstrates the most growth in parenting skills, and they agree to nominate one member as "Parent of the Year" in the community newspaper contest. After stabilization occurs and the system achieves a new equilibrium, the change agent–client system relationship can be terminated for this specific change effort.

Applying Planned Change to Larger Aggregates

We have viewed the planned-change process primarily in the context of introducing change to smaller aggregates. Community health nurses also use these eight steps when managing change at organization, population group, community, and larger aggregate levels. For example, a nurse may suspect that there is a widespread lack of confidence among young parents. This hypothesis could be tested through a survey using a mailed questionnaire to determine parenting needs among the entire community's population of young parents. If symptoms are present (step 1), the nurse, in collaboration with health department personnel or other appropriate professionals, could analyze the symptoms and reach a diagnosis (step 2), perhaps that many young parents in the community are lacking in confidence and knowledge of parenting skills. Several approaches to meeting this need could be considered, such as instituting a parenting center in the community with satellite clinics, organizing churches or clubs to sponsor parenting support groups, or working through the community college system to hold workshops and classes on parenting skills (step 3). The most feasible and useful alternative could be selected (step 4), and a parenting program for the community could be planned (step 5) and implemented (step 6). The nurse, with parents and other professionals involved, then would evaluate the outcomes (step 7) and make necessary adjustments in the parenting program before finally stabilizing it (step 8), making certain that this change, undertaken to meet a population group need, remains an established and effectively functioning service.

Planned-Change Strategies

Here we focus on the three major change strategies: (1) empiric-rational, (2) normative-reeducative, and (3) power-coercive. In a given situation, the change agent may use one or a combination of these strategies to effect a change.

Empiric-Rational Change Strategies

Empiric-rational change strategies are used to effect change based on the assumption that people are rational and, when presented with empiric information, will adopt new practices that appear to be in their best interest. To use this approach, which is common in community health, new information is offered to people. For instance, most family planning programs use empiric-rational strategies. Clients are given basic information (communication-related strategy) on reproductive anatomy and physiology, and they are told about the benefits of contraception with an explanation of a variety of family planning methods. Health workers hope that once clients have this information, they will adopt some method of family planning. Some clients respond well to this approach, and others do not. The difference lies in client ability and interest in self-help. The nurse/change agent uses empiric-rational strategies with clients who can assume a relatively high degree of responsibility for their own health.

Normative-Reeducative Change Strategies

Normative-reeducative change strategies are used to influence change that not only presents new information but also directly influences people's attitudes and behaviors through persuasion. It is a sociocultural reeducation. This approach assumes that people's attitudes and practices are determined by sociocultural norms and that they need more than presentation of information to change behavior. This approach strengthens client self-understanding, self-control, and commitment to new patterns through direct urging and influence. For example, a health education program that aims to increase safety practices in an industrial setting not only provides safety information, such as posters and warning signs, but also uses persuasive tactics, such as individual rewards for safe practices, division recognition for minimum number of accidents, or discipline for noncompliance. Nurses use normative-reeducative strategies with clients who have a measure of self-care skill but at the same time need external assistance to effect lasting behavioral change. This type of client is found in teaching, counseling, and therapy situations.

Power-Coercive Change Strategies

Power-coercive change strategies use coercion based on fear to effect change. Change agents may derive power from the law (e.g., health regulations, administrative policies), from position (e.g., political, social, or managerial), from a group (social, work, or professional), or from personal power (e.g., personal charisma, competence, respect of followers). They use this power to coerce change; the result is forced compliance on the part of the client system. Some situations, particularly those that are life-threatening, may require power-coercive strategies. In community health practice, power-coercive strategies may be used with people who cannot help themselves or in situations that threaten individuals' safety or the public's health. An example is the stringent enforcement of infection control policies regarding the treatment of contaminated objects such as used needles and the safe disposal of infectious wastes. In another example, if officials find a restaurant to be in violation of health codes, they will either force compliance with the code or close the restaurant. Occasionally, clients cannot exercise responsibility because of temporary or permanent physical or psycho-

logical incapacitation; examples may include mentally ill individuals, abusive parents, or developmentally disabled persons. In such cases, the nurse may need to use the power of the law to effect changes that are in clients' best interests. Although power-coercive strategies are appropriate in some situations, they should be used with caution because they can rob people of opportunities to grow in autonomy and capacity for self-care.

Planned-change strategies may be combined; for instance, a normative-reeducative approach might have a power-coercive backup. This combination is evident in programs that educate and persuade groups of people to be immunized against an impending epidemic or to keep their garbage contained to avoid insect and rodent infestation. Behind this normative-reeducative strategy is an implied coercive threat of official disapproval, or worse, if the clients are noncompliant.

The effectiveness of a change strategy, then, varies with each situation and particularly with the degree of client capacity for self-care. The community health nurse, as a change agent must adapt strategies to fit each change situation. It is important to remember that "the central issue in change is not just strategy, structure, culture, or systems change, but how people see the proposed change and how it affects their feelings about the changes proposed" (Rowitz, 2006, p. 437).

Principles for Effecting Positive Change

Community health nurses introduce change every day that they practice. Every effort to solve a problem, prevent another problem from occurring, meet a potential community need, or promote people's optimal health requires changes. For these changes to be truly successful, so that desired outcomes are reached, they must be managed well. The following six principles provide guidelines for effecting positive change: (1) principle of participation, (2) principle of resistance to change, (3) principle of proper timing, (4) principle of interdependence, (5) principle of flexibility, and (6) principle of self-understanding.

Principle of Participation

Persons affected by a proposed change should participate as much as possible in every step of the planned change process (Cherry & Jacobs, 2005). This involvement is important for several reasons. Collaboration with those who have a vested interest in the change can produce a wealth of ideas and insights that can greatly improve the change plan. Furthermore, such participation can help remove obstacles and reduce resistance. Participation ensures a greater likelihood that the change will be accepted and maintained. One nurse, for instance, when planning with a school's parent–teacher association for a drug education program, involved students as well as teachers and parents. As a result, the nurse secured all this group's support and cooperation, gained many helpful suggestions that had not been previously considered, and discovered that students were more responsive to the program because the change plan was specifically tailored to their needs.

Principle of Resistance to Change

Because all systems instinctively preserve the status quo, the change agent can expect people to resist change (Cherry & Jacob, 2005). The homeostatic mechanism operating in any system seeks to maintain equilibrium; change poses a threat to that stability and security. Furthermore, all systems experience inertia; that is, they resist beginning movement. People do not undertake a change until they are convinced of its worth. Resistance may also come from a conflict over goals and methods or from misunderstanding about what the change will mean and require. Involving people in the planned change process, as discussed in the previous section, is one way to overcome resistance. Another way is establishing and maintaining open lines of communication to make ideas clearly understood and to resolve disagreements quickly. The nurse must prepare clients thoroughly for the change, provide support and patience during the change process, and encourage response and expression of feelings (Tiffany & Lutjens, 1998).

Principle of Proper Timing

Sometimes a change, even a well-designed and much-needed one, should be postponed because it is not the right time to introduce it. For example, perhaps the client system is experiencing too many other changes to handle the stress of this one. Other projects or activities in which the client system is currently engaged may compete for energy and other resources, depleting the energy and resources needed to make the proposed change successful. For example, in November, some middle-aged women, eager to start a book club that focused on discussion of preparing for midlife changes (including menopause, "empty-nest" syndrome, and planning for retirement), had to postpone the project because the holidays were approaching. Shopping, entertaining, and vacations made it impossible to give the kind of time and energy needed to make the book club effective.

Proper timing is as important to a planned change as well-timed seed planting is to a good harvest. The change idea must be appropriate, the change recipient prepared, the climate right, and the resources available before the change can be fostered to grow into full maturity and usefulness.

Principle of Interdependence

Every system has many subsystems that are intricately related to and interdependent on one another. A change in one part of a system affects its other parts, and a change in one system may affect other systems. For example, a county community nursing agency made a change in its use of home health aides. Because many homebound clients needed more care than the agency staff could provide, the agency contracted with a private home-care service for extra home health aides. These paraprofessionals worked in the homes of agency clients, supplementing the care given by agency staff. The private company preferred to supervise its own aides, whereas the county agency had a policy of using community health nurses to supervise aides. The county agency was legally responsible and professionally accountable for the quality of care given to clients. The private company wanted to retain control of its workers. The matter was resolved by contracting with a different private service that would accept the county agency's supervision. The change, however, had affected the roles of nurses and aides within the system, as well as the relationships between the two systems.

This principle of interdependence reminds the nurse that change does not take place in a vacuum. When workers learn new health and safety practices associated with their jobs, their relationships with one another, and their bosses, their overall productivity in the organization may easily be affected. One must anticipate and prepare for the impact of the proposed change on the clients involved, other persons, departments, organizations, or even geographic areas.

Principle of Flexibility

Unexpected events can occur in every situation. This fifth principle—flexibility—emphasizes two points. First, the nurse needs to be able to adapt to unexpected events and make the most of them. Perseverance and flexibility are the marks of a creative change manager (Clampitt & DeKoch, 2001; Roussel et al., 2006). One community health nurse had tried unsuccessfully to contact a young mother who was reportedly abusing her 2-year-old son. After several phone calls and visits to an empty house, the nurse finally found the mother and son at home with a neighbor who insisted on staying for the entire visit. At first, the nurse was irritated by the neighbor's presence and viewed it as interfering with the goal of getting to know the mother and child. When the nurse realized that the neighbor's presence offered an opportunity to learn more about the situation through the neighbor's input, the nurse viewed it as an opportunity to influence another client as well. She asked whether the neighbor had children, and began to include both women in the discussion, explaining what could be offered in terms of health teaching and support. This nurse was flexible in her approach to this situation.

The second point to remember about flexibility is that a good change planner anticipates possible blocks or problems by preparing strategies and alternative plans. During step 3 of the planned change process, it is helpful to rank the alternative solutions considered. Then, if the first choice does not work out for some reason, an alternative is ready to be put into action. Flexibility involves a willingness to consider a variety of options and suggestions from many sources (Clampitt & DeKoch, 2001).

Principle of Self-Understanding

Self-understanding is essential for an effective change agent (Hersey, Blanchard, & Johnson, 2008). The community nurse (as change agent) should be able to clearly define his role and learn how others define it. It is important to understand one's values and motives in relation to each change that one might ask people to make. Nurses also should understand their own personality traits, so that they can capitalize on or alter them to be more effective change agents. Understanding oneself is crucial to learning to make use of one's best qualities and skills to effect change.

Change is inevitable. It can be seen as the "process of moving from what has become an obsolete present into a revitalized present with an eye on the future . . . the old rules do not seem to be working anymore, and new rules and procedures need to be developed for the changing context in which we live today" (Rowitz, 2006, p. 431). Understanding the principles of planned change can assist the community health nurse in guiding individuals, families, and communities toward achieving the highest level of health.

CHANGE THROUGH HEALTH EDUCATION

Early in this chapter, you were introduced to one definition of health promotion, with a clear focus on individual and aggregate behavior (Pender et al., 2006). Consider another definition: "any combination of educational, organizational, environmental, and economic supports for behavior and conditions of living that are conducive to health" (Ottoson & Green, 2008, p. 614). This definition points out the need for a system-wide approach to promoting healthy behaviors, one that includes education. For the community health nurse, health education is a foundation of practice. Whether the nurse is providing one-on-one education to a new mother about the benefits of breast-feeding or briefing county officials on the need to maintain breast-feeding support centers, educational techniques are being used to promote health in the community. Knowledge of educational theories and teaching methods can assist the nurse to frame these "health messages" for the greatest impact and chance of success.

Teaching is a specialized communication process in which desired behavior changes are achieved. The goal of all teaching is learning. Learning is thought to mean gaining knowledge, comprehension, or mastery. These are nebulous terms, and a more acceptable definition suggests that **learning** is a process of assimilating new information that promotes a permanent change in behavior. All people have been presented with information that was not interesting, relevant to their needs, or comprehensible. In such situations, learning is difficult, if not impossible. The nurse as teacher seeks to transmit information in such a way that the client demonstrates a relatively permanent change in behavior. After learning, clients are capable of doing something that they could not do before learning took place. Effective teaching is a cause; learning becomes the effect. To teach effectively, especially in the community where teaching is the focus of care, nurses need to understand the various domains of learning and related learning theories.

DOMAINS OF LEARNING

Learning occurs in several realms or domains: cognitive, affective, and psychomotor. Understanding of the differences among the domains and of the related roles of the nurse provides the background necessary to teach effectively.

Cognitive Domain

The **cognitive domain** of learning involves the mind and thinking processes. When the meaning and relationship of a series of facts is grasped, cognitive learning is experienced. The cognitive domain deals with the recall or recognition of knowledge and the development of intellectual abilities and skills (Bloom, 1956). There are six major levels in the cognitive domain (Gronlund, 1970; Gronlund & Linn, 1990): knowledge, comprehension, application, analysis, synthesis, and evaluation. To **operationalize** these levels (i.e., put these ideas or concepts into words that can be used), verbs are used. As the goal of the learning or behavioral objective changes, so do the verbs, indicating the learning to be accomplished within that particular level of the cognitive domain. Notice that the objectives at the beginning of each chapter in this text follow this format, using a variety of verbs to indicate the expected level of learning. A representative sample of behavioral objectives focusing on nutrition and appropriate cognitive-level verbs is included in the discussion of each level.

Knowledge

Knowledge, the lowest level of learning according to Bloom's taxonomy (1956), involves recall. If students remember material previously learned, they have acquired knowledge. This level may be used with clients who are unable to understand underlying reasons or rationales, such as young children or people who have had strokes. Stroke clients may need to remember that medication should be taken daily, that regular exercise restores function, and that drinking alcohol should be avoided, although they may not grasp the reasons behind these measures. Five-year-olds may need to identify healthful foods rather than understand why they are nutritious.

A knowledge-level behavioral objective might be, "The client can *recall* the names of six fruits to eat as nutritious snacks." Other knowledge-level verbs include *define, repeat, list,* and *name.*

Comprehension

The second level of cognitive learning, comprehension, combines remembering with understanding. Teaching aims at instilling at least a minimal understanding. Nurses want clients to grasp the meaning and to recognize the importance of suggested health behaviors.

An example of a comprehension-level behavioral objective might be, "The pregnant client will *describe* a well-balanced diet during pregnancy." Other appropriate verbs at the comprehension level include *discuss, explain, identify, tell,* and *report.*

Application

Application is the third level of cognitive learning, in which the learner can not only understand material but also apply it to new situations. Application approaches the possibility of self-care when clients use their knowledge to improve their own health. The test of application is a transfer of understanding into practice. Therefore, to encourage application, the nurse can design teaching plans that provide clients with knowledge that can be put into practice. In the home setting, a nurse may suggest that a diabetic client write down glucometer readings to show the nurse at the next visit. A school nurse could ask adolescents in a weight-loss group to keep a diet record for a week, draw up a diet plan, and share this plan with the group at the next meeting. In contrast, the construction worker who understands on-the-job hazards but seldom wears a protective hat in the work area has yet to transfer knowledge and comprehension into practice or application.

An example of an application-level behavioral objective might be, "The client will *practice* eating well-balanced meals at least two times a day." Other verbs at this level include *apply, use, demonstrate,* and *illustrate.*

Analysis

The fourth level of cognitive learning is analysis; at this level, the learner breaks down material into parts, distinguishes between elements, and understands the relationships among the parts. This level of learning becomes a preliminary step toward problem-solving. The learner carefully scrutinizes all of the variables or elements and their relationships to each other to explain the situation. A family that studies its own communication patterns to identify sources of conflict is using analysis. A mother analyzes when she seeks to determine the cause of an infant's crying. After viewing the total situation, she breaks it down into variables such as hunger, pain, overstimulation, loneliness, type of crying, and intensity of crying. She examines these parts and draws conclusions about their relationships. In health teaching, community health nurses foster clients' analytic skills by (a) demonstrating how to isolate the parts in a situation, and (b) encouraging the clients to consider the relationships among the parts and to draw conclusions from their thinking.

An analysis-level behavioral objective for senior citizens trying to learn more about low-fat foods might be, "The seniors should be able to *compare* the fat content in a variety of packaged foods." Other verbs at the analysis level include *differentiate, contrast, debate, question,* and *examine.*

Synthesis

Synthesis, the fifth level of cognitive learning, is the ability not only to break down and understand the elements of a situation, but also to form elements into a new whole. Synthesis combines all of the earlier levels of cognitive learning to culminate in the production of a unique plan or solution. Clients who achieve learning at this level not only analyze their problems but also find solutions for them. For example, a nurse may assist mental health clients in a therapy group to examine their frequent depression and then to generate their own plan for alleviating it. A young couple who want to toilet train their 2-year-old child may learn the physiologic and psychological dimensions of toilet training, analyze their own situation, and then develop strategies (their own plan) for training the child. Nurses facilitate synthesis by assisting and encouraging clients to develop their own solutions with specific plans. After a problem is identified, the client should be asked, "What are some possible causes? Do you see anything that has been overlooked about the problem?" If the client asks for a solution, the nurse should encourage synthesis by asking, "What are some possible solutions to this problem that you might carry out?"

An example of a synthesis-level behavioral objective for a client on a sodium-restricted diet might be, "The client will be able to *prepare* an enjoyable meal using low-sodium foods." Other verbs at this level include *compose, design, formulate, create,* and *organize.*

Evaluation

The highest level of cognitive learning is evaluation: at this level, the learner judges the usefulness of new material compared with a stated purpose or specific criteria (Gronlund & Linn, 1990). Clients can learn to judge their own health behavior by comparing it with standards established by others—such as complete abstinence from smoking, maintenance of normal weight, or exercising three times a week. Alternatively, clients may establish their own criteria. For example, a parent support group might design activities to enhance parent–child communication, then judge their performance by using their desired outcomes as evaluation criteria. When nurses aim for this level of client learning, they have made self-care a concrete objective. Evaluation, because it goes beyond attempts at problem-solving, enables the client to judge the adequacy of solutions, to critique lifestyle and health-related behaviors, and to anticipate needed improvements.

An example of a behavioral objective at the evaluation level might be, "The clients in a nutrition class will be able to *measure* the cholesterol content in one portion of the low-cholesterol dish they brought to share." Other verbs at this level include *judge, rate, choose,* and *estimate.*

How to Measure Cognitive Learning

Cognitive learning at any of the levels described can be measured easily in terms of learner behaviors. Nurses know, for instance, that clients have achieved teaching objectives for the application of knowledge if their behavior demonstrates actual use of the information taught. Client roles in cognitive learning range from relatively passive (at the knowledge level) to active (at the evaluation level). Conversely, as clients become more active, the nurse's role becomes less directive. Notice that not all clients need to be brought through all levels of cognitive learning, nor does every client need to reach the evaluation level for each aspect of care. For some clients and situations, comprehension is an adequate and effective level; for others, the nurse should focus on the application level as the level of achievement. Table 11.2 illustrates client and nurse behaviors for each cognitive level.

Affective Domain

The **affective domain** in which learning occurs involves emotion, feeling, or *affect.* This kind of learning deals with changes in interest, attitudes, and values (Bloom, 1956). Here, nurses face the task of trying to influence what clients value and feel. Nurses want clients to develop an ability to accept ideas that promote healthier behavior patterns, even if those ideas conflict with the clients' own values.

Attitudes and values are learned. They develop gradually, as the way an individual feels and responds is molded

TABLE 11.2 Cognitive Learning: Case Study in Controlling Diabetes

Level	Illustrative Client Behavior	Illustrative Nurse Behavior
Knowledge (recalls, knows)	States that insulin, if taken, will control own diabetes	Provides information
Comprehension (understands)	Describes insulin action and purpose	Explains information
Application (uses learning)	Adjusts insulin dosage daily to maintain proper blood sugar level	Suggests how to use learning
Analysis (examines, explains)	Discusses relationships between insulin, diet, activity, and diabetic control	Demonstrates and encourages analysis
Synthesis (integrates with other learning, generates new ideas)	Develops a plan, incorporating above learning, for controlling own diabetes	Promotes client formulation of own plan
Evaluation (judges according to a standard)	Compares degree of diabetic control (outcomes) with desired control (objectives)	Facilitates evaluation

by family, peers, experiences, and cultural influences (Hollinger, 2005). These feelings and responses are the result of imitation and conditioning. In this way, clients acquire their health-related beliefs and practices. Because attitudes and values become part of the person, they are difficult to change unless the nurse is aware of how they develop.

Affective learning occurs on several levels as learners respond with varying degrees of involvement and commitment. At the first level, learners are simply receptive; they are willing to listen, to show awareness, and to be attentive. The nurse aims at acquiring and focusing learners' attention (Gronlund & Linn, 1990). This limited goal may be all that clients are ready for during the early stages of the nurse–client relationship.

At the second level, learners become active participants by responding to the information in some way. Examples are a willingness to read educational material, to participate in discussions, to complete assignments (e.g., keeping a diet record), or to voluntarily seek out more information.

At the third level, learners attach value to the information. Valuing ranges from simple acceptance through appreciation to commitment. For example, a nurse taught members of a therapy group several principles concerning group effectiveness. An explanation of the importance of a democratic group process and ways to improve group skills was given. Members showed acceptance when they acknowledged the importance of these ideas. They showed appreciation of the ideas by starting to practice them. Commitment came when they assumed responsibility for having their group function well.

The final level of affective learning occurs when learners internalize an idea or value. The value system now controls learner behavior. Consistent practice is a crucial test at this level. Clients who know and respect the value of exercise but only occasionally play tennis or go for a walk have not internalized the value. Even several weeks of enthusiastic jogging is not evidence of an internalized value. If the jogging continues for 6 months, 12 months, or longer, learning may have been internalized.

Affective learning often is difficult to measure (Rankin, Stallings, & London, 2005). This elusiveness may influence community health nurses to concentrate their efforts on cognitive learning goals instead. Yet, client attitudes and values have a major effect on the outcome of cognitive learning—desired behavioral changes. Therefore, both cognitive and affective domains must remain linked in teaching, otherwise, results quickly fade.

Attitudes and values can change in the same way that they were first learned, that is, through imitation and conditioning (Redman, 2001). Role models, particularly individuals from the client's peer group who practice the desired health behaviors, can be a strong influence. Support groups, such as mastectomy clubs or chemical dependency support groups, can have a powerful role-model effect. Frequently, the nurse is viewed as a role model by clients; for this reason, nurses should be careful to demonstrate healthy behaviors.

Attitudes often change when the nurse provides clients with a satisfying experience during the learning process. The nurse who recognizes clients' participation in a group, praises them for completing assignments, or commends them for sticking to diet plans will have more success than the nurse who only criticizes failures. Another point to remember is that clients can develop a close relationship with the nurse during the teaching–learning process. When this occurs, some limited sharing of the nurse's experiences in managing personal health issues may be appropriate to let clients know that the nurse, too, is human. This can be an effective addition to teaching strategies if it feels comfortable and is used wisely. Table 11.3 shows client and nurse behaviors for each level of affective learning.

To influence affective learning requires patience. Values and attitudes seldom change overnight. Remember that other forces continue to reinforce former values. For example, a middle-aged housewife may want to pursue a career for self-fulfillment, but she might not do so because she has children in high school and feels that their needs come first. A young man who can verbalize to the nurse the importance of safe sex may be uncomfortable discussing the subject with his partner, thus jeopardizing his compliance with the nurse's instruction.

TABLE 11.3   Affective Learning: Case Study in Family Planning

Level	Illustrative Client Behavior	Illustrative Nurse Behavior
Receptive (listens, pays attention)	Attentive to family planning instruction	Directs client's attention
Responsive (participates reacts)	Discusses pros and cons of various methods	Encourages client involvement
Valuing (accepts, appreciates, commits)	Selects a method for use	Respects client's right to decide
Internal consistency (organizes values to fit together)	Understands and accepts responsibility for planning for desired number of children	Brings client into contact with role models
Adoption (incorporates new values into lifestyle)	Consistently practices birth control	Positively reinforces healthy behaviors

Psychomotor Domain

The **psychomotor domain** includes visible, demonstrable performance skills that require some kind of neuromuscular coordination. Clients in the community need to learn skills such as infant bathing, temperature taking, breast or testicular self-examination, prenatal breathing exercises, range-of-motion exercises, catheter irrigation, walking with crutches, and how to change dressings.

For psychomotor learning to take place, three conditions must be met: (1) learners must be capable of the skill, (2) learners must have a sensory image of how to perform the skill, and (3) learners must practice the skill.

The nurse must be certain that the client is physically, intellectually, and emotionally capable of performing the skill. An elderly diabetic man with tremulous hands and fading vision should not be expected to give his own insulin injections; it could frustrate and harm him. An accessible person who is more physically capable should be enlisted and taught the skill. Clients' intellectual and emotional capabilities also influence their capacity to learn motor skills. It may be inappropriate to expect persons of limited intelligence to learn complex skills. The degree of complexity should match the learners' level of functioning. However, educational level should not be equated with intelligence. Many clients have had limited formal schooling but are able to learn complex skills for themselves or as caregivers after thorough instruction. Developmental stage is another point to consider in determining whether it is appropriate to teach a particular skill. For example, most children can put on some article of clothing at 2 years of age but are not ready to learn to fasten buttons until well past their third birthday.

Learners also must have a sensory image of how to perform the skill through sight, hearing, touch, and sometimes taste or smell. This sensory image is gained by demonstration. To teach clients motor skills effectively, the nurse has to provide them with an adequate sensory image. The nurse must demonstrate and explain slowly, one point at a time, and sometimes repeatedly, until clients understand the proper sequence or combination of actions necessary to carry out the skill.

The third necessary condition for psychomotor learning is practice. After acquiring a sensory image, clients can start to perform the skill. Mastery comes over time as clients repeat the task until it is smooth, coordinated, and unhesitating. During this process, the nurse should be available to provide guidance and encouragement. In the early stages of practice, the nurse may need to use hands-on guidance to give clients a sense of how the performance should feel. When clients give return demonstrations, the nurse can make suggestions, give encouragement, and thereby maximize the learning. For example, a nurse demonstrates passive range-of-motion exercises on a client's wife to show her how the exercises should feel (giving her a sensory image). The wife then learns to perform the exercises on her husband. During practice, feedback from the nurse enables the wife to know whether the skill is being performed correctly.

The psychomotor domain, like the cognitive and affective domains, ranges from simple to complex levels of functioning. It is necessary to exercise judgment in assessing a client's ability to perform a skill. Even clients with limited ability often can move to higher levels once they have mastered simple skills. Nurse behavior that influences psychomotor learning is shown in Table 11.4.

TABLE 11.4   Nurse Behaviors in Psychomotor Learning

The Nurse	Provides Sensory Image	Encourages Practice
Determines capability: Assesses client's physical, intellectual, and emotional ability	Demonstrates and explains	Uses guidance and positive reinforcement

LEARNING THEORIES

A *learning theory* is a systematic and integrated look into the nature of the process whereby people relate to their surroundings in such ways as to enhance their ability to use both themselves and their surroundings more effectively. Each nurse has and uses a particular theory of learning, whether consciously or unconsciously, and that theory, in turn, dictates his way of teaching. It is useful to discover what each nurse's learning theory is and how it affects his role as health educator.

Some of the learning theories developed by educational psychologists in the 20th century remain influential. They are grouped into four categories: behavioral, cognitive, social, and humanistic. Recently, the adult learning theory of Malcolm Knowles (1980, 1984, 1989) has influenced client teaching. A brief examination of these categories and the specific theories of each follows.

Behavioral Learning Theories

Behavioral theory (also known as stimulus-response or conditioning theory) approaches the study of learning by focusing on behaviors that can be observed, measured, and changed. Developed early in the 20th century, behavioral theory work is associated primarily with three famous names: Ivan Pavlov (1957), Edward Thorndike (1932, 1969), and B. F. Skinner (1974, 1987). To a behavioralist, learning is a behavioral change—a response to certain stimuli. Therefore, the behavioristic teacher seeks to significantly change learners' behaviors through a series of selected stimuli.

The stimulus-response "bond" theory proposes that, with conditioning, certain causes (stimuli) evoke certain effects (responses). The teacher promotes acquisition of the desired stimulus-response connections so that transfer of learning can occur in another situation having the same stimulus-response elements. Pavlov's early work with stimulus-response and involuntary reflex actions is the best-known application of this theory. Pavlov conditioned a dog to anticipate food by ringing a bell at feeding time. Initially, the dog would salivate as the food was brought to the cage. However, after time, the dog would salivate at hearing the bell, before seeing or smelling the food.

Two other behavioral theories are conditioning with no reinforcement (Thorndike) and conditioning through reinforcement (Skinner). No-reinforcement theorists focus on the learner's innate reflexive drives to accomplish the desired response after conditioning, such as when the nurse repeatedly emphasizes to a group of pregnant women that their prenatal classes promote a positive delivery experience and healthy newborns. In contrast, the reinforcement theorists use successive, systematic changes in the learner's environment to enhance the probability of desired responses. For example, a school nurse might give rewards (balloons, coloring books, crayons) to children who attend each class on safety.

Cognitive Learning Theories

Jean Piaget is the most widely known cognitive theorist. His theory of cognitive development contributed to the theories of Kohlberg (moral development) and Fowler (development of faith). Piaget (1966, 1970) believed that cognitive development is an orderly, sequential, and interactive process in which a variety of new experiences must exist before intellectual abilities can develop. His work with children led him to develop five phases of cognitive development, from birth to 15 years of age (Table 11.5).

Each stage signifies a transformation from the previous one, and a child must move through each stage sequentially. The three abilities of **assimilation** (reacting to new situations by using skills already possessed), **accommodation** (being sufficiently mature so that previously unsolved problems can now be solved), and **adaptation** (the ability to cope with the demands of the environment) are used to make the transformation. Nurses must understand their audience's learning stage to ascertain how to approach teaching for that developmental stage. The nurse can see how the use of puppets with 3-year-olds may be a beneficial addition to a presentation on safety, whereas a group of young teens with diabetes may respond to information on the consequences of taking or not taking their insulin.

The **Gestalt-field** family of cognitive theories assumes that people are neither good nor bad—they simply interact with their environment, and their learning is related to perception (Wertheimer, 1945/1959, 1980). A principal assumption of this approach is that "each person perceives, interprets, and responds to any situation in his or her own way" (Braungart, & Braungart, 2008, p. 61).

The first Gestalt-field theory, called *insight theory,* regards learning as a process in which the learner develops new insights or changes old ones. Learners sense their way intuitively and intelligently through problems. However, the "insight" is useful only if the learner understands its significance. For example, Lana dropped out of high school after the birth of her daughter; after attending a career planning class offered by a community health nurse, she realizes that

TABLE 11.5 Piaget's Five Phases of Cognitive Development		
Age	**Stage**	**Behavior**
Birth to 2 yr	Sensorimotor stage	The child moves focus from self to the environment (rituals are important).
2—4 yr	Preconceptual stage	Language development is rapid and everything is related to "me."
4—7 yr	Intuitive thought stage	Egocentric thinking diminishes, and words are used to express thoughts.
7—11 yr	Concrete operations stage	Child can solve concrete problems and recognize others' viewpoints.
11—15 yr	Formal operations stage	Child uses rational thinking and can develop ideas from general principles (deductive reasoning) and apply them to future situations.

she has limited job skills and that if she knew how to use a computer she could get a better job. This learner understood the significance of her insight.

The second theory, *goal-insight,* is similar to the insight theory but goes beyond intuitive hunches to tested insights. Teachers subscribing to this theory promote insightful learning but assist learners in developing higher-quality insights. For example, Lana takes a beginning and then an advanced computer class and is offered a higher-paying job. The community health nurse discusses Lana's successes with her, asks Lana whether she ever thought about going to college, and mentions the added benefits of college-level course work. Lana reflects on this for a while and begins to think about completing the requirements to go to junior college, because if she had an associate degree she could be promoted to supervisor.

In the third theory, *cognitive-field theory,* the learner is seen as purposive and problem-centered. Teachers seek to help learners gain new insights and restructure their lives accordingly. For example, Lana confers with the community health nurse about her choices and has changed her thinking about herself so much that she is planning to get an apartment in a neighborhood that is better for her child, and she may continue taking classes "for the fun of it" after she completes her degree in a few months.

Social Learning Theories

The aim of social learning theory is to explain behavior and facilitate learning. An important social theorist, Bandura (1977, 1986), pointed out that apparent but not real relationships often are dysfunctional, producing undesirable or inappropriate behavior. He described three ways that dysfunctional beliefs develop:

1. In *coincidental association*, outcomes typically are preceded by numerous events, and the client selects the wrong events as predictors of an outcome. For example, Juanita had a negative experience with a man who wore a hearing aid. Afterward, all of her experiences with men who wore hearing aids were negative. She reached the conclusion that all men who wear hearing aids were undesirable. This client's beliefs became a self-fulfilling prophecy.

2. In *inappropriate generalization*, one negative experience provokes negative feelings for future experiences. For example, Shauna had a purse snatched by a teenager and generalized that all teenagers are bad. Three-year-old Ryan accidentally drank some spoiled milk. He generalized that milk tastes bad and now refuses to drink it.

3. In *perceived self-inefficacy*, "Persons who judge themselves as lacking coping capabilities, whether the self-appraisal is objectively warranted or not, will perceive all kinds of dangers in situations and exaggerate their potential harmfulness" (Bandura, 1986, p. 220). For example, an older client, William, tells the community health nurse about two missing Social Security checks, but he refuses to take a bus to the post office. He states that he does not know what to say to the postal clerk and has read about senior citizens getting mugged on buses. He refused to follow up on his lost income.

Social learning theory focuses on the learners. They are benefitted by role models, building self-confidence, persuasion, and personal mastery. Self-efficacy can lead to the desired behaviors and outcomes. Juanita may begin to separate her negative experiences with men from their hearing disabilities after attending a class on building self-esteem suggested by the nurse. Through some positive experiences with teenagers organized by the nurse, Shauna may learn that not all teenagers are bad. The nurse can suggest to Ryan's mother that he may be persuaded to drink chocolate milk. She then can slowly reintroduce plain milk. William might find the courage and self-confidence to solve future problems after the nurse introduces him to another gentleman in the apartment complex who feels confident in the neighborhood.

Humanistic Learning Theories

Humanistic theories assume that people possess a natural tendency to learn and that learning flourishes in an encouraging environment. Two of the best-known humanists are Abraham Maslow and Carl Rogers. Abraham Maslow developed the classic hierarchy of human needs in the 1940s. It suggests that a person's first needs are physiologic (e.g., air, food, water). Once these needs are met, people work to fulfill safety and security needs. Next is the need for love and a sense of belonging; then come self-esteem needs (positive feelings of self-worth). Only after these needs are met do people work toward self-actualization or "becoming all that we can be" (Maslow, 1970).

In community health nursing, the clients' needs must be considered when planning health education programs. For example, it would be difficult for a group of young mothers to concentrate on learning about proper infant nutrition if they are worried about their babies crying in the next room or about an abusive partner who doesn't want them out of the house. Their need to care for their children (need for love and belonging) or for their personal well-being (security and safety) would be greater than the need to learn about future health considerations (self-esteem, self-actualization). Likewise, it is impossible for learning to take place if a room is so warm that the participants are falling asleep (i.e., physiologic needs are not being met).

Carl Rogers developed the client-centered counseling approach that has long been important in psychotherapy. He believed the role of the therapist should be nondirective and accepting, and proposed approaching clients in a warm, positive, and empathetic manner to get in touch with their feelings and thoughts. Rogers soon applied his beliefs to education, suggesting that the learning environment be learner-centered (1969, 1989). The outcome of a learner-centered educational environment is that students become more self-directed and guide their own learning. Rogers believed that the learner is the person most capable of deciding how to find the solutions to problems. The client identifies the problem and, given time and space, can find a way through the problem to a solution. The nurse acts as a facilitator in this learning process, as for example, when a 55-year-old man wants to quit smoking after a prolonged upper respiratory tract infection, aggravated by his habit, and comes to a stop-smoking class conducted by a nurse in the county health department.

| DISPLAY 11.2 | CHARACTERISTICS AND IMPLICATIONS FOR KNOWLES' ADULT LEARNING THEORY |

Characteristics	Learning Implications
Self-Concept Adult learners are self-directed.	Openness and respect between teacher and learner. The learner plans and carries out own learning activities. Learner evaluates own progress toward self-chosen goals.
Experience Adults have a lifetime of experience and define self in terms of this experience.	Teaching methods focus on experiential activities. Discovering how to learn from experience is key to self-actualization. Mistakes are opportunities for learning.
Readiness to Learn Learning is focused on social and occupational roles.	Experiential learning opportunities focus on requirements for occupational and social roles. Learning peaks when there is a need to know. Adults can best assess own readiness to learn and teachable moments.
Need to Learn Adults have a problem-centered time perspective.	Teaching needs to be problem-centered rather than theoretically oriented. Teacher needs to teach what the learners need to learn. Learners need to apply and try out learning quickly.

Knowles' Adult Learning Theory

In the last 20 to 30 years, a variety of techniques have been developed to help adults learn. One of the main discoveries is that adults as learners are different from children. They do not learn differently, but rather are a different kind of learner. Knowles (1984) suggested that there are four characteristics of adult learners, and these characteristics have implications for adult learning. Adults are self-directed in their learning; they have a lifetime of experience to draw on when learning; their readiness to learn is focused on requirements for their personal and occupational roles; and adults have a problem-centered time perspective, in that the learners have a need to learn so that it can be applied and tried out quickly. Display 11.2 describes the characteristics of adult learners and implications for nurses working with adults in more detail.

HEALTH TEACHING MODELS

Theories on learning provide a general understanding of how people learn. In addition, various health teaching models specifically focus on explaining individual health experiences, behaviors, and actions. These models fit with the learning theories to give nurses a more accurate picture of the client and the clients' learning needs. Five useful models are described here: the Cloutterbuck Minimum Data Matrix (CMDM), the Health Belief Model (HBM), Pender's Health Promotion Model (revised) (HPM), and the PRECEDE and PROCEED models.

The Cloutterbuck Minimum Data Matrix

The Cloutterbuck Minimum Data Matrix (CMDM) generates a comprehensive base of client information. This information is prerequisite to the in-depth level of critical analysis and synthesis needed to produce quality health care outcomes in the 21st century. It assumes an interdisciplinary perspective and educates the nurse to recognize and incorporate client diversity into care. In teaching, it assists the nurse in conceptualizing clients beyond the institutional, individual, and biomedical perspectives (Cloutterbuck & Cherry, 1998). The model helps the nurse to discern the life circumstances or chain of events that have jeopardized a client's health (Fig. 11.3).

The model comprises a set of empiric variables that are "known to influence consumer health status, behavior, and outcomes" (Cloutterbuck & Cherry, 1998, p. 386). For example, in the personal variables dimension are items such as age, ethnicity, level of education, and self-care practices. These variables are distributed across three dimensions: personal, situational, and structural. Information generated by the CMDM creates a more comprehensive profile than information gathered in the traditional biomedical health care system. This information, such as client health beliefs and practices and a broad range of personal factors, can be instrumental in helping the nurse design and implement health education programs to promote positive changes in clients' health. Although community health nurses have a long tradition of considering the client holistically, this matrix helps the nurse visualize the complexity of factors

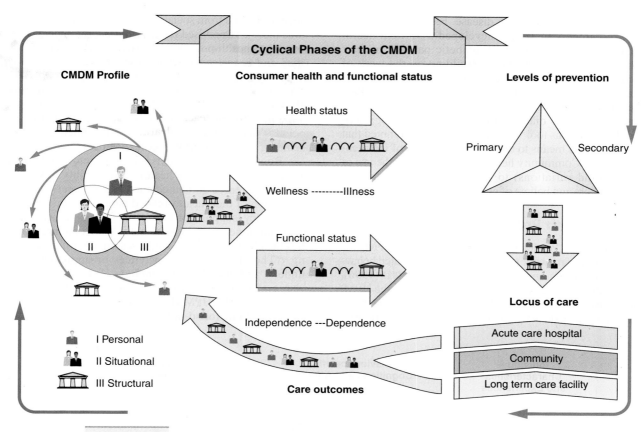

FIGURE 11.3   The Cloutterbuck Minimum Data Matrix, a tool to promote health education.

influencing clients' health. It helps to identify and challenge assumptions, recognize the importance of context, imagine and explore alternatives, and use reflective skepticism. When the nurse approaches individuals, families, and groups prepared with complete information, all of the caregiving—especially the appropriateness and effectiveness of the teaching—is enhanced.

This model has been found to be particularly useful in helping undergraduate nursing students to differentiate between individual- and population-focused practice (Dalton, 2008; Dalton & Cloutterbuck, in press). The model provides an "opportunity for critical analysis of the multiple variables that affect health and the provision of health care" (Dalton, 2008) and can be used in a wide variety of community settings (e.g., elementary schools, homeless shelters, home care settings, home visiting programs for new mothers and their infants, and community senior service centers). An expected student outcome of the use of this particular model is an enhanced awareness of the need for advocating for social change in the communities served. In addition, health promotion and learning needs of the target populations can be more easily identified with this approach.

The Health Belief Model

This section and the next describe two closely associated health models. The HBM, which was developed by social

psychologists and brought to the attention of health care professionals by Rosenstock (1966), has undergone much empiric testing. The HBM is useful for explaining the behaviors and actions taken by people to prevent illness and injury. It postulates that readiness to act on behalf of a person's own health is predicated on the following (Strecher & Rosenstock, 1997):

Perceived susceptibility to the condition in question
Perceived seriousness of the condition in question
Perceived benefits to taking action
Barriers to taking action
Cues to action, such as knowledge that someone else has the condition or attention from the media
Self-efficacy—the ability to take action to achieve the desired outcome.

For example, using concepts from this model, researchers looked at beliefs about the ability to control diabetes and beliefs about the degree to which family members supported a targeted Mexican American population in following their diabetes treatment regimen (Brown, Becker, Garcia, Barton, & Hanis, 2002). Unable to find many tools to measure diabetes-related health beliefs, the researchers took ideas from some older tools and designed a culturally sensitive education and group support intervention (Brown & Hanis, 1999). They realized how influential health beliefs are in managing one's health, whether in promoting or improving health or in trying to control a disease. Facing similar challenges, researchers in Turkey developed a 33-item health belief model scale for use with diabetic patients in their country (Kartal & Ozsoy, 2007). Building on the work of Schwab, Meyer, and Merrell (1994) with Mexican Americans and Tan's (2004) work with Chinese individuals, they studied the validity and reliability of the tool with 352 patients with type 2 diabetes mellitus. Their findings supported the use of this tool with this population and noted that it could provide a means to test the effectiveness of intervention strategies. Community health nurses may find the use of the HBM (and variations) to be helpful in assessing the health behaviors and beliefs of culturally diverse populations.

Pender's Health Promotion Model

First published by Pender in the early 1980s, the HPM was envisioned as a framework for exploring health-related behaviors within a nursing and behavioral science context (1996). Reflecting the growing body of literature relevant to the HPM, Pender revised the model to reflect a number of major theoretical changes. Consistent with the original, the revised

model is derived from social cognitive theory and expectancy-value theory. The revised HPM includes three general areas of concern to health-promoting behavior: *Individual characteristics and experiences* are seen to interact with *behavior-specific cognitions and affect* to influence specific *behavioral outcomes* (Pender, Murdaugh, & Parsons, 2006). The revised HPM modifies the HBM and focuses on predicting behaviors that influence health promotion. In addition, the HPM includes the variable of interpersonal influence of others, including family and health professionals.

Being able to predict health promotion behaviors enhances the community health nurse's ability to work with clients. Awareness of their characteristics, experiences, comprehension of their health-related issues, perceived barriers, self-efficacy, support (or lack of it) from significant others, and commitment provides the nurse with a picture that clarifies the client–nurse role and gives direction for action-taking. "The HPM is a competence- or approach-oriented model . . . [and] does not include 'fear' or 'threat' as a source of motivation for health behavior" (Pender, et al., 2006, p. 48). The HPM (Fig. 11.4) is based on the theoretical propositions found in Display 11.3.

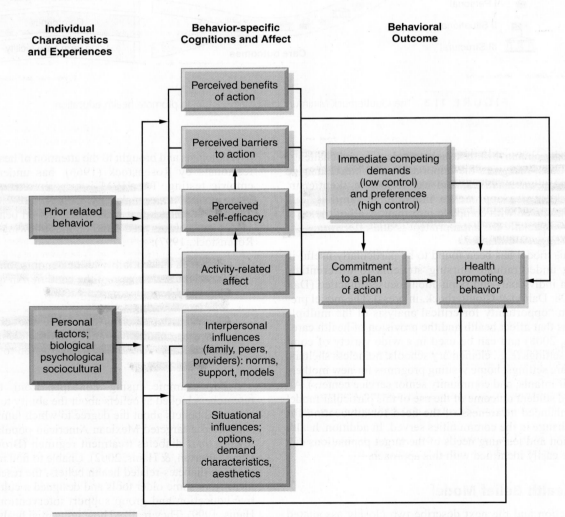

FIGURE 11.4　Health Promotion Model. From Pender, N.J., Murdaugh, C.L., & Parsons, M.A. (2006). *Health promotion in nursing practice*, 5th ed. Upper Saddle River, NJ: Pearson Education, Inc., p. 50, with permission.

DISPLAY 11.3   THEORETICAL PROPOSITIONS OF THE HEALTH PROMOTION MODEL

1. Inherited and acquired characteristics along with prior behavior influence beliefs, affect, and health-promoting behavior.
2. People engage in behaviors from which they anticipate deriving personally valued benefits.
3. Perceived barriers can constrain action to change behavior and the behavior itself.
4. Perceived self-efficacy to embrace a given behavior increases the likelihood to commit to action and implementing the behavior.
5. Greater perceived self-efficacy results in fewer perceived barriers.
6. Positive affect toward a behavior results in greater perceived self-efficacy, which can result in increased positive affect.
7. When positive affect is associated with a behavior, commitment and action are increased.
8. People are more likely to commit to and participate in health-promoting behaviors when significant others model the behavior, expect it, and provide assistance and support for the behavior.
9. Others—family members, peers, and health care providers—are important sources of influence that can positively or negatively influence commitment to and implementation of health-promoting behavior.
10. Situational influences can positively or negatively influence commitment to and implementation of health-promoting behavior.
11. The greater the commitment to a behavior change, the more likely the change will be maintained over time.
12. Distracting demands over which the person has little control may affect commitment to a behavior change.
13. Commitment to a behavior change is less likely to be maintained when other actions are more attractive and preferred.
14. People can modify the interpersonal and physical environments to create incentives for behavior changes.

Adapted from Pender, N.J., Murdaugh, C.L., & Parsons, M.A. (2006). *Health promotion in nursing practice* (5th ed.). Upper Saddle River, NJ: Pearson Education, Inc.

Using these propositions, researchers explored clients' health behaviors in many studies conducted in the 1980s, 1990s, and into the 21st century. Examples of some of the most recent uses of the model include surveying health-promoting behavior among low-income elderly Korean women (Shin, Kang, Park, Cho, & Heitkemper, 2008), and surveying health promotion in adolescents (Srof & Velsor-Friedrich, 2006), in older Iranian adults (Morowatisharifabad et al., 2006), and low-income pregnant minority women (Esperat, Feng, Zhang, & Owen, 2007). The model was even used in a pilot study of farm accidents in children (Conway, McClune, & Nosel, 2007).

The PRECEDE and PROCEED Models

First published by Green in 1974, the PRECEDE model was developed for educational diagnosis. The acronym PRECEDE has been slightly revised from the original to stand for *P*redisposing, *R*einforcing, and *E*nabling *C*onstructs in *E*ducational/*E*cological *D*iagnosis and *E*valuation (Green & Kreuter, 2005).

The PROCEED model (1991) works in tandem with the PRECEDE model as the community health nurse proceeds to plan, implement, and evaluate health education programs. This acronym stands for *P*olicy, *R*egulatory, and *O*rganizational *C*onstructs for *E*ducational and *E*nvironmental *D*evelopment. The entire PRECEDE-PROCEED model includes eight phases in the formulation and evaluation of health educational programs. The first five of these phases are included in the PRECEDE portion of the model and include: (1) social, (2) epidemiologic, and (3) education/ecological assessments, followed by (4) administrative and policy assessment and intervention alignment, and (5) implementation. The PROCEED model is emphasized in the last three phases: (1) process evaluation, (2) impact evaluation, and (3) outcome evaluation.

A hallmark of the PRECEDE-PROCEED model is the emphasis on the desired outcome. The model both begins and ends with *quality of life,* which includes "subjectively defined problems and priorities of individuals and communities" (Green, & Kreuter, 2005, p. 11). The emphasis on what the individual or community perceives as the problem, not what the professional believes it to be, is crucial. Outcome evaluation is logically linked back to that same individual or community in assessing achievement of the desired change.

The steps in this model are similar to those of the nursing process. Because of this familiarity, the model has become a useful tool for nurses teaching in the community. The nurse builds on the assessment formulated from the PRECEDE model, determines the best interventions, and then proceeds to evaluate the outcome of those interventions. The emphasis on the perceived needs of the individual or community as the starting point for all community efforts is consistent with community health nursing practice. The model reminds us of the importance of an organized approach to health educational programs, one that that begins and ends with the "experts"—the individuals, families, and communities we hope to help through our efforts. The PRECEDE-PROCEED model can be seen in Figure 11.5.

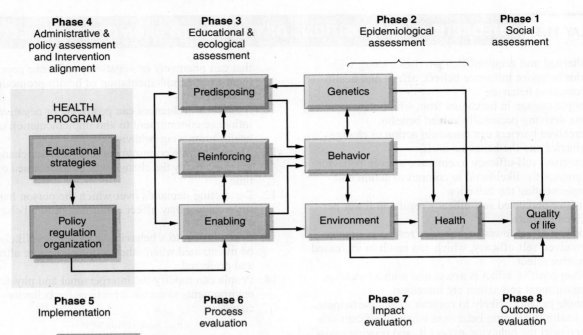

FIGURE 11.5 The PRECEDE-PROCEED model. From Green, L.W., & Kreuter, M.W. (2005). Health program planning: An educational and ecological approach, 4th ed., p.10. New York: McGraw-Hill, with permission.

TEACHING AT THREE LEVELS OF PREVENTION

Nurses should develop teaching programs that coincide with the level of prevention needed by the client. The three levels of primary, secondary, and tertiary prevention are demonstrated in the Levels of Prevention Pyramid for nurses who teach clients, families, aggregates, or populations.

Ideally, the community health nurse focuses teaching at the primary level. If nurses were able to reach more people at this level, it would help to diminish years of morbidity and limit subsequent infirmity. Many people experience disabilities that could have been prevented if primary prevention behaviors had been incorporated into their daily activities.

Because the primary level of prevention is not possible in all cases, a significant share of the nurse's time is spent teaching at the secondary or tertiary level. An example is an 88-year-old woman with a fractured hip who has returned home after 3 weeks of physical therapy at a skilled nursing facility. The nurse assesses the client's environment, gait, functional limitations, safety, and adherence to medication, and initiates needed referrals. The teaching focuses on rehabilitation and prevention of a secondary problem that may affect the healing process and the client's health and safety in general.

EFFECTIVE TEACHING

Teaching is an art. It was described in the classic book *The Educational Imagination* by E.W. Eisner (1985). Teaching can be performed with such skill and grace that the client becomes part of a well-orchestrated event, with learning as the natural outcome. Instead of relying on prescribed teaching methods, the skillful nurse can make judgments based largely on client qualities, situations, and needs that guide the experience to fruition. The desired changes emerge in the course of the interaction rather than at a level conceived before the teaching. Before the community health nurse can reach this level of artistry, there is much to learn about being an effective teacher.

Teaching–Learning Principles

Teaching lies at one end of a continuum. At the other end is learning. Without learning, teaching becomes useless in the same way that communication does not occur unless a message is both sent and received. Both the teacher and the learner have responsibilities on that continuum. Learners must take responsibility for their own learning (Braungart & Braungart, 2008). Teachers obstruct that process if they assume complete responsibility for bringing about changed behavior. Clients can be directed toward health knowledge, but they will not learn unless they have the desire to learn. Teaching, then, becomes a matter of facilitating both the desire and the best conditions for satisfying it. Teaching in community health nursing means to influence, motivate, and act as a catalyst in the learning process. Nurses bring information and learners together and stimulate a reaction that leads to a change (Rankin et al., 2005). Nurses facilitate learning when they make it as easy as possible for clients to change. To do this, the nurse needs to understand the basic principles underlying the art and science of the teaching–learning process and the use of appropriate materials to influence learning (Table 11.6).

LEVELS OF PREVENTION PYRAMID

SITUATION: Several examples of teaching at three levels of prevention.
GOAL: Using the three levels of prevention, negative health conditions are avoided, or promptly diagnosed and treated, and the fullest possible potential is restored.

Tertiary Prevention

Rehabilitation

- Restore function: a nurse teaches a stroke survivor about home safety, alternative housing options, physical therapy, and retraining opportunities

Primary Prevention

Health Promotion & Education
- Health teaching: a nurse teaches about the importance of diet, rest, and exercise to prevent a secondary health problem

Health Protection
- Maintenance: a nurse observes clients with tuberculosis where they live while taking their oral medication on a daily basis (DOT therapy)

Secondary Prevention

Early Diagnosis

- Screening and case-finding: a nurse takes blood pressure measurements from all family members at each home visit and teaches them the importance of maintaining a healthy blood pressure reading

Prompt Treatment

- Treatment: a nurse teaches clients how to navigate through the complexities of the health care delivery system to receive prompt treatment

Primary Prevention

Health Promotion & Education

- Health education: a nurse teaches a class on sensible weight control for teenagers

Health Protection

- Immunizations: a nurse teaches about the importance of pneumonia and flu vaccines for seniors, followed by an immunization clinic

---

TABLE 11.6 Seven Principles for Maximizing the Teaching-Learning Process

Teaching Principles	Learning Principles
1. Adapt teaching to clients' level of readiness.	1. The learning process makes use of clients' experience and is geared to their level of understanding.
2. Determine clients' perceptions about the subject matter before and during teaching.	2. Clients are given the opportunity to provide frequent feedback on their understanding of the material taught.
3. Create an environment that is conducive to learning.	3. The environment for learning is physically comfortable; offers an atmosphere of mutual helpfulness, trust, respect, and acceptance; and allows for free expression of ideas.
4. Involve clients throughout the learning process.	4. Clients actively participate. They assess needs, establish goals, and evaluate their learning progress.
5. Make subject matter relevant to clients' interest and use.	5. Clients feel motivated to interest and learn.
6. Ensure client satisfaction during the teaching-learning process.	6. Clients sense progress toward their goals.
7. Provide opportunities for clients to apply material taught.	7. Clients integrate the learning through application.

Adapted from Knowles, M. (1980). *The modern practice of adult education. Androgogy versus pedagogy* (2nd ed.). Chicago: Follett.

Client Readiness

Clients' readiness to learn influences teaching effectiveness (Kitchie, 2008; Rankin et al., 2005). Four facets of client readiness have been identified (Kitchie) and must be assessed by the nurse: (1) physical readiness, which deals with ability, complexity of the task, environment, health status, and gender; (2) emotional readiness, which deals with the state of receptivity to learning; (3) experiential readiness, which reflects the learner's past experiences with learning; and (4) knowledge readiness, which encompasses the learner's knowledge and understanding. For instance, one community health nurse found that a young primipara was not ready for prenatal teaching on fetal growth and development. She had strong fears, the nurse discovered, that "losing her figure" would make her sexually unattractive to her partner. Until these anxieties had subsided, the teaching would remain ineffective. Clients' needs, interests, motivation, stress, and concerns determine their readiness for learning.

Another factor that influences readiness is educational background. If a group of women who never completed grade school meet to learn how to care for a sick person in the home, material should be presented simply, factually, and in terms that they understand. To discuss complex concepts of health, illness, and scientific research would be above their level of readiness. However, increasingly complex concepts can be introduced as the nurse works with the women and assesses their readiness to assimilate advanced concepts.

Maturational level also affects readiness. An adolescent mother who is still working on the normal developmental tasks of her age group, such as seeking independence or selecting a career path, may not be ready to learn parenting skills. Readiness of the client determines the amount of material presented in each teaching session. The pace or speed with which information is presented must be manageable. A moderate amount of anxiety often increases client receptivity to learning; however, high or low levels of anxiety can have the opposite effect.

Client Perceptions

Clients' perceptions also affect their learning, serving as a screening device through which all new information must pass. Individual perceptions help people interpret and attach meaning to things. A wide range of variables affects human perception. These variables include values, past experiences, culture, religion, personality, developmental stage, educational and economic level, surrounding social forces, and the physical environment. One client may view the experience of parenting as a positive, growth-producing relationship; another may see it as a conflict-ridden, unhappy experience to avoid. Each kind of perception has a different consequence for teaching and learning. In another example, the nurse working with adolescents to educate them about the dangers of substance abuse should understand that adolescents seeking independence need to feel that they have options and choices and do not want to be told what to do.

Frequently, clients use selective perception. They screen out some statements and pay attention to those that fit their values or personal desires. For example, a nurse is teaching a client about the various risk factors in coronary disease; the individual screens out the need to quit smoking and lose weight, paying attention only to factors that would not require a drastic change in lifestyle. Nurses must know their clients, understand their backgrounds and values, and learn about their perceptions before health teaching can influence their behavior.

Educational Environment

The setting in which the educational endeavor takes place has a significant impact on learning (Kitchie, 2008). Students probably have had the experience of sitting in a cold room and trying to concentrate during a lecture or of being distracted by noise, heat, or uncomfortable seating. Physical conditions such as ventilation, lighting, decor, room temperature, view of the speaker, and whispering must be controlled to provide the environment most conducive to learning.

Equally important for learning is an atmosphere of mutual respect and trust. The nurse needs to convey this attitude both verbally and nonverbally. The way the nurse addresses clients, shows courtesies, and gives recognition makes a considerable difference in establishing clients' respect and trust. Both nurse and clients need to be mutually helpful and considerate of one another's needs and interests. All participants in the educational experience should feel free to express ideas, should know that their views will be heard, and should feel accepted despite differences of opinion and perspective. According to Knowles, this requires that the nurse refrain from seeming judgmental or inducing competitiveness among learners. Knowles adds that the teachers should share their own feelings and knowledge "as a co-learner in the spirit of inquiry" (1980, p. 58).

Client Participation

The degree of participation in the educational process directly influences the amount of learning. One nurse discovered this principle while working with a group of clients who were nearing retirement. After talking to them about the changes they would face and receiving little response, the nurse shifted to a different method of teaching. Pamphlets on Social Security benefits were distributed, and everyone was asked to read them during the week and come the next week with questions generated by the pamphlets. This strategy prompted the group to slowly begin to participate in their own learning.

When the nurse works with clients in a learning context, one of the first questions to discuss is, What does the client want to learn? As Carl Rogers (1969, p. 159) stated:

Learning is facilitated when the student participates responsibly in the learning process. When he chooses his own directions, helps to discover his own learning resources, formulates his own problems, decides his own course of action, lives with consequences of each of these choices, then significant learning is maximized.

The amount of learning is directly proportional to the learners' involvement. In another example, a group of senior citizens attended a class on nutrition and aging, yet made few changes in eating patterns. It was not until the members became actively involved in the class, encouraged by the nurse to present problems and solutions for food purchasing and preparation on limited budgets, that any significant behavioral changes occurred.

Contracting, in which the client participates in the process as a partner to determine goals, content, and time for learning, can contribute to client learning (see Chapter 10). Contracting in the context of teaching assists clients to develop a sense of accountability for their own learning (Rankin et al., 2005).

Subject Relevance

Subject matter that is relevant to the client is learned more readily and retained longer than information that is not meaningful (Lorig, 2000). Learners gain the most from subject matter that is immediately useful to their own purposes. This is particularly true for adult learners, who have more life experiences that can be related to learning and who tend to see the immediate relevance of the material taught (Knowles, 1980).

Consider two middle-management men taking a physical fitness course offered by their employer. One, the father of a Boy Scout, has agreed to co-lead his son's troop on a 2-week backpacking trip in the mountains. He wants to get in shape. The second man is taking the course because it is required by the company. Its only relevance to his own purposes is that it prevents incurring the disfavor of his boss. There is little question about which man will learn and retain the most. The course has considerable relevance and meaning to the first man and little to the second.

Relevance also influences the speed of learning. Diabetic clients who must give themselves daily injections of insulin to live, learn that skill quickly. When clients see considerable relevance in the learning, they accomplish it with speed. According to Rogers (1969), 65% to 85% of the time allotted for learning various subjects could be deleted if learners perceived the material to be related to their own purposes. This is seen in the short period of time that it takes for families to learn the skills needed to provide home care for a family member in need (Baltazar, Ibe, & Allender, 1999).

When the subject matter is relevant to the learner, more knowledge is retained. On seeing the usefulness of the material, the learner develops a strong motivation to acquire and use it, and he is less likely to forget it. Even in instances when a previously learned motor skill has not been used for years, it often is quickly recaptured when it is needed.

Client Satisfaction

To maintain motivation and increase self-direction, clients must derive satisfaction from learning (Lorig, 2000). Learners need to feel a sense of steady progress in the learning process. Obstacles, frustrations, and failures along the way discourage and impede learning. Many clients who have had strokes and who have potential for rehabilitation give up trying to regain speech or move paralyzed limbs because they become frustrated, discouraged,

and dissatisfied. On the other hand, clients who experience satisfaction and progress in their speech and muscle retraining maintain their motivation and work on exercises without prompting (Diamantopulos, 1999). Nurses can promote client satisfaction through support and encouragement.

Realistic goals contribute to learner satisfaction. Objectives should be set within the learner's ability, thereby avoiding the frustration resulting from a task that is too difficult and the loss of interest resulting from one that is too easy. Setting objectives requires agreement on goals, periodic reviews, and revision of goals if they become too easy or too difficult. Nurses further promote clients' learning satisfaction by designing tasks with rewards. One school nurse led a class for obese adolescents, and together they set the goal of a weekly 2-lb weight loss. The nurse helped the group to design a plan that included counting calories, reducing fat in their diets, increasing physical activity, and a buddy system to bring about behavior change. As members in the group achieved monthly goals, they were encouraged to reward themselves with a pair of earrings, new nail polish, or a special outing as a group. These students found this learning experience satisfying because goals were attainable, and their progress was rewarded. Instead of competing with one another, the group members set out to help each member achieve the goal. As a result, most kept the weight off after the class finished.

Client Application

Learning is reinforced through application (Lorig, 2000). Learners need as many opportunities as possible to apply the learning in daily life. If such opportunities arise during the teaching–learning process, clients can try out new knowledge and skills under supervision. Learners are given an opportunity to begin integrating the learning into their daily lives at a time when the teacher is there to help reinforce that pattern. Take a prenatal class as an example. The learning begins with explanations of proper diet, exercise, breathing techniques, hygiene, and avoidance of alcohol and tobacco. More learning occurs as the group members discuss these issues and apply them intellectually, exploring ways to practice them at home. Additional reinforcement comes by demonstrating how to do these activities. Sample diets, demonstrations of exercises, posters, pamphlets, or models may be used. The group can begin application in the classroom by making diet plans, exercising, role-playing parenting behavior, or engaging in group problem-solving. The members then can be encouraged to apply these activities on a daily basis at home and to share their results with the group at future sessions.

Frequent use of newly acquired information fosters transfer of learning to other situations. The major goal of illness prevention and health promotion depends on such a transfer. For instance, mothers who learn and practice a well-balanced diet that is free of non-nutritious snacks can be encouraged to offer more nourishing foods to other family members. A family that practices asepsis and good handwashing techniques when caring for a family member's postsurgical wound can learn to transfer this same principle to prevention of infection in daily living.

Teaching Process

The process of teaching in community health nursing follows steps similar to those of the nursing process:

1. *Interaction:* Establish basic communication patterns between clients and nurse.
2. *Assessment and diagnosis:* Determine clients' present status and identify clients' need for teaching (keeping in mind that clients should determine their own needs).
3. *Setting goals and objectives:* Analyze needed changes and prepare objectives that describe the desired learning outcomes.
4. *Planning:* Design a plan for the learning experience that meets the mutually developed objectives; include content to be covered, sequence of topics, best conditions for learning (place, type of environment), methods, and materials (e.g., visual aids, exercises). A written plan is best; it may be part of the written nursing care plan.
5. *Teaching:* Implement the learning experience by carrying out the planned activities.
6. *Evaluation:* Determine whether learning objectives were met and if not, why not. Evaluation measures progress toward goals, effectiveness of chosen teaching methods, or future learning needs.

Interaction

Reciprocal communication must occur between nurse and client. It is essential in the nurse–client relationship and requisite to effective use of the nursing process. Community health nurses need to develop good questioning techniques and listening skills to determine clients' learning needs and levels of readiness.

Assessment and Diagnosis

Identifying clients' learning needs presents a challenge to the nurse. Too often, teaching occurs based on the nurse's assumption of what the learner needs to know. In client education, nurses have a responsibility to tailor their teaching to clients' real and perceived needs. Knowles (1980, 1984, 1989) described educational needs as gaps between what people know and what they need to know to function effectively. He related that the potential learners, the sponsoring organization, and the community all help to determine the needs to be addressed in the teaching–learning situation.

Assessing educational needs may be accomplished in several ways. The nurse can use surveys, interviews, open forums, or task forces that include representative clients as members. The principle to remember is that clients should be involved in identifying what they want to learn. When a "need" to learn something, such as the importance of immunizing children, is identified by the nurse rather than by clients, the nurse may need to "sell" clients on the importance of the topic. Nurses need to use approaches that assist clients toward their own awareness of the need.

Setting Goals and Objectives

Once a need has been clearly identified, the nurse and clients can establish mutually agreed-on goals and objectives. *Goals* are broad statements of intent, and *objectives* are more specific descriptions of intended outcome (Mager, 1975). Sometimes, in a teaching situation, an objective may be broken down into short- and long-term goals. For example, the nurse may have identified a group's desire to stop smoking. The need and teaching goals might be stated as follows:

Need: A group of smokers wish to end their addiction to nicotine.
Short-term goal: All members of the group will stop smoking within 1 month.
Long-term goal: Ninety percent of group members will remain tobacco-free for 6 months.

Objectives should be stated in measurable behavioral terms, using a grammatical structure that contains a subject, verb, condition/criterion, and time frame. That is, each objective should include a single idea that describes an outcome that can be measured within a certain time frame. To accomplish the short- and long-term goals of smoking cessation, educational objectives are developed from the levels of cognitive learning covered earlier in this chapter. Each behavioral objective is stated in measurable terms and includes a verb that coincides with one of the six levels within the cognitive domain (Display 11.4). Objectives might appear as follows:

At the end of the program all clients should be able to:

1. *List* three reasons why smoking is unhealthy.
2. *Identify* at least two factors that influenced their smoking habit.
3. *Apply* a series of action steps leading to smoking cessation within 1 month.
4. *Examine* the steps as they contribute to living tobacco-free in the first 3 months.
5. *Design* a way to live a fulfilled, tobacco-free life.
6. *Evaluate* successful strategies to remain tobacco-free for 6 months.

Each of these objectives (a) refers to a subject; (b) can be readily measured, because each describes a specific outcome, condition, criterion, or expected behavior; (c) uses a verb for stating cognitive outcomes; and (d) includes a specific time frame. Well-written objectives meet these four criteria and enhance evaluation of the success of the educational effort.

Planning

Teaching preparation and the planning of it are all-important (Bastable & Doody, 2008). Although nurses teach individuals and families informally, it is generally best to have a written plan when teaching. The formalization of creating a written plan provides a framework within which the nurse can function securely, knowing that the topic is well thought out and presented and individualized for a specific client group. This plan should include the following eight items: (1) purpose; (2) statement of the overall goal; (3) list of objectives; (4) outline of the related

DISPLAY 11.4 SAMPLE VERBS FOR STATING COGNITIVE OUTCOMES

Knowledge	Comprehension	Application	Analysis	Synthesis	Evaluation
Define	Translate	Interpret	Analyze	Compose	Judge
Repeat	Restate	Apply	Distinguish	Plan	Appraise
Record	Describe	Employ	Appraise	Propose	Evaluate
List	Discuss	Use	Calculate	Design	Rate
Recall	Recognize	Practice	Experiment	Formulate	Value
Name	Explain	Operate	Differentiate	Arrange	Revise
Relate	Express	Schedule	Test	Assemble	Score
Underline	Identify	Sketch	Compare	Collect	Select
	Locate	Shop	Contrast	Construct	Choose
	Report	Practice	Criticize	Create	Assess
	Review	Demonstrate	Diagram	Set up	Estimate
	Tell		Inspect	Organize	Measure
			Debate	Manage	
			Inventory	Prepare	
			Question		
			Relate		
			Categorize		
			Examine		

content; (5) instructional methods; (6) time allotted for the teaching of each objective; (7) instructional resources; and (8) evaluation methods and criteria (Bastable & Doody).

Teaching

The class, seminar, workshop, or small-group teaching should be conducted according to the plan described earlier. Even with one-on-one teaching, these eight steps should be planned in advance, because each client has a different cultural background, education, intellectual level, and learning need. Use of a variety of teaching methods addresses the unique needs of learners and makes the teaching interesting. Include and combine such methods as lectures, discussions, role-playing, demonstrations, and videos (see Teaching Methods and Materials).

If necessary, assignments can be made, such as readings, presentations, journaling, practice experiences, or return demonstrations can be designed to reinforce and synthesize the learning. The teaching methods used and activities selected are important parts of the teaching plan. The teacher will find that a well-designed plan enhances the smoothness and effectiveness of the teaching situation. Problems in teaching often can be related to a poorly developed plan.

Evaluation

The final step of evaluation is critical in the teaching–learning process. According to Tyler (1949, p. 106), "evaluation is the process for determining the degree to which changes in behavior are actually taking place." At this point, the nurse determines whether the goals and objectives for the educational experience have been met and, if not, why not. Clear, measurable objectives facilitate evaluation.

If objectives have not been met or have been met only partially, this too requires attention. The nurse should explore this outcome with his clients to determine what factors hindered their success and what actions might be helpful. Partially met objectives give the nurse a place to begin with the group at follow-up sessions and should not be considered a failure.

Teaching Methods and Materials

Teaching occurs on many levels and incorporates various types of activities. It can be formal or informal, planned or unplanned. Formal presentations, such as group lectures, usually are planned and fairly structured. Some teaching is less formal but still planned and relatively structured, as in group discussions in which questions stimulate the exploration of ideas and guide thinking. Informal levels of teaching, such as counseling or **anticipatory guidance** (in which the client is assisted in preparing for a future role or developmental stage), require the teacher to be prepared, but there is no defined plan of presentation. Perhaps the nurse uses a pamphlet or agency protocol steps as a guide. All nurses use one or a combination of methods and a variety of materials to facilitate the teaching–learning process. However, nurses need to expand their repertoire of teaching methods and avoid relying on only one or two methods. Generating a variety of teaching methods stimulates creative thinking. Nurses use knowledge from physiology, pathology, sociology, and psychology in their practice, and, when teaching, nurses can benefit from using concepts, principles, and teaching methods derived from education, especially adult education. This chapter closes by discussing four commonly used teaching methods (lecture, discussion, demonstration, and role playing), teaching materials for enhanced learning, and how to effectively teach the client with special learning needs.

Lecture

The community health nurse sometimes presents information to a large group, such as a local parent–teacher association, a women's club, or a county board of commissioners. Under such circumstances, the lecture method, a formal kind of presentation, may be the most efficient way to communicate general health information. However, lecturers tend to create a passive learning environment for the audience unless strategies are devised to involve the learners. Many individuals are visual rather than auditory learners. To capture their attention, slides, overhead projections, computer-generated slide presentations, or videotapes can supplement the lecture. Allowing time for questions and discussion after a lecture also actively involves learners. This method is best used with adults, but even they have a limited attention span, and a break at least midway through a presentation of 1 hour or longer will be appreciated. Distributing printed material that highlights and summarizes the content shared, or supplements it, also reinforces important points.

Discussion

Two-way communication is an important feature of the learning process. Learners need an opportunity to raise questions, make comments, reason out loud, and receive feedback to develop understanding. When discussion is used in conjunction with other teaching methods, such as demonstration, lecture, and role playing, it improves their effectiveness. In group teaching, discussion enables clients to learn from one another as well as from the nurse. The nurse must exercise leadership in controlling and guiding the discussion so that learning opportunities are maximized and objectives are met. Discussions that are organized around specific questions or topics are most fruitful.

Demonstration

The demonstration method often is used for teaching psychomotor skills and is best accompanied by explanation and discussion, with time set aside for return demonstration by the client or caregiver. It gives clients a clear sensory image of how to perform the skill. Because a demonstration should be within easy visual and auditory range of learners, it is best to demonstrate in front of small groups or a single client. Use the same kind of equipment that clients will use, show exactly how the skill should be performed, and provide learners with ample opportunity to practice until the skill is perfected.

This is an ideal method to use in a client's home as well as in groups. The materials and supplies that the client will use when unaided by the nurse should be used in the demonstration. This might be the time when the nurse uses improvising skills. Helping families figure out ways to accomplish goals with materials found at home often becomes the hallmark of an experienced community health nurse. The new mother learns how to bathe her baby safely in the kitchen sink. The nurse assists several low-income parents in using household items to make inexpensive toys (e.g., mobiles from plastic coat hangers, string, and pictures from a magazine; bean bags using dry beans and scraps of fabric). The husband learns how to change dressings over his wife's central venous line site using sterile technique while conserving supplies purchased on their fixed income. Each activity takes a different type of psychomotor skill and ingenuity on the part of the nurse.

Role-playing

At times, having clients assume and act out roles maximizes learning. A parenting group, for example, found it helpful to place themselves in the role of their children; their feelings about various ways to respond became more apparent. Reversing roles can effectively teach spouses in conflict better ways to communicate. To prevent role-playing from becoming a game with little learning, plan the proposed drama with clear objectives in mind. What behavioral outcomes should be achieved? Define the context (the "stage") clearly, so that everyone shares in the situation. Then define each role ahead of time, making sure that participants understand their performance roles. Emphasize that no wrong or right performance exists, and that participants should behave the way people behave in everyday life. Avoid having people play themselves, because it can embarrass them and make it difficult for them to achieve objectivity. After the drama has concluded, elicit discussion with carefully prepared questions. This technique can be used with staff, co-workers, young children, teenagers, and adults. However, it can be a risk-taking experience for some people, and they may be reluctant to participate. The nurse should use judgment, begin with volunteers, and avoid pushing this technique on unwilling or nonreceptive people. Build up to full participation.

Teaching Materials

Many different kinds of teaching materials are available to the nurse. They often are used in combination and are useful during the teaching process. Visual images—such as PowerPoint presentations, pictures, slides, posters, chalkboards, flannel boards, DVDs, bulletin boards, flash cards, pamphlets, flyers, charts, and gestures—can enhance most learning. Some tools, such as tapes and compact disks, provide an auditory stimulus as well. Americans readily learn from television; it appeals to vision and hearing senses and more or less grabs attention. Learning of both positive and negative health behaviors through television can be more effective and efficient than traditional teaching methods. Other tools, such as anatomic models and improvised or purchased equipment, provide clients with both visual and tactile learning experiences. Still others, such as interactive computer games or instruction, actively involve the learners.

The choice of teaching materials varies with the clients' interests and abilities and the resources available. Teaching often occurs in casual conversations, spontaneously in situations in which clients raise unexpected questions, or when a crisis arises. In these instances, nurses draw on their background of knowledge and exercise professional judgment in their selection of content, methods, and materials.

Several different types of printed educational support materials are available, such as pamphlets, brochures, booklets, flyers, and informational sheets. Each should be evaluated for its appropriateness and effectiveness with particular individuals, families, or groups. Many come from state and local official sources. Nurses can create their own handouts by using the Internet and a computer, customizing them to the needs of individual clients. The Internet has vast health resources that can be combined with the desktop publishing capabilities of the nurse's computer to create one-of-a-kind materials for clients. The nurse can get educational information from state, federal, and international health agencies such as state health departments, the U.S. Food and Drug Administration (FDA), the Centers for Disease Control and Prevention (CDC), the National Institutes of Health (NIH), and the World Health Organization (WHO). Other materials come from nonprofit national agencies such as the American Diabetes Association (ADA), the March of Dimes, the American Association for Retired Persons (AARP), and the American Heart Association (AHA). Materials from these sources can be acquired in large quantity for free or at a nominal cost to the nurse or agency. Major manufacturers of infant formulas, foods, diapers, and toys are good sources for literature on growth and development, safety, and caring for infants and children. Pharmaceutical companies develop educational materials for the public, as do the manufacturers of in-home supplies and equipment. Usually, these are excellent sources of information for families or groups; however, the nurse needs to assess the material for appropriateness. Also, be sure that the commercial message in the literature does not outweigh the educational impact, thus making it misleading or confusing to the client.

Factors to be considered with all educational literature include the material's content, complexity, and reading level. There are several ways to assess the readability of the printed word. One easy way is to use the Fog Index. It is a rough way of determining the years of schooling needed to understand printed material. It works by analyzing words and sentence length. The higher the Fog Index, the more difficult the reading level. A Fog Index of 6 is a sixth-grade reading level, and 11 is the junior year in high school (Bastable, 2008). Fortunately, most word processing programs now include a feature to allow assessment of the reading level in text. Another very common tool is the Fleish Reading Ease program, which evaluates the material on a 100-point scale, with 90 to 100 being rated as very easy to read, and 60 to 70 as the standard; a rating of under 59 indicates a more difficult level (Bastable, 2008). Similar to the Fog Index, the Flesch-Kincaid Grade Level readability score rates the material in terms of typical grade level; a score of 8 would indicate that an 8th grade student should be able to read and understand the material. For most health promotion materials, a reading level of 6th grade is normally sufficient (Doak, Doak, & Root, 1996). The nurse should always consider the population when selecting a reading level, as many individuals cannot understand materials at that high a grade level. (For a related discussion on a research project that studied how reading levels affect understanding and behavior, see the Evidence-based Practice box.)

Culturally appropriate health education materials must be acquired or developed for the predominant cultural and linguistic minority populations taught by the nurse. Developing printed materials is an important first step, but the development of video, audio, and public service announcements in community-appropriate languages is also necessary. When translating printed materials from English into another language, it is strongly suggested that a separate translator, "back-translate" the materials. This added step helps assure that the meaning from the original has not been distorted or lost in the translation. Essentially one person or

EVIDENCE-BASED PRACTICE

Advance directives allow individuals to legally express their end-of-life wishes. These forms are typically written at the 12th grade reading level (or higher) and are often difficult to understand, especially for those with limited literacy skills. In a study involving over 200 English- and Spanish-speaking individuals, aged 50 years and older, researchers sought to determine if a redesigned advance directive form would be more useful, especially for individuals with limited literacy skills. The redesigned form was written at the 5th grade level. The researchers cited the relatively low rate of completion of advance directives, especially among disadvantaged populations, as impetus for this study. Approximately 40% of the study participants had limited literacy skills.

Results from this study demonstrated that the redesigned form was more acceptable and useful when compared to the typical form. Of particular importance was that 19% of the participants assigned the redesigned form had completed it at 6 months, as compared to the only 8% of completed forms using the standard format. The researchers suggest that these findings support the redesign of advance directive forms that can meet the literacy needs of most adults.

Nursing Implications
The community health nurse is often in a position to inform individuals about end-of-life decisions and the need for preparing advance directives well in advance of life-threatening illness or injury. Typical advance directive forms are often difficult to understand and may not be in the native language of the individual. This study points out the need for a variety of forms that can be used with individuals with either limited literacy or language needs. The forms should be both easily understood by the client and be clear to the care provider or hospital should the need arise for these documents. Increased use of advance directives may be achieved with options addressing the needs of particular individuals.

Sudore, R.L, Landefeld, C.S., Barnes, D.E., Linquist, K., Williams, B.A., Brody, R., et al. (2007). An advance directive redesigned to meet the literacy level of most adults: A randomized trial. *Patient Education and Counseling, 69*, 165–195.

group translates the material and another individual or group translates it back into English. This can add time and cost to the project, but it may prevent inaccuracies in the final material.

Finally, nurses teach by example. Actions speak louder than words. If a nurse teaches the importance of washing hands to reduce disease transmission and then begins a newborn assessment without hand-washing, the message of observed actions carries more impact than the words. Nurses who exhibit healthy practices use themselves as teaching tools and serve as role models as well as health teachers.

Clients with Special Learning Needs

At times, the nurse experiences a challenging teaching situation with an individual, family, or group. These challenges may involve clients who have cultural or language differences, hearing impairments, developmental delays, memory losses, visual perception distortions, problems with fine or gross motor skills, distracting personality characteristics, or demonstrations of stress or emotions. Regardless of the situation, the nurse will feel most comfortable and confident if he is prepared to deal with these situations before they are experienced.

Before beginning to teach a client, family, or aggregate, thorough preparation is important for successful learning to occur. This includes finding out whether it is possible to teach in English or whether other modifications are needed as the teaching plan is being developed. Nurses should never assume anything, including the primary language spoken by clients, their visual or hearing ability, or their capacity to understand. When teaching unfamiliar groups, the nurse can obtain information regarding the interests and abilities of the members from a center manager, caretaker, or program director. These human resources are invaluable in planning any teaching when English may be a second language or when other barriers exist that may impede success if they are not known by the nurse. The phases of the nursing process continue to guide the nurse as a teacher.

Another difficulty that can arise is unexpected behavior from a client who disrupts the group process. The client may monopolize the discussion, answer questions asked of others, burst out with personal experiences that have no relevance to the topic, become irate at the comments of others, or sit silently and never speak. This can be unnerving to even the most experienced nurse. Any behavior that has the potential to distract the other learners must be diffused by the nurse. This is accomplished by caringly giving the recognition sought by the person while also setting limits.

Summary

The purpose of health education is to effect change, which alters the equilibrium in a system. Change may occur gradually, with time for people involved to adjust, or it may occur in a drastic fashion, such as in a crisis or natural disaster. Change occurs in three stages: *unfreezing* when the system is ready for change, *changing* when the innovation is implemented, and *refreezing* when the change is stabilized.

Planned or managed change is a purposeful, designed effort to effect improvement in a system with the help of a change agent. It involves a process of eight steps, similar to the nursing process, which nurses can use to create change. These steps include assessing symptoms, diagnosing need, analyzing alternative solutions, selecting a change, planning the change, implementing the change, evaluating the change, and stabilizing the change. During planned change, the nurse can use one or a combination of several change strategies. However, the three major change strategies—a rational approach of providing information to influence people to change, an educative approach of combining new information with persuasion to effect change, and a coercive approach of enforcing compliance—are encompassing strategies. Several important principles serve as guidelines for community health nurses to effect change. They include involving all persons affected by the change, introducing change in a timely fashion, considering the impact of the change on other systems, being flexible, and understanding oneself and one's own qualities, which can be groomed to provide the most effective leadership.

Much of community health nursing practice involves teaching. More than simply giving health information to clients, the purpose of teaching is to change client behavior to healthier practices. If these practices are internalized and implemented regularly, years of morbidity and premature mortality can be avoided, thus contributing to the quality and length of the human lifespan. *Healthy People 2010* focuses on teaching to improve the quality of life.

Understanding the nature of learning contributes to the effectiveness of teaching in community health. Learning occurs in three domains: cognitive, affective, and psychomotor. The cognitive domain refers to learning that takes place intellectually. It ranges in levels of learner functioning from simple recall to complex evaluation. As learners move up the scale of cognitive learning, they become more self-directed; the nurse then assumes a more facilitative role.

Affective learning involves the changing of attitudes and values. Learners may experience several levels of affective involvement, from simple listening to adopting the new value. Again, as the client increases involvement, the nurse becomes less directive.

Psychomotor learning involves the acquisition of motor skills. Clients who learn psychomotor skills must meet three conditions: they must be capable of the skill, they must develop a sensory image of the skill, and they must practice the skill.

Learning theories can be grouped into four broad categories: (1) behaviorist theories, which view learning as a behavioral change accomplished through stimulus-response or conditioning; (2) cognitive learning theories, which seek to influence learners' understanding of problems and situations through promoting their insights; (3) social learning theories, which explain dysfunctional behavior and facilitate learning; and (4) humanistic theories, which assume that people have a natural tendency to learn and that learning flourishes in an encouraging environment. Knowles' adult learning theory provides a framework for understanding adult characteristics and appropriate teaching interventions.

Health teaching models work together with the learning theories to give nurses a more accurate picture of the client and the client's learning needs. Five models were explored in this chapter. The CMDM is designed as a teaching mechanism to create a comprehensive base of client information that enhances all care, including client teaching. The HBM is useful in explaining the behaviors that are triggered by people with an interest in preventing diseases, and the revised

HPM modifies the HBM and focuses on predicting behaviors that influence health promotion. The PRECEDE-PROCEED model is designed to guide health educational program development. The model has a strong focus on the perceived problems and priorities of a particular individual or group as they impact quality of life. Educational interventions are developed following a thorough assessment, which includes administrative and policy issues, and evaluation is conducted at three levels: process, impact, and outcome.

Teaching in community health nursing is the facilitation of learning that leads to behavioral change in the client. Ideally, this is done at the primary level of prevention. However, much of the nurse's work is done at the secondary and tertiary levels. The nurse uses several teaching–learning principles to facilitate the learning process, such as clients' readiness for learning, clients' perceptions, learners' physical and emotional comfort within an educational setting, degree of client participation, relevant subject matter, allowing clients to derive satisfaction from learning, and reinforcing learning through application.

The teaching process in community health nursing is similar to the nursing process, including steps of interaction, assessment and diagnosis, goal setting, planning, teaching, and evaluation. The teaching may be formal or informal, planned or unplanned, and methods may range from structured lecture presentations and discussions to demonstration and role-playing.

Selection of teaching materials depends on how well they suit learners and help to meet the desired objectives. Sources of teaching materials that are free or inexpensive can enhance the nurses' teaching efforts, but need to be evaluated for effectiveness and appropriateness. The nurse needs to know how to help learners with special needs, those with physical or mental disabilities, those who are from a different culture or who speak a different language, and those who monopolize the discussion, become emotional, or are hostile. The nurse must be prepared for each situation to effectively teach the individual, family, or group. ■

ACTIVITIES TO PROMOTE CRITICAL THINKING

1. As a staff community health nurse, you have been asked to chair an ad hoc committee in your health department made up of interdisciplinary colleagues and community members. The committee's task is to plan a health fair for the local community.
   a. Outline the specific planned change steps that your committee needs to ensure a successful health fair with outcomes that promote improved levels of community health.
   b. Select one specific objective of your health fair (e.g., cholesterol screening of an at-risk aggregate with the goal of reduced cholesterol levels in a year). Does the proposed objective require an evolutionary or revolutionary change in citizens' health-related behaviors? Justify your choice of the type of change.
   c. Explain the strategies that you would use to effect the change.
   d. Six principles for effecting positive change are presented in this chapter. Briefly discuss how you would use each one as you and your committee develop the health fair.

2. What learning theories discussed in this chapter most closely reflect your own position? How can they be applied in your practice?

3. A child day care center is in your service area. What populations in this setting are potential recipients of health teaching? How would you assess each group's learning needs?

4. Your city governmental officials often make decisions that appear to reflect a lack of knowledge regarding health and health care. How might you "educate" them using the concepts and principles described in this chapter?

5. Discuss the differences between cognitive, affective, and psychomotor learning. Why do cognitive and affective learning need to be linked in health teaching?

6. Using behavioral objectives that match the learning level desired, develop a flyer or program for an educational presentation for clients.

7. Select one of the health-teaching models. Use the model to plan an educational program for a group of teenagers. How did the use of the model enhance your teaching?

8. You are teaching an aggregate of middle-aged women about menopause. One woman monopolizes the class by telling stories and talking negatively about her husband. The other women are getting upset with her. How do you resolve the situation?

9. Using the list of Internet resources at the end of this chapter, review the type and quality of free or low-cost educational materials that they offer. Try to locate additional resources from other companies, public service agencies, and voluntary health agencies. Either request useful material to be used with clients now or bookmark a selection of sites to refer to later as needed, developing a resource file.

References

Baltazar, V., Ibe, O.B., & Allender, J.A. (1999). Maintaining optimum nutrition among elderly clients at home. In S. Zang & J.A. Allender (Eds.), *Home care of the elderly* (pp. 98–121). Philadelphia: Lippincott Williams & Wilkins.

Bandura, A. (1977). *Social learning theory.* Englewood Cliffs, NJ: Prentice-Hall.

Bandura, A. (1986). *Social foundations of thought and action: A social cognitive theory.* Englewood Cliffs, NJ: Prentice-Hall.

Bastable, S.B. (2008). Literacy in the adult client population. In *Nurse as educator: Principles of teaching and learning for nursing practice* (3rd ed., pp. 229–283). Boston: Jones & Bartlett.

Bastable, S.B., & Doody, J.A. (2008). Behavioral objectives. In S.B. Bastable, *Nurse as educator: Principles of teaching and learning for nursing practice* (3rd ed., pp. 383–427). Boston: Jones & Bartlett.

Bloom, B. (Ed.). (1956). *Taxonomy of educational objectives: The classification of educational goals. Handbook I: Cognitive domain.* New York: Longman.

Braungart, M.M., & Braungart, R.G. (2008). Applying learning theories to healthcare practice. In S.B. Bastable, *Nurse as educator: Principles of teaching and learning for nursing practice* (3rd ed., pp. 51–89). Sudbury, MA: Jones & Bartlett.

Brown, S.A., Becker, H.A., Garcia, A.A., Barton, S.A., & Hanis, C.L. (2002). Measuring health beliefs in Spanish-speaking Mexican Americans with type 2 diabetes: Adapting an existing instrument. *Research in Nursing and Health, 25,* 145–158.

Brown, S.A., & Hanis, C.L. (1999). Designing a culturally-referenced intervention for Mexican Americans with type 2 diabetes: The Starr County diabetes education study. *The Diabetes Educator, 25,* 226–236.

Cherry, B., & Jacob, S.R. (2005). *Contemporary nursing: Issues, trends, & management* (3rd ed.). St. Louis, MO: Elsevier.

Clampitt, P.G., & DeKoch, R.J. (2001). *Embracing uncertainty: The essence of leadership.* Armonk, NY: M.E. Sharpe.

Cloutterbuck, J.C., & Cherry, B.S. (1998). The Cloutterbuck Minimum Data Matrix: A teaching mechanism for the new millennium. *Journal of Nursing Education, 37*(9), 385–393.

Conway, A.E., McClune, A.J., & Nosel, P. (2007). Down on the farm: Preventing farm accidents in children. *Pediatric Nursing, 33*(1), 45–48.

Dalton, J.M. (2008). *Application of the Cloutterbuck Minimum Data Matrix to a community health nursing course.* Presented at the 2008 Association of Community Health Nursing Educators annual meeting.

Dalton, J.M., & Cloutterbuck, J.C. (in press). Application of the Cloutterbuck Minimum Data Matrix to a community health nursing course. *Journal of Nursing Education.*

Diamantopulos, D. (1999). Caring for the elderly client with neurological deficits. In S. Zang & J.A. Allender (Eds.), *Home care of the elderly* (pp. 388–411). Philadelphia: Lippincott Williams & Wilkins.

Doak, C.C., Doak, L.G., & Root, J.H. (1996). *Teaching patients with low literacy skills* (2nd ed.). Philadelphia: J.B. Lippincott Company.

Eisner, E.W. (1985). *The educational imagination* (2nd ed.). New York: Macmillan.

Esperat, C., Feng, D., Zhang, Y., & Owen, D. (2007). Health behaviors of low-income pregnant minority women. *Western Journal of Nursing Research, 29,* 284–300.

Green, L.W., & Kreuter, M.W. (1991). *Health promotion planning: An educational and environmental approach* (2nd ed.). Mountain View, CA: Mayfield.

Green, L.W., & Kreuter, M.W. (2005). *Health program planning: An educational and ecological approach* (4th ed.). Mountain View, CA: Mayfield.

Gronlund, N.E. (1970). *Stating behavioral objectives for classroom instruction.* New York: Macmillan.

Gronlund, N.E., & Linn, R. (1990). *Measurement and evaluation in teaching* (6th ed.). New York: Macmillan.

Hersey, P., Blanchard, K., & Johnson, D.E. (2008). *Management of organizational behavior: Leading human resources* (9th ed.). Upper Saddle River, NJ: Prentice-Hall.

Hollinger, B. (2005). Integration of cultural systems and beliefs. In S.H. Rankin, K.D. Stallings, & F. London, *Patient education in health and illness* (5th ed., pp. 47–71). Philadelphia: Lippincott Williams & Wilkins.

Kartal, A., & Ozsoy, S.A. (2007). Validity and reliability study of the Turkish version of Health Belief Model Scale in diabetic patients. *International Journal of Nursing Studies, 44,* 1447–1458.

Kitchie, S. (2008). Determinants of learning. In S.B. Bastable, *Nurse as educator: Principles of teaching and learning for nursing practice* (3rd ed., pp. 93–145). Boston: Jones & Bartlett.

Knowles, M. (1980). *The modern practice of adult education: Androgogy versus pedagogy* (2nd ed.). Chicago: Follett.

Knowles, M. (1984). *The adult learner: A neglected species* (3rd ed.). Houston, TX: Gulf.

Knowles, M. (1989). *The making of an adult educator: An autobiographical journey.* San Francisco: Jossey-Bass.

Knowles, M. (1990). *The adult learner: A neglected species* (4th ed.). Houston, TX: Gulf Publishing.

Lewin, K. (1947). Frontiers in group dynamics: Concept, method, and reality in social science; social equilibria and social change. *Human Relations, 1*(1), 5–41.

Lewin, K. (1951). *Field theory in social science: Selected theoretical papers.* New York: Harper & Row.

Lippitt, G.L. (1973). *Visualizing change: Model building and the change process.* La Jolla, CA: University Associates.

Lippitt, R., Watson, J., & Westley, B. (1958). *The dynamics of planned change.* New York: Harcourt.

Lorig, K. (2000). *Patient education: A practical approach* (3rd ed.). Thousand Oaks, CA: Sage.

Mager, R.F. (1975). *Preparing instructional objectives* (2nd ed.). Belmont, CA: Pitman Learning.

Maslow, A.H. (1970). *Motivation and personality* (2nd ed.). New York: Harper and Row.

Morowatisharifabad, M.A., Ghofranipour, F., Heidarnia, A., Ruchi, G.B., & Ehrampoush, M.H. (2006). Self-efficacy and health promotion behaviors of older adults in Iran. *Social Behavior and Personality, 34,* 759–768.

Ottoson, J.M., & Green, L.W. (2008). Public health education and health promotion. In L.F. Novik, C.B. Morrow, & G.P. Mays, *Public health administration: Principles for population-based management* (2nd ed., pp. 589–619). Sudbury, MA: Jones & Bartlett.

Pavlov, I.P. (1957). *Experimental psychology and other essays.* New York: Philosophical Library.

Pender, N.J. (1996). *Health promotion in nursing practice* (3rd ed.). Stamford, CT: Appleton & Lange.

Pender, N.J., Murdaugh, C.L., & Parsons, M.A. (2006). *Health promotion in nursing practice* (5th ed.). Upper Saddle River, NJ: Pearson Education, Inc.

Piaget, J. (1966). *The origin of intelligence in children.* New York: Norton.

Piaget, J. (1970). Piaget's theory. In P.H. Mussen (Ed.), *Charmichael's manual of child psychology* (Vol. 1). New York: Wiley.

Rankin, S.H., Stallings, K.D., & London, F. (2005). *Patient education in health and illness* (5th ed.). Philadelphia: Lippincott Williams & Wilkins.

Redman, B.K. (2001). *The practice of patient education* (9th ed.). St. Louis: Mosby.

Rogers, C. (1969). *Freedom to learn.* Columbus, OH: Merrill.

Rogers, C. (1989). *Freedom to learn for the eighties.* Columbus, OH: Merrill.

Rosenstock, I.M. (1966). Why people use health services. *Milbank Memorial Fund Quarterly, 44,* 94–127.

Roussel, L., Swansburg, R.C., & Swansburg, R.J. (2006). *Introductory management and leadership for nurses* (4th ed.). Sudbury, MA: Jones & Bartlett.

Rowtiz, L. (2006). *Public health for the 21st century: The prepared leader.* Sudbury, MA: Jones & Bartlett.

Schwab, T., Meyer, M., & Merrell, R. (1994). Measuring attitudes and health beliefs among Mexican-Americans with diabetes. *The Diabetes Educator, 20,* 221–227.

Shin, K.R., Kang, Y., Park, H.J., Cho, M.O., & Heitkemper, M. (2008). Testing and developing the health promotion model in low-income, Korean elderly women. *Nursing Science Quarterly, 21,* 173–178.

Skinner, B.F. (1974). *About behaviorism.* New York: Knopf.

Skinner, B.F. (1987). *Upon further reflection.* Englewood Cliffs, NJ: Prentice-Hall.

Spradley, B.W. (1980). Managing change creatively. *Journal of Nursing Administration, 10*(5), 32–37.

Spradley, J., & McCurdy, D. (1994). *Conformity and conflict: Readings in cultural anthropology* (8th ed.). New York: Harper Collins.

Strecher, U.J., & Rosenstock, I.M. (1997). The health belief model. In K. Glanz, F.M. Lewis, & B.K. Rimer (Eds.), *Health behavior and health education: Theory, research and practice* (2nd ed., pp. 41–59). San Francisco: Jossey-Bass.

Srof, B.J., & Velsor-Friedrich, B. (2006). Health promotion in adolescents: A review of Pender's health promotion model. *Nursing Science Quarterly*, 19, 366–373.

Tan, M.Y. (2004). The relationship of health beliefs and complications prevention behaviors of Chinese individuals with Type 2 diabetes mellitus. *Diabetes Research and Clinical Practice*, 66, 71–77.

Thorndike, E.L. (1932). *The fundamentals of learning.* New York: Teachers College Press.

Thorndike, E.L. (1969). *Educational psychology.* New York: Arno Press.

Tiffany, C.R., & Lutjens, L.R.J. (1998). *Planned change theories for nursing: Review, analysis, and implications.* Thousand Oaks, CA: Sage.

Tyler, R.W. (1949). *Basic principles of curriculum and instruction.* Chicago: University of Chicago Press.

U. S. Department of Health and Human Services. (2000). *Healthy people 2010: Understanding and improving health* (2nd ed.). Washington, DC: U.S. Government Printing Office.

Wertheimer, M. (Ed.). (1945/1959). *Productive thinking.* New York: Harper & Row.

Wertheimer, M. (1980). Gestalt theory of learning. In G.M. Gazda, & R.H. Corsini (Eds.), *Theories of learning: A comparative approach.* Ithasca, IL: Peacock.

Seligman, H.K., Wallace, A.S., DeWalt, D.A., Schillinger, D., Arnold, C.L., Shilliday, B.B., et al. (2007). Facilitating behavior change with low-literacy patient education materials. *American Journal of Health Behavior*, 31(Suppl. 1), S69–S78.

Shinitzky, H.E., & Kub, J. (2001). The art of motivating behavior change: The use of motivational interviewing to promote health. *Public Health Nursing 18*(3), 178–185.

Skybo, T., & Polivka, B. (2006). Health promotion model for childhood violence prevention and exposure. *Journal of Clinical Nursing, 16*, 38–45.

Thomson, M.D., & Hoffman-Goetz, L. (2007). Readability and cultural sensitivity of web-based patient decision aids for cancer screening and treatment: A systematic review. *Medical Informatics and the Internet in Medicine, 32*, 263–286.

Trifiletti, L.B., Sheilds, W.C., McDonald, E.M., Walker, A.R., & Gielen, A.C. (2006). Development of injury prevention materials for people with low literacy skills. *Patient Education and Counseling, 64*, 119–127.

Wallace, L.S., Keenum, A.J., Roskos, S.E., Blake, G.H., Colwell, S.T., & Weiss, B.D. (2008). Suitability and readability of consumer medical information accompanying prescription medication samples. *Patient Education and Counseling, 70*, 420–425.

Wilson, F.L., Baker, L.M., Nordstrom, C.K., & Legwand, C. (2007). Using the teach-back and Orem's Self-care Deficit Nursing theory to increase childhood immunization communication among low-income mothers. *Issues in Comprehensive Pediatric Nursing, 31*, 7–22.

Wolf, M.S., Davis, T.C., Shrank, W., Rapp, D.N., Bass, P.T., Conner, U.M., et al. (2007). To err is human: Patient misinterpretations of prescription drug label instructions. *Patient Education and Counseling, 67*, 293–300.

Selected Readings

Conobbio, M. M. (2006). *Mosby's handbook of patient teaching* (3rd ed.). St. Louis: Mosby.

Fisher, N.T., & Schneider, L.C. (2007). Literacy education and the workforce: Bridging a critical gap. *Journal of Jewish Communal Service, 82*(3), 210–215.

Health Resources and Services Administration. (2002). *Web teaching materials: Compendium to how to start a youth web advisory program.* Washington, DC: Department of Health and Human Services.

Lee, J.W., Jones, P.S., Mineyama, Y., & Zhang, X.E. (2002). Cultural differences in responses to a Likert scale. *Research in Nursing & Health, 25*, 295–306.

Mack, S.E., Spotts, D., Hayes, A., & Warner, J.R. (2006). Teaching emergency preparedness to restricted-budget families. *Public Health Nursing, 23*, 354–360.

Murray, R.B., Zenter, J.P., & Yakimo, R. (2009). *Health promotion strategies through the life span* (8th ed.). Upper Saddle River, N.J.: Prentice-Hall.

O'Bryant, S.E., Lucas, J.A., Willis, F.B., Smith, G.E., Graff-Radford, N.R., & Ivnik, R.J. (2007). Discrepancies between self-reported years of education and estimated reading level among elderly community-dwelling African-Americans: Analysis of the MOAANS data. *Archives of Clinical Neuropsychology, 22*, 327–332.

Redman, B.K. (2007). *The practice of patient education: A case study approach* (10th ed.). St. Louis: Mosby.

Internet Resources

American Association for Health Education: *http://www.aahperd.org/AAHE/*

American Public Health Association—Public Health Education and Health Promotion Section: *http://www.apha.org/membergroups/sections/aphasections/phehp/*

Californian Journal of Health Promotion: *http://www.cjhp.org/*

Center for the Advancement of Health: *http://www.cfah.org/*

Centers for Disease Control and Prevention—*Healthy Living*: *http://www.cdc.gov/healthyliving/*

Cochrane Public Health Group: *http://ph.cochrane.org/en/index.html*

Health Literacy Initiative [National Institutes of Health]: *http://www.nih.gov/icd/od/ocpl/resources/improvinghealthliteracy.htm*

Health Promotion and Disease Prevention for Older Adults—*Live Well, Live Long*: *http://www.asaging.org/CDC/index.cfm*

Institute of Medicine—Health Literacy: *http://www.iom.edu/?id=31489*

National Center for Health Education: *http://www.nche.org/*

Office of Disease Prevention and Health Promotion: *http://odphp.osophs.dhhs.gov/*

Society for Public Health Education: *http://www.sophe.org/*

SMOG Simple Measure of Gobbledygoop: *http://www.harrymclaughlin.com/SMOG.htm*

Stanford Health Promotion Resource Center: *http://hprc.stanford.edu/*

World Health Organization—Health Promotion: *http://www.who.int/topics/health_promotion/en/*

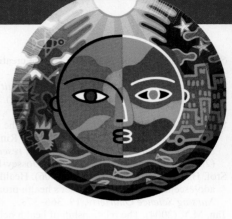

12

Planning and Developing Community Programs and Services

LEARNING OBJECTIVES

Upon mastery of this chapter, you should be able to:

◆ List sources of information that can be used to identify group and community health problems.

◆ Identify change strategies that maximize cooperation of target populations.

◆ Identify methods to gain input from target populations to define the scope of a health problem.

◆ Identify and evaluate the effectiveness of intervention methods targeting health problems.

◆ Classify health problems based on their changeability.

◆ Identify barriers to solving health problems.

◆ Discuss the role of the nurse within quality measurement and improvement programs in community health nursing.

◆ Recognize the role of social marketing in health promotion programs.

◆ Locate appropriate grant funding sources for select health promotion programs.

"*True genius resides in the capacity for evaluation of uncertain, hazardous, and conflicting information.*"

—Winston Churchill (1874–1965), British Prime Minister during World War II

KEY TERMS

Advisory group
Authoritative knowledge
Benchmarking
Enabling factors
Geographic information system (GIS)
Grant
Letter of inquiry
Predisposing factors
Reinforcing factors
Request for Proposal (RFP)
Social marketing

A public health nurse (PHN) collaborates with the county housing authority to implement a comprehensive fall-prevention program for community dwelling seniors; another nurse works into the night to complete a multimillion-dollar grant to fund comprehensive HIV educational programs in Kenya; community health nursing students volunteer to do a weekly radio program on health issues. The efforts described may seem very different, but each represents a health promotion program targeting populations, not just individuals. A fall-prevention program could potentially reduce the number of hospitalizations in the community resulting from serious falls, the HIV program may ultimately save tens of thousands from contracting this dreaded disease, and the radio program may reach thousands in the community, prompting them to think about their own health habits. Each of these examples represents the emerging role of the community health nurse and argues for the acquisition of a new set of skills. The skills of grant writing, radio programming, and collaborating with county officials all require new abilities that may require additional training or work with a mentor. These roles may seem foreign to you now, as you begin your career, but they may be the very skills needed to help bring vital health promotion programs to fruition.

In many communities across the country, local health departments struggle to recruit nurses to provide much-needed services. With shrinking budgets, many communities are forced to change long-held views on the scope and nature of services provided by PHNs. The home visiting model, once a mainstay of public health nursing, has been eliminated in many communities. Increasingly, community nurses/PHNs find themselves providing health promotion and educational programs to larger and larger audiences. To meet this need, community health nurses must become skilled at planning and implementing health promotion programs. As with any activity, the need for the program must be justified and, with limited resources, the benefit to the community must be demonstrated. Additionally, communities are rarely in a position to fund the entire realm of needed health programs and must turn to outside agencies for funding, either through grants or contracts. The responsibility for locating, securing, and maintaining grant funding is often assumed by the community health nurse.

Whether the program is funded by the county or an outside agency, results must be assessed. Evaluation of programs is vital for their continuation and is a requirement of most funders, whether public or private. A nurse who receives $500 to start an emergency preparedness program with low-income families may not be expected to provide the level of evaluation data that a million-dollar effort to address methamphetamine use in the community would likely require. However, some level of evidence showing the impact of the program will be needed. Even the populations served want to know whether the programs were successful, and why. For instance, a mother agrees to have her daughter enrolled in an after-school program to increase self-esteem. At the end of the first 6-week session, the mother is asked to give permission for her daughter to attend the second session. Her daughter says she enjoys the sessions but would also like to go to a dance class that is held at the same time. With competing demands on the daughter's time, the mother may ask for details on what was accomplished in the first session and what expectations the providers have for this second session. With this information, she can discuss various options with her daughter. The funders, consumers, and the nurse all need to be aware of the demonstrated outcomes of programs.

In Chapter 11, you were introduced to the concept of change—how it influences the adoption of health behaviors and what factors impede change in individuals. Educational methods are often used to influence change in behaviors and play a vital role in those efforts. In this chapter, we build on the concepts of change and appropriate educational techniques, and apply them to larger groups and populations. The discussion of the PRECEED-PROCEED model (Green & Kreuter, 2005) will be expanded upon as you are introduced to the basics of health program planning, intervention, and evaluation to maximize successful results. *Social marketing*, a relatively new tool for reaching large audiences with health information will be presented. Several well-known models familiar to nurses will be explored in terms of facilitating the evaluation of programs and services. Finally, as the need for grant funding becomes increasingly important, information on the various types of available funding will be provided.

PROGRAM PLANNING: THE BASICS

Ottoson and Green (2008, p. 590) define public health education programs as interventions "designed to inform, elicit, facilitate, and maintain positive health practices in large numbers of people." Even the American Nurses Association (ANA), *Public Health Nursing: Scope and Standards of Practice* (2007) is centered on the role of the nurse in planning, implementing, and evaluating population-focused health promotion/health education programs. Specifically, Standard 5B calls on the PHN to "employ multiple strategies to promote health, prevent disease, and ensure a safe environment for populations" (p. 23), through programs and services that include appropriate teaching–learning methods, that are culturally and age-appropriate, and that include an evaluation component.

With so much emphasis on planning and developing health education/health promotion programs, the process can seem overwhelming to the new community health nurse, or even to the acute-care nurse who may be involved in some aspect of health initiatives development within her agency. The first part of this chapter is designed to take some of the mystery out of the process. You will be guided through the complex problem of obesity in school-aged children. This particular issue is of great importance to the health of our children, and the principles applicable to this example can be utilized in other situations and other programs, even those that are very broad in scope and involve many practice partners. In your nursing program, you may even have been tasked with developing a health program, working on an existing community program, or simulating the process in a written assignment. Whatever your experience level, the essential elements are the same. As you begin this next section, think about past experiences you have had such as taking blood pressures at a local health fair or developing a pamphlet on the need for prostate screening in non–English speaking residents. Did these actions have the impact you hoped for? Successful health promotion programs do not occur by accident; they take skill, time, patience, and most of all listening to and understanding the needs and opinions of the individuals who are the focus of your program (the target population).

IDENTIFYING GROUP OR COMMUNITY HEALTH PROBLEMS

Nursing education emphasizes practice with a focus on individuals, families, and communities, yet nurses often practice at the individual and family level. When is it appropriate for a nurse to expand her practice to the community level? Perhaps the most natural time is when a nurse identifies an ongoing issue that does not change with traditional interventions. Examples might include overuse of the emergency room for urgent care; recurrent hospitalization of the elderly from several nursing homes for dehydration, sepsis, and malnutrition; or hospitalization of 6- to 8-year-olds for injuries caused by insufficient car seat restraint. These types of recurrent problems might lead the nurse to investigate the feasibility of a community-based intervention.

Individually or in a group, identify a possible issue to explore—one that you believe is leading to poor health outcomes in your community. How do you know if this problem is widespread or if others also find it to be a problem? Several methods can be used to validate the importance of the issue. One method would be to consider *Healthy People 2010* objectives for the nation (U.S. Department of Health and Human Services [USDHHS], 2000). What are the major issues that are of concern to improving health outcomes for the United States? What are the priorities of the state in which you live? You might take some time to review websites for federal agencies to identify the programs they are promoting to meet the *Healthy People 2010* goals and objectives. Your state department of health may also have a website with information on achievement of *Healthy People 2010* objectives, including those objectives that remain challenging. Local communities also establish priorities that reflect the *Healthy People 2010* objectives for the nation. As *Healthy People 2020: The Road Ahead* is being developed, the public is invited to submit comments on all aspects of the effort, including the mission, vision, and overarching goals (USDHHS, 2008). The comments submitted by others may provide information on current health concerns across the country, and are available for review on the Healthy People website.

Community agencies and organizations frequently network to establish community-wide goals. This work is often spearheaded by the local health department. It may also be organized by community-based health agencies and volunteer organizations. Improved outcomes for individuals who have diabetes or asthma are issues a local community might want to address. Another topic of concern is childhood obesity. Nurses can work collaboratively with these types of special interest groups to find solutions for individuals and families with identified problems.

As a specific problem is identified, it is crucial to analyze the extent to which individuals and families are affected by the problem. It is a poor use of resources to set up a program if there is a very small incidence of the condition or situation. For example, it would be a waste of resources to establish a program on diabetes and pregnancy for a local homeless shelter that only serves 35 women a year. Of those 35 women, none may be pregnant, and since 2.5% of the population of pregnant women develops gestational diabetes (Xiong, Saunders,

Wang, & Demianczuk, 2001), it may be a number of years before an eligible client is found. A better use of resources would be to target a community with a higher proportion of individuals at risk for diabetes and pregnancy. An example might be a program targeting a community with a large population of young Hispanic or Southeast Asian families, as the incidence of gestational diabetes is higher in these populations than in the general population (up to 11% of Southeast Asian pregnant women) (Dabelea et al., 2005; Thorpe et al., 2005).

There are many ways a nurse can decide if a problem has affected a sufficient percentage of the population to warrant intervention. The best way to start is by reviewing the local, state, and national data available through government repositories. This can be done through the Internet, by going to a university library for assistance, and by asking for sources of specific data from your local health and social service agencies, police and judicial departments, and local school districts. Hospital discharge data is also reported to state agencies, and this information is sometimes available at the local level. As nurses and other community groups narrow their focus, they can often map data by zip codes and neighborhoods, which helps to identify the best places to target groups and communities. Currently, many organizations have this ability and are able to identify target groups by race, age, and family status. This type of data, known as **geographic information system (GIS)** information is widely available. At the federal level, the National Center for Health Statistics (NCHS) website maintains GIS maps on the major causes of mortality in the country (NCHS, 2008).

Another effective approach is to talk to other nurses and other health care professionals within and outside of your organization. Get their ideas about the problem, and ideas about what should be done to alleviate the problem. In addition, find out what has been tried in the past, and get their input on why past interventions failed. One very helpful source of information is the *Guide to Community Preventive Services: Systematic Reviews and Evidence-based Recommendations* (2008), a federally sponsored initiative that provides recommendations regarding population-based interventions, including which are recommended, which need more evidence to determine effectiveness, and which are not recommended. The interventions with limited evidence may actually be very effective, but they need to be demonstrated by more studies; perhaps your idea is among those listed. Publication of program results is not only professionally gratifying, but adds to the body of evidence on which health promotion programs can be evaluated.

The next step of intervention is the most important of all, as it will determine whether your interventions succeed or fail. A nurse may think, "I know what the problem is—now I will think up an intervention to alleviate it!" This approach may be well-intentioned, but will lead the nurse down the path of failure. At this point, only part of the assessment is completed; the most important part of the assessment is to find out the views of the target population about the identified problem. What do they think causes it? What ideas do they have about solving it? Which approaches do they think will work, and which are doomed to failure? These are all important questions the nurse needs to ask. It is crucial that the views of the target population be heard and respected. Anthropologists talk about a concept called **authoritative knowledge**. This is "whose knowledge is respected," not "whose knowledge is right" (Davis-Floyd & Sargent, 1997). Nurses may think that they know more about a topic, such as diabetes, than their target population does, and therefore their solutions are better than the target population's solutions. Members of a target population hold just as strongly to their own belief systems. If nurses don't learn about the target population's beliefs, and only consider their own, they will not be able to work out an acceptable and appropriate solution with the target population. Interventions that fail to engage the target population will likely be unsuccessful because of this. It is crucial that interventions utilize health resources effectively, and that positive working relationships be established with high-risk target communities.

Getting Started

When working with target groups it's important to get as much information about the population as possible. Start by asking those whom you know as colleagues and as patients/clients about their local community. What do they see as issues regarding the problem about which you are concerned? What do they think about the quality of services currently available? What do they see as barriers to services? What about barriers to adherence to treatment and other health care recommendations?

Additional issues to explore include: Who else do they think you should speak with to gain insight about the issues relevant to this problem? Who are key people with whom you should build relationships? What are their customs in regard to health care? Who are the leaders within a family? If you want to establish linkages with this population, what is the best method? Who are their *formal* and *informal leaders*? What types of events bring them together? What are the roles of family, church, and health care providers within their community? Should you go through church groups, school groups, or other organizations? What radio stations do they listen to, and what television stations are they most likely to watch? This information will not only help you gain insight into factors influencing the health problem, it will also give you information about how most effectively to reach out to the target population.

As you start to gain insight into the environmental and social factors that influence the problems about which you are concerned, you are also building interest in the issue. As you participate in discussions with others, be open to their input. It may be that the ideas you start out with need to change in response to feedback from members of the target and service communities. For example, an experienced PHN was involved in a project developed to serve Hispanic women with gestational diabetes. When interviewed, the monolingual Spanish-speaking women expressed concern that they were told to go on a diabetic "diet" and were then chastised for not eating enough. To these women, going on a "diet" meant they should eat less. They were also told that if they followed the diabetic diet they wouldn't have such "big babies." They thought a "big" baby was a healthy baby and couldn't understand why they were being told to avoid having a larger baby. These were simple issues to fix, but required knowledge of how the "diabetic teaching plan" was interpreted by the target audience. Another key factor was

that the clinic was a family event, thus all of the children were brought along. The clinic staff had been consistently irritated by the presence of large groups of children, but learned that they needed to alter the clinic set-up and resources to accommodate the expectations of their clients. Modifications were made based on dialogue with members of the target population that positively influenced the eventual success of the clinic's program.

This example demonstrates how use of *local knowledge* can increase the effectiveness of a community-based intervention. The participation of members of the target population also builds greater community capacity for resolution of health problems within target communities. Working with community partners, including members of target populations, is a technique that has been used in work within developing countries. This type of approach ensures community *buy-in* for an intervention. It also builds networks that can continue to increase the capacity of communities to resolve other health care issues, both current and emerging (Goodman et al., 1998; Poole, 1997).

It is essential to review literature regarding health problems, factors influencing the outcomes of interventions, and the role of families and communities in adherence to interventions. The literature review can offer the opportunity to develop additional insights that may shape interviews with members of the target and service communities. How does this target group compare to other target groups? What else should be addressed that wasn't found in the literature? Another PHN conducted a study that addressed use of the emergency room for after-hours urgent care. The literature focused heavily on "mis-use" of emergency rooms by parents to treat urgent ambulatory care health problems, such as otitis media. Based on input from an emergency room nurse, families were asked what their doctors had told them to do if their child became ill at night. The families indicated that they were told to take their children to the emergency room! None of the literature addressed what the families had been told to do for after-hours care. This is an example of how being open to information from a variety of sources (in this case the emergency room nurse) enhanced the researcher's understanding of the problem beyond what could be learned by solely relying on the literature.

As nurses work with community members to identify factors contributing to a health problem, individuals will begin to stand out because of their knowledge, their network capabilities, and their interest in the subject. A key factor for ensuring the success of any intervention is to appoint an **advisory group** that includes representatives from the target and service communities. Findings from interviews, literature reviews, and data analyses need to be reviewed with this advisory group. To ensure success of the advisory group, all meetings should be carefully planned, so that they are well organized, punctual, and efficient. Strategies to encourage input from the advisory group should be employed; meetings should focus on getting the advisory group to interpret findings and community feedback, and to develop possible solutions. Contributions from each member should be sought and valued equally. Depending on the size of the group, it may be most effective to have some break-out sessions, as well as larger group sessions. An evaluation should be done by each member after each meeting, so that any problems can be addressed before the next meeting. Maintaining a record of these meetings—either in the form of minutes or a brief written overview—is also very helpful. Be certain to also keep a record of attendees. Maintaining a *paper trail* is always important.

Delineating the Problem to Be Addressed

With the help of the advisory group, it's important to delineate the problem or problems to be addressed. The following is a case example. A group of nurses identified childhood obesity as a problem. Input from community members, as well as a review of data, demonstrated a higher rate of childhood obesity in a local elementary school, where a high proportion of the children were African American. Although the original plan made by the nurses was to establish a special educational program for overweight children, ages 10 to 12, input from members of the service and target community indicated major problems with this approach:

1. It would be embarrassing for any child identified as needing the program.
2. Children this age usually don't pick the menu for their home or school.
3. Diet is culturally dependent, and the nurses knew very little about the dietary practices of African American families within the targeted community.

The use of an advisory group helped the nurses first identify what behavioral factors contributed to childhood obesity in the target population. These behavioral factors included the following:

- School breakfasts and lunches served were high in fat and salt, with limited fresh vegetable and fruit choices.
- Physical education classes were conducted for 45 minutes, once a week.
- No sports equipment was available for use during school recess and lunch periods.
- Participation in after-school sports cost $150 per student for uniforms and fees.
- The students aged 10 to 12 preferred to drink sodas and eat French fries for lunch.
- Most parents were working and often bought "fast food" for their children for dinner.
- Local parks were unsafe for children to play in, and there were no outdoor recreational activities that were free (no cost).
- Children in the target group described feeling very stressed due to high homework demands and expectations to score well on national tests.
- Children in the target group indicated that they went home after school and watched TV or played video games because their parents wouldn't allow them to play outside while they were at work.
- When asked what they did when stressed, children in the target group indicated they watched TV, listened to music, played videogames, and had snacks.
- The favorite after-school snacks eaten by children in the target group were macaroni and cheese from a box or packaged noodles—both of which are high in fat, carbohydrates, and salt.

Rating the Importance and Changeability of Identified Behavioral Factors

To achieve success, programs must narrow their focus to a limited number of health behaviors that can be addressed successfully within a specific timeframe (Green & Kreuter, 1999, 2005). To prioritize which behaviors to address, Green and Kreuter (2005) suggest that they be rated in terms of importance and changeability. The final list should include problems that are both important and easy to change.

Importance is determined by rating how frequently the identified behavior occurs and how strongly it is linked to a health problem. The advisory group for childhood obesity ranked the importance of the identified behaviors; their ranking and rationale (basis) for the ranking can be seen in Table 12.1. For instance, the lack of available sports equipment was not rated very highly since the advisory group observed that children can be physically active without sports equipment. A highly rated item was the poor quality of the school-provided breakfasts and lunches; as a primary source of nutrition for many of the school's children, it could contribute to obesity in this population.

The advisory group was then asked to rate the changeability of the behaviors. Green and Kreuter (1999, p. 138) indicate that those that are easiest to change:

- Are still in the developmental stages
- Have only recently been established
- Are not deeply rooted in cultural patterns or lifestyle
- Have been found to change in previous attempts

The advisory group's changeability ratings for the behaviors can be seen in Table 12.2. In this round of assessments, the advisory group found that the lack of sports equipment, although not as important, could be potentially changed. This rating was based on the fact that the underfunding of the play equipment was a relatively new occurrence, and funding might be redirected if attention was brought to the problem. The poor nutritional quality of the breakfasts and lunches was seen as less changeable due to existing contracts with outside businesses to provide the meals.

After rating the identified problems based on changeability and importance, the nurses and advisory group sought to narrow their focus to specific goals. Green and Kreuter (1999) suggest ranking the behaviors in a simple table, as seen in Table 12.3. This effort yielded a table with the problems categorized in four groups: more important/more changeable, less important/more changeable, more important/less changeable, and less important/less changeable. The issues seen as most important and changeable included fifth and sixth grade students choosing high fat, high sugar foods for lunch and breakfast; children feeling stressed by homework demands; and children engaging in sedentary activities.

The use of this grid enabled the advisory group to focus on more changeable and important issues. They wrote behavioral objectives for each identified factor they hoped to change. These objectives identified *who* was targeted, *what* they hoped would change or what action would be taken, *how* the change would be measured, and what the *timeframe*

TABLE 12.1   Importance of Behaviors Contributing to Childhood Obesity at Stevens Place Elementary School

Important	Basis for Rating
• School breakfasts and lunches were served that were high in fat and carbohydrate, with limited fresh vegetable and fruit choices.	A number of children ate their main meals at school, and studies have shown that high fat, high carbohydrate diets contribute to childhood obesity.
• Physical education classes were conducted for 45 minutes once a week.	Increasing exercise frequency will increase muscle mass as well as metabolic rates.
• The students aged 10–12 preferred to drink sodas and eat French fries for lunch.	Peer pressure can adversely influence food choices.
• Most parents were working and often bought "fast food" for their children for dinner.	Fast foods are high in carbohydrates and fat.
• Children in the target group described feeling very stressed due to high homework demands and expectations to score well on national tests.	High stress levels in adults contribute to obesity by increasing cortisol levels.
• Children in the target group indicated they went home after school and watched TV or played video games because their parents wouldn't allow them to play outside while they were at work.	Sedentary activities contribute to childhood obesity.
• When asked what they did when stressed, children in the target group indicated they watched TV, listened to music, played videogames, and had snacks.	Sedentary activities contribute to childhood obesity.
• The favorite after-school snacks eaten by children in the target group were macaroni and cheese from a box or packaged noodles—both of which are high fat, high carbohydrate and high salt.	These foods are high in fat and carbohydrates.
Less Important	
• There was no sports equipment available for use during school recess and lunch periods.	Children can be physically active without sports equipment.
• Participation in after-school sports cost $150 per student for uniforms and fees.	High costs for participation in sports are a deterrent for low-income children.
• Local parks were unsafe for children to play in and there were no outdoor recreational activities that were free.	Although important, there isn't a direct linkage between the lack of safe parks and free recreation and childhood obesity.

---

was for achieving the expected outcome. The following are their behavioral objectives:

1. By the end of the fall semester, 75% of the fifth and sixth grade students will choose a breakfast and lunch diet that includes fruit, vegetables, protein, dairy, and starch (bread, potatoes) at each meal.
2. By the end of the school year, the teachers will schedule homework that can easily be done by a low-average student within a half-hour.
3. By the end of the fall semester, all fifth and sixth grade students who have the support equipment will be provided physically interactive games free of charge (such as Wii).

Factors That Influence Behavior Change: Predisposing, Reinforcing, and Enabling Factors

Green and Kreuter (1999, 2005) suggest that three categories of factors affecting individual behavior be addressed, as they can break down factors that contribute to successful behavioral change and create barriers to behavioral change. These factors are:

Predisposing factors are antecedents to behavior that provide the rationale or *motivation* for the behavior.

Reinforcing factors are factors following a behavior that provide the continuing reward or incentive for the persistence or repetition of the behavior.

Enabling factors are antecedents to behavior that allow a motivation to be realized. (1999, p. 153)

Predisposing factors include the knowledge, beliefs, values, attitudes, and confidence of the target population that influence their behavioral choices. **Reinforcing factors** include the knowledge, values, beliefs, and attitudes of the family and friends of the target population. It also includes authority figures such as teachers or managers, as well as agency and community decision makers, as these individuals also influence the target population. Finally, **enabling factors** include the availability of resources, the accessibility of

TABLE 12.2 Changeability Ratings of Behaviors Contributing to Childhood Obesity at Stevens Place Elementary School

More Changeable	Basis for Rating Behavior
There was no sports equipment available for use during school recess and lunch periods.	Trends in under-funding school play equipment are relatively recent.
The students aged 10–12 preferred to drink sodas and eat French fries for lunch.	Peer pressure often changed student behavior, and could be used to encourage healthy choices.
Children in the target group described feeling very stressed due to high homework demands and expectations to score well on national tests.	Pressure for children to perform well on standardized tests is a recent phenomenon of questionable value.
When asked what they did when stressed, children in the target group indicated they watched TV, listened to music, played videogames and had snacks.	This was rated as easier to change due to the newer interactive video games that include movement.

Less Changeable	
Physical education (PE) classes were conducted for 45 minutes once a week.	Trends to decrease PE time per week are relatively recent—limited funding creates barriers to PE.
School breakfasts and lunches were served that were high in fat and salt, with limited fresh vegetable and fruit choices.	For a number of years schools have contracted out for lunch services from businesses based on bids.
Participation in after-school sports cost $150 per student for uniforms and fees.	Sports have been privately funded for a number of years.
Most parents were working and often bought "fast food" for their children for dinner.	Most parents are working, and fast food restaurants have become part of the American culture.
Local parks were unsafe for children to play in and there were no outdoor recreational activities that were free.	Funding for parks and recreation have steadily declined for a number of years.
Children in the target group indicated they went home after school and watched TV or played video games because their parents wouldn't allow them to play outside while they were at work.	This has become common place in the modern culture.
The favorite after-school snacks eaten by children in the target group were macaroni and cheese from a box or packaged noodles—both of which are high fat, high carbohydrate and high salt.	These are cheap and easy foods to fix.

resources, laws, and government support for the health behaviors or for the health program, as well as skills (Green & Kreuter, 2005).

The advisory group, following the Green and Kreuter model, identified the predisposing, enabling, and reinforc-ing factors that affected each behavioral objective. Table 12.4 shows the grid they developed for the first behavior objective—"By the end of the fall semester, 75% of the fifth and sixth grade students will choose a breakfast and lunch diet that includes fruit, vegetables, protein, dairy and

TABLE 12.3 Rankings of Behaviors Contributing to Childhood Obesity at Stevens Place Elementary School by Importance and Changeability

	More Important	Less Important
More Changeable	Fifth and sixth grade students chose high fat, high sugar foods for lunch and breakfast Children stressed by homework demands Children engaged in sedentary activities (watch TV, play videogames) after school	Limited sports equipment
Less Changeable	High-fat and high-carbohydrate school food Limited physical education classes Favorite after-school snacks high fat, high carbohydrate, and high salt	Participation in after-school sports cost $150 per student Parents often bought "fast food" for dinner Local parks unsafe; lack of free recreational activities

TABLE 12.4 Predisposing, Enabling, and Reinforcing Factors That Influence Meal Choices of Fifth and Sixth Grade Students Attending Stevens Place Elementary School

Factors That Support the Change	Factors That Inhibit the Change
Predisposing	
Fifth and sixth grade students tend to believe what they are taught by teachers, thus educating them on food choices could positively affect their choices	Fifth and sixth grade students are beginning to feel some independence from adults and may like to eat what they want versus what adults tell them they should do
Fifth and sixth grade students like to be similar to other children their age	Students like the taste of sodas and French fries more than balanced food choices
Reinforcing	
Students emulate behavior of popular students	Media shows teens eating French fries and drinking sodas
Teachers and parents are concerned about poor food choices being made by fifth and sixth grades students	
Local community leaders expressed outrage about the obesity rates of African American children at Stevens Place Elementary School	
Enabling	
A local community-based organization has offered to provide incentives to students who model positive food choices	The school has no funding for educational intervention programs for obese children
The principal has offered to allow time for the nurses to work with an identified group of student leaders to educate them about modeling better food choices	
The local Parent Teacher Association has offered to help monitor student behavioral changes.	

starch (bread, potatoes) at each meal." For example, one enabling factor that supported the change was the identification of a community group that agreed to provide incentives to students making positive food choices. On the other hand, the lack of school funding for educational intervention programs for obese children was seen as inhibiting change.

The advisory group decided to establish a peer mentoring program, in which student leaders would work with the advisory group and model food choices from all food groups. The advisory group had teachers nominate students for this intervention. The principal allowed the nominated students to attend special educational classes conducted by the nurses to increase their knowledge about the food groups. The nurses worked collaboratively with the students to ensure their teaching approaches were effective. Students suggested rewards that the students could work for that would encourage them to eat more balanced meals. One of the rewards students felt should be offered is sports equipment for student use during recess and lunch periods. One local community-based organization offered to sponsor a fund raising event that would allow them to purchase sports equipment for the school.

Grids similar to that shown in Table 12.4 were developed for the remaining two objectives. This process allowed the nurses and the advisory group to develop program intervention strategies that maximized their potential to achieve desired outcomes. Working with the advisory group, the nurses developed a program plan map outlining activities for each objective, as well as who was responsible for the activity, date by which the activities were to be accomplished, and how outcomes would be documented. Display 12.1 shows

the program plan that was developed for the first objective. This type of mapping allows the group to stay focused, share responsibilities, and monitor outcomes. For instance, student leaders were tasked with modeling balanced food choices at breakfast and lunch and completing a checklist of their food choices each day. The nurses were tasked with meeting each week with the student leaders to provide peer mentoring training sessions.

Working with the advisory group allowed the nurses to contextualize the problem about which they were concerned within the target community. The advisory group ensured that the nurses identified solutions that were culturally acceptable, appropriate, and ultimately effective. This process also helped them to develop outcome measures that were consistent with the concerns of the community. As data were gathered, findings could be interpreted with input from the advisory group. This approach grounded the findings and ensured that interpretations were culturally consistent with the target population. Evaluation was facilitated by clearly defined goals that could be measured against actual results.

This particular case study is an example of the program development needed in schools to address obesity and overweight. The Guide to Community Preventive Services (2005) systematic review of published school-based programs indicated that more evidence was needed to determine the effectiveness of these programs. Although they noted some positive effects in the studies reviewed, the results were too varied to make any conclusions. Their review supports continued efforts to demonstrate program effectiveness in school-based programs. Clear and verifiable outcome measures are needed.

DISPLAY 12.1	SAMPLE PROJECT PLAN MAP

Goal: Fifth and sixth grade students attending Stevens Elementary School will engage in behaviors designed to decrease their obesity levels.

Objective	Activity	Who Responsible	Due Date	Evaluation
1. By the end of the Fall semester, 75% of the fifth and sixth grade students will choose a breakfast and lunch diet that includes fruit, vegetables, protein, dairy, and starch (bread, potatoes) at each meal	1a. Teachers will identify student leaders from the fifth and sixth grade classes who can participate in leadership training for peer mentoring	1a. J. Jamison, school principal	September 20, 2008	1a. A list of student leaders will be available for review
	1b. Students will be approached to participate in the program	1b. J. Jamison, school principal	September 25, 2008	1b. Student response will be documented
	1c. Permission slips for student leaders to participate will be sent home to parents	1c. J. Jamison, school principal	September 27, 2008	1c. Copies of permission slips will be maintained by the principal
	1d. Nurses will meet with the student leaders weekly during the designated time period to provide them training for their peer mentoring	1d. Nurses	September 28–October 31, 2008	1d. Copies of the meeting notes and educational plans will be maintained by the nurses
	1e. Student leaders will model balanced food choices during breakfast and lunch meals	1e. Student leaders	November 1–December 22, 2008	1e. Student leaders will provide a check list of their food choices to the principal at the end of each day
	1f. A check list of possible food choices for students' breakfast and lunch meals using the school menus will be developed	1f. Nurses	December 1, 2008	
	1g. PTA volunteers will monitor student food choices during breakfast and lunch meals one day each week for 3 weeks	1g. PTA volunteers	December 3, 12, 17, 2008	1g. Results of checklists will be tabulated and available for review

EVALUATION OF OUTCOMES

The Institute of Medicine (IOM) report, *The Future of the Public's Health in the 21st Century* (2002), called for examining the benefits of accrediting governmental public health departments (Benjamin, Fallon, Jarris, & Libbey, 2006; IOM, 2002). Responding to this challenge, the Exploring Accreditation Steering Committee published *Final Recommendations for a Voluntary National Accreditation Program for State and Local Public Health Departments* in 2006, outlining this first-ever accreditation program for health departments (Benjamin et al., 2006). The benefits of this program were described as:

- Promoting high performance and continuous quality improvement.
- Recognizing high performers that meet nationally accepted standards of quality.
- Clarifying the public's expectations of state and local health departments.
- Increasing the visibility and public awareness of governmental public health, leading to greater public trust, increased health department credibility and accountability, and ultimately a stronger constituency for public health funding and infrastructure (p. 4).

In 2008, 16 states were selected to "lead a national initiative to advance accreditation efforts and quality improvement strategies in public health departments" (National Network of Public Health Institutes, 2008, p. 1). Areas explored by these states in the initiative included culturally appropriate services, use of health data, and integration of customer service into health programs. Made clear in both the IOM report and the voluntary accreditation program under development is the effort to assure quality through measurable outcomes and standards of practice in the programs and services provided by both state and local health departments. The previous section of this chapter discussed the issues of program planning, implementation, and evaluation as they related to a small health program. This section focuses on the programs and services provided by the agencies. Although the scope of the effort to address outcome evaluation is understandably broader, the concepts are essentially the same. The accreditation initiative has raised the issue of demonstrating in real and objective terms the outcomes resulting from health promotion programs provided through public health agencies. The principles discussed have relevance in many community settings and should be considered whenever health promotion programs and services are provided. PHNs are instrumental to many of the health promotion programs and services offered through health departments; their expertise with and understanding of the communities served is invaluable to assuring ongoing quality assurance and outcome evaluation.

Setting Measurable Goals and Objectives

Planned programs should have specific goals to help identify who the program is supposed to serve, what services are provided, the length of time the services are to be provided, and the resources that are needed. Then, measurable objectives are developed that describe the expected outcomes.

Use of selected verbs indicates the expected level of achievement, such as "clients will be able to demonstrate safe administration of insulin after three home visits," or "parents will have their infants' recommended immunizations up to date by 24 months of age." Goal setting is imperative when developing an educational program (see Chapter 11) for an entire health program or service. These statements of measurable goals are then examined during the program evaluation. Without such statements, accurate evaluations cannot be conducted.

In evaluating programs and care, outcomes must be measured against certain standards. *Standards* are generic guidelines of expected functioning. They can focus on the client, the caregiver, or the organization (finances). All care and services must also be measured against these guidelines. The core standards of care, practice, and finance must be integrated and compatible if they are to ensure quality care.

Evaluating Outcomes

The outcomes or results of care (having the right things happen) are the desired effect of the structure (having the right things) and the processes (doing the right things). The focus on client outcomes demands continued analysis of structure and process, because these two components produce the desirable or undesirable outcomes. With the focus on outcomes, there has been an impetus to include positive outcome terms such as improved health status, functional ability, perceived quality of life, and client satisfaction. Client satisfaction is measured by how closely a client's expectations of nursing care match the perception of the nursing care actually received (Gordon, 1998). Client satisfaction, as one outcome measurement, can be determined by a telephone survey or a mailed questionnaire (Donabedian, 1969).

If the responses indicate that a program is meeting its goals, maintaining set standards, and having positive client outcomes and satisfied clients, the program is providing quality care. However, the accuracy of using outcomes as a primary measure of quality care is limited, because some clients have unsatisfactory outcomes despite receiving good care. Factors other than specific health interventions influence outcomes. These factors include a client's adherence to medically prescribed treatments; the progress of chronic or terminal disease beyond the capabilities of medicine, nursing care, or client behaviors; and the client's ability to respond to care as a result of such situations as a compromised immune system. Community health nurses need to keep such factors in mind when evaluating care.

Quality indicators of client outcomes are the quantitative measures of a client's response to care (Gordon, 1998). Defining and quantifying client outcomes from these indicators are worthwhile processes that enable the nursing staff to evaluate the results of the care they provide. The goal of care in the community is successful client outcomes. By starting with measurable indicators, successful outcomes can be demonstrated in quantifiable terms. When client care meets the standards set, client satisfaction—another quality outcome indicator—is greater.

Quality indicators are part of the broader quality management program and are used to determine goal achievement. A chart audit is a useful method by which to measure the frequency of quality indicator occurrence. For example,

DISPLAY 12.2	QUANTIFYING OUTCOME INDICATORS

$$\text{Outcome indicators} = \frac{\text{Number of patient care events}}{\text{Total number of clients of total number of times at risk for event during a given period}}$$

Example:

$$\text{Occurrence of urinary tract infections in clients with indwelling urinary catheters} = \frac{\text{Number of clients experiencing urinary tract infections related to long-term use of indwelling urinary catheters from January 1 to March 1, 2008}}{\text{Number of clients with long-term indwelling urinary catheters from January 1 to March 1, 2008}}$$

an agency may have a quality indicator such as, "all infants younger than 6 months of age are weighed on each home visit." Every fifth chart of infants visited in March, June, September, and December during a designated year is audited for documentation of the number of home visits and the number of infant weights recorded. A sampling of charts is sufficient to measure goal achievement and specific quality indicators. It is generally accepted that a sample of 20 randomly selected cases will provide useful information. If the population to be sampled numbers more than 200, some sources recommend that the sample include more than 20 cases.

Quantifying the indicators also can be accomplished through a rate or ratio of events for a defined population and timeframe. Such indicators can be tailored to express almost any patient outcome (Williams, 1991). For example, in Display 12.2, the nursing staff sets a standard for the number of urinary tract infections (UTIs) the agency will tolerate in clients with indwelling urinary catheters (perhaps 5% to 7%, depending on client age, diagnosis, family support, and home environment). In another situation, a public health nursing service has a standard to make home visits within 5 days of delivery to first-time mothers and babies born at one hospital 95% of the time. To evaluate this goal, the dates of initial home visits to first-time mothers and the birth dates of the infants are measured from a sample of client records during several measurement periods. These are both examples of assessing quality outcome indicators.

It is necessary to have indicators when setting standards in order to measure the success and quality of programs at home or in the community. The same types of indicators are used in acute care settings, with the focus appropriate to that population. If the standards are being met, but client outcomes are unacceptable, the process indicators are explored for possible areas of weakness. Such areas may need further study to identify the cause of the poor client outcomes. For example, a process indicator such as the catheter-care protocol used by an agency or the communication system between hospital and health department nurses may be examined to determine, respectively, the cause of infections or the reason why initial home visits are delayed. In addition, Medicaid and Medicare regulations in some states mandate that a percentage of records be audited each year.

While striving for excellence and best practices, agencies use the benchmarking process. **Benchmarking** uses continuous, collaborative, and systematic processes for measuring and examining internal programs' strengths and weaknesses; benchmarking includes studying another's processes in order

to improve one's own (Lewis & Latney, 2002). Internal benchmarking occurs within the organization, between departments or programs. External benchmarking occurs between similar agencies providing like services. For example, a home care agency may have developed a clinical pathway that has proved useful with clients with congestive heart failure; another agency could benefit by using the same clinical pathway. In another example, an agency may use clinical practice guidelines obtained from a specialty organization along with information from a national database; another agency could benefit from this knowledge. In this way, an agency identifies what is achievable while comparing and contrasting how others provide quality services.

Role of the Nurse in Quality Measurement and Improvement

Although nurses who deliver care directly to clients are not managers as such, improving quality is a "management" activity, not only of administration personnel but of the practicing nurses, as members of the team. Community health nurses may not be responsible for a staff or agency budget and functioning, but they may be responsible for managing a caseload of clients with needs of varying degrees of urgency. With judicious use of the resources available, they must provide priority services that promote the highest possible level of personal and group functioning and health. Any activities the community health nurse engages in to realize these goals contribute to the quality management program.

Some quality improvement activities for community health nurses include daily prioritizing of care needs for a caseload of clients, seeking supervision or skills development for a difficult case, systematizing charting so that needed documentation is efficiently completed (e.g., using flow sheets to chart maternal–child health visits), proposing better ways to organize care of chronically ill clients, and establishing new agency procedures. All of these actions demonstrate that nurses are evaluating their work and looking for ways to improve care. Staff meetings, peer review, and case conferences are common settings for nurses to bring the lessons of their practices to the larger group for examination and potential adoption.

It is the role of nursing administration to develop a formalized quality management program that includes a three-pronged focus, based on a classic approach to quality management: (1) review organizational structure, personnel, and environment; (2) focus on standards of nursing care and methods of delivering nursing care (process); and (3) focus on the outcomes of that care (Donabedian, 1985). These formal evaluations include peer review audits (documented care delivered by peers), client satisfaction assessments, review of agency policies and procedures, analysis of demographic information, and the like (Ellis & Hartley, 2001).

Nurses who are new to formal quality improvement activities in the work setting need to recognize the value of these efforts and their part in ensuring that quality care is being delivered. Direct service providers are the best judges of care problems and their potential solutions. For this reason, it is critical that quality assurance reviews and other quality improvement activities focus on issues relevant to staff and client concerns and be structured so that they can be accomplished quickly and with minimal effort. When these activities are clear, concise, and well-integrated into daily routines, they become less time-consuming, and staff members can see the positive client outcomes as rewards for their contributions to the process. Moreover, when health care providers have the opportunity to systematically examine the care they provide, they can generate useful ideas for improving that care and can identify care issues sooner.

Whether small or large, health care agencies are complex organizations with interrelated components. The nursing staff has input into or some control over the quality of care delivered to clients who use the services of the agency. The following paragraphs review the nurse's role in each of the three areas of structure, process, and outcomes.

Structure

The organizational structure and financial stability of the agency should allow the mission statement or philosophy to be realized. The agency should be client-focused, with sufficient resources to maintain present services and introduce additional services as needed. Public agencies need to operate within budget and also have a well-developed system of acquiring additional funding for new services through grants and contract expansion. Private agencies should operate efficiently enough to realize a profit that encourages the owners and boards of directors to continue to support the services. They should look for additional ways to solicit clients, in addition to employing highly motivated and qualified staff.

Process

The agency should maintain standards set by the professional staff that comply with or surpass those recommended by the relevant accrediting bodies. The staff is encouraged to contribute to the evaluation of the standards and to revise them as needed. Staff members need to keep themselves current by attending in-service training sessions and acquiring additional education appropriate to their job requirements. The staff members work collaboratively with others across disciplines to improve the quality of care given in the community by using a variety of participative management tools (e.g., audit instruments, peer review). The agency is supportive of its staff and the needs of individuals. Staff turnover is minimal because employee values are compatible with the goals of the agency. Administration and staff have a compatible working relationship. A system of quality review is in place, and each staff member contributes to this process

as a member of a peer review committee or quality improvement or assurance committee. Staff members also listen to clients and provide an outlet to evaluate the care received (e.g., questionnaires, surveys, interviews), and the agency acts on client suggestions and comments.

Outcomes

All services an agency provides should be reviewed periodically to determine whether standards are meeting the present needs of the population and whether the nursing staff are implementing these standards. The nursing services used most frequently, such as well-child care, self-care education with chronically ill adults, and various screening programs, are excellent places to begin the review. Usually, these services involve the entire nursing staff and consume a significant amount of nursing care time.

The focus on commonly served high-risk groups presents an opportunity to optimize care delivery as well as to benefit high-risk clients. Children living in neighborhoods that are known to have high lead toxicity rates from leaded paint in older homes stand to benefit tremendously from a consistently implemented lead screening, treatment, and advocacy program. Without review, such a program may not achieve its goals of decreasing toxic levels of lead in area children.

Incidents of poor client outcomes are important areas for further study. Through clinic or home visit records, community nurses can routinely review documentation of deceased or hospitalized clients to assess whether any aspect of the clinic's care or home visit activities might have prevented these occurrences. For instance, the case of a child with repeated high serum lead levels who requires hospitalization for chelation might stimulate a clinic's examination of the adequacy of parent education regarding environmental sources of lead. The clinic could also explore the effectiveness of its advocacy with the area's lead-abatement staff to ensure needed repairs in leaded homes and the removal of families to safe housing while repairs are being made.

As another example, a review of the charts of hospitalized clients who take multiple medications can be conducted to ascertain whether teaching or compliance issues regarding medication contributed to each client's hospitalization. The results may prompt a change in home-visit teaching techniques, an increase in the frequency of visits, or a change in vital-sign parameters for notifying a physician. Persistence of problems and deficiencies could be a clue that the community health nurse needs additional education in this area or that the nurse's caseload is too heavy and therefore exceeds the ability of the nurse to provide minimally expected care. Once the cause is determined, implementation of appropriate changes can commence, after allowing adequate time for the staff to address critical issues. Should additional education be needed, it is the responsibility of the coordinating, in-service, or staff education nurse to provide or arrange for the needed education.

Given adequate resources, including sufficient time, information, and support, good care is the norm. Occasionally, quality-of-care problems result from an individual provider's performance. Recommendations are made for counseling or another type of intervention by that person's supervisor, and appropriate corrective action should be taken to resolve the problem and preserve the employee's potential contributions as a successful team member.

Identification of quality health care characteristics and "checkpoints" for quality helps the community health care practitioner recognize the quality indicators of best practice. These also give community health nurses direction for their role in quality measurement and improvement. This role is grounded in the structure, process, and outcomes of caregiving and services provided.

MODELS USEFUL IN PROGRAM EVALUATION

Models of client caregiving are based on structure, process, and outcome; ideally, they provide *structure* to guide nurses through the *nursing process* to reach desired *client outcomes*. Each of the following models has all three components; some work more effectively than others, depending on the agency and its philosophy.

Donabedian Model

Donabedian (1966, 1969, 1981, 1985, 2002), the country's premier researcher on health care quality, proposed a model for the structure, process, and outcome of quality that has been widely used over the past 35 years as the framework for more elaborate models. The care environment structure—from philosophy, to facility resources, to personnel—is the first component. Next are the processes responsible for improving or stabilizing the client's health status, such as standards, attitudes, and effectiveness of tools used in caregiving (e.g., nursing care plans). Finally, the resultant outcomes are causally linked indicators of quality, such as client health care goals and effectiveness of service. The Donabedian model is recognized as a simplistic and basic method of measuring quality. Structure, process, and outcome can be depicted in a box-shaped model (Fig. 12.1).

Quality Health Outcomes Model

Mitchell and colleagues (1998) took the time-tested Donabedian model a step further. The Quality Health Outcomes model includes the client in the model and proposes a two-dimensional relationship among components. Interventions always act through the system and the client, creating a dynamic model. The uniqueness of this model is the postulate

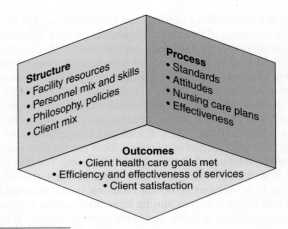

that there are "dynamic relationships with indicators that not only act upon, but reciprocally affect the various components" (Mitchell, Ferketich, & Jennings, 1998, p. 43). A major criticism of other models is that they do not lend themselves to the population focus of community health nursing. However, this model includes community as a client. Figure 12.2 depicts the Quality Health Outcomes model.

American Nurses Association Model

The ANA provides a quality improvement model based on standards of care and quality indicators within the Donabedian framework of structure, process, and outcome. Adopted by the ANA in 1975, the model was developed by Lang to depict the multiple components of evaluation of client care (ANA, 1975). The ANA model has changed as more information has been gathered through research and as the profession of nursing has grown; however, it has proved beneficial over time (Bull, 1996). This circular and continuous model suggests ongoing evaluation. Its core includes the agency's philosophy or mission statement, which identifies the values of the agency and reflects its views of clients, nursing, the community, and health. Defining the beliefs of the agency is the first step in improving quality. The three components of structure, process, and outcome are depicted as pie-shaped wedges located around this central core. Specific nursing actions are added to more closely interrelate

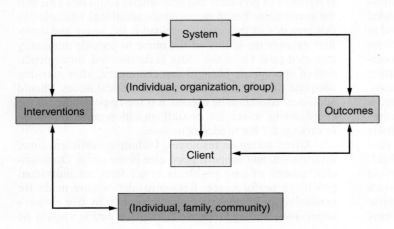

FIGURE 12.2   Quality Health Outcomes model.

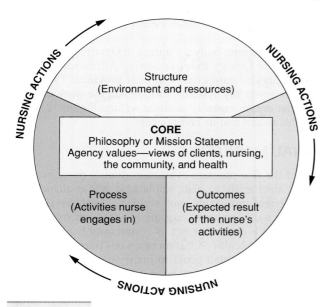

FIGURE 12.3 The American Nurses Association quality assurance model.

each section and make the transition to the next section smoother (Fig. 12.3).

Although each component is important, agencies rely on positive client outcomes as key indicators of success. Successful outcomes are the purpose of the agency's existence and the key to positive evaluation by accrediting bodies. Moreover, continued reimbursement by third-party payers, such as private insurance companies, Medicare, and Medicaid, depends on successful outcomes.

Omaha System

Also discussed in Chapter 14, the Omaha System has measurement approaches that make it a useful model for determining the quality of nursing care provided to individuals, families, and communities. Evaluation focuses on process indicators, client outcome measures, and satisfaction with care (Bowles & Naylor, 1996; Martin, Leak, & Aden, 1997). With the use of this multifocal approach, measurement of nursing practice becomes comprehensive. Although originally designed to evaluate care to individuals and families, the model has been modified to include the community (Martin, 2005). This revision was prompted by the wider use of the model to document population-based and community-level interventions. The inclusion of community as a modifier is seen as a work in progress, awaiting further research and testing.

Community is defined as "groups, schools, clinics, neighborhoods, or other larger geographic areas that share a common physical environment and ownership of a health-related problem" (Martin, 2005, p. 464). In this model, outcomes are rated in terms of knowledge (what the client knows), behavior (what the client does), and status (how the client is). This approach allows for quantifying a range of severity, as well as progress toward or away from optimal health. Ongoing monitoring of these aspects as they relate to individual, family, or community problems allows for evaluation of nursing interventions—a necessary component of

both quality assurance and outcome assessment. For instance, individuals enrolled in a 6-week health promotion program on weight management can be assessed initially for their knowledge of healthy eating and exercise, their current behaviors relative to both, and their current health status (e.g., body mass index [BMI]). The outcome of the program can be assessed by measuring those same indicators and then comparing the initially obtained individual and aggregated data with data collected after the program is concluded. Whereas individual positive changes, such as decreased BMI, are a positive indicator, the impact on the entire group is of even more importance in terms of community-level health status.

The following is a case study exemplifying another use of the Omaha System. A group of county health department community health nurses conducted an assessment of a community's need for a satellite health clinic in a rural part of the county. The nurses gathered data on population needs, age, health status, and accessibility to health care by surveying clients who lived in rural zip code areas and used the main health department. They also conducted a survey by mail of additional residents who were not presently using the health department clinic system for immunizations, screening for tuberculosis or sexually transmitted diseases, or well-baby visits, to see whether these people had unmet needs. After carefully analyzing the data, they began operating three 4-hour clinics during the first week of each month in an empty storeroom of the community pharmacy.

After funding the clinics for 6 months, the health department evaluated the effectiveness of this nursing service. The number of emergency-room visits for infants in the area was compared with the number of visits during a similar period before the satellite clinic was established, as was the number of cases of influenza and pneumonia among residents older than 65 years of age. Finally, clients were surveyed in regard to their satisfaction with nursing care and services and were asked if there were any additional services they needed. Survey outcomes were supportive of continuing the clinics and adding an additional well-baby clinic, a dental clinic, and a prenatal clinic. Clients liked the convenience—older residents did not have to drive the 35 miles to the main clinic, parents were able to keep more closely to the recommended schedule for their children's immunizations, and they liked the shorter wait. Follow-up after human immunodeficiency virus (HIV) screening included the formation of an HIV/AIDS support group for clients and families in the rural area, meeting a need that no one had previously identified. The nurses combined clinic responsibilities with home visits in the area on clinic days and were able to do case finding, thus improving the overall health of this rural area.

The nurses were evaluated and their charts were audited with the use of traditional tools, and clients received the same periodic surveys. Case conferences continued to be held among the nurses serving the rural area and, at times, cases were presented among the larger group of nurses. By utilizing the comprehensive Omaha Visiting Nursing Association measurement approaches, they met the quality measurement needs of a population. The Omaha System provides an organized method to assess individual-, family-, and community-level health. With ongoing research efforts, the utility of the model with respect to program evaluation will be enhanced.

The Quality Practice Setting Attributes Model

This model, developed by the College of Nurses of Ontario in Canada, provides the foundational framework for a unique quality improvement approach to creating quality practice environments. The College of Nurses of Ontario is the regulatory body for registered nurses and registered practical nurses in the Province of Ontario, Canada; it has functions similar to those of the Boards of Registered Nursing in each state in the United States. The Quality Practice Setting Attributes Model is used as a tool to assist in ensuring the quality of nursing practice and the nursing profession by promoting continuing competence among nurses in Canada (Mackay & Risk, 2001).

This nurse-centered model of quality improvement is designed to contribute to the best possible health outcome for the client, regardless of health care setting. The components of this quality assurance program include reflective nursing practice, practice review, and practice setting consultation. The first two components focus on the nurse's individual responsibility for maintaining competence throughout her careers; the practice setting consultation focuses on the practice environment in which nursing care is delivered.

The governing body for nurses in Ontario, Canada, has relied on the Quality Practice Setting Attributes Model to improve nursing care quality in their province. The model identifies seven key systems attributes in the work environment that create a quality practice setting. Figure 12.4 portrays this model and its components.

SOCIAL MARKETING

Each of the five program evaluation models presented provides a mechanism to plan, implement, and evaluate community-based programs and services. Emphasizing the importance of demonstrating quality through measurable outcomes is a crucial aspect of community health. Health promotion and health education programs must demonstrate achievement of stated goals to justify continuation. Likewise, the overall program, be it a health department or a community-based health center staffed by volunteers, is challenged to demonstrate quality outcomes through ongoing evaluation efforts. Community health services are also

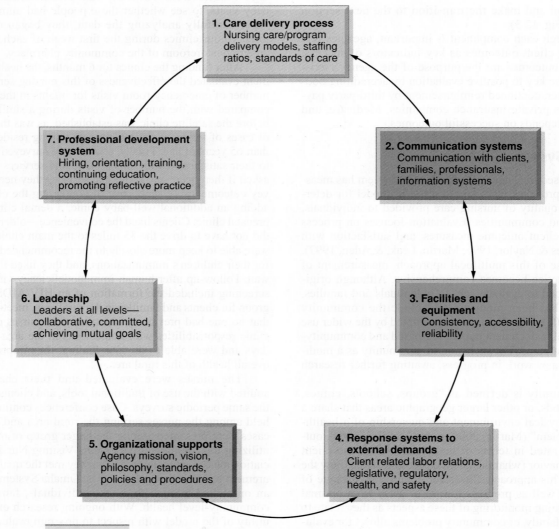

FIGURE 12.4 The quality practice setting attributes model.

challenged to provide programs in ways that reach and engage their target populations. In this section, the role of social marketing is explored as an additional tool for community health care professionals to influence health behaviors and lifestyle choices. These methods must be selected carefully and evaluated against the same standards as previously presented, perhaps more so, due to the potentially higher costs of this type of intervention.

Are you of an age that when you hear the words *"Smoky the Bear,"* your mind finishes the phrase with *"only you can prevent forest fires!"*? Or, perhaps, when you see two golden arches you start craving a hamburger and fries? The ideas that are imbedded in your psyche are all due to marketing. Businesses have long recognized that providing "catchy" advertisements in a way that is memorable to the potential customer is vital to their success. Marketing can literally make or break their business. If the message is effective, they often have more business; if not, they may lose customers. The military has even begun to recognize the effectiveness of these advertising methods, using those same techniques in television and print advertising to increase recruitment. Children as young as 2 years have been found to be "branded" with current fast food items and beverages, meaning they recognize and prefer one particular brand or logo over another. The techniques used by some of these businesses and corporations have in many ways contributed to health issues we currently face as a nation (i.e., obesity in children; teenage smoking).

The public health care sector has only recently begun to recognize the power of marketing health messages. Although used in some capacity since the 1960s, not until the 1990s—when federal agencies, such as the Centers for Disease Control and Prevention (CDC) spearheaded efforts—did it gain the attention it now has in addressing health issues (Andreasen, 2006). The term **social marketing** refers to "influencing the behavior of target audiences" (Andreasen, p. vii). Lotenberg and Siegel go on to explain that in "the public health context, marketing efforts are undertaken to improve societal health, either through influencing changes in health behaviors of individuals, in policies that impact health behaviors, or in perceptions of and support for public health as an institution" (2008, pp. 621–622). The integration of marketing with public health practice is seen as a useful method to increase the effectiveness of public health practitioners (Lotenberg & Siegel).

Concepts that are important in marketing are applicable to social marketing as well. The following concepts are outlined by Lotenger and Siegel (2008):

◆ Exchange: An individual gives something to get something; the person weighs the cost and the perceived benefits.
◆ Self-interest: People act in their own interests in most cases.
◆ Behavior change: Change in behavior is the focus; thoughts and ideas may also need to change but are not the ultimate goal.
◆ Competition: Selecting one option (or action) inherently involves giving up another option (or action).
◆ Consumer orientation: Problem-solving process is directed at the target—the consumer (could be an individual, group, or organization).

◆ Product, price, place, and promotion: Also called the marketing mix; each can be altered to increase market share.
◆ Partners and policy: Other organizations that share similar interests and could provide opportunities to work together; identification of policy changes necessary for behavioral change, those supportive of the change, and those that the organization could help influence.

These principles seem rather straightforward, yet public health practitioners are often at a disadvantage when attempting to implement social marketing campaigns (Lotenger & Siegel, 2008). They often lack training in the necessary skills, may be outspent by the competition (e.g., the fast food industry), or have limited access for the distribution of their message (e.g., public service announcements). One example of a very successful social marketing campaign is the *Go Red for Women* initiative begun in 2004 by the American Heart Association (2008). Using a red dress as the symbol of the program, the initiative seeks to raise awareness of heart disease among women. Another less well known campaign was the American Cancer Society's *Polyp Man* campaign, designed to bring awareness to the need for colon cancer screening. The 2002 campaign featured the funny little polyp-shaped man with the line: "Get the test, get the polyp, get the cure" (Cohen & Falco, 2002). These health issues are equally important, but one has a more broadly recognized campaign; the other was humorous but not necessarily well received. Ultimately, the issue is whether or not behaviors have been changed and health outcomes improved as a result of these social marketing campaigns. Time will be the judge of all these efforts.

One international example of social marketing was an effort to increase consumption of iron-fortified soy sauce among women in China (Sun, Guo, Wang, & Sun, 2007). Nearly 400 women living in both urban and rural areas of Guizhou province participated in this study. Using the marketing techniques of product, price, place, promotion, policy, and partnership, they demonstrated that mass-media campaigns can be effective. In the study, availability of the iron-fortified soy sauce increased in all areas and purchases were increased by nearly 30% more in the intervention groups as compared to the control groups. The researchers point to the feasibility of the campaign and the impact it had on knowledge, intention to purchase, and actual consumption as justification for use of other mass-media campaigns. For health care providers, use of mass-media is an option, but for cost reasons it is not always practical.

How can social marketing principles be utilized when you have a limited budget, limited time, and limited creativity? University campuses hold a wealth of oft-untapped expertise. For nursing students working on a health promotion program, the substance of the effort (the health issue) is often pretty straightforward, but the presentation is more challenging. Many schools of nursing are providing collaborative experiences for students, supporting partnering with non-nursing students and faculty in addressing health education needs. The following is one example of how collaboration can be effective: Two nursing students recognized that off-campus housing lacked sufficient smoke detectors due to a loophole in state and local building codes. This meant that students living in the most high-risk housing for fires (older buildings) might only have one smoke detector in the entire apartment; this was clearly inadequate. After discussing the issue with their faculty member, they sought input from several student organizations. From those discussions they identified a low level of knowledge about the issue and modest concern by the students present. Recognizing that college students are not prone to worrying about how many smoke detectors they have, the nursing students sought help from the university housing department. The staff of housing agreed that this was an important issue, and they were willing to post information on the housing website regarding the need to install additional smoke detectors. The students didn't know how to develop online materials but, based on input from the student groups, they knew that it had to be eye-catching and quickly present a message. In conjunction with their faculty advisor, they contacted the graphic arts department and found an instructor who was willing to include the development of an online smoke detector campaign as part of a class assignment. The nursing students provided the educational information that needed to be included, and the graphic arts students proceeded to develop a campaign within those parameters. In the end, several outstanding examples were submitted, and one was selected and posted on the housing website. The campaign was particularly effective with parents who saw the campaign on the website as they helped in apartment searches. Many messages were sent to the website by the parents regarding the campaign, and the responses were handled by the nursing students. The campaign was not expensive, identified the most skilled individuals for each task (health information: nursing students; web-based campaign: graphic arts students), and provided much-needed health and safety information to the university students and their parents. Even though they had targeted the college students, the nursing students found that the parents were much more interested in the campaign. The results of this initial effort provided vital information for future campaigns that might target parents, students, apartment management, and the local building code enforcement office.

Social marketing is not a panacea, but it does provide techniques that can support health education and health promotion programs. The method can be very expensive and very elaborate, or it can provide simple, straightforward messages. The point is that well-presented marketing can be the difference in whether behavior changes are made or not. Media messages are not a replacement for a sound health promotion program; they are just one tool that can be used for great impact.

GRANTS

Grants are a reality in public health efforts. They are not easy to locate, easy to secure, or easy to manage once you have one, but they are vital to providing a wide range of programs and services in the community. Many local and county health departments see them as an integral part of their service delivery, even hiring grant writers and grant managers in some cases. For most health departments, community agencies, and volunteer service providers, the task of locating grant funds, writing the grant application, and doing the work stipulated by the grant all falls on the nurses and other professionals within those agencies. On the positive side, it provides an opportunity for community health nurses to explain to others what they can provide to the community in terms of services and

programs targeting the community's health. Some basic knowledge about grants can demystify the topic.

Even if you aren't ever required to write a grant, you will likely be involved in some part of a programmatic grant at some point in your career, either in the delivery of services stipulated by the grant (product) or in evaluating the outcomes of the services provided (i.e., satisfaction surveys). You may even be asked to provide ideas for specific services to be included in the grant application; take advantage of these opportunities. The experience you gain will enhance your knowledge of the process and may prove instrumental in future efforts you may be involved with. The grant process, although arduous, provides the opportunity to focus clearly on what you intend to accomplish, why it is needed, and what part you will play in the successful outcome of the project. This is similar to a job interview, in which your prospective employer asks you *"Why should we hire you? What will you contribute to this organization?"* You have a limited amount of time to express your worth. You have to be very specific and concise about what you and your organization or group will be doing to address a specific need. You are making the case that providing you with support is the best choice.

What exactly is a grant? A **grant** is, very simply, one individual or group providing another individual or group the support (i.e., money) for a specified purpose. In health promotion and education, it generally means funding for program development or project support. These types of grants fall into the following common categories: planning grants (i.e., initial project development), start-up grants (i.e., seed money), management or technical assistance grants (e.g., for fund raising or marketing), and facilities or equipment grants (e.g., money for a building, computer, or van) (Minnesota Council on Foundations, 2008). This money doesn't typically need to be paid back; however, it is a contractual agreement and the terms and conditions are usually clearly delineated. For federal grants, the following definition applies: "award of financial assistance from a federal agency to a recipient to carry out a public purpose of support or stimulation authorized by a law of the United States" (Grants.gov, 2008). Federal grants are available from 26 grant-making agencies. The funding categories most applicable to community health include community development, disaster preparation and relief, food and nutrition, and health. Federal grants are available to a wide variety of groups, but typically health-related grants are available to state or local governments, which includes public health departments, public housing organizations, educational organizations, and nonprofit organizations.

What is a *nonprofit organization*? Nonprofit means that the organization was not established to earn a profit (Agnes & Guralnik, 2004). This does not mean that it doesn't generate income, only that there are restrictions on how those funds can be used. Of particular importance to the discussion of grants is the term *501c3*. This is a designation that refers to the Internal Revenue Service (IRS) tax-exempt status granted to certain nonprofit organizations. To be granted this designation, an organization must be organized and operated exclusively for specific purposes, which include charity, science, education, or the prevention of cruelty to children or animals (Internal Revenue Service [IRS] – Department of the Treasury, 2008). Some grants are only available to 501c3 organizations, and the funders will request proof of this in the grant application. Only corporations, community chests, funds, or foundations can receive this designation; individuals or partnerships do not qualify (IRS, 2008). Essentially, the 501c3 organization can be the provider of the grant funding or the organization seeking the funding.

Grants are available from government sources, private philanthropic sources, and corporations. Federal grants can be found on the website www.grants.gov or on individual federal agency websites. Private organizations often have sections on their websites with information on available grant funding. This is likewise the case with corporations. This broad search approach is not a terribly effective way to find grants; to improve search efficiency, a number of proprietary grant-locating programs are available. These programs are very expensive and, because of cost considerations, often are licensed only to large organizations, such as universities and medical centers. They allow the user the ability to limit the search (e.g., type of funder, health issue, age group, program or research grant, funding limits, and timeframe for submission). For the small nonprofit organization seeking funding, one effective approach is to partner with a local university, which allows for more access to grant-locating programs, as well as the expertise offered on the campuses (e.g., content area experts, experienced researchers, statisticians, business plan experts). In a discussion of academic/community partnerships, Chorpita and Mueller (2008) caution that these relationships can be complicated and "projects should be based on a win-win-win proposition, in which consumers, researchers, and service agencies all stand to benefit" (pp. 144–145). Sieber (2008) notes that "productive collaboration requires long-term commitment by the academic researcher despite all the conditions that make this difficult" (p. 137). The community organization and the academic institution both stand to gain from these types of arrangements as do, of course, the target populations.

Some grant funders allow letters of inquiry to be submitted prior to an actual full grant application. The letter of inquiry may be by invitation-only or be part of the original advertisement of the grant funding. In any case, this letter is normally only two or three pages in length and includes a concise overview of the project. For example, a **letter of inquiry** would likely include an overview of your organization and its purpose, the reason for the funding request, clearly stated need or problem to be addressed, overview of the proposed project or program, and other funding sources for your project or program (prospective and committed) (Non-profit Guides, 2008). This letter is brief, yet clearly lays out your plan. Your goal is to be invited to submit a full proposal for consideration. If this approach is successful, you will be asked to complete the organization's application process (the proposal), which can vary in length and complexity depending on the organization.

Crucial to either the letter of inquiry or the full proposal is that you have selected a funder that is a good match for your organization and your program/project. For instance, applying to a faith-based organization that supports abstinence-only educational programs would not be a good fit for your program to provide contraceptive information in an after-school program for teens. Before you spend valuable time and energy writing a letter of inquiry or a grant application, be sure to do your homework. The Internet provides a quick method for reviewing potential funders, their vision, mission, and types of previous funding. You may even be able to find out the monetary range of grants funded by the organization. Perhaps you have a small grant request and find that the organization you are reviewing only funds large multimillion-dollar projects; it might be best to look for other options. The website will likely have contact information; making a phone call can assure you that this organization is a good match for your project and can give you an opportunity to start building a relationship with their staff.

Grants are most often competitive—which means you can expect to have competition from other deserving groups—so be prepared. A well prepared grant—one that carefully follows the application guidelines specified in the Request for Proposals (RFP) and very clearly describes the program you are seeking support for—is more likely to be funded. The **Request for Proposals (RFP)** outlines the specific requirements of the application, the information to include and in what order, and what supplemental forms to include, if any. Submitting a grant after the deadline and not including all required items will mean that your grant application is not likely to be reviewed. If your grant is not selected, make certain to contact the funder to see if they will provide you with a review of your submission; this is common with government-sponsored grants. With knowledge of what hampered your selection, you will be in a much better position to resubmit to this funding source again, or to be more prepared for other grant opportunities. Another suggestion for new grant writers is to seek the help of an experienced mentor—someone who has been successful in grant writing—as they can critique your proposal prior to submission and offer suggestions.

The following tips may be helpful as you begin the process of seeking grant funding (Corporation for Public Broadcasting, 2008):

1. Define your project:
   - Clarify the purpose of your project and write a concise mission statement.
   - Define the scope of work to focus your funding search.
   - Determine the broad project goals, then identify the specific objectives that define how you will focus the work to accomplish those goals.
2. Identify the right funding sources.
3. Contact the funders; think of the funder as a resource.
4. Acquire proposal guidelines.
5. Know the submission deadline.
6. Determine personnel needs.
7. Update your timeline.

One reality of grant funding is that experience counts. If you have a proven record in securing grants and completing the requirements specified in those grants, you or your organization will have an easier time securing additional funding. For the new grant seeker, this can be a bit discouraging. So, where to begin? Don't start with the most complicated grants available. Look for small local grants with a proven track record in grant management, and build your reputation. Work with partners. A school of nursing could partner with a home health agency to write a grant to provide worksite wellness programs for uninsured agricultural workers. Or, several faith-community groups could partner in a grant application to provide free health screenings for uninsured adults in their area. Finally, be certain that the grant will allow you to meet the mission and goals of your program. The grant funder will also be looking to see if their support will enable you to provide a service that you have both the skill and expertise to accomplish. With limited funds available, funders are looking for proof of the sustainability of your program after their support ends. For instance, a breast-feeding support program sought funding in a high-risk area where there was a clear need. Although the need was demonstrated, the agency had no plan for continuing the program after the funding ended; they did not receive funding. Grant support is often seen as funding to get programs started—not to provide for long-term operations.

Many courses are available to assist you in understanding how to locate grants, write them, and be successful in your attempts. Your local library is another source of information, and a wide variety of information is available on the Internet. Some examples of helpful websites are included in the Internet Resources at the end of this chapter.

Summary

Successful community health programs require that the nurse listen to the target population, and not determine the problem and solution without their assistance. Awareness of predisposing, reinforcing, and enabling factors facilitates the assessment of health-related behaviors. Importance and changeability are important considerations when determining priorities among competing behavioral targets. An advisory group, with representation from the target and service communities, is an effective tool in helping to identify the problem, select appropriate interventions to address the problem, and evaluate the outcomes of the interventions chosen. Outcome measures should be consistent with the concerns of the community. Evaluation can be facilitated by clearly defined goals that can be measured against actual results.

The multiple models or frameworks on which quality management systems are based include a classic way of looking at programs through organizational structure, process, and outcomes, along with the interrelatedness of each component. The five models presented in this chapter are structured in unique ways that enable them to meet the differing needs of community agencies. Whether quality measurement and improvement techniques are formally or informally practiced, whenever nurses monitor, assess, and judge the quality and appropriateness of care as measured against professional standards, the interests of clients are being served.

Social marketing is one tool that can enhance health promotion efforts in the community. Media messages are particularly helpful in reaching large audiences. The basis of social marketing is similar to product marketing to consumers. The goal of consumer marketing is not necessarily to change the way people think, but the way they behave. Social marketing seeks to first change behavior and then to influence how people think about health, lifestyle, and the choices they make every day that influence their health. One example of social marketing is the American Heart Association, *Go Red for Women* campaign, which seeks to bring attention to heart disease risk among women. Social marketing, like any consumer-focused marketing, must consider the target population in the design, implementation, and evaluation of the effort. Successful outcomes are imperative for continuation of this type of program, as with any other health promotion campaign.

Grants are increasingly vital to providing health promotion programs and services in the community. Community health nurses frequently are involved in some aspect of a grant program, whether in the writing, implementation of the

program or services stipulated in the grant, or in the evaluation of the outcomes for the grant. Grants are available from government sources, private philanthropic sources, and corporations. Successful grant proposals comply with the instructions provided in the Request for Proposals. Community agencies and academic programs can collaborate in providing community services and evaluation research that seeks to improve the lives of the target population. Mastering the grant process, from formulating the goal to defining the evaluation methods, is a skill that can benefit all manner of health promotion programs, whether funded or not.

Community health nurses are in a key position to plan, implement, and evaluate all types of health promotion/health education programs. Knowledge of the target population and engaging the target population in determining the problem and solutions is vital to successful outcomes. Ongoing use of quality measurement techniques and application of recognized professional standards helps assure effective and appropriate service delivery. Social marketing is a tool that can be effective in reaching large audiences with valuable health messages. Finally, the skills gained in working on any portion of a grant effort can be utilized in future programmatic efforts, whether supported through funding or not. ■

 ACTIVITIES TO PROMOTE CRITICAL THINKING

1. A group of student PHNs are approached by a faculty member who teaches acute care nursing. She informs them that there is a high incidence of chlamydia infection in a local community among Spanish-speaking people. The hospital where she has students wants to do something to reduce the incidence of chlamydia. The faculty member has found a pamphlet online that describes chlamydia infection, how it's diagnosed, and how it's treated. She thinks it would be a wonderful idea for the student PHNs to translate the pamphlet into Spanish.
   a. Is this the appropriate intervention?
   b. What data should be gathered? What literature should be reviewed?
   c. What agencies, organizations, and groups should the students contact?
   d. Who is the target population?
   e. What outreach should be done with this population? What information should be gathered from the population prior to developing any educational materials?
   f. What steps should the students take to ensure that the target population finds the educational materials they develop to be appropriate, acceptable, and understandable?

2. A school nurse works in a rural agricultural community. The main crop is rice. Every year after harvesting the rice, the local farmers burn their rice fields. The school nurse notes a significant increase in absences during this period for respiratory problems, especially asthma. She notes that even the teachers have increasing respiratory problems. She believes that the respiratory problems are aggravated by the

burning rice fields. She mentions her concerns about the relationship between the fields burning and increased respiratory-related illnesses to the school principal. He responds that while it may be true, the local farmers control the local community—without them, the community would collapse. He states that kids and adults will just have to adjust.

   a. What can the nurse do to find out if the burning rice fields are a threat to the health of children and adults in the local area? (What data should be gathered, what literature should be reviewed, to whom should she talk?)

   b. What steps should she take to increase interest in addressing this problem?

   c. What agencies, organizations, and groups should she contact?

3. Identify a health-related social marketing campaign that you viewed recently on the television or in a store or billboard advertisement. Has this campaign effectively reached out to the target audience?

References

Agnes, M., & Guralnick, D.B. (Eds.). (2004). *Webster's new world college dictionary* (4th ed.). Cleveland, OH: Wiley Publishing, Inc.

American Heart Association. (2008). *Food retailers*. Retrieved June 17, 2008 from http://www.americanheart.org/presenter.jhtml?identifier=760.

American Nurses Association. (1975). *A plan for implementation of the standards of nursing practice*. Kansas City, MO: Author.

American Nurses Association. (2007). *Public health nursing: Scope and standards of practice*. Silver Spring, MD: Nursesbooks.org.

Andreasen, A.R. (2006). *Social marketing in the 21st century*. Thousand Oaks, CA: Sage Publications, Inc.

Benjamin, G., Fallon, M., Jarris, P.E., & Libbey, P.M. (2006). *Final recommendations for a voluntary national accreditation program for state and local public health departments*. Retrieved June 25, 2005 from http://www.phaboard.org/Documents/finalrec.pdf.

Bowles, K.H., & Naylor, M.D. (1996). Nursing intervention classification systems. Image. *Journal of Nursing Scholarship, 28*(4), 303–308.

Bull, M.J. (1996). Past and present perspectives on quality of care in the United States. In J. A. Schmele (Ed.), *Quality management in nursing and health care* (pp. 141–157). Albany, NY: Delmar.

Chorpita, B.F., & Mueller, C.W. (2008). Toward new models for research, community, and consumer partnerships: Some guiding principles and an illustration. *Clinical Psychology: Science & Practice, 15,* 144–148.

Cohen, E., & Falco, M. (2002). *Ad campaign uses humor to fight colon cancer*. Retrieved June 17, 2008 from http://archives.cnn.com/2002/HEALTH/conditions/01/30/polyp.man.ad/.

Corporation for Public Broadcasting. (2008). *Grant proposal writing tips*. Retrieved June 17, 2008 from http://medi-smart.com/grant2.htm.

Dabelea, D., Snell-Bergeon, J.K., Heartsfield C.L, Bischoff, K.J., Hamman, R.F., & McDuffie, R.S. (2005). Increasing prevalence of gestational diabetes mellitus (GDM) over time and by birth cohort. *Diabetes Care, 28,* 579–584.

Davis-Floyd, R.E., & Sargent, C.F. (1997). *Childbirth and authoritative knowledge: Cross-cultural perspectives*. Berkeley, CA: University of California Press.

Donabedian, A. (1966). Evaluating the quality of medical care. *Milbank Memorial Fund Quarterly, 44,* 166–206.

Donabedian, A. (1969). Medical care appraisal: Quality and utilization. In *Guide to medical care administration*. New York: American Public Health Association.

Donabedian, A. (1981). *The criteria and standards of quality*. Ann Arbor, MI: Health Administration Press.

Donabedian, A. (1985). *Explorations in quality assessment and monitoring* (Vol. 3). Ann Arbor, MI: Health Administration Press.

Donabedian, A. (2002). *An introduction to quality assurance in health care*. New York: Oxford University Press.

Ellis, J.R., & Hartley, C.L. (2001). *Nursing in today's world: Challenges, issues, and trends* (7th ed.). Philadelphia: Lippincott Williams & Wilkins.

Goodman, R., Speers, M., McLeroy, K., Fawcett, S., Kegler, M., Parker, E., et al. (1998). Identifying and defining dimensions of community capacity to provide a basis for measurement. *Health Education Behavior, 25,* 258–278.

Gordon, M. (1998, September 30). Nursing nomenclature and classification system development. *Online Journal of Issues in Nursing*. Retrieved June 25, 2008 from http://nursingworld.org/ojin.

Grants.gov. (2008). *Who is eligible for a grant?* Retrieved June 25, 2008 from http://www.grants.gov/.

Green, L.W., & Kreuter, M.W. (1999). *Health program planning: An educational and environmental approach* (3rd ed.). Mountain View, CA: Mayfield Publishing Company.

Green, L.W., & Kreuter, M.W. (2005). *Health program planning: An educational and ecological approach* (4th ed.). New York: McGraw-Hill.

Guide to Community Preventive Services. (2005, June). *More evidence is needed to determine the effectiveness of school-based programs to control overweight or obesity*. Retrieved June 16, 2008 from http://www.thecommunityguide.org/obese/obese-int-schools.pdf.

Guide to Community Preventive Services. (2008). *The community guide*. Retrieved June 16, 2008 from http://www.thecommunityguide.org/.

Institute of Medicine. (2002). *The future of the public's health in the 21st century*. Washington, DC: National Academies Press.

Internal Revenue Service—Department of the Treasury. (2008). *Tax-exempt status for your organization*. Retrieved June 25, 2008 from http://www.irs.gov/pub/irs-pdf/p557.pdf.

Lewis, P.S., & Latney, C. (2002). Achieve best practice with an evidence-based approach. *Nursing Management, 33*(12), 24, 26–29.

Lotenberg, L.D., & Siegel, M. (2008). Using marketing in public health. In L.F. Novick, C.B. Morrow, & G.P. Mays (Eds.). *Public health administration: Principles for population-based management* (2nd ed., pp. 621–656). Sudbury, MA: Jones & Bartlett Publishers.

Mackay, G., & Risk, M. (2001). Building quality practice settings: An attributes model. *Canadian Journal of Nursing Leadership, 14*(3), 19–27.

Martin, K.S. (2005). *The Omaha System: A key to practice, documentation, and information management* (2nd ed.). St. Louis, MO: Elsevier.

Martin, K., Leak, G., & Aden, C. (1997). The Omaha system: A research-based model for decision making. In B.W. Spradley & J.A. Allender (Eds.), *Readings in community health nursing* (5th ed., pp. 316–324). Philadelphia: Lippincott-Raven.

Minnesota Council on Foundations. (2008). *Common types of grants*. Retrieved June 25, 2008 from http://www.mcf.org/MCF/whatis/common.htm.

Mitchell, P.H., Ferketich, S., & Jennings, B.M. (1998). Quality health care outcomes model. *Image: Journal of Nursing Scholarship, 30,* 43–46.

National Center for Health Statistics. (2008). *GIS and public health*. Retrieved June 25, 2008 from http://www.cdc.gov/nchs/about/otheract/gis/gis_atnchs.htm.

National Network of Public Health Institutes. (2008). *MLC-3: Lead states in public health quality improvement*. Retrieved June 25, 2008 from http://www.nnphi.org/home/section/1-15/view/view/39/.

Non-profit Guides. (2008). *Grant-writing tools for non-profit organizations*. Retrieved June 25, 2008 from http://www.npguides.org/.

Ottoson, J.M., & Green, L.W. (2008). Public health education and health promotion. In L.F. Novick, C.B. Morrow, & G.P. Mays (Eds.). *Public health administration: Principles for population-based management* (2nd ed., pp.). Sudbury, MA: Jones & Bartlett Publishers.

Poole, D.L. (1997). Building community capacity to promote social and public health: Challenges for universities. *Health and Social Work, 22*, 163–170.

Sieber, J.E. (2008). When academicians collaborate with community agencies in effectiveness research. *Clinical Psychology: Science & Practice, 15*, 137–143.

Sun, X., Guo, Y., Wang, S., & Sun, J. (2007). Social marketing improved the consumption of iron-fortified soy sauce among women in China. *Journal of Nutrition Education & Behavior, 39*, 302–310.

Thorpe, L.E., Berger, D., Ellis, J.A., Bettegowda, V.R., Brown, G., Matte, T., et al. (2005). Trends and racial/ethnic disparities in gestational diabetes among pregnant women in New York City, 1990–2001. *American Journal of Public Health, 95*, 1536–1539.

U.S. Department of Health and Human Services. (2000). *Healthy People 2010: Understanding and Improving Health* (2nd ed.). Washington, DC: U.S. Government Printing Office. Retrieved June 16, 2008 from http://www.healthypeople.gov/.

U.S. Department of Health and Human Services. (2008). *Healthy People 2020: The road ahead*. Retrieved June 16, 2008 from http://www.healthypeople.gov/hp2020/Comments/.

Williams, A.D. (1991). Development and application of clinical indicators for nursing. *Journal of Nursing Care Quality, 6*(1), 1–5.

Xiong, X., Saunders, L.D., Wang, F.L., & Demianczuk, N.N. (2001). Gestational diabetes mellitus: Prevalence, risk factors, maternal and infant outcomes. *International Journal of Gynecology & Obstetrics, 75*, 221–228.

Selected Readings

Baptiste-Roberts, K., Gary, T.L., Beckles, G.L.A., Gregg, E.W., Owens, M., Porterfield, D., et al. (2007). Family history of diabetes, awareness of risk factors, and health behaviors among African Americans. *American Journal of Public Health, 97*, 907–912.

Craib, K.J.P., Hackett, G., Back, C., Cvitkovich, Y., & Yassi, A. (2007). Injury rates, predictors of workplace injuries, and results of an intervention program among community health workers. *Public Health Nursing, 24*, 121–131.

Cramer, M.E., Chen, L., Roberts, S., & Clute, D. (2007). Evaluating the social and economic impact of community-based prenatal care. *Public Health Nursing, 24*, 329–336.

Farris, R.P., Will, J.C., Khavjou, O., & Finkelstein, E.A. (2007). Beyond effectiveness: Evaluating the public impact of the WISEWOMAN program. *American Journal of Public Health, 97*, 641–647.

Lee, C.V. (2008). Public health data acquisition. In L.F. Novick, C.B. Morrow, & G.P. Mays (Eds.). *Public health administration: Principles for population-based management* (2nd ed., pp. 297–328). Sudbury, MA: Jones & Bartlett Publishers.

Macnee, C.L, Edwards, J., Kaplan, A., Reed, S. Bradford, S., Walls, J., et al. (2006). Evaluation of NOC standardized outcome of "health seeking behavior" in nurse-managed clinics. *Journal of Advanced Care Quality, 21*, 242–247.

Mayer, J.A., Slymen, D.J., Clapp, E.J., Pichon, L.C., Eckhardt, L., Eichenfield, L.F., et al. (2007). Promoting sun safety among U.S. Postal Service letter carriers: Impact of a 2-year intervention. *American Journal of Public Health, 97*, 559–565.

Pechmann, C., & Reibling, E.T. (2006). Antismoking advertisements for youths: An independent evaluation of health, counter-industry, and industry approaches. *American Journal of Public Health, 96*, 906–913.

Public Health Accreditation Board. (2008). *Public Health Accreditation Board (PHAB): Begin to prepare for national accreditation now!* Retrieved June 25, 2008 from http://www.phaboard.org/.

Seligman, H.K., Wallace, A.S., DeWalt, D.A., Schillinger, D., Arnold, C.L, Shilliday, B.B., et al. (2007). Facilitating behavior change with low-literacy patient education materials. *American Journal of Health Behavior, 31*(Suppl. 1), S69–S78.

Sin, M., Belza, B., LoGerfo, J., & Cunningham, S. (2005). Evaluation of a community-based exercise program for elderly Korean immigrants. *Public Health Nursing, 22*, 407–413.

Valente, T.W., Chou, C.P., & Pentz, M.A. (2007). Community coalitions as a system: Effects of network change on adoption of evidence-based substance abuse prevention. *American Journal of Public Health, 97*, 880–886.

Zotti, M.E., Graham, J., Whitt, A.L., Anand, S., & Replogle, W. (2006). Evaluation of a multi-state faith-based program for children affected by natural disaster. *Public Health Nursing, 23*, 400–409.

Internet Resources

California Department of Public Health (Healthy People 2010 Goals & Objectives): *http://ww2.cdph.ca.gov/data/indicators/goals/Pages/default.aspx*

Federal Grants: *http://www.grants.gov/*

Federal Health Information Centers & Clearinghouses: *http://www.health.gov/NHIC/Pubs/2008clearinghouses/clearinghouses.htm*

Guide to Community Preventive Services (CDC): *http://www.thecommunityguide.org/*

Health Finder (USDHHS—Office of Health Promotion & Disease Prevention): *http://www.healthfinder.gov/organizations/*

Health Resources & Services Administration (Shortage Designation): *http://bhpr.hrsa.gov/shortage/*

National Center for Health Marketing (CDC): *http://www.cdc.gov/healthmarketing/*

National Center for Health Statistics (GIS and Public Health): *http://www.cdc.gov/nchs/gis.htm*

National Center for Health Statistics (Other sites): *http://www.cdc.gov/nchs/sites.htm*

National Center for Health Statistics (Research & Development): *http://www.cdc.gov/nchs/rd.htm*

National Center for Health Statistics (Surveys & Data Collection Systems): *http://www.cdc.gov/nchs/express.htm*

National Committee for Quality Assurance: *http://www.ncqa.org/*

National Quality Measures Clearinghouse: *http://www.qualitymeasures.ahrq.gov/*

Network for a Healthy California—GIS Map Viewer: *http://www.cnngis.org/*

Oklahoma State Department of Health: *http://www.ok.gov/health/Data_and_Statistics/index.html*

Public Health Accreditation Board: *http://www.phaboard.org/*

Public Health Foundation (National Public Health Performance Standards Program [NPHPSP]): *http://www.phf.org/performance.htm*

U.S. Public Health Service Grant—Application: *http://grants1.nih.gov/grants/funding/phs398/phs398.html*

U.S.A. Grants.gov (non-profits): *http://www.usa.gov/Business/Nonprofit.shtml*

13

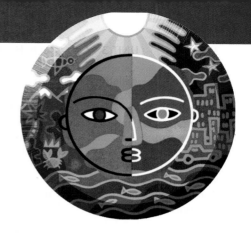

Policy Making and Community Health Advocacy

KEY TERMS

Advocacy
Community health
  advocacy
Distributive health
  policy
Empowerment
Grassroots
Health policy
Lobbying
Lobbyists
Polarization
Policy
Policy analysis
Political action
Political action committee
  (PAC)
Politics
Power
Public policy
Redistributive health policy
Regulatory health policy
Social justice
Special interest groups

LEARNING OBJECTIVES

Upon mastery of this chapter, you should be able to:

- ◆ Define health policy and explain how it is established.
- ◆ Analyze the influence of health policy on community health and nursing practice.
- ◆ Explain the role of special interest groups in health care reform and policy making.
- ◆ Explain the role that professional organizations play in public policy.
- ◆ Define power and empowerment and the roles these concepts play in policy development.
- ◆ Identify the four stages in the policy process and briefly explain what each entails.
- ◆ Explain the concepts of policy analysis and strategy development.
- ◆ Explain the role of community health nurses in determining a community's health policy needs.
- ◆ Discuss the difference between advocacy and lobbying and the influence of both on policy.
- ◆ Identify the 10 steps in mobilizing a community for political action.
- ◆ Describe the steps involved in how a bill becomes law.
- ◆ Discuss several methods of communicating with legislators on policy issues.

"Genuine politics—even politics worthy of the name—the only politics I am willing to devote myself to—is simply a matter of serving those around us: serving the community and serving those who will come after us. Its deepest roots are moral because it is a responsibility expressed through action, to and for the whole."

—Vaclav Havel

Behind all legislation and health care regulation lie power struggles. Only the very naive think that others will be persuaded by facts alone. In all legislative activities and reforms, social and political factions are at work—special interest groups, business, and industry each bring their power into play. Because the outcomes of these struggles determine the availability and quality of all health and social services, nurses need to develop an operational knowledge of health policy and the political process in order to protect the individuals, families, and communities they serve, as well as their own nursing practice. This chapter examines health policy, the political process involved in determining health policy, and the role of community health nursing in the process. Community health nurses should provide not only input to policy circles through advocacy, but also leadership at decision-making tables. Community health nurses must understand and emphasize their powerful role in providing an essential influence and unique perspective in health care.

EVOLUTION AND EFFECTS OF CURRENT U.S. HEALTH POLICIES

The United States is often touted as having the best health care system in the world. It is recognized worldwide for achievements in the medical and auxiliary sciences that have contributed to the mapping of the genome, advances in biomedical technologies, and increasing numbers of pharmaceuticals that hold promise for addressing the myriad chronic and acute illnesses that affect the world's populations. People often come from other countries to the United States to access our high-quality medical care.

Uninsured and Underinsured

Conversely, and as discussed in Chapter 6, more than 45 million U.S. citizens are uninsured and many millions more are underinsured. A major reason for bankruptcy filings is the inability to pay medical bills. Millions of citizens suffer death and disease because of ethnic disparities (Smedley, Stith, & Nelson, 2003), and there continues to be an imbalance in the ethnic makeup of our professional caregivers—nurses, physicians, dentists, and others (Sullivan Commission, 2004). Our medical care system is the most expensive in the world, but our longevity is lower than in countries that spend much less than we do for health care, and these countries are still able to provide care for their entire populations (Commonwealth Fund, 2004).

In the United States, infant mortality rates—a marker for quality of health care—are near the bottom of industrialized nations, with a rate of 6.4 per 1,000 births (State of the World's Mothers Index, 2006). Our publicly financed health system—Medicaid and Medicare—is constantly under siege, and increasing numbers of medical errors are harming 1.5 million patients per year (Institute of Medicine, 2000, 2006). The changing demographics of our society, along with other issues such as immigration, shortages of professional health care workers, the increased use of alternative medicine and, most importantly, the shift from a nonprofit to a for-profit health care system, affects our society in innumerable ways (Leape & Berwick, 2005; Milstein & Smith, 2006).

Economic Effects

The 1990s ushered in an era of health care reform, and with it came downsizing—registered nurses (RNs) in the acute care setting were thought to be dispensable and were replaced by less-prepared staff (American Nurses Association, 1994; Seago, Spetz, & Mitchell, 2004). The core functions of public health—assessment, assurance, and policy development—became underfunded and underappreciated by local and state governments. As this is written, health departments continue to be in crisis as a result of economic downturns that have necessitated nursing staff layoffs. Also, due to the normal attrition of licensed staff, a substantial reduction in programs and services has occurred (Hall, 2006). More critically, schools of nursing have closed or been reduced in size (Kovner, Fairfield, & Jacobson, 2006). We have yet to recover from this dramatic downsizing, and these problems are further exacerbated by the current nursing shortage. The cyclical changes in health workforce patterns are accentuated by the aging of our health care workforce—the average age of public health employees is 47 (National Council of State Legislators, 2004). Additionally, the shortages of nursing faculty hinder our nursing schools from accommodating students interested in entering nursing (National League for Nursing, 2006).

Federal nursing programs, including the Nurse Reinvestment Act, Title VIII funding of the Public Health Service Act, and various state funding programs are attempting to address these issues. For example, California and Florida have loan forgiveness programs in return for a commitment to work in designated areas, notably state facilities or underserved areas, for a designated period of time. Additionally, California is offering loan forgiveness for graduate students to become nursing instructors for 3 to 5 years. Many other states are offering various incentives to attract and retain their public health personnel (American Association of Colleges of Nursing, 2006).

The reality of today's health care arena is managed care, which when first developed, offered a population-based approach to care that included the assurances of preventive care and early intervention necessary for maintaining a healthy patient (Barr, 2004). Physicians within this system were paid based on an agreed-upon fee (per member, per month) to provide all needed services. This system, then called *prepaid group practice*, was first developed by Kaiser Permanente in the 1920s to care for its employees in remote locations and later refined in 1973 when the federal government passed the *Health Maintenance Organization Assistance Act*. Prepaid group practice was touted as an example of wellness care, not sick care. It was to be a combination of insurance and health care, quite different from indemnity plans, which would lower health care costs. Signed into law by President Nixon, the plan was seen by one of its proponents—Representative Ted Kennedy—as the first step toward universal care. However, as this model evolved, its emphasis shifted from prevention to cost containment. Reductions in reimbursement, particularly for disadvantaged patients (e.g., those covered under Medicaid and Medicare), reductions in the choice of practitioners, and limitations on the types of care available drastically transformed the system from its original concept. Most managed care today is for profit, thus setting up a dichotomy between the insured and the owners/investors (Baker, 2000; Friedman, 1999; Kovner & Knickman, 2005; Robinson, 2001).

Health care coverage and access are ongoing policy discussions in the United States, with the cost of care high and growing each year, according to the latest information from the National Coalition on Health Care (2004). Health care insurance coverage is often provided through employers, and as costs rise, employers are passing on more costs to the worker. Co-pays and deductibles have increased, with workers paying an increase of 10% over 2004 (see Chapter 6). As the numbers of elderly Americans increase, costs to provide health coverage for them are growing exponentially.

Need for Action to Change

Most people agree that health care policy in the United States must change, but there is little agreement among policy makers and citizens about how this should occur (Gordon, 2003). Some believe market forces should be allowed to work this problem out, others believe the government should assume responsibility—as in other countries—and ensure that all have access to health care coverage. Public health activists believe that if every person adhered to healthful lifestyles, the need for medical care would lessen.

Policy discussions at the state and local level determine access to care for their residents; other issues, such as high rates of unemployment, health care allotments in state and local budgets, and increasingly incendiary discussions on the role that undocumented residents play in the costs of health care, affect how health care is delivered. The latter issue is a discussion that occurs more frequently in those states with significant numbers of undocumented workers (see Chapter 29). Nonetheless, the numbers of uninsured or underinsured result in patients who lack access to primary care, or who delay care, thus resulting in higher morbidity, mortality, and expense. Disadvantaged populations are more likely to be uninsured because of unemployment or underemployment, resulting in low or no income, health disparities, poor housing, and neighborhoods that may be unsafe (see Chapter 25). Recent studies document that uninsured or underinsured patients have difficulty maintaining economic and social stability (Himmelstein, Warren, Thorne, & Woolhandler, 2005; Institute of Medicine, 2002a, 2003).

Himmelstein, Warren, Thorne, and Woolhandler (2005) reported that over half of personal bankruptcy filings were the result of medical bills and/or loss of health coverage. "These were working-class or middle-class people, and 76% of them had health insurance when they first got sick . . . (although) many lost this coverage because the insurance was through their jobs, so it disappeared when they couldn't work. Half of the bankruptcies were caused, in part, by illness and medical debt . . . and the major part of that debt was payments to doctors and hospitals. Families initially tried to pay the debt for several months . . . 61% went without needed medical care to make payments, 30% had a utility shut off, and 22% percent cut back on their food" (p. 6).

Larger employers complain that they are subsidizing those firms that don't provide coverage, and this also drives up the cost of the premiums they have to pay. Loss of insurance coverage leads to increases in charity care which, in turn, impacts health care facilities' ability to continue to provide care. People with health insurance pay higher deductibles and co-pays as a result of the lack of universal health coverage.

Disproportionate-share hospitals are closing, while others are implementing diversion policies to ensure greater equity in the care of patients without sufficient health care insurance.

As an example of a deteriorating health care system, despite advances in caring for and addressing infectious diseases, one of the scourges of an earlier time, tuberculosis (TB), has resurfaced. Although the increased incidence of AIDS accounts for some of this resurgence, drug resistance to the TB bacillus and the influx of immigrants from endemic areas, coupled with budget cuts, have impeded the labor-intensive measures of tracking patients, directly observing therapy, and providing continuous follow-up for these patients (see Chapter 8).

Despite the availability of vaccines against childhood diseases, the numbers of children fully vaccinated is inadequate—only about 76% of 2-year-olds are appropriately immunized (Centers for Disease Control and Prevention [CDC], 2006). Because of a complicated vaccination schedule, coupled with access issues, many youngsters are not fully immunized; consequently, periodic outbreaks of childhood diseases (e.g., mumps, pertussis, meningitis) occur. With the increased emphasis on terrorism, public health departments are being called on to provide the critical disaster preparedness plans that each state and local jurisdiction will need in the event of a major disaster (Khan, Morse, & Lillibridge, 2000; Geberding, Hughes, & Koplan, 2002).

With the health care arena in a state of flux, nurses are beginning to take on more of a role in influencing health policy. Currently, three former RNs are in Congress: Lois Capps (D-CA); Eddie Bernice Johnson (D-TX), the first nurse to be elected to U.S. House of Representatives; and Carolyn McCarthy (D-NY). These representatives carry on the legacy of nurses involved in influencing health policy in the United States since the 19th century. They have proved, as others before them, to be instrumental in the introduction and passage of policies that affect the health of all Americans (Roberts & Group, 1995).

FOUNDATIONS OF POLITICAL ACTION AND ADVOCACY

The basic concepts of public health have evolved over the last 150 years. From an emphasis on the individual to a population focus, policy development aims for a broader effect encompassing "healthy policies—education, adequate and affordable housing, living wage, and environmental concerns" (Institute of Medicine [IOM], 2002b, p. 46).

Public Health

The concept of social justice is seen as the very foundation of public health nursing (Fahrenwald, 2003; Keller, Strohschein, Lia-Hoagberg, & Schaffer, 1998). The American Association of Colleges of Nursing (2003) emphasizes that the guiding values of nursing include social justice, and the American Nurses Association (ANA) *Code of Ethics with Interpretive Statements* (2001, preface) states that "nurses should act to change those aspects of society that detract from health and well-being." The many definitions of social justice depend on the discipline involved; for purposes of this chapter, **social justice** is "both a process and a goal which includes a vision of society that is equitable and all members are physically and psychologically safe and secure" (Adams,

Bell, & Griffin, 1997, p. 1). However, it has been noted that nurses "lack a multi-disciplinary vocabulary to discuss, critique and strategize about injustice" (Boutain, 2005, p. 10). You may be caught in a "Catch-22," working within a market-based system that is inherently unfair and often leads to health and social disparities for ethnic and other disadvantaged groups, while having pledged to alleviate suffering within the groups you serve (Fahrenwald, 2003).

As a community health nurse, you are expected to give voice to the disparities found in the communities you serve (e.g., substandard housing, high rates of unemployment, death and disability)—disparities that often could be prevented or alleviated at early stages. Your efforts through nursing interventions can address not only health issues but also the educational, social, and economic issues that give rise to these disparities (Cohen, de la Vega, & Watson, 2001). The Minnesota Department of Public Health Nursing Section has developed a public health interventions model that gives a broad overview of public health nursing. The model is based on the type of intervention and level of practice that allows a range of activities, such as advocacy, community organizing, coalition building, case management, and policy development, that you as a public health practitioner can activate (see Chapter 14). The nexus between social justice, advocacy, and policy is interesting, complex, and one that will affect every aspect of your community health nursing career.

History of Public Health Nursing Advocacy

Nurses have a long history of action in social justice and **advocacy**, which can be defined as pleading the case of another or championing a cause. A more encompassing definition has been proposed by the Advocacy Institute in its publication *Advocacy for Social Justice: A Global Action and Reflection Guide* (Cohen, de la Vega, & Watson, 2001, p. 7): "Advocacy is the pursuit of influencing outcomes—including public policy and resource allocation decisions within political, economic, and social systems and institutions—that directly affect people's lives. . . ."

Advocacy is a process, not an outcome, one that includes identifying an issue, collecting information, identifying who can be influenced/who can make the decision sought, building support, and taking action. Advocacy can present itself in a variety of ways—self-advocacy, which is advocating for one's self; individual advocacy, which is pleading the case of others; and legislative advocacy, which is changing or modifying state or federal laws. Advocacy also includes litigation and public education campaigns. Finally, advocacy is also the process of empowering those less able to present their views or needs, with the goal of giving them a voice and/or achieving their objectives. Nurses have long been advocates for their patients, and advocacy can and does affect the larger systems of care (Diers, 2004). **Community health advocacy** refers to efforts aimed at creating awareness of and generating support for meeting the community's health needs. Both nurses and communities have a common goal—the best possible health services for all.

The term and concept of *public health nursing* was coined in 1893 by Lillian Wald, who described public health nurses (PHNs) as "those nurses working outside the hospital in poor and middle-class communities" (Jewish Women's Archive, 2006 ¶ 2). These nurses "specialized in both preventative care and the preservation of health, these nurses responded to referrals from physicians and patients, and received fees based on the patient's ability to pay" (¶ 2). In 1893, Lillian Wald and Mary Brewster established the Visiting Nurses Service, and a year later the famed Henry Street Settlement House was established (see Chapter 2).

Public health as a concept grew out of Wald's exposure to the plight of newly arrived immigrants to the lower east side of Manhattan and their appalling living conditions. She was determined that these immigrants and other poor people, regardless of ethnicity or religious affiliation, would have access to health care and adequate housing. Remarkably, Henry Street Settlement (2006) still provides many of the services established by Wald and her associates—currently, the organization advocates for the homeless, builds AIDS awareness, fights illiteracy and domestic violence, and provides youth and senior programs. Understanding the critical concepts of primary care, prevention, and early intervention, and the role they played in assuring a healthy childhood, Lillian Wald advocated for the hiring of public school nurses. In 1902, Lina Rogers became the first school nurse in New York City "as a one month experiment," and within 1 year's time New York City had hired an additional 12 school nurses (Woodfill & Beyrer, 1991, p. 5). Wald also went on to encourage the establishment of the Department of Nursing and Health at Columbia University's Teachers College through a series of lectures she presented starting in 1910. She also was instrumental in creating the U.S. Children's Bureau in 1912, an agency that oversaw fair child labor laws.

The importance of these nurses—Lillian Wald and her compatriots, Sojourner Truth, Margaret Sanger, Clara Barton, Mary Seacole, Susie King Taylor, Mary Mahoney, and others—is that they wielded influence at a time when women were not even allowed to vote. In fact, many women in the 1800s, regardless of socioeconomic status, did not attend school. African American women in the early 20th century were legally forbidden to learn to read and write (Hall-Long, 1995).

Historically, women—both Black and White—volunteered their services during crises (Carnegie, 1986), although nursing as a profession didn't exist. For these women to be successful and influential during the 19th century is a tribute to their ability to take on the system in which they lived and to triumph over it. Women during these times rarely, if ever, voiced their opinions about issues affecting their lives, the lives of their children, their families, or their communities; it was neither expected nor accepted. These early pioneers also are seen as feminists, and the entrance of these women into the political arena opened the way for others. By 2006, 23% of state elected officials were women, and 82 women had been elected to the U.S. Congress, 14 in the Senate and 68 in the House of Representatives (Center for American Women & Politics, 2006). Despite nursing's early history of political activism and the fact that nurses are the largest group of health care providers in the United States, widespread political involvement has yet to be realized (Feldman & Lewenson, 2006; Sapp & Bliesmer, 1995; Des Jardin, 2001). Nor is nursing thought of as a major player in Washington when discussing health care policy (Sharp, 1997; Des Jardin, 2001).

Professional Advocacy

Membership in professional organizations has provided the most important way for nurses to advocate for change. The late 19th century may be seen as the beginning of nurse activism. The National Associated Alumnae of the United States and Canada and the American Society of Superintendents of Training Schools of the United States and Canada were formed in the 1890s. Out of these groups came the ANA and the National League for Nursing (Woodfill & Beyrer, 1991). Large professional organizations have the resources, relationships with policy makers, success at coalition building, and reputation for the ability to compromise needs to assure viable outcomes. Being a part of your professional organization demonstrates your professionalism, promotes your organization's viability, and demonstrates your social responsibility to advocate for the needs of your patients. Nurses must take advantage of how the public views the profession: a 2006 Harris Poll ranked nurses highly for trustworthiness (Donelan, Buerhaus, Desroches, Dittus, & Dutwin, 2008).

The pursuit of personal agendas over the common good results in a piecemeal approach to problems and promotes polarization. **Polarization** is the process by which a group is severely split into two or more factions over a political issue. Polarization can be so intense that people perceive one another as good or wicked, depending on their ideological opinions. One of the primary goals of a professional nursing association is to build a collective voice for nurses. A strong professional association limits polarization by developing the political skills of its members and ensuring that its structure and processes equitably meet the needs of its constituencies. This is the essence of politics: people must listen to one another, learn from others' viewpoints, and compromise to ensure the most positive outcomes from their endeavors (Mason & Leavitt, 2006).

Despite criticism about special interest and professional organizations "protecting their turf," professional nursing organizations demonstrate how a critical mass can be influential and successful in moving the discussion forward on health care. These organizations have raised the level of professionalism in nursing, given voice to the inequities that affect our society, and developed the paradigms that influence and affect public health at the institutional, state, and national level in the 21st century (Hein, 2001). A united voice on public policy is more powerful than individual nurses pleading with their legislators.

CURRENT PUBLIC HEALTH NURSING ADVOCACY

Representatives Lois Capps, Eddie Bernice Johnson, and Carolyn McCarthy, all ran for Congress because of their commitment to improving the lives of their constituents. How they came to serve in Congress exemplifies the history of dedicated people wanting to make a difference for their communities. For example, when Carolyn McCarthy's husband was killed and her son badly injured by the same gunman, she began to work on the assault weapons ban—and when her congressman voted against it, she was so outraged she decided to run for office. She won with strong **grassroots** support (defined as a political movement driven by community members, a bottom-up rather than a top-down process). Eddie Bernice Johnson ran for office because she believed her work as a volunteer in a low-income immunization program could be expanded, and again, with a grassroots movement behind her, she won and is now serving her seventh term in the House of Representatives. Lois Capps' story is similar. Her husband, who was the representative for California's 23rd Congressional district, died suddenly and she was drafted to run in his place. Capps, a former school nurse, and the 91-member Congressional Nursing Caucus that she founded, supported the National Nurse Act HR 4903. According to her, this legislation "will improve public awareness of health issues and the role of nurses in improving healthcare" (Polick, 2006, p. 3). A national nurse would be an "advocate for nursing issues at a time when our profession faces growing demands for its skills and an increasing shortage of qualified personnel to meet those challenges" (Polick, 2006, p. 3). Therese Polick and Teri Mills, both RNs, are the impetus behind HR 4903. In a desire to do something about the health care crisis, Teri Mills called for an Office of the National Nurse in a *New York Times* Op-Ed piece; after reading it, Polick joined with her to form the National Nurse Team. Together, they headed to Capitol Hill (Polick, 2006).

What Teri and Therese engaged in is called **lobbying**—the process of influencing legislators or other policy makers to make decisions on policy issues. Professional organizations or other **special interest groups**—individuals who share a common interest and work politically to make their goals a reality—may have paid lobbyists on staff. **Lobbyists**—professionals who engage in lobbying—know the rules governing the state or federal political process, have or develop relationships with policy makers, provide guidance for members of the organizations employing them on how to impact public policy decisions, and work behind the scenes to influence policy discussions and outcomes. States and the federal government have laws and regulations that determine the legal actions of lobbyists as well as the organizations that employ them (Mason & Leavitt, 2006; Milstead, 1999).

Universal health and social issues affecting communities include health care access, affordable housing, safe neighborhoods, domestic and youth violence, safe schools, gun control, and many others. Dr. Deborah Prothrow-Stith, a young physician in the mid-1980s, was weary of seeing young victims of violence in the emergency rooms of inner-city Boston, so she started a movement that swept across the country. She changed the way youth violence was viewed by recognizing that youth violence was a public health issue, not merely a criminal issue. She believed that applying public health principles of prevention could decrease the incidence of violence. She wrote about this in her groundbreaking book *Deadly Consequences: How Violence Is Destroying Our Teenage Population and a Plan to Begin Solving the Problem*. Because of her belief in prevention and early intervention, she developed a discipline that is now recognized and taught throughout the country and the world—*violence prevention*. Dr. Prothrow-Stith also developed the precursor to violence prevention curricula for schools and communities. *The Violence Prevention Curriculum for Adolescents* (Biography, 2006) is still used by many today.

POLICY

Community health nursing, as it has evolved, puts nurses where the people are—in schools, homes, neighborhood centers, and churches. Community health nurses are in a position to see and understand the issues affecting people at an individual and group level. With this access to information and the issues affecting the communities they serve, who better than nurses to advocate for policy changes in the health care system? **Policy** is defined as a plan of action or an agenda that outlines steps or actions to implement a stated goal or objective. Policies are laws, regulations, or administrative rulings; when issued by national, state, or local governments they are called **public policy**. **Health policy** refers to specific policies involving health care. The legislative and regulatory process may start with lofty goals, but the final product is usually the result of compromise often encouraged by special interest groups, coalition groups, political realities, or the current economic environment. Although the study of politics has a long history, the systematic study of public policy, on the other hand, can be said to be a 20th century creation. According to Daniel McCool, in his classic treatise on policy (1995), study of public policy dates to 1922, when political scientist Charles Merriam sought to "connect the theory and practices of politics to understanding the actual activities of government, which is public policy" (p. 4).

Health policies can be distributive or regulatory. A **distributive health policy** promotes nongovernmental activities that are thought to be beneficial to society as a whole. An example of a distributive policy is the Nurse Training Act, Title VIII of the Public Health Service Act, which was established in 1965 and provided federal subsidies for nursing education in an effort to address the need for more nurses. A **redistributive health policy** changes the allocation of resources from one group to another, usually to a broader or different group. Medicare is an example of redistributive policy, in that provisions under Medicare were expanded to provide a broader range of benefits and coverage to needy groups—such as those older than age 65 and the permanently disabled of any age (Wieczorik, 1985).

A **regulatory health policy** is one that attempts to control the allocation of resources by directing those agencies or persons who offer resources or provide public services. For example, certain government regulations set standards for the licensure of health care organizations (e.g., hospitals) and health care providers (e.g., nurses). Regulatory public health policy is often used to protect the health of the community (Kovner & Knickman, 2005). In the United States, one example is the mandatory reporting of certain communicable diseases. On the international level, regulatory health policy has a broad scope, including areas such as international communicable disease control, trade, human rights, armed conflict and arms control, and the environment (Fidler, 1999; Gunn, Mansourian, Davies, Piel & Sayers, 2005; also see Chapter 16).

Regulatory policy can be further categorized as either competitive or protective. *Competitive regulation* limits, or structures, the provision of health services by designating who can deliver them. *Protective regulations* set conditions under which various private activities can be undertaken. Although professional licensure is most commonly identified as having the primary purpose of protecting the public, such policy is really competitive regulation in terms of its

social impact. Protective regulation is more clearly evident in utilization review organizations, regulatory bodies that critically examine health agency utilization patterns, or certificates of need, the legal requirement that a potential provider agency demonstrate the need for its services before a license to practice is granted (see Chapter 6).

As the medical system slowly moves from an emphasis on diagnosis and treatment to prevention and health promotion, nurses are uniquely situated to provide guidance in developing health policy. The aforementioned activities are fundamentally nursing functions, and we must realize that public policy affects nursing practice regardless of venue (Murphy, Canales, Norton, & DeFilippis, 2005). Nurses must have a voice in the development of policy (Conn & Armer, 1996; Spenceley, Reutter, & Allen, 2006).

Policy can also be viewed as the key interests of professional organizations (e.g., *Nursing's Agenda for Healthcare Reform,* American Nurses Association, 1994); government agencies (e.g., *Healthy People 2010*); think tanks, such as the Heritage Foundation (e.g., *Massachusetts Health Plan: Lessons for the States,* Woolhandler & Himmelstein, 2006); or advocacy groups, such as the Children's Defense Fund—the originators of the *Leave No Child Behind®* movement that advocates for legislation and policies that ensure every child a "healthy start, a head start, a fair start, a safe start, and a moral start"(2007, ¶1). These disparate groups reflect various political persuasions that influence which policies are debated at the national and state levels (Murphy, Canales, Norton, & DeFilippis, 2005). How effective these groups are in influencing policy development and implementing change is also tied to the political environment, or more specifically, to who is in power. Each major political party has differing political agendas that impact the policies that eventually become law.

Workplaces also implement policy, such as workplace rules and regulations that affect how the workplace functions and what is required of an employee (e.g., dress code, policies and procedures manual, hours of work, who has access to e-mail, what is acceptable behavior in the workplace, and so forth). One of the most contentious issues recently, the roles and responsibilities of unlicensed versus licensed personnel, is also a health care workplace issue that generates policy development (see Display 13.1, A Ruling Affecting Nursing).

Policies affect our daily lives, regardless of whether they are health- or work-related. So, community health nurses must have an understanding of health policy to better understand the issues affecting the communities they serve. It must be recognized that nurses have differing opinions on health policy, even down to the basic premise of whether nurses should become involved in political issues and the political process. According to Plato, "One of the penalties for refusing to participate in politics is that you end up being governed by your inferiors."

Process of Public Policy

The development of public policy is rarely easy, straightforward, or even rational. Myriad concerns determine whether one is successful with any attempt to make policy. Increasingly, the complexity of public–private interactions play a strong role in how policy is developed, both because of the privatization of health care and the increased consolidation of

---

DISPLAY 13.1   A RULING AFFECTING NURSING

An October 2006 ruling by the National Labor Relations Board (NLRB) determines which employees are seen as "supervisors" or staff employees. This ruling has been interpreted by one nursing union as a policy that will severely impact who can belong to a union, based on their job classification. This ruling grew out of a 2001 Supreme Court case that stated that an NLRB ruling in a Kentucky nursing facility case was flawed. The board at that time, comprised mainly of Democrats, ruled that the RNs at the

nursing home were not supervisors because they did not "exercise independent judgment." The Supreme Court, in reviewing the case, sent it back to the board, stating that the role and duties of a supervisor should be more carefully reviewed. At the time of the ruling, the NLRB was comprised mainly of Republicans. The American Hospital Association is in favor of the decision.

From George Raine, San Francisco Chronicle, July 13, 2006.

---

health care providers and insurers. As noted earlier, managed care that is regulated by federal and state policies has a direct effect on how health care is delivered at the local level. Many states have applied for waivers that allow them to demonstrate how they can better provide access, save money, and increase the numbers of people covered if they don't have to follow the existing federal regulations. This has, in some cases, created unforeseen problems. For example, during the 1990s, 27 states under the federal state children's health insurance program (SCHIP) established new non-Medicaid programs and, as a result, the states were not able to collect Vaccines for Children (VCF) funds for those in managed care because the Centers for Medicare and Medicaid Services interpreted the new laws to mean that these children were in private health plans. The providers of vaccines for children, who obtained their care through Medicaid's Early Periodic Screening Diagnosis and Treatment (EPSDT), were eligible to acquire vaccines through the VFC program, as were

providers of care to Native Americans, the uninsured, and rural or federally qualified health clinics. The states were not eligible to capture VFC funds and were financially responsible for paying for immunizations for those children enrolled in the non-Medicaid plans. This demonstrates the unintended consequences of regulatory and legislative changes if all aspects are not known or adequately investigated or if disagreement arises regarding interpretation.

The public policy process is similar to advocacy or **political action** and involves a number of steps that are synonymous with the nursing process. The policy/advocacy process may appear linear, but it involves overlap, reordering of priorities, mobilization of resources, and development of stakeholders. The overarching issues in advocacy or public policy development are timing, funding, and politics. Each year, thousands of measures at the state and federal level are introduced, but only a fraction of them complete the legislative process (see Figs. 13.1 and 13.2). This fall off can be attributed to a number of

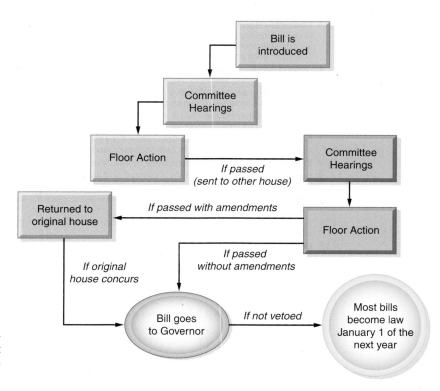

FIGURE 13.1   How a bill becomes a law—state process. The process may vary by state, but generally the schematic shows how the process unfolds. Source: California Legislative Counsel.

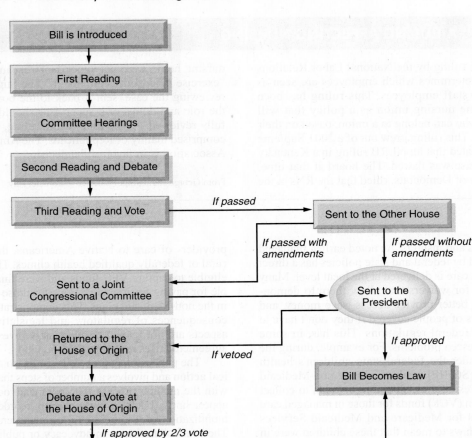

1. **Bill is Introduced.** Ideas for laws can come from a legislator, constituent, staff member, or organization.
2. **First Reading.** A legislator introduces the bill, and sends it to the clerk of his or her corresponding body (Senate or House), who gives it a number and title. This is the *first reading*, and the bill is referred to the proper committee.
3. **Committee Hearings.** The committee may decide the bill is unwise or unnecessary and *table* it, thus killing it at once. Or it may decide the bill is worthwhile and hold hearings to listen to facts and opinions presented by experts and other interested persons. After members of the committee have debated the bill and perhaps offered amendments, a vote is taken; if the vote is favorable, the bill is sent back to the floor of the house.
4. **Second Reading and Debate.** The clerk reads the bill sentence by sentence to the house; this is known as the *second reading*. Members may then debate the bill and offer amendments.
5. **Third Reading and Vote.** The *third reading* is by title only, and the bill is put to a vote, which may be by voice or roll call, depending on circumstances and parliamentary rules.
6. **Sent to the Other House.** The bill then goes to the other house of Congress, where it may be defeated or passed, with or without amendments.
7. **Sent to a Joint Congressional Committee.** If the bill is passed with amendments, a joint congressional committee must be appointed by both houses to resolve the differences.
8. **Sent to the President.** After its passage by both houses, the bill is sent to the president.
9. **Returned to the House of Origin.** If the president *vetoes* the bill, it is sent back to the house of origin with his reasons for the veto.
10. **Debate and Vote at the House of Origin.** The president's objections are read and debated, and a roll-call vote is taken.
11. **Second House Vote.** If the bill receives a two-thirds vote or greater in the house of origin, it is sent to the other house for a vote.
12. **Bill Becomes Law.** If the president approves the bill, or if his veto is overridden by a 2/3 vote in both houses, the bill becomes a law.

<u>Note:</u> Should the president desire neither to sign nor to veto the bill, he may retain it for ten days (Sundays excepted) after which time it automatically becomes a law without signature. However, if Congress has adjourned within those ten days, the bill is automatically killed, that process of indirect rejection being known as a *pocket veto*.

FIGURE **13.2** How a bill becomes a law—federal process.

reasons: conflicting sides of the issue with the strongest side winning out, timing of bill introduction or an unwillingness to put it on the agenda based on other influences or competing issues, or the inability to identify a funding source.

How and Where to Start

It can be very tricky to come into a community and determine that a problem exists that can be addressed politically. If you are aware of the problems, there are no doubt others who are also aware. It would be incumbent on you to identify the leaders or elders of the community and determine if they have previously addressed the issue and, if so, what the outcome was. It is helpful to ask if they feel that the issue is something that should be reopened if they were not successful, or if they were satisfied with the previous outcome. It helps to know how these problems relate to the priorities of the city or county, and if there are stakeholders who are willing to become engaged in the issue. Costs or possible effects of addressing these issues must be considered. These are by no means exhaustive questions, but should be considered prior to assuming leadership in addressing the issues or problems affecting a community.

If you determine you are on safe ground and others are willing to be involved, various steps can be used to put forth the agenda of issues or problems the community will be addressing and may agree to take forward to their political representatives. Nurses can take several approaches when analyzing a policy that affects the health of a community or target population (Diers, 2004). They can look at the reasons for policy formulation, the groups of people affected by the policy, or the policy's possible long-range consequences. When analyzing policy, nurses need to answer two general questions: Who benefits from this policy? Who loses from this policy? Whether the policy should be advocated by the community as a whole depends on the degree to which the policy benefits the community without being detrimental to individuals or the country.

Figure 13.3 provides a simple model for studying health policy. If nurses know something about the forces shaping health policy and the policy process, they are in a better position to influence policy outcomes. The model identifies four major stages in the policy process: formulation, adoption, implementation, and evaluation.

◆ *Policy formulation* involves identifying goals, problems, and potential solutions.
◆ *Policy adoption* involves the authorized selection and specification of means to achieve goals, resolve problems, or both.

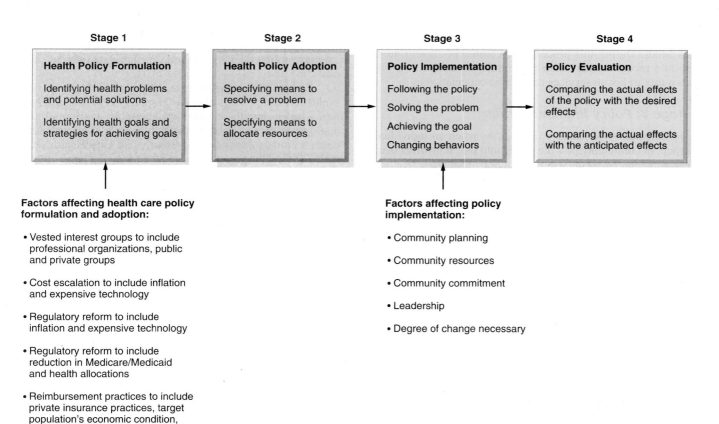

FIGURE 13.3 Policy analysis model.

◆ *Policy implementation* follows adoption and occurs when the policy is put to use.

◆ *Policy evaluation* compares policy outcomes or effects with the intended or desired effects.

Stages 1 and 2: Policy Formulation and Adoption

Health policy formulation is the stage at which a policy is conceptualized and ultimately defined. It is approached in at least two ways. Most commonly, a health problem is identified, such as the increased infant mortality rate associated with teenage pregnancy, and health policy is developed to correct that particular problem. Another approach to policy formulation emphasizes health planning more than corrective actions, at least initially (Murphy, Canales, Norton, & DeFilippis, 2005). This is a goal-oriented approach. Health goals and strategies for achieving the goals are identified. In this more proactive approach, resources may be created as well as allocated for health services. Although either approach to policy formulation may lead to the solution of a health problem, the goal-oriented approach is less reactive in that it does not require problem identification before creating health policy.

The social and political conditions that affect policy formulation are limitless, but public need and public demand *should* be the strongest influences (Kovner & Knickman, 2005). Health care providers can stimulate a community to identify its health needs and demand health policies to fulfill its needs. During this process, the community health nurse should recognize that each community is unique, with its own mix of health services and public expectations.

Stage 3: Policy Implementation

Implementation of health policy occurs when an individual, group, or community puts the policy into use. It involves overt behavior changes as the policy is put into nursing practice. The extent of compliance with a policy is the most direct measure of the policy's implementation (Harrington & Estes, 2004). *Noncompliance* refers to conscious or unconscious refusal to follow the policy directives. Community health nurses have always been health policy implementers and, recently, evaluators, regardless of whether these roles were consciously chosen.

Implementation of health policy is an essential part of effective, comprehensive client care for many documentable reasons. It should now be apparent that policies come in many forms and can have statutory or nonstatutory origins. Nurses are most cognizant of the latter, in the form of procedure manuals and institutional guidelines. Communities are most aware of policies that limit or restructure their activities and growth, such as curfews and zoning regulations.

Once a health policy is written and adopted, its successful implementation depends heavily on the manipulation of many variables. For example, the implementation of day care standards depends, in part, on how they are interpreted and what resources are available to enforce them. As an implementer, the community health nurse assesses the capacity of the community to formulate and define strategies that will enhance the community's compliance with the policy. This phase of policy analysis does not focus on the merits or shortcomings of the policy, in contrast to policy formulation, adoption, and evaluation.

Stage 4: Policy Evaluation

Comparing what a policy does with what it is supposed to do is *evaluation*. Evaluation of a policy should result in continuation of the policy in its original form, revision or modification of the policy, or termination of the policy. Laws and policies are created to express the collective and powerful interests of the political system that generated them (Kovner & Knickman, 2005; Murphy, Canales, Norton, & DeFilippis, 2005). The need for a particular health policy may be temporary, but a policy is difficult to change once it is adopted and implemented. Once a policy system is in operation, vested interests evolve as a result and become political influences. These vested interests, under the guise of jobs, positions, titles, and wealth, are perceptibly jeopardized by any change in the health policy that helped create them. Hence, tradition, in the form of old policies, tends to prevail.

One form of policy evaluation examines the health outcomes that are believed to be attributable to the health policy. Indicators such as mortality and morbidity statistics are used. However, the manner in which the outcomes are defined and measured is highly political and is more subjective than many recognize. For example, mortality statistics are often treated as objective data, yet the way in which the data are collected and the formulas used can often render them subjective. For example, if data regarding driving under the influence of alcohol or drugs are not included in data on deaths from motor vehicle crashes, or if smoking data are left out of data on deaths from lung cancers, policy decisions based on such data may be seriously misdirected.

Perhaps the major premise that should underlie policy evaluation is that the goal of health policy is to design a system wherein health services are equitably distributed and appropriate care is given to the right people at a reasonable cost (National Association of County and City Health Officials, 2002). This premise leads to the following basic criteria for evaluation:

1. Are the health services appropriate and acceptable to the population?
2. Are the health services accessible (physically and financially)?
3. Are the health services comprehensive?
4. Is there continuity of care?
5. Is the quality of the services adequate?
6. Is the efficiency of the services adequate?
7. Is there an ongoing (formative) evaluation of the services?
8. Is there a final (summative) evaluation of the services?
9. Is appropriate action taken based on the findings of the evaluations?

Regardless of the factors that affect policy evaluation, continual comparison is necessary between what a community believes and wants in health care and what it is getting. Nurses have a responsibility to increase community awareness of health issues. They help the community make sure that its health needs are met through productive, desirable health policies. See Display 13.2 for steps in policy analysis and development, and places where influence can be applied.

| DISPLAY 13.2 | STEPS IN POLICY ANALYSIS AND DEVELOPMENT |

A number of models can be used to address these issues; the following steps are an amalgamation of models available for policy/advocacy development:

Policy Analysis. Looking at public problems and determining the appropriate solution—may consist of the following steps:

1. **Define the problem.** What is the problem and how will you solve it? It should be succinctly worded, so that those not familiar with the issue can understand it. A concept or issue paper may assist in clarifying the ideas and thoughts of the group.
2. **Gather information.** Be sure that information is accurate. Can you identify trends—increase or decrease over time, demographics? There must be agreement on the analysis of the facts and data.
3. **Find alternatives to your approach.** Don't reinvent the wheel. Have other communities solved this problem? How did they address it? Will their approach work in this community? If not, what is necessary to make it workable in your situation? There should be multiple alternatives, but the fewer the better to make it more manageable. There should also be agreement on consequence.
4. **Choose the most appropriate approach.** Which objectives will work, either long- or short-term? What is the cost of your approach and where will you get the funding? Can you determine the consequences of your actions? The approach must be strong and the message clear and understandable.

Strategy development will tell you where you are, where you want to go, and how to get there. It is best to determine:

1. **Objective.** Clear and concise goals and objectives as determined by the policy analysis process. Objectives must be measurable.
2. **Audience.** Who is the audience that you must influence? Is this an issue addressed by local authorities—city, (city council) or county (board of supervisors)—or by state (legislature, state agencies) or federal (Congress, federal agencies) authorities? Is this an issue that warrants people's attention?
3. **Message.** Frame the discussion. The message should be accurate and reflect the self-interest of the receiver. Receptivity also depends on whether the people are ready to hear the message. Messages should be tailored to each audience. Get the message out in various ways, e.g., press conferences, letter writing, public presentations, and the like. Timing is critical in getting the message out.
4. **Messenger.** The messenger must be creditable—a member of the community or someone with ties to the community. Messengers can be seen as "experts" or speaking from experience. How does the group assist the messenger?
5. **Resources.** What do you already have, and what do you need to be successful? Build on the resources you currently have and determine what gaps exist.

How can resources be increased if necessary? Are your coalitions reflective of the groups within the community and if not, how can others be brought aboard? Maintain open communication with all involved.

6. **Evaluation.** Is this working? Is your message meeting with success, and how is the audience responding? Review the goals and objectives and change if necessary. Ask what isn't working? Are we getting support on these issues?

How to Influence Public Policy. Several arenas exist in which one can influence public policy:

1. **Legislative.** Influence in this arena is done through bills or measures introduced by our representatives but may be the result of issues brought to them by individuals, professional organizations, or state/federal agencies. If these measures can complete the legislative process and be signed by the governor or president, these measures become law. This is a process for the development and passage of the majority of our laws or statutes. The process whereby this occurs is called the *legislative process,* and the public must be involved to ensure that the needs of various communities are met. Laws/policies determine how the society functions, how services and programs are distributed, and who can access them. Public comment and involvement allow for the development of sound public policy, hopefully with few unintended consequences. Each state has a nurse practice act that determines the roles and responsibilities of RNs and how they can legally function. One approach to addressing the nursing shortage was initiated by the National Council of Boards of Nursing–Nurse Licensure Compacts. By changing the laws and regulations of each state it allows nurses licensed and in good standing to practice in another state if both are "compact states." These nurses have "multi-state licenses." Currently, more than 20 states have changed their laws to allow nurses to move from one state to another while licensed in only one state.
2. **Judicial.** In the judicial arena, disputes relating to laws and/or regulations are brought before the court for affirmation or invalidation. Scope of practice and licensing laws, many times, are played out judicially. Professional organizations, employers, and unions may be more likely than individuals to use the courts for rulings on licensing, scope of practice, and workplace rules. However, there have been rulings on controversial health and social issues, such as minors' access to abortions and same-sex marriages, as well as findings relating to medical malpractice.
3. **Regulatory.** The regulatory arena involves implementation of existing laws. Codes of Regulations are issued by the agency that has oversight of the laws passed by the legislature. Regulations provide the specificity of the statute; for example, regulations accompanying a state nurse practice act provide the

(continued)

detail of how the act is to be implemented. The process allows for public comment prior to implementation; it is critical for nurses be involved in the regulatory process, as many have a direct effect on individual nursing practice. For example, a California regulation—California Standards of Competence, Title 16, Section 1443.5 (6)— states that nurses must be patient advocates.

4. **Executive Order.** This order can be issued only by presidents or governors. President Bush in August 2006 issued an executive order that instructed administrative agencies to increase the use of health information technology and transparency in measuring the quality of health services as well as the more efficient administration of health programs.

5. **Initiative.** An initiative is also called a *referendum* or *proposition*. It is a local process in which groups can qualify an issue for the ballot by collecting a percentage of names of voters, usually based on the numbers of voters in the last election. This is an example of direct democracy by voters bypassing our representative process. As an example, in 2006, four states placed tobacco initiatives on the ballot that would increase tobacco taxes to fund health and education programs.

6. **Budgetary.** The budgetary arena involves federal or state plan/legislation for funding services and programs. The federal or state budgets are reflective of what policy makers or those who are influential deem important. Being involved in the budget process is important for the implementation of various policies, as *most* policies require funding to be effective. The state–federal health programs of Medicaid and Medicare are affected by the funding appropriated in the state budgets. The SCHIP is a children's health program instituted to cover those children who qualify based on certain criteria. This is a state–federal program; the amount of money coming from the federal government is based on the amount of money allocated by the state, this is called a "match."

POLITICS AS USUAL

Communities are the places of employment for community health nurses and, as such, any advocacy on your part and/or policy changes will affect those within the communities you serve (Deschaine & Schaffer, 2003). Your role is to be responsive to the needs of the community you serve and its attendant politics. **Politics** is defined as the art or science of government, or governing of a political entity. It can be and is often defined as the art of using influence to bring about change. However, you may already be aware that politics can represent the machinations in which groups or individuals engage to influence, gain power, or get their way. Politics can also be labeled as the relationships between elected officials and their constituents; it can also be seen as the interplay between staff nurses and their head nurse or nursing supervisor. Aroskar, Moldow, and Good (2004) see politics as the practice of public ethics. A clear example of this is the conflict between individual needs and the needs of a community—such as the debate around assisted suicide or the continuing debate regarding universal health care. Within communities, it may be the debate on whether to have and/or where to locate a family planning clinic, or the most appropriate and effective methods to address teen pregnancy issues. As stated by the late Massachusetts congressman and former Speaker of the House, Tip O'Neill, "*All politics is local.*"

Public health practice is inherently political because it involves the different values and worldviews that exist in communities because of their specific ethnicities, languages, and cultures. The primacy of these perspectives influences the community's needs and what will be done about public policy issues. Be aware that issues change over time; for example, chronic disease management and safety and quality issues take front stage currently, but in the 1970s substance abuse was a high priority and in the 1990s, it was violence prevention. These shifts reflect the dynamic nature of public health policy and how differing policies attract public attention and funding. The funding issues for public health have also changed over time with private funding (e.g., managed care) now providing much of the care for low-income populations. This funding shift has also encouraged a swing back to the primary mission of public health—assurance, assessment, and policy development (see Chapter 1). It is imperative to understand that policy and politics go hand in hand; neither exists without the other.

POWER AND EMPOWERMENT

Eliciting services and programs for unserved or underserved populations is a never-ending issue. Citizen participation is never particularly easy in communities that are excluded from political or economic resources. Sherry Arnstein, in her classic 1969 treatise *A Ladder of Citizen Participation*, stated that "citizen participation is citizen power," and without access to information about how the system functions, these populations cannot obtain the resources they need to make their communities livable and nurturing (p. 217). Arnstein goes on to point out that those in power prevent those in need from accessing the process:

> The idea of citizen participation is a little like eating spinach: no one is against it in principle because it is good for you. Participation of the governed in their government is, in theory, the cornerstone of democracy—a revered idea that is vigorously applauded by virtually everyone. The applause is reduced to polite hand claps, however, when this principle is advocated by the have-not Blacks, Mexican Americans, Puerto Ricans, Indians, Eskimos, and Whites. When the have-nots define participation as redistribution of power, the American consensus on the fundamental principle explodes into many shades of outright racial, ethnic, ideological, and political opposition (p. 216).

Although Arnstein writes about the anger disenfranchised populations feel, she does offer possible solutions that allow each party to "share power through partnership," as outlined by engaging in the process discussed in her treatise (p. 217). **Power** can be defined as the ability to act or produce an effect, possession of control, or authority or influence over others. As public health professionals, nurses have a commitment to social justice and working with disadvantaged communities. This means that nurses have a responsibility to ensure community participation in issues affecting them, and they must continually examine the relationship and position they hold within these communities. The term **empowerment** has been used to explain a process of assisting communities to come together to express their values and ideas to those outside the community (Bernstein, Wallerstein, Braithwaite, et al., 1994; Weis, Schank, & Matheus, 2006). Generally, the issue of empowerment comes up when outside forces are behaving in a way that the community considers detrimental to its well-being. The various definitions of empowerment and the expansion of the definition of health, which now includes the social, political, and economic determinants of health, have changed our thinking on how best to interact with the communities we serve. Theorists have suggested that if power is the ability to control, predict, and participate in one's environment, then empowerment is the process whereby individuals and communities take power and transform their lives (Robertson & Minkler, 1994; Hooser, 2002) (see Perspectives: Student Voices). This also suggests a change in the relationship between professionals and communities; a change from the customary hierarchical patient–provider relationship to one of a partnership (Robertson & Minkler, 1994; Yoo et al., 2004; Messias, DeJong, & McLoughlin, 2005). However, one must be mindful that professionals hold the power and authority by virtue of their place in the bureaucracy. They have access to information, are better connected politically, and are more cognizant of how to make the system positively respond to the issues they bring forth.

How does one make sure that preconceived ideas about what should be the community's concerns are not forced on the community in order to meet the goals and objectives of the public health agency? Some may argue that "much of current health promotion practice meets the bottom rung of Arnstein's ladder by using the rhetoric of community participation but in fact the professionals are setting the agenda for the community" (Labonte, 1990, p. 7). Robertson and Minkler state "that health promotion practitioners facilitate empowerment by assisting individuals and communities in articulating their problems and solutions to address them . . . by providing access to information, supporting indigenous leadership, and by assisting them to overcome bureaucratic hurdles to action, they are truly increasing the communities' problem-solving abilities" (1994, p. 301). This is a concept also enforced in the Institute of Medicine (2002b) report, *The Future of the Public's Health in the 21st Century*.

INFLUENCING POLICY

So, how can community health nurses influence policies that affect the communities they serve? We have discussed how you, as a professional, can empower your communities, based on your knowledge of how to influence others and your ability to encourage those within your communities to join with you in advocating policies that positively impact their lives. Health care policies are usually the result of legislative action at the state and federal levels, and the regulations that are implemented as a result of this legislation provide the specifics of how each law is to be carried out. So, how do we influence policy makers to hear our concerns and act on them?

Seasoned advocates have developed skills in influencing policy decisions; ground rules also exist by which to play the game. Some call them the "ten commandments of lobbying" or the "ten commandments of politics" (Dodd, 1997, p. 417). However these steps are

---

PERSPECTIVES
STUDENT VOICES

Advocacy for the Ages

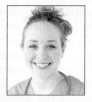

I remember being told in nursing school that we needed to become "politically active" and should be prepared to "legislatively advocate for our clients." I always thought that it would be up to someone else—someone older, more experienced, more eloquent, and knowledgeable. I didn't really think they were talking about me. Well, I realize now that *anyone* can be a political advocate! I just read about Bria Brown, a 12-year-old girl from Florida who was diagnosed with osteosarcoma at age 6. She was an inpatient at Miami Children's Hospital for a year, and she still has regular visits there. But despite all of this, she and her family have found the time and energy to go to Washington, D.C., and meet with their congressman in order to seek help for children with cancer. What an inspiring story! She told Congressman Meek about 17 of her friends who died of cancer, and the congressman said that she was "one of the best spokespersons" he had ever seen and that he was "committed to this effort" (Meek, 2006, ¶ 2). If a young girl can be a political advocate and can lobby for health issues, I certainly need to rethink my priorities and get to work! After all, I have a wealth of knowledge and experiences I can share to help persuade my legislator to vote for issues and policies that I believe are important.

Cara, Age 24, Oncology Nurse

described, advocates adhere to the basic ideas inherent in the following:

1. **Honesty is the best policy.** Being known as someone who has integrity is a lasting virtue. Never mislead a legislator or someone who is likely to support your interests, as it is difficult to regain credibility once you lose it. Speaking beyond your level of expertise gets advocates into trouble. If you don't know the answer, say so; but if you promise to get the answer, then do so. Do not promise what you can't deliver.

2. **Start early.** Planning always takes longer than you think it will. Your interests are not everyone's interests and convincing others they should be involved always involves time. If you are planning policy change at the state or federal level, it is vital to know the legislative process and the critical time lines.

3. **Know what you want.** Be aware of all sides of the issue prior to approaching a policy maker; know the pros and cons, and be prepared to answer questions and provide data on both sides of the issue. Understand the role politics plays in getting what you want and how policy makers may respond to your issue. Targeting your story to the goals, emotions, and interests of the legislator is important and may result in a positive outcome. Be *clear* about what you are asking the legislator for—to carry legislation, or to vote no or yes on specific legislation. Asking your legislator to vote a certain way is perfectly legitimate, and if you don't ask, the opposition will.

4. **KISS** (Keep it simple, stupid). Be able to articulate your issues in a clear and concise manner. Do not confuse possible supporters with complicated arguments. Key issues should be concise and clear and on one page, no more than two. Leave behind an informational packet with pertinent information about the community and/or services and programs.

5. **No permanent enemies, no permanent friends.** Political affiliation doesn't always determine what interests a person has or whether they are likely to support your interests. It behooves you to speak with everyone on your issue; if nothing else, you may find out who they are and why they may oppose your concerns. Remember, in politics, there are only permanent interests.

6. **Know your opponents.** Visit with all possible supporters—just because someone opposed you in the past, doesn't mean they won't support you on a current issue. Respectful disagreement keeps the door open for future agreement and compromise.

7. **Compromise.** Ask for much more than you think you can get. When negotiating, you can give up something without hurting your priorities or your bottom line. In politics, rarely does anyone get all they want, but priority setting is key: What do we expect to accomplish with this activity?

8. **There is strength in numbers.** The more groups involved, the more likely you are to be successful. Any opportunity for networking is an opportunity to enlarge your coalition. Including disparate groups means you may have accessed conflicting political persuasions. Additionally, having groups who can speak with those who are not seen as "friends" is useful. Cross-fertilization of groups is politically expedient, but understand that next time you or they may be in opposition.

9. **Work at the local level.** Legislators are interested in their constituents—these are the people who elected them to office and who will keep them in office. To be noticed by policy makers, sharing information with them about their constituents is the surest way to capture their attention. Information sharing should occur on issues both in the community where you live and the one where you work.

10. **Thank you.** Everyone loves to be told, "Job well done." To maintain your coalitions, always recognize the work of others. Spreading the credit is like sowing seeds: the wider the spread, the more bountiful the crop.

Finally, it is important for those new to policy development and influencing to understand one major influence on policy—*money*. Nurses must become more actively involved in the process of influencing policy. How many nurses understand that their practice acts, or portions thereof, are developed by legislators or special interest groups who don't have a background in health care? How many nurses know who their legislators are at either the state or federal level? How many nurses have written their legislators about pending health care legislation or legislation that affects nursing (e.g., Nurse Reinvestment Act or the National Nurse Act)? See Display 13.3.

In the 2006 midterm elections, much discussion was held about campaign finance reform because of the Abramoff scandal. Kickbacks, bribery, paying off legislators for their votes, or giving lucrative government contracts to those who gave large campaign contributions captured our attention (*Washington Post*, 2006). This was seen as the lobbying process run amuck. Although this was not a new occurrence, the amounts of money and the numbers of legislators and lobbyists caught in the web were one of the highest in U.S. history. Nonetheless, money is important in assuring that your legislator or candidate can maintain or win a seat—whether at the state or federal level. Campaign financing is important because TV ads, direct mailers, campaign staff (volunteers notwithstanding), and political consultants all require adequate funding. Anyone running for a political position knows that, in order to compete, money is required; those with the most financing can get their message out and encourage potential voters to elect them. Although spending the most money doesn't always guarantee success, without sufficient financing, you can be assured your message will *not* be heard. As stated by Jesse Unruh, the Speaker of the California Assembly in the 1960s, *"Money is the mother's milk of politics."*

Political Action Committees

One reason why nurses are less politically active can be tied to a lack of money. Nurses don't earn as much money or appear

DISPLAY 13.3 HOW TO HELP YOUR LEGISLATOR KNOW THE COMMUNITY

1. **Know who your legislators are—local, state, and federal:**
   - Include their contact information on your e-mail and regular mailing lists.
   - Develop a relationship with them or their staff.
2. **Assign a constituent to the legislator:**
   - Keep all critical information on legislators up to date.
   - What are the key committees they sit on?
3. **Keep legislators and staff informed:**
   - Keep them aware of any actions occurring in the community.
   - Share any printed materials.
   - Provide them with updated, current promotional information.
   - Send copies of news articles, radio interviews, alerts.
   - If you have a website, blog, podcasts, etc., send URL.
   - Invite legislators to your facility or community tour for "show and tell."
4. **When passing out awards, think of your legislators:**
   - Recognize any actions by legislators that benefit the community in which you serve.
   - Invite legislators to award ceremonies and/or community events.
5. **Communicate with your policy maker:**
   - Write your policy maker about issues important to the communities in which you serve or issues important to your profession.
   - Provide real stories or examples of the issue.
   - Use personal letters; postcards, phone calls, form letters, and e-mail are not always the most effective way to deliver your message.

not to have access to as much money as other health care interests (e.g., hospitals, physicians, insurance companies, and health care plans), and as such there is much less money for nursing organizations to use for lobbyists or to assist chosen candidates. The ANA has a **political action committee** (PAC) that supports federal candidates on a nonpartisan basis; candidates must demonstrate an interest in and willingness to vote for nursing issues or issues that nurses support (Dodd, 1997). To participate in the PAC, you must be a member of ANA (this also allows your family to contribute to the PAC). By giving to the ANA-PAC, one maximizes the contribution by joining with other nurses—this power in numbers increases our influence with those candidates we choose to endorse. However, giving to your personal legislator can keep you on their mailing list, and it may get you invited to local legislative activities. It also

lets your legislator know you are interested in whether she remains in office. Being in regular contact with your legislators provides an avenue for introducing legislation that impacts nursing or other health-related issues, and when you call to ask for a vote "for" or "against" an issue, the legislator is more likely to entertain your request. Aren't you more likely to respond to someone you know, rather than someone who comes to you out of the blue to ask for a favor?

Volunteering

Money is *not* the only way to build a relationship with your legislator. Volunteering your time can be just as important (see Perspectives: Voices from the Community). Candidates for office need bodies to get things done (e.g., phone

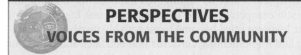

PERSPECTIVES
VOICES FROM THE COMMUNITY

Volunteer Service for the Long Term

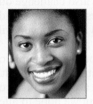

An RN who had been through what I called the women's legislative career ladder—School Board, City Council, County Board of Supervisors—was now posed to run for the state legislature. Because we had had numerous contacts and I believed she would make a good state legislator and a voice for nursing and health care, I volunteered to work in her campaign office. I primarily answered the phones on the evenings I worked, but I met the office staff—many of whom were much younger than I. And, even once, she came in while I was

there. I talked with the staff about some of my experiences as a lobbyist, and they shared their experiences; many of them were fresh out of college.

She was successful in her run for office, and whenever I needed to meet with her or her staff, I was shown right in. I was also asked my opinion about the hiring of certain staff. Her staff knew me by name—many of them did not work on her campaign, but they were told about me by those campaign staff who were still around. After 3 years in office, she was appointed chairperson of a key committee, and I maintained access to her committee consultants and to her when necessary. We were able to work together quite successfully and, although we didn't always agree on every policy issue, I think the weeks I put in volunteering 3 years earlier really paid off for the clients and the issues I was representing.

L.B., Professional Lobbyist

banking, stuffing mailers, answering phones, putting up flyers and campaign posters, walking door to door to spread the message, and assisting in the development of issue papers). Candidates develop issue papers to tell their constituents where they stand on key campaign concerns. Nurses have the expertise to assist legislators in developing an agenda on health care policy, or at the least to review and comment on issue papers.

Relationships are key in policy development. As demonstrated earlier, being a friend can reap huge benefits when health care policy is on the line. Being involved in local and state elections can take many forms. Voting, for instance, is vital—RNs represent one in 45 potential voters (Waldron, 2003). Joining your local and state professional organizations is vital to having the voice of nursing heard at all levels. You can become more actively involved by writing legislators about the health care issues that impact the communities, both where you live and work. It is also vital to understand the importance of critically timing those communications. Effective communications with legislators should be tied to times when the issues are being heard in policy committee—thus, you must know when your issue is scheduled to be discussed in committee. For example, it is prudent to send letters on your issue—via fax or regular mail—close to the time of the committee hearing. Holding a press conference or getting other media coverage when the bill is introduced, or on the day it will be heard in committee, is quite effective in drawing attention to your issue. Writing letters to the editor of your local newspaper on health issues, as well as writing articles for various publications, are also effective methods of persuading others to back your issue. Other methods for influencing health policy or nursing issues include applying for positions on boards and commissions; each local area has advisory committees for their locally elected officials at the city and county level. The state board of registered nurses needs nurses willing to sit on their board or to serve on various advisory committees and task forces. At your state capitols, there are usually vacancies on policy committees, or legislators may be looking for new staff—either personal or policy. And, who better to serve in this capacity than a nurse! Who else has more knowledge about health issues than nurses? When all else fails, *run for office*.

A Call to Action

The need for health care reform has become critical as the costs of health care continue to rise. The United States spends a disproportionate percentage of the national budget on health care, yet major segments of the population still do not have adequate access to quality health services. Because of these economic concerns, health care reform and policy making have become politically charged issues involving many groups and factions, including not only health care providers and health care professionals but also government, third-party payers, insurance companies, and others with vested interests.

Many people are just beginning to realize that health care is a business. It has always been a business—we are just more aware of it now because of the scarcity of resources. Many believe that business interests and efforts to curb rising costs may divert public services away from community health issues, such as preventive and primary care. Because community health nurses know community needs and the value of such services, they need to be a major force in the political arenas where health policy decisions are being made. Community health nurses need to become politically aware and active to ensure quality health services by working as community health advocates. They must collaborate with community constituents and with nurses and other professionals to ensure the safety and well-being of groups and populations at risk.

Health care is the talk of the nation, and nurses must be involved in the process of setting policy for themselves and their communities. Although nursing's influence has been limited in the recent past, we must learn how to empower our own profession, ourselves, and the communities with whom we work by becoming politically active and aware. If we are to fulfill our mission of promoting, protecting, and preserving the health of aggregates, we must become policy makers as well as policy implementers. We must learn to use policy systems and the political process, so that our voice is heard and we have influence in policy decision making. We must learn to formulate, implement, and evaluate health policies. We must understand the legislative process and how to influence that process. The politically involved nurse should aim to accomplish three primary goals: (1) generate support for one's views by communicating ideas effectively and getting to know and influence representatives at local, state, and national levels; (2) create professional legitimacy by keeping abreast of current issues in health care and nursing and becoming involved in professional nursing organizations, community boards or committees, or political office at the local, state, or national level; and (3) resolve conflict and effectively negotiate and compromise.

We have a rich history of advocacy, of using data and statistics to influence public policy, of speaking out about the injustices in our society and providing leadership in the development of services and programs that uplift and enrich the lives of the least among us. The inequities in our system, both socially and politically, add to the existing health disparities (National Association of County and City Health Officials, 2002).

Chapters 5 and 10 highlighted the need for cultural and linguistic competency, and it is clear that our institutions of higher learning must become more actively involved in developing and implementing curricula that educates and trains our health care providers with an understanding of, appreciation for, respect for, and competency in dealing with diverse cultures and languages. These programs must also challenge our individual values relating to other cultures and their worldviews. After all, these are the populations with whom you will work, and they will look to you for advice and leadership.

We also must do a better job of encouraging people of color to enter and complete courses of study in the health professions, for it is only when we have a critical mass of diverse providers and educators that we can we hope to alleviate some of the health inequities that challenge us today. *It is not enough to be clinically competent; one must be culturally competent.*

Nurses, despite their numbers and past history of public health nursing advocacy, have not really challenged the society in which they function. This duality has also hindered nurses' development as policy developers and advocates. Because of pressing health care concerns and the nursing shortage, we have begun to realize and encourage our profession to become politically aware and active. We are still gaining knowledge and experience in empowering the communities we serve by working with them to identify their strengths, examining the system rather than blaming the individual, and engaging with them in the development and implementation of preventive and health promotional behaviors that allow communities to grow and to become independent and self-reliant. When we "work with" communities, and do not "direct" them, we achieve personal growth as well.

Finally, community health nursing is a proud discipline with a rich foundation of helping the less fortunate and addressing issues that impact poorer communities. We are continually working toward empowering ourselves, our profession, and the larger communities that often suffer because of societal inequities. Community health nurses must honor this mandate to become policy advocates, to influence policy, and to learn how the policy process works, so that their voices and the voices of their communities are heard.

Summary

This chapter has reviewed the political processes inherent in the development of health policies and the community health nurse's policy and advocacy roles within those processes. The foundations of political action and advocacy stem from a rich history of public health nurses, like Lillian Wald, who strived to provide a voice for vulnerable and disenfranchised populations. Social justice remains a pillar of our current practice.

Advocacy for our clients is always important, but professional advocacy through affiliation and activity in our professional nursing organizations, is also vital so that we, as PHNs, may have a "collective voice." This chapter highlighted examples of nurses who have recently served or are still serving as elected officials—many of whom came to power through grassroots efforts. Politics may be uncomfortable and foreign to many of us, yet it provides the methods for needed change through lobbying or influencing legislators. Nurses and special interests groups can gain access to legislators individually or through the services of a professional lobbyist or PACs.

Policies are actions or agendas that can be used to implement important goals and objectives, such as the health objectives found in *Healthy People 2010*. Distributive, redistributive, and regulatory health policies were defined and discussed, along with the processes that can be used by PHNs to impact policy formulation, adoption, implementation, and evaluation. Tips on how to influence policy makers were outlined, and nurses may consider volunteering time to a candidate of their choice as a means of gaining greater access to the political process.

Community and public health nursing are, by nature, political because we deal with many issues that affect the health and well-being of diverse populations. Power and empowerment are important concepts to both public health nursing and politics, and the skills of political action and advocacy should be honed by every community health nurse. ■

ACTIVITIES TO PROMOTE CRITICAL THINKING

1. Investigate a major health policy system in your community or state; discover how it works, and determine whether community health nurses are represented in this system. Areas to investigate include the boundaries of the system, the authority by which the system generates health policy, how the system receives input (formally and informally), resources the policy system uses and allocates to others, and the system's output over the past few years.

2. Describe a legislative bill related to community health at either the state or federal level and the issues involved in it. Identify who is sponsoring the bill, who is opposing it, and why. Determine who will be affected by the bill if it passes and in what ways they will be affected. Discuss what you, as a community health nurse, could do to be involved in this bill, and then develop a political action plan to support or oppose the bill. Write a letter to your legislator regarding your position.

3. Carefully review your own health care plan and determine whether you believe it is an adequate and equitable plan. Describe the plan and the issues involved in it. Include what health services are covered and who is authorized to provide services and receive direct reimbursement. Also determine who qualifies for the plan, who is excluded, and what conditions can disqualify a person or a family once they have been covered by the plan. Compare the cost of this plan to one proposed by a political candidate.

4. Attend a meeting of a professional organization, board of directors, government agency, or council when a health policy or health care issue is on the agenda. Analyze the positions of the major interest groups involved and describe to what extent economics comes into the discussion. Describe who controls the discussion and how this is done.

5. Interview a health care administrator in your local area and determine this person's position on health care reform and the rationale for his position. Determine at what levels this administrator is politically active and involved in influencing policy.

6. Several websites for government agencies and organizations are shared in this chapter. Contact two or three of them. What resources can you get from these sites? How can you use the political advocacy information as a community health nurse? Did these sites lead you to other sites? If they did, contact these additional sites and write down the additional website addresses in the margin of the chapter for future reference.

7. What issues or events occurred in the United States that lessened the willingness of nurses to speak out about health care issues? Examine the years starting with the 1930s. What events or issues changed, if

any, to reinvigorate nurses serving as political activists?

8. Are nurses the most qualified group to articulate national health care issues? If so, why? If not, why not?

9. Do you consider it an ethical or human rights issue to provide appropriate and accurate health information? If yes, why? If not, why not?

10. Who are your state legislators? What are the critical health issues in your state, and how have your legislators responded to the issues? If there has been health care-related legislation introduced:
    • What is the issue?
    • What party introduced the bill?
    • Where is the bill in the legislative process?
    • What groups support or oppose the legislation?
    • What is the reasoning for the groups' support or opposition?

11. How active is your state professional nursing organization in policy issues?

    Are you a member of the organization? If not, why not?

    What are the public policy issues the organization is involved in?

    How successful have they been?

    Does the group have a paid lobbyist or does it rely on volunteer lobbyists?

References

Adams, M., Bell, L.A., &, Griffin, P. (1997). *Teaching for diversity & social justice: A sourcebook.* New York: Routledge.

American Association of Colleges of Nursing. (2003). *White paper on the role of the clinical nurse leader.* New York: Author.

American Association of Colleges of Nursing. (2006). *Scholarships and financial aid resources for nursing students.* Retrieved August 4, 2008 from http://www.aacn.nche.edu/Education/financialaid.htm.

American Nurses Association. (1994). *Nursing's agenda for healthcare reform.* Washington, DC: Author.

American Nurses Association. (2001). *Code of ethics for nurses with interpretive statements.* Retrieved August 4, 2008 from http://www.nursingworld.org/ethics/code/protected _nwcoe303.htm.

Arnstein, S. (1969). A ladder of citizen participation. *Journal of American Planning Association, 35*(4), 216–224.

Aroskar, M., Moldow, D., & Good, C. (2004). Nurses' voices: Policy, practice & ethics. *Nursing Ethics, 11*(3), 266–276.

Baker, M. (2000, January). The HMO system takes over—the Nazi model from the pamphlet "Ban the HMOs". *American Almanac.* Retrieved September 28, 2008 from http://american_almanac.tripod.com/hmotakeo.htm.

Barr, D., Fenton L., & Edwards, D. (2004). Politics and health. *QJM, 97*(2), 61–62.

Bernstein, E., Wallerstein, N., Braithwaite, R., Guiterrez, L., Labonte, R., & Zimmerman, M. (1994). Empowerment Forum: A dialogue between guest editorial board members. *Health Education Quarterly, 21*(3, Part 11), 281–294.

Biography. (2006). *Deborah Prothrow-Stith.* Harvard School of Public Health. Retrieved October 19, 2006 from http://www.hsph.harvard.edu/faculty/DeborahProthrow-Stith.htm.

Boutain, D.M. (2005). Social justice as a framework for professional nursing. *Journal of Nursing Education, 44*(9), 404–408.

Carnegie, M.E. (1986). *The path we tread: Blacks in nursing, 1854–1984.* Philadelphia: J. B. Lippincott Company.

Center for American Women & Politics. (2006). State University of New Jersey. *Fact sheet.* Retrieved October 31, 2006 from http://cawp.rutgers.edu/Facts/officeholders/elective.pdf.

Centers for Disease Control and Prevention, National Center for Health Statistics. (2006). *National Immunization Survey.* Retrieved August 4, 2008 from http://www.cdc.gov/nis/.

Children's Defense Fund. (2007). *Policy areas.* Retrived September 29, 2008 from http://www.childrensdefense.org/site/PageServer?pagename=How_CD_F_Works.

Cohen D., de la Vega, R., & Watson, G. (2001). *Advocacy for social justice: A global action and reflection guide.* Sterling, VA: Kumarian Press, Inc.

Commonwealth Fund (2006). US Health Performance: A National Scorecard. Retrieved August 4, 2008 from http://www.cmf.org/publications/publications_show.htm?doc_id=403925\.

Conn, V., & Armer, J. (1996). Meta-analysis & public policy: Opportunity for nursing impact. *Nursing Outlook, 44*(6), 267–271.

Des Jardin, K. (2001). Political involvement in nursing—Politics, ethics, and strategic action. *AORN Journal.* Retrieved August 4, 2008 from http://www.findarticles.com/p/articles/mi_mOFSL/is_5_74/ai_81161374/print.

Deschaine, J., & Schaffer, M. (2003). Strengthening the role of public health nurse leaders in policy development. *Policy, Politics & Nursing Practice, 4*(4), 266–274.

Diers, D. (2004). *Speaking of nursing*: Narratives of practice, research, policy and the profession. Sudbury, PA: Jones & Bartlett Publishers.

Dodd, C. (1997). Can meaningful health policy be developed in a political system? In: C. Harrington & C. Estes, (Eds.). *Health policy & nursing* (pp. 416–434). Sudbury, MA: Jones & Bartlett Publishers.

Donelan, K., Buerhaus, P., Desroches, C., Dittus, R., & Dutwin, D. (2008). Public perceptions of nursing careers: The influence of the media and nursing shortages. *Nursing Economics, 26*(3), 143–150, 165.

Drevdahl, D. (2002). Partnerships with managed care. *Public Health Nursing, 19*(3), 161–167.

Drevhahl, D., Kneipp, S.M., & Canales, M.K. (2001). Reinvesting in social justice: A capitol idea for public health nursing? *Advances in Nursing Science, 24*(2), 19–31.

Fahrenwald, N. (2003). Teaching social justice. *Nurse Educator, 28*(5), 222–226.

Feldman, H.R., & Lewenson, S.B. (2000). *Nurses in the political arena: The public face of nursing.* New York: Springer Publishing.

Fiddler, D.P. (1999). *International law and infectious diseases.* Oxford: Clarendon Press.

Freire, P. (1968). *Pedagogy of the oppressed.* New York: Seabury Press.

Friedman, E. (1999). Managed care: Devils, angels and the truth in between. *Health Progress, 80*(3), 22–26.

Geberding, J.L., Hughes, J.M., & Koplan, J.P. (2002). Bioterrorism preparedness and response: Clinicians and public health agencies as essential partners. *Journal of the American Medical Association, 287*(7), 898–900.

Gordon, C. (2003). *Dead on arrival: The politics of health care in 20th century America.* Princeton, NJ: Princeton University Press.

Gunn, S.W., Mansourian, P.B., Davies, A.M., Piel, A., & Sayers, B.M. (Eds.). (2005). *Understanding the global dimensions of health.* New York: Springer.

Hall, M. (2006, December 12). US health system unprepared, report says. *USA Today.*

Hall-Long, B.A. (1995). Nursing's past, present & future political experience. *Nursing & Healthcare: Perspectives on Community, 16*(1), 24–28.

Harrington, C., & Estes, C.L. (2004). *Health policy & nursing: Crisis & reform in the US healthcare delivery system* (4th ed.). Boston: Jones & Bartlett Publishing.

Harris Poll 37. (May 10, 2006). Retrieved October 13, 2006 from http://harrisinteractive.com/harris_poll.index.asp?PID=661.

Hein, E.C. (2001). *Nursing issues in the 21st century*. Philadelphia: Lippincott Williams & Wilkins.

Henry Street Settlement. (2006). About Henry Street settlement. Retrieved August 4, 2008 from http://www.henrystreet.org/site/PageServer?JServSessionIdr012=7t7bgvq6t1.app25a&pagename=abt_home.

Himmelstein, D., Warren, E., Thorne, D., & Woolhandler, D. (2005). Illness & injury as contributors to bankruptcy. *Health Affairs–Health Tracking Market Watch*.

Hooser, D. (2002). Public health nurses used 4 strategies to facilitate client empowerment. *Evidence Based Nursing, 5*, 94.

Institute of Medicine. (2000). *To err is human: Building a safer health system*. Washington, DC: The National Academies Press.

Institute of Medicine. (2002a). *Health insurance is a family matter*. Washington, DC: The National Academies Press.

Institute of Medicine. (2002b). *The future of the public's health in the 21st century*. Washington, DC: The National Academies Press.

Institute of Medicine. (2003). *A shared destiny: Community effects of uninsurance*. Washington, DC: The National Academies Press.

Institute of Medicine. (2006). *Preventing medication errors: Quality chasm series*. Washington, DC: The National Academies Press.

Jewish Women's Archive. (2006). Lillian Wald Introduction. Retrieved from http://www.jwa.org/exhibits/wov/wald/index.html.

Keller, L.O., Strohschein, S., Lia-Hoagberg, B., & Schaffer, M. (1998). Population-based public health nursing intervention: A model from practice. *Public Health Nursing, 15*(3), 207–215.

Khan, A., Morse, S., & Lillibridge, S. (2000). Public-health preparedness for biological terrorism in the USA. *The Lancet, 356*(9236), 1179–1182.

Kovner, A.R., & Knickman, J.R. (Eds.). (2005). *Jonas and Kovner's health care delivery in the United States* (8th ed.). New York: Springer Publishing.

Kovner, C., Fairchild, S., & Jacobson, L. (2006). *Nurse educators 2006: A report of the faculty census survey on RN and graduate programs*. New York: National League of Nursing.

Labonte, R. (1990). Empowerment: Notes on professional & community dimensions. *Canadian Review of Social Policy, 26*, 1–12.

Leape, L., & Berwick, D. (2005). Five years after to err is human: What have we learned? *Journal of the American Medical Association, 293*(13), 2384–2390.

Mason, J., & Leavitt, J. (2006). *Policy & politics in nursing & healthcare* (5th ed.). Philadelphia: W.B. Saunders Co.

McCool, D. (1995). *Public policy theories, models and concepts: An anthology*. Old Tappan, NJ: Prentice Hall.

Meek, K.B. (2006, September 22). *Meek welcomes young Miami Gardens cancer survivor to US capitol*. Retrieved August 4, 2008 from http://www.kendrickmeek.house.gov/press/2006.09.22.shtml.

Messias, D., DeJong, M., & McLoughlin, K. (2005). Being involved and making a difference: Empowerment and well-being among women living in poverty. *Journal of Holistic Nursing, 23*, 70–88.

Milstead, J.A. (1999). *Health policy and politics–A nurse's guide*. Gaithersburg, MD: Aspen Publishers.

Milstein, A., & Smith, M. (2006). America's new refugees—Seeking affordable surgery offshore. *New England Journal of Medicine, 355*, 1637–1640.

Murphy, N., Canales, M., Norton, S., & DeFilippis, J. (2005). Striving for congruence: The interconnection between values, practice, and political action. *Policy and Politics in Nursing Practice, 6*, 20–29.

National Association of County & City Health Officials. (2002). *Testimony of Adewale Troutman, MD, MPH before the IOM on the creation of an Annual Report on Health Disparities*.

Retrieved October 10, 2006 from http://archive.naccho.org/Documents/Testimony/Troutman-testimony-03-20–02.pdf.

National Coalition on Health Care. (2004). *Facts on health care cost*. Retrieved August October 16, 2006 from http://www.nchc.org/facts/cost.shtml.

National Council of State Legislators. (November 2004). *Trends alert: Public health worker shortages*. Retrieved October 13, 2006 from http://www.csg.org/pubs/documents/TA411HealthWork.pdf.

National League for Nursing. (2006). *Nurse educators 2006: A report of the faculty census survey of RN programs and graduate programs*. New York: Author.

Polick, T. (2006, October 16). Grassroots nursing. *Advance Online Editions for Nurses*. Retrieved October 19, 2006 from http://nursing.advanceweb.com/common/Editorial.

Roberts, J.I., & Group, T.M. (1995). *A historical perspective on power, status, and political activism in the nursing profession*. Westport, CT: Praeger Publishing.

Robertson, A., & Minkler, M. (1994). New health promotion movement: A critical examination. *Health Education Quarterly, 2*(3), 295–312.

Robinson, J. (2001). The end of managed care. *Journal of the American Medical Association, 285*, 2622–2628.

Sapp, M., & Bliesmer, M. (1995). A health promotion/prevention approach to meeting elders' health care needs through public policy and standards of care. In M. Stanley & P. Beare, (Eds.), *Gerontological nursing*. Philadelphia: Davis Co.

Seago, J.A., Spetz, J., & Mitchell, S. (2004). Nurse staffing and hospital ownership in California. *Journal of Nursing Administration, 34*(5), 228–237.

Sharp, N. (1997). Politics, power and vested interests: Washington at work. In: C. Harrington & D. Estes (Eds.), *Health policy & nursing*, pp. 453–461. Sudbury, MA: Jones & Bartlett Publishers.

Smedley, B., Stith, A., & Nelson, A. (Eds). (2003). *Unequal treatment: Confronting racial and ethnic disparities in health care*. Washington, DC: The National Academies Press.

Spenceley, S., Reutter, L., & Allen, M. (2006). The road less traveled: Nursing advocacy at the policy level. *Policy, Politics & Nursing Practice, 7*(3), 180–194.

State of the World's Mothers Index. (2006). *Mothers 2006: Saving the lives of mothers & newborns*. Washington, DC: Save the Children.

Sullivan Commission. (2004). *Missing persons: Minorities in the health professions*. Washington, DC: Institute of Medicine.

U.S. Department of Health & Human Services. (2000). *Healthy People 2010: Understanding & improving health*. Atlanta, GA: National Center for Chronic Disease Prevention & Health Promotion.

Waldron, T. (2003). Nurses vote. *Johns Hopkins Nursing–Online edition*, (1), 2.

Washington Post. (January 4, 2006). *Abramoff pleads guilty to 3 counts*. Retrieved August 4, 2008 from http://www.washingtonpost.com/wp-dyn/content/article/2006/01/03/AR2006010300474_pf.html.

Weiss, D., Schank, M.J., & Matheus, R. (2006). The process of empowerment: A parish nurse perspective. *Journal of Holistic Nursing, 24*, 17–24.

Wieczorik, R. R. (1985). *Power, politics & policy in nursing*. New York: Springer Publishing.

Woodfill, M.M., & Beyrer, M.K. (1991). *The role of the nurse in the school setting: A historical perspective*. Kent, OH: American School Health Association.

Woolhandler, S., & Himmelstein, D. (October 2006). The new Massachusetts health reform: Half a step forward and three steps back. *Medscape*. Retrieved November 1, 2006 from http://www.medscape.com/viewarticle/545565.

Yoo, S. et al. (2004). Collaborative community empowerment: An illustration of a six-step process. *Health Promotion Practice, 5*, 256–265.

Selected Readings

Aufderheide, T., et al. (2006). Community lay rescuer automated external defibrillation programs: Key state legislative components and implementation strategies: A summary of a decade of experience for healthcare providers, policy makers, legislators, employers, and community leaders from the American Heart Association Emergency Cardiovascular Care Committee, Council on Clinical Cardiology, and the Office of State Advocacy. *Circulation, 113*, 1260–1270.

Barnes, L.E., Asajara, L., Davos, A., & Konishi, E. (2002). Questions of distributive justice: Public health nurses' perceptions of long-term care insurance for elderly Japanese people. *Nursing Ethics, 9*(1), 67–79.

Caulfield, T., Knowles, L., & Meslin, E.M. (2004). Law and policy in the era of reproductive genetics. *Journal of Medical Ethics, 30*, 414–417.

Christoffel, K.K. (2000). Public health advocacy: Process and product. *American Journal of Public Health, 90*, 722.

Cody, W., & Mitchell, G. (2002). Nursing knowledge and human science revisited: Practical and political considerations. *Nursing Science Quarterly, 15*, 4–13.

Galer-Unti, R.A., Tappe, M.K., & Lachenmayr, S. (2004). Advocacy 101: Getting started in health education advocacy. *Heath Promotion Practice, 5*, 280–288.

Gillan, J.S. (2006). Legislative advocacy is key to addressing teen driving deaths. *Injury Prevention, 12*, 144–148.

Gomm, M., Lincoln, P., Pikora, T., & Gtiles-Corti, B. (2006). Planning and implementing a community-based public health advocacy campaign: A transport case study from Australia. *Health Promotion International, 21*, 284–292.

Goodley, D. (2005). Empowerment, self-advocacy and resilience. *Journal of Intellectual Disabilities, 9*, 333–343.

Gruen, R.L., Campbell, E.G., & Blumenthal, D. (2006). Public roles of US physicians: Community participation, political involvement, and collective advocacy. *Journal of the American Medical Association, 296*, 2467–2475.

Hansen, A., & Gunter, B. (2006). Constructing public and political discourse on alcohol issues: Towards a framework for analysis. *Alcohol and Alcoholism*. Retrieved August 4, 2008 from http://alcalc.oxfordjournals.org/cgi/content/abstract/agl114v1.

Harwood, E., Witson, J., Fan, D., & Wagenaar, A. (2005). Media advocacy and underage drinking policies: A study of Louisiana news media from 1994 through 2003. *Health Promotion Practice, 6*, 246–257.

Jabbour, S., El-Zein, A., Nuwayhid, I., & Glacaman, R. (2006). Can action on health achieve political and social reform? *British Medical Journal, 333*, 837–839.

Kumanyika, S.K., Morssink, C.B., & Nestle, M. (2001). Minority women and advocacy for women's health. *American Journal of Public Health, 91*, 1383.

Sohier, R. (1992). Feminism & nursing knowledge: The power of the weak. *Nursing Outlook, 40*(2), 62–93.

Williams, L., Labonte, R., & O'Brien, M. (2003). Empowering social action through narratives of identity and culture. *Health Promotion International, 18*, 33–40.

Woodhouse, L.D., Sayre, J.J., & Livingood, W.C. (2001). Tobacco policy and the role of law enforcement in prevention: The value of understanding context. *Qualitative Health Research, 11*, 682–692.

Internet Resources

American Nurses Association: *http://www.nursingworld.org*
American Public Health Association: *http://www.apha.org/* and *http://www.apha.org/legislative/*
Center on Budget & Priorities: *http://www.cbpp.org/*
Citizen Joe: *http://www.citizenjoe.org*
Families USA: *http://www.familiesusa.org/*
National Association of School Nurses: *http://www.nasn.org/*
National Coalition on Health Care: *http://www.nchc.org/*
Public Health Nursing Section: *http://www.apha.org/extranet/phn/default.htm*
US House of Representatives: *http://www.house.gov/*
US Senate: *http://www.senate.gov/*

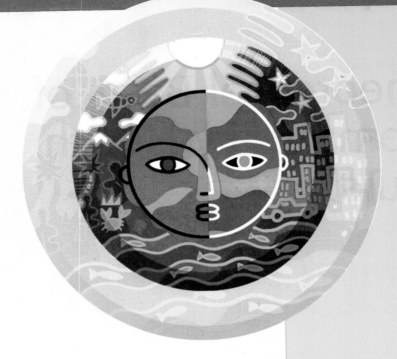

THE COMMUNITY AS CLIENT

14

Theoretical Basis of Community Health Nursing

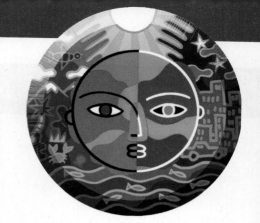

LEARNING OBJECTIVES

Upon mastery of this chapter, you should be able to:

◆ Discuss two essential characteristics of nursing service when a community is the client: community-oriented, population-focused care, and relationship-based care.

◆ Describe the contributions of at least five models of nursing practice to community health nursing practice.

◆ Explain the benefits of applying the eight principles of public health nursing to community health nursing.

◆ Identify at least five social issues that influence contemporary community health nursing care.

"*We know a great deal more about the causes of physical disease than we do about the causes of physical health.*"

—M. Scott Peck, *The Road Less Traveled*

When you open the door of a senior center where you will be promoting cardiovascular fitness, advocating for exercise equipment, and suggesting changes in the on-site meal program, how might theories of community health nursing contribute to your success? When you approach your city council about the need to increase staffing of public health services, what models of community health nursing practice might support your argument? What is meant by *theories, models,* and *principles,* and what is their relevance to day-to-day community health nursing practice? These are the key issues explored in this chapter. First, however, we revisit some of the fundamental characteristics of community health nursing that we began to explore in Unit 1.

WHEN THE CLIENT IS A COMMUNITY: CHARACTERISTICS OF COMMUNITY HEALTH NURSING PRACTICE

Nursing exists to address people's health care needs, and nurses fulfill this purpose through their work in various specialty areas. Specialties are characterized by the unit of care for which the specialty is responsible and by the goal of the specialty. Each specialty requires a particular area of knowledge and a set of skills for excellence in practice.

Community health nursing is a specialty in which the unit of care is a specific community or aggregate, and the nurse has responsibility to promote group health. The goal of this specialty is health improvement of the community. The skills required for excellence in community health nursing practice include epidemiology, research, teaching, community organizing, and interpersonal relational care, as well as many others.

In summary, community health nursing is characterized by community-oriented, population-focused care and is based on interpersonal relationships. In the following sections, each of these characteristics is examined in more depth.

Community-Oriented, Population-Focused Care

As was discussed in Chapter 1, a *community* is a group of people who have some characteristics in common, are bounded by time, interact with one another, and feel a connection to one another. For example, members of an Internet-based support group for people with colitis are a community. They share similar experiences and concerns, and they often influence one another's behavior. For instance, they may recommend food choices or complementary therapies to one another. Members of a class of community health nursing students are also a community. Because they begin and end their studies in a particular month and year, they are bonded by time, and they certainly share certain values and feel a sense of connection to one another.

Community orientation is a process that is actively shaped by the unique experiences, knowledge, concerns, values, beliefs, and culture of a given community. For example, when an outbreak of hepatitis occurs, the community health nurse does more than simply treat infection in individuals. The nurse also

◆ Uses disease-investigation skills to locate possible sources of infection.

◆ Determines how the community's knowledge, values, beliefs, and prior experiences with infectious disease may influence its interpretation of the disease, response to the outbreak, and treatment preferences.

◆ Uses knowledge and suggestions gathered from the community to develop, in collaboration with other health professionals, a community-specific program to prevent future outbreaks.

A community-oriented nurse who provides education about sexually transmitted diseases to a group of students at a Catholic college includes consideration of community values regarding sexual behavior. Similarly, a community-oriented nurse who provides nutritional counseling to a community of Hispanic seniors considers the meaning of food in this culture, the types of food most commonly consumed, and the cooking methods most commonly used.

A *population* is any group of people who share at least one characteristic, such as age, gender, race, a particular risk factor, or disease. Smokers and breast cancer survivors are two populations. The concept of population may also include delineation by time (e.g., all children born in the year 2008). The nurse's place of employment commonly limits the population that the nurse serves. For example, a nurse who works for a county health department is limited professionally to caring for the population of that county.

A *population focus* implies that a nurse uses population-based skills such as epidemiology, research in community assessment, and community organizing as the basis for interventions. For example, a population-focused nurse employed by an autoworkers' union may study all cases of repetitive-use injury occurring in the auto industry in the United States in the past 5 years, develop a program for reducing repetitive-use injury, and lobby industry executives for adoption of the program.

Community-oriented, population-focused care employs population-based skills and is shaped by the characteristics and needs of a given community. Community health nurses provide community-oriented, population-focused care when they count and interview homeless people sleeping in a park and, based on these data, help develop a program to provide food, clothing, shelter, health care, and job training for this population.

Relationship-Based Care

Relationship-based care incorporates the value of establishing and maintaining a reciprocal, caring relationship with the community. It is a necessary and feasible aspect of community health nursing practice and is foundational to caring effectively for the community's health. A reciprocal, caring relationship with the community involves listening, participatory dialogue, and critical reflection, and it may also involve sociopolitical elements of practice such as advocacy, community empowerment, and movement to action (Shields & Lindsey, 1998).

Community health nurses provide relationship-based care when they meet regularly with groups of female inmates to learn about their physical and psychosocial health care needs and the needs of their families, and then use the information gathered to advocate for this population with prison officials and other professionals in the community. A nurse also provides relationship-based care when working with parents of children with cancer, a psychologist, and a hospital chaplain to determine the needs of each family and to facilitate formation of a self-help group. In both these examples, community health nurses are working to establish and maintain ongoing relationships with other professionals in the community and with their communities of clients.

THEORIES AND MODELS FOR COMMUNITY HEALTH NURSING PRACTICE

A **theory** is a set of systematically interrelated concepts or hypotheses that seek to explain or predict phenomena. For example, the "big bang theory" seeks to explain the series of events that occurred during the earliest moments in the history of our universe. The evolution of theory development in nursing dominated the last half of the 20th century. The scholarly and creative efforts of these nurse leaders and researchers resulted in broad and often abstract theories explaining what nursing is and how it influences individuals, families, or communities. These early theories, also termed *grand theories* or **conceptual models** (Walker & Avant, 2005), provided a basis for building nursing knowledge. One feature separating **nursing theory** from other professional theories is the use of the nursing metaparadigm concepts: nursing, client/patient, health, and environment (Fawcett, 1989; Walker & Avant, 2005). As you read through the descriptions of the theories and models, see if you can determine which ones conform to the nursing metaparadigm and which ones can be used by nurses as well as other health care professionals.

From these early efforts came more testable theories, many from those same nurse researchers; these theories are typically referred to as middle-range theories. Although less abstract than the grand theories, the need for an even more practical approach to theory use and testing led ultimately to practice-based theories. Walker and Avant note that "the essence of practice theory was a desired goal and prescriptions for action to achieve the goal" (p. 14), clearly emphasizing the goal directiveness of nursing practice. Most significantly, the focus on practice has opened up new opportunities for generalist nurses to both understand and use nursing theories.

To more fully understand the elements inherent in a nursing theory, a pictorial representation, or **model**, is often used. These models provide a visual means to understand the relationships between, for instance, the nurse and the environment, the nurse and the client, or the stress factors experienced by the client. However complex these models, comprehension of the entire work can only be derived from reading the theorist's descriptions of the model and the use of the theory by others. Both theories and models have been developed to describe, clarify, and guide nursing practice. Theories and models that have particular relevance to the practice of community health nursing are described here.

Nightingale's Theory of Environment

Florence Nightingale's environmental theory has great significance to nursing in general and to community health nursing specifically, because it focuses on preventive care for populations. While organizing and supervising a nursing service for soldiers in the Crimean War, Nightingale kept meticulous records. Her observations suggested that disease was more prevalent in poor environments, and that health could be promoted by providing adequate ventilation, pure water, quiet, warmth, light, and cleanliness. The crux of her theory was that poor environmental conditions are bad for health and that good environmental conditions reduce disease (Nightingale, 1859/1992).

There is no consensus of opinion on specific conditions that ensure people's health. Some people believe that, in addition to a clean environment, social services such as public transportation, education, and health care are necessary. In thinking about services that promote the health of communities, it is useful to consider

- ◆ Why these services were created.
- ◆ Who benefits from the services.
- ◆ Who pays for the services.
- ◆ The cost to the people using the services.
- ◆ The public's perception of the services.

For example, if ventilation in a city's homeless shelter is inadequate, the community health nurse who plans to advocate for capital improvements to the shelter needs to consider who pays for the shelter as well as the public's perception of the shelter.

One contemporary example of the utility of Nightingale's theory is the work of Shaner-McRae, McRae, and Jas (2007), who sought to bring attention to the need for nurses to optimize environments for healing. Although they specifically focused on the health care setting, describing ways to manage both "upstream and downstream waste (solid, biohazard, and hazardous chemical wastes)" (p. 1), their premise can be easily applied to the home, community, or even the public health department. Controlling environmental contaminants and protecting the environment are important goals in a wide variety of settings. Nightingale's influence on the way we approach health issues impacting our communities remains a powerful force.

Orem's Self-Care Model

Dorothy Orem, a nurse administrator and educator, focused on the concept of *self-care*—learned, goal-oriented actions to preserve and promote life, health, and well-being. She described people who need nursing care as those who lack ability in self-care (Orem, 2001). If a demand for self-care exceeds the client's ability, the client experiences a self-care deficit, and nursing intervention becomes appropriate. The goal of nursing action is to help people recognize their self-care demands and limitations and increase their self-care ability. Nursing care also functions to meet clients' self-care needs until they are able to care for themselves.

Orem further described three types of requirements that influence people's self-care abilities:

- ◆ Universal requirements, common to all human beings, are self-care activities essential to meet physiologic and psychosocial needs.
- ◆ Developmental requirements are activities necessary to help people progress developmentally.
- ◆ Health-deviation requirements are activities needed to help people deal with a diminished level of wellness.

Although Orem's model focused primarily on individuals, it can be applied to community health nursing. Populations and communities can be considered to have a collective set of self-care actions and requirements that affect the well-being of the total group. If an aggregate's demands for self-care exceed its ability, the aggregate experiences a self-care deficit, and community health nursing intervention is indicated. According to this interpretation, the goal of community health nursing is to promote a community's collective independence and self-care ability.

For example, a riverside community that ingests large quantities of fish contaminated with heavy metals might have self-care deficits related to the lack of awareness that eating local fish is dangerous and that some subpopulations, such as pregnant women and young children, are especially vulnerable. The community health nurse should help the community become aware of the risk and identify other food sources. The nurse should also help the community lobby government and industry to reduce pollution and clean up the river.

Three specific theories have been derived from the original model: the self-care deficit theory, the theory of self-care, and the theory of nursing system (Gast & Montgomery, 2005). The applicability of the self-care deficit theory to public health nursing was demonstrated in a study of adherence to latent tuberculosis therapy among Latino immigrants (Ailinger, Moore, Nguyen, & Lasus, 2006), and in a pilot study of mother's knowledge of childhood immunizations (Wilson, Baker, Nordstrom, & Legwand, 2008). The theory of self-care was utilized to identify self-care behaviors of school-aged children with heart disease (Fan, 2008). Clearly the model and the derived theories have shown applicability to public health practice directed at improving health outcomes in the community setting.

Neuman's Health Care Systems Model

Betty Neuman, a leader in mental health nursing and nursing education, proposed a systems model (Neuman, 1982; Neuman & Fawcett, 2002) that can be adapted to view clients as aggregates. In this model, people are seen as open systems that constantly and reciprocally interact with their environments. Each system is greater than the sum of its parts, and wellness exists when the parts of the system interact in harmony with each other and with the system's environment. Four sets of variables, or influences, make up each system's "whole." These are physiologic, psychological, sociocultural, and developmental variables. Given these variables, each system has a unique response to stressors and to those tension-producing stimuli that may cause disequilibrium or illness.

A system's response to stressors may be envisioned as a series of concentric circles (Fig. 14.1). In the center is a core of basic survival abilities, such as a community's ability to make the best use of its natural resources. Surrounding this core are three boundaries. The innermost boundary is a flexible line of resistance that encompasses internal defenses, such as a community's collective sense of responsibility for raising healthy children. The second boundary is the system's normal line of defense, such as a community's police force or voluntary fire brigade. The third boundary is a dynamic, flexible line of defense, a buffer that prevents stressors from invading the system's normal line of defense. An example is regular maintenance of a community's roads and bridges.

In Neuman's model, stressors can originate from the internal environment or the external environment. Examples of internal stressors include a high proportion of low-income residents or an inadequate system of water purification.

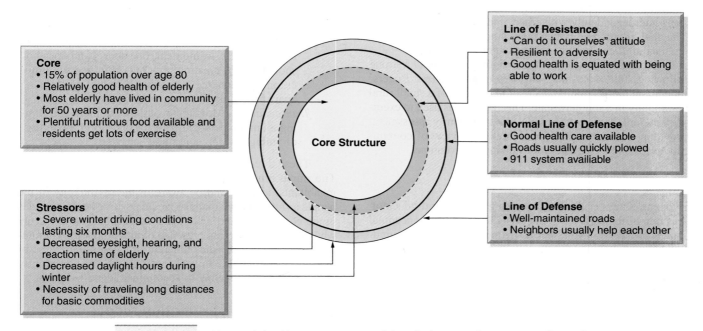

Line of Resistance
• "Can do it ourselves" attitude
• Resilient to adversity
• Good health is equated with being able to work

Core
• 15% of population over age 80
• Relatively good health of elderly
• Most elderly have lived in community for 50 years or more
• Plentiful nutritious food available and residents get lots of exercise

Normal Line of Defense
• Good health care available
• Roads usually quickly plowed
• 911 system availiable

Core Structure

Stressors
• Severe winter driving conditions lasting six months
• Decreased eyesight, hearing, and reaction time of elderly
• Decreased daylight hours during winter
• Necessity of traveling long distances for basic commodities

Line of Defense
• Well-maintained roads
• Neighbors usually help each other

FIGURE 14.1 Neuman's health care systems model applied to a rural county regarding traffic safety issues concerning the elderly by D. Block, from Allender, J., & Spradley, B. (2001). *Community health nursing: Concepts and Practice* (5th ed.). Philadelphia: Lippincott, with permission.

External stressors might include natural disasters, war, or a downturn in the global economy. The role of community health nursing, then, is to assist communities in remaining stable within their environments. The applicability of the Neuman model to community health nursing was clearly demonstrated in a comprehensive literature review of published studies between 1983 and 2005 (Skalski, DiGerolamo, & Gigliotti, 2006). This review yielded 13 studies dealing with stressors in client populations; the vast majority were pertinent to community health nursing practice (i.e., spousal alcoholism, long-term cancer survivors, informal caregivers of head-injured adults, and telephone counseling).

Rogers' Model of the Science of Unitary Beings

Not typically linked with community health nursing practice, Martha Rogers (1915–1994) established the first visiting nursing service in Arizona in the mid 1940s; it was one of the first in the nation (Tomasson, 1994). A nursing administrator and long-time nurse educator, Rogers is responsible for modern nursing's emphasis on the whole person (Hemphill & Muth Quillin, 2005). In 1970, she developed a nursing conceptual model based on systems theory. Her model emphasized that the whole is greater than the sum of its parts; that is, focusing on the parts of a community, such as its health care or housing, does not provide an adequate picture of its totality.

Rogers also incorporated developmental theory into her model by describing the development of "unitary" persons or systems according to three principles: (1) life proceeds in one direction along a rhythmic spiral, (2) energy fields follow a certain wave pattern and organization, and (3) human and environmental energy fields interact simultaneously and mutually, leading to completeness and unity (Rogers, 1990). Using this model, the community health nurse can focus on community–environment interaction; the community functions interdependently with others and with the environment. The goal of community health nursing is to promote holistic and healthful community–environment interaction.

Even after her death, Rogers continues to garner a strong following. Talley, Rushing, and Gee (2005) utilized Rogers' model as a framework in the creation a profile of a small rural community in a southern state. This profile was used to exemplify the link between the model and community assessment, providing a comprehensive and thoughtful view of community needs and a clear basis for nursing interventions.

King

Imogene King (1923–2007), nursing scholar and educator, was one of the early nurse theorists to provide a conceptual model of nursing (Messmer & Palmer, 2008). Her groundbreaking work *Toward a Theory for Nursing* (1970) and the subsequent *A Theory for Nursing: Systems, Concepts, Process* (1981) were designed to "promote conceptual learning in undergraduate and graduate nursing programs" (1981, p. vii). From the original general systems model, which demonstrated the interrelationship between social, interpersonal, and personal systems (Killeen & King, 2007), King formulated the *theory of goal attainment*. The theory focuses on the personal and interpersonal systems of the model. The basis of the theory is that, in any nurse–client encounter, each comes to the situation with her own goals and expectations. Optimal success at goal achievement is only possible when the nurse and the client work together to set goals, thus recognizing the expectations of both parties rather than the preeminence of one over the other. For instance, a community health nurse may have planned to speak to a teen mother about birth control on a home visit. The teen, however has nearly run out of formula and has exhausted all her cash. In this instance, the teen's priorities are to locate formula or the resources to obtain formula, while the nurse may be concerned that the teen has resumed sexual activity and may become pregnant again. The priority would clearly be the formula, but the nurse can also provide birth control information within that context after the teen is aware that a solution to the formula issue can be found. King's theory is a reminder of the importance of the reciprocal relationship between the nurse and the client. Negotiation is a skill inherent in the theory; only through recognition of the perceived needs and goals of the client can the community health nurse help maintain or improve the client's health and well-being. The principles of public health nursing discussed later in this chapter (ANA, 2007) also emphasize the need to treat the client as an equal partner—a strong reminder of King's legacy to nursing practice.

Parse's Human Becoming Theory

Rosemarie Rizzo Parse developed her theory, initially called the "man-living-health" theory, in 1981. In 1992, she changed the name to "Human Becoming Theory" to better reflect all people. The theory posits quality of life from each person's own perspective as the goal of nursing practice. The theory is structured around three themes (Parse, 1981, 1998):

Meaning. People coparticipate in creating what is real for them through self-expression by living their values in their own chosen way.

Rhythmicity. The unity of life encompasses apparent opposites in rhythmic patterns of relating. While living moment-to-moment, one shows and does not show the self, creating both opportunities and limitations that emerge as moving with and moving apart from others.

Transcendence. Moving beyond the moment and forging a unique personal path for oneself in the midst of ambiguity and continuous change.

These three themes apply effectively to the community. The nurse must know what the community means to its inhabitants, identify and be aware of the rhythmicity of the people as attempts are made to create positive health changes in the community, and realize the transcendence that occurs when people work in the presence of ambiguity and continuous change, characteristics inherent in a community. Use of this model as a guide enhances the ability of community members to work together to accomplish identified goals.

Pender's Health Promotion Model

As we have noted throughout this text, health promotion is a priority in community health nursing practice. Pender defined health promotion as actions that are directed toward increasing the level of well-being and self-actualization in individuals or groups (Pender, Murdaugh, & Parsons, 2006). It is a proactive set of behaviors in which people act on their environment rather than react to stressors arising from the environment.

Pender's *health promotion model* seeks to explain this proactive behavior. The model, based on social learning theory, stresses cognitive processes that help regulate behavior such as perceptions people have that directly influence their motivation to begin or continue health-promoting behaviors. These include, for example, perceptions of control of health, health status, benefits of health-promoting behaviors, and barriers to engaging in health-promoting behaviors.

Five types of modifying factors influence people's perceptions about pursuing health-promoting behaviors:

◆ Demographic factors, such as age and race
◆ Biologic characteristics, such as height and weight
◆ Interpersonal influences, such as the expectations of others
◆ Situational factors, such as availability of healthful foods
◆ Behavioral factors, such as stress-coping patterns

Using Pender's model, a community health nurse might interview the residents of a low-income housing project to determine their perceptions about improving health and safety. Research of demographic, situational, and other factors that might influence the residents' motivation and ability to change their circumstances could then be conducted. Pender's model is being increasingly used as a framework in studies of health promotion in diverse populations: preventing farm accidents in children (Conway, McClune, & Nosel, 2007), self-efficacy and health-promoting behaviors in older adults in Iran (Morowatisharifabad, Ghofranipour, Heidarnia, Ruchi, & Ehrampoush, 2006), adolescent health-promoting behavior (Srof & Velsor-Friedrich, 2006), and health-promoting behaviors of low-income elderly Korean women (Shin, Kang, Park, Cho, & Heitkemper, 2008). Pender's model is further discussed in relation to client education in Chapter 11.

Roy's Adaptation Model

Sister Callista Roy's model describes people as open and adaptive systems that experience stimuli, develop coping mechanisms, and produce responses. These responses, which may be adaptive or maladaptive, provide feedback that influences the amount and type of stimuli that can be handled in the future (Andrews & Roy, 1991; Roy & Andrews, 1999).

Roy describes two response processes. In the *regulator* process, stimuli from the internal and external environments are received, and this combination of information is then processed to produce a response. In the *cognator* process, perceptions, learning, judgment, and emotion are considered in formulating a response to stimuli. For example, a regulator process might begin with a community's desire to keep adolescents from smoking (internal stimulus) and new state regulations prohibiting the sale of tobacco products to minors (external stimulus). These combined stimuli lead to a city ordinance that prevents the sale of cigarettes to minors (coping mechanism), resulting in reduced levels of smoking (response) among this population. A cognator process might begin with the stimulus of heavy rainfall in a riverside community. Residents' perceptions of the amount of rainfall, memories of past floods, insights about preventing or managing floods, and the level of anxiety all contribute to their plans for evacuation, sandbagging, and soliciting county or state assistance.

In applying Roy's model to community health nursing, it is important to remember that communities are made up of many parts and are influenced by many variables. The community's collective adaptation level is constantly changing. The community health nurse must assess a community's coping mechanisms and help its members use these collective abilities in adapting to challenges. For example, if a community is doing nothing to respond to the increased number of teen pregnancies, nursing actions can be designed to encourage more healthful coping patterns and adaptive responses. Roy's model has been utilized in a number of studies with direct applicability to community health: bulimia nervosa (Hannon-Engel, 2008), self-concept of children with HIV/AIDS in the United States and Kenya (Waweru, Reynolds, & Buckner, 2008), and as the basis for developing a new conceptual framework explaining the coping processes of Taiwanese families following the hip fracture of an elderly family member (Li & Shyu, 2007).

Salmon's Construct for Public Health Nursing

Marla Salmon, a leader in public health nursing administration, nursing education, and public health policy in the United States, proposed a model to guide community health nursing practice. In *Construct for Public Health Nursing*, Salmon (1982) described public health as an organized societal effort to protect, promote, and restore the health of people, and public health nursing as focused on achieving and maintaining public health.

The model describes three practice priorities. Not surprisingly, these are prevention of disease and poor health, protection against disease and external agents, and promotion of health. There are three general categories of nursing intervention:

◆ Education directed toward voluntary change in the attitudes and behavior of the subjects
◆ Engineering directed at managing risk-related variables
◆ Enforcement directed at mandatory regulation to achieve better health

The scope of practice spans individual, family, community, and global care. Interventions target determinants in four categories: human/biologic, environmental, medical/technologic/organizational, and social. Using Salmon's approach, a community health nurse attempting to reduce the transmission of tuberculosis would use education, engineering, and enforcement in working with the population of affected individuals and families. The nurse would also collaborate with the client community on a variety of interventions, from medications to teaching to social support, to prevent further disease in the community and to promote global health.

A decade later, Salmon's editorial entitled *Public Health Nursing: The Opportunity of a Century* again stressed the importance of the central functions of public health nursing practice: "assessment, surveillance, policy, and health promotion and disease and injury prevention activities" (1993, p. 1674). In the revised *Public Health Nursing: Scope and Standards of Practice* (ANA, 2007) the Salmon model is cited as an exemplar of an ecological approach to public health nursing interventions.

Minnesota Wheel—The Public Health Interventions Model

The Minnesota Department of Health, Division of Community Health Services, Public Health Nursing Section, has devised a model that depicts public health interventions and applications for public health practice. In the form of a wheel, the model shows 17 different interventions within three levels of public health practice: population-based community-focused practice, systems-focused practice, and individual-focused practice. The "Minnesota Wheel" (2001) is depicted in Figure 14.2.

The intervention wheel was first proposed in 1998 (Keller, Strohschein, Lia-Hoagberg, & Schaffer) as a practice model for population-based public health nursing. It is currently used in a

variety of venues including public health practice, nursing education, and management. Keller and colleagues emphasize that "use of the Wheel has empowered nurses to explain in a better way how their practice contributes to the improvement of population health (Keller, Strohschein, Lia-Hoagberg, & Schaffer, 2004, p. 454). The wheel is useful for community health nurses because it visually depicts the comprehensive list of interventions nurses must consider in the scope of practice. Saewyc, Solsvig, and Edinburgh (2007) utilized the Minnesota Wheel in an evaluation of "a coalition formed to address a growing issue of young Hmong girls in a Midwest state running away from home, being truant from school, and experiencing subsequent sexual exploitation" (p. 69). The outcomes of the task force were assessed relative to best practices identified in the model. This example shows just one of the many ways the model can assist both the novice nurse and the expert practitioner, as well as other public health disciplines.

Public Health Nursing Practice Model

The need for a model that could blend public health nursing practice and the principles of public health, and could be applicable to both the generalist nurse and nurses working in specific programs, was the impetus for development of the Public Health Nursing Practice Model (Smith & Bazini-

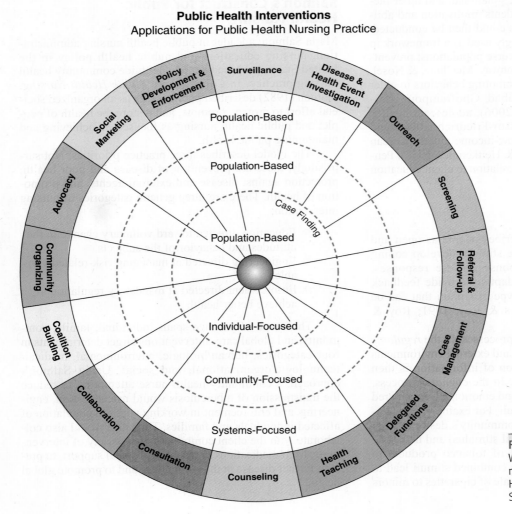

Public Health Interventions
Applications for Public Health Nursing Practice

FIGURE 14.2 The Minnesota Wheel. (*Source:* Minnesota Department of Health, Division of Community Health Services, Public Health Nursing Section.)

Barakat, 2003). The model was created by Los Angeles County, Department of Health Services (LAC-DHS), Public Health Nursing with input from the California Conference of Local Health Department Nursing Directors (CCLHNDN) Southern Region and other public health nurse leaders. Referred to as the LAC PHN Practice Model, it is described as integrating the Public Health Nursing Standards of Practice, the 10 Essential Public Health Services, the 10 Leading Health Indicators from *Healthy People 2010*, and the Minnesota Public Health Nursing Interventions Model. "The LAC PHN Practice Model provides a conceptual framework that assists in clarifying the role of the public health nurse and presents a guide for public health practice applicable to all public health disciplines" (Smith & Bazini-Barakat, p. 42).

As described by Smith and Bazini-Barakat (2003), the principles of population-based practice are included in the LAC PHN Practice Model. The public health nurse integrates assessment, policy development, and assurance into her work. The three levels of population-based practice—individuals and families, community, and systems—are addressed, with the nursing process applied throughout the model. Seventeen interventions, as first presented in the Minnesota Public Health Nursing Model, are also incorporated into the LAC PHN Practice Model. The LAC PHN Practice Model promotes the concepts of an interdisciplinary public health team working together, with an emphasis on primary prevention. It also recognizes the importance of active participation of the individual, family, and community. See Figure 30.2 for a depiction of the LAC PHN Model.

Omaha System

The Omaha System was developed and refined during four research projects conducted between 1975 and 1992 in the Omaha Visiting Nursing Association. It was designed to increase the effectiveness and efficiency of nursing practice in the agency (Bowles & Naylor, 1996; Martin, Leak, & Aden,

1997). The system is now finding increasing utility in facilitating evidence-based practice, documentation, and information management (Martin, 2005), all of which are critical to contemporary public health care systems. It is a comprehensive system, including the following components (Martin, 2005):

- ◆ Problem classification scheme. Offers nurses a holistic, comprehensive method for identifying clients' health-related concerns. It includes domains, problems, modifiers, and signs/symptoms. Problems can be identified at the individual, family, or community level.
- ◆ Intervention scheme. Provides a framework for documenting plans and interventions in the client record in the areas of health teaching, guidance, and counseling; treatments and procedures; case management; and surveillance
- ◆ Problem rating scale for outcomes. Consists of a Likert-type scale that is a systematic and recurring method used to document the progress of clients in the record and in case conferences during their time of service in the agency. It is used in conjunction with any problem in the Problem Classification Scheme. Central to problem rating is quantifying outcomes in three dimensions: knowledge (what the client knows), behavior (what the client does), and status (how the client is).

The Omaha System is based on universal principles of nursing practice. The model was judged to be consistent with the Nightingale model of environmental health (Zurakowki, 2005). Citing some variations in language use, Gast and Montgomery (2005) found that Orem's model of self-care was also consistent with the premises of the Omaha System. The *Omaha System model of the problem solving process* (Fig. 14.3) shows the interrelationship between the practitioner and the client in addressing health problems. The model guides the nurse through the six steps in the

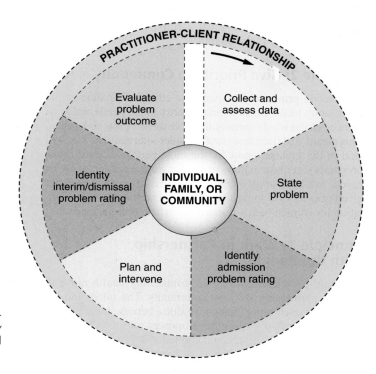

FIGURE 14.3　Omaha System Model of the Problem Solving Process. From Martin, K.S. (2005). *The Omaha System: A Key to Practice, Documentation, and Information Management,* 2nd ed. St. Louis: Elsevier, with permission.

process: (1) collecting and assessing data, (2) stating the problem, (3) identifying the problem rating on admission, (4) planning and actual interventions, (5) identification of interim or dismissal problem rating, and finally, (6) evaluating problem outcome. The model is applicable to individuals, families, and communities, and provides a mechanism to evaluate both individual and group change over time. Of particular concern to many public health departments is tangibly demonstrating what changes have resulted following interventions with clients.

The system is now available in a Web-based format. This automated version of the model is currently being used in home care agencies, public health departments, and residential long-term care, as well as in schools and universities (Martin, 2005). The Omaha System website provides links to a wide variety of resources for those interested in the system (see Internet Resources). For students and practicing nurses, case studies are available that demonstrate the use of the system with a variety of client types. An extensive list of references is continually updated to provide the most up-to-date evidence regarding the system and its impact on nursing practice.

PRINCIPLES OF PUBLIC HEALTH NURSING

The word **principle** can be defined variably as rule of conduct, a quality that produces a specific effect, or even the method of operation of a thing (Webster's, 2004). Whatever the definition, there are universals in practice that can guide public health nursing practice in a way that can help achieve the most beneficial outcomes. The goals of community health nursing, to promote and protect the health of communities, are facilitated by adhering to the eight principles of public health nursing summarized in Display 14.1 (ANA, 2007).

Principle 1: Focus on the Community

The first principle reminds us that the ultimate responsibility of public health nursing is to direct services to the population as a whole. Even though public health nurses may intervene to address individual, family, or group needs, the entire community is the client.

Principle 2: Give Priority to Community Needs

The second principle deals with the ethical obligation of the community health nurse to give priority to the needs and preferences of the whole community over those of one individual. This means that the nurse must consider interventions that will lead to the greatest good for the most people. For example, programs that make mammograms for early detection of breast cancer available to all women regardless of income level are given priority over those that provide bone marrow transplantation for women with advanced metastatic breast cancer.

Principle 3: Work in Partnership With the People

The third principle requires the community health nurse to work in partnership with the community. The nurse and the community each bring their own values, beliefs, and expertise to the partnership. Policy development and assurance are more likely to be accepted and applied if there is mutual consideration of and respect for these elements. Developed policies need to be communicated in language that reflects an understanding of the community. For these reasons, an essential part of establishing a partnership with a community is getting to know the members and groups within that community.

Principle 4: Focus on Primary Prevention

The fourth principle of public health nursing underscores the importance of primary prevention in promoting the health of people. Most fields of medicine, including acute care nursing, are primarily concerned with illness, and with efforts to prevent complications from and reoccurrence of the illness. In contrast, community health nursing has an obligation to prevent health problems and to promote a higher level of wellness. Community health nurses take initiative to seek out high-risk groups, potential health problems, and situations that contribute to health problems. They then institute preventive programs. For example, if community assessment revealed a large number of new mothers with postpartum depression, community health nurses would address secondary prevention by establishing mental health programs. Equally as important, they would attend to primary prevention by working to change the conditions in the community that increase the risk for postpartum depression.

DISPLAY 14.1   PRINCIPLES OF PUBLIC HEALTH NURSING

1. **Focus on the Community.** The client or unit of care is the population.
2. **Give Priority to Community Needs.** The primary obligation is to achieve the greatest good for the greatest number of people or the population as a whole.
3. **Work in Partnership With the People.** The processes used by public health nurses include working with the client as an equal partner.
4. **Focus on Primary Prevention.** Primary prevention is the priority in selecting appropriate activities.
5. **Promote a Healthful Environment.** Public health nursing focuses on strategies that create healthy environmental, social, and economic conditions in which populations may thrive.
6. **Target All Who Might Benefit.** A public health nurse is obligated to actively identify and reach out to all who might benefit from a specific activity or service.
7. **Promote Optimum Allocation of Resources.** Optimal use of available resources to assure the best overall improvement in the health of the population is a key element of the practice.
8. **Collaborate with Others in the Community.** Collaboration with a variety of other professions, populations, organizations, and other stakeholder groups is the most effective way to promote and protect the health of the people.

Adapted from American Nurses Association. (2007). *Public health nursing: Scope and standards of practice.* (pp. 7–9). Silver Spring, MD: Nursesbooks.org.

Principle 5: Promote a Healthful Environment

The fifth principle recognizes the importance of ensuring that people live in conditions conducive to health. Therefore, it is aligned with Nightingale's environmental theory of health. People are less likely to be healthy if they live in a community with high unemployment, crowded housing, and dirty air, or where it is difficult to obtain inexpensive, healthful food. They are also less likely to be healthy if the community's norms include acceptance or even encouragement of activities such as smoking, binge drinking, drug use, or unsafe sex. To change these conditions requires commitment, perseverance, patience, resourcefulness, and a long-range view.

Principle 6: Target All Who Might Benefit

The sixth principle involves outreach strategies to meet the obligation to serve all people who might benefit from an intervention. This tenet requires that the nurse examine policies or programs to determine whether they are accessible and acceptable to the entire population in need and advocate for change if necessary.

In one community, families with young children had a high (80%) rate of compliance with regulations requiring the use of infant and toddler car seats, but assessment revealed that more than 90% of the seats were being used incorrectly. For example, the harness straps were too loose, the seats were not properly installed, or the model used had been recalled because of safety problems. A coalition of community health nurses and law enforcement officials implemented a summer-long, monthly car seat checkup service in the parking lot of a local mall and advertised the service in a media campaign. In evaluating the program, the coalition acknowledged that the campaign had not affected the transport of children born after the intervention period had expired, nor residents who were out of town for the summer, nor had it increased the knowledge of car seat safety among expectant parents or the community in general.

The questions in Display 14.2 can help the nurse evaluate a planned program's success in reaching people who might benefit. These questions should guide the design, implementation, and evaluation of outreach strategies.

DISPLAY 14.2	DETERMINING WHETHER PROGRAMS SERVE INTENDED POPULATIONS

- Is the service offered in a manner that encourages utilization?
    - Are the services located conveniently?
    - Do the hours of the service fit with the work or school life of the people?
    - Are the services offered in a manner that is respectful of the values, beliefs, mores, and traditions of the people?
    - What kind of marketing strategies have been used to inform the people of the service?
- What is the satisfaction level of users of the service?
- Why are some people not using services?

Principle 7: Promote Optimum Allocation of Resources

The seventh principle addresses resource-allocation decisions. In most communities, the available resources are not sufficient to meet all the needs of all the people. The nurse must ensure that the community is using limited resources in ways that lead to the greatest improvement in health. To promote optimum allocation of resources, the nurse must

- Know the latest research on the effectiveness of various programs in addressing needs
- Collect information about the short- and long-term costs of programs
- Evaluate existing programs and policies for ways to improve or discontinue them
- Communicate this information to community decision makers, so that they can make resource-allocation decisions that are most likely to improve the community's health

Principle 8: Collaborate with Others in the Community

The eighth principle underscores the importance of collaboration with other nurses, health care providers, social workers, educators, spiritual leaders, business leaders, and government officials within the community. This interdisciplinary collaboration is essential to establish and maintain effective programs. Programs that are planned and implemented in isolation can lead to fragmentation, gaps, and overlaps in health services. For example, without collaboration, a well-child clinic may be started in a community that already has a strong developmental screening program but does not have community prenatal services. Without collaboration, programs may also fail to be effective. For instance, a Saturday-morning cardiovascular fitness program designed without consultation with spiritual leaders may be totally ineffective in a devout Jewish community, where members devote Saturdays to religious observances.

SOCIETAL INFLUENCES ON COMMUNITY-ORIENTED, POPULATION-FOCUSED NURSING

Society is constantly changing. The community health nurse needs to stay abreast of these changes for several reasons.

Social changes influence a community's health. Community health nurses need to continually adapt their strategies to respond to changing conditions. For example, increased international air travel means increased levels of communicable disease in a small city with a new international airport. Community health nurses in this city must be proactive in developing strategies to control the spread of communicable disease.

Social changes affect the availability of resources necessary to ensure that effective intervention strategies are available. For example, a downturn in the stock market may prompt closure of a community business that once generously supported local community services.

Contemporary community health nurses must be especially aware of the mutual interaction between nursing and technology. The term **technology** refers to the application of science to change processes of production or industry. Ideally, technologic innovations lead to improvements in processes for creating products or services. The 20th century was filled with technologic innovations that simultaneously disrupted old patterns of production and created new opportunities to increase production. Two technologic changes that are highly relevant to contemporary community health nursing are communication technology and genetic engineering.

Communication Technology

Changes in communication technology present new opportunities and challenges for community-oriented, population-focused care. Because of advances in satellite and telecommunications technology, communication is possible anywhere in the world where resources are available to purchase equipment and services. This means that a community health nurse, whether working in the Australian outback or at a public health clinic in Anchorage, Alaska, can contact clients, consultants, and agencies worldwide, if resources are available to take advantage of the technologies.

In addition, Internet technology has made it possible to access local, state, national, and international data for community assessment, planning, and evaluation. Nurses who require data for a new intervention strategy, for example, can search the Internet for information from consumer groups, researchers, and other experts worldwide. To keep apprised of emerging issues and trends in public health, the nurse can join numerous Internet-based electronic discussion groups or listservs (electronic discussions distributed by way of e-mail). The challenge to the nurse is to manage the volume of information and to weigh its worth.

Health care consumers face similar opportunities and challenges. Most diseases and disabilities can be researched online; information is available on the Internet, and consumers are increasingly searching the Net for health-related data. Certainly, the validity and reliability of information on the Internet vary widely. Research is needed to understand how people decide what information to use from the Internet, how they use it, and how its use affects their health. As health educators, community health nurses can provide guidelines to help people decide how to use health information found on the Internet (Display 14.3). Additionally, community health nurses need to

DISPLAY 14.3	DETERMINING WORTH OF HEALTH INFORMATION ON THE INTERNET

- What are the credentials and affiliation of the author?
- Is it easy to determine who is the publisher or sponsor of the web site? Evaluate how the publisher or sponsor might gain economically through your use of the information.
- Is the date of publication of the web site included? Is the information current?
- Are both sides of an issue described? Does the author discuss pros and cons of information presented?
- What references are included to substantiate the information in the article?

participate in studies to determine whether regulation of health information on the Internet is feasible and desirable.

At the same time, community health nurses need to be actively involved in creating their own Internet sites to provide health information specific to their targeted communities. Such sites can include interactive chat sessions, listserv discussions, and asynchronous communications in which community health nurses interact with community members to improve their health (Goldsmith, 2001).

The Internet is a superb vehicle for rapidly tracing the international spread of infectious diseases. For example, the World Health Organization has developed an Internet site for countries to report epidemiologic and laboratory data on influenza. The Centers for Disease Control and Prevention (CDC) offers current data on communicable diseases through the online publication, *Morbidity and Mortality Weekly Report.*

With so much technology at our finger tips, we often forget that not everyone has access to, or regularly uses the internet. A study by Rains (2008) supported the notion that younger, more educated individuals living in urban areas utilize the Internet at much higher rates than do other groups. Access to broadband (rather than dial-up connections) is one likely explanation. The public health nurse must be vigilant, so that access issues do not impede access to health information for the many poor and elderly clients who are less likely to have access to computers.

Genetics, Genomics, and Genetic Engineering

Genetics, the science of heredity and **genomics**, the study of the entire genome, are terms that have gained increased attention from nurses over the past decade. An outgrowth of this knowledge is **genetic engineering**, which can be defined as gene manipulation in a laboratory setting. The development of the field was made possible by the discovery of certain enzymes that can "cut" DNA from two or more different sources into pieces that can be recombined in a test tube. Gene manipulation also required the development of methods for inserting these recombinant DNA molecules into cells by the use of so-called *vectors* such as viruses.

Genetic engineering allows scientists to alter the herbicide-, pest-, and stress-resistance of crops and to increase the nutrition and attractiveness of the foods we eat. Genetic engineering also allows scientists to develop new kinds of medicines and to cure diseases by replacing absent or faulty genes. Mapping of the DNA sequence that makes up the "genetic blueprint" of human beings has provided new opportunities for protecting human health (Ellsworth & Manolio, 1999; Jenkins & Calzone, 2007). In addition to increasing understanding of the contribution of genetic material to health and disease, genetic research has created new opportunities for early identification, prevention, and treatment of people at risk for disease. For example, techniques for DNA screening of newborns allows early detection of risk for certain diseases and disabilities, thereby permitting early intervention. Genetic counseling, previously only available to a limited population, is being used increasingly by women in the preconception and prenatal periods (Dolan, Biermann, & Damus, 2007).

Despite the enthusiasm of many groups, especially commercial concerns, genetic engineering has generated much controversy. The controversy emerges from a number of different concerns. One concern is the inability to know for certain the long-term consequences of genetic alteration of foods or organisms such as bacteria, insects, or human beings. For example, the release of a genetically altered weed or insect could be catastrophic if that weed or insect reproduces prolifically and damages the ecosystem. Fears of negative effects of engineered gene transfers between species in genetically engineered food include allergic reactions, spread of diseases across crop species, and emergence of new diseases because of unpredictable mutations in the genetic code.

The Human Genome Project has opened dramatic possibilities for health and well-being, as well as creating ethical challenges in the near future. The potential scientific capacity to alter methods of human reproduction raises concerns about creating unintended consequences for the human race. Another source of concern is that science is "playing God." For some people, the possibility of being able to select the gender, intelligence, or eye color of a child raises concerns about interfering with nature and creates conflict with religious or ethical views. In addition, genetic screening could be used to deny rights and opportunities to people. For example, someone who is found to carry a gene that increases the risk for heart disease might be denied health insurance coverage. Another source of concern is the distrust many people have of government, large commercial enterprises, and the scientific community. Some people believe that they are not being told the truth about scientific or other issues. Because genetic alteration of food or humans can affect the survival of individuals, groups, or society as a whole, this distrust results in some strong opposition to any type of genetic engineering.

In dealing with these concerns, it is the community health nurse's responsibility to be aware of the latest scientific information when educating communities, so that the decisions made best fit the community's value system. Advocating for the highest scientific rigor in genetic engineering research is another important role of community health nurses. Community health nurses need to advocate for research that not only maps DNA but also identifies interventions that can change the outcome for people at risk for genetic disorders. Nurses need to balance what is good for the community as a whole against potential costs to people at risk, advocating for policies and regulations that ensure such a balance. Despite growing evidence of the need to establish essential nursing competencies in this area, Jenkins and Calzone (2007) note that "the relevance of genetics and genomics to nursing practice is not fully appreciated and many nurses still consider it a subspecialty that is not relevant to the entire profession" (p. 11).

Global Economy

Hundreds of years ago, the economies of communities were largely local. If drought led to a reduction in crop yield in one region, only that region and perhaps its closest neighbors would be affected. Since World War II, however, there has been a consistent trend toward international trade, investment, travel, and ownership of information and ideas (Moller, 1999). This increasingly **global economy** is evidenced by the creation of the European Economic Community and passage of the North American Free Trade Agreement. It has contributed to a strong economy for many developed nations, including the United States, but has also led to increased instability of all economies as problems in markets in distant countries affect markets worldwide.

This interrelationship was made clear after the terrorist attacks in the United States on September 11, 2001. Key markets in the world experienced downturns, as did the economies of the United States and other nations. The United States and other countries are still experiencing the effects of that day, compounded by the effects of the "war on terrorism." The toll worldwide—a dramatic increase in refugees and poverty, and the long-term expense of infrastructure repair and redevelopment—is further evidence that national economies are interrelated. Added to this stress on world economic health is the rising cost of fuels, predominately oil. As world economies grow, so too does their need for oil. Fueled by increasing demand and limited growth in production capacity, the price of a barrel of oil is no longer a discussion only on Wall Street, but on Main Street as well.

A global economy also permits rich countries in need of skilled workers to recruit them from developing countries, causing a shortage of skilled labor in those countries that need it most. In countries able to recruit labor, the presence of new immigrant groups may be seen as a threat to the local culture or economy, causing an increase in ethnic, racial, and religious tensions. Even people with jobs that pay well may react negatively because they see their world changing and their own future as more uncertain. At the same time, when citizens in developing nations perceive their country or its citizens as suffering unjustly because of unfair economic changes, there may be an increase in nationalism and even international terrorism.

More recently, the national economy has been impacted by a major decline in U.S. home values, precipitated by imprudent and possibly illegal lending practices by some residential mortgage lenders. The result has been thousands of home mortgage foreclosures, as families found they were unable to afford the escalating costs of mortgages with adjustable interest rates. With rising foreclosures, others who were continuing to pay their mortgages on time found their homes' values decreasing at an alarming rate, due in part to the large inventory of foreclosed houses in their neighborhoods. Fear that the housing market could decline further has kept many prospective buyers out of the market. The resulting impact on available and affordable rental properties is felt most by those with limited incomes. As more and more people compete for limited rental housing options, the prices rise accordingly. The impact on the international community of the U.S. housing decline is just starting to be realized.

Finally, the economic trends of the late 20th century have contributed to greater worldwide disparities in wealth, health, and *relative poverty,* a measurement of an individual's income against the average for the society in which that individual lives. In the United States, economic disparity has been fueled by increased demand for skilled workers and decreased demand for unskilled laborers. When the demand for skilled workers (e.g., software engineers) exceeds the supply, these workers can demand increased wages, resulting ultimately in increased costs for housing, health care, products, and services, even for those unskilled laborers whose wages have decreased proportionately.

Reducing income disparity and its numerous effects is a challenge for all people who work in service to humanity. Community health nurses have an obligation to read the latest research, so that they can better understand the relationship of poverty to health. At the same time, they need to advocate for policies that will reduce adverse effects of poverty and income disparities.

Migration

Migration is the act of moving from one region or country to another, either temporarily, seasonally, or permanently. Throughout history, people have migrated from place to place to seek improved opportunities or to escape intolerable conditions in their home countries. In the late 20th century and the early years of the 21st century, a dramatic increase occurred in the number of *refugees* who migrated from their homes to escape invasion, oppression, or persecution. We also saw an increased reliance on migrant farm workers, people who move from one region to another seasonally, following the crops.

The health care needs of migrants and migrant refugees are enormous. Environmental factors are a primary reason for compromised health, and include inadequate waste disposal, crowded and often unsanitary living conditions, lack of access to healthful foods, and air pollution from an increased concentration of vehicles used for moving refugees. The potential detriments to health associated with migration require that community health nurses ensure that surveillance systems able to detect emerging health problems are in place; programs to prevent health problems and treat existing conditions also need to be developed.

Terrorism and Bioterrorism

Terrorism is one way in which a small number of people who perceive that they have been unfairly treated can exert influence on a larger group or nation. Groups wishing to harm other countries need sophisticated skills and coordination for most conventional weapons. Terrorists may also use unconventional weapons when highly motivated such as flying planes into buildings, strapping bombs to their bodies, or hiding bombs in their shoes.

Some methods of bioterrorism may be even cheaper and easier to use. **Bioterrorism** is the use of living organisms, such as bacteria, viruses, or other organic materials, to harm or intimidate others, in order to achieve political ends. Some of the possible biologic agents used include *Bacillus anthracis,* smallpox virus, *Brucella,* and botulinum toxin (see Chapter 17).

Because of escalating concerns about bioterrorism, public health workers increasingly recognize the need for skills in dealing with a bioterrorist attack. They need to do the following (CDC, 2008):

◆ Ensure that adequate surveillance systems are in place for early detection.
◆ Educate emergency and other health personnel about symptoms, treatment, and prevention of further spread.
◆ Establish coordinated response plans with health and law-enforcement officials.

Perhaps more importantly, community health nurses need to be involved in primary prevention of bioterrorism through advocating for the elimination of biologic weapons and addressing the root causes of terrorism, such as poverty, hunger, poor housing, limited educational opportunities, lack of clean water, and inadequate or no health care.

Climate Changes

Climate changes can be considered societal changes because they may be influenced by economics. Since the Industrial Revolution, increased amounts of carbon dioxide, methane, and nitrous oxide created by manufacturing industries, automobile emissions, and consumer products have been introduced into the earth's atmosphere. These increases have contributed to climate changes that are expected to affect sea level; the production of food, fiber, and medicines; and the spread of infectious diseases. Conversely, significant increases in fuel efficiency and efforts to reduce pollution could avoid millions of deaths around the world. Population-focused nurses need to educate the public about the potential dangers of continuing to contaminate the environment and to advocate for changes in public policy that reduce air and water contaminants. Chapter 9 explores health-related environmental issues in detail.

Summary

Community health nursing is a community-oriented, population-focused nursing specialty that is based on interpersonal relationships. The unit of care is the community or population rather than the individual, and the goal is to promote healthy communities.

Theories and models of community health nursing aid the nurse in understanding the rationale behind community-oriented care. Florence Nightingale's environmental theory emphasizes the importance of improving environmental conditions to promote health. Orem's self-care model provides a framework, within which the community health nurse can promote a community's collective independence and self-care ability. Neuman's health care systems model describes the nurse's role as one of assisting clients to remain stable within their environment, whereas Rogers' model of the science of unitary man focuses on client–environment interaction and holistic health. King's Theory of Goal Attainment reminds us to work in partnership with clients to achieve the best health outcomes. Parse's Human Becoming Theory posits quality of life from each person's own perspective as the goal of nursing practice. Pender's model focuses on the promotion of health behaviors in people; the goal of nursing is to enhance the likelihood that people will engage in health-promoting behaviors by assessing and influencing perceptual and modifying factors. Roy's adaptation model describes the nurse's goal as one that promotes healthful coping mechanisms and adaptive responses to stressors. Salmon's construct for public health nursing prescribes education, engineering, and enforcement with individuals, families, communities, and nations. Finally, the models used in public health nursing practice, the Minnesota Intervention "Wheel," the Los Angeles County–Public Health Nursing Practice Model, and the Omaha System Model of the Problem Solving Process provide a mechanism for public health nurses to assess, plan, intervene, and evaluate the care they provide in their communities.

The eight principles of public health nursing applied to community health nursing provide a framework within which the nurse works to promote and protect the health of populations. They emphasize the primacy of prevention, the need for outreach, and the importance of working in collaboration for the greatest good of the greatest number of people.

Nurses need to anticipate and adapt to societal changes in order to fulfill their mission of promoting the health of all people. Contemporary societal influences on community health nursing include communication technology, genetic engineering, the global economy, migration, terrorism, and climate changes. ■

 ACTIVITIES TO PROMOTE CRITICAL THINKING

1. Interview a community health nursing director to determine what population-focused programs are offered in your locality. Explore nursing's role in the assessment, development, implementation, and evaluation of these programs. Discuss with the director how community health nurses might expand their population-focused interventions.

2. Describe a situation in community health nursing practice in which the use of an educational intervention would be most appropriate. Do the same with engineering and enforcement interventions. Discuss what made you match each situation with that intervention.

3. Assume you have been asked to make a home visit to a 75-year-old man, living alone, whose wife recently died. In addition to assessing his individual needs, what factors should you consider for assessment and intervention that would indicate an aggregate- or community-focused approach?

4. Select one of the societal influences on community or population. How would the theories or models for community health nursing practice that were discussed in this chapter guide your practice concerning that societal issue? Choose three models or theories to discuss.

5. Explore one of the societal influences on community or population using the Internet. Using the information in Display 14.3, try to determine the worth of the information available on several Internet sites.

References

Ailinger, R.L., Moore, J.B., Nguyen, N., & Lasus, H. (2006). Adherence to latent tuberculosis infection therapy among Latino immigrants. *Public Health Nursing, 23*, 307–313.

American Nurses Association. (2007). *Public health nursing: Scope and standards of practice.* Silver Spring, MD: Nursesbooks.org.

Andrews, H.A., & Roy, C. (1991). *The Roy adaptation model: The definitive statement.* Norwalk, CT: Appleton-Lange.

Bowles, K.H., & Naylor, M.D. (1996). Nursing intervention classification systems. Image. *Journal of Nursing Scholarship, 28*(4), 303–308.

Centers for Disease Control and Prevention. (2008). *CDC Emergency Preparedness and Response.* Retrieved June 2, 2008 from http://www.bt.cdc.gov/.

Conway, A.E., McClune, A.J., & Nosel, P. (2007). Down on the farm: Preventing farm accidents in children. *Pediatric Nursing, 33*(1), 45–48.

Dolan, S., Biermann, J., & Damus, K. (2007). Genomics for health in preconception and prenatal periods. *Journal of Nursing Scholarship, 39*, 4–9.

Ellsworth, D.L., & Manolio, T.A. (1999). The emerging importance of genetics in epidemiologic research. I. Basic concepts in human genetics and laboratory technology. *Annals of Epidemiology, 9*(1), 1–16.

Fan, L. (2008). Self-care behaviors of school-age children with heart disease. *Pediatric Nursing, 34*, 131–138.

Fawcett, J. (1989). *Analysis and evaluation of conceptual models of nursing,* 2nd ed. Philadelphia: F.A. Davis.

Gast, H.L., & Montgomery, K.S. (2005). Orem's model of self-care. In J.J. Fitzpatrick, & A.L. Whall (Eds.). *Conceptual models of nursing: Analysis and application,* 4th ed. (pp. 104–145). Upper Saddle River, NJ: Pearson Education, Inc.

Goldsmith, J. (2001). How will the Internet change our health system? In E.C. Hein (Ed.). *Nursing issues in the 21st century: Perspectives from the literature.* (pp. 295–308). Philadelphia: Lippincott Williams & Wilkins.

Hannon-Engel, S.L. (2008). Knowledge development: The Roy Adaptation Model and bulimia nervosa. *Nursing Science Quarterly, 21*, 126–132.

Hemphill, J.C., & Muth Quillin, S.I. (2005). Martha Rogers' model: Science of unitary beings. In J.J. Fitzpatrick, & A.L. Whall (Eds.). *Conceptual models of nursing: Analysis and application,* 4th ed. (pp. 247–272). Upper Saddle River, NJ: Pearson Education, Inc.

Jenkins, J., & Calzone, K.A. (2007). Establishing the essential nursing competencies for genetics and genomics. *Journal of Nursing Scholarship, 39*, 10–16.

Keller, L.O., Strohschein, S., Lia-Hoagberg, B., & Schaffer, M.A. (1998). Population-based public health interventions: A model from practice. *Public Health Nursing, 15*, 207–215.

Keller, L.O., Strohschein, S., Lia-Hoagberg, B., & Schaffer, M.A. (2004). Population-based public health interventions: Practice-based and evidenced-supported. Part I. *Public Health Nursing, 21*, 453–468.

Killeen, M.B., & King, I.M. (2007). Viewpoint: Use of King's conceptual system, nursing informatics, and nursing classification systems for global communication. *International Journal of Nursing Terminologies and Classifications, 18*(2), 51–57.

King, I.M. (1970). *Toward a theory for nursing.* New York: John Wiley & Sons.

King, I.M. (1981). *A theory for nursing: Systems, concepts, process.* Albany, NY: Delmar Publishers, Inc.

Li, H., & Shyu, Y.L. (2007). Coping processes of Taiwanese families during the postdischarge period for an elderly family member with hip fracture. *Nursing Science Quarterly, 20*, 273–279.

Los Angeles County, Department of Public Health. (2007). *Public health nursing practice model.* Retrieved June 2, 2008 from http://admin.publichealth.lacounty.gov/PHN/docs/NarrativePH-NModela2007.pdf.

Martin, K.S. (2005). *The Omaha System: A key to practice, documentation, and information management,* 2nd ed. St. Louis, MO: Elsevier.

Martin, K., Leak, G., & Aden, C. (1997). The Omaha System: A research-based model for decision making. In B.W. Spradley, & J.A. Allender (Eds.). *Readings in community health nursing,* 5th ed. (pp. 316–324). Philadelphia: Lippincott-Raven.

Messmer, P., & Palmer, J. (2008, First Quarter). In honor of Imogene M. King. *Refections on Nursing Leadership.* Retrieved May 25, 2008 from http://nursingsociety.org/RNL/Current/in_touch/tribute_king.html.

Minnesota Wheel. (2001). *Public health interventions.* Minneapolis, MN: Minnesota Department of Health,

Division of Community Health Services, Public Health Nursing Section.

Moller, J.O. (1999). The growing challenge to internationalism. *The Futurist, 33*(3), 22–27.

Morowatisharifabad, M.A., Ghofranipour, F., Heidarnia, A., et al. (2006). Self-efficacy and health promotion behaviors of older adults in Iran. *Social Behavior and Personality, 34,* 759–768.

Neuman, B. (1982). *The Neuman systems model: Application to nursing education and practice.* Norwalk, CT: Appleton-Lange.

Neuman, B., & Fawcett, J. (2002). *The Neuman systems model,* 4th ed. Upper Saddle River, NJ: Prentice Hall.

Nightingale, F. (1859/1992). *Florence Nightingale's notes on nursing* [Edited with an introduction, notes, and guide to identification by V. Skretkowicz]. London: Scutari Press.

Orem, D.E. (2001). *Nursing: Concepts of practice,* 6th ed. St Louis, MO: Mosby.

Parse, R.R. (1981). *Man-living-health: A theory of nursing.* New York: Wiley & Sons.

Parse, R.R. (1998). *The human becoming school of thought: A perspective for nurses and other health professionals.* Thousand Oaks, CA: Sage.

Pender, N.J., Murdaugh, C.L., & Parsons, M.A. (2006). *Health promotion in nursing practice,* 5th ed. Upper Saddle River, NJ: Pearson Education, Inc.

Rains, S.A. (2008). Health at high speed: Broadband internet access, health communication, and the digital divide. *Communication Research, 35,* 283–297.

Rogers, M. (1990). Nursing: Science of unitary, irreducible human beings: Update 1990. In E.A.M. Barrett (Ed.). *Visions of Rogers' science-based nursing.* (pp. 5–11). New York: National League for Nursing.

Roy, C., & Andrews, H.A. (1999). *The Roy adaptation model.* Stamford, CT: Appleton-Lange.

Saewyc, E.M., Solsvig, W., & Edinburgh, L. (2007). The Hmong youth task force: Evaluation of a coalition to address the sexual exploitation of young runaways. *Public Health Nursing, 25,* 69–76.

Sakamoto, S., & Avila, M. (2004). The public health nursing practice manual: A tool for public health nurses. *Public Health Nursing, 21,* 179–182.

Salmon, M.E. (1982). Construct for public health: Where is it practiced, in whose behalf, and with what desired outcome. *Nursing Outlook, 30*(9), 527–530. (Originally published under the author name Marla Salmon White.)

Salmon, M.E. (1993). Public health nursing: The opportunity of a century. *American Journal of Public Health, 83*(12), 1674–1675.

Shaner-McRae, H., McRae, G., & Jas, V. (2007). Environmentally safe health care agencies: Nursing's responsibility, Nightingale's legacy. *Online Journal of Nursing Issues, 12*(2),1.

Shields, L.E., & Lindsey, A.E. (1998). Community health promotion nursing practice. *Advances in Nursing Science, 20,* 23–36.

Shin, K.R., Kang, Y., Park, H.J., et al. (2008). Testing and developing the health promotion model in low-income, Korean elderly women. *Nursing Science Quarterly, 21,* 173–178.

Skalski, C.A., DiGerolamo, L., & Gigliotti, E. (2006). Stressors in five client populations: Neuman systems model-based literature review. *Journal of Advanced Nursing, 56,* 69–78.

Smith, K., & Bazini-Barakat, N. (2003). A public health nursing practice model: Melding public health principles with the nursing process. *Public Health Nursing, 20,* 42–48.

Srof, B.J., & Velsor-Friedrich, B. (2006). Health promotion in adolescents: A review of Pender's health promotion model. *Nursing Science Quarterly, 19,* 366–373.

Talley, B., Rushing, A., & Gee, R.M. (2005). Community assessment using Cowling's Unitary appreciative inquiry: A beginning exploration. *Visions: The Journal of Rogerian Nursing Science, 13*(1), 27–40. Retrieved May 25, 2008 from http://drtcbear.servebbs.net:81/Visions/.

Tomasson, R.E. (May 24, 1994). *Martha Rogers, 79, an author of books on nursing theory.* The New York Times. Retrieved June 1, 2008 from http://www.nytimes.com/.

Ume-Nwagbo, P.N., DeWan, S.A., & Lowry, L.W. (2006). Using the Neuman systems model for best practices. *Nursing Science Quarterly, 19,* 31–35.

Walker, L.O., & Avant, K.C. (2005). *Strategies for theory construction in nursing,* 4th ed. Upper Saddle River, NJ: Pearson Education, Inc.

Waweru, S.M., Reynolds, A., & Buckner, E.B. (2008). Perceptions of children with HIV/AIDS from the USA and Kenya: Self-concept and emotional indicators. *Pediatric Nursing, 34*(2), 117–124.

Webster's. (2004). *Webster's New World College Dictionary,* 4th ed. Cleveland, OH: Wiley.

Wilson, F.L, Baker, L.M., Nordstrom, C.K., & Legwand, C. (2008). Using the teach-back and Orem's self-care deficit nursing theory to increase childhood immunization communication among low-income mothers. *Issues in Comprehensive Pediatric Nursing, 31,* 7–22.

Zurakowski, T.L. (2005). In J.J. Fitzpatrick, & A.L. Whall (Eds.). *Conceptual models of nursing: Analysis and application,* 4th ed. (pp. 21–45). Upper Saddle River, NJ: Pearson Education, Inc.

Selected Readings

Avila, M., & Smith, K. (2003). The reinvigoration of public health nursing: Methods and innovations. *Journal of Public Health Management Practice, 9*(1), 16–24.

Esperat, C., Feng, D., Zhang, Y., & Owen, D. (2007). Health behaviors of low-income pregnant minority women. *Western Journal of Nursing Research, 29,* 284–300.

Frey, M.A. (2005). King's conceptual system and theory of goal attainment. In J.J. Fitzpatrick, & A.L. Whall (Eds.). *Conceptual models of nursing: Analysis and application,* 4th ed. (pp. 225–246). Upper Saddle River, NJ: Pearson Education, Inc.

Kartal, A., & Ozsoy, S.A. (2007). Validity and reliability study of the Turkish version of Health Belief Model Scale in diabetic patients. *International Journal of Nursing Studies, 44,* 1447–1458.

Keller, L.O., Strohschein, S., Schaffer, M.A., & Lia-Hoagberg, B. (2004). Population-based public health interventions in practice, teaching, and management. Part II. *Public Health Nursing, 21,* 469–487.

King, I.M. (2007). King's conceptual system, theory of goal attainment, and transaction process in the 21st century. *Nursing Science Quarterly, 20,* 109–116.

King, I.M. (2008). Adversity and theory development. *Nursing Science Quarterly, 21,* 137–138.

Los Angeles County Department of Public Health. (2006). *Public health nursing practice exercises.* Retrieved May 26, 2008 from http://www.lapublichealth.org/phn/phn_practice_exercises.htm.

McNaughton, D. (2005). A naturalistic test of Peplau's theory of home visiting. *Public Health Nursing, 22,* 429–438.

Neuman, B., & Reed, K.S. (2007). A Neuman Systems Model perspective on nursing in 2050. *Nursing Science Quarterly, 20,* 111–113.

Nme-Nwagbo, P.N., DeWan, S.A., & Lowry, L.W. (2006). Using the Neuman Systems Model for best practice. *Nursing Science Quarterly, 19,* 31–35.

Parse, R.R. (1999). Nursing science: The transformation of practice. *Journal of Advanced Nursing, 30,* 1383–1387.

Roy, C. (2008). Adversity and theory: The broad picture. *Nursing Science Quarterly, 21,* 138–139.

Roy, C., & Jones, D. (2007). *Nursing knowledge development and clinical practice.* New York: Springer Publishing.

Swenson, M.J., Salmon, M.E., Wold, J., & Sibley, L. (2005). Addressing the challenges of the global nursing community. *International Nursing Review, 52*, 173–179.

U.S. Department of Health and Human Services (USDHHS). (2001). *Healthy people in healthy communities: A community planning guide using Healthy People 2010*. Washington, D.C.: U.S. Government Printing Office. Retrieved May 25, 2008 from http://www.healthypeople.gov/Publications/.

Wood, M.E. (2008). Theoretical framework to study exercise motivation for breast cancer risk reduction. *Oncology Nursing Forum, 35*(1), 89–95.

World Health Organization (WHO). (2002). *Healthy villages: A guide for communities and community health workers*. Geneva, Switzerland: Author. Retrieved May 25, 2008 from http://www.who.int/water_sanitation_health/hygiene/settings/hvintro.pdf.

Internet Resources

AACN'S Institutional Data Systems and Research Center (IDS): *http://www.aacn.nche.edu/IDS/index.htm*

Department of Public Health Nursing Administration: *http://admin.publichealth.lacounty.gov/PHN/whatphn.htm*

Interagency Council on Information Resources for Nursing (ICIRN): *http://icirn.org*

Minnesota *http://dhfs.wisconsin.gov/phnc/index.htm*

National League for Nursing: *http://www.nln.org*

Neuman Systems Model: *http://neumansystemsmodel.org/*

NurseScribe—Nursing Theory Page: *http://www.enursescribe.com/nurse_theorists.htm*

Nursing Theory & Theorists (Flinders University): *http://www.lib.flinders.edu.au/resources/sub/healthsci/a-zlist/nursingtheory.html*

Omaha System: *http://www.omahasystem.org/*

Sr. Calista Roy—Professor and Nurse Theorist at the William F. Connell School of Nursing at Boston College: *http://www.bc.edu/schools/son/faculty/theorist.html*

The Nursing Theory Page (Hahn School of Nursing, University of San Diego): *http://www.sandiego.edu/ACADEMICS/nursing/theory/*

Theory Art Gallery—Understanding the Work of Nurse Theorists, a Creative Beginning: *http://nursing.jbpub.com/sitzman/artgallery.cfm*

Visions—The Journal of Rogerian Nursing Science: *http://drtcbear.servebbs.net:81/visions/*

Welcome to Nursing Theories A–Z: *http://www.nurses.info/nursing_theory.htm*

15

Community as Client: Applying the Nursing Process

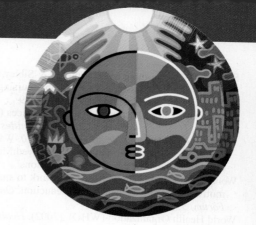

LEARNING OBJECTIVES

Upon mastery of this chapter, you should be able to:

◆ Describe the characteristics of a healthy community.

◆ Describe the meaning of community as client.

◆ Articulate three specific considerations of each of the three dimensions of the community as client.

◆ Explain methods the community health nurse might use to interact with the community.

◆ Discuss methods of community needs assessment.

◆ Compare and contrast five types of community needs assessment.

◆ Delineate five sources of community data.

◆ Describe the role of the community health nurse as a catalyst for community development.

"A community needs a soul if it is to become a true home for human beings. You, the people, must get it this soul."

—Pope John Paul II (1920–2005)

KEY TERMS

Assets assessment
Coalition
Community as client
Community development
Community diagnoses
Community needs assessment
Community subsystem assessment
Comprehensive assessment
Descriptive epidemiologic study
Evaluation
Familiarization assessment
Goals
Implementation
Interaction
Key informants
Location variables
Objectives
Outcome criteria
Partnerships
Planning
Population variables
Priority setting
Problem-oriented assessment
Social class
Social system variables
Survey
Windshield survey

Although community health nursing practice involves the care of individuals, families, and groups, the care of communities is vital to promoting health and preventing disease. The terms community health nurse and public health nurse (PHN) will be used synonymously in this chapter as both roles require specialized knowledge and skills to work with populations. The American Public Health Association (APHA) (1996) defines public health nursing as "the practice of promoting and protecting the health of populations using knowledge from nursing, social, and public health sciences" (p. 1).

The term community has been well defined in the nursing literature. A community is a collection of people interacting with one another because of geography, common interests, characteristics, or goals. These interactions include social institutions, such as schools, government agencies, and social services. The concept of **community as client** refers to a group or population of people as the focus of nursing service (Anderson & McFarlane, 2004). Understanding the concept of the community as client is a prerequisite for effective service at every level of community nursing practice, as described in Chapter 1. It is this population-focused practice that distinguishes community health nursing from other nursing specialties (APHA, 2003; Williams, 1977). The Quad Council of Public Health Nursing Organizations, building on the work of the Council on Linkages Between Academia and Public Health Practice (COL) developed a list of "Core Competencies for Public Health Nurses." These competencies help clarify the role of the community health nurse within the context of community as client (Quad Council, 2003). See Display 15.1.

DISPLAY 15.1 — QUAD COUNCIL CORE COMPETENCIES OF PUBLIC HEALTH NURSING

1. **Analytic Assessment Skills.** Define a problem, select and define relevant variables, identify sources of appropriate data and information, identify gaps in data, partner with community to assess meaning of data, make relevant inferences from data, interpret risk and benefits for community, recognize overall public health issues and ethical, scientific, economic, and political implications.

2. **Policy Development and Program Planning Skills.** Collect and interpret relevant information regarding a specific issue; write policy statements; identify, interpret, and implement policies, laws, and regulations specific to programs; determine feasibility and expected outcomes of policy options; decide on appropriate course of action; develop action plan to implement policy; translate policies into organizational structures and programs, including monitoring and evaluation components to determine effectiveness and quality.

3. **Communication Skills.** Communicate effectively; solicit individual and organizational input; serve as advocate for public health programs and resources; lead and participate in groups to address specific needs and issues; use the media, technology, and community networks to disseminate information; effectively present information to professional and lay audiences; listen to others in an unbiased manner, respecting others' viewpoints; promote expression of diverse perspectives and opinions.

4. **Cultural Competency Skills.** Interact professionally and effectively with persons from diverse cultures, socioeconomic, educational, and racial/ethnic backgrounds, as well as with persons of different lifestyle preferences and ages; utilize culturally, socially, and behaviorally appropriate methods of delivering public health services; appreciate the importance of a diverse public health workforce.

5. **Community Dimensions of Practice Skills.** Establish and maintain linkages with key stakeholders; build partnerships in the community through the use of team building, leadership, conflict resolution, and negotiation; collaborate with community partners in promoting population health; identify operations of public and private community organizations; engage effectively with the community; develop, implement, and evaluate community public health assessments; understand government's role in the delivery of community health services.

6. **Basic Public Health Sciences Skills.** Identify individual and organizational responsibilities related to essential public health services and core functions; define, assess, and understand the health status of populations, determinants of health and illness, factors that contribute to disease prevention, health promotion, and the use of health services; understand the historical development of public health; apply basic public health sciences (e.g., social and behavioral sciences, epidemiology and biostatistics, environmental health, prevention of infectious and chronic diseases, injuries); identify and retrieve current relevant scientific evidence and understand the limitations of research; develop a lifelong commitment to critical thinking.

7. **Financial Planning and Management Skills.** Develop and present a budget; manage programs within budget constraints; monitor program performance; determine budget priorities; prepare proposals for external funding sources; apply basic human relations skills in managing organizations, motivating personnel, and resolving conflicts; manage collection, retrieval, and use of data for decision making; negotiate and develop contracts and other documents for population-based services; conduct cost–benefit, cost-effectiveness, and cost–utility studies.

8. **Leadership and Systems Thinking.** Create a culture of ethnical standards within communities and organizations; help create key values and shared vision and use these principles to guide actions; identify internal and external issues that could impact essential public health service delivery; facilitate collaboration with internal and external groups to facilitate participation of key stakeholders; promote organizational and team learning; contribute to development, implementation, and monitoring of organizational performance standards; use legal and political system to effect change.

Adapted from Quad Council (2003, April 3). Quad Council PHN competencies. Retrieved from http://www.resourcecenter.net/image/ACHNE/Files/Final_PHN_competencies.pdf.

WHAT IS A HEALTHY COMMUNITY?

What is a healthy community? Just as health for an individual is relative and will change, all communities exist in a relative state of health. A community's health can be seen within the context of health being more than the absence of disease, and "includes those elements that enable people to maintain a high quality of life and productivity" (USDHHS, 2001). A key vision for healthy communities is presented in *Healthy People 2010*, the national health promotion and disease prevention agenda published by the U.S. Department of Health and Human Services (USDHHS). *Healthy People 2010* presents two overarching goals for the health of the nation: to increase quality and years of healthy life and to eliminate health disparities (USDHHS, 2000). "These two goals are supported by specific objectives in 28 focus areas. Each objective was developed with a target to be achieved by the year 2010" (¶ 2). (See Chapter 1 describing *Healthy People 2010*.) These objectives and targets provide guidelines for communities to follow to promote the health of their members USDHHS, n.d. "Motivating individuals to act on just one of the indicators can have a profound effect on increasing the quality and years of healthy life and on eliminating health disparities—for the individual, as well as the community overall" (USDHHS, 2001, ¶ 4).

DIMENSIONS OF THE COMMUNITY AS CLIENT

The health of a community can be characterized through a number of perspectives. One such view is by examining three dimensions: status, structure, and process (Shuster & Goeppinger, 2004).

Status is the most common measure of the health of a community. It typically comprises morbidity and mortality data identifying the physical, emotional, and social determinants of health. Physical and social indices include vital statistics, leading causes of death and illness, suicide rates, and rates of drug and alcohol addiction. Social determinants can be identified by crime rates and functional ability level, or by high school dropout rates or average income levels.

Structure of a community refers to its services and resources. Adequacy and appropriateness of health services can be determined by examining patterns of use, number and types of health and social services, and quality measures. Classification as a medically underserved area is indicative of a lack of sufficient health care providers (e.g., nurses, physicians, dentists). Demographic data, such as socioeconomic and racial distribution, age, gender, and educational level, are also important indicators of community structure. These measures provide key information and correlate to health status.

Process reflects the community's ability to function effectively. In a classic work, Cottrell (1976) describes *community competency* as a key component to the process dimension. Just as nurses assess the strengths and limitations of clients when working with individuals, the community health nurse must assess the strengths and limitations of the community when working with the community as client. Strengths must be enhanced and limitations addressed to achieve agreed-upon goals. Characteristics of a competent community follow. A competent community can:

- ◆ Collaborate effectively in identifying community needs and problems

- ◆ Achieve a working consensus on goals and priorities
- ◆ Agree on ways and means to implement the agreed-upon goals
- ◆ Collaborate effectively to take the required actions.

These characteristics will be discussed in more detail later in the discussion on "Planning to Meet the Health Needs of the Community." See Chapter 1 for more information on healthy communities.

Addressing community health by examining the process in addition to the structure and status dimensions provides a broader view into the complexities of community health and community actions for change. It is key to examine not only the individual components of the community, but also the sum of all the parts—*the whole*—including interactions among all the constituents (Schulte, 2000).

Another perspective identifies the community as having three features: a location, a population, and a social system. Figure 15.1 presents a visual interpretation of this perspective. Each of these features has several components that need to be addressed and represents further information that must be collected and analyzed when assessing the health of a community. These are detailed in Tables 15.1, 15.2, and 15.3.

Location

Every physical community carries out its daily existence in a specific geographic location. The health of a community is affected by location, because placement of health services, geographic features, climate, plants, animals, and the human-made environment are intrinsic to geographic location. The location of a community places it in an environment that offers resources and also poses threats (Skelly, et al., 2002; Neuman & Fawcett, 2001). The healthy

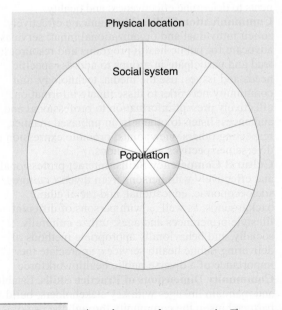

FIGURE 15.1　Three features of a community. The community has (1) a physical location, represented here by the square boundary; (2) a population, shown here by the central circle; and (3) a social system, divided here into subsystems.

community is one that makes wise use of its resources and is prepared to meet threats and dangers. In assessing the health of any community, it is necessary to collect information not only about variables specific to location but also about relationships between the community and its location. Do groups cooperate to identify threats? Do health agencies cooperate to prepare for an emergency such as a flood or earthquake? Does the community make certain that its members are given available information about resources and dangers? Table 15.1 describes the location perspective of the Community Profile Inventory, including the six **location variables**: community boundaries, location of health services, geographic features, climate, flora and fauna, and the human-made environment.

Community Boundaries

To talk about the community in any sense, one must first describe its boundaries (Tatalovich, Wilson, Milam, Jerrett, & McConnell, 2006). Measurements of wellness and illness within a community depend on defining the outer geographic limits of the unit under consideration (Chappell, Funk, & Allan, 2006). Nurses need to be clear, for example, that a target community of the elderly includes a description of age and location (e.g., all persons age 65 and older in a given city or county). Some communities are distinctly separate, such as an isolated rural town, whereas others are closely situated to one another, such as the suburbs of a large metropolis. Therefore, it is important for the

TABLE 15.1   Community Profile Inventory: Location Perspective

Location Variables	Community Health Implications	Community Assessment Questions	Information Sources
Boundary of community	Community boundaries serve as basis for measuring incidence of wellness and illness, and for determining spread of disease.	Where is the community located? What is its boundary? Is it a part of a larger community? What smaller communities does it include?	(For all—various Internet sites) Atlas State maps County maps City maps Telephone book City directory Public library
Location of health services	Use of health services depends on availability and accessibility.	Where are the major health institutions located? What necessary health institutions are outside the community? Where are they?	Telephone book Chamber of commerce State health department County or local health departments Maps Public library
Geographic features	Injury, death, and destruction may be caused by floods, earthquakes, volcanoes, tornadoes, or hurricanes. Recreational opportunities at lakes, seashore, mountains promote health and fitness.	What major landforms are in or near the community? What geographic features pose possible threats? What geographic features offer opportunities for healthful activities?	Atlas Chamber of commerce Maps State health department Public library
Climate	Extremes of heat and cold affect health and illness. Extremes of temperature and precipitation may tax community's coping ability.	What are the average temperature and precipitation? What are the extremes? What climatic features affect health and fitness? Is the community prepared to cope with emergencies?	Weather atlas Chamber of commerce State health department Maps Local government Weather bureau Public library
Flora and fauna	Poisonous plants and disease-carrying animals can affect community health. Plants and animals offer resources as well as dangers.	What plants and animals pose possible threats to health?	State health department Poison control center Police department Emergency rooms Encyclopedia Public library
Human-made environment	All human influences on environment (housing, dams, farming, type of industry, chemical waste, air pollution, and so forth) can influence levels of community wellness.	What are the major industries? How have air, land, and water been affected by humans? What is the quality of housing? Do highways allow access to health institutions?	Chamber of commerce Local government City directory State health department University research reports Public library

nurse to know the nature of each location and explicitly define its boundaries.

Location of Health Services

If the members of a town must travel 200 miles to the nearest clinic or dental office, the health of the community will be affected. When assessing a community, the community health nurse needs to identify the major health centers and know where they are located (Schulte, 2000). For example, an alcoholism treatment center for indigent alcoholics was located 30 miles outside one city. This location presented transportation problems and profoundly affected the willingness of clients to voluntarily seek treatment and the length of time they remained at the center. If a well-baby clinic is located on the edge of a high-crime district, parents may be deterred from using it. It is often enlightening to plot the major health institutions, both inside and outside the community, on a map that shows their proximity and relationship to the community as a whole.

Geographic Features

Communities have been constructed in every conceivable physical environment, and environment certainly can affect the health of a community (see Chapter 9). A healthy community is one that takes into consideration the geography of its location, identifies possible problems and likely resources, and responds in an adaptive fashion (Neuman & Fawcett, 2001). For example, both Anchorage, Alaska, and San Francisco, California, are located on a geologic fault line and subject to major earthquakes. In such places, the health of the community is determined, in part, by its preparedness for an earthquake and its ability to cope and respond quickly when such a crisis occurs. In Ontario, Canada, a series of lakes called the Lac la Croix is a valuable food resource for Ojibway Indian communities because they depend on fish from the lakes for their livelihood. Over the years, acid rain generated from coal-burning power plants in the United States and Canada has begun to affect the lakes and the fish, thus contaminating a major food supply of the Ojibway communities. In another example, naturally occurring high levels of arsenic are found in the ground and surface water and are linked to diarrheal illness among the people living in the Kanker District of India (Pandey, Sharma, Roy, Roy, & Pandey, 2006). Although this is not a human-made hazard that can be controlled by compliance with environmental regulations, it must be addressed in order to prevent disease.

Climate

The climate also has a direct influence on the health of a community (Dixon, 2002; Knowlton et al., 2007). When Buffalo, New York, is blanketed with deep winter snows, members of the community sometimes are immobilized for days. Deaths from coronary occlusion increase as people attempt to shovel their sidewalks and uncover their cars. Falls in the elderly have been associated with colder climate (Stevens, Thomas, & Sogolow, 2007). The intense summer heat of a location such as Phoenix, Arizona, can create many health problems (e.g., heat stroke, heat exhaustion). Asthma and other lung diseases are exacerbated in the Central San Joaquin Valley of California because the area is surrounded by mountains that create an air inversion, trapping vehicle and agricultural by-products in what can be described as a "large bowl" and causing smog during many months of the year. In Costa Rica, higher asthma prevalence has been linked to the warm, humid, tropical weather and the presence of mites and cockroach allergens (Soto-Quiros, Soto-Martinez, & Hanson, 2002). Skin cancer incidence is associated with unprotected sun exposure, which increases the risk for people who live in warm, sunny regions (Saraiya, Glanz, Briss, Nichols, & White, 2003).

A healthy community encourages physical activity among its members, but the climate affects this activity. Although long, cold winters can restrict activity, one community, St. Paul, Minnesota, holds an annual Winter Carnival. Sporting events, parades, ice sailing, dogsledding, a treasure hunt, and hot air balloon races bring thousands of Minnesotans outdoors at a time when they might otherwise be confined by the weather.

Flora and Fauna

Plant and animal populations in a community are often determined by location. The way a community responds to these populations, whether wild or domesticated, can affect the health of the community. The asthma study, mentioned earlier, not only dealt with climate, but also with the preponderance of tropical plants and animals and the high exposure to mites and cockroaches (Soto-Quiros et al., 2002). Poison oak, ivy, and sumac can be found across the United States, and these plants produce an allergic contact dermatitis in many people who come in contact with it (Gladman, 2006). In the Sierra foothill communities of central California, black widow and tarantula spiders, scorpions, and rattlesnakes are resident populations that pose potential health threats. The poison from a single bite may cause injury or death (Diaz, 2005). In the south-central Midwest, the bite of the brown recluse spider injects a toxin that can lead to necrotic skin ulcers as well as systemic symptoms (Rhoads, 2007). In the Northeast and Midatlantic states, increased deer populations—and consequently deer ticks—bring with them an increased incidence of Lyme disease.

The community health nurse needs to know about the major sources of danger from plants and animals affecting the community under study. Are there community agencies that provide educational information about these dangers? Does the populace understand their significance? Are emergency services, such as a poison control center, available to community members?

Human-Made Environment

Every community is located in the midst of an environment created and transformed by human ingenuity. People build houses and factories, dump wastes into streams or vacant lots, fill the air with gases, and build dams to control streams. All of these human alterations of the environment have important implications for community health (Sattler & Lipscomb, 2003). A community health nurse might improve the health of a community by working for legislation to prevent disposal of waste chemicals into water or landfills. Such legislation might have prevented the disaster at Love Canal in New York state, where groundwater contaminated with toxic wastes continued to seep into residential areas for many years, severely affecting the community's health and spurring community activism that led to the creation of the federal Superfund program to clean up areas with hazardous wastes (Brown & Clapp, 2002).

Population

When one considers the community as the client, examining the health status of the total population in a given community is a critical component. Population consists not of a specialized aggregate, but of all the diverse people who live within the boundaries of the community.

The health of any community is greatly influenced by the attributes of its population. Various features of the population suggest health needs and provide a basis for health planning (Oleske, 2001; Hutchings, Raine, Brady, Wildman, & Rowan, 2004). A healthy community has leaders who are aware of the population's characteristics, know its various needs, and respond to those needs. Community health nurses can better understand any community by knowing about its **population variables**: size, density, composition, rate of growth or decline, cultural characteristics, social class structure, and mobility. Table 15.2 presents the population perspective section of the Community Profile Inventory.

Size

The town of Dover, Delaware, with approximately 35,000 people, and the city of Los Angeles, California, with around 4 million people, have radically different health problems. If a single case of *Salmonella* poisoning occurred in Dover, health officials would probably quickly learn of it. It would be relatively easy to trace the course, check the few restaurants in town, and interview people about sanitation practices. However, many cases might occur in Los Angeles without the health department's knowledge. Moreover, once the cases were discovered, tracing the source of contamination might involve a long and complicated search. This is only one small way in which population size can affect the health of a community. The size of a community also influences the presence of inadequate housing, the heterogeneity of the population, and almost every conceivable aspect of health needs and services. Knowing a community's size provides community health nurses with important information for planning. See Chapter 29 for issues related to rural and urban health of populations.

Density

In some communities, thousands of people are crowded into high-rise apartment buildings. In others, such as farm communities, people live at great distances from one another. The full impact of living in high-density communities is being researched, and some research has already shown that crowding affects individual and community health. Motor vehicle exhaust from highways has been shown to be associated with higher risk of asthma and reduced lung function in children, as well as higher pulmonary and cardiac mortality in adults (Brugge, Durant, & Rioux, 2007). Fine particulate matter in urban areas is linked to higher rates of hospital admissions (Dominici et al., 2006). When compared with rural populations, urban populations in Ireland have a higher incidence of lung cancer and respiratory disease, thought to be associated with higher air pollution levels (O'Reilly, O'Reilly, Rosato, & Connolly, 2007). A Michigan study found that urban residents had higher risk of mortality when compared with rural residents, even when health and sociodemographic variables were controlled (House et al., 2000).

A low-density community, however, may have problems. When people are spread out, health care provision can become difficult. There may not be enough resources in the form of taxes to support public health services. Rural communities often suffer from inadequate distribution of health care personnel, including private physicians and community health nurses. A large national survey indicated that rural residents reported fewer visits with their health care provider than those living in urban areas (Larson & Fleishman, 2003). A Canadian study found that "rural residents are increasingly less likely to receive personal care assistance" (Forbes & Janzen, 2004, p. 227). Other rural health risks include greater rates of injuries from traffic accidents (Tiesman, Zwerling, Peek-Asa, Sprince, & Cavanaugh, 2007) and illnesses related to agricultural pesticide exposure (Calvert et al., 2004)

A healthy community takes into consideration the density of its population. It organizes to meet the differing needs created by its density levels (e.g., it recognizes differences in density between the inner city and the suburbs and allocates services accordingly). See Chapter 29 for more on health risks specific to rural and urban areas.

Composition

Communities differ in the types of people who live within their boundaries. A retirement community in Florida whose members are mostly older than age 65 has one set of interests and concerns, whereas a city with a large number of women in their childbearing years will have another set of concerns. A healthy community is one that takes full account of its constituents and provides for their differences. Age, sex, educational level, occupation, and many other demographic variables affect health concerns (Smedley, Stith, & Nelson, 2003). In communities with a high proportion of low-income families, considerations must be made to accommodate the needs of the poor (Kumanyika & Grier, 2006). Occupation can also affect health. For example, in a town where 75% of the workers are employed in a textile mill, the community lives with the threat of brown lung disease, which is caused by cotton dust. In areas where tobacco is the main source of income and a large proportion of the population is engaged in its production, green tobacco sickness—or acute nicotine poisoning—is a concern because workers can absorb nicotine through the skin, and precautions must be taken to prevent this from happening (McKnight & Spiller, 2005). Understanding a community's composition is an important early step in determining its level of health.

TABLE 15.2 Community Profile Inventory: Population Perspective

Population Variables	Community Health Implications	Community Assessment Questions	Information Sources
Size	The number of people influences number and size of health care institutions. Size affects homogeneity of the population and its needs.	What is the population of the community? Is it an urban, suburban, or rural community?	(For all—various Internet sites) State health department Census data Maps City or town officials Chamber of commerce
Density	Increased density may increase stress. High and low density often affect the availability of health services.	What is the density of the population per square mile?	Census data State health department
Composition	Composition of the population often determines types of health needs.	What is the age composition of the community? What is the sex composition of the community? What is the marital status of community members? What occupations are represented and in what percentages?	Census data State health department Chamber of Commerce U.S. Department of Labor Statistics
Rate of growth or decline	Rapidly growing communities may place excessive demands on health services. Marked decline in population may signal a poorly functioning community.	How has population size changed over the past two decades? What are the health implications of this change?	Census data State health department
Cultural differences	Health needs vary among sub-cultural and ethnic populations. Utilization of health services varies with culture. Health practices and extent of knowledge are affected by culture.	What is the ethnic breakdown of population? What racial groups are represented? What subcultural populations exist in the community? Do any of the subcultural groups have unique health needs and practices? Are different ethnic and cultural groups included in health planning?	Census data State health department Social and cultural research reports Human rights commission City government Health planning boards
Social class	Class differences influence the utilization of health services. Class composition influences cost of public health services.	What percentage of the population falls into each social class? What do class differences suggest for health needs and services?	State health department Census data Sociological reports
Mobility	Mobility of the population affects continuity of care. Mobility affects availability of service to highly mobile populations.	How frequently do members move into and out of the community? How frequently do members move within the community? Are there any specific populations, such as migrant workers, that are highly mobile? How does the pattern of mobility affect the health of the community? Is the community organized to meet the health needs of mobile groups?	State health department Census data Health agencies serving migrant workers Farm labor offices Program serving transients and the homeless

(continued)

TABLE 15.2   Community Profile Inventory: Population Perspective (*Continued*)

Population Variables	Community Health Implications	Community Assessment Questions	Information Sources
Poverty Level	Economic disparities may lead to health disparities.	What percentage of the population is below federal poverty levels? How many children qualify for free or reduced cost school lunch?	Census data State data Local data (schools)
Education level	Education disparities may lead to health disparities.	What percentage of the population has less than high school education? What is the literacy rate?	State data Local data (schools)
Unemployment rate	Health insurance is often tied to employment. Lack of regular income can be a family stressor. Both can lead to health disparities.	What is the rate of unemployment? How variable is this rate?	U.S. Department of Labor State data Local data
Population by age	A high proportion of children and elderly can overburden health care and social systems.	What is the dependency ratio? Has this rate changed dramatically? What is the trend?	Census data State data Local data
Health status	Community members' status relative to the 10 Leading Health Indicators can impact overall community health.	What is the rate of obesity/overweight? What are the rates of tobacco use and substance abuse? What is the immunization rate? What are rates of injury and violence? What are the STD and HIV/AIDS rates?	State data Local data CDC data Vital Statistics—Numbers of births, deaths, marriages, and infant mortality rate. (Compare local to state data; state to national data.)
Environmental health status	Poor environmental health (e.g. presence of coliform bacteria in well water, toxic chemicals or poor air quality) can lead to increased incidence of communicable or chronic diseases.	What are rates of communicable or chronic diseases (e.g., *E. coli* infections, asthma)? What is the Toxic Release Inventory?	CDC data State data Local data

Rate of Growth or Decline

Community populations change over time. Some grow rapidly. The unparalleled recent growth of Las Vegas, Nevada, as a popular place to live has placed extreme demands on the environment, along with the provision of health care and other services. Other populations may experience a decline because of economic change, for example those areas of the United States where steel manufacturing has declined (Aeppel, 2007). Any significant fluctuation in population size can affect the health of the community. As people leave to find new employment or better living conditions, consumption of goods and services drops. Community morale may suffer, and community leadership may decline. Even a stable community can have problems (e.g., members may resist needed change because they notice little fluctuation in their population; commercial and residential properties may be abandoned or left vacant).

Cultural Characteristics

A community may be composed of a single cultural group, such as Ojibway Indians on their reservation in Wisconsin, or it may be made up of many cultures or subcultures. For instance, if a city has a large Hispanic population, along with a group of Native Americans living in the inner city and a cluster of Vietnamese refugees, the cultural differences among these members will influence the health of the community. These differences can create conflicting or competing demands for resources and services or create intergroup hostility. A healthy community is aware of such cultural differences and acts to promote understanding among cultural subgroups (Spector, 2009).

Social Class and Educational Level

Social class refers to the ranking of groups within society by income, education, occupation, prestige, or a combination of these factors. There is no absolute agreement on income levels or other criteria to designate social class categories (upper, middle, lower), other than the government formula used to compute poverty level (U.S. Department of Health & Human Services, 2007). Although class distinctions are not clearly defined, class rankings based on occupation, education, and wealth (income plus assets) seem to correlate with many different social patterns and are used frequently in research (Cargan, 2007). Occupational level, in particular, has historically and consistently proven to be a reliable measure, with surprisingly similar rankings among all societies for which data exist (Adcock & Brown, 1957). This classic research has shown that people with higher occupational levels generally have higher incomes and education, exert greater political influence, and are more highly esteemed by others.

Healthy People 2010 identified the relationship between education, income, and health status:

> "Inequalities in income and education underlie many health disparities in the United States . . . in general, population groups that suffer the worst health status also are those that have the highest poverty rates and the least education. Disparities in income and education levels are associated with differences in the occurrence of illness and death, including heart disease, diabetes, obesity, elevated blood lead level, and low birth weight. Higher incomes permit increased access to medical care, enable people to afford better housing and live in safer neighborhoods, and increase the opportunity to engage in health-promoting behaviors" (USDHHS, 2000, p.12).

Typically, health promotion and preventive health services are most needed by low-income groups and people with fewer years of education, although a good number of community residents will benefit from community health efforts (Clark, 2002).

It is generally known that different social classes have different health problems, as well as a variety of resources for coping with illness and diverse ways of using health services. A healthy community recognizes these differences and creates health care services to meet these varied needs.

Mobility

Americans are a mobile population; between 2002 and 2003, more than 40 million residents moved (Population Reference Bureau, 2005). People move to go to college, take a new job, join other family members or friends, or seek a new climate after retirement. This mobility has a direct effect on the health of communities (Dong et al., 2005). If the population turnover is extensive, continuity of services may suffer. Leadership for improving the health of the community may change so frequently that concerted action becomes difficult. High turnover may necessitate special attention to health education about local conditions.

Population groups may arrive and depart in seasonal swings; fluctuations in the number of migrant farm workers, tourists, or college students can affect a community. Border health issues are of special concern, as people continually move across borders, bringing with them health issues such as communicable diseases (National Latino Research Center, 2004). Immigrants and refugees may represent a significant population subgroup in many areas of a country, and public health officials must meet their unique needs. The community health nurse also needs to identify those populations that are seasonally mobile. These subgroups present special health needs and place an added burden on a community (e.g., migrant workers). If a town of 3,000 people has an annual influx of 10,000 students who disappear in the summer, residents must prepare to meet this population instability. The small towns of the San Juan Islands in Puget Sound, Washington, can command such high prices for accommodations in the summer that some low-income, year-round residents camp in tents during those months because they are unable to pay the high rents. Thus, the lives of many families are disrupted each year. A healthy community neither ignores nor overreacts to this kind of mobility. Rather, it identifies the nature of the population change, determines the needs created by such change, and organizes to meet those needs.

Social System

In addition to location and population, every community has a third feature—a social system. The various parts of a community's social system that interact and influence the health of a community are called **social system variables**. These variables include health, family, economic, educational, religious, welfare, political, recreational, legal, and communication. Whether assessing a community's health, developing new services for the mentally ill within the community, or promoting the health of the elderly, the community health nurse needs to understand the community as a social system. A community health nurse working in a tiny village in Alaska needs to understand and work with the social system of that village no less than a nurse practicing in New York City. Table 15.3 guides the nurse in assessing a community's social system variables.

The Concept of a Social System

A social system is an abstract concept and can be more readily understood by first considering the people who make up the community's population. Each person enacts multiple roles, such as parent, spouse, employee, citizen, church member, and political volunteer. People in certain roles tend to interact more closely with others in related roles, such as a nursing supervisor with a staff nurse or a customer with a sales clerk. The patterns and communication that emerge from these interactions form the basis of organizations. Some organizations are informal (e.g., an extended family group). Other organizations, such as a city police department or a software business, are more formal. However, all organizations are constructed from roles that are enacted by individual citizens. Organizations, in turn, interact with one another, forming linkages. For example, a medical equipment company and a laboratory establish contracts (linkages) with a home care agency. When a group of organizations are linked and have similar functions, such as all those providing social services, they form

TABLE 15.3 Community Profile Inventory: Social System Perspective

Social System Variables	Community Health Implications	Community Assessment Questions	Information Sources
Health system Family system Economic system Educational system Religious system Welfare system Political system Recreational system Legal system Communication system	Each system must fulfill its functions for a healthy community. Collaboration among the systems to identify goals and problems affects health of community. Undue influence of one system on another may lower the health of the community. Agreement on the means to achieve community goals affects community health. Communication among organizations in each system affects community health.	What are the functions of each major system? What are the major subsystems of each system? What are the major organizations in each subsystem? How well do the various organizations function? Are the subsystems in each major system in conflict? Is there adequate communication among the major systems? Is there agreement on community goals? Are there mechanisms for resolving conflict? Do any parts of the total system dominate the others? What community needs are not being met?	(For all—various Internet sites) Chamber of Commerce Telephone book City directory Organizational literature Officials in organizations Community self-study Community survey Local library Key informants

a community system or subsystem (Fig. 15.2). The various community systems have a profound influence on one another. Because this interaction among parts determines the health of the whole, it is the total social system that concerns community health nurses.

Community Systems

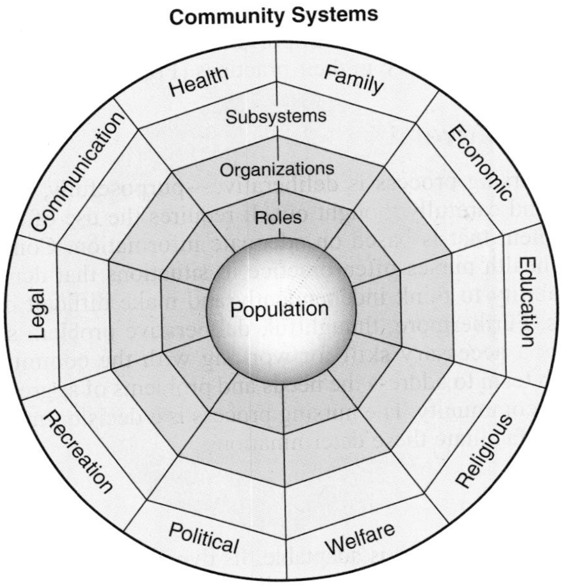

FIGURE 15.2 The community as a social system. Each of the 10 major systems of a community includes a number of subsystems that are made up of organizations. Members of the community occupy roles in these organizations.

The Health Care Delivery System as Part of the Social System

Although community health nurses must examine all the systems in a community and must understand how they interact, the health system is of particular importance. The major function of the health system is to promote the health of the community. Community assessment asks not only whether, but also how well, the system is functioning. What is the level of health promotion carried out by the health system of a community? To answer this question, one that can be applied to any system, the PHN needs a clear notion about the subsystems, organizations, and roles that make up the system. Any evidence of inadequate functioning becomes a warning signal for more careful assessment. For example, a high rate of teenage pregnancies in a city may signal inadequate functioning of several systems (e.g., family, educational, religious, health), so a closer look is in order. What community values influence sexual behavior among adolescents? What sex education programs are available to this population? Does the health system provide information and counseling?

The components of the health system, described in Figure 15.3, include eight major subsystems—each with one or more organizations. Although the community health nurse must be aware of all the systems in a community, the health system is of central importance.

THE NURSING PROCESS FOR THE COMMUNITY AS CLIENT

Consisting of a systematic, purposeful set of interpersonal actions, the nursing process provides a structure for change that remains a viable tool employed by the community health

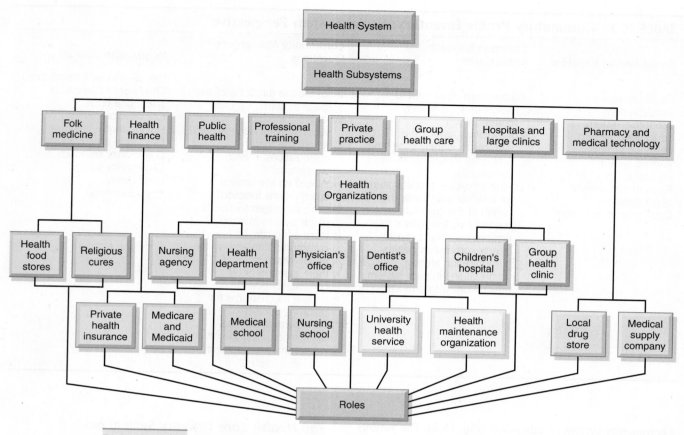

FIGURE 15.3 Components of the health system. This figure shows some representative types of organizations for each of the major subsystems. In turn, each of these organizations also has members with many different roles, and the health of the entire system depends, in part, on how well these roles are carried out.

nurse. This chapter examines the use of the nursing process as applied at the aggregate or community level. Five components—assessment, diagnosis, planning, implementation, and evaluation—give direction to the dynamics for solving problems, managing nursing actions, and improving the health of communities and community health nursing practice.

NURSING PROCESS CHARACTERISTICS APPLIED TO COMMUNITY AS CLIENT

Three characteristics support the use of the nursing process in community health nursing. First, the nursing process is a problem-solving process that addresses community health problems at every aggregate level with the goals of preventing illness and promoting public health. Second, it is a management process that requires situational analysis, decision making, planning, organization, direction, and control of services, as well as outcome evaluation. As a management tool, the nursing process addresses all aggregate levels. Third, it is a process for implementing changes that improve the function of various health-related systems and the ways that people behave within those systems.

The nursing process provides a framework or structure on which community health nursing actions are based. Application of the process varies with each situation, but the

nature of the process remains the same. Certain characteristics of that process are important for community health nurses to emphasize in their practices (Fig. 15.4).

Deliberative

The nursing process is deliberative—purposefully, rationally, and carefully thought out. It requires the use of sound judgment that is based on adequate information. Community health nurses often practice in situations that demand the ability to think independently and make difficult decisions. Furthermore, thoughtful, deliberative problem solving is a necessary skill for working with the community health team to address the needs and problems of aggregates in the community. The nursing process is a decision-making tool to facilitate these determinations.

Adaptable

The nursing process is adaptable. Its dynamic nature enables the community health nurse to adjust appropriately to each situation and to be flexible in applying the process to aggregate health needs. Furthermore, its flexibility is a reminder to the nurse that each client group and each community situation is unique. The nursing process must be applied specifically to the

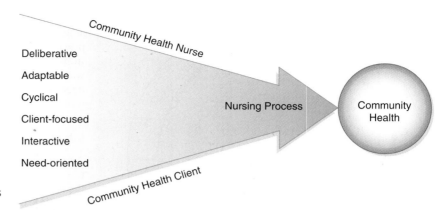

FIGURE 15.4   Nursing process characteristics emphasized in community health.

individual situation and group of people. Based on assessment and sound planning, the nurse adapts and tailors services to meet the identified needs of each community client group.

Cyclic

The nursing process is cyclic and is in constant progression. Steps are repeated over and over in the nurse–aggregate client relationship. The nurse engages in continual interaction, data collection, analysis, intervention, and evaluation. As interactions between nurse and client group continue, various steps in the process overlap with one another and are used simultaneously. The cyclic nature of the nursing process enables the nurse to engage in a constant information feedback loop: The information gathered and lessons learned at each step of the process promote greater understanding of the group being served, the most effective way to provide quality services, and the best methods of raising this group's level of health.

Client-focused

The nursing process is client-focused; it is used for and with clients. Community health nurses use the nursing process for the express purpose of addressing the health of populations. They are helping aggregate clients, directly or indirectly, to achieve and maintain health. Clients as total systems—whether groups, populations, or communities—are the PHN's target of the nursing process.

Interactive

The nursing process is interactive, in that nurse and clients are engaged in a process of ongoing interpersonal communication. Giving and receiving accurate information is necessary to promote understanding between nurse and clients and to foster effective use of the nursing process. Furthermore, because of the movement toward informed use of medical care, demands for clients' rights and the concept of self-care have gained emphasis. Client groups and community health nurses have increasingly joined forces to assume responsibility for promoting community health. The nurse–aggregate client relationship can and should be a partnership, a shared experience by professionals (nurses and others) and client groups (Chrisman, 2007; Schulte, 2000).

Need-oriented

The nursing process is need-oriented. A long association with problem solving has tended to limit the focus of the nursing process to the correction of existing problems. Although problem solving is certainly an appropriate use of the nursing process, the community health nurse can also use the nursing process to anticipate client needs and prevent problems. The nurse should think of nursing diagnoses as ranging from health problem identification to primary prevention and health promotion opportunities. This focus is needed if the goals of community health—to protect, promote, and restore the people's health—are to be realized.

Interacting with the Community

All steps of the nursing process depend on **interaction**, reciprocal exchange and influence among people. Although nurse–client interaction is often an implied or assumed element in the process, it is an essential first consideration for community health nursing (see Chapter 10 for more details). Listening to a group of elderly people, teaching a class of expectant mothers, lobbying in the legislature for the poor, working with parents to set up a dental screening program for children—all these involve relationships, and relationships require interaction. Mutual give and take between nurse and clients—whether a family, a group of mothers on a Native American reservation, or a population of school children—is an expected and much needed skill that should be integrated throughout the nursing process (Fig. 15.5).

Need for Communication

When a community health nurse initially contacts a group of community leaders, for example, any information the nurse may have in advance can give only partial clues to that group's needs and wants. Unless everyone involved talks and listens, the steps of the nursing process will go awry.

Interaction Requires Communication

Through open, honest sharing, the nurse (and others on the health team) will begin to develop trust and establish lines of effective communication. For instance, the nurse explains

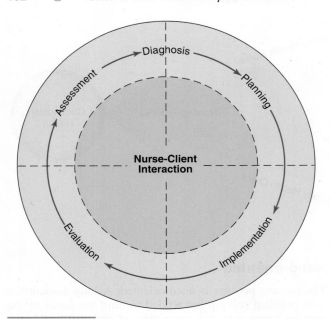

FIGURE 15.5 Nursing process components. Nurse–client interaction, a preamble structure, forms the core of the process. As a nurse and client maintain a reciprocal exchange of information and trust through interaction, they can effectively assess client needs, diagnose needs, and plan, implement, and evaluate care.

who he is and why he is there. The nurse encourages the group members to talk about themselves. Nurse and group members together discuss their relationship and clarify the desired nature of that alliance (Badger, Gagan, & McNiece, 2001). Does the group want help to identify and work on its health needs? Would its members like this nurse to continue regular contacts? What will their respective roles be? Effective communication, as a part of interaction, is essential to develop understanding and facilitate a free exchange of information between nurse and client.

Interaction Is Reciprocal

Sharing of information, ideas, feelings, concerns, and self goes both ways. Nurses must avoid the temptation either to do all the talking or merely to listen while a few group members monopolize the conversation (Stone, 2002). A dynamic exchange must exist between two systems. The community health nurse (and other collaborating health professionals) represents one system and the client group represents the other. Health care professionals tend to prioritize based on their own perspective and many times neglect to take the clients' wishes into account. Whether the client is a parent group, a homeless population, or an entire community, this exchange involves a two-way sharing between the nurse and client group. The key elements of interaction are mutuality and cooperation.

Consider the following example: A dozen junior high school boys, most of whom were on the football team, met for several weeks with the school nurse to discuss physical fitness, nutrition, and other health topics. After their agreed-upon goals had been accomplished, the nurse wondered whether further meetings were needed. The nurse raised the

question and offered several topics for possible future sessions, such as the use of steroids and other drugs and injury prevention. The boys were not interested in these suggestions, but, after more discussion, they decided that they wanted help with talking to girls. Renewed interaction was a necessary first step in reapplying the nursing process and redefining the goals for the group.

Interaction Paves the Way for a Helping Relationship

As nurse and client interact, each learns about the other. A test period occurs before trust can be fully established. For the school nurse, establishing interaction was more difficult at the time of the initial contact with the boys. They had been reluctant to talk and felt embarrassed to discuss personal subjects with an adult they did not know. Nonetheless, their interests in bodybuilding and personal appearance were strong enough to attract them to these optional sessions. Interaction began with a friendly exchange on nonthreatening topics and gradually deepened as the boys seemed ready to discuss personal subjects. Eventually, it was relatively simple to talk about a new "problem" (and start the nursing process over again), because a helping relationship had already been developed. The nurse had a track record. The boys trusted, respected, and liked the nurse, so they were happy to interact around a newly stated need.

Aggregate Application

As noted in earlier chapters, community health practice focuses largely on the health of population groups; therefore, interaction goes beyond the one-on-one with individual patients. The challenge that the community health nurse faces is a one-to-aggregate approach. A group of parents concerned about teenage alcoholism, handicapped people needing access ramps, and a neighborhood's elderly population frightened by muggings and thefts are all aggregates or clients with different concerns and opinions. As defined in Chapter 1, an aggregate refers to a mass or grouping of distinct individuals who are considered as a whole and who are loosely associated with one another. Each person in an aggregate is influenced by the thoughts and behavior of other group members. Nursing interaction with an aggregate client demands an understanding of group behavior, group dynamics, and group-level decision-making. It requires interpersonal communication at the group level. Interaction is more complex with an aggregate than with an individual, but it also can be challenging and rewarding. Once community health nurses acquire an understanding of aggregate behavior, they can capitalize on the potential of group influence to make a far-reaching impact on the health of the total community. Chapter 10 examines communication and interaction with groups more closely.

Forming Partnerships and Building Coalitions

Another important consideration in community-level nursing practice requires teamwork. The job of planning for the health of an entire community or a community subsystem requires that the nurse collaborate with other professionals. Usually, the nurse is part of an organized team, separate from the agency that employs the nurse. The team is brought together with the goal of improving the health of the community. Each group member brings expertise and a particular view of the problem. These interprofessional work groups are often formed as either partnerships or coalitions.

Partnerships are agreements between people (and agencies) that support a joint purpose (Zahner, Kaiser, & Kapelke-Dale, 2005). A partnership can be large (e.g., a multinational corporation and several high schools; a city government and the county jail system), or it can be a more modest endeavor (e.g., a group of senior citizens and a preschool program; a Girl Scout troop and a community recycling program). Community-wide partnerships require more planning and coordination than do small partnerships. For example, because of increased student enrollment, a college may need two additional temporary and part-time faculty members who can teach the community health nursing course. The county public health department is interested in more new graduate nurses coming to work in the agency. The nursing program and the health department form a partnership and design a plan to solve both problems. The health department selects two staff nurses who have master's degrees and are qualified to teach undergraduate clinical laboratories in community health nursing one day a week for two semesters. The benefits for everyone are numerous. The nursing program solves a temporary staffing problem; the nurses from the health department share their expertise with students, enhancing their practice and the students' learning experience; and the health department successfully introduces a pool of students who may be potential staff members to the agency and the services that it provides for the community.

A **coalition** is an alliance of individuals or groups that work together to influence the outcomes of a specific problem (Green, Daniel, & Novick, 2001; Seng et al., 2005). Coalitions are an effective means to achieve a collaborative and coordinated approach to solving community problems (Chrisman, 2007). Steps to coalition building include defining goals and objectives, conducting a community assessment, identifying key players or leaders, and identifying potential coalition members. Once these steps have been accomplished, the leader needs to keep the coalition active. This is best done by knowing and staying in touch with the coalition members, running effective meetings, and keeping every participant involved.

Sound public health practice depends on pooling resources—including people—in ways that will best serve the public. Whether health service is aimed at families, groups, subpopulations, populations, or communities, the consumers of that service are equally important members of the team. In planning for a community's health, the community (represented by appropriate individuals and agencies) must be involved (Badger, Gagan, & McNiece, 2001). Community health nurses cannot lose sight of the need for client involvement at all levels and in all stages of community health practice.

Types of Community Needs Assessment

After considering the importance of community partnerships and coalitions, the community health nurse is ready to determine the community's needs. Assessment is the key initial step of the nursing process. Assessment for nurses means collecting and evaluating information about a community's health status to discover existing or potential needs

and assets as a basis for planning future action (Heinemann & Zeiss, 2002).

Several models or frameworks can be used for assessment. Three such models are Assessment Protocol for Excellence in Public Health (APEXPH), Planned Approach to Community Health (PATCH), and Mobilizing for Action through Planning and Partnerships (MAPP). All three of these models have been developed through partnerships involved in meeting *Healthy People 2010* goals (Kalos, Kent, & Gates, 2005; Lenihan, 2005). *Healthy People 2010* also provides a *Tool Kit* for health planning in local communities (see Internet Resources at end of chapter). These are all valuable resources that provide specific guidelines focusing on local-level strategies to improve the health of communities.

Assessment involves two major activities. The first is collection of pertinent data, and the second is analysis and interpretation of data. These actions overlap and are repeated constantly throughout the assessment phase of the nursing process. While assessing a community's ability to enhance its health, the nurse may simultaneously collect data on community lifestyle behaviors and interpret previously collected data on morbidity and mortality.

Community needs assessment is the process of determining the real or perceived needs of a defined community. In some situations, an extensive community study may be the first priority; in others, all that is needed is a study of one system or even one organization. At other times, community health nurses may need to perform a cursory examination or "windshield survey" to familiarize themselves with an entire community without going into any depth (Laraia, 2006).

Familiarization or Windshield Survey

A familiarization assessment is a common starting place in evaluation of a community. **Familiarization assessment** involves studying data already available on a community, then gathering a certain amount of firsthand data in order to gain a working knowledge of the community. Such an approach may utilize a **windshield survey**—an activity often used by nursing students in community health courses and by new staff members in community health agencies. Nurses drive (or walk) around the community of interest; find health, social, and governmental services; obtain literature; introduce themselves and explain that they are working in the area; and generally become familiar with the community and its residents. This type of assessment is needed whenever the community health nurse works with families, groups, organizations, or populations. The windshield survey provides a knowledge of the context in which these aggregates live and may enable the nurse to better connect clients with community resources (Table 15.4). See an example in From the Case Files I.

Problem-Oriented Assessment

A second type of community assessment, **problem-oriented assessment**, begins with a single problem and assesses the community in terms of that problem. Suppose that Jean, the nurse who explored services available for the Angelo family's deaf child in From the Case Files I, had discovered that there

TABLE 15.4 Windshield Survey*

	Observations	Data
I. Community Core 1. History—What can you glean by looking (e.g., old, established neighborhoods; new subdivision)? Ask people willing to talk: How long have you lived here? Has the area changed? As you talk, ask if there is an "old-timer" who knows the history of the area. 2. Demographics—What sorts of people do you see? Young? Old? Homeless? Alone? Families? What races do you see? Is the population homogeneous? 3. Ethnicity—Do you note indicators of different ethnic groups (e.g., restaurants, festivals)? What signs do you see of different cultural groups? 4. Values and Beliefs—Are there churches, mosques, temples? Does it appear homogeneous? Are the lawns cared for? With flowers? Gardens? Signs of art? Culture? Heritage? Historical markers?		
II. Subsystems 1. Physical Environment—How does the community look? What do you note about air quality, flora, housing, zoning, space, green areas, animals, people, human-made structures, natural beauty, water, climate? Can you find or develop a map of the area? What is the size (e.g., square miles, blocks)? 2. Health and Social Services—Evidence of acute or chronic conditions? Shelters? "Traditional" healers (e.g., *curanderos*, herbalists)? Are there clinics, hospitals, practitioners' offices, public health services, home health agencies, emergency centers, nursing homes, social service facilities, mental health services? Are there resources outside the community but accessible to them? 3. Economy—Is it a "thriving" community or does it feel "seedy?" Are there industries, stores, places for employment? Where do people shop? Are there signs that food stamps are used/accepted? What is the unemployment rate? 4. Transportation and Safety—How do people get around? What type of private and public transportation is available? Do you see buses, bicycles, taxis? Are there sidewalks, bike trails? Is getting around in the community possible for people with disabilities? What types of protective services are there (e.g., fire, police, sanitation)? Is air quality monitored? What types of crimes are committed? Do people feel safe? 5. Politics and Government—Are there signs of political activity (e.g., posters, meetings)? What party affiliation predominates? What is the governmental jurisdiction of the community (e.g., elected mayor, city council with single member districts)? Are people involved in decision making in their local governmental unit? 6. Communication—Are there "common areas" where people gather? What newspapers do you see in the stands? Do people have TVs and radios? What do they watch/listen to? What are the formal and informal means of communication? 7. Education—Are there schools in the area? How do they look? Are there libraries? Is there a local board of education? How does it function? What is the reputation of the school(s)? What are major educational issues? What are the dropout rates? Are extracurricular activities available? Are they used? Is there a school health service? A school nurse? 8. Recreation—Where do children play? What are the major forms of recreation? Who participates? What facilities for recreation do you see?		
III. Perceptions 1. The Residents—How do people feel about the community? What do they identify as its strengths? Problems? Ask several people from different groups (e.g., old, young, field worker, factory worker, professional, minister, housewife) and keep track of who gives what answer. 2. Your Perceptions—General statements about the "health" of this community. What are its strengths? What problems or potential problems can you identify?		

Note: Supplement your impressions with information from the census, police records, school statistics, chamber of commerce data, health department reports, and so on to confirm or refute your conclusions. Tables, graphs, and maps are helpful and will aid in your analysis.

*This survey form was renamed "Learning about the Community on Foot" to underscore the necessity of walking around the community. Also, when one of the authors (Elizabeth T. Anderson) used it in rural Mexico, the area being assessed was not accessible by automobile. For ease of citation and referral, we will continue to use "windshield survey" as its title.

Source: Anderson, Elizabeth T., & McFarlane, Judith. (2006). *Community as Partner: Theory and Practice in Nursing* (5th ed.) Philadelphia: Lippincott, Williams & Wilkins.

From the Case Files I

The Angelo Family and a Familiarization Assessment

A community health nurse named Jean visited the Angelo family on the outskirts of Philadelphia. During the initial visit, she gathered information, learning that the family was Italian American and that there were four children, ranging in age from 13 to 3. The father had been out of work for 6 months; the mother worked on weekends as a maid in a motel; the oldest boy had been in trouble with the juvenile authorities; a younger child was deaf; and their house appeared rundown. Jean assessed this family, trying to determine its coping ability and its level of health. Furthermore, because community health nursing is population focused, her concern was not only for the Angelo family but also for the population of families with similar problems that this family represented.

However, the nurse's assessment was almost impossible without further knowledge of the community. Was theirs an Italian-American neighborhood with specific cultural influences? What was the extent of unemployment in this city? What were the services for the deaf? Were all the houses in this part of town old and in need of repair? Once the nurse began working with the family, familiarity with the community became even more imperative. She discovered that, as a result of the Angelos' low income, family conflicts were intense. The family members seldom got out; they made almost no use of the community's recreational system. Before she could help them make use of it, however, the nurse had to find out what resources were available. As she familiarized herself with the community, she discovered Friends of the Deaf, which sponsored a group for parents of deaf children. The nurse could now help Mr. and Mrs. Angelo become part of that group. A quick survey of the religious system in the community revealed two job-transition support groups, one of which would welcome Mr. Angelo. In the meantime, the nurse chose to find out about the welfare system and how this family and other similar families could benefit from its services. Even her own attitude changed as she studied the community. For instance, she discovered that a strike had closed down the plant where Mr. Angelo worked for 20 years, and so could view his and others' unemployment from a broader perspective. Using a familiarization assessment helped this nurse to enhance her practice.

Whatever role nurses play in community health promotion, they will want to be making a continuous study, an ongoing assessment. Whether nurses become client advocates, work with the local government, or operate from a nursing agency serving the elderly, a familiarization assessment is prerequisite for their work.

were none. Confronted with this problem—one family with one deaf child—she could make a problem-oriented community assessment. Her first step would be to discover the incidence of childhood deafness, both in the community and in the state. Second, she might begin interviewing officials in the schools and health institutions to find out what had been done in the past to assist deaf children. She could check the local library or the Internet to locate available resources on the subject of deafness. Are there interpreters available for people who use sign language? How do hospitals and courts approach deafness? Are there any clubs or other organizations for deaf people? Are there school programs for the deaf, and, if so, where are they located?

The problem-oriented assessment is commonly used when familiarization is not sufficient and a comprehensive assessment is too expensive. This type of assessment is responsive to a particular need. The data collected will be useful in any kind of planning for a community response to the specific problem.

Community Subsystem Assessment

In **community subsystem assessment**, the community health nurse focuses on a single dimension of community life. For example, the nurse might decide to survey churches and religious organizations to discover their roles in the community. What kinds of needs do the leaders in these organizations believe exist? What services do these organizations offer? To what extent are services coordinated within the religious system and between it and other systems in the community?

Community subsystem assessment can be a useful way for a team to conduct a more thorough community assessment. If five members of a nursing agency divide up the ten systems in the community and each person does an assessment of two systems, they could then share their findings to create a more comprehensive picture of the community and its needs.

Comprehensive Assessment

Comprehensive assessment seeks to discover all relevant community health information. It begins with a review of existing studies and all the data presently available on the community. A survey compiles all the demographic information on the population, such as its size, density, and composition. **Key informants** are interviewed in every major system—education, health, religious, economic, and others.

Key informants are experts in one particular area of the community or they may know the community as a whole. Examples of key informants would be a school nurse, a religious leader, key cultural leaders, the local police chief or fire captain, a mail carrier, or a local city council person. Then, more detailed surveys and intensive interviews are performed to yield information on organizations and the various roles in each organization. A comprehensive assessment describes not only the systems of a community but also how power is distributed throughout the system, how decisions are made, and how change occurs (Blewett, Casey, & Call, 2004; Gandelman, Desantis, & Rietmeijer, 2006).

Because comprehensive assessment is an expensive, time-consuming process, it is not often undertaken. Performing a more focused study, based on prior knowledge of needs, is often a better and less costly strategy. Nevertheless, knowing how to conduct a comprehensive assessment is an important skill when designing smaller, more focused assessments.

Community Assets Assessment

The final form of assessment presented here is **assets assessment**, which focuses on the strengths and capacities of a community rather than its problems (Sharpe, Greaney, Lee, & Royce, 2000). The type of assessment depends on variables such as the needs that exist, the goals to be achieved, and the resources available for carrying out the study (Pan, Littlefield, Valladolid, Tapping, & West, 2005). Although it is difficult to determine the type of assessment needed in advance, the decision will be facilitated by understanding several different types of community assessment. Based on a classic model developed by McKnight and Kretzmann in the 1980s (Kretzman & McKnight, 1993), the assets assessment provides a framework with which to conduct a complete functional community assessment and serves as a guide to the community for the nurse, as well as the foundation for community development. The previously mentioned methods are needs-oriented and deficit-based—in other words, they are *pathology* models, in which the assessment is performed in response to needs, barriers, weaknesses, problems, or perceived scarcity in the community. This may result in a fragmented approach to solutions for the community's problems rather than an approach focused on the community's possibilities, strengths, and assets. The assets assessment also provides the community the ability to "identify a variety and richness of skills, talents, knowledge, and experience of people" and "provides a base upon which to build new approaches and enterprises" (p. 4).

Assets assessment begins with what is present in the community (Davis, Cook, & Cohen, 2005). The capacities and skills of community members are identified, with a focus on creating or rebuilding relationships among local residents, associations, and institutions to multiply power and effectiveness. This approach requires that the assessor look for the positive, or see the glass as half full. The nurse can then become a partner in community intervention efforts, rather than merely a provider of services. Assets assessment has three levels:

1. Specific skills, talents, interests, and experiences of individual community members such as individual businesses, cultural groups, and professionals living in the community.

2. Local citizen associations, organizations, and institutions controlled largely by the community such as libraries, social service agencies, voluntary agencies, schools, and police.
3. Local institutions originating outside the community controlled largely outside the community such as welfare and public capital expenditures (p. 14).

The key, however, is linking these assets together to enhance the community from within. The community health nurse's role is to assist with those linkages.

COMMUNITY ASSESSMENT METHODS

Community health needs may be assessed using a variety of methods. Regardless of the assessment method used, data must be collected. Data collection in community health requires the exercise of sound professional judgment, effective communication techniques, and special investigative skills. Four important methods are discussed here: surveys, descriptive epidemiologic studies, community forums or town meetings, and focus groups.

Surveys

A **survey** is an assessment method in which a series of questions is used to collect data for analysis of a specific group or area. Surveys are commonly used to provide a broad range of data that will be helpful when used with other sources or if other sources are not available. To plan and conduct community health surveys, the goal should be to determine the variables (selected environmental, socioeconomic, and behavioral conditions or needs) that affect a community's ability to control disease and promote wellness. The nurse may choose to conduct a survey to determine such things as health care use patterns and needs, immunization levels, demographic characteristics, or health beliefs and practices. The survey method involves three phases that are needed to ensure an adequate design and appropriate collection of data (Polit & Beck, 2007).

Descriptive Epidemiologic Studies

A second assessment method is a **descriptive epidemiologic study**, which examines the amount and distribution of a disease or health condition in a population by person (Who is affected?), by place (Where does the condition occur?), and by time (When do the cases occur?). In addition to their value in assessing the health status of a population, descriptive epidemiologic studies are useful for suggesting which individuals are at greatest risk and where and when the condition might occur. They are also useful for health planning purposes and for suggesting hypotheses concerning disease etiology. Their design and use are detailed in Chapter 7.

The choice of assessment method varies depending on the reasons for data collection, the goals and objectives of the study, and the available resources. It also varies according to the theoretical framework or philosophical approach through which the nurse views the community. In other words, the community health nurse's theoretical basis for approaching community assessment influences the purposes for conducting the assessment and the selection of methodology. For example, Neuman's health care systems model forms the basis for the "community-as-partner" assessment model developed by Anderson and McFarlane (2004, p. 85). Additional resources on methodologies for assessing community health are available in the list of References and Selected Readings at the end of this chapter.

Community Forums or Town Hall Meetings

The community forum or town hall meeting is a qualitative assessment method designed to obtain community opinions. It takes place in the neighborhood of the people involved, perhaps in a school gymnasium or an auditorium. The participants are selected to participate by invitation from the group organizing the forum. Members come from within the community and represent all segments of the community that are involved with the issue. For instance, if a community is contemplating building a swimming pool, the people invited to the community forum might include potential users of the pool (residents of the community who do not have pools and special groups such as the Girl Scouts, elders, and disabled citizens), community planners, health and safety personnel, and other key people with vested interests. They are asked to give their views on the pool: Where should it be located? Who will use it? How will the cost of building and maintaining it be assumed? What are the drawbacks to having the pool? Any other pertinent issues the participants may raise are included. This method is relatively inexpensive, and results are quickly obtained. A drawback of this method is that only the most vocal community members, or those with the greatest vested interests in the issue, may be heard. This format does not provide a representative voice to others in the community who also may be affected by the proposed decision.

This method is used to elicit public opinion on a variety of issues, including health care concerns, political views, and feelings about issues in the public eye, such as gangs. Frequently, local cable television channels air important city government or school board meetings. Local news programs may hold town meetings, soliciting public opinion on regional issues. Other methods of opinion gathering include e-mailing (e.g., to a television news program) to support a particular view, Web-based survey sites (e.g., Survey Monkey), and using a toll-free phone number set up especially for text messaging a Yes or No vote on an issue. Now commonplace, chat rooms are available for a host of topics and interests. Electronic town meetings are designed to elicit grassroots opinions from local community members, and have been utilized by many entities, including the Minnesota Senate (2006). Even presidential debates are available over the Internet, with citizens sending in e-mail questions for candidate responses in real time (Gough, 2007).

Focus Groups

This fourth assessment method, focus groups, is similar to the community forum or town hall meeting in that it is designed to obtain grassroots opinion. However, it has some differences. First, only a small group of participants, usually 5 to 15 people (Polit & Beck, 2007), is present. The members chosen for the group are homogeneous with respect to specific demographic variables. For example, a focus group may consist of female community health nurses, young women in their first pregnancy, or retired businessmen. Leadership skills are used in conjunction with the small group process to promote a supportive atmosphere and to accomplish set goals. The interviewer guides the discussion according to a predetermined set of questions or topics.

Major advantages of focus groups are their efficiency and low cost, similar to the community forum or town hall meeting format. A focus group can be organized to be representative of an aggregate, to capture community interest groups, or to sample for diversity among different population groups. One example is a research study involving Hmong youths and adults. Eight focus groups were held to determine perceptions of healthy diet and exercise among parents and children (Pham, Harrison, & Kagawa-Singer, 2007). Whatever the purpose, however, some people may be uncomfortable expressing their views in a group situation (Polit & Beck, 2007).

SOURCES OF COMMUNITY DATA

The community health nurse can look in many places for data to enhance and complete a community assessment. Data sources can be primary or secondary, and they can be from international, national, state, or local sources. Websites for many primary and secondary data sources are included at the end of this chapter.

Primary and Secondary Sources

Community health nurses make use of many sources in data collection. Community members, including formal leaders, informal leaders, and community members, can frequently offer the most accurate insights and comprehensive information. Information gathered by talking to people provides primary data, because the data are obtained directly from the community. Secondary sources of data include people who know the community well and the records such people create in the performance of their jobs. Specific examples are health team members, client records, community health (vital) statistics, census bureau data, reference books, research reports, and community health nurses. Because secondary data may not totally describe the community and do not necessarily reflect community self-perceptions, they may need augmentation or further validation through focus groups, surveys, and other primary data collection methods.

International Sources

International data are collected by several agencies, including the World Health Organization (WHO) and its six regional offices and health organizations, such as the Pan-American Health Organization. In addition, the United Nations and global specialty organizations that focus on certain populations or health problems, such as the United Nations Children's Fund, are major sources of international health-related data (WHO, 2008a). The WHO publishes an annual report of their activity, and international statistics for diseases and illness trends can be found on the Internet (WHO, 2008b). Information from these official sources can give the nurse in the local community information about immigrant and refugee populations he serves. More information on international health agencies can be found in Chapter 16.

National Sources

Community health nurses can access a wealth of official and nonofficial sources of national data (see Chapter 6 for more information). Official sources develop documents based on data compiled by the government. The following are the major official agencies:

♦ **U.S. Department of Health and Human Services, (USDHHS).** This is the main agency from which data can be retrieved, and its agency, the National Center for Health Statistics (NCHS), was specifically established for the collection and dissemination of health-related data. This agency is the nation's principal health statistics agency, compiling data from many sources. These data provide information for many functions, including health status for various populations and subgroups, identification of disparities, monitoring trends, identifying health problems, and supporting research.

USDHHS also published *Healthy People 2010* (USDHHS, 2000), which was designed to focus America's attention on the major national health problems, including realistic goals for national, state, and local agencies to work toward over one decade.

♦ **U.S. Bureau of the Census.** This agency undertakes a major survey of American families every 10 years, gathering data on health, socioeconomic, and environmental conditions. This information is available on the Web or on a CD-ROM, allowing numerous variables to be viewed in combination, for easier development of a community profile.

♦ **National Institutes of Health (NIH).** This system of 27 Institutes and Centers, a part of the USDHHS, focuses on improving the health of the nation. An emphasis is placed on discovery of new cures or treatments and preventing disease. Employees of these agencies prevent, diagnose, and treat diseases and conduct research and disseminate research findings (NIH, 2007).

Nonofficial agencies have data sources generated from research they conduct that focuses on the population, disease, or condition they were developed to serve. Each agency collects data at the national level; however, the more accessible arm for services function at state and local levels. Examples of these agencies are the American Cancer Society (ACS), the American Association of Retired Persons (AARP), Mothers Against Drunk Drivers (MADD), and Students Against Drunk Drivers (SADD). Information from such national sources allows community health assessment teams to compare local data with national and state statistics and trends—a very valuable function.

State and Local Sources

For nurses, the most significant state source of assessment data comes from the state health department. This official agency is responsible for collecting state vital statistics and morbidity data. The Behavioral Health Surveillance System (BRFSS) is the world's largest telephone health survey that monitors health risk at the state level (Centers for Disease Control & Prevention [CDC], 2007). Supported by the CDC, the information is used at various levels to identify risk and prevent disease. As a resource to local health departments, the state health department provides invaluable support services and it is the main source of health-related data on the state level. Nonofficial agencies have state chapters or headquarters and compile their information at the state level. Local nonofficial agency chapters have documents of compiled state and national data on the population, disease, or condition they address.

Many sources of information may be obtained at the local level. Some key sources are the local visitor's bureau, city Chamber of Commerce, city planner's office, health department, hospitals, social service agencies, county extension office, school districts, universities or colleges, libraries, clergy, business and service organizations, and community leaders and key informants. Some of these sources compile their own statistics, but all have views of the community particular to their discipline, interest, or knowledge base. Some agencies at the local level develop city or county directories. These are updated periodically and are valuable resources for community health assessment teams and community health nurses. More detailed information on national, state, and local health agencies can be found in Chapter 6.

DATA ANALYSIS AND DIAGNOSIS

This stage of assessment requires analysis of the information gathered, so that inferences or conclusions may be made about its meaning. Such inferences must be validated to determine their accuracy, after which a nursing diagnosis can be formed.

The Analysis Process

First, the data must be validated: Are they accurate? Several validation procedures may be used:

1. Data can be rechecked by the community assessment team.
2. Data can be rechecked by others.
3. Subjective and objective data can be compared.
4. Community members can consider the findings and verify them.

Validated data are then separated into categories such as physical, social, and environmental data. In many instances, data spreadsheets are used to provide a structure for data organization. Next, each category is examined to determine its significance. At this point, there may be a need to search for additional information to clarify the meaning of the data. Only then can inferences be made and a tentative conclusion about the meaning of the data be reached (Anderson & McFarlane, 2004; Gandelman, Desantis, & Rietmeijer, 2006).

Some computer programs are designed to analyze community assessment data. For large, complex, or ongoing community assessment plans, this may be the best method. For smaller, one-time assessments, the paper-and-pencil method may be sufficient and less unwieldy. Some communities may hire an outside professional assessment service. These teams often use the latest technology when analyzing data. Not all communities can afford such a service, and if key leaders become familiar with assessment, analysis, and diagnostic processes, an investment in a computer program may be worthwhile. Geographic information systems (GIS) technology is proving very useful in community assessment. These tools are becoming more user friendly and cost effective, and have been used to pinpoint incidences of various diseases, display environmental risks, note the location of health care facilities, and determine accurate community boundaries (Faruque, Lofton, Doddato, & Mangum, 2003; Choi, Afzal, & Sattler, 2006). Regardless of the analysis method used, data interpretation remains a critical phase of the process.

In data interpretation, the ever-present danger exists of making inaccurate assumptions and diagnoses. The importance of validation cannot be overemphasized. Before making a diagnosis, all assumptions must be validated: Are they sound? Community members should participate actively in validation efforts by clarifying perceptions, explaining the circumstances surrounding the situation, and acting as sounding boards for testing assumptions. Other resources, such as the health team members and community leaders, are used to explore and confirm inferences. Data collection, data interpretation, and nursing diagnosis are sequential activities, with validation serving as the bridges between them (Table 15.5). When performed thoroughly, these steps lead to accurate diagnoses.

Community Diagnosis Formation

The next step of the nursing process, after analysis, is the development of the community diagnosis. "Community diagnoses clarify who gets the care (the community as opposed to the individual), provide a statement identifying problems faced by who is getting care (i.e., the community), and identify the factors contributing to the identified problem" (Shuster & Goeppinger, 2004, p. 360). Various taxonomies and classification systems are used in nursing

to describe specific nursing problems and each one has its limitations when dealing with community-level diagnoses. The North American Nursing Diagnosis Association (NANDA) is much more oriented to nursing diagnoses of individuals and families than to community-level problems. Nursing Outcomes Classification (NOC) is also generally individual-oriented. The Omaha System, originally designed by the Omaha Visiting Nurse Association, is again primarily used in nursing diagnoses of individuals, families, and small groups, although some community health applications have been developed (Omaha System, 2005; Mantas & Hasman, 2001).

This chapter discusses nursing diagnosis as characterized by Neufeld and Harrison (1996), based on the classic work of Mundinger and Jauron (1975). These authors proposed the use of nursing diagnoses in the community by substituting the term *client, family, group,* or *aggregate* for the word *patient.* Their definition of a nursing diagnosis is (Neufeld & Harrison, 1996, p. 221):

> The statement of a [client's] response which is actually or potentially unhealthful and which nursing intervention can help to change in the direction of health. It should also identify essential factors related to the unhealthful response.

Neufeld and Harrison built on this work to form a wellness diagnosis by using the phrase *healthful response* instead of *unhealthful response.* Their definition of a wellness diagnosis is (p. 221):

> The statement of a client's [community's] healthful response which nursing intervention can support or strengthen. It should also identify the essential factors related to the healthful response.

Stolte (1996) developed a manual for nursing wellness diagnosis. By substituting the term *community* for client, family, group, or aggregate, the nursing or wellness diagnosis can be applied to the community as a whole. These diagnoses identify the conclusion the nurse draws from interpretation of collected data and describe a community's healthy or

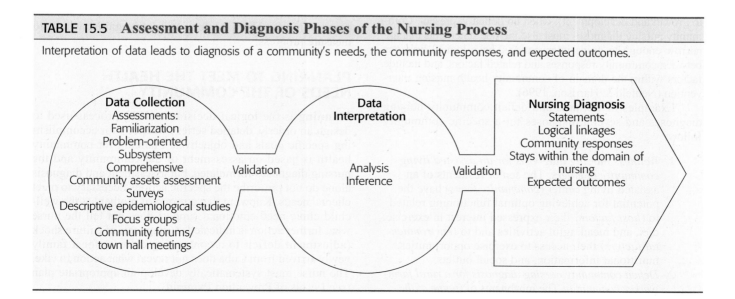

TABLE 15.5   Assessment and Diagnosis Phases of the Nursing Process

Interpretation of data leads to diagnosis of a community's needs, the community responses, and expected outcomes.

Data Collection
Assessments:
Familiarization
Problem-oriented
Subsystem
Comprehensive
Community assets assessment
Surveys
Descriptive epidemiological studies
Focus groups
Community forums/
town hall meetings

Validation

Data Interpretation
Analysis
Inference

Validation

Nursing Diagnosis
Statements
Logical linkages
Community responses
Stays within the domain of nursing
Expected outcomes

unhealthy responses that can be influenced or changed by nursing interventions. Change comes about through collaboration with other community and health team members.

In community health, nurses do not limit their focus to problems; they consider the community as a total system and look for evidence of all kinds of responses that may influence the community's level of wellness. Responses encompass the whole health–illness continuum, from specific deficits, such as a lack of senior centers or day care programs, to opportunities for maximizing a community's health, such as promoting improvement of police protection or the safety of the roadways. The statement of community response—the diagnosis—can focus on a wide range of topics.

Community Diagnoses

Data have been gathered from a variety of sources and have been validated by several means. The data have been recorded, tabulated, analyzed, and synthesized, so that patterns and trends can be seen. The use of charts, graphs, and tables assists in visualizing the synthesized data. The community assessment team should present their findings to peers and colleagues, and use their expertise to assist in the formulation of the community diagnoses.

Continuing with the nursing process format, nursing diagnoses for the community are developed. **Community diagnoses** refer to nursing diagnoses about a community's ineffective coping ability and potential for enhanced coping. The statements about the community should include the strengths of the community and possible sources for community solutions, as well as the community's weaknesses or problem areas. Using the standard nursing diagnosis format, community-level diagnoses can be developed (Carpenito-Moyet, 2007). These diagnoses are used as tools as the community begins to plan, intervene, and evaluate outcomes. Diagnostic categories for individuals (e.g., knowledge deficit of senior services, high risk for injury or falls) can often be applied at the community level. Community-level nursing diagnoses should portray a community focus, include the community response, and identify any related factors that have potential for change through community health nursing. These may also include wellness diagnoses, which indicate maintenance or potential change responses (due to growth and development), when no deficit is present. Community nursing diagnoses must also include statements that are narrow enough to guide interventions, have logical linkages between community responses and related factors, and include factors within the domain of community health nursing intervention (Neufeld & Harrison, 1996).

Examples of wellness and deficit community nursing diagnoses and several diagnoses for a specific community follow:

1. *Wellness nursing diagnosis for an assisted living community of elders.* The senior residents of an assisted living center (*community focus*) have the potential for achieving optimal functioning related to (*host factors*) their expressed interest in exercise, diet, and meaningful activities and to (*environmental factors*) their access to exercise opportunities, nutritional information, and social outlets.
2. *Deficit community nursing diagnosis for a rural farmworker community.* The inhabitants of (*name of the*

town) in (*name of the state*) are at risk for illness and injury related to (*host factors*) exposure to pesticides, lack of motivation to add or use safety devices on farm machinery, lack of safety knowledge, choice to take unnecessary risks (*environmental factors*), lack of family income to purchase newer equipment and long hours of work that lead to stress and exhaustion.
3. *Community diagnoses for Anytown, Kansas.* Anytown, Kansas, is experiencing an increase in crime, a problem compounded by the small size of the police force and an influx of many new community members. The community has worked together constructively in the past, communicates well, and has strong recreational outlets for community members. The community:
    - Has expressed vulnerability and feels overwhelmed related to threats to community safety
    - Has failed to meet its own expectations related to inadequate law enforcement services
    - Has expressed difficulty in meeting the demands of change related to an influx of new community members
    - Has a successful history of coping with a previous crisis of teenage pregnancy
    - Has positive communication among community members
    - Has a well-developed program for recreation and relaxation

Such diagnoses can guide communities toward maximizing or improving their health as they plan, implement, and evaluate changes to be measured by established outcome criteria. **Outcome criteria** are measurable standards that community members use to measure success as they work toward improving the health of their community. Outcome-based or evidence-based nursing practice applies to aggregates in the community as well as to patients in acute-care settings.

The nursing diagnosis changes over time because it reflects changes in the health status of the community; therefore, diagnoses need to be periodically reevaluated and redefined. The changing diagnosis can be a useful means of moving a community toward improved health because it gives community members a clear standard against which to measure progress.

PLANNING TO MEET THE HEALTH NEEDS OF THE COMMUNITY

Planning is the logical decision-making process used to design an orderly, detailed series of actions for accomplishing specific goals and objectives. Planning for community health is based on assessment of the community and the nursing diagnoses formulated, but assessment and diagnosis alone do not prescribe the specific actions necessary to meet clients' needs. Knowing that a group of mothers at the well-child clinic need emotional support does not tell the nurse what further action is indicated. A diagnosis of culture shock (adjustment deficit to a contrasting culture) for a family newly arrived from Cuba does not reveal what action to take. The nurse must systematically develop an appropriate plan (see Levels of Prevention Pyramid).

LEVELS OF PREVENTION PYRAMID

SITUATION: Desire to reduce the incidence of child abuse in a given community by 50% within 2 years.

GOAL: Using the three levels of prevention, negative health conditions are avoided, or promptly diagnosed and treated, and the fullest possible potential is restored.

Tertiary Prevention

Rehabilitation	**Primary Prevention**	
	Health Promotion & Education	
• Establish rehabilitation programs for abused children, including safe home placement, physical and emotional treatment, and self-esteem building • Rebuild the family unit if appropriate or possible	• Provide family life education programs for families • Develop resources to support health promotion programs	**Health Protection** • If unable or inappropriate to rehabilitate the abuser or family, keep abuser away from victim through incarceration or court order

Secondary Prevention

Early Diagnosis	**Prompt Treatment**
• Develop early detection programs through schools, clinics, and physicians' offices • Promote enforcement of child protection laws	• Establish programs to provide prompt treatment for abused children and abusing parents

Primary Prevention

Health Promotion & Education	**Health Protection**
• Assess factors contributing to child abuse • Institute family life education programs through schools and community groups • Develop community resources to support health promotion programs	• Identify families in the community who are at greatest risk (e.g., parents with history of child abuse, families under great stress) • Develop community resources to support health protection programs

Tools to Assist with Planning

Planning for community health care provision and programs can be enhanced by using various tools, including operational definitions of objectives and activities, conceptual frameworks, and models (Epstein et al., 2002; Kalos, Kent, & Gates, 2005). Such tools help to identify target population characteristics, clarify program goals, specify nursing interventions, and anticipate client outcomes. Tools that assist with planning also enable the nurse to test ideas and adjust solutions before actual implementation. Finally, the use of standardized tools enhances the planning process and promotes effectiveness of services, as well as professional standards of practice.

In addition to using tools, a systematic approach to planning guides the community health nurse to list needs in order of priority, establish goals and objectives, and record the plan. As they do in the rest of the nursing process, community health nurses collaborate with clients and other appropriate professionals throughout each of these planning activities.

The Health Planning Process

The health planning process is a four-stage system used to design new health-related programs or services in the community. It is often used by health educators when designing educational programs, or by administrators in community health agencies when initiating new services, and it can be used by other people who are not nurses when developing services. The nursing process is similar to the health planning process (Table 15.6). Each model helps to promote service effectiveness in addition to maintaining standards of practice. Community health

TABLE 15.6 Comparison Between the Health Planning Process and the Nursing Process

Health Planning Process	Nursing Process
1. ASSESSMENT STAGE Determine data needed and collect data. Interpret data and identity needs. Set goals based on needs.	**1. ASSESSMENT**
2. ANALYSIS AND DESIGN Analyze findings and set specific objectives. Design alternative interventions. Analyze and compare pros and cons of various solutions.	**2. DIAGNOSIS** Formulate nursing diagnoses.
Create a plan.	**3. PLANNING** List needs in order of priority. Establish goals and objectives. Write an action plan.
3. IMPLEMENTATION STAGE Describe how to operationalize the plan. Design a method for monitoring progress.	**4. IMPLEMENTATION**
4. EVALUATION STAGE Examine costs and benefits of proposed solution. Judge the potential outputs, outcomes, and impact of plan. Modify to achieve the best plan. Present plan to sponsoring group or agency. Obtain acceptance (and funding).	**5. EVALUATION**

nurses familiar with both the health planning process and the nursing process should be able to work collaboratively with community health professionals using either model.

Setting Priorities

Priority setting involves assigning rank or importance to the identified needs to determine the order in which goals should be addressed. There are numerous ways to set priorities in the planning process. The WHO (1976) and later, Shuster and Goeppinger (2004) identified useful criteria that can guide ranking problems for order of action. They are presented here as a combination of criteria:

1. Significance of the problem or the number of people affected in the community
2. Level of community awareness of the problem
3. Community motivation to act on the problem (or, Is this important to the community?)
4. Nurse and partnership's ability to reduce risk and/or influence the solution
5. Cost of risk reduction in terms of financial, social, and ethical capital
6. Ability to identify a specific target population for an intervention
7. Availability of expertise to solve the problem within the partnership, coalition, or community
8. Severity of the outcome if left unresolved or the consequences of inaction
9. Speed with which the problem can be resolved

For example, a community assessment revealed that a group of elderly residents living within a specific zip code were fearful of crime, but also identified the lack of public transportation as issues to be addressed. Using the above criteria, the community health nurse working in this community identified that 85% of residents of the community had fears about crime but did not see transportation as an issue. The residents saw crime as an important concern and were also motivated to act on the crime issue, but were not willing to explore the transportation issue at the current time. The nurse, along with the community coalition partners, would be better able to influence the crime problem by helping to form Town Watch groups and getting the local police district to provide increased patrols during evening hours when robberies were more likely to occur. However, the partners had little influence to extend the hours of operation on buses or influence the creation of new bus routes. Members of the coalition included the local police chief, and chamber of commerce director. If the crime problem was left unchecked, more people could be adversely affected, including businesses, because people would not be willing to leave their homes to shop or might even be forced to move away. Finally, these initiatives could be put in place rather quickly and inexpensively after the formation and training of volunteer Town Watch groups. There certainly are no adverse social, economic, or ethical consequences attached to addressing this problem. Therefore, it would seem that the crime issue would take priority over the transportation issue. It is important to remember that each community diagnosis is examined separately and then compared. Priorities for action are discussed, ranked, and then prioritized for action. Criteria for prioritizing health problems in the community include:

◆ Numbers of community members affected by the problem
◆ Community awareness of the problem
◆ Ability of team to reduce risk or influence the problem
◆ Cost of risk reduction (social, economic, and ethical)
◆ Ability to clearly identify a target or risk population

- Availability of expertise
- Consequences of inaction
- Speed of resolution (WHO 1976; Shuster & Goeppinger, 2004)

Establishing Goals and Objectives

Goals and objectives are crucial to planning and should be feasible and specific (Anderson, Guthrie, & Schirle, 2002). The diagnosis that identifies needs must be translated into goals to give focus and meaning to the nursing plan. **Goals** are broad statements of desired outcomes. **Objectives** are specific statements of desired outcomes, phrased in behavioral terms that can be measured. Target dates for expected completion of each objective are also stated. Objectives are the stepping-stones to help one reach the end results of the larger goal. For the elderly group concerned about crime in the neighborhood, the need, the goal, and the objectives were defined as follows:

- *Need:* The group of elderly people has altered coping ability related to their fear of crime.
- *Goal:* Within 6 months, this group of elderly people will be free to walk the streets of their neighborhood without experiencing any incidents of criminal assault.
- *Objectives:*
  1. By the end of the first month, a safety committee (composed of senior citizens, nurses, police, and other appropriate community members) will be established to study the crime patterns in the neighborhood.
  2. The safety committee will develop strategies for crime reduction and elder protection, which will be presented to the city council for approval by the end of the third month.
  3. Safety strategies, such as increased police surveillance, Town Watch patrols, and escort services, will be implemented by the end of the fifth month.
  4. By the end of the sixth month, nursing assessment will determine that senior citizens feel free to walk about the neighborhood.
  5. By the sixth month, there will be no reported incidents of criminal assault.

Development of objectives depends on a careful analysis of all the ways in which one could accomplish the larger goal. One should first select the course of action that is best suited to meet the goal and then build objectives. For the group of elderly people, other alternatives, such as staying indoors or always walking in pairs, were considered and rejected. The ultimate choice was to find a way to make their environment safe and enjoyable.

Some rules of thumb are helpful when writing objectives. First, each objective should state a single idea. When more than one idea is expressed—as in an objective to both obtain equipment and learn procedures—it is more difficult to measure the completion of the objective. Second, each objective should describe *one* specific behavior that can be measured. For instance, the fourth objective from the list states that the seniors will report feeling free to walk outdoors within 6 months. It describes a behavior that can be measured at some point in time. One can more readily evaluate objectives that include specifics—such as what will be done, who will do it, and when it will be accomplished. Then it is clear to everyone involved exactly what has to be done and within what time frame. Writing measurable objectives makes a tremendous difference in the success of planning. (See Chapter 11 for more information on writing behavioral objectives.)

Planning means thinking ahead. The nurse looks ahead toward the desired end and then decides what intermediate actions are necessary to meet that goal. Sometimes, an objective itself describes the intermediate actions. At other times, an objective may be further broken down into several activities. For example, the second objective states that the safety committee will be charged with developing strategies, presenting them to the city council, and gaining their approval. Good planning requires this kind of detail.

Making decisions is an important part of planning. Decisions must be made during the process of establishing priorities. Decisions are necessary for selecting goals and for choosing the best course of action from many possible courses. Further decision making is involved in selecting objectives and taking action to accomplish the objectives.

To facilitate planning and decision making, the community health nurse involves other people. Clients must be included at every step because they are the ones for whom the planning is being done. Without their insight and cooperation, the plan may not succeed. Additionally, the involvement of other nurses may be important. Team meetings, nurse–supervisor conferences, and nurse–expert consultant sessions are all useful resources for planning. In addition, you may wish to confer with members of other health and professional disciplines (e.g., teachers, social workers, mental health professionals, city planners). Interdisciplinary team conferences are valuable for gaining a broader perspective and enlisting wider support for the evolving plan.

IMPLEMENTING PLANS FOR PROMOTING THE HEALTH OF THE COMMUNITY

Implementation is putting the plan into action. The activities delineated in the plan are carried out by the nurse, other professionals, or clients. Implementation is often referred to as the action phase of the nursing process. In community health nursing, implementation includes not just nursing action or nursing intervention but collaboration with clients and perhaps other professionals. When bringing about change in a community organization, "implementation involves preparing a timeline for completion of each program objective, obtaining the necessary funding, collaborating with agencies outside the community as needed, recruiting additional community volunteers needed for program implementation, and actually putting into action the interventions designed during the planning phase" (Anderson, Guthrie, & Schirle, 2002, p. 44). Certainly, the nurse's professional expertise and judgment provide a necessary resource to the client group. The nurse is also a catalyst and facilitator in planning and activating the action plan. However, a primary goal in community health is to help people learn to help themselves in achieving their optimal level of health. To realize this goal, the nurse must constantly involve clients in the deliberative process and encourage their sense of responsibility and autonomy. Other health team members may also participate in carrying out the plan. All are partners in implementation.

Preparation

The actual course of implementation, outlined in the plan, should be fairly easy to follow if goals, expected outcomes, and planned actions have been designed carefully. Professionals and clients should have a clear idea of *who, what, why, when, where,* and *how.* Who will be involved in carrying out the plan? What are each person's responsibilities? Do all understand why and how to do their parts? Do they know when and where activities will occur? As implementation begins, nurses should review these questions for themselves, as well as for clients. This is the time to clarify any doubtful areas, thereby facilitating a smooth implementation phase.

Even the best planning may require adjustments. For example, some nurses who planned a health fair for seniors discovered that the target group would not have transportation to the site because the volunteering bus company had withdrawn its offer. To smoothly implement the plan, the nurses arranged for volunteers from local churches to pick up the seniors, bring them to the health fair, and deliver them afterward to their homes. Implementation requires flexibility and adaptation to unanticipated events.

Activities or Actions

The process of implementation requires a series of nursing actions or activities:

1. The nurse applies appropriate theories, such as systems theory or change theory, to the actions being performed.
2. The nurse helps to facilitate an environment that is conducive to carrying out the plan (e.g., a quiet room in which to hold a group teaching session or solicitation of support from local officials for an environmental cleanup project).
3. The nurse and other health team members prepare clients to receive services by assessing their knowledge, understanding, and attitudes and by carefully interpreting the plan to clients. This interaction nurtures open communication and trust between nurse and clients. Professionals and clients (or representatives if the aggregate is large) form a contractual agreement about the content of the plan and how it is to be carried out.
4. The plan is carried out, or modified and then carried out, by professionals and clients. Modification requires constant observation and interchange during implementation, because these actions determine the success of the plan and the nature of needed changes.
5. The nurse and the team monitor and document the progress of the implementation phase by process evaluation, which measures the ongoing achievement of planned actions.

EVALUATING IMPLEMENTED COMMUNITY HEALTH PLAN

Evaluation is usually seen as the final step, but since the nursing process is cyclic in nature, the nurse is constantly evaluating throughout the entire process. For instance, in the assessment phase, the nurse must evaluate whether the collected data are sufficient and appropriate to beginning planning. Evaluation methods must be addressed "in the planning phase, when goals and measurable objectives are established" and interventions are identified (Shuster & Groeppinger, 2004, p. 369). **Evaluation** refers to measuring and judging the effectiveness of goal or outcome attainment. Too often, emphasis is placed primarily on assessing client needs and on planning and implementing service. The nursing process is really not complete until evaluation takes place. Actually, if you look at the nursing process as cyclical instead of linear, then the evaluation guides the next assessment (Tembreull & Schaffer, 2005). How effective was the service? Were client needs truly met? How has health status changed? Professional practitioners owe it to their clients, themselves, and other health service providers to fully and effectively evaluate a program (see From the Case Files II).

As stated earlier, evaluation is an act of appraisal in which one judges value in relation to a standard and a set of criteria. Evaluation requires a stated purpose, specific standards and criteria by which to judge, and judgment skills.

Types of Evaluations

To determine the success of their planning and intervention, community health nurses use two main types of evaluation: formative and summative evaluation. The focus of *formative* evaluation is on process during the actual interventions. *Summative* evaluation focuses on the outcome of the interventions: Did you meet your goals? In formative evaluation, performance standards are developed and used to determine what is and is not working throughout the process (Anderson, Guthrie, & Schirle, 2002). They could include the physical and organizational structure of the agency, as well as resources that provide a foundation for any interventions. Formative evaluation essentially looks at the step-by-step process of program implementation. Could I do anything better or differently to increase my desired outcome? An example would occur when looking at the poor attendance at two sessions of an evening health-promotion class for senior citizens. The nurse identifies the reason for poor attendance as being seniors' reluctance to attend an evening class because they either don't drive at night or fear coming out in the dark. The class is rescheduled for mid-morning, and the attendance dramatically increases.

Summative evaluation examines outcomes of the interventions. The *effect,* or degree to which an outcome objective has been met, informs the agency or program leader of the program's impact on clients' health. As an example, one manufacturing company had an 80% adherence rate for employees who were supposed to wear proper protective devices (goggles, safety shoes, and hard hats) in the plant. Noncompliance on the part of some workers was a concern to union representatives, the health and safety team, and the company management. They were concerned that 20% of their

From the Case Files II

Evaluating Outcomes of a Home Care Postpartum Program

Scenario

As a nurse working as the liaison between Capitol City Hospital and its home health agency, you are given the job of reviewing your early postpartum discharge program. Your program has been in effect for 18 months. Client satisfaction is high. The program has increased revenue for the hospital as many clients choose to deliver at Capitol City Hospital because of the early discharge program.

The protocol for your early discharge program includes a postpartum home visit by an RN from the home health agency. These visits are provided as a service to the client. In some cases, visits are billable to insurance companies. Medicaid authorizes payment for one postpartum visit.

You have gathered the following information about the early discharge program:

I. Protocol: Standard is one visit within 48 hours after discharge which includes:
   A. Education
      1. Newborn care
      2. Breast-feeding
      3. Warning signs warranting follow-up (mother and baby)
         —Infection
         —Hemorrhage
      4. Comfort
      5. Parenting
      6. Sexuality
         —Resumption of sexual activity
         —Contraception
      7. Community resources
      8. Nutrition
      9. Well and sick baby care
   B. Assessment
      1. Infant: Jaundice (heel stick performed if necessary)
         Mother: Hemorrhage, perineal lacerations, hematomas
         Both: Nutrition
         —Weight
         —Hydration
         —Breast-feeding
      2. Elimination

II. Cost:
   A. Fully reimbursed by some insurance companies
   B. All mother/baby dyads receive postpartum visits, regardless of insurance coverage
   C. Optional or additional methods of reimbursement have not been explored by the agency
   D. Agency makes money on reimbursed visits, loses money on non-reimbursed, but additional revenue generated by clients choosing the hospital because of the positive public perception. The program is thought to balance out cost of nonreimbursed visits.

Outcomes. Outcomes of postpartum early discharge with accompanying home visit (as compared to traditional length of postpartum stay)

I. Positive
   A. Higher percentage of successful (at least 2 months) breast-feeding
   B. Higher rate of immunization compliance
   C. Fewer inappropriate emergency room visits
   D. High client satisfaction
   E. Lower levels of maternal stress reported to pediatricians

II. Negative
   A. Higher incidence in jaundice in babies whose mothers participated in the early discharge program

Questions

1. What, if any, additional information do you need to make a recommendation regarding the program?
   - How will you obtain this information?
2. As the nurse making a recommendation for the continuation or termination of the postpartum early discharge program, what are your recommendations?
   - Should the program be abandoned?
   - Should the program be maintained?
3. What, if any, alterations would you make in the following areas:
   - Funding
   - Protocol
     —Client education
     —Assessment
     —Timing of visit
4. Outcome measurements are critical to demonstrate the efficacy of this program.
   - What will you evaluate?
   - How often?
   - Why?

employees were at risk for injury that would cause pain, suffering, loss of work time, disruption to the manufacturing process, and reduced profitability. The occupational health nurse along with the safety officer began a month-long safety campaign that included safety mini-classes, posters, and incentives for departments with 100% safety equipment adherence. Three months after the program, 95% of the employees were adhering to the safety regulations. This 15% increase was attributed to the effect of the safety program. See Chapter 12 for more on program evaluation.

The *impact* of a program determines how close it comes to attaining its goals. In the earlier example, the objective of the safety campaign was to increase safety equipment use, and use was significantly increased as a result of the program. However, if the goal of the program had been to decrease accidents and save the company money, the result could be determined only with additional information. Were there fewer injuries caused by accidents? Were there fewer days lost to injuries? Did the company save money as the direct result of employee safety adherence? Depending on the answers to these questions, the overall goal of the program may or may not have been met, even though the objective of the program was met. The full impact of the program cannot be determined without additional data. See Chapter 12 for more on program evaluation.

Community Development Theory

An outcome of effective community level nursing practice is community development. **Community development** is the process of collaborating with community members to assess their collective needs and desires for positive change and to address these needs through problem-solving, the use of community experts, and resource development (Seng et al., 2005; Fawcett et al., 2000; Green, 2000; Green, Daniel, & Novick, 2001). A community development perspective assumes that community members participate in all aspects of change—assessment, planning, development, delivery of services, and evaluation. With

this approach, the focus is on healthful community changes generated from within the community, as a partnership between health care providers and inhabitants, rather than a commodity dispensed by health care providers (McLennan & Lavis, 2006; Tembreull & Schaffer, 2005; Zahner, Kaiser, & Kapelke-Dale, 2005). Chapter 11 details community change theory.

The outcomes are more positive when community members have a sense of ownership in the health programs and services that address their needs (Sharpe, Greaney, Lee, & Royce, 2000; Timmons et al., 2007). This enhances empowerment among members of the community and enables them to more effectively control and participate in transforming their environment and their personal circumstances. This implies that health care agency infrastructures are appropriate additions to services that are planned and delivered in an acceptable manner to the community (see Fig. 15.6, Arnstein's Ladder). See Chapter 13.

When applying community development theory, the agent of change (often the community health nurse) is considered a partner rather than an authority figure responsible for the community's health. To achieve acceptance as a partner, the nurse must listen and learn from the community members, because they are the experts with respect to their health care needs, culture, and values (Timmons et al., 2007; Kreuter, Lezin, & Young, 2000; Pan et al., 2005). They have mastered adaptation to the community, and they have first-hand knowledge of prevention methods and interventions that are appropriate to their lifestyles. For example, a study was conducted with 690 women from 18 impoverished inner-city neighborhoods in five cities. Women who were considered by peers to be opinion leaders conducted human immunodeficiency virus (HIV) risk-reduction workshops and community HIV prevention events. There was evidence that significant changes in health behaviors to prevent HIV infection occurred among the women who attended these events (Sikkema et al., 2000). The principles of community-based participatory research also

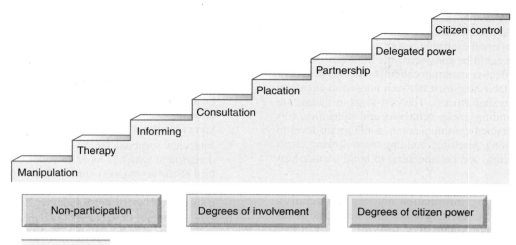

Citizen control

Delegated power

Partnership

Placation

Consultation

Informing

Therapy

Manipulation

| Non-participation | Degrees of involvement | Degrees of citizen power |

FIGURE 15.6 Arnstein's Ladder—Eight steps of citizen participation. Adapted from Arnstein, S.R. (July 1969). A ladder of citizen participation. *Journal of the American Institute of Planners,* 217–224.

involve this type of partnership (see Chapters 13 and 25 for more information on this subject). Members of the community are engaged as co-researchers, and time is spent building trust and developing collaborative relationships with community members, stakeholders, and neighborhood health care providers. The expertise of community members is valued and can be useful in designing recruitment strategies, as well as in data analysis (Savage et al., 2006). This experience can enrich the community as a whole, as well as the actual participants.

The outcomes of the services provided by any organization can be benchmarked against those of other groups. *Benchmarking* involves comparing an organization's outcomes against those of a similar organization or an organization that is known for its excellence in a particular area of client care (Nolan & Mock, 2000; Wojner, 2001). Information from this comparison can be used to identify an organization's areas of weakness and to focus attention on specific outcomes. The establishment of *best practice* activities entails "continuous, collaborative, and systematic processes for measuring and examining internal programs' strengths and weaknesses" (Lewis & Latney, 2002, p. 24).

From a global perspective, the Conference on Primary Health Care held at Alma-Ata in 1978 concluded that people have little control over their own health care services and that the emphasis should be on health problems identified by the members of the community in their attempts to attain a state of wellness (WHO, 1998). Since that time, the WHO, along with other agencies and groups, has been providing leadership in the use of community development methods to improve global health, based on the following concepts (Community Development Society, 2007):

◆ Promote active, representative participation to influence decisions affecting community members' daily lives
◆ Engage community members in economic, social, political, environmental, psychological, and other issues that impact them

◆ Interest them in learning more about alternative courses of action
◆ Incorporate diverse cultures, ethnic and racial groups, and varied interests in the process of community development
◆ Refrain from supporting efforts that are likely to adversely affect disadvantaged members of the community
◆ Actively work to build leadership capacity of community leaders and groups, and individuals
◆ Work toward long-term sustainability and community well-being

Summary

Characteristics of healthy communities include those elements that enable people to maintain a high quality of life and productivity by increasing health and decreasing disease and disparities in health and health care delivery. The effectiveness of community health nursing practice depends on how well the nursing process is used as a tool to enhance aggregate health. The nursing process involves appropriate application of a systematic series of actions with the goal of helping clients achieve their optimal level of health. The components of this process are assessment, diagnosis, planning, implementation, and evaluation.

The concept of community as client refers to a group or population of people as the focus of nursing service. The community's health is reflected in its status (e.g., morbidity and mortality rates, crime rates, educational and economic levels), structure (availability, use and quality of services and resources), and processes (how well it functions in regard to its strengths and limitations). The dimensions of a community's health may be seen in regard to its location (e.g., climate, vegetation, boundaries), population (e.g., diversity or homogeneity, old, young, pregnant, addicted, or academic members), and social systems (e.g., schools, businesses, communications, health care, and religious organizations, among others).

Interaction is deeply integrated in the nursing process. Because nurse and clients must first establish a relationship of reciprocal influence and exchange before any change can take place, interaction could be considered the most essential step in the process. Effective communication is inherent in assessing needs and establishing trust between nurse and clients as partners in the nursing process. The first steps in interacting involve understanding group behaviors and dynamics, followed by interpersonal communication at the group level in the form of listening, teaching, building trust, seeking client involvement, sharing, and collaborating to build partnerships and teams.

Assessment for community health nurses means collecting and evaluating information about a community's health status to discover existing or potential needs and assets as a basis for planning future action. Assessment involves two major activities. The first is collection of pertinent data, and the second is analysis and interpretation of that data.

Community health nurses may use various assessment methods to determine a community's needs. They include *familiarization assessments*, such as windshield surveys, which involves studying data already available on a community; *problem-oriented assessment*, which focuses on a single problem and looks at the community in terms of that problem; *community subsystem assessment,* by which the community health nurse focuses on a single dimension of community life; a complicated and time-consuming *comprehensive assessment,* to discover *all* relevant community health information; or an *assets assessment* that focuses on the strengths of a community as opposed to its deficits.

Community data may be provided by surveys, descriptive epidemiologic studies, community forums or town meetings, focus groups, and primary and secondary sources, such people who are familiar with the community and its character and history, websites, government departments and agencies that compile statistics, such as the Bureau of the Census, the county health department and others. Sources can include national international, state, county, and local agencies, as well as business and social organizations.

Using the nursing process in the community would not be complete without looking at the role of the community health nurse as a catalyst for community development. Community development theory is the foundation that supports citizen empowerment and use of key players in the community to plan for the health and safety of that community. ∎

ACTIVITIES TO PROMOTE CRITICAL THINKING

1. Explain to a colleague why it is important to understand and work with the community as a total entity.
2. How does defining the community as the client change the community health nurse's practice? List some specific examples of how this concept can be applied.
3. If you were part of a health planning team concerned about the health needs of the elderly people in your community, what are some location, population, and social system variables you would want to assess? Name some of the sources from which you might collect the data.
4. Discuss under what circumstances you might choose to conduct a problem-oriented community health assessment. What method would you consider using to conduct this assessment, and how would you carry it out?
5. Interview someone from your state or local health department who has recently conducted a community needs assessment survey. Analyze the process used, and compare it with the steps for conducting a survey described in this chapter.
6. Use the Internet to contribute your ideas in response to a health-related survey taken by a television show, newspaper, or magazine, or share your opinions in a health-related chat room.

References

Adcock, C., & Brown, L. (1957). Social class and the ranking of occupations. *The British Journal of Sociology, 8*(1), 26–32.

Aeppel, T. (2007, May 4). *Youngstown thinks small as its population declines.* The Wall Street Journal Online. Retrieved July 24, 2008 from http://www.homes.wsj.com/bysell/regionalnews/20070504-aeppel.html.

American Public Health Association, Public Health Nursing Section. (October 1996). *The definition and role of public health nursing: A statement of APHA nursing section.* Washington, DC: Author.

Anderson, D., Guthrie, T., & Schirle, R. (2002). A nursing model of community organization for change. *Public Health Nursing, 19*(1), 40–46.

Anderson, E.T., & McFarlane, J. (2004). *Community as partner: Theory and practice,* 4th ed. Philadelphia: Lippincott, Williams & Wilkins.

Badger, T., Gagan, M.J., & McNiece, C. (2001). Community analysis for health planning with vulnerable populations. *Clinical Nurse Specialist, 15*(3), 95–102.

Blewett, L., Casey, M., & Callk, K. (2004). Improving access to primary care for a growing Latino population: The role of safety net providers in the rural Midwest. *Journal of Rural Health, 20*(3), 237–245.

Brown, P., & Clapp, R. (2002). Looking back on Love Canal. *Public Health Reports, 117,* 95–98.

Brugge, D., Durant, J., & Rious, C. (2007). Near-highway pollutants in motor vehicle exhaust: A review of epidemiologic evidence of cardiac and pulmonary health risks. *Environmental Health, 6,* 23.

Calvert, G., Plate, D., Das, R., et al. (2004). Acute occupational pesticide-related illness in the US, 1998–1999: Surveillance findings from the SENSOR-pesticides program. *American Journal of Industrial Medicine, 45*(1), 14–23.

Cargan, L. (2007). *Doing social research.* Lanham, MD: Rowman & Littlefield.

Carpenito-Moyet, L.J. (2007). *Handbook of nursing diagnosis,* 12th ed. Philadelphia: Lippincott, Williams & Wilkins.

Centers for Disease Control & Prevention (CDC). (2007). *Behavioral Risk Factor Surveillance System: Turning information into health.* National Center for Chronic Disease Prevention & Health Promotion. Retrieved July 24, 2008 from http://www.cdc.gov/brfss/.

Chappell, N., Funk, L., & Allan, D. (2006). Defining community boundaries in health promotion research. *American Journal of Health Promotion, 21*(2), 119–126.

Choi, M., Afzal, B., & Sattler, B. (2006). Geographic information systems: A new tool for environmental health assessments. *Public Health Nursing, 23*(5), 381–391.

Chrisman, N.J. (2007). Extending cultural competence through systems change: Academic, hospital, land community partnerships. *Journal of Transcultural Nursing, 18*(Suppl. 1), S68–S76, discussion S77–S85.

Clark, C.C. (Ed.). (2002). *Health promotion in communities: Holistic and wellness approaches.* New York: Springer.

Community Development Society. (2007). Principles of good practice. Retrieved July 24, 2008 from http://www.comm-dev.org.

Cottrell, L.S., Jr. (1976). *The competent community.* In B.H. Kaplan, R.N. Wilson, & A.H. Leighton (Eds.). *Further explorations in social psychiatry.* (pp. 195–209). New York: Basic Books.

Davis, R., Cook, D., & Cohen, L. (2005). A community resilience approach to reducing ethnic and racial disparities in health. *American Journal of Public Health, 95*(12), 2168–2173.

Diaz, J.H. (2005). The epidemiology, syndromic diagnosis, management, and prevention of spider bites in the South. *Journal of the Louisiana Medical Society, 157*(1), 32–38.

Dixon, J.K. (2002). Kids need clean air: Air pollution and children's health. *Family and Community Health, 24*(4), 9–26.

Dominici, F., Peng, R., Bell, M., et al. (2006). Fine particulate air pollution and hospital admission for cardiovascular and respiratory diseases. *JAMA, 295*(10), 1127–1134.

Dong, M., Anda, R., Felitti, V., et al. (2005). Childhood residential mobility and multiple health risks during adolescence and adulthood. *Archives of Pediatric & Adolescent Medicine, 159*(12), 1104–1110.

Epstein, L., Gofin, J., Gofin, R., & Neumark, Y. (2002). The Jerusalem experience: Three decades of service, research, and training in community-oriented primary care. *American Journal of Public Health, 92*(11), 1717–1721.

Faruque, F., Lofton, S., Doddato, T., & Mangum, C. (2003). Utilizing geographic information systems in community assessment and nursing research. *Journal of Community Health Nursing, 20*(3), 179–191.

Fawcett, S.B., Francisco, V.T., Paine-Andrews, A., & Schultz, J.A. (2000). A model memorandum of collaboration: A proposal. *Public Health Reports, 115,* 199–204.

Forbes, D., & Janzen, B. (2004). Comparison of rural and urban users and non-users of home care in Canada. *Canadian Journal of Rural Medicine, 9*(4), 227–235.

Gandelman, A., Desantis, L., & Rietmeijer, C. (2006). Assessing community needs and agency capacity: An integral part of implementing effective evidence-based interventions. *AIDS Education & Prevention, 18*(4 Suppl. A), 32–43.

Gladman, A.C. (2006). Toxicodendron dermatitis: Poison ivy, oak, and sumac. *Wilderness Environmental Medicine, 17*(2), 120–128.

Gough, P.J. (2007). *Presidential candidates to debate over Internet.* The Hollywood Reporter. Retrieved July 24, 2008 from http://www.hollywoodreporter.com/hr/content_display/news/e3i af82321e51c9ae093c3c40caeeba91eo0.

Green, L.W. (2000). Caveats on coalitions: In praise of partnerships. *Health Promotion Practice, 1,* 191–197.

Green, L., Daniel, M., & Novick, L. (2001). Partnerships and coalitions for community-based research. *Public Health Reports, 116*(Suppl. 1), 20–31.

Heinemann, G.D., & Zeiss, A.M. (2002). *Team performance in health care assessment and development.* Norwell, MA: Kluwer Plenum.

House, J., Lepkowski, J., Williams, D., et al. (2000). Excess mortality among urban residents: How much, for whom and why? *American Journal of Public Health, 90*(12), 1898–1904.

Hutchings, A., Raine, R., Brady, A., et al. (2004). Socioeconomic status and outcome from intensive care in England and Wales. *Medical Care, 42*(10), 943–951.

Kalos, A., Kent, L., & Gates, D. (2005). Integrating MAPP, APEXPH, PACE-EH, and other planning initiatives in Northern Kentucky. *Journal of Public Health Management Practice, 11*(5), 401–406.

Knowlton, K., Lynn, B., Goldberg, R., et al. (2007). Projecting heat-related mortality impacts under a changing climate in the New York City region. *American Journal of Public Health,* (ePub ahead of print).

Kretzman, J., & McKnight, J. (1993). *Building communities from the inside out: A path toward finding and mobilizing a community's assets.* Chicago, IL: ACTA Publications.

Kreuter, M.W., Lezin, N.A., & Young, L.A. (2000). Evaluating community-based collaborative mechanisms: Implications for practitioners. *Health Promotion Practice, 1,* 49–63.

Kumanyika, S., & Grier, S. (2006). Targeting interventions for ethnic minority and low-income populations. *Future of Children, 16*(1), 187–207.

Laraia, B., Messer, L., Kaufman, J., et al. (2006). Direct observation of neighborhood attributes in an urban area of the US south: Characterizing the social context of pregnancy. *International Journal of Health Geography, 17,* 5–11.

Larson, S., & Fleischman, J. (2003). Rural-urban differences in usual source of care and ambulatory service use: Analyses of national data using Urban Influence Codes. *Medical Care, 41*(Suppl. 7), III65–III74.

Lenihan, P. (2005). MAPP and the evolution of planning in public health practice. *Journal of Public Health Management Practice, 11*(5), 381–388.

Lewis, P.S., & Latney, C. (2002). Achieve best practice with an evidence-based approach. *Nursing Management, 33*(12), 24–30.

Mantas, J., & Hasman, A. (2001). *Textbook in health informatics: A nursing perspective.* Amsterdam: IOS Press.

McKnight, R., & Spiller, H. (2005). Green tobacco sickness in children and adolescents. *Public Health Reports, 120*(6), 602–605.

McLennan, J., & Lavis, J. (2006). What is the evidence for parenting interventions offered in a Canadian community? *Canadian Journal of Public Health, 97*(6), 454–458.

Minnesota Senate. (2006). *Town meeting internet forums.* Retrieved July 25, 2008 from http://www.senate.leg.state. mn.us/caucus/dem/demforums.htm.

Mobilizing for Action through Planning and Partnerships (MAPPS). Retrieved August 5, 2007 from http://www.naccho. org/topics/infrastructure/MAPP/mappbasics.cfm.

Mundinger, M.O., & Jauron, G.D. (1975). Developing a nursing diagnosis. *Nursing Outlook, 23*(2), 94–98.

National Institutes of Health. (2007). *About NIH.* Retrieved July 25, 2008 from http://www.nih.gov/about/index.html.

National Latino Research Center. (October 2004). *The border that divides and units: Addressing border health in California.* San Marcos, CA: Author.

Neufeld, A., & Harrison, M.J. (1996). Educational issues in preparing community health nurses to use nursing diagnosis with population groups. *Nurse Education Today, 16,* 221–226.

Neuman, B., & Fawcett, J. (2001). *The Neuman systems model,* 4th ed. Stamford, CT: Appleton & Lange.

Oleske, D.M. (2001). *Epidemiology and the delivery of health care services: Methods and applications* (2nd ed.). NY: Springer Publishing.

Omaha System. (2005). *The Omaha System: An overview.* Retrieved July 25, 2008 from http://www.omahasystem.org/systemo.htm.

O'Reilly, G., O'Reilly, D., Rosato, M., & Connolly, S. (2007). Urban and rural variations in morbidity and mortality in Northern Ireland. *BMC Public Health, 7,* 123.

Pan, R., Littlefield, D., Valladolid, S., et al. (2005). Building healthier communities for children and families: Applying asset-based community development to community pediatrics. *Pediatrics, 115*(Suppl. 4), 1185–1187.

Pandey, P., Sharma, R., Roy, M., et al. (2006). Arsenic contamination in the Kanker district of central-east India: Geology and health effects. *Environmental & Geochemical Health, 28*(5), 409–420.

Pham, K., Harrison, G., & Kagawa-Singer, M. (2007). Perceptions of diet and physical activity among California Hmong adults and youths. *Prevention of Chronic Disease, 4*(4), A93.

Polit, D., & Beck, C.T. (2007). *Nusing research: Generating and assessing evidence for nursing practice.* Philadelphia, PA: Lippincott, Williams & Wilkins.

Population Reference Bureau. (2005). *People on the move. Activity 2: Population mobility is changing my state.* Retrieved July 25, 2008 from http://www.prb.org/Educators/LessonPlans/2005/PeopleontheMove/Activities/Activity2.aspx.

Quad Council. (2003). Quad Council PHN Competencies. Retrieved on July 3, 2007 from http://www.resourcecenter.net/image/ACHNE/Files/Final_PHN_competencies.pdf.

Rhoads, J. (2007). Epidemiology of the brown recluse spider bite. *Journal of the American Academy of Nurse Practitioners, 19*(2), 79–85.

Saraiya, M., Glanz, K., Briss, P., et al. (2003). Preventing skin cancer: Findings of the Task Force on Community Preventive Services on Reducing Exposure to Ultraviolet Light. *Morbidity & Mortality Weekly Report, 54*(RR15), 1–12.

Sattler, B., & Lipscomb, J. (Eds.). (2003). *Environmental health and nursing practice.* New York: Springer.

Savage, C., Xu, Y., Lee, R., et al. (2006). A case study in the use of community-based participatory research in public health nursing. *Public Health Nursing, 23*(5), 472–478.

Schulte, J. (2000). Finding ways to create connections among communities: Partial results of an ethnography of urban public health nurses. *Public Health Nursing, 17*(1), 3–10.

Seng, P., Acorda, E., Carey-Jackson, J., et al. (2005). AANCART best practices: Cancer awareness activities for Seattle's Cambodian community. *Cancer, 104*(Suppl. 12), 2916–2919.

Sharpe, P., Greaney, M., Lee, P., & Royce, S. (2000). Assets-oriented community assessment. *Public Health Reports, 115*(2–3), 205–211.

Shuster, G. F., & Goeppinger, J. (2004). Community as client. In M. Stanhope, & J. Lancaster (Eds.). *Community and Public Health Nursing.* St. Louis: Mosby.

Sikkema, K.J., Kelly, J.A., Winett, R.A., et al. (2000). Outcomes of a randomized community-level HIV prevention intervention for women living in 18 low-income housing developments. *American Journal of Public Health, 90*(1), 57–63.

Skelly, A.H., Arcury, T.A., Gesler, W.M., et al. (2002). Sociospatial knowledge networks: Appraising community as place. *Research in Nursing and Health, 25,* 159–170.

Smedley, B., Stith, A., & Nelson, A. (Eds.). (2003). *Unequal treatment: Confronting racial & ethnic disparities in health care.* Washington, DC: Institute of Medicine, The National Academies Press.

Soto-Quiros, M., Soto-Martinez, M., & Hanson, L. (2002). Epidemiological studies of the very high prevalence of asthma and related symptoms among school children in Costa Rica from 1989 to 1998. *Pediatric Allergy & Immunology, 13*(5), 342–349.

Spector, R.E. (2009). *Cultural diversity in health and illness* (7th ed.). Upper Saddle River, NJ: Prentice-Hall Allied Health.

Stevens, J., Thomas, K., & Sogolow, E. (2007). Seasonal patterns of fatal and nonfatal falls among older adults in the U.S. *Accidents: Annals of Prevention, 39*(6), 1239–1244.

Stolte, K.M. (1996). *Wellness: Nursing diagnosis for health promotion.* Philadelphia: Lippincott, Williams & Wilkins.

Stone, J. (2002). Race and healthcare disparities: Overcoming vulnerability. *Theoretical Medicine, 23,* 499–518.

Tatalovich, Z., Wilson, J., Milam, J., et al. (2006). Competing definitions of contextual environments. *International Journal of Health Geography, 7*(5), 55.

Tembreull, C., & Schaffer, M. (2005). The intervention of outreach: Best practices. *Public Health Nursing, 22*(4), 347–353.

Tiesman, H., Zwerling, C., Peek-Asa, C., et al. (2007). Non-fatal injuries among urban and rural residents: The National Health Interview Survey, 1997–2001. *Injury Prevention, 13*(2), 115–119.

Timmons, V., Critchley, K., Campbell, B., et al. (2007). Knowledge translation case study: A rural community collaborates with researchers to investigate health issues. *Journal of Continuing Education in the Health Professions, 27*(3), 183–187.

U.S. Department of Health and Human Services. (n.d.). *Healthy people 2010 tool kit.* Retrieved July 25, 2008 from http://www.healthypeople.gov/state/toolkit/overview.htm.

U.S. Department of Health and Human Services. (2000). *Healthy people 2010: Understanding and improving health,* 2nd ed. Washington, DC: U.S. Government Printing Office.

U.S. Department of Health and Human Services. (February 2001). *Healthy people in healthy communities.* [Electronic version.] Washington, DC: U.S. Government Printing Office.

U.S. Department of Health and Human Services. (n.d.). *Planned approach to community health: Guide for the local coordinator.* Retrieved August 7, 2007 from http://www.cdc.gov/nccdphp/publications/PATCH/pdf/00patch.pdf.

U.S. Department of Health & Human Services. (2007). *The 2005 HHS poverty guidelines.* Retrieved July 25, 2008 from http://aspe.hhs.gov/poverty/05poverty.shtml.

Williams, C.A. (1977). Community health nursing: What is it? *Nursing Outlook, 25*(4), 250–254.

Wojner, A.W. (2001). *Outcomes management: Applications to clinical practice.* St. Louis: Mosby.

World Health Organization (WHO). (2008a). Data and statistics. Retrieved October 1, 2008 from http://www.who.int/research/en/.

World Health Organization (WHO). (2008b). The world health report. Retrieved October 1, 2008 from http://www.who.int/whr/en/.

World Health Organization. (n.d.). Retrieved August 17, 2007 from http://www.who.int/whr/en/.

World Health Organization. (n.d.). Retrieved August 17, 2007 from http://www.who.int/research/en/.

World Health Organization. (1976). Community health nursing report of a WHO expert committee. Technical Report Series No. 555. Geneva: Author.

World Health Organization. (1998). *Primary health care in the 21st century is everybody's business.* Geneva: Author.

Zahner, S., Kaiser, B., & Kapelke-Dale, J. (2005). Local partnerships for community assessment and planning. *Journal of Public Health Management Practice, 11*(5), 460–464.

Selected Readings

Clark, L., Barton, J.A., & Brown, N.J. (2002). Assessment of community contamination: A critical approach. *Public Health Nursing, 19*(5), 354–365.

Eide, P., Hahn, L., Bayne, T., et al. (2006). The Population-Focused Analysis Project for teaching community health. *Nursing Education Perspectives, 27*(1), 22–27.

Farquhar, S., Poarker, E., Schulz, A., & Israel, B. (2006). Application of qualitative methods in program planning for health promotion interventions. *Health Promotion Practice, 7*(2), 234–242.

Gilbertson, M., Carpenter, D., & Upshur, R. (2001). Methodology for assessing community health in areas of concern: Measuring the adverse effects on human health. *Environmental Health Perspectives, 109* (Suppl. 6), 811–812.

Gushulak, B., & MacPherson, D. (2006). The basic principles of migration health: Population mobility and gaps in disease prevalence. *Emerging Themes in Epidemiology, 3*(3), doi:

10.1186/1742-7622-3-3. Retrieved from http://www.ete-online.com/content/3/1/3.

Keller, L., Schaffer, M., Lia-Hoagberg, B., & Strohschein, S. (2002). Assessment, program planning, and evaluation in population-based public health practice. *Journal of Public Health Management & Practice, 8*(5), 30–43.

MacPherson, D., & Gushulak, B. (2001). Human mobility and population health. New approaches in a globalizing world. *Perspectives in Biological Medicine, 44*(3), 390–401.

McClellan, C.S. (2005). Utilizing a national performance standards local public health assessment instrument in a community assessment process: The Clarendon County Turning Point Initiative. *Journal of Public Health Management & Practice, 11*(5), 428–432.

Olivia, G., Rienks, J., & Chavez, G. (2007). Evaluating a program to build data capacity for core public health functions in local maternal child and adolescent health programs in California. *Maternal Child Health Journal, 11*(1), 1–10.

Omaha System. (2005). *Solving the clinical data-information puzzle: Julie B., 18-year-old pregnant teen.* Retrieved July 25, 2008 from http://www.omahasystem.org/julieb.htm.

Plescia, M., Joyner, D., & Scheid, T. (2004). A regional health care system partnership with local communities to impact chronic disease. *Prevention of Chronic Disease, 1*(4), A16.

Plescia, M., Koontz, S., & Laurnet, S. (2001). Community assessment in a vertically integrated health care system. *American Journal of Public Health, 91*(5), 811–814.

Strauss, R.P., Sengupta, S., Quinn, C., et al. (2001). The role of community advisory boards: Involving communities in the informed consent process. *American Journal of Public Health, 91*(12), 1938–1943.

U.S. Department of Health & Human Services. (2000). *Community health status report: Data sources, definitions, and notes.* Retrieved July 25, 2008 from http://www.phf.org/CHSI-notes.pdf.

Wells, R., Ford, E., Holt, M., et al. (2004). Tracing the evolution of pluralism in community-based coalitions. *Health Care Management Review, 29*(4), 329–343.

Yoshioka-Maeda, K., Murashima, S., & Asahara, K. (2006). Tacit knowledge of public health nurses in identifying community health problems and need for new services: A case study. *International Journal of Nursing Studies, 43*(7), 819–826.

Zahner, S., Kaiser, B., & Kapelke-Dale, J. (2005). Local partnerships for community assessment and planning. *Journal of Public Health Management & Practice, 11*(5), 460–464.

Zust, B.L., & Moline, K. (2003). Identifying underserved ethnic populations within a community: The first step in eliminating health care disparities among racial and ethnic minorities. *Journal of Transcultural Nursing, 14*(1), 66–74.

Internet Resources

Agency for Toxic Substances & Disease Registry: *http://www.atsdr.cdc.gov/*

Agency for Toxic Substances & Disease Registry: (neighborhood public health assessment): *http://www.atsdr.cdc.gov/HAC/pha/NewhallStreet/newhall-p3.html*

Champions for Inclusive Communities (state snapshots of children/family services, etc.): *http://www.championsinc.org/main/ctb.cfm*

Child Health Care Quality (community assessment tool): *http://www.ahrq.gov/chtoolbx/*

Community Assessment & Planning Process (CAPP): *http://www.cpc.unc.edu/measure/publications/html/ms-00-08-tool12.html*

Community/Coalition Assessment Tools: *http://www.udetc.org/surveyandcommunity.asp*

Community Development Tool Box: *http://www.communitydevelopment.uiuc.edu/toolbox/*

Community Tool Box (tools for building healthier communities): *http://ctb.ku.edu/en/*

Contra Costa County (community health indicators): *http://www.cchealth.org/health_data/hospital_council_2007/*

Florida Community Health Assessment Resource Tool Set (CHARTS): *http://www.floridacharts.com/charts/chart.aspx*

Health Finder (health information guide; screening tools): *http://www.healthfinder.gov/*

Healthy Communities Tool Kit: *http://www.mihealthtools.org/documents/HealthyCommunitiesToolkit_web.pdf*

Healthy People 2010 Tool Kit: *http://www.healthypeople.gov/state/toolkit*

Healthy People in Healthy Communities (planning guide for HP2010): *http://www.healthypeople.gov/Publications/HealthyCommunities2001/healthycom01hk.pdf*

Multnomah County Health Assessment & Evaluation: *http://www.co.multnomah.or.us/health/hra/haq.shtml*

National Alliance for Hispanic Health: *http://www.hispanichealth.org/*

National Association of City & County Health Officials/CDC (MAPP toolkit): *http://www.naccho.org/pubs/documents/na30_mappfieldguide.pdf*

National Center for Health Statistics: *http://www.cdc.gov/nchs/*

National Health Information Center (health information resource database; list of national health observances): *http://www.health.gov/nhic/*

National Institute of Environmental Health Sciences: *http://www.niehs.nih.gov/*

National Safety Council (accidental injury/death prevention): *http://www.nsc.org*

National Vital Statistics System (CDC): *http://www.cdc.gov/nchs/nvss.htm*

Office of Disease Prevention: *http://www.odphp.osophs.dhhs.gov/*

Suicide Prevention Community Assessment Tool: *http://www.sprc.org/library/catool.pdf*

U.S.D.A. Economic Research Service (food insecurity community assessment tools): *http://www.ers.usda.gov/Publications/EFAN02013/*

U.S.D.A. Rural Development (community tool box resource links): *http://www.rurdev.usda.gov/rbs/ezec/Toolbox/index.html*

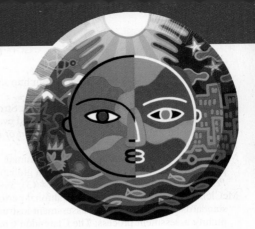

16

Global Health and International Community Health Nursing

LEARNING OBJECTIVES

Upon mastery of this chapter, you should be able to:

◆ Describe a context and framework for delivering community based nursing within the context of international community health nursing.

◆ Describe the major health care conditions currently affecting the world's populations and the types and preparation of health care workers addressing them.

◆ Describe the community health nursing interventions and strategies commonly used within an international context.

◆ Recognize the factors that influence populations' perceptions of health and health status and their receptivity to community health nursing programs.

◆ Describe the personal and professional perceptions and biases you bring to providing community health nursing interventions within an international context.

◆ Identify the major international, national, regional, and local organizational structures and organizations that affect the ways in which community health nursing is practiced.

◆ Locate relevant resources as a basis for planning the assessment, implementation, and evaluation of community health nursing within an international context.

"Our country is the world—our countrymen are mankind."
—William Lloyd Garrison, American abolitionist (1805–1879)

KEY TERMS

Community health worker (CHW)
Control
Disability-adjusted life year (DALY)
Elimination
Era of Chronic, Long-Term Health Conditions
Era of Infectious Diseases
Era of Social Health Conditions
Eradication
Global burden of disease (GBD)
Global nursing
Health for All
Integrated Management of Childhood Illness (MCI)
Multilateral agencies
Oral rehydration therapy (ORT)
Pluralistic health care systems
Primary Health Care (PHC)
Universal Imperatives of Care
World Bank (WB)
World Health Assembly (WHA)
World Health Organization (WHO)
World Health Organization Collaborating Centers

Let us suppose that you have completed your schooling and are ready to embark on a career in global community health nursing. **Global nursing** can range from providing clinical services to policy making at an international level. Perhaps you engaged in several years of successful clinical practice and are interested in pursuing an international opportunity to practice nursing in another country. You undertake a search of the World Wide Web, you talk to professional colleagues, and you read articles in nursing and other professional and popular journals.

You quickly realize that researching health care is a rather awesome undertaking, and the search for health care opportunities within a global context is even more of a challenge. You also learn that health care is complex, and that it affects and is affected by multiple factors that have to do with geography, history, politics, culture, religion, and a nation's wealth. You also learn that some countries' data are difficult to access, and you realize this may be because a country has been involved in a long, protracted civil war, or has experienced continuous cycles of disasters or financial collapse.

In your search, you also find that people's conception of health, wellness, and illness varies from culture to culture, and that the ways in which they view nurses and other health care providers is affected by their culture and belief systems. You will also notice patterns across countries and regions regarding who lives, who dies, the way people function on a day-to-day basis, the health care decisions they make, and the cost of the care they receive (Display 16.1).

In your search, you also will learn a great deal about the health care providers that countries look to for nursing care and medical treatment. You will notice a disparity between the health status and health conditions of people in a country, as well as the kind of health care providers educated and practicing in that country. You may become sensitized to the difference between your kind of nursing education and that of the nurses in countries different from your own. The ways in which one is recruited and educated do vary from country to country, as does legislation regarding licensure and entry to practice.

You will come across hundreds of references to international, national, and regional agencies that work in health care internationally. These references will be organized according to international agencies, national governments, churches, and nongovernmental organizations, including those with religious affiliations and universities.

Finally, you will see that the ways in which community health nursing is practiced in an international context are influenced by all these factors and by your own orientation, values, cultural beliefs, and education. These factors and issues constitute a global framework for community health nursing, and they are the foci of this chapter.

This chapter begins with a framework you can use to organize your thinking and around which you can structure your search as you expand your repertoire of knowledge and understanding. Those of us who work abroad need this kind of framework in which to place our searches, professional dialogues, and readings. We also need a way of thinking about the regions of the world or countries in which we would like to practice and about the kinds of community health nursing interventions a country may need, given the elements described here.

A FRAMEWORK FOR GLOBAL COMMUNITY HEALTH NURSING

The Three P's

To guide your thinking, consider a global framework bounded by a context and including three parts, the three "P's." These are: the population, the provider, and the procedure. In community health nursing, we speak about populations rather than about patients. The provider refers to the health care team which may include a community health nurse, a physician, a midwife, an "injector" (someone who is trained to only give injections), or a community health worker (CHW). The procedure refers to the interventions health care providers implement for or with populations.

Three Eras of Health Conditions

In this global framework, alongside the three P's, think about three *eras* of health and health conditions. During our ancestors' time, people easily contracted the plague, tuberculosis, puerperal fever, and other infectious diseases. Entire populations were sometimes eliminated through these infections. During this first era, families had many children, as they knew that most children would die before adulthood and without any form of social security, children were their parents' only source of livelihood. This is referred to as the **Era of Infectious Diseases**. With the advent of antibiotics, it became usual for people to survive common infections. Children began to survive much longer than did their parents, but often they suffered from chronic, long-term illnesses such as heart disease, cancer, and debilitating arthritis (Cox, 2005). This is referred to as the **Era of Chronic, Long-Term Health Conditions**. Despite changes and advances in health care, people continued to produce large families because of the cost or absence of birth control measures, persistent religious beliefs that influenced families regarding birth, and the intent of countries—such as Romania (before 1989)—to increase their populations for financial reasons. More recently, a new array of health conditions is affecting world populations, including addictions and obesity, and social conditions such as prostitution and deviant behavior. These are examples from the **Era of Social Health Conditions**. The popular press has exposed many of these conditions through documentaries on the effects of methamphetamine on entire communities, the obesity epidemic sweeping countries throughout the world, and the slave trade of young children (Medical News Today, 2005).

Continuing Emerging Health Conditions

Today, the communities of the world are experiencing all three eras of health conditions. In one community, a population may be dealing simultaneously with avian (bird) influenza, heart

---

DISPLAY 16.1	DEFINITION OF HEALTH

Health is a state of complete physical, mental, and social well-being and not merely the absence of disease or infirmity.

Source: World Health Organization Constitution

disease, cancer, and adolescent prostitution. Most of these health conditions have been present for many years, some for thousands of years. Twenty-five years ago, public health specialists believed that infectious diseases would soon play a minor role in health. However, they are still the world's leading cause of death, and some of the newly identified infectious agents have developed into public health challenges that confront countries worldwide (WHO, 1998b). This chapter examines the context in which these conditions occur, the health care providers who work with them, and the ways in which interventions are applied through the work of many sponsoring global health organizations.

Universal Imperatives of Care

In addition to the three P's and the three eras of health conditions, community health nurses need to consider the current status of health in the community of interest. The **Universal Imperatives of Care** is one useful paradigm. These imperatives include: mortality, morbidity, daily functioning, decision-making, and cost. This paradigm underscores the notion of *first things first*. That is, one must be alive and well before interventions focus on functioning or decision-making (Fig. 16.1).

Mortality

A government's first priority is to keep its population alive and free from illness. This is critical if a country is to survive, protect itself, and feed its population. In this regard, community health nurses may be frustrated that the disabled are going without community resources, or programs are not created to help couples make informed decisions about abortion and birth control. However, when countries are poor, they will focus on mortality and the evidence-based interventions that will ensure the survival of the people (Farrell, 2006). When mortality is a priority, the physician will be the valued health care provider.

Morbidity

When people are not dying, a country will focus on its population morbidity—the conditions that make people sick—and will look to physicians and nurses for assistance. Sickness derives from infectious diseases, long-term chronic health conditions, and the social conditions (discussed in upcoming sections).

Daily Functioning

In many countries, the ability to care for oneself—to bathe, secure food, and carry out other activities of daily living—are the purview of social services and social workers, or, for the elderly, of nursing homes. However, in some countries, social workers are not part of the health care team and these functions are left entirely to the family. This is not because the government is negligent. It is because the universal imperatives in a country with constrained resources must focus on the necessities first.

Decision-Making

In order to choose, one needs options. In countries where there is only one health care delivery provider, there are no options. As countries have expanded to include privatization, and as people increasingly have access to the World Wide Web, they have generally evolved in their decision-making processes about the providers they will use and the sources of their health information.

Cost

In many countries in the past, the state provided all health care, and all costs were the burden of the community. Increasingly, these health services are being rationed, restricted, or placed under insurance schemes. Nations are forced to weigh the cost of managing some health conditions over others. Most of the time, they opt for those that can be addressed with the least input and the maximum benefit. This is, in part, the reason that the Era of Social Conditions is not being addressed in many countries. The interventions that will reduce the incidence of these conditions are largely unknown, and the knowledge and research needed to access them are well beyond many countries' resources, thus encouraging these countries to work increasingly with the international community. Many countries do not have the resources to support the necessary research and programming to address the issues that may involve them and their border countries.

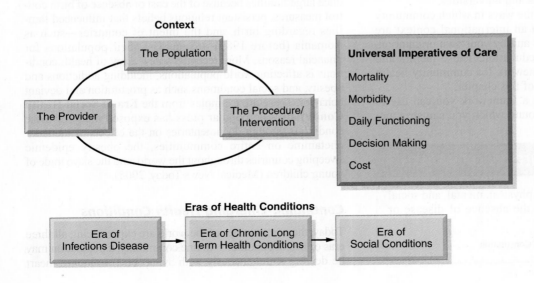

Context

The Population

The Provider

The Procedure/ Intervention

Universal Imperatives of Care

Mortality

Morbidity

Daily Functioning

Decision Making

Cost

Eras of Health Conditions

Era of Infections Disease → Era of Chronic Long Term Health Conditions → Era of Social Conditions

FIGURE 16.1 Framework for global community health nursing (M. Farrell, 2006).

THE CONTEXT

A Context of Interdependency

The context of community health nursing suggests considering one planet of interdependent nations. This interdependence relates to virtually all areas of life, including health. As systems theory suggests, what happens in one country affects many others in important ways (Friedman, 2005). For example, air travel can transport health problems from a country halfway around the world to new communities in less than a day.

Human immunodeficiency virus/acquired immunodeficiency disease (HIV/AIDS) began in Africa and is now pandemic because communicable diseases know no geographic boundaries. In New York, in the fall of 1999, 61 severe cases and seven deaths were reported from a mysterious viral illness later identified as the West Nile virus, which had not previously been reported in the United States. Researchers now speculate that the virus may have traveled to the United States in smuggled exotic birds. The virus was closely related genetically to strains found in the Middle East (Centers for Disease Control and Prevention [CDC], 2000). Within two years, 3,737 cases of West Nile Virus and 214 deaths had occurred in 39 states. Evidence of infections in birds, humans, mosquitoes, and other animals has been documented in 43 states and the District of Columbia (CDC, 2002a).

The globalization of food commodities and food safety also affects health. For example, researchers suggest that a causal relationship exists between ongoing outbreaks in Europe of bovine spongiform encephalopathy, or *mad cow disease*, and the human disease called new variant Creutzfeldt-Jakob disease (vCJD). Of the worldwide total of 153 vCJD cases, 143 of these have occurred in the United Kingdom. Cattle are considered the only source of the disease (CDC, 2006). Global health issues become everyone's issues when they spread within or beyond one's borders, when we commit resources to a country in need, when we make a personal commitment to improve the health of a population beyond our shores, and when we import or export food.

The community health nurse works with populations that live in particular parts of the world. These localities are unique, with their own geography and environment, history, cultural traditions, religion, and ideas about health, wellness, disease, and death. Each of these elements constitutes entire disciplines of study and require years of interacting with people to understand the ways in which they affect health care in a particular country.

Geography and Environment

The environment in which people live includes air, climate, soil, and water, and each of these may undergo changes that turn natural elements into hazardous ones. Humans are exposed to pollutants in two basic ways: by exposure to the source or by release of the pollutant into air or water.

When people use streams and rivers to dispose of body wastes and then use the same body of water for cleaning and washing their clothes, they expose themselves to infections from those waters. When people in villages build their homes around sources of water, they also invite mosquitoes that carry malaria, for instance. In this environment, community health nurses' interventions might include teaching people the steps to preventing malaria, such as placing netting around a bed during the night, cleaning pools of stagnant water around the home, and covering the body with light cotton clothes (Heymann, 2004).

People throughout the world are affected by the impact of major developments that may occur in their communities over which they have no control. Governmental authorities may build a dam, create a waterway, or move populations to clear land for crops (Reuters News Service, 2006). For example, populations in Ethiopia were moved from one part of the country to another as colonial rulers developed crops for their own use. In the process, they displaced farmers to other areas to grow crops about which they knew little and which were not appropriate for the soil and weather conditions.

Environmental experts have focused on these and other issues, such as the effects on communities when climate changes occur or when weather conditions affect entire regions. The Tsunami in Asia and Hurricane Katrina in the United States are recent examples, sweeping away entire communities (National Geographic News, 2005). Most recently, former United States Vice President Al Gore has brought the world's attention to global warming through his provocative and moving film, *An Inconvenient Truth,* in which he examines the ways in which our current habits and beliefs are affecting the world's temperature and environmental conditions (Bender, David, Chilcott, & Burns, 2006).

Sometimes change is intentional and is made in the interests of survival and daily functioning. For example, when governments address energy concerns for transportation and industry, they may move to nuclear sources of that energy—clearly as an effort to secure a local resource, but also with some risk. The people of Chernobyl found their beloved home a wasteland when the nuclear plant disaster polluted the region with caesium and iodine (*Chernobyl Accident: Information and Issue Briefs*, March 2006). In a follow-up meeting in the Netherlands, representatives spoke of the population's fears and actions, including possessing machines that would measure the radioactivity near their homes. This accident prompted the discussion at this meeting of disaster-preparedness strategies to evacuate entire cities of people after a nuclear environmental accident.

Classification of Environmental Hazards

The Organization for Economic Co-operation and Development (OECD), World Health Organization (WHO), and others have classified the environmental hazards affecting communities that include the impact of local climate changes on weather patterns and agriculture (OECD, 2006). The Blumenthal Classification lists classes of environmental hazards. They include: infectious agents (e.g., bacteria and viruses), respiratory fibrotic agents (e.g., coal dust), asphyxiates (e.g., carbon monoxide), poison (e.g., pesticides), physical agents (e.g., noise), psychological agents (stressful synergisms such as crowding combined with noise), mutagens (e.g., dioxin), teratogens (e.g., cadmium), and carcinogens (e.g., cigarette smoke).

Contamination of Water Sources

In places such as Peru, Egypt, Bangladesh, India, Indonesia, and Thailand, raw sewage is released into rivers that are used for drinking and bathing. Such practices often result in

DISPLAY 16.2 ENVIRONMENTAL HAZARDS THAT KILL CHILDREN

1. Inadequate drinking water and sanitation
2. Indoor air pollution and accidents
3. Injuries and poisonings

These are just three of the causes of the approximately 3 million deaths suffered annually by children younger than 5 years of age as a result of environmental hazards. Research suggests that more than 40% of the global burden of disease due to environmental risk factors may fall on such young children, who constitute only about 10% of the world's population.

(World Health Organization [2002, March 3], Environmental hazards kill at least 3 million children aged under 5 every year. *Press Release WHO/12*. Geneva: WHO.)

diarrheal diseases, including cholera. In 1991, a cholera outbreak was identified at the port of Chancoy in Peru; it rapidly spread along the coast, over the Andes, and into the Amazon basin, resulting in 400,000 reported cases and 4,000 reported deaths in 13 countries (Whaley & Hashim, 1995). The International Center for Diarrhea Disease Control (ICDDR) in Bangladesh specializes in those illnesses, including cholera, that result from these practices, for which residents know of no alternative.

Five million people die annually from illnesses linked to unsafe drinking water, poor household hygiene, and improper human and animal waste disposal. Every 8 seconds, a child dies of a water-related disease. Half of the population in the poor countries of the world suffers from one or more of the five main diseases associated with water and sanitation—diarrhea, ascariasis, hookworm, schistosomiasis, and trachoma—and one-fourth of the world's population is without proper access to water and sanitation (WHO, 1996) (see Display 16.2).

Water-related diseases arise from the ingestion of pathogens in contaminated water or food and from insects or other water-associated vectors. However, overall progress in reaching people deprived of adequate water and sanitation services has been poor since 1990 (Jamison et al., 2006).

The Ozone Layer

As the challenge of a depleted ozone layer is addressed, the incidence of cataracts and cancer (especially melanoma and basal cell carcinoma) is reduced. It is believed that human activities are contributing to the depletion of the ozone layer; these activities include the use of chlorofluorocarbons (CFCs) (used in the manufacture of air conditioners, refrigerators, aerosol propellants, and other products) and methyl bromides (found in pesticides and herbicides). Efforts are underway to phase out CFCs in 13 countries, including the United States (The Ozone Hole, 2006).

History

If you have tea with a group of health care providers in Moscow, the conversation inevitably turns to the devastating effects of the major historical event that faced that country—World War II. Despite the fact that this war occurred over 60 years ago, it remains in the collective memory of the Soviet people, their leaders, and many others in Eastern Europe, as 20 million Russians died along with thousands of people in other countries. That war, and the war that involved Bosnia–Herzegovina and Serbia, will affect people for decades to come and will influence the ways in which the health care systems of these countries will partner and collaborate with each other in the future.

Throughout the past century, countries throughout the world have been colonized, and they continue in their relationships with former or current colonizing countries. These political relationships also affect the ways in which community health nurses might be recruited and practice. For example, given a country's history, health care providers with particular nationalities or religious backgrounds might not be acceptable to a country. While people in one country might consider these biases unacceptable, they remain as policy in other places, determining whether or not care providers of a particular nationality are allowed to enter and work in a country. These biases are often unexpected and may be puzzling. At first glance, one may wonder why Italy might want to support a disaster preparedness program in Ethiopia. But a review of the historical relationship between Italy and Ethiopia reveals a relationship that preceded the program initiative.

Community health nurses are involved in designing and implementing projects in collaboration with international governmental organizations and non-governmental organizations. The historical context of a country is paramount as people are selected for international positions and projects, for interventions that a community is willing to adopt, and organizations are chosen to intervene in a region.

Language

Often a language connection exists between countries, and this linkage prompts health officials to seek nurses who speak the same language. For example, common history and language often connect Mozambique, Portugal, and Brazil, which are all Portuguese-speaking countries. Many people from Mozambique immigrated to Portugal during the 1970s, and the shared historical past affects current perceptions about the two countries' relationship with each other. Knowing that a shared language exists among countries may suggest ways of gathering existing health-related teaching and learning materials and can reduce the costs of production and language validation.

A country's political orientation and practices affect the ways in which community health nurses are educated and function daily. For example, in some countries, nurses and midwives were not exposed to the emerging knowledge and practices concerning the HIV/AIDS epidemic. This happened, in part, because countries whose economies depended on tourism were fearful that high numbers of HIV-infected people would frighten away tourists. Consequently, national health policies and announcements denied the presence of the virus, and nurses and midwives were not protected as they collected blood samples, administered injections, and delivered babies.

Cultural and Religious Context

The culture and religion of a community represent the frame within which people understand who they are, why they are on the earth, and what their purposes are in life (Spector, 2004). Culture and religion influence the knowledge, attitudes, and practices of people about what they think will kill them or make them sick, will help them function or make decisions, or will affect their financial status. People in different cultures manage these in ways that may seem peculiar, ill-advised, immoral, or even criminal to someone outside the society. For example, Illyes, (1969) in the classic book *People of the Puszta*, discusses the cultural practice of suicide in a part of Hungary, the Puszta, where people are characterized as "dirt poor." Yet, suicide is not a socially accepted option for people in other cultures. In the Philippines, some prostitutes see their activities as their daily work, not as a moral act. Efforts to dismantle the country's prostitution business have met with negative reactions from the prostitutes themselves, as this is their way of feeding their children and caring for their families (The Official Website of the Republic of the Philippines, 2006).

Community health nurses will face their own beliefs when confronting female circumcision, the use of nonlicensed personnel to carry out medical treatments, and the use of Western interventions used simultaneously with local treatments. For example, in Chad, clients in a Chadian hospital received Western style medical treatment and nursing care through the interventions of French physicians and nurses while lines snaked around the grounds of the hospital to the offices of the two Chinese acupuncturists.

Cultural issues are of concern when individuals and groups of a particular background from one country are often fiercely committed to "helping" their homeland. Here, both donors and recipients need to understand each other and their reasons for entering collaborative relationships. When this is thought through, the results can be most positive. In this regard, Armenian communities benefited enormously from the fundraising efforts of American community health nurses and physicians who knew well the Armenian communities in Boston, parts of Canada, and Los Angeles (Armenia Fund USA, 2006).

Women and Culture

Women in most societies are viewed in ways that require close scrutiny. They are seen as Madonnas, superheroes, warriors, nurturers, slaves, income producers, objects of sexual desire, concubines, negotiators, angels of mercy, and assistants. Although these characterizations may be repulsive to some, to others, women in their communities have played these roles for so long that they are considered immutable and acceptable. In many countries, nurses are exclusively women and experience these projections as they carry out their daily work. In some places, women have no or little voice and are viewed as weak or ineffectual, despite their physiological hardiness and ability to survive above their male counterparts (Valadian & Farrell, 1995).

Community health nurses may perceive themselves as excellent practitioners with excellent theoretical and clinical backgrounds, and expect to be respected for these qualities. Yet, in another country, their nursing notes may be torn up (who will read them?), their projects taken over by others (a nurse can't possibly lead a project), and their research may be published under someone else's name (anyone can write hypotheses, so what makes these so special?). In some countries, women (and nurses) are not expected to argue with authority, assume a team leadership role, or attend important meetings at high levels (Valadian & Farrell, 1995).

These are challenging situations, some of which become teachable moments. Some may be events that alter the duration of one's assignment, or provide an opportunity to reframe interactions with others of differing persuasions, beliefs, and practices. Community health nurses need to determine their own position on these issues and come to terms with being placed in subservient positions or in roles that detract from their level of academic preparation, expectations for learning and developing, an ultimately, their sense of self.

Armed Conflict, Uprisings, Wars, and Humanitarian Emergencies

An armed conflict is defined as major if the number of deaths has reached 1,000. Increasingly, conflicts are internal rather than between states. In their quest for economic and political power, the combatants target the lives and livelihoods of civilians associated with opposing factions. Typically, armed conflicts and uprisings initially cause governments and agencies to place a high priority on health care, but their ability to sustain health care is reduced as time goes on. Countries engaged in armed conflict form internal factions, including those supporting the government and those in conflict against them. Most conflicts occur between states for economic and political power, and approximately 90% of those affected by such conflicts are civilians of all ages (Toole, Waldman, & Zwi, 2001). Sometimes, outside nations support a country's factions, and fighting escalates and continues until the supporting powers win, lose interest, change their political orientation, or exhaust their source of finance. In this regard, community health nurses need to be aware of those involved in the immediate situation and of those who are influencing the situation from abroad. In turn, funding and sustaining nursing projects may depend ultimately on the local population and on those external sources of support.

Countries that have longstanding conflicts suffer as current health care needs are unaddressed, and the long-term health status of an entire country may be affected—sometimes for decades. For example, Mozambique has endured a national conflict for over two decades. Entire generations of young people have had no formal education and are prepared only to fight. Countries in conflict deflect resources to the battlefield, and those fighting receive whatever resources are available. These conflicts are extremely complex social phenomena, for which the most rooted causes are inequity, cultural and religious intolerance, and ethnic discrimination (Mulli, 1996). The health infrastructure during conflicts and uprisings becomes vulnerable because of the instability. Often, opposing factions raid hospitals and clinics. During the 1989 Romanian uprising, health providers told of instances in which the underground secret police feigned injury, transported themselves in rigged ambulances, and entered the emergency room areas of the capitol's major hospitals, all in an effort to kill or wound the hospitals' health care providers.

Between the end of World War II and the end of the Cold War, most conflicts occurred in developing countries in Africa, the Middle East, Asia, and Latin America. After the dissolution of the Soviet Union, major conflicts occurred in the emerging European states, most recently in Yugoslavia (Glenny, 1992; Hall, 1994; Samary, 1995). Wars in other areas of the world also were reignited, such as that between Eritrea and Ethiopia (Global Issues, 2000). We now see similar situations in Iraq (Drum, 2005).

The community interventions that nurses develop are informed by the situation and the layers of conflict that have occurred in the past and those that may be continuing (see From the Case Files I). During national conflicts, health services become disorganized and experience decreased resources. Outside help is needed in these instances, and international help is often available. For example, during the Romanian uprising, members of WHO/EURO's International Disaster Preparedness Team, along with the country's health officials, established an Interim Ministry of Health and identified key areas that required attention. Members of the team, including the Regional Nursing Advisor, met with NATO and COMECON ambassadors in the capitol and communicated the health needs of the population. They remained in Romania and established a WHO office, participating with groups, universities, and organizations to assist the country during this difficult period.

During wars, epidemics are almost inevitable. As conflict goes on, the health care needs of the combatants often take priority over those of civilians; consequently, thousands of children may be injured, orphaned, and at risk for disease. Additionally, conflict disrupts food cultivation, harvest, and distribution, leaving populations at risk for malnutrition and setting the stage for disease. Refugees from such events have special health and social needs. Often refugee camps are developed by international organizations on the fringe of such conflicts to temporarily assist refugees with shelter, food, and the rudiments of health care. Such camps place a strain on the resources of neighboring countries, as illustrated during the recent war in Sudan (United States Fund for UNICEF, 2006).

All of these factors can lead to complex humanitarian emergencies. The Centers for Disease Control (CDC) describes complex humanitarian emergencies as situations that involve large civilian populations, and factors related to war or civil strife, shortage of necessities such as food, and the dislocation of local populations. These situations and these factors result in mortality beyond that expected under normal circumstances (Burkholder & Toole, 1995; United Nations High Commissioner for Refugees [UNHCR], 2006).

Recovery after war is a long-term project. Any post war recovery effort must deal with the disabled, the mentally ill, prisoners, widows, orphans, abandoned children, homeless and displaced persons, refugees, and the unemployed (Mulli, 1996; Siegel & Watson, 2006). These issues are complex; for example, in some African countries, if a family loses its land and its members cannot plant and harvest crops, the family dies. During the long conflict in that region, many women lost their husbands and their land. They required care from others who had very little to offer them.

In these environments, populations are displaced and people find themselves living in war zones that are strewn with the remnants of the war (Farrell, 1992a; Farrell 1992b; UNHCR, 2006). Land mines have continued to injure or kill long after hostilities have ceased. This issue received international attention from Princess Diana of Wales, who made their removal one of her major projects before her untimely death (The Work Continues, 2006).

Health Care Systems

Countries throughout the world have developed health care systems that they organize and structure in particular ways. When community health nurses find themselves in locations different from their own, they notice differences immediately, and their ability to focus on these differences, and even to document them, is critical. The capacity to reflect on one's consciousness is an essential skill as one considers the ways in which people expect to govern others, to provide people with what they need, determine who gets served and who does not, establish lines of authority and communication, and establish payment systems for health care services.

Important questions arise as one delivers community health nursing services within a country's health care system. For example, if a client has to wait 6 months for an elective operation, what does she do in the meantime? If a government provides all prenatal and obstetrical services, but will not instruct couples on birth control, how do couples manage, and how do health authorities deal with prevalent practices that result in an abortion rate that is three times the birth rate (Farrell, M. et al., 1994) or that allow *under the table* reimbursement for these services? If a ministry of health is administered in a centrally governed model of decision making, how do

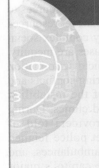

From the Case Files I

During the war in Yugoslavia, Bosnians and Serbs worked with the European Regional Office of the World Health Organization (WHO/EURO) in Copenhagen, Denmark, to develop interventions for women and children's health. WHO/EURO developed the training program to be held in Denmark, but was not certain that the roads between Sarajevo and the coast would be open and safe for travel, as snipers continued to operate out of the mountains surrounding Sarajevo and along the roads to the country's borders. The workshop the nurses, physicians, and midwives attended in Copenhagen included both Bosnians and Serbs in the breakout sessions, but the facilitator had to ensure separate dining spaces, as the workshops occurred during the latter part of the war—a time during which communications were difficult and awkward.

WHO Regional Advisor

decisions get made that require local—rather than district or national—answers? If a local nursing group is interested in developing community health nursing standards of practice, and yet all nursing actions are reviewed by only a medical board of physicians, on what are the nursing standards based?

Pluralistic health care systems are found in many countries. They often consist of traditional healing systems, lay practices, household remedies, transitional health workers, and practitioners of Western medicine (Kloos, 1994; Carr, 2004). Traditional healing may be all that is available to populations in most rural areas and in some cities.

Western medicine was introduced to other countries during colonial times, and systems were operated either by colonial administrations or by missions. After independence, health systems tended to vary in their development. Some continue their colonial practices; others followed tax-financed government insurance or socialist health care systems (Carr, 2004).

During the second half of the 20th century, curative health care expanded rapidly in urban areas, and the level of health care was raised in those areas. In the late 1970s, many countries adopted the primary health care (PHC) approach as they sought to serve their urban and rural populations. Four major types of health care systems are currently operational throughout the world. These systems are: entrepreneurial, welfare-oriented, comprehensive, and socialist systems.

◆ *Entrepreneurial health care systems.* A country's health care system is based, in part, on its political economy. An entrepreneurial health system is typically found in industrialized countries with free-market economies; abundant resources, large amounts of money allocated to health care, and decentralized governments. These countries operate from a highly individualistic perspective. For example, the health care system in the United States is typical of the entrepreneurial system.

◆ *Welfare-oriented health care systems.* Statutory programs drive these systems that support the cost of health care for all, or almost all, of the population through their "national health insurance." In these, half of the health-related expenditures are covered by government sources, but most physicians and dentists remain in private practice. Western Europe, Japan, and Australia subscribe to welfare-oriented health care systems.

◆ *Comprehensive health care systems.* These systems are a step away from the welfare-oriented types in that substantial modifications exist in delivery and financing that result in universal entitlements. These systems abandon the separate and complex sources of financing found in the previous two systems. The Scandinavian countries, Great Britain, and New Zealand use a comprehensive health care delivery system.

◆ *Socialist health care systems.* These systems came about through social revolutions that abolished free-market economies and replaced them with socialism, in which the health care system is also socialized. The first overthrow of capitalism was in Russia in 1917, followed by Eastern Europe, Albania, Bulgaria, Czechoslovakia, East Germany, Hungary, Poland, Romania, Yugoslavia, and later China. In these

systems, health services are viewed as a social entitlement and a government responsibility. They emphasize prevention engage in central planning for health resources and services with one central health authority, prioritize special groups such as industrial workers and children, and base health care work on scientific principles. Nonscientific and cultist practices are not permitted. Some of these countries are now in the process of democratization and are attempting to redesign their health care systems.

The four health systems described above apply to industrialized countries. Roemer (1993) applies the same typology to transitional and very poor countries. (Countries that are in the process of development are referred to as "transitional.") Such countries and their health care systems are moving effectively toward economic and social development. The global median gross national product (GNP) of these countries is $1,500 per capita. (It should be noted that some might object to this classification system that considers being financially poor synonymous with being socially underdeveloped. This suggests a bias in thinking and a Western perspective that determines what is developed and what needs developing.)

Very poor countries are even less economically developed and have lower per-capita GNPs than do the industrialized or transitional countries. Examples of very poor countries are Ethiopia, Kenya, Ghana, Myanmar, Sri Lanka, Mozambique, and China. Other countries that do not easily fit into the health care system matrix are the oil-rich developing countries. In just a few years, the wealth in such countries exploded upward, from low levels typical of Africa and some Asian countries to levels equal to or greater than those of highly industrialized countries. Examples are Gabon, Libya, Saudi Arabia, and Kuwait. The governments of these countries use their income to extend and improve health services for the general population. Entrepreneurial or socialist systems are not found in these countries. Gabon and Libya are classified as welfare-oriented because they have different schemes of social insurance for health services for a large percentage of the population. Saudi Arabia and Kuwait are universal and comprehensive systems that use government funding to provide complete health services to everyone.

Trends Affecting Health Care Systems

Health care systems are affected by major social influences such as urbanization, industrialization, education, government structure, international trade, and demographic changes. Many national health systems have undergone major changes during the 1980s and 1990s. Specifically, these health care systems have changed the way they organize and are managed. For example, in England, health services were traditionally led by health care professionals. In the mid 1980s, the emerging view was that one did not have to be a health provider to manage the health services of the country. Increasingly, health care administrators who were not from the health service ranks assumed these positions, and the composition of health teams changed among its leadership ranks.

Health care systems also expanded their resources and added personnel, facilities, and equipment. Meanwhile, populations grew, migrated, and became more educated. They demanded more and better health care services. Over the past decade, hospitals worldwide have shifted to outpatient services and home care, expanding the roles and positions of community health nurses. For example, hospitals in Denmark benefited from a surgical procedure for hip replacement that would allow a patient to be discharged from hospital to home in a much shorter time period than previously experienced. This meant that home care had to be ready to accept the patient within an abbreviated time frame, thus requiring innovations in discharge planning and teaching protocols. In addition to these advances, the PHC movement supported efforts to reduce the number of hospital buildings and to increase community based nursing services (Carr, 2004). Technological advances occurred to support this move, and ways of thinking about health promotion emerged with a variety of quality measures and, more recently, evidence-based practices that support nursing interventions on an outpatient basis and at lowered costs.

Most importantly, people have begun to educate themselves through the Internet and World Wide Web. Ministries of health are training community care workers in communication, observation, and technical skills for telemedicine systems that link remote areas to academic and health centers. For example, the PHC Center in Almaty, SSR is now connected through the Internet, even though it began as a relatively isolated Center in what was referred to Alma Ata. Now groups with relatively rare health care conditions can receive support and information from others in parts of the world formerly unknown to them.

THE POPULATION

The populations that community health nurses serve are complex and include their concerns, values, beliefs, physical symptoms, and health history. As described earlier, the framework that provides some boundaries for considering these issues focuses on the three eras of health conditions and the universal imperatives of care.

Era of Infectious Diseases

Infectious diseases and conditions have killed people, made them sick, altered their daily functioning, influenced their decision making, and affected the costs of care. Thus, these infections and infectious processes involve all the universal imperatives of care, but do so differently, depending on a variety of factors (Carr, 2004). These factors include the climate, geography, and other conditions infectious organisms need to survive and thrive, and the populations the infectious agents invade–often infants and children. Thus, it is not surprising that 98% of all deaths in children younger than 15 years of age are in those countries in which infectious diseases are rampant. Eighty-three percent of deaths of those aged 15 to 59 years are in these countries as well. The probability of death before age 15 ranges from 22% in sub-Saharan Africa to only 1.1% in countries with established market economies. Five of the 10 leading causes of death are communicable, perinatal, and nutritional maladies that largely affect children. Most of these are preventable. The major preventive measure, immunization, is described here, followed by brief descriptions of the major infectious diseases. See Display 16.3 for a ranked listing of the leading causes of death worldwide.

DISPLAY 16.3 RANKED LEADING CAUSES OF DEATH WORLDWIDE, FOR HIGH, LOW, AND MIDDLE INCOME COUNTRIES IN 2001

High Income Countries
1. Heart disease
2. Stroke
3. Lung cancer
4. Lower respiratory infections
5. Chronic obstructive pulmonary disease
6. Colon and rectum cancers
7. Alzheimer's disease and other dementias
8. Type 2 diabetes
9. Breast cancer
10. Stomach cancer

Low and Middle Income Countries
1. Heart disease
2. Stroke
3. Lower respiratory infections
4. HIV/AIDS
5. Perinatal conditions
6. Chronic obstructive pulmonary disease
7. Diarrhea
8. Tuberculosis
9. Malaria
10. Road traffic accidents

From Lopez, A. (May 27, 2006). Top 10 causes of death worldwide. *The Lancet, 367*, 1747–1757.

Immunization

The WHO estimates that 3 million more lives could be saved each year with immunizations. One of the most cost effective interventions available has been developed through the WHO Expanded Program on Immunization (EPI) (Reingold & Phares, 2001). Vaccines are one of the most cost-effective interventions found in public health. Today, almost three-fourths of the world's children are being reached with essential vaccines, but many barriers make it difficult to maintain high levels of immunization in low- and middle-income countries. In sub-Saharan Africa, for example, only one-half of the children have access to basic immunization against common diseases (WHO, 2002i).

Barriers persist and include limited finances, lack of trained health care workers, physical obstacles to reaching remote areas, and civil wars; these factors have prompted the development of an interagency vaccine initiative entitled the Global Alliance for Vaccine and Immunizations. This initiative seeks to protect every child against vaccine-preventable diseases (Reingold & Phares, 2001). Strategies include funding, research, development, distribution of vaccines, and program sustainability. These approaches are expected to result in more immunized children and to move newer vaccines into developing countries more quickly.

Maternal and Perinatal Morbidity and Mortality

The WHO estimates that 500,000 women die yearly from complications of pregnancy and childbirth. Ninety-nine percent of these deaths are in economically poor countries. Pregnant women living in parts of Africa face a one in 16 risk of death because they do not receive needed prenatal care. In comparison, the risk in Europe and North America is one in 4,000 (WHO, 1999g). The death of a mother profoundly affects the well-being of the entire family.

Early pregnancy, high fertility, and close child spacing are common in developing countries, and are known to be major determinants of poor health for mothers and children. Poverty, illiteracy, poor nutrition, low weight gain, maternal age (younger than 20 or older than 34 years of age), infections, smoke in the home, smoking, and poor health care are some of the major determinants associated with high health risks to mothers and children in the poorest nations of the world.

Prevention strategies include better general health for women through poverty alleviation, education, family planning guidance, prenatal care including food supplementation, immunization, local and regional care with referrals for complications, training of traditional birth attendants (TBAs), and effective postpartum care (Walsh, Feifer, Measham, & Gertler, 1993; WHO, 2001b; Carr, 2004).

Measles

Measles is a vaccine-preventable communicable disease. In 2000, the number of measles deaths was 800,000 (WHO/EIP, 2006). The largest number of deaths occurred in Africa and in Southeast Asia (WHO, 2006). The intervention considered to have the greatest impact in reducing measles is the **Integrated Management of Childhood Illness (MCI)**. This intervention promotes wide immunization coverage, rapid referral of serious cases, prompt recognition of secondary conditions, improved nutrition including breastfeeding, and vitamin A supplementation (WHO, 1998c). A WHO/UNICEF Measles Mortality Reduction and Regional Elimination Strategic Plan sought a 50% reduction in measles mortality worldwide by 2005–hoping eventually to eradicate the disease (WHO, 2002d).

Poliomyelitis

In 1988, there were 35,000 annual cases of poliomyelitis (polio) in the world (WHO, 1999e). By 1991, polio was eliminated from the Western hemisphere. Polio is now almost eliminated worldwide, even in densely populated and wartorn countries. Since the inception of the Global Polio Eradication initiative, cases have fallen by 99.8% to only 483 (in 2001), and the number of polio-infected countries dropped from 125 to 10. These 10 polio-endemic countries are classified as areas of high-intensity or low-intensity transmission. India, Pakistan/Afghanistan, and Nigeria/Niger are the areas with high-intensity transmission, and together they accounted for 85% of new polio cases in 2001. All have large populations, low immunization rates, poor sanitation, and a wide distribution of the wild virus. Somalia, Sudan, Ethiopia, Angola, and Egypt are areas with low-intensity transmission; they have lower-density populations and smaller focal areas of wild poliovirus. Global priorities for polio eradication include closing the funding gap, maintaining access and political commitment to the initiative, implementing the *polio endgame* strategies including laboratory containment, certificating polio eradication, and developing of a post certification polio immunization policy. The estimated cost of eradication is $1 billion (WHO, 2002f).

Diarrheal Diseases

Diarrhea is defined as the passage of more than three stools during a 24-hour period for individuals older than 3 months of age. The incidence of diarrheal diseases is somewhat elusive because it depends on the definition of diarrhea used, the frequency of surveillance, and the population. Sometimes public health professionals use the term *diarrhea* to mean dysentery, although the latter is usually characterized by the presence of blood in the stool, with or without looseness or specified frequency.

Among other causes, a host of enteric pathogens can result in diarrhea; these pathogens are most significant in countries where there is poverty, poor personal and domestic hygiene, infected water, low maternal education, and lower occupational status. These factors have been associated with diarrheal morbidity and mortality (Martines, Phillips, & Feachem, 1993; Heymann, 2004).

The risk is highest among infants who are not breastfed. In 2000, an estimated 1.3 million children younger than 5 years of age in developing countries died from diarrheal diseases caused by unsafe water supply, lack of sanitation, and poor hygiene (WHO, 2002).

Reductions in mortality rates have occurred; in some areas as many as 90% fewer deaths have been reported. This was largely the result of the promotion of **oral rehydration therapy (ORT)**, a simple treatment that mothers may administer to their children in order to replace lost fluid and electrolytes (Kosek, Bern, & Guerrant, 2003), (Display 16.4). Actions need to prevent diarrheal disease include community programs that promote personal and domestic hygiene, water supply and sanitation facility improvements, breast-feeding promotion and improved weaning practices, and immunizations for cholera and measles (Schlein, 2002d, 2007).

Countries have the possibility to reduce deaths and illness from 20% to 80% simply by improving water and sanitation (WHO, 1996; Carr, 2004). No single type of intervention has greater overall impact on national development and public health than does the provision of safe drinking water and proper disposal of human excreta.

DISPLAY 16.4	**HOW TO PREPARE HOMEMADE ORAL REHYDRATION SOLUTION (ORS)**

If ORS sachets are available: dilute one sachet in 1 L of safe water.
Otherwise, use 1 L of safe water and add
　　Salt—1/2 small teaspoon (3.5 g)
　　Sugar—4 big spoons (40 g)
In addition, try to compensate for loss of potassium (e.g., eat bananas or drink green coconut water).

World Health Organization. (2003). First steps for managing an outbreak of acute diarrhea. WHO Global Task Force on Cholera. Global health security: Epidemic alert and response, Box 2. Geneva: WHO.

Acute Respiratory Tract Infections

The most common illness in the world and a leading cause of mortality is acute respiratory tract infection (ARI). Three million deaths annually are attributed to ARI among children younger than 5 years of age, usually from pneumonia. Risk factors include low birth weight, poverty, crowding, lower educational levels, poor nutrition, inadequate childcare practices, and a lack of health education about ARI. Additional risk factors include smoking and indoor and outdoor air pollution. Indoor air pollution is 20 times higher in villages in poor areas than in homes in those countries of the world where two packs of cigarettes are smoked per day (Stansfield & Shepard, 1993; Schlein, 2002g, 2007). The source of pollution is largely indoor cookstoves that use organic fuel (Ezzati, Utzinger, Cairncross, Cohen, & Singer, 2005). A threat to the reduction of pneumonia, however, is the increase in drug-resistant organisms. Measures to better control ARI include: immunizations, birth spacing, and improvement in nutrition and living conditions (including use of smokeless cooking stoves). A global commitment to reduce ARI was realized by a resolution at the World Summit for Children in 1990 that called for a one-third reduction in deaths from the condition. This goal has been difficult to achieve because of the varying clinical symptoms and causative organisms of pneumonia (see Levels of Prevention Pyramid).

Human Immunodeficiency Virus Infection and Acquired Immunodeficiency Syndrome

An estimated 42 million people worldwide are living with the human immunodeficiency virus infection (HIV) and acquired immunodeficiency syndrome (AIDS). Almost 95% of these people live in developing or transitional countries where health care, resources, and drugs are scarce (WHO/Food and Agriculture Organization, 2003). Asia and Eastern Europe are experiencing epidemic rates of HIV/AIDS cases. Russia reported a 15-fold increase in just 3 years, and HIV is beginning to spread among high-risk populations in some Middle Eastern countries (WHO, 2001c). The pandemic could claim an additional 68 million lives by 2020–55 million of them in Africa (Fleshman, 2002). It is predicted that life expectancy in those countries is likely to decline by as much as 27%.

The virus attacks young adults in productive age groups, requiring older people to care for and support their terminally ill adult children and, later, their orphaned grandchildren. Often these elders are themselves impoverished and in poor health, and are left without caregivers when they require assistance in their later years. The HIV/AIDS epidemic threatens to upset and destabilize entire societies in Africa. Reduced productivity of adult workers and early death are counterproductive to economic and social development (WHO, 2002l).

Recently, an expanded global response to the pandemic offered 12 essential interventions to reduce HIV transmission: mass media campaigns, public sector condom promotion and distribution, condom social marketing, voluntary counseling and testing programs, prevention of mother-to-child transmission, school-based programs, programs for out-of-school youth, workplace programs, treatment of sexually transmitted infections, peer counseling for sex workers, outreach to men who have sex with men, and harm reduction programs for injection drug users. It is estimated that if these interventions were enacted by 2005, 29 million new HIV infections among adults could be prevented by 2010. The estimated cost for the large-scale prevention program is $27 billion (WHO, 2002c).

There is also hope regarding treatment. In 2002, the International AIDS Society launched new international guidelines to treat AIDS in resource-poor areas. Simplified and less expensive antiretroviral therapy has become available, and is expected to extend life expectancy and productivity of those persons living with AIDS (WHO, 2002b). Other research has demonstrated the effectiveness of circumcision for adult males in decreasing the spread of HIV (The Boston Globe, 2006), and the importance of protecting HIV-positive patients from malaria, as they become "super-contagious" and are more likely to spread HIV after contracting malaria (International Herald Tribune, 2006, p. 2).

Tuberculosis

Tuberculosis (TB) is an infectious disease caused by the tubercle bacillus. The disease has been known for hundreds of years and was commonly referred to as consumption. The tubercle bacillus has become resistant to the medications used to treat it, and currently a worldwide TB epidemic is underway. Two million die from TB each year, accounting for more than one-quarter of all preventable adult deaths in developing countries. Someone in the world is newly infected with TB every second. More than 8 million people around the world become sick with the condition each year; of these, 2 million cases occur in sub-Saharan Africa, 3 million in Southeast Asia, a 250,000 in Eastern Europe. Tuberculosis is one of the illnesses that disproportionately affect poor people around the world (Carr, 2004).

Tuberculosis and Human Immunodeficiency Virus

Tuberculosis alone is a pernicious illness. When TB and HIV occur in one individual, the combination is lethal, with each speeding the other's progress. Tuberculosis is the leading cause of death among people who are HIV-positive. Poorly managed TB programs are threatening to make TB incurable, and the movement of people through travel and relocation is helping to spread the disease. In the United States, almost 40% of TB cases are among foreign-born people (WHO, 2002e).

Malaria

Malaria is a disease caused by the presence of the protozoan parasite Plasmodium in human red blood cells; the parasite is usually transmitted to humans by the bite of an infected female mosquito. "Humans are the only important reservoir of human malaria" (Heymann, 2004, p. 325). Fifty percent of the world population lives in malaria endemic areas. During the 1990s, 200 million new cases were diagnosed yearly, and 2 million deaths were reported from the disease (Kaneko, 1998). Over 1 million deaths occur per year due to malaria (Heymann, 2004). In 2003, it was reported that sub-Saharan Africa accounted for 90% of the deaths due to malaria (WHO, 2003).

LEVELS OF PREVENTION PYRAMID

SITUATION: Prevent acute respiratory tract infections (ARIs) in children in developing countries.

GOAL: Using the three levels of prevention, negative health conditions are avoided or promptly diagnosed and treated, and the fullest possible potential is restored.

Tertiary Prevention

Rehabilitation	Primary Prevention

	Health Promotion & Education	Health Protection
• Restore child to optimal level of functioning through the recovery period	• Continue to promote educational programs and individual teaching regarding practices that promote health and prevent diseases among family members	• Educate on the prevention of recurrence and spread of disease

Secondary Prevention

Early Diagnosis	Prompt Treatment
• Get a prompt diagnosis of an acute ARI	• Collaborate with families to combine the best of folk and home remedies with established Western medical practices • Treat early with antibiotics (if indicated and available) • Provide culturally appropriate symptomatic care • Teach caregiver signs and symptoms of complications

Primary Prevention

Health Promotion & Education	Health Protection
• Promote general health education among community members • Good prenatal care • Advocate breast-feeding, child spacing, and adequate nutrition • Teach good hygiene and child care practices • Teach when to seek medical attention • Eliminate poverty and household crowding	• Administer appropriate immunizations • Eliminate indoor contaminants such as smoke from cookstoves without chimneys and cigarette, cigar, or pipe smoking • Ventilate rooms to eliminate indoor smoke and allow fresh air in

The global disease burden from malaria is estimated to be greater than 300 million acute illnesses and 1 million deaths per year. Ninety percent of the world's malaria cases occur in Africa, south of the Sahara. Malaria and the deaths it causes mainly affect two vulnerable groups–young children and pregnant women.

Malaria is resistant to multidrug therapy, and the mosquito, its tenacious vector, persists. Malaria is highly endemic in some areas, and its eradication depends on pesticides such as DDT. In addition, human and economic resources are not available to fully implement a malaria program. Perhaps the major contributors to lack of success have been failure to integrate the malaria eradication effort into basic health services, inadequate efforts to exploit the effective involvement of communities, and the absence of political will.

Health authorities who have reduced their expectations and are now focusing on programs of control, joined the WHO in a control strategy (Trigg & Kondrachine, 1998). This strategy includes the following elements (Jamison, Mosley, Measham, & Bobadilla, 1993; Heymann, 2004):

1. Early case finding and treatment
2. Reduction of contact with mosquitoes
3. Destruction of adult mosquitoes and larvae
4. Source detection
5. Destruction of malaria parasites
6. Community education programs

The WHO, UNICEF, UNDP, and the World Bank have partnered to launch an initiative entitled the Roll Back Malaria Program (RBM) the goal of which is to halve the incidence of malaria-related deaths throughout the world by 2010. The RBM initiative focuses on four major actions (WHO, 2002a):

1. Prompt access to treatment
2. Use of insecticide-treated bed nets
3. Prevention and control of malaria in pregnant women
4. Malaria epidemic and emergency response

The CDC, based in Atlanta, Georgia, continues work on developing an antimalaria vaccine using recombinant gene techniques. India and Kenya also have vaccine studies under way (WHO, 1999f).

Decreased effectiveness of antimalaria drugs due to development of drug resistance, particularly for the parasite of the most deadly form of the disease (*Plasmodium falciparum*), has brought attention to the need for new antimalaria medications. This problem is most acute on the Thai-Myanmar border in Southeast Asia, but it is also widespread in Africa. The WHO Tropical Disease Research Program (TDR), the Swiss Medicines for Malaria Venture (MMV), and Shin Poong Pharmaceuticals, Co. Ltd. in Seoul, Korea have collaborated in developing and producing a new combination antimalaria medicine, pyronaridine-artesunate, which is proving effective and affordable. One component of this medicine is a natural plant, *Artemesia annua,* whose antimalarial properties were first discovered centuries ago by the Chinese (WHO, 2002j).

Illustrating the spillover effect of disease from an endemic country to a nonendemic country are statistics on malaria in the United Kingdom. In 1996, 2,500 cases of malaria were reported—the largest number of cases in over 25 years (Bradley, Warhurst, Blaze, Smith, & Williams, 1998). Researchers found that 46% of the infected people had traveled to West or Central Africa on oil-related business (Nathwani & Spiteri, 1997). This spike in cases has declined due to community health education efforts.

River Blindness (Onchocerciasis)

Onchocerciasis or River Blindness destroys vision and causes significant damage to other tissues. This centuries-old infection is transmitted by the bites of black flies that appear near rivers. Hundreds of thousands were affected by this condition, which has now been eliminated. Officials announced its eradication in Ouagadougou, Burkina Faso, on December 6, 2002. A 30-year effort was required to eliminate this scourge as a public health threat in West Africa. When the program began, 10% of the infected population in high-impact areas was blind, and 30% had severe visual handicaps that caused loss of livelihood and autonomy (WHO, 2002k).

Health authorities carried out massive aerial spraying of *larvicide* to eliminate the vector, the black fly, in an area of 1.3 million square kilometers with a population of 30 million people. In 1991, the program delivered Ivermectin, the medication used to treat river blindness, to at least 80% of those living in endemic areas to maintain coverage for 10 to 15 years (Miri, 1998). The evidence of the elimination of the condition was the return of people to fertile areas formerly left unoccupied because of the debilitating disease. The resulting economic benefits are now dramatically enhancing the well-being of the population.

Leprosy

Leprosy is a chronic granulomatous infection caused by *Mycobacterium leprae* (Hansen's bacillus). It affects various parts of the body including the skin (*Stedman's Medical Dictionary*, 1995). Leprosy is curable, and in the last two decades of the 20th century, the prevalence of leprosy was reduced by 90%; today, it is found mainly in Africa, Asia, and Latin America, with 70% of the world's registered leprosy patients living in India (WHO, 2003a). People with leprosy have had access to free effective drug treatment since 1995. The global health community has set a goal of leprosy elimination by 2005. Communities can help others meet this goal through proper diagnosis and treatment and provision of care without stigma or isolation. Interventions require that communities make political commitments, integrate the treatment protocols into the everyday practices of the PHC systems, and change in the image of leprosy, so that people with the condition will more readily present themselves for treatment (WHO, 2003b).

Guinea Worm Disease (Dracunculiasis)

Dracunculiasis or Guinea Worm Disease is a parasitic disease that is transmitted to humans when a person drinks water containing a worm's intermediate host, a water flea that can ingest and harbor guinea worm larvae. Once in a human body, the larvae migrate through the tissue and the mature adult worm attempts to emerge, usually from the lower leg. Farmers are the most commonly affected. Although there is no cure, once the larvae are ingested, the eradication strategy includes interruption of transmission, surveillance, health education, and certification.

It is expected that Guinea Worm Disease will be completely eradicated soon. It is prevalent in 17 countries, 16 of which are in Africa. Cases decreased from 1 million to 80,000 between 1989 and 1997, demonstrating great promise for eradication. Interruption of transmission includes measures such as protecting drinking water by keeping infected persons out of it, filtering drinking water, and chemically treating water to eliminate the intermediate host. Geographical Information Systems (GIS) monitor guinea worm cases. There is interagency collaboration for the Dracunculiasis Eradication Program; the estimated cost to reach the ultimate goal of eradication is $40 million (WHO, 1998a). In 2000, over 75,000 cases were reported by WHO (2006b).

Era of Infectious Disease and the Universal Imperatives of Care

The infectious diseases and processes carry the potential for death, illness, and compromised functioning. When addressed promptly, some diseases, such as measles, can be prevented. When left unmanaged, they can result in sickness and lifelong consequences to daily functioning. Some of these conditions involve decision making. For example, when national governments do not provide clear national policies or funding for immunization programs, entire populations are at risk for the consequences of diphtheria, pertussis, typhoid, measles, and polio. When families and communities insist on living in areas with infectious agents, or do not clear their land as needed, they expose their members to the ravages of malaria. When community health programs do not include sanitation and the building of latrines, the result is diarrheal diseases that affect an entire community (Carr, 2004).

Eradication, Elimination, and Control of Communicable Diseases

The primary global health goals related to communicable disease are eradication, elimination, and worldwide control. **Eradication** means interruption of person-to-person transmission and limitation of the reservoir of infection so that no further preventive efforts are required; it indicates a status whereby no further cases of a disease occur anywhere. At times, the term **elimination** is used when a disease has been interrupted in a defined geographic area. In 1991, WHO defined elimination as a reduction of prevalence to less than one case per 1 million population in a given area. In contrast, the term **control** indicates that a specific disease has ceased to be a public health threat. Control programs are aimed at reducing the incidence and prevalence of communicable and some noncommunicable conditions.

Although eradication is always the desired effect, extensive funding and much international cooperation are usually required to achieve such a goal (see What Do You Think?). The successful eradication of smallpox from the world in 1977 came about because of the leadership of the WHO, and it was a tremendous accomplishment in public health. In 1967, smallpox was endemic in 31 countries, with 10 to 15 million individuals infected. Remarkably, within 10 years, there were no cases in the world (Whaley & Hashim, 1995). Clearly, if global eradication programs are to be successful, collaboration and partnerships are essential. Certification of river blindness elimination has now joined the growing list of global public health accomplishments (WHO, 2002k). These programs are dependent on commitment from involved governments, international bodies, NGOs, and the affected communities themselves. Global eradication and elimination programs that are close to meeting the goal include poliomyelitis and Guinea Worm Disease. Eradication programs for leprosy and measles are continuing. Additional major efforts have increased to reduce, control, and prevent malaria, tuberculosis, HIV/AIDS, diarrheal diseases, and respiratory infections. Unfortunately, international terrorism threatens to reintroduce smallpox through acts of bioterrorism; smallpox vaccination programs have had to be reestablished to protect health workers and the populations at risk (Connolly, 2003).

What Do You Think?

Imagine today's world without any international cooperation related to communicable disease knowledge or control. What would be some of the health, social, and economic consequences of such inaction?

New and Emerging Infectious Diseases and Conditions

Despite the advances made, new and emerging diseases, conditions, and syndromes have appeared in parts of the world. Health authorities thought that some of these were under control. Since 1973, a number of previously unknown diseases have emerged, among them Ebola hemorrhagic fever, Lassa fever, Hantavirus, Lyme disease, Legionnaires' disease, and toxic shock syndrome (see Table 16.1). Most recently, severe acute respiratory syndrome (SARS), an atypical pneumonia thought to be caused by a coronavirus, has been recognized (WHO, 2003e). SARS has been reported to have a mortality rate of up to 15%, and up to 50% for seniors and infants.

The development of antimicrobial-resistant organisms, mainly as a result of the overuse and misuse of antibiotics, has fueled a resurgence of some diseases that were under control, such as TB. Anti-TB medications are no longer effective in up to 20% of patients in some parts of the world. Two leading antimalaria medicines have become ineffective in many Asian countries, and a third is effective in only half of the world. The easy availability of global air travel and subsequent rapid transmission of microbes pose real health threats (Howard, Scott, Packard, & Jones, 2003).

Another factor related to emergence of new and recycling conditions is urbanization, which serves to concentrate large numbers of people in small geographic areas. With urbanization, deforestation continues, and the two phenomena may permit the infestation of microbes into human populations, as humans who move into the cleared forests may encounter previously unknown pathogens. Changes in agricultural practices, such as new dams and irrigation schemes, also present potential transmission scenarios (Shannon, 2001). The ability of microbes to change and adapt rapidly is a persistent threat as well.

Era of Chronic Long-term Health Conditions

Despite the programs of control, many infectious diseases persist. But populations now survive and also experience chronic, long-term conditions. These conditions affect mortality and morbidity, daily functioning, decision-making, and cost. Thus, the longevity that has resulted from meeting the challenges of the Era of Infectious Diseases compounds the more recent emergence of chronic diseases in the many countries. For countries in development, an interesting transition occurs. As infectious diseases decrease, life expectancy lengthens and the population experiences the degenerative diseases seen in developed countries. The concept of epidemiologic transition explains the replacement of

TABLE 16.1 Examples of Emerging Pathogens Identified Since 1973

Year	Microbe	Disease
1973	Rotavirus	Major cause of infantile diarrhea globally
1976	*Cryptosporidium parvum*	Acute and chronic diarrhea
1977	Ebola virus	Ebola hemorrhagic fever
1977	*Legionella pneumophilia*	Legionnaires' disease
1977	Hantaan virus	Hemorrhagic fever with renal syndrome
1977	*Campylobacter jejuni*	Enteric diseases distributed globally
1980	Human T-lymphotropic virus 1 (HTLV-1)	T-cell lymphoma-leukemia
1981	Toxin producing strains of *Staphylococcus aureus*	Toxic shock syndrome
1982	*Escherichia coli 0157:H7*	Hemorrhagic colitis; hemolytic uremic syndrome
1982	HTLV-II	Hairy cell leukemia
1982	*Borrelia burgdorfei*	Lyme disease
1983	HIV	AIDS
1983	*Helicobacter pylori*	Peptic ulcer disease
1988	Hepatitis E	Enterically transmitted non-A, non-B hepatitis
1990	Guanarito virus	Venezuelan hemorrhagic fever
1991	*Encephalitozzon hellem*	Conjunctivitis, disseminated disease
1992	*Vibrio cholerae 0139*	New strain associated with epidemic cholera
1992	*Bartonella henselae*	Cat-scratch disease; bacillary angiomatosis
1994	Sabia virus	Brazilian hemorrhagic fever
1995	Hepatitis G virus	Parenterally transmitted non-A, non-B hepatitis
1995	Human herpesvirus-8	Associated with Kaposi sarcoma in AIDS patients
1996	TSE-causing agent	New variant Creutzfeldt-Jakob disease
1997	Avian influenza (Type A [H5N1])	Influenza
1999	Nipah virus	Influenza-like symptoms, high fever, myalgia; may progress to encephalitis, convulsions, coma; 50% mortality rate
2002	SARS	Severe acute respiratory syndrome

(World Health Organization. [1998d]. Examples of pathogens recognized since 1973. *WHO Fact Sheet No. 97, 4*. Geneva: WHO; World Health Organization. [2001]. Nipah virus. WHO Fact Sheet, 262, 1–2. Geneva: WHO; World Health Organization [2003, 12 March]. WHO issues a global alert about cases of atypical pneumonia. *Press Release WHO/22*. Geneva: WHO.)

infectious disease morbidity and mortality with that of chronic disease. How people in remote areas will manage their heart disease or cope with the stigma of a disability is yet to be understood. Formerly, those with disabilities or compromised activities of daily living were cared for by the family, and were often hidden from the community. This was often due to religious and cultural beliefs and lack of knowledge.

As families change their composition, the care of those who require daily assistance will also have to change. It will require a change in the response of the health care system in terms of provision of care, planning, and allocation of resources. Addressing these concerns is considered a cost-effective investment in a nation's human capital (McQueen, McKenna, & Sleet, 2001).

Era of Social Health Conditions

The WHO researchers suggest that dramatic changes in health-related needs will occur within the next 20 years. There is evidence that noncommunicable diseases are rapidly replacing infectious diseases as the major causes of disability and premature death. Noncommunicable diseases are expected to account for seven of every 10 deaths in developing countries, compared with fewer than five of every 10 today (Display 16.5).

Mental Health Conditions

The burden of mental illness was previously unseen. Now recognized, it accounts for almost 11% of disease burden worldwide. Unipolar major depression is expected to be a

DISPLAY 16.5	THE TOP TEN PREVENTABLE HEALTH RISKS WORLDWIDE

Childhood and maternal underweight
Unsafe sex
High blood pressure
Tobacco
Alcohol
Unsafe water
Sanitation and hygiene
High cholesterol
Indoor smoke from solid fuels
Iron deficiency
Overweight/obesity

World Health Organization. (2002h). October 28. Years of life can be increased 5–10 years. *Press Release WHO/84*, Geneva. Author.

leading cause of disability-adjust life years (DALYS) by 2020 (WHO, 2002h).

Tobacco

Tobacco is expected to develop into the single largest killer and to cause the greatest burden of disease in the 21st century, with deaths increasing from 4.9 million to 10 million per year by the late 2020s (WHO, 2002g). The WHO has predicted that tobacco will be the leading cause of disease burden in the world by the year 2030, accounting for one in eight deaths, with 70% of them in poor countries (WHO, 1999a). With a decline of tobacco use in Western countries, the tobacco industry has aggressively marketed in low- and middle-income countries (Kickbusch & Buse, 2001). As a result, the prevalence of smoking among adult men is high and troublesome. For example, more than 50% of men in Bangladesh, China, Japan, Korea, Russia, Indonesia, and Vietnam smoke tobacco (McQueen, McKenna, & Sleet, 2001).

The aim of WHO's Tobacco Free Initiative is to prevent and control the global spread of tobacco use in the 21st century. By 2003, 171 member states completed a groundbreaking public health treaty to control tobacco supply and consumption (WHO, 2003c). The treaty's signatory parties agreed to implement comprehensive tobacco control programs and strategies. Some of its central control components are tobacco taxation and pricing, health warning labels, restriction of advertising and promotion, holding the tobacco industry liable for tobacco-related costs, financial support for national tobacco control programs, and funding for treatment programs. This legally binding treaty and international effort represents an important step in global public health and is expected to reduce the impact of tobacco use in the decades to come.

Global Burden of Disease (GBD)

If a member of your family dies, what does it cost? What does it cost if you miss a month of work or school due to an illness? What does it cost a country when the majority of adults smoke a package of cigarettes a day or when adults eat beetle nut several times a day? These questions

are often irritating and are sometimes considered in poor taste. Yet governments and community members do ask these questions—as they must carry the financial burden for them. But how does one go about putting a value on a life? Or, a value on the cost of a disability? To capture these concerns, WHO coined the term: the *global burden of disease* (GBD).

WHO's GBD numerically verified numerous long-held assumptions about disparities in the burden of disease worldwide, especially in regard to children, through landmark studies by Murray and colleagues that revealed startling statistics:

◆ 98% of all child and deaths (younger than 15 years) are in the developing world.
◆ 83% of deaths between ages 15 and 19 are in the developing world (Murray & Lopez, 1997).

In addition to causes of mortality, the GBD study quantified the burden of disease with a measure that could be used for cost-effectiveness analysis. To compare across conditions and risk factors, researchers developed a measure called the **disability-adjusted life year (DALY)**, which are the combination of years of life lost due to premature mortality and years of life lived with disability adjusted for the severity of disability. The GBD study ranked the leading causes of DALYs in 1990 and projected changes by the year 2020 (see Table 16.2). Chronic disease, unipolar major depression, and accidents were expected to be the three top DALYs by that time, replacing respiratory infections, diarrheal diseases, and perinatal disorders.

Within the first 10 years of this period, changes in the rankings were evident. The three leading causes of DALYs in 2001 were acute respiratory infections, HIV/AIDS, and conditions related to the perinatal period (WHO, 2003d). The GBD study grouped diseases and injuries into three clusters: Group 1 represents communicable diseases, maternal causes, conditions arising in the perinatal period, and nutritional conditions; Group 2 lists noncommunicable diseases; and Group 3 lists all types of injuries (see Table 16.3).

The information obtained from the GBD and its analysis guides current decisions related to investments in health, research, human resource development, and physical infrastructure. Reassessment of global and regional information on diseases and injuries is expected to occur every 3 to 5 years.

PROVIDERS OF HEALTH CARE

The implications for community health nursing concerning the three eras of health conditions are many. The health provider most appropriate when death is a common occurrence, as it was during the Era of Infectious Diseases, is a physician. This category of health worker is best suited for saving lives and for delivering the medical interventions that keep people alive. Nursing and nursing personnel are health care providers who have traditionally served populations that experience long-term chronic illnesses. Nursing personnel worldwide serve populations in nursing homes, long-term care facilities, and in community-based programs for the elderly and disabled. The nursing services in Slovenia and Germany are excellent examples of this kind of practice in Europe.

TABLE 16.2	Seventeen Leading Causes of Disability-adjusted Life Years (DALYs) in the World in 1990 and Projected to 2020	
Disease or Injury	Rank: 1990	Rank: 2020
Lower respiratory tract infections	1	6
Diarrheal diseases	2	9
Conditions arising during the perinatal period	3	11
Unipolar major depression	4	2
Ischemic heart disease	5	1
Cerebrovascular disease	6	4
Tuberculosis	7	7
Measles	8	25
Road traffic accidents	9	3
Congenital anomalies	10	13
Malaria	11	24
Chronic obstructive pulmonary disease	12	5
Falls	13	19
Iron deficiency anemia	14	39
Protein-energy malnutrition	14	37
War	16	8
Self-inflicted injuries	17	14
Violence	19	12
Human immunodeficiency virus (HIV) infection	28	10
Trachea, bronchus, and lung cancers	33	15

(Murray, C.J. & Lopez, A.D. [1996]. Evidence-based health policy—Lessons from the Global Burden of Disease Study. *Science, 274,* 740–743.)

TABLE 16.3	Distribution of Death by Specific Causes in 1990	
Group 1	Group 2	Group 3
Infectious and parasitic diseases	Malignant neoplasms	Unintentional injuries
Respiratory infections	Other neoplasms	Intentional injuries
Maternal disorders	Diabetes mellitus	
Perinatal disorders	Endocrine disorders	
Nutritional deficiencies	Neuropsychiatic disorders	
	Sense organ disorders	
	Cardiovascular disorders	
	Respiratory disorders	
	Digestive disorders	
	Genitourinary disorders	
	Skin disorders	
	Musculoskeletal disorders	
	Congenital anomalies	
	Oral disorders	

(Murray, C.J. & Lopez, A.D. [1996]. Evidence-based health policy—Lessons from the Global Burden of Disease Study. *Science, 274,* 740–743.)

The caregiver needed for the Era of Social Conditions is evolving. For example, community health nurses and primary care physicians are developing new competencies for HIV/AIDS prevention among adolescent prostitutes, but a host of other interventions that require collaboration with other social service and educational personnel is needed. In addition, some communities, because of their former political persuasion and cultural beliefs, have not created networks and other mechanisms to address their emerging social health conditions. For example, during the earthquake in Armenia, international workers recognized the need for social supports for those whose homes and community had been destroyed. At that time, these social structures, as they existed in North America, were not available to that population. In Mizoram, India, the burgeoning drug trade from Myanmar has had a profound impact on this Christian, family-centered, close-knit community in the northeast part of India (Segor, 2006).

In the future, community health care will be increasingly collaborative, and experienced as participatory partnerships with clear shifts in ownership and leadership. Formerly, international workers and consultants went to a country as outsiders and delivered their ideas, programs, and projects. The philosophy, beliefs, practices, and values of this dominant group of outsiders prevailed, and the recipient groups were considered a success to the extent that they adopted the dominant groups ways of being, living, and caring for their health.

In the future, partnerships that are sensitive to the dynamics of power and oppression, and which honor the need for local groups to be in control of their own projects and the resources that are used to implement them, will prevail. Freire's (1970) advocacy for using *generative themes* that support education and critical consciousness are being adopted as collaborative projects demonstrate innovative ways of learning and conducting research. For example, in many countries, local experts and community members are forming partnerships with outside consultants and are insisting on striking changes in responsibility, authority, and ownership of data and innovations. In these emerging models, the community becomes the initiator of action.

Health Providers at District Levels

In earlier forms of primary health care (PHC), the locus of decision-making was at the village level. However, after many years of effort, the WHO and other organizations realized that the power to sustain change required more than village-level involvement. Thus, the move to the district level of implementation is currently being practiced in many places.

Regardless of level, however, the essential point is the adage: Think globally, act locally. Specifically, this means that expertise is needed from those at international, national, regional, and district levels; but the ways in which communities interpret the issues and their solutions belongs to them. In local areas, communities adopt the health centers or organizations created to address community concerns. For example, in one Greek community, a local mayor sat through a week of deliberations on ways to bring PHC to his island. He heard the comments of members of the local community, its health workers, and an international WHO PHC team. Ultimately, the mayor realized that rooms for health providers would be needed, and he declared the community's full support to provide these rooms to further the work of the health center. In this way, his community was fully active and responsible for its own health status.

Community Health Workers

In some countries, particularly those in which professional health providers are scarce, the community identifies a local, respected, responsible person most often called the **community health worker (CHW)**. This person is selected from the village and is approved by the committee to serve the village people in health matters. CHWs usually provide 1 to 2 hours of health service per day, for which they may or may not be compensated by the community.

The CHW is trained in the fundamentals of promoting health and preventing and treating the most common health care conditions (Lewin et al., 2004). This includes basic first aid, advice and assistance on simple treatments, and health teaching on personal hygiene, safe water supplies, safe disposal of human waste and refuse, and nutrition. Community health nurses often serve as consultants to the CHW and, in some places, are expected to supervise their work and provide ongoing education. These CHWs have demonstrated their effectiveness in controlling communicable diseases, for example, in the malaria control programs in Ethiopia (Gebreyesus et al., 2000).

Village Midwife

The village midwife receives training in obstetrics and childcare. This person provides basic antenatal, intrapartum, and postnatal care and makes referrals as required (McInerney, 2004). In India, the village midwife is referred to as a trained *dais*. These are most often older women who may have had training from professional nurses and who are expected to call on professionals when needed. However, they often make their own decisions even though they have a referral source to professionals. Many times, adverse effects occur because cultural practices take precedence over knowledge-based practices that require collaborative decision-making.

In some countries, traditional health practitioners receive formal training and return to their villages to continue their services with new knowledge and skills to enhance their effectiveness. Countries such as Bangladesh implemented programs to train workers who would practice in ways similar to the "barefoot doctors" of China (Valentine, 2005). The Ministry of Health in Bangladesh was challenged in its efforts

during the 1980s, as women would not leave their homes for training and, if they did, would rarely allow themselves to be posted in a village other than their own. This is because women are viewed as wayward if they are not with their families in their home environments. This issue also occurred in Indonesia, when community health nurses were placed in villages away from home. They did not have the respect of the local community, were not seen as experts, and were considered to be in dubious moral standing. This cultural barrier presents challenges to nursing education programs that focus on community- rather than hospital-based experiences.

Community Health Nurses

Background and Age at Entry to Nursing Education

When community health nurses join their colleagues in a country other than their own, they often assume that "a nurse is a nurse, is a nurse." Nothing could be further from the truth. The ways in which women and men are socialized, recruited into, advanced through, and graduated from nursing school varies considerable from country to country. So does the age at entry, the exposure that nursing students have to the social and behavioral sciences, the theoretical and clinical applications studied, and the kind and extent of supervision they receive. For example, in some countries, young people begin their study of nursing at age 15, studying nursing in programs designed, sequenced, and financed by the government. These graduates are expected to practice as fully experienced community health nurses by age 18.

Curricula of Nursing Programs

The practice of controlling and designing nursing curricula at central levels carries opportunities and risks. The opportunity it provides is consistency of teaching and learning and the possibility to produce teaching learning materials in a uniform way, and in the language of the country. The risks are that local conditions are not included, and care practices essential for a region of a country may not be addressed. For example, during the earthquake in Armenia, nurse leaders requested that content related to earthquakes and disaster preparedness be added to the curriculum. Authorities refused, showing the consulting team and local nurse leaders the detailed content and hours developed for the curriculum designed in Moscow. No opportunities, at that time, were possible for this content to be added, despite the fact that 25,000 people had lost their lives in the natural disaster.

Nursing educational programs may be based in a hospital, technical school, or university. Specialty areas may be introduced as part of the basic curriculum, as is the practice in Denmark where midwifery is a basic program offered and is seen as a discipline different from nursing. This design differs from other countries in which nursing is the basic preparation upon which mental health, midwifery, and other areas are built and considered as advanced practice.

Development of Nursing Programs Globally

Nursing is a discipline that takes many forms and often requires champions to support its contributions. Nursing education's development history has been checkered, in part, because of this need for champions. The reasons are many. Modern nursing was launched by Florence Nightingale, who began her work during the war in the Crimea, within the context of a military hospital system (see Chapter 2). Since that time, nurses—who are predominately women—have had to demonstrate the difference between curing and caring, between a hierarchy of disciplines under physicians—who are predominately men at the top of the hierarchy—and a horizontal organizational structure that recognizes nursing and other health care disciplines as equal contributors to the health care team.

Forces That Support Nursing Development

In many places, nursing has yet to distinguish itself with its own body of research, knowledge, managerial practices, standards of practice, and ethical tenets. However, it appears that nursing has thrived as a respected discipline in countries where women, in general, are respected and where those in leadership positions understand the value of the caring process and are willing to champion nursing at all levels, including at the national level. For example, Turkey stands out as a country with a cadre of doctorally prepared nurses who were able to secure their education abroad thanks to Dr. Ihsan Dogramaci, an international figure, pediatrician, and child health specialist (2006). Dr. Dogramaci sponsored nurses in Turkey, so that they were able to pursue higher education through the doctoral level of preparation. Nursing has developed in unusual ways in other countries as well. For example, conversations with Portuguese nurses reveal that many of the leaders of nursing in that country came from wealthy families and were committed to a contemporary view of nursing practice.

In Indonesia, many types of nursing personnel had proliferated, and 25 categories of nursing personnel practiced in the country until the mid-1980s. The WHO worked diligently with the Ministry of Health to introduce PHC nursing, a transformation that was clearly a challenge in a country peppered with hundreds of islands, where providing community learning experiences requires time and financial resources to travel to clinical sites. This situation is exacerbated by the limited availability of qualified faculty and the nature of the clinical experiences available in remote locations.

A major challenge to community health nurses who have undergone theory and clinical experiences as learners is working with nurses who have not had community health experience. As is well understood, functioning well in a fully equipped hospital is different from working in a community or village where resources are not easily available. Exploring these differences is an essential part of one's own needs assessment as one embarks on an experience with a team from locations other than one's own.

THE PROCEDURES/INTERVENTIONS

Community health nurses consider the population as their patient or client. A population might refer to all those living in a catchment area, in a neighborhood, village, a district, or city. Countries might refer to their populations at national, regional, or international levels. Regardless of location or level, community health nurses practice within the context of some kind of health care system or organization.

Nurses and midwives constitute 80% of the qualified work force in most national health care systems, and they represent a powerful force for bringing health care to all populations. Nurses provide the spectrum of PHC services and conduct health research (International Council of Nurses [ICN], 1999).

The interventions that community health nurses provide depend on the context in which they are working, and on the population, its health status, and the health conditions it presents. These interventions also depend on how nursing is practiced in a country and on the organizations in which community health nurses are employed or with which they are collaborating.

The key issue here is that community health nurses need to know the mission of the agencies with which they are working and the kinds of services and resources their employing organizations provide. This section describes selected organizations that provide interventions to address community health care issues and the ways in which community health nurses work within them.

Providing an intervention that "works" constitutes an achievement. Providing an intervention in community health constitutes a remarkable achievement. This is because interventions are complex, often costly, and involve considerable knowledge, planning, and expert execution and evaluation skills. This section also focuses on the interventions community health nurses provide in a context different from their own within the context of a sponsoring organization.

As noted, the first step is to understand who is involved, the roles they play, and the contributions they are able to bring to the issue. Again, knowing the context in which one is working, and understanding the population and their health status and health conditions are also critical elements (and have been addressed earlier). A second, but often-overlooked step, is to understand the reasons the interventions are being delivered, and one's reasons for being involved. Specifically, what does the donor agency believe is its mission, and why now, why here? What do the recipients have to say? Do they see themselves as recipients of donations or as partners and collaborators? How do they see the intervention? Did they identify the need and ask for assistance? Have the recipients been involved in identifying the issue, in planning strategies for the intervention? Are they committed to the issue and to the outcome? What is their level of involvement in the issue?

Questions you need to ask yourself are: Why are you there? What motivates you and what is your commitment? How does this fit with the scope of the work you will be undertaking, and will your time commitment see the project through, and if not, what effect will your leaving have on its success?

Criteria for Support of Interventions

Most donor groups want to know if the recipient unit, a village health center, a district hospital, a regional health office, has the capacity to manage projects, and if they are able to sustain the project after external funds are no longer available. Some organizations want to know if the project and its principles and practices might be applied to other areas in the country or throughout the world. These questions address three critical criteria that organizations use to determine funding. These are: sustainability, absorptive capacity, and transferability.

An example of these criteria was made clear in a project the WHO was asked to develop in several African countries. The donor indicated that no project under $5 million would be supported, as the paperwork and administration of the project would not be worth the cost of resources. The office of the Maternal Child Health Section in the country's Ministry of Health included a full-time staff member and one half-time staff member. These two staff members worked with no computer, no typewriter, and no bookkeeping staff. Clearly, the criteria of sustainability and absorptive capacity could not be met, as they would not have any way of managing the many written papers and financial accounting documents required for a $5 million dollar international project. In addition, the unique situation of a project developed for this Ministry of Health would have to be tailored to such an extent that its transferability, or use in another country, would be minimal.

When considering a project's funding, questions need to be asked about gender, political, and cultural issues. For example, if an organization plans to support the elimination of the practice of female circumcision, how will that be seen by the population? If a donor agency insists on a democratic process of decision-making, how do leaders implement this process when they have no background or skills in the democratic process, and their positions are tied to their ability to make decisions without team input? How do community health workers implement sanitation programs that place farm animals in places segregated from humans when villagers see their cows as sacred and want to have them in the family compound? How does the community health nurse reduce the fever of a newly delivered woman when the village midwife, the dais, insists "you sponge her only on day three"?

These and many other questions challenge the underlying assumptions about the process of change and the unplanned effects a well-intentioned intervention is designed to deliver. Yet another question relates to the way community health services are organized. Many communities throughout the world have adopted a form of organization that is presented here.

The most commonly involved organizations that provide health-related interventions and support are described here. An overall umbrella agency is the United Nations (UN). Most people know of the UN's work in peacekeeping. This body also focuses on working conditions through the International Labor Organization (ILO), educational issues through the United Nations Educational Scientific and Cultural Organization (UNESCO) and health issues, specifically, through WHO and UNICEF.

The World Health Organization (WHO)

The leading global agency that focuses specifically on health is the **World Health Organization (WHO)**. The organization has regional offices in six parts of the world with its headquarters in Geneva, Switzerland. The six regional offices include: WHO Regional Office for Americas (PAHO), WHO Regional Office for the Eastern Mediterranean (EMRO), WHO Regional Office for Europe (EURO), WHO Regional Office for Southeast Asia (SEARO), WHO Regional Office for Africa (AFRO), and WHO Regional Office for the Western Pacific (WPRO). The WHO established special offices in

Addis Ababa, Ethiopia, to work with the new African Union (formerly the Organization of African Unity), and in Moscow to work with Eastern European countries and the newly independent states of Central Asia. These regional offices recruit and place community health nurses in their many projects throughout their regions.

The WHO, Its History and Its Work

The WHO began in 1945. It developed its own charter, although it has been closely associated with the UN since its inception. It is responsible for its own programs, funded by regular and extra budgetary funds, and also for health-related initiatives sponsored and funded by UN agencies and other international bodies. The WHO carries out its work through the policies it creates with its member states throughout the world. It does this initially at its annual May meeting, the World Health Assembly.

The World Health Assembly

The World Health Assembly (WHA) is the highest governing body within the WHO and includes 193 member countries. Representatives from each of the world's regions attend this Assembly and bring the policies and recommendations to their respective regional offices for implementation and expression at regional and local levels. Staff members at the regional offices then work with their member countries through their annual September Regional Committee Meeting held each year after the World Health Assembly.

The WHO provides technical support and advises member states on strategies to meet their health care needs. The WHO serves as a catalyst to mobilize the resources of national governments, financial institutions and endowments, and bilateral partners for health development (WHO, 2002m). The WHO is not the organization of choice when vehicles, equipment, and medicines are required; the WHO can help a member state determine the drugs that are essential, and will assist in developing health policy, project plans, and programs.

The WHO employs many types of professionals, including nurses. However, the organization does not focus on professional issues to support the development of particular health-related practitioners, such as nurses, midwives, social workers, or physicians. Nurses interested in these types of issues should explore opportunities with the ICN or nursing organizations at national or state levels. In the United States, these would include the American Association of Colleges of Nursing, the American Nurses Association, or National Council of State Boards of Nursing.

The WHO does focus on the interventions these health professionals deliver, and for these, considerable effort is expended on developing nursing, midwifery, social work, and physician-related knowledge and skills that are basic to the interventions they deliver. However, the WHO works closely with the ICN and with national nursing organizations on policies and programming issues.

WHO Collaborating Centers

The WHO uses a 5-year planning cycle that is divided into 2-year cycles of projects, documentation, publications, and the development of information systems. Community health nurses are employed at the international level in Geneva, and they hold regional level positions as Regional Nursing Advisors. However, one or two Regional Nursing Advisors cannot possibly carry out the work of a region that might be the home to thousands of nursing personnel. To address this issue, WHO has developed a network of **World Health Organization Collaborating Centers** in nursing and other fields. These Centers focus on specific areas of expertise and carry out the work of the member countries in these areas. For example, the Collaborating Center network in nursing of the European Region has focused on primary health care and information systems, and the network in the United States has worked through universities in their respective areas of excellence. In the United States, early pioneer universities included the University of Illinois, the University of Pennsylvania, the University of Texas, the University of Alabama, and the University of California. Student nurses in these universities have the opportunity to participate in the research, nursing projects, and other international activities their universities sponsor, both in the United States and in their partnering countries. Sometimes these collaborating centers represent the WHO and their countries at national and international meetings. They provide critical services that are recognized by, but cannot be funded or staffed by the WHO. They also bring credibility to projects, as they come from the communities they represent, and they know the issues and interventions that have the greatest chances of succeeding.

WHO and Its Collaborators

The WHO works closely with national governments, its collaborating center network, its universities, research centers, and nongovernmental organizations. Experts from member countries are recruited throughout the year to deliberate on global health and health-related issues. For example, during the Chernobyl disaster, WHO/EURO called five internationally recognized nuclear experts to an emergency meeting to examine the issues and assist the member countries with next-step actions to protect their populations, livestock, and agricultural industries. Historically, the WHO has collaborated with centers of excellence throughout the world, including the CDC in the United States.

WHO As a Multilateral Agency

The WHO and other UN agencies are sometimes referred to as *multinational* or **multilateral agencies**. They support development efforts of governments and organizations in countries throughout the world. The WHO regional offices also collaborate with each other to address issues on which they can partner and provide resources. For example, during the civil wars in Africa, Chad, Angola, and Mozambique, WHO/AFRO and WHO/EURO collaborated to develop projects on rehabilitation for the countries with no medical schools and no comprehensive programs for the disabled. The WHO intervenes through its own staff's efforts and through those of its partnerships. In another example, the WHO's Health Promoting Schools is a collaborative effort with UNESCO and UNICEF. Still another example is the Human Reproduction Program, a global research program on reproductive health. It collaborates with two programs of the UN as well as the WB. Similarly, the WHO has joined with several other organizations to fight

---

DISPLAY 16.6 **HEALTH PROMOTION**

Health is created and lived by people within the settings of their everyday life; where they learn, work, play and love. Health is created by caring for oneself and others, by being able to make decisions and have control over one's life circumstances; and by ensuring that the society one lives in creates conditions that allow the attainment of health by all its members.

World Health Organization. (1997). Promoting health through schools: Report of a WHO expert committee on comprehensive school health education and promotion. *WHO Technical Report Series, 180, 5.* Geneva: WHO.

---

hunger and improve food standards, and has collaborated in a *Solar Alert Campaign* to alert people about the harmful effects of solar radiation (WHO, 1999d) (Display 16.6).

Health for All: A Primary Health Care Initiative

In its earlier years, the WHO personnel watched as hospitals and costly health establishments were built throughout the world. One of the world's leading economists, Dr. Brian Abel Smith, noted that countries could not afford to erect costly buildings, nor could they add numbers of health professional to their cadres of personnel. Rather, he suggested that the health personnel available work with the population to manage their health care needs. His major assertion is that health care needs and wants may expand infinitely, but resources do not, and all must manage with the resources currently available. Many health leaders throughout the world recognized the trends emerging and believed that a major change in thinking and practice was needed. They met together in Alma Ata, Kazakhstan, in the former Soviet Union and created a sweeping set of declarations that became the *Declaration of Alma-Ata* (see Chapter 1) or **Health for All**. The world body of 134 countries called on all members to reframe their expectations and implement primary health care (PHC). In Europe, the 32 member countries developed its 38 Regional Targets for Health. In the United States, health care professionals launched *Healthy People 2000*. Since then, the 2000 year mark has passed, and *Healthy People 2010* is now the blueprint for the future (United States Department of Health and Human Services, 2000).

Primary Health Care (PHC) is sometimes called a philosophy, a movement, a way of thinking, a way of working, a setting for health services, or a set of principles. Making it operational at the national level, however, meant that communities would focus on health care services at the local level rather than building large, tertiary hospitals that cater exclusively to urban, financially secure populations. This also meant that the education of health care providers would be located at this level with a de-emphasis on high-cost medical interventions and technology available only to a few members of the population.

Health for All emphasizes PHC that is affordable, culturally acceptable, appropriate, accessible, and delivered through partnerships between national health services system

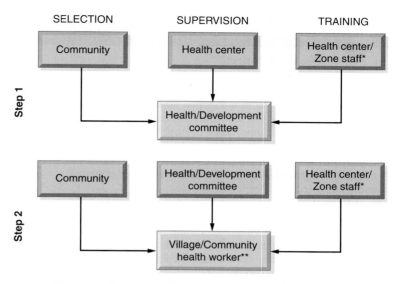

SELECTION   SUPERVISION   TRAINING

FIGURE 16.2   Community-based primary care.

*Nurse, sanitarian, midwife, health education assistant
**Assistant midwife, traditional birth attendant, traditional practitioner

and local communities. The communities take the leading responsibility for identifying their own priority health concerns and planning and implementing their own PHC service. These PHC services include prevention, health promotion, and curative and rehabilitative care provided by the people themselves (WHO, 1998e). (See Figure 16.2 for an illustration of the organizational pattern of community-based PHC.)

Functions of Public Health Care

Article VII of the *Declaration of Alma-Ata* lists the eight basic elements of PHC (*Primary Health Care*, 1978).

1. Education concerning prevailing health problems and the methods of preventing and controlling them
2. Promotion of food supply and proper nutrition
3. An adequate supply of safe water and basic sanitation
4. Maternal and child health, including family planning
5. Immunization against major infectious diseases
6. Prevention and control of locally endemic diseases
7. Appropriate treatment of common diseases and injuries
8. Provision of essential drugs

Public health care also involves related sectors concerned with national and community development, including agriculture, animal husbandry, food, industry, education, housing, public works, and communication (Article VI, section 4).

Deterrents to Public Health Care

Fostering a PHC approach is one thing, implementing it is another. Initially, there were political reactions from professional groups who saw their incomes being funneled to the local level in a health care system. Universities and teaching institutions did not know how to educate professionals for PHC. Textbooks were based on education for treating diseases and assumed the back-up of well-equipped hospital environments. Nursing faculty adopted community health nursing textbooks from North America but continued to teach students as if PHC did not exist. Faculty was virtually nonexistent in rural areas and, if they were available, clients were not. Stationing young women in villages without supervision was seen in some countries as ill-advised, and clients refused to appear at these health centers. Inadequate supervision and follow-up led to misapplication of theory learned, and those in rural areas were not prepared for the situations they faced daily. Health care workers did not understand their responsibilities for maintaining, restocking, and securing medical supplies on a regular basis, and many had no knowledge of community-based principles of case finding, record keeping, community monitoring of immunizations, prenatal care, disease prevention, health promotion, and basic measures to ensure community sanitation.

In many places, referral systems to nearby hospitals were not effective, and health care workers were reluctant to place themselves in responsible positions without back-up and accessible secondary and tertiary facilities.

Natural environmental phenomena such as rain, floods, and poor or absent communication facilities periodically isolated areas and prevented transport of patients to nearby facilities. Other problems arose when expensive drugs were dispensed in place of less expensive generic brands (or in some cases were given first to the family and friends of the health care workers) and when health centers failed to refer patients back to the referring CHW (see Evidence-Based Practice).

Achievements of Public Health Care

A renewal took place in 1994 regarding the strategy of Health for All by WHO members and acknowledged significant global accomplishments. The worldwide infant mortality rate decreased from 90 per 1000 live births in 1975, to 59 per 1000 in 1995—a 34% decrease. Immunization coverage for children

EVIDENCE-BASED PRACTICE

The Uferi Project

Despite an increasing number of high-technology assessments or interventions in developed countries, many villages throughout the world continue to rely on the creativity of nurses and the most basic of health care principles. This study of tropical leg ulcer treatment demonstrated one way in which village health workers can be taught by nurses to improve health in the community in an effective and economical manner.

Painful, debilitating leg ulcers are not uncommon for children in many developing countries. A group of five schoolchildren in the village of Chiba, in the Democratic Republic of Congo, requested treatment for such leg ulcers. Their request triggered a successful treatment project in 1996 that continues today.

Tropical leg ulcers primarily affect school age children and are painful and often debilitating. There is no causative organism for these ulcers: rather, they are caused by poor nutrition and lack of sanitation. Because they are more frequent in times of food scarcity, improved nutrition may not be available. Left untreated, tropical ulcers progress to open, weeping sores, 2 to 3 inches in diameter, that attract flies, eventually exposing tendons and bones. Such ulcers can remain for months or years. If healing occurs, it is often the site for future breakdown. These ulcers can lead to septicemia, osteomyelitis, or even death.

A house-to-house survey was conducted in the village to determine the underlying causes of the ulcers. Open-ended questions regarding overall health as well as the leg ulcers were included. The survey revealed an even higher incidence of ulcer than was initially projected.

Tissue biopsies were performed to diagnose the cases. If no causative organisms were found, the diagnosis of "tropical leg ulcers" was made. The design of the treatment plan included cost, availability of material, and sustainability for the project. The researcher served as a consultant to the village health workers who implemented the treatment. Pictures were designed for teaching children and mothers, and captions were translated into Swahili. Volunteers in the United States prepared bandages (made from sheets), washcloths, and bars of soap, and raised money for antibiotic ointments that were subsequently sent to Africa.

Word of mouth alerted the villagers about the project. Parents and children were invited to a teaching session to learn about causes of the ulcers and intervention. Each affected child was given supplies and an identification number. Once treatment began, a patient's response to treatment was tracked. The treatment consisted of cleaning the ulcers with a traditional tea made from guava leaves, applying antibiotic ointment to the most severe ulcers, and covering them with bandages. The traditional antiseptic solution made from guava tea has been reported to be effective in several nations, was readily available, and had no cost because villagers could make it themselves from local resources.

Mothers were taught to wash their hands and the wound with soap, apply the antiseptic solution, and cover each wound with a dressing and bandages. Each patient was given a replacement dressing for use while the other was washed and dried in the sun for "sterilization."

The sores responded rapidly to treatment. The ulcers were dubbed "uferi" after a local political party that had the same characteristics of "emerging and flourishing overnight." Many patients saw dramatic improvement in 1 week. A review of the records 6 months later revealed that volunteer health workers treated more than 600 uferi that had successfully healed. Eight failures were attributed to patients' lack of compliance.

News of the successful treatment traveled for several hundred miles and into the neighboring Zambia. Volunteer caregiver health care workers became consultants to neighboring communities. The development of self-esteem and leadership skills was a side benefit of the Uferi project. Both the treatment and the community leadership of health care workers continue today despite recent civil war and political difficulties. This is an excellent example of operationalization of the Primary Health Care model supported by the World Health Organization.

1. Do you think the results of the Uferi project would be the same if a nurse had conducted the intervention rather than the village health care worker? Why or why not?
2. How does the village health care worker fit into the Primary Health Care scheme? What were the advantages of the village health care workers in the Uferi project?
3. What factors do you think might affect a mother's compliance with the treatment of tropical leg ulcers?
4. If you were the nurse researcher, how would you go about determining indigenous, effective treatment interventions?
5. Could something like the Uferi project work in the United States?
6. Why do you think the health care workers developed increased self-esteem and leadership skills because of this project?

Reference:

Kirkpatrick, S.M. (2000). The Congo children's weeping sores. *Reflections on Nursing Leadership, 26(2)*. 10–16,45.

younger than 1 year of age rose from 20% to 80% between 1980 and 1990. Access to safe drinking water in developing countries increased from 38% to 66%, and adequate improved sanitation moved from 32% to 38% between the mid-1970s and 1990.

Future action regarding PHC calls for strengthened collaboration among governmental agencies and NGOs in both the public and private sectors. Only then will the world have a realistic chance of achieving all the goals set out in the *Declaration of Alma-Ata* (1978) (Display 16.7).

DISPLAY 16.7 · WHO'S TEN GOALS TOWARD HEALTH FOR ALL

- To increase the span of healthy life for all people in such a way that health disparities between social groups are reduced.
- To ensure universal access to an agreed upon set of essential health-care services of acceptable quality, comprising at least the eight essential elements of primary health care.
- To ensure survival and healthy development of children.
- To improve the health and well being of women.
- To ensure healthy population development.
- To eradicate, eliminate, or control major diseases constituting global health problems.
- To reduce avoidable disabilities through appropriate preventive and rehabilitative measures.
- To ensure continued improvements in nutritional status for all population groups.
- To enable universal access to safe and healthy environments and living conditions.
- To enable all people to adopt and maintain healthy lifestyles and health behavior.

Lanza, R. (1996). *One world: The health and survival of the human species in the 21st century.* Santa Fe, NM: Health Press.

The Way Forward

One of the greatest achievements of WHO has been the eradication of smallpox. In 1967, when smallpox was endemic in 31 countries, 13 million cases were estimated worldwide. It is projected that 20 million people would have died in the next two decades if smallpox had not been eradicated. The WHO, with Dr. D.A. Henderson of Johns Hopkins University, is credited with eliminating smallpox (Henig, 1997). The WHO's other accomplishments include reduction of malaria, standardization of data-collection systems, adoption of international standards for the control and reporting of morbidity and mortality, and publication of classic works for the prevention and management of disease (Whaley & Hashim, 1995). In addition, the WHO has been credited with preventing hundreds of millions of cases of tropical diseases. As the 21st century begins, new eradication/elimination programs are under way for polio, leprosy, Guinea Worm Disease, and measles. Other initiatives include:

1. Reducing transmission and incidence of HIV/AIDS
2. Launching the *Roll Back Malaria* program
3. Stopping the transmission of tuberculosis
4. Increasing access to essential pharmaceuticals
5. Improving the poor quality of some pharmaceuticals
6. Preventing and treating iron deficiency
7. Reducing maternal morbidity and mortality
8. Promoting healthful lifestyles for all age groups, including elders

Dr. Gro Harlem Brundtland, former Director General of WHO, characterized the 20th century as one encompassing the biggest social transformations of history. Living conditions, she noted, have dramatically improved for the large majority of human beings, and she identified health as the key to improving the productivity of people and nations. She noted the persistence of excess mortality and morbidity that disproportionately affect poor people, and underscored the need to focus on those interventions that can achieve the greatest health gains possible using available resources (Newsday, 2001).

International Governmental Organizations with National Governments

Sometimes, the WHO is the first to describe a health-related situation requiring international support. It then contacts other groups or organizations with the requisite expertise, assembling members of its international disaster-preparedness teams from governmental organizations that represent various nations. Organizations such as church-related groups, universities, researchers, and governments provide international assistance.

Countries throughout the world are structured to fund within-country health issues and to contribute to the international agenda. The United States contributes internationally through its United States Agency for International Development (USAID). Some other countries' international arms include Denmark's DANIDA and Italy's Italian Cooperation. The European Union (EU) is an organization that provides funding for many health-related projects.

United States Agency for International Development

The United States Agency for International Development (USAID) is an independent, bilateral agency of the executive branch that is under the guidance of the Secretary of State. It works to enhance long-term and equitable economic growth and to advance U. S. foreign policy by supporting countries in their efforts to recover from disaster, escape poverty, and engage in democratic reforms. The Agency provides support to developing countries for economic development, agriculture and trade, global health, democracy, conflict prevention, and humanitarian assistance and does this through its collaboration with many governmental and private agencies to implement its programs (Natsios, 2002). This agency also hires nurses and other health care providers, and often provides workshops to brief grant writers on the interventions currently under exploration.

American International Health Alliance

The USAID often collaborates with other organizations to implement its programs. The American International Health Alliance (AIHA) is one of these, and operates under a cooperative agreement with USAID. It establishes and manages hospital partnerships between health care institutions in the United States and their counterparts in central and Eastern Europe and in the newly independent states of Central Asia. The AIHA is reportedly the U.S. hospital sector's most coordinated response to health care issues in those areas. In 2002, AIHA managed more than 90 partnerships in 21 countries (AIHA, 2002).

World Bank

The **World Bank (WB)** is an agency that focuses on economic development, and it includes a health component. It partners with countries, the WHO, and other organizations to address poverty, build capacity, transfer knowledge, provide resources, and forge partnerships in the public and private sectors (Display 16.8).

Nongovernmental Organizations

Countries throughout the world provide interventions through formal governmental organizations and through nongovernmental organizations (NGOs). These organizations are not under government sponsorship or control. In the United States, they are designated as private voluntary organizations (PVOs) that focus on humanitarian and professional issues related to global health. Examples of PVOs are the Global Health Council, the Center for International Health and Cooperation, CARE, the Carter Center, and the International Council of Nurses (ICN).

These organizations contribute in their particular areas of expertise and work with other international organizations, research centers, and universities. Some focus on children, such as Save the Children; some on medically focused interventions, such as Doctors Without Borders; and some on logistics and supplies, such as Direct Relief International.

Global Health Council

The Global Health Council (GHC), (formerly known as the National Council for International Health), is the world's largest membership alliance dedicated to saving lives by improving health throughout the world. The GHC advocates for needed policies and resources, builds networks and alliances among those working to improve health, and shares innovative ideas, knowledge, and best practices in health (Global Health Council, 1999b).

The GHC's membership includes hundreds of private and public organizations around the world, as well as several thousand professionals involved in global health. It is staffed by a multidisciplinary, cross-cultural board of directors, health professionals, student interns, volunteers, and members (GHC, 1999b).

Center for International Health and Cooperation

The Center for International Health and Cooperation (CIHC), founded in 1992, promotes healing and peace in countries shattered by war, regional conflicts, and ethnic violence. Its belief is that health and other basic humanitarian actions often provide the only common ground for initiating dialogue and cooperation among warring parties (CIHC, 2002).

CARE

The Cooperative for American Remittances to Europe (CARE) was founded in 1945, when 22 American organizations joined together to rush life-saving *care packages* from individual American citizens, churches, clubs, and businesses to survivors of World War II. Millions of CARE packages followed in the next two decades. In the 1950s, CARE expanded its program to developing nations, using surplus American food to feed the hungry. In the 1960s, it pioneered PHC. Now renamed the Cooperative for Assistance and Relief Everywhere, CARE is affiliated with an international confederation of 11 member organizations. CARE intervenes by responding to famines and disasters worldwide with emergency food, supplies, and rehabilitative efforts. It delivers programs in education, health, population, water and sanitation, agriculture, environmental preservation, economic development, and community building (CARE, 2002).

The Carter Center

Former United States President, Jimmy Carter, and his wife Roselyn, founded the Carter Center in 1986. The Carter Center intervenes in disease prevention and agriculture throughout the world. The particularly successful interventions include the Guinea Worm Disease eradication program in Africa and parts of Asia in the areas served by the Carter Center, and the program to eradicate River Blindness, which has been eliminated in Africa and Latin America. Its Trachoma Control Program continues to fight blindness in Africa and Yemen.

The Carter Center also sponsors the Ethiopia Public Health Training Initiative, designed to strengthen teaching capacities of faculty members at five major universities of Ethiopia. Staff members of the Carter Center collaborate with Ethiopians to develop curriculum materials specifically created to meet the learning needs of rural and urban health center team personnel (Carter Center, 2002).

International Council of Nurses

As noted earlier, the ICN represents the global interests and concerns of the nursing profession. ICN's mission is to maintain the role of nursing in health care through its global voice (Vance, 1999). Its current membership includes nursing organizations from 120 countries and 1.5 million nurses.

National Governments Working Alone

Individual nations have considerable experience working across agencies and organizations, and they have traditions that they honor as they intervene. For example, the Federal Republic of Germany has one of the largest voluntary sectors in the world and is known for its work with the International Red Cross. The Finnish Nursing Organization has an outstanding international reputation for its work during the Armenian earthquake and in other international efforts throughout Europe. The Danish Nurses Organization has provided funds, leadership, and expertise to numerous projects in collaboration with the WHO and with the ICN.

At times, however, governments facing a crisis or disaster prefer to operate alone, without international assistance. This position must be respected and, because of this expectation, international organizations will not appear in a country until a formal request is received from representatives of the country in crisis. Furthermore, some countries are more receptive to certain kinds of assistance than others. Some countries do not welcome foreign professionals, as they believe they have enough of their own. They may prefer help in the form of equipment, transport, medications, or vital supplies, such as water and food. Those in disaster preparedness are well aware of what some refer to as the "second disaster," when well-intentioned groups send in truckloads of used clothing and articles that are useless in some environments. At times, governments would prefer to work alone, but do not have the resources to do so, nor can their authorities provide the personnel to sort the kinds of contributions donors provide during emergencies.

Organizations with Religious Affiliations

Many organizations are sponsored by religious groups, some of which include a religiously oriented agenda along with their interventions. Some, however, do not. Often, the work of these groups is similar to those with a nonreligious focus, and the source of funding for a particular project may be the only overt connection to any religious group. Catholic Charities and other Christian organizations provide critical interventions, as do Moslem, Jewish, and other religiously oriented organizations. These organizations often recruit community health nurses and other health care providers for short- and long-term assignments.

COMMUNITY HEALTH NURSING OPPORTUNITIES

Let us suppose that, after reading this chapter and some of its references, you have decided to work in a location other than your own. In all probability, you would begin your work at a local level, at a local health center in a village. You would be aware of your own issues and reasons for wanting this experience, and you would have selected the location because of some factors that draw you to it. How then might you go about preparing for the experience? In what kind of activities might you be involved? What might be the expectations and commitments you would make regarding the assignment?

Community health nurses, as shown in this chapter, carry major responsibility for managing health services in health centers, clinics, schools, workplaces, and community settings that range in population density and complexity from remote areas to major centers in large metropolitan areas. This work includes providing education, guidance, and professional supervision to other cadres of health care providers.

Before you travel, conduct your own preliminary needs assessment. You can use the logic of the thinking process developed in this chapter and move through the framework as a guide. Begin, as this chapter suggests, with a review of the context. Here you would examine the location, climate, temperatures, weather conditions, travel routes, living arrangements, languages spoken, cultural patterns, religious beliefs, and religious holidays. Locate novels and literature from the country, as this source of data is often more revealing that many of the statistical charts and information available from official sources (Illyes, 1967; Dizdarevic, 1993; Cooke, 1967; Barzini, 1983; Rushdie, 1995; McCourt, 1999). Interacting with people from the country often provides valuable insights not available from reading materials. In all probability, you will find enclaves of people living in the United States from the country in which you plan to work. For example, Armenian communities are located in Watertown, Massachusetts and Los Angeles, California. There are many Ethiopian communities in Atlanta, Georgia; New York City, New York; and Los Angeles, California. There are groups and organizations of Albanian Americans, Polish Americans, Hungarian Americans, Romanian Americans, and Indian Americans. These groups maintain close contact with their mother country, and receive and give support to their family members and organizations in those countries.

Next, examine the population's health status, at the regional levels (e.g., Europe, Asia, Africa) the country level (Chad, Nepal, India) and at the local level (Tete Provinces and villages in Tete Provinces, Mozambique). Here you would review the data to identify the universals of care; that is, the causes of mortality and morbidity, the level of functioning in the community, decision making (if available), and cost of health care (Farrell, Gehring, & Howe, 2000).

Then, move on to review evidence of the three eras of health conditions in the country and determine the age of the population and the health conditions they experience, given their history, location, and experiences with natural or man made disasters. Look at birth rates, death rates, infant mortality rates, and maternal mortality rates, asking: How many infants are born? How many of these die at birth, during the first month of life, during the first year of life? How long do people live? What kills them? What makes them sick? How do people function everyday? What kinds of decisions do they have to make and how do they make them? What community supports exist to help people with these processes? What is the average income per capita? What do people buy with their money?

Review the conditions that account for the three eras of health conditions as described in this chapter, and determine the prevailing health conditions that you will encounter. Review the kinds of health conditions that are reported both in the professional literature and in the popular literature and media.

Next, it's helpful to review the organization with which you will be associated. Examine its philosophy, its mission, its ways of working, its relationship to the community of interest, and the ways in which community health nurses are considered, placed, and function. Query the nature of the health care team of which you would become a member, those to whom you report and those who would report to you. Review their scope of practice, the interventions they provide, and their ways of delivering health services.

It is helpful to identify the international governmental and NGOs working in the area and obtain their publications for review, and their addresses and contact numbers (when you arrive in the area, visit these organizations and request a briefing). Review the projects currently under way, and examine their track record for the factors that suggest ill-conceived outcomes and evidence of those that produced successful outcomes.

You cannot build a strong country on the backs of sick people.

Dr. Mohammad Akhter, Executive Director,
American Public Health Association

Nurses and midwives play a crucial and cost-effective role in reducing excess mortality, morbidity, and disability and in promotion of healthy lifestyles.

Dr. Gro Harlem Brundtland, Director-General,
World Health Organization

Global health nurses always receive far more than they give.

Cydne, former Peace Corps nurse

The developing world may be poor materially, but it is rich in hope and spirit.

Edith, missionary nurse

Nurses working in foreign lands make a big difference through their training and support of local nurses and others. Their professional dedication to quality health care and promotion of healthful living among their patients, families, and communities serves as an effective role model and has a profound impact on the well-being of the people they work with.

Tom, physician

Living overseas for many years was a challenging and rewarding experience. Raising a family was not always easy, but our six children, now adults, value the exposure they had to other cultures and the many interesting friendships they made.

Inez, spouse of a global health administrator

Nurses play an important role ministering to the health care needs of not only the indigenous population, but also the sometimes-sizable population of expatriates and their families.

Jennifer, teacher

There is nothing so powerful as seeing a community that has changed through individuals taking responsibility for themselves and their own community.

Lydia, volunteer PHN with Medical Ambassadors

Following this review, identify and remediate gaps in your knowledge of theory and practice. Most importantly, take the time to plan, to take care of yourself and your health, as your own health status is critical to your functioning in what may be a very different context from your own.

To explore specific opportunities, contact the organization of interest (see the listing of selected organizations at the end of the chapter). Some of the larger organizations, such as the WHO, require graduate education and at least 5 years of experience, but many organizations do not. Nurses can participate in numerous smaller organizations that are involved in health programs. Among such groups seeking nurses are the U.S. Peace Corps, religious and lay organizations, and

private and governmental agencies, societies, and foundations. Health Volunteers Overseas (HVO) is an example of a private, nonprofit organization that seeks to improve health care quality and access in developing countries through education. Twelve professional organizations sponsor HVO, including the American Association of Colleges of Nursing (Health Volunteers Overseas, 2003). The GHC provides information on career opportunities in global health for community health nurses and others. It also offers career seminars and provides suggestions from global health experts for nurses interested in entering the field (Global Health Council, 1999b). University student nurses can also contact their campus Office of Global Affairs for opportunities available overseas (see Perspectives: Voices from the Community).

Summary

Community health nursing is practiced throughout the world and can be considered within a useful, worldwide framework. This framework considers first the context within which the population, the provider, and the procedures interact.

The context reflects a location's geography, history, weather, culture, religious patterns, and belief systems. This context is a critical element that community health nurses appreciate for its influences on the populations, the providers, and the interventions they are able to deliver.

Community health nurses work with populations that vary from country to country, and to serve them appropriately requires an understanding of the ways in which the context in which they are located interacts with their health status and health histories. In this regard, an examination is required to assess the universal imperatives of care, to identify the population's current health status, and to determine the focus of nursing interventions. That is, when a population is experiencing high mortality, the interventions must be targeted to that level, and not, say, at the level of functioning.

Community health nurses also examine the population to assess the kinds of health conditions they experience, and the three eras are helpful guides in this assessment. These are: the Era of Infectious Diseases, the Era of Chronic Long Term Health Conditions, and the Era of Social Conditions. The three P's (Population, Providers, and Procedures) relate to the interventions community health nurses deliver as they serve populations and are informed by the organization with which the community health nurse works. A number of international, national, and local organizations intervene in communities. Some of these agencies are intergovernmental and multilateral, such as the United Nations and WHO; others are bilateral, such as the USAID and the Peace Corps. Many NGOs (or PVOs) also assist with global health.

The focus remains on delivering PHC to populations throughout the world. The world's communities deliver health care in different ways, depending on their political economies. The entrepreneurial, welfare-oriented, comprehensive, and socialist systems provide for the health of their citizens in unique ways.

Variations of these systems exist, depending on whether the country is considered industrialized, transitional, or very poor. The GBD study has provided important quantifiable information about morbidity and mortality in the world, as well as disability measurements. Primary global health concerns include the eradication, elimination, or control of communicable disease, as well as immunization, maternal and perinatal morbidity and mortality, tobacco-related diseases, chronic disease, environmental illness, and malnutrition. In addition to these age-old health problems, there are new, emerging, and re-emerging diseases. Armed conflicts and political upheavals also adversely affect health; this is an important consideration because of the number of major armed conflicts occurring at any given time.

Community health nursing services are critical to the ultimate health of a community. They provide important primary, secondary, and tertiary levels of care and prevention throughout the world. In the future, community health nurses will continue as major contributors to global health. ■

ACTIVITIES TO PROMOTE CRITICAL THINKING

1. Identify a country or community in which you would like to practice community health nursing. Before you being a review of this community, bracket your own knowledge, attitudes, and beliefs about the country, the people, and the culture. Examine your own reasons for wanting this experience. Identify the way you might feel if you were the recipient rather than the donor of the services you plan to provide?

2. Conduct your own needs assessment using the framework provided in this chapter. Given what you have found, what would you prioritize as the major focus of a community nursing intervention for that community? Provide your rationale for your choices.

3. Given what you have found, what organizations, groups, or references would you access before you left on your assignment?

4. Based on your examination, what questions would you want to ask of the employing agency before you left on your assignment? What additional actions would you take to protect yourself and your health, given the review you conducted?

5. What sources of information appear to be most informative? What data are you seeking that is not reported? Why do you think this is the case?

6. Identify a person or a group from the community in which you plan to work. Develop an interview protocol that includes questions that address the framework developed in this chapter. What are the most appropriate questions these individuals or groups can answer?

References

American International Health Alliance. (2002). *About AIHA*. Retrieved August 7, 2008 from http://www.aiha.com/printversion.jsp?+=1081436351174.

Armenia Fund USA. (October 5, 2006). *I Love Armenia! I love Artsakh! 9th International Armenia Fund telethon is approaching*. Retrieved August 7, 2008 from http://www.armenia fundusa.org/new/20061005-telethon-2006.htm.

Barzini, L. (1983). *The Europeans*. N.Y.: Simon and Schuster.

Bender, L., David, L., Chilcott, L., & Burns, S.Z. (Producers) & Guggenheim, D. (Director) (2006). *An Inconvenient Truth* [Film]. United States: Paramount Home Entertainment.

Bradley, D., Warhurst, D., Blaze, M., et al. (1998). Malaria imported into the United Kingdom in 1996. *European Surveillance, 3*(4), 40–42.

Burkholder, H.H., & Toole, M.J. (1995). Evolution of complex disease. *Lancet, 346*, 1012–1015.

CARE. (2002). *About CARE*. Retrieved August 7, 2008 from http://www.CARE.ORG/about/history.html.

Carlaw, R. (1988). Community-based primary health care: Some factors in its development. In R.W. Carlaw, & W.B. Ward (Eds.). *Primary health care: The African experience*. (pp. xx–xi). Oakland, CA: Third Party Publishing Company.

Carr, D. (2004). *Improving the health of the world's poorest people. Health Bulletin 1*. Washington, DC: Population Reference Bureau.

Carter Center. (2002). *Health programs*. Retrieved August 7, 2008 from http://www.cartercenter.org/healthprograms/.

Center for International Health and Cooperation. (2002). *About CIHC: The Center for International Health and Cooperation*. New York, NY: Author.

Centers for Disease Control and Prevention. (2000). *Division of Vector-borne Infectious Diseases: West Nile virus*. Retrieved August 7, 2008 from http://www.cdc.gov/ncidod/dvbidarbpr/West_Nile_QA.htm.

Centers for Disease Control and Prevention. (2002a). *Surveillance and control of the West Nile virus*. Retrieved August 7, 2008 from http://www.CDC.gov/ncidoddvbid/westnile/surv/contol.htm.

Centers for Disease Control and Prevention. (2006). *Preliminary investigation suggests BSE-infected cow in Washington State was likely imported from Canada*. Retrieved November 27, 2006 from http://www.cdc.gov/ncidod/dvrd/bse/bse_washington_2003.htm.

Chernobyl Accident: Information and issue briefs. (2006). Retrieved November 27, 2006 from http://www.worldnuclear.org/info/chernobyl/inf07.htm.

Connolly, C. (March 16, 2003). Smallpox vaccine comes full circle: A trusty immunization is called out of retirement to face a new threat. *Washington Post*, p. A28.

Cooke, D.C. (1967). *Dera: A village in India*. New York, NY: W.W. Norton & Co.

Cox, C.B. (2005). *Community care for an aging population: Issues, policies, and services*. New York, NY: Springer Publishing.

Dizdarevic, L. (1993). *Sarajevo: A war journal*. New York, NY: Henry Holt and Co.

Dogramaci, I. (2006). *Family Health Foundation Fellowship and Prize*. Retrieved November 27, 2006 from http://www.who.int/governance/awards/dogramaci/en/.

Drum, K. (2005). *Civil war*. The Washington Monthly. Retrieved August 7, 2008 from http://www.washingtonmonthly.com/archives/individual/2005_10/007329.php.

Ezzati, M., Utzinger, J., Cairncross, S., et al. (2005). Environmental risks in the developing world: Exposure indicators for evaluating interventions, programmes, and policies. *Journal of Epidemiology in Community Health, 59*, 15–22.

Farrell, M. (1992). After war: The long term effects on people, their health and the health system. *Nursing Administration Quarterly, 16*(2), 4–7.

Farrell, M. (1992). The price of war. *Nursing and Health Care, 13*, 414–417.

Farrell, M. (2006). Living evidence: Translating research into practice. In T. Porter-O-Grady, & K. Malloch (Eds.). *Evidence-based practice: A professional resource*. Boston: Jones and Bartlett.

Farrell, M., Gehring, L., & Howe, C. (2000). Child and family international consulting: The Web Way. *Journal of Child and Family Nursing, 3*(1), 71–76.

Farrell, M., Harkless, G., Orzack, L.H., et al. (1994). Hungarian midwives and their practice: A national survey. *Midwifery, 10*, 67–72.

Fleshman, M. (2002). A grim prognosis for AIDS in Africa. *Africa Recovery, 16*, 7–8.

Freire, P. (1970). *Pedagogy of the oppressed*. New York: Continuum Publishing Company.

Friedman, T.L. (2005). *The world is flat: A brief history of the 21st*. New York, NY: Farrar, Straus & Giroux.

Gebreyesus, A.M., Witten, K.H., Getachew, A., et al. (2000). The community-based malaria control programme in Tigray, Northern Ethiopia: A review of programme set-up, activities, outcomes, and impact. *Parassitologia, 42*(34), 255–290.

Glenny, M. (1992). *The fall of Yugoslavia: The third Balkan war*. New York, NY: Penguin Books.

Global Health Council. (1999a). Speech delivered by Dr. Gro Harlem Brundtland, Director General, World Health Organization. Washington, DC: Global Health Council. Retrieved November 4, 1999 from http://www.who.int/directorgeneral/speeches/1999/english/19990621_arlington.html.

Global Health Council. (1999b). *The Global Health Council, May 1, 1999*. Retrieved August 7, 2008 from http://www.globalhealth.org/view_topphp3?id+25.

Global Issues. (2000). *Conflicts in Africa: Conflict between Ethiopia and Eritrea*. Retrieved August 7, 2008 from http://www.globalissues.org/Geopolitics/Africa/EthiopiaEritrea.asp.

Grad, F.P. (2002). Public health classics: The preamble of the constitution of the World Health Organization. *Bulletin of the World Health Organization, 80*(12), 981–984.

Hall, B. (1994). *The impossible country: A journey through the last days of Yugoslavia*. New York, NY: Penguin Books.

Health Volunteer Overseas. (2002). *Volunteering with HVO* [Brochure]. Washington, D.C.: Author.

Henig, R.M. (1997). *The people's health: A memoir of public health and its evolution at Harvard*. Washington, DC: Joseph Henry Press.

Heymann, D.L. (Ed.). (2004). *Control of communicable diseases manual*, 18th ed. Washington, DC: American Public Health Association.

Howard, D., Scott, R.D., Packard, R., & Jones, D. (2003). The global impact of drug resistance. *Clinical Infectious Diseases, 36*, S4–S10.

Illyes, G. (1979*). People of the Puszta*. Budapest, Hungary: Franklin Printing House.

International Council of Nurses. (2000). *Nursing N Line*. Retrieved December 29, 2003 from http://www.icn.ch.

International Herald Tribune. (2006). *The AIDS-malaria link*. Retrieved August 7, 2008 from http://www.iht.com/articles/2006/12/18/opinion/edaids.php.

Jamison, D.T., Breman, J.G., Measham, A.R., et al. (Eds.). (2006). *Disease control priorities in developing countries*, 2nd ed. New York, NY: Oxford University Press.

Kaneko, A. (1998). Malaria on the global agenda: Control and chemotherapy of malaria in Vanuatu. *Rinsho Yori, 46*(7), 637–644.

Kickbusch, I., & Buse, K. (2001). Global influences and global responses: International health at the turn of the twenty-first century. In M.H. Merson, R.E. Black, & A.J. Mills (Eds.). *International public health diseases, program, system, and policies*. (pp. 710–711). Gaithersburg, MD: Aspen.

Kirkpatrick, S.M. (2000). The Congo children's weeping sores. *Reflections on Nursing Leadership, 26*, 10–16, 45.

Kloos, H. (1994). The poorer third world: Health and health care in areas that have yet to experience substantial development. In D.R. Phillips, & Y. Verhasselt (Eds.). *Health and development*. (pp. 199–215). New York: Routledge.

Kosek, M., Bern, C., & Guerrant, R.L. (2003). The global burden or diarrhoeal disease, as estimated from studies published between 1992 and 2000. *Bulletin of the World Health Organization, 81*(3), doi: 10.1590/S004296862003000300010. Retrieved October 1, 2008 from http://www.scielosp.org/scielo.php?pid=S004296862003000300010&script=sci_arttext&tlng=en.

Lewin, S.A., Dick, J., Pond, P., et al. (2004). *Lay health workers in primary and community health care*. The Cochrane Library. Retrieved August 7, 2008 from http://www.cochrane.org/reviews/en/ab004015.html.

Lopez, A. (May 27, 2006). News release. *The Lancet, 367,* 1747–1757.

Martines, J., Phillips, M., & Feachem, R.G. (1993). Diarrheal diseases. In D.T. Jamison, W.H. Mosley, A.R. Measham, & J.L. Bobdilla (Eds.). *Diseases control priorities in developing countries*. (pp. 91–116). New York, NY: Oxford University Press.

McCourt, F. (1999). *Angela's ashes*. New York, NY: Scribner.

McInerney, P.A. (2004). Evidence-based nursing and midwifery: The state of the science in South Africa. *Worldviews in evidence-based nursing, 1*(4):207–208.

McQueen, D.V., McKenna, M.T., & Sleet, D.A. (2001). Chronic diseases and injury. In M.H. Merson, R.E. Black, & A.J. Mills (Eds.). *International public health diseases, program, system, and policies*. (p. 293). Gaithersburg, MD: Aspen.

Medical News Today. (2005, August 25). Over 100 groups urge Bush to enforce anti-prostitution policy to aid sexually exploited women and children. Retrieved October 1, 2008 from http://www.medicalnewstoday.com/articles/28834.php.

Miri, E.S. (1998). Problems and perspectives of managing an onchocerciasis control programme: A case study from Plateau state, Nigeria. *Annals of Tropical Medicine and Parasitology, 68E*(92), 121–128.

Mulli, J.D. (1996). War and health. In R. Lanza (Ed.). *One world: The health and survival of the human species in the 21st century*. (pp. 149–160). Santa Fe, NM: Health Press.

Murray, C.J., & Lopez, A.D. (1996). Evidence-based health policy: Lessons from the Global Burden of Disease Study. *Science, 274,* 740–743.

Murray, C.J., & Lopez, A.D. (1997). Mortality by cause for eight regions of the world: Global Burden of Disease Study. *Lancet, 349,* 1269–1347.

Nathwani, D., & Spiteri, J. (1997). Information about anti-malarial chemoprophylaxis in hospitalized patients: Is it adequate? *Scottish Medical Journal, 42*(1), 13–15.

National Geographic News. (2005). *Tsunami in Southeast Asia: Full coverage*. Retrieved August 7, 2008 from http://www.nationalgeographic.com/news/2005/01/0107_050107_tsunami_index.html.

Natsios, A.S. (2002). *This is USAID*. USAID, Washington, D.C. Retrieved August 7, 2008 from http://www.usaid.gov/about_usaid/.

Newsday. (2001). WHO to unveil 14-year world health strategy. Retrieved August 7, 2008 from http://www.cid.harvard.edu/cidinthenews/articles/newsday_122001.html.

Organization for Economic Cooperation and Development (OECD). (2006). *Chemicals classification and labeling*. Retrieved November 27, 2006 from http://www.oecd.org/department/0,2688,en_2649_34371_1_1_1_1_1,00.htm.

Phillips, D.R. (1990). *Health and health care in the third world*. New York: Longman Scientific & Technical with Wiley and Sons.

Primary Health Care. (1978). (Alma Ata, 1978). *Health for All Series No. 1*. Geneva: World Health Organization. Retrieved August 7, 2008 from www.euro.who.int/AboutWHO/Policy/20010827_1.

Reingold, A.L., & Phares, C.R. (2001). Infectious diseases. In M.H. Merson, R.E. Black, & A.J. Mills (Eds.). *International public health diseases, program, system, and policies*. (pp. 710–711). Gaithersburg, MD: Aspen.

Reuters News Service. (2006). *Amazon dam project draws heated opposition in Brazil*. Retrieved August 7, 2008 from http://www.plantark.org/avantgo/dailynewsstory.cfm?newsid=39379.

Roemer, M.I. (1993). *National health systems of the world*, Vols. I & II. New York: Oxford University Press.

Rushdie, S. (1995). *The moor's last sigh*. New York, NY: Pantheon Books.

Samary, C. (1995). *Yugoslavia dismembered*. New York, NY: Monthly Review Press.

Schlein, L. (2007, July 28). WHO says environmental hazards kill millions of children. *Voice of America News*. Retrieved October 1, 2008 from http://www.voanews.com/english/archive/2007-07/2007-07-28-voa27.cfm?CFID=48545824&CFTOKEN=37283846.

Segor, D. (2006). *Living the unimaginable in Mizo country: Women's stories of how they survive independence movement, counter-insurgency and forced village groupings in the State of India*. [Unpublished doctoral dissertation]. Santa Barbara, CA: Fielding Graduate University.

Siegel, R., & Watson, I. (2006). *Lebanon begins post-war recovery effort*. National Public Radio broadcast. Retrieved August 7, 2008 from http://www.npr.org/templates/story/story.php?storyid=5671702.

Shannon, J.B. (Ed.). (2001). *Worldwide health sourcebook*. (pp. 104–113). Detroit, MI: Omnigraphics.

Spector, R.E. (2004). *Cultural diversity in health and illness*, 6th ed. Upper Saddle River, NJ: Pearson Education Inc.

Stansfield, S.K., & Shepard, D.S. (1993). Acute respiratory infection. In D.T. Jamison, W.H. Mosley, A.R. Measham, & J.L. Bobadilla (Eds.). *Disease control priorities in developing countries*. (pp. 67–90). Oxford: Oxford University Press.

Stedman's medical dictionary, 26th ed. (1995). Baltimore, MD: Williams & Wilkins.

The Boston Globe. (2006). *A surgical strike against AIDS*. Retrieved August 7, 2008 from http://www.boston.com/news/globe/editorial_opinion/editorials/articles/2006/12/17/a_surgical_strike_against_aids/.

The Official Website of the Republic of the Philippines (2006). *Forum*. Retrieved August 7, 2008 from http://www.gov.ph/forum/thread.asp?rootID=29670&catID=9.

The Ozone Hole. (September 16, 2006). *Montreal Protocol on ozone-depleting substances effective, but work still unfinished says Secretary General in message for International Day*. Retrieved August 7, 2008 from http://www.theozonehole.com/ozoneday2006.htm.

The Work Continues. (2006). Diana, Princess of Wales: Championing causes. Retrieved August 7, 2008 from http://www.theworkcontinues.org/causes/index.asp.

Toole, M.J., Waldman, R.J., & Zwi, A. (2001). Complex humanitarian emergencies. In M.H. Merson, R.E. Black, & A.J. Mills (Eds.). *International public health: Diseases, programs, systems, policies*. (pp. 439–513). Gaithersburg, MD: Aspen.

Trigg, P.I., & Kondrachine, A.V. (1998). Commentary: Malaria control in the 1990s. *Bulletin of the World Health Organization*, 76(1), 11–16.

United Nations High Commissioner for Refugees (UNHCR). (2006). Health: familiar images. *Refugees Magazine*, Issue 105 (Life in a refugee camp), Retrieved from http://www.unhcr.org/publ/PUBL/3b582839c.html.

United States Department of Health and Human Services. (2000). *Healthy people 2010: Understanding and improving health*, 2nd ed. Washington, DC: Author.

United States (U.S.) Fund for UNICEF. (November 20, 2006). *Camps swell as women and children flee fighting in south Darfur*. Retrieved October 1, 2008 from http://www.unicef.org/infobycountry/sudan_36600.html.

Valadian, I., & Farrell, M. (1995). Women's health: An international perspective. *Armenian women in a changing world*. Boston, MA: AIWA Press.

Valentine, V. (November 4, 2005). *Health for the masses: China's "barefoot doctors."* National Public Radio. Retrieved August 7, 2008 from http://www.npr.org/templates/story/story.php?storyid=4990242.

Vance, C. (1999). Nursing in the global arena. In E.J. Sullivan (Ed.). *Creating nursing's future*. (p. 335). St. Louis: Mosby.

Walsh, J.A., Feifer, C.N., Measham, A.R., & Gertler, P.J. (1993). Maternal and perinatal health. In D.T. Jamison, W.H. Mosley, A.R. Measham, & J.L. Bobdilla (Eds.). *Disease control priorities in developing countries*. (pp. 363–390). Oxford: Oxford University Press.

Wenzel, E. (1998). *WHO Constitution: Article 2*. Retrieved August 7, 2008 from http://www.ldb.org/vl/top/whoconst.htm.

Whaley, R.F., & Hashim, T.J. (1995). *A textbook of world health: A practical guide to global health care*. New York, NY: Parthenon.

World Bank. (2002). *What is the World Bank?* Retrieved August 7, 2008 from http://www.worldbank.org.

World Health Organization. (November 1996). Water and sanitation. *WHO Fact Sheet, 112*, 2. Geneva: Author. Retrieved August 7, 2008 from http://www.who.int/inf-fs/en/fact112.html.

World Health Organization. (1998a, March). Dracunculiasis eradication. *WHO Fact Sheet, 98*, 1–2. Geneva: Author.

World Health Organization. (1998b, August Revised). Emerging and re-emerging infectious diseases. *WHO Fact Sheet 97*, 1–7. Geneva: Author.

World Health Organization. (1998c, September). Reducing mortality from major killers of children. *WHO Fact Sheet 178*, 3. Geneva: WHO. Retrieved August 7, 2008 from http://www.who.int/inf-fs/en/fact178.html.

World Health Organization. (1998d). Examples of pathogens recognized since 1973. *WHO Fact Sheet, 97*, 4. Geneva: Author.

World Health Organization. (1998e, November). Primary health care in the 21st century is everybody's business. *Press Release WHO/89*, 1–2. Geneva: Author.

World Health Organization. (1999a, February). WHO executive board gives green light to framework convention on tobacco control. *Press Release WHO/6*. Geneva: Author.

World Health Organization. (1999b). Highlights of the 52nd World Health Assembly. *Bulletin of the World Health Organization, 77*(7), 612–613. Geneva: Author.

World Health Organization. (1999d, August 3). Solar alert '99. *Press Release WHO/40*, 1–2. Geneva: Author.

World Health Organization. (1999e, April 5). Polio outbreak in Central Africa. *Press Release WHO/21*, 102. Geneva: Author.

World Health Organization. (1999f). Malaria vaccine progress. *Bulletin of the World Health Organization, 77*(4), 361–362.

World Health Organization. (1999g, October 28). UN agencies issue joint statement for reducing maternal mortality. *WHO Press Release*. Geneva: Author.

World Health Organization. (2001). Nipah virus. *WHO Fact Sheet, 262*, 1–2. Geneva: Author.

World Health Organization. (2001a). Vaccines against diarrheal diseases. *WHO/GPV Strategic Plan 1998–2001*. Geneva: Author.

World Health Organization. (2001b). Surveillance for neonatal tetanus. *WHO/GPV Strategic Plan 1998–2001* (pp. 29, 46). Geneva: Author.

World Health Organization. (2001c, November). AIDS epidemic faster in eastern Europe than in rest of world: New figures. *Joint UNAIDS/WHO Press Release/53*, 1–2. Geneva: Author.

World Health Organization. (2002a). Roll back malaria: 2001–2010 United Nations decade to roll back malaria. *RBM Infosheet 2 of 11, March 2002*. Geneva: Author. Retrieved from http://www.rbm.who.int

World Health Organization. (2002b, July 9). Three million HIV/AIDS sufferers could receive antiretroviral therapy by 2005. *WHO Press Release/58*, 1–2. Geneva: Author.

World Health Organization. (2002c, July 4). Scaling up interventions could prevent 29 million new HIV infections among adults by 2010. *WHO Press Release/57*, 1–2. Geneva: Author.

World Health Organization. (2002d, July 12). *WHO-UNICEF measles mortality reduction and regional elimination strategic plan 2001–2005*. Geneva: WHO. Retrieved August 7,

2008 from http://www.who.int/mediacentre/releases/2003/pr76/en/.

World Health Organization. (2002e, August Revised). Tuberculosis. *WHO Fact Sheet, 104*, 1–3. Retrieved from http://www.who.int/mediacentre/factsheets/who104/en/

World Health Association (WHO). (2003). *Global Polio Eradication Initiative: strategic plan 2004–2008*. Geneva, Switzerland: Author.

World Health Organization. (2002g, October). WHO atlas maps global tobacco epidemic. *Press Release WHO/82*. Geneva: Author.

World Health Organization. (2002h, October 28). Years of life can be increased 5–10 years. *Press Release WHO/84*. Geneva: Author.

World Health Organization. (2002i, November). Low investment in immunization and vaccines threatens global health. *Press Release WHO/87*. Geneva: Author.

World Health Organization. (2002j, November 25). TDR, Medicines for Malaria Venture and Shin Poong Pharmaceuticals sign agreement for development of pyronaridine-artesunate for treatment of malaria. *Notes for the Press WHO/8*. Geneva: Author.

World Health Organization. (2002k, December 6). River blindness campaign ends: West Africans return to fertile farmlands. *Press Release WHO/93*. Geneva: Author.

World Health Organization. (2002l, December 11). WHO study reveals harsh realities for older persons caring for orphans and people living with AIDS. *Press Release WHO/95*, 1–2. Geneva: Author.

World Health Organization. (2002m, December). *About WHO*. Retrieved August 7, 2008 from http://www.who.int/about/en/.

World Health Organization. (2003a, January). Leprosy. *WHO Fact Sheet, 101*, 1–3. Retrieved August 7, 2008 from http://www.who.int/mediacentre/factsheets/fs101/en/.

World Health Organization. (2003b, February). Leprosy: Urgent need to end stigma and isolation. *Press Release WHO/7*, 1–2. Geneva: Author.

World Health Organization. (2003c, March). Agreement reached on global framework convention on tobacco control. *Press Release WHO/21*. Geneva: Author.

World Health Organization (2003, 12 March). WHO issues a global alert about cases of atypical pneumonia. *Press Release WHO/22*. Geneva: Author.

World Health Organization. (2003d, March). *Burden of disease project*. Geneva: Author. Retrieved August 7, 2008 from http://www.who.int/whr/2003/en/Annex3-en.pdf.

World Health Organization. (2003e, May). *Severe acute respiratory syndrome (SARS)*. Retrieved August 7, 2008 from http://www.who.int/csr/sars/en/.

World Health Organization. (2003). First steps for managing an outbreak of acute diarrhea. WHO global task force on cholera. Global health security: Epidemic alert and response, Box 2. Geneva: Author.

World Health Organization (2006). *Immunization, vaccine and biologicals*. Retrieved August 7, 2008 from http://www.who.int/vaccines-document/DoxGen/H3DoxList.htm.

World Health Organization (2006b). *Dracunculiasis: Recent epidemiological data*. Retrieved August 7, 2008 from http://www.who.int/ctd/dracun/epidemio.htm.

Worley, H. (2006, July). Best buys and challenges for malaria prevention in subsaharan Africa. *Population Reference Bureau*. Retrieved October 1, 2008 from http://www.prb.org/Articles/2006/BestBuysandChallengesforMalariaPreventioninSubSaharanAfrica.aspx.

Selected Readings

Berlinguer, G. (1999). Health and equity as a primary global goal. *Development, 42*, 17–21.

Fiddler, D.P. (2007). SARS: Political pathology of the first post-Westphalian pathogen. *Journal of Law & Medicine, 31*(4), 485–505.

Flood, C.M., Gable, L., & Gostin, L.O. (2005). Introduction: Legislating and litigating health care rights around the world. *The Journal of Law, Medicine & Ethics, 33*(4), 636–640.

Forman, L. (2005). Ensuring reasonable health: Health rights, the judiciary and South African HIV/AIDS policy. *The Journal of Law, Medicine & Ethics, 33*(4), 711–724.

Garrett, L. (2000). *Betrayal of trust: The collapse of global public health*. New York: Hyperion.

Kikuchi, J.F. (2005). Cultural theories of nursing responsive to human needs and values. *Journal of Nursing Scholarship, 37*(4), 302–307.

Mayer, K.H., & Pizer, H.F. (Eds.). (2000). *The emergence of AIDS: The impact on immunology, microbiology and public health*. Washington DC: American Public Health Association.

Merson, M.H., Black, R.E., & Mills, A.J. (Eds.). (2001). *International public health: Diseases, programs, systems and policies*. Gaithersburg, MD: Aspen.

Rosskam, E. (Ed.). (2006). *Winners or losers? Liberalizing public services*. Geneva: International Labour Office.

Salvatierra-Gonzalez, R., & Benguigui, Y. (Eds.). (2000). *Antimicrobial resistance in the Americas: Magnitude and containment of the problem*. Washington, DC: Pan American Health Organization.

Stapleton, D. (2004). Lessons of history? Anti-malaria strategies of the International Health Board and the Rockefeller Foundation from the 1920s to the era of DDT. *Public Health Reports, 119*(2), 206–215.

World Health Organization. (1986). *The Ottawa charter for health promotion*. Geneva: Author.

World Health Organization. (March 2003). *Burden of disease project*. WHOIS: Geneva. Retrieved August 7, 2008 from http://www3.int/whois/menu.cfm?path=whosis,burden%language=english.

Internet Resources

American Red Cross, and International Red Cross and Red Crescent Societies: *http://www.red-cross.org*
Career Network: Global Health Council (GHC): *http://www.globalhealth.org*
Doctors of the World: *http://www.doctorsoftheworld.org*
Doctors Without Borders: *http://www.doctorswithoutborders.org*
Global Volunteers: Partners in Development: *http://www.globalvolunteers.org*
Health Volunteers Overseas (HVO): *http://www/hvousa.org*.
International Center for Equal Health care Access: *http://www.iceha.org*
International Jobs: *http://www.internationaljobs.org*
Medical Ambassadors International: *http://www.medicalambassadors.org*
Peace Corps: *http://www.peacecorps.gov*
Unite for Sight: *http://www.uniteforsight.org*

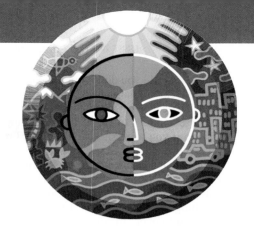

17

Being Prepared: Disasters and Terrorism

LEARNING OBJECTIVES

Upon mastery of this chapter, you should be able to:

◆ Describe a variety of characteristics of disasters, including causation, number of casualties, scope, and intensity.
◆ Discuss a variety of factors contributing to a community's potential for experiencing a disaster.
◆ Identify the four phases of disaster management.
◆ Describe factors involved in disaster planning.
◆ Describe the role of the community health nurse in preventing, preparing for, responding to, and supporting recovery from disasters.
◆ Use the levels of prevention to describe the role of the community health nurse in relation to acts of chemical, biologic, or nuclear terrorism.

"Dig a well before you are thirsty."

—Chinese Proverb

What would you do if your local news station broadcast an announcement that your community was directly in the path of a hurricane that earlier in the day had caused extensive damage and loss of life in a neighboring state? What would you do if you were shopping at a local mall, suddenly heard an explosive noise followed by shouts and cries for help, then noticed that a pungent odor was filling the air? What *did* you do on the morning of September 11, 2001, when the world of each American, especially those in New York City, in Washington, D.C., and on a plane over rural Pennsylvania, changed forever? In August of 2007, were you glued to your television set as the frantic search for survivors of the I-35W bridge collapse in Minneapolis, MN, took place? When you heard news of the massive loss of life and property from the 2008 cyclone that devastated Myanmar (Burma), could you even imagine the plight of the survivors whose lives hung in the balance? Even today, the impact of the 2005 hurricanes Katrina and Rita on the Gulf Coast continues to affect the lives of the residents of those communities devastated by the storms. As distant as some of these scenarios might seem from your own life, natural disasters and terrorism are ever-present possibilities, and nurses and other health care professionals have an obligation to respond appropriately. This chapter will increase your understanding of the community health nurse's role in preparing for, responding to, and recovering from natural disasters and terrorism.

DISASTERS

A **disaster** is any natural or man-made event that causes a level of destruction or emotional trauma exceeding the abilities of those affected to respond without community assistance. The crash of a private plane over the Pacific Ocean in which no bodies are recovered and no environmental impact is felt is not a disaster by this definition, because no specific community-based response is required or even possible. Such a tragedy may however, be felt for a lifetime by family members and friends, who need emotional support and possibly long-term financial assistance. If a plane with 150 passengers crashes over land, destroying several homes in its path, the community affected is unable to cope with the resulting injuries, deaths, and property destruction without assistance; by the definition used here, this constitutes a disaster.

The geographic distribution of disasters varies because certain types of disasters are more common in some parts of the world. For example, California is associated with earthquakes and Florida with hurricanes. Similarly, it is not surprising to hear of drought in Ethiopia or floods in India during the monsoon season. When certain types of disasters are anticipated, communities are usually better prepared for them. For instance, California has strict building codes to prevent destruction of structures in the event of earthquakes, but most California homes lack the basements and insulation that characterize homes in regions often visited by tornados or winter storms. Similarly, residents of Germany, Austria, and Russia are better prepared for blizzards than for heavy rain, which probably explains in part the devastation caused in some communities by floods there in 2002.

Because the local media in the United States do not typically report on disasters unless there are mass casualties, one may be unaware of the frequency and variety of both natural and technologic disasters worldwide. Here is a brief sampling of major disasters that occurred in 2007–2008 (Infoplease, 2008; International Charter, 2008):

May 2007
◆ **Russia:** Explosion killed 38 coal miners in Yubileinaya, 2 months after a similar explosion in a nearby town killed 110.

June 2007
◆ **Pakistan:** More than 200 people died during severe storms in Karachi, Pakistan's biggest city.

August 2007
◆ **Greece:** Over 220 separate fires ravaged the Greek countryside, threatening ancient Olympic sites around Athens. At least 59 people died in the blazes.

September 2007
◆ **Sudan:** Over 20 people died, 65 people were injured, and thousands of livestock were lost by flooding in central Sudan.

October 2007
◆ **California:** Wildfires burned more than 516,000 acres in southern California. Seven died, and nearly 90 people were injured. Over 500,000 people were forced to evacuate their homes; 2,000 homes were destroyed.

November 2007
◆ **Bangladesh:** Cyclone killed nearly 3,500 people in southern Bangladesh; millions of people were left homeless.

February 2008
◆ **U.S. South:** Violent tornadoes strike Kentucky, Tennessee, Alabama, Mississippi, and Arkansas with little warning, resulting in 54 deaths and hundreds of injured, with widespread damage reported.

May 2008
◆ **China:** Earthquake struck eastern Sichuan, northwest of Chengdu. The tremor was felt throughout the region, with the death toll exceeding 65,000.

Characteristics of Disasters

Disasters are often characterized by their cause. A **natural disaster** is caused by natural events, such as the floods in Namibia or the earthquake in China in 2008. A **man-made disaster** is caused by human activity, such as the 2007 bombings in India on a train headed to Pakistan, the bombing of the World Trade Center in New York City in 2001, the displacement of thousands of Kosovars during their war with Serbia in 1999, or the riots in Los Angeles in the early 1990s. Other man-made disasters include nuclear reactor meltdowns, industrial accidents, oil spills, construction accidents, and air, train, bus, and subway crashes.

A **casualty** is a human being who is injured or killed by or as a direct result of an accident. Although major disasters sometimes occur without any injury or loss of life, disasters are commonly characterized by the number of casualties involved. If casualties number more than two people but fewer than 100, the disaster is characterized as a *multiple-*

casualty incident. Although multiple-casualty incidents may strain the health care systems of small or mid-sized communities, a **mass-casualty incident**—involving 100 or more casualties—often completely overwhelms the resources of even large cities. Preparedness for mass-casualty incidents is essential for all communities.

The possibility of being prepared is another characteristic that varies with different types of disasters. For instance, the path and time of landfall of a hurricane can be tracked, so that residents in the storm's path can be evacuated and families and businesses can be protected. Communities can also minimize devastation from flooding by building reservoirs or refusing to grant building permits in flood-prone areas, and by reinforcing areas around waterways with sandbags during rainy weather. In fire-prone areas, communities can post notices to heighten awareness of fire danger and enforce regulations to cut back vegetation near structures in forested areas.

On the other hand, some disasters strike without warning. For example, the terrorist attacks in New York City caught thousands of civilians unaware. They were trapped in buildings with limited escape routes and very little time to retreat to safety. For employees in the Pentagon on 9/11, survival depended on being in the right place at the right time. The number of fires in southern California in 2007 was unanticipated and uncharacteristically large, and control was hindered by heat and high winds. Residents were barred from reentering their communities for weeks, without any knowledge of whether they would have homes when they were allowed to return.

The **scope** of a disaster is the range of its effect, either geographically or in terms of the number of victims. The collapse of a 500-unit high-rise apartment building has a greater scope than does the collapse of a bridge that occurs while only two cars are crossing.

The **intensity** of a disaster is the level of destruction and devastation it causes. For instance, an earthquake centered in a large metropolitan area and one centered in a desert may have the same numeric rating on the Richter scale, yet have very different intensities in terms of the destruction they cause.

Victims of Disasters

Because disasters are so variable, there is no typical victim in a disaster. Nor can anyone predict whether he will ever become a victim of a disaster. However, once disaster strikes, victims may be characterized by their level of involvement. **Direct victims** are the people who experience the event, whether fire, volcanic eruption, war, or bomb. They are the dead and the survivors, and even if they are without physical injuries, they are likely to have health effects from their experience. Some may be without shelter or food, and many experience serious psychological stress long after the event is over (Display 17.1).

Depending on the cause and characteristics of the disaster, some direct victims may become displaced persons or refugees. **Displaced persons** are forced to leave their homes to escape the effects of a disaster. Usually, displacement is a temporary condition and involves movement within the person's own country. A common example is relocation of residents of flooded areas to schools, churches, and other shelters on higher ground. Typically, the term **refugee** is reserved for people who are forced to leave their homeland because of war or persecution. For example, over 2.5 million displaced people live in camps in Darfur after fleeing ethnic cleansing by Sudanese government forces and militia. The United Nations (U.N.) estimates that an additional 2 million have been impacted by the conflict, resulting from the damage to local economies and trade (Human Rights Watch, 2008). Also of concern to the world community is the 4.5 million Iraqis believed to have been displaced by violence in their country, over 2 million of

---

| DISPLAY 17.1 | **DIRECT AND INDIRECT VICTIMS OF A DISASTER** |

On September 11, 2001, almost 3,000 people died in the terrorist attacks on the World Trade Center in New York City. Although all of the employees and visitors in the two buildings were direct victims of this disaster, the entire population of Manhattan can be considered indirect victims. Hotels, businesses, and apartments for blocks surrounding the Twin Towers suffered structural damage, blown-out windows, and interiors covered with inches of powdered cement and other debris. A year after this disaster, many residents in the surrounding areas still were unable to return home.

Many rescue workers who were survivors have lasting psychological effects from their own survival experiences and from losing close friends and colleagues. In addition, many rescuers inhaled the dust in the air for days and now suffer respiratory damages, which changes their status from indirect to direct victims of the disaster.

All people working or visiting in Manhattan that day were affected by the closing of the bridges and tunnels and were stranded in New York City until transportation routes opened again, thus becoming indirect victims. Other indirect victims included children attending school and living within sight of the Twin Towers. They received counseling in school for months, and in some cases years, after the disaster.

For 1 year after the attack, volunteer construction workers and rescue workers who lost fellow police officers, paramedics, or firefighters worked 24 hours a day. First, the efforts were geared to find survivors. Shortly after, workers knew that they were looking for the bodies or body parts of victims while removing thousands of tons of building pieces. Thousands of people involved in the recovery efforts can still be considered indirect victims.

Family members of the 2,980 deceased victims, who have been affected for a lifetime, also are indirect victims. Thousands of children lost a parent, some parents lost multiple children, and, in some cases, both spouses were lost because husband and wife worked in the World Trade Center. The ripples of tragedy extended beyond the borders of the United States, because there were hundreds of people working in the Twin Towers from many different countries whose family members remain indirect victims.

whom now live in neighboring countries, such as Jordan and Syria (United Nations Refugee Agency, 2008). Often, the displacement of refugees is permanent, with lasting impact to both the country of origin and the host country.

Indirect victims are the relatives and friends of direct victims. Although these people do not experience the stress of the event itself, they often undergo extreme anguish from trying to locate loved ones or accommodate their emergency needs. If bodies cannot be found or are unidentifiable, indirect victims experience even greater anguish and may not be able to accept that their loved one has died. For example, many of the mothers of young Argentineans who disappeared in the 1970s still march daily in downtown Buenos Aires, demanding public acknowledgment of the murders of their daughters and sons. Family members of victims from 9/11 in New York City have worked with architects to develop a complex of buildings and a memorial that meets the expectations of most of the indirect victims and honors their loved ones. This effort, along with the Flight 93 National Memorial (Shanksville, PA) and the Pentagon Memorial Project, will help with the long healing process. They also serve as a reminder of the impact that day had on each of our lives.

Factors Contributing to Disasters

It is useful to apply the host, agent, and environment model to understand the factors contributing to disasters, because manipulation of these factors can be instrumental in planning strategies to prevent or prepare for disasters.

Host Factors

The *host* is the human being who experiences the disaster. Host factors that contribute to the likelihood of experiencing a disaster include age, general health, mobility, psychological factors, and even socioeconomic factors. For instance, elderly residents of a mobile home community may be unable to evacuate independently in response to a tornado warning if they no longer can drive. Impoverished residents of a low-income apartment complex in a large city may notice that their building is not compliant with city fire codes but may avoid alerting authorities for fear of being forced to move to more expensive housing.

Agent Factors

The *agent* is the natural or technologic element that causes the disaster. For example, the high winds of a hurricane and the lava of an erupting volcano are agents, as are radiation, industrial chemicals, biologic agents, and bombs. The Station Nightclub fire and the apartment deck collapse in Chicago (both in 2003) demonstrated that the irresponsibility of contractors and inspectors and failure to adhere to safety policies, can act as agents of disaster, resulting in death and destruction.

Environmental Factors

Environmental factors are those that could potentially contribute to or mitigate a disaster. Some of the most common environmental factors are a community's level of preparedness; the presence of industries that produce harmful chemicals or radiation; the presence of flood-prone rivers, lakes, or streams; average amount of rainfall or snowfall; average high and low temperatures; proximity to fault lines, coastal waters, or volcanoes; level of compliance with local building codes; and presence or absence of political unrest.

Agencies and Organizations for Disaster Management

Among disaster-relief organizations, perhaps none is as famous as the Red Cross, the name commonly used when referring to the American Red Cross, the Federation of Red Cross and Red Crescent Societies, and the International Committee of the Red Cross. The American Red Cross was founded in 1881 by Clara Barton and was chartered by the U.S. Congress in 1905. It is authorized to provide disaster assistance free of charge across the country through its more than 1 million volunteers. A common misconception is that the Red Cross is supported by the federal government; this is not the case. The American Red Cross provides services solely on donations from individuals, groups, and corporations. The duties assumed by the Red Cross in the event of a disaster are to provide sheltering, food, basic health and mental health services, and distribution of emergency supplies (American Red Cross, 2008).

The Federal Emergency Management Agency (FEMA), established in 1979, is the federal agency responsible for assessing and responding to disaster events in the United States. It also provides training and guidance in all phases of disaster management. In 2003, FEMA became part of the Department of Homeland Security (DHS). The DHS was organized in 2002, and incorporates many of the nation's security, protection, and emergency response activities into a single federal department. Other agencies that fall under the DHS include: Directorate for Preparedness, Domestic Nuclear Detection Office, Federal Law Enforcement Training Center, Office of the Inspector General, and the more widely known agencies—the Transportation Security Administration (TSA), U.S. Customs and Border Protection, U.S. Immigration and Customs Enforcement (ICE), U.S. Coast Guard, and the U.S. Secret Service (DHS, 2006). Under the oversight of FEMA is the National Incident Management System (NIMS), which was developed to allow responders from different jurisdictions and disciplines to work more cohesively in response to natural disasters, emergencies, and terrorist acts. "NIMS benefits included a unified approach to incident management; standard command and management structures; and emphasis on preparedness, mutual aid and resource management" (FEMA, 2008). Nurses and other health care professionals must understand this system and are encouraged to take courses dealing with the incident command system; these courses are available free online from FEMA.

The World Health Organization's (WHO) Emergency Relief Operations provide disaster assistance internationally, and the Pan American Health Organization works to coordinate relief efforts in Latin America and the Caribbean. In addition, various international nongovernmental organizations (such as Doctors Without Borders, the International Medical Corps, and Operation Blessing), religious groups, and other volunteer agencies provide needed emergency care.

Governments often send their military personnel and equipment in response to international disasters. For example, in May 2008, the U.S. Navy attempted for 3 weeks to provide much-needed supplies to the cyclone survivors in Myanmar (Burma). With limited options, the Navy had helicopters and landing craft on standby to deliver food, water, and medical supplies to the most remote areas of the country. The military junta in Myanmar refused to allow the shipments; further risking the lives of the millions of survivors. U.S. military planes were eventually allowed to land with supplies in the country's largest city, Rangoon (Washington Post, 2008). Transport of vital supplies to the rural areas was conducted by the government, with questionable results.

When natural or man-made disasters within the United States are accompanied by civil disturbance, looting, or violent crime, the resources of local police departments may be overwhelmed. In such cases, the National Guard is often called in to restore order. This action is typically accomplished within each individual state, under the jurisdiction of the governor.

In this situation, political agendas prevented the aid so typically accepted by countries experiencing catastrophe. Fortunately, nurses from the Commissioned Corps of the U.S. Public Health Service (USPHS) were allowed to provide aid in 2004/2005 for the tsunami and earthquake victims in Indonesia, as well assist in the 2006 medicine contamination in Panama, which ultimately claimed the lives of over 100 (USPHS, 2008). Chapter 30 contains additional information about the role of the USPHS Commissioned Corps Nurses and their role in emergency preparedness.

Phases of Disaster Management

In developing strategies to address the problem of disasters, it is helpful for the community health nurse to consider each of the four phases of disaster management: prevention, preparedness, response, and recovery. Additionally, some knowledge of the language typically used in disaster preparedness may be helpful and is included in Display 17.2.

DISPLAY 17.2   COMMON TERMS USED IN EMERGENCY PREPAREDNESS AND RESPONSE

All-hazards preparation: Preparedness for domestic terrorist attacks, major disasters, and other emergencies.

Chain of command: A series of command, control, executive or management positions in hierarchical order of authority.

Credential: A health volunteer's qualifications. Credentials are used to determine a health volunteer's emergency credentialing level (i.e., nursing license).

Designated equivalent source: Selected agencies that have been determined to maintain a specific item or items of credential information that is identical to the information at the primary source.

Disaster, major (federal): Any natural catastrophe, or regardless of cause, any fire, flood, or explosion, in any part of the United States, which in the determination of the President, causes damage of sufficient severity and magnitude to warrant major disaster assistance to supplement the efforts and available resources of states, local governments, and disaster relief organizations.

Emergency declaration: Refers to the State (or local) government's capacity to declare a general emergency or public health emergency, or state of disaster.

Emergency Management Assistance Compact (EMAC): An interstate mutual aid agreement that allows States to assist one another in responding to all types of natural and man-made disasters.

Just-in-Time **training:** Concise, targeted training, normally provided on-site after a disaster or emergency has occurred. It provides a minimum level of exposure for volunteers to select issues in disaster response. Examples could be use of self-protection equipment, documentation, mental health triage, or registration of casualties.

Hospital Emergency Incident Command System (HEICS): An emergency management system that employs a logical management structure, defined responsibilities, clear reporting channels, and a common nomenclature to help unify hospitals with other emergency responders.

Incident Command System (ICS): The combination of facilities, equipment, personnel, procedures, and communications operating within a common organizational structure, designed to aid in the management of resources during incidents.

National Electronic Disease Surveillance System (NEDSS): A CDC initiative promoting the use of data and information systems standards to improve disease surveillance systems at federal, state, and local levels.

National Incident Management System (NIMS): The single all-hazards incident management system required by Homeland Security Presidential Directive 5 that governs the management of the National Response Plan.

Public Health Information Network (PHIN): A framework providing the basis for information technology projects for CDC-funded programs including NEDSS, Health Alert Network (HAN), and others.

Strategic National Stockpile: A national cache of drugs, vaccines, and supplies that can be deployed to areas struck by disasters, including bioterrorism.

Surge capacity: The accommodation by the health system to a transient sudden rise in demand for health care following an incident with real or perceived adverse health effects.

Adapted from U.S. Department of Health and Human Services–HRSA. (2005). ESAR–VHP interim technical and policy guidelines, standards, and definitions (Ver. 2) (Appendix 8: ESAR–VHP Guidelines glossary of terms). Washington, DC: U.S. Government Printing Office.

Prevention Phase

During the *prevention phase,* no disaster is expected or anticipated. The task during this phase is to identify community risk factors and to develop and implement programs to prevent disasters from occurring. Task forces typically include representatives from the community's local government, health care providers, social services providers, police and fire departments, major industries, local media, and citizens' groups. Programs developed during the prevention phase may also focus on strategies to mitigate the effects of disasters that cannot be prevented, such as earthquakes, hurricanes, and tornadoes.

The United States has strengthened this phase of disaster management since September 2001. This can be seen especially at airports, where airline passengers must now go through a more rigorous security screening before boarding the plane. Nonpassengers cannot go beyond the security area. Photographic identification is required at two or more points before boarding. Strict limits have been placed on liquids that can be in carry-on baggage. Random searches of hand-carried luggage occur, and passengers are screened with wands that detect metal. In some states, luggage is tested for radioactive material, police officials with trained dogs patrol the airport, or people are asked to remove their shoes for examination as part of the screening process. All of these measures have been initiated to prevent a disaster.

Preparedness Phase

Disaster *preparedness* involves improving community and individual reaction and responses, so that the effects of a disaster are minimized. Disaster preparedness saves lives and minimizes injury and property damage. It includes plans for communication, evacuation, rescue, and victim care. Any plan must also address acquisition of equipment, supplies, medicine, and even food, clean water, blankets, and shelter. Semiannual disaster drills and tests of the Emergency Broadcast System are examples of appropriate activities during the preparedness phase.

Disaster preparedness activities occur locally, regionally, and nationally. A town keeps its warning system working and tests it each month. Sections of the country coordinate larger warning systems to notify communities in the path of a tornado or hurricane, and the country has a plan to stockpile vital pharmaceuticals such as smallpox vaccine for mass immunization. The Centers for Disease Control (CDC) reports that the Strategic National Stockpile (SNS) contains enough doses of smallpox vaccine to vaccinate every person in the U.S. should biological warfare become a threat (CDC, 2007). The last case of smallpox in the United States occurred in 1949, and routine immunization was halted in 1972 (CDC, 2007). With a largely unvaccinated population, most people in the nation would need the vaccine. Having the vaccine ready is a demonstration of disaster preparedness.

Response Phase

The *response phase* begins immediately after the onset of the disastrous event. Preparedness plans take effect immediately, with the goals of saving lives and preventing further injury or damage. Activities during the response phase include rescue, triage, on-site stabilization, transportation of victims, and treatment at local hospitals. Response also requires recovery, identification, and refrigeration of bodies, so that notification of family members is possible and correct, even weeks after a disaster. This care of the dead is demanding and time-consuming work that is often overlooked by people unfamiliar with disaster response. Persons trained in mortuary services are an essential part of any emergency planning efforts. Supportive care, including food, water, and shelter for victims and relief workers is also an essential element of the total disaster response. The extent of care provided for animals is an additional area of concern that should be addressed in the overall plan. Many shelters will not accept pets; those that do need to be identified as soon as possible to avoid unnecessary confusion and delays in sheltering.

Recovery Phase

During the *recovery phase,* the community takes actions to repair, rebuild, or relocate damaged homes and businesses and restore health and economic vitality to the community. Psychological recovery must also be addressed. The emotional scars from witnessing a traumatic event may last a lifetime. Both victims and relief workers should be offered mental health services to support their recovery (see Perspectives: Voices from the Community).

Role of the Community Health Nurse

The community health nurse has a pivotal role in preventing, preparing for, responding to, and supporting recovery from a disaster. After a thorough community assessment for risk factors, the community health nurse may initiate the formation of a multidisciplinary task force to address disaster prevention and preparedness in the community.

Preventing Disasters

Disaster prevention may be considered on three levels: primary, secondary, and tertiary. These are applied to a natural disaster in the Levels of Prevention Pyramid.

Primary Prevention

Primary prevention of a disaster means keeping the disaster from ever happening by taking actions that completely eliminate its occurrence. This is the first aspect of primary disaster prevention. Although it is obviously the most effective level of intervention, both in terms of promoting clients' health and containing costs, it is not always possible. Tornadoes, earthquakes, and other disasters often strike without warning, despite the use of every available technologic device for prediction and tracking.

If possible, primary prevention of disasters can be practiced in all settings: in the workplace and home with programs to reduce safety hazards, and in the community with programs to monitor risk factors, reduce pollution, and encourage nonviolent conflict resolution. Primary

PERSPECTIVES
VOICES FROM THE COMMUNITY

It was 5:00 p.m. on October 17, 1989, in Santa Cruz, CA, a day that would change my view of life forever. I had just fed my newborn son and was rocking him in a soft, comfortable chair when the house began to shake. Without even thinking or being aware of what I was doing, I jumped up with my baby in my arms and headed for the nearest doorway, as I had done so many times before in an earthquake. I stood there holding my son in one arm and braced myself against the door jamb with the other one as the house continued to shake all around us. It was not until the shaking stopped that I began to feel fear and worry as I surveyed the damage to my house.

In my kitchen, all of the cupboard doors were flung open and their contents spilled onto the floor, which was now a mess of spilled food, sticky sauces, dented tin cans, and broken glass. Tears came to my eyes as I saw my son's infant seat, where he had been seated only moments before the quake, covered with glass shards and fallen tin cans. I realized he could have been killed, and I had no control over it. I became afraid for the safety of my 10-year-old daughter, who was at dancing lessons across town. Fortunately, when I got to her, she was safe.

The next few days continued to be very stressful. We had no gas or electricity and no running water that was safe to drink. I went to the drug store in a panic to buy premixed formula to feed my son, since I could not boil the water to mix with the powdered formula. Both the drug store and the grocery store were "trashed," all of the items were thrown off of the shelves and laying on the debris-strewn floors. The grocery store was giving away the ice cream because they had no power to keep it frozen. But who could eat ice cream?

There was something about seeing my favorite grocery store in such a disastrous condition that made me realize how little control I had over the consequences of what insurance companies call "acts of God." I couldn't just run to the grocery store for what I needed; it wouldn't be there for me. My family and I felt very unsafe as we all huddled together in the master bedroom at night. My son was in his bassinet at the foot of the bed and my daughter slept with me until she felt safe enough to return to her own room. I was attempting to regain control of my life as I cleaned up my house and waited for the water and electricity to be restored. Of all the losses, the greatest loss was the illusion of safety and the illusion that I had control over my life.

Over the next week, I experienced the loss of many services and products that made up my comfortable and safe lifestyle: homes were damaged, with their chimneys strewn across front lawns, there was no phone service for days, and a normal 10-minute drive took an hour and a half on clogged highways provided as an alternative route to highways and bridges damaged by the quake. As a community mental health nurse, I wanted to volunteer to help others who were experiencing the same feelings as I was, but I was told that they were not taking mental health volunteers from the immediate area because we, too, were victims of the disaster, and needed to care for ourselves first. I think they were right, since I had many feelings that took a long while to heal, and I have lost the illusion of control forever.

---

disaster prevention efforts should take into account a community's physical, psychosocial, cultural, economic, and spiritual needs. The community health nurse has a role in each of these areas. As a teacher, the community health nurse educates people at home, at work, at school, or in a faith community about safety and security focused on preventing a disaster. The community health nurse can teach community members how to protect themselves from the effects of a natural disaster. The nurse can be a part of a safety team, if working as a school nurse or occupational health nurse. If working for a health department, the nurse can determine during home visits whether a family has a personal disaster plan and help them develop one if none exists. Nursing students can work with low-income community dwelling elders to assure that they have enough food, water, and medical supplies to "shelter in place" for at least several days. There are many actions the nurse can initiate.

The second aspect of primary disaster prevention is anticipatory guidance. Disaster drills and other anticipatory exercises help relief workers experience some of the feelings of chaos and stress associated with a disaster before one occurs. It is much easier to do this when energy and intellectual processes are at a high level of functioning. Anticipatory work can dissipate the impact of a disastrous event. The community health nurse has a role in these disaster drills through committee membership, organization of drills at the place of employment, or activism at the grassroots level to assist in holding community-wide disaster drills on a regular basis.

Secondary Prevention

Secondary disaster prevention focuses on the earliest possible detection and treatment. For example, a mobile home community is devastated by a tornado, and the local health department's community health nurses work with the American Red Cross to provide emergency assistance. Secondary prevention corresponds to immediate and effective response. In a post-Katrina study of the emergency planning and response by home health providers serving the poor in New Orleans during the emergency (Kirkpatrick & Bryan, 2007), the successes and challenges of these providers were identified. Agencies that provided early evacuation, identified shelters for special-needs patients outside the high risk area, implemented volunteer cascading communication systems,

LEVELS OF PREVENTION PYRAMID

SITUATION: A natural disaster—tornado.

GOAL: By using the three levels of prevention, negative health conditions are avoided, promptly diagnosed and treated, and/or the fullest possible potential is restored.

Tertiary Prevention

Rehabilitation

- Remain safe during the immediate recovery period
- Accept help from others—friends, family, and community services
- Rebuild family lives through counseling and other services to reestablish stable life physically, emotionally, spiritually, and financially

Primary Prevention

Health Promotion & Education

- Educate community members about the need to enhance planning against damage from future natural disasters, based on experiences with the current disaster

Health Protection

- Keep recommended immunizations current
- Community physical structures need rebuilding, with infrastructure planning and supports that improve ability to withstand natural disasters

Secondary Prevention

Early Diagnosis

- Remain in your position of safety until a community all-clear warning signal is sounded or until rescued
- Leave a damaged building cautiously, if able and not seriously injured, and do not return until it is declared safe

Prompt Treatment

- Rescue individuals promptly and get appropriate care for those injured as soon as possible
- The infrastructure of the community becomes/remains intact, keeping community members safe from hazards such as live wires, broken gas lines, and fallen debris

Primary Prevention

Health Promotion & Education

- Increase community awareness
- Increase community preparation through education
- Each person is as prepared as possible both physically and emotionally

Health Protection

- Community members know what to do and where to go, whether at home, work, school, or elsewhere in the community
- Get to safety before the impact—southwest corner of a home's basement or an interior room away from windows and under heavy furniture

---

conducted pre-event mock evacuation plans, and those that included volunteers in their disaster plan were most successful. Recommendations to improve response include identification of patients who may be reluctant to evacuate, the provision of adequate security at special-needs shelters and, most importantly, practice drills (Kirkpatrick & Bryan, 2007). With appropriate planning, sound and easily understood emergency response can provide optimal care and services to those impacted by the disaster.

Tertiary Prevention

Tertiary disaster prevention involves reducing the amount and degree of disability or damage resulting from the disaster.

Although it involves rehabilitative work, it can help a community recover and reduce the risk of further disasters. In this sense, it becomes a preventive measure.

An example from September 11, 2001, comes from a nurse living in the Boston area who, after that date, began to lose a sense of hope for her future. She often found it difficult to assist her patients with their needs because of her own insecurities and fears. She and a peer responded to a request from the Logan Airport Employee Assistance Program (EAP) asking for help with crisis counseling for United Airlines survivors of 9/11. The planes used in the attacks were from American and United Airlines, and the community of employees felt like survivors because they lived while fellow employees were lost in the disaster.

Employees were in turmoil, and their ability to function was affected. "The terrorists had taken away their colleagues, friends and sense of security" (DiVitto, 2002, p. 21).

The most important interventions the nurses provided were a listening ear and validation that what the employees were feeling and experiencing was normal, and often essential, for healthy grieving. Some employees needed to talk about good times, others were quiet and sad, and others expressed a fear of flying again but did so with the support of family and friends. All demonstrated courage and an ability to continue their lives with a sense of strength and hope. Working with these employees enabled the nurse to recapture the essence and true meaning of her life (DiVitto, 2002).

Preparing for Disasters

Disaster planning is essential for a community, business, or hospital. It involves thinking about details of preparation and management by all involved, including community leaders, health and safety professionals, and lay people. A disaster plan need not be lengthy. Two weeks after the April 1995 Oklahoma City bombing of the Murrah Federal Building by two American citizens, one hospital distilled its 44-page manual into a 5-page disaster response guide. Such a concise plan should still contain information on the elements discussed in this and the following section. See Display 17.3 for a summary of these elements.

Personal Preparation

The preparation of a disaster plan for a community should be preceded by the need for all nurses to address their own personal preparedness to respond in a disaster. Display 17.4 describes the tragic outcome of one nurse's lack of preparation when she attempted to provide nursing care at the scene of the Oklahoma City bombing.

Personal preparedness means that the nurse has read and understood workplace and community disaster plans and has developed a disaster plan for his own family. The prepared nurse also has participated in disaster drills and knows cardiopulmonary resuscitation and first aid. Finally, nurses preparing to work in disaster areas should bring

---

DISPLAY 17.3	ELEMENTS OF A DISASTER PLAN

A disaster plan should address all of the following:
Chain of authority
Lines of communication
Routes and modes of transport
Mobilization
Warning
Evacuation
Rescue and recovery
Triage
Treatment
Support of victims and families
Care of dead bodies
Disaster worker rehabilitation

DISPLAY 17.4	NURSES AT DISASTER SITES: HELP OR HINDRANCE?

On April 19, 1995, 37-year-old Rebecca Anderson, a registered nurse working in Oklahoma City, after hearing a televised report of the bombing of the Federal Building, went to the site wearing jeans and a sweatshirt. Along with firefighters and other rescue workers in hardhats and other protective gear, she was allowed to enter the scene. Within a short time, Rebecca was struck on the back of the head by a concrete slab that fell from the building's wreckage. She died 5 days later of massive cerebral edema. Nurses can learn the following lessons from this tragedy:

- Never enter a disaster scene unless you are directed to do so by an emergency medical technician, fire, or law enforcement official.
- Contact local hospitals and clinics to offer your help; your medical expertise is more useful in the clinical environment.
- Take courses in first aid and emergency care. Contact your local Red Cross for a list of courses.
- Contact your local health department to learn more about your community's disaster plan and how you can contribute in the event of a disaster in your area.

---

copies of their nursing license and driver's license, durable clothing, and basic equipment, such as stethoscopes, flashlights, and cellular phones. In the event of an emergency, many who are unprepared or untrained often present at the site of a disaster or at local hospitals to volunteer. These "spontaneous volunteers" can be an additional burden to those in charge (Display 17.5).

To increase understanding of and the ability to work within an emergency situation, every nurse should become familiar with the National Incident Command System (NIMS). The NIMS offers a "unified approach to incident management; standard command and management structures; and emphasis on preparedness, mutual aid, and resource management" (FEMA, 2008). In essence, it provides a common language for disaster response, to reduce confusion as much as possible. Free

---

DISPLAY 17.5	SPONTANEOUS VOLUNTEERS

Volunteers represent a potential resource to a community affected by a disaster, whether of natural or man-made origin. However, individuals who respond spontaneously and without appropriate training and verifiable qualifications can easily overwhelm the capabilities of local government and other agencies.

From Warner, K., & Hanna, B. (2007, October). *Disasters happen: Do you know your role?* Presented at 21st Century Nursing Challenges, Kappa Omicron Chapter STTI, Chico, CA.

online courses are offered through FEMA (see Display 17.6). Additionally, every nurse should have up-to-date vaccinations; many biologic threats have the same initial presentations, and reducing susceptibility to common illnesses such as influenza can help with initial identification.

Assessment for Risk Factors and Disaster History

As noted earlier in the chapter, the community health nurse is uniquely qualified to perform a community assessment for risk factors that may contribute to disasters. In addition, the nurse should review the *disaster history* of the community. Have earthquakes, tornadoes, hurricanes, floods, blizzards, riots, or other disasters occurred in the past? If so, what (if any) were the warning signs? Were they heeded? Were people warned in time? Did evacuation efforts remove all people in danger? What were the community's onsite responses, and how effective were they? What programs were put in place to rehabilitate the community?

Establishing Authority, Communication, and Transportation

In addition to assessing for preparedness, the effective disaster plan establishes a clear chain of authority, develops lines of communication, and delineates routes of transport. Establishing a clear and flexible chain of authority is critical for successful implementation of a disaster plan. Usually, the chain is hierarchical, with, for example, the community's governmental head (e.g., mayor) initiating the plan, alerting the media to broadcast warnings, authorizing the police to begin evacuations, and so on. Within each level of the organization, the hierarchy continues. For example, at the local hospital, the hospital administrator may be responsible for alerting nurse managers to call in additional personnel. Flexibility is essential, because key authority figures may themselves be victims of the disaster. If the home of the chief of police is destroyed in an earthquake, his second-in-command must have equal knowledge of the community's disaster plan and be able to step in without delay.

Effective communication is often a point of breakdown for communities attempting to cope with major disasters. After the terrorist attacks in Oklahoma City and New York City, phone lines were damaged and cellular sites were overwhelmed, making communication difficult. Communication was possible only through handheld radios or by way of couriers on foot. At times of heightened chaos and stress, as well as after physical damage to communication facilities and equipment, misinformation and misinterpretation can flourish, leading to delayed treatment and increased loss of life.

Again, clarity and flexibility are the watchwords for establishing lines of communication. How will warnings be communicated? What backups are available if the normal communication systems are destroyed in the disaster? How will communication between relief workers at the disaster site, hospital personnel, police, and governmental authorities be maintained? What role will local media play, both in keeping information flowing to the outside world and in broadcasting needs for assistance and supplies? Finally, how will friends and family members of victims be informed of the whereabouts or health status of their loved ones? The characteristics of effective communication during disasters are summarized in Display 17.7.

Closed or inefficient routes of transportation can also increase injury and loss of life. For example, if a single, narrow mountainous road is the only means of transporting firefighters to or evacuating residents from the scene of a forest fire, then disaster planners should propose widening the road or clearing a second road. Disaster planners must also consider what routes emergency vehicles will take when transporting disaster victims to local and outlying hospitals or health care workers to the disaster site. What if the chosen routes are inaccessible because of floodwaters, advancing fires, mountain slides, or building rubble? Are alternative routes designated?

Mobilizing, Warning, and Evacuating

In many natural disasters, local weather service personnel, public works officials, police officers, or firefighters have the earliest information indicating an increasing potential for a disaster. These officials typically have a plan in place for providing community authorities with specific data indicating increased risk. They may also advise the mayor's office or other community leaders of their recommendations for warning or evacuating the public. Additionally, they may recommend actions the community can take to mitigate damage, such as spraying rooftops in the path of fires, sandbagging the banks of rising rivers, or imposing a curfew in times of civil unrest.

Disaster plans must specify the means of communicating warnings to the public, as well as the precise information that should be included in warnings. Planners should never assume that all citizens can be reached by radio or television or that broadcast systems will be unaffected by the disaster. Broadcast media may indeed be a primary means of communicating warnings, but alternative strategies, such as police or volunteers canvassing neighborhoods with loudspeakers, should also be in place. In multilingual communities, messages should be broadcast in multiple languages. Not only homes but also businesses must be informed. Information that should be communicated includes the nature of the disaster; the exact geographic region affected, including street names if appropriate, and the actions citizens should take to protect themselves and their property.

An evacuation plan is an essential component of the total disaster plan. The plan should cover notification of the police, local military personnel, or voluntary citizens' groups of the need to evacuate people, as well as methods of notifying and transporting the evacuees. A plan should also be made for responding to citizens who refuse to evacuate. For example, will police authorities forcibly remove an elderly citizen from his home to a shelter? Will evacuation plans include household pets? If farms or ranches are in the path of fires or floods, will animals be evacuated?

Responding to Disasters

At the disaster site, police, firefighters, nurses, and other relief workers develop a coordinated response to rescue, triage, and treat disaster victims. One of the first obligations of relief workers is to remove victims from danger.

Rescue

The job of rescue typically belongs to firefighters and personnel with special training in search and rescue. Depending on the disaster agent, protective gear, heavy equipment, and special vehicles may be needed, and dogs trained to locate dead bodies may be brought in (Fig. 17.1). Usually, the immediate disaster site is not the best place for the disaster nurse, who can be far more effective in triage and treatment of victims. One of the lessons of the World Trade Center

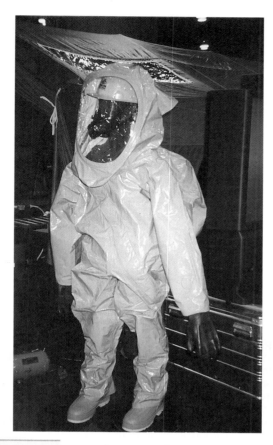

FIGURE 17.1 Hazardous materials suit used by the military and most fire departments. (Photo by Cynthia Tait.)

bombing was that the greatest need for medical professionals was at the local hospitals, not at the disaster site.

Rescue workers face the logistically and psychologically difficult task of determining when to cease rescue efforts. Some factors to consider include increasing danger to rescue workers, diminishing numbers of survivors, and diminishing possibilities for survival. For example, after a plane crash on a snowy mountain, rescue efforts may cease if it is deemed that anyone who might have survived the crash would subsequently have died of exposure.

Triage

Whereas emergency nurses daily determine which clients require priority care, the community health nurse may be at a loss as to where to start when faced with multiple victims of a disaster. Knowing the principles and practice of triage allows the nurse to offer nursing skills most effectively. **Triage** is the process of sorting multiple casualties in the event of a war or major disaster. It is required when the number of casualties exceeds immediate treatment resources. The goal of triage is to effect the greatest amount of good for the greatest number of people. Figure 17.2 shows the four basic categories of the international triage system, as well as a triage tag.

Prioritization of treatment may be very different in a mass-casualty event as opposed to an average day in a hospital emergency department. Under normal circumstances, a person presenting to a hospital emergency department with a

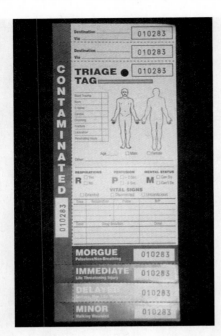

1. **Red:** Urgent/Critical
   Victims in this category have injuries or medical problems that will likely lead to death if not treated immediately (e.g., an unconscious victim with signs of internal bleeding).
2. **Yellow:** Delayed
   Victims in this category have injuries that will require medical attention; however, time to medical treatment is not yet critical (e.g., a conscious victim with a fractured femur).
3. **Green:** Minor/Walking Wounded
   Victims in this category have sustained minor injury or are presenting with minimal signs of illness. Prolonged delay in care most likely will not adversely effect their long-term outcome (e.g., a conscious victim with superficial cuts, scrapes, and bruises).
4. **Black:** Dead/Non-salvageable
   Victims in this category are obviously dead or have suffered mortal wounds because of which death is imminent (e.g., an unconscious victim with an open skull fracture with brain matter showing). Life-saving heroics on this group of victims will only delay medical care on more viable victims.

FIGURE 17.2   Victim triage tag recommended by the California Fire Chiefs Association. Four basic categories are all applied when a medical system is overwhelmed with victims. (Photo by Cynthia Tait.)

myocardial infarction and showing no pulse or respirations would receive immediate treatment and have a chance of recovery. At a disaster site, a victim without a pulse or respirations would most likely be placed in the nonsalvageable category.

The term *mass casualty* refers to a number of victims that is greater than that which can be managed safely with the resources the community has to offer (such as rescue vehicles and emergency facilities available to serve disaster victims while also meeting the needs of the rest of the community). Frequently, in mass-casualty occurrences, the broader community needs to become involved, which necessitates calling in rescue vehicles, firefighters, and police officers from neighboring towns, or the use of neighboring hospitals. This adds another layer of disaster management coordination that must be considered.

DISPLAY 17.8   MOBILE FIELD HOSPITAL

On August 25, 2007, we attended a statewide disaster-training exercise featuring the first state-owned mobile field hospital. The tent hospital is one of three 200-bed hospitals purchased by California and prepositioned around the state in the event of a major emergency. The hospital can be deployed and onsite within 72 hours, and comes equipped for 7 days of full patient care. Used together, the hospitals can even be reconfigured into a 400- or 600-bed hospital, if needed. This is the same type of mobile field hospital used by the military, and it was modeled after the hospitals used by the Air Force and Navy. The various units within the hospital mirror services provided in any modern facility including emergency room, surgical suite, laboratory, x-ray, surgical intensive care, and even a pediatric unit. The exercise included personnel from the Medical Reserve Corps (MRC), federal Disaster Medical Assistance Team (DMAT), state Medical Assistance Team, Mental Health Response Team, Ambulance Strike Team, California Air National Guard, and the California Highway Patrol. "Victims" were provided by a local nursing program.

From Warner, K., & Hanna, B. (2007, October). *Disasters happen: Do you know your role?* Presented at 21st Century Nursing Challenges, Kappa Omicron Chapter STTI, Chico, CA.

Immediate Treatment and Support

Disaster nurses provide treatment onsite at emergency treatment stations, at mobile field hospitals, in shelters, and at local hospitals and clinics (see Display 17.8). In addition to direct nursing care, onsite interventions might include arranging for transport once victims are stabilized and managing the procurement, distribution, and replenishment of all supplies. Disposable items might be in short supply, requiring resterilization procedures that may be unfamiliar to a nurse not accustomed to field work. These procedures may pose a challenge even to an experienced nurse because of the field environment. The nurse may also manage provision or distribution of food and beverages, including infant formulas and rehydration fluids, and arrange for adequate, accessible, and safe sanitation facilities, either onsite or in a shelter. Finally, the nurse often must also arrange for psychological and spiritual care of victims of disasters.

Some victims who seem physically uninjured may, in fact, be suffering from major injuries but be unable to relate their symptoms to a relief worker because of shock or anxiety. For instance, a father pulling debris away from his collapsed house after a tornado may be so worried about a missing child that he does not realize that he has a broken arm.

Other victims may be so emotionally traumatized by a disaster that they act out, disrupting efforts to assist them and other victims and even engaging in dangerous activities. This may cause relief workers to focus on emotional care; however, such victims must be assessed for head trauma and internal injuries, because their behavior may have a physical cause. If they are physically able, such victims may be given a simple, repetitive task to perform, which serves as both a distraction and a means to restore, to a small extent, their sense of control over their environment.

Care of Bodies and Notification of Families

Identification and transport of the dead to a morgue or holding facility are crucial, especially if contagion is feared. Toe tags make documentation visible and accessible. Records of deaths must be made and maintained, and family members should be notified of their loved ones' deaths as quickly and compassionately as possible. If feasible, a representative from each of the area's faith communities should be available to assist families awaiting news of missing loved ones. As stated earlier, a family's recovery from loss is often delayed when notification of relatives (indirect victims) is not possible because the victims' bodies are badly damaged or not found.

Supporting Recovery from Disasters

Disasters do not suddenly end when the rubble is cleared and the victims' wounds are healed. Rather, recovery is a long, complex process. It often includes long-term medical treatment, physical rehabilitation, financial restitution, and psychological and spiritual support.

Long-term Treatment

Long-term treatment may be required for many victims of disasters, straining the local rehabilitative-care facilities and resources. Children who were victims may have to deal with lifelong disabilities or scars from their ordeal, and families may be without adequate financial support for their child's medical care. Elderly citizens who had been in excellent health but who sustained serious injuries in the disaster might suddenly find that they can no longer live independently and must move to a long-term care facility. After floods, landslides, fires, or earthquakes, extensive property damage may cause some residents or businesses to relocate rather than rebuild on land they now deem to be disaster prone. A disaster that creates numerous victims in a small community may alter the entire social fabric of that community permanently.

Long-term Support

Disaster victims may need funding to repair or rebuild their homes or to reopen businesses, such as stores, restaurants, and other services needed by the community. Insurance settlements, FEMA funding, and private donations may assist in financing community rehabilitation. Health care workers may be required to assist victims with necessary paperwork. Immediately after a disaster, some victims may be unable to concentrate on anything beyond fulfilling their immediate needs and those of their family.

Psychological support is often required after a disaster, both for victims and for relief workers. Some individuals may experience posttraumatic stress disorder (PTSD) (discussed later). Many victims, especially elderly persons displaced from their homes, may quietly lose their will to live and drift into apathy and malaise. Individuals whose belief in God was unshakable before the incident may now question their faith, wondering how a loving God could have let this happen, espe-

cially if they lost a loved one. These victims often require not only empathic listening but also long-term skilled spiritual counseling. In assessing a community's citizens for counseling needs after a disaster, the nurse should not forget to include children. Often, children do not have words to express their feelings or fears and may act out in ways adults find difficult to understand, unless age-appropriate psychological intervention is provided.

Need for Self-care

Self-care, including stress education for all relief workers after a disaster, helps to reduce anxiety and put the situation into proper perspective. **Critical incident stress debriefing (CISD)** provides relief workers with professional debriefing in small groups or individually and becomes a mechanism for emotional reconciliation. The ideal time for CISD is between 24 and 72 hours after the disaster event. CISD typically produces positive effects by

- Accelerating the healing process
- Equipping participants with positive coping mechanisms
- Clearing up misconceptions and misunderstandings
- Restoring or reinforcing group cohesiveness
- Promoting a healthy, supportive work atmosphere
- Identifying individuals who require more extensive psychological assistance.

A CISD addresses all components of the human response to trauma, including physiologic effects, emotions, and cognition. Studies show that CISD allows individuals to regain a sense of normalcy much sooner than those not involved in CISD. Self-care comes in many forms and is part of a prescription for emotional healing after a traumatic event. Self-care is not just for rescue workers but for everyone touched by trauma. Keep in mind the following self-care points (Peeke, 2002):

- *Give yourself time to heal.* You need time to adjust. Even though you want the pain to be over immediately, it is healthier to realize that this is a long-term recovery process.
- *Ask for emotional support.* Talk with family and friends around the country. It feels good to be connected with others. You listen and support one another as you share your feelings.
- *Take care of yourself;* it will improve your ability to deal with stress. Eat regularly, avoid alcohol, maintain sleep patterns, follow your exercise routine, and embrace each day as a gift.
- *Reestablish daily routines.* Getting back to your regular routine is important and gives you a sense of security and normalcy.
- *Use your time wisely.* A significant traumatic event gives you an opportunity to reprioritize how you spend your time each day. Are you living your dreams and passions? Traumatic events remind us of our fragile nature and that each moment should be savored and enjoyed.
- *Give something back.* Your life goes on. Demonstrate your gratefulness by becoming part of a global healing process. Donate to charities and give time to causes you have ignored. Seek ways to reach out to those who are in need of help.

Psychological Consequences of Disasters

In addition to physical injury, potential loss of life, and destruction of property that can occur from a disaster, people affected by the disaster can also suffer from psychological consequences, such as acute stress disorder, depression, and PTSD. The community health and community mental health nurses, through education, screening, assessment, and referral, have an important role in the primary, secondary, and tertiary prevention of psychological disturbances due to a disaster.

Primary Prevention

Although a disaster, by its very nature, is often unforeseen, people's ability to cope with the disaster can be determined in part by their previous level of coping and the resources available to help them. Stuart and Laraia (2005) explain that primary prevention in behavioral health care has two basic objectives:

◆ To help people avoid stressors or cope with them more adaptively
◆ To change the resources, policies, or agents of the environment so that they no longer cause stress but rather enhance people's functioning (pp. 208–209).

A community health nurse can engage in many activities to promote mental health and strengthen adaptive coping skills in individuals and the community. He can teach health education classes in positive stress adaptation, positive ways of coping, self-efficacy, and **resilience**, an important quality that enables people to cope with disaster. A definition of resilience is offered by the President's New Freedom Commission on Mental Health in their 2003 report *Achieving the Promise: Transforming Mental Health Care in America*:

Resilience means the personal and community qualities that enable us to rebound from adversity, trauma, tragedy, threats, or other stresses—and to go on with life with a sense of mastery, competence, and hope. We now understand from research that resilience is fostered by positive individual traits, such as optimism, good problem-solving skills, and treatments. Closely knit communities and neighborhoods are also resilient, providing supports for their members (p. 5).

According to Stuart and Laraia (2005), the building of competency or resilience may be the most important primary prevention strategy, since a competent person or community can make informed decisions based on availability of resources and problem-solving skills. In a phone survey of more than 2,700 New York City residents (after September 11, 2001), Bonanno, Galea, Bucciarelli, and Vlahov (2007) found that the strongest variables associated with resilience pertained to the absence of additional life stressors, pointing to the need for more research on the role of resilience in recovery from extreme incidents.

In addition to working with individuals within the community to enhance their resilience, community health nurses can contribute to primary prevention in the face of disaster by being active advocates for improving the social structure of the community, including housing, work, and economic conditions for community members. At a time when governments are reducing spending and services, it is important for the community health nurse to advocate for the resources necessary for the community to meet both the physical and psychological challenges of a disaster.

Secondary Prevention

Despite community education and intervention, people involved in a disaster often feel anxious and overwhelmed. They are in a *mental health crisis*, defined as a state when people's usual coping mechanisms no longer are effective in the face of the overwhelming disaster (Stuart & Laraia, 2005). A crisis or disaster, an event that is out of the ordinary in magnitude and personal experience, is called an *adventitious crisis*. Examples of adventitious crises are natural disasters, such as floods, earthquakes, and fires, and national disasters such as terrorist attacks, war, riots, and airplane crashes (Varcarolis, Carson, & Shoemaker, 2006). When the stress of these disasters causes overwhelming anxiety, *crisis intervention* is a secondary prevention intervention that the trained community heath or community mental health nurse can employ to minimize the psychological consequences of the disaster.

Crisis intervention is a short-term intervention, no longer than 6 weeks, designed to return an individual or community to its predisaster level of functioning and solve immediate psychological problems. Interventions are provided on several levels: environmental manipulation, general support, generic approach, and the individual approach (Stuart & Laraia, 2005). *Environmental manipulation* results in the change of a person's physical or interpersonal situation, providing situational support to relieve stress. An example of environmental manipulation is when a community health nurse coordinates the reunification of family members separated by the disaster. *General support* is defined as the caring, warmth, and concern the community health nurse conveys to the client as he delivers services (Stuart & Laraia, 2005).

The *generic approach* is an aspect of crisis intervention that is particularly well suited to the community health nurse. This approach is designed to reach high-risk individuals and large groups who have experienced the same disaster, teaching them about the expected emotional reactions to the type of disaster they have experienced and promoting adaptive responses. Grief reactions follow a known pattern, and large groups can be taught what to expect in the face of severe loss while giving individual members of the group an opportunity to express their feelings of loss. This generic approach is sometimes called *debriefing*. Individual crisis intervention is reserved for high-risk individuals who need special treatment because of the severity of their symptoms and is best provided by nurses trained in mental health treatment and crisis intervention (Stuart & Laraia, 2005).

Tertiary Prevention

People who have experienced or witnessed a disaster and have been unable to adequately cope with its consequences can develop long-term effects, such as *acute stress disorder* or **post-traumatic stress disorder (PTSD)**. According to the fourth edition of *Diagnostic and Statistical Manual of Mental Disorders,* text revision (DSM-IV-TR) (American Psychiatric Association [APA], 2000), both acute stress disorder and PTSD can occur after any traumatic event in which a person responds with intense fear, helplessness, or horror to an actual or threatened death or serious injury to oneself or others. Both natural and man-made disasters fit into this definition (see Evidence-based Practice).

EVIDENCE-BASED PRACTICE

Posttraumatic Stress Disorder and Physical Health

What is the relationship between posttraumatic stress disorder (PTSD) and physical health? Researchers in the Netherlands (Dirkzwager et al., 2007) asked this question and conducted a longitudinal study of 876 survivors of a man-made disaster to look for answers.

In 2000, a fireworks depot in a residential neighborhood in Enschede, Netherlands, exploded, leaving 1,000 people injured and 23 people (including four firefighters) dead. Five hundred houses were uninhabitable and 1,000 more houses were damaged. Twelve hundred residents were left homeless and had to be relocated.

The researchers examined survivors' medical records from 1 year before until 4 years after the disaster. They also surveyed the survivors at 3 weeks and 18 months after the disaster. A self-rating scale for PTSD symptoms, a Dutch version of the Symptom Checklist-90-R, and a Dutch translation of the Short Form Health Survey-36 (RAND-36) were administered to survivors 18 months post disaster. The data were examined using multiple regression

analysis and adjusting for demographics, predisaster health status, and smoking behavior. Results showed a significant relationship between PTSD and vascular, musculoskeletal, and dermatologic problems, as recorded in the medical record and between PTSD and all self-reported physical health problems.

Nursing Implications

The results of this study indicate that a relationship exists between PTSD and physical problems. Nurses assessing people for PTSD should be aware of physical symptoms as well as psychological ones. Nurses assessing physical symptoms in people who have survived a disaster should be aware of the possible comorbidity of PTSD.

Reference:

Dirkzwager, A.J., Van der Velden, P.G., Grievink, L., & Yzermans, C.J. (2007). Disaster- related posttraumatic stress disorder and physical health. *Psychosomatic Medicine, 69*, 435–440.

The DSM IV-TR (APA, 2000) defines acute stress disorder as occurring within 1 month of the disaster and resolving within 4 weeks. A person experiencing acute distress disorder must have three symptoms of dissociation during or after the disaster:

◆ A subjective sense of numbing, or absence of emotional responsiveness
◆ A reduction of awareness of his or her surroundings (e.g., "being in a daze")
◆ Derealization (a sense of unreality regarding one's environment)
◆ Depersonalization (sense of unreality or self-estrangement)
◆ Dissociative amnesia (i.e., inability to recall an important aspect of the trauma) (p. 432)

If an acute reaction to the disaster lasts longer than 4 weeks, it can develop into the more chronic disorder of PTSD. According to the DSM-IV-TR (APA, 2000), the symptoms for both acute stress disorder and PTSD include the following:

◆ The traumatic event is persistently reexperienced in one (or more) of the following ways:
1. Recurrent and intrusive distressing recollections of the event, including images thoughts, or perceptions
2. Recurrent distressing dreams of the event
3. Acting or feeling as if the traumatic event were recurring (includes a sense of reliving the experience, illusions, hallucinations, and dissociative flashback episodes, including those which occur on awakening or while intoxicated)

4. Intense psychological distress at exposure to internal or external cues that symbolize or resemble an aspect of the traumatic event
5. Physiological reactivity on exposure to internal or external cues that symbolize or resemble an aspect of the traumatic event
◆ Persistent avoidance of stimuli associated with the trauma and numbing of general responsiveness (not present before trauma) as indicated by three (or more) of the following:
1. Efforts to avoid thoughts, feelings, or conversations associated with the trauma
2. Efforts to avoid activities, places, or people that arouse recollections of the trauma
3. Inability to recall an important aspect of the trauma
4. Markedly diminished interest or participation in significant activities
5. Feelings of detachment or estrangement from others
6. Restricted range of affect (e.g., unable to have loving feelings)
7. Sense of a foreshortened future (e.g., does not expect to have a career, marriage, children, or normal life span)
◆ Persistent symptoms of increased arousal (not present before the trauma), as indicated by two (or more) of the following:
1. Difficulty in falling or staying asleep
2. Irritability or outburst of anger
3. Difficulty concentrating
4. Hypervigilance
5. Exaggerated startle response (p. 428)

It is important for the community health nurse to be aware of the symptoms of these disorders so that he can refer the client for treatment, which should be left to the advanced practice mental health nurse and other mental health professionals.

TERRORISM

At the start of the 21st century, the world is a global community. This is particularly evident in the increased incidence and sophistication of terrorist threats and acts around the world. Incidents occurring on U.S. soil, such as the bombing of the World Trade Center in 1993 and its destruction on September, 11, 2001, alerted us to our vulnerability and dramatically emphasized the need for increased preparedness within our communities.

The July 2005 bombings in London that struck multiple transportation system sites, which killed 56 and injured over 700; the February 2008 bombings in Baghdad by remotely controlled bombs carried by two mentally disabled women, which killed 98 and wounded 200; and the 2007 bombings in Karachi, Pakistan, which killed 136 and injured 387, all confirm that our vulnerability exists in many areas. Biologic, chemical, and nuclear terror are tragically possible.

The U.S. Federal Bureau of Investigation (FBI) defines **terrorism** as "the unlawful use of force and violence against persons or property to intimidate or coerce a government, the civilian population, or any segment thereof, in furtherance of political or social objectives" (Evans, Crutcher, Shadel, Clements, & Bronze, 2002). A terrorist is overzealous and obsessed with an idea. Terrorism and terrorist acts are not new. The term *terrorism* can be traced to 1798, and the use of terrorist tactics precedes this date. A highly organized religious sect called the *sicarii* attacked crowds of people with knives during holiday celebrations in Palestine at about the time of Christ. During the French and Indian War of 1763, British forces gave smallpox-contaminated blankets to Native Americans. During World War I, the German bioweapons program developed anthrax, glanders, cholera, and wheat fungus as weapons targeting cavalry animals. In World War II, the Japanese tested biologic weapons on Chinese prisoners.

Three major countries operated offensive bioweapons programs in recent years: the United Kingdom until 1957, the United States until 1969, and the former Soviet Union until 1990. Iraq started its bioweapons program in 1985 and continued to develop weapons until 2003. At least 17 other nations are currently suspected of operating offensive bioweapons programs (Evans et al., 2002). Bioweapons include mustard gas, sarin and VX gas, and anthrax. Terrorists typically use biologic, or chemical agents and explosives or incendiary devices to deliver the agents to their targets.

Nuclear warfare involves the use of nuclear devices as weapons, and can take several forms. Terrorists who gain access to nuclear power plants could cause a chain of events that lead to a meltdown of the nuclear core, thereby releasing radioactive particles for hundreds of miles around the site. Nuclear accidents have occurred, but no known terrorist attacks have yet involved the use of nuclear power plants as weapons. A terrorist attack using nuclear weapons or destruction of a nuclear plant would cause multiple and prolonged deaths with extensive damage and negative effects for decades.

Chemical warfare involves the use of chemicals such as explosives, nerve agents, blister agents, choking agents, and incapacitating or riot-control agents to cause confusion, debilitation, death, and destruction (Yergler, 2002). Terrorists in the Middle East, willing to sacrifice their own lives, strap bombs to themselves and detonate the explosives in or near targets. Others crash vehicles loaded with explosives into crowds of people or into a building.

The aircraft used on September 11, 2001, were huge chemical weapons because they were carrying thousands of tons of jet fuel. The success of the mission depended on the surprise of the attack, severe damage to recognizable buildings, and the deaths of many people. The collapse of the buildings was unplanned. If the planes had been low on fuel, the damage would not have been as severe. The liquid fuel burned at such a high temperature that the internal structures of the buildings were weakened (National Institute of Standards and Technology, 2006).

Biologic warfare involves using biologic agents to cause multiple illnesses and deaths. Typical biologic agents are anthrax, botulinum, bubonic plague, Ebola, and smallpox. These agents could be used to contaminate food, water, or air. Deliberate food and water contamination remains the easiest way to distribute biologic agents for the purpose of terrorism (Khan, Swerdlow, & Juranek, 2001). The U.S. Office of Technology Assessment has speculated that the release of 220 pounds of anthrax spores from a crop-duster over the Washington, D.C., area on a calm, clear night could kill between 1 and 3 million people (U.S. Army Chemical and Biological Defense Command, 1998).

The United States is very concerned about the possibility of biologic warfare or bioterrorism, as nations should be. The anthrax infections and deaths that occurred after September 11, 2001, added to these concerns. For years, it was not known if these incidents were committed by an organized foreign or domestic terrorist group, or a single disturbed citizen. In 2008 the investigation led to an army scientist as the cause of this terroristic act. Although charges were never filed due to the individual's suicide, the Federal Bureau of Investigation believes that he was solely responsible for this act of domestic terrorism (FBI, 2008). Regardless of the source of terrorism, the outcomes are the same: fear, death, and destruction.

Factors Contributing to Terrorism

Political factors are the most common contributors to terrorism. Anti-American sentiment runs high in many foreign countries, especially those that perceive the United States as a threat to their military, economic, social, or religious self-determination. Terrorist acts against American military installations abroad, in airports, in airplanes, at American embassies, and even on American soil have occurred frequently in the last decade as an expression of political unrest. The war in Iraq in 2003 was based on information about suspected bioterrorism weapons and reports that Iraq was harboring anti-Western terrorists; these two pieces of information resulted in the toppling of the Saddam Hussein political regime. However, hundreds of military lives were lost, and no weapons of mass destruction were found. As of September 2008, more than 4,000 U.S. military have lost their lives, and some 30,000 are dealing with injuries in the ongoing military campaign (Associated Press, 2008).

Within the United States, violence-prone members of militia movements, violent anti-abortion activists, racial desegregation advocates, and other radical groups have performed terrorist acts, such as the bombing of health clinics offering abortions. In 1984, members of a religious cult, the Rajneeshees, lived in Wasco County, Oregon, and followed a self-proclaimed guru exiled from India. In an attempt to reduce voter turnout in an upcoming county election, they sprinkled *Salmonella* bacteria over items on salad bars in local restaurants and in the produce sections of grocery stores. They hoped that, with a reduced voter turnout, representatives friendlier to their group would win the election. Their attack failed to affect the election and killed no one; however, 751 people became sick (Bernett, 2006; McDade & Franze, 1998). The media underreported this event because domestic terrorism was not a topic of concern at that time in U.S. history.

Role of the Community Health Nurse

Community health nurses need to be prepared for the possibility of terrorist activity. They have a role in primary, secondary, and tertiary prevention.

Primary Prevention

Community health nurses are in ideal situations within communities to participate in surveillance. They must look and listen within their communities for anti-group sentiments, for example, anti-religion, anti-gay, or anti-ethnic feelings. The nurse should report any untoward activities accordingly.

Nurses should be alert to signs of possible terrorist activity. Specific indicators of possible chemical or biologic terrorism include unusual numbers of dead or dying animals; unexplained serious illnesses or deaths; an unusual liquid, spray, vapor, or odor; and low-lying clouds or fog unrelated to weather. Unusual swarms of insects might also indicate the use of biologic agents for terrorism. "Many nurses currently employed have little knowledge regarding the potential pathogens that could be released or how to respond to a chemical or biologic attack" (Veenema, 2002, p. 63). Additionally, Secor-Turner and O'Boyle (2006) noted a lack of studies of nurses' responses to bioterrorism events in a literature review of studies between 2002 and 2004. They emphasized the need for bioterrorism plans that "incorporate strategies to support nurses and address their physical, psychological, and emotional issues" (p. 414). Less subtle forms of terrorism include bombings, mass shootings, and hijackings, which are more difficult to uncover in time to prevent injury or death.

Secondary and Tertiary Prevention

Although prevention of terrorist incidents is primarily the responsibility of the Department of Defense, the Department of Homeland Security, and public health and law enforcement agencies, community health nurses must be ready to handle the secondary and tertiary effects of such attacks. Knowing the lethal and incapacitating chemical weapons that may be used by terrorists is important. Many of the communicable disease organisms that could be used by terrorists were discussed in Chapter 8.

Realizing that terrorist attacks may result in large numbers of casualties, the community health nurse must be prepared to act safely, access information rapidly, and use resources effectively. Specifically, the community health nurse may be called on to provide direct care to victims, to volunteer as a hospital–community liaison, to set up and administer mass immunizations, to make home visits to affected families, or to serve on committees responding to terrorist acts. Formulating, updating, and following a disaster plan is one of the most effective community-based strategies to minimize injury and mortality from terrorism.

Most community health nurses will not be on the front line of uncovering or immediately responding to terrorist activities, but their skills will be needed with groups, families, or individuals who experience a terrorist-related event. Some of the activities listed earlier in this chapter to help people deal with the aftermath of a disaster would also be appropriate if terrorism is the cause of the disaster. In addition, community health nurses may work with people who need help coping or who want to do something to help. After experiencing a traumatic event such as a terrorist attack, people do not know how to cope. We are warned to expect more attacks. We are told to be vigilant. The terror we are fighting is often our own. This is a new experience for most people, and assistance from the community health nurse can help them cope effectively. The following 10 tips were gathered from experts in many fields by Foley (2002) and are common-sense approaches to fighting anxiety:

- *Be a little afraid.* A certain level of fear is healthy if you learn to use it as positive energy. Use your pinch of anxiety to be more vigilant about your safety and that of your family, especially when you travel, and in taking care of your health.
- *Keep a courage journal.* Fear immobilizes, and courage takes action. Every time you take action, you are getting past fear. Even small steps are an opportunity to build more courage. Every time you take a courageous step—getting on a plane, opening your mail—write it down.
- *Reassure your children.* In the act of reassuring your children, you will reassure yourself.
- *Hang out with children.* Do things with your children—most young people carry a charge of positive energy that is infectious. If you do not have young children, volunteer at a school or read to children at a nearby day care center.
- *Cook something hearty, healthy, and large, and invite lots of people in to eat it.* The process of cooking is good for the soul. The aromas are good for the soul. And the chopping and dicing make you feel that you are doing something useful and concrete.
- *Give kindness to others.* We all need each other. Make a point of chatting with the woman at the checkout counter or letting a pedestrian cross the street when you are driving. Wave hello to strangers. You will be amazed how much it is true that in giving, we receive.
- *Get spiritual.* Reach out and participate in your faith community or get involved in one, if so inclined. Believing in a power greater than yourself can be comforting.
- *Laugh.* Laughter is the best medicine for fear. Spend evenings in good company—group laughter is better than laughing alone.

◆ *Get back to nature.* Spending interactive time with nature is a remedy for just about any soul sickness. Go to the park, take a walk, or work in your garden.

◆ *Find reasons to believe the sky is not falling.* All the unpleasant facts and figures get our "anxiety juices" flowing. Seek out positive people, and read literature that encourages positive thinking. Do not feed the "dark side." Turn off the news and opt for a funny movie or an inspirational story.

Community health nurses can make major differences in grassroots efforts to bring about change, but on a day-to-day basis, the little things they say and do with peers and clients can make just as big a difference.

Current and Future Opportunities

There are many ways in which nurses, and most especially nursing students, can prepare themselves both personally and professionally for emergency events in their own communities. Various governmental and educational programs have been developed to provide free online training covering a broad range of topics. A summary of some of those training opportunities is provided in Display 17.6. For the novice nurse, or nursing student, an important issue is your role, if any, in your local response plan. Many schools of nursing have now begun to formalize their emergency preparedness plans in coordination with local hospitals, public health departments, or faith institutions. Take some time to discuss with your faculty what role you have in the event of a local emergency. If no organized plan exists, then perhaps you can work with the nursing faculty or your local student nurses association to prepare one. Knowing your role in an emergency will give you the peace of mind of knowing where you should go and what you are expected to do. Doing a little extra work by completing some of the online courses listed will help you to feel more involved and less fearful if the unimaginable were to happen. FEMA offers four particular courses within the Incident Command System (ICS 100, ICS 200, IS700, & IS800B); these are recommended for all health care personnel. Students who are also employed at local hospitals as interns or salaried employees should find out what role they have in the hospital's emergency plan.

Increasingly, communities are conducting emergency preparedness exercises (for example, mass casualty exercises and table-top exercises; see Display 17.9) in response to the need to prepare local resources to coordinate emergency response efforts for maximum effectiveness (Center for Public Health Preparedness, 2007). As a student, you may be asked to participate in one of these exercises as a "victim." Take the opportunity. The knowledge you gain from this experience will enhance your understanding of the process, and you may be able to help identify gaps in services or areas in need of improvement. With your expertise in nursing, you are a much greater asset to the exercise than untrained individuals. You may be asked to have **moulage** applied to simulate injuries, and you will likely be given a brief description of your trauma (see Display 17.10). Your assigned health problem may be emotional and not physical, allowing you to utilize your understanding of behavioral health issues and crisis intervention. Whatever your capacity, the experience will provide as close to a realistic event as possible. Just as

---

DISPLAY 17.9   WHAT IS A TABLE-TOP EXERCISE?

A table-top exercise is a drill typically used by emergency planners and responders. It is designed to allow personnel to gather in a semi-formal setting, so that they can participate in open discussions regarding their role in the event of an emergency situation. Participants typically assume their own role, but may be required to assume other key positions. A simulated disaster/emergency event is provided, called the *scenario*. This type of drill:
• Does not require complete plans and procedures.
• Allows for practice in coordinated emergency problem solving.
• Permits discussion of the decisions reached.
• Prepares personnel for larger, more costly exercises (i.e., mass casualty exercises).

Adapted from Placer County Department of Health and Human Services (2005). *Table Top Exercises: What are they? Why do we have them?* Auburn, CA.

---

immunizations help fight against infections, participating in an emergency preparedness drill can build your tolerance for responding appropriately in a real event.

Many organizations, both private and governmental, are seeking volunteers. As a student, you have more limited options; however, two major opportunities are available to you. Both require initial and ongoing training, but if you wish to become more active in emergency preparedness volunteer efforts, the American Red Cross and your local Medical Reserve Corps are two options. You can continue your relationship with these organizations after you receive your nursing license, and your role with them will likely evolve.

With your registered nurse license in hand, many more options are open to you. Each state is developing plans for a database of licensed health care providers who may be willing to volunteer in the event of local, state, or national emergencies. The exact criteria being developed for registration by each

---

DISPLAY 17.10   WHAT IS MOULAGE?

Pronounced *mü-läzh,* the term *moulage* comes from the French word *mouler,* which means "to mold." In emergency preparedness training, moulage refers to the art of applying mock injuries for use in mass-casualty exercises. These injuries can be very simple or more complex, depending on available resources and the skills of the person applying the moulage. The use of moulage typically provides a more realistic experience for personnel participating in mass casualty exercises.

Of the many online resources for information regarding equipment needed and how-to advice, one such website is Community Emergency Response Team (CERT) Los Angeles–*Moulage Information* at: http://www.cert-la.com/education/moulage.htm.

state may vary slightly, but as a licensed health care professional you may add your name to the registry along with your specialty training and contact information. Registration does not obligate you to any service; you agree only to be contacted if the need arises. The guidelines for these state-run databases were generated by the U.S. Department of Health and Human Services, and can be reviewed in the document *Emergency Systems for Advance Registration of Volunteer Health Professionals* (ESAR-VHP) (USDHHS Health Resources Services Administration, 2005). The professional volunteer registry in Wisconsin is named WEAVR (*Wisconsin Emergency Assistance Volunteer Registry*). Using similar guidelines, California launched its version of the registry (*California Medical Volunteers*). Mississippi has the *Volunteers in Preparedness Registry* (VIPR), and Arkansas nurses can register with the *Arkansas Volunteer Registry*. Check with your state's office of emergency preparedness and response for the link to your particular registry or information on availability.

As you progress in your career, many other high-intensity efforts are available for your involvement. At both the national and state level are Disaster Medical Assistance Teams (DMAT), groups of highly trained health professionals who can rapidly respond to emergencies within a state or nationally. The DMATs operate as part of the National Disaster Medical System (NDMS). Each DMAT has a sponsoring organization (i.e., major medical center, public health agency, nonprofit organization). Check to see if your organization has sponsored a DMAT; if so, you might want to interview one of the members to learn more about his training and experiences.

For those assuming roles in public health nursing, competencies formulated by Gebbie and Qureshi (2002, 2006) provide a sound basis for practice. The work of Gebbie and Qureshi was included in the 2007 position paper *The Role of Public Health Nurses in Emergency Preparedness and Response* (Jakeway, LaRosa, Cary, & Schoenfisch, 2008). The specific competencies can serve as an emergency preparedness guide for students and practicing public health nurses. They include the following:

1. Describe the public health role in responding to a range of likely emergencies.
2. Describe the agency's chain of command in emergency response.
3. Identify and locate the agency's emergency response plan.
4. Describe one's functional roles and responsibilities in emergency response and demonstrate those roles in regular drills.
5. Demonstrate the correct use of equipment (including personal protective equipment) and the skills required in emergency response during regular drills.
6. Demonstrate the correct use of all equipment used for emergency communication.
7. Describe communication role(s) in emergency response.
8. Identify the limits of one's own knowledge, skills, and authority, and identify key system resources for matters that exceed these limits.
9. Apply creative problem-solving skills and flexible thinking to unusual challenges within one's func-

tional responsibilities, and evaluate the effectiveness of all actions taken.
10. Recognize deviations from the norm that might indicated an emergency and describe appropriate action.
11. Participate in continuing education to maintain up-to-date knowledge in areas relevant to emergency response.
12. Participate in planning, exercising, and evaluating drills.

Many options are available to you as both a student and a practicing nurse. What is important is that you are prepared. Assuring that you understand the role you may assume in the event of a local disaster or emergency situation is critical to your own welfare as well as to your community. You decide your level of participation, but resources are available for you to become as prepared as possible.

Healthy People 2010

The past decade of *Healthy People* has been devoted to increasing quality and years of healthy life and to eliminating health disparities (USDHHS, 2000). Formulated in the years before January 2000, many disasters, both natural and man-made, had yet to occur. The United States had not yet faced the national failures in the response to the hurricanes Katrina and Rita. We would also learn 18 months after the publication of *Healthy People 2010* that our nation was not immune from acts of terrorism. The objectives of *Healthy People 2010* do not directly address issues of emergency preparedness and response, but rather document a plan to support and strengthen the public health structure of this country. In the ensuing years, many of those objectives originally seen as less significant to the public's health received new and invigorated attention. Objective 23 deals with issues relevant to a robust public health structure at the local, state, and national levels (see Display 17.11). Those

---

DISPLAY 17.11   HEALTHY PEOPLE 2010

Data and Information Systems
23-1   Public health employee access to the Internet
23-2   Public health access to information and surveillance data
23-3   Use of geocoding in health data systems

Workforce
23-8   Competencies for public health workers
23-9   Training in essential public health services
23-10   Continuing education and training by public health agencies

Public Health Organizations
23-11   Performance standards for essential public health services
23-13   Access to public health laboratory services
23-14   Access to epidemiology services
23-15   Model statutes related to essential public health services

specific objectives provide the support needed to enhance public health surveillance activities, training, development of professional competencies, and performance standards for public health organizations. With enhanced funding and increased attention to the emerging needs of the coming decade, the issue of emergency preparedness is already on the list of proposed goals for *Healthy People 2020: The Road Ahead* (USDHHS, 2008).

Summary

A disaster is any event that causes a level of destruction that exceeds the abilities of the affected community to respond without assistance. Disasters may be caused by natural or man-made/technologic events and may be classified as multiple-casualty incidents or mass-casualty incidents.

The scope of a disaster is its range of effect, and its intensity is the level of destruction it causes. Victims of disasters include direct victims (those injured or killed) and indirect victims (the loved ones of direct victims). Displaced persons are those who are forced to flee their homes because of the disaster, and refugees are those who are forced to leave their homelands, usually in response to war or political persecution.

Host factors that contribute to the likelihood of experiencing a disaster include age, general health, mobility, psychological factors, and socioeconomic factors. The disaster agent is the fire, flood, bomb, or other cause. Environmental factors are those that could potentially contribute to or mitigate a disaster.

In developing strategies to address the problem of disasters, it is helpful for the community health nurse to consider each of the four phases of disaster management: prevention, preparedness, response, and recovery.

Primary prevention of disasters means keeping the disaster from ever happening by taking actions to eliminate the possibility of its occurrence. Secondary prevention focuses on earliest possible detection and treatment. Tertiary prevention involves reducing the amount and degree of disability or damage resulting from the disaster.

In addition to assessing for preparedness, an effective disaster plan establishes a clear chain of authority, develops lines of communication, and delineates routes and modes of transport. Plans for mobilizing, warning, and evacuating people are also critical elements of the disaster plan. At the disaster site, police, firefighters, nurses, and other relief workers develop a coordinated response to rescue victims from further injury, triage victims by seriousness of injury, and treat victims on-site and in local hospitals. Care and transport of dead bodies must also be managed, as well as support for the loved ones of the injured, dead, or missing. Long-term support includes both financial assistance and physical and emotional rehabilitation.

In addition to the physical injuries resulting from disasters, people also suffer psychological trauma that can affect them for life. The importance of prevention, early crisis intervention, and ongoing treatment for those in need is evident. The community health nurse plays a key role in assessing individuals for symptoms of psychological trauma and intervening to prevent long-term consequences. Self-care, including stress education for all relief workers after a disaster, helps to lower anxiety and put the situation into perspective. CISD provides relief workers with a mechanism for emotional reconciliation and healing.

Terrorism is the unlawful use of force or violence against persons or property to intimidate or coerce a government or civilian population in the furtherance of political or social objectives. Terrorism may be nuclear, biologic, or chemical, and may involve the use of nerve agents and explosive devices. The community health nurse should be alert to signs of possible terrorist activity and prepared to address the secondary or tertiary effects of such attacks. Preparation includes knowledge of the effects of specific biologic or chemical agents and how to help people cope with the terror they personally feel.

Many opportunities are available for both student nurses and experienced community health nurses to become involved in emergency preparedness and response efforts. Agencies such as the American Red Cross and the Medical Reserve Corps are options available to students and at a higher level of involvement, once licensed. Natural and man-made disasters are a too frequent occurrence. It is the obligation of all nurses to be involved in emergency preparedness and to seek training that will enable them to provide the best possible service if the unthinkable happens. With the development of *Healthy People 2020*, ongoing efforts to help communities prepare for disasters and emergencies will require more nurses willing and able to respond to a call for action. ■

ACTIVITIES TO PROMOTE CRITICAL THINKING

1. Think about your own community and its residents. What are some host factors that might increase its risk of experiencing a disaster? What environmental factors might be significant? In each case, identify the likely agent. What interventions could be included in a disaster plan to reduce these risk factors?

2. The nightly news on TV shows that at least 200 people have been injured in an explosion in a neighboring community. At the disaster site, victims are still being recovered from the wreckage, and local hospitals are overwhelmed with patients who have fractures, lacerations, and burns. You want to offer your assistance as a registered nurse. How should you go about volunteering your services?

3. Access one or more of the Internet sites listed in this chapter. Report on the change in statistics for disasters or terrorism since the year 2005. Have rates increased or decreased? What factors might be involved in this change?

References

Associated Press. (2008, September 29). *US military deaths in Iraq war at 4,176.* Retrieved October 2, 2008 from http://ap.google.com/article/ALeqM5gqgQCcv26kB1dkgZRZNHmbn_1J8gD93HBG481.

American Psychiatric Association. (2000). *Diagnostic and statistical manual of mental disorders,* 4th ed. [Text revision]. Washington, DC: Author.

American Red Cross. (2008). *Disaster services.* Retrieved August 7, 2008 from http://www.redcross.org/services/disaster/0,1082,0_319_,00.html.

Bernett, B.C. (2006). *U.S. biodefense and homeland security: Toward detection and attribution.* Unpublished master's thesis. Naval Postgraduate School, Monterey, California. Retrieved October 3, 2008 from http://www.ccc.nps.navy.mil/research/theses/bernett06.pdf.

Bonanno, G.A., Galea, S., Bucciarelli, A., & Vlahov, D. (2007). What predicts psychological resilience after disaster? The role of demographics, resources, and life stress. *Journal of Consulting and Clinical Psychology, 75,* 671–682.

Center for Public Health Preparedness. (2007). *Conducting a BT-Table Top: A "how-to" guide.* Decatur, GA: DeKalb County Board of Health. Available from NACCHO (toolbox) website, http://www.naccho.org/toolbox/.

Centers for Disease Control and Prevention. (2007). *What You Should Know About a Smallpox Outbreak.* Retrieved October 2, 2008 from http://www.bt.cdc.gov/agent/smallpox/basics/outbreak.asp.

Department of Homeland Security. (2006). *Department of Homeland Security. Freedom of Information Act. Operational review and improvement plan.* Retrieved June 12, 2008 from http://www.dhs.gov/xlibrary/assets/foia/privacy_rpt_foia_improvement-plan.pdf.

DiVitto, S. (2002). Giving hope, she found hope. *Reflections on Nursing Leadership, 28*(3), 21.

Evans, R.G., Crutcher, J.M., Shadel, B., Clements, B., & Bronze, M.S. (2002). Terrorism from a public health perspective. *American Journal of the Medical Sciences, 323,* 291–298.

Federal Bureau of Investigation. (2008). *Anthrax investigation: Closing a chapter.* Retrieved October 2, 2008 from http://www.fbi.gov/page2/august08/amerithrax080608a.html.

Federal Emergency Management Agency. (2008). *National Incident Management System.* Retrieved August 7, 2008 from http://www.fema.gov/emergency/nims/.

Foley, D. (2002). Fight terror: Your own. *Prevention, 54*(2), 126–133, 174–176.

Gebbie, K.M., & Qureshi, K. (2002). Emergency and disaster preparedness: Core competencies for nurses. *American Journal of Nursing, 102*(1), 46–52.

Gebbie, K.M., & Qureshi, K. (2006). A historical challenge: Nurses and emergencies. *Online Journal of Issues in Nursing, 11*(3), 6.

Human Rights Watch. (2008). *Q & A: Crisis in Darfur.* Retrieved August 7, 2008 from http://hrw.org/english/docs/2004/05/05/darfur8536.htm.

Infoplease. (2008). *2007 disasters.* Boston, MA: Pearson Education. Retrieved August 7, 2008 from http://www.infoplease.com/ipa/A0934966.html.

International Charter. (2008). *Charter activations.* Retrieved August 7, 2008 from http://www.disasterscharter.org/new_e.html.

Jakeway, C.C., LaRosa, G., Cary, A., & Schoenfisch, S. (2008). The role of public health nurses in emergency preparedness and response: A position paper of the Association of State and Territorial Directors of Nursing. *Public Health Nursing, 25,* 353–361.

Khan, A.S., Swerdlow, D.L., & Juranek, D.D. (2001). Precautions against biological and chemical terrorism directed at food and water supplies. *Public Health Reports, 116,* 3–14.

Kirkpatrick, D.V., & Bryan, M. (2007). Hurricane emergency planning by home health providers serving the poor. *Journal of Health Care for the Poor & Underserved, 18,* 299–314.

McDade, J.E., & Franze, D. (1998). Bioterrorism as a public health threat. Retrieved October 2, 2008 from http://www.cdc.gov/ncidod/eid/vol4no3/mcdade.htm.

National Institute of Standards and Technology. (2006). *Federal building and fire safety investigation of the World Trade Center disaster: Answers to frequently asked questions.* Retrived October 3, 2008 from http://wtc.nist.gov/pubs/factsheets/faqs_8_2006.htm.

Peeke, P.M. (2002). Reclaim your peace of mind. *Prevention, 54*(1), 92–97.

President's New Freedom Commission on Mental Health. (2003). *Achieving the promise: Transforming mental health care in America. Final report.* Retrieved August 7, 2008 from http://www.mentalhealthcommission.gov/reports/FinalReport/toc.html.

Secor-Turner, M., & O'Boyle, C. (2006). Nurses and emergency disasters: What is known. *American Journal of Infection Control, 34,* 414–420.

Stuart, G., & Laraia, M. (2005). *Principles and practice of psychiatric nursing,* 8th ed. St. Louis, MO: Elsevier-Mosby.

United Nations Refugee Agency. (2008). *Iraqi crisis fuels rise in asylum seekers in industrialized world.* Retrieved August 7, 2008 from http://www.unhcr.org/news/NEWS/47de99982.html.

U.S. Army Chemical and Biological Defense Command. (1998). *Domestic preparedness program: Hospital provider course.* McLean, VA: Booz-Allen & Hamilton, Inc. and SAIC, Inc.

U.S. Department of Health and Human Services. Health Resources Service Administration. (2005). *Emergency systems for advance registration of volunteer health professionals (ESAR-VHP) program. Interim technical and policy guidelines, standards, and definitions (Version 2).* Washington, DC: U.S. Government Printing Office.

U.S. Department of Health and Human Services. (2000). *Healthy People 2010: Understanding and improving health,* 2nd ed. Washington, DC: U.S. Government Printing Office.

U.S. Department of Health and Human Services. (2008). *Healthy People 2020: The road ahead.* Retrieved August 7, 2008 from http://www.healthypeople.gov/hp2020/.

U.S. Public Health Service, Commissioned Corps. (2008). *About the Commissioned Corps. Disaster response.* Retrieved August 7, 2008 from http://www.usphs.gov/AboutUs/emergencyResponse.aspx.

Varcarolis, E., Carson, V., & Shoemaker, N. (2006). *Foundations of psychiatric mental health nursing: A clinical approach.* St. Louis, MO: Elsevier-Mosby.

Veenema, T.G. (2002). Chemical and biological terrorism: Current updates for nurse educators. *Nursing Education Perspectives, 23*(2), 62–71.

Washington Post. (June 5, 2008). *U.S. Navy ends bid to ferry storm relief into Burma.* Retrieved August 7, 2008 from http://www.washingtonpost.com/.

Yergler, M. (2002). Nerve gas attack. *The American Journal of Nursing, 102*(7), 57–60.

Selected Readings

Bushberg, J., Telles, S., Wagner, B., et al. (2005). *Are you prepared? A guide to emergency preparedness for Sacramento County.* Sacramento, CA: U.C. Davis Health System.

Federal Emergency Management Agency & American Red Cross. (2004). *Preparing for disaster for people with disabilities and other special needs.* Jessup, MD: FEMA.

Fothergill, A., Palumbo, M.V., Rambur, B., et al. (2005). The volunteer potential of inactive nurses for disaster preparedness. *Public Health Nursing, 22,* 414–421.

Kumar, M.S., Murhekar, M.V., Hutin, Y., et al. (2007). Prevalence of posttraumatic stress disorder in a coastal fishing village in Tamil Nadu, India, after the December 2004 Tsunami. *American Journal of Public Health, 97,* 99–101.

Kuntz, S., Frable, P., Qureshi, K., & Strong, L. (2008). *Disaster preparedness white paper for community/public health nursing educators.* Wheat Ridge, CO: Association of Community Health Nursing Educators.

Landesman, L.Y. (2005). *Public health management of disasters: The practice guide,* 2nd ed. Washington, DC: American Public Health Association.

Landesman, L.Y. (2006). *Public health management of disasters: The pocket guide.* Washington, DC: American Public Health Association.

Langan, J.C., & James, D.C. (2005). *Preparing nurses for disaster management.* Upper Saddle River, NJ: Pearson Education, Inc.

Macario, E., Benton, L.D., Yuen, J., et al. (2006). Preparing public health nurses for pandemic influenza through distance learning. *Public Health Nursing, 24*, 66–72.

Mack, S.E., Spotts, D., Hayes, A., & Rains Warner, J. (2006). Teaching emergency preparedness to restricted-budget families. *Public Health Nursing, 23*, 354–360.

McKinney, W.P., Wesley, G.C., Sprang, M.V., & Troutman, A. (2005). Educating health professionals to respond to bioterrorism. *Public Health Reports, 120*[Suppl. 1], 42–47.

Moss, W.J., Ramakrishnan, M., Storms, D., et al. (2006). Child health in complex emergencies. *Bulletin of the World Health Organization, 84*(1), 58–64.

Phillips, S., & Lavin, R. (2004). Readiness and response to public health emergencies: Help needed now from professional nursing organizations. *Journal of Professional Nursing, 20*, 279–280.

Polivka, B.J., Stanley, S.A.R., Gordon, D., et al. (2008). Public health nursing competencies for public health surge events. *Public Health Nursing, 25*, 159–165.

Rosenkoetter, M.M., Covan, E.K., Cobb, B.K., et al. (2007). Perceptions of older adults regarding evacuation in the event of a natural disaster. *Public Health Nursing, 24*, 160–168.

Stanley, S.A.R., Polivka, B.J., Gordon, D., et al. (2008). The ExploreSurge Trail Guide and Hiking Workshop: Discipline-specific education for public health nurses. *Public Health Nursing, 25*, 166–175.

Tracy, L. (2007). *Muddy waters: The legacy of Katrina and Rita. Health care providers remember and look ahead.* Washington, DC: American Public Health Association.

Wisniewski, R., Dennik-Champion, G., & Peltier, J.W. (2004). Emergency preparedness competencies: Assessing nurses' educational needs. *Journal of Nursing Administration, 34*, 475–480.

Wu, P., Duarte, C.S., Mandell, D.J., et al. (2006). Exposure to the World Trade Center attack and the use of cigarettes and alcohol among New York City public high-school students. *American Journal of Public Health, 96*, 804–807.

Zerwekh, T., McKnight, J., Hupert, N., et al. (2007). Mass medication modeling in response to public health emergencies: Outcomes of a drive-through exercise. *Journal of Public Health Management Practice, 13*(1), 7–15.

Zotti, M.E., Graham, J., Whitt, A.L., et al. (2006). Evaluation of a multistate faith-based program for children affected by natural disaster. *Public Health Nursing, 23*, 400–409.

Internet Resources

Agency for Healthcare Research and Quality (AHRQ) [Public Health Emergency Preparedness]: *http://www.ahrq.gov/prep/index.html*

American College of Physicians [Bioterrorism Resources]: *http://www.acponline.org/clinical_information/resources/bioterrorism/*

American Red Cross: *http://www.redcross.org/*

Association of State and Territorial Nursing Directors (ASTDN): *http://www.astdn.org/*

Citizen Corps: *http://www.citizencorps.gov/*

Community Emergency Response Teams (CERT): *http://www.citizencorps.gov/cert/index.shtm*

Disaster Preparedness Information (American Red Cross): *http://www.prepare.org/*

Emergency Preparedness & Response (CDC): *http://www.bt.cdc.gov/*

Federal Emergency Management Agency (FEMA): *http://www.fema.gov/*

FEMA online training: *http://training.fema.gov/IS/NIMS.asp*

FEMA for Kids: *http://www.fema.gov/kids/*

Home Safety Council [Get Ready with Freddie]: *http://www.homesafetycouncil.org/index.aspx*

International Committee of the Red Cross: *http://www.icrc.org/eng*

International Council of Nurses [Disaster Preparedness]: *http://www.icn.ch/disasterprep.htm*

Medical Reserve Corps: *http://www.medicalreservecorps.gov/HomePage*

National Association of County & City Health Officials: *http://www.naccho.org/*

National Center for Disaster Preparedness [Columbia University]: *http://www.ncdp.mailman.columbia.edu/*

National Disaster Search Dog Foundation: *http://searchdogfoundation.org*

National Humane Society [National Disaster Animal Response Team: Volunteer Opportunities]: *http://www.hsus.org/*

National Voluntary Organizations Active in Disaster (NVOAD): *http://www.nvoad.org/*

Nursing Emergency Preparedness Education Coalition: *http://www.nursing.vanderbilt.edu/incmce/*

Points of Light Institute: *http://www.pointsoflight.org/programs/disaster/resources.cfm*

Salvation Army: *http://www.salvationarmyusa.org/*

United Nations: *http://www.un.org/english/*

U.S. Department of Health and Human Services [National Disaster Medical System]: *http://www.hhs.gov/aspr/opeo/ndms/index.html*

U.S. Food & Drug Administration [counterterrorism]: *http://www.fda.gov/oc/opacom/hottopics/bioterrorism.html*

U.S. Public Health Service Commissioned Corps [Emergency Response]: *http://www.usphs.gov/AboutUs/emergencyResponse.aspx*

World Health Organization [Emergency and Humanitarian Action]: *http://www.searo.who.int/en/Section1257/Section2263.htm*

World Health Organization [Emergency Preparedness and Response Commitments in Emergencies]: *http://www.searo.who.int/en/Section1257/Section2263/Section2299.htm*

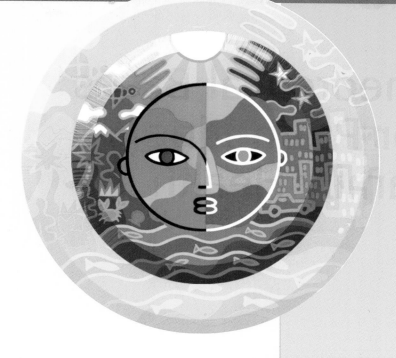

THE FAMILY AS CLIENT

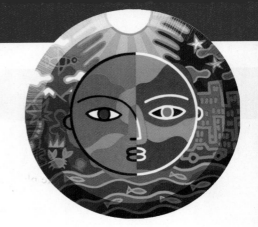

18

Theoretical Bases for Promoting Family Health

LEARNING OBJECTIVES

Upon mastery of this chapter, you should be able to:

◆ Analyze changing definitions of family.
◆ Discuss characteristics all families have in common.
◆ Identify five attributes that help explain how families function as social systems.
◆ Discuss how a family's culture influences its values, behaviors, prescribed roles, and distribution of power.
◆ Compare and contrast the variety of structures that make up families.
◆ Describe the functions of a family.
◆ Identify the stages of the family life cycle and the developmental tasks of a family as it grows.
◆ Analyze the role of the community health nurse in promoting the health of the family unit.

❝*Call it a clan, call it a network, call it a tribe, call it a family. Whatever you call it, whoever you are, you need one.* ❞

—Jane Howard, *"Families"*

Community health nurses are intimately involved with families. Whether the client is an individual within the context of the family or the family is the unit of care, the family plays a critical role in the health of its members. Health habits, such as preventive care, diet, exercise, and physical activity, are developed within the context of the family (Campbell, 2006). Health beliefs, genetic influences, and care of the ill family member all take place within the family environment.

The community health nurse is in a unique position to influence and promote family health while facing a multitude of challenges. The family is a separate entity with its own structure, functions, and needs. Throughout history, the family has been the most basic unit. Among one of the biggest controversies facing the community health nurse is defining what constitutes a family. This definition is important because how nurses define a family influences the care they give and, at the most basic level, how they interact with the family. When you hear the word *family*, what do you think of? How would you define your own family? Is your grandfather a member of your family? Your niece? Your neighbor? A friend? A family pet?

The definition of a **family** varies by organization, discipline, and individual. The World Health Organization (1976) characterized the family as "the primary social agent in the promotion of health and well-being" (p. 17). Many family theorists suggest that a family consists of two or more individuals who share a residence or live near one another; possess some common emotional bond; engage in interrelated social positions, roles, and tasks; and share cultural ties and sense of affection and belonging (Anderson & Sabatelli, 2006; Friedman, Bowden, & Jones, 2003; Hanson, Gedaly-Duff, & Kaakinen, 2005; McBride, 2006; Murray & Zentner, 2000). The common thread in the definitions is the recognition that the family itself defines who its members are (Bomar, 2004).

Today's community health nurse needs to understand and work with many types of families, each of which has unique health problems and needs. For example, a young single mother who is homeless seeks help in caring for her sick infant. A 55-year-old grandfather provides care for his elderly mother, who was recently discharged from the hospital after a stroke. A group of parents, siblings, cousins, and children, all refugees from Laos, need instruction on the purchase and preparation of food. Why is it important for the community health nurse to understand and respect the unique characteristics, cultures, structures, and functions of each of these families? Do families as basic units of a community have characteristics that affect community health nursing service? The answer is an unqualified yes. The effectiveness of the community health nurse depends on knowing how to work with a family as a unit of care.

This chapter examines the nature of families, family functioning, and family health. It draws from various theories to strengthen the student's understanding and appreciation of families as clients. This information will promote the effectiveness of interventions with families at the primary, secondary, and tertiary levels of preventions (see Levels of Prevention Pyramid). **Family functioning** is defined as those behaviors or activities by family members that maintain the family and meet family needs, individual member needs, and society's views of family. The interdependence of family members involves a set of internal relationships that influence the effectiveness of family functioning (Friedman et al., 2003). There is a complex communication pattern of functioning among family members, and the quality of the pattern contributes to the health of the family.

Family health is concerned with how well the family functions together as a unit. It involves not only the health of the members and how they relate to other members, but also how well they relate to and cope with the community outside the family. In fact, family health, like individual health, ranges along a continuum from wellness to illness. A family may be at one point on that continuum now and at a much different point 6 months from now. Family health refers to the health status of a given family at a given point in time (Hanson et al., 2005). It includes all the attitudes, beliefs, knowledge, and habits that families use to obtain, sustain, or regain maximum health (Fiese, 2006; McBride, 2006).

UNIVERSAL CHARACTERISTICS OF FAMILIES

Several observations can be made about families in general. First, each family is unique, with its own distinct problems and strengths. When you approach the door of a house or push the buzzer of an apartment, you cannot assume what the family inside will be like. Consequently, you will have to gather information about each particular family to achieve nursing objectives.

Second, every family shares some universal characteristics with every other family. These universal characteristics provide an important key to understanding each family's uniqueness. Five of the most important family universals for community health nursing are:

1. Every family is a small social system.
2. Every family has its own cultural values and rules.
3. Every family has structure.
4. Every family has certain basic functions.
5. Every family moves through stages in its life cycle.

No matter how many families a nurse might visit or serve in the course of a year, each one will have these universal features; it is important for community health nurses to know each family's unique manifestation of these features and their effects on family health. These five universals of family life, which provide the framework of this chapter, are based on systems theory, sociologic theories, and theories of family development. In addition to considering the universals of family life, this chapter covers the unique family features and structures that characterize our changing world.

ATTRIBUTES OF FAMILIES AS SOCIAL SYSTEMS

Many Americans fall into the habit of viewing families merely as collections of individuals. Caused partly by the strong cultural emphasis on individualism, this error also occurs because families are often encountered through the individual members. When a community health nurse sits in a living room talking with a young mother about her new infant, it is difficult to keep in mind that all the other family members are present by way of their influence. Systems

LEVELS OF PREVENTION PYRAMID

SITUATION: The family will provide the emotional and material resources necessary for its members' growth and well-being.

GOAL: Using the three levels of prevention, negative health conditions are avoided, promptly diagnosed and treated, and/or the fullest possible potential is restored.

Tertiary Prevention

Rehabilitation		Primary Prevention
	Health Promotion & Education	
		Health Protection
• After the family suffers a crisis, the members recognize the need for help and accept that help • Families draw on personal resources to rebuild relationships and heal the family unit	• The family continues using resources that enhance the growth and well-being of individuals and the family as a unit	• Engage in family strengthening practices to protect the family from possible inhibitors to growth and well-being

Secondary Prevention

Early Diagnosis	Prompt Treatment
• Identification of a family member's personal problems that affect the family as a whole • Early recognition that problems exist in the relationship among or between family members	• The family seeks out the appropriate resources that bring the family to the highest level of wellness possible

Primary Prevention

Health Promotion & Education	Health Protection
• Adults are well prepared for the responsibilities of their union. • Adults enter the relationship with the personal resources necessary to promote the growth and development of their family unit.	

theory offers some insights about how families operate as social systems. Knowing the attributes of living systems or open systems can help strengthen understanding of family structure and function. There are five attributes of open systems that help explain how families function: (1) families are interdependent, (2) families maintain boundaries, (3) families exchange energy with their environments, (4) families are adaptive, and (5) families are goal-oriented.

Interdependence Among Members

All the members of a family are interdependent; each member's actions affect the other members, and what affects the family system affects each family member. For example, consider the changes a father might make to reduce his risk of coronary heart disease. If he cuts back on working overtime, the family's income will be reduced. If he begins to eat different foods, food preparation and eating patterns in the

family will be altered. If he starts a new exercise program three evenings a week, this may upset other family routines. Even his ability to carry out his usual roles as husband and father may be affected if, for instance, he has less time to help his children with their homework or share household chores with his wife.

It is possible to illustrate the pattern of interactions between members using a **family map** (Fig. 18.1). This tool can reveal a great deal about the interdependence of family members. The way parents relate to each other, for instance, influences the quality of their parenting. When the interactions between them are frequent, honest, and nurturing, they have more to offer their children. Marital, parent–child, and sibling relationships all significantly influence family functioning. They determine how well the family as a system handles conflict, provides a support system for its members, copes with crises, solves daily problems, and capitalizes on its own resources.

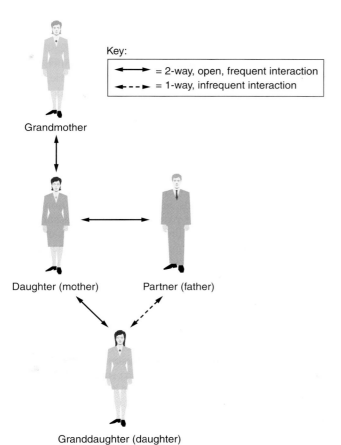

Key:

←——→ = 2-way, open, frequent interaction

←- - -► = 1-way, infrequent interaction

Grandmother

Daughter (mother)   Partner (father)

Granddaughter (daughter)

FIGURE 18.1 Family map. This map indicates that the mother is a key figure for family interaction. The maternal grandmother, father, and daughter communicate primarily to her, rather than directly to one another.

Family Boundaries

Families as systems set and maintain boundaries that include some people as members while excluding others (Denham, 2005; McBride, 2006). These boundaries, which result from shared experiences and expectations, link family members together in a bond that excludes the rest of the world. Also, a greater concentration of energy exists within the family than between the family and its external environment, thereby creating a **family system boundary**.

For example, the Salazar extended family gathers for a Sunday afternoon backyard cookout. The distinctiveness of this family from all the others in the neighborhood is noticeable, as would be that of any other family. The elders in the family were born in Mexico, and they sit together reminiscing in Spanish. The food is traditional and plentiful. It is prepared and served by the women: Aunt Rosa's tamales, Cousin Teresa's tortillas, and flan for dessert from Grandma Lupe's own recipe. While the women prepare the food, some of the men play ball and others listen to Uncle Gilberto play the guitar and discuss the future of the family grape-growing business. The children gather in small groups and play loudly. Several of them, prompted by their parents, display their musical talent later in the day by singing some old favorite songs and doing some traditional Mexican dances. Because of the things they have in common, the Salazars set

and maintain boundaries that unite them and also differentiate them from others.

Energy Exchange

Family boundaries are semipermeable; although they protect and preserve the family unit, they also allow selective linkage with the outside world. To function adequately as open systems, families exchange materials or information with their environment (Friedman et al., 2003). This process is called **energy exchange**. All normally functioning living systems engage in such an input–output relationship. This energy exchange promotes a healthy ecologic balance between the family system and the environment that is its immediate community.

A family's successful progress through its developmental stages depends on how well the family manages this energy exchange. For example, a child-bearing family needs adequate food, shelter, and emotional support, as well as information on how to accomplish its developmental tasks. The family also needs community resources, such as health care, education, and employment, all of which are forms of environmental input. In return, the family contributes to the community by working and by consuming goods and services. If a family does not have adequate income or emotional support or does not use community resources, that family does not experience a proper energy exchange with its environment. An inadequate exchange can lead to dysfunction and poor health (Neuman, 2001).

Adaptive Behavior

Families are adaptive, equilibrium-seeking systems. In accordance with their nature, families never stay the same. They shift and change in response to internal and external forces. Internally, the family composition changes as new members are added or members leave through death or divorce. Roles and relationships change as members advance in age and experience; normative expectations change as members resolve their tensions and differing points of view. Externally, families are bombarded by influences from sources, such as school, work, peers, neighbors, religion, and government; consequently, they are forced to accommodate to new demands. Adapting to these influences may require a family to change its behaviors, its goals, and even its values. Like any system, the family needs a state of quasi-equilibrium to function (Neuman, 2001). With each new set of pressures, the family shifts and accommodates to regain balance and maintain a normal lifestyle.

Sometimes a family's capacity for adaptation may be stressed beyond its limits. At this point, the system may be in danger of disintegrating; that is, family members may leave or become dysfunctional because of unresolved stress. This is an indication that some form of intervention may be needed to help restore family equilibrium. These interventions may take the form of extended family mediation or external professional help. Community health nurses play an influential role in family equilibrium-seeking. Neuman described the major goal of nursing as keeping the individual and family client systems stable within their environments (Neuman, 2001). Chapter 19 explores the community health nurse's stabilizing interventions with families in detail.

Goal-Directed Behavior

Families as social systems are goal directed. Families exist for a purpose—to establish and maintain a milieu that promotes the development of their members. To fulfill this purpose, a family must perform basic functions, such as providing love, security, identity, a sense of belonging; assisting with preparation for adult roles in society; and maintaining order and control. In addition to these functions, each family member engages in tasks to maintain the family as a viable unit. Duvall and Miller (1985) described specific functions and tasks for each stage of the family's development. These functions and tasks are examined in more detail later in this chapter.

FAMILY CULTURE

Family culture is the acquired knowledge that family members use to interpret their experiences and to generate behaviors that influence family structure and function. The concept of family culture arises from a significant body of literature in the social and behavioral sciences. Cross-cultural comparisons and in-depth analyses demonstrate that each family has a "culture" that strongly influences its structure and function. Culture explains why families behave as they do (Leininger, 2001; Pender, Murdaugh, & Parsons, 2006; Spector, 2000). Family culture also gives the community health nurse a basis for assessing family health and designing appropriate interventions. Three aspects of family culture deserve special consideration: (1) family members share certain values that affect family behavior, (2) certain roles are prescribed and defined for family members, and (3) a family's culture determines its distribution and use of power.

Shared Values and Their Effect on Behavior

Although families share many broad cultural values drawn from the larger society in which they live, they also develop unique variants. Every family has its own set of values and rules for operation that can be considered as family culture (Stewart & Goldfarb, 2007). Some values are explicitly stated: "Family matters must always stay within the family." Such values may give rise to specific operating rules: "Don't tell anyone about our problems."

Like all cultural values, many family values remain outside the conscious awareness of family members. These values, often not verbalized, become powerful determinants of what the family believes, feels, thinks, and does. Family values include those beliefs transmitted by previous generations, religious influences, immediate social pressures, and the larger society. Values become an integral part of a family's life and are very difficult to change. A family that values free expression for every member engages comfortably in loud, noisy debates. Another family that values quietness, order, and control does not tolerate its members' raising their voices. One family uses birth control based on beliefs about human life and parental responsibility; another family chooses not to use birth control because the members hold a different set of values. How a family views education, health care, lifestyle, courtship, marriage, child-rearing, sex roles, or any of the myriad other issues requiring choices depends on the cultural values of that family.

Prescribed Roles

Roles, the assigned or assumed parts that members play during day-to-day family living, are bestowed and defined by the family (Denham, 2005; Hanson et al., 2005; McBride, 2006). For instance, in one family the father role may be defined as an authoritative one that includes establishing rules, judging behavior, and administering punishment for violation of rules. In another family, the father role may be defined primarily as that of a loving benefactor. If there is an absence of an immediate male parent, a grandfather, uncle, friend, or mother may take over the father role. Selection of specific roles to be played in any given family varies depending on the family's structure, needs, and patterns of functioning. In a single-parent family, the parent may need to assume the roles of mother, father, and breadwinner, as well as others.

Families distribute among their members all the responsibilities and tasks necessary to conduct family living. The responsibilities of breadwinner and homemaker, with their accompanying tasks, may belong to husband and wife, respectively, or may be shared if both husband and wife hold jobs outside the home. Older children may help younger ones with homework or entertain them. This releases parents for other tasks and increases the responsibility of older children.

Family members play several roles at the same time. This **intrarole functioning** can be exceptionally taxing. A woman may play the role of wife to her husband, daughter to her mother who lives with her, and mother to each of her children. The mother role may involve taking on several additional roles and responsibilities, and varies with each child's needs. In a family in which the mother is seriously ill, many of the roles she held must be assumed by others. A single parent often takes on the roles of both father and mother but may distribute responsibilities and tasks more widely. A grandmother or a child may assume responsibility for some chores and thereby relieve the demands placed on the single parent. Among families, there is great variation in expectations for each role and in the degree of flexibility in role prescriptions. A family may place great demands on some members, but those same members may interpret the expectations placed on them and their roles differently. Confusion and conflict can develop unless roles are clarified.

Other roles of family members extend beyond the immediate family. There may be extended family members nearby who interact with the family on a regular basis or only on special occasions such as birthdays. If both parents are employed, they may have an expansive social network from work or from within the neighborhood. Friendships are often made with the parents of the childrens' friends, particularly if their children participate in the same activities. Many families enjoy the fellowship of organized religious or cultural groups. This fellowship can be a source of support and comfort, as well as an additional role function for the family members. Another intrarole function is that of community participant in activities separate from the family. These roles may involve local or regional politics, community improvement, volunteerism for nonprofit agencies, or any other service outside the home that the community may offer. These diverse role relationships should enrich and energize the participants. However, many people become overcommitted, creating an imbalance of role responsibilities that is draining and causes friction and stress. The community health nurse must work with families to achieve a balance of activities and roles that promotes family health.

Power Distribution

Power—the possession of control, authority, or influence over others—assumes different patterns in each family. In some families, power is concentrated primarily in one member; in others, it is distributed on a more egalitarian basis. The traditional *patriarchal family*, in which the father holds absolute authority over the other members, is rare in American society. However, the pattern of husband as head of the household and dominant member of the family is still frequently seen. Whether male or female, the dominant partner holds the majority of the decision-making power, particularly over more important family matters such as employment and finances. Other areas of decision making, including choices about vacations, housing, leisure activities, household purchases, and child rearing, may be shared or delegated. With changing societal influences, however, the present trend among American families is toward *egalitarian power distribution*.

Rudolf Dreikurs (1964) advocated that families form a "family council" for shared decision making and distribution of tasks. Today, many families practice joint decision making and equal participation by all members, and the community health nurse may suggest this activity for families not using such a method. Role-playing this technique can be incorporated during a home visit or as a teaching technique with an aggregate group.

Roles often influence power distribution within the family. Along with the responsibilities attached to a role, a family may assign decision-making authority. The mother role frequently includes decision making with respect to household management. Responsibility related to a son's role, such as lawn-mowing, may be enhanced as a learning activity if he is allowed to decide when and how often he does the job.

Family power structure is also influenced by the amount of personal power residing in each member (Friedman et al., 2003). A mother or eldest son, for example, can exercise considerable influence over the family by virtue of personality and position, rather than by delegated authority. Even a child who throws temper tantrums can wield considerable power in a family.

FAMILY STRUCTURES

Globally, families—in all their varied forms—are the basic social unit. The meaning of family among the Hmong of northern Laos may include hundreds of people who make up a clan. In Mexico, families remain close, are large, and extend into multiple generations. In Germany and Japan, families are small and tend to the needs of their elders at home. In the United States, where families come from many cultural groups, many variations coexist within communities.

For many people in the United States, the term *family* used to evoke a picture of a husband, wife, and children living under one roof, with the man as breadwinner and the woman as homemaker. In the past, this nuclear family was often seen as the norm for everyone. Changes in social values and cultural lifestyles (e.g., women working outside the home) combined with acceptance of alternative lifestyles has changed the definition of family. Today, definitions of family include unmarried adults living together with or without children, single-parent households, divorced couples who combine households with children from previous marriages (the blended family), and homosexual couples with or without children.

It must be considered a privilege to gain entrance into a family's home. This is a uniquely private space belonging to the family. The people who are members of this household interact, care for one another, and bond in ways that may never be fully understood by anyone outside the family. Therefore, being granted entrance into this system gives the community health nurse an opportunity to work with the family that few other professionals experience. Each type of household requires recognition and acceptance by community health nurses, who must help families achieve optimal health (see Display 18.1).

Families come in many shapes and sizes. The varying **family structures** or compositions comprise the collective characteristics of individuals who make up a family unit (age, gender, and number). A growing body of research on family structure and function shows that families have changed dramatically because of a decrease in the number of marriages, an increase in unmarried couples living together, divorce rates, and an increase in births outside of marriage (Hofferth, 2003; McBride, 2006). Family structures fall into two general categories: traditional and contemporary.

DISPLAY 18.1   A LOOK AT AFRICAN AMERICAN FAMILIES

Much academic attention on the African American family focuses on pathologies. However, there is information from cultural equivalent or emergent models to recognize positive, adaptive features that is not always discussed. Three family types are described as predominant models among African American families—nuclear, single-parent, and augmented families, which are described in this chapter.

African American families can reflect other dimensions that provide broader ways to describe them. The *cultural equivalent model* demonstrates that African American families share mainstream values similar to those of Whites but do not have the same access. In the *emergent model*, the family is rooted in African culture rather than American and reflects similarities that include religion, special care of children, strong kinship ties, dance, language, stability, unity, and security as a foundation of their expression. And to some degree, the *pathological model* is represented among families who experience structural problems, symptoms of stress, physical and emotional illness, and inadequate housing. However, it is felt that the pathological model is a response to societal pathologies such as racism and discrimination, and is not a model exclusive to African Americans.

Barnes, S.L. (2001). Stressors and strengths: A theoretical and practical examination of nuclear, single-parent, and augmented African American families. *Families in Society: The Journal of Contemporary Human Service, 82*(5), 449–460.

Traditional Families

Traditional family structures are those that are most familiar to us. They include the **nuclear family**—husband, wife, and children living together in the same household. In nuclear families, the workload distribution between the two adults can vary. Both adults may work outside the home; one adult may work outside the home while the other stays at home and assumes primary responsibilities for the household; or partners may alternate, constantly renegotiating work and domestic responsibilities. A **nuclear-dyad family** consists of a husband and wife living together who have no children or who have grown children living outside the home. Traditional families also include **single-adult families**, in which one adult is living alone by choice or because of separation from a spouse or children or both. Separation may be the result of divorce, death, or distance from children. Some 4% of U.S. households are **multigenerational families**, in which several generations or age groups live together in the same household (Cohn, 2001). A household in which a widowed woman lives with her divorced daughter and two young grandchildren is an example of a multigenerational family, as is one in which adult children live with aging parents. Such arrangements are increasing in number, according to the 2000 U.S. Census. Sometimes, particularly in close-knit ethnic communities, families form a **kin-network**, in which several nuclear families live in the same household or near one another and share goods and services. They may own and operate a family business, sharing work and child care responsibilities, income and expenses, and even meals. Variations of this trend are increasing among all groups as children postpone leaving home because of economic conditions or educational plans or an elderly parent moves into an adult child's home to recover from a recent illness. A variation of the kin-network is the **augmented family**. This is a family group in which extended family members or nonrelatives or both live with and provide significant care to the children (Barnes, 2001).

Another variation of the traditional nuclear family is the **blended family**. In this structure, single parents marry and raise the children from each of their previous relationships together. They may be custodial parents who have the children except during planned visits with the noncustodial parent, or they may share custody, so that the children live in the blended arrangement only part-time. This family may include children from the couple's union, in addition to the children brought into this relationship.

Single-parent families include one adult (either father or mother) caring for a child or children as a result of a temporary relationship, a legal separation or divorce, or the death of a spouse. In single-parent families, the parent may or may not be employed. Other contempary single-parent family situations are described in the next section.

One contemporary variant of the traditional family is the **commuter family**. Both partners in this family work, but their jobs are in different cities. The pattern is usually for one partner to live, work, and perhaps raise children in the "home" city, while the second partner lives in the other city and commutes home. Sometimes this arrangement is short-term; for example, one partner may be transferred through work, and the couple chooses not to move the rest of the family for one or several reasons (e.g., waiting until the end of the school year, making sure the new job is secure, locating the right housing, or selling the old home). At other times, commuting may continue for years. For example, the family home may be in a town where the cost of living is reasonable, but one parent works in a financially and personally rewarding career several hundred miles away and commutes home on weekends. In other instances, one parent may be on military assignment in another country for 6 months or longer, leaving the other parent alone for months at a time. Clearly, these arrangements influence family roles and functions, challenging a family's ability to maintain healthy relationships. A traditional family in which one partner is required to travel often (e.g., for business, to care for an ill family member at a distant location) may experience similar problems and stressors. Table 18.1 lists a number of traditional family structures.

Nontraditional or Contemporary Families

The traditional nuclear family has been a fundamental part of the European cultural heritage shared by many Americans, and reinforced by religion, education, and other influential social institutions. Variations from this pattern often were treated as deviant and abnormal, even in relatively recent studies of the family (Olson et al., 1989). Nonetheless, infants born to unwed mothers made up 26.6% of the births in 1990 and 37% in 2005 (National Center for Health Statistics [NCHS], 2007). The number of unmarried people living together continues to increase, as does the never-married population. In 1980, 20.3% of the population were never married, increasing to 22.2% in 1990 and 23.9% in 2000 (U.S. Census Bureau, 2008b). In addition, the proportion of single-parent families has continued steady over the past decade with a slight shift toward more father-headed households. Forty-eight percent of African American children, 26% of Hispanic children, and 16% of White children live in mother-headed households, while 5.8% of African American children, 4.4% White children, and 1.5% of Hispanic children live in father-headed households (U.S. Census Bureau, 2008a). There is every indication that the upward trend for unmarried family units, single-parent households, and female heads of households will continue in the 21st century and will represent important contemporary family units in American society.

Society has begun to accept nontraditional definitions of family. The concept of **wider family** was initially presented by Marciano (1991) and is defined as a family that "emerges from lifestyle, is voluntary, and independent of necessary biological or kin connections" (p. 160). "With today's wide variety of family types and structures, the most advanced definition of family may be 'the family is who the client says it is'" (Bell & Wright, 1993, p. 391).

Divorce changes family structures. Half of all marriages now end in divorce (the rate is higher for teenage marriages), and the median duration of marriages is approximately 7 years. In the United States, the divorce rate in 2005 was 5.4 per 1,000. This number has decreased slightly since 1990, but remains higher than in other industrialized nations (Germany, 4.0 per 1,000; United Kingdom, 3.9 per 1,000; Japan, 3.1 per 1,000; Italy, 1.2 per 1,000) (U.S. Census Bureau, n.d.).

Some **contemporary family** structures are becoming more common and are generally accepted by society. Other arrangements are still regarded as unacceptable. Table 18.1

TABLE 18.1   The Traditional and Nontraditional American Family

Structure	Participants	Living Arrangements
TRADITIONAL		
Nuclear dyad	Husband Wife	Common household
Nuclear family	Husband Wife Child(ren)	Common household
Commuter family	Husband Wife Children (sometimes)	Household divided between two cities
Single-parent family	One adult (separated, divorced, widowed) Children	Common household
Divorced family (shared custody of children)	One adult parent, children part-time	Two separate households
Blended family	Husband Wife (His and/or hers, and possibly their children)	Common household
Single adult	One adult (at times not considered a "Family")	Living alone
Multigenerational family	Any combination of the traditional family structures	Common household
Kin network	Two or more reciprocal households (related by birth or marriage)	Close geographic proximity
Augmented family	Extended family group or nonrelatives who provide significant child care	Common household or close geographic proximity
NONTRADITIONAL		
Unmarried single-parent family	One parent (never married) Children	Common household
Cohabitating partners	Two adults (heterosexual, homosexual, or "just friends") Children (possibly)	Common household
Commune family	Two or more monogamous couples Sharing children	Common household
Group marriage commune family	Several adults "married" to each other Sharing childrearing	Common household
Group network	Reciprocal nuclear households or single members	Close geographic proximity
Homeless families	Any combination of family members previously mentioned	The streets and shelters
Foster families	Husband and wife or single adult Natural children (possibly) Foster children	Common household
Gangs	Males and females usually of same cultural or ethnic background	Close geographic proximity (same neighborhood)
"Loose shirt" families	Parents work from home via the personal computer (word processing, e-mail, faxing, cellular telephone—"telecommuting")	Common household

lists some of the more common nontraditional and contemporary family structures.

The approach used by Scanzoni and colleagues (1989) is to consider the **primary relationship** of two or more persons interacting in a continuing manner within the greater environment. This primary relationship encompasses all the possible family structures. In 1981, Stein suggested the idea of a "life spiral," rather than a life cycle, to describe the fluctuations of contemporary nontraditional families. The spiral more realistically depicts the fluid movement within family structures than does a cycle, which suggests continuous curvilinear movement along a path. Traditional functions and structures of the family continue to evolve as new combinations of people live together and consider themselves a "family."

One of the most common nontraditional family structures is the single-parent family headed by a woman. Sometimes, single women choose to adopt or have children without being married. Sometimes, an unplanned pregnancy without marriage creates this family unit. Statistics indicate that single-parent families are being headed increasingly by teenagers, some of whom become pregnant while in junior high school. Although the birth rate among teens 15 to 19 years old declined in 2005 for the 14th consecutive year, the rate of 40.4 births per 1,000 teenage women remains high (NCHS, 2007). The implications for the role of the community health nurse are greatest with this population. For example, nurses work with young teens through schools or clinics to ensure healthy pregnancies and to teach parenting skills to the youthful parents and grandparenting skills to the teen's parents. Nurses can also ensure that the infant receives immunizations and primary health care services as needed and can provide family planning information to the new parents. On a broader scale, community health nurses collaborate with other professionals to make sure that the community has resources for all levels of prevention, with a focus on primary prevention.

Many adult couples form a family alliance outside of marriage or in a private ceremony not legally recognized as marriage. **Cohabitating couples** may range from young adults living together to an elderly couple sharing their lives outside of marriage to avoid tax penalties or inheritance issues. Cohabitating couples may be heterosexual or homosexual; they may or may not share a sexual relationship. In some instances, these couples have their own biologic or adopted children.

Another nontraditional family form is the **commune family**, a group of unrelated couples who are monogamous (married or committed to one person) but who live together and collectively rear their children. Perhaps more popular in the 1960s and 1970s, this type of family may presently exist among people with similar life-views or spiritual beliefs. A **group-marriage family** involves several adults who share a common household and consider that all are married to one another; they share everything, including sex and child rearing. Group-marriage families usually center on a patriarch who designates responsibilities and dictates to the other members some religious or social ideology. The Branch Davidians, who lived together outside of Waco, Texas, until their compound was destroyed by fire in 1993, was a tragic example of this family type. Another disturbing situation was the removal in 2008 of more than 450 children from a polygamist sect in Texas. Although the practice of polygamy is illegal in the United States, Texas officials cited concern over sexual abuse of minors as the basis for separating the children from their parents. In a ruling by the Texas Supreme Court, the children were ordered to be returned to their parents with the stipulation that they remain in Texas and the parents take parenting classes (Ayres, 2008). The ultimate resolution to this sect's activities and others like it remains unclear.

A **group-network family** is made up of unrelated nuclear families that are bound by a common set of values, such as a religious system. These families live close to one another and share goods, services, and child-rearing responsibilities. Some commune and group-network families select one of their members, usually a man, to be their leader or head.

Many children are removed from their homes of origin because of abuse, violence, or neglect. In most communities, these children are housed with families known as **foster families**. These families take a variety of forms, but all foster families have had formal training to accept unrelated children into their homes on a temporary basis, while the children's parents receive the help necessary to reunify the original family. Although this arrangement is not ideal, most foster families provide safe and loving homes for these children in transition. Often foster children have emotional and physical health problems, and they may never have experienced the positive structure that foster families provide. These problems, which can cause stress for everyone involved, are typically ones that the community health nurse can help to solve.

Some families, because of lack of marketable skills, negative economic changes, or chronic mental health problems including substance abuse, find themselves without permanent shelter. **Homeless families** are increasing in numbers, and their characteristics are changing. In 2005, about 41% of the counted homeless population were families with children (National Alliance to End Homelessness, 2007). This does not include families that are homeless but live with friends or relatives. The community health nurse may provide services to shelters or drop-in clinics frequented by the homeless. Because this population is increasing, it has many implications for the nurse.

A destructive form of "family" that occurs in many cities is gangs. **Gangs** are formed by young people who are searching for emotional ties and turn to one another as a substitute for an absent or dysfunctional family. Gang members consider themselves family; they rely on one another and the group for support that they do not receive from their families of origin. Obviously, gangs are a dysfunctional and destructive form of family. Typically, members are drawn into drugs and violence; frequent injury, abuse, and even death to gang members, their associates, and innocent bystanders may be the result. Nurses who serve in urban areas may be working with families and groups who are involved with gangs, and they should be prepared to deal with the issues that gangs create.

Implications for the Community Health Nurse

The variety of family structures raises three important issues for consideration. First, community health nurses can no longer hold to a myth that idealizes the traditional nuclear family. They must be prepared to work with all types of families and accept them as valid. Unless the community health nurse can accept the full array of family lifestyles and address the special problems and needs of each, she may not be able to help the family, and may even create additional problems.

Second, the structure of an individual's family may change several times over a lifetime. A girl may be born into a kin-network, shift to a nuclear family when her parents move, and become part of a single-parent family when her parents are divorced. As she matures, she may become a single adult living alone, then become a part of a cohabitating couple. Still later, she may marry and have children in a nuclear family. For the individual, each family form involves changes in roles, interaction patterns, socialization processes, and links with external resources. The community health nurse must learn to address clients' needs throughout these

DISPLAY 18.2	FACTS ABOUT FAMILIES IN AMERICA

- On any given night in the United States, there are 500,000 to 600,000 homeless men, women, and children (National Alliance to End Homelessness, 2007).
- Some 500,000 children go missing each year.
- More than 3 million children live with their grandparents as the primary care providers.
- Approximately 500,000 children are in foster homes.
- Almost 8% of girls between 15 and 19 years of age get pregnant each year, producing 750,000 pregnancies annually (National Center for Health Statistics, 2006).
- Ten percent of the population has significant problems related to substance abuse (Reilly, 1998).
- At least 4% of U.S. households include three generations; approximately 78,000 homes include four generations (Cohn, 2001).
- In California, gay adoptions, or "second-parent" adoptions, number 10,000 (Kravets, 2003).

life changes, equipping people with the skills needed to deal with the inevitability of changing structures.

Finally, each type of family structure creates different issues and problems that, in turn, influence a family's ability to perform basic functions. Each particular structure determines the kind of support needed from nursing or other human service systems (Eliopoulos, 2001). A single adult living alone may lack companionship or a sense of being needed by other family members. A kin-network family provides extended family support and security but may have problems with power distribution and decision making. An unmarried couple raising a child may be parenting well but may feel isolated from married couples in the community; they may need more peer support and socialization. Variations in structure create variations in family strengths and needs, an important consideration for community health nurses. Display 18.2 lists additional facts about families in America.

FAMILY FUNCTIONS

Families in every culture throughout history have engaged in similar functions: families have produced children, physically maintained their members, protected their health, encouraged their education or training, given emotional support and acceptance, and provided supportive and nurturing care during illness. Some societies have experimented with separation of these functions, allocating activities such as child care, socialization, or social control to a larger group. The Israeli kibbutz and Chinese commune are examples. In U.S. society, certain social institutions help perform some aspects of traditional family functions. Schools, for example, help socialize children, professionals supervise health care, and religious organizations influence values.

Six functions are typical of American families today and are essential for the maintenance and promotion of family health: (1) providing affection, (2) providing security, (3) instilling identity, (4) promoting affiliation, (5) providing socialization, and (6) establishing controls (Duvall & Miller,

1985). These tasks help promote the growth and development of family members. Understanding these functions and how well individual families provide them enables the community health nurse to work effectively with each family at its level of functioning.

Providing Affection

The family functions to give members affection and emotional support. In Western societies, love brings couples together. In some other cultures, affection comes after marriage. Continued affection creates an atmosphere of nurturance and care for all family members, which is necessary for health, development, and survival. It is common knowledge that infants require love to thrive. Indeed, human beings of any age require love as sustenance for growth and find it most often in their families. Families, unlike many other social groups, are bound by affectionate ties, the strength of which determines family happiness and closeness. Consider how sharing of gifts on a holiday or loving concern for a sick member draws a family together.

Positive sexual identity and sexual fulfillment are also influenced by a loving atmosphere. Early studies of the family emphasized sexual access and procreation as basic family functions. It is now recognized that families exist not only to regulate the sex drive and perpetuate the species, but also to sustain life and foster human potential through a strong affectional climate.

Providing Security and Acceptance

Families meet their members' physical needs by providing food, shelter, clothing, health care, and other necessities; in so doing, they create a secure environment. Members need to know that these basics will be available and that the family is committed to providing them. The stability of the family unit also gives members a sense of security. The family offers a safe retreat from the competition of the outside world and provides a place in which its members are accepted for themselves. They can learn, make mistakes, and grow in a secure environment. Where else does a toddler, after repeated falls, receive the encouragement to keep trying to walk; or a child, teased by a bully, regain his courage; or a parent, feeling burned out by a job, find comfort and renewal? The dependability of the family unit promotes confidence and self-assurance among its members. This contributes to their mental and emotional health and equips them with the skills necessary to cope with the outside world.

Instilling Identity and Satisfaction

The family functions to give members a sense of social and personal identity. Like a mirror, the family reflects back to its members a picture of who they are and how valuable they are to others. Positive reflections provide the individual with a sense of satisfaction and worth such as that experienced by a girl when her family applauds her efforts in a swim meet or by a boy whose family praises the bird house he builds in Cub Scouts. Needs fulfillment in the home determines satisfaction in the outside world; it particularly affects other interpersonal relationships and career choices. Roles learned within the family also give members a sense of identity. A boy growing up and learning his family's expectations for the male role quickly develops a sense of the kind of person he must strive to be; often, he is expected to be strong, competitive, successful, and unemotional. As a girl grows up, she often learns what is expected of her from her mother: to defer her needs to those of the family, be flexible and nurturing, and have homemaking skills. In other families, all children may have equal expectations of achievement and success. Families influence their members' positions in society by instilling values and goals. For some families, the emphasis may be on higher education; for others, it may be to work at a skill or trade. Still other families may be influenced by religious or political affiliations. Whatever the family influence, it is certain to shape each member's identity.

Promoting Affiliation and Companionship

The family functions to give members a sense of belonging throughout life. Because families provide associational bonds and group membership, they help satisfy their members' needs for belonging. Each person knows that she is *integral*—that she belongs—to the family. However, the quality of a family's communication influences its closeness. If communication patterns are effective, then affiliation ties are strong and needs for belonging are met. One family handles conflict over financial expenditures, for instance, by discussing differences and making compromises; this promotes affiliation. In another family, financial conflicts go unacknowledged; members keep spending selfishly and never discuss compromises.

The family, unlike other social institutions, involves permanent relationships. Long after friends from school, the old neighborhood, work, or the religious center have come and gone, the family remains. The family provides its members with affiliation and fellowship that remain unbroken by distance or time. Even if scattered across the country, family members gather to support one another and to share a holiday, wedding, graduation, or funeral. It is to the family that its members turn in times of happiness, tragedy, or need. This family affiliation remains a resource for life.

Providing Socialization

The family functions to socialize the young. Families transmit their culture—their values, attitudes, goals, and behavior patterns—to their members. Members, socialized into a way of life that reflects and preserves the family's cultural heritage, pass that heritage on, in turn, to the next generation. Starting in infancy, children learn to control bodily functions, eat with utensils, dress themselves, manage emotions, and behave according to sociocultural prescriptions for their age and sex. Through this process, members also learn their roles in the family. Lifestyle, food preferences, relationships with other people, ideas about child rearing, and attitudes about religion, abortion, equal rights, or euthanasia are all strongly influenced by the family. Although experiences outside the family also have a strong influence, they are filtered through the perceptions acquired during early socialization.

The socialization process also influences the degree of independence experienced by growing children. Some families release their maturing members by degrees, preparing them gradually but steadily for adult roles. Other families promote dependent roles and find release painful and difficult.

Establishing Controls

The family functions to maintain social control. Families maintain order through establishment of social controls both within the family and between family members and outsiders. Conduct of members is controlled by the family's definition of acceptable and unacceptable behaviors. From minor etiquette rules such as keeping elbows off the table to larger issues such as standards of home cleanliness, appropriate attire, children's behavior toward adults, or a teenager's curfew, the family imposes limits. It then maintains those limits by a system of rewards for conformity and punishments for violations. Children growing up in a family quickly learn what is "right" and what is "wrong" by family standards. Gradually, family control shifts to self-control as members learn to discipline their own behaviors; later on, they adopt or modify many of the same standards to use with their own children.

Division of labor is another aspect of the family's control function. Families allocate various roles, responsibilities, and tasks to their members to ensure the provision of income, household management, child care, and other essentials. Families also regulate the use of internal and external resources. The family identifies and directs the use of internal resources, such as member abilities, financial income, or material assets. For instance, if a man has artistic skills, he may be chosen to landscape the yard; if a woman has mechanical aptitude, she may be designated to repair appliances. One family may choose to drive an old car, rather than buy a new one, in order to spend more on entertainment.

Families also determine the external resources used by their members. Some families take advantage of the religious, health, and social services available to them in the community. They seek regular medical care, encourage their children to use the public library, become involved in religious activities, or join a bowling league. Other families, either because they do not know about potential external resources or because they do not recognize those resources as having any value, limit their members' use of them.

FAMILY LIFE CYCLE

Many of the characteristics and defined developmental stages of individual growth also apply to families. For example, it is known that families, while maintaining themselves as entities, change continuously. Families inevitably grow and develop as the individuals within them mature and adapt to the demands of successive life changes. A family's composition, set of roles, and network of interpersonal relationships change with the passage of time (Friedman et al., 2003). Family structures, too, vary with each stage of the family life cycle.

Consider the following example. The Jordans, a young married couple, concentrated on learning their respective roles of husband and wife and building a mutually satisfying marriage. With the birth of their first child, Scott, the family composition and relationships changed and role transitions occurred. The Jordans were not only husband and wife but also father, mother, and son; the family had added three new roles. Within the next 4 years, two daughters, Lisa and Tammy, were born. The introduction of each new member not only increased family size but also significantly reorganized family living. As Duvall and Miller (1985) pointed out, no two children are ever born into precisely the same family. The children entered school; Mrs. Jordan returned to work as a florist, and soon, Scott was leaving for college. The Jordans, like every family, were moving through a predictable and sequential pattern of stages known as the *family life cycle.*

Community nurses who are knowledgeable about this cycle can provide anticipatory guidance to families. For instance, while teaching prenatal care to a pregnant teen, the nurse can help the soon-to-be mother anticipate the responsibility and costs of raising her child by helping her calculate child care needs that must be met while she finishes school. The nurse can suggest that she figure out the monthly costs of breast-feeding versus buying formula; disposable diapers versus cloth or a diaper service; and the clothing, equipment, and medical costs of infant care. When working with the middle-aged parents of a brain-injured adult son living at home, the nurse can discuss what arrangements the parents have made for their son's care after they are older and unable to provide care themselves, or after one or both of them die.

Stages of the Family Life Cycle

There are two broad stages in the family life cycle: one of *expansion* as new members are added and roles and relationships are increased, and one of *contraction* as family members leave to start lives of their own or age and die. Within this framework of the expanding–contracting family are more specific phases, such as launching of children and retirement of parents. In some families, expansion and contraction are repeated as various members are added, return home with their children and perhaps a partner, or leave home permanently.

Family Developmental Tasks

To progress through the stages of the life cycle, a family must carry out its basic functions and the developmental tasks associated with those functions. Unlike individual developmental tasks, which are specific to each age level, family developmental tasks are ongoing throughout the life cycle. All families, for instance, must provide for the physical needs of their members at every stage. The manner and degree to which each function is carried out varies depending on how well members accomplish individual developmental tasks and meet the demands of each particular stage. Physical maintenance, for example, is affected by the parents' ability to accept responsibility and procure the necessary resources to provide food, clothing, and shelter for their children. At early stages, children are dependent on their parents for meeting these needs; at the school, teenage, and launching stages, children may increasingly contribute to home management and family income. The responsibility for these tasks shifts from just the parents to other family members as well.

Some functions require greater emphasis at certain stages. Socialization, for example, consumes much of a family's time during the early years of child development. These same functions and their associated developmental tasks can be further broken down into actions specific to certain stages. While carrying out its function of maintaining controls, a family sets clearly defined limits for children at the preschool stage: "Do not cross the street." "You may have dessert only after you finish your vegetables." "Bedtime is at 8 o'clock." During the school stage, control activities may center on allocating responsibilities and division of labor within the family: "Feed the dog." "Clean your room." "Take out the trash." When a family reaches the teenage stage, its control function increasingly focuses on the relationships between family members and outsiders. The family may regulate some activities by setting limits: "Be home by midnight." In areas such as moral conduct, controls may involve family values and therefore may be more subtle. A family at this stage must recognize the need for young people to assume increasing responsibility for their own behavior and acknowledge its own diminishing control over members who are exploring independence. Duvall and Miller (1985) described these activities as "stage-critical" family developmental tasks that must be completed before moving onto the next stage. Sample community health nursing actions with the family at different stages are presented in Table 18.2.

EMERGING FAMILY PATTERNS

Up to this point, the discussion of the family life cycle has focused primarily on the nuclear family. Because the nurse encounters many nuclear families in community health, the family life cycle provides a useful means of analyzing their growth and development. Not all families progress through the family life cycle in the same way or sequence. Because of gradual changes in American society, community health nurses face increasing numbers of adolescent unmarried mothers, gay and lesbian families, blended families, elderly couples, and individuals living alone. They need to recognize the impact that emerging diverse family patterns have on society and available resources. To be effective, nurses must equip themselves with an appropriate knowledge base to provide needed services.

Adolescent Unmarried Parents

Teen parenthood is an important social issue, with distinct medical and nursing ramifications. Teens are still developing emotionally. They have limited parenting skills and need a tremendous amount of education and support. Even with much media attention, availability of family planning methods, and a social environment open to discussing sexuality and pregnancy, teen pregnancy rates have remained high, especially among teens of color and those in lower socioeconomic situations.

Infants born to teen mothers are at risk for low birth weight, developmental delay, and death before 1 year of age. The infant mortality rate among mothers younger than 15 years is twice as high as for women between ages 20 and 24 years, and 20% higher among teens between ages 15 and 19 years than for women in their twenties (U.S. Department of Health and Human Services, 2000). In addition, children born to teen mothers face high rates of poverty, educational underachievement, and inadequate health care.

Teen fathers are often left out of the bevy of services that communities provide for the teen mother and infant. However, paternal involvement contributes positively to the physical, social, and cognitive development of children.

TABLE 18.2 Selected Stage-Critical Family Developmental Tasks

Stage of Family Life Cycle	Family Position	Stage-Critical Family Developmental Tasks	Role of the Community Health Nurse
Forming a partnership	Female partner Male partner	Establishing a mutually satisfying relationship	Interact with family where they are at
Childbearing	Partner-mother Partner-father Infant child(ren)	Adjusting to pregnancy and the promise of parenthood Fitting into the kin network Having and adjusting to infants, and encouraging their development Establishing a satisfying home for both parents and infant(s)	Assist them in developing strong relationships
Preschool-age	Partner-mother Partner-father Child, siblings	Adapting to the critical needs and interests of preschool children in stimulating, growth-promoting ways Coping with energy depletion and lack of privacy as parents	Assist in preparing for family expansion through education and anticipatory guidance
School-age	Partner-mother Partner-father Child, siblings	Fitting into the community of school-age families in constructive ways Encouraging children's educational achievement	Encourage time for each other as adults in a relationship separate from parenting role
Teenage	Partner-mother Partner-father Child, siblings	Balancing freedom with responsibility as teenagers mature and emancipate themselves Establishing outside interests and careers as growing parents	Provide anticipatory guidance for the school-age children as they grow into adulthood
Launching center	Partner-mother-grandmother Partner-father-grandfather Child, sibling, aunt or uncle	Releasing young adults into work, military service, college, marriage, etc., with appropriate rituals and assistance Maintaining a supportive home base	Provide anticipatory guidance for the contracting family as children leave home
Middle-aged parents	Partner-mother-grandmother Partner-father-grandfather	Rebuilding the relationship Maintaining kin ties with older and younger generations	Prepare adults for grandparenting role
Aging family members	Widow or widower Partner-mother-grandmother Partner-father-grandfather	Adjusting to retirement Coping with bereavement and living alone Closing the family home or adapting it to aging	Assist aging adults with emotional and financial security as they approach retirement Prepare the aging adults with ways to cope with the losses of old age, including changes in space, work, health, status, and loss of friends and family members

Children with absent fathers are at increased risk for behavioral difficulties and poor academic performance. A father who is emotionally supportive of the mother and provides child care and financial support directly and indirectly affects the well-being of his child.

With so many high-risk factors for pregnant teens and their children, it is imperative that community health nurses be knowledgeable about needed services, available resources, and the accessibility of each. In addition, because of the high-risk nature of teen pregnancy, prevention should be a priority. Nurses must collaborate in caregiving with other professionals and key players in teens' lives to provide the supportive services that young families need. *Healthy People*

2010 provides a number of national objectives relative to teen pregnancy prevention, family planning, and delayed sexual activity in younger teens, along with increased male involvement in healthy choices (see Display 18.3).

Gay and Lesbian Families

Another emerging family pattern is the gay or lesbian family. Whether the unions between two same-sex individuals are legitimate in the eyes of the law (such civil unions are legal in some states and marriages in California in 2008) or are based on strong emotional attachments without legal sanction, gay and lesbian families may include natural

DISPLAY 18.3	*HEALTHY PEOPLE 2010: OBJECTIVES RELATED TO FAMILY PLANNING AND CONCEPTION*

9-1   Increase the proportion of pregnancies that are intended.

9-2   Reduce the proportion of births occurring within 24 months of a previous birth.

9-3   Increase the proportion of females at risk of unintended pregnancy (and their partners) who use contraception.

9-6   (Developmental) Increase male involvement in pregnancy prevention and family planning efforts.

9-7   Reduce pregnancies among adolescent females.

9-8   Increase the proportion of adolescents who have never engaged in sexual intercourse before age 15 years.

9-9   Increase the proportion of adolescents who have never engaged in sexual intercourse.

9-12   Reduce the proportion of married couples whose ability to conceive or maintain a pregnancy is impaired.

9-13   (Developmental) Increase the proportion of health insurance policies that cover contraceptive supplies and services.

Source: U.S. Department of Health and Human Services. (2000). *Healthy People 2010: Understanding and Improving Health* (2nd ed.). Washington, DC: U. S. Government Printing Office. Retrieved May 30, 2008 from http://www.healthypeople.gov/Document/HTML/Volume1/09Family.htm

children from previous heterosexual relationships, artificial insemination, or adoption (Kravets, 2003). Although the exact number of families is not known, this emerging family pattern is increasing. It is estimated that there are between 2 and 14 million children with lesbian or gay parents in the United States (Tasker, 2005).

Although much progress has been made in accepting people with values and beliefs different from those of the mainstream, pervasive homophobia and heterosexism persist (Kravets, 2003; Silvestre, 2001). Nurses must confront and set aside their own biases in order to provide nonjudgmental and comprehensive care to these emerging families.

Gay and lesbian families have all the fears and concerns regarding parenting that any family a community health nurse visits may have. In addition, they experience the stress that accompanies being stigmatized by much of society. The nurse can become a valued resource for the family. Through education and anticipatory guidance, the nurse can assist the parents to successfully navigate the growth and developmental stages of their children, as well as the varied issues faced by families. Research has shown that the psychosocial development of the children of gay or lesbian parents is the same as that of children with heterosexual parents (American Academy of Pediatrics, 2002; Tasker, 2005).

Divorced and Blended Families

Divorce and remarriage are more frequent occurrences today than in previous generations. Divorces have gone from fewer than 20% of all marriages in the 1960s to almost 50% in 2000 (U.S. Census Bureau, 2008b). It is estimated that close to half of all children will experience living with divorced or single parents before they reach adulthood (Gunsberg & Hymowitz, 2005).

Adjusting to divorce involves a series of transitions and reorganizations for all family members. For children, it may require coping with a new geographic location and a new school, as well as adjusting to changes in the mental and physical health of family members. In addition to the normal growth and developmental changes, children of divorce may face an absent father or mother, interparental conflict, economic distress, parental adjustment, multiple life stressors, and short-term crises.

Not all divorced adults stay single. Most remarry or cohabitate with another adult who may or may not have children. This new couple may have children from their union, creating an even more complex family. Merged or blended families require considerable adjustment and relearning of roles, tasks, communication patterns, and relationships (Friedman et al., 2003).

Identifiable phases occur in divorce, remarriage, and the blending of families; each phase has its own emotional transitions and developmental issues. Table 18.3 shows the phases of a divorce, and Table 18.4 shows the phases of remarriage and blending families.

Because this emerging family pattern has become so prominent in such a short period, it is very possible that the community health nurse is familiar with this pattern or lives in such a family. Nursing skills that are needed when working with divorced or blended families include the ability to listen and be empathic, as well as a nonjudgmental attitude. The nurse can be a rich resource for the family. Support groups for adults and children are excellent resources and provide invaluable services at a time of emotional instability in the family. Peer support groups for children and adolescents and support from within the schools should be used, if available, or started if they do not exist. The community health nurse can have a significant role in community-wide planning if services are needed but unavailable.

Older Adults

Elderly individuals are the fastest growing segment of the population. From 1950 to 2005, the population of those 65 years of age and older increased from 12 to 37 million persons (NCHS, 2007). Most elders live independently well into their 80s and maintain healthy contacts with family and friends. Others feel isolated because of chronic health problems that limit mobility, thereby reducing or eliminating the ability to interact or contribute meaningfully in society.

The community health nurse needs to understand the complex dynamics of such situations and offer support and encouragement as family members work through these problems. Often, a nurse serves an entire community of elders, in a senior apartment complex, an assisted living center, or a mobile home community, for whom maintaining wellness is the focus. Keeping physically active, eating healthy

TABLE 18.3   When Families Divorce

Phase	Emotional Responses	Transitional Issues
1. Stressor leading to marital differences	Reveal the fact that the marriage has major problems	Accepting fact that marriage has major problems
2. Decision to divorce	Accepting the inability to resolve marital differences	Accepting one's own contribution to the failed marriage
3. Planning the dissolution of the family system	Negotiating viable arrangements for all members within the system	Cooperating on custody visitation, and financial issues Informing and dealing with extended family members and friends
4. Separation	Mourning loss of intact family Working on resolving attachment to spouse	Develop coparental arrangements/relationships Restructure living arrangements Adapt to living apart Realign relationship with extended family and friends Begin to rebuild own social network
5. Divorce	Continue working on emotional recovery by overcoming hurt, anger, or guilt	Giving up fantasies of reunion Staying connected with extended families Rebuild and strengthen own social network
6. Post-divorce	Separate feeling about ex-spouse from parenting role Prepare self for possibility of changes in custody as child(ren) get older, be open to their needs Risk developing a new intimate relationship	Make flexible and generous visitation arrangements for child(ren) and noncustodial parent and extended family members Deal with possibilities of chaning custody arrangements as child(ren) get older Deal with child(ren)s' reaction to parents establishing relationships with new partners

TABLE 18.4   Remarriage and Blending Families

Phase	Emotional Responses	Developmental Issues
1. Meeting new people	Allowing for the possibility of developing a new intimate relationship	Dealing with child(ren)s' and ex-family members' reactions to a parent "dating"
2. Entering a new relationship	Completing an "emotional recovery" from past divorce Accepting one's fears about developing a new relationship Working on feeling good about what the future may bring	Recovery from loss of marriage is adequate Discovering what you want from a new relationship Working on openness in a new relationship
3. Planing a new marriage	Accepting one's fears about the ambiguity and complexity of entering a new relationship such as: New roles and responsibilities Boundaries; space, time, and authority Affective issues: guilt, loyalty, conflicts, unresolvable past hurts	Recommitment to marriage and forming a new family unit Dealing with stepchild(ren) as custodial or noncustodial parent Planning for maintenance of coparental relationships with ex-spouses Planning to help child(ren) deal with fears, loyalty conflicts, and memberships in two systems Realignment of relationships with ex-family to include new spouse and child(ren)
4. Remarriage and blending of families	Final resolution of attachment to previous spouse Acceptance of new family unit with different boundaries	Restructuring family boundaries to allow for new spouse or stepparent Realignment of relationships to allow inter-mingling of systems Expanding relationships to include all new family members Sharing family memories and histories to enrich members lives

meals regularly, receiving appropriate medical care and immunizations, and establishing and maintaining social contacts are some of the tasks elders should focus on to stay healthy well into old age, and these are some of the areas in which the community health nurse can intervene as teacher, counselor, and clinician (Gavan, 2003). Reaching 100 years of age is not an unusual occurrence today, and more people will live to see advanced age in the 21st century.

Summary

The family as the unit of service has received increasing emphasis in nursing over the years. Today, family nursing has an important place in nursing practice, particularly in community health nursing. Its significance results from recognizing that the family itself must be a focus of service, that family health and individual health strongly influence each other, and that family health affects community health. A community health nurse's effectiveness in working with families depends on an understanding of family theory and characteristics, in addition to changing family structures.

Every family on the globe is unique; its needs and strengths are different from those of every other family. At the same time, each family is alike because of certain shared universal characteristics. Five of these universals have particular significance for community health nursing: every family is a small social system, has its own cultural values and rules, has structure, has certain basic functions, and moves through stages in its life cycle.

Every family is a small social system. The members within a family are interdependent; what one does affects the others and, ultimately, influences total family health. Families, as social systems, set and maintain boundaries that unite them and preserve their autonomy, while also differentiating them from others. Because these boundaries are semipermeable, families engage in an input–output energy exchange with external resources. Families are equilibrium-seeking, adaptive systems that strive to adjust to internal and external life changes. Like other systems, families are goal directed. They exist for the purpose of promoting their members' development.

Every family has its own culture, its own set of values, and rules for operation. Family values influence member beliefs and behaviors. These same values prescribe the types of roles that each member assumes. A family's culture also determines its power distribution and decision-making patterns.

Every family has a structure that can be categorized as either traditional or nontraditional (contemporary). The most common traditional family structure is the nuclear family, consisting of husband, wife, and one or more children living together. Other traditional structures include husband and wife living as a couple alone, single-parent families, single-adult families, multigenerational families, kin-networks, and blended families. Nontraditional or contemporary family structures incorporate many family forms, not all of which are readily accepted by society. These variations include commune families, group marriages, and group networks. Unmarried single-parent families, unmarried gay or straight couples living together with or without children, and unmarried older adults living together are examples of emerging contemporary family structures. As less typical families become more common, they receive more recognition and acceptance. These diverse family structures remind us that the nuclear family is now in the minority, that people experience many family structures during their lifetimes, and that a family's ability to perform its basic functions is influenced by its structure.

Every family has six basic functions: (1) to provide members with affection and emotional support; (2) to promote security by providing members with an accepting, stable environment in which physical needs are met; (3) to provide members with a sense of social and personal identity and influence their placement in the social order; (4) to provide members with affiliation, a sense of belonging; (5) to socialize members by teaching basic values and attitudes that determine behavior; and (6) to establish social controls to maintain order. Community health nurses use this information to assess a family's functioning. This information enables the nurse to work with the family and assist in improving the quality of its functioning.

Every family moves through stages in its life cycle. Families develop in two broad stages: a period of expansion when new members and roles are added, and a period of contraction when members leave. Some families demonstrate a spiraling pattern with repeated expansion and contraction.

Emerging family patterns influence the role of the community health nurse. The single adolescent parent in particular needs the community health nurse's knowledge of family developmental theory. Gay and lesbian families with children may also have special needs. More complex interaction patterns and living arrangements are created by divorce, remarriage, the blending of families, and the unique relationships these arrangements create. Older adults are living longer and will soon make up 20% of the population. The multiple needs of elders from age 65 to 100 years or older are more varied than those of any other population group. Today, community health nurses see many more families expressing one of these emerging family patterns. Understanding their different needs will help the nurse provide appropriate services. ■

ACTIVITIES TO PROMOTE CRITICAL THINKING

1. Within a small group of your peers, individually define *family* and then compare each of your definitions. How similar and how different is each definition? What in each person's background contributes to the differences in the definitions? Was each of the peers in nursing? If not, how did that contribute to any differences in the definitions?

2. Analyze two families (other than your own) that you know well, one traditional and the other nontraditional (contemporary), and answer the following questions:
   - If the major breadwinner in this family became permanently disabled and unable to work or lost his or her income, how would the family most likely respond immediately and in the long term?

- What are some of this family's rules for operation and the values underlying the rules?
- Structurally, what kind of family is this?
- What are the strongest and weakest functions performed by this family, and why do you think this is so?
- In what developmental stage is this family, and how does it affect their functioning?

3. Talk with the members of a blended family and discuss with each member his or her relationships with stepchildren or siblings, half-siblings, and stepparents. What problems can they identify? What problems have they overcome? What do they see as the positive elements of the union?

4. Gay and lesbian couples often seek parenting opportunities. How do you feel about this? What makes you feel this way? What are the positive and negative aspects of a child's being raised by a homosexual couple?

5. Use the Internet and find information at various websites on family structural patterns in other countries. Many families in developing and some industrialized countries live in clans, tribes, groups, and kin-networks. In what countries do you find such family structures? What are the benefits and drawbacks of such systems?

References

American Academy of Pediatrics. Committee on Psychosocial Aspects of Child and Family Health. (2002). Coparent or second-parent adoption by same-sex parents. *Pediatrics, 109*, 339–340.

Anderson, S.A., & Sabetelli, R.M. (2006). *Family interaction: Multigenerational developmental perspective,* 4th ed. Boston: Allyn & Bacon.

Ayres, C. (2008). *Polygamist sect leader faces DNA test over alleged sex attacks on girls.* TimesOnline. Retrieved August 7, 2008 from http://www.timesonline.co.uk/tol/news/world/us_and_americas/article4036201.ece.

Barnes, S.L. (2001). Stressors and strengths: A theoretical and practical examination of nuclear, single-parent, and augmented African American families. *Families in Society: The Journal of Contemporary Human Service, 82*(5), 449–460.

Bell, J.M., & Wright, L.M. (1993). Flaws in family nursing education. In G. Wegner, & R. Alexander (Eds.) *Readings in family nursing.* (pp. 390–394). Philadelphia: Lippincott Williams & Wilkins.

Bomar, P. (2004). *Promoting health in families: Applying family research and theory to nursing practice,* 3rd ed. Philadelphia: Saunders.

Campbell, T.L. (2006). Improving health through family interventions. In D.R. Crane, & E.S. Marshall (Eds.). *Handbook of families & health: Interdisciplinary perspectives.* (pp. 379–395). Thousand Oaks, CA: Sage Publications.

Cohn, D. (September 7, 2001). 4% of U.S. homes are multigenerational: Culture, finances dictate lifestyles. *Washington Post,* p. A8.

Denham, S.A. (2005). Family structure, function, and process. In S.H. Hanson, V. Gedaly-Duff, & J.R. Kaakinen (Eds.). *Family health care nursing: Theory, practice, and research,* 3rd ed. (pp. 119–156). Philadelphia: F. A. Davis.

Dreikurs, R. (1964). *Children: The challenge.* New York: Meredith.

Duvall, E.M., & Miller, B. (1985). *Marriage and family development,* 6th ed. New York: Harper & Row.

Eliopoulos, C. (2001). *Gerontological nursing,* 5th ed. Philadelphia: Lippincott Williams & Wilkins.

Fiese, B.H. (2006). *Family routines and rituals.* New Haven: Yale University Press.

Friedman, M.M., Bowden, V.R., & Jones, E. (2003). *Family nursing: Research, theory, and practice,* 5th ed. Upper Saddle River, NJ: Prentice-Hall.

Gavan, C.S. (2003). Successful aging families: A challenge for nurses. *Holistic Nursing Practice, 17*(1), 1–18.

Gunsberg, L., & Hymowitz, P. (Eds.). (2005). *Divorce and custody: Forensic, developmental, and clinical perspectives.* Hillsdale, NJ: The Analytic Press, Inc.

Hanson, S.M.H., Gedaly-Duff, V., & Kaakinen, J.R. (2005). *Family health care nursing: Theory, practice, and research,* 3rd ed. Philadelphia: F.A. Davis.

Hofferth, S.L. (2003). The American family: Changes and challenges for the 21st century. In H.M. Wallace, G. Green, & K.J. Jaros (Eds.). *Health and welfare for families in the 21st century.* (pp. 71–79). Boston: Jones and Bartlett Publishers.

Kravets, D. (May 8, 2003). High court weighs gay adoptions. *The Fresno Bee,* p. B3.

Leininger, M.M. (2001). *Culture, care, diversity, and universality: A theory of nursing.* New York: NLN Press.

Marciano, T. (1991). A postscript on wider families: Traditional family assumptions and cautionary notes. *Marriage and Family Review, 17,* 159–163.

McBride, J.L. (2006). *Family behavioral issues in health and illness.* New York: The Haworth Press.

Murray, R.B., & Zentner, J.P. (2000). *Health promotion strategies through the life span,* 7th ed. Upper Saddle River, NJ: Prentice-Hall.

National Alliance to End Homelessness. (2007). *Homelessness counts.* Retrieved August 7, 2008 from http://www.endhomelessness.org.

National Center for Health Statistics, U.S. Department of Health and Human Services. (2006). *Recent Trends in Teenage Pregnancy in the United States, 1990–2002.* Retrieved October 10, 2008 from http://www.cdc.gov/nchs/products/pubs/pubd/hestats/teenpreg1990–2002/teenpreg1990–2002.htm.

National Center for Health Statistics, U.S. Department of Health and Human Services. (2007*). Health, United States, 2007 with chartbook on trends in the health of Americans.* Hyattsville, MD: U.S. Government Printing Office.

Neuman, B. (2001). *The Neuman systems model,* 4th ed. Upper Saddle River, NJ: Prentice-Hall.

Olson, D.H., McCubbin, H.I., Barnes, H.L., et al. (1989). *Families: What makes them work.* Newbury Park, CA: Sage.

Pender, N.J., Murdaugh, C.L., & Parsons, M.A. (2006). *Health promotion in nursing practice,* 5th ed. Upper Saddle River, NJ: Prentice-Hall.

Scanzoni, J., Polonko, K., Teachman, J., & Thompson, L. (1989). *The sexual bond: Rethinking family and close relationships.* Newbury Park, CA: Sage.

Silvestre, A.J. (Ed.). (2001). *Lesbian, gay, bisexual, and transgender health issues.* Washington, DC: American Public Health Association.

Spector, R.W. (2000). *Cultural diversity in health and illness,* 5th ed. Upper Saddle River, NJ: Prentice-Hall.

Stein, P.J. (Ed.). (1981). *Single life: Unmarried adults in social context.* New York: St. Martin's.

Stewart, P., & Goldfarb, K.P. (2007). Historical trends in the study of diverse families. In B.S. Trask, & R.R. Hamon (Eds.). *Cultural diversity and families.* (pp 3–19). Thousand Oaks, CA: Sage Publications.

Tasker, F. (2005). Lesbian mothers, gay fathers, and their children: A review. *Developmental and Behavioral Pediatrics, 26*(3), 224–240.

U.S. Census Bureau. (2008a). *The 2008 Statistical Abstract.* Retrieved August 7, 2008 from http://www.census.gov/compendia/statab/brief.html.

U.S. Census Bureau. (2008b). *Statistical Abstract of the United States. Statistical Abstract: Historical Statistics.* Retrieved August 7, 2008 from http://www.census.gov/compendia/statab/hist_stats.html.

U.S. Census Bureau. (n.d.). *Marriage and divorce rates by country: 1980 to 2005.* Retrieved May 1, 2008 from http://www.census.gov/compendia/statab/tables/08s1302.pdf.

U.S. Department of Health and Human Services. (2000). *Healthy People 2010: Understanding and Improving Health,* 2nd ed. Washington, DC: U.S. Government Printing Office.

World Health Organization. (1976). *Statistical indices of family health* (Rep. No. 589). Geneva, Switzerland: WHO Press.

Selected Readings

Crewe, S.E., & Wilson, R.G. (2007). Kinship care: From family tradition to social policy in the African American community. *Journal of Health and Social Policy, 22*(3/4), 1–7.

Doucet, F., & Hamon, R.R. (2007). A nation of diversity: Demographics of the United States of America and their implications for families. In B.S. Trask, & R.R. Hamon (Eds.). *Cultural diversity and families.* (pp. 20–43). Thousand Oaks, CA: Sage Publications.

Erikson, E. (1963). *Childhood and society,* 2nd ed. New York: Norton.

Hamilton, L., Cheng, S., & Powell, B. (2007). Adoptive parents, adaptive parents: Evaluating the importance of biological ties for parental investment. *American Sociological Review, 72,* 95–116.

Hernandez, D.J., Denton, N.A., & Macartney, S.E. (2007). Family circumstances of children in immigrant families. In J.E. Lansford, K. Deater-Deckard, & M.H. Bornstein (Eds.). *Immigrant families in contemporary society.* (pp. 9–29). New York: The Guilford Press.

Humphreys, J., & Campbell, J.C. (2004). Family violence and nursing practice. Philadelphia: Lippincott Williams & Wilkins.

Mays, R.M. (2006). Culturally responsive care. In M. Craft-Rosenberg, & M.J. Krajicek (Eds.). *Nursing excellence for children and families.* (pp. 57–76). New York: Springer Publishing Company.

Omariba, D.W.R., & Boyle, M.H. (2007). Family structure and child mortality in Sub-Saharan Africa: Cross-national effects of polygyny. *Journal of Marriage and Family, 69,* 528–543.

Piaget, J. (1973). *The psychology of intelligence.* Totowa, NJ: Littlefield Adams.

Internet Resources

American Academy of Child and Adolescent Psychiatry—Facts for Families, Foster Care: *http://www.aacap.org/cs/root/facts_for_families/foster_care*

Centers for Disease Control and Prevention (Family Health): *http://www.cdc.gov/Family/*

Child Welfare League of America—The Adoption History Project: *http://www.uoregon.edu/~adoption/people/cwla.html*

Children's Aid Society—Adoption and Foster Care: *http://www.childrensaidsociety.org/adoption?gclid=COLut8Cn0JMCFSLOIgodglc5iQ*

Family Health International: *http://www.fhi.org/en/index.htm*

Healthy People 2010—Health Finder: *http://www.healthfinder.gov/justforyou/*

Medline Plus: *http://www.nlm.nih.gov/medlineplus/parenting.html*

National Alliance to End Homelessness: *http://www.endhomelessness.org/section/policy/focusareas/families*

National Institutes of Health—Adventures in Parenting: *http://www.nichd.nih.gov/publications/pubs/adv_in_parenting/index.cfm*

U.S. Department of Health and Human Services—U.S. Surgeon General's Family History Initiative: *http://www.hhs.gov/familyhistory/*

19

Working with Families: Applying the Nursing Process

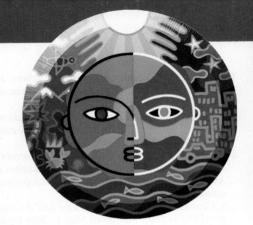

LEARNING OBJECTIVES

Upon mastery of this chapter, you should be able to:

- Describe the components of the nursing process as they apply to enhancing family health.
- Identify the steps in a successful family health intervention.
- Describe useful activities and actions when intervening on family health visits.
- List at least six specific safety measures the community health nurse should take when traveling to a home or making a home visit.
- Describe the effect of family health on individual health.
- Describe individual and group characteristics of a healthy family.
- Identify five family health practice guidelines.
- Describe three conceptual frameworks that can be used to assess a family.
- Describe the 12 major assessment categories for families.
- List the five basic principles the community health nurse should follow when assessing family health.
- Discuss the two foci of family health visits: Education and Health Promotion.
- Describe three types of evaluations that are necessary after family health interventions.

KEY TERMS

Conceptual Framework
Developmental Framework
Eco-map
Family health
Family nursing
Genogram
Interactional framework
Outcome evaluation
Referral
Resource directory
Strengthening
Structural-functional
   framework

"If the family were a fruit, it would be an orange, a circle of sections, held together but separable—each segment distinct."

—Letty Cottin Pogrebin

Chapter 18 explored the theoretical basis of family formation and the variety of family structures. Other chapters have stressed that families come in all sizes, consist of members of many ages and biologic relationships, and experience the world filtered through their unique cultures. There are many theoretical approaches and roles to consider when caring for families. This chapter explores the nursing process as it applies to working with families as a unit of service.

Community health nurses deliver care to families in their homes, their work settings, classrooms, clinics and outpatient departments, neighborhood centers, and homeless shelters. Although community health nursing emphasizes the family as a unit of service, a gap exists between family nursing theory, development, and practice (Friedman, Bowden, & Jones, 2003). The problem, in part, is derived from a health care system that fosters individual services, often to the exclusion of family. This is evident in many third-party payer and reimbursement policies that impose limits to the kinds of services funded, in public health agencies' tendencies to organize services around individuals, and in government requirements that agencies keep statistics for specific diseases or service categories that reflect individual rather than family or aggregate data.

The family has been the main unit of service in communities for more than a century (Schorr & Kennedy, 1999). It is with the family in mind that the bulk of health care and related services are provided in the community. Immunization programs exist for infants and children. Parks, recreational services, organized team sports, and social centers exist for the physical and emotional well-being of families. Pregnant women can attend childbirth education classes and receive medical care from their health care providers. Growing families can access parenting classes and support groups for help with developmental crises and in the management of chronic illness. Senior centers exist for the older adults in families, and myriad social and recreational activities offer senior discounts. What all these clients have in common is they are members of families.

Think about how your family has influenced you. Did family members sway your career choice or where you are attending school? What about your value system, or how you view your health? What about the friendships you've formed? What about the foods you eat; would those choices be different if you had grown up with vegetarian parents versus a parent who took you out every fall to hunt deer?

Just as each family is unique, so too are their homes and communities. Some families live in homes that look very much like yours, where you will feel comfortable almost immediately, whereas others live in places that may not feel so comfortable to you. To a novice community health nurse, it can be daunting to enter a small cluttered apartment or a sparsely furnished single room, or a home in disrepair. Families live in mobile homes, in high-rise inner-city apartments, in rural cabins, and on farm labor camps. Each home and neighborhood can bring its own set of unique challenges, as well as strengths, to the families you are visiting.

Family-level problem-solving techniques are needed to deal with important health issues including health promotion, pregnancy and childbirth, acute life-threatening illness, chronic illness, substance abuse, and terminal illness (Chambers, 2004; Gavan, 2003; Kitzman et al., 2000; Pinelli, 2000;

Saunders, 2003). The first step is to develop family assessment skills. This is foundational to the development of a database on which to formulate nursing diagnosis, an essential step before planning, implementation, and evaluation of services can occur. This chapter focuses on the nursing process: assessing, planning, implementing, and evaluating to enhance family health.

NURSING PROCESS COMPONENTS APPLIED TO FAMILIES AS CLIENTS

Assessing, planning, implementing, and evaluating nursing care are steps used to deliver care to clients in acute care settings and in the extensive clinic system. These same steps are used with families and aggregates in community health settings. The steps do not change, but the context and client focus are different, and external variables that have not been encountered in other contexts must now be considered.

Working with Families in Community Health Settings

Family visits need not be limited to homes. Family members may be visited in school or at work during a lunch break, in a day care or senior center, in a group home, or myriad after-work or after-school and recreational settings. The nurse must be creative in accommodating various family schedules and routines. In general, if a visit is all right with the family, school, or employer, it should be all right with the nurse (see Perspectives: Voices from the Community). Families appreciate the individualized effort and respond more positively when nurses are willing to work with family member schedules.

When making visits in public places, such as worksites or schools, be mindful of confidentiality and respect the family's wishes. A client may agree to your visit during lunch break in a department store on a Tuesday, which is the boss's day off, or after the lunch crowd in a fast-food restaurant disperses and the client can take a break. Seek out a place for the visit where other employees or customers cannot overhear your conversation with the client.

Sometimes, visiting clients where they spend their time during the day helps to enhance family assessment. In families with a child in day care or an elderly family member in an adult day care program, your assessment of that individual's

---

PERSPECTIVES
VOICES FROM THE COMMUNITY

"I couldn't believe it when she [the community health nurse] said she could visit me during my lunch break. I have been so worried about Ben's hearing and with my new work hours I kept missing her—I got her notes she left in the screen door. She actually drove all the way out to my work to tell me about his hearing test at school and the teacher's classroom changes. I can't afford to lose this job—and she came here!"

Beth, 34, Ben's mother

ability to manage, participate, and interact in the situation can give insight into problems the family is referring to when you make a home visit. Visiting children during the school day often gives insight into health problems the parents may be concerned about. Such visits can offer the community health nurse an excellent opportunity to consult with the principle, teachers, school nurse, counselor, and school psychologist. The community health nurse may suggest a team meeting of school professionals and the parents, coordinate the meeting, and act as liaison and client advocate during the meeting.

Working with Families Where They Live

Depending on the setting for community health nursing practice, the nurse encounters most clients in their homes and neighborhoods. Some see families in transition, who are living on the streets, in homeless shelters, or with relatives or friends. Regardless of the family's location, the client is the family; the family is the unit of service in family nursing (Friedman et al., 2003).

The Home Visit

Working in the community and being able to visit families in their homes is a privilege. In this unique setting you are permitted into the most intimate of spaces we, as human beings, have. Our homes are our creations, our private spaces; they hold our personal treasures and our memories. To let a stranger into our home takes a certain amount of trust. To enter a client's family home also takes trust on the part of the nurse. Once the door is shut behind you, the rules change; you are in the client's world where they are the experts, and you are the guest and may feel like a stranger.

Nursing Skills Used During Home Visits

Many skills, in addition to expert nursing skills, are needed when assessing, planning, implementing, and evaluating services in the home to families at a variety of functional levels (Tapia, 1997). Expert interviewing skills and effective communication techniques are essential for effective family intervention (see Chapter 10). The following paragraphs describe special skills required when making home visits.

Acute Observation Skills

The environment is new to you, and observation of environment and client are equally important. In addition to focusing on the family members' concerns and the purpose of the visit, you need to be observant about the neighborhood, travel safety, home environmental conditions, number of household members, client demeanor, and body language, as well as other nonverbal cues.

Travel in new neighborhoods and attempts to locate a family can cause distress to even the most experienced nurse. Often clients are difficult to locate because the house or apartment number is missing. The residence may be situated behind another house, or it may be a basement apartment without a number. Many anomalies in the layout of a building or a neighborhood may make it difficult for the nurse to locate a client. Addresses on referrals may have numbers transposed such as 123 Hickory instead of 132 Hickory.

Perhaps there is a North Hickory that is miles away from South Hickory, or there is a Hickory Boulevard, Drive, Road, Street, Court, Lane, or Way. There is always the chance that the address is fictitious, given by a client who, for whatever reason, prefers to remain as anonymous as possible.

Assessment of Home Environmental Conditions

Conditions in the neighborhood and home environments reveal important assessment information that can guide planning and intervention with families. While traveling to and arriving at the family home, you have been gathering information about resources and barriers encountered by the family. This information is used during planning with the family. It is important to remember that neighborhood conditions and even the physical appearance of the apartment or house may contradict the family's values, resources, and goals. They may have little control over the neighborhood or the building they live in, especially if they are renting. For instance, the family may be a young couple with a baby who can afford $475 in rent; the only apartment available to them for that amount is in a deteriorating low-income neighborhood with dilapidated buildings occupied by renters and owned by absentee landlords, who may own several buildings, mainly for profit. A manager who may not know the landlord and is employed through the owner's management company handles the property. Yet, when you enter the apartment, you may see a well-furnished, neat, and clean home that is opened to you with pride by the family.

In another situation, you may plan to visit an older couple who lives in their own home in an upscale suburban neighborhood. On approaching the house, however, you barely manage to squeeze through a pathway made in the living room, which is piled ceiling-high with boxes, newspapers, and furniture. This continues throughout the house and even into a back bedroom, where half the bed is covered with papers, books, and a few cats. An older woman is in the bed. The husband moves very slowly, and after showing you in, he leaves the bedroom and heads toward the backyard.

Many environmental clues in each of these situations help the nurse begin an assessment that will lead to a plan to assist each family. Most neighborhoods and homes do not present such extremes. However, if you are unprepared for the extremes, they may overwhelm you, and you may become so distracted that you cannot focus wholly on the family and incorporate these important observations into the plan.

Assessment of Body Language and Other Nonverbal Cues

After you have knocked on the door or rung the doorbell and are in the home (see What Do You Think?), or even while greeting the people in the doorway, you are gathering data. Being human, you may form opinions or make judgments about the family from the initial meeting. Know that they are doing the same. Be aware of all household members; acknowledge and greet them. If some are absent, inquire about them. Make this a habit on all visits. Each family member is important and has opinions and health care needs, even if you only see certain members of the family on each visit.

Be observant of family body language and demeanor. These nonverbal cues provide information that must not be

What Do You Think?

HOW YOU KNOCK HELPS FAMILIES OPEN THE DOOR

At first this may seem trite, but how do you knock on the door when you visit a family? Do you use the "I don't want to be here and if they don't hear the knock I can quietly leave" type of knock that even Superman can't hear? Or do you knock like, "I'm a bill collector and YOU BETTER open this door!" During this knock, the entire family is leaving through the back door! We suggest a knock that is loud enough to be heard, yet friendly and nonthreatening. If necessary, practice "your knock" until you can create this beneficial combination.

With some families, it is helpful to call toward the door as you knock or ring the bell with, "Mrs. Smith, this is Jenny from the Health Department—remember I was coming by today" or, "Ms. Jiminez, it's the student community health nurse, Terry Guara, and I brought those pamphlets for you" or, "Hello, it's James from the neighborhood clinic, we planned to meet today." Using such a greeting allows the family to know who is at the door and choose to open the door if they want. It will get you into more homes than the "quiet-as-a-mouse" or "bill-collector" knocks.

overlooked. Observations such as, "You seem anxious today," or "Did I come at a bad time? You seem distracted," are openings that allow family members to express what is on their minds. If you are not open to body language while making a visit, you may overlook important cues and continue with your agenda, without realizing that the family is distracted by another, more pressing issue.

On a related note, it is important to be aware of your own body language. If you fidget with car keys during the entire visit, noisily chew gum, give minimal eye contact while continuously looking at your paperwork, appear rushed, or refuse to sit on any of the furniture, your behavior with tell the family a great deal about you, including how you feel about being in their home.

PLANNING TO MEET THE HEALTH NEEDS OF FAMILIES DURING HOME VISITS

The greatest barrier to a successful family health visit is lack of planning and preparation. A visit is not successful just because the nurse enters a home or other setting where clients are present. A successful family health visit takes much planning and preparation and requires accurate documentation and follow-up. In addition, safety measures must be followed not only while traveling in the neighborhood, but also in the home.

Components of the Family Health Visit

The structure of family health visits can be divided into four components that follow the nursing process (Display19.1). Pre-visit preparation steps (assessment and planning) are necessary to ensure that the actual family health visit (implementation) is complete. The documentation and planning for the next visit (evaluation) concludes the responsibilities for one visit and prepares the nurse for the next action needed.

Pre-visit Preparation

Community health nurses design a plan for the initial family health visit based on a referral coming into the agency. A **referral** is a request for service from another agency or person. This request is formalized by use of a form or information that the originating agency has transferred to the receiving agency. Referrals may be formal, coming from complementary agencies, or they may be informal, resulting from verbal or telephone referrals from friends or relatives who believe that someone needs help. Referrals are the source of new cases for the agencies, and they need timely responses. Referrals could be from labor and delivery units, requesting service for low-birth-weight babies and teen mothers. They could be from social service agencies, requesting a home assessment for a child being returned to parents after previous removal from the home. A referral could come via a telephone call from a woman in a city 500 miles away, requesting that a nurse check on an elderly relative who lives alone in the community and has recently exhibited slurred speech. Follow-up visits are made to these families based on need and agency protocol.

Nurses must have a physical place to work, with access to a telephone and any other supportive resources deemed necessary, such as educational material (pamphlets, brochures, computer, and related website addresses to access educational information), charting tools, and other supplies required for home visits. Nurses also need a **resource directory**, which is a published list of resources for the broader community, or a nurse-made directory of resources created over years of working with people in the community. Some agencies issue a nursing bag to their nurses but if not, many community health nurses become creative and devise their own carry-all for supplies. The supplies needed depend on the type of visit; some nurses have several totes for different types of visits. Think about what basic supplies you would need to visit a new mother and her infant, or an elderly man with hypertension.

Once the nurse is prepared, contact with the family is needed. For a home visit, ideally, the referral contains a correct telephone number for the family, a relative, or a neighbor. If the referral or chart does not contain this information, the nurse makes an unannounced visit. During this visit, it is important to get a contact number for the family. When calling for the first time, introduce yourself, explain the reason for the call, and why the family was referred, what the visit consists of, and determine when a visit would be convenient for the family and the nurse. Some people become defensive or suspicious of the nurse's intentions. For example, a new young mother may think, "What did they see me doing wrong with my baby in the hospital?" In this kind of situation, it is very important that the nurse explain that

- ◆ The visit is a service provided by the agency to all mothers.
- ◆ The visit is paid for by taxes (or donations) or by the client's health maintenance organization (if applicable), so there is no direct charge to the family.

DISPLAY 19.1 — GUIDELINES FOR MAKING HOME VISITS: 30 STEPS TO SUCCESS

The following guidelines can be followed to evaluate yourself after making a home visit; or it can be a tool used when you are evaluated by another nurse (peer or instructor). Rate yourself using the following scale: 0 = does not apply, 1 = unsatisfactory, 2 = satisfactory.

Rating Assessment

_____ 1. Studies referral, record, or other available data about the family.
_____ 2. Gathers community resource information potentially appropriate to the family.
_____ 3. Obtains appropriate supplies or educational material in anticipation of family needs.

Planning

_____ 4. Contacts family to set up an appropriate time for the home visit.
_____ 5. Ascertains correct address and directions to the family for the home visit.
_____ 6. Formulates a written plan for nursing intervention with each family member.
_____ 7. Organizes a chart with forms and charting tools based on the focus of the visit.
_____ 8. Plans a route to the family's home that is the most direct, being resource efficient.

Implementation

_____ 9. Travels the community with safety, locating the family home with ease.
_____ 10. Knock on the door loudly enough to be heard and in a friendly manner.
_____ 11. Introduces self to family members in an appropriate manner.
_____ 12. Clearly states the reason for the visit.
_____ 13. Allows a few moments of socialization before beginning the visit.

_____ 14. Smiles, speaks in a pleasant, friendly tone of voice, and maintains eye contact.
_____ 15. Uses aseptic technique when providing nursing care.
_____ 16. Respects the dignity, privacy, safety, and comfort of family members.
_____ 17. Listens attentively to ascertain what family members are saying or implying.
_____ 18. Converses with family members during the home visit.
_____ 19. Communicates accurate and meaningful information to family members.
_____ 20. Responds to family members in a way that encourages them to continue talking.
_____ 21. Uses appropriate words of explanation for family member understanding.
_____ 22. Utilizes opportunities for incidental teaching.
_____ 23. Commends progress made by individual family members.
_____ 24. Explains nursing measures before, during, and after each procedure.
_____ 25. Shares the results of nursing measures with family members when indicated.
_____ 26. Closes the home visit by summarizing the main points of the visit.
_____ 27. Makes plans for the next visit, considering family member wishes.

Evaluation

_____ 28. Utilizes information gathered on the home visit to plan care for next visit.
_____ 29. Documents home visit in an appropriate and timely manner.
_____ 30. Completes a self-evaluation of the home visit.

◆ Young mothers often have lots of questions about their new babies. Having a nurse come to the home provides an opportunity for the mother to ask questions and for the nurse to show the mother things she may not know about her baby.

The nurse needs to ask explicit directions to where the family is staying. The referral may have a different address, and the family may forget to mention that they are staying elsewhere.

Making the Visit

On locating and meeting the family, the following guidelines for initial contact should be used (Allender, 1998):

◆ Introduce yourself and explain the value to the family of the nursing services provided by the agency.
◆ Spend the first few minutes of the visit establishing cordiality and getting acquainted (a mutual discovery or "feeling out" time).

◆ Use acute observational skills.
◆ Be sensitive to verbal and nonverbal cues.
◆ Be adaptable and flexible (you may be planning a prenatal visit, but the woman delivered her baby the day after you made the appointment, and now there is a newborn).
◆ Use your "sixth sense" as a guide regarding family responses, questions they ask, and your personal safety (trust your feelings).
◆ Be aware of your own personality; balance talking and listening, and be aware of your nonverbal behaviors.
◆ Be aware that most clients are not acutely ill and have higher levels of wellness than are generally seen in acute care settings.
◆ Become acquainted with all family and household members if you are making a home visit.
◆ Encourage each person to speak for himself.
◆ Be accepting and listen carefully.
◆ Help the family focus on issues and move toward the desired goals.

◆ After the body of the visit is over, review the important points, emphasizing family strengths.
◆ Plan with the family for the next visit.

The length and primary focus of the visit will vary depending on its purpose. As a general guide, if the visit is shorter than 20 minutes, it probably should be folded into another visit (unless you are offering a piece of very important information, providing supplies, or have come at the family's request). On the other hand, if the visit exceeds 1 hour, it should be conducted over two visits. Families have routines that are important to them, and taking a large portion of time out of their day may lead to resentment, putting future visits in jeopardy. Similarly, if nothing of value (according to the family) occurs on a visit, family members may not continue to make themselves available for future visits. This becomes a balancing act for the family and the nurse, and it is an area in which using your sixth sense and picking up on nonverbal cues is helpful (Zerwekh, 1997). In addition, home visits are an expensive way to provide community health nursing services, which are community-based. The outcome of better health for family members must be demonstrated in order to support the value of such costly services (see Evidence-Based Practice).

Concluding and Documenting the Visit

After planning for the next visit, saying goodbye to the family members terminates the home visit. This is a good time to put away the paperwork, materials, and supplies from this visit and retrieve items needed for the next visit on your schedule. It is always safer to open your trunk in front of this home and get out what is needed for the next family's visit than to open your trunk in front of the next family's home. You do not want to give community members information about what is stored in your car's trunk while it is unattended and you are in the family's home.

Most typically, the documentation of each home visit is completed as soon as the nurse returns to the agency. Some agencies provide their nurses with laptop computers and electronic charting forms, and charting is encouraged at the end of the visit before leaving for the next one. Sometimes, time is allowed for the nurse to chart at home after the last visit of the day. For the most part, you will be expected to complete the charting by hand, using agency forms, as soon as is practically possible. Most agencies expect all charting to be completed by the end of each workday or not later than the end of the work week.

Agencies use a variety of forms that assist the nurse to document fully and succinctly. On some forms, the nurse uses code numbers, letters, or checkmarks on developmental or disease-specific care plans that are devised in a checklist format. For example, a packet of four pages may be used to document a postpartum visit and newborn assessment: two narrative forms to chart the expectations for the mother and baby, and postpartum newborn assessment forms on which head-to-toe assessment information is documented. These forms contain a place to document parent or client teaching according to expected parameters and a place for listing other professional's involvement with the family. Similar developmentally focused forms may be used in the agency for high-risk infants, high-risk children, adolescents, and older adults. Other packets of

EVIDENCE-BASED PRACTICE

Prenatal and Infancy Home Visits

The Nurse–Family Partnership (NFP) has a long history of providing prenatal and infancy home visits by nurses to first time at-risk mothers. The goal of this program is to prevent child abuse and neglect, children's mental health problems, and infant mortality through home visiting during the first 2 years of the child's life. Through randomized trials, the program has demonstrated positive results in various ethnic and racial groups and in a variety of living contexts.

To test the long-term effectiveness of this program, mothers enrolled in an earlier randomized trial who had received nurse visits ($n = 191$) and a control group ($n = 436$) were compared. By age 9 (7 years following the intervention), the nurse-visited women used welfare and food stamps for fewer months, had reduced rates of subsequent births along with increased intervals between births, and had more stable partner relationships. The children who received the nurse visits also demonstrated higher academic adjustment and a lower rate of preventable deaths prior to age 9. Both mother and child had demonstrable benefits from the nursing intervention.

Nursing Implications

Home visiting can be a costly effort for a community. The NFP has demonstrated that comprehensive home visiting by nurses can have a positive impact on both the mothers and the children. The cost savings in terms of reduced use of public assistance programs, reduced pregnancy rates, and delayed pregnancy can offset the operating costs of the program. In addition, the academic achievement of these children may ultimately prove beneficial to the long-term economic prospects of these at-risk children and the communities in which they live. Communities considering reducing or eliminating home visiting programs may want to consider retaining them or possibly implementing the NFP program.

Reference:

Olds, D.L., Kitzman, H., Hanks, C., Cole, R., Anson, E., Sidora-Arcoleo, K., et al. (2007). Effects of nurse home visiting on maternal and child functioning: Age-9 follow-up of a randomized trial. *Pediatrics, 120*, e832–e845.

forms may focus on chronic illness, such as chronic obstructive pulmonary disease, hypertension, diabetes, alcoholism, acquired immunodeficiency syndrome (AIDS), or cancer that are common in the agency client base.

Focus of Family Health Visits

The focus of family health visits depends on the mission and resources of the agency providing the service and the needs of the families being served. Some agencies provide education, recreational activities such as summer camps, and support groups for families of people with specific health problems such as Alzheimer's disease, asthma, diabetes, or neurologic disorders. Other agencies provide services directed toward those with special social or economic needs, such as immigrant families, people living in poverty, or the homeless. Home visits may be a part of the service being provided and are best conducted and received in the comfort and privacy of a family's home. In general, family health visits are designed to be educational, to provide anticipatory guidance, and to focus on health promotion or prevention.

Family Education and Anticipatory Guidance

Official agencies, such as county or city health departments, distribute their services based on the broader community's needs. For example, if there is a large population of teen pregnancies and high-risk infants, the health department may contract with hospitals and private doctors' offices to provide home or clinic visits to all teens and women with high-risk pregnancies and their newborns after delivery. On these visits, the community health nurse teaches prenatal, postpartum, and newborn care, and provides anticipatory guidance (information needed in the future regarding the child and the need for regular infant health care provider visits, immunizations, and safety awareness). Another community may have a significant number of older adults who need to learn how to manage a chronic illness, enhance their nutrition, and practice safety measures to prevent injuries and falls.

Family Promotion and Illness Prevention

All populations, regardless of age, income, culture, or nation of origin, need the fundamental protection immunization gives to protect themselves and the health of the larger community. In addition, providing the means for families to receive required immunizations is a responsibility of health departments. Usually, immunization services are not brought into the home, but the nurse can provide information about immunizations, teach the importance of following an immunization schedule, and follow up with the client during home visits.

Teaching people how to prevent illness and how to remain healthy is basic to community health nursing (see Chapter 11). Even within the limitations of chronic illnesses, family members can be taught health promotion activities to live as healthfully as possible (Denham, 2002; Pender, Murdaugh, & Parson, 2006). Health promotion activities may include screening for hypertension and elevated cholesterol, performing a physical assessment, and teaching about nutrition and safety. The American Nurses Association's 2007 *Public Health Nursing: Scope and Standards of Practice* highlights this role in the following statement: "When public health nurses partner with individuals, the focus becomes the promotion of knowledge, attitudes, beliefs, practices, and behaviors that support and enhance health, with the ultimate goal of improving the overall health of the population" (p. 7).

Such activities can occur during a family health visit; while family members are at their place of work, school, or recreation; or at self-help group meetings. Community health nurses provide health promotion services to couples during prenatal classes by teaching about the expected changes during pregnancy and providing anticipatory guidance for safe infant care. They may also screen older adults

at senior centers for hypertension or elevated cholesterol, or teach family members who attend support groups, such as Alcoholic Anonymous.

Personal Safety on the Home Visit

As mentioned earlier in this chapter, personal safety while traveling throughout the community is essential. In addition, continuation of personal safety while on the home visit must be considered.

Personal Safety While Traveling and in the Neighborhood

On leaving your "base of operation," such as the health department office, neighborhood clinic, homeless shelter, or campus classroom, have with you all the necessary tools to travel in the community with safety. Most importantly, leave an itinerary of your planned travels, the telephone numbers of families you will attempt to visit, and your cellular phone number. Traveling in the community takes a variety of forms and means different things to different people.

If you are traveling in an agency or private car, you need:

- ◆ A full gas tank
- ◆ A city/county map
- ◆ A cellular phone
- ◆ The family addresses
- ◆ Money for lunch or telephone calls (in case you are in an area where your cellular phone does not work)

If you are using public transportation, plan to

- ◆ Have exact change for each bus trip
- ◆ Carry a bus schedule
- ◆ Exit the bus as near as possible to your client's home
- ◆ Know where to get the bus for the return trip or to the next home visit
- ◆ Carry a cellular phone

If you are walking or riding a bicycle to a home visit, you still need to travel safely. In some neighborhoods, it is best to call ahead to the family you plan to visit, give them an approximate time of your arrival, and if necessary, ask them to watch out for your arrival. When walking in neighborhoods, walk with direction and purpose; do not look lost even if you are. Use neighborhood shopkeepers as resources for direction and information and as refuge if you feel uncomfortable or threatened. If you need to ask for directions, and you are not near any stores, look for another professional, such as a social worker, a public service employee (postal or utility worker), or an apartment manager. If you need to approach a stranger for information, select a woman. If you see a group of people that makes you feel uncomfortable, cross the street, limit eye contact, and continue to the home you are intending to visit. Always avoid walking through alleys or along buildings that open onto alleys, and stay in the middle of the sidewalk or closer to the street. It might be helpful to carry a whistle on your key ring.

It is always safest to avoid compromising situations by staying alert and using safe traveling methods whenever you are in public, no matter how "safe" the area appears. However, if an individual or group accosts you, immediately try to break free and run to a public place while making loud noises. Yell "Fire!" This response gets more attention than "Help!" If a criminal wants your nursing bag, purse, or wallet, freely give it up; the contents are not worth your safety. Some nurses feel safer after they have attended self-defense classes, which are offered by police departments, as employee in-service programs in some agencies, and on some university campuses.

In some rough inner-city neighborhoods, professionals visiting families travel only in pairs (usually with at least one male in the pair) or with a security guard or police escort. Know whether these resources are necessary or available to you before venturing into a crime-ridden community. In some inner-city neighborhoods, community health nurses refuse to visit people living on one block or in one apartment building. Similar issues are found in rural areas known for drug manufacturing and distribution. Know and do not challenge important safety measures that are used by expert nurses and are followed for personal safety. Safety issues are unique to each community.

Another focus of concern is the perceived risk to self when making a home visit. An individual's cognition and perception of a situation, his views on risk taking, and the time, setting, and coping process all factor into feelings of safety when traveling in a community, entering a family's home, or conducting a home visit (Kendra & George, 2001). What one person sees as a risk, another sees as a challenge or an opportunity. Yet another may see nothing. We each perceive risks differently based on knowledge, experience, and personality.

Arriving at the Home

Make sure you are at the right house, and do not go into the home until you are assured that the family you are intending to visit does live there and is home. For example, you may be planning to visit 16-year-old Jennifer and her 5-day-old infant, Marcus. However, when you knock, a 50-year-old man answers the door. Do not enter the house without asking whether Jennifer can come to the door or you can see her, even if he invites you in. Remain outside the home and go inside only after you talk to Jennifer at the door. This precaution ensures that the family members you want to visit are really home and that this is the right address.

Friction Between Family Members

During a home visit, two or more family members may begin to argue or physically fight with one another. Immediately remove yourself from the home visit, let the family know that with such distraction it is not a good time to visit, and that you will return at another time. Never step in and offer to assist an adult family member when two people are physically fighting; you may be the next victim. If necessary, call 911 from your cellular phone once you are out of the house. Depending on the type of altercation, it may be appropriate to discuss the friction in the family at a later visit.

Family Members Under the Influence

If the focus of the visit is on two family members and a third member is demonstrating behaviors that indicate drug or alcohol use, you must use your judgment as to the best action to take. The agency you work for or the school you attend has guidelines you should follow. If the intoxicated person goes to another room, it might be appropriate to continue the visit and perhaps discuss your observations with the remaining family members. If the person becomes abusive, remains in the room, or interrupts the visit it is best to terminate the visit and reschedule when the family member is not under the influence or is not present. You do not want to put yourself in the middle of a situation that could deteriorate rapidly and compromise your safety.

The Presence of Strangers

In some families, the coming and going of many extended family members, neighbors, and friends is common; it is the norm and is not distracting to them, but it may be to the nurse. For example, what would you do if you arrived at a home and five teenage boys were sitting on the front porch steps, so that you had to edge your way past them to the door? What if you found three men sleeping on the living room floor in the small apartment of a teenage mother and her infant, or four neighbor children riding their tricycles inside the house during a teaching visit to two young parents who do not seem fazed by the commotion? These situations may not be indicative of danger, but they can make you feel vulnerable, uncomfortable, or distracted from the purpose of the visit. Inquire about the people you observe in the periphery of the home visit; ask about their relationship to the family and whether they should be included in the visit. The family may suggest that you ignore the other people or say they are transient family members. It may be important to learn who they are and if they have unmet health care needs or their presence influences the health of the family you are visiting.

EFFECTS OF FAMILY HEALTH ON THE INDIVIDUALS

The health of each family member affects the other members and contributes to the level of **family health.** For example, a woman whose husband has had a stroke may cope successfully with the resulting physical and emotional demands of his care but may have inadequate reserves for effectively meeting the needs of her children. The level at which a family functions—how well it is able to solve problems and help its members reach their potential—significantly affects the individual's level of health (Early, 2001). A healthy family fosters individual growth and resistance to ill health and sustains members during times of crisis such as serious illness, emotional dilemmas, divorce, or death of a family member. On the other hand, a family with limited coping skills or an underdeveloped capacity for problem solving, self-management, or self-care is often unable to promote the potential of its members or assist them in times of need (Barnes, 2001; Donnelly, 2002; Reutter, 1997).

Family health standards and practices also influence each member's health. For instance, many individuals, even as adults, adhere to cultural and family patterns of eating, exercise, and communication. Cultural (see Chapter 5) and family values influence decisions about utilizing preventative health care as well as access to services such as immunizations, regular health assessments, or family planning. Family patterns also dictate whether members participate in their own health care and how they follow through and comply with professional advice. Individuals influence family health, and the family can either obstruct or facilitate individual health. The family becomes an important focus for community health nursing assessment and intervention.

CHARACTERISTICS OF HEALTHY FAMILIES

How does the community health nurse determine family health status? Analysis of how basic functions are met does not give a satisfactory picture of a family's health status. More definitive criteria are needed. Although it is difficult to define a "normal" family, studies have provided some standards that characterize a healthy family (Barker, 1998; Thompson, 1998). Over the years, research on families and on family health behavior has produced a growing body of data with which to assess family health.

In looking at families over the years, researchers have found many similar characteristics. Otto (1973) identified characteristics of family unity, loyalty and interfamily cooperation, support and security, role flexibility, and constructive relationships with community. Olson, McCubbin, Barnes, and colleagues (1983) identified seven major family strengths that are important for family functioning and coping with crisis: family pride, family support, cohesion, adaptability, communication, religious orientation, and social support. Becvar and Becvar (2003) listed the following characteristics: (a) a legitimate source of authority that is supported and consistent over time, (b) a stable and consistent system of rules, (c) consistent and regular nurturing behaviors, (d) effective child-rearing practices, (e) stable and well-maintained marriages, (f) a set of agreed-upon goals toward which the family and individuals work, and (g) sufficient flexibility to change in the face of both expected and unexpected stressors. Parachin (1997) identified six signs of a healthy family: maintaining a spiritual foundation, making the family a top priority, asking for and giving respect, communicating and listening, valuing service to others, and expecting and offering acceptance. Rucibwa, Modeste, and Montgomery (2003) found significant relationships between family characteristics and sexual attitudes and behaviors among Black and Hispanic adolescent males.

Six important characteristics of healthy families that consistently emerge in the literature (Becvar & Becvar, 2003; Freidman et al., 2003; Parachin, 1997) are:

1. A facilitative process of interaction exists among family members.
2. Individual member development is enhanced.
3. Role relationships are structured effectively.
4. Active attempts are made to cope with problems.
5. There is a healthy home environment and lifestyle.
6. Regular links with the broader community are established.

Healthy Interaction Among Members

Healthy families communicate. Their patterns of interaction are regular, varied, and supportive. Adults communicate with adults, children with children, and adults with children (Anderson & Sabatelli, 2003). These interactions are frequent and assume many forms. Healthy families use frequent verbal communication. They discuss problems, confront each other when angry, share ideas and concerns, and write or call each other when separated. They also communicate frequently through nonverbal means, particularly those families from cultural or subcultural groups that are less verbal. There are innumerable ways to convey feelings and thoughts without words, including smiling encouragingly, embracing warmly, frowning disapprovingly, being available, withdrawing for privacy, doing an unsolicited favor, serving refreshments, and giving a gift. The family that has learned to communicate effectively has members who are sensitive to one another. They watch for cues and verify messages to ensure understanding. This kind of family recognizes and deals with conflicts as they arise. Its members have learned to share and to work collaboratively with each other.

Effective communication is necessary for a family to carry out basic functions. Family members must communicate to demonstrate affection and acceptance, to promote identity and affiliation, and to guide behavior through socialization and social controls. Just as there is a correlation between a high degree of communication and a high degree of effectiveness in organizational functioning, facilitative communication patterns within a family promote the health and development of its members. Healthy families are more likely than unhealthy families to negotiate topics for discussion, use humor, show respect for differences of opinion, and clarify the meaning of one another's communications.

Enhancement of Individual Development

Healthy families are responsive to the needs of individual members and provide the freedom and support necessary to promote each member's growth. If a father in a healthy family loses his job, the family will work to support his ego and help him use his energy constructively to adjust and find new work. The healthy family recognizes and fosters the growing child's need for independence by increasing opportunities for the child to try new things alone. This kind of family can tolerate differences of opinion or lifestyle. Each member is accepted unconditionally, and the right to be an individual is respected. Within an appropriate framework of stability and structure, the healthy family encourages freedom and autonomy for its members (Friedman et al., 2003).

Patterns of promoting individual member development vary from one family to another depending on cultural orientation. The way in which autonomy is expressed in an Italian American family differs from its expression in a Native American family, yet each family can promote freedom and autonomy. The result is an increase in competence, self-reliance, social skills, intellectual growth, and overall capacity for self-management among family members (Wright & Leahey, 2005) (see From the Case Files).

Effective Structuring of Relationships

Healthy families structure role relationships to meet changing family needs over time (Hanson, 2001). In a stable social context, some families establish member roles and tasks (e.g., breadwinner, primary decision-maker, homemaker) that are maintained as workable patterns throughout the life of the family. Families in rural areas, isolated communities, or religious and subcultural groups are more likely than others to retain role consistency, because they face little or no external pressure or need to change. For example, the Amish

From the Case Files

A Family Assessment: Meeting Hector's Needs

You are a home health nurse working in Smithville. You have been given a referral for a new client, Hector. Hector is being released from the rehabilitation unit of Metropolis Hospital. Although he lives in Smithville, Metropolis Hospital was the only facility willing to accept a Medicaid client with a severe spinal cord injury.

Hector is a 19-year-old Hispanic man who sustained major injury to his spinal cord (T-4 injury) in a motorcycle accident. The injury occurred approximately 6 weeks ago. Hector has been diagnosed as paraplegic with some residual limitation of upper body strength and mobility.

Your job is to facilitate Hector's transition from the hospital to the home environment. You will be teaching Hector and his caregivers about the following:

1. Nutrition and fluid intake
2. Signs and symptoms warranting follow-up
3. Medication administration
4. Bowel and bladder care
5. Skin care
6. Activities of daily living (ADLs), self-care with sensory-motor deficits
7. Safety/injury prevention
8. Community resources
9. Rehabilitative services
10. Anticipatory guidance about grief, anger, and suicidal ideations; sexual function; fear of abandonment, role change, and social isolation; and altered family processes.

Following is a synopsis of information obtained during your initial visit with Hector and his family in their home.

Visit One. Hector lives in a migrant labor camp located on the outskirts of Smithville. His family has resided in the camp for 18 years. Living in the two-bedroom cabinlike home are:

- Hector
- Hector's uncle Manuel (32 years old). Manuel's job is seasonal; he has been offered a temporary job for a much higher salary, working out of state.
- Hector's brother Efran (16 years old). Efran is considering dropping out of high school in order to assist with the care of his family. His goal is to become an auto mechanic. He is fluent in both Spanish and English.
- Manuel's wife Micaela (29 years old). Micaela was a teacher in Mexico. She is extremely supportive of her family. She is concerned about the possibility of another pregnancy but does not believe in the use of birth control.
- Manuel and Micaela's children, Arturo (5 years old) and Jasmin (6 months old). Arturo begins a Head Start Program soon and will be gone for 5 hours each day. Jasmin is a healthy baby; she continues to be breast fed and is thriving at home.
- Hector's 74-year-old paternal grandmother (Abuela), who has recently arrived from Mexico and plans on assiting in Hector's care. Abuela has congestive heart failure and arthritis. She is not a legal resident of the United States and is not eligible for medical assistance.

The whereabouts of Hector's mother are unknown; she moved from their village in Mexico shortly after Efran was born. She has remarried and started another family. She has had no contact with Hector or Efran. Hector's father lives in their home village in Mexico. Although he lived in the migrant camp in Smithville for many years, he recently remarried and has two young daughters in Mexico. Hector's father is aware of Hector's injury and has no plans to return to the United States.

Your ability to speak fluent Spanish has enabled you to solicit the above information. Manuel has provided you with most of the information. He has been very involved in Hector's recovery through daily visits to the rehabilitation unit and frequent discussions with Hector's health care providers. Manuel tells you that "Hector is like a son to me . . . I have a responsibility to my older brother to watch over his son. My brother watched out for me when I was young . . . he even left school to work to help support our family." Manuel adds, "We don't have much but we will take care of Hector . . . we'll all work together."

You begin your discussion by explaining your role as home health nurse. You inform the family about the type of education and interventions you are able to provide. You ask Hector and the family to tell you what they have learned from the health care team at the rehabilitation unit and what plans have been developed by the family to address Hector's medical and psychosocial needs. As you begin the visit you notice that Hector's grandmother is sitting quietly in the corner of the room rocking Jasmin. You learn that Efran is working in the fields. Arturo is in school. Manuel, Micaela, and Abuela are participating in the home visit this morning. The conversation is as follows.

Nurse: Hector, can you tell me how you feel about being home?

(continued)

Hector (looks at Micaela): Okay, I guess.

Micaela: He's a little scared, I think. He feels like it's going to be too much for us to deal with.

Nurse (looking at Hector): There's so much happening right now, so much to think about . . .

Hector: Uh-huh.

(Hector is maintaining eye contact with Manuel and Micaela only; since this is your initial visit to the home you feel that Hector may be more comfortable in the role of observer.)

Nurse (looking at Manuel and Micaela): Do you have any questions before we begin?

Micaela: They gave us a lot of information at the hospital... I'm most afraid about if the phone doesn't work and Hector needs help. What if something happens to Hector and I can't call anyone? That's the only thing I worry about.

Abuela: If anything happens to him I'll be right here with you, "mija." We can do this, we can take care of Hector if we work together.

Manuel: There is a store with a phone only two blocks away, if you needed to you could call from there. What I want to know is how we can get Hector into school or something that will help him to be around kids his own age. His English is good enough, he even finished high school. He needs to be ready to make a future for himself.

Hector (grins and looks at Manuel): Right, uncle, that is what I want, too.

You continue the conversation by revisiting Micaela's concerns about access to a telephone in case of an emergency. You ask specific questions about her concerns and use this as an opportunity to educate the family about circumstances warranting immediate follow-up. Together you decide that Micaela will develop a list of specific concerns that you will review together at a subsequent visit planned for 2 days from today.

Today's visit consists of:
- I. Assessment
  - A. Home environment
    1. Safety
    2. ADLs
  - B. Knowledge of disease processes
  - C. Fluid volume balance
  - D. Nutritional resources of family
    1. Food availability
    2. Food preparation
  - E. Insurance and financial status
- II. Education
  - A. Medications
  - B. Warning signs and symptoms and appropriate follow-up procedures
  - C. Bowel and bladder care
  - D. Hygiene prior to and following patient care

The plan for your visit in 2 days includes:
- I. Referrals
  - A. Community resources
  - B. Educational opportunities
  - C. Support groups (Spanish speaking)
  - D. Peer group opportunities for Hector
- II. Assessment
  - A. Continuation of above
- III. Education
  - A. Continuation of above

Questions
1. What is the social structure of this family (traditional versus nontraditional)? Be specific about the type of traditional or nontraditional family system that exists in this scenario.
2. Discuss an example of triangulation in this scenario.
3. What essential functions are present within this family system?
4. What developmental stages appear to have been achieved?
5. What steps will you take in order to empower the family to make their own decisions?
6. List the strengths of the family.
7. Prioritize Hector's issues—medical and psychosocial.
8. Prioritize issues facing the other family members.
9. Identify mutual goals for this family:
   Immediate
   Mid-range
   Long-term
10. What community health nursing interventions will you utilize to achieve these mutual goals?

community in Pennsylvania has maintained marked differentiation in family roles for more than 100 years.

In a technologically advanced society such as the United States, most families must adapt their roles to changing family needs created by external forces. As women enter the workforce, family roles, relationships, and tasks change to meet the demands of the new situation. Many husbands assume more homemaking responsibilities; fathers engage in child rearing, children along with adults in their families share decision-making and a more equal distribution of power. The latter may be essential for the survival of a single-parent family, in which the children must assume adult responsibilities while the parent works to support the family (Baris et al., 2001).

Changing life cycle stages require alterations in the structure of relationships. The healthy family recognizes members' changing developmental needs and adapts parenting roles, family tasks, and controls to fit each stage (Anderson & Sabatelli, 2003). For example, household chores of increasing complexity and responsibility are assigned as children become capable of handling them. Rules of conduct relax as members learn to govern their own behavior.

Active Coping Effort

Healthy families actively attempt to overcome life's problems and issues. When faced with change, they assume responsibility for coping and seek energetically and creatively to meet the demands of the situation (Becvar & Becvar, 2003; Olson et al., 1983). Coping skills are needed to deal with emotional tragedies such as substance abuse problems, serious illness, or death. If a family member has a substance abuse problem, the family may seek counseling and treatment opportunities involving all family members. If a family member is seriously ill, the family may ask for and accept assistance from extended family members or community health care workers. In the event of death in the family, receiving consolation and support from one another and from relatives and friends is an important step in the healing process. The healthy family recognizes the need for assistance, accepts help, and pursues opportunities to eliminate or decrease the stressors that affect it.

More frequently, healthy families cope with less dramatic, day-to-day changes. For instance, one family may cope with the increased cost of food by cutting down on meat consumption, substituting other protein foods, and eating in restaurants less frequently. Healthy families are open to innovation, support new ideas, and find ways to solve problems. One family may try to solve the problem of spending too much on transportation by cutting down on daily travel; this may cause additional problems if three members have jobs in different areas of town or need to go to school functions and meetings. Another family, responding to environmental concerns and a personal need for a healthier lifestyle, may explore and arrive at new ways to reach destinations by walking, bicycling, skating, or car-pooling to school or work. Healthy coping may go beyond finding a simple, obvious solution. Members may try to rearrange schedules to avoid frequent trips to regular destinations and plan ahead to avoid last-minute trips to stores. Healthy families actively seek and use a variety of resources to solve problems. They may discover these resources within the family or externally; they engage in self-care. For example, a professional couple, faced with the unaffordable expense of daytime baby-sitting, arranged their work schedules so that they could share childcare during the first 2 years. Later, they joined a cooperative preschool that allowed their child to attend daily, but required parental participation only 1 day a week. In another example, a single parent of five children, who was also a full-time nursing student, was able to finance two or three family outings each year by recycling aluminum cans that everyone in the family collected.

Healthy Environment and Lifestyle

Another sign of a healthy family is a healthy home environment and lifestyle. Healthy families create safe and hygienic living conditions for their members. For instance, a healthy family with young children "childproofs" the home by removing potential hazards such as exposed electric outlets and cleaning solvents from the child's reach. A healthy family with an older adult who is prone to falls installs lighting and handrails (Farren, 1999). A healthy home environment is one that is clean and reduces the spread of disease-causing organisms.

A healthy family lifestyle encourages appropriate balance in the lives of its members. In an ideal family, there is activity and rest sufficient for the energy needs of daily living; the diet offered is varied and nutritionally sound, physical activity maintains ideal weight while promoting cardiac health; preventative hygiene habits are taught and followed by family members; emotional and mental health are encouraged through a support network of caring others; and family members seek out and use health care services and demonstrate adherence to recommended regimens.

The emotional climate of a healthy family is positive and supportive of growth. Contributing to this healthful emotional climate is a strong sense of shared values, often combined with a strong religious orientation (Olson et al., 1983; Parachin, 1997). A healthy family demonstrates caring, encourages and accepts expression of feelings, and respects divergent ideas. Members can express their individuality in the way they dress or decorate their rooms. The home environment makes family members feel welcome and accepted.

Regular Links with the Broader Community

Healthy families maintain dynamic ties with the broader community. They participate regularly in external groups and activities, often in a leadership capacity. They may join in local politics, participate in a church bazaar, or promote the school's paper drive to raise money for science equipment. They use external resources suited to family needs. For example, a farm family with teenagers, recognizing the importance of peer group influences on adolescents, becomes very active in the local 4-H Club. Another family, in which the father is out of work, joins a job transition support group. Healthy families also know what is going on in the world around them. They show an interest in current events and attempt to understand significant social, economic, and political issues. This ever-broadening outreach gives families knowledge of external forces that might influence their lives. It exposes them to a wider range of alternatives and a variety of contacts, which can increase options for finding resources and strengthen coping skills.

An unhealthy family has not recognized the value of establishing links with the broader community. This may be because of knowledge deficits regarding community resources, previous negative experiences with community services, or a lack of connection with the community due to family expectations or cultural practices.

It is important for the community health nurse to assess the family's relationship with the broader community, in addition to structural and developmental variations, interaction, coping strategies, and lifestyle. With a comprehensive family assessment, the nurse has a base from which to begin a plan of care.

FAMILY HEALTH PRACTICE GUIDELINES

Family nursing is a kind of nursing practice in which the family is the unit of service (Friedman et al., 2003). It is not merely a family-oriented approach, in which family concerns that affect the health of an individual are taken into account. Family nursing asks how one provides health care to a collection of people. It does not mean that nursing must relinquish the service to individuals. One of the distinct contributions of the nursing profession is its holistic approach to individual needs. Community health nurses rise to the challenge of adding a service to populations that include families.

Five principles guide and enhance family nursing practice: (1) work with the family collectively, (2) start where the family is, (3) adapt nursing interventions to the family's stage of development, (4) recognize the validity of family structural variations, and (5) emphasize family strengths.

Work with the Family Collectively

To practice family nursing, nurses must set aside their usual focus on the individual and remind themselves that several people together have a collective personality, collective interests, and a collective set of needs. Viewing a group of people as one unit may seem less strange if one considers the way in which business organizations are perceived. For example, you may think of a particular corporation as conservative or liberal. You may hear that a women's group has taken a stand on abortion or that a government agency needs to become better organized. In each case, the group is viewed collectively as a single entity with attributes and activities in common. So it is with families. A family has its own personality, interests, and needs.

As much as possible, community health nurses want to involve all the family's members during nurse–client interactions (Wallace, Green, Jaros, Paine, & Story, 1999; Wright & Leahey, 2005). This approach reinforces the importance of each individual member's contributions to total family functioning. Nurses want to encourage everyone's participation in the work that the nurse and the family jointly agree to do. Like a coach, the nurse wants to help family members work together as a team for their collective benefit. Consider how a nurse might work collectively with the Beck family (Display 19.2).

Start Where the Family Is

When working with families, community health nurses begin at the present, not the ideal level of functioning. To discover where a family is, the community health nurse first conducts a family assessment to ascertain the members' needs and level of health and then determines collective interests, concerns, and priorities. The accompanying description of the Kovac family illustrates this principle (Display 19.3).

DISPLAY 19.2	THE BECK FAMILY

A community health nurse had an initial contact with Mr. and Mrs. Beck and their youngest child at the well-baby clinic. The 9-month-old child was over the 95th percentile for weight and at the 40th percentile for height. The nurse also noted that both parents were obese. The nurse asked about the eating patterns in the family and of the baby in particular and suggested a home visit to determine whether the Becks were interested in family nursing. The nurse explained the purpose of home visits (to assess all family members, coping patterns, eating patterns, and food purchasing choices) and the importance of including all family members, and asked for a time that would be good for the family as a whole. The nurse explained that each person should be involved and committed to the agreed-upon goals; that, like a team of oarsmen, the family would have to pull together to accomplish the purpose of the visits. To help the Beck family improve its nutritional status, the nurse might suggest a session of brainstorming to uncover many causes of poor nutrition. More brainstorming might result in solutions and plans for action. On each visit the nurse would view the Becks as a group. Group responses and actions would be expected. Evaluation of outcomes would be based on what the family did collectively. The Becks were interested, and a home visit date was made.

Adapt Nursing Intervention to the Family's Stage of Development

Although every family engages in the same basic functions, the tasks necessary to accomplish these functions vary with each stage of the family's development. A young family, for instance, can appropriately meet its members' affiliation needs by establishing mutually satisfying relationships and meaningful communication patterns. As the family enters later stages, bonds change with the release of some members into new families and the loss of others through death. Awareness of the family's developmental stage enables the nurse to assess the appropriateness of the family's level of functioning and to tailor interventions accordingly. Nurses are often adept at family assessment, but interventions need to be the focus (Hanson, 2001; Wright & Leahy, 2005). A nurse's work with the Ravina family illustrates this need (Display 19.4).

Recognize the Validity of Family Structure Variations

Many families seen by community health nurses are nontraditional, such as single-parent families and unmarried couples (Baris et al., 2001; Scanzoni, 1999). Other families are organized around nontraditional patterns, for example both parents may have careers, a husband may care for children at home while his wife financially supports the family, or both parents may telecommute and work at home. Such variations in structure and organizational patterns have resulted from social and technologic changes in employment practices, welfare programs, economic conditions, gender roles,

DISPLAY 19.3 THE KOVAC FAMILY

Marcia Kovac brought her baby. Tiffany, to the well-child clinic once but failed to keep further appointments. Concerned that the family might be having other difficulties, Sara Villa, a community health nurse, made a home visit. The mobile home was cluttered and dirty; the baby was crying in her playpen. Marcia seemed uninterested in the nurse's visit. She listened politely but had little to say. She repeated that everything was okay and that the baby was doing fine, explaining that she was just fussy because she was teething. As they talked, Marcia's husband Henry, a delivery van driver, stopped by to pick up a sports magazine to read on his lunch hour. The three of them discussed the problems of inflation and how expensive it was to raise a child. Sara reminded them that the clinic was free and that they could at least get good health care without extra cost. They agreed without enthusiasm. After Henry left, the nurse spent the remainder of the visit discussing infant care with Marcia, particularly emphasizing regular checkups and immunizations.

The next visit also focused on the baby, but Sara had an uncomfortable feeling that this family was not really interested in her help. After consulting her supervisor, the nurse did what she wished she had done in the first place. She asked to talk with Marcia and Henry together and explained frankly why she had come to their home and what she could offer in the way of counseling, teaching, support, and referral to other community resources. She then asked them what problems or concerns they had. The Kovacs were more than responsive and described their financial difficulties and feelings of isolation from family and friends. They were new in the city, and both their families lived some distance away on farms. The neighbors were friendly but not close enough to confide in. They believed they would eventually overcome their problems if they just had "someone to lean on," as they put it.

Now Sara could address the Kovacs' primary needs and concerns for friends and emotional support. The nurse began to address the Kovacs' social needs first and introduced them to a young couples' group that met at the community center. Sara continued to make periodic home visits and shared additional information about community services that the Kovacs might find helpful. She praised Marcia and Henry for following up on immunizations for Tiffany. Over time, Sara saw differences in the family's interest in their relationship with the community and their connection to its services. Sara realized that before she could address the issue of Tiffany's health, she needed to address the emotional health of the parents.

status of women and minorities, birth control, incidence of divorce, and even war. Such variations in family structure and organization lead to revised patterns of family functioning. Member roles and tasks often differ dramatically from our expectations. Examples are a family with a single parent who works full-time while raising children or a dual-career marriage in which both partners have undifferentiated roles. Community health nurses, many of whom are accustomed to traditional family patterns, must learn to understand and accept these variations in family structure and organization in order to address the needs of the families.

There are two important principles to remember. First, what is normal for one family is not necessarily normal for another. Each family is unique in its combination of structures, composition, roles, and behaviors. As long as a family carries out its functions effectively and demonstrates the characteristics of a healthy family, one must agree that its form, no matter how variant, is valid.

DISPLAY 19.4 THE RAVINA FAMILY

The Ravinas, a couple in their early 70s, recently moved to a retirement complex. They received nursing visits after Mrs. Ravina's stroke 3 years earlier but requested service now because Mr. Ravina was feeling "poorly" all the time. He though that perhaps his diet and lack of activity might be the cause and hoped the nurse would have some helpful suggestions. The couple had eagerly awaited Mr. Ravina's retirement from teaching, planning to be lazy, travel, visit all their children, and do all those things they never had time to do when they were young. Now neither of them seemed to have enough energy or the capacity to enjoy their new life. The move from their home of 28 years had been difficult: they were still trying to find space in the tiny apartment for their cherished books and mementos, although they had given many of them away.

Ronald Bell, a community health nurse, recognized that the Ravinas were experiencing a situational crisis (leaving their home of 28 years), a developmental crisis (aging and entering retirement), and perhaps some underlying health problems. Many of the Ravinas' expectations for this new life stage were unrealistic; they had not adequately prepared themselves for the adjustments that the loss of their home and retirement would demand. Through discussion Ronald was able to help the Ravinas understand their situation and express their feelings. He competed physical assessments on the Ravinas and encouraged regular follow-up with their health care provider. He also helped them join a support group of retired persons who were experiencing some of the same difficulties. Because this nurse was able to help the Ravinas through their crisis in a supportive and nonjudgmental manner, he found them receptive later to discussing preparation for the inevitable loss and bereavement that would occur when one of them died. He was adapting his nursing intervention to this family's stage of development.

Second, families are constantly changing. Marriage transforms two people into a married couple without children. Adding children changes the family structure. Divorce alters the structure and roles. Remarriage with the addition of children from another family changes the family again. Children grow up and leave the home while the parents, together or singly, are left to adjust to yet another family structure. Throughout the life cycle, a family seldom stays the same for very long. Each of these changes forces a family to adapt to its circumstances. Consider the young women with a baby whose husband deserts her: she has no choice but to assume a single-parent role. Each change also creates varying degrees of stress and demands considerable adaptive energy on the family's part. Many family changes are predictable and part of the normal life-cycle growth. Some changes are not predictable or may have a less traditional structure. The nurse's responsibility is to help families cope with the changes while remaining nonjudgmental and accepting of variations in family structure. For example, homosexual unions may be difficult for some nurses to deal with, particularly if they conflict with the nurse's own set of values. Yet the nurse's responsibility remains the same—to help promote the collective health of that family. The nurse should view all families as unique groups, each with its own set of needs and whose interests can best be served through unbiased care. Consider the nurse's work with James Cutler and Brian Hoag (Display 19.5).

DISPLAY 19.5	JAMES CUTLER AND BRIAN HOAG

James Cutler and Brian Hoag have a 6-year monogamous relationship. A homosexual couple, they worked with an attorney to privately adopt a child. The arrangements were completed and their 2-week-old son, Adrian, arrived in their home last week. Helen Jeffers, a community health nurse, receives a referral from the county hospital where Adrian was born. The request is for an assessment of the home situation and parenting skills. The baby tested positive for cocaine with Apgar scores of 6 and 8 and had some inital difficulty sucking. Birth weight was 2,900 g. Discharge weight, at 3 days, was 2,850 g. At her first home visit Helen finds a neat and orderly two-bedroom condominium, well-equipped with baby supplies. The infant has gained 200 g and is being well cared for by two fatigued parents who had had limited contact with infants previously. James and Brian have many questions and are anxious learners. Helen plans with the couple to make weekly home visits to assess infant growth and development, provide support, and answer questions. She also suggests a neighborhood parenting class and finding a reliable babysitter, and she helps James and Brian develop an infant care work schedule. After 6 weeks of intervention, Adrian is thriving; Helen closes the case to home visits, feeling confident that the parents' goal of becoming knowledgeable and confident has been achieved.

Empowering Families

Throughout the family visit, you must remember that the ultimate goal is to assist the family in becoming independent of your services. This is accomplished through the approach used in conducting the visit. How you structure the nurse–client relationship also influences the outcomes. Four thoughts will help to clarify your working relationship with families:

◆ The family functioned in a manner that worked for them before you ever met them.
◆ If you ever feel obliged to do something for a family, consider who did this before you were available.
◆ Find family strengths even in the most deprived family situation.
◆ If you were in a similar situation, would you manage, cope, or function as well as the members of this family?

Many families have strengths that some middle-class nurses may overlook or interpret as weaknesses. It is the nurse's job to recognize the strengths in families and to help families recognize them as well. For example, some families borrow needed items (diapers, food, clothes) from each other, whereas others do not even recognize their next-door neighbors by sight. Children from large families often learn to physically care for one another and entertain themselves, whereas in some families with only one or two children the youngsters must constantly be entertained. The members of one family may take public transportation or walk to accomplish errands.

Too often, community health nurses tend to focus their attention on family weaknesses, looking for and referring to them as *needs* or *problems*. This negative emphasis can be devastating to a family and can undermine any hope of a therapeutic relationship between nurse and client. Families need their strengths reinforced. Emphasizing a family's strengths fosters a positive self-image, promotes self-confidence, and often helps a family feel better able to address other problems.

At times, community health nurses want to help families by taking one of the members to a doctor or to the store or by bringing a supply of formula or diapers. It might be a simple task, because you will be driving by the clinic anyway or there are extra cans of formula in the agency office, but will it promote the family's independence and self-sufficiency? It is a much better gift to promote the skill of planning ahead, so that the family may meet its own transportation needs (neighbors, family members, loose change saved for the bus, or even walking) or find ways to use formula supplies wisely. For example, bottles can be filled with only the amount the baby consumes, so that ounces are not wasted at each feeding. Unused formula should be kept refrigerated, so that it does not spoil, and care should be taken to make sure that infants are not overfed. The amount of formula consumed in 24 hours by the baby can be determined to ensure that the correct quantity is being provided. After a child reaches the appropriate age, foods and fluids other than formula may be provided. A can of powdered formula may be kept on hand for emergencies, and families may wish to switch to powdered formula if they are using the more expensive premixed or concentrated formulas. Once families learn these skills, crises will occur less frequently or will be managed more effectively.

Finally, you should always look for ways to genuinely praise families for managing in difficult situations. On a home visit, you can empower families by pointing out the positive aspects of their self-care and care giving, rather than pointing out what they do not do or have (Renpenning, Taylor, & Eisenhandler, 2003).

One helpful communication technique is **strengthening**. Verbally list the positive aspects of an otherwise negative situation in a natural and conversational manner. For example, a young woman, who is holding her baby, greets you at the door. You note that she has a dresser drawer on the floor next to her mattress for the baby to sleep in. They live in a sparsely furnished one-room apartment. She has two baby bottles and a limited assortment of baby clothes. Later during the first visit, you say, "Carlo looks so happy when you cuddle him in your arms, and you are considering his safety by letting him sleep in the dresser drawer next to your mattress. I notice you wash each bottle before making the formula, and you keep him warm in the sleeper and blanket. I think you are managing Carlo very well." In this brief scenario, you have mentioned, in a positive way, bonding, infant health and safety, and proper infant clothing. You have not mentioned the absence of furniture, a full set of bottles, or a layette of clothing. During the remainder of the visit, you discuss the services your agency can provide and assess whether any of them would be of interest to the young mother. This strengthening technique helps the nurse approach the family positively rather than with a condescending or punitive approach. And, in the above example, you have empowered this young mother to make decisions for her family and to use you as a resource and guide (Wright & Leahey, 2005).

If there is nothing positive the nurse can honestly say, he should be able at the very least to say that the family seems to be managing as best it can. This is not to say that the nurse should ignore problems. On the contrary, assessment should explore all aspects of family functioning to determine both strength and weaknesses. The nurse needs a total picture to achieve an adequate perspective in nursing care planning and to know when the family is ready to begin work on problems. Even as the nurse becomes more aware of a family's unhealthy behaviors, the emphasis should remain on the positive ones. Emphasizing strengths indicates to the clients they are important to the nurse.

Family strengths are traits that facilitate the ability of the family to meet the members' needs and the demands made by systems outside the family unit. Not all traits that appear positive are necessarily strengths. Before the nurse selects a trait to emphasize, the behavior should be examined closely to determine whether it is actually facilitating family functioning. A strong work orientation may be a strength when balanced with play and relaxation, but a family obsessed by work experiences this trait as a weakness. Whether a trait is considered a strength or weakness is determined by the amount of free choice, as opposed to compulsive drive, being exercised.

Some traits a nurse may consider as possible strengths are basic family functions, family developmental tasks, and characteristics of family health. For instance, a nurse might wish to note when a family meets its members' physical,

DISPLAY 19.6   THE STEVENSON FAMILY

The community health nurse, Keith Dow, made an initial home visit after referral by an outpatient physician who was concerned about possible child abuse. Alice Stevenson had brought her baby to the emergency room for treatment of a laceration on the baby's forehead. He had fallen off the table while she was changing him, she claimed. A bruise on his arm made the physician suspicious, but Alice explained it was caused by his older brother's rough play. The nurse opened the visit by stating that he was simply following up on the emergency room treatment and wanted to see how the baby was progressing. Keith made no mention of child abuse. He observed the mother and children closely, looking for small things to compliment Alice on (strengthening) while learning all he could about the family's background. Because the nurse appeared approving rather than suspicious or judgmental, Alice agreed to further visits. During a later visit, Alice admitted to the nurse that she had slapped the baby and her ring cut his forehead. She could not get him to stop crying, no matter what she did; she just could not endure it any longer, she said. There had been other times when she grabbed him roughly to pull him away from things he wasn't allowed to touch, causing bruises on his arms. Alice told the nurse that she had not planned this baby; when her husband found out she was pregnant, he had left her shortly before the baby was born. Like many abusive parents, Alice had unrealistic expectations of her children's behavior as well as very inadequate self-esteem (Ryan, 1997; Taylor & Kemper, 1998). Realizing that Alice would be particularly vulnerable to any criticism, the nurse concentrated on her strengths. Keith complimented her on how well she managed her home and dressed the children, on maintaining her job, and on reading to her 3-year-old son. It took many visits before Alice trusted the nurse, but in time they were able to discuss her feelings frankly and work toward improving this family's health. Keith got her to attend a support group for single parents and she began counseling. Emphasizing strengths had provided a bridge for Alice and assisted in bringing her into a helping relationship.

emotional, and spiritual needs; shows respect for members' various points of view; or fosters self-discipline in its children. An illustration of this principle is found in the family nursing care of the Stevensons (Display 19.6).

FAMILY HEALTH ASSESSMENT

The focus of each family visit is different. On a first visit, initial assessment data must be obtained in addition to helping the family set goals they want to accomplish. On subsequent visits, action and activities are taken to reach the goals. To assess a family's health in a systematic way, three tools are needed: (1) a conceptual framework on which to base the assessment, (2) a clearly defined set of assessment categories for data collection, and (3) a method for measuring a family's functional level.

Conceptual Frameworks

A **conceptual framework** is a set of concepts integrated into a meaningful explanation that helps one interpret human behavior or situations. Several conceptual frameworks have been used historically to study families (Hill & Hansen, 1960; Kantor & Lehr, 1975; Reiss, 1981). Beavers and Hampton (1990) and Anderson and Sabatelli (2003) have also published models describing family functioning. Three frameworks that are particularly useful in community health nursing are presented here: the interactional, structural–functional, and developmental frameworks.

The **interactional framework** describes the family as a unit of interacting personalities and emphasizes communication, roles, conflict, coping patterns, and decision-making processes. This framework focuses on internal relationships but neglects the family's interactions with the external environment.

The **structural–functional framework** describes the family as a social system relating to other social systems in the external environment, such as church, school, work, and the health care system. This framework examines the interacting functions of society and the family, considers family structure, and analyzes how a family's structure affects its function.

The **developmental framework** studies the family from a life-cycle perspective by examining members' changing roles and the tasks in each progression of life-cycle stage. This framework incorporates elements from interactional and structural–functional approaches, so that family structure, function, and interaction are viewed in the context of the environment at each stage of family development.

Others have combined these concepts in various ways to design family assessment and intervention models that focus on human–environmental interactions, interactional and structural-functional frameworks, self-care, responses to stressors, and a developmental framework.

The six characteristics of healthy families already discussed serve as an initial framework for assessing family health by a combination of interactional, structural–functional, and developmental concepts.

Data Collection Categories

When using a conceptual framework for family health assessment, the community health nurse selects specific categories for data collection. The amount of data that one can collect about any given family may be voluminous, perhaps more than necessary for the purposes of the assessment. The assessment process is lengthy, time-consuming, and ongoing. The nurse must gather the most essential on the first visit. By selecting one or two priority concerns of the family and the nurse, it is possible to focus assessment on these identified areas. The nurse then uses this information as a guide to obtaining additional information needed on subsequent visits.

Certain basic information is needed, however, to determine a family's health status and to design appropriate nursing interventions. From many sources in the family health literature, particularly Turk and Kerns (1985), Edelman and Mandle (2002), and Friedman and co-workers (2003), a list of 12 data collection categories has been generated. Table 19.1 lists the 12 categories, each grouped into one of three data sets: family strengths and self-care capabilities, family stresses and problems, and family resources.

1. *Family demographics* refer to such descriptive variables as a family's composition, its socioeconomic status, and the ages, education, occupation, ethnicity, and religious affiliations of members.
2. *Physical environment* data describe the geography, climate, housing, space, social and political structures, food availability and dietary patterns, and any other elements in the internal or external

TABLE 19.1 Categories of Data Collection for Family Health Assessment

Assessment Categories	Family Strengths and Self-care Abilities	Family Stresses and Problems	Family Resources
1. Family demographics			
2. Physical environment			
3. Psychological and spiritual environment			
4. Family structure/roles			
5. Family functions			
6. Family values and beliefs			
7. Family communication patterns			
8. Family decision-making patterns			
9. Family problem-solving patterns			
10. Family coping patterns			
11. Family health behavior			
12. Family social and cultural patterns			

physical environment that influence a family's health status.

3. *Psychological and spiritual environment* refers to affective relationships, mutual respect, support, promotion of members' self-esteem and spiritual development, and life satisfaction and goals.

4. *Family structure and roles* include family organization, socialization processes, division of labor, and allocation and use of authority and power.

5. *Family functions* refer to a family's ability to carry out appropriate developmental tasks and provide for members' needs.

6. *Family values and beliefs* influence all aspects of family life. Values and beliefs might deal with raising children, making and spending money, education, religion, work, health, and community involvement.

7. *Family communication patterns* include the frequency and quality of communication within a family and between the family and its environment.

8. *Family decision-making patterns* refer to how decisions are made in a family, by whom they are made, and how they are implemented.

9. *Family problem-solving patterns* describe how a family handles problems, who deals with them, the flexibility of a family's approach to problem-solving, and the nature of solutions.

10. *Family coping patterns* encompass how a family handles conflict and life changes, the nature and quality of family support systems, and family perceptions and responses to stressors.

11. *Family health behavior* refers to familial health history, current physical health status of family members, family use of health resources, and family health beliefs.

12. *Family social and cultural patterns* comprise family discipline and limit-setting practices; promotion of initiative, creativity, and leadership; family goal setting; family culture; cultural adaptations to present circumstances; and development of meaningful relationships within and outside the family.

Assessment Methods

Many different methods are used to assess families. These methods serve to generate information about selected aspects of family structure and function; the methods must match the purpose for assessment and are done in conjunction with the family. Assessing family health may be done informally through observation and occasional questioning, or it can take a more formal approach. Specific questions may be asked of each family member, and information such as health data and family history may be included. Physical data such as height, weight, pulses, temperature, and blood pressure are recorded on an assessment tool. The developmental level of the family will guide specific assessment questionnaires, tools, or tests that the community health nurse can use for gathering information on individuals within the family, for example, the use of developmental screening tests for young children or a high-risk infant flow sheet (Fig. 19.1) for a newborn with an identified or potential health problem (e.g., high-risk newborn, drug-exposed newborn, failure-to-thrive, birth-defect).

Two assessment tools are the eco-map and the genogram. The **eco-map** is a diagram of the connections between a family and the other systems in its ecologic environment. It was originally devised to depict the complexity of the client's story. Developed by Ann Hartman in 1975 to help child welfare workers study family needs, the tool visually depicts dynamic family–environment interactions. The nurse involves family members in the map's development. A central circle is drawn to represent the family, and smaller satellite circles on the periphery represent people and systems, such as school or work, whose relationships with the family are significant. The lines to and from the central circle to the satellite circle depicts the strength of the relationship (Fig. 19.2). The map is used to discuss and analyze these relationships (Hanson, Gedaly-Duff, & Kaakinen, 2005; Hartman, 1978; Wright & Leahey, 2005).

The **genogram** displays family information graphically in a way that provides a quick view of complex family patterns. It is a rich source of hypotheses about a family over a significant period of time, usually three or more generations (McGoldrick & Gerson, 1985). Family relationships are delineated by genealogic methods, and significant life events are included (e.g., birth, death, marriage, divorce, illness). Identifying characteristics (e.g., race, religion, social class), occupations, and places of family residence are also noted (Meyer, 1993). Again, this tool is used jointly with the family. It encourages family expression and sheds light on family behavior and problems (Fig. 19.3). Recognizing the value of this type of assessment, the *U.S. Surgeon General's Family History Initiative* was launched in 2005. This ongoing initiative seeks to bring awareness of the familial links between health outcomes and the need to develop prevention strategies based on potential health risks (U.S. Department of Health and Human Services [USDHHS], 2005). Using the downloadable materials provided on the website, families can create their own family heath portrait; this is also a valuable tool for the nurse to use with the family.

Community health nurses use several different family assessment instruments to gather data on family structure, function, and development. Public health nursing agencies usually develop their own tools, often in the form of questionnaires, checklists, flow sheets, or interview guides. The format varies to fit organizational needs. For example, most agencies have changed to computerized information management systems and have adjusted data collection to be technologically compatible. Two sample assessment tools are shown in Figures 19.4 and 19.5. Figure 19.4 shows a checklist format with scores and dates of assessment gathering. It is useful over a span of time for observing family growth or decline, especially for the novice community health nurse, who can document assessment data as rapport with the family is established or as the comfort level with home visits increases.

Figure 19.5 offers an open-ended assessment tool. Such a tool may be useful in a teen perinatal program or a senior support program, in which a primary nurse makes the home visits and an additional nurse visits occasionally. The open-ended format is brief and lends itself to subjectivity. The goal is to create a document that is informative for all who use it while limiting subjective observations—a difficult

FLOW SHEET——HIGH-RISK INFANT

Pt's Name _____ Address _____ Phone _____

At Birth: Weight _____ Length _____ Head Circ. _____ APGARS _____

	Date								
Irritability									
Lethargic									
Vomiting									
Diarrhea									
Feedings									
• Amount									
• Frequency									
• Suck									
Seizures/Convulsions									
Stools									
• Color									
• Consistency									
• Frequency									
Urine Output									
Edema									
Eyes Roll									
Temperature									
Pulse									
Respiration									
Weight									
Length									
Femoral Pulses									
Reflexes									
Muscle Tone									
Skin									
• Color									
• Condition									
Auscultate Chest									
Edema									
Output-Concentration									
Respiratory Function									
• Nasal Flaring									
• Grunting									
• Sternal Retracting									
• Tachycardia									
Head Circumference									
Chest Circumference									
Initials									

O - Normal   X - Problem (See Narrative)   C - Counseled for prevention

FIGURE 19.1   High-risk infant flow sheet.

Immunization (Circle & Date)

DTaP 1 2 3 4 _____ PPD _____ MMR _____ Hib _____

Polio 1 2 3 _____ Hep B _____ Varicella _____ PCV _____ RV _____ Flu _____

Instruction	Instruction Date	Pt. Understanding Date	Pamphlets Given Date	Comments	Initials
Review Disease Process					
Temperature Technique					
Feeding & Technique					
Bonding					
General Care					
• Bath					
• Hygiene					
• Formula Preparation					
• Cord Care					
Prevention of Infection					
Environment—Temperature Control					
Position					
Growth & Development					
Safety					
Stimulation					
Immunizations					
Referred to:					
Medical App./Date/M.D.					
S/S of Sick Child					

Initials	Signature

FIGURE **19.1** *Continued.*

task with open-ended tools. However, there may be an agency or program for which this tool fits best.

Other methods may use assessment tools or technology (e.g., videotaping family interactions, structured observation, analysis of life-changing events). The Self-Care Assessment Guide (Cleveland & Allender, 1999) measures a family member's ability to provide self-care (Fig. 19.6). In a public health nursing agency or other community-based agency, documentation is completed for individuals after family assessment information data are gathered. Useful information can be gathered about stressors and self-care practices, including prescription medicines, over-the-counter (OTC) medicines, herbal remedies, nutritional supplements, and other complementary therapies. Such tools are useful adjuncts, especially for families coming from cultural groups different from that of the health care provider. They are often used in combination with other tools to enhance the breadth of data collection and understanding of the family.

GUIDELINES FOR FAMILY HEALTH ASSESSMENT

An assessment of family health will be most accurate if it incorporates the following five guidelines:

1. Focus on the family as a total unit.
2. Ask goal-directed questions.
3. Collect data over time.
4. Combine quantitative and qualitative data.
5. Exercise professional judgment.

Focus on the Family, Not the Member

Family health is more than the sum of its individual members' health. If the health of each person in a family were rated and the scores combined, the total would not show how healthy that family is. To assess a family's health, the nurse must consider the family as a single entity and appraise its

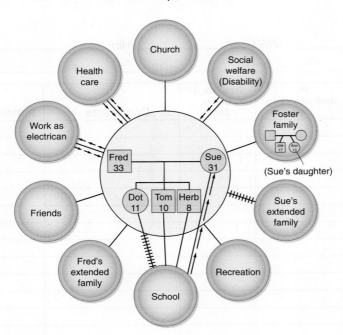

FIGURE 19.2 Eco-map of family's relationship to its environment. Lines indicate types of connections: *solid lines*, strong: *dotted lines*, tenuous; *lines with crossbars*, stressful. *Arrows* signify energy or resource flow, and absence of lines indicates no connection.

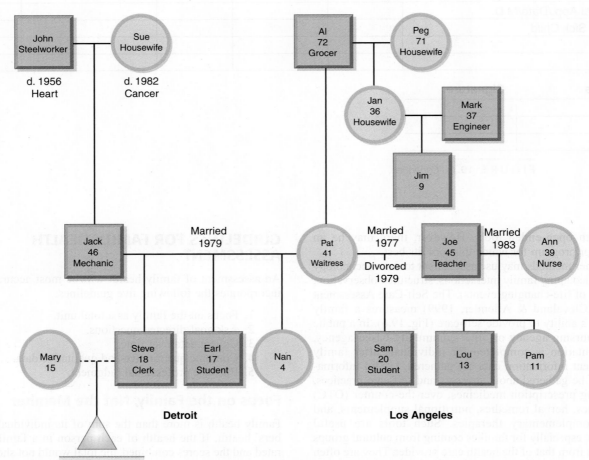

FIGURE 19.3 A genogram depicting three generations of family history. *Square*, male; *circle*, female; *triangle*, infant; *solid line*, married; *broken line*, not married.

aggregate behavior (Centers for Disease Control and Prevention, 2008; Wright & Leahey, 2005). As each criterion in the assessment process is considered, the community health nurse asks, "Is this typical of the family as a whole?" Assume that the nurse is assessing the communication patterns of a family. The nurse observes supportive interaction between two members in the family. What about the others? Further observation shows good communication among all but one member. It may be decided that, despite that one person, the family as a whole has good communication. If individual behavior deviates from that of the aggregate, the nurse notes the differences. They can influence total family functioning and need to be considered in nursing care planning.

Ask Goal-directed Questions

The activities of any investigator, if fruitful, are guided by goal-directed questions. When solving a crime, a detective has many specific questions in mind. So, too, does the physician attempting a diagnosis, the teacher trying to discern a student's

Family Assessment

Family Name ______________________________

Family Constellation

Member	Birth Date	Sex	Marital Status	Education	Occupation	Community Involvement

Financial Status ______________________________

Using the following scale, score the family based on your professional observations and judgement:

0 = Never 3 = Frequently
1 = Seldom 4 = Most of the time
2 = Occasionally N = Not observed

	score	date	score	date	score	date	score	date
Facilitative Interaction among Members								
a. Is there frequent communication among all members?								
b. Do conflicts get resolved?								
c. Are relationships supportive?								
d. Are love and caring shown among members?								
e. Do members work collaboratively?								
Comments ______________________________								
Totals								
Enhancement of Individual Development								
a. Does family respond appropriately to members' developmental needs?								
b. Does it tolerate disagreement?								
c. Does it accept members as they are?								
d. Does it promote member autonomy?								
Comments ______________________________								
Totals								

FIGURE 19.4 Family assessment using questions based on characteristics of healthy families. *(continued)*

	score	date	score	date	score	date	score	date
Effective Structuring of Relationships								
a. Is decision making allocated to appropriate members?								
b. Do member roles meet family needs?								
c. Is there flexible distribution of tasks?								
d. Are controls appropriate for family stage of development?								
Comments _____								
Totals								
Active Coping Effort								
a. Is family aware when there is a need for change?								
b. Is it receptive to new ideas?								
c. Does it actively seek resources?								
d. Does it make good use of resources?								
e. Does it creatively solve problems?								
Comments _____								
Totals								
Healthy Environment and Life-style								
a. Is family life-style health promoting?								
b. Are living conditions safe and hygienic?								
c. Is emotional climate conducive to good health?								
d. Do members practice good health measures?								
Comments _____								
Totals								
Regular Links with Broader Community								
a. Is family involved regularly in the community?								
b. Does it select and use external resources?								
c. Is it aware of external affairs?								
d. Does it attempt to understand external issues?								
Comments _____								
Totals								

FIGURE 19.4 *Continued.*

knowledge level, or the mechanic repairing a car. Similarly, the nurse determining a family's level of health has specific questions in mind. It is not enough to make family visits and merely ask members how they are. If relevant data are to be gathered, relevant questions must be asked. The family assessment tool shown in Figure 19.4 provides a sample set of questions that community health nurses use to assess a family's health. Built on the framework of the characteristics of a healthy family, these questions guide thinking and observations. They direct attention to specific aspects of family behavior to facilitate the goal of discovering a family's level of health.

Consider the characteristic, "Active Coping Effort." When visiting a family, the community health nurse watches for signs of the family's response to change and its problem-solving ability. The nurse asks, "Does this family recognize when it needs to make a change?" or "How does it respond

when a change is imposed?" Perhaps a health problem has arisen; for instance, the baby has diarrhea. Does the family assume responsibility for dealing with the problem? Do family members consider a variety of ways to solve it? How do they respond to the nurse's suggestions? Do they seek out resources on their own, such as reading about causes of infant diarrhea, using home remedies, or consulting with the community health nurse, the doctor, or a nurse practitioner? How well do they use resources, once identified? Do they try creative methods for solving the problem and see it through to resolution? As the nurse focuses on these behaviors, he is asking goal-directed questions aimed at finding out the family's coping skills. This investigation is one part of the nurse's assessment of the family's total health picture.

The set of questions presented in Figure 19.4 is one useful way to appraise family health. Another, more

FAMILY ASSESSMENT

Family Name _____

Family Constellation

Member names	Occupation	Educational background

_____

_____

_____

_____

Significant change in family life —

Coping ability of family —

Energy level —

Decision-making process within the family —

Parenting skills —

Support systems of the family—

Use of health care (include plans for emergencies) —

Financial status —

Other impressions —

Signature of Nurse _____   Date _____

FIGURE **19.5**   Open-ended family assessment.

open-ended format is used by some community health nursing agencies. This approach, displayed in Figure 19.5, proposes assessment categories as stimuli for nursing questions. When exploring family support systems, for example, the nurse asks, "What internal resources or strengths does this family have?" "Who outside the family can they and do they turn to for help?" "What agencies such as churches, clubs, or community services do they use?" The open-ended style of this assessment tool allows questions aimed at determining family health to be raised.

Allow Adequate Time for Data Collection

Accurate family assessment takes time. The assessment initiated on the first or second visit will most likely give only a partial picture of how a family is functioning. Time is needed to accumulate observations, make notes, and see all the family members interacting together in order to make a thorough assessment. To appraise family communication patterns, for instance, the nurse needs to observe the family as a group, perhaps at mealtime or during some family activity. The family needs to feel comfortable in the nurse's presence, so that they will respond freely; time and patience are needed for such rapport to develop.

Consider one nurse's experience. Jolene Burns had talked with the Olson family twice, first in the clinic, and then at home. Because Mr. Olson had not been present either time, Jolene asked to see the family together and arranged an early evening visit. The Olsons were receiving nursing services for health promotion. They were particularly interested in discussing discipline of their young children. They contracted with Jolene for six weekly visits to be held in the late afternoon, when Mr. Olson was home from work. Jolene's assessment began with her first contact with the Olsons. She made notes on their chart and, guided by questions similar to those in Figure 19.5, kept a brief log. After the fourth visit, she filled out an assessment form to keep as a part of the family record. It was not until then that Jolene felt she had collected enough data to make valid judgments about this family's level of health.

Combine Quantitative with Qualitative Data

Any appraisal of family health must be qualitative. That is, the nurse must determine the presence or absence of essential characteristics in order to have a database for planning nursing actions. To guide planning more specifically, the nurse can also determine the degree to which various signs of health are present. This is a quantitative measure. The nurse asks whether a family does or does not engage in some behaviors and how often. Is this behavior fairly typical of the family, or does it occur infrequently? Figures 19.4 and 19.5 demonstrate ways to measure family health quantitatively.

For example, if the nurse were to use the tool in Figure 19.4 to assess the Beck family's ability to enhance individuality, he could score behavior on a scale from 0 (never) to 4 (most of the time). After several observations, the nurse

SELF-CARE ASSESSMENT GUIDE

Name _____ Birth date _____

Address _____ Phone number _____

Names of health care providers visited in past year:

Name	Discipline	Address	Phone number	Times visited past year
1.				
2.				

Surgeries (Include date)

1. _____

2. _____

Major acute illnesses (Include date; indicate whether hospitalization was necessary)

1. _____

2. _____

Chronic illnesses (Include date)

1. _____

2. _____

Age of parents (If deceased, indicate date of death, age at death, and cause of death)

Mother _____ Father _____

Age of grandparents (If deceased, indicate age at death and cause of death)

MGM _____ MGF _____ PGM _____ PGF _____

Natural teeth   Y   N

Dentures or partials   Y   N

Dental care: _____ Brush teeth/Frequency _____

_____ Floss teeth/Frequency _____

Women/men over 50 Sigmoidoscopy/colonoscopy Date _____

Women

Breast self-exam   Y   N   Frequency _____

Mammograms   Y   N   Frequency _____

Pap smears   Y   N   Frequency _____

Men

Testicular self-exam   Y   N   Frequency _____

PSA   Y   N   Date _____ Results _____

TB skin test (Date) _____ Results _____

Immunizations

Td/Tdap _____

Flu vaccine _____

Hepatitis vaccine _____

Zoster _____

Other _____

Weight (At age 25) _____Current weight _____Normal weight _____

Height (At age 25) _____Current height _____

Dietary practices (24-hour dietary recall)

First meal (Time) _____ Contents (Include amount) _____

_____

Second meal (Time) _____ Contents (Include amount) _____

_____

Third meal (Time) _____ Contents (Include amount) _____

_____

Snacks (Include time, contents, and amount) _____

_____

Usual food eaten (not mentioned above) _____

Foods not eaten at all (by preference) _____

Food allergies _____

Medicine allergies _____

Food taboos _____

Religious practices that affect health (prayer, special practices or services) _____

_____

Exercise patterns (Include sample activities, duration, frequency, problems or side effects):

1. _____

2. _____

Medications and therapies

OTC drugs (Include name, length of treatment, frequency of use, side effects):

1. _____

2. _____

3. _____

4. _____

Prescription drugs (Include name, length of treatment, frequency of use, side effects):

1. _____

2. _____

3. _____

4. _____

Folk medicine/home remedies (e.g., postpartum isolation, mustard poultice for chest congestion):

1. _____

2. _____

3. _____

4. _____

Complementary therapies (e.g., biofeedback, imagery, herbalism)

1. _____

2. _____

3. _____

4. _____

Plan for self-care improvement

Overall goal _____

Areas needing modification (e.g., enhancement, moderation, deletion; include short- and long-term goal for each area):

1. _____

STG: _____

LTG: _____

2. _____

STG: _____

LTG: _____

Client role to reach long-term goals

Nurse's role(s) to reach long-term goals (e.g., collaboration, teaching, evaluation)

_____

Others' roles in reaching goals (Include discipline, name, address and phone number)

1. _____

2. _____

Comments

_____

_____

_____

FIGURE **19.6** Self-care assessment guide. Adapted from Cleveland, L., & Allender, J. A. (1999). Environment: Self-care issues. In L. Cleveland, D. S. Aschenbrenner, S. J. Veneable, & J. A. P. Yensen, *Nursing management in drug therapy*. Philadelphia: Lippincott Williams & Wilkins, with permission.

would probably conclude that responses to the members' developmental needs were appropriate most of the time (*a* under "Enhancement of Individual Development"). Opposite *a* on the assessment form, the nurse would write the numeral 4 and the date of assessment.

The value of developing a quantitative measure is to have some basis for comparison. The nurse can assess a family's progression or regression by comparing its present score with its previous scores. For instance, had the nurse conducted a family health assessment of the Kovacs 6 months ago and compared it with their present level of health, he would probably have discovered a drop in their scores in several areas. Many of their communication patterns, role relationships, and coping skills, in particular, would show signs of deterioration. A scored assessment gives a vivid picture of exactly which areas need intervention. For this reason, it is useful to conduct periodic assessments when a case is reopened, or every 3 to 6 months if it is kept open for an extended period. The nurse can monitor the progress of high-risk families through early introduction of preventive measures when a trend or regressive behavior is observed. Periodic quantitative assessments also provide a means of evaluating the effectiveness of nursing action and can point to documented signs of growth.

Quantitative data serve another useful purpose. The nurse can compare one family's health status with that of another family as a basis for priority setting and nursing care planning. The difference in the level of health between the Becks and the Kovacs, for example, shows that the Kovacs need considerably more attention right now.

Exercise Professional Judgment

Although nurses seek to validate data, their assessment of families is still based primarily on their own professional judgment. Assessment tools can guide observations and even quantify those judgments, but, ultimately, any assessment is subjective. Even though it may be observed that a family makes good use of a community agency, the decision that use of this external resource contributes to the health of the family is a subjective one. This determination is not bad. Indeed, effective health care practice depends on sound professional judgment. However, nurses must be cautious about overemphasizing the value or infallibility of an assessment tool. It is only a tool, and should be used as a guide for planning, not as an absolute and irrevocable statement about a family's health status. Caution is particularly important when dealing with quantitative scores, which may seem to be objective.

Ordinarily, assessment of a family is best conducted unobtrusively. An assessment tool used by the nurse is not a questionnaire to be filled out in the family's presence but rather a way to guide the nurse's observations and judgments. Before going into a family's home, the community health nurse may wish to review the questions. He may find it helpful to keep the assessment tool in a folder for easy reference during the visit. Depending on the nurse's relationship with the family, notes may be made during or immediately after the encounter. Like Jolene, the nurse may choose to keep a short log—an accumulation of notes—until enough data have been collected to complete the assessment form. Occasionally, a family with high self-care capability may be involved in the assessment. The nurse should introduce the idea carefully and use professional judgment to determine when the family is ready to engage in this kind of self-examination.

EDUCATION AND HEALTH PROMOTION

Teaching health promotion activities should begin only after family members express an interest and recognize a need. If the family is not at a level of functioning that enables members to use anticipatory guidance and teaching, the nurse can provide more basic services, such as gathering resources and acting as a counselor (Tapia, 1997). If family members are ready to learn ways to improve their health status, the nurse needs to assess the best teaching approach to use (see Chapter 11). Consideration of language barriers, previous knowledge and experience, family and community resources, and time available will influence the choice of approach.

EVALUATING IMPLEMENTED FAMILY HEALTH PLANS

The final step in the nursing process is evaluation. The evaluation process leads to a reassessment of your work with the family and a determination of what is needed in preparation for the next visit. This reassessment helps you in further individualizing services to the family. Evaluation of the structure-process of the visit and your self-evaluation can be done informally in a reflective manner. Outcomes are documented in the client record, and the evaluation becomes formalized. A thorough evaluation also assists you in making the most appropriate referrals and contacting key resources to meet family needs.

Types of Evaluations

Each family visit should be evaluated in three ways: structure-process, outcome, and self-evaluation. Each provides a different piece of information about the success of the visit. If the visit was not successful, what part made it less than successful? Most importantly, were the outcomes achieved? If not, is there something about the structure-process or your own preparedness or behavior that needs to be changed? When conducting an evaluation of the home visit, you are looking for answers to these questions.

Structure-Process

The structure-process of a visit should be analyzed first. Were there aspects of the organization, timing, environment, or sequencing of the components that needed to be changed or modified to make it a more effective visit? What could you have done about these factors? Were you organized? Would better preparation help with your organization? Were there distractions in the home that influenced organization? Ask yourself questions such as these, and then make plans to avoid or reduce disorganizing distractions. For example, if you made the visit based on limited information from a referral, you now have additional family data and can be better prepared for the next visit. If transportation schedules made the family late to the clinic, perhaps other transportation could be arranged. If the distraction on a home visit occurred because children were arriving home from school, visits could be made earlier in the day. If the television was playing loudly, you could make it a point to ask the family whether they would mind turning down the volume, or visit at a time when they do not watch television. Make the modifications that you can to assist with the visit process.

Outcome Evaluation

Second and most important is evaluation of the outcomes of the visit. Were the anticipated outcomes achieved? If not, why? If so, what made it possible? The **outcome evaluation**, or the assessment of change in the family's (client's) health status based on mutually agreed activities, is a formal process demonstrated in the documentation of the home visit. The agency may use the Nursing Outcomes Classification (NOC) System along with the Nursing Intervention Classification (NIC) System, or it may use the Omaha System discussed in Chapters 12 and 14. Alternatively, there may be agency-driven criteria for success and expectations for each client category or visit type. On a visit-by-visit basis, the changes observed in the family may be small; progress toward an expected outcome is noted. At the conclusion of agency services to the family, the cumulative changes in the client's health and the success or failure to achieve various outcomes are evaluated. Depending on the conclusions that can be drawn, the decision to terminate services may need to be reevaluated. It is possible that continuance of service is required, and the terms must be renegotiated. Whatever the decision, the family must be included in the decision-making process.

Self-evaluation

The third component of evaluation is self-evaluation. What aspect of your performance as a community health nurse during the home visit facilitated the achievement of a desired outcome? Were you prepared? Did you gather all the data needed to assist the family on the next visit? What would you do differently if you could do the visit over? What went right? What went wrong? What are you going to do on the next visit to make it better? This closer look at yourself is important for your own growth and effectiveness as a community health nurse.

Sometimes, we cannot see our own strengths or flaws, and evaluations by others are helpful. In some agencies, regular peer evaluations are conducted. An agency staff nurse makes a family visit with the community health nurse and provides feedback based on her observations. This is a useful technique to use even at times other than planned evaluations of all staff members in the agency. You might ask a colleague to accompany you on a home visit to a family that has not made progress toward outcome achievement or to a family you have not been able to "reach" or find difficult to work with (Drummond, Weir, & Kysela, 2002). For a variety of reasons, consultation with peers regarding certain visits and how best to conduct them can assist you in being better prepared or more focused. It can improve your interaction with families from different cultures or in difficult situations (Spector, 2000; Walsh, 1999).

Planning for the Next Visit

Part of the evaluation of one family visit is planning for the next. Use what occurred on the previous visit to guide you toward activities on subsequent visits. Goals may need to be modified, or family situations may change and specific outcomes become irrelevant. For example, you may plan to visit a prenatal family one last time before the baby is born to reinforce prior teaching about when to leave for the hospital with a second pregnancy. You intend to remind the parents to arrange babysitting for the older child and to assess the pregnant woman's rising blood pressure and complaints of backache. When you arrive for the visit, the husband is home alone with the younger child and is about to leave to bring his wife and new baby home from the hospital. He asks you about the diaper rash that just appeared on the 2-year-old. He also asks how to secure the new car seat into the car, because the instructions do not seem to make sense for his make of car. Outcomes for a problem-free pregnancy and healthy birth are no longer relevant; there are new outcomes to be formulated and worked on with this young family.

More frequently, planning for subsequent visits is relatively predictable and is done to ensure that steps toward outcome accomplishment are achieved on the visit. Being totally prepared each time is the best predictor of a successful family visit. Once you have met and gotten to know a family during a visit, the planning can be individualized and tailored to meet the family's unique needs. This information is not available from a paper referral, which makes planning for a first home visit important. The tone set during the first visit can affect your continued success with the family.

Referrals

A referral in written or verbal form (by agency-created form, telephone, fax, or e-mail) initiates contact with a family. In addition to responding to a referral, which begins the relationship with a family, the nurse makes referrals on behalf of the family. Families often need access to services beyond the agency's scope, and the nurse's knowledge of other resources can mean the difference between their having and not having access to additional services. Therefore, nurses must have information available to them about the eligibility requirements and availability of services provided by a bevy of official, voluntary, religious, and neighborhood organizations. If this information is not readily at hand, community health nurses need to know how to locate needed services. This is a daunting challenge, because the services are many, and organizations frequently change telephone numbers, services, and the populations they serve. Networking with colleagues on a regular basis helps keep nurses up to date with community services from which they can generate referrals for clients.

Contacting Resources

At times, community health nurses implement their roles as client advocates by facilitating easier access to services for the family. Community health nurses know how to access key personnel in agencies and can eliminate some of the red tape involved in obtaining services. Nurses can provide pointers that may help families procure needed services; for example, clients may have an advantage if they go to an agency early in the morning in the middle of the week. The fact that they should have all forms completely filled out and should bring their last 3 month's rent and utility receipts, or that they should ask to speak with a certain worker, may also be helpful information.

When nurses seek informal services for families, a relationship with the director of the agency can help them gain services for the clients. For example, a client family has a personal crisis and needs a donation of food and a volunteer to stay with a handicapped child for 3 days while a spouse undergoes surgery. The nurse telephones the religious leader of a neighborhood church and shares the family's requests, clarifies the situation, and gets a donation of food from the church's food pantry. The name of a member of the church who can stay with the child is also provided. The family may not have been aware that such services were available to them, and the links provided by the nurse are as important as other community health nursing functions.

Summary

The family unit remains the focus of service in community health nursing. Family health and individual health strongly influence each other, and family health also affects community health. Assessing, planning, implementing, and evaluating nursing care are steps used to deliver care to clients in acute care settings, in the extensive clinic system, and in the home.

It is important for the nurse to understand healthy family characteristics and to use a variety of tools so that family assessments are thorough.

Healthy families demonstrate six important characteristics:

1. A facilitative process of interaction exists among family members.
2. Individual member development is enhanced.
3. Role relationships are structured effectively.
4. Active attempts are made to cope with problems.
5. There is a healthy home environment and lifestyle.
6. Regular links with the broader community are established.

To assess a family's health systematically, the nurse needs a conceptual framework on which to base the assessment, a clearly defined set of categories for data collection, and a method for measuring the family's level of functioning. The six characteristics of a healthy family provide one assessment framework that community health nurses can use. Assessment tools to aid the nurse in appraising the health of families include the eco-map and the genogram.

There are 12 main categories of family dynamics for which the nurse must collect data: family demographics, physical environment, psychological/spiritual environment, family structure and roles, family functions, family values and beliefs, family communication patterns, family decision-making patterns, family problem-solving patterns, family coping patterns, family health behaviors, and family social and cultural patterns.

Community health nurses enhance their practices with families by observing five principles: work with the family collectively, start where the family is now, fit nursing interventions to the family's stage of development, recognize the validity of family structural variation, and emphasize family strengths.

During assessment, the nurse should focus on the family as a total unit, use goal-directed assessment questions, allow adequate time for data collection, combine quantitative with qualitative data, and exercise professional judgment.

Making family health visits is a unique role for nurses and is one of the activities common to most community health nurses. In some agencies, family health visits are conducted for only the most high-risk families. In other agencies, a visit is the method of choice for most care.

When nurses visit families, they must use acute observational skills, good verbal and nonverbal communication, assessment skills, and a "sixth sense" to guide them safely in the community and with the families they visit. Some visits are conducted with families in settings other than their homes. Neighborhood clinics, schools, work places, or recreational settings may be the preferred or the only locations in which you can gather most of the family members for the visit. Other families may be in transition and living in homeless shelters or with relatives or neighbors. These settings are familiar to the family and provide a unique environment for the nurse in which to visit the family.

Pre-visit preparation, conduct of the visit, and post-visit documentation are the main components of a family health visit. Each step is important and has value for the success of the next step. Being well prepared for a visit is the first concern (e.g., know the location, have family health status information and needed materials). The visit should be conducted in an orderly and organized fashion. Time should be allowed for getting acquainted, for the body of the visit, including teaching and anticipatory guidance, and for any other nursing care that may be a part of the visit. Concluding with a summary of the important parts of the visit and planning for the next visit ensures an appropriate ending.

Being safe in a neighborhood is important for all people. Community health nurses spend a great part of the day in the community, and safe travel is of constant importance. Use of a personal or agency car, public transportation, or walking to visit families each has its own set of precautions for personal safety. Even in a family's home, personal safety must be a consideration. If family members are arguing or under the influence of drugs or alcohol, the situation may deteriorate rapidly and become unsafe; at this point, it is best to terminate the visit.

During the implementation phase of the family health visit, the nurse establishes a verbal or written contract with the family. This permits understanding by both the family and the nurse of the personal roles and responsibilities in the relationship. Empowerment of family members is significant for clients. People who are empowered can help themselves for a lifetime and can make independent decisions about their own health.

Evaluation and preparation for the next visit completes the family health visit cycle. Three types of evaluation can be conducted at the end of a visit. Recall of the structure-process assists the nurse in reflecting on the physical aspects of the visit that were positive or negative. Discovering these factors can help enhance the positive and eliminate the negative. Evaluating whether the outcomes of the visit were achieved is done in a more formal way with agency documentation. Because the purpose of conducting family health visits is to bring about positive changes in family behaviors, it is necessary to evaluate the achievement of mutual goals made by the nurse and the family. The hardest part of evaluation is looking at yourself and how you conduct home visits. Often, peer evaluation is a helpful way to obtain feedback, because people tend to minimize their own strengths and overlook their weaknesses.

Conducting family health visits involves making referrals to other agencies and services on behalf of the family. One agency cannot provide all the services that a family needs. Written or verbal forms of communicating a need involve contacting resources available in the community. Community health nurses have unique skills in knowing and locating both official and voluntary services within their community. Such skills come with experience. ■

ACTIVITIES TO PROMOTE CRITICAL THINKING

1. Construct an eco-map of your family. Ask a peer to do the same thing. Assess the balance between your family and the resources in its environment. How does your eco-map compare with that of your peer? What changes are needed in each family system? Are you able to influence the changes that are needed?

2. Draw a genogram of your family and ask a peer to discuss it with you. Make your drawing of the genogram as complete as possible. Then analyze your thoughts and feelings. How did you feel while tracing your family history? Did you learn anything new about your family? Did any family trends or traits appear? Did any uncomfortable or suppressed information come to the surface? Do you have any new insights about your family?

3. Assess a family (other than your own) that you know well by completing a family assessment guide. You may use one of the forms in this chapter or an available form from another source. Based on your assessment, determine as many nursing interventions as you can think of that could be used to promote this family's health as practically as possible.

4. Invite a peer to go on a family health visit with you, and be open to feedback regarding your strengths and weaknesses. How does it make you feel to have someone else on a family health visit with you, knowing they are observing your skills? Offer to do the same for a peer and provide him with feedback. Discuss your experience.

5. Go on several family-health visits with an experienced community health nurse and observe the nurse's visiting techniques. Observe how he contacts the family, knocks on the door, greets the family, conducts, summarizes, and concludes the visit, and makes plans for the next visit. Discuss the various techniques used, and ask questions about your observations to get a better idea of why things are done as they are. Use some of this information on your next home visit.

6. Initiate a small group discussion among your peers about safety on your school campus and in your community. Encourage each person to share the safety habits used. How are these techniques different from safety techniques used when making home visits in the community? If they are different, why? Should they be different?

References

Allender, J.A. (1998). *Community and home health nursing.* Philadelphia: Lippincott-Raven.

American Nurses Association. (2007). *Public health nursing: Scope and standards of practice.* Silver Spring, MD: Nursesbooks.org.

Anderson, S.A., & Sabatelli, R.M. (2003). *Family interaction: A multigenerational developmental perspective* (3rd ed.). Boston: Allyn & Bacon.

Baris, M.A., Coates, C.A., Duvall, B.B., Garrity, C.B., Johnson, E.T., & Lacrosse, E.R. (2001). *Working with high-conflict families of divorce: A guide for professionals.* Northvale, NJ: Jason Aronson.

Barker, P. (1998). *Basic family therapy* (4th ed.). New York: Oxford University Press.

Barnes, S.L. (2001). Stressors and strengths: A theoretical and practical examination of nuclear, single-parent, and augmented African American families. *Families in Society: The Journal of Contemporary Human Services, 82*(5), 449–460.

Beavers, W.R., & Hampton, R.B. (1990). *Successful families: Assessment and intervention.* New York: Basic Books.

Becvar, D.S., & Becvar, R.J. (2003). *Family therapy: A systematic integration* (5th ed.). Boston: Allyn & Bacon.

Centers for Disease Control and Prevention—National Center for Health Statistics. (2008). *National survey of family growth.* Retrieved June 26, 2008, from http://www.cdc.gov/nchs/about/major/nsfg/cycledescript.htm.

Chambers, C. (2004). *The holistic nursing approach to chronic disease.* New York: Springer.

Cleveland, L., & Allender, J.A. (1999). Environment: Self-care issues. In L. Cleveland, D.S. Aschenbrenner, S.J. Veneable, & J.A.P. Yensen (Eds.), *Nursing management in drug therapy.* Philadelphia: Lippincott Williams & Wilkins.

Denham, S.A. (2002). *Family health: A framework for nursing.* Philadelphia: F.A. Davis.

Donnelly, T.T. (2002). Contextual analysis of coping: Implications for immigrants' mental health care. *Mental Health Nursing, 23,* 715–732.

Drummond, J.E., Weir, A.E., & Kysela, G.M. (2002). Home visitation practice: Models, documentation, and evaluation. *Public Health Nursing, 19,* 24–29.

Early, T.J. (2001). Measures for practice with families from a strengths perspective. *Families in Society: The Journal of Contemporary Human Services, 82*(3), 225–232.

Edelman, C., & Mandle, C.L. (Eds.). (2002). *Health promotion throughout the life span* (5th ed.). St. Louis: Mosby.

Farren, M. (1999). Ensuring safety for the elderly client at home. In S. Zang & J.A. Allender (Eds.), *Home care of the elderly* (pp. 59–77). Philadelphia: Lippincott Williams & Wilkins.

Friedman, M.M., Bowden, V.R., & Jones, W. (2003). *Family nursing: Research, theory and practice* (5th ed.). Upper Saddle River, NJ: Prentice-Hall.

Gavan, C.S. (2003). Successful aging families: A challenge for nurses. *Holistic Nursing Practice, 17*(1), 11–18.

Hanson, S.M.H. (Ed.). (2001). *Family health care nursing: Theory, practice, and research* (2nd ed.). Philadelphia: F.A. Davis.

Hanson, S.M., Gedaly-Duff, V., & Kaakinen, J. (2005). *Family health care nursing* (3rd ed.). Philadelphia: F.A. Davis.

Hartman, A. (1978). Diagrammatic assessment of family relationships. *Social Casework, 59*(10), 59–64.

Hill, R., & Hanson, D. (1960). The identification of conceptual frameworks utilized in family study. *Marriage and Family Living, 22,* 299–311.

Kantor, D., & Lehr, W. (1975). *Inside the family: Toward a theory of family process.* San Francisco: Jossey-Bass.

Kendra, M.A., & George, V.D. (2001). Defining risk in home visiting. *Public Health Nursing, 18,* 128–137.

Kitzman, H., Olds, D.L., Sidora, K., Henderson, C.R., Hanks, C., Cole, R., et al. (2000). Enduring effects of nurse home visitation on maternal life course: A 3-year follow-up of a randomized trial. *Journal of the American Medical Association, 283,* 1983–1989.

McGoldrick, M., & Gersen, R. (1985). *Genograms in family assessment.* New York: Norton.

Meyer, C.H. (1993). *Assessment in social work practice.* New York: Columbia.

Olds, D.L., Kitzman, H., Hanks, C., Cole, R., Anson, E., Sidora-Arcoleo, K., et al. (2007). Effects of nurse home visiting on maternal and child functioning: Age-9 follow-up of a randomized trial. *Pediatrics, 120,* e832–e845.

Olson, D., McCubbin, H.I., Barnes, H., et al. (1983). *Families: What makes them work?* Beverly Hills, CA: Sage.

Otto, H.A. (1973). A framework for assessing family strengths. In A. Reinhardt & M. Quinn (Eds.), *Family-centered community nursing: A sociocultural framework.* St. Louis: Mosby.

Parachin, V.M. (1997, March/April). Six signs of a healthy family. *Vibrant Life,* 5–6.

Pender, N.L., Murdaugh, C.L., & Parson, M.A. (2006). *Health promotion in nursing practice* (5th ed.). Upper Saddle River, NJ: Pearson.

Pinelli, J. (2000). Effects of family coping and resources on family adjustment and parental stress in the acute phase of the NICU experience. *Neonatal Network, 19*(6), 27–37.

Reiss, D. (1981). *The family's construction of reality.* Cambridge, MA: Harvard University Press.

Renpenning, K.M., Taylor, S.G., & Eisenhandler, S.A. (2003). *Self-care theory in nursing: Selected papers of Dorothea Orem.* New York: Springer.

Reutter, L. (1997). Family health assessment: An integrated approach. In B.W. Spradley & J.A. Allender (Eds.), *Readings in community health nursing* (5th ed., pp. 329–342). Philadelphia: Lippincott Raven.

Rucibwa, N.K., Modeste, N., & Montgomery, S. (2003). Exploring family factors and sexual behaviors in a group of Black and Hispanic adolescent males. *American Journal of Health Behavior, 27*(1), 63–74.

Saunders, J.C. (2003). Families living with severe mental illness: A literature review. *Mental Health Nursing, 24,* 175–198.

Scanzoni, J. (1999). *Designing families: The search for self and community in the information age.* Thousand Oaks, CA: Pine Forge.

Schorr, T.M., & Kennedy, M.S. (1999). *100 years of American nursing.* Philadelphia: Lippincott Williams & Wilkins.

Spector, R.E. (2000). *Cultural diversity in health and illness* (5th ed.). Upper Saddle River, NJ: Prentice-Hall.

Tapia, J.A. (1997). The nursing process in family health. In B.W. Spradley & J.A. Allender (Eds.), *Readings in community health nursing* (5th ed., pp. 343–350). Philadelphia: Lippincott Raven.

Thompson, P. (1998). Adolescents from families of divorce: Vulnerability to physiological and psychological disturbances. *Journal of Psychosocial Nursing and Mental Health Services, 36*(3), 34–39.

Turk, D.C., & Kerns, R.D. (Eds.). (1985). *Health, illness and families: A life span perspective.* New York: John Wiley.

U.S. Department of Health & Human Services. (2005). *U.S. Surgeon General's Family History Initiative.* Retrieved June 25, 2008, from http://www.hhs.gov/familyhistory/.

Wallace, H.M., Green, G., Jaros, K., Paine, L., & Story, M. (1999). *Health and welfare for families in the 21st century.* Boston: Jones & Bartlett.

Walsh, M. (1999). Dealing effectively with physically and verbally abusive elderly clients and families. In S. Zang & J.A. Allender (Eds.), *Home care of the elderly* (pp. 190–206). Philadelphia: Lippincott Williams & Wilkins.

Wright, L., & Leahey, M. (2005). *Nurses and families: A guide to family assessment and intervention* (4th ed.). Philadelphia: F.A. Davis.

Zerwekh, J.V. (1997). Making the connection during home visits: Narratives of expert nurses. *International Journal for Human Caring, 1*(1), 25–29.

Selected Readings

Aston, M., Meagher-Stewart, D., Sheppard-Lemoine, D., Vukic, A., & Chircop, A. (2006). Family health nursing and empowering relationships. *Pediatric Nursing, 32,* 61–67.

Crewe, S.E., & Wilson, R.G. (2007). Kinship care: From family tradition to social policy in the African American community. *Journal of Health and Social Policy, 22*(3/4), 1–7.

Hohashi, N., Honda, J., & Kong, S.K. (2008). Validity and reliability of the Chinese version of the Feetham Family Functioning Survey (FFFS). *Journal of Family Nursing, 14,* 201–223.

Humphreys, J., & Campbell, J.C. (2004). *Family violence and nursing practice.* Philadelphia: Lippincott Williams & Wilkins.

Leddy, S. (2006). *Health promotion: Mobilizing strengths to enhance health, wellness, and wellbeing.* Philadelphia: F.A. Davis.

Leininger, M., & McFarland, M. (2006). *Culture care diversity and universality: A worldwide nursing theory* (2nd ed.). Boston: Jones & Bartlett.

McNaughton, D.B. (2008). Nurse home visits during pregnancy and early childhood improved maternal life course 7 years later. *Evidence-based Nursing, 11*(2), 41.

Miller, S.M., McDaniel, S.H., Rolland, J.S., & Feetham, S.L. (Eds.). (2007). *Individuals, families, and the new era of genetics: Biopsychosocial perspectives.* New York: Norton.

Olds, D.L. (2006). The Nurse-Family Partnership: An evidence-based preventive intervention. *Infant Mental Health Journal, 27*(1), 5–25.

Running, A., Martin, K., & Tolle, L.W. (2007). An innovative model for conducting a participatory community health assessment. *Journal of Community Health Nursing, 24,* 203–213.

Wigle, D.T. (2003). *Child health and the environment.* New York: Oxford University Press.

Internet Resources

Bright Futures (Prevention & health promotion for infants, children, adolescents and their families): *http://brightfutures.aap.org/3rd_Edition_Guidelines_and_Pocket_Guide.html*

Center for Children and Families (The Brookings Institute): *http://www.brookings.edu/ccf.aspx*

Center for Research on Child Well Being: *http://crcw.princeton.edu/*

Centers for Disease Control and Prevention (Family Health): *http://www.cdc.gov/family/*

Children's Bureau (Administration for Children & Families—USDHHS): *http://www.acf.hhs.gov/programs/cb/*

Eunice Kennedy Shriver—National Institute of Child Health and Human Development (NIH): *http://www.nichd.nih.gov/*

Family Health International: *http://www.fhi.org/en/index.htm*

The Future of Children: *http://www.futureofchildren.org/info-url2815/info-url.htm*

Guide to Clinical Preventive Services: *http://www.ahrq.gov/clinic/cps3dix.htm*

Harvard Medical School—Family Health Guide: *http://www.health.harvard.edu/fhg/*

Nurse-Family Partnership: *http://www.nursefamilypartnership.org/index.cfm?fuseaction=home*

U.S. Surgeon General's Family History Initiative (USDHHS): *http://www.hhs.gov/familyhistory/*

World Health Organization (Family and Community Health Cluster): *http://www.who.int/fch/en/*

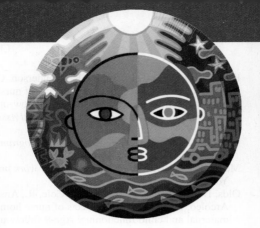

20

Violence Affecting Families

" *The right things to do are those that keep our violence in abeyance; the wrong things are those that bring it to the fore.* "

—Robert J. Sawyer (1960–), *Calculating God*

A **family crisis** is a stressful and disruptive event (or series of events) that comes with or without warning and disturbs the equilibrium of the family. A family crisis can also result when usual problem-solving methods fail. All families experience periods of crisis: a toddler is diagnosed with a serious illness; a teenager discovers she is pregnant; a father and sole breadwinner in a family loses his job; a mother's social drinking becomes habitual after her children go off to college; or a family's home is destroyed in a hurricane, earthquake, flood, or fire. If you think back on your family's history, you probably can identify one or more periods of crisis that you and your family members experienced. If so, how directly were you affected? How did the crisis resolve? As a result of the crisis, did any permanent changes occur in your family's dynamics or individual behaviors?

People respond to crises differently. Some people approach crises as a challenge, an event to be reckoned with, while others may feel overwhelmed and defeated or give up. Some individuals seek help if needed and come through the experience unscathed or as survivors, perhaps even stronger than before. Other individuals who are unable to cope with the crisis, or who do not cope well, may suffer severe psychological damage or may inflict their feelings of rage, frustration, or powerlessness onto their children, partners, or elders. This chapter focuses on families that have responded to stressors with violence, neglect, or abuse and those that have experienced stress and loss as a result of violence initiated by others.

Regardless of their responses, families in crisis need help, and community health nurses have a unique opportunity and responsibility to provide that help in a broad variety of situations. For example, in one family, an 8-year-old boy begins doing poorly in school; he wets his pants during class twice in one week and starts a small fire in the schoolyard. The school nurse is astute enough to begin an investigation into the family dynamics that may be contributing to these symptoms. In another family, a pregnant woman reschedules her appointment at a community clinic twice, then arrives at the appointment with multiple faded bruises on her face and arms. The clinic nurse uses sensitivity and caring while screening her for domestic violence.

Primary and secondary prevention measures used by community health nurses that help prevent crises include teaching families parenting skills, coping strategies, and informing them about community resources. In addition to assessment and education, community health nurses provide tertiary responses with direct assistance during times of crisis. This chapter discusses the knowledge and skills that community health nurses use in their practice of crisis prevention and intervention aimed at promoting improved health for families in the community.

DYNAMICS AND CHARACTERISTICS OF A CRISIS

Researchers have studied the nature of crises and have developed a body of knowledge called **crisis theory**. Initially limited to the field of mental health, crisis theory now influences every field of health care. The theory helps to explain why people respond in certain ways during a crisis and predicts phases people go through during and after a crisis. These responses and phases are important ideas for the community health nurse to understand before working in prevention or management of crises.

How does a crisis occur? Each of us is a dynamic system living within a given environment under circumstances unique to us alone. Our behavior—both consciously and subconsciously—is gauged to maintain a balance within ourselves and in our relations with others. When some internal or external force disrupts our system's balance and alters its functioning, a loss of equilibrium occurs. The individual then attempts to restore equilibrium by using whatever resources are available to him, in an effort to cope with the situation. **Coping** refers to those actions and ways of thinking that assist people in dealing with and surviving difficult situations. If individuals cannot readily cope with a stressful event—for example, if one's home is destroyed by fire, or one fails a final examination—the person experiences a crisis.

Crises are precipitated by a specific identifiable event that becomes too much for the usual problem-solving skills of those involved. Often, a single distressing event follows a host of previous difficulties and becomes the "straw that breaks the camel's back." For example, a wife who suffers years of spousal abuse finally becomes unable to cope and shoots her husband during a violent attack. Occasionally, tragic events occur suddenly without previous stressors, as when a father is killed in a plane crash or a child drowns in the family swimming pool.

Crises are normal in that all people feel overwhelmed occasionally. A person intervening in a crisis today may well be tomorrow's crisis victim. No individual is immune from sudden overwhelming difficulties. For example, Barbara, a hospice nurse, assists families through crises as part of her job, and suddenly her own spouse is diagnosed with cancer. Her coping skills are strained as she feels overwhelmed with personal and increased demands that require her support and attention.

Often a crisis is not an event per se, but rather a person's perception of the event. Each person reacts in his own way. A situation that throws one person off course may merely create an interesting detour for another (Display 20.1). It is usually the individual's interpretation of the event, rather than the event itself, that is crucial. At other times, a community crisis occurs on a large scale or is so unexpected that the crisis directly involves people who are known by others hundreds of miles away, causing distant friends and relatives shock and sorrow. Examples of such crises are Hurricane Katrina, or a night-club fire that kills dozens of people, or the terrorist attacks on September 11, 2001. Even strangers, knowing no one involved directly, are affected and experience signs and symptoms of stress (Levy & Sidel, 2002).

Crises are resolved, either positively or negatively, within a brief period, usually 4 to 8 weeks (Aguilera, 1998; Hoff, 2001). People's strong need to regain homeostasis and the intense nature of crises contribute toward making the crisis a temporary condition that will not continue indefinitely. In the family in which the wife shot her abusive husband, as shocking as the event might seem, life returns to a recognizable pattern within a few weeks. Even though family members will feel the change for years, the crisis soon subsides. The husband is hospitalized and recovers from his wound; the wife's case goes to trial, and she is sentenced to 2 years in prison; the children stay with relatives and attend school.

TWO FAMILIES' RESPONSE TO CRISIS

The Redondos and the Fosters will be moving to a town in another state, 900 miles away, because of a job change. The Redondos are in crisis over the move. They have never lived in any other town. They will have to leave relatives and lifelong friends who live nearby and a community in which they have been very involved. Mrs. Redondo is the secretary at her family's house of worship. Their teenage daughter, a cheerleader, just started high school. Their son is in kindergarten; Grandma happily watches him in the mornings before school. Everyone is upset because of how the move will affect them. The family is stressed and argues each evening. They don't want to put their house up for sale or even to visit the new community to which they will be moving. Mr. Redondo is second guessing his decision to move, but his choices were limited as his company is relocating. The Redondos, in crisis, are not exploring alternatives that may allow them to stay in their present community. One possible alternative might be for Mrs. Redondo to work while Mr. Redondo looks for another job. When people perceive that they are in crisis, decision making and problem solving become more difficult.

The Fosters, however, are excitedly looking forward to their move. They have two young children who are not yet in school. The move will bring them only 50 miles from old college friends. They hope to realize a significant profit on their house, which they recently remodeled. They can't wait to go "house hunting" in the new town. Everyone is enjoying planning the anticipated move; their two children, aged 3 and 4, have been playing "moving day" with their favorite toys.

Both families are experiencing the same event. The difference is each person's situation and perception of the event. The Redondos' equilibrium is being disrupted. They have not developed previous coping skills and do not see the move as a positive experience. They are at a different time in their family life cycle than are the Fosters. Although the move upsets their equilibrium, too, the Fosters experience it as an exciting event that conjures positive feelings; they are passing these feelings on to their children. They see this move as an opportunity.

Crisis resolution can be an adaptive process in which growth and improved health occur, or it can be maladaptive, resulting in illness or even death. The battered wife reevaluates her life, gets divorced, learns employment skills in jail, becomes more assertive, with stronger self-esteem; after she is paroled, she returns to her children, now able to support them financially and emotionally. She finds personal growth and health while successfully resolving the crisis. The children settle into their aunt's home with minimal difficulty, start a new school, and visit their mother and father regularly. After release, the mother finds an apartment near her sister's home, so that the children can continue in the same school district. The husband recovers from his wounds, gets counseling, relocates to another town, and sees his children frequently. The

crisis situation is resolved at a higher level of wellness for all members than existed before the crisis. In this example, the members are determined to improve their situation by working with skilled health care professionals. By using the resources within the community, this family is healthier after the crisis.

Developmental Crises

Developmental crises are periods of disruption that occur at transition points during normal growth and development (Display 20.2). When developmental crises occur, people feel threatened by the demands placed on them and have difficulty making the changes necessary to fit the new stage of development.

During the process of normal bio-psycho-social growth, people go through a succession of life cycle stages, from birth through old age. Each stage differs from the previous one, and transitions from one stage to the next require changes in roles and behavior. Popular and classic authors such as Levinson (1978), Bridges (1980, 2001), Sheehy (1976, 1992, 1999), and Sheehy and Delbourgo (1996) have called these periods "passages" and "transitions." These transitions are times when developmental or maturational crises occur.

Most family developmental crises have a gradual onset. The change is evolutionary rather than revolutionary. People usually anticipate and even prepare to start school, enter adolescence, leave home, marry, have a baby, retire, or die. Individuals move into and through each transitional period knowing in advance that some kind of change will be required. In many instances, people have already seen others experience these transitions. As a result, developmental crises have a degree of predictability. These developmental crises offer a time for anticipation and adjustment.

Developmental crises arise from both physical and social changes. Each new life stage confronts people with changed relationships, responsibilities, and roles. The transition to parenthood, for example, demands a change in role from caring for oneself and one's mate to include nurturing, caring for, and protecting a completely helpless infant. Relationships with adults, children, and even one's parents also change. Parenthood is an entrance into a previously inexperienced part of the adult world.

MAJOR DIFFERENCES BETWEEN TYPES OF CRISES

Developmental Crisis
Part of normal growth and development that can upset normalcy
Precipitated by a life transition point
Gradual onset
Response to developmental demands and society's expectations

Situational Crisis
Unexpected period of upset in normalcy
Precipitated by a hazardous event
Sudden onset
Externally imposed "accident"

| DISPLAY 20.3 | A DEVELOPMENTAL CRISIS |

DISPLAY 20.3 A DEVELOPMENTAL CRISIS

Marcia Sand is 39 years old. Married for 22 years, she has been a capable homemaker and mother of four children. Her husband, Lou, a construction worker for the past 20 years, thinks Marcia does a "super job at home." In the past, Marcia's time was filled with cooking, laundry, cleaning, shopping, and meeting the endless demands of the family. Their limited income prompted her to adopt many money-saving strategies. She made most of her own and the children's clothes, did all her own baking, and raised vegetables in her backyard garden. Now the youngest of the children, Tommy, has just left home to join the Navy. Her husband spends much of his spare time at the local bar with his friends, leaving Marcia alone. With a nearly empty house and little need for cooking, baking, and sewing, Marcia has lost her sense of usefulness. She thinks of taking a job, but knows her choices are limited because she has only a high school education. Marcia has not slept well in weeks; she wakes up tired and drags through the day barely able to manage the simplest task. She cries frequently but does not know why. Her hair, always neat and attractive in the past, looks bedraggled, and her shoulders slump. "I just can't seem to get on top of things any more," she complains.

Marcia has entered a developmental crisis that is sometimes called the "empty nest syndrome." She faces a turning point in her life, a time when parenting has seemingly ended. Leaving her satisfying homemaker role, she faces a new life stage filled with unknowns, changes, and a seeming lack of purpose. The transition came about gradually, almost imperceptibly, but now she must deal with it. Yet she feels unable to cope and wishes to turn to someone who would understand and lend her strength. She can be helped, but her crisis could also have been prevented at the pre-crisis phase. Anticipatory planning could have prevented the dilemma Marcia finds herself in now.

New parents may fear the unknown. Will this infant develop normally? Can I give adequate care? Parents often feel anxiety about the responsibility of shaping this new person's life, satisfying society's expectations for their child's proper education and training, or bringing children into a world that is in crisis and already overpopulated. Parents may worry about the increased financial burden while struggling with mixed feelings about giving up a large measure of freedom. These transitions put people under considerable stress, which contributes to tension, feelings of helplessness, and resultant crisis. Some people adapt quickly; others cannot cope, probably because earlier developmental crises went unresolved. If people lack a repertoire of adaptive skills, even positive and planned changes can develop into crises (Display 20.3).

Situational Crises

A **situational crisis** is a stressful, disruptive event arising from external circumstances that occur suddenly, often without warning, to a person, group, aggregate, or community. Typically, the external event requires behavioral changes and coping mechanisms beyond the abilities of the people involved.

Such events are not predicted, expected, or planned. The crisis occurs to people because of where they are in time and space. For instance, a baby grabs her mother's hot cup of tea and burns her chest; a college student is raped in the library parking lot; an older adult falls and fractures a hip; a mother with a van full of Little League baseball players has a crash at a busy intersection; or a hurricane devastates a state. These events, which involve loss or the threat of loss, represent life hazards to those affected. Some crisis-precipitating events can be positive, such as a significant job promotion or sudden acquisition of great wealth; however, the change still makes increased demands on individuals who must make major life adjustments. Even positive events involve a modified grieving process, because the individuals involved may be losing or giving up old, familiar, and comfortable situations and facing stressful changes.

Community health nurses see an almost infinite variety of situational crises, including debilitating disease, economic misfortune, unemployment, physical abuse, divorce, unwanted pregnancy, drug and alcohol abuse, sudden death of a loved one, tragic accidents such as a drowning or plane crash, and many others. In each situation, people feel overwhelmed and need help to cope. Skilled intervention can make the difference between a healthy or an unhealthy outcome.

Multiple Crises

Different kinds of crises can overlap in actual experience, compounding the stress felt by the persons involved. For example, a couple may experience a developmental crisis (birth) and a situational crisis (birth defect) simultaneously, thus compounding the resulting stress. The developmental crisis of midlife may be complicated by situational crises such as a divorce or job change. With older adults, the developmental crisis of retirement may be compounded by the situational crisis of a fire that destroys the family home. The transition a child faces entering school may occur at the same time the family moves to a new neighborhood and a new infant joins the family. The child must share the parent's attention and affection with a new sibling at a time when all the child's resources are needed to cope with starting school and adjusting to the new neighborhood. Classic research shows that accumulated stresses can lead to ill health (Holmes & Rahe, 1967). Those who normally work through one crisis in a healthy way may find that compounding events overwhelm them, causing more stress than they can handle.

HISTORY OF FAMILY VIOLENCE

Family crisis is not limited to the developmental crises people experience or the situational crises that come upon us suddenly, usually from forces—such as nature—that are external to the family. Many women and children in the world also experience the crisis of domestic violence. The terms **domestic violence**, **family violence**, and **interpersonal violence** refer to morbidity and mortality attributable to violence within the home setting, involving action by a family member or intimate partner. Domestic violence involves "a systematic pattern of assaultive and coercive behaviors, including physical, sexual, and psychological attacks and economic coercion, that adults or adolescents use against their intimate partner" (Kramer, 2002, p. 190). This type of violence occurs worldwide and is becoming more of a global public health burden.

Global History

Family violence is not new. For centuries, children were thought of as the property of their parents, and any treatment doled out by the parents was their prerogative. In fact, most countries had animal welfare laws long before child welfare laws were adopted. In addition, the ideology of childhood that emerged in the Western world in the late 1800s assumed that only "abnormal" children needed protection. These children were casualties of an urban-industrial society, and were abandoned, dependent, or delinquent—the products of social dislocation such as orphans or refugee children.

In the early 1900s, sensitive leaders concerned with child welfare issues emerged. Several international agencies were created designed to positively affect the health of children. The British Children's Act was passed in 1908, and the first White House Conference on children was held in 1909. These were early attempts to define a role for the state in the welfare of children. The U.S. conference was the forerunner of the United States Children's Bureau (USCB) and a national voluntary organization, later known as the Child Welfare League of America, was established to complement federal agency efforts (Bolen, 2001). The USCB became a model for other countries, with well-developed programs targeting infant mortality. In one innovative program of the early 1900s, a heated, mobile, child welfare center was used in rural communities and was staffed by a female physician and a public health nurse to improve health care to children.

Other international organizations emerged in the early 1900s including the International Association for the Promotion of Child Welfare (IAPCW), the League of Red Cross Societies (LRCS), the Save the Children Fund (SCF), and the Save the Children International Union (SCIU). The latter two agencies were immensely successful in raising funds for children in Germany, Austria, France, Hungary, and Serbia. As these organizations began serving the needs of children internationally, they moved from a sentimental depiction of victims to a medico-social-scientific view of children at risk, expanding and uncovering the concepts of child victimization, exploitation, and abuse (Bolen, 2001).

By the mid-1920s, the work of these agencies began to focus on children from non-European countries. The first conference on children from non-European countries focused on African children in 1931 and included such issues as infant mortality, child labor, education, and child slavery. In 1924, the League of Nations adopted the Declaration of the Rights of the Child, which would influence the League of Nation's successor, the United Nations, in the years to come in the form of the Declaration of the Rights of the Child (1959) and the Convention on the Rights of the Child (1989). The United Nations continues to hold annual hearings on the Rights of the Child, and has addressed global concerns, such as children without parental care, indigenous children, violence against children, HIV/AIDS, children with disabilities, and the economic exploitation of children (Office of the United Nations High Commissioner for Human Rights, Committee on the Rights of the Child, 2007).

Children are not the only victims of family morbidity and mortality from violence. Historically, women were also treated as property and often suffered physical and psychological damage. **Gender-based violence**, or **violence against women** (VAW), has global public health and human rights ramifications (World Health Organization [WHO], 2007a). Between 16% and 52% of women in some parts of the world experience domestic violence and other forms of violence ranging from emotional abuse to rape and genital mutilation. One in five women worldwide experience rape or attempted rape in their lifetime, and an estimated 100 to140 million girls and women alive today have undergone genital mutilation (WHO, 1998, 2007a). As with children, the rights of women are socially, culturally, and religiously influenced, with change coming slowly.

United States History

The history of treatment of children, women, and elders in the United States began with emigration in the 1500s and has been influenced by the cultural and religious practices of early settlers. In addition, necessity, attitudes of the time, and the stress and hardship of life in the colonies and on the frontier influenced how people were treated.

Children were born into families to help with the chores of an agricultural society. Families had many children, infant mortality rates were high, and it was not uncommon for half of the children in a family to die before their second birthday. Older people did not retire; they contributed to family survival until they died. There were no special considerations for children, women, or elders. The best a woman could hope for was that the man she married would not abuse her emotionally, physically, sexually, or fiducially (taking advantage of a person's financial resources). Women had limited or no education, resources, or rights, and children had none. If a woman married "poorly," she would have to live with the consequences. Separation and divorce were either unheard of or were a "death sentence" for the woman and her children, because there was nowhere they could go and no way for the woman to support her family.

Public Laws and Protection

It took many years for the United States to establish laws that benefited women and children. Nonetheless, the United States began earlier than many other countries to protect children, women, and elders. The Children's Bureau began to focus on child abuse in the 1960s, supporting development of a child abuse mandatory reporting law in 1962 to be used as a model by the states. The law required health professionals and child care workers to report suspected child abuse to appropriate officials.

In 1974, the Child Abuse Prevention and Treatment Act was passed, becoming Public Law 93-247 (PL 93-247). This law served to reinforce the earlier mandatory reporting law model and was aimed at solving the growing problem of child abuse in the country. Public Law 93-247 has been amended several times since 1974. The Child Abuse Prevention and Treatment and Adoption Reform Act of 1978 was followed by the Family Violence Prevention and Services Act of 1984. Later, all three acts were consolidated into the Child Abuse Prevention, Adoption, and Family Services Act of 1988 (Public Law 100-294), and most recently, the Act was amended and reauthorized as the Keeping Children and Families Safe Act of [Public Law 108-36] (Child Welfare Information Gateway, 2004).

Public Law 108-36 supports funding to states in their efforts to prevent violence in families and to identify and treat victims. The funding comes in the form of the Child Abuse Prevention and Treatment Act (CAPTA) and state grants that meet eligibility requirements (Administration for Children & Families, 2006b). One aspect of the funding supports the National Child Abuse and Neglect Data System (NCANDS) that tracks reports of child abuse and neglect, and all fatalities from child abuse or neglect in the United States. In 2006, NCANDS reported an estimate of 1,530 child deaths "caused by an injury resulting from abuse or neglect, or where abuse or neglect was a contributing factor" (Child Welfare Information Gateway, 2008a, para. 2). Information on adoption, out-of-home care for children, preventing and responding to child abuse and neglect, supporting and preserving families, and resources are available via the Child Welfare Information Gateway, a program under the United States Department of Health and Human Services (USDHHS), Administration of Children and Families. The Administration on Aging, also under the USDHHS, supports similar programs including the National Center on Elder Abuse that works to educate and assist families, seniors, and health care and legal providers regarding elder abuse (2006).

Healthy People 2010 *Goals*

The goal for *Healthy People 2010* regarding violence and abuse is to reduce injuries, disabilities, and death due to violence among all people of the United States. On an average day in America, 70 people die from homicide, 87 people commit suicide, as many as 30,000 people attempt suicide, and a minimum of 18,000 people survive interpersonal assaults. The problem of violence is pervasive, affecting the victim directly and family members indirectly. Selected violence and abuse objectives for *Healthy People 2010* include the following:

◆ Reduce maltreatment and maltreatment fatalities of children from 13.9 victims per 1,000 by the year 2010
◆ Reduce physical assault by current or former intimate partners from 4.5 per 1,000 people to 3.6 per 1,000 by 2010
◆ Reduce the annual rate of rape or attempted rape of persons aged 12 years and older to less than 0.7 per 1,000 persons by 2010, down from 0.8 per 1,000 in 1998
◆ Reduce sexual assault other than rape to less than 0.2 per 1,000 people in 2010, down from 0.6 in 1998
◆ Reduce weapon carrying by adolescents on school property (grades 9 through 12) from 8.5% in 1997 to 6% by 2010 (USDHHS, 2000)

Injury and violence prevention, one of the 28 identified focus areas in *Healthy People 2010,* is also in the top 10 high-priority leading health indicators (LHI) chosen to track national progress toward meeting the *Healthy People 2010* national health goals (Office of Disease Prevention and Health Promotion, n.d.). Types of injury and violence prevention tracked for *Healthy People 2010* include motor vehicle accidents, firearm injuries, poisonings, suffocation, falls, fires, and drownings. In the *Healthy People 2010 Midcourse Review* of violence and abuse prevention, four objectives—sexual assault other than rape in those 12 and older, physical assault of those older than 12 years, physical fighting in 9th to 12th grade students, and carrying weapons on school property by students in grades 9–12—demonstrated a 40% or higher improvement (Office of Disease Prevention and Health Promotion, *Healthy People 2010: Midcourse Review*, 2005, p. 15-6).

Some injury and violence prevention objectives did not demonstrate improvement in the *Healthy People 2010 Midcourse Review* including firearm-related deaths (–2%), nonfatal poisonings (–89%), deaths from poisonings (–38%), deaths from suffocation (–22%), deaths from unintentional injuries (–9%), deaths from homicides (–3%), and maltreatment fatalities for those under 18 (–100%) (pp. 15-11–15-14). Gender, education, race/ethnicity, and location are identifiers used in tracking and measuring *Healthy People 2010* injury and violence objectives. Of particular concern in these identifiers are findings that: (1) males are three times more likely than females to be a victim of homicide; (2) a person with a high school education or less is four times more likely to be a homicide victim than an individual who had at least some college; and (3) American Indian, Alaska Native, Hispanic, and Black non-Hispanic populations were three to seven times higher than White non-Hispanic populations to be victims of homicide (p. 15-20). Firearm related deaths reflected the lowest rate in Asian or Pacific Islander populations (p. 15-19), whereas nonfatal firearm injuries notably decreased in the Hispanic population between 1997 and 2001 "from 39.4 injuries per 100,000 population to 21.8 injuries per 100,000 population" (p. 15-19). Ongoing data collection and review of the *Healthy People 2010* goals promote identification of issues for specific populations and an opportunity to revise and update objectives reflecting current science, data gathering, and presentation of information (Office of Disease Prevention and Health Promotion, *Healthy People 2010, Midcourse Review, Executive Summary*, 2005). This review process allows new programs and approaches to be planned and implemented, such as the Positive Parenting Program (Triple P), a parent education program that addresses the risks of child mistreatment (p. 15-17), or advocacy for legislation that supports increased domestic violence services, a finding that has been linked to decreased intimate partner homicides, and possibly to a reduction in intimate partner physical assaults (p. 15-24). More importantly, this review and attention to new measures support the overarching goals of *Healthy People 2010*: to increase quality and years of healthy life, and to eliminate health disparities.

Myths and Truths About Family Violence

Many myths about family violence need to be dispelled. Strongly held myths by members of society, including community health nurses and other health care providers, may interfere with their ability to help families in crisis get the

TABLE 20.1   Common Myths and Truths About Abuse in Families

Myth	Truth
Violence in families is rare	Family violence is common and increasing
Violence occurs most frequently among low-income families	Family violence occurs across all incomes
Violence occurs more frequently in some racial and cultural groups	Family violence occurs across all racial and cultural groups
Violence in families does not coexist with love	Love may exist but is unable to be displayed appropriately due to conflicting emotions
Men who batter women are mentally ill	The percentage of batterers who are mentally ill is the same as in the general population
Women who accept battering are mentally ill	The percentage of battered women who are mentally ill is the same as in the general population; however, they have low-esteem and a damaged spirit
Violence occurs only in heterosexual relationships	Domestic violence has no gender or sexual boundaries; it can occur among all people
Abused women instigate the battering	Quite the contrary, they go out of their way not to agitate or confront the abuser
Abuse occurs when the abuser is under the influence of drugs or alcohol	It can, but many abusers do not drink or use drugs
Children should not be taken from their parents	In some violent families, the safest place for the child is with another family member or a foster home (temporarily or permanently)
Even abusive parents are better for a child than a child living elsewhere	Children must be protected, and living away from abusive parents may save their lives
Abused children become abusive adults	Some may, but most can learn how to channel their emotions positively if the cycle of violence is broken

help they need. Table 20.1 displays some common myths and truths about family violence.

FAMILY VIOLENCE AGAINST CHILDREN

Communicable diseases, as a cause of morbidity among children, "are coming under control through a combination of health promotion, prevention, and simplified standard treatment regimens. At the same time, the healthy growth and development of many children is threatened by very rapid, often disruptive social, cultural, and economic changes" (WHO, 1998, p. 71). This emerging new morbidity is psychosocial in nature and is associated with behavioral problems that are more difficult to prevent than the diseases known for centuries. In 2001, the World Health Organization (WHO)'s Committee on the Rights of the Child stated, "Globally, around 40 million children are subjected to child abuse each year . . . violence [that] results from individual, family, community, and structural factors" (para. 5-6), yet this violence directed at children is preventable.

Child abuse defined by the federal Child Abuse Prevention and Treatment Act (CAPTA; 42.U.S.C.A., 5106g) from the *Keeping Children and Families Safe Act* of 2003, is "at minimum: any recent act or failure to act on the part of a parent or caretaker which results in death, serious physical or emotional harm, sexual abuse or exploitation; or an act or failure to act which presents an imminent risk of serious harm" (Child Welfare Information Gateway, 2008b, para. 1). More commonly, child abuse is defined in identifying categories of maltreatment toward a child that may include physical, emotional, general neglect, medical or educational neglect, physical punishment or battering, emotional or sexual maltreatment and exploitation, or a combination of these mistreatments.

Child abuse and the associated psychosocial developmental problems are taking a toll globally in human costs and economically in health care services. Countries vary in risk toward children; for example the homicide rate for children in Japan is 0.6 per 100,000, yet 7 per 100,000 in the United States, to a high of 25 per 100,000 in Estonia (WHO, Committee on the Rights of the Child, 2001, para. 8). Worldwide, fatal abuse of infants and very young children is nearly double that of children who are between 5 and 14 years old and varies with lower rates of child homicide in countries with higher levels of income (WHO, 2007b, chap. 3, p. 60). Identifying and gathering worldwide data about child abuse is difficult because many cases are not investigated and death reports may not be classified as the result of abuse or homicide.

Another concern for children is their role in families that may require very young children to aid the family financially. A child's "chores" may include spending the whole day scrounging around city dumps gathering bits of food, clothing, or other useful or saleable items. Some children are sold for sexual favors to whomever asks, while others spend all day working in fields, home businesses, or "sweat shops" for the equivalent of pennies a day. In some societies, female children are not valued and are killed at birth, given away, or sold into slavery for a pittance.

Child abuse in the United States has seen a slight increase over the past few years from "1.96 per 100,000 in 2001, increasing to 1.98 in 2002, 2.00 in 2003, 2.03 in 2004, decreasing back to 1.96 in 2005, and increasing to 2.04 in 2006" (Child Welfare Information Gateway, 2008a, p. 2). Many researchers think child abuse cases are underreported due in part to variation in reporting requirements, state investigation requirements, and the amount of time an investigation may require, along with difficulty in coding and sharing information between agencies and jurisdictions. The National Child Abuse and Neglect Data System (NCANDS) estimated 1,530 child fatalities in the United States in 2006 (Child Welfare Information Gateway, 2008a, para. 2). Most of these fatalities were in children under 3 years old, with 45% of the fatalities in children under 1 year (para. 9). The dependence of small children makes them vulnerable to abuse and neglect, as reflected in the 2004 child fatalities rate, when 35.5% died as the result of neglect, 28.3% died of physical abuse, and 30.2% of multiple types of abuse (para. 11).

Representation of children of color is higher in child abuse data. "While there were 10.6 cases of substantiated maltreatment for every 1,000 white children, the rates for Black, Hispanic, and Indian/Alaskan Native children were 25.2, 12.6, and 20.1 cases per 1,000 children, respectively" (Lane, Rubin, Monteith, & Christian, 2002, p. 1603). These rates may give a false picture of the actual rates among racial groups. It may be that minority children are abused more frequently, or that abuse of minority children is more likely to be reported, or that reports among minority groups are more likely to be substantiated. Mandated reporters may have biases that contribute to the differences, while characteristics of the community in which the child resides have also been cited as a factor in the over-representation of children of color in abuse reporting (United States Children's Bureau, 2003).

Of the four types of reportable child abuse—physical, emotional, sexual, and neglect—the majority of reports in the United States are for neglect. The National Child Abuse and Neglect Data System (NCANDS) reported in 2006, "approximately 905,000 children were found to be victims of child abuse or neglect," and of that number 64.2% suffered from neglect, 16% were physically abused, 8.8% were sexually abused, 6.6% were emotionally or psychologically maltreated, 2.2% were medically neglected, while 15% were victims of "other" types of maltreatment such as abandonment, threat of harm to the children, and congenital drug addiction (Administration for Children & Families [ACF], 2006a, pp. iii, 27). Similar to the worldwide data, younger children were at greater risk, as 38.6 per 1,000 children under 3 years were victims, with 13.5 per 1,000 in the 4 to 7 year old range, decreasing to 10.8 per 1,000 in 8-11 year olds, 10.2 in 12-15 year olds, and 6.3 in those 16-17 years (ACF, 2006a).

Nationally, measures have been taken to improve data gathering and information about violence toward children, as well as outcomes for these children. The *National Survey of Child and Adolescent Well-Being* (NSCAW) is a longitudinal study on the well-being of children who have encountered the child welfare system (ACF, 2007). Another important source of tracking child maltreatment occurs in conjunction with the *Healthy People 2010* goals that set a target for a 20% improvement in reducing child (under 18 years old) maltreatment and maltreatment fatalities from the 1998 baseline of 12.9 child victims per 1,000 children (USDHHS, 2000, *Healthy People 2010*: 15 Injury and Violence Prevention, 15-33).

Child Neglect

Neglect occurs when the physical, emotional, medical, or educational resources necessary for healthy growth and development are withheld or unavailable. Neglect is obvious to an observer if a very young child is playing unattended outside, is not dressed appropriately for the weather, or has an unkempt appearance. However, neglect is not always so obvious. Parents may refuse to buy eyeglasses for a child who needs them or to access dental care for severely decayed teeth (medical neglect). An 8-year-old may get to school only 3 days a week, possibly without breakfast and no lunch money or packed lunch (educational neglect). A family with three children may live in a sparsely furnished apartment with very little food available and only intermittent heat and multiple people coming and going in the residence, while the children may appear at school unwashed and without coats in winter weather (general neglect). Emotional neglect may be seen when demands placed on a child are excessive or inappropriate for her development, or the caretaker berates or verbally humiliates a child frequently and without reason.

Thousands of children in the United States experience neglect each day. They are frequently "invisible" victims. At times, sensational stories of severe child neglect are reported in the media and cause public outrage. Examples include 12 children found among piles of garbage in an abandoned apartment building during a drug raid; parents vacationing in Florida while their two daughters, aged 6 and 4, were left unattended at home; or three young children found barely alive, kept in a basement closet. However, most children suffering from neglect do not make newspaper headlines or television reports. They go to school like others. If they are fortunate, their plight is uncovered by a community health nurse, a teacher, neighbor, or counselor. Because of the invisibility of neglect, its prevalence is hard to estimate. Often cases of neglect are brought to the attention of the proper authority only during the investigation of other forms of abuse or family issues (Display 20.4).

DISPLAY 20.4   SIGNS AND SYMPTOMS OF NEGLECT

Neglect may be suspected if one or more of the following conditions exist:

- The child lacks adequate medical or dental care.
- The child is often sleepy or hungry.
- The child is often dirty, demonstrates poor personal hygiene, or is inadequately dressed for weather conditions.
- There is evidence of poor or inadequate supervision for the child's age.
- The conditions in the home are unsafe or unsanitary.
- The child appears to be malnourished.
- The child is depressed, withdrawn, or apathetic; exhibits antisocial or destructive behavior; shows fearfulness; or suffers from substance abuse or speech, eating, or habit disorders (e.g., biting, rocking, whining).

Physical Abuse

Physical abuse is intentional harm to a child by another person that results in pain, physical injury, or death. The abuse may include striking, biting, poking, burning, shaking, or throwing the child. **Corporal punishment**, which involves violence against a child as a form of discipline, was an acceptable form of discipline earlier in our country's history and is still condoned in some subgroups. Many parents today were raised in families in which physical punishment was used as a form of discipline. Even today, it is not unusual to see a parent slap the hand of a toddler to get his attention after he has been told not to do something several times or to prevent him from touching something that would hurt him more than a slap on the hand. Most families know where to draw the line. Others—especially if they were raised with "the belt" or "the switch"—see no harm in using the same physical disciplinary practices with their children.

Some parents cannot control the degree of physical punishment they give their child. In one case in 2002, a mother repeatedly physically assaulted her young daughter while getting her into the car. The mother's behavior was recorded by the store's parking lot surveillance camera. Intervention and follow-up occurred, including incarceration and counseling for the mother and foster home placement for the child. If physical punishment is administered in anger, while the parent is under the influence of mind-altering substances or out of a sense of frustration, the punishment may cross over to become battering of the child.

C. Henry Kempe identified the **battered child syndrome** in the 1960s, now defined as "the collection of injuries sustained by a child as a result of repeated mistreatment or beating" (United States Department of Justice [USDOJ], 2002, p. 1). Battered child investigations require thorough follow-up and interviews with caretakers, medical personnel, family members, and school personnel. Investigators should be aware that "A major trait of abusive caretakers is either the complete lack of an explanation for critical injuries or explanations that do not account for the severity of injuries" (p. 4). Display 20.5 lists behavioral indicators of physical abuse (USDOJ, 2002).

Sexual Abuse

Sexual abuse of children includes acts of sexual assault or sexual exploitation of a minor and may consist of a single incident or many acts over a long period. Sexual assault includes rape, gang rape, incest, sodomy, lewd or lascivious acts with a child younger than 14 years of age (in most states), oral copulation, fondling of the child's genitals, penetration of the genital or anal opening by a foreign object, and child molestation. **Sexual exploitation** of children includes conduct or activities related to pornography that depict minors in sexually explicit situations and promotion of prostitution by minors (USDOJ, 2007). **Incest** is sexual abuse among family members who are related by blood (e.g., parents, grandparents, older siblings, aunts and uncles); it constitutes the most hidden form of child abuse. **Intrafamilial sexual abuse** refers to sexual activity involving family members who are not related by blood (e.g., stepparents, boyfriends).

More than 88,000 children were confirmed victims of sexual abuse in 2002, while studies cite victimization as 12% to 25% of girls and 8% to 10% of boys under the age of 18 (Kellogg, 2005). In most reported cases, the father or male caretaker is the initiator, and the victim is a female

---

DISPLAY 20.5	SIGNS AND SYMPTOMS OF PHYSICAL ABUSE

Types of Injuries
Types of physical abuse injuries include bruises, burns, bite marks, abrasions, lacerations, head injuries, internal injuries, and fractures.

Behavioral Indicators of Physical Abuse
The following behaviors are often exhibited by physically abused children:

- The child is frightened of parents/caretakers or, at the other extreme, is overprotective of parent or caretakers.
- The child is excessively passive, overly compliant, apathetic, withdrawn or fearful or, at the other extreme, excessively aggressive, destructive, or physically violent.
- The child and/or parent or caretaker attempts to hide injuries; child wears excessive layers of clothing, especially in hot weather; child is frequently absent from school or misses physical education classes if changing into gym clothes is required; child has difficulty sitting or walking.
- The child is frightened of going home.
- The child is clingy and forms indiscriminate attachments.
- The child is apprehensive when other children cry.
- The child is wary of physical contact with adults.

- The child exhibits drastic behavioral changes in and out of parental/caretaker presence.
- The child is hypervigilant.
- The child suffers from seizures or vomiting.
- The adolescent exhibits depression, self-mutilation, suicide attempts, substance abuse, or sleeping and eating disorders.

Other indicators of physical abuse may include the following:
- A statement by the child that the injury was caused by abuse (chronically abused children may deny abuse).
- Knowledge that the child's injury is unusual for the child's specific age group (e.g., any fracture in an infant).
- Knowledge of the child's history of previous or recurrent injuries.
- Unexplained injuries (e.g., parent is unable to explain reason for injury; there are discrepancies in explanations; blame is placed on a third party; explanations are inconsistent with medical diagnosis).
- A parent or caretaker who delays seeking or fails to seek medical care for the child's injury.

child; however, boys are victims more often than previously believed, and adolescents were reported as "perpetrators in at least 20% of reported cases" (Kellogg, 2005). The initial sexual abuse may occur at any age, from infancy through adolescence. However, the largest number of cases involves girls younger than 11 years of age. Regardless of how gentle, trivial, or coincidental the first approach may have seemed, sexual coercion tends to be repeated and to escalate over a period of years. The child may blame himself or herself for tempting or provoking the abuser.

The mother, who is expected to protect the child, may purposely isolate herself from a problem of sexual abuse. Sometimes the mother is distant, uncommunicative, or so disapproving of sexual matters that the child is afraid to speak up. Sometimes she is extremely insecure, and feels confrontation may cause anger or the loss of her husband or boyfriend, or the mother's economic security may depend on her partner/spouse. The mother may feel threatened or feel that she cannot allow herself to believe or even to suspect that her child is at risk. She may have been a victim herself of child abuse and may not trust her judgment or her right to challenge the man's authority in the home. Some mothers consciously acknowledge that their children are being sexually abused but, for whatever reason, choose to "look the other way." Until the victim is old enough to realize that incest or intrafamilial sexual abuse is not a common occurrence or is strong enough to obtain help outside the family, there is little chance of escape unless the abuse is reported (Crime and Violence Prevention Center, 2003b).

Indicators of sexual abuse are seen in various ways, and attention should be given to a history of sexual abuse; sexual behavior indicators; behavioral indicators in younger children, and behavioral indicators of sexual abuse in older children and adolescents, and physical symptoms of sexual abuse (see Display 20.6). As mandated reporters, community health nurses should be aware that sexual abuse of a child may surface through a broad range of physical, behavioral, and social symptoms. Some of these indicators, taken separately, may not be symptomatic of sexual abuse and should be examined in the context of other behaviors or situational factors.

Community health nurses can be part of the (SART). This group's responsibilities include obtaining the evidence and providing support to the victim and family after an episode of sexual abuse has been reported. Sexual abuse response team members include nurses, physicians, social workers, police, laboratory personnel, lawyers, and district attorney staff. Care for children who have been sexually abused varies, as the duration of the molestation, the age, and symptoms of the child will influence their care measures. "Poor prognostic signs include more intrusive forms of abuse, more violent assaults, longer periods of sexual molestation, and closer relationship of the perpetrator to the victim" (American Academy of Pediatrics, Committee on Child Abuse and Neglect, 1999, para. 24). Parents may also need counseling and support following the investigation and proceedings involving their child's victimization.

The sexual assault nurse examiner (SANE) role is more explicit in assisting the victim and appropriate family members immediately after the victim presents to the police or to an emergency department setting. The nurse has very specific actions to take to promote trust, obtain needed speci-men evidence, and treat the sexual abuse victim. The victim has already been significantly traumatized, and the nurse can be effective in this role only if trust can be established during this critical time after the sexual assault. The SANE is trained to work with victims of all ages, both genders, and under all sexual abuse situations.

Although there are several classifications of child molesters, pedophiles present the greatest danger. A **pedophile** is an adult whose main sexual interest is a child. A pedophile tends to be well-liked by children. Pedophiles, who most often are men, frequently choose to work in professions or volunteer organizations that allow them easy access to children, where they can develop the trust and respect of children and their parents. The pedophile believes that sex with children is appropriate and often lures children into sexual relationships with love, rewards, promises, and gifts. He may be among a child's family members (e.g., grandfather, father, uncle, cousin) or a trusted community leader the child knows (e.g., next-door neighbor, teacher, coach, or religious leader). Recent reports of pedophiles among clergy in the Roman Catholic Church have clearly rocked the church's status and stability. As of July 2006, the National Sex Offender Public Registry (NSOPR), sponsored through the Department of Justice, is used in all 50 states, thereby improving efforts to safeguard all children (Rape, Abuse, & Incest National Network [RAINN], 2006). This resource provides information regarding the more than 500,000 registered sex offenders throughout the United States.

Emotional Abuse

Emotional abuse of children involves psychological mistreatment or neglect, such as when parents do not provide the normal experiences that produce feelings of being loved, wanted, secure, and worthy (Crime and Violence Prevention Center, 2003c). This type of abuse is commonly associated with other types of abuse, and may involve verbal abuse, such as name calling, belittling, or threatening. A mother may shout at the child, "You're just like your father, a good-for-nothing, lazy bum." A father may say, "You're ugly. You look just like your mother." If the child spills some juice, a parent may scream, "Everything you do, you do wrong. Can't you do anything right?"

Emotional abuse may also take the form of emotional abandonment. Some parents "shun" their children as a form of punishment. They will not speak to them and do not look at them; they behave as if their child does not exist. This behavior may continue for a day or longer, whenever a child displeases the parent. In some cases, the shunning lasts for days.

Verbal threats, although a common discipline practice, are also a form of emotional abuse. Examples of verbal threats include, "Take your feet off the furniture of I'll chop your feet off" and "Do that again, and you'll really know what my belt feels like." In the first instance, the child might realize that the parent wouldn't really chop her feet off, but hearing the parent say such a violent thing can be emotionally scarring. In the second instance, the parent may have beaten the child with a belt in the past, so merely threatening to use the belt again causes emotional trauma.

Emotional abuse alone is rarely reported because it is another "hidden" form of abuse. However, **mandated reporters**, people who have a responsibility for the welfare

DISPLAY 20.6	INDICATORS OF SEXUAL ABUSE

I. History of Sexual Abuse

- A child confides to a friend, classmate, teacher, a friend's mother, or other trusted adult that she/he has experienced sexual abuse.
- A child may disclose information indirectly by such statements as:
  "I know someone . . ."
  "What would you do if . . .?"
  "I heard something about somebody..."
- The child has torn, stained, or bloody underclothing (among her/his clothing or is wearing it).
- Knowledge that a child's injury/disease (vaginal trauma, sexually transmitted disease) is unusual for the specific age group.
- Unexplained injuries/diseases (parent/caretaker unable to explain reason for injury/disease); there are discrepancies in explanation; blame is placed on a third party; explanations are inconsistent with medical diagnosis.
- A very young girl is pregnant or has a sexually transmitted disease. Pregnancy alone does not constitute sexual abuse, but if there are indications of coercion or significant age disparity between the minor and her partner, this may lead to reasonable suspicion of sexual abuse that must be reported.

II. Sexual Behavioral Indicators of Sexually Abused Children

- Detailed and age-inappropriate understanding of sexual behavior (especially among very young children).
- Sexually explicit language.
- Inappropriate, unusual, or aggressive sexual behavior with peers or toys.
- Compulsive indiscreet masturbation.
- Excessive curiosity about sexual matters or genitalia (self or others).
- Unusually seductive or flirtatious behavior with classmates, teachers, and other adults.
- Excessive concern about homosexuality, especially by boys.

III. Behavioral Indicators of Sexual Abuse in Younger Children

- Enuresis (wetting pants or bedwetting).
- Fecal soiling.
- Eating disturbances such as overeating or undereating.
- Fears or phobias.
- Overly compulsive behavior.
- School problems or significant change in school performance (attitude and grades).
- Age-inappropriate behavior that includes pseudomaturity or regressive behavior such as bedwetting or thumb sucking.
- Inability to concentrate.
- Sleeping disturbances (nightmares, fear of falling asleep, fretful sleep pattern, sleeping long hours).

- Drastic behavior changes.
- Speech disorders.
- Frightened of parents/caretaker or of going home or being at home.

IV. Behavioral Indicators of Sexual Abuse in Older Children and Adolescents

- Withdrawal.
- Chronic fatigue.
- Clinical depression, apathy.
- Overly compliant behavior.
- Over or under reaction (hysteria or cavalier attitude) to a genital exam.
- Poor hygiene or excessive bathing.
- Poor peer relations and social skills; inability to make friends.
- Acting out, running away, aggressive, antisocial or delinquent behavior.
- Alcohol or drug abuse.
- Prostitution or excessive promiscuity.
- School problems, frequent absences, sudden drop in school performance.
- Refusal to change clothes for physical education class.
- Nonparticipation in sports and social activities.
- Fearful of showers or restrooms.
- Fearful of home life as demonstrated by arriving at school early and leaving late.
- Suddenly fearful of other things (going outside or participating in familiar activities).
- Extraordinary fear of males (in cases of male perpetrator and female victim).
- Self-consciousness of body beyond that expected for age.
- Sudden acquisition of money, new clothes, or gifts with no reasonable explanation.
- Suicide attempt or other self-destructive behavior.
- Crying without provocation.
- Setting fires.

V. Physical Symptoms of Sexual Abuse

- Sexually transmitted diseases, especially in pre-pubescent girls.
- Genital discharge or infection.
- Physical trauma or irritation to the anal/genital area (pain, itching, swelling, bruising, bleeding, lacerations, abrasions), especially if injuries are unexplained or there is an inconsistent explanation.
- Pain during urination or defecation.
- Difficulty in walking or sitting due to genital or anal pain.
- Psychosomatic symptoms (stomach aches, headaches, chronic pain).

Adapted from the Crime and Violence Prevention Center. (1996). *Child abuse: Educator's responsibilities.* Sacramento, CA: California Attorney General's Office.

DISPLAY 20.7   SIGNS AND SYMPTOMS OF EMOTIONAL ABUSE OR DEPRIVATION

Emotional abuse should be suspected if the child displays the following behavioral indicators:

- Is withdrawn, depressed or apathetic.
- Is clingy and forms indiscriminate attachments.
- "Acts out" and is considered a behavior problem.
- Exhibits exaggerated fearfulness.
- Is overly rigid in conforming to instructions of teachers, doctors, and other adults.
- Suffers from sleep, speech, or eating disorders.
- Displays signs of emotional turmoil that include repetitive, rhythmic movements (rocking, whining, picking at scabs).
- Pays inordinate attention to details or exhibits little or no verbal or physical communication with others.
- Suffers from enuresis and fecal soiling.
- Unwittingly makes comments such as "Mommy always tells me I'm bad."
- Experiences substance abuse problems.

Emotional deprivation should be suspected if the child

- Refuses to eat adequate amounts of food and therefore is very frail.
- Is unable to perform normal learned functions for a given age (e.g., walking, talking).
- Displays antisocial behavior (aggression, disruption) or obvious delinquent behavior (drug abuse, vandalism); conversely, the child may be abnormally unresponsive, sad, or withdrawn.
- Constantly "seeks out" and "pesters" other adults such as teachers or neighbors for attention and affection.
- Displays exaggerated fears.

---

of children, including public and private school employees; administrators and employees of youth centers and recreation programs; child welfare employees; foster parents; group home and residential facility personnel; social workers; probation workers; health care workers including nurses, doctors, and chiropractors; animal control workers; and personnel working in film development laboratories, are required by law to report *suspected* cases of severe emotional neglect or abuse or deprivation in addition to *suspected* neglect and physical or sexual abuse (Crime and Violence Prevention Center, 2003a, 2003c) (see Display 20.7).

Specific Abusive Situations

The previous information addressed the major types of child abuse in families, yet other patterns of abuse against children need to be discussed. Shaken baby syndrome and Munchausen syndrome by proxy are fairly rare, but by the time the condition is discovered it is often too late, with the diagnosis made during subsequent visits to the emergency department or at autopsy.

In addition, Internet crimes against children, child abduction, and crimes against children by babysitters are an increasingly common fear of parents. These types of abuse are occurring more often as children and adolescents have increased time and access to computers, and because both parents (or a single parent) must work, children are spending more time alone or with babysitters. Community concern regarding child abductions by family members or strangers has resulted in the institution of Amber Alert systems in many states. School violence is also an area of increasing concern for families and will be addressed.

Shaken Baby Syndrome

Shaken baby syndrome is the intentional abusive action of violently shaking an infant or toddler, usually child of 2 years or younger (National Institute of Neurological Disorders and Stroke, 2007). The type of damage that occurs to these infants very seldom occurs through play, as in minor falls at play, or as a result of tossing a baby in the air. The classic medical symptoms associated with infant shaking are bilateral retinal hemorrhage, subdural or subarachnoid hematomas, absence of other external signs of abuse, and symptoms that may include breathing difficulties, seizures, dilated pupils, lethargy, and unconsciousness (USDOJ, 2002). These injuries occur from a violent, sustained action in which the infant's head, which lacks muscular control, is violently whipped forward and backward, hitting the chest and shoulders. According to experts, an observer would describe the shaking as being "as hard as the shaker was humanly capable of shaking the baby" or "hard enough that it appeared the baby's head would come off" (USDOJ, 2002). Within minutes to hours after the injury, the baby begins to show symptoms such as irritability, lethargy, vomiting, breathing problems, seizures, or unconsciousness. A typical explanation given by the parents or caretakers is that the baby was "fine" and then suddenly went into respiratory arrest or began having seizures—both common symptoms of shaken baby syndrome. Children who survive shaken baby syndrome may require lifelong care (National Institute of Neurological Disorders and Stroke, 2007).

Munchausen Syndrome by Proxy

Munchausen syndrome is a psychological disorder in which a client fabricates the symptoms of a disease in order to undergo medical tests, hospitalization, or even medical or surgical treatment. Clients with this disorder may intentionally injure themselves or induce illness in themselves. In cases of **Munchausen syndrome by proxy**, a parent or caretaker attempts to bring medical attention to herself by injuring or inducing illness in her child. The following scenarios are typical of these cases:

- The child's parent or caretaker brings the child to the emergency department or calls paramedics repeatedly for alleged problems that have no medical basis.
- The child experiences "seizures" or "respiratory arrest" only when the parent or caretaker is present—never in the presence of a neutral third party or when hospitalized, unless the parent or caretaker reports that the incident occurred in her presence.

◆ While the child is hospitalized, the parent or caretaker shuts off intravenous tubes or life-support equipment, causing the child distress, and then turns everything back on and summons help.

◆ The parent or caretaker induces illness by introducing a mild irritant or poison into the child's body; chronic ingestion of such substances may cause the child's death.

Health providers, mental health professionals, and attorneys may be involved in working with such cases, requiring careful attention to the history of the illness/injury, the treatment, documentation, and communication with the parent/caretaker. Attention to the child's safety is paramount, although the parent may remove the child from care or take the child to another facility if the caregiver's suspicions are aroused (Stirling, 2007).

Internet Crimes Against Children

Internet crimes are insidious because they come right into the home. A recent national survey found that annually, one in five youth had been sexually solicited over the Internet (Finkelhor, Mitchell, & Wolak, 2000). Children either unintentionally or intentionally may access an Internet chat room or website developed or used by pedophiles. The perpetrator establishes contact, usually passing himself off as a teen or young man who has similar interests, and states affection for and understanding of the youth's "problems." Eventually, the pedophile either sets up a meeting time and place or engages in sexually explicit dialogue with the minor (USDOJ, 2001b). Many minors find the attention from this stranger inviting or exciting and make plans to meet the person. When this happens, the minor falls victim to this individual who preys on children, putting the child/adolescent at great risk. This computer-based child abuse risk has led the United States Attorney General to authorize a federal awareness and justice program focusing solely on technology-facilitated sexual exploitation and abuse against children, named *Project Safe Childhood* (USDOJ, 2006).

Community health nurses can assist families to prevent such Internet crimes in various ways by:

◆ Encouraging placement of "blocks" on computers via the Internet server
◆ Urging parents to discuss with their children the dangers of online "friendships" that seek face-to-face meetings
◆ Establishing parent–child contracts for Internet use
◆ Monitoring the time and Internet sites a child uses
◆ Keeping the computer in a high-traffic area in the home, affording easy observation
◆ Setting the Internet browser security feature to "high"
◆ Installing a firewall, antivirus, and anti-adware/spyware programs that increase privacy
◆ Discouraging downloading of games and other media that might contain Trojan or worm programs that enable remote access by unauthorized users (Dombrowski & Gischlar, 2004)

Furthermore, parents can contact the Cyber Tip Line at (800) 843-5678 or www.cybertipline.com if they suspect

that an online predator has contacted their child (Dombrowski & Gischlar, 2004, para. 5).

Child Abduction

Child abduction is a crime that every parent fears, and although stranger abduction happens infrequently, it remains the greatest fear for parents. However, intense media coverage gives the impression that such crimes occur frequently, and this causes great stress among parents and community members. Nationally, the Amber Alert program and the Child Abduction Response Teams (CART) were established to provide a prompt and professional response to child abduction (USDOJ, 2005).

Child abduction by family members or intimate partners, such as a divorced mother, father, step-parent, boyfriend, or grandparents, is more common. Nonetheless, the parent from whom the child was taken may be unaware that the abduction was by a relative or known person and may experience the same type of stress and loss as parents who lose a child by stranger abduction. In some cases, knowing the relative or person who abducted the child causes just as much fear, because the abductor may have a history of violence or sexual abuse crimes.

Prevention of child abduction is difficult, and at times parents who think they have taught their children well may have a false sense of security. Some studies assessed the effects on children of taking a "stranger awareness" class. The class included lessons on avoiding strangers, not talking to strangers, identifying who is a stranger, saying "no" to strangers, and running away and screaming if addressed by a stranger. Yet, researchers found that when the children left the classroom, if an unknown person (a stranger sent in by the researcher) asked the child to help him find a lost puppy or go help them get candy, many of the children responded readily without using any of the actions learned in the stranger awareness class. Parents who watched their children on tapes of these studies could not believe what they saw. Children are trusting and curious, and they may not consider people who look like their parents as *strangers*.

Community health nurses can help parents improve their child's safety by promoting close supervision of young children and practicing behaviors that promote anonymity. Ideas that help improve the child's safety include:

◆ Holding the child's hand while in malls or stores
◆ Keeping the child in the seat of a shopping cart
◆ Keeping a young child in sight at all times when playing outside
◆ Sharing parental supervision with another mother when children play, so that an adult is always supervising the children
◆ Not putting the child's name or initials on clothing or backpacks
◆ Teaching the child a "password" that only the parents and child know to use when a different person is picking them up from a neighborhood activity

Older children and teens who go outside the home unattended by parents should be encouraged to use the following behaviors that promote safety: staying with groups of other children or teens, having a cell phone, leaving an itinerary with the parents, and not changing their plans without contacting parents. Other measures that can benefit older children and adolescents are attending a self-defense class and carrying a whistle and/or pepper spray.

Crimes Against Children by Babysitters

Crimes against infants and young children by babysitters have been given attention by the media in recent years (USDOJ, 2001a). Some parents who have suspected mistreatment of their children by caretakers have used hidden cameras to reveal the problem. Abuse by caretakers is a fear of parents who must work and leave their children with others.

The community health nurse can help parents assess day care settings by providing them descriptors for finding good day care providers. Parents who use neighbors as babysitters should get references and should drop by the home or day care setting at various times during the day. They should assess their infants and follow-up on any bruises, rashes, burns, conditions, or behaviors they observe that are not normal for their child. With older children, parents need to listen to them and ask about their day and activities. Parents must not ignore signs, such as a child's fear of going to the babysitter or reports of spankings, being shouted at, or other inappropriate treatment. Day care centers and many home day care programs are licensed by the state. Programs for which parent complaints have been filed with licensing agencies are monitored more closely, and the state is mandated to make changes or close the facility if necessary. Parents need to know that their child is safe and cared for when they leave them to pursue their employment or educational activities.

School Violence

An area of growing concern regarding violence against children has been in school settings. Random shootings and hostage situations in schools over the past decade have fueled fears about the safety of students and promoted research into how to prevent this type of community violence affecting children. The United States Department of Education, Department of Health and Human Services, and Department of Justice have collaborated to provide funding, programs, and trainings that improve school safety through the *Safe Schools Healthy Students* initiative. Six areas identified for attention in building safe school climates are:

- ◆ Creating a safe school environment
- ◆ Providing alcohol, drug, and violence prevention and early-intervention programs
- ◆ Supporting school and community mental health prevention and treatment intervention services
- ◆ Providing early childhood psychosocial and emotional development programs
- ◆ Addressing education reform
- ◆ Designing safe school policies (Safe Schools Healthy Students Initiative, 2006).

PARTNER/SPOUSAL ABUSE

Adult violence is rooted in childhood violence. A father hits a mother. The mother hits her son. The son hits his sister. The sister hits her little brother. The little brother sets fire to the cat, pulls wings off butterflies, and grows up to be a spouse

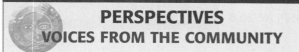

PERSPECTIVES
VOICES FROM THE COMMUNITY

Family Violence

My family was always shouting at each other—it was just the way it was. The hitting—well, that happened, but it wasn't nearly as bad as all that yelling. Now here I am in the same boat all over again—the yelling, the hitting, and I've got this new baby to take care of. I'm just so tired. When the nurse showed up today to check on the baby and me, I swore to myself I wouldn't tell her about the fight we had last night (anyway it wasn't nearly as bad as the other times). Then she looked at me and asked if I felt safe and that was it . . . I said NO before I realized my mouth was even open. I told her that he punched me in the side while I was changing the baby's diaper. She was so kind—she didn't tell me how stupid I was for staying with him, but she did help me look at my options. Since I was holding the baby when he hit me, she said she was required to make a report of child abuse. That was awful news, and I started to cry; but like she said, I could have dropped her or he could have missed me and hit her. I knew he'd be furious when he found out—then I was really in a panic. Well, she told me about a place in town I can stay for a time with the baby, and she helped me make arrangements. I'm so tired and scared, but I know now that I need to keep my baby safe. I still don't know what made me tell the nurse—I guess it was because she asked. I know I'm doing the right thing for me and the baby.

batterer. Although abused girls may grow up to be abusing mothers, more often they grow up to be abused wives. Researchers operationalize domestic violence as punching, grabbing, shoving, slapping, choking, kicking, biting, hitting with a fist or some other object, being beaten, or being threatened with a knife or gun by a spouse or cohabiting partner. See Perspectives: Voices from the Community.

Partner violence often begins during adolescent dating or dating at any age, with a push or shove that at first is overlooked by the girlfriend (Hanson, 2002). As these minor episodes of violence continue, the victim typically feels that she is doing something wrong and attempts to modify her behavior. She also assumes wrongly that once she and her boyfriend are married, these physical assaults will stop automatically or that in time she will be able to "change" him, yet the cycle of violence has already begun.

Cycle of Violence

The **cycle of violence** is a repetitive, cyclic pattern of abuse seen in domestic violence situations. This theory of family violence was first described as a three-phase cycle by Walker in 1979, after she studied more than 1,000 battered women and a smaller group of battering men. The cycle includes the tension-building phase, the acute battering incident, and the

DISPLAY 20.8   THE CYCLE OF VIOLENCE

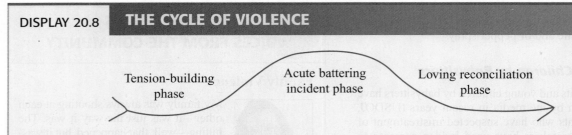

Tension-building phase   Acute battering incident phase   Loving reconciliation phase

Tension-Building Phase

The woman senses her partner's increasing tension. She may or may not know what is wrong. The partner is "edgy" and lashes out in anger. He challenges her, calls her names, and tells her she is stupid, incompetent, and unconcerned about him. She "tries hard" not to make any "mistakes" that may upset him. She takes the responsibility for making him feel better, and begins to set herself up to feel guilt when he eventually explodes in spite of her best efforts to calm and please him. During the increasing tension, the woman is rarely angry even at the most outrageous demands or blame. Rather, she internalizes her appropriate anger at the partner's unfairness and, instead, experiences depression, anxiety, and a sense of helplessness. As the tension in the relationship increases, minor episodes of violence increase, such as pinching, tripping, or slapping. The batterer knows his behavior is inappropriate, and he fears the woman will leave him. This fear of rejection and loss increases his rage at the woman and his need to control her.

Acute Battering Incident

The tension-building phase ends in an explosion of violence. The incident that sets off the man's violence is often trivial or unknown, leaving the woman confused and feeling helpless. The woman may or may not fight back. She may try to escape the violence or call for help. If she cannot escape the beating, she may have a sense of unreality—as if it is a dream. Following the battering, the woman is in a state of physical and psychological shock. She may be passive and withdrawn or hysterical and incoherent. She may not be aware of the seriousness of her injuries and may resist help. The man discounts the episode and also underestimates the woman's injuries. He may not summon medical help even when her injuries are life-threatening.

Loving Reconciliation

The loving reconciliation phase may begin a few hours to several days following the acute battering incident. Both partners have a profound sense of relief that "it's over." Although the woman is initially angry at the man, he begins an intense campaign to "win her back." Just as his tension and violence were overdone, his apologies, gifts, and gestures of love may also be excessive. Showering her with love and praise helps her repair her shattered self-esteem. It is nearly impossible for her to leave him during this phase as he is meeting her desperate need to see herself as a competent and lovable woman. The woman's feelings of power and romantic ideals are nurtured. She believes this gentle, loving person is her "real" lover. She believes that if only she can find the key, she can stop him from further violent episodes. She believes that, no matter how often it has happened before, somehow this episode seems different this time and it will never happen again.

The Increasing Spiral of Violence

One aspect of the cycle of violence of particular concern is its progressive and spiraling nature. Once violence has begun, every study indicates that it not only continues but over time increases in both frequency and severity. As the violence continues, the three-phase cycle begins to change. The tension-building phase becomes shorter and more intense, the acute battering incidents become more frequent and severe, and the loving reconciliation phase becomes shorter and less intense. After many years of battering, the man may not apologize at all.

loving reconciliation (Jenkins & Davidson, 2001). The psychological dynamics of these three phases help explain why women feel so guilty and ashamed of their partner's violence toward them, and why they find it so difficult to leave, even when their lives are in danger (see Display 20.8). Often, as the cycle of violence continues, the frequency of the cycle increases, with the tension-building phase and the acute battering incident occurring more often, and elimination of the loving reconciliation phase. Without intervention, this shorter, more violent cycle becomes increasingly risk-filled for outcomes that may lead to injury or maiming of a partner, incarceration, or death of a partner.

The Domestic Abuse Intervention Project in Duluth, Minnesota, developed a wheel of violence, identifying power and control at the center, and citing eight categories of perpetrator behaviors. This model is a useful tool for visu-alizing the multidimensional nature of abuse in which threats, coercion, isolation, blaming, intimidation, and use of children, male privilege, and economics convene to control the victim (Fig. 20.1).

Dating Violence

Dating violence in adolescent relationships is a serious and prevalent problem. Because of its prevalence, community health nurses should include screening for dating violence in all encounters with teens. **Adolescent dating violence (ADV)** includes physical, sexual, emotional, and verbal abuse between teenagers who are or have been in a casual or serious dating relationship (Hanson, 2002). Adolescent dating violence begins on average at age 15 years. About 50% of rape victims are between 10 and 19 years old, which indicates

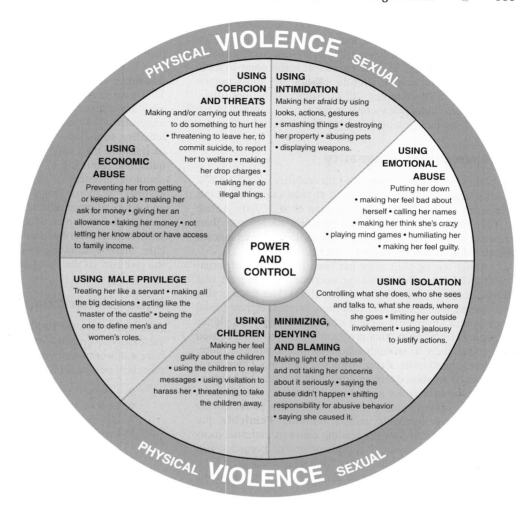

FIGURE 20.1 Wheel of Violence.

that teenage girls are vulnerable to the violence of sexual abuse (Jackson, Cram, & Seymour, 2000).

Partner/Spousal Abuse

Spousal abuse is violence against an intimate partner and is pervasive globally. The WHO reported in a multistudy review that 10% to 52% of women reported being physically abused by an intimate partner at some point in their lives, and 10% to 30% of women had experienced sexual violence by an intimate partner (WHO, 2005, p. 1). Because of the nature of **intimate partner violence (IPV)**, the problems are difficult to study and believed to be under-reported. Much remains unknown about factors that increase or decrease the likelihood that men will behave violently toward women, factors that endanger or protect women from violence, and the physical and emotional consequences of partner violence on women and their children.

The United States Department of Justice defines domestic violence as "a pattern of abusive behavior in any relationship that is used by one partner to gain or maintain power and control over another intimate partner" (USDOJ, Office of Violence Against Women, n.d., para. 1). Although domestic violence is categorized as physical abuse, sexual abuse, emotional abuse, economic abuse, or psychological abuse, the victim commonly experiences a combination of these abuses or threats of abuse in these areas. Intimidation and threats create an atmosphere of fear for the victim and may include humiliation, isolation, terrorizing, coercing, blaming, manipulating, stalking, and/or destruction of property or pets valued by the partner.

Domestic violence is a leading cause of morbidity and mortality in women nationwide, as battering exceeds rapes, muggings, and motor vehicle crashes combined as the leading cause of injury to women age 15 to 44 years (Sheehy, 2000a). Intimate partner violence resulted in nearly 2 million injuries and 1,300 deaths in 2003; while Fox and Zawitz (2004), cited by the CDC, found females accounted for 76% of IPV homicides and males were 24% of IPV homicides (Centers for Disease Control [CDC], 2006a). It is important to note that of those who died from IPV homicide, 44% had been to an emergency department within the last 2 years, and, of those, 93% had at least one injury at that time (Crandall, Nathens, Kernic, Holt, & Rivara, 2004; CDC, 2006a). Health care providers have a responsibility and opportunity to assess and initiate a safety plan when these patients are seen in the emergency room. A compendium of assessment tools for IPV can be found on the CDC website.

Healthy People 2010 identified the reduction of physical assault by current or former intimate partners as one of the nation's health objectives (USDHHS, 2000). In a 1998 survey by the Commonwealth Fund, almost one-third of American women (31%) reported having been physically or sexually abused by a husband or male partner at some point in their lives, whereas for women with disabilities, the abuse ranges from 33% to 83% (Kramer, 2002). Additionally, more than 25% of female homicide victims in the general population are killed by a husband, ex-husband, boyfriend, or ex-boyfriend.

Violence During Pregnancy

Pregnancy increases a woman's vulnerability, as 4% to 8% of all pregnant women are abused at least once during the pregnancy (CDC, 2006a; Gazmararian et al., 2000). Abuse is more likely to be reported by pregnant adolescents than pregnant adults and by women with unplanned pregnancies compared with other pregnant women.

Abuse during pregnancy has been linked with maternal health problems such as smoking, decreased weight gain, and substance use (Cokkinides & Coker, 1998). The fetus is also endangered, with spontaneous abortion, preterm delivery, fetal distress, and lower birth weight often seen. Curry, Doyle, & Gilhooley (1998) found that pregnant teens who were abused were more likely to be high school dropouts, smoked more, and experienced more second-trimester bleeding. Once born, the infant of an abused teen or adult is at risk for child abuse.

The most serious aspect of domestic violence as a threat to a woman's safety is the link between abuse during pregnancy and homicide, called femicide. **Femicide**, the killing of women, is now the leading cause of maternal mortality, rather than medical complications of pregnancy in several cities in the United States. Men who abuse their partners during pregnancy are more likely to own guns or knives or both, which puts the women at greater risk, and batterings that occur during pregnancy tend to have increased severity (Campbell, 1998, 1999).

Studies indicate that the prenatal care visit is one of the few times when women are seen by the helping professions. This visit is an important opportunity to identify women who are abused and therefore at risk for homicide. It is imperative that nurses conduct an assessment for danger and lethality, so that the women can be aware of their own level of risk and take safety precautions as needed. A series of questions requiring a "yes" or "no" response and inquiries about occurrences of abuse, escalation of abuse, frequency, severity, weapons, drugs or alcohol use by the perpetrator, and safety of other children should be incorporated into prenatal home visit assessments. This is especially important with women who have not followed through with prenatal care, thereby allowing health care professionals to monitor the progress of their pregnancies (Display 20.9).

Batterer Characteristics

Although men who batter come from all walks of life educationally, culturally, and socioeconomically, perpetrators have some common characteristics. The following attributes represent personal characteristics often seen in batterers:

- ◆ Low self-esteem
- ◆ Low income
- ◆ Low academic achievement
- ◆ Involvement in aggressive or delinquent behavior as youth
- ◆ Heavy alcohol and drug use
- ◆ Depression

DISPLAY 20.9	**DOMESTIC VIOLENCE RISK ASSESSMENT TOOL**

Frame the Questions

"Because abuse and violence are common in the lives of women, I have begun to ask about it with all women (or all pregnant women). I don't know if this is a problem for you, but I would like to ask you some questions, talk about ways to reduce your risk of being hurt, and give you some information and phone numbers that might be helpful to you."

Universal Questions

	Yes	No
1. Do you feel safe in your current relationships? Comments: _____	_____	_____
2. Have you ever been physically abused (pushed, shoved, hit, punched, bitten, burned, etc.)? Comments: _____	_____	_____
3. Have you ever been emotionally abused (neglected, called names, controlled, threatened, had your activities or decisions hindered,	_____	_____

been denied resources to meet your physical or financial needs)? Comments: _____

4. Have you ever been sexually abused _____ _____ (forced to have an unwanted sexual act)? Comments: _____

5. Do you want to talk to someone about _____ _____ receiving help? Comments: _____

Resources
National Domestic Violence Hotline:
1-800-799-SAFE (7233)
Local Battered Women's Shelter _____
Local Department of Women's Health Services _____
Other resources _____

Adapted from Sheehy, G. (2000b). *Violence against women.* Fairfax, VA: The National Women's Health Information Center; Kramer, A. (2002). Domestic violence: How to ask and how to listen. *Nursing Clinics of North America, 37*(1), 189–210; and Davis, R.E., & Harsh, K.E. (2001). Confronting barriers to universal screening for domestic violence. *Journal of Professional Nursing, 17*(6), 313–320.

◆ Anger and hostility
◆ Personality disorders
◆ Prior history of being physically abusive
◆ Having few friends and being isolated from other people
◆ Unemployment
◆ Emotional dependence and insecurity
◆ Belief in strict gender roles (e.g., male dominance and aggression in relationships)
◆ Desire for power and control in relationships
◆ Being a victim of physical or psychological abuse (consistently one of the strongest predictors of perpetration) (CDC, 2006a, para. 24).

Relationship, community, and societal factors have also been identified that affect a perpetrator's risk for battering. Identified relationship factors include: marital fights and tension, divorce and separations, money problems, and problematic and difficult family relationships, as well as the male's need for dominance and control in the relationship. Societal factors associated with increased risk are strict role stereotyping about the roles the husband and wife should follow in a relationship. Aspects identified within a community that lead to increased risks for IPV may be a lack of resources in the community, a failure or unwillingness of others to intervene or contact authorities when they are aware of the abuse, and factors associated with poverty, such as overcrowding and unemployment (CDC, 2006a).

Victim Characteristics

Studies have also revealed risk factors associated with victims. Increasing the victim's abilities to manage and improve their behaviors and understanding of relationship patterns and abuse allows victims to change their risk of being a victim. Individual risk factors for IPV victims include:

◆ A prior history of IPV
◆ Being female
◆ Young age
◆ Heavy alcohol and drug use
◆ High-risk sexual behaviors
◆ Witnessing or experiencing violence as a child
◆ Being less educated
◆ Unemployment
◆ For men, having a different ethnicity from their partner
◆ For women, having a greater education level than their partner
◆ For women, being American Indian/Alaska Native or African American
◆ For women, having a verbally abusive, jealous, or possessive partner (CDC, 2006, para. 19).

Marked differences between partner's incomes, levels of education, or job status places a victim more at risk for IPV. Community characteristics are similar to those of the perpetrator, revealing that those communities with fewer available resources, in areas of poverty, and having a lack of sanctions against violent behaviors increases one's risk. Traditional gender roles, such as a belief that men work and women are submissive and should stay home, are societal risk factors associated with higher IPV risk (CDC, 2006a, para. 19).

Effects of Violence on Children

Children who are exposed to family violence are more at risk for abuse and for violence later in their life as either a perpetrator or victim. Although domestic violence may not be directed at a child, that child may become a victim as a bystander or when trying to protect a parent. Effects of family violence are often seen in emotional, cognitive, physical, and/or behavioral manifestations of the child. Symptoms to be aware of in children are anxiety, hostility, depression, guilt, impaired concentration, confusion, fear of losing control or of a reoccurrence of the violence, sleep disturbances, nightmares, an exaggerated startle response, psychosomatic symptoms, social withdrawal, distrust, avoidance, or substance abuse (Volpe, 1996).

Most often, wife abuse and child abuse occur together. Literature reviews consistently suggest that a positive correlation exists between children's witnessing IPV and some aspects of impaired child development (Lemmey et al., 2001). Young children are particularly vulnerable to the effects of violence, as they lack the ability to understand the trauma and are likely to exhibit somatic complaints (headaches, eating or sleep problems) and/or behavior regression (clinging, whining, or becoming nonverbal) (Volpe, 1996). Meanwhile, school-age children and adolescents are more likely to either act out with delinquent behaviors or withdraw. It is more common for girls to become withdrawn and an important reason for health care providers to include an assessment for family violence concerns. Children in families with domestic violence are at risk for depression, negative mental health effects, and consequences that last far into their adult lives. These maladjustments may be behavioral (aggression and conduct problems), emotional (withdrawal, anxiousness, fearfulness), social, cognitive (learning disabilities), and/or physical. Providers who work with children need to listen in a sincere, nonjudgmental manner, and provide ongoing support when assisting the child and family with resources, such as counseling, education, or community violence prevention programs (Fig. 20.2).

MISTREATMENT OF ELDERS

It is estimated that as many as 10% of older adults are victims of abuse (Gray-Vickrey, 2001). **Elder abuse**, the mistreatment or exploitation of older adults, may involve neglect; physical, sexual, emotional, or fiduciary abuse; or any combination of these mistreatments. Among substantiated cases of elder abuse, 25% involve physical abuse, 49% intentional or unintentional neglect, 35% emotional abuse, and 30% financial or material exploitation. Elders are abused by family members in similar ways that younger family members are abused: by abandonment or neglect (physical or emotional); by physical, sexual, or emotional abuse; or by exploitation. Two-thirds of elder abuse is perpetrated by family members (Kramer, 2002). Adult children, divided between males and females equally, are the most frequent abusers of the elderly. However, spouses who were batterers do not stop at age 65; they commit about 14% of the reported cases of elder abuse in the United States. Victims of elder abuse have a median age of 76.5 years, and 65% of them are White.

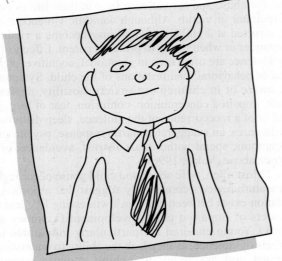

My Daddy is a Monster

He hurts my mommy
He hurts me too
Sometimes he hits
Sometimes he says things
That scare me and
make my mommy cry
after he leaves
Sometimes I wish he
won't come back ...ever.
I love my daddy.

National Coalition Against Domestic Violence • P.O. Box 34103 • Washington, DC 20043-4103 • 1-800-799-SAFE

FIGURE 20.2 Poster of "My Daddy Is a Monster."

Abuse against elders is not new, but research on elder abuse is new. Until recently, the reasons for elder abuse were extrapolated from the literature on abuse in younger populations. But, by the mid-1980s, more research was being conducted about elder abuse, and the findings indicated that elder abuse results from multiple, interrelated variables associated with the perpetrator or the victim (Menzey, 2001).

Forms of physical abuse were found to include rough handling during caregiving, pinching, hitting, and slapping. Emotional abuse, which can take many forms, included being shouted at or threatened, and having needed care withheld. More rarely, elders are sexually abused, which may include rape. Some elders are neglected by those they depend on to meet their caregiving needs. Elders with dementia and those requiring assistance for all activities of daily living (ADLs) are more at risk because of caregiver stress or burnout, which increases an elder's risk for abuse and neglect. With neglect, the elder may appear unwashed and unkempt or may suffer from malnutrition and dehydration, or even pressure sores. Elders who are dependent on others for their care often do not report abuse for fear of being abandoned. They feel powerless and at a loss about how to change a bad situation. They often fear reprisal from the perpetrator if they tell others about the abuse.

Older adults are frequently exploited in a variety of ways. Family members may take their Social Security retirement money, savings, or investments and use these funds on themselves. Criminals often approach elders with get-rich-quick schemes, sham investment opportunities, overpriced home repairs, or as collectors for illegitimate charities, thereby preying on the trusting nature of older adults.

Perpetrator and Victim Characteristics

The dominant underlying factors that contribute to abuse of an elder by a family member are social isolation and pathology on the part of the perpetrator. Research has identified emotional or financial dependence on the victim, alcohol use, and isolation or few external contacts as major contributing factors. Men are more likely to exploit or physically abuse elders, whereas women are more likely to neglect elders physically or abuse them psychologically. Because women are more frequently the caretakers of elders, they are in a position to provide either appropriate or neglectful care to frail older adults (Menzey, 2001).

Some characteristics of older people appear to increase their risk of abuse. These risks include dementia and poor health (Menzey, 2001). Newly diagnosed cognitive impairment correlates with occurrences of abuse. If violence or threats of violence by the elder toward the caregiver accompany dementia, this contributes to elder's risk for abuse. The failing health of an elder may also contribute to self-neglect or diminished ability for self-defense or escape from maltreatment. Finally, if the abuser and victim live together, the close proximity can bring up unresolved family conflicts or create new conflicts and tension (Menzey, 2001).

Risk Factors

Regardless of the type of abuse an elder suffers or the motivation of the abuser, two factors are common to all elder abuse situations. The first factor is the *invisibility* of elders in general and of abused elders specifically. It is estimated that fewer than 10% of elder abuse cases are reported. In 1988, Pillemer and Finkelhor found that only one of every 14 cases of elder abuse came to public attention in Massachusetts, a state with model reporting laws. Reasons for invisibility among the elderly are multifaceted. Older people usually have less contact with the community. They are no longer in the workforce or in public on a regular basis, which keeps their problems hidden longer. In addition, older adults are reticent to admit to being abused or neglected. Because the abuser is most often a family member, the elder desires to protect the abuser; without this abusing family member, the elder may be entirely alone. On the other hand, the elder may fear reprisal from the abuser for coming forward with a self-report of abuse or telling someone about the home situation. Cultural and societal values also contribute to keeping "family matters" private, while shame and embarrassment make it difficult for many elders to tell others of the abuse (American Psychological Association, 2007).

The second risk factor is the *vulnerability* of older adults. Many elders who are frail are dependent on others for some aspect of their day-to-day survival. At first, they may need to rely on others for transportation, shopping, and housekeeping. Later, they may need help with financial affairs, cooking, and laundry. In time, the elder may need help managing medications, bathing, and eating. The degree to which an elder needs assistance is often kept hidden from others because the elder person fears being removed from his present living situation and being placed in a more restrictive environment. Additionally, vulnerability in elders is increased when any of the following characteristics are present: (a) impairment and isolation, (b) poverty and pathologic caregivers, (c) learned helplessness and living in a violent subculture, and (d) living in deteriorating housing and crime-ridden neighborhoods.

Prevention of Elder Abuse

Awareness of elder abuse and education about the types of abuse via media campaigns has improved community awareness of the problem. The unique care needs for elders, resources for the elderly, along with recognition of the need for respite for caregivers has also received increased attention and services. Training for caregivers as well as health care and social service providers that focus on recognizing stress and initiating measures for intervening has developed new understanding of effective interventions (e.g., use of physical therapists, occupational therapists, and geropsychiatrists). Statutory requirements for reporting abuse and providing crisis hotlines for reporting elder abuse are also integral aspects of a community's response to the problem of elder abuse (American Psychological Association, 2007).

OTHER FORMS OF FAMILY VIOLENCE

Three other forms of violence that directly affect families are suicide, homicide, and rape. These three forms of violence demonstrate the ultimate extreme of violence to the victim and are the most traumatic to the surviving family members.

Suicide

Suicide is taking action that causes one's own death. In the United States, suicide is the 11th leading cause of death, as more than 31,000 people kill themselves each year (CDC, 2006b). Not all suicide attempts are successful and each year over 425,000 people are treated in emergency rooms from self-inflicted injuries (CDC, 2006b). These attempts to cause or actually cause self-harm are known as *parasuicidal acts*. Gender has an influence on suicide rates and fatalities—men are four times more likely than women to die, yet women are three times more likely than men to report a suicide attempt (CDC, 2006b). The *Healthy People 2010* goal is to reduce suicides to not more than 6.0 per 100,000 people, yet in 2004, there were 32,439 suicides, a rate of 89 suicides/day, or one suicide every 16 minutes (American Association of Suicidology, 2006).

Worldwide, the suicide rate has been increasing for the past 45 years. In 2000, "a global mortality rate of 16 per 100,000 people, or one death every 40 seconds" occurred, which translates to nearly 1 million people (WHO, n.d., Suicide prevention [SUPRE], para. 1). The estimate for suicide

attempts is up to 20 times more frequent than the fatality rate. Older men have traditionally had the highest suicide rate, although a noted increase in younger people is occurring in both developed and developing countries (WHO, para. 3). Ninety percent of suicides are associated with mental disorders, the most common are depression and substance abuse, which commonly occur during times of individual or family crisis (e.g., loss of a loved one, loss of employment) (WHO, para. 4).

It is important to be aware of warning signs of potential suicide when working with people in crisis. Threats or comments that indicate a plan or giving personal items away are potential indicators of a person contemplating suicide. Access to guns increases one's risk regardless of age, gender, or ethnicity because firearms are the most utilized method of suicide. Health providers and others may find *IS PATH WARM*, a mnemonic from the American Association of Suicidology (AAS), is helpful when looking at possible warning signs for suicide. These signs are:

I— ideation
S— substance abuse

P— purposelessness
A— anxiety
T— trapped
H— hopelessness

W— withdrawal
A— anger
R— recklessness
M— mood change
(American Association of Suicidality [AAS], n.d.)

Completed suicides are carried out in a variety of ways, some more violent than others. Women usually choose less violent methods, such as overdosing on medications. Men choose more violent forms of suicide, such as hanging, use of firearms, or vehicle crashes. Deaths from suicide are under-reported because of a tendency to group them as accidental deaths or deaths from undetermined causes.

Community awareness campaigns and education programs are needed to help a person recognize the risks and the importance of initiating prevention for someone who is suicidal. Crisis hotlines with 24-hour access are a vital resource for a distraught individual, friend, or loved one to contact and find help during a crisis and to learn about local resources to contact. Appropriate and consistent treatment, most often a combination of antidepressants and psychotherapy approach, is needed for those suffering from depression, because individuals with a major depressive disorder have approximately a 20 times higher risk for suicide than the general population (AAS, 2007). The surviving loved ones require attention to their grief and bereavement. Support groups often provide benefits, allowing the bereaved to share their intense feelings of guilt and learn how to deal with any sense of a stigma, embarrassment, or shame felt by the survivors.

Homicide

Homicide is any non–war-related action taken to cause the death of another person. Violence has historically been associated with crime and is generally categorized by the method or age group affected. The WHO cites, "On an average day,

1,424 people are killed in acts of homicide, almost one person every minute" (2002b, para. 2). More shocking is the report that violence is the leading cause of death for those from ages 15 to 44 years, and precipitating factors are often fighting, bullying, and drunkenness (para. 5).

In the *Healthy People 2010 Midcourse Review,* the homicide rate between 1999 and 2002 increased to 6.1 deaths per 100,000 population (up from 6.0 deaths/100,000), while leading researchers and public health providers continue their efforts toward understanding these trends (Office of Disease Prevention and Health Promotion, n.d., p. 15-8). In the United States, homicide was the 15th leading cause of death in 2004, with 17,357 deaths (Minino, Heron, Murphy, & Kochanek, 2007, Table 2). Many homicide casualties are victims of domestic abuse as the cycle of violence escalates; a partner may be killed during a violent episode or by a recruited third party. Homicide in young infants and children is most often perpetrated by the parent, step-parent, or caregiver. Conflict between adolescent males may escalate if weapons or guns are available, resulting in homicide.

Evidence suggests that violence can be prevented by measures aimed at individuals, families, and communities. Although biologic and personal factors may influence one's predisposition to violence, an interaction between one's family, community, cultural, and other factors combine to create violence (WHO, 2002b). The WHO cites four key steps in developing a public health approach to violence; these steps are:

◆ Uncovering as much knowledge as possible about all aspects of violence
◆ Investigating why it occurs
◆ Exploring ways to prevent violence
◆ Taking action, which includes disseminating information, and evaluating programs' effectiveness (WHO, 2002a, p. 1)

Prevention methods include education programs for preschool, school-age children, and adolescents to decrease bullying and improve social skills; parent education courses and parent resources such as advice lines, support groups, or a crisis nursery; and community measures that improve firearm safety and reduce firearm injuries (WHO, 2002b).

Rape

Rape is an act of aggression in which the perpetrator is motivated by a desire to dominate, control, and degrade the victim. Once considered an act of sexuality, rape is now believed to be a combination of domination and sexuality, or defined as a "sexual expression of aggression." The National Violence Against Women Survey (NVAWS) working with the CDC and National Institute of Justice, reports that 302,091 women and 92,748 men are raped each year in the United States. Furthermore, the survey estimates that one in six women and one in 33 men have been a rape victim at some time during their life, with over half of all rapes occurring before the age of 18, and one-third of the rapes occurring before age 12 (CDC, 2004). Rape, in more than eight of ten cases (83%), is perpetrated by someone the victim knows (CDC, 2004).

The violence of rape creates physical and psychological harm for the victim and those close to them. Health problems for the victim may include head, pelvic, back or facial pain, depression, suicidal ideation, eating disorders, gastrointestinal disorders, or substance abuse (CDC, 2004). Fear, anxiety, or shame may become debilitating for the victim. Counseling and professional care are necessary for the rape victim from the time the rape is reported through any legal process that may result.

Community measures useful in preventing rape include rape prevention education (RPE) programs for adolescents and college students, date rape education, hotlines staffed to provide help for victims of rape or violence against women, and having trained professionals, such as a sexual assault response teams (SART) on hand (CDC, 2004). SART members are trained to understand the psychological and physical assessment needs of the victim, as well as the legal requirements for an investigation and court proceeding. Rape crisis centers and state sexual assault coalitions work together with law enforcement, health care providers, and community-based organizations (CBOs) to provide community education, and care and support to victims.

LEVELS OF PREVENTION: CRISIS INTERVENTION AND FAMILY VIOLENCE

Family violence is a family crisis and needs intervention. Community health nurses are in a unique position to prevent, identify, and intervene during crisis situations. Because community health nurses encounter people in their own settings, a more accurate assessment with direct observation, discussion, and intervention can occur. The community health nurse's assessment skills, familiarity with the community, and access to resources, enhances her ability to help families in crisis. By using the three levels of prevention, the nurse can begin to assist families in a variety of ways to counter problems arising from domestic violence.

Primary Prevention

The cycle of violence within the family can be interrupted. Even when partners, spouses, or parents have been brought up in violent homes by abusive parents, they can learn to rechannel and control their emotions and behaviors and use more appropriate coping strategies. Primary prevention is the most effective level of intervention in terms of promoting clients' health and containing costs. Primary prevention reflects a fundamental human concern for well-being and includes planned activities undertaken by the nurse to prevent an unwanted event from occurring, to protect current health and healthy functioning, and to promote improved states of health for all members of a community. For the community health nurse, any activity that fosters healthful practices will counteract unhealthful influences, thereby empowering an individual or family help prevent a crisis. Health promotion must take into account the physical, psychological, sociocultural, and spiritual needs of the individual and family.

Opportunities for families to improve relationships with their partner or spouse and children may begin with learning social problem-solving skills. Both partners benefit by participating in these learning sessions/opportunities. Assertiveness skills for women provide a foundation on which additional empowerment can build. Many people have not learned positive problem-solving skills that are socially acceptable, while women may have learned passivity and submissiveness in response to their own childhood parenting or from an abusive upbringing.

Healthy self-esteem improves education and occupational success. If poverty is a factor related to the violence, adequate educational preparation and having a successful employee role may eliminate this stressor. Violence occurs across all socioeconomic levels; however, if a family is so impoverished that its basic needs cannot be met, stress can lead vulnerable family members to seek illegal ways to solve their financial problems. Living in neighborhoods where criminal activity is common often leads to increased violence and risk of abuse.

Parenting, one of life's most difficult roles, influences children in their coping strategies, decision making, and sense of self-confidence. Parenting classes are an important resource to assist parents, particularly parents who are at high risk, such as teens, people with no exposure to children in their upbringing, and people raised in violent and abusive families. Parenting classes offer an opportunity for parents to share information and the stresses of parenting, while learning new strategies for managing their children's behaviors and appropriate physical, emotional, and developmental expectations for their children's ages.

Community health nurses often make home visits to families based on referrals from hospital perinatal departments. During the mother's postpartum stay, a nurse may have noted some inappropriate parenting behaviors or that the parents may meet high-risk parameters set by the hospital, such as being age 17 or younger, being a single parent, or having a history of substance abuse. On the first few visits to the family, the nurse can assess parenting skills and need for further teaching. If a parenting class is recommended, the course should cover age-appropriate content, such as safety, breast-feeding, formula preparation, food progression, anticipatory guidance for growth and development, discipline techniques including behavior modification and time-out, well-baby care, and immunizations. Additional benefits for the parents are the social support they receive from participating with other parents and having the opportunity to share their needs and concerns about child-rearing.

Home visiting has been formalized into public health nursing model programs around the country, based on two decades of work by David Olds and others. This model program has shown that nurse follow-up and interventions during the pregnancy and for the first 2 years of the child's life was effective in preventing child abuse, decreasing the mother's reliance on government assistance, having mothers with longer spacing between their children and fewer subsequent pregnancies, and improving health habits, such as less smoking by mothers (Olds et al., 1988, 1997, 1999, 2004). In these programs, a nurse visits the mother and child on a regular basis over 1 to 3 years, teaching and role-modeling parenting techniques, providing needed support, and initiating necessary referrals.

The interrelatedness between families and communities cannot be overlooked or underestimated. Neighborhoods need to be enfranchised, developed, and attentive to the needs for health and safety for all community members. Empowered families can take back their neighborhoods from criminals, and their empowerment acts as a source of growth for other families.

Secondary Prevention

Early diagnosis and prompt treatment of the effects of family crisis or violence is the focus at a secondary level of prevention. Secondary prevention seeks to reduce the intensity and duration of a crisis and to promote adaptive behavior. By creating a positive relationship with family members and seeing them in their homes, the community health nurse can often uncover and intervene in a crisis or stop abusive situations.

People in crisis need help. Often they desperately want help. The crisis or violence and its associated disequilibrium has a twofold effect on the individuals involved: it renders them temporarily helpless and unable to cope on their own, and it makes them especially receptive to outside influence. Community health nurses can implement crisis resolution models to assist clients at the secondary level. The following process has been used successfully in the mental health field by those working on crisis hot lines, in mental health centers, or in emergency departments. These steps are:

1. Establish rapport.
2. Assess the individual and the problem for lethality.
3. Identify major problems and intervene.
4. Deal with feelings.
5. Explore alternatives and coping mechanisms.
6. Develop an action plan.
7. Follow up, including anticipatory planning for coping with future crises (Aguilera, 1998).

People in crisis will seek and generally receive some kind of help, but the nature of that help may act in favor of or against a healthy outcome from which the participants can grow and evolve. A client's desire for assistance gives the helping professional a prime opportunity to intervene; this opportunity also presents a challenge to make the intervention as effective as possible. Behaviors found to be helpful in these interventions include the following:

◆ *Respect confidentiality.* Discussions must occur in private, without other family members present or in within the proximity for hearing. Confidentiality is essential to build trust and ensure the client's safety.
◆ *Believe and validate the client's experiences.* Listen to and believe him. Acknowledge the client's feelings and validate that many others have had similar experiences.
◆ *Acknowledge any injustice.* In the case of violence, acknowledge that no one deserves to be abused.
◆ *Respect clients' autonomy.* Respect their right to make life decisions, particularly regarding whether to involve the police. Validate and respect clients' choices. They are the experts in their lives.
◆ *Help the client plan for future safety.* What past strategies have been successful for self-protection? Does the client have a safe place to escape to if necessary? If children are involved, what plans are available to protect them? Help clients to recognize danger in their lives.
◆ *Promote access to community services.* Know the resources in your community. Is there a shelter for battered or homeless clients? A domestic violence

hotline? A rape crisis center? Give clients the appropriate phone numbers (Davis & Harsh, 2001; Kramer, 2002).

One goal of crisis intervention should be to help clients reestablish a sense of safety and security while allowing them to ventilate their feelings and have those feelings validated. This process helps reestablish equilibrium at as healthy a level as possible and can result in client change and growth. Minimally, the goal is to resolve the immediate crisis and restore clients to their pre-crisis level of functioning. Ultimately, however, intervention seeks to raise their functioning to a healthier, more mature level that will enable them to cope with and prevent future crises. As discussed earlier, crises tend to be self-limited; intervention time generally lasts from 4 to 8 weeks, with resolution, one way or another, within 2 or 3 months (Aguilera, 1998). The urgency of the situation represents a window of opportunity that invites prompt, focused attention by the client and nurse in working together to achieve intervention goals.

Special programs for children who live in homes where crises and violence are chronic include Head Start programs for pre-kindergarten children who meet certain socioeconomic characteristics. These programs are designed to give children social and academic stimulation, thereby increasing their skills for when they enter kindergarten. Other programs for social skills development may include a Special Friends program explicitly for children who have survived abusive situations, or primary intervention programs (PIP), in which the child works with a trained, supportive, and caring adult.

Abuse survivors and those living in homes with domestic violence experience multiple developmental and psychological problems. Children who are experiencing academic and social failure should receive ongoing services as needed through their elementary, middle, and high school grades. Early identification and intervention with conduct-disordered youth ensures that appropriate resources are obtained and, hopefully, that behavior outbursts and violence will be eliminated. School nurses are important interprofessional team members in providing assessments and programs for these youth.

Intervention at the secondary level for adults who experience abuse focuses on women and their children. Shelters for women and children are available in most communities and offer a variety of services, including counseling, classes in self-esteem building and assertiveness training, referrals to or programs for job training, and even money/budgeting and time management classes. Some shelters offer programs that last up to 2 years with progressive independence and employment skill development while the women and their children live in a protected home environment with their addresses kept confidential from abusers.

Depending on the situation that brings the woman to a shelter, the perpetrator may or may not be incarcerated or on probation. If arrested during the most recent violent episode, the abuser may be released, on parole, or incarcerated. Even while incarcerated, the abuser may be able to take part in an anger-management class, psychological counseling, substance abuse treatment, Alcoholics Anonymous (AA) meetings, or Narcotics Anonymous (NA) meetings. Visits between the abuser and the children are supervised, if that is part of a court order.

At times, the nurse may be responding to a referral regarding suspected abuse; at other times, an abusive or neg-lectful situation may be uncovered on a home visit made for another reason. In any case, the community health nurse has an important role in reporting suspected abuse and encouraging the child, partner/spouse, or elder to go to the appropriate facility to seek care and to file required documentation about the abuse (see From the Case Files).

Reporting Abuse

All states have reporting laws for suspected abuse, although states differ on aspects of the timeline for reporting, who to notify, and the sequence of events. The following steps represent one state's guidelines for reporting suspected child abuse (Crime and Violence Prevention Center, 2003b):

1. All mandated reporters must report known or suspected abuse.
2. Immediately, or as soon as reasonably possible, a local child protective agency (police department after normal working hours) must be contacted and given a verbal report. During this verbal report, mandated reporters must give their name—which is kept confidential and may be revealed only in court or if the reporter waives confidentiality (others can give information anonymously)—the name and age of the child, the present location of the child, the nature and characteristics of the injury, and any other facts that led the reporter to suspect abuse or that would be helpful to the investigator.
3. Within 2 working days, a written report must be completed by the mandated reporter and filed. If a mandated reporter fails to report known or suspected instances of child abuse, she may be subject to criminal liability, punishable by up to 6 months in jail or a fine of $1,000.

Similar steps are required for nurses when reporting elder abuse. Cases of maltreatment and neglect among elders are reported to a local area agency on aging, Adult Protective Services, or to the police, and a screening/documentation form is used to gather and record pertinent information. Guidelines for filing the report and agency notification are specific within each state.

In cases of partner/spousal abuse, adults who are mentally competent cannot be removed involuntarily from the abusive situation. The community health nurse can encourage the victim to leave the perpetrator for the victim's safety until the perpetrator gets professional help, and can give information regarding community resources, such as a shelter for women and children. If the adult has a life-threatening injury or illness, medical follow-up must be encouraged; however, the victim may still be reluctant to seek help. At times, another family member or neighbor who witnesses the abusive event calls 911; when the police and paramedics arrive, the victim may have support to seek care and needed protection. A domestic violence screening/documentation form is completed by the nurse as a part of the official health records for the client.

Tools

Assessment of suspected abuse cannot be overemphasized. The community health nurse may be the only person entering the home of a family in crisis where abuse is occurring.

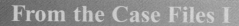

From the Case Files I

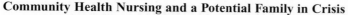

Community Health Nursing and a Potential Family in Crisis

You are a community health nurse working for Smithville Health Department. You are following up on a referral from a community clinic's family planning clinic. The referral was made for a 19-year-old woman, Sandy, who presented in clinic and exhibited inappropriate behaviors with her 6-month-old daughter. In their referral, staff stated that they observed the mother shouting at the child, accusing her of "being spoiled rotten." They added that the mother appeared quite anxious and seemed to have difficulty waiting the 15 minutes for her examination. Although the behaviors described in this referral were insufficient to warrant a report to social services, the staff felt that this young mother would benefit from intervention on the part of the nurse.

You prepare for this home visit by reviewing the medical records of both Sandy and her child to determine whether the family has had previous involvement with social service agencies such as child protective services. You find that the maternal grandparents made a referral to Child Welfare on behalf of Sandy when she was 15, They were concerned about the relationship between Sandy and her step-father. The report cited suspected sexual involvement between the two. An investigation occurred but was inconclusive, and the charges were never pursued.

You also discuss the case with family planning and immunization clinic staff, since the family receives services at both clinics. The staff advise you that they are familiar with Sandy and her husband Nick. They state that their only interaction with Nick was during a family planning clinic 2 months ago. They report that Sandy appeared anxious and in a hurry on that day, stating, "I really need to hurry, Nick is waiting in the car and he gets impatient." Shortly after that, the staff tells you, Nick came running into the clinic shouting, "What the hell is taking you people so long?" He reportedly glared at Sandy, and the two quickly exited the clinic.

You phone the client and advise her that you are a nurse with the local health department. You inform her that nurses often visit new mothers to assist them in finding resources. You add that as a community health nurse, you will be available to talk with her about her child's growth and development.

The client expresses interest in the visit and states, "I want you to show me some things about feeding her and stuff. I need help figuring out what to do at night, she still isn't sleeping much and it's driving me crazy." You advise the client that you will be happy to discuss those issues with her, that you will bring information which you will review with her. You add that you noted in her medical record that the father of the baby is living in the home and assure her that she may involve other family members, including the father of the baby, in the home visit. You jointly decide that the visit will occur the following day at 10:30 a.m. and that the father of the baby will be present if his work schedule allows.

On the day of the visit, as you walk up the stairs toward the apartment, you notice someone looking at you through the curtains. As you near the apartment door the curtains close. Your repeated knocking on the door is met with no response. You call the client's name but there is no answer.

Questions

1. Would this scenario provoke anxiety for you? How would you deal with your reaction?
2. How is this different from a scenario in the acute care setting in which a supervisor would be readily available?
3. Given this scenario, what actions will you take?
4. If you had been working in the family planning clinic on the day that Nick came in, what, if anything, would you have done differently?
5. As young parents, Nick and Sandy are part of an aggregate that has unique risk factors for parenting. List as many of these risk factors as you can think of and brainstorm about possible community health nursing interventions for each.
6. What methods would you suggest the clinic staff utilize to detect signs and symptoms of physical, sexual, or emotional abuse among this aggregate?

Asking the right questions, being a careful observer, and following the correct reporting process and recording procedures may mean the difference between life and death for a victim of violence.

Displays 20.10, 20.11, and 20.12 consist of three sample tools that the community health nurse and other advocates use in their role as a mandated reporter. These forms include a Suspected Child Abuse Report, a two-page Medical Report of Suspected Child Abuse, and a Domestic Violence Screening/Documentation Form.

Tertiary Prevention

Tertiary prevention focuses on the rehabilitation of the family from the violence and crisis they have sustained. The family may never again have the same connections because

DISPLAY 20.10 | **SUSPECTED CHILD ABUSE REPORT**

SUSPECTED CHILD ABUSE REPORT
To Be Completed by Reporting Party
Pursuant to Penal Code Section 11166

A. CASE IDENTI-FICATION

TO BE COMPLETED BY INVESTIGATING CPA
VICTIM NAME: _____
REPORT NO./CASE NAME: _____
DATE OF REPORT: _____

B. REPORTING PARTY

NAME/TITLE

ADDRESS

PHONE ( )　　DATE OF REPORT　　SIGNATURE

C. REPORT SENT TO

☐ POLICE DEPARTMENT　☐ SHERIFF'S OFFICE　☐ COUNTY WELFARE　☐ COUNTY PROBATION

AGENCY　　ADDRESS

OFFICIAL CONTACTED　　PHONE ( )　　DATE/TIME

D. INVOLVED PARTIES

VICTIM

NAME (LAST, FIRST, MIDDLE)　　ADDRESS　　BIRTHDATE　SEX　RACE

PRESENT LOCATION OF CHILD　　PHONE ( )

SIBLINGS

	NAME	BIRTHDATE	SEX	RACE		NAME	BIRTHDATE	SEX	RACE
1.					4.				
2.					5.				
3.					6.				

PARENTS

NAME (LAST, FIRST, MIDDLE)　BIRTHDATE　SEX　RACE　　NAME (LAST, FIRST, MIDDLE)　BIRTHDATE　SEX　RACE

ADDRESS　　ADDRESS

HOME PHONE ( )　BUSINESS PHONE ( )　　HOME PHONE ( )　BUSINESS PHONE ( )

E. INCIDENT INFORMATION

IF NECESSARY, ATTACH EXTRA SHEET OR OTHER FORM AND CHECK THIS BOX. ☐

1. DATE/TIME OF INCIDENT　　PLACE OF INCIDENT　　(CHECK ONE)　☐ OCCURRED　☐ OBSERVED

IF CHILD WAS IN OUT-OF-HOME CARE AT TIME OF INCIDENT, CHECK TYPE OF CARE:
☐ FAMILY DAY CARE　☐ CHILD CARE CENTER　☐ FOSTER FAMILY HOME　☐ SMALL FAMILY HOME　☐ GROUP HOME OR INSTITUTION

2. TYPE OF ABUSE: (CHECK ONE OR MORE)　☐ PHYSICAL　☐ MENTAL　☐ SEXUAL ASSAULT　☐ NEGLECT　☐ OTHER

3. NARRATIVE DESCRIPTION:

4. SUMMARIZE WHAT THE ABUSED CHILD OR PERSON ACCOMPANYING THE CHILD SAID HAPPENED:

5. EXPLAIN KNOWN HISTORY OF SIMILAR INCIDENT(S) FOR THIS CHILD:

SS 8572 (Rev. 1/93)

INSTRUCTIONS AND DISTRIBUTION ON REVERSE

DO NOT submit a copy of this form to the Department of Justice (DOJ). A CPA is required under Penal Code Section 11169 to submit to DOJ a Child Abuse Investigation Report Form SS-8583 if (1) an active investigation has been conducted and (2) the incident is **not** unfounded.

Police or Sheriff-WHITE Copy;　County Welfare or Probation-BLUE Copy;　District Attorney-GREEN Copy;　Reporting Party-YELLOW Copy

DISPLAY 20.11   **MEDICAL REPORT—SUSPECTED CHILD ABUSE**

DOJ 900   84 89220

MEDICAL REPORT—SUSPECTED CHILD ABUSE	HOSPITAL

INSTRUCTIONS: ALL PROFESSIONAL MEDICAL PERSONNEL ARE REQUIRED BY SECTION 11166 OF THE PENAL CODE TO COMPLETE THIS FORM IN CONJUNCTION WITH THE SS 8572 SUSPECTED CHILD ABUSE REPORT WHERE CHILD ABUSE, AS DEFINED BY SECTION 11165 OF THE PENAL CODE, IS SUSPECTED. THE REPORTS, DOJ 900 AND SS 8572, MUST BE SUBMITTED TO A POLICE OR SHERIFF'S DEPARTMENT, OR A COUNTY PROBATION OR WELFARE DEPARTMENT WITHIN 36 HOURS. PROFESSIONAL MEDICAL PERSONNEL MEANS ANY PHYSICIAN AND SURGEON, PSYCHIATRIST, PSYCHOLOGIST, DENTIST, RESIDENT, INTERN, PODIATRIST, CHIROPRACTOR, LICENSED NURSE, DENTAL HYGIENIST OR ANY OTHER PERSON WHO IS CURRENTLY LICENSED UNDER DIVISION 2 (COMMENCING WITH SECTION 500) OF THE BUSINESS AND PROFESSIONS CODE. EACH PART OF THE FORM MUST BE COMPLETED UNLESS INAPPLICABLE. IN FILLING OUT THIS FORM, NO CIVIL LIABILITY ATTACHES AND NO CONFIDENTIALITY IS BREACHED.

I. GENERAL INFORMATION   Print or type

PATIENT'S NAME   HOSPITAL ID NO.

ADDRESS   CITY   COUNTY   STATE   PHONE

AGE | BIRTHDATE | RACE | SEX | DATE AND TIME OF ARRIVAL | MODE OF TRANSPORTATION | DATE AND TIME OF DISCHARGE

ACCOMPANIED TO HOSPITAL BY: NAME   ADDRESS   CITY   STATE   RELATIONSHIP

PHONE REPORT MADE TO   ID NO.   DEPARTMENT   PHONE   RESPONDING OFFICER/AGENCY

NAME OF: ☐ FATHER   ☐ STEPFATHER   ADDRESS   CITY   COUNTY   HOME PHONE   BUS. PHONE   AGE/DOB

NAME OF: ☐ MOTHER   ☐ STEPMOTHER   ADDRESS   CITY   COUNTY   HOME PHONE   BUS. PHONE   AGE/DOB

SIBLINGS: LAST NAME, FIRST   DOB   LAST NAME, FIRST   DOB   LAST NAME, FIRST   DOB

II. MEDICAL EXAMINATION

A. History   1. EXPLANATION OF INJURIES BY PARENT OR PERSON ACCOMPANYING CHILD (LOCATION; DATE, TIME AND CIRCUMSTANCES)

2. PATIENT'S STATEMENT EXPLAINING INJURY (PARAPHRASE)

3. PATIENT'S EMOTIONAL REACTION TO EXAMINATION (SUBMISSIVE, COMPLIANT, ETC.)

4. PREVIOUS HISTORY OF CHILD ABUSE (IF KNOWN)

B. Sexual Assault   Perform exam only if necessary.

1. ACTS COMMITTED: NOTE—COITUS, FELLATIO, CUNNILINGUS, SODOMY

2. DURING ASSAULT
☐ VAGINAL PENETRATION (HOW)   EJACULATION: ☐ VAGINAL ☐ ORAL ☐ ANAL ☐ OTHER:
☐ ANAL PENETRATION (HOW)   ☐ CONDOM USED   ☐ VOMITED   ☐ LOSS OF CONSCIOUSNESS   ☐ OTHER:

3. AFTER ASSAULT:
☐ WIPED/WASHED   ☐ BATHED   ☐ DOUCHED   ☐ VOMITED   ☐ CHANGED CLOTHES   ☐ BRUSHED TEETH   ☐ DEFECATED   ☐ OTHER:

C. Physical Examination   DATE AND TIME OF EXAM   DATE AND TIME OF ASSAULT   BP   PULSE   RESP.   TEMP

HEIGHT | WEIGHT | HEAD CIRCUM | LAST TETANUS | KNOWN ALLERGIES   CURRENT MEDICATION

DIAGNOSTIC DATA

Check if indicated and incorporate results in written examination at left

☐ X-rays (skull, chest, longbone, full skeletal)
☐ Bleeding, coagulation, tourniquet, tests
☐ Funduscopic
☐ Other

DISPLAY 20.11   **MEDICAL REPORT—SUSPECTED CHILD ABUSE (Continued)**

DOJ 900

DATE	HOSPITAL ID NO.	HOSPITAL

PHYSICAL EXAMINATION (CONTINUED) LOCATE AND DESCRIBE IN DETAIL ANY INJURIES OR FINDINGS: TRAUMA, BRUISES, ERYTHEMA, EXCORIATIONS, LACERATIONS, WOUNDS. TRACE OUTLINE USED AND INDICATE LOCATION OF WOUNDS/LACERATIONS USING 'X' FOR SUPERFICIAL, 'O' FOR DEEP; SHADE FOR BRUISES OR BURNS. BESIDE EACH INJURY INDICATED NOTE COLOR, SIZE, PATTERN, TEXTURE, AND SENSATION. WRITE OVER UNUSED OUTLINES. DESCRIBE IN DETAIL SHAPE OF ARM OR OTHER BRUISES WHICH MAY INDICATE FORCE.

D. PELVIC   A PELVIC EXAMINATION SHOULD NOT BE PERFORMED UNLESS THE PARENT, GUARDIAN OR MINOR CONSENT OR UNLESS NECESSARY AS PART OF TREATMENT. SEE DEPARTMENT OF HEALTH REGULATIONS TITLE 22, DIVISION 2, VICTIMS OF SEXUAL ASSAULT. SAME INSTRUCTIONS AS GENERAL PHYSICAL; IN ADDITION, NOTE PUBIC HAIR COMBINGS WHERE INDICATED, DRIED SECRETIONS AND RECENT INJURIES TO HYMEN. TRACE AND OUTLINE AS ABOVE.

V. SPECIMENS

STAINS/FOREIGN MATERIALS (WHEN INDICATED)

LOOSE HAIR	____	FINGERNAIL SCRAPINGS	____
BLOOD	____	DIRT OR GRAVEL	____
THREADS	____	VEGETATION	____
GRASS	____	CLOTHING	____
DRIED SECRETIONS	____		

	SLIDES	SWABS
VAGINAL	____	____
RECTAL	____	____
ORAL	____	____
ASPIRATES/ WASHINGS	____	____
BITE MARKS	____	____
OTHER:	____	____

III. DIAGNOSTIC IMPRESSION OF TRAUMA AND INJURIES

IV. TREATMENT/DISPOSITION OF PATIENT

A. ☐ GC CULTURE   ☐ VDRL   ☐ PREGNANCY TEST   ☐ POST COITAL ESTROGEN   ☐ VD PRO-PHYLAXIS   ☐ OTHER:

☐ MOTILE SPERM: ☐ PRESENCE   ☐ ABSENCE   ☐ NOT TAKEN   ☐ FAMILY ASSESSMENT BY: ☐ NOT ORDERED

B. ORDERS:

C. DISPOSITION: ☐ ADMIT   TRANSFERRED TO:

☐ RELEASED   ACCOMPANIED BY: NAME   ADDRESS   RELATIONSHIP

I HAVE RECEIVED THE INDICATED ITEMS AS EVIDENCE AND A COPY OF THIS REPORT.

OFFICER: ID NO.:   DATE:

NURSE   SIGNATURE OF EXAMINATION PHYSICIAN

PATIENT'S SAMPLES. TIME OF COLLECTION AT MD DISCRETION

BLOOD	____
HAIR FROM HEAD	____
SALIVA	____
HAIR FROM PUBIC AREA	____

D. FOLLOW-UP WITHIN:

☐ MEDICAL
____ HRS   ____ DAYS

☐ SOCIAL SERVICES
____ HRS   ____ DAYS

☐ PRIVATE MD
____ HRS   ____ DAYS

☐ OTHER
____ HRS   ____ DAYS

DISPLAY 20.12 **DOMESTIC VIOLENCE SCREENING/DOCUMENTATION FORM**

DV SCREEN
- ☐ Screened
  - ☐ Yes
  - ☐ No
  - ☐ Probable/Suspected DV
- ☐ Not Screened

Date _____ Patient ID# _____
Patient Name _____
Provider Name _____
Patient Pregnant? Yes ____ No ____

Describe frequency and severity of present and past abuse (use direct quotes as much as possible)
_____
_____
_____
_____
_____

Routinely Screen at Each Visit
"Because violence is so common in women's lives, I've begun to ask about it routinely."

Ask Direct Questions
"I'm concerned that your injuries/symptoms may have been caused by someone hurting you. Is this what happened to you?"
-OR-
"Has your intimate partner or ex-partner ever physically hurt you? Have they ever *threatened* to hurt you or someone close to you?"

Describe location and extent of injury
_____
_____
_____
_____
_____

Assess Patient Safety

- ☐ Yes ☐ No Is patient afraid to go home?
- ☐ Yes ☐ No Has physical violence increased in severity over past years?
- ☐ Yes ☐ No Have threats of homicide been made?
- ☐ Yes ☐ No Have threats of suicide been made?
- ☐ Yes ☐ No Is alcohol or substance abuse also a problem?
- ☐ Yes ☐ No Is there a gun in the house?
- ☐ Yes ☐ No Is patient afraid of their partner?
- ☐ Yes ☐ No Was safety plan discussed?

Indicate where injury was observed

Referrals
- ☐ hotline number given
- ☐ legal referral made
- ☐ shelter number given
- ☐ in-house referral made
- ☐ discharge instructions given

☐ Yes ☐ No Photographs taken?
☐ Yes ☐ No Consent to be photographed?
(Attach Photographs) + Appropriate Form

partners may separate—by choice, motivated by fear or hatred; by court order, if the perpetrator is incarcerated; or by death. If the family chooses to stay together, long-term intervention for all family members is needed to establish a climate more conducive to family normalcy. Many of the services discussed as part of the secondary level of prevention are continued into the tertiary prevention phase to promote healing and to restore and promote family growth.

If incarceration is a part of tertiary prevention, the effects of having one family member living in this environment must be factored into the services and support provided by the community health nurse to the family as a whole (see Chapter 30 for information on correctional facilities). Even if the partner/spouse has separated from the perpetrator emotionally and/or legally, the perpetrator usually has legal rights to see the children. This may mean that other family members, usually from the abuser's side of the family, can bring the children to the prison to visit their parent. Just making arrangements for these visits can cause stress to the visitors. The community health nurse needs to be aware of the complicated dynamics and emotional stress such difficult situations can produce for all family members. The victim–perpetrator relationship is as complex as the forces that created the violence and abuse.

FAMILIES FACING VIOLENCE FROM OUTSIDE THE FAMILY

The concern of violence coming into the family from outside the home, often beyond the family's control, is a relatively new phenomenon in the United States. There has always been some degree of violence that affects families in their homes, such as burglaries, or at times murder, or abduction. Increasingly, however, home invasion, a form of forced entry to terrorize family members, is a violent crime perpetrated most frequently by strangers. Other forms of violence of which families are more aware include the potential for terrorist activities through planned community violence (such as the plane crashes on September 11, 2001), biologic, chemical, or radioactive actions (see Chapter 17). Communities have developed resources such as the National Organization for Victim Assistance (NOVA) and crisis response teams (CRT), to assist individuals and groups experiencing a disaster or violent event (e.g., child murder or school shootings).

Home invasion is an increasing new form of terror. It occurs mainly in large cities, although rural areas are not immune. **Home invasion** is the purposeful and sudden entry into a home by force while the family is home and awake. The effectiveness of this form of terror relies on surprise. Motivation may be material or thrill; household belongings are frequently stolen while family members are incapacitated by being bound, blindfolded, and/or gagged. In some cases, family members are killed. Often the perpetrators are under the influence of drugs or alcohol, and at times the violence may be gang related.

The community health nurse most likely will not encounter families who have experienced such violence. However, nurses may work with extended family members of the victims or families who have reported such a happening in their neighborhood and are now fearful of a reoccurrence. Fear of violence can create psychological and physi-

ologic stress reactions similar to the sensations that occur when one actually experiences the violence. These fears should not be ignored. The role of the nurse includes four steps discussed in the generic approach to crisis intervention (see discussion in "Generic Approach").

METHODS OF CRISIS INTERVENTION

Crisis intervention in community health nursing uses either a generic or individual approach, or both. For the majority of crisis encounters, the generic approach is more appropriate. Family violence is a major situational crisis in which community health nurses intervene. However, many other situational and developmental crises affect families, and these families are benefited by the skills of the community health nurse. Newly recognized crises include community violence coming into the home and the potential of terrorism at home.

Generic Approach

The generic approach creates interventions to fit a particular type of crisis, focusing on the nature and course of the crisis rather than on the psychodynamic of each client (Aguilera, 1998). Crisis intervention using the generic approach is tailored to a specific kind of crisis, situational or developmental, and comprises four important elements: (1) use of adaptive behavior and coping strategies, (2) support of the individual/family, (3) preparation for the practical and emotional future, and (4) anticipatory guidance.

As an example, the generic approach is used with families experiencing child abuse. The child may be in foster care while the family receives needed services and rebuilds itself. The nurse encourages the parents to discuss and analyze their feelings, teaches stress-reduction techniques and positive coping skills, and creates a supportive, caring atmosphere, especially through self-help groups such as Parents Anonymous. The nurse can help individual family members strengthen their self-esteem by encouraging positive interpersonal relationships. The community health nurse also teaches needed parenting skills, providing anticipatory guidance, so that parents are prepared to raise their children with consistent and age-appropriate discipline techniques.

The generic approach does not require advanced professional psychotherapy skills. More importantly, this approach works well with families, groups, and even communities in crisis. The community health nurse may work with a group of cancer clients, abused elders, adolescents struggling with developmental crisis, or an entire community recovering from a natural or man-made disaster. The generic approach allows the nurse to intervene with any group of people who have a crisis in common. This approach also offers a broad base of support, because the crisis group members can provide resources for one another beyond those brought by the nurse.

Individual Approach

The individual approach is used for clients who do not respond to the generic approach or who need special therapy. Individual crisis intervention should not be confused with individual psychotherapy, which tends to focus on a client's developmental past. In contrast, crisis intervention directs treatment toward the immediate state of disequilibrium, identifying its causes and developing coping mechanisms. Family members or significant others are included during the process of crisis resolution. An entire group may need this type of intervention. If this approach is needed, clients should be referred to a professional with specialized training.

ROLE OF THE COMMUNITY HEALTH NURSE IN CARING FOR FAMILIES IN CRISIS

Crisis intervention in community health assumes that clients have resources. If their potential for managing stressful events can be tapped, people in crisis will need minimal direct assistance. In accordance with the self-care concept, crisis intervention seeks to identify and build on client strengths. Aguilera (1998) outlined a series of four steps for intervention during crisis: assessment, planning, intervention, and resolution. Interventions to promote crisis resolution are presented using the three levels of prevention in Table 20.2.

Assessment and Nursing Diagnosis

Initially, the nurse must assess the nature of the crisis and the client's response to it. How severe is the problem, and what risks are the clients facing? Are other people also at risk? Assessment must be rapid but thorough and focused on specific areas.

First, the nurse concentrates on the immediate problem during the assessment. Why have clients asked for help right now? How do they define the problem? What precipitated the crisis? When did it occur? Was it a sudden accidental or situational event, or a slower developmental one?

Next, the nurse focuses on the clients' perceptions of the event. What does the crisis mean to them, and how do they think it will affect their future? Are they viewing the situation realistically? When a crisis occurs to a family or group, some members see the situation differently from others. During intervention, all family members should be encouraged to express themselves, to talk about the crisis, and to share their feelings about its meaning. Acceptance of the wide range of feelings is important.

Determine who is available to offer support to the individual or family. Consider family, friends, clergy, other professionals, community members, and agencies. Who are the clients close to, and who do they trust? One advantage of group intervention is that the members provide some of this support for one another. In subsequent sessions, the quality of support should be evaluated. Sometimes a well-meaning individual can worsen the situation or deter clients from facing and coping with reality.

Finally, the nurse assesses the clients' coping abilities. Have they had similar kinds of experiences in the past? What techniques have they tried in this situation, and if they did not work, why not? Clients should be encouraged to think of other stress-relieving techniques, perhaps ones they have used in the past, and to try them.

The nurse gathers all of this data and mentally begins to form nursing diagnoses. As a plan of care is developed for the client, these nursing diagnoses are formalized in writing. Standardized nursing diagnoses are available for reference, or the agency where the nurse works may have a preferred format for nursing diagnoses. These nursing diagnoses are effective tools for the nurse to begin planning interventions.

Planning Therapeutic Interventions

Several factors influence clients' reaction to crises. Nurses should try to determine what factors are affecting clients before making intervention plans. The major balancing factors—clients' perceptions of the event, situational supports, human resources, and clients' coping skills—have been assessed in the first step (Aguilera, 1998). While continuing to explore these, the nurse now also considers the clients' general health status, age, past experiences with similar types of situations, sociocultural and religious influences, and the actual assets and liabilities of the situation. This assessment helps clarify the situation and gives the nurse an

TABLE 20.2   Levels of Prevention to Promote Crisis Resolution

Phase	Goals	Interventions
		PRIMARY PREVENTION
Precrisis	Health promotion	Anticipatory guidance
	Disease prevention	Reduce factors that increase vunerability
	Education	Reduce hazards in some events (safety and multiplicity of stressors)
		Reinforce positive coping strategies
		Mobilize social support and other resources
		SECONDARY PREVENTION
Crisis	Reduction of stress load	Assist with reaction to the event and functioning
	Cure or restoration of function	Allow behavior: dependence, grief
		Set goals with client
		Refer to resources
		TERTIARY PREVENTION
Postcrisis	Rehabilitation and maintenance	Promote adaptation to a changed level of wellness
		Promote interdependence
		Reinforce newly learned behaviors, lifestyle changes, coping strategies
		Explore application of leamed behaviors to new situations
		Identification and use of additional resources

opportunity to further encourage the clients' participation in the resolution process. If clients are defensive, resistant, and rigid, they are not processing clearly and can complete only simple tasks. It will take time before these clients can begin to solve problems related to the effects of the crisis on themselves and the loss they are experiencing, but the nurse will want to encourage them to reach this level.

A therapeutic plan is based on multiple factors:

◆ The kind of crisis (situational or developmental, acute or chronically recurring)
◆ The effect the crisis is having on clients' lives (can they still work, go to school, and keep house, or are they secured within their home for an indefinite period, not knowing whether other family members have survived a major natural or manmade crisis?)
◆ Where they are in coming to resolution of the crisis
◆ The ways in which significant others are affected and respond
◆ Their level of preparation for such a crisis
◆ The clients' strengths and available resources

Using this problem-solving process, the nurse and clients develop a plan. They review the event that precipitated the crisis, obvious symptoms, and the disruption in the clients' lives. The plan may focus on several areas. For instance, clients may need to grasp intellectually the meaning of the crisis, to engage in greater expression of feelings, or work both on the intellectual and emotional aspects. Part of the plan may be directed toward finding appropriate and safe shelter, counseling, or physical care. Another part may focus on helping clients identify and use more effective coping techniques or locate supportive agencies and resources. The plan may also include development of realistic goals for the future.

Implementation

During implementation, communication between the nurse and clients is important. Discussions about what is happening, reviewing the family's plan and rationale for this approach, and making appropriate changes are necessary parts of this communication. Assigning definite activities at the end of each session will help clients try out different solutions and evaluate various coping behaviors. Implementation is enhanced by using the following guidelines (Levy & Sidel, 2002; Vastag, 2001):

1. *Demonstrate acceptance of clients.* A crisis often shatters the ego. Clients need to feel the support of a positive, caring person who does not judge their feelings or behavior. Some negative expressions, such as anger, withdrawal, and denial, are normal aspects of the crisis phase. Accept them as normal.
2. *Help clients confront crisis.* Clients need to face and discuss the situation. Expressing their feelings reduces tension and improves reality perception. Recounting what has actually occurred may be painful, but it helps clients confront the crisis. Do not assume that once clients have told about the event, no further recounting is necessary. Each time the story is told, the client comes closer to dealing realistically with the crisis.

3. *Help clients find facts.* Distorted ideas and unknown factors of the situation create additional tension and may lead to maladaptive responses. For instance, it would help inexperienced parents to know that children younger than 2 years of age cannot deliberately misbehave. Facts about childhood development and parenting training may be important for preventing crisis.
4. *Help clients express feelings openly.* Suppressed feelings can be harmful. For instance, a widow may feel guilty that she is glad her husband is gone. Expression of such feelings helps reduce tension and gives clients an opportunity to deal with them.
5. *Do not offer false reassurance.* Clients need to face reality, not avoid it. A statement such as "Don't worry, it will all work out" is demeaning and meaningless. Instead, make positive statements about faith in the clients' ability to cope: "It is a very difficult situation, but I believe you will be able to deal with it."
6. *Discourage clients from blaming others.* Clients often blame others as a way to avoid reality and the responsibility for problem solving. Withhold judgment when clients blame others, but point out other causal factors and avenues for dealing with the situation.
7. *Help clients seek out coping mechanisms.* Explore and test old and new techniques to reduce stress and anxiety. Ask questions. What are the things that need to be done? What do clients think they can do? This assistance gives clients more adaptive energy to work toward resolution.
8. *Encourage clients to accept help.* Denial in the early phases of crisis cuts off help. Encouraging clients to acknowledge the problem, is a first step toward acceptance of help. Often clients fear the loss of their independence and the invasion of their privacy. A client may say, "We ought to be able to handle this problem." At this point, the community health nurse can reassure clients that people in a crisis of this sort almost always need help. Preparing people to accept help enables them to make the best use of what others have to offer.
9. *Promote development of new positive relationships.* Clients who have lost significant others through unintentional or intentional death, divorce, incarceration, or an act of perpetrated violence should be encouraged to find new connections, purpose, and people to fill the void and provide needed supports and satisfactions.

Evaluation of Crisis Resolution and Anticipatory Planning

In the final step, clients and the nurse evaluate, stabilize, and plan for the future. Evaluating the outcome of the intervention might address the following:

◆ Are the clients using effective coping skills and exhibiting appropriate behavior?
◆ Are adequate resources and support persons available?

◆ Is the diagnosed problem solved?

◆ Have the desired results been accomplished?

Analysis of these outcomes will provide a greater understanding for coping with future crises.

To stabilize the change that has occurred, identify and reinforce all of the positive coping mechanisms and behaviors. Discuss why they are effective, and explore ways to use them in future stressful situations. Summarize the crisis experience, emphasizing the clients' successes with coping, reconfirm their progress, and reinforce their self-confidence. It is especially important to point to the evidence that the client has reached their pre-crisis level, or an even higher level of functioning.

Clients' plans for the future should include setting realistic goals and means to implement them. Review with clients how their handling of the present crisis can help them cope with, minimize, or preferably prevent future crises.

Summary

Crisis is a temporary state of severe disequilibrium for persons who face a threatening situation. A crisis is a state that individuals can neither avoid nor solve with their usual coping abilities, and occurs when some force disrupts normal functioning, thereby causing a loss of balance or normalcy in life. Crises create tension; subsequently, efforts are made to solve the problem and reduce the tension. If such efforts meet with failure, people feel upset, redefine the situation, try other solutions, and, if failure continues, the person eventually reaches the breaking point.

Two main types of crisis are developmental and situational. Developmental crises are disruptions that occur during transitional periods in normal growth and development. These transitions usually have a gradual onset and are often predictable. Situational crises are precipitated by an unexpected external event and occur suddenly, sometimes without warning.

Family violence constitutes a unique crisis for the victim and the entire family and is becoming disturbingly prevalent in the world. Historically, family violence is not new. Only in the last half century of our nation's history have laws and societal concerns been raised about the treatment of spouse/partners, children, and seniors. Although advances in human rights have been made, abuses against women and children remain socially and culturally accepted in some countries, and attitudes have been slow to change.

Child abuse occurs among children of all ages, from infancy through the teen years, and may be physical, emotional, and/or sexual. Neglect and sexual exploitation are additional forms of child abuse. Neglect may be described as general neglect or specific, such as medical or educational neglect. Child abuse, such as shaken baby syndrome or Munchausen syndrome by proxy, is sometimes identified only on autopsy. Teen dating violence, violence during pregnancy, and violence against women in general constitutes partner/spousal abuse. Finally, a most unsettling form of violence—elder abuse, neglect, and exploitation—is occurring with an increased frequency than previously suspected.

New and unexpected forms of violence are becoming a reality in our unsettled world. Within communities, violence comes into the home in the form of Internet crimes against children, child abductions, and home invasions. Globally, terrorist groups threaten attacks on civilians in the United States and abroad. For people in the United States, this form of terror is a new reality. Preparation against and survival of such attacks is a new concern for most Americans, and the community health nurse has an important role to play (see Chapter 17).

Community health nurses use three levels of prevention when working with families. Primary prevention focuses on providing people with the skills and resources to prevent violent situations. Secondary prevention involves immediate intervention at the time of the violent episode. This secondary level includes providing different services for each family member, such as medical attention, emotional support, and police involvement. Tertiary prevention offers family rebuilding services and helps the family establish equilibrium with a structure that may be different, but healthier.

People in crisis need and often seek help. Crisis intervention builds on these two phenomena to achieve its primary goal—reestablishment of equilibrium. The two major methods of crisis intervention are the generic and the individual approaches. The generic approach is used with groups of people involved in the same type of crisis, such as rape victims, mothers who have lost children because of drunken driving, or a family experiencing child abuse. The individual approach is used if clients do not respond to the generic approach or need additional therapy. Crisis intervention begins with assessment of the situation, followed by planning a therapeutic intervention. The nurse then implements and carries out the intervention, building on the strengths and self-care ability of clients. Crisis intervention concludes with resolution and anticipatory planning to avert possible future crises.

Regardless of the method of intervention the community health nurse uses, the steps of the nursing process provide a framework within which to intervene. Assessing the family's assets and liabilities, their willingness to change, and the nature of the violence helps the nurse form a nursing diagnosis. With this diagnosis, the nurse can begin to plan appropriate interventions and implement plans in concert with the family. Evaluation of the intervention techniques provides the nurse with new data to assist with ongoing assessment of the family's progress and additional anticipatory guidance needs. ∎

ACTIVITIES TO PROMOTE CRITICAL THINKING

1. What are the major differences between a developmental and a situational crisis? Give examples of each from personal experiences.

2. Describe a developmental crisis experienced by a family. What was this family's response? Describe some actions a community health nurse might have taken (alone or within an interdisciplinary team) to help the family cope with the crisis.

3. Watch a news station on television. Listen for examples of developmental or situational crises occurring to families in the world. Analyze the situations and

anticipate what the role of a community health nurse would be during the crises selected.

4. Family violence is a significant public health problem. Assume that a battered wife becomes a community health nurse's client, and the nurse suspects there may be more women with this problem in the community. Describe how the nurse might provide assistance using the crisis intervention steps. Then discuss how a three-level preventive program might be instituted in the community.

5. Using the Internet, select a situational crisis, such as spousal abuse, adolescent sexual exploitation, or neglect of the elderly and read the most current information on this topic. Depending on your personal interests or current community health nursing experiences, develop a file of articles you have uncovered using the Internet. This file can be useful to you, to agency staff in your clinical setting, and to families you visit.

References

Administration for Children and Families. (2006a). *Child maltreatment 2006.* Retrieved October 12, 2008 from http://www.acf.hhs.gov/programs/cb/pubs/cm06/cm06.pdf.

Administration for Children and Families. (2006b, March 15). *Modifications to the CAPTA State Grant Program by the Keeping Children and Families Safe Act of 2003 (Public Law 108-36).* Washington D.C.: U.S. Department of Health and Human Services. Retrieved http://www.acf/hhs/gov/programs/cb/laws_policies/policy/im/im0304.htm.

Administration for Children and Families. (2007a, February 28). *How many children are abused and neglected each year?* Retrieved from http://faq.acf.hhs.gov/cgi-bin/acfrightnow.cfg/php/enduser/std_adp.php?p_faqid.

Administration for Children and Families. (2007b). National Survey of Child and Adolescent Well-Being (NSCAW), 1997-2010. Retrieved October 12, 2008 from http://www.acf.hhs.gov/programs/opre/abuse_neglect/nscaw/nscaw_overview.html#overview.

Aguilera, D.C. (1998). *Crisis intervention: Theory and methodology,* 8th ed. St. Louis: Mosby.

American Academy of Pediatrics, Committee on Child Abuse and Neglect. (1999). Guidelines for the evaluation of sexual abuse of children: Subject review. *Pediatrics, 103*(1), 186–191. Retrieved July 25, 2008 from http://pediatrics.aappublications.org/cgi/content/full/pediatrics;103/1/186.

American Association of Suicidology. (n.d.). *Warning signs: IS PATH WARM?* Retrieved July 25, 2008 from http://www.suicidology.org/associations/1045/files/Mnemonic.pdf.

American Association of Suicidology. (2006). *Suicide in the U.S.A. based on current (2004) statistics.* Retrieved December 28, 2006 from http://www.suicidology.org/associations/1045/files/Suicide InThe US.pdf.

American Association of Suicidology. (2007). *Facts about suicide and depression.* Retrieved January 2, 2007 from http://www.suicidology.org/associations/104/files/Depression.pdf.

American Psychological Association. (2007). *Elder abuse and neglect: In search of solutions.* Washington DC: Office on Aging. Retrieved July 25, 2008 from http://www.apa.org/pi/aging/eldabuse.html.

Bolen, R.M. (2001). *Child sexual abuse: Its scope and our failure.* Norwell, MA: Kluwer Plenum.

Bridges, W. (1980). *Transitions: Making sense of life's changes,* 2nd ed. Cambridge, MA: Perseus Publishing.

Bridges, W. (2001). *The way of transition: Embracing life's most difficult moments.* Cambridge, MA: Perseus Publishing.

Campbell, J. (1998). *Empowering survivors of abuse: Health care, battered women and their children.* Thousand Oaks, CA: Sage.

Campbell, J.C. (1999). If I can't have you no one can: Murder linked to battery during pregnancy. *Reflections, 25*(3), 8–12.

Centers for Disease Control and Prevention (2004). *CDC's rape prevention and education grant program: Preventing sexual violence in the United States 2004.* Centers for Disease Control and Prevention, National Center for Injury Prevention and Control, Atlanta, GA. Retrieved July 25, 2008 from http://www.cdc.gov/ncipc/pub-res/pdf/RPE%20AAG.pdf.

Centers for Disease Control and Prevention. (2006a, August, 26). *Intimate partner violence: Overview.* Retrieved July 25, 2008 from http://www.cdc.gov/ncipc/factsheets/ipvfactshtm.

Centers for Disease Control and Prevention. (2006b). *Understanding suicide.* Retrieved July 25, 2008 from http://www.cdc.gov/ncipc/pub-res/Suicide%20Fact%.

Child Welfare Information Gateway. (2004). *About CAPTA: A legislative history.* Retrieved October 12, 2008 from http://www.childwelfare.gov/pubs/factsheets/about.cfm.

Child Welfare Information Gateway. (2008a). *Child abuse and neglect fatalities: Statistics and interventions.* Retrieved October 12, 2008 from http://www.childwelfare.gov/pubs/factsheets/fatality.cfm.

Child Welfare Information Gateway. (2008b). *What is child abuse and neglect?* Retrieved October 12, 2008 from http://www.childwelfare.gov/pubs/factsheets/whatiscan.pdf.

Cokkinides, V.E., & Coker, A.L. (1998). Experiencing physical violence during pregnancy: Prevalence and correlates. *Family Community Health, 20*(4), 19–37.

Crandall, M., Nathens, A.B., Kernic, M.A., et al. (2004). Predicting future injury among women in abusive relationships. *Journal of Trauma-Injury Infection and Critical Care, 56*(4), 906–912.

Crime and Violence Prevention Center. (2003a). *Child abuse: Educator's responsibilities.* Sacramento, CA: California Attorney General's Office. Retrieved July 25, 2008 from http://www.safestate.org/shop/files/CAEd.Resp.pdf.

Crime and Violence Prevention Center. (2003b). *Child abuse and neglect reporting law, condensed version.* Sacramento, CA: California Attorney General's Office. Retrieved July 25, 2008 from http://www.safestate.org/shop/files/CA_Child_Abuse_Rep.pdf.

Crime and Violence Prevention Center. (2003c). *Child abuse prevention handbook.* Sacramento, CA: California Attorney General's Office. Retrieved January 16, 2004 from http://www.safestate.org/shop/files/child abuse handbook chap_1-3.pdf, .../child abuse handbook chap_4-6.pdf, and .../child abuse handbook appen3-7.pdf.

Curry, M.A., Doyle, B.A., & Gilhooley, J. (1998). Abuse among pregnant adolescents: Differences by developmental age. *Maternal and Child Nursing, 23*(3), 144–150.

Davis, R.E., & Harsh, K.E. (2001). Confronting barriers to universal screening for domestic violence. *Journal of Professional Nursing, 17*(6), 313–320.

Dombrowski, S.C., & Gischlar, K.L. (2004). Keeping children safe on the Internet: Guidelines for parents. Retrieved July 25, 2008 from http//www.nasponline.org/publications/cq/cq342internetsafety_ho.aspx.

Finkelhor, D., Mitchell, K.J., & Wolak, J. (2000). *Online victimization: A report on the nation's youth.* Alexandria, VA: National Center for Missing and Exploited Children.

Fox, J.A., & Zawitz, M.W. (2004). *Homicide trends in the United States.* Washington DC: Department of Justice.

Gazmararian, J.A., Petersen, R., Spitz, A.M., et al. (2000). Violence and reproductive health: Current knowledge and future research directions. *Maternal and Child Health Journal, 4*(2), 79–84.

Gray-Vickrey, P. (2001). Protecting the older adult. *Nursing Management, 32*(10), 36–40.

Hanson, R.F. (2002). Adolescent dating violence: Prevalence and psychological outcomes. *Child Abuse and Neglect, 26*, 449–453.

Hoff, L.A. (2001). *People in crisis: Clinical and public health perspectives,* 5th ed. Indianapolis, IN: Jossey-Bass.

Holmes, T., & Rahe, R. (1967). The social readjustment rating scale. *Journal of Psychosomatic Research, 11,* 213–217.

Jackson, S.M., Cram, F., & Seymour, F.W. (2000). Violence and sexual coercion in high school students' dating relationships. *Journal of Family Violence, 15,* 23–36.

Jenkins, P.J., & Davidson, B.P. (2001). *Stopping domestic violence: How a community can prevent spousal abuse.* Norwell, MA: Kluwer Academic/Plenum.

Kellogg, N. (2005). The evaluation of sexual abuse in children. *Pediatrics, 116* (2), 506–512.

Kramer, A. (2002). Domestic violence: How to ask and how to listen. *Nursing Clinics of North America, 37*(1), 189–210.

Lane, W.G., Rubin, D.M., Monteith, R., & Christian, C.W. (2002). Racial difference in the evaluation of pediatric fractures for physical abuse. *Journal of the American Medical Association, 288*(13), 1603–1609.

Lemmey, D., Malecha, A., McFarlane, J., et al. (2001). Severity of violence against women correlates with behavioral problems in their children. *Pediatric Nursing, 27*(3), 265–270.

Levinson, D.J. (1978). *The seasons of a man's life.* New York: Knopf.

Levy, B.S., & Sidel, V.W. (2002). *Terrorism and public health: A balanced approach to strengthening systems and protecting people.* New York: Oxford University Press.

Menzey, M.D. (2001). *The encyclopedia of elder care: The comprehensive resource on geriatric and social care.* New York: Springer Publishing.

Minino, A.M., Heron, M., Murphy, S.L., & Kochanek, K.D. (2007). *Deaths: Final data for 2004.* Centers for Disease Control, National Center for Health Statistics. Hyattsville, MD. Retrieved January 11, 2007 from http://www.cdc.gov/nchs/products/pubs/pubd/hestats/finaldeaths04.htm.

National Center on Elder Abuse. (2006). *Help for elders and families.* Washington DC: National Center on Elder Abuse. Retrieved September 28, 2006 from http://www.elderabusecenter.org/default.cfm?p=worried.cfm.

National Institute of Neurological Disorders and Stroke. (2007). *NINDS Shaken baby syndrome information page.* Retrieved February 14, 2007 from http://www.ninds.nih.gov/disorders/shakenbaby/shakenbaby.htm.

Office of Disease Prevention and Health Promotion. (n.d.). *Healthy People 2010: Midcourse review, executive summary.* Retrieved July 25, 2008 from http://www.healthypeople.gov/data/midcourse/html/introduction.htm.

Office of Disease Prevention and Health Promotion. (2005). *Healthy People 2010: Midcourse review, Injury and violence prevention.* Retrieved July 25, 2008 from http://www.healthypeople.gov/data/midcourse/pdf/FA15.pdf.

Office of Disease Prevention and Health Promotion. (n.d.). *Leading health indicators.* Rockville, MD: U.S. Department of Health and Human Services. Retrieved July 25, 2008 from http://www.healthypeople.gov/LHI/Priorities.htm.

Office of the United Nations High Commissioner for Human Rights. (2007). Committee on the Rights of the Child. Retrieved July 25, 2008 from http://www.ohchr.org/english/bodies/crc/discussion.htm.

Olds, D.L., Eckenrode, J., Henderson, C.R., et al. (1997). Long-term effects of home visitation on maternal life course and child abuse and neglect: Fifteen-year follow-up of a randomized trial. *Journal of the American Medical Association, 276*(8), 637–643.

Olds, D.L., Henderson, C.R., Tatelbaum, R., & Chamberlin, R. (1988). Improving the life-course development of socially disadvantaged mothers: A randomized trial of nurse home visitation. *American Journal of Public Health, 78*(11), 1436–1445.

Olds, D.L., Kitzman, H., Cole, R., et al. (2004). Effects of nurse home-visiting on maternal life course and child development: Age 6 follow-up results of a randomized trial. *Pediatrics, 114,* 1550–1559.

Olds, D.L., et al. (1999). Prenatal and infancy home visitation by nurses: Recent findings. *The Future of Children, Home Visiting: Recent Program Evaluations, 9*(1), 44–65.

Pillemer, K., & Finkelhor, A. (1988). The prevalence of elder abuse: A random sample survey. *The Gerontologist, 28,* 51–57.

Rape, Abuse, & Incest National Network. (2006). *All 50 states now included in national sex offender public registry.* Retrieved July 25, 2008 from http://www.rainn/org.news/national-sex-offender-registry.index.html.

Safe School Healthy Students Initiative. (2006). About the Safe Schools/Healthy Students (SS/HS) initiative: A comprehensive approach to youth violence prevention. Retrieved September 25, 2006 from http://www.sshs.samhsa.gov/initiative/about.aspx.

Sheehy, G. (1976). *Passages: Predictable crises of adult life.* New York: Dutton.

Sheehy, G. (1992). *The silent passage.* New York: Ballantine.

Sheehy, G. (1999). *Understanding men's passages: Discovering the new map of men's lives.* New York: Ballantine Books.

Sheehy, G. (2000a, March). Oklahoma monitors intimate partner violence. *The Nation's Health, 30*(2), 1, 7.

Sheehy, G. (2000b). *Violence against women.* Fairfax, VA: U.S. Department of Health and Human Services, National Women's Health Information Center.

Sheehy, G., & Delbourgo, J. (1996). *New passages: Mapping your life across time.* New York: Ballantine Books.

Stirling, J., & Committee on Child Abuse and Neglect. (2007). Beyond Munchausen Syndrome by Proxy: Identification and treatment of child abuse in a medical setting. *Pediatrics, 119,* 1026–1030.

U.S. Children's Bureau. (2003). *Children of color in the child welfare system: Perspectives from the child welfare community.* Child Welfare Information Gateway. Retrieved July 25, 2008 from http://www.childwelfare.gov/pubs/otherpubs/children/findings.cfm.

U.S. Department of Health and Human Services. (2000). *Healthy People 2010,* 2nd ed. Part B: Focus Areas 15–28. Washington, DC: U.S. Government Printing Office. Retrieved July 25, 2008 from http://www.healthypeople.gov/document/HTML/Volume2/15Injury.htm#_Toc490549392.

U.S. Department of Justice (2001a). *Crimes against children by babysitters* (NCJ 189102). Washington, DC: U.S. Department of Justice, Office of Justice Programs.

U.S. Department of Justice (2001b). *Internet crimes against children* (NCJ 184931). Washington, DC: U.S. Department of Justice, Office of Justice Programs.

U.S. Department of Justice. (2002). *Battered child syndrome: Investigating physical abuse and homicide.* Retrieved July 25, 2008 from http://www.ncjrs.gov/pdffiles1/ojjdp/161406.pdf.

U.S. Department of Justice. (2005). Department of Justice launches initiative to train child abduction response teams. Retrieved November 30, 2005 from http://www.ojp.gov/newsroom/2005/OJP06010.htm.

U.S. Department of Justice. (2006). *Project safe childhood: Protecting children from online exploitation and abuse.* Retrieved July 25, 2008 from http://www.projectsafechildhood.gov/introductionwcover.pdf.

U.S. Department of Justice. (2007). *Commercial sexual exploitation of children: What do we know and what do we do about it?*

Retrieved October 10, 2008 from http://www.ojp.usdoj.gov/nij/pubs-sum/215733.htm.

U.S. Department of Justice, Office of Violence Against Women. (n.d.). *About domestic violence*. Retrieved July 25, 2008 from http://www.usdoj.gov/ovw/domviolence.htm.

Vastag, B. (2001). Experts urge bioterrorism readiness. *Journal of the American Medical Association, 285*, 30–31.

Volpe, J.S. (1996). *Effects of domestic violence on children and adolescents: An overview.* American Academy of Experts in Traumatic Stress, Inc. Retrieved July 25, 2008 from http://www.aaets.org/article8.htm.

World Health Organization. (n.d.). *Suicide prevention (SUPRE).* Retrieved July 25, 2008 from http://www.who.int/mental_health/prevention/suicide/suicide prevent/en/.

World Health Organization. (1998). *Report of the Director-General: The world health report 1998. Life in the 21st century: A vision for all.* Geneva: World Health Organization.

World Health Organization, Committee on the Rights of the Child. (2001). *Prevention of child abuse and neglect: Making the links between human rights and public health.* Retrieved September 28, 2001 from http://www.who.int/child-adolescent-health/New_Publications/Rights/CRC-statement_rev_III.htm.

World Health Organization. (2002a, October 3). *Public health and violence: European facts and trends.* Retrieved July 25, 2008 from http://www.euro.who.int/document/mediacentre/fs1.

World Health Organization. (2002b, October 3). *First ever global report on violence and health released.* Geneva. Retrieved July 25, 2008 from http://www.who.int/mediacentre/news/releases/pr73/en/.

World Health Organization. (2005). *WHO Multi-country study on women's health and domestic violence against women: Initial results on prevalence, health outcomes and women's responses.* Retrieved October 12, 2008 from http://www.who.int/gender/violence/who_multicountry_study/summary_report/en/index.html.

World Health Organization. (2007a). *Gender-based violence.* Geneva: World Health Organization. Retrieved July 25, 2008 from http://www.who.int/gender/violence/en/.

World Health Organization. (2007b). *World report on violence and health: Child abuse and neglect by parents and other caregivers.* Retrieved July 25, 2008 from http://www.who.int/violence_injury_prevention/violence/global_campaign/en/chap3.pdf.

Selected Readings

Crosson-Tower, C. (2007). *Understanding Child Abuse and Neglect.* Upper Saddle River, NJ: Pearson.

Fontes, L.A., & Conte, J.R. (2008). *Child abuse and culture: Working with diverse families.* New York: Guilford Publications, Inc.

Giardino, A.P., & Giardino, E.R. (2002). *Recognition of Child Abuse for the Mandated Reporter.* St. Louis, MO: G W Medical Publishing.

Hardt, J., Sidor, A., Nickel, R., Kappis, B., Petrak, P., & Egle, U. (2008). Childhood adversities and suicide attempts: A retrospective study. *Journal of Family Violence, 23*,713–718.

Lapierre, S. (2008). Mothering in the context of domestic violence: The pervasiveness of a deficit model of mothering. *Child and Family Social Work, 13,* 454–463.

Mam, S. (2008). *The road of lost innocence: The true story of a Cambodian heroine.* New York: Random House.

Pelzer, D. (1995). *A Child Called It.* Deerfield Beach, FL: Health Communications, Incorporated.

Pelzer, D. (1997). *Lost boy: A foster child's search for the love of a family.* Deerfield Beach, FL: Health Communications, Incorporated.

Pelzer, D. (2000). *A man named Dave: A story of triumph and forgiveness.* New York: Penguin Group, Incorporated.

Poole, A., Beran, T., & Thurston, W. (2008). Direct and indirect services for children in domestic violence shelters. *Journal of Family Violence, 23,* 679–686.

Internet Resources

American Academy of Child and Adolescent Psychiatry: *http://www.aacap.org/cs/root/facts_for_families/child_abuse_the_hidden_bruises*

American Association of Poison Control Centers: *http://www.aapcc.org/DNN/*

American Professional Society on the Abuse of Children (APSAC): *http://www.apsac.org/mc/page.do*

Centers for Disease Control and Prevention, Division of Violence Prevention: *http://www. cdc.gov/ncipc/dvp/dvp. htm*

Child Abuse Prevention Network: *http://child.cornell.edu/*

Child Welfare Information Gateway: *http://www.childwelfare.gov/*

Convention on the Rights of the Child: *http://www. unicef.org/crc/*

Domestic Violence Resources: *http://www.growing.com/nonviolent/*

Mothers Against Guns: *http://mothersagainstguns.org/*

National Center for the Prosecution of Child Abuse, American Prosecutors Research Institute: *http://www.ndaa.org/apri/programs/ncpca/ncpca_home.html*

National Criminal Justice Reference Service: *http://www.ncjrs.org/*

National Latino Alliance for the Elimination of Domestic Violence: *http://www.dvalianza*.org

Prevent Child Abuse America: *http://www.preventchildabuse.org/index.shtml*

United Nations Background Note on Children's Rights: *http://www.un.org/rights/dpi1765e.htm*

Violence Research Resources on the Web: *http://www1.umn.edu/cvpc/linksviolence.html*

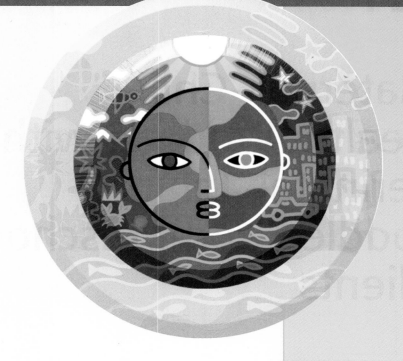

PROMOTING AND PROTECTING THE HEALTH OF AGGREGATES WITH DEVELOPMENTAL NEEDS

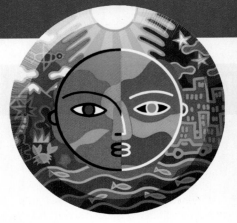

21

Maternal–Child Health: Working with Perinatal, Infant, Toddler, and Preschool Clients

LEARNING OBJECTIVES

Upon mastery of this chapter, you should be able to:

◆ Identify major health problems and concerns for infant, toddler, and preschool populations globally and in the United States.

◆ Identify the *Healthy People 2010* goals established for the maternal child population.

◆ Discuss major risk factors and special complications for childbearing families.

◆ Describe the important considerations in developing effective health promotion programs to fit the needs of diverse maternal child populations.

◆ Describe various roles of a community health nurse in serving the maternal child population.

◆ Describe a variety of programs that promote and protect health and prevent illness and injury of infant, toddler, and preschool populations.

◆ State the recommended immunization schedule for infants and children, and give the rationale for the timing of each immunization.

◆ Give examples of methods and interventions the community health nurse might use in working with infants, toddlers, and preschool populations to help promote their health.

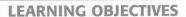

❝*Be gentle with the young.*❞

—Juvenal (55–127 AD)

KEY TERMS

Alcohol-related birth defects
Alcohol-related neurodevelopmental disorder
Child abuse
Drug dependent
Drug exposed
Environmental tobacco smoke
Fetal alcohol effects
Fetal alcohol spectrum disorders
Fetal alcohol syndrome
Gestational diabetes mellitus
Head Start
High-risk families
Infant
Low-birth-weight
Preconception care
Preschooler
Shaken baby syndrome
Smokeless tobacco products
Sudden infant death syndrome (SIDS)
Toddler
Very-low-birth-weight

Many of the community health nurse's clients are pregnant teens and women, along with infants and young children. Working with maternal and infant populations is a primary facet of community health nursing. Often, more than half of nursing practice in official health agencies involves primary preventive work with mothers and infants, as well as provision of prenatal care. Maternal child expenses are a large part of the health care dollar. The average cost of maternity care in 2004 was $7,737 for vaginal deliveries and $10,958 for cesarean section deliveries, with facility costs and professional fees accounting for the largest proportion of expenses (Thomson Healthcare, 2007). Why should maternal/infant populations require this amount of attention from community health nursing? Despite advanced technology and availability of excellent perinatal services in the United States, certain segments of the maternal and infant populations, such as adolescent mothers and those who are economically disadvantaged, remain at high risk for disease, disability, and even death. Although some women receive excellent prenatal care and benefit from diagnostic and technological resources, many others are without access to prenatal care and adequate nutrition. The Save the Children (2008, p. 31) report on maternal–child health notes that:

> The United States spends more money on health care per capita than nearly any other country in the world, yet has the highest rates of child poverty and the lowest levels of child health and safety of the rich countries. As a result, infant and child mortality rates in the United States are higher than in any other industrialized country, the only exceptions being Latvia, Lithuania, and Slovakia.

For an example of a country that has implemented successful policies to eliminate maternal child inequities, see Evidence-Based Practice: How Sweden Achieved Maternal–Child Health Equity.

Historically, the health of U.S. women and children has largely fallen under the umbrella of Title V of the Social Security Act, enacted in 1935. (For more on the Social Security Act see Chapter 6.) Funding for state Maternal and Child Health and Crippled Children programs were part of this original legislation, as was some provision for child welfare services. Title V is "the longest-standing public health legislation in American history," and came to fruition after other legislation established a National Birth Registry; provided *Infant Care,* the first educational pamphlet; established the Children's Bureau; and enacted the first Child Labor Law of 1916 (Maternal Child Health Bureau [MCHB], 2008, para 4). For an illustration of MCHB functions and programs see Display 21.1.

In 1909, formal prenatal care was first provided in Boston by the Instructive District Nursing Association, and spread across the country to outpatient clinics (MCHB, 2008). Since the inception of Title V, other legislation has included Emergency Maternity and Infant Care Program (1943) that funded maternity and infant care for the wives of lower-income servicemen in the early days of the Baby Boom, and the 1970 Family Planning Act that provided the first federal funds for birth control to prevent unintended pregnancies. In 1976, the Improved Pregnancy Outcome Projects sought to decrease the levels of infant mortality by strengthening the efforts of states to better plan and implement maternal child health programs, and Healthy Start programs were begun in 1991—starting with 15 demonstration project sites exhibiting

EVIDENCE-BASED PRACTICE

How Sweden Achieved Maternal Child Health Equity

For mothers and children of any income level, Sweden is a wonderful place to live. However, this was not always the case; the poorest infants were 3.5 times more likely to die before age 1 in the 1920s. In the 1930s, due to public concern about the "child survival gap" (p. 32), the government instituted a set of comprehensive new policies that included free prenatal and other maternal–child health services, along with housing reforms and welfare support—including financial support for low-income families. Around 60% of pregnant women and 80% of infants were covered by 1950. Currently, the inequity related to infant morality rates has virtually been eliminated, and the decreases in social inequality have led to "one of the lowest rates of child mortality in the world" (p. 32). This case study highlighting how government policies can affect population health outcomes is an example for other countries, such as the United States, that struggle with less than adequate maternal–child health indicators and significant disparities in health outcomes.

Reference:

Save the Children. (2008). *State of the world's mothers 2008.* Westport, CN: Author.

DISPLAY 21.1 TYPES OF SERVICES OFFERED THROUGH FEDERAL MCH FUNDING

Direct Health Care Services (gap filling)
Examples: Basic Health Services, and Health Services for CSHCN

Enabling Services
Examples: Transportation, Translation, Outreach, Respite Care, Health Education, Family Support Services, Purchase of Health Insurance, Case Management, Coordination with Medicaid, WIC, and Education

Population-Based Services
Examples: Newborn Screening, Lead Screening, Immunization, Sudden Infant Death Syndrome Counseling, Oral Health, and Injury Prevention

Infrastructure Building Services
Examples: Needs Assessment, Evaluation, Planning, Policy Development, Coordination, Quality Assurance, Standards Development, Monitoring, Training, Applied Research, Systems of Care, and Information Systems

U.S. Department of Health and Human Services. (2008). *State MCH-Medicaid Coordination: A Review of Title V and Title XIX Interagency Agreements* (2nd ed). Retrieved August 13, 2008 from http://mchb.hrsa.gov/IAA/appendices.htm.

high infant mortality rates and growing to 96 within two decades—to provide preconception, postpartum, and infant care to at-risk women (MCHB, 2008). Evaluation of Healthy Start programs reveals that almost all programs provide home visitation to clients, and most continued these visits to infants and toddlers. Health education, smoking cessation counseling, services for perinatal depression, and involvement of male partners are hallmarks of most programs. Barriers to success of Healthy Start include mobility of clients and unstable housing, along with lack of transportation (MCHB, 2006).

Preconception care seeks to improve the health and well-being of adolescents and women before they become pregnant. Its goal is to decrease birth defects through health education, screening, and interventions that reduce risk factors for the future mother and infant (Association of State & Territorial Health Officials [ASTHO], 2006). The community health nurse has always had a prominent role in planning, implementing, and evaluating these programs.

This chapter addresses major areas of concern regarding the health of maternal–infant populations. It also explores the global needs of and related services available to the youngest and most vulnerable of society's members. Health services that are commonly available in the United States for pregnant and postpartum women, infants, toddlers, and the preschool population are examined, and the role of the community health nurse in providing those services is explored.

HEALTH STATUS AND NEEDS OF PREGNANT WOMEN AND INFANTS

Community health nurses constitute a key group of health care workers involved in both program planning and the actual delivery of services to mothers and babies. A solid understanding of vital statistics and other data regarding mothers and infants serves nurses as they determine the appropriateness and the effectiveness of programs and services. A review of some global and national vital statistics of the past decade provides insight into the key problems facing this population.

Global Overview

In 2005, an estimated half million women died of maternal causes, 88% of them in sub-Saharan Africa and South Asia. In these areas, maternal mortality rate (MMR) exceeds 1,000 per 100,000 live births, but it is less than 10 per 100,000 live births in Canada, Australia, New Zealand, Japan, and most European countries—a very wide disparity. The U.S. maternal mortality rate was 13 in 2004. Ireland's MMR is one, making it a very good place for mothers (World Health Organization [WHO], 2008a). The MMR is a measure of obstetric risk and is determined by dividing the number of maternal deaths by the number of live births per 100,000. Most maternal deaths are the result of direct causes (complications of pregnancy, labor, and delivery), interventions, omissions, or incorrect treatment, or of the chain of events resulting from any one of these. Eclampsia, hemorrhage, sepsis, and unsafe abortions account for 70% of maternal deaths (Graham & Hussein, 2006; WHO, 2008b).

Infant Mortality

Globally, 3.5 to 4 million neonatal deaths and 3.3 to 4 million stillbirths occur each year; they are largely caused by the same factors that result in death and disability for mothers. Causes include poor maternal health, inadequate care, poor hygiene, and inefficient management of delivery, as well as lack of essential newborn care (Ten Hoope-Bender, Liljestrand, & MacDonagh, 2006; Tinker, Paul, & Ruben, 2006; WHO, 2008b). For example, two 20-cent injections given to mothers during or before pregnancy can prevent the deaths of 250,000 infants from neonatal tetanus each year (Tinker, Paul, & Ruben, 2006). Infant mortality rate is regarded as a valid indicator of population health worldwide. Sadly, a substantial number of neonatal deaths or stillbirths are likely due to hypoxia/asphyxia because of failure to establish effective breathing at birth resulting from lack of appropriate neonatal resuscitation (Reidpath & Allotey, 2003; Spector & Daga, 2008). Infections and low-birth-weight (LBW) or premature birth account for 64% of neonatal deaths, and most newborns die at home, without the presence of a skilled health care provider. Of the total of neonatal deaths, 99% are found in low- and middle-income nations, and 66% occur in Africa and Asia (Tinker, Paul, & Ruben, 2006). A mother from sub-Saharan Africa is 83 times more likely to have her child die before age 5 than a mother from an industrialized nation, and almost four of every five mothers there will lose a child during their lifetime (Save the Children, 2008). In the United States, Black infant mortality rates (13.6) are 2.4 times higher than the rate for Whites (5.7), and the rate for American Indian/Alaska Native infants is 1.5 to 2 times higher (Save the Children, 2008). About 1.3 million infants would survive annually if mothers were able to exclusively breast-feed their infants for 6 months. The lack of breast-feeding is related to decreased survival and increased morbidity from infections, lower intelligence test scores, increased cardiac risk factors, and inadequate nutrition (Labbok, 2006).

Across the world, 6.5 million children die before age 5, and there are great disparities between nations: a child is 40 times more likely to die in the country with the highest rate than a child in the country with the lowest rate (WHO, 2008b). Worldwide, over 200 million children under age 5 cannot get the basic health care they need, and 26,000 of them die each day from such preventable and easily treatable illnesses as respiratory infections and diarrhea (Save the Children, 2008; WHO, 2008b). Although bleak, these figures actually represent substantial gains in reducing the rate of under-5 child deaths worldwide. Ten million children die each year, the lowest number in recorded history, because of the efforts of international groups promoting basic health care interventions targeted to vulnerable infants and children. Over 11% of all U.S. children have no health insurance, public or private, and 20% of Hispanic children are uninsured (Save the Children, 2008).

Teenage Pregnancy

About 10% of all births worldwide are to adolescent mothers (Hanna, 2001). Teenage mothers have a higher rate of pregnancy-related complications, and their infants are more likely to have LBW or to be premature, injured at birth, or stillborn. Mortality rates for infants born to adolescent mothers are higher than for those born to older women. Long-term problems for both mother and child may result typically from educational and employment limitations for moms and less cognitive stimulation and emotional support for babies. In 2005, the U.S. birth rate for 15 to 17 year olds was 21 per 1,000 (for Hispanics the rate was 48)—a record low rate, having declined from a rate of 39 per 1,000 in 1991 (Forum on Child & Family Statistics, 2007).

HIV/AIDS

Worldwide, human immunodeficiency virus (HIV) rates are rising faster among women than men; in 2005, about 17.5 million women were estimated to have HIV (Mehta, 2006). Perinatal transmission of HIV is a global health issue: 1,600 infants every day acquire HIV from their mothers and the HIV/AIDS pandemic has orphaned 12 million children (Greene, 2007). Most children with acquired immunodeficiency syndrome (AIDS) are children of HIV-positive mothers. Mother-to-child transmission (MTCT) of HIV can be reduced by a stunning 67% with a single antiretroviral drug taken for a short time, and combination therapies are even more effective in reducing MTCT (Bassett, 2001; Harris, Fowler, Sansom, Ruffo, & Lampe, 2007). However, even after 25 years of the HIV/AIDS pandemic, only 20% of all persons who need antiretroviral medications and who live in low- and middle-income nations can receive them (Merson, 2006). Worldwide, HIV/AIDS is among the leading causes of death for women. In poor areas of the world, the death of a mother often means that her children, especially those under age 5, will die also (Bellamy, 2004). To reduce MTCT, it is important to prevent HIV infection among women of childbearing age—but, in some areas, girls are six times more likely to be infected than boys. Women must seek prenatal care early enough in their pregnancies for the antiretroviral drug to be effective. Also, breast-feeding benefits and risks must be weighed (Bellamy, 2004). In Botswana, routine HIV testing began in 2004 and rates of HIV transmission from mother to baby dropped from 35% to 40% down to 5% to 10% due to intervention with maternal antiretroviral therapy and infant formula feeding (Seipone, et al., 2004). Most of the population favors routine HIV testing, and women are more likely to be tested and understand that treatment can help their unborn children (Cockcroft, Andersson, Milne, Mokoena, & Masisi, 2007).

National Overview

In the United States, 4.1 million women gave birth in 2005; these numbers remained constant from the previous year. The birth rate was 14 per 1,000 and birth rates declined in all ethnic/racial groups except for Hispanics and American Indian/Alaska Native groups. For the 25- to 29-year-old group, the overall birth rate was highest at 115.6, with rates for Hispanic mothers at 148.8, White mothers at 109.3, Black mothers at 103, and Asian/Pacific Islander mothers at 108 per 1,000. Almost 37% of births were to unmarried women (U.S. Department of Health and Human Services [USDHHS], 2007). It is estimated that about 49% of pregnancies are unintended (Centers for Disease Control [CDC], 2006a). Many of these women do not have the financial or social resources to sustain minimal health levels for themselves and their infants.

Teenage Mothers

In 1991, after a steady 5-year upward trend, the United States reached a 20-year high in the number of children born to teen mothers (aged 15 to 17 years). That trend then declined until 2005, when it rose ever so slightly to a rate of 21 per 1,000. Ninety percent of these births are to unmarried mothers (Forum on Child & Family Statistics, 2007). The downward trend for teen pregnancy rates has been attributed largely to better use of contraception (77%) rather than to less sexual activity (23%)

(Santelli, Lindberg, Finer, & Singh, 2007). Although most pregnant adolescents are of European-American descent, the rate of pregnant adolescents is higher among Black (35) and Hispanic (48) populations, and lower among Asians/Pacific Islanders (8) and Whites (12) (Forum on Child & Family Statistics, 2007). For older age groups (ages 25 to 44), the pregnancy rate has increased since 1991, but the rate for younger teens (10 to 14 age group) declined at about the same rate as older teens (Hamilton, Martin, Sutton, & Menacker, 2005). Additionally, there continues to be an increasing trend for unwed teenage mothers to keep their babies. These "children having children" with limited educational and economic advantages will affect the health of society well into the future. See Chapter 22 for more on adolescent pregnancy.

Substance Use and Abuse

Another area of concern is substance use and abuse among the childbearing population. The range of adverse consequences associated with the use of tobacco, alcohol, and illicit drugs during pregnancy is wide and includes preterm birth, LBW, and fetal alcohol syndrome (described later in this chapter). Two studies showed that many women who abuse drugs while pregnant do not receive prenatal care (Armstrong et al., 2003; Chasnoff et al., 2001). This puts these women and their unborn children in double jeopardy: not only are they at risk from the consequences of alcohol or drug use, but they also do not receive the preventive prenatal care that can eliminate or reduce other obstetric complications. Mothers who smoke also are at risk of having premature or lower birth weight babies, along with other sequelae (Mercer, Merlino, Milluzzi, & Moore, 2008).

Violence

Violence is often the cause of injuries and death for pregnant and postpartum women, as well as their unborn and infant children (Janssen et al., 2003), and homicide is the leading cause of injury death for women who are pregnant and 1-year postpartum (Chang, Berg, Saltzman, & Herndon, 2005). It is not uncommon for physicians to note injuries consistent with blunt trauma in women who are pregnant; however, they may be explained away as accidentally self-inflected (Grossman, 2004). One large-scale retrospective study of pregnant and postpartum women in Massachusetts from 2001 to 2005 found that in 1,675 hospital visits for assault, 1,528 physical injuries were diagnosed—largely to the head and neck (42.2%) for the total sample and torso (21.5%) in pregnant women; the percentage dropped to 8.7% in the postpartum sample (Nannini et al., 2008). Victims of intimate partner violence have high levels of stress and higher rates of smoking during pregnancy, as well as inadequate utilization of prenatal care services (Chambliss, 2008).

Prenatal care is crucial to ensure good outcomes of pregnancy. The crisis surrounding professional liability insurance has been especially critical in the case of physicians specializing in obstetrics and gynecology (OB-GYN). Over the past decade, insurance costs have risen dramatically. In some instances, premiums have equaled the obstetrician's income. For example, average liability insurance premiums in Miami, Florida, were $147,621 in 2000, but rose to $277,241 just 4 years later (Hale, 2006). OB-GYNs have either moved to states where lawsuits have limits set by legislation and insurance rates are reasonable, or they reduce the number of high-risk obstetrical cases (22%) or total deliveries (9.2%) in an effort to reduce their premium costs. Some of them chose to stop practicing altogether (14%), leaving many pregnant women without convenient access to appropriate prenatal care (Hale, 2006). Because most lawsuits involve neurologic impairment of a newborn (34.4%) and these injuries are amortized over the life of the individual, awards or settlements are often quite large (see Perspectives: Student Voices).

The *Healthy People 2010 (HP 2010)* document encompasses specific goals and objectives for the maternal child population, based on the previous achievements in the same or similar areas, and have been revised during the midcourse review (USDHHS, 2006). (See Table 21.1 for selected maternal–child health objectives and progress toward goals.) After years of working toward improving maternal–child health, the United States has made limited progress. One objective, however, has been met: 70% of infants are now being put to sleep on their backs (up from 35% baseline), largely due to public health educational efforts and reminders (USDHHS, 2006). Although the infant mortality rate (IMR, or deaths for all babies up to 1 year of age) has dropped substantially, from 20.0 per 1,000 live births in 1970 to 7.1 per 1,000 in 1999, it remained high at 6.79 in 2004—higher than in many other industrialized nations. In addition, the IMR for African-American infants remains more than twice that of White infants (Hamilton, Minino, Martin, Kochanek, Strobino, & Guyer, 2007; Save the Children, 2008).

Birth Weight and Preterm Birth

Low-birth-weight (LBW) babies are those weighing less than 2,500 g (or less than 5.5 lbs) at birth; **very-low-birth-weight** (VLBW) babies weigh less than 1,500 g (or less than 3 lbs 4 oz) at birth (Child Trends Databank, 2006). Premature births account for 67% of LBW babies, and others are considered small-for-gestational age or may have been exposed to tobacco or another growth-retarding substance, for instance (March of Dimes, 2005a,b). Maternal mortality, LBW, and VLBW births are three areas requiring attention. Birth weight is one of the most important predictors of infant mortality (Tinker, Paul, & Ruben, 2006). Ethnic differences exist in the rates of infant mortality, largely as a result of ethnic differences in the rate of LBW (Hessol & Fuentes-Afflick, 2005). Congenital deformities, premature birth, LBW, newborn demise from maternal complications, and unintentional injuries were responsible for over half of all 2004 infant deaths (Hamilton, Minino, Martin, Kochanek, Strobino, & Guyer, 2007). The rate of LBW infants dropped between 1970 and 1980, but has continued to rise since then (Child Trends Databank, 2006). In 2005, the rate for LBW infants rose from 8.1% in the previous year to 8.2%, and for preterm births there was also an increase from 12.5% to 12.7%; objectives for LBW, VLBW, and preterm births all moved away from their *HP 2010* targets (UDHHS, 2006). Objectives for LBW, VLBW and preterm birth are not being met; rather they are moving away from target levels (USDHHS, 2006).

PERSPECTIVES
STUDENT VOICES

I began working as a nurse's aide at our local hospital when I started nursing school. I learned first-hand the dangers of childbirth and the long-term consequences that can result. One night, a single young female reported to the Emergency Room in labor and was admitted to the Labor and Delivery Department and seen by the nurse midwife who had provided prenatal care for the mother in the clinic. The young mother-to-be was very excited. Her contractions continued, and she did not progress with the labor process, so she was to be started on Pitocin to increase the effectiveness of her labor. The nurse midwife checked on her patient frequently, but problems began after the first 8 hours of labor. As the Pitocin dosage was increased, the fetus reacted with bradycardia, and the nurse midwife did not notify the physician. The Pitocin dosage was decreased and then the heart rate stabilized; this process continued for three cycles. The nurse midwife signed off her 12-hour shift and handed care of the patient over to the nurse midwife coming on shift. Again, whenever the Pitocin dosage was increased to the point of becoming effective, the fetus would respond with bradycardia. Report was given, and the physician in charge was still not notified. The first two times, the fetus recovered. The third time, the fetus did not recover; instead the bradycardia increased. By this time, the mother had been in labor for over 24 hours and the fetus was in irreversible distress. The physician was notified of an emergency, and reported to the

bedside within 5 minutes. An emergency cesarian section was performed, and the Apgar scores at delivery were 0 at 1 minute, 0 at 5 minutes, 0 at 10 minutes, and 3 at 15 minutes. The infant was severely neurologically damaged. I found out later that the infant was diagnosed with severe cerebral palsy and will never walk, talk, or feed normally. She cannot swallow and will require suctioning, gastrostomy tube feeding, and total care throughout her lifetime. She is also cortically blind. The hospital and physician were sued. The nurses and the nurse midwives in the labor and delivery room were found negligent in not reporting to the physician when the patient's labor failed to progress. The nurse midwives from both shifts were found negligent for failure to recognize fetal distress and summon the physician. A multimillion dollar award was given, and the nurses and nurse midwifes employed by the hospital were fired. It is sad to think that this tragedy could have been avoided with prudent nurse–patient advocacy, reporting, and appropriate documentation—the things our nursing instructors are always drumming into our heads. I know that as a new graduate, I am now in a position of responsibility to make decisions to notify the physician or not. I have decided that the choice should always be to notify the physician. Even though it may seem inconvenient, it really should be done. I will never forget this case and its long-reaching consequences for the child and family, as well as for the nursing staff and nurse midwives.

Linda Marie, Student Nurse

TABLE 21.1   *Healthy People 2010:* **Selected Maternal Child Objectives and Progress Toward Targeted Goals**

Objective	1997–1998 Baseline	2010 Target	% Change
Reduction in fetal & infant deaths	7.3 rate/1,000	4.4 rate/1,000	+14%
Reduction in child deaths (ages 1–4)	34.1 rate/100,000	20.0 rate/100,000	+21%
Reduction in maternal deaths	9.9 rate/100,000	4.3 rate/100,000	+18%
Reduction in cesarean births among low-risk women (first birth)	18% live births	15% live births	−133%
Reduction in low-birth-weight infants	7.6% live births	5.0% live births	−8%
Reduction in very-low-birth-weight infants	1.4% live births	0.9% live births	−20%
Reduction in total preterm births	11.6% live births	7.6% live births	−13%
Reduction in occurrence of cerebral palsy	33.3 rate/10,000	31.6 rate/10,000	−388%
Reduction in occurrence of spina bifida and other neural tube defects	6.0 new cases/ 10,000 live births	3.0 new cases/ 10,000 live births	+33%
Increase in percentage of infants put to sleep on their backs	35%	70%	100% met
Increase in proportion of mothers breast-feeding at 6 months	29%	50%	+19%

The rate of preterm births has risen over 30% since 1981. The reasons for this steady increase are complex and "require multifaceted solutions" (Behrman & Stith-Butler, 2007, p. 4). Individual medical, psychosocial, and behavioral factors (e.g., chronic health conditions, substance abuse, infertility treatments), along with sociodemographic influences (e.g., poverty, lack of education) and neighborhood characteristics (e.g., lack of easy access to prenatal care providers, unsafe areas) overlap to influence birth outcomes. Infant complications of preterm birth include hearing and vision problems, acute respiratory, gastrointestinal and immunologic problems, and central nervous system, motor, cognitive, behavioral, and socioemotional disorders. A variety of growth concerns, as well as acute and chronic health and developmental problems, often occur, and the families of these infants are burdened with additional economic and emotional costs. In 2005, it was estimated that preterm births in the United States represented $26.2 billion in economic burden (Behrman & Stith-Butler, 2007). As preschoolers, children born preterm were more likely than peers to have poor social, emotional, and physical functioning, indicating some continuing effects (Zwicker & Harris, 2008).

In addition to infant deaths and LBW, the effects of pregnancy and childbirth on women are other important indicators of health and reflect discrepancies in access to reproductive health care. Great strides have been made in this area over the past century, with 99% decreases in maternal deaths; however, 29 developed nations have lower MMRs (Berg et al., 2005). In the United States, the MMR is higher than in other developed countries, mostly due to the disparities found among women of color. The MMR for Blacks (36.1 per 100,000 live births) is four times greater than that for Whites (9.8), and the gap has continued to widen since 2000 (Save the Children, 2008) (Fig. 21.1). The United States is not ranked among the top 10 countries on the *2008 Mother's Index.* It is ranked 27th out of the 41 more developed countries listed, largely due to poor maternal and

under age 5 mortality rankings, as well as fewer children enrolled in preschool and limited maternal leave policies compared with other nations. Latvia, Lithuania, the Czech Republic, and Hungary rank higher than the United States

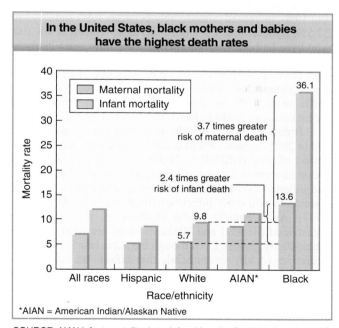

SOURCE: AIAN infant mortality data: *Infant Mortality Statistics from the 2004 Period Linked Birth/Infant Death Data* Set. National Vital Statistics Reports. Vol. 55, No. 14; AIAN Maternal mortality data: U.S. Department of Health and Human Services: Indian Health Service. *Indian Health Disparities;* All others: National Center for Health Statistics. *Health, United States, 2007 With Chartbook on Trends in the Health of Americans.*

FIGURE 21.1 U.S. Mother/Infant Death Rate Disparities by Ethnicity. In the United States, infant mortality rates among Blacks are 2.4 times higher than those of Whites, and maternal mortality rates are 3.7 times higher. Note: Infant mortality is reported per 1,000 live births, maternal mortality per 100,000 live births.

(Save the Children, 2008). Pregnancy-related death risk increases with age and with lack of prenatal care for women of every race, but the risk of pregnancy-related death for Black women is three to four times greater than for White women. Sixty percent of maternal deaths occur after giving birth to a living child, and are usually related to embolism and pregnancy-induced hypertension or preeclampsia (Chang, Elam-Evans, Berg et al., 2003). Other studies indicate that cardiomyopathy (21%), hemorrhage (14%), and pregnancy-induced hypertension (10%) were the most common causes of pregnancy-related deaths—even though 90% of deaths from chronic disease and hemorrhage are largely preventable (Berg et al., 2005). However, some progress has been made toward the *HP 2010* target for MMR: it is 18% closer to meeting the target (USDHHS, 2006).

Great progress has been made toward the year 2010 goals in several areas. The neonatal mortality rate (deaths for all infants up to 28 days old) has moved 5% closer to its target level, as has perinatal deaths (28 weeks gestation to less than 7 days after birth—14% progress) and fetal deaths (over 20 weeks' gestation—15% closer to target). Progress is also being made in early prenatal care, with over 81% of Medicaid clients and over 91% of commercial care clients receiving timely prenatal care or beginning care in the first trimester (National Committee for Quality Assurance, 2006). Movement toward *HP 2010* goals is evidenced for objectives related to first trimester prenatal care and also early and adequate prenatal care (USDHHS, 2006).

Progress in other areas has been mixed. The percentage of cesarean section deliveries, while dropping between 1990 and 1996, increased considerably between 1996 and 2003 to 23.5%, representing a one third increase. Women at low risk who have had one cesarean delivery are now more likely to have repeat cesarean sections, as the rate for vaginal births after cesarean section decreased by 63% over the same time period (Menacker, 2005). These figures represent dramatic shifts away from *HP 2010* targets for both primary and repeat cesarean births to low-risk women (USDHHS, 2006).

Breast-feeding is beneficial to both mother and infant, and in 2005, almost 73% of infants were breast-fed for some period of time (USDHHS, 2007). The risk of ovarian and breast cancers is decreased among women who breast-feed, and infants who are breast-fed have a lowered risk of upper respiratory and other infections (Ip et al., 2007; USDHHS, 2007). Asian/Pacific Island mothers are more likely to breast-feed (81.4%) and Black mothers are least likely to breast-feed (55.4%). Even though the American Academy of Pediatrics (AAP) recommends that infants be exclusively breast-fed for the first 6 months of life, less than 14% of infants fell into that category in 2005. Older mothers are more likely to breast-feed their infants than younger mothers and are also more likely to breast-feed for a longer period of time (USDHHS, 2007). However, breast-feeding objectives—including the rates for early postpartum period, 6 months of age, and at age 1 year—have all moved toward their *HP 2010* targets (USDHHS, 2006).

The success in reaching the year *HP 2010* objectives for abstinence from alcohol, tobacco, and drug use during pregnancy was not assessed at the midcourse review. However, the rate of abstinence from tobacco has improved steadily since 1989 when 19.5% of pregnant women smoked. In 2000, 12.2% of women reported smoking during pregnancy, and this was highest for non-Hispanic white women (15.6%). In 2003, approximately 11 million women were estimated to smoke during pregnancy, revealing progress toward the 1% target from the 13% baseline (CDC, 2006b).

Risk Factors for Pregnant Women and Infants

Most pregnant women in the United States are healthy; they have normal pregnancies and produce healthy babies. Many factors contribute to the health problems of those mothers and babies who figure in the statistics on infant mortality and LBW. The factors associated with LBW and infant mortality can be grouped into three categories (MacDorman, Minino, Strobino, & Guyer, 2002):

1. Lifestyle: Smoking, inadequate nutrition, low pre-pregnancy weight, high alcohol consumption, narcotic addiction, environmental toxins, prolonged standing, strenuous work, stress, and lack of social support
2. Sociodemographic: Low maternal age, low educational level, poverty, and unmarried status
3. Medical and gestational history: Primiparity, multiple gestation, short interpregnancy intervals, premature rupture of the membranes, uterine abnormality, febrile illness during pregnancy, abortion, genetic factors, gestation-induced hypertension, and diabetes

It is in the realm of lifestyle choices that community health nurses can have the most significant impact.

Drug Use

Substance abuse during pregnancy is a problem with staggering social and medical implications, because preterm birth is associated with a number of modifiable risk factors, including the use of illicit drugs during pregnancy (Armstrong et al., 2003; Chasnoff et al., 2001). The precise rate of substance abuse among pregnant women is difficult to determine. Nevertheless, current estimates of the number of women who are **drug exposed** (use drugs intermittently) and give birth to crack- or cocaine-exposed newborns range from 30,000 to 100,000 or greater annually. Other illicit substances may be abused in combination, contributing to higher numbers of exposed women and infants. Another 5,000 to 10,000 infants each year are born to women who are **drug dependent** (physically and psychologically require use of drugs to function). Many pregnant addicts do not receive prenatal care, and it is not until their newborns exhibit signs of withdrawal after birth that many of these women are identified (USDHHS, 2000).

In the United States, almost 90% of substance-abusing women are of reproductive age and are most commonly reported to abuse cocaine, amphetamines, opioids, alcohol, marijuana, and tobacco. Also, the use of several substances—or polysubstance abuse—is fairly common in this population (Kuczkowski, 2007). Data is not always current or complete, but 44 states reporting on pregnant women seeking substance abuse treatment during 2002 indicated that about 4% of 15- to 44-year old women admitted for treatment were pregnant. They reported cocaine/crack (22%), amphetamine/methamphetamine (21%), or marijuana (17%) as their primary drug of choice. Although 31%

of nonpregnant women reported primarily abusing alcohol, only 18% of pregnant women did. Also, pregnant women less often used their substance of abuse during the month prior to treatment admission or reported recent daily use—an indication that pregnancy may have been a consideration (Substance Abuse & Mental Health Services Administration [SAMHSA], 2004). However, this change in drug use may not happen until the pregnancy is diagnosed, exposing their unborn children to illicit drug use or substance abuse (Rayburn, 2007). Pregnant substance abusers were more likely to enter residential/rehabilitative (22%) and ambulatory services (71%) than detoxification treatment centers (7%), and were more likely to be younger and unmarried (SAMHSA, 2004).

Often associated with drug use are limited prenatal care, inadequate nutrition, low pre-pregnancy weight, hypertension and more rapid heart rate, preterm labor and birth, higher rates of depression, physical abuse, and HIV/AIDS and other STDs, as well as sometimes alcohol consumption and smoking (Alexander & Kotelchuck, 2001; National Institute of Drug Abuse, 2006). Increased risk of intrauterine fetal death is associated with maternal drug dependence, as is prematurity, LBW, increased chance of infections, birth defects, neurological problems, learning disabilities, and HIV/AIDS (McDonald, Vermeulen, & Ray, 2007; National Institute for Drug Abuse, 2006).

Specifically, maternal methamphetamine use is associated with fetal growth restriction; infants exposed in utero were 3.5 times more likely to be small-for-gestational-age than infants who were not exposed to methamphetamines (Smith, et al., 2006). Opiate-exposed infants are at increased risk of perinatal morbidity and mortality, and are more likely than healthy infants to have neurodevelopmental impairment at 18 months and 3 years of age (Hunt, Tzioumi, Collins, & Jeffery, 2008). Longer-term developmental deficiencies have also been found (Steinhausen, Blattmann, & Pfund, 2007). In addition, cocaine use during pregnancy is associated with impaired fetal growth, neonatal seizures, and congenital anomalies. Cocaine-exposed infants demonstrate dysregulation of autonomic nervous system functions (e.g., heart rate, respiratory sinus arrhythmias) within the first year of life, and this alteration of response to stressors continues into later childhood (Schuetze, Eiden, & Coles, 2007; Kable, Coles, Lynch, & Platzman, 2008). Furthermore, learning problems have been found in 8- to 10-year old children who were exposed to cocaine in utero (Mayes, Snyder, Langlois, & Hunter, 2007). Infants exposed to marijuana during pregnancy were found to have altered neurobehavioral performance when compared to those who were not exposed. This large-scale study noted altered arousal, regulation, and excitability in marijuana-exposed infants (deMoraes-Barros, Guinsberg, de Araujo-Peres, Mitsuhiro, Chalem, & Laranjeira, 2006). A longitudinal study found that marijuana exposure before birth is a predictor of that child's later use of marijuana at age 14, even after controlling for other variables, such as family history of drug use, home environment, delinquency, peer drug use, and sexual activity (Day, Goldschmidt, & Thomas, 2006).

Neonatal withdrawal is characterized by abnormal functions of the gastrointestinal tract, the central nervous system, and the respiratory system. Poor feeding, abnormal sleep patterns, long-term learning disabilities, and delayed language development may be observable results of maternal drug use. In addition, the child faces a high risk of infectious diseases,

including hepatitis B and HIV (March of Dimes, 2008). Infants prenatally exposed to opiates are also more likely to succumb to sudden infant death syndrome (SIDS) (Kahlert et al., 2007).

A lifestyle choice that includes the use of drugs during pregnancy has placed millions of children at risk. These children are seen in neonatal intensive care units, foster care, special-education programs in the public schools, and later in the juvenile court system. Maternal alcohol and substance abuse can predict child maltreatment and subsequent foster care placement (Smith, Johnson, Pears, Fisher, & DeGarmo, 2007). Family structure patterns are altered because grandparents may find themselves primary caregivers for their grandchildren. A woman who is an intravenous drug user or who engages in high-risk sexual behaviors introduces another public health problem, that of acquisition of HIV infection and possible spread of the virus to the fetus or others (De Genna, Cornelius, & Cook, 2007; Minkoff, 2003). The primary, secondary, and tertiary prevention roles of the community health nurse cannot be underestimated when drug use takes such a high toll on every aspect of society.

Alcohol Use

Another societal problem is the use and especially addiction to alcohol, and it is often the substance of choice. Because alcohol is a legal and socially acceptable substance, it is often the drug most commonly abused by pregnant women (Weber, Floyd, Riley, & Snider, 2002). It is difficult to establish accurate statistics on the number of women who drink during pregnancy, because inquiries about drinking habits trigger denial or minimization of intake, especially in heavy drinkers (Barr & Streissguth, 2001). However, alcohol use can cause devastating effects in the fetus, even when limited to early pregnancy and in the absence of addiction, and can lead to an array of neurocognitive and behavioral disorders, sometimes with structural anomalies, now described as **fetal alcohol spectrum disorders** (FASD). For example, regular intake of alcohol during pregnancy, especially in the first trimester, can cause the most recognizable form of the disorder, **fetal alcohol syndrome** (FAS), which is characterized by structural abnormalities of the head and face (e.g., microcephaly and flattening of the maxillary area), intrauterine growth retardation, decreased birth weight and length, developmental delays related to central nervous system abnormalities that can cause intellectual impairment, hyperactivity, altered sleep patterns, feeding problems, perceptual difficulties, impaired concentration, mood problems, and language dysfunction (Manning & Eugene-Hoyme, 2007).

What was once termed **fetal alcohol effects** (FAE) syndrome, characterized as causing some but not all of the symptoms of FAS, is now separated into the more descriptive categories of **alcohol-related birth defects** (ARBD), indicating problems with hearing, bones, or heart and kidneys, and **alcohol-related neurodevelopmental disorder** (ARND), represented by mental or functional problems, including cognitive and/or behavioral abnormalities (National Center for Birth Defects [NCBDDD], 2006). Recent research has helped to better classify the fetal effects of alcohol, and may continue to lead to more specific classifications (Manning & Eugene-Hoyme, 2007). These conditions occur in children whose mothers have used varying amounts of alcohol while pregnant, and physical signs are often much more subtle than in cases of

FAS. However, those with FASD may have one or more of the following behaviors or characteristics (NCBDDD, 2006):

- Small size for gestational age, or small stature in relation to peers
- Facial abnormalities such as small eye openings
- Poor coordination
- Hyperactive behavior
- Learning disabilities
- Developmental disabilities (e.g., speech and language delays)
- Mental retardation or low IQ
- Problems with daily living
- Poor reasoning and judgment skills
- Sleep and sucking disturbances in infancy

This completely preventable leading cause of birth defects has been estimated to cost more than $4 billion annually (Hoyme et al., 2005). FAS is estimated to occur at a rate of 0.2 to 1.5 per 1,000 live births, and the rates of FASD may be triple those of FAS (NCBDDD, 2006). Among the Native American population, the incidence of FAS is four times higher than in the general U.S. public (Struck, 2003). Common in alcohol consumption research is the underreporting of consumption by subjects (Del Boca & Darkes, 2003; Hankin, McCaul, & Heussner, 2000; Kaskutas, 2000). For example, participants may report one or two drinks a day, but when asked to show the vessel used, it is frequently a beverage container of large capacity (standard measurements of alcohol are 1 beer = 12 oz, 1 glass of wine = 4 oz, 1 drink of liquor = 1 oz). The containers from which they drink may hold 16 to 24 oz per "drink." A large-scale survey reported that 2% of pregnant women engaged in binge drinking, and 28.5% of women of childbearing age reported drinking 5 or more drinks on "typical drinking days," and 21.4% had at least 45 drinks in an average month. More binge-drinking women with high levels of usual alcohol consumption were found in the 18- to 24-year old age group or among women who were current smokers (Tsai, Floyd, Green, & Boyle, 2007, p. 437).

A study using volumetric MRI to examine brain volumes in 10- to 14-year-old children exposed in utero to cocaine, alcohol, cigarettes, and marijuana found that each substance was individually related to decreased head circumference and cortical gray matter, and that "these substances may act cumulatively during gestation to exert lasting effects on brain size and volume" (Rivkin et al., 2008, p. 741).

It is important to provide evidence-based primary prevention before pregnancy and to reach women before a lifestyle of drinking becomes such a part of their lives that they are unable or unwilling to abstain during pregnancy. For example, the Pregnancy Risk Assessment Monitoring System (PRAMS) is a surveillance system developed by the Centers for Disease Control and Prevention (CDC) and state health departments to collect population-based information on maternal preconception, prenatal, pregnancy, and postpartum behaviors and experiences (CDC, 2007a). Recent data collection revealed that prior to conception, 23.2% of women used tobacco, over 50% used alcohol, and 53.1% of women who were not trying to become pregnant did not use any form of birth control. Also, only 35.1% took a multivitamin tablet at least four days a week, 10.2% were anemic, and 3.6% reported physical abuse (D'Angelo et al., 2008). Working with women of childbearing age to improve their general health behaviors and promote better preparation for pregnancy is essential. For those pregnant women and mothers already using substances, maternal drug and alcohol treatment programs that focus on supportive parent–child attachment, enhancement of parenting and childrearing capabilities, and encouragement of the use of support systems that can improve child health and cognitive development are needed. In-home family skills training and parenting education programs that are evidence-based and promote public health nurse (PHN) and client rapport are very effective methods of working with substance-abusing mothers and their at-risk children (Kumpfer & Fowler, 2007).

Tobacco Use

Tobacco use has increased dramatically among women, especially since the women's movement of the 1970s, inevitably affecting maternal and newborn health. The nicotine in tobacco is a major addictive substance, and smoking is an addiction that many people find difficult to stop. Although the risk factors of smoking are well documented, many pregnant women continue to smoke. Smoking during pregnancy is one of the most studied risk factors in obstetric history. It has been associated with ectopic pregnancy, spontaneous abortions, intrauterine growth retardation, preterm birth, stillbirths, higher perinatal mortality, small-for-gestational-age (SGA) birth, LBW birth, neonatal anomalies, and lower Apgar scores (Duncan, 2002; Weck, Paulose, & Flaws, 2008). For pregnant women, an education level below high school graduation and those with a current nicotine-dependence were at higher risk of smoking (90.5%) than college-educated women without nicotine dependence (3.9%), according to a recent Harvard study (Gillman, Breslau, Subramanian, Hitsman, & Koenen, 2008). Smoking is "one of the strongest predictors of both LBW and preterm birth" and is "often linked to stress and depression" (Hobbell, Goldstein, & Barrett, 2008, p. 345). For instance, women who may have started smoking as adolescents often continue to smoke in response to life stressors. Health problems do not end once the infant is born. Infants of women who smoked during pregnancy continue to be at higher risk for LBW, preterm birth, poor fetal growth, SIDS, respiratory infections, asthma, ear infections, and decreased lung function (Mercer, Merlino, Milluzzi, & Moore, 2008; Wang & Pinkerton, 2008; Wigle et al., 2008). As the children get older, they are at higher risk for activity and attention problems (Cornelius, Goldschmidt, DeGenna, & Day, 2007).

Passive smoking or **environmental tobacco smoke (ETS)**—exposure to tobacco smoke from other people smoking in one's environment—also puts a person at risk for smoking-related disease. The smoke from a burning cigarette sitting on an ashtray, inhaled passively by the nonsmoker, contains a higher concentration of toxins and carcinogens than the smoke inhaled directly by the smoker; physical distance between infant and smoker correlates with the amount of cotinine (the chief metabolite of nicotine) in the baby's urine (Blizzard, Ponsonby, Dwyer, Venn, & Cochrane, 2003). If a pregnant woman lives with a smoker, she and her fetus can be negatively affected by the other person's addiction. Passive or environmental tobacco smoke has been associated with decreased head circumference, depressed cognitive development, and lower birth weight. When ETS is present along with poverty (e.g., deficits in housing, food, clothing), even greater cognitive deficits occur (Perera et al., 2005). The use of **smokeless tobacco products**, such as snuff and chewing tobacco, has led to an increase in oral cancers related to tobacco exposure. Maternal smokeless tobacco use has been associated with lower birth weight and gestational age (Gupta & Sreevidya, 2004).

Community health nurses and other health care professionals must be involved in the control of tobacco products on many levels, especially in health policy development. It is also important to have skills in client assessment, planning, and intervention, to serve as positive role models, and to be active in research implementation. In the case of tobacco control, health policy development has made important strides at the grassroots level (see Chapter 13). A top priority of health care policy development is to reduce access of youth to tobacco products by restricting tobacco product advertising and promotion. Some significant steps that have been taken to discourage young people from smoking include imposing substantial cigarette excise taxes; requiring that public places such as malls, restaurants, and even bars, be smoke free; monitoring tobacco retailers for illegal sales to minors; and keeping cigarettes in locked cases. Most smokers become addicted to tobacco use in their early teens. One study of tobacco use among Wisconsin adolescents found that 31.6% were current users, although 38% of the general adolescent population currently smoked (Sims & Sims, 2005). If fewer adolescents begin smoking, there will be fewer women of childbearing age who smoke in the future.

An initial health history of a pregnant woman should always include the assessment of tobacco use, smoking status, and exposure to smoke in the personal environment. Stress should also be assessed (e.g., unintended pregnancy; nutrition; chronic stress and daily hassles; levels of social support; mental health issues, such as depression or anxiety, work stressors, racism or discrimination; and any significant life events, such as death or other significant losses) (Hobbell, Goldstein, & Barrett, 2008). The PHN must not only advise clients to quit smoking but also offer supportive and empathetic approaches to stress reduction and smoking cessation, including methods or interventions that can help. For example, the community health nurse may counsel clients individually, suggest behavioral therapy, provide self-help manuals, or recommend nicotine replacement therapy or medication. Other approaches, such as support groups, can be helpful. Any permanent reduction in the number of cigarettes smoked, amount of secondhand smoke inhaled, or amount of smokeless tobacco used is helpful in improving the health of the mother and her fetus.

Nurses can be positive role models for health and demonstrate health-promotion strategies to clients by their own behavior—if a nurse has struggled with smoking cessation, his admission of failures or explanation of successful strategies offers an opportunity to enhance his believability with clients. They recognize that he struggles with some of the same health issues as they do.

Sexually Transmitted Diseases

In the United States, an estimated 880,000 pregnant women annually are infected with herpes simplex virus 2, and 100,000 have *Chlamydia*. Fewer than 1,000 annually contract syphilis and 13,200 are estimated to have gonorrhea. Hepatitis B is estimated in 16,000 pregnant women and around 6,400 women are diagnosed with HIV annually (CDC, 2008a).

Sexually transmitted diseases (STDs) can pass from mother to baby. Syphilis can cross the placenta and infect the fetus, as can HIV—which can also be passed to the infant through breast-feeding (CDC, 2008a). Other STDs (e.g., gonorrhea, hepatitis B, *Chlamydia*, genital herpes) can infect the baby as it passes through the birth canal during delivery. LBW, stillbirth, conjunctivitis, blindness, deafness, neurological damage, chronic liver disease and cirrhosis, along with neonatal sepsis and pneumonia, are possible infant complications of maternal STDs. Mothers may have premature rupture of membranes and resultant infection, or may have a premature onset of labor. Some STDs can lead to cervical and other cancers, pelvic inflammatory disease, infertility, chronic hepatitis, and many other health problems (CDC, 2008a).

Adolescent girls who are pregnant and who use marijuana or other substances may be more at risk for STDs (De Genna, Cornelius, & Cook, 2007). A pregnant woman who discovers she has an STD often feels ashamed, betrayed, embarrassed, and angry. Those who are asymptomatic may not realize they are infected or deny the existence of the disease and fail to carry out the treatment plan after diagnosis. Although educating the pregnant client about the effects of STDs is critical, providing information alone is not enough. The community health nurse has a pivotal role in enhancing the empowerment of women so they can act on the information they receive. The PHN engages with the pregnant clients and helps them understand that they have control over their bodies. Usually, STDs are first discovered in pregnancy during routine prenatal screening, which places the clinic nurse and the nurse who may make home visits in the position to take an affirmative approach to treatment and follow-up.

HIV and AIDS

The HIV epidemic is the great tragedy of the final two decades of the 20th century. In 2005 in the United States, 111 infants born to HIV-infected mothers positively tested for HIV, one third the amount reported in 1994. This is related to the growing use of prophylaxis during the perinatal period in an effort to decrease virus transmission (USD-HHS, 2007). HIV/AIDS infection in Black infants diminished almost 66%, and infection was reduced for Hispanic infants by over 40%. However, the largest decline was found for White infants (81.8%): 77 to 14 cases (USDHHS, 2007). Mothers who transmitted the virus to their newborn infants reported contracting it through sex with an infected partner, injection drug use, or other unspecified methods.

In a large-scale New York study, HIV prevention interventions between 1994 and 2003 were examined and researchers found that 83% of mothers of HIV-exposed infants received prenatal care and were diagnosed with HIV before delivery. Also, the use of prenatal antiretroviral agents by these mothers increased from 63% to 82%. However, 45% of mothers with infected infants had not participated in perinatal HIV prevention interventions. Prenatal, intrapartum, or neonatal antiretroviral drugs were lacking, largely due to maternal illicit drug use, and were associated with LBW babies (Peters et al., 2008).

An HIV-positive woman who is pregnant or who has delivered a baby requires special nursing management of the pregnancy and of the family after the birth of the newborn. There are many teaching opportunities for the community health nurse during a high-risk pregnancy such as helping the client identify, change, or curtail high-risk behaviors. Success in changing behaviors often requires an interdisciplinary approach of health care, social, emotional, and financial resources.

In the United States and other developed nations, HIV-infected women are advised not to breast-feed their infants, because there is a 15% chance that the infants will become infected with HIV from breast milk (Shearer, 2008). The community health nurse focuses teaching on providing a safe, available form of infant formula. In developing countries, the lack of clean water still makes formula feeding dangerous, and breast-feeding is usually recommended. The infection rate for HIV from breast-feeding and the mortality rate from formula made with impure water are about the same, resulting in a dilemma for women and health care providers in developing countries.

Poor Nutrition, Weight Gain, and Oral Health

Nutrition is very important to the unborn child, and mothers' choices, even before conception, can affect the baby's health and development. At about three weeks' gestation—often before the woman recognizes that she is pregnant—the infant's neural tube is forming, and poor nourishment during this period is associated with "incomplete interconnection between brain regions" (House, 2007). Hormones and nutrients set gene-switches that affect later life. Nutrients that are particularly important in reproductive health and that have been shown to lower the risk of obesity and childhood cancers, as well as neural tube defects, autism, and dyslexia, include B vitamins (especially B_1, B_6, B_{12}, and folate), antioxidants (especially E and C vitamins), minerals (especially iron, zinc, selenium, iodine, magnesium, and copper), and essential fatty acids (Katzen-Luchenta, 2007). Important nutrients specifically associated with fetal and infant brain development include vitamin A, choline, folate, selenium, iodine, copper, zinc, and iron. Protein and certain fats are also important, and functioning of specific brain regions is associated with particular nutrients (Georgieff, 2007). Diets rich in protein, nuts, seeds, legumes, and whole grains, along with colorful fruits and vegetables, promote health for both the mother and the fetus. One Harvard University study found that women who ate more fish during pregnancy had infants who demonstrated better cognition, but researchers cautioned that fish high in mercury contamination was detrimental and should be avoided (Oken et al., 2005).

Research has demonstrated a positive correlation between weight gain during pregnancy and normal birth weight in the babies. During 2004, one-third of U.S. women reported weight gains that were outside the recommendations: 13% of women gained less than 16 lbs (19% of Black women) and 20% gained more than 40 lbs (most often White women, at 22.2%). Inadequate weight gain is related to LBW, premature births, and perinatal mortality (USDHHS, 2007). Gaining large amounts of weight can also cause problems at birth, including increased numbers of cesarean deliveries, large-for-gestational-age babies, and the mother's retention of excessive weight. Weight gain between 15 and 35 lbs during pregnancy is recommended for women with body mass indexes (BMIs) ranging from 19.8 to 25; the recommendation is 28 to 40 lbs for underweight women with a BMI under 19.8 and no standard recommendations exist for overweight

women with a BMI over 29.1 (USDHHS, 2007). Obese women have a higher incidence of gestational diabetes, urinary tract infections, wound infection, thromboembolism, pregnancy-induced hypertension, fetal monitoring difficulties, prolonged labor, and birth trauma (Sherwen, Scoloveno, & Weingarten, 2001). Some studies show that, compared with women of normal weight, women who were obese or overweight before pregnancy faced double the risk of having babies with heart defects and multiple birth defects (Watkins et al., 2003). Community health nurses who work with morbidly obese pregnant women can help them most by emphasizing good nutrition and by encouraging them to maintain their pre-pregnant weight without drastically reducing caloric intake. This can be accomplished primarily by a marked decrease in consumption of "empty calories" from junk food and replacing with increased intake of fruits and vegetables. Pregnancy is never a time for dieting. Following nutritional guidelines ensures the proper number of servings and portion sizes. Nutritional counseling can have an additional benefit in that it may ultimately decrease the risk of obesity or eating disorders in the client's children.

Underweight women have twice as many LBW babies as women whose weight is within normal range. Low maternal weight gain is associated with LBW infants who have higher incidences of growth problems, developmental delays, central nervous system disorders, and mental retardation (USDDHS, 2007).

Nutritional teaching is part of the community health nurse's role when working with a pregnant woman who has difficulty gaining the recommended weight during pregnancy. Finding ways to add calories to foods and increasing the woman's desire to eat are effective methods to improve maternal weight gain. Insufficient caloric intake in pregnant adolescents (who themselves are still growing) is an additional concern. For women who are prone to gaining too much weight, nutrition-rich, low-calorie foods are recommended. Exercise during pregnancy is also beneficial, and can reduce maternal weight gain and improve cardiovascular fitness (Gavard & Artal, 2008). After assessment, the community health nurse can determine whether the unwanted weight gain is related to the consumption of additional calories, to limited activity, or to fluid retention. Each cause must be managed differently.

Oral health during pregnancy is also very important to assess. Periodontal infection may affect around 40% of women of childbearing age, and is especially common among disadvantaged and ethnic or racial minorities who may not have adequate access to dental health care (Boggess et al., 2008). Maternal periodontal disease has also been linked to preterm birth, LBW, preeclampsia, and early fetal loss (Ferguson, Hansen, Novak, & Novak, 2007). High maternal levels of the bacteria that cause cavities has been associated with a greater chance of subsequent dental caries in the infant (Silk, Douglass, Douglass, & Silk, 2008).

Public health nurses should teach women of childbearing age the importance of regular dental health checkups and proper dental hygiene, along with making referrals for dental treatment when needed. Dental health procedures have generally been found to be effective and safe for pregnant women, especially during the second trimester (Dasanayake, Gennaro, Hendricks-Munoz, & Chghun, 2008; Silk et al., 2008). Sugar-free gums that contain xylitol and chlorhexidine may be helpful in reducing the maternal child transmission of caries-causing bacteria (Silk et al., 2008). Dental health is not only important during pregnancy, but poor dental hygiene and disease have been linked to health conditions, such as cardiovascular disease and diabetes. Dental health should be a part of general primary preventive education for all public health clients (Ferguson et al., 2007).

Socioeconomic Status and Social Inequality

As noted earlier, poverty plays a role in pregnancy and birth outcomes. Social and economic disparities are factors in preterm birth in both developed and developing nations. This relationship may be more indirect, as poorer women often lack health insurance, have less access to quality prenatal care services, and are exposed to more situational and psychological stressors. Even Canada, noted for universal health care coverage, has been noted to have inadequate levels of prenatal care related to socioeconomic status (SES) disparities (Weck, Paulose, & Flaws, 2008). Employment-related stress has been associated with risk of preterm delivery, and prolonged sitting or standing, heavy lifting, and long work hours are often associated with the type of low-paying jobs available to women living in poverty (Pompeii et al., 2005). Other factors, outlined in more detail in Chapter 25, may also affect the health of both mothers and babies.

Teenage Pregnancy

The United States leads most developed nations in the rates of teenage pregnancy, abortion, and childbearing. Among 46 developed countries, the United States has the second highest teen pregnancy and birth rates, largely because U.S. adolescents are less likely to consistently use contraception (Darroch, Singh, Frost, & the Study Team, 2001; Singh & Darroch, 2000). There is a strong association between young maternal age and high IMR, and infants born to teenagers are at increased risk for preterm delivery, and for neonatal and postneonatal mortality (Briggs, Hopman, & Jamieson, 2007; March of Dimes, 2007; Usta, Zoorob, Abu-Musa, Naassan, & Nassar, 2008). These adverse birth outcomes are independent of education level, use of cigarettes and alcohol during pregnancy, or prenatal care. Simply being an adolescent puts pregnant teens and their offspring at risk (Chen, Wen, Fleming, Demissie, Rhoads, & Walker, 2007). Infants born to Black adolescents are more likely to be LBW babies than are infants of White teens. Infants born to very young adolescents (aged 10 to 14 years) are at very high risk for neonatal mortality. Teen mothers have increased psychological risks, such as isolation, powerlessness, depressive disorders, and increased somatic complaints. Developmental and maturational processes are disrupted or compromised, and young mothers face diminished prospects for completing their education. It is important for PHNs to assess each pregnant adolescent's situation (e.g., family support and living situation, relationship with the father of the baby and other supportive friends), as well as her hopes, goals, strengths, weaknesses, in order to effectively plan interventions (Rentschler, 2003).

The markers for successful pregnancy outcomes and future life events are more complex. The mother's educational attainment, marital experiences, subsequent fertility behavior, labor force experience, occupational attainment, and experiences with poverty and public assistance are all directly related to the adolescent pregnancy and are often negatively affected (Boden, Fergusson, & Horwood, 2008).

The issues of adolescent parenting are complex. They encompass many areas, including emotional, physical, and social issues, and the life experiences of adolescent mothers often are characterized as unequal to those of their peers who delayed childbirth (Smithbattle, 2007).

Pregnant adolescents are less likely to receive early and continuous prenatal care and they are more likely to use alcohol and to smoke during their pregnancies. Moreover, their diets are often lacking in essential vitamins and minerals (Moran, 2007; USDHHS, 2000). As an aggregate, their infants are at risk for lower 5-minute Apgar scores, LBW, neonatal mortality, and preterm birth (Chen et al., 2007).

The community health nurse has a unique challenge when teaching teens about pregnancy-related changes, accompanying needs, and preparation for the important role of parent. In a Virginia study, adolescent mothers felt that they were not "plainly informed" about the advantages of breast-feeding, and postpartum education classes were recommended to support breast-feeding teen mothers who only got instruction while in the hospital (Spear, 2004, p. 106). A British study of adolescent breast-feeding mothers noted that the teens felt "watched and judged, reported that they lacked confidence, complained of fatigue and discomfort, and recognized the need for both emotional and instrumental/informative support (Dykes, Moran, Burt, & Edwards, 2003, p. 391). Development of a trusting relationship helped teens to continue breast-feeding. Emotional support is provided by relationships that engender love and appreciation, and instrumental support is more concrete (e.g., a ride to the clinic, help with homework, or money to buy food). Informational support is the provision of information or advice (Orr, 2004).

Another issue with pregnant adolescents is the problem of repeated pregnancies. One Texas study found that 42% of teen mothers had another pregnancy within 2 years' time, 73% of these teens went on to deliver an infant (Child Trends, 2006a; Raneri & Wiemann, 2007). Predictors identified in the study included "not being in a relationship with father of the first child three months later," being more than 3 years younger than the father of the first baby, "experiencing intimate partner violence" within 3 months of the first birth, not being in school 3 months after the first child's birth, and "having many friends who were adolescent parents" (p. 39). Second pregnancies during adolescence have been associated with "worse outcomes" when compared to first-time teen mothers (Reime, Schucking, & Wenzlaff, 2008, p. 4). Public health nurses can provide needed interventions to postpone subsequent pregnancies and encourage the effective and consistent use of contraception (Kershaw, Niccolai, Ickovics, Lewis, Meade, & Ethier, 2003).

Emotional Needs

Teenagers who become pregnant deal with this change in their life in a variety of ways. Some have such a strong denial system that they deny the pregnancy, even to themselves. They may be 3 or 4 months into the pregnancy before they can admit it and seek a physician's diagnosis. Often, their parents are the last to know. What is difficult about this scenario is that prenatal care is delayed into the second trimester of pregnancy. If the teen chooses to continue with the pregnancy, the delayed prenatal care could compromise the well-being of both the young mother and the fetus. Holub and colleagues (2007) studied the effects of prenatal and parenting stress on a large group of 14-

to 19-year-olds and found that those who had high levels of both stressors exhibited lower maternal adjustment (i.e., positive attitude toward being a mother, care of the infant, competent parenting) and higher emotional distress after giving birth. They concluded that early interventions for both prenatal and parenting support are needed. In a small study of pregnant Hispanic teens, Lloyd (2004, p. 239) noted "poor communication and unstable relationships with parents" prior to pregnancy, and a hesitancy to communicate with parents about becoming pregnant. However, most adolescents reported improved communication and relationship with parents after talking with them. Parents and grandparents often provide emotional support. They not only serve as parents to the adolescent, but also compensate for the inadequate parenting skills of the teen with their infant (Dallas, 2004). It takes time for adolescent mothers to begin to understand the role of parent and to get to "know their baby" (Smithbattle, 2007, p. 261).

Caring and supportive parents and community health or school nurses can be instrumental in guiding an adolescent through this difficult time. Teen parents have difficult choices to make, including decisions about continuing with the pregnancy, keeping the baby, or finding adoptive parents. Some may choose abortion. These choices are difficult and are fraught with emotion. Adolescents and supportive parents, in consultation with professionals, can explore all options. This may be the time that the community health nurse first begins to work with the teen, perhaps at school or in a school-based clinic. First contact may also occur in a clinic or physician's office, or on a home visit resulting from a referral from a health care provider. Home visiting programs for adolescent mothers have been effective in improving prenatal care parenting scores and school continuation rates. They have also contributed to reducing preterm births (Barnet, Liu, DeVoe, Alperovitz-Bichell, & Duggan, 2007; Flynn, Budd, & Modelski, 2008; Nguyen, Carson, Parris, & Place, 2003). The nurse can offer educational services, emotional support, and referrals for services as needed. Because postpartum depression is not uncommon, and adolescents are at increased risk, it may be important for PHN visitation to continue periodically for 1 to 2 years postpartum (Mayberry, Horowitz, & Declercq, 2007; Reid & Meadows-Oliver, 2007).

The goal of any pregnancy is positive maternal–infant outcomes, including a positive relationship. For some teen mothers, positive relationships are more difficult to achieve than for older mothers. Positive relationships and self-esteem have an impact on the quality of mothering and positive responses to infant distress. Typically, older adolescents have higher self-esteem than younger mothers: this was observed in classic studies conducted by Olds and colleagues (1999, 2000) and by Koniack-Griffin and colleagues (2000, 2002, 2003). These significant studies demonstrated the benefits of intensive intervention programs. Community health nurses who have special training can provide each participant with services that promote the overall health of the mother and maternal–infant bonding. Results of these studies can further guide nurses in their work with pregnant adolescents.

Physical Needs

Pregnant teens have a gamut of physical needs that can be addressed by routine prenatal care and education, but there is need for continuity if such endeavors are to be successful.

Routine prenatal care is one of the most important needs, and teens may require assistance in recognizing the value of monitoring the pregnancy. Some may feel embarrassed and uncomfortable with male health care providers and refuse to keep appointments or may want to be accompanied by the baby's father or a girlfriend. Whatever it takes to get the teen to prenatal appointments should be encouraged, including making arrangements for transportation (e.g., procuring bus tokens, calling a taxi, or arranging for a friend or social worker to drive the teen to her appointments) (Michels, 2000). Where feasible, specially focused clinics for pregnant and parenting teens may be most effective; a multi-center Australian study found that teens attending a specialized teen prenatal clinic had significantly lower rates of preterm births (Quinlivan & Evans, 2004). School-based clinics have shown promise in providing easily accessible prenatal care, lowering the risk of giving birth to LBW infants and reducing school dropout rates (Barnet, Arroyo, Devoe, & Duggan, 2004; Barnet, Duggan, & Devoe, 2003; Strunk, 2008).

The pregnant teen needs education regarding changes in her emotional state and her body, the growth and development of the fetus, dietary requirements, and rest and relaxation needs. She also needs anticipatory guidance for care giving and parenting. Teaching can take place as part of each prenatal appointment, in specific classes at school for pregnant teens, in the health department clinic, or during home visits. In each setting, the community health nurse can modify the teaching methods to the setting and the individual needs of the teen. Studies show that PHN home visits and preparation-for-motherhood classes are effective in promoting better outcomes for adolescents and their infants, including better use of resources (e.g., prenatal visits), fewer hospital days, lower school dropout rates, fewer repeat pregnancies 2 years postpartum, and decreased infant mortality (Flynn, Budd, & Modelski, 2008; Koniak-Griffin et al., 2000; Koniak-Griffin et al., 2003).

Changing teen behavior during pregnancy can be challenging, and PHNs must keep in mind the developmental differences between early, middle, and late adolescents with regard to intentions and health habits (Phipps, Rosengard, Weitzen, Meers, & Billinkoff, 2008). The community health nurse may focus on one important and seemingly less complex issue of nutrition during pregnancy. However, it is a more difficult task to change the eating habits of teens than it is to change those of adults. In their stage of development, teens usually are more concerned with body image than with fetal growth and development. Fad diets, peer pressure, and personal control are all issues with which the pregnant teen is struggling. If a teen has been raised in poverty, a multiplicity of other issues can affect her motivation to make dietary changes during pregnancy. Teens are more often concerned with present needs and respond better to relaxed, informal group approaches to education that involve topics of their choosing and do not resemble the school setting. Pregnancy diaries, creative activities (crafts, drawing, making snacks), small group activities and games, videos with discussions, and visits to local community resources (hospital delivery rooms, social services, lactation counselors) are more appealing than classroom lectures (Robertson, 2003). Programs that offer empowerment and group prenatal care are helpful (Klima, 2003). Also, teaching and support groups may be helpful in promoting healthy prenatal behaviors and preparing for motherhood (National Clearinghouse on Families & Youth, 2007; Quinlivan, 2004).

Social Needs

Pregnant teens are dealing with two stages of their own growth and development at the same time, which makes their social needs complex. They are struggling with the normal adolescent challenges along with the responsibilities of pregnancy and parenting (young adulthood stage of development).

There may be changes in acceptance by social groups or in types of activities (e.g., surfboarding, mountain climbing). The group may participate in activities that the pregnant teen should not participate in, such as smoking, drinking, or taking illicit drugs. This causes conflict for a pregnant teen who has a strong need to be accepted by her peer group and who also knows that she has a responsibility to her unborn child. The community health nurse can help the teen solve her dilemma by providing a social support system among the attendees at prenatal classes. The nurse can also convince the teen's parents or other adults in her life to offer her more support. Often, a developmental crisis such as a teen pregnancy can help cement the mother-daughter relationship. It takes time and work on the part of the parents and the teen. The teen will need the support of her parents after the baby is born, and strengthening the relationship during pregnancy is an important start.

Another social outlet and an important resource is school. The teen should be encouraged to continue her studies, with the goal of graduation. The health and welfare of children are related to the educational levels of their parents. Higher educational levels increase the likelihood that children will receive adequate medical care and live in a safe and supportive environment with adults who are responsive to their needs (Koniack-Griffin et al., 2000). Internet support groups organized and monitored by nurses are beginning to provide another means of social support for pregnant and parenting adolescents (Hudson, Campbell-Grossman, Keating-Lefler, & Cline, 2008). Computer and Internet-based interventions have demonstrated success in providing knowledge and promoting delayed sexual activity in Appalachian high schools (Roberto, Zimmerman, Carlyle, & Abner, 2007). Greater self-efficacy in negotiating condom use was also noted in participants, and the majority of high school students (88.5%) participated in at least one activity aimed at preventing teen pregnancy and transmission of STDs and HIV. Teen pregnancy and education are discussed more thoroughly in Chapter 22.

Maternal Developmental Disability

For couples who are developmentally disabled, having a child puts increased stress on a system that is already burdened. Past studies have shown that child abuse, neglect, and child behavior problems, along with poor academic achievement and inadequate home environments, accompany the parenting style of developmentally disabled parents (Feldman & Walton-Allen, 1997; Morch, Skar, & Andersgard, 1997). However, more recent research has found that children with an IQ at or above 85 were not at greater risk of exhibiting behavior problems, regardless of the mother's IQ level (Chen, Schwarz, Radcliffe, & Rogan, 2006). Children are still at risk, however, for understimulation and environmental insecurity, but parent training/child-care skills programs and careful home monitoring can reduce the risk of child abuse and neglect and promote more effective parenting (Bager, 2003; Feldman, Ducharme, & Case, 1999; Nitzkin & Smith, 2004).

Much of the pediatric literature discusses the needs of developmentally disabled infants and children and the roles of nurses and health care professionals in assisting the families of these children. Developmentally disabled adults, however, are rarely represented in studies of disability, so there is limited information about their success as parents. Over the past 20 years, studies identified that a primary problem affecting the children of developmentally disabled mothers is the poor quality of maternal–infant/child interaction. The parenting style of mothers with developmental disabilities is often nonstimulating, punitive, and restrictive (Feldman, Case, Towns, & Betel, 1985). In addition, unusual and sometimes bizarre behaviors can occur because the parent does not understand basic concepts regarding normal child development. Better cognitive outcomes for infants have been documented when developmentally delayed or mentally retarded parents were more responsive and involved (Feldman et al., 1985). Periodic developmental screening, infant stimulation and home visitation programs, and special health care instruction have demonstrated evidence-based results (Nitzkin & Smith, 2004). How does the community health nurse work with developmentally disabled parents effectively? Most importantly, nursing support must enhance the natural resilience of the family. Extended family support systems, along with community agencies that provide services to mentally disabled adults and children, can improve the outcomes for these families. The success of family support depends on immediate and continuing health promotion visits. The goal is to establish safe parenting routines that will serve as a foundation for parenting skills needed when the infant begins to walk and explore—a time when the infant's safety is more in jeopardy.

The establishment of a trusting relationship between the nurse and the family is of foremost importance. Teaching by demonstration with many visual aids and prompts, along with games and creative approaches to engage and sustain attention, can challenge the nurse's creativity. Modeling of appropriate parenting behavior needs to occur on each visit. Supervision and monitoring of family functioning must continue until the child reaches adulthood. Many agencies employing PHNs cannot provide the intensive follow-up that such a family requires. It is then necessary to make referrals to organizations that can provide support, such as the American Association of Retarded Citizens (AARC) or Exceptional Parents Unlimited. The nurse may stay involved as a consultant to the paraprofessionals or make periodic home visits at times of developmental or situational crisis.

Complications of Childbearing

Some maternal deaths are not preventable (e.g., amniotic fluid embolism), but one large study in North Carolina found that 40% of pregnancy-related deaths were preventable, either through better preconception care, improved system factors, better quality of care, or patient actions (Berg et al., 2005). Morbidity is also a factor, and although some major risk factors among pregnant women and infants have been discussed, several common complications of childbearing bear mentioning. The effects of hypertensive disease in pregnancy, gestational diabetes, postpartum depression, and grief in families who have lost a child are important areas in which the community health nurse can intervene successfully.

Hypertensive Disease in Pregnancy

Blood pressure measurements in all people show daily variation, regardless of physical and mental activities. Hypertension in pregnancy may be chronic or related specifically to pregnancy. In 2004, chronic hypertension during pregnancy was found in 9.6 per 1,000 births, and was more often found in Black women than in White and Hispanic women. The rate for pregnancy-related hypertension was markedly higher at 37.9, with lower rates for Hispanic mothers. Severe hypertension, due to either cause, is associated with premature birth, fetal growth restriction, abruption of the placenta, and stillbirth (USDHHS, 2007).

Preeclampsia is an "idiopathic multisystem disorder" related to disease of the placenta (Norwitz, Hsu, & Repke, 2002, p. 308); or, a "vascular endothelial disease" resulting in placental dysfunction (Van Pampus & Aarnoudse, 2005, p. 489). It results in new-onset high blood pressure and protein in the urine, along with nondependent edema, and can result in eclampsia (characterized by convulsions and/or coma), pulmonary edema, liver rupture, renal failure, disseminated intravascular coagulopathy (DIC), and cortical blindness (Van Pampus & Aarnoudse, 2005). Preeclampsia/eclampsia is the second leading cause of maternal death (15%), and often occurs in adolescent pregnancies or with mothers older than 35 (Norwitz et al., 2002). HELLP syndrome (named for hemolysis, elevated liver enzymes, and low platelet count) is a severe form of preeclampsia and can lead to bleeding tendencies and other complications (Matchaba & Moodley, 2001). The effects from pregnancy-induced hypertension on infants are often serious because placental health is associated with fetal growth (Salafia, Charles, & Maas, 2006), but long-term maternal consequences can also be significant. A woman who has experienced preeclampsia is at increased risk of cardiovascular disease and chronic hypertension later in life (Van Pampus & Aarnoudse, 2005).

Various methods are employed to attempt to prevent and control hypertension during pregnancy, namely, a diet rich in fresh fruits and vegetables, adequate fluid intake, weight gain limitations, rest, and regular exercise. These remain the most common preventive suggestions that community health nurses, in collaboration with the clients' primary health care providers, can give to their pregnant clients. A calm environment, along with periods of rest with the pregnant woman either elevating her feet or reclining in a left side-lying position, are also recommended. Additional assessment data may guide the nurse to focus teaching on stress reduction techniques and modification or elimination of smoking. Public health nurses can provide frequent monitoring of blood pressure and encourage the client to be vigilant in keeping prenatal appointments. However, medication or even hospitalization may be necessary. The nurse can offer support and understanding while continuing to be a resource for the client as the pregnancy progresses and the infant is born. Calcium supplements have shown some promise in reducing the risk for preeclampsia in those women at increased risk (e.g., previous preeclampsia, mother and/or female relatives with history of preeclampsia), and in reducing the risk of death or serious problems in women with preeclampsia (Hofmeyr, Atallah, & Duley, 2005). Low-dose aspirin therapy also can prevent preeclampsia and subsequent infant complications (Meads et al., 2008).

Gestational Diabetes

Gestational diabetes mellitus (GDM) is defined as "glucose intolerance of variable degree with onset or first recognition during pregnancy." GDM occurs in about 7% of pregnancies (American Diabetes Association [ADA], 2003, p. s103). For the mother with GDM, there is a higher risk of hypertension, preeclampsia, urinary tract infections, cesarean section, and future risk of type 2 diabetes (ADA, 2003). The infant is at increased risk for fetal death because GDM has been associated with large-for-gestational-age (LGA) babies, which puts them at risk especially during delivery (Mondestin, Ananth, Smulian, & Vintzileos, 2002). An Iranian study using a 75-g glucose tolerance testing (GTT) protocol found a 6.1% incidence of GDM and a correlation between 1-hour blood glucose levels and neonatal birth weights (Shirazian et al., 2008). In 2004, the rate of GDM was 35.8 per 1,000 live births (USDHHS, 2007). Pathophysiologically, GDM is similar to type 2 diabetes, and more than one-third of women with GDM eventually develop type 2 diabetes during their lifetimes.

Because growth and maturation of the fetus are closely associated with the delivery of maternal nutrients, particularly glucose, maintenance of appropriate glucose levels is essential to the health of the fetus. Daily self-monitoring of blood glucose levels is recommended (ADA, 2003). Glucose control is most crucial in the third trimester because of fetal growth at that stage, and is directly related to the duration and degree of maternal glucose elevation.

The community health nurse can help in the control of GDM by encouraging early prenatal care, adequate nutrition, rest and exercise, and adherence to the particular regimen suggested by the woman's health care provider. A structured walking program was shown to regulate glucose levels in women with GDM effectively, while reducing daily insulin levels (Davenport, Mottola, McManus, & Gratton, 2008). Although earlier recommendations were restricted to human insulin, a comprehensive review of current research on GDM management and outcomes found both maternal and infant benefits and a low likelihood of fetal harm with either the use of insulin or oral diabetes medications (ADA, 2003; Nicholson et al., 2008). Waist circumference measurements and a family history of diabetes along with GDM are associated with development of later type 2 diabetes (Nicholson et al., 2008; Lee, Jang, Park, Metzger, & Cho, 2008). Women should be encouraged to monitor blood glucose levels regularly 6 weeks postpartum and periodically throughout their life (ADA, 2003). Those PHNs working with pregnant women should provide education on early warning signs for GDM and the importance of regular prenatal care and follow up.

The infants of women with GDM often weigh significantly more than other full-term infants, and a large-scale Harvard study found that higher birth weight babies, as well as those born to mothers with GDM, were at higher risk of being overweight in adolescence (Gillman, Rifas-Shiman, Berkey, Field, & Colditz, 2003). Some women who have such large babies may expect more of the infant because, at birth, the baby weighs the same as a 2- to 3-month-old child. Teaching and anticipatory guidance become particularly important for these women.

Thyroid disease, the second most common endocrine disorder in pregnancy next to diabetes, is also an important consideration in women of childbearing age as thyroid hormones factor strongly into fetal brain development (Neale, Cootauco, & Burrow, 2007).

Postpartum Depression

Although most people recognize the common fleeting mood swings immediately after childbirth known as "baby blues," high-profile cases like Andrea Yates, who suffered from postpartum psychosis and drowned her five small children, are rare (1 or 2 per 1,000 births) but nonetheless tragic (Williams, 2002). The actress Brooke Shields discussed her postpartum depression and treatment with antidepressant medications, making this condition more visible and less stigmatizing (National Institutes of Health [NIH], 2005).

Depressive disorders during a woman's lifetime are fairly common phenomena; 20.6% of women and 11% of men were diagnosed in 2006 (Heo, Murphy, Fontaine, Bruce, & Alexopoulos, 2008). In the postpartum period, approximately 10% to 15% of women are affected by postpartum depression for a period of 1 month up to 1 year (NIH, 2005). About 20% of women are estimated to suffer from depression during pregnancy, but about half the time health care providers do not recognize it (Bennett, Einarson, Taddio, Koren, & Einarson, 2004). Depression can affect anyone, even women without a history of prior depression. Perinatal depressive symptoms may not indicate major clinical depression. Nevertheless, symptoms may cause considerable psychological distress, such as irritability and restlessness; feeling hopeless, sad, and overwhelmed; having little energy or motivation and crying unexpectedly; sleeping and eating too little or too much; problems with cognition (memory, decision-making, focus); loss of pleasure or interest in usually pleasant activities; and withdrawal from family and friends (National Women's Health Information Center [NWHIC], 2005).

Through numerous studies over the years, researchers have identified specific risk factors associated with perinatal depression and have developed a profile of women with postpartum depression (NWHIC, 2005). Risk factors for depression during pregnancy include a personal or family history of depression, substance abuse or mental illness, lack of social support, anxiety about the fetus, marital or financial problems, recent death of family member, and problems with previous pregnancies or births, along with young maternal age. Rapid hormonal shifts within the first 24 hours after giving birth may lead to postpartum depression. Sometimes, thyroid levels drop after childbirth, and low levels can cause depressed mood, fatigue, difficulties with concentration, weight gain, and sleep problems (NWHIC, 2005).

Most depressed postpartum women experience low self-esteem, which can be reinforced by the infant's temperament. Moreover, the demands of an irritable infant on a new mother who is fatigued and has limited support from a spouse or significant other can increase the depressive symptoms. Other mothers, who have babies who are not irritable, may feel guilty because of the apathy they feel toward their babies, or they may experience anxiety about hurting their infants or themselves (NIH, 2005). In addition, stressful life events combined with a lack of social support and everyday stressors, the greatest of which is interpersonal conflict, are etiologic factors in postpartum depressive symptoms. Postpartum depression affects maternal–infant bonding (NIH, 2005; NWHIC, 2005).

The value of confidants to new mothers is evident, and mothers should be encouraged to ask for help from family and friends or to talk with other new mothers or join support groups. Group and individual therapy are helpful, as is medication. Public health nurses can encourage new mothers with depressive symptoms to get adequate rest (nap while baby is sleeping), be realistic and not try to be the perfect homemaker, ask for help from her partner with feedings during the night and with household chores, get out of the house periodically, and spend quality time with her partner (NWHIC, 2005).

There are several nonpharmacologic interventions the community health nurse can initiate in addition to the ones mentioned above. First, caffeine can lead to sleep disturbance, and alcohol is a depressant that has been implicated in depression. The elimination of both is a simple yet helpful suggestion. Getting adequate sleep is important because sleep deprivation exacerbates psychiatric symptoms. Napping when the baby naps, resting when possible throughout the day, and going to bed early (albeit with the knowledge that sleep may be interrupted two or more times to feed the infant) will provide more hours of rest and sleep. Anxiety symptoms often coexist with depression. Relaxation techniques that reduce anxiety can be helpful, including listening to relaxing music, doing yoga, or performing a simple exercise routine. Participation in a support group allows women to identify with others who may be experiencing similar difficulties. Through discussion, women provide each other with both emotional and practical support.

A final area of assistance is client education. A woman with postpartum depression is more likely to manage her depression successfully if she is aware of the symptoms of depression; the need for a support system; the importance of adequate rest, sleep, and nutrition; and the possibility of supportive psychological or pharmacologic therapy. The critical nature of postpartum depressive symptoms and the potential negative ramifications for mothers and their children are evident. Depression during pregnancy can result in lower birth weight or premature infants, and postpartum depression can affect parenting and infant stimulation that can lead to delays in infant language development, emotional bonding, lower activity levels, and behavior and sleep problems (NWHIC, 2005). Untreated depression can lead to substance abuse, inadequate prenatal care and nutrition, poor pregnancy outcomes, family disruption, and inadequate mother-infant bonding. However, the safety of antidepressants in pregnant and breast-feeding women is not clear (Boucher, Bairam, & Beaulac-Baillargeon, 2008; Maschi, Clavenna, Campi, Schiavetti, Bernat, & Bonati, 2008; Mian, 2005; Oberlander, Warburton, Misri, Riggs, Aghajanian, & Hertzman, 2008; Pearson et al., 2007).

Even though psychotropic medications have been shown to cross the placental barrier and have been found both in amniotic fluid and breast milk, the American College of Obstetricians & Gynecologists (ACOG) cautions against leaving mental illnesses untreated and recommends that the use of antidepressants be individualized and that further research be conducted (ACOG Committee on Practice Bulletins, 2008).

Community health nurses can intervene by initiating primary preventive measures that promote health throughout pregnancy and the postpartum period. Assessment of the pregnant woman for factors that contribute to depression with standardized questionnaires or one developed by the nursing agency is a beginning (Beck & Gable, 2001). If women with compromised mental health resources can be identified, then positive mental health outcomes may be fostered by supporting their self-esteem, optimizing the quality of their primary intimate relationships, and reducing day-to-day stressors. At times, the nurse's efforts alone are not sufficient and a referral to community mental health services is essential for the women and their children.

Fetal or Infant Death

An infrequent role for community health nurses in maternal–child health is that of grief counselor. A couple may experience a miscarriage or ectopic pregnancy, stillbirth, or the death of an infant from SIDS. **Sudden infant death syndrome (SIDS)** is "the sudden death of an infant less than one year of age that cannot be explained after a thorough investigation is conducted, including a complete autopsy, examination of the death scene, and review of the clinical history" (CDC, 2008b). More than 2,250 infants die annually from SIDS, making it the leading cause of death for 1- to 12-month-old infants. Since 1990, the rate of SIDS has dropped over 50% (CDC, 2008b).

In each situation of loss, the nurse has an important supportive role. People respond to grief in a variety of ways: some express deep sadness, shock, or disbelief; some weep and are unable to talk; and others talk incessantly about regrets or guilt. Even if a miscarriage occurs early in a pregnancy, the bonding between the mother and fetus has begun and expressions of grief may be as intense as with the loss of an infant or child. Women have described feeling a sense of abandonment and bereavement, and thinking that "they are the cause of the miscarriage through something they have done, eaten, or thought" (Adolfsson, Larsson, Wijma, & Betero, 2004, p. 543). Although grief reactions vary, the grief experienced by women after a miscarriage has been described as "similar in intensity to grief after other types of major losses." The sense of grief usually begins to diminish by around 6 months (Brier, 2008). Increased anxiety levels are also found, sometimes more frequently than depression, and can last for about the same amount of time, leaving some women more at risk for post-traumatic stress disorder (PTSD) and obsessive-compulsive disorder (OCD) (Brier, 2004; Cumming et al., 2007). Psychological counseling has been associated with greater decreases over time in levels of worry, grief, and self-blame (Nikcevi, Kuczmierczyk, & Nicolaides, 2007). When parents are unable to identify the exact cause of their fetal loss, they have a more difficult time letting go of grief and anxiety (Nikcevi et al., 2007).

For couples who have delivered a stillborn baby, the shock is compounded by the experience of carrying the pregnancy to full term, along with the anticipation of an imminent delivery and the expectation of an addition to the family. This is especially true if all signs before the birthing event itself were positive. They may say such things as, "we felt him move just yesterday and now he's dead—what did I do wrong?" or "I did everything right during this pregnancy. Why did this happen?" These are questions for which there may be no answers, even from the family's health care provider. Frequently, a stillbirth is related to birth defects (15% to 20%), fetal entanglement in the umbilical cord (15%), placental problems (10% to 20%), reduced fetal growth (20%), or to an infection (10% to 20%). Trauma and *Rh* disease can also lead to stillbirths (March of Dimes, 2005b).

Mothers who experience stillbirths recognize the need for spiritual and psychosocial support from professional caregivers, and relate that they struggle to find meaning through their grief, which is often "emotionally complex" and long lasting (Cacciatore & Bushfield, 2007). Families must acknowledge the death of the child and integrate the loss into their family lives through "significant and meaningful family practices" (Gudmundsdottir & Chesla, 2006, p. 143). Sharing their stories of loss, facilitating sociocultural rituals regarding the loss, having a "sensitive presence," and validating the loss are helpful nursing interventions (Callister, 2006, p. 227).

Often, the family needs reassurance that they did nothing wrong or that there is nothing they could have done differently to prevent the stillbirth. Tenderly encouraging the family to talk about the baby and the sadness they feel is important. Home visitation and simply being there for the family and listening well are invaluable nursing interventions. Referral to mental health counseling or support groups specific to parents of stillborn children where they can share their feelings may be very helpful (March of Dimes, 2005b).

When a family experiences loss of an infant after the baby has been brought home from the hospital, grief and guilt are compounded by the loss of an anticipated future and the disrupted continuity in family life. An infant may die of SIDS, a congenital anomaly, an infection, or an accident. There are constant reminders of the infant's presence in the home from memories, photos, videos, and accumulated possessions. This death disrupts family homeostasis and the psychological and physiologic equilibrium of the family. In many cases, the police are involved and an autopsy is required, contributing to the anguish of the grieving family. This promotes both guilt and loss of self-esteem and can even threaten the marriage. The lack of a clear causative factor, especially in the case of SIDS, can be very frightening to parents (Yiallourou, Walker, & Horne, 2008).

The nurse's presence at this time is important. Often, families are inundated with visits from supporters immediately after a death and during the burial ceremony. Thereafter, the parents are visited less frequently or not at all, although this is usually a very lonely and critical time for them. Providing continuity and support to the family for months after the death of an infant gives the PHN an opportunity to assess the family for signs of unresolved grief. After the loss of a child, ruminative coping (rather than distractive coping) style puts the mother at greater risk of major depression, and the incidence of depression in cases of child loss have been reported to be as high as 69% (Ito et al., 2003). Grieving families may find comfort, support, and helpful information from support groups and resources such as Compassionate Friends or First Candle.

Maternal grief can encompass the emotions of envy, jealousy, shame, and guilt. This can occur after miscarriage, stillbirth, or sudden death of an infant (Barr & Cacciatore, 2007). Thinking about and planning for subsequent pregnancies may induce feelings of "ambivalence, doubts, and insecurities," and influence parenting of subsequent children (Lamb, 2002). Couples may experience significant distress; fathers also experience grief after the perinatal deaths (Vance, Boyle, Najman, & Thearle, 2002). The nurse should encourage the parents to express their feelings by using supportive statements and open-ended questions. The parents may have doubts about actions or behaviors that they believe may have caused the miscarriage, stillbirth, or sudden death of their child. Reassurance and clarification of any misconceptions may alleviate the parents' feelings of guilt and help them cope with their grief in a healthy manner.

INFANTS, TODDLERS, AND PRESCHOOLERS

Healthy children are a vital resource to ensure the future well-being of nations. They are the parents, workers, leaders, and decision makers of tomorrow, and their health and safety depend on today's decisions and actions. Their futures lie in the hands of those people responsible for their wellbeing, including the community health nurse.

The well-being of children has been a subject of great concern globally and in the United States. Its importance has been emphasized through development of numerous laws and services, yet the needs of many children continue to go unmet. Many young children often go to bed hungry; some infants and toddlers do not receive even the most basic immunizations before they reach school age. Accidents and injuries are a leading cause of death; preventable communicable diseases increase mortality among the very young. For a country that leads in many areas, the failure to protect and promote the health of its youngest citizens represents a significant breakdown. However, in many other nations— mostly less developed countries—infant health and well-being are in even greater jeopardy.

Global History of Children's Health Care

Only recently in the history of the world have children been considered valuable assets, even in countries where there are now well-developed programs of infant health promotion and protection, infant and child day care services, and strict educational expectations for all children. In some countries today, however, female infants and children or those born with congenital anomalies are not valued. Countries such as India and China provide inequitable care for male and female children. Gender-selective abortions or infanticide also occur. Some birth, growth, and developmental rituals are harsh and would be considered illegal if judged by Western standards. Cultural practices that are fostered by political forces prevent many countries from improving the health of infants and young children (Save the Children, 2008).

The health of children in one country can affect that of children in other countries, including the United States. Major natural disasters place whole populations at risk, especially the very young and the very old. Examples include the severe acute respiratory syndrome (SARS) epidemic in 2003; the 2004 earthquake and tsunami that affected families from Sri Lanka, India, Indonesia, and Somalia to Thailand; and the Chinese earthquake of 2008 (International Save the Children Alliance, 2008).

NATIONAL PERSPECTIVE ON INFANTS, TODDLERS, AND PRESCHOOLERS

The **infant** (birth to 1 year), **toddler** (ages 1 and 2 years), and **preschooler** populations (ages 3 and 4 years) are generally healthy, and most of them have a usual source of health care (96%). For children age 4 and younger, 87% were reported by their parents to be in excellent or very good health (National Center for Health Statistics [NCHS], 2005). The major causes of death among the 1- to 4-year-old population are unintentional injuries (motor vehicle crashes, falls, drowning, fires, and burns), followed by birth defects and cancer (NCHS, 2005). Assault (homicide) and diseases of the heart are also among the five leading causes of death for this age group (Hamilton, Minino, Martin, Kochanek, Strobino, & Guyer, 2007).

Accidents and Injuries

Toddlers and preschoolers are vulnerable to many types of accidents and unintentional injuries, such as those caused by unsafe toys, falls, burns or scalding, drowning, motor vehicle crashes, and poisonings. These injuries may result in death or significant disability. The loss of children's lives resulting from all injuries combined represents a staggering number of years of productive life lost to society. Childhood injuries lead to about 16,000 deaths each year, and 70% of these are the result of unintentional injuries. Over 20 million nonfatal injuries occur yearly to children, resulting in 300,000 hospital admissions and costing over $347 billion (Schnitzer, 2006).

Suffocation is the leading cause of death in infants (66%). Most causes of suffocation death are related to either prone sleeping position, wedging between the wall and mattress, soft bedding or sleeping surface obstructing the nose and mouth, head entrapment, hanging, and "overlaying by another person" (Schnitzer, 2006, p. 1867). Infants should go to sleep on their backs, in a crib or child-friendly bed without soft bedding or pillows, and parents should be cautioned about risk factors for SIDS and the potential dangers of sleeping with their babies (Kemp, Unger, Wilkins, et al., 2000; Lahr, Rosenberg, & Lapidus, 2005). Information about the SIDS prevention campaign *Back to Sleep* should be provided to all parents of infants and education should begin with hospital nurses and continue with PHNs in the community (Association of Maternal & Child Health Programs, n.d.).

Infants and toddlers are at risk of falling when they are not adequately supervised. Falls are a leading cause of nonfatal injuries and hospitalizations for infants, toddlers, and preschoolers (Schnitzer, 2006). Falls from stairs, a bed, or other furniture can cause permanent injury or death. Public health nurses should teach families that infants should never be left unattended when not in a crib or play yard. As the infant grows and learns to walk, frequent falls are common and continuous supervision and childproofing the home are essential activities. Pointing out to parents the potential dangers related to falls and teaching them about effective preventive measures they can take (e.g., window guards, dangers of infant walkers) are viable means of preventing serious injuries (Committee on Injury & Poison Prevention, 2001a; 2001b). Young children are curious, and their explorations can lead to injuries from other sources (e.g., burns, drowning, poisoning).

Burn injuries can affect children of all ages. Over 116,000 children are treated yearly for burn- and fire-related injuries. Spilled hot liquids or foods cause most scald burns for 6 month olds to 2 year olds (Safe Kids Worldwide, 2007). Bath water that is too hot can also cause serious scalding injuries. Scalding is the most common cause of burns requiring hospitalization in toddlers; reducing water heater temperature settings to below 130°F is an effective preventive measure that PHNs can promote (Schnitzer, 2006). Infants are often burned by touching a parent's cigarette or by reaching for a cup of hot coffee or the handle of a pot on the stove. A crawling or toddling child can pull an iron cord, causing the iron to topple on him, resulting in a burn or injury. Electrocution can result from inserting a finger or toy into an electrical outlet. Young children playing with lighters and matches often cause house fires; proper installation and maintenance of smoke alarms help to prevent deaths and injuries (Istre, McCoy, Carlin, & McClain, 2002. Cigarette lighters and matches are fascinating to young children. Toddlers or preschoolers may be able to start a flame, injuring or killing themselves or others. The sound of a smoke alarm may frighten young children, and it is important for community health nurses to instruct parents not only to teach their young children about fire prevention, but also to be aware of the sound of the alarm and know what actions to take when they hear it (Schnitzer, 2006).

Preventing the sources of injury or death from burns may be accomplished by eliminating opportunity and source. Through child supervision, safe storage of matches and lighters, and keeping children away from stoves and electrical outlets, burns can be prevented. Adults can protect children from burns by keeping pot handles turned toward the center of the stove, by not using stove burners or ovens to heat their homes, by reducing the temperature setting on water heaters, by always testing bath water with an elbow before placing a child in the bath, and by keeping electrical outlets covered with inexpensive plastic inserts. Many local fire departments and public health programs offer safety education in this area. Such programs emphasize the use of heat- and smoke-detecting systems; fire drills; home evacuation plans; use of less flammable structural materials, furnishings, and clothing; and not permitting smoking inside the house. Child-resistant cigarette lighters, which have been mandated by the U.S. Consumer Product Safety Commission, have resulted in a 58% decline in the number of fires caused by children playing with lighters and a 31% reduction in deaths (Safe Kids Worldwide, 2007; Smith, Greene, & Singh,

2002). Flame-resistant sleepwear for children and anti-scald plumbing for new construction have also been developed.

The rates of drowning are highest for children between the ages of 1 and 3. One-fourth of all injury-related deaths of toddlers are due to drowning (Schnitzer, 2006). Brief lapses in supervision can have disastrous consequences. Young children are at risk for drowning wherever water occurs in depths exceeding a few inches—such as in toilet bowls, bathtubs, mop buckets or cans filled with rainwater, puddles, ponds, spas, and swimming pools. Lakes, rivers, streams, and irrigation ditches or canals are other water hazards. Infants, toddlers, and preschool-aged children are especially vulnerable because they are not aware of water dangers and they explore without fear. Parents need to provide a drown-free environment. Guidelines include the following:

◆ Bathe young children in shallow water
◆ Never leave young children unattended during a bath
◆ Keep toilet lids down and bathroom doors closed—preferably secured with childproof safety handles
◆ Never leave full mop buckets unattended
◆ Eliminate water-collection sites around the home by turning over or removing empty buckets, containers, flower pots, and other items that can collect rainwater
◆ Fence swimming pool areas and install childproof locks or alarm devices that sound when the water is disturbed
◆ Promote water safety measures, including teaching young children to swim
◆ Vigilantly observe young children at play to protect them from wandering off toward neighborhood water sources

The AAP recommends that while supervising children in or around bathtubs, spas, or pools, adults remain within an arm's length and not be distracted by other activities (Brenner, 2003). The real dangers of accidental drowning are related in From the Case Files I.

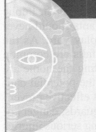

From the Case Files I

Mop Bucket Drowning

I am a Head Start nurse, and one of my assigned centers is located within a farm labor camp. There are many large, hardworking families in the camp. Older siblings often watch over young children and help with household chores. Most families keep their cinderblock homes tidy and clean, and floors are constantly being mopped (no one has carpeting—it is a bare-minimum type of accommodation). One day, several children were absent from school, and when I made home visits to determine the cause of the absences, I discovered that one of the Garcia family's children, a toddler named Miguel, had unexpectedly died. Because many of the absent children were cousins, parents had kept them home while attending to the family. I knew the Garcia family well, and when I stopped by to check on them they told me that Miguel had fallen into a large mop bucket the older sister had been using to clean the kitchen floor. She had gone outside for just a minute to separate the 5-year-old twins who were fighting, and when she returned she found Miguel head first in the bucket. She tried to revive him, but could not. The parents were working, trying to earn extra money for an elderly grandmother who needed surgery, and only learned of the tragedy when they returned home at the end of a long day. It was a very sad situation, and it reminded me of how even an everyday item can become deadly. Safety and prevention of unintentional injuries, especially with curious toddlers and preschoolers, is extremely important to teach all families.

Myra, Head Start Nurse

Injuries and deaths from motor vehicle crashes continue to be a major safety problem in the United States. Approximately one third of injury-related deaths of toddlers and 58% of those for school-age children are a result of motor vehicle crashes (Schnitzer, 2006). Some families do not use infant safety seats or child booster seats consistently, even though these devices have been required by law for decades. Other families have them and use them regularly, but do not install them properly, placing the child at as much risk as if there were no restraint. A study found that of almost 3,500 child-restraint systems inspected, 72% were not placed or used correctly and could increase the risk of child injury if a crash occurred (National Highway Traffic Safety Administration, 2006). Children under age 12 are generally safer in the back seat (CDC, 2007b). There is much opportunity in this area for the community health nurse to educate the public and ensure that parents have the information and skills to secure their children properly when traveling by car. Safety seat clinics, where installations are checked and corrected, can help to promote the correct use of age-appropriate child restraints. See Evidence-Based Practice: Getting Families to Use Child Booster Seats for an example of effective interventions.

EVIDENCE-BASED PRACTICE

Getting Families to Use Child Booster Seats (Carrot or Stick?)

Many health departments, law enforcement, and social service agencies educate parents about the laws and benefits related to the use of child safety seats. Still, not every family consistently uses them. What is the best method to use to ensure compliance with laws? Should we offer incentives (carrots), or should we rely on tickets and fines (sticks)?

Researchers conducted a systematic review of research involving the "acquisition and use of booster seats," those child safety seats that should be used for children up to 80 pounds and 58 inches. They found five quality studies with a total of 3,070 participants, and concluded that interventions which included incentives—like gift certificates or discount coupons for booster seats—or gifts of booster seats, along with education about their proper use, were the most effective. They only found one study that looked at enforcement of laws related to use of booster seats, and it was without significant findings. Therefore, researchers concluded that public health professionals could be more effective in their use of carrots rather than sticks when promoting the use of booster seats or, possibly, other child safety seats or restraints.

Reference:

Ehiri, J., Ejere, H., Magnussen, L., Emusu, D., King, W., & Osberg, W. (2006). Interventions for promoting booster seat use in four to eight year olds traveling in motor vehicles. *Cochrane Database of Systematic Reviews*, Issue 1, Art. No.: CD004334. Retrieved August 13, 2008 from http://www.cochrane.org/reviews/en/ab004334.html.

Poisoning is a constant safety concern for young children, and toddlers are most often at risk. Poisoning is one of the leading causes of injury-related hospitalization in this age group (Schnitzer, 2006). Sources of poisoning include household plants, prescription medications, over-the-counter drugs, unintentional medication overdoses, household cleaning products, other chemicals stored within a child's reach, and lead. "Mr. Yuk," a sticker displaying a scowling green face with a protruding tongue, has not proved effective in preventing toddler poisonings, and the Poison Prevention Packaging Act of 1970 has also failed to reduce poisoning cases significantly (Schnitzer, 2007). However, PHNs can provide parents with the number for the Poison Help Hotline (1-800-222-1222) and encourage them to post it next to each telephone and call immediately in the event of a suspected poisoning or overdose (American Association of Poison Control Centers [AAPCC], 2008a).

Childproofing the home to eliminate major sources of poisoning is the best way to keep children safe. This includes keeping plants out of a child's reach or eliminating them from the home until the child is older, locking up household chemicals (e.g., toilet bowl cleaner, bleach, mouthwash, oven and drain cleaners, pesticides, gasoline, paint thinner, hair products) and storing them out of a child's sight and reach, using childproof medication containers, and storing all medicines in a locked box with a key that is kept out of reach (AAPCC, 2008b). Alcoholic beverages should also be kept out of reach, as should tobacco products. Outside hazards, such as wild mushrooms and poisonous plants, flowers, and berries, must also be considered (AAPCC, 2008b). It is also important to eliminate sources of lead in and around the home.

Lead is a major cause of childhood poisoning. There is no safe level of lead, and the elimination of elevated blood lead levels in children is a *Healthy People 2010* objective. During the three decades between 1970 and 1999, new state and federal regulations to control lead exposure were enacted and enforced, and resulted in the reduction of blood lead levels. The primary sources of lead exposure in preschool-aged children continue to be lead-based paint and lead-contaminated soil and house dust. The critical age of exposure (or peak level) is thought to be between 18 and 36 months. Levels generally begin to decline after age 3. High blood levels of lead in children between 6 and 24 months of age are correlated with lower IQ levels at older ages (CDC, 2005a). Children who live in poverty and play in substandard housing areas remain at risk for direct exposure to significant sources of lead. For example, in Louisville, Kentucky, 35% of all children with high blood lead levels were found to reside in just 79 housing units—representing less than 1% of units in that community (CDC, 2005a). Lead safety and housing code enforcement, along with periodic monitoring to detect new lead hazards, can help prevent future lead exposures. Community health nurses, working together with environmental health sanitarians, should promote opportunities for blood lead screening, especially if it is suspected that children in certain homes, apartments, or neighborhoods are at risk for lead poisoning. Children have also been exposed to lead in some toys, candies, cosmetics, traditional medicines, and eating or drinking utensils imported from other countries. Many of these have been tested and revealed to have high levels of lead. Thirty five percent of children with elevated blood lead levels were found to have this type of exposure (CDC, 2005a).

Education and public awareness campaigns can help prevent this type of lead poisoning.

Among infants aged 1 year or younger, American Indian/Alaska Natives and Blacks have had higher total injury death rates over the past few years than other racial and ethnic populations—two times the rate of injury death compared with White infants. Black infants were affected by the highest rate of homicide (Bernard, Paulozzi, & Wallace, 2007). The percentage of children under 1 year of age who have died violent deaths is 1.6%, almost twice the percentage for children below the age of 15 (Karch, Lubell, Friday, Patel, & Williams, 2008). Almost 20% of child maltreatment deaths occur to infants under age 1 (CDC, 2008c).

Child Maltreatment

Child abuse and neglect are major concerns for the United States. Abuse and neglect comprise the third leading cause of death for young children under the age of 3 and the fifth leading cause of death for those between the ages of 1 and 9. Almost 20% of child maltreatment deaths occur to infants under age 1 (CDC, 2008c). **Child abuse** is the maltreatment of children, which may include any or all of the following: physical abuse, emotional abuse, neglect (physical, medical, or educational), and sexual abuse (including sexual exploitation and child pornography) (Goldman, Salus, Wolcott & Kennedy, 2003). In 2006, an estimated 91,000 infants were abused or neglected before age 1, almost 40% of them within the first month of life. About 30,000 were maltreated during their first week of life. Of these, 13% were physically abused and 68.5% were neglected (CDC, 2008c). Exposure of infants to drugs in utero is a form of neglect (ScoutNews, 2008). In recent years, there has been an increase in reported cases of physical and sexual abuse in day care centers, nursery schools, children's organizations, and churches. However, only about 10% of abuse cases involve nonparental perpetrators, such as foster care staff or day care personnel—80% of child abuse perpetrators are parents (USDHHS, 2008).

A large, national prospective cohort study following at-risk children from birth to age 8 recently determined that children who are victims of neglect in the first 2 years of life are more likely to have symptoms of childhood aggression than those who were physically abused or neglected later in life (Kotch et al., 2008). It is believed that many more children also suffer from forms of abuse and neglect, but thousands of cases are not reported and not reflected in the statistics. The problem is often difficult to detect and is underreported (ScoutNews, 2008). One example of an often-overlooked form of abuse is shaken baby syndrome. **Shaken baby syndrome**, suspected in infants or toddlers who exhibit traumatic brain injuries caused by violent shaking or impact, is characterized by a triad of symptoms: retinal hemorrhage, subdural hemorrhage, and/or subdural hemorrhage with few signs of external trauma (Gutierrez, Clements, & Averill, 2004; Altimer, 2008). The soft brain tissues are injured as they move violently against the rough cranial bones as the infant is shaken or thrown against a hard object. Failure to thrive (FTT), or "inadequate physical growth diagnosed by observation of growth over time using a standard growth chart," is a condition that derives from a variety of causes, such as poor sucking and appetite, poor feeding techniques, organic diseases, and mother-infant attachment problems. However, it

can also be related to neglect (Krugman & Dubowitz, 2003, p. 879). Risk factors that point to child neglect as the basis for FTT include those most often cited for abuse and neglect, along with specific concerns about parents intentionally withholding food, being resistant to recommended interventions, and having rigid beliefs about nutrition and health regimens that may jeopardize the infant (Block et al., 2005). Growth problems in the first 2 months of life may result in IQ deficits in later childhood, and early intervention programs that involve home visitation have been effective in attenuating the long-term effects of FTT (Black, Dubowitz, Krishnakumar, & Starr, 2007; Emond, Blair, Emmett, & Drewett, 2007).

Child abuse is seldom the result of any single factor, but rather a combination of chaotic environments, stressful situations, and parents who have difficulty coping with problems and stress. Risk factors for child maltreatment are found in four areas:

- Parent or caregiver behaviors
- Family characteristics
- Child factors
- Environment

Parental factors may include personality characteristics that include an external locus of control and poor self-esteem, along with problems with impulse control and anti-social behavior. Depression and anxiety may also play a role, and about one third of parents who had a childhood history of abuse or neglect will go on to maltreat their children (Goldman, Salus, Wolcott, & Kennedy, 2003). Substance abuse is a factor in roughly one-third to two-thirds of child abuse and neglect cases. Alcohol and drug abuse often lead to neglect, as parents use money meant for household expenses on substances. Little knowledge of normal child development can result in unrealistic expectations. Holding negative attitudes toward their children, viewing them as property, exhibiting harsh parenting styles and verbal aggression, not knowing how to handle children's behaviors, and being easily frustrated are parental characteristics that have also been associated with risk of child maltreatment. Young parental age is also a factor, although this may be because it is also associated with poverty, lower levels of social support, and higher levels of stress (Goldman et al., 2003).

Family characteristics that include domestic violence and marital conflict, financial stress and unemployment, and social isolation may lead to increased risk of child maltreatment. Children living with single parents (most often mothers) are at higher risk of physical and sexual abuse, as well as neglect; they are also more likely to live in poverty. Single parents have the sole caretaker burden and experience more stress than parents who have joint responsibilities. Children from single parent homes are 77% more likely than those living with both parents to experience physical abuse, and are 80% more at risk of a resultant injury. Families in which child neglect occurs often are characterized by greater numbers of children or report a larger number of people living in the household. The household is frequently more chaotic, with constantly changing players—e.g., mothers and children living on and off with grandmothers, aunts, boyfriends, or others (Goldman et al., 2003). Families at high risk for child abuse may be those that are either chronically troubled or temporarily stressed.

Slightly more girls than boys were reported to be victims of maltreatment in 2006 (51.5% versus 48.2%), and rates were highest for the youngest children (24.4 per 1,000 for birth to age 1; 14.2 for ages 1 to 3; 13.5 for ages 4 to 7). Almost 75% of children from birth to age 3 were neglected, and American Indian/Alaska Native and Black children had the highest rates of maltreatment (15.9/15.4 and 19.8, respectively) when compared to White and Hispanic children (10.7 and 10.8 per 1,000) (USDHHS, 2008). Children who are premature or LBW may be at greater risk of maltreatment because of the greater maternal stress engendered by more demands on the caregiver. Significant relationships between child maltreatment and LBW, unintended pregnancy, and developmental problems or poor health in infancy have been found (Sidebotham & Heron, 2003). Children with difficult temperaments or behavior problems, or whose parents perceive them to have problems, could be at greater risk of abuse or neglect, but some research has noted that these child characteristics are probably less significant than negative parental attitudes (Sidebotham & Heron, 2003). Disabled children have higher rates of maltreatment than those without disabilities, and may be at risk for repeated abuse or neglect. If bonding or attachment has been disrupted by infant hospitalizations or parental incarcerations, for instance, the child may be at risk of maltreatment (Goldman et al., 2003).

The environment can play a part, along with parental, family, and child factors, in determining risk for child abuse and neglect. Parents who maltreat their children have reported more loneliness, greater isolation, and lower levels of social support. Social isolation may indicate a lack of positive role models to help them better understand parenting and the consequences of child maltreatment. Unemployment, poverty, and neighborhood factors such as crime, violence, and substance use play a part in the stress placed on families. Strong, significant relationships have been found between unemployment, poverty, and child maltreatment, especially child neglect. Certainly, this is not true in all cases—not every poor and/or unemployed parent abuses or neglects his children—however, these stressors can interact with others (e.g., substance abuse, depression) to amplify the likelihood of abuse. Theories of how poverty may contribute to higher levels of child abuse and neglect include higher levels or perceptions of stress, inability to provide basic needs, and disproportionate reporting of child abuse because of more frequent contact with those who are mandated reporters (Goldman et al., 2003). Although poverty and lack of education are often linked with child abuse and neglect, no socioeconomic level is immune. Parent training programs can help teach parents to cope with fussy infants and difficult toddlers, and child sexual abuse prevention programs may also be helpful. However, PHN home visitation programs, like the Nurse Family Partnership, have been researched and found to be "the most effective and longest enduring intervention for high-risk families" (Krugman, Lane, & Walsh, 2007, p. 711). See Display 21.2. See also Chapters 20 and 22 for more on child abuse and neglect.

DISPLAY 21.2 REPORTS OF AN EMERGENCY FOSTER HOME

The following are examples of the various situations from which abused and neglected children come, as reported by a couple who had an emergency foster home for the county department of social services. The examples represent children placed with them over a 2-year period in which they cared for 256 children.

- Two-week-old Jose was taken to their home because the parents (under the influence of drugs) were found swinging Jose upside down in circles in an infant carrier as they walked along a downtown street at 3 a.m. After being returned to his parents, he returned to foster care 1 month later after being found abandoned in an infant carrier at the county fair.
- Andre, Otis, and Selma, ages 8, 5, and 4, went to the foster home when the social services agency discovered they had been living with their father in an abandoned car for 2 years. They stayed for 3 weeks while the social worker found suitable housing for this family and counseling for the father.
- Victoria, 5 years old, a loving and passive child, arrived wearing a diaper and appeared developmentally delayed. She had a history of being physically and sexually abused. Her family was very dysfunctional, and it took the social worker several weeks to sort out relatives and their intentions before placing Victoria in a long-term foster home.
- Ronald and Randall, 6-year-old twin boys who were forced to "sexually please their mother" for several years, came to the emergency foster home before being placed with relatives while their mother underwent psychiatric treatment. The boys began counseling during their stay in the emergency foster home.
- Antoinette, age 7, had severe asthma and was very withdrawn. She came to the emergency foster home because her mother (and the mother's boyfriend) refused to care for her. The child came with every photograph of herself and personal mementos because the mother wanted no reminders of the child. The social worker located a grandmother who would be the child's guardian.
- Thirteen-year-old Robert came home from school one day and found his mother and all their furniture gone. After a few weeks of Robert living in the basement of the apartment building, someone alerted the social services agency and he was placed in the emergency foster home for 2 months. His mother finally called social services after 6 weeks, saying Robert was too difficult for her to handle, but she may want to see him again someday. Robert was eventually placed in a group home for boys.
- Quyn, a 17-year-old Laotian girl, came into foster care after being referred by the school nurse because of wounds observed on her wrists and ankles. Quyn reported being strapped to a chair for 12 or more hours at a time by her father because she was not following the old ways and was shaming the family by being seen in public, unchaperoned, with a boy. Several meetings were held between the parents, a Southeast Asian community leader, and the social worker to resolve this situation so that Quyn could go home safely.

Communicable Diseases

Infants, toddlers, and preschool-aged children experience a high frequency of acute illnesses, more than any other age group. Common types of acute conditions seen from birth to age 5 include fever, respiratory infections (including ear infections, colds, influenza), conjunctivitis (pink eye), and gastrointestinal problems (Kwok, Vazquez, & Isaacman, 2006). Communicable diseases are prevalent in these age groups, as very young children are building an immune system and are just beginning to come in contact with a greater number of people outside their families. In 2008, Yorita, Holman, Sejvar, Steiner, and Schonberger found that almost 43% of infant hospitalizations were due to infectious diseases; about 1 in every 14 infants were hospitalized. Males and non-White infants were most at risk, and the annual cost of hospitalization of U.S. infants was almost $700 million. The most common diagnoses were infections of the lower respiratory tract (59%) and upper respiratory tract (6.5%), septicemia (6.5%), and urinary tract, kidney, and bladder infections (76%). The incidence of pneumonia in North America is about 35 to 40 cases per 1,000 children under age 5, but most are handled with outpatient care and medication (Durbin & Stille, 2008).

Acute respiratory illnesses (ARIs) are common in children under age 5. In a community-based prospective cohort study tracking children from birth through age 5, researchers found that before age 2, an average of four ARIs occurred each year. Between ages 2 and 5, the number of ARIs dropped to two or three episodes yearly. Most of the infections were upper respiratory, but about half of the children had at least one lower respiratory infection during their first year of life. They also noted that symptoms generally lasted for 4 weeks and resolved with or without the use of cough and cold medications and antibiotics (Kusel, de Klerk, Holt, Landau, & Sly, 2007). This information is especially helpful for community health nurses who need to emphasize that over-the-counter cough and cold medications should not be used for children under age 2. The U.S. Food and Drug Administration (FDA) deemed them unsafe and ineffective and most manufacturers took them off the market in fall of 2007 in response to emergency room visits and deaths linked to their toxic effects. However, parents may be uninformed about this, and may use old bottles or try to give smaller doses of adult medications to their infants and toddlers. Public health nurses should inform parents of the dangers and suggest safer interventions that may help alleviate symptoms, such as use of a bulb syringe and saline nose drops, a cool-mist humidifier, or petroleum jelly under the nose (Dowshen, 2008).

Bronchiolitis is the most common type of lower respiratory infection among infants. It is the leading cause of hospitalization in this age group. The majority of hospitalizations for bronchiolitis are for infants 6 months and younger. Respiratory syncytial virus (RSV) is the cause in 70% of cases, and can rise to 100% during winter epidemics. Although wheezing, tachypnea, and chest retractions can be frightening to parents, most healthy infants survive (95%). However, PHNs working with at-risk infants need to work with parents and pediatricians to ensure that palivizumab (monoclonal antibody) or RSV immunoglobulin are given to preterm infants, or those born closer to term but exposed to environmental pollution or to other children (Worrall, 2008). An effective RSV vaccine has not yet been found.

As with older children and adults, air pollution may make infants and children under age 5 more susceptible to bronchitis and other respiratory illnesses. Preschool-age children are thought to be especially "vulnerable to air pollution-induced illnesses" (Hertz-Picciotto, Baker, Yap, et al., 2007, p. 1510). Public health nurses can inform families who live in areas where air pollution is significant to take the necessary precautions.

Vaccines are one of the greatest achievements of public health. Since 1980, there has been a 99% or greater decrease in deaths due to the vaccine-preventable diseases of mumps, pertussis, tetanus, and diphtheria, and 80% or greater decline in deaths associated with vaccines instituted since 1980: hepatitis A and B, *Haemophilus influenzae* type B (HiB), and varicella (Roush, Murphy, & the Vaccine-Preventable Disease Table Working Group, 2007). Smallpox has been eradicated worldwide, and the viruses for polio, rubella, and measles are no longer endemic in the United States. The decline in the number of cases of measles, mumps, rubella, pertussis, and tetanus has been dramatic (99.9%, 95.9%, 99.9%, 92.2%, and 92.9%, respectively), and cases of varicella have declined 88%. Intensive campaigns have promoted immunizations that stimulate "protective immune responses against acute and chronic infectious diseases, as well as some infectious diseases that result in cancer" (Roush et al., 2007, p. 2155). Their immature immune systems and lack of exposure to antigens, along with somewhat porous physical barriers to microbes, put infants at high risk of infection. By 4 to 6 months, however, a brisker antibody response to vaccines becomes possible (Nadel, 2008). Successful infant and childhood immunization programs have been responsible for high vaccine coverage and the subsequent decline in morbidity and mortality from these preventable diseases (Roush et al., 2007).

The CDC's Advisory Committee on Immunization Practices develop policies and guidelines, based on review of current scientific research, recommending "specific licensed vaccines for infants, children, adolescents, and adults" (Roush et al., 2007, p. 2156). The committee provides suggestions for available immunizations for the 17 vaccine-preventable diseases through the Vaccines for Children Program, a federal program providing uninsured and low-income families vaccines at no charge through their primary care providers and local health department clinics. The National Immunization Survey provides surveillance for this program, and the *Healthy People 2010* goal regarding immunization administration was met and exceeded in 2004 when more than 80% of children received all recommended vaccines (CDC, 2008e). State level immunization registries help track vaccine coverage at all age levels. Because day care centers and schools require proof of immunization, vaccination rates have improved over the last two decades (Roush et al., 2007).

The financing of immunizations for infants and children has significantly improved as a result of two major initiatives. The Vaccines for Children Program and the Child Health Insurance Program (CHIP) cover children on Medicaid, uninsured children, and American Indian/Alaska Native children. In addition, underinsured children who receive immunizations at federally qualified health centers and rural health clinics are covered. Additional state programs and funds help provide free or low-cost vaccines for children who are not covered by the other programs. There are several ways for community health nurses to help all families obtain free or low-cost immunizations.

Even if financial barriers are removed, there are other barriers. Transportation is a significant problem for some parents, especially in rural areas and for families in urban areas who have several children and need to take public transportation. All 50 states provide for medical exceptions to mandatory vaccination, and 49 allow religious exemptions; 20 permit philosophical or personal exemptions (Steele, 2005). Despite public health announcements in the media, some mothers remain unaware of the disabling consequences of diseases such as polio and do not realize the importance of fully vaccinating their children. In a survey of parents, 25% of them believed that receiving too many vaccines would weaken their child's immune system (Offit & Jew, 2003). Also, as more vaccines become available and the deadly diseases they prevent become a distant memory in the public's mind, more concerns about the safety of vaccines emerge. Numerous websites have emerged that advise against childhood immunizations and provide graphic horror stories about the handful of severe reactions to vaccination. Media coverage about vaccine adverse events also contributes to decreased compliance on the part of parents in getting their children immunized (Steele, 2005). Specifically, antivaccine individuals and groups have been very vocal and have appeared on television programs such as *Oprah* and *Larry King Live* to "make strong emotional appeals" against vaccinating children (Parikh, 2008, p. 622). They have linked childhood immunizations to their children's autism, even though extensive scientific research has failed to find any significant association. Parikh (2008) notes that, logical or not, people "do not forget this kind of emotional prowess," and notes that scientific and medical experts only counter these emotion-laden arguments with dry evidence and statistics that "do not resonate with many parents" (p. 622). Public health nurses and other health professionals are encouraged to provide parents of very young children with meaningful stories of preventable deaths due to these diseases, and to "defend our beliefs . . . more strongly" rather than relying solely on dispassionate facts and figures (Parikh, 2008, p. 622).

Chronic Diseases

Infants and young children can be afflicted with chronic diseases that affect their quality of life. For instance, the most common chronic disease in early childhood is *dental caries*, which is five times more common than asthma (Douglass, Douglass, & Silk, 2004). Some children begin to show signs and symptoms of cavities by the age of 10 months, and decay can begin to develop as soon as teeth erupt. Enamel defects, and subsequent caries, are more prevalent in children living in poverty and in preterm or LBW infants (Douglass et al., 2004).

Asthma symptoms may begin in infants and toddlers. Asthma is considered by some to be the most common chronic disease of childhood, with 13% of children younger than age 18 years diagnosed with asthma in 2003 (Forum on Child and Family Statistics [FCFS], 2005). Inner city, low-income, and minority children are disproportionately affected, and asthma hospitalizations are common (Jacobson et al., 2008). Public health nurses can assist families in finding appropriate health care providers and encourage proper administration of asthma medications and treatments. They can also teach families to reduce the presence of asthma triggers in their homes (see Chapter 22 for more information on asthma and other chronic diseases of childhood and adolescence).

Autism is a developmental spectrum disorder that is often first noticed in toddlers. Parents become aware that the child's communication and interaction with others is different, and that the child may also display obsessive and narrow interests. The CDC estimates the prevalence of autism at 1 in 150 children, and boys are four times more likely than girls to develop autism (2007). What causes autism is unclear, but some theories suggest faulty early neural patterning and overgrowth as a possible explanation (Courchesne et al., 2007). Families may need to be referred to early educational intervention programs and social services agencies for assistance.

Sickle cell anemia, an inherited blood disorder, affects thousands of children in the United States, most often those of African or Hispanic Caribbean ancestry. The characteristic chronic and severe anemia is common in young children with this condition, and it can affect memory, learning, and behavior (Schatz & Roberts, 2007). When both parents have the genetic mutation, the newborn will be afflicted with the disease. Those with the sickle cell trait have no symptoms of the disease, but can pass it on to their offspring. In many states, routine newborn screening for sickle cell anemia is offered. Because sickle cell anemia can lead to splenic sequestration (or pooling of blood in the spleen), many children have either nonfunctioning spleens or have had them surgically removed. Risk of infection is always a concern when this occurs before age 5 (University of Maryland Medical Center, 2007). Public health nurses working with populations at risk for this disease can educate and refer families for diagnosis and treatment.

The incidence of *food allergies* is increasing in the population. Infants with close family members who have atopic diseases are at risk for development of allergies. Prolonged breast-feeding for 1 year is recommended for these infants, or the use of hypoallergenic infant formula, and delayed introduction of solid foods is also important: i.e., dairy foods after age 1, eggs after age 2, nuts and fish after age 3 (Kleinman, 2000). Fortunately, once allergies are diagnosed, they can be managed through dietary changes and by avoidance of allergy-producing foods. Parents need to be educated, so that they can consistently read food labels and alert family members to the young child's allergy so that inappropriate foods are avoided.

Other chronic illnesses can have a profound effect on child and family. *Muscular dystrophy* (MD) and *cystic fibrosis* (CF) are two diseases that not only affect quality of life, but also severely shorten the child's life. Muscular dystrophy is a constellation of 30 genetic diseases characterized by progressive atrophy and weakening of skeletal muscles. The onset of some forms of MD begins in infancy or early childhood, and MD is more common in boys than in girls. *Duchenne MD* usually begins between ages 3 and 5, and progresses rapidly until most boys are wheelchair bound and require a ventilator (Emory University, 2007). Genetic testing can determine who is a carrier of the gene, and can aid in confirming the clinical diagnosis.

Cystic fibrosis usually begins in infancy and is characterized by a persistent cough or wheeze, shortness of breath, poor weight gain despite a good appetite, and a salty taste to the skin. Greasy and bulky stools are also common, as are respiratory infections that become increasingly more frequent with age (American Lung Association, 2006). It is the major cause of severe chronic lung disease in children. Cystic fibrosis occurs in 1 in 3,200 White and 1 in 11,500 Hispanic live births. About 80% of new cases are diagnosed before age 3, often by the "sweat test." Routine newborn screening is recommended (Grosse, Boyle, Botkin, et al., 2004).

Chest physiotherapy to help mobilize secretions is performed daily, usually by the parents. Aerosolized antibiotic treatments and mucus-thinning medications help to improve lung function and reduce respiratory infections. Community health nurses reinforce these techniques and teach the family to avoid exposure to respiratory infections and to initiate prescribed antibiotic prophylaxis promptly. As much as feasible, the young child should be involved in his own care, offered valid choices, and encouraged to participate in decision making. The family needs emotional support as members work through feelings of anticipatory grief.

Antecedents for a number of chronic diseases that develop in adolescence and adulthood may be found in infancy and early childhood. Some evidence of the influence of fetal or infant birth weight, weight gain, and nutrition in later development of specific chronic diseases has been studied (Kleinman, 2000). For instance, a protein in cow's milk formula has been linked to greater risk of later type 1 diabetes, and a longitudinal Canadian study is underway to determine if delaying the introduction of cow's milk formulas may prevent or delay the development of diabetes in at-risk children (American Chemical Society, 2008; Canadian Diabetes Association, 2003; Kleinman, 2000). A systematic review of the literature found that infants who experience rapid growth or who have higher BMIs are at greater risk for later obesity (Baird, Fisher, Lucas, et al., 2005). Some evidence also demonstrates a relationship between adult hypertension and LBW with rapid weight gain between the ages of 1 and 5, with "part of the risk of adult hypertension . . . set in fetal life" (Law et al., 2002, p. 1088). More epidemiologists are beginning to recognize the importance of a life course approach to chronic disease and the societal costs of disadvantaged fetal and child health and development (Ben-Shlomo & Kuh, 2002; Guyer et al., 2008). Among other variables, diet and nutrition play an important role in later health.

Poor Nutrition and Dental Hygiene

Other health problems found in the birth to preschool age group include nutritional problems (underfeeding or overfeeding, overeating, and inappropriate food choices) and poor dental health. Nutritional and dental health needs are great during this period of rapid growth. Many factors contribute to early nutritional and dental problems.

A healthy start is foundational to well-being later in life. Nutrition is basic in strengthening this foundation. Bonding between mother and infant and overall maternal health are predictors of infant weight gain. Both nutrition and bonding can be accomplished by breast-feeding. Some of the benefits of breast-feeding include (Goldman, Hopkinson, & Rassin, 2007; Office of Women's Health, 2005; Wiggins, 2001):

Convenience: Milk is always at the perfect temperature, and no preparation is needed; the infant can instantly begin feeding when hungry.
Cost: No formula or bottles to buy; costs are limited to healthy diet for the mother, breast pads, nursing bras, and (possibly) a breast pump.
Nutrition: Breast milk is species specific; the proteins are easily digested, and fats are well absorbed; it is the most complete form of nutrition for human infants.

Anti-infective and anti-allergic properties: Breast milk contains immunoglobulins, enzymes, and leukocytes that protect against pathogens, and it decreases the incidence of allergy by eliminating exposure to potential antigens; babies exclusively breast-fed for 6 or more months have fewer respiratory illnesses, ear infections, and cases of diarrhea.
Infant growth: Breast-fed babies usually gain weight at a more moderate rate and are leaner than bottle fed babies; rapid weight gain in infancy has been associated with later chronic diseases.
Long-term health effects: Breast-feeding exclusively for at least 6 months is associated with reduced risk of overweight in later life, and breast-fed infants have slightly higher IQ scores.
Benefits for mothers: Breast-feeding burns extra calories, helps to reduce postpartum bleeding, and delays ovulation and menstruation; it also lowers the risk of later ovarian and breast cancers.

The benefits of breast-feeding for the infant are well-established and include protection against respiratory infections and diarrhea, long-term increased cognitive development through adolescence, and some improvement in blood pressure and total cholesterol (Klein et al., 2008; Martin, Gunnell, & Davey-Smith, 2005; Office of Women's Health, 2005; Turck, 2007). Higher levels of docosahexaenoic acid, important to brain development, are found in breast milk, and its benefits are correlated with the duration of breast-feeding (Turck, 2007). Several systematic reviews have found that the longer a mother breast-feeds her infant, the greater the protection against later obesity. This is thought to be due to the "growth acceleration hypothesis" that associates faster growth in infancy with later obesity levels and the fact that breast milk permits slower growth when compared to infant formulas (Singhal, 2007, p. 15).

Public health nurses can encourage pregnant women to consider the benefits of breast-feeding their infants carefully, and provide education and interventions to assist them with the most common barriers: concern about insufficient supply of breast milk, problems with the baby latching onto the breast, painful nipples, and scheduling problems (Lewallen, et al., 2006; McCann, Baydar, & Williams, 2007). Women often choose to breast-feed their babies when they fully understand the health effects for their infants and themselves and when they receive positive influence from family and friends (Brodribb, Fallon, Hegney, & O'Brien, 2007). The community health nurse can join with labor and delivery nurses and lactation consultants in promoting breast-feeding among mothers in the community. Nurses can lobby local hospitals to educate new mothers about the benefits of breast-feeding and stop the routine distribution of free samples of infant formula (Kaplan & Graff, 2008). It is important to establish breast-feeding early, as 70% of women in a nationwide study made the same feeding choice (bottle or breast) for subsequent infants (Taylor, Geller, Risica, Kirtania, & Cabral, 2008).

Overfeeding of an infant can lead to childhood obesity and becomes a risk factor for heart disease, hypertension, and diabetes. Eleven percent of school-age children are overweight, with the foundation begun in the preschool years (Hodges, 2003). The propensity for obesity begins as early as infancy and by childhood for most people. Obesity is a contributing factor to the worldwide increase in type 2 diabetes and has been reported to result in lower health-related quality of life (Kimm & Obarzanek, 2002; Schwimmer, Burwinkle, & Varni, 2003).

Although overfeeding can lead to problems, poor infant growth is also problematic. Small body size at age 1 and poor rates of growth through infancy are predictive of later coronary heart disease. The risk was threefold for those weighing less than 8 kg at age 1 (Forsen, Eriksson, Osmond, & Barker, 2004). The pattern of growth may also be important, as growth problems in infancy along with overweight in later childhood has been associated with adult development of hypertension and elevated serum lipid and glucose levels (Stein, Thompson, & Waters, 2005).

The most common sources of energy and nutrients for infants and toddlers are breast milk, formula, and milk. For toddlers, juices and fruit-flavored juice drinks are the next two sources of nutrition. Fortified foods (e.g., grain-based foods with added vitamin A, folate, and iron) become increasingly more significant in diets of toddlers, as do supplements (multivitamins). Dieticians recommend feeding older infants and toddlers a "wide variety of fruits, vegetables, and whole grains, as well as food naturally rich in iron" (Fox, Reidy, Novak, & Ziegler, 2006, p. s28). Generally, inadequate intake of vitamins and minerals for infants and toddlers is rare (fewer than 1% to 2%), and the recommendation of dietetic professionals is to allow infants and toddlers to use food, rather than supplements, as the primary source of these nutrients (Briefel, Hanson, Fox, Novak, & Ziegler, 2006). The Continuing Survey of Food Intakes by Individuals and Feeding Infants and Toddlers Study shows that over time, infants and toddlers demonstrate a gradual increase in portion size of most foods which are generally comparable to recommended portions for formula, juice, meats, and cheese and a bit higher than recommended portions for milk, breads, cereal, fruits, and vegetables. Researchers advised against "clean-your-plate" admonitions. They suggested that offering a wide variety of foods—especially whole grains, vegetables, and fruits—and allowing infants and toddlers to eat until they are satiated was the best approach (Fox, Reidy, Karwe, & Ziegler, 2006). A large-scale study comparing Hispanic and non-Hispanic infants and toddlers found that between age 12 and 24 months 80% to 90% of toddlers ate an afternoon snack, and that Hispanic toddlers' snacks were higher in fiber and lower in saturated fats. Researchers discouraged the use of fruit drinks, crackers, and cookies, and encouraged more culturally appropriate whole grains, fruits and vegetables. They also noted that new foods might need to be introduced to toddlers 8 to 10 times before they are accepted and healthy eating habits are established (Ziegler, Hanson, Ponza, Novak & Hendricks, 2006). Public health nurses can encourage parents to continue to introduce new healthy foods to their toddlers and not give up or give in too soon. Home visiting programs that promote fruit and vegetable consumption in preschoolers have been shown to be effective in increasing the number of servings for both children and parents (Haire-Joshu et al., 2008).

Young children's diets, often unreasonably high in sugar, increase the incidence of dental caries in this population group. The combination of sugar, bacteria that cause dental disease, and the composition of the teeth determines the severity of dental caries (Douglass, Douglass, & Silk, 2004). Also, passive exposure to tobacco smoke increases the risk of dental caries, and bacteria responsible for caries can be transmitted from mother to infant (Aligne, Moss, Auinger, & Weitzman, 2003;

Douglass, Douglass, & Silk, 2004). The practice of allowing infants to feed from the bottle beyond 15 to 16 months, or to fall asleep with a bottle, can lead to *baby bottle tooth decay* or *nursing caries*. This causes the decay of the front teeth and, eventually, the molars, requiring extraction of the affected teeth (American Academy of Pediatrics [AAP], 2003). Mothers may persist in giving toddlers and preschoolers bottles filled with milk, juice, or sugared drinks in an effort to buy time by assuaging crying children, who often cease crying when they see the bottle (Freeman & Stevens, 2008). Frequent snacking and sippy cups filled with juice or sugary drinks can also lead to cavities. It is recommended that sugary foods be eaten at mealtimes and not as snacks, and that regular snack times be established. Also, between ages 6 and 12 months, sippy cups are often used to wean infants from the breast or bottle, but between-meal drinks should consist of water or milk. Juice should be given only with meals (American Academy of Pediatrics Committee on Nutrition, 2001; Douglass, Douglass, & Silk, 2004).

Parents of infants older than 6 months who have several erupted teeth should be instructed to rub the infant's gums with a damp, clean cloth and to begin tooth brushing, using a soft pediatric toothbrush with a very small amount of fluoride toothpaste—about the size of a grain of rice. It is best done while the parent stands behind the child, supporting his head, and the area where the teeth and gums meet should be the main focus (Douglass, Douglass, & Silk, 2004). It is also important to address parents' misconceptions about dental health and question them about their cultural beliefs and practices related to dental health and hygiene (Horton & Barker, 2008; Schroth, Brothwell, & Moffatt, 2007).

Fluoride supplementation may be needed by 6 months of age if local water supplies are not fluoridated. Generally, breast-feeding infants do not require supplemental fluoride, and liquid or chewable fluoride supplements should not be given with formula or milk because absorption will be decreased (Douglass, Douglass, & Silk, 2004). As children reach the toddler years, they are able to brush their own teeth with enthusiasm. Toothpaste should be used sparingly, and adults should continue to supervise tooth brushing. Children of this age can get overzealous with the amount of toothpaste they use and it should not be ingested. Some physicians and dentists suggest that parents need to assist children with tooth brushing until age 8 (Douglass, Douglass, & Silk, 2004). The American Academy of Pediatric Dentistry recommends an initial dental visit at 12 months of age. However, the AAP recommends that only children at risk for caries be referred to a dentist at this age (Hale et al., 2003). Children at lower risk are typically referred to a dentist at around age 3 years (Douglass, Douglass, & Silk, 2004).

Dental caries is a preventable condition that can be addressed with proper nutrition and hygiene. Reducing consumption of sugar-sweetened beverages in childhood not only helps to decrease cavities but also reduces the risk of chronic disease later in life. One recent study found an association between higher intake of sugary beverages in childhood and an increased risk of developing metabolic syndrome in adolescence (Snider, 2007). Untreated early dental caries can lead to self-esteem issues and body-image disorders when children live with teeth that are discolored, misshapen, or missing. Beyond that, poor dental health can interfere with the young child's growth and nutrition, as well as cognitive development (Sheiham, 2006). The younger the age when dental caries first appear, the more the child is at risk for future tooth decay that sets up inflammatory responses leading to chronic health conditions, such as heart disease and stroke, in adulthood (Smoots, 2008; Yost & Li, 2008). Significant untreated dental disease is especially harmful in children who are medically fragile (Foster & Fitzgerald, 2005).

Many health departments are using fluoride varnishes as a means of preventing dental caries in young children. Dental hygienists and PHNs may be trained to apply the varnishes while making home visits, or children and families may visit clinics for treatment. Systematic reviews have found that fluoride varnishes can substantially reduce decay in both deciduous and permanent teeth (Marinho, Higgins, Logan, & Sheiham, 2002).

HEALTH SERVICES FOR INFANTS, TODDLERS, AND PRESCHOOLERS

A variety of programs that directly or indirectly serve the health needs of very young children may be found in most communities. Community health nurses play a major and vital role in delivering these services. In community health, programs fall into three categories, which approximate the three priorities of public health nursing practice: prevention, protection, and promotion.

Preventive Health Programs

Neighborhood community centers found in urban and rural settings provide families with parenting education, health and safety education, immunizations, various screening programs, and family planning services. In some areas, nurse-run clinics are established at local schools or community centers to assist in outreach services to the community. Community health nurses, in collaboration with an interdisciplinary team, are often the primary care providers in these programs. The major goals are to keep communities healthy by focusing on primary and secondary prevention services. Three examples of preventive health programs for infants and young children are immunization programs, parent training programs, and quality day care services.

Immunization Programs

Health departments, community clinics, and private health care providers continue to offer immunizations against the major childhood infectious diseases—measles, mumps, rubella, varicella, polio, diphtheria, tetanus, pertussis, Hepatitis A and B, and HiB—some of which can cause permanent disability and even death. Pneumococcal, meningococcal, and influenza vaccines are also recommended, as is the vaccine for rotavirus (CDC, 2008d; Committee on Infectious Diseases, 2008). Many of these diseases no longer plague infants and children, and newer vaccines offer even greater promise of health. Pneumococcal conjugate vaccine has been associated with reductions in the incidence of otitis media and insertion of pressure-equalizing tubes in children under age 5, resulting in reduced expense for antibiotic prescriptions and ambulatory medical visits (Grijalva et al., 2006; Poehling et al., 2007; Zhou, Shefer, Kong, & Nuorti, 2008). See Figures 21.1 and 21.2.

Although the threat of these diseases has been substantially reduced, vigilance is still essential. Low immunization levels in many areas, particularly among the poor and medically underserved, and increased disease rates signal the need for constant surveillance, outreach programs, and innovative educational efforts (Rosenthal et al., 2004; Roush et al., 2007; Stringer, Ratcliffe, & Gross, 2006). A study comparing vaccination coverage among 19- to 35-month-old children found that those children with special health care needs had roughly the same rate of coverage as children in the general population. However, White, affluent children were more likely to be underimmunized, and poor, Hispanic children on Medicaid were more likely to be immunized (O'Connor & Bramlett, 2008). This was one case of disadvantaged populations having an advantage over those with access to private health care and insurance. One large study, examining the rates of underimmunization of 3 month olds in underserved areas of Manhattan, Detroit, San Diego, and rural Colorado, found that vaccination coverage varied between 70.5% and 82.4%. The most commonly cited reasons involved missed opportunities for immunization; other factors involved either no insurance or public insurance, two or more children in the household, and living with an unmarried parent (Bardenheier et al., 2004). Whenever infants and young children come in contact with public health and other community clinics, it is always important to check immunizations and provide the necessary vaccines. Community health nurses are deeply involved in preventive activities that promote immunizations. Health departments and day care centers often work collaboratively to provide vaccinations. However, a study of inner-city, subsidized child care centers found that only 73.3% of 3 month olds were up to date on vaccines, and 12 month olds had even worse compliance at 44.2% (McCaskill et al., 2008). A compulsory immunization law, varying in its application from state to state, has enabled public health personnel to carry out these preventive services.

Parent Training Programs

Parent education and training programs have been useful in providing parents with the tools needed to deal with the stresses and challenges of parenting effectively. A meta-analysis of 77 program evaluations revealed that effective programs consist of teaching parents to use time-out rather than corporal punishment as a means of discipline; promoting consistency in discipline; encouraging emotional communication skills and positive parent–child interaction; and requiring that parents practice these skills during classroom sessions (Kaminski, Valle, Filene, & Boyle, 2008). An effective training program for parents of preschool children is the Incredible Years Parent Training Program. Parent participants report decreased levels of stress and positive changes in their children after participating in this program (Levac, McCay, Merka, & Reddon-D'Arcy, 2008). Some health and social service agencies offer this program for high-risk families of young children, and some evaluation studies have found this program to improve behavior and reduce symptoms of attention-deficit hyperactivity disorder (ADHD) in preschool age children (Jones, Daley, Hutchings, Bywater, & Eames, 2007; 2008).

Quality Day Care and Preschool Programs

Quality child care provides a significant avenue for preventing illness and injury among young children. In 2005, 66% of children younger than age 6 spent time in the care of someone

Catch-up Immunization Schedule

for Persons Aged 4 Months–18 Years Who Start Late or Who Are More Than 1 Month Behind

The table below provides catch-up schedules and minimum intervals between doses for children whose vaccinations have been delayed. A vaccine series does not need to be restarted, regardless of the time that has elapsed between doses. Use the section appropriate for the child's age.

CATCH-UP SCHEDULE FOR PERSONS AGED 4 MONTHS–6 YEARS

Vaccine	Minimum Age for Dose 1	Minimum Interval Between Doses			
		Dose 1 to Dose 2	Dose 2 to Dose 3	Dose 3 to Dose 4	Dose 4 to Dose 5
Hepatitis B[1]	Birth	4 weeks	8 weeks (and 16 weeks after first dose)		
Rotavirus[2]	6 wks	4 weeks	4 weeks		
Diphtheria, Tetanus, Pertussis[3]	6 wks	4 weeks	4 weeks	6 months	6 months[3]
Haemophilus influenzae type b[4]	6 wks	4 weeks if first dose administered at younger than 12 months of age / 8 weeks (as final dose) if first dose administered at age 12-14 months / No further doses needed if first dose administered at 15 months of age or older	4 weeks[4] if current age is younger than 12 months / 8 weeks (as final dose)[4] if current age is 12 months or older and second dose administered at younger than 15 months of age / No further doses needed if previous dose administered at age 15 months or older	8 weeks (as final dose) This dose only necessary for children aged 12 months–5 years who received 3 doses before age 12 months	
Pneumococcal[5]	6 wks	4 weeks if first dose administered at younger than 12 months of age / 8 weeks (as final dose) if first dose administered at age 12 months or older or current age 24–59 months / No further doses needed for healthy children if first dose administered at age 24 months or older	4 weeks if current age is younger than 12 months / 8 weeks (as final dose) if current age is 12 months or older / No further doses needed for healthy children if previous dose administered at age 24 months or older	8 weeks (as final dose) This dose only necessary for children aged 12 months–5 years who received 3 doses before age 12 months	
Inactivated Poliovirus[6]	6 wks	4 weeks	4 weeks	4 weeks[6]	
Measles, Mumps, Rubella[7]	12 mos	4 weeks			
Varicella[8]	12 mos	3 months			
Hepatitis A[9]	12 mos	6 months			

CATCH-UP SCHEDULE FOR PERSONS AGED 7–18 YEARS

Vaccine	Minimum Age for Dose 1	Dose 1 to Dose 2	Dose 2 to Dose 3	Dose 3 to Dose 4	Dose 4 to Dose 5
Tetanus, Diphtheria/ Tetanus, Diphtheria, Pertussis[10]	7 yrs[10]	4 weeks	4 weeks if first dose administered at younger than 12 months of age / 6 months if first dose administered at age 12 months or older	6 months if first dose administered at younger than 12 months of age	
Human Papillomavirus[11]	9 yrs	4 weeks	12 weeks (and 24 weeks after the first dose)		
Hepatitis A[9]	12 mos	6 months			
Hepatitis B[1]	Birth	8 weeks (and 16 weeks after first dose)			
Inactivated Poliovirus[6]	6 wks	4 weeks	4 weeks	4 weeks[6]	
Measles, Mumps, Rubella[7]	12 mos	4 weeks			
Varicella[8]	12 mos	4 weeks if first dose administered at age 13 years or older / 3 months if first dose administered at younger than 13 years of age			

1. Hepatitis B vaccine (HepB).
- Administer the 3-dose series to those who were not previously vaccinated.
- A 2-dose series of Recombivax HB® is licensed for children aged 11–15 years.

2. Rotavirus vaccine (Rota).
- Do not start the series later than age 12 weeks.
- Administer the final dose in the series by age 32 weeks.
- Do not administer a dose later than age 32 weeks.
- Data on safety and efficacy outside of these age ranges are insufficient.

3. Diphtheria and tetanus toxoids and acellular pertussis vaccine (DTaP).
- The fifth dose is not necessary if the fourth dose was administered at age 4 years or older.
- DTaP is not indicated for persons aged 7 years or older.

4. Haemophilus influenzae type b conjugate vaccine (Hib).
- Vaccine is not generally recommended for children aged 5 years or older.
- If current age is younger than 12 months and the first 2 doses were PRP-OMP (PedvaxHIB® or ComVax® [Merck]), the third (and final) dose should be administered at age 12–15 months and at least 8 weeks after the second dose.
- If first dose was administered at age 7–11 months, administer 2 doses separated by 4 weeks plus a booster at age 12–15 months.

5. Pneumococcal conjugate vaccine (PCV).
- Administer one dose of PCV to all healthy children aged 24–59 months having any incomplete schedule.
- For children with underlying medical conditions, administer 2 doses of PCV at least 8 weeks apart if previously received less than 3 doses, or 1 dose of PCV if previously received 3 doses.

6. Inactivated poliovirus vaccine (IPV).
- For children who received an all-IPV or all-oral poliovirus (OPV) series, a fourth dose is not necessary if third dose was administered at age 4 years or older.

- If both OPV and IPV were administered as part of a series, a total of 4 doses should be administered, regardless of the child's current age.
- IPV is not routinely recommended for persons aged 18 years and older.

7. Measles, mumps, and rubella vaccine (MMR).
- The second dose of MMR is recommended routinely at age 4–6 years but may be administered earlier if desired.
- If not previously vaccinated, administer 2 doses of MMR during any visit with 4 or more weeks between the doses.

8. Varicella vaccine.
- The second dose of varicella vaccine is recommended routinely at age 4–6 years but may be administered earlier if desired.
- Do not repeat the second dose in persons younger than 13 years of age if administered 28 or more days after the first dose.

9. Hepatitis A vaccine (HepA).
- HepA is recommended for certain groups of children, including in areas where vaccination programs target older children. See MMWR 2006;55(No. RR-7):1–23.

10. Tetanus and diphtheria toxoids vaccine (Td) and tetanus and diphtheria toxoids and acellular pertussis vaccine (Tdap).
- Tdap should be substituted for a single dose of Td in the primary catch-up series or as a booster if age appropriate; use Td for other doses.
- A 5-year interval from the last Td dose is encouraged when Tdap is used as a booster dose. A booster (fourth) dose is needed if any of the previous doses were administered at younger than 12 months of age. Refer to ACIP recommendations for further information. See MMWR 2006;55(No. RR-3).

11. Human papillomavirus vaccine (HPV).
- Administer the HPV vaccine series to females at age 13–18 years if not previously vaccinated.

Information about reporting reactions after immunization is available online at http://www.vaers.hhs.gov or by telephone via the 24-hour national toll-free information line 800-822-7967. Suspected cases of vaccine-preventable diseases should be reported to the state or local health department. Additional information, including precautions and contraindications for immunization, is available from the National Center for Immunization and Respiratory Diseases at http://www.cdc.gov/vaccines or telephone, 800-CDC-INFO (800-232-4636).

DEPARTMENT OF HEALTH AND HUMAN SERVICES • CENTERS FOR DISEASE CONTROL AND PREVENTION • SAFER • HEALTHIER • PEOPLE

CS113897

FIGURE 21.2 Catch-up Immunization Schedule for persons 4 months to 18 years of age.

other than their parents; relatives cared for 22%, nonrelatives cared for 14%, and child care center-based programs cared for 36% (Child Trends, 2006b). Only half of child care centers meet standards set by the American Public Health Association and the AAP—and most quality ratings are moderate to poor (Patten & Ricks, 2003). Working mothers need quality child care services: 85% of children under age 6 whose mothers worked at least 35 hours a week were in some form of non-parental care in 2005 (Child Trends, 2006b).

Although safe, affordable child care is important, the long-term benefits of early childhood education are numerous. They include higher rates of high school completion, college attendance, and full-time employment; lower rates of felony arrests, convictions, and incarcerations; and fewer reports of depressive symptoms (Reynolds et al., 2007). Higher incomes, more positive outcomes for mental health, higher levels of health efficacy, and more positive health behaviors have been noted in adults who participated in early childhood education programs (Palfrey et al., 2005). More than half of 3- to 5-year-old children in the United States were enrolled in half- or full-day preschool programs in 2003 (Child Trends, 2004). Quality preschool program attendance can provide children with language and pre-academic skills that may lead to better learning outcomes in kindergarten (National Institute of Child Health & Development [NICHD] Early Child Care Research Network, 2002). **Head Start**, a federally funded program that offers early childhood education to low-income children between ages 3 and 5, has consistently demonstrated significant improvements in preschoolers' social-emotional and cognitive development, and those attending Head Start do better on several developmental measures than children who did not attend Head Start (Love, Tarullo, Raikes, & Chazan-Cohen, 2006). Those attending Head Start were found to be significantly more likely to finish high school and go on to attend college than their siblings who did not attend Head Start (Garces, Thomas, & Currie, 2002). Head Start children are also more likely to receive dental and health screenings, to have up-to-date immunization coverage, to have better school attendance, and to be less likely to be held back in school. The benefits of Head Start extend to families because more Head Start parents read more frequently to their children than do parents of children not enrolled in the program. Because parents of preschoolers in Head Start must demonstrate parent involvement in the program, they are more likely to demonstrate upward mobility and positive growth. These parents also report less depression, anxiety, and illness and more life satisfaction and increased coping skills (National Head Start Association, 2006).

Many states provide preschool programs, but Head Start programs generally offer higher quality, more comprehensive services than those found in state preschool programs (Barnett, 2002). The availability of affordable, quality, licensed day care facilities is recognized as one long-term solution for the prevention of child abuse. When their young children are safely cared for, two parents or a single parent can work and provide more resources for the family, thereby decreasing the stress that may precipitate abuse. The quality of day care and preschool programs varies considerably; licensing laws can regulate only minimum safety and health standards. In addition, numerous child care operations are too small to require licensing, leaving quality and compliance unevaluated. Community health nurses can influence the quality of day care and preschool programs through active educational efforts, monitoring of health and safety standards, and working to improve the state's role in passing stronger licensing laws.

Health Protection Programs

Health protection programs for infants and young children are designed to protect them from illness and injury. Ultimately, these programs may even protect their lives.

Safety and Injury Protection

Accident and injury control programs serve a critical role in protecting the lives of children. Efforts to prevent motor vehicle crashes, a major cause of death, may include driver education programs, better highway construction, improved motor vehicle design and safety features, and continuing research into the causes of various types of crashes. Injury prevention and reduction have been addressed through strategies such as state laws requiring the use of safety restraints (e.g., seatbelts, child safety seats), availability of front and side driver and passenger airbags, substitution of other modes of travel (air, rail, or bus), lower speed limits, stricter enforcement of drunk driving laws, safer automobile design, and helmets for motorcyclists, bicycle riders, and skaters.

For infants, toddlers, and preschool-aged children to be safe when traveling in vehicles, they must be restrained in an approved infant carrier, child restraint seat, or booster seat. These must be positioned and secured as described by the manufacturer; used at all times, even for the shortest distances; placed in the back seat, never in the front seat; and installed in the appropriate position (facing rear or front) based on the weight or age of the infant or young child. It is recommended that booster seats be used until the child is 58 inches tall and weighs around 80 lbs (Ehiri et al., 2006). Programs that provide training, education, and child safety seats have been shown to improve child safety seat use (Letourneau, Crump, Bowling, Kuklinski, & Allen, 2008). A systematic review of booster seat intervention studies found that incentives (e.g., coupons, gift certificates), free booster seats, and educational interventions were most effective. Legislation and enforcement of laws may also be beneficial (Ehiri et al., 2006).

Protection from Child Abuse and Neglect

Services to protect children from abuse are not as well developed or effective as safety and injury prevention programs, an observation accounted for by a variety of factors. Most child abuse occurs in the home, so only the most blatant situations become evident to outsiders. Community health nurses and physicians who see injured children may find parents' explanations plausible and may not suspect or want to believe that abuse might be responsible. Avoidance of legal involvement keeps others from reporting suspected cases. Fortunately, this attitude is changing among professionals who work with children and other community members.

For many years, states have had mandatory reporting laws. The Child Abuse Prevention and Treatment Act, enacted in 1974, provides funding to states to aid in preventing and investigating child abuse and neglect (Child Welfare Information Gateway, 2004). Over the years, numerous amendments have expanded the definition of child abuse and the persons who are required to report. People mandated to report suspected child abuse include all those who work with children:

day care providers, teachers, social workers, nurses, doctors, clergy, coaches, and so forth. In addition, animal humane workers and commercial photograph developers are mandated reporters. Procedures for reporting categories of child abuse have also been clarified, and 1990 updates included services for homeless children and families. Today, professionals and the public are more aware of the problem, and there has been an increase in reporting. In 1974, the National Center for Child Abuse and Neglect was established as a result of the Child Abuse Prevention and Treatment Act. The center collects and analyzes information on child abuse and neglect, serves as an information clearinghouse, publishes educational materials on the subject, offers technical assistance, and conducts research into the problem. The Adoption and Safe Families Act, enacted in 1997, gives further direction in working with families and promotes the safety of children, while recognizing the child's need for a permanent home.

Child and family well-being are also a concern of child protection agencies (Goldman, Salus, Wolcott, & Kennedy, 2003). In addition, these acts spurred all of the states to pass mandatory reporting laws and design procedures for investigation of suspected cases of child abuse and neglect. All states have some form of child protective services or family services, whose charge is to protect children and strengthen families. They often work with law enforcement and the judicial system, but health professionals and educators are also important team members. The basic dilemma facing those who work in this area is maintaining the family unit and still providing a safe environment for the child (Goldman et al., 2003). Most professionals adopt the *levels of prevention* model to describe child abuse and neglect prevention efforts.

Primary Prevention

Primary prevention measures include the use of public service announcements that promote positive parenting, family support groups, and public awareness campaigns about child maltreatment and how to report it, along with establishing community education to enhance the general well-being of children and their families (Thomas, Leicht, Hughes, Madigan, & Dowell, 2003). Educational services are designed to enrich the lives of families, to improve the skills of family functioning, and to prevent the stress and problems that might lead to dysfunction and abuse or neglect (Feinberg & Kan, 2008; Melnyk et al., 2007).

Prevention should focus on parent preparation during the prenatal period; practices that encourage parent–child bonding during labor, delivery, the postpartum period, and early infancy; and provision of information regarding support services for families with newborns. It is also helpful to provide parents of children of all ages with information regarding child-rearing and community resources (Goldman et al., 2003). Child sexual abuse prevention curricula, such as *Good Touch/Bad Touch*, teach children skills to avoid victimization and promote discussion. They have been found effective in utilization of protective strategies and some evidence suggests they may afford some protection against physical abuse (Thomas et al., 2003).

Secondary Prevention

Services are designed to identify and assist high-risk families to prevent abuse or neglect. **High-risk families** are those families that exhibit the symptoms of potentially abusive or neglectful behavior or that are under the types of stress associated with abuse or neglect. These can include families living in poverty, exhibiting substance abuse or mental health problems, and parents or children with disabilities. Early intervention with high-risk families can improve emotional and functional coping and help prevent further problems (Melnyk et al., 2004). High school parent education programs for pregnant adolescents, home visitation programs targeted to at-risk families, and respite care for families with special needs children are all examples of secondary prevention actions. Family resource centers in schools or community centers located in low-income neighborhoods can offer resource and referral services to families who may be dealing with multiple sources of stress (Thomas et al., 2003). Home visitation programs, such as the Nurse Family Partnership, Early Head Start, and Healthy Families America, provide parent support and education, and promote healthier family functioning (Olds et al., 2004a; 2004b; 2007; Thomas et al., 2003). Some home visitation programs to high-risk mothers and families have demonstrated decreased rates of child abuse and neglect (Black et al., 2007; Thomas et al., 2003).

Tertiary Prevention

Intervention and treatment services are designed to assist a family in which abuse or neglect has already occurred, so that further abuse or neglect may be prevented and the consequences of abuse or neglect may be minimized. Often, families are referred to mental health counselors for "intensive family preservation services" to improve family communication and functioning (Thomas et al., 2003, p. 8). Some families may require crisis respite when they feel they cannot manage the stresses of child care. Role models, through the use of parent mentor programs, provide support and nonjudgmental coaching to parents who have sometimes been the victims of abuse themselves (Thomas et al., 2003).

The community health nurse has a major role in primary prevention of child maltreatment. In addition, the nurse is in a unique position to detect early signs of neglect and abuse. The PHN must establish rapport with families and assist with appropriate interventions and referrals at the secondary and tertiary levels of prevention. An interdisciplinary approach with teachers, the department of social services, foster families, and other health care providers is needed (Goldman et al., 2003; Thomas et al., 2003). The effectiveness of local programs depends, in large measure, on the willingness of community health professionals to increase their awareness and work as a team to detect, report, and develop interventions for the perpetrators and victims of abuse and neglect. Ongoing education of health care providers is recommended to increase awareness of changing child abuse patterns, new reporting laws, and resources available to families.

Health Promotion Programs

Early childhood development and intervention programs are designed to have positive effects on the outcomes of children's cognitive and social development. Some health promotion programs have considered children's physical health, and fewer have focused on parent–child interaction and child social development. All are considered important health promotion programs from birth through preschool years.

Infant Brain Development Research and Parent–Child Interactions

New research into the normal brain development of infants and toddlers has revealed that brain maturation in the first few years of life is very rapid: the brain grows to 80% of adult size by age 3, and the myelination pattern of an 18- to 24-month-old child is similar to that of an adult (Almli, Rivkin, & McKinstry, 2006; Zero to Three, n.d.). The prefrontal cortex of 4 year olds is already functional and becomes more organized throughout later adolescence (Tsujimoto, 2008). Maturation of the corpus callosum begins after birth, signaling a potential for vulnerability to environmental stimuli and stress (Gilmore, Lin, & Gerig, 2006). Early environment exerts a lasting influence on brain development, even in the womb (Nava-Ocampo & Koren, 2007; Rees & Inder, 2005; World Bank, 2008). Appropriate early environment and stimulation promotes healthy development.

Because brain development is thought to be "activity-dependent," and *pruning* or selection of only the most active neural circuits occurs in early childhood, parents are encouraged to provide appropriate nutrition, avoid potentially harmful substances, and provide appropriate stimulation for their infants, toddlers, and preschoolers (Zero to Three, n.d.). During the first 2 years, when rapid myelination is taking place, 50% of total calories should come from fat, but after age 2, 1% or 2% milk should be the norm. Harmful substances, such as tobacco (cigarettes), chemicals, and radiation, should be avoided during pregnancy, as should contact with people who have infectious diseases. Meaningful parent–child interactions should be established early; they include holding, rocking, comforting, touching, talking, and singing. When parents talk to infants and read to young children, children later demonstrate more advanced language and literacy skills. Providing a caring and supportive environment, with opportunities to learn and explore, is supportive of healthy brain development and promotes secure infant attachment (Duursma, Augustyn, & Zuckerman, 2008; Jeppson & Myers-Walls, 2003; Roisman & Fraley, 2008; Zero to Three, n.d.).

Young children who do not have early exposure to this type of environment—for example, those who are in institutional care—exhibit delays in cognitive and social development, as well as attachment disorders (Johnson, Browne, & Hamilton-Giachritsis, 2006). However, when placed with foster families who provide a warm, stimulating environment, children's cognitive development improves—especially for those who made the change at younger ages (Nelson et al., 2007).

Gazing into an infant's eyes, paying attention to and interacting with toddlers, and listening to and answering preschoolers' questions are important parental behaviors that promote social development (Chouinard, 2007; Grossman & Johnson, 2007; Jeppson & Myers-Walls, 2003). Providing infants and young children with secure, learning-rich environments where they can use their senses to discover new things helps them to maximize their potential. Emotional comfort and a secure environment ensure that young children will better deal with their feelings. Early social experiences affect oxytocin and vasopressin neuropeptide systems that aid in establishing social bonds and attachment, and these systems continue to regulate emotional functions throughout adult life (Fries, Ziegler, Kurian, Jacoris, & Pollak, 2005). Public health nurses can provide resources and work with young families to encourage quality parent–child interactions that promote cognitive and social development.

Developmental Screening

With the emphasis on infant and early childhood development, community health nurses often routinely carry out developmental screenings. Tools such as the Ages and Stages Questionnaire (ASQ), Parents' Evaluation of Developmental Status (PEDS), and the Denver II are often used by PHNs as they make routine home visits to follow at-risk infants, children, and families (Gaines, Jenkins, & Ashe, 2005; Wagner, Jenkins, & Smith, 2006). Those working with high-risk or medically vulnerable infant programs periodically screen their clients to determine gaps in development and provide suggestions to parents that promote advancement.

Developmental screening tools are also helpful in educating parents about normal child development and can provide a means of anticipatory guidance on developmental milestones and future safety issues. *Bright Futures*, an important resource for nurses and parents, provides tools to help families determine appropriate developmental milestones and expected behaviors, along with suggestions about when to seek help from professionals (Mayer, Anastasi, & Clark, 2006). A variety of screening tools available to nurses and other health professionals, ranging from parent report instruments to those that involve direct assessment of behaviors and skills, can examine overall physical and cognitive development, or screen for such things as temperament, behavior, autism, and speech and language (AAP, Committee on Children with Disabilities, 2001). Early identification of problems can lead to interventions that help children with school readiness (Wold & Nicholas, 2007). A study of preschool children born to low-risk mothers concluded that 10% of the children screened were at high risk for developmental problems, indicating that routine developmental screening can not only promote health but also provide secondary prevention through early detection of potential problems (Tough et al., 2008).

In the last decade, more than 70% of children with disabilities were not first detected by their health care providers, but the AAP now recommends developmental screening and surveillance during preventive health care visits (AAP, 2008; Glascoe, 2000). Developmental screenings can provide parents with information on their child's development and can assist in early detection of possible developmental delays and earlier access to interventions that may provide better outcomes (CDC, 2008e; Harris & Handleman, 2000; Rydz et al., 2006).

Programs for Children with Special Needs

Many children have special needs. They may have a congenital or acquired developmental disability, birth defect, or a chronic emotional, mental, or physical disease. Approximately 16% of children have a developmental disability, and between 12% and 16% have some type of behavioral or developmental disorder (AAP Committee on Children with Disabilities, 2001; Wagner, Jenkins, & Smith, 2006). About 3% of U.S. infants are born with a birth defect. The most

From the Case Files II

A Case of Kernicterus

A young mother was hospitalized for the birth of her second daughter, a beautiful little girl born without incident. The infant was taken to the mother for feeding and care by the nursing staff, and the mother noticed that her daughter was not very active. The infant had difficulty latching on for breast-feeding. The mother told her obstetrical nurse that the infant seemed very different from her first child. The infant was irritable, but the nurse reassured the mother that the baby was fine and "not all babies are alike." Still, the new mother was concerned.

By the second day, the mother noticed that the baby was not very alert and did not want to feed. She also noticed that the baby's color was "yellowish," and the mother notified the nurse. Again, the nurse reassured the mother that this was "normal" for infants of Asian descent. The baby still was not feeding well, and there was yellowish-orange color stool in the baby's diaper. The mother notified the nurse, and asked the nurse to call the doctor. The nurse refused and told the mother that she was "overreacting." The nurse again reassured the mother that the baby was "fine" and no action was taken. The mother felt that the nurse was not listening to her concerns. The baby continued to be irritable, and the nurse said that the baby just needed to breast-feed and was very insistent that the new mother was "not breast-feeding properly." The new mother was instructed not to give the baby water or additional fluids, so that the baby would breast-feed. No additional fluids were offered. The young mother was not satisfied with the nursing care and was offended that the nurse would not listen to her. A referral was made to the breast-feeding specialist at the hospital to help the new mother feed her infant. There were no phone calls documented to the physician, or documentation of the "yellowish-orange" stool. (The young mother kept the diaper for further proof of her concerns, though.) There was no documentation of irritability, inability to breast-feed, lethargy, or jaundiced appearance of the skin. The physician discharging the infant did not receive any information regarding irritability or yellowish stool. The nursing emphasis postpartum was on breast-feeding and the nurses documented that the young mother had an "uncooperative attitude."

The young mother and infant were discharged home on the second postpartum day. No blood work was done for the "yellowish" color of the baby's skin, even though the yellowish tone to lower extremities and abdomen was documented in the nurse's notes and on the discharge summary. No referrals were made to Home Health or Public Health for follow-up.

Within 48 hours of discharge, the young mother brought her lethargic baby to the hospital's Emergency Room. On day 4 of life, the infant's bilirubin was 46. The infant was severely neurologically damaged, and the brain damage that resulted was irreversible. She was diagnosed with severe cerebral palsy, secondary to kernicterus (excessive bilirubin). The child will never be able to walk or talk. She will be fed through a gastrostomy tube for the rest of her life. She has normal intelligence, but it is locked into a dysfunctional body. The patient and family were devastated.

The physician and hospital (nurses) were sued. The nurses on duty could not defend their actions with their charting, or lack thereof. The attorneys for the hospital, representing the physician and nurses, could not defend the actions of their clients. A multimillion dollar settlement was granted, and the nurses were fired. Unfortunately, this is not an isolated case. The irreversible brain damage that occurs as a result of untreated hyperbilirubinemia should not occur in the 21st century. This was a no-win situation that could have been avoided with proper nursing intervention. Hyperbilirubinemia should always be in the forefront of newborn assessment during the first few days of life.

The nurses involved in this case were not acting as the patient's advocate. The young mother tried to tell the nurses, and the nurses should have listened to their patient. The physician should have been notified immediately when signs and symptoms were first noted. Incorrect assumptions were made due to the nationality of the patient, an indication of lack of cultural competence. Home Health Nursing or Public Health Nursing should have been arranged for infant follow-up after discharge, but these interventions did not happen.

Linda O., Certified Life Care Planner, Nurse Consultant

common birth defects involve the heart, or are classified as neural tube defects (e.g., spina bifida) or orofacial clefts (e.g., cleft palate, cleft lip), and a substantial number of birth defects, such as hypospadia or hearing loss, are generally not life threatening (CDC, 2005b). Some children suffer injuries after birth (see From the Case Files II). Autism and other mental or behavioral disorders develop after infancy and may require special services. Educational, health, and social or recreational services should be available for all children.

Federal law mandates early identification and intervention services for those with a variety of developmental disabilities. Developmental delays are characterized by slower development in one or more areas. The Individuals with Disabilities Education Act (IDEA) provides early intervention services, usually at home, for those from birth to age 2 who have developmental delays in physical, cognitive, communication, emotional, social, and adaptive development. Intervention services are also available to children with a mental or physical problem that is likely to result in a developmental delay. Newborns can receive infant stimulation services at home or in some schools specially designed to meet the needs of the very young. These programs are offered on a part-time basis for 1 to 2 hours, two to three times a week. Special education preschools are available for young children from ages 3 to 5. By preschool age, children may advance to half-day programs (Kupper, 2005; National Dissemination Center for Children with Disabilities [NICHCY], 2002). Additional services can be provided to assist the families in getting children to the programs. Door-to-door bus service in specially equipped small buses or vans safely transport young children who arrive at school in wheelchairs or with other assistive devices. Early stimulation programs, such as the Infant Health and Development Program targeted to preterm and LBW infants, have demonstrated improved parent–child interactions, along with greater motor skill and cognitive development (Bonnier, 2008).

Availability of health services for children with special needs varies with the size of the community. In small rural communities, children and their parents may have to travel long distances to receive specialized services, and in inner-city neighborhoods, lack of money for transportation can make even nearby services equally inaccessible. Accessibility is also influenced by lack of knowledge, attitudes, and prejudices. Community health nurses must recognize the power of these immobilizing factors and be able to deal with them effectively to make positive changes. See Chapter 25 for more on barriers to health care.

Most communities offer additional social and recreational programs for children with special needs. For example, American Lung Association affiliate offices sponsor camping programs for children with asthma or other lung diseases. Often, these are camps for school-aged children that may last up to 1 week and be located in mountain or beach areas, but they may also be day camps, with parents in attendance for preschoolers. Nationwide programs such as the Special Olympics offer recreational competition for children with special needs in a variety of sports, such as bowling, track and field, skiing, and swimming.

The community health nurse best serves families as a resource for such programs. Some parents are not aware of the rights or services available for their special needs children. Nurses can advocate for parents and help establish services in communities where needed services are lacking.

Nutritional Programs

Adequate nutrition must begin before birth. One of the most productive health promotion programs is the Special Supplemental Food Program for Women, Infants, and Children (WIC). In addition to supporting women and young children with nutritious foods and achieving the initial goals of decreasing the rates of preterm and LBW babies, increasing the length of pregnancy, and reducing the incidence of infant and child iron deficiency anemia, WIC also increases breast-feeding rates and improves pregnant women's nutritional status. Children enrolled in WIC demonstrate improved cognitive skills and vocabulary, and for each dollar spent on WIC, between $1.77 and $3.13 are saved in health care costs (Parraga & Doughten, 2007).

WIC provides information to parents about eating healthfully and promoting healthy rates of growth. Parents become more aware of the need to reduce consumption of saturated fat, salt, sugar, and over-processed foods. The community health nurse, through nutrition education and reinforcement of positive practices, plays a significant role in promoting the health of infants and young children (see Levels of Prevention Pyramid). For more information about WIC, see Chapter 22.

ROLE OF THE COMMUNITY HEALTH NURSE

Community health nurses face the challenge of continually assessing each population's current health problems, as well as determining available and needed services. Community health nursing interventions with maternal, infant, toddler, and preschool populations are focused on health promotion and early intervention. They may include work in family planning or high-risk clinics, telephone information services and hotlines, or home visitation programs. The nurse uses educational interventions when teaching family planning, nutrition, safety precautions, or child care skills. Such interventions involve providing information and encouraging client groups (parents and young children) to participate in their own health care. Other interventions include strategies in which the nurse uses a greater degree of persuasion or positive manipulation, such as conducting voluntary immunization programs, encouraging smoking cessation during pregnancy, preventing communicable diseases, and encouraging appropriate use of child safety devices such as car seats. Finally, the nurse may use interventions that coerce people into compliance with laws that require certain immunizations or mandate reporting of suspected child abuse and environmental health standards violations, such as sanitation issues.

The community health nurse acts as an advocate and a resource for families of young children. The PHN may be called upon to provide information to young mothers about infant temperament, sleep schedules, colic, parenting, discipline, toilet training, television or video choices, and nutrition and feeding (Dopkins-Stright, Canley-Gallagher, & Kelley, 2008; Gurian, n.d.; Klassen et al., 2006; Rideout, Vandewater, & Wartella, 2003; Tempfer, 2005). The PHN should be aware of federal, state, and local laws that preserve and protect the rights of children and families. Availability of educational, medical, social, and recreational services needed by young families is a necessity. The nurse helps to secure these services in the community she or he serves. Ensuring that families have the resources to provide a safe and healthy environment for their children can take many forms. The nurse may lobby to change existing laws, initiate the effort needed to establish programs and services in the community, and teach families about infant safety or the importance of immunizations.

LEVELS OF PREVENTION PYRAMID

SITUATION: Desire for a healthy, full-term infant
GOAL: Using the 3 levels of prevention, negative health conditions are avoided, promptly diagnosed and treated, and/or the fullest possible potential is restored.

Tertiary Prevention

Rehabilitation

Primary Prevention

- The parents and significant others begin to bond with the newborn
- Parents get to know the newborn and establish a successful breast- or bottle-feeding routine
- The infant returns home in an age-appropriate infant car seat, which is used properly when traveling
- The infant's birth is celebrated according to cultural and religious preferences
- Parents resume sexual intercourse using a family planning method of their choice
- The parents enjoy the new life they have created

Health Promotion & Education
- Appointments are made and kept for postpartum and newborn visits to health care providers

Health Protection
- Exposure to people with infectious diseases is avoided
- Infant immunization schedule begins on time and continues through childhood

Secondary Prevention

Early Diagnosis

Prompt Treatment

- The mother starts prenatal care early in the first trimester, and continues care at regular intervals throughout the pregnancy

- The mother does not use alcohol, tobacco, or other mood-altering substances during the pregnancy
- The mother takes a daily prenatal vitamin with folic acid
- Parents avoid exposure to people with infectious disease
- The mother has adequate nutrition, rest, sleep, and exercise
- The mother begins supportive services if eligible (WIC, Temporary Assistance for Needy Families)
- Family and significant others continue to be supportive
- The parents attend labor preparation, infant care, and parenting classes
- Name(s) are selected for the infant
- Delivery method and location are selected
- The home is prepared for the infant: e.g., adequate infant furnishings and supplies are acquired within the parents' budget
- Preparations and plans are made regarding breast or bottle feeding

(continued)

LEVELS OF PREVENTION PYRAMID (*Continued*)

Secondary Prevention

Early Diagnosis	Prompt Treatment
	• A pediatrician or pediatric nurse practitioner is selected • An infant car seat is acquired and properly installed • Plans are made to get to the chosen health care facility when in labor

Primary Prevention

Health Promotion & Education	Health Protection
• The pregnancy is planned • Pregnancies are spaced 2 years (or more) apart • Mother has a positive attitude going into the pregnancy • A health care provider is chosen • There are financial resources to meet the expanding family's needs • Family and significant others are supportive • Mother's weight is as close to ideal as possible before conception	• Parents do not use alcohol, tobacco, or other mood-altering substances when planning to conceive • The mother begins a vitamin regimen containing folic acid before the pregnancy

Summary

Maternal–child health clients are an important population group to community health nurses, because their physical and emotional health is vital to the future of society. The United States does not fare well in comparison to other developed nations on maternal–child health indicators. *Healthy People 2010* objectives for maternal child populations have shown mixed results at midcourse review. Some have moved away from their targets, such as those for low-birth-weight (LBW), very-low-birth-weight (VLBW), and preterm births, and others, like the maternal mortality rate (MMR), have moved closer to the target rate. The target for childhood immunization coverage has been met.

Problems of substance abuse, sexually transmitted diseases, and teen pregnancy can lead to less than optimal outcomes for newborns. Complications of pregnancy and childbirth, such as hypertension, gestational diabetes, postpartum depression, and fetal or infant death, offer opportunities for community health nurses to provide education and support.

Infant mortality rates are no longer declining. Toddler and young child mortality and morbidity are often related to unintentional injuries. Worldwide, toddlers and preschoolers are at risk for accidents (falls, drowning, burns, and poisoning); acute illnesses, particularly respiratory illnesses; and nutritional, dental, and emotional ailments. Violence against children and deaths from homicide elicit valid concerns. These problems create major challenges for the community health nurse who seeks to prevent illness and injury among children and to promote health.

Health services for children span three categories: preventive, health protecting, and health promoting. The community health nurse plays a vital role in each. Preventive services include immunization programs, along with quality day care and preschool. Health protection services include accident and injury prevention and control, as well as services to protect children from child abuse. Health promotion services include infant development through effective parent–child interaction, developmental screening, and services to children with special needs.

The role of community health nurses include providing interventions to serve young children's health needs, such as educational interventions for the young child that include nutrition teaching to provide information and encourage parents to act responsibly on behalf of their children to assist in healthy habit formation for a lifetime. Other interventions involve encouraging age-appropriate immunizations or cessation of smoking during pregnancy, and PHNs may employ persuasive tactics to move clients toward more positive health behaviors. With reporting and intervening in child abuse, nurses practice a form of coercion to protect children from threats to their health. ■

ACTIVITIES TO PROMOTE CRITICAL THINKING

1. What specific objectives has your local health department developed for mothers and infants to help achieve the goals listed in the U.S. *Healthy People 2010* document? How do your county's statistics compare with those of others in your state on (1) infant mortality rates (collectively and by specific ethnic groups), (2) incidence of LBW and VLBW infants, and (3) incidence of birth defects?

2. Using the Internet, locate national websites that give you current information about progress toward meeting some of the *Healthy People 2010* goals with infants, toddlers, and preschool-aged children. Are we making progress? Will we meet or have we met the 2010 goal with these populations? What can a community health nurse do locally to promote meeting these goals? What needs to be done on the regional, state, or national level?

3. Describe three different maternal child populations in your county. What are their most pressing health needs? Do any existing services target these populations? How well, in your judgment, are clients' needs being met? Interview a city or county community health nurse and other public health professionals to help you find answers.

4. Sonia, an 18-year-old woman, is single and 14 weeks pregnant. Her first prenatal visit was made at the urging of her aunt, who uses the clinic. Sonia reluctantly admitted to the clinic nurse that the pregnancy was unplanned. She consumes alcohol two to three times a week, frequently as much as six 12-oz cans of beer and 16 oz of wine, and she smokes one pack of cigarettes a day. She has tried a variety of street drugs in the last 3 months but does not use any on a regular basis. The clinic nurse believed that Sonia might not return for regular prenatal care and made a referral to the PHN for follow-up home visits to assess Sonia's home environment and teach prenatal care and preparation for the infant. You have been assigned the case. Design a plan of care to address Sonia's needs. What specific services and programs might you recommend? What barriers might exist? How would the prenatal and postpartum teaching delivered to Sonia differ from care needed by other single teens?

5. What is the major cause of death among infants, toddlers, and preschool-aged children? What community-wide interventions could be initiated to prevent these deaths? Select one intervention for each age group, and describe how you and a group of community health professionals might develop this preventive measure.

6. Describe one health promotion program that you as a community health nurse could initiate and carry out to improve the health of children in a day care center or preschool program.

References

ACOG Committee on Practice Bulletins. (2008). ACOG practice bulletin: Clinical management guidelines for obstetrics & gynecology No. 92. Use of psychiatric medication during pregnancy and lactation. *Obstetrics & Gynecology, 111*, 1001–1020.

Adolfsson, A., Larsson, P., Wijma, B., & Bertero, C. (2004). Guilt and emptiness: Women's experiences of miscarriage. *Health Care of Women International, 25*(6), 543–560.

Alexander, G.R., & Kotelchuck, M. (2001). Assessing the role and effectiveness of prenatal care: History, challenges, and directions for future research. *Public Health Reports, 116*, 306–316.

Aligne, C., Moss, M., Auinger, P., & Weitzman, M. (2003). Association of pediatric dental caries with passive smoking. *JAMA, 289*(10), 1258–1264.

Almli, C., Rivkin, M., McKinstry, R., & Brain Development Cooperative Group. (2007). The NIH MRI study of normal brain development (objective-2): Newborns, infants, toddlers, and preschoolers. *NeuroImage, 35*, 308–325.

Altimer, L. (2008). Shaken baby syndrome. *Journal of Perinatal & Neonatal Nursing, 22*(1), 68–76.

American Academy of Pediatrics Committee on Nutrition. (2001). The use and misuse of fruit juice in pediatrics. *Pediatrics, 107*(5), 1210–1213.

American Academy of Pediatrics. Committee on Injury and Poison Prevention. (2001a). Injuries associated with infant walkers. *Pediatrics, 108*, 790–792.

American Academy of Pediatrics Committee on Injury and Poison Prevention. (2001b). Falls from heights: windows, roofs, and balconies. *Pediatrics, 107*, 1188–1191

American Academy of Pediatrics (AAP). (2008). *Developmental/ behavioral.* The National Center of Medical Home Initiatives for Children with Special Needs. Retrieved August 18, 2008 from http://www.medicalhomeinfo.org/screening/cdc_rev1.html.

American Academy of Pediatrics (AAP) Committee on Children with Disabilities. (2001). Developmental surveillance and screening of infants and young children. *Pediatrics, 108*(1), 192–196.

American Association of Poison Control Centers. (2008a). *Poison centers can help.* Retrieved August 18, 2008 from http://www.aapcc.org/dnn/PoisoningPrevention/FAQ/tabid/117/Default.aspx.

American Association of Poison Control Centers. (2008b). *You can prevent poisonings at home.* Retrieved August 18, 2008 from http://www.aapcc.org/dnn/PoisoningPrevention/PoisonProofYour Home/tabid/118/Default.aspx.

American Chemical Society. (May 7, 2008). *New insights on link between early consumption of cows' milk and Type 1 diabetes.* Retrieved August 18, 2008 from http://portal.acs.org:80/portal/acs/corg/content?_nfpb=true&_pageLabel=PP_ARTICLE MAIN&node_id=223&content_id=WPCP_008872&use_sec= true&sec_url_var=region1#P50_3380.

American Diabetes Association. (2003). Gestational diabetes. *Diabetes Care, 26*[Suppl. 1], S102–S105.

American Lung Association. (November 2006). *Cystic fibrosis (CF) fact sheet.* Retrieved August 18, 2008 from http://www.lungusa.org/site/pp.asp?c=dvLUK900E&b=35042.

Armstrong, M.A., Osejo, V.G., Lieberman, L., et al. (2003). Perinatal substance abuse intervention in obstetric clinics decreases adverse neonatal outcomes. *Journal of Perinatology, 23*, 3–9.

Association of Maternal & Child Health Programs. (n.d.). *Best practices in maternal & child health: Back to Sleep training for nursery room nurses.* Retrieved August 18, 2008 from http://www.amchp.org/best_practices/Downloads/Best%20Practice%20Posters.pdf.

Association of State & Territorial Health Officials (ASTHO). (February 2006). *Fact sheet: Preconception care.* Arlington, VA: Author.

Bager, B. (2003). Children of mentally-retarded mothers: An inventory. Small group at risk with considerable need of assistance during an insecure childhood. *Lakartidningen, 100*(1–2), 22–25.

Baird, J., Fisher, D., Lucas, P., et al. (2005). Being big or growing fast: Systematic review of size and growth in infancy and later obesity. *BMJ: British Medical Journal, 22,* 929–931.

Bardenheier, B., Yusuf, H., Rosenthal, J., et al. (2004). Factors associated with underummunizaiton at 3 months of age in four medically underserved areas. *Public Health Reports, 119*(5), 479–485.

Barnet, B., Arroyo, C., Devoe, M., & Duggan, A. (2004). Reduced school dropout rates among adolescent mothers receiving school-based prenatal care. *Archives of Pediatric & Adolescent Medicine, 158*(3), 262–268.

Barnet, B., Duggan, A., & Devoe, M. (2003). Reduced low birth weight for teenagers receiving prenatal care at a school-based health center: Effect of access and comprehensive care. *Journal of Adolescent Health, 33*(5), 349–358.

Barnett, W.S. (September 13, 2002). *The battle over Head Start: What the research shows.* Presentation at a Science and Public Policy Briefing sponsored by the Federation of Behavioral, Psychological, and Cognitive Sciences.

Barnet, B., Liu, J., Devoe, M., Alperovitz-Bichell, K., & Duggan, A. (2007). Home visiting for adolescent mothers: Effects on parenting, maternal life course, and primary care linkage. *Annals of Family Medicine, 5*(3), 224–232.

Barr, H.M., & Streissguth, A.P. (2001). Identifying maternal self-reported alcohol use associated with fetal alcohol spectrum disorders. *Alcoholism: Clinical and Experimental Research, 25*(2), 283–287.

Barr, P., & Cacciatore, J. (2007). Problematic emotions and maternal grief. *Omega, 56*(4), 331–348.

Bassett, M.T. (2001). Keeping the M in MTCT: Women, mothers, and HIV prevention. *American Journal of Public Health, 91*(5), 701–703.

Beck, C.T., & Gable, R.K. (2001). Further validation of the postpartum depression screening scale. *Nursing Research, 50*(3), 155–164.

Behrman, R., & Stith-Butler, A. (Eds.). (2007). *Preterm birth: Causes, consequences, and prevention.* Washington, DC: National Academies Press.

Bellamy, C. (2004). Globalization and infectious diseases in women. *Emerging Infectious Diseases, 10*(11), 2022–2024.

Ben-Shlomo, & Kuh, D. (2002). A life course approach to chronic disease epidemiology: Conceptual models, empirical challenges and interdisciplinary perspectives. *International Journal of Epidemiology, 31,* 285–293.

Bennett, H., Einarson, A., Taddio, A., et al. (2004). Depression during pregnancy: Overview of clinical factors. *Clinical Drug Investigations, 24*(3), 157–179.

Berg, C., Harper, M., Atkinson, S., et al. (2005). Preventability of pregnancy-related deaths: Results of a statewide review. *Obstetrics & Gynecology, 106*(6), 1228–1234.

Bernard, S., Paulozzi, L., Wallace, D., & Centers for Disease Control and Prevention (CDC). (2007, May). Fatal injuries among children by race and ethnicity—United States, 1999–2002. *MMWR Surveillance Summary 18, 56*(5), 1–16.

Black, M., Dubowitz, H., Krishnakumar, A., & Starr, R. (2007). Early intervention and recovery among children with failure to thrive: Follow-up at age 8. *Pediatrics, 120*(1), 59–69.

Blizzard, L., Ponsonby, A., Dwyer, T., et al. (2003). Parental smoking and infant respiratory infection: How important is not smoking in the same room with the baby? *American Journal of Public Health, 93*(3), 482–488.

Block, R., Krebs, N., & the Committee on Child Abuse & Neglect & the Committee on Nutrition. (2005). Failure to thrive as a manifestation of child neglect. *Pediatrics, 116*(5), 1234–1237.

Boden, J.M., Fergusson, D.M., & Horwood, L.J. (2008). Cigarette smoking and suicidal behaviour: results from a 25-year longitudinal study. *Psychological Medicine, 38*(3), 433–439.

Boggess, K., & Society for Maternal-Fetal Medicine Publications Committee. (2008). Maternal oral health in pregnancy. *Obstetrics & Gynecology, 111*(4), 976–986.

Bonnier, C. (2008). Evaluation of early stimulation programs for enhancing brain development. *Acta Paediatrica, 97*(7), 853–858.

Boucher, N., Bairam, A., & Beaulac-Baillargeon, L. (2008). A new look at the neonate's clinical presentation after in utero exposure to antidepressants in late pregnancy. *Journal of Clinical Psychopharmacology, 28*(3), 334–339.

Brenner, R., Trumble, A., Smith, G., Kessler, E., & Overpeck, M. (2001). Where children drown, United States, 1995. *Pediatrics, 108*(1), 85–89.

Briggs, M.M., Hopman, W.M., & Jamieson, M.A. (2007). Comparing pregnancy in adolescents and adults: Obstetric outcomes and prevalence of anemia. *Journal of Obstetrics and Gynaecology Canada, 29*(7), 546–555.

Briefel, R., Hanson, C., Fox, M., et al. (2006). Feeding Infants and Toddlers Study: Do vitamin and mineral supplements contribute to nutrient adequacy or excess among US infants and toddlers? *Journal of the American Dietetic Association, 106*[1 Suppl. 1], S52–S65.

Brier, N. (2004). Anxiety after miscarriage: A review of the empirical literature and implications for clinical practice. *Birth, 31*(2), 138–142.

Brier, N. (2008). Grief following miscarriage: A comprehensive review of the literature. *Journal of Women's Health, 17*(3), 451–464.

Brodribb, W., Fallon, A., Hegney, D., & O'Brien, M. (2007). Identifying predictors of the reasons women give for choosing to breastfeed. *Journal of Human Lactation, 23*(4), 338–344.

Cacciatore, J., & Bushfield, S. (2007). Stillbirth: The mother's experience and implications for improving care. *Journal of Social Work in End-of-Life & Palliative Care, 3*(3), 59–79.

Callister, L. (2006). Perinatal loss: A family perspective. *Journal of Perinatal & Neonatal Nursing, 20*(3), 227–234.

Canadian Diabetes Association. (2003). *Are wheat and cow's milk triggers for Type 1 diabetes?* [News release.] Retrieved August 18, 2008 from http://www.diabetes.ca/section_main/NewsReleases.asp?ID=85.

Centers for Disease Control & Prevention (CDC). (2008e). *Statistics and surveillance: Immunization coverage in the in U.S.* Retrieved October 14, 2008 from http://www.cdc.gov/vaccines/stats-surv/imz-coverage.htm

Centers for Disease Control & Prevention (CDC). (2005a). *Preventing lead poisoning in young children.* Atlanta, GA: Author.

Centers for Disease Control & Prevention (CDC). (2005b). *Basic facts about birth defects.* Retrieved August 18, 2008 from http://www.cdc.gov/ncbddd/bd/facts.htm.

Centers for Disease Control & Prevention (CDC). (2006a). *Pregnancy Risk Assessment Monitoring System (PRAMS): PRAMS and unintended pregnancy.* Retrieved August 18, 2008 from http://www.cdc.gov/PRAMS/UP.htm.

Centers for Disease Control & Prevention (CDC). (2006b). *2002 PRAMS surveillance report. Multi-state exhibits, prenatal care counseling: Smoking during pregnancy.* Retrieved August 18, 2008 from http://www.cdc.gov/PRAMS/2002PRAMSSurvReport/MultiStateExhibits/Multistates4.htm.

Centers for Disease Control & Prevention (CDC). (2007a). *Pregnancy Risk Assessment Monitoring System (PRAMS): Home.* Retrieved August 18, 2008 from http://www.cdc.org/PRAMS/index.htm.

Centers for Disease Control & Prevention (CDC). (2007b). *Child passenger safety: Fact sheet.* Retrieved August 18, 2008 from http://www.cdc.gov/ncipc/factsheets/childpas.htm.

Centers for Disease Control & Prevention (CDC). (2008a). *STDs & pregnancy: CDC fact sheet.* Retrieved August 18, 2008 from http://www.cdc.gov/STD/STDFactSTDs&Pregnancy. htm#Common.

Centers for Disease Control & Prevention (CDC). (2008b). *Sudden infant death syndrome (SIDS): Home.* Retrieved August 18, 2008 from http://www.cdc.gov/SIDS/index.htm.

Centers for Disease Control & Prevention (CDC). (2008c). Nonfatal maltreatment of infants: United States, October 2005–September 2006. *Morbidity and Mortality Weekly Report, 57*(13), 336–339.

Centers for Disease Control & Prevention (CDC). (2008d). *Recommended immunization schedule for persons aged 0–6 years, United States 2008.* Retrieved August 18, 2008 from http:// www.cdc.gov/vaccines/recs/schedules.

Centers for Disease Control & Prevention (CDC). (2008e). *Statistics and surveillance: Immunization coverage in the U.S.* Retrieved October 14, 2008 from http://www.cdc.gov/vaccines/ stats-surv/imz-coverage.htm.

Chambliss, L.R. (2008). Intimate partner violence and its implication for pregnancy. *Clinical Obstetrics & Gynecology, 51*(2), 385–397.

Chang, J., Berg, C., Saltzman, L., & Herndon, J. (2005). Homicide: A leading cause of injury deaths among pregnant and postpartum women in the United States, 1991–1999. *American Journal of Public Health, 95*(3), 471–477.

Chang, J., Elam-Evans, L., Berg, C., et al. (2003). Pregnancy-related mortality surveillance: United States, 1991–1999. *Morbidity and Mortality Weekly Report, Surveillance Summaries, 52*(SS–2), 1–12.

Chasnoff, I.J., Neuman, K., Thornton, C., & Callaghan, M.A. (2001). Screening for substance use in pregnancy: A practical approach for the primary care physician. *American Journal of Obstetrics and Gynecology, 184,* 752–758.

Chen, A., Schwarz, D., Radcliffe, J., & Rogan, W. (2006). Maternal IQ, child IQ, behavior, and achievement in urban 5–7 year olds. *Pediatric Research, 59*(3), 471–477.

Chen, X., Wen, S., Fleming, N., et al. (2007). Teenage pregnancy and adverse birth outcomes: A large population-based retrospective cohort study. *International Journal of Epidemiology, 36*(2), 368–373.

Child Trends. (2004). *Preschool and pre-kindergarten programs.* Retrieved August 18, 2008 from http://www.childtrendsdatabank. org/indicators/103prekindergarten.cfm.

Child Trends. (April 2006a). *Facts at a glance: Teen birth rate.* [Publication # 2006–03]. Washington, DC: Author.

Child Trends. (2006b). *Child care.* Retrieved August 18, 2008 from http://www.childtrendsdatabank.org/indicators/21ChildCare.cfm.

Child Trends Databank. (2006). *Low and very low birthweight infants.* Retrieved August 18, 2008 from http://www. childtrendsdatabank.org/pdf/57_PDF.pdf.

Child Welfare Information Gateway. (2004). *About CAPTA: A legislative history factsheet.* Retrieved August 18, 2008 from http://www.childwelfare.gov/pubs/factsheets.about.cfm.

Chouinard, M.M. (2007). Children's questions: A mechanism for cognitive development. *Monographs of the Society for Research in Child Development, 72*(1), vii–ix, 1–112; discussion 113–126.

Cockcroft, A., Andersson, N., Milne, D., et al. (2007). Community views about routine HIV testing and antiretroviral treatment in Botswana: Signs of progress from a cross sectional study. *BMC: International Health & Human Rights, 7,* 5.

Committee on Infectious Diseases. (2008). Prevention of influenza: Recommendations for influenza immunization of children, 2007–2008. *Pediatrics, 121*(4), 1016–1031.

Cornelius, M., Goldschmidt, L., DeGenna, N., & Day, N. (2007). Smoking during teenage pregnancies: Effects on behavioral problems in offspring. *Nicotine & Tobacco Research, 9*(7), 739–750.

Courchesne, E., Pierce, K., Schumann, C., et al. (2007). Mapping early brain development in autism. *Neuron, 56*(2), 399–413.

Cumming, G., Klein, S., Bolsover, D., et al. (2007). The emotional burden of miscarriage for women and their partners: Trajectories of anxiety and depression over 13 months. *BJOG: British Journal of Obstetrics & Gynecology, 114*(9), 1139–1145.

Darroch, J., Singh, S., & Frost, J. (2001). Differences in teenage pregnancy rates among five developed countries: The roles of sexual activity and contraceptive use. *Family Planning Perspectives, 33*(6), 244–250, 281.

Dallas, C. (2004). Family matters: How mothers of adolescent parents experience adolescent pregnancy and parenting. *Public Health Nursing, 21*(4), 347–353.

D'Angelo, D., Williams, L., Morrow, B., et al. (2008). Preconception and interconception health status of women who recently gave birth to a live-born infant: Pregnancy Risk Assessment Monitoring System (PRAMS), United States, 26 reporting areas, 2004. *Morbidity and Mortality Weekly Report, Surveillance Summaries, 56*(10), 1–35.

Dasanayake, A., Gennaro, S., Hendricks-Munoz, K., & Chun, N. (2008). Maternal periodontal disease, pregnancy, and neonatal outcomes. *MCN: American Journal of Maternal & Child Nursing, 33*(1), 45–49.

Davenport, M., Mottola, M., McManus, R. & Gratton, R. (2008). A walking intervention improves capillary glucose control in women with gestational diabetes mellitus: A pilot project. *Applied Physiology, Nutrition & Metabolism, 33*(3), 511–517.

Day, N., Goldschmidt, L., & Thomas, C. (2006). Prenatal marijuana exposure contributes to the prediction of marijuana use at age 14. *Addiction, 101*(9), 1313–1322.

De Genna, N., Cornelius, M., & Cook, R. (2007). Marijuana use and sexually transmitted infections in young women who were teenage mothers. *Women's Health Issues, 17*(5), 300–309.

Del Boca, F., & Darkes, J. (2003). The validity of self-reports of alcohol consumption: State of the science and challenges for research. *Addiction, 98*[Suppl. 2], 1–12.

deMoraes-Barros, M., Guinsburg, R., deAraujo-Peres, C., et al. (2006). Exposure to marijuana during pregnancy alters neurobehavior in the early neonatal period. *Journal of Pediatrics, 149*(6), 781–787.

Dopkins-Stright, A., Cranley-Gallagher, K., & Kelley, K. (2008). Infant temperament moderates relations between maternal parenting in early childhood and children's adjustment in first grade. *Child Development, 79*(1), 186–200.

Douglass, J., Douglass, A., & Silk, H. (2004). A practical guide to infant oral health. *American Family Physician, 70*(11), 2113–2120.

Dowshen, S. (January 2008). *FDA officially nixes cough and cold meds for babies and toddlers.* Rady Children's Hospital of San Diego. Retrieved August 18, 2008 from http://kidshealth.org/ PageManager.jsp?dn=chsd&article_set=59678&lic= 102&cat_id=5.

Duncan, C. (2002). Smoking and pregnancy: An update. *Women and Reproductive Nutrition Report, 3*(2), 1–3.

Durbin, W., & Stille, C. (2008). Pneumonia. *Pediatrics in Review, 29,* 147–160.

Duursma, E., Augustyn, M., & Zuckerman, B. (May 2008). Reading aloud to children: The evidence. *Archives of Disease in Childhood,* doi:10.1136/adc.2006.106336.

Dykes, F., Moran, V., Burt, S., & Edwards, J. (2003). Adolescent mothers and breastfeeding: Experiences and support needs: An exploratory study. *Journal of Human Lactation, 19*(4), 391–401.

Ehiri, J., Ejere, H., Magnussen, L., et al. (2006). Interventions for promoting booster seat use in four to eight year olds traveling in motor vehicles. *Cochrane Database of Systematic Reviews.* Retrieved August 18, 2008 from http://www.cochrane.org/ reviews/en/ab004334.html.

Emond, A., Blair, P., Emmett, P., & Drewett, R. (2007). Weight faltering in infancy and IQ levels at 8 years in the Avon Longitudinal Study of Parents and Children. *Pediatrics, 120*(4), E1051–E1058.

Emory University. (2007, April/May). Take the genetic challenge: Test your knowledge of clinical genetics. *Emory Genetics Newsletter Fax.* Retrieved August 15, 2008 from http://www.genetics.emory.edu/newsletter/files/newsletter63.pdf.

Feinberg, M., & Kan, M. (2008). Establishing family foundations: Intervention effects on coparenting, parent/infant well-being, and parent-child relations. *Journal of Family Psychology, 22*(2), 253–263.

Feldman, M., Case, L., Towns, F., & Betel, J. (1985). Parent Education Project. I: Development and nurturance of children of mentally retarded parents. *American Journal of Mental Deficiency, 90*(3), 253–258.

Feldman, M., Ducharme, J., & Case, L. (1999). Using self-instructional pictorial manuals to teach child-care skills to mothers with intellectual disabilities. *Behavior Modification, 23*(3), 480–497.

Feldman, M., & Walton-Allen, N. (1997). Effects of maternal mental retardation and poverty on intellectual, academic, and behavioral status of school-age children. *American Journal of Mental Retardation, 101*(4), 352–364.

Ferguson, J., Hansen, W., Novak, K., & Novak, M. (2007). Should we treat periodontal disease during gestation to improve pregnancy outcomes? *Clinical Obstetrics & Gynecology, 50*(2), 454–467.

Flynn, L., Budd, M., & Modelski, J. (2008). Enhancing resource utilization among pregnant adolescents. *Public Health Nursing, 25*(2), 140–148.

Forsen, T., Eriksson, J., Osmond, C., & Barker, D. (2004). The infant growth of boys who later develop coronary heart disease. *Annals of Medicine, 36*(5), 389–392.

Forum on Child & Family Statistics. (2007). *America's children: Key national indicators of well-being, 2007: Adolescent births.* Retrieved August 18, 2008 from http://www.childstats.gov/americaschildren/famsoc6.asp.

Foster, H., & Fitzgerald, J. (2005). Dental disease in children with chronic illness: Community child health, public health, and epidemiology. *Archives of Disease in Childhood, 90*(7), 703–708.

Fox, M., Reidy, K., Karwe, V., & Ziegler, P. (2006). Average portions of foods commonly eaten by infants and toddlers in the United States. *Journal of the American Dietetic Association, 106*[1 Suppl. 1], S66–S76.

Fox, M., Reidy, K., Novak, T., & Ziegler, P. (2006). Sources of energy and nutrients in the diets of infants and toddlers. *Journal of the American Dietetic Association, 106*[1 Suppl. 1], S28–S42.

Freeman, R., & Stevens, A. (2008). Nursing caries and buying time: An emerging theory of prolonged bottle feeding. *Community Dental & Oral Epidemiology*, doi: 10.1111/j.1600-0528.2008.00425.x.

Fries, A., Ziegler, T., Kurian, J., et al. (2005). Early experience in humans is associated with changes in neuropeptides critical for regulating social behavior. *Proceedings of the National Academy of Sciences, 102*(47), 17237–17240.

Gaines, C., Jenkins, S., & Ashe, W. (2005). Empowering nursing faculty and students for community service. *Journal of Nursing Education, 44*(11), 522–525.

Garces, E., Thomas, D., & Currie, J. (2002). Longer-term effects of Head Start. *The American Economic Review, 92*(4), 999–1012.

Gavard, J., & Artal, R. (2008). Effect of exercise on pregnancy outcome. *Clinical Obstetrics & Gynecology, 51*(2), 467–480.

Georgieff, M.K. (2007). Nutrition and the developing brain: Nutrient priorities and measurement. *American Journal of Clinical Nutrition, 85*(2), S14–S20.

Gillman, S., Breslau, J., Subramanian, S., et al. (2008). Social factors, psychopathology, and maternal smoking during pregnancy. *American Journal of Public Health, 98*(3), 448–453.

Gillman, M., Rifas-Shiman, S., Berkey, C., et al. (2003). Maternal gestational diabetes, birth weight, and adolescent obesity. *Pediatrics, 111*(3), E221–E226.

Gilmore, J., Lin, W., & Gerig, G. (2006). Fetal and neonatal brain development. *American Journal of Psychiatry, 163*(12), 2046.

Glascoe, F.P. (2000). Detecting and addressing developmental and behavioral problems in primary care. *Pediatric Nursing, 26*(3), 251–257.

Goldman, A., Hopkinson, J., & Rassin, D. (2007). Benefits and risks of breastfeeding. *Advances in Pediatrics, 54*, 275–304.

Goldman, J., Salus, M., Wolcott, D., & Kennedy, K. (2003). *A coordinated response to child abuse and neglect: The foundation for practice.* USDHHS. Washington, DC: U.S. Government Printing Office.

Graham, W., & Hussein, J. (2006). Universal reporting of maternal mortality: An achievable goal? *International Journal of Gynecology & Obstetrics, 94*, 234–242.

Greene, W.C. (2007). A history of AIDS: Looking back to see ahead. *European Journal of Immunology, 37*[Suppl. 1], S94–S102.

Grijalva, C., Poehling, K., Nuorti, J., et al. (2006). National impact of universal childhood immunization with pneumonococcal conjugate vaccine on outpatient medical care visits in the United States. *Pediatrics,118*(3), 865–873.

Gross, S.D., Boyle, C.A., Botkin, J.R., et al. (2004). Newborn screening for Cystic Fibrosis: Evaluation of benefits and risks and recommendations for state newborn screening programs. *Morbidity and Mortality Weekly Report, 53*(RR13).

Grossman, N.B. (2004). Blunt trauma in pregnancy. *American Family Physician, 70*(7), 1303–1310.

Grossman, T., & Johnson, M. (2007). The development of the social brain in human infancy. *European Journal of Neuroscience, 25*(4), 909–919.

Gudmundsdottir, M., & Chesla, C. (2006). Building a new world: Habits and practices of healing following the death of a child. *Journal of Family Nursing, 12*(2), 143–164.

Gupta, P.C., & Sreevidya, S. (2004). Smokeless tobacco use, birth weight, and gestational age: Population-based, prospective cohort study of 1217 women in Mumbai, India. *BMJ: British Medical Journal, 328*, 1538–1542.

Gurian, A. (n.d.). *Parenting styles/children's temperaments: The match.* New York University Child Study Center. Retrieved August 18, 2008 from http://www.aboutourkids.org/articles/parenting_styleschildren039s_temperaments_match?print=1.

Gutierrez, F., Clements, P., & Averill, J. (2004). Shaken baby syndrome: Assessment, intervention & prevention. *Journal of Psychosocial Nursing & Mental Health Services, 42*(12), 22–29.

Guyer, B., Ma, S., Grason, H., et al. (2008). *Investments to promote children's health: A systematic literature review and economic analysis of interventions in the preschool period.* Baltimore, MD: Johns Hopkins Bloomberg School of Public Health.

Haire-Joshu, D., Elliott, M., Caito, N., et al. (2008). High 5 for kids: The impact of a home visiting program on fruit and vegetable intake of parents and their preschool children. *American Journal of Preventive Medicine*, Epub ahead of print, PubMed PMID: 18486203.

Hale, R.W. (2006). Legal issues impacting women's access to care in the United States: The malpractice insurance crisis. *International Journal of Gynecology & Obstetrics, 94*, 382–385.

Hale, K.J., & American Academy of Pediatrics Section on Pediatric Dentistry. (2003). Oral health risk assessment timing and establishment of the dental home. *Pediatrics, 111*(5 pt 1), 1113–1116.

Hamilton, B., Minino, A., Martin, J., et al. (2007). Annual summary of vital statistics: 2005. *Pediatrics, 119*, 345–360.

Hamilton, B., Martin, J., Ventura, S., et al. (2005). Births: Preliminary data for 2004. *National Vital Statistics Reports, 54*(8). Hyattsville, MD: National Center for Health Statistics.

Hankin, J., McCaul, M., & Heussner, J. (2000). Pregnant, alcohol-abusing women. *Alcoholism: Clinical and Experimental Research, 24,* 1276–1286.

Hanna, B. (2001). Negotiating motherhood: the struggles of teenage mothers, *Journal of Advanced Nursing, 34*(4), 456–464.

Harris, N., Fowler, M., Sansom, L., et al. (2007). Use of enhanced perinatal human immunodeficiency virus surveillance methods to assess antiretroviral use and perinatal human immunodeficiency virus transmission in the United States, 1999–2001. *American Journal of Obstetrics & Gynecology, 197*[3 Suppl.], S33–S41.

Harris, S., & Handleman, J. (2000). Age and IQ at intake as predictors of placement for young children with autism: A four- to six-year follow up. *Journal of Autism & Developmental Disorders, 30,* 137–142.

Heo, M., Murphy, C., Fontaine, K., et al. (2008). Population projection of U.S. adults with lifetime experience of depressive disorder by age and sex from year 2005 to 2050. *International Journal of Geriatric Psychiatry*, doi: 10.1002/gps.2061.

Hertz-Picciotto, I., Baker, R., Yap, P., et al. (2007). Early childhood lower respiratory illness and air pollution. *Environmental Health Perspectives, 115*(19), 1510–1518.

Hessol, N., & Fuentes-Afflick, E. (2005). Ethnic differences in neonatal and postneonatal mortality. *Pediatrics, 115*(1), E44–E51.

Hobbell, C., Goldstein, A., & Barrett, E. (2008). Psychosocial stress and pregnancy outcome. *Clinical Obstetrics & Gynecology, 51*(2), 333–348.

Hofmeyr, G., Atallah, A., & Duley, L. (2005). Calcium supplementation during pregnancy for preventing hypertensive disorders and related problems. *Cochrane Database of Systematic Reviews.* Retrieved August 18, 2008 from http://www.cochrane.org/reviews/en/ab001059.html.

Holub, C., Kershaw, T., Ethier, K., et al. (2007). Prenatal and parenting stress on adolescent maternal adjustment: Identifying a high-risk subgroup. *Maternal Child Health Journal, 11*(2), 153–159.

Horton, S., & Barker, J. (2008). Rural Latino immigrant caregivers' conceptions of their children's oral disease. *Journal of Public Health Dentistry, 68*(1), 22–29.

House, S.H. (2007). Nurturing the brain nutritionally and emotionally from before conception to late adolescence. *Nutrition & Health, 19*(1–2), 143–161.

Hoyme, H., May, P., Kalberg, W., et al. (2005). A practical clinical approach to diagnosis of fetal alcohol spectrum disorders: Clarification of the 1996 Institute of Medicine criteria. *Pediatrics, 115*(1), 39–47.

Hudson, D., Campbell-Grossman, C., Keating-Lefler, R., & Cline, P. (2008). *Issues in Comprehensive Pediatric Nursing, 31*(1), 23–35.

Hunt, R., Tzioumi, D., Collins, E., & Jeffery, H. (2008). Adverse neurodevelopmental outcome of infants exposed to opiate in-utero. *Early Human Development, 84*(1), 29–35.

International Save the Children Alliance. (2008). *Three years on from the tsunami: Rebuilding lives: Children's road to recovery.* London, UK: Author.

Ip, S., Chung, M., Raman, G., et al. (April 2007). *Breastfeeding and maternal and infant health outcomes in developed countries.* Evidence Report/Technology Assessment No. 153. AHRQ Publication No. 07-E0007. Rockville, MD: Agency for Healthcare Research and Quality.

Istre, G., McCoy, M., Carlin, D., & McClain, J. (2002). Residential fire-related deaths and injuries among children: fireplay, smoke alarms, and prevention. *Injury Prevention, 8,* 128–132.

Ito, T., Tomita, T., Hasui, C., et al. (2003). The link between response styles and major depression and anxiety disorders after child-loss. *Comprehensive Psychiatry, 44*(5), 396–403.

Jacobson, J., Goldstein, I., Canfield, S., et al. (2008). Early respiratory infections and asthma among New York City Head Start children. *Journal of Asthma, 45*(4), 301–308.

Janssen, P., Holt, V., Sugg, N., et al. (2003). Intimate partner violence and adverse pregnancy outcomes: A population-based study. *American Journal of Obstetrics & Gynecology, 188*(5), 1341–1347.

Jeppson, J., & Myers-Walls, J. (2003). *Brain development.* West Fayetteville, IN: Purdue University.

Johnson, R., Browne, K., & Hamilton-Giachritsis, C. (2006). Young children in institutional care at risk of harm. *Trauma Violence & Abuse, 7*(1), 34–60.

Jones, K., Daley, D., Hutchings, J., et al. (2007). Efficacy of the Incredible Years Basic Parent Training Programme as an early intervention for children with conduct problems and ADHD. *Child Care, Health & Development, 33*(6), 749–756.

Jones, K., Daley, D., Hutchings, J., et al. (2008). Efficacy of the Incredible Years Programme as an early intervention for children with conduct problems and ADHD: Long-term follow-up. *Child Care, Health & Development, 34*(3), 380–390.

Kable, J., Coles, C., Lynch, M., & Platzman, K. (2008). Physiological responses to social and cognitive challenges in 8-year olds with a history of prenatal cocaine exposure. *Developmental Psychobiology, 50*(3), 251–265.

Kahlert, C., Rudin, C., Kind, C., et al. (2007). Sudden infant death syndrome in infants born to HIV-infected and opiate-using mothers. *Archives of Diseases in Children, 92*(11), 1005–1008.

Kaminski, J., Vale, L., Filene, J., & Boyle, C. (2008). A meta-analytic review of components associated with parent training program effectiveness. *Journal of Abnormal Child Psychology, 36*(4), 567–589.

Kaplan, D., & Graff, K. (2008). Marketing breastfeeding: Reversing corporate influence on infant feeding practices. *Journal of Urban Health*, doi: 10.1007/s11524-008-9279-6.

Karch, D., Lubell, K., Friday, J., et al. (2008). Surveillance for violent deaths: National Violent Death Reporting System, 16 states, 2005. *Morbidity and Mortality Weekly Report, Surveillance Summaries, 57*(SS03), 1–43, 45.

Kaskutas, L.A. (2000). Understanding drinking during pregnancy among urban American Indians and African Americans: Health messages, risk beliefs, and how we measure consumption. *Alcoholism: Clinical and Experimental Research, 24*(8), 1241–1250.

Katzen-Luchenta, J. (2007). The declaration of nutrition, health, and intelligence for the child-to-be. *Nutrition & Health, 19*(1–2), 85–102.

Kemp, J., Unger, B., Wilkins, D., et al. (2000). Unsafe sleep practices and analysis of bedsharing among infants dying suddenly and unexpectedly: results of a four-year, population-based, death-scene investigation study of sudden infant death syndrome and related deaths. *Pediatrics, 106*(3), E41.

Kershaw, T., Niccolai, L., Ickovics, J., et al. (2003). Short and long-term impact of adolescent pregnancy on postpartum contraceptive use: Implications for prevention of repeat pregnancy. *Journal of Adolescent Health, 33*(5), 359–368.

Kimm, S., & Obarzanek, E. (2002). Childhood obesity: A new pandemic of the new millennium. *Pediatrics, 110*(5), 1003–1007.

Klassen, T., Kiddoo, D., Lang, M., et al. (2006). The effectiveness of different methods of toilet training for bowel and bladder control. *Evidence Report/Technology Assessment, 147,* 1–57.

Klein, M., Bergel, E., Gibbons, L., et al. (2008). Differential gender response to respiratory infections and to the protective effect of breast milk in preterm infants. *Pediatrics, 121*(6), E1510–E1516.

Kleinman, R.E. (2000). Complementary feeding and later health. *Pediatrics, 106*(5), 1287–1291.

Klima, C.S. (2003). Centering pregnancy: A model for pregnant adolescents. *Journal of Midwifery & Women's Health, 48*(3), 220–225.

Koniack-Griffin, D., Anderson, N.L.R., Brecht, M.L., et al. (2002). Public health nursing care for adolescent mothers: Impact on infant health and selected maternal outcomes at 1 year post-birth. *Journal of Adolescent Health, 30,* 44–54.

Koniack-Griffin, D., Anderson, N.L.R., Verzemnieks, I., & Brecht, M.L. (2000). A public health nursing early intervention program for adolescent mothers: Outcomes from pregnancy through 6 weeks postpartum. *Nursing Research, 49,* 130–138.

Koniack-Griffin, D., Verzemnieks, I.L., Anderson, N.L.R., et al. (2003). Nurse visitation for adolescent mothers: Two-year infant health and maternal outcomes. *Nursing Research, 52*(2), 127–136.

Kotch, J., Lewis, T., Hussey, J., et al. (2008). Importance of early neglect for childhood aggression. *Pediatrics, 121*(4), 725–731.

Krugman, S., & Dubowitz, H. (2003). Failure to thrive. *American Family Physician, 68*(5), 879–884, 886.

Krugman, S., Lane, W., & Walsh, C. (2007). Update on child abuse prevention. *Current Opinions in Pediatrics, 19*(6), 711–718.

Kuczkowski, K.M. (2007). The effects of drug abuse on pregnancy. *Current Opinions in Obstetrics & Gynecology, 19*(6), 578–585.

Kumpfer, K., & Fowler, M. (2007). Parenting skills and family support programs for drug-abusing mothers. *Seminar in Fetal & Neonatal Medicine, 12*(2), 134–142.

Kupper, L. (2005). *Finding help for young children with disabilities (birth-5).* Washington, DC: NICHCY.

Kusel, M., de Klerk, N., Holt, P., et al. (2007). Occurrence and management of acute respiratory illnesses in early childhood. *Journal of Paediatrics & Child Health, 43*(3), 139–146.

Kwok, M., Vazquez, H., & Isaacman, D. (May 23, 2006). *Fever in the toddler.* Retrieved August 18, 2008 from http://www.emedeicine.com/ped/topic3009.htm.

Labbok, M. (2006). Breastfeeding: A woman's reproductive right. *International Journal of Gynecology & Obstetrics, 94,* 277–286.

Lahr, M., Rosenberg, K., & Lapidus, J. (2005). Bedsharing and maternal smoking in a population-based survey of new mothers. *Pediatrics, 116*(4), E530–E542.

Lamb, E.H. (2002). The impact of previous perinatal loss on subsequent pregnancy and parenting. *Journal of Perinatal Education, 11*(2), 33–40.

Law, C., Shiell, A., Newsome, C., et al. (2002). Fetal, infant, and childhood growth and adult blood pressure. *Circulation, 105,* 1088–1092.

Lee, H., Jang, H., Park, H., et al. (2008). Prevalence of type 2 diabetes among women with a previous history of gestational diabetes mellitus. *Diabetes: Research & Clinical Practice, 81*(1), 124–129.

Letourneau, R., Crump, C., Bowling, J., et al. (2008). Ride Safe: A child passenger safety program for American Indian/Alaska Native children. *Maternal Child Health Journal,* Epub ahead of print, PubMed, PMID: 18340516.

Levac, A., McCay, E., Merka, P., & Reddon-D'Arcy, M. (2008). Exploring parent participation in a parent training program for children's aggression: Understanding and illuminating mechanisms of change. *Journal of Child & Adolescent Psychiatric Nursing, 21*(2), 78–88.

Lewallen, L., Dick, M., Flowers, J., et al. (2006). Breastfeeding support and early cessation. *Journal of Obstetrical, Gynecological, & Neonatal Nursing, 35*(2), 166–172.

Lloyd, S.L. (2004). Pregnant adolescent reflections of parental communication. *Journal of Community Health Nursing, 21*(4), 239–250.

Love, J., Tarullo, L., Raikes, H., & Chazan-Cohen, R. (2006). Head Start: What do we know about its effectiveness? What do we need to know? In K. McCartney, & D. Phillips (Eds.). *Blackwell handbook of early childhood development.* (pp. 550–575). Malden, MA: Blackwell Publishing.

MacDorman, M.F., Minino, A.M., Strobino, D.M., & Guyer, B. (2002). Annual summary of vital statistics: 2001. *Pediatrics, 110*(6), 1037–1052.

Manning, M., & Eugene-Hoyme, H. (2007). Fetal alcohol spectrum disorders: A practical clinical approach to diagnosis. *Neuroscience & Biobehavioral Reviews, 31*(2), 230–238.

March of Dimes (2008). *Databook for policymakers: Maternal, infant and child health in the United States 2008.* Washington, DC: Author.

March of Dimes. (2005a). *Professionals & researchers quick reference & fact sheets: Low birthweight.* Retrieved August 18, 2008 from http://www.marchofdimes.com/printableArticles/14332_1153.asp.

March of Dimes. (2005b). *Professionals & researchers quick reference & fact sheets: Stillbirth.* Retrieved August 18, 2008 from http://www.marchofdimes.com/printableArticles/14332_1198.asp.

Marinho, V., Higgins, J., Logan, S., & Sheiham, A. (2002). Fluoride varnishes for preventing dental caries in children and adolescents. *Cochrane Database of Systematic Reviews.* Retrieved August 18, 2008 from http://www.cochrane.org/reviews/en/ab002279.html.

Martin, R., Gunnel, D., & Davey-Smith, G. (2005). Breastfeeding in infancy and blood pressure in later life: Systematic review and meta-analysis. *American Journal of Epidemiology, 161*(1), 15–26.

Maschi, S., Clavenna, A., Campi, R., et al. (2008). Neonatal outcome following pregnancy exposure to antidepressants: A prospective controlled cohort study. *BJOG: British Journal of Obstetrics & Gynecology, 115*(2), 283–289.

Matchaba, P., & Moodley, J. (2004). More research is needed to determine if corticosteroids can improve outcomes for women and babies affected by HELLP syndrome in pregnancy. *Cochrane Database of Systematic Reviews.* Retrieved August 18, 2008 from http://www.cochrane.org/reviews/en/ab002076.html.

Maternal Child Health Bureau (MCHB). (2006). *Maternal & child health: A profile of Healthy Start: Findings from phase I of the evaluation 2006.* Health Resources & Services Administration. Retrieved August 18, 2008 from http://mchb.hrsa.gov/healthystart/phase1report/.

Maternal Child Health Bureau (MCHB). (2008). *Historical timeline.* Health Resources and Services Administration. Retrieved August 18, 2008 from http://www.mchb.hrsa.gov/timeline/.

Mayberry, L., Horowitz, J., & Declercq, E. (2007). Depression symptoms prevalence and demographic risk factors among U.S. women during the first 2 years postpartum. *Journal of Obstetrical, Gynecological & Neonatal Nursing, 36*(6), 542–549.

Mayer, R., Anastasi, J., & Clark, E. (2006). *What to expect & when to seek help: A Bright Futures developmental tool for families and providers.* Washington, DC: National Technical Assistance Center for Children's Mental Health, Georgetown University Center for Child & Human Development, in collaboration with the National Center for Education in Maternal & Child Health.

Mayes, L., Snyder, P., Langlois, E., & Hunter, N. (2007). Visuospatial working memory in school-aged children exposed in utero to cocaine. *Child Neuropsychology, 13*(3), 205–218.

McCann, M., Baydar, N., & Williams, R. (2007). Breastfeeding attitudes and reported problems in a national sample of WIC participants. *Journal of Human Lactation, 23*(4), 314–324.

McCaskill, Q., Livingood, W., Crawford, P., et al. (2008). Immunization levels among inner city children enrolled in subsidized childcare. *Journal of Healthcare for the Poor & Underserved, 19*(2), 596–610.

McDonald, S., Vermeulen, M., & Ray, J. (2007). Risk of fetal death associated with maternal drug dependence and placental abruption: A population-based study. *Journal of Obstetrics & Gynaecology Canada, 29*(7), 556–559.

Meads, C., Cnossen, J., Meher, S., et al. (2008). Methods of prediction and prevention of preeclampsia: Systematic reviews of accuracy and effectiveness literature with economic modeling. *Health & Technology Assessment, 12*(6), 1–270.

Mehta, S. (2006). The AIDS pandemic: A catalyst for women's rights. *International Journal of Gynecology & Obstetrics, 94,* 317–324.

Melnyk, B., Alpert-Gillis, L., Feinstein, N., et al. (2004). Creating opportunities for parent empowerment: Programs effects on the mental health/coping outcomes of critically ill young children and their mothers. *Pediatrics, 113*(6), E597–E607.

Melnyk, B., Feinstein, N., Alpert-Gillis, L., et al. (2007). Reducing premature infants' length of stay and improving parents' mental health outcomes with the Creating Opportunities for Parent Empowerment (COPE) neonatal intensive care unit program: A randomized, controlled trial. *Pediatrics, 118*(5), E1414–E1427.

Menacker, F. (2005, September 22). Trends in cesarean rates for first births and repeat cesarean rates for low-risk women: United States, 1990–2003. *National Vital Statistics Reports, 54*(4), 1–5.

Mercer, B., Merlino, A., Milluzzi, C., & Moore, J. (2008). Small fetal size before 20 weeks' gestation: Associations with maternal tobacco use, early preterm birth, and low birthweight. *American Journal of Obstetrics & Gynecology, 198*(6), 673–678.

Merson, M.H. (2006). The HIV-AIDS pandemic at 25: The global response. *New England Journal of Medicine, 354*(23), 2414–2417.

Mian, A.L. (2005). Depression in pregnancy and the postpartum period: Balancing adverse effects of untreated illness with treatment risks. *Journal of Psychiatric Practice, 11*(6), 389–396.

Michels, T.M. (2000). "Patients like us": Pregnant and parenting teens view the health care system. *Public Health Reports, 115*(6), 557–575.

Minkoff, H. (2003). Human immunodeficiency virus infection in pregnancy. *Obstetrics and Gynecology, 101*(4), 797–810.

Mondestin, M.A.J., Ananth, C.V., Smulian, J.C., & Vintzileos, A.M. (2002). Birth weight and fetal death in the United States: The effect of maternal diabetes during pregnancy. *American Journal of Obstetrics and Gynecology, 187*, 922–926.

Moran, V.H. (2007). A systematic review of dietary assessments of pregnant adolescents in industrialized countries. *British Journal of Nutrition, 97*(3), 411–425.

Morch, W., Skar, J., & Andersgard, A. (1997). Mentally-retarded persons as parents: Prevention & the situation of their children. *Scandinavian Journal of Psychology, 38*(4), 343–348.

Nadel, S. (Ed.). (2007). *Infectious diseases in the pediatric intensive care unit.* London, UK: Springer Publishing.

Nadel, S. (Ed.). (2008). *Infectious diseases in the pediatric intensive care unit.* London: Springer-Verlag.

Nannini, A., Lazar, J., Berg, C., et al. (2008). Physical injuries reported on hospital visits for assault during the pregnancy-associated period. *Nursing Research, 57*(3), 144–149.

National Center for Birth Defects & Developmental Disabilities. (2006). *Fetal alcohol spectrum disorders.* Retrieved August 18, 2008 from http://www.cdc.gov/ncbddd/fas/fasask.htm.

National Center for Health Statistics (NCHS). (2005). *NCHS data on infant and toddler health.* Retrieved August 18, 2008 from http://www.cdc.gov/nchs/data/factsheets/infanthlth.pdf.

National Clearinghouse on Families & Youth. (2007). *YES! Youth empowerment strategies for all working with pregnant and parenting youth.* Retrieved August 18, 2008 from http://wwwncfy.acf.hhs.gov/publications/esworkingparting.htm.

National Committee for Quality Assurance. (2006). HEDIS measures of perinatal care, by payer, 2001–05. *The state of health care quality 2006.* Washington, DC: Author.

National Dissemination Center for Children With Disabilities (NICHCY). (2002). *Disabilities that quality infants, toddlers, children, and youth for services under the IDEA.* Retrieved August 18, 2008 from http://www.nichcy.org/pubs/genresc/gr3.htm.

National Head Start Association. (2006). *Research bites: Head Start research.* Retrieved August 18, 2008 from http://www.nhsa.org/research/research_re_bites_detail.htm.

National Highway Traffic Safety Administration (NHTSA). (2006). *Traffic safety facts research note 2005: Misuse of child restraints.* Washington, DC: Author.

National Institute of Drug Abuse. (2006). *Women and drug abuse.* Retrieved August 18, 2008 from http://www.nida.niuh.gov/womendrugs/Women-DrugAbuse2.html.

National Institutes of Health. (2005). *Understanding postpartum depression: Common but treatable.* News In Health. Retrieved August 18, 2008 from http://newsinhealth.nih.gov/2005/December2005/docs/01features_02.htm.

National Institute of Child Health & Development (NICHD). Early Child Care Research Network. (2002). Early child care and children's development prior to school entry: Results from the NICHD study of early child care. *American Educational Research Journal, 39*(1), 133–164.

National Women's Health Information Center (NWHIC). (2005). *Frequently asked questions: Depression during and after pregnancy.* Retrieved August 18, 2008 from http://www.4woman.gov/gov/FAQ/postpartum.htm.

Nava-Ocampo, A., & Koren, G. (2007). Human teratogens and evidence-based teratogen risk counseling: The Motherisk approach. *Clinical Obstetrics & Gynecology, 50*(1), 123–131.

Neale, D., Cootauco, A., & Burrow, G. (2007). Thyroid disease in pregnancy. *Clinical Perinatology, 34*(4), 543–557.

Nelson, C., Zeanah, C., Fox, N., et al. (2007). Cognitive recovery in socially deprived young children: The Bucharest Early Intervention Project. *Science, 318*(5858), 1937–1940.

Nguyen, J., Carson, M., Parris, K., & Place, P. (2003). A comparison pilot study of public health field nursing home visitation program interventions for pregnant Hispanic adolescents. *Public Health Nursing, 20*(5), 412–418.

Nicholson, W., Wilson, L., Witkop, C., et al. (2008). Therapeutic management, delivery, and postpartum risk assessment and screening in gestational diabetes. *Evidence Report/Technology Assessment AHRQ, 162*, 1–96.

Nikcevi, A., Kuczmierczyk, A., & Nicolaides, K. (2007). The influence of medial and psychological interventions on women's distress after miscarriage. *Journal of Psychosomatic Research, 63*(3), 283–290.

Nitzkin, J., & Smith, S. (2004). *Clinical preventive services in substance abuse and mental health update: From science to services.* [DHHS Pub. No. (SMA) 04–3906]. Rockville, MD: Center for Mental Health Services, Substance Abuse and Mental Health Services Administration.

Norwitz, E., Hsu, C.D., & Repke, J. (2002). Acute complications of preeclampsia. *Clinical Obstetrics & Gynecology, 45*(2), 308–329.

Oberlander, T., Warburton, W., Misri, S., et al. (2008). Major congenital malformations following prenatal exposure to serotonin reuptake inhibitors and benzodiazepines using population-based health data. *Birth Defects Research B: Developmental & Reproductive Toxicology, 83*(1), 68–76.

O'Connor, K., & Bramlett, M. (2008). Vaccination coverage by special health care needs status in young children. *Pediatrics, 121*, E768–E774.

Office of Women's Health. (2005). *Benefits of breastfeeding.* USDHHS. Retrieved August 18, 2008 from http://www.4woman.gov/Breastfeeding/index.cfm?page=227.

Offit, P., & Jew, R. (2003). Addressing parents' concerns: Do vaccines contain harmful preservatives, adjuvants, additives or residuals? *Pediatrics, 112*, 1394–1397.

Oken, E., Wright, R., Kleinman, K., et al. (2005). Maternal fish consumption, hair mercury, and infant cognition in a U.S. cohort. *Environmental Health Perspectives, 113*(10), 1376–1380.

Olds, D., Henderson, C., Kitzman, H., et al. (1999). Prenatal and infancy home visitation by nurses: Recent findings. *Future of Children, 9*, 44–65.

Olds, D., Hill, P., Robinson, J., et al. (2000). Update on home visiting for pregnant women and parents of young children. *Current Problems in Pediatrics, 30*, 109–141.

Olds, D., Kitzman, H., Cole, R., et al. (2004b). Effects of nurse home-visiting on maternal life course and child development:

Age 6 follow-up results of a randomized trial. *Pediatrics, 114*(6), 1550–1559.

Olds, D., Kitzman, H., Hanks, C., et al. (2007). Effects of nurse home-visiting on maternal and child functioning: Age 9 follow-up of a randomized trial. *Pediatrics, 120*(4), E832–E845.

Olds, D., Robinson, J., Pettitt, L., et al. (2004a). Effects of home visits by paraprofessionals and by nurses: Age 4 follow-up results of a randomized trial. *Pediatrics, 114*(6), 1560–1568.

Orr, S.T. (2004). Social support and pregnancy outcome: A review of the literature. *Clinical Obstetrics & Gynecology, 47*(4), 842–855.

Palfrey, J., Hauser-Cram, P., Bronson, M., et al. (2005). The Brookline Early Education Project: A 25-year follow-up study of a family-centered early health and development intervention. *Pediatrics, 116*(1), 144–152.

Parikh, R.K. (2008). Fighting for the reputation of vaccines: Lessons from American politics. *Pediatrics, 121*, 621–622.

Parraga, I., & Doughten, S. (2007). *WIC.* Retrieved August 18, 2008 from: http://www.faqs.org/nutrition/Smi-Z/WIC-Program.html.

Patten, P., & Ricks, O. (2003). *Child care quality: An overview for parents.* Clearinghouse on Early Education and Parenting. Retrieved August 1, 2008 from http://ceep.crc.uiuc.edu/eecearchive/digests/2000/patten00.html.

Pearson, K., Nonacs, R., Viguera, A., et al. (2007). Birth outcomes following prenatal exposure to antidepressants. *Journal of Clinical Psychiatry, 68*(8), 1284–1289.

Perera, F., Rauh, V., Whyatt, R., et al. (2005). A summary of recent findings on birth outcomes and developmental effects of prenatal ETS, PAH, and pesticide exposures. *Neurotoxicology, 26*(4), 573–587.

Peters, V., Liu, K., Robinson, L., et al. (2008). Trends in perinatal HIV prevention in New York City 1994–2003. *American Journal of Public Health*, doi: 10.2105/AJPH.2007.110023.

Phipps, M., Rosengard, C., Weitzen, S., et al. (2008). Age group differences among pregnant adolescents: Sexual behavior, health habits and contraceptive use. *Journal of Pediatric & Adolescent Gynecology, 21*(1), 9–15.

Poehling, K., Szilagyi, P., Grijalva, C., et al. (2007). Reduction of frequent otitis media and pressure-equalizing tube insertions in children after introduction of pneumococcal conjugate vaccine. *Pediatrics, 119*(4), 707–715.

Pompeii, L., Savitz, D., Evenson, K., et al. (2005). Physical exertion at work and the risk of preterm delivery and small-for-gestational age birth. *Obstetrics & Gynecology, 106*, 1279–1288.

Quinlivan, J.A. (2004). Teenagers who plan parenthood. *Sexual Health, 1*(4), 201–208.

Quinlivan, J.A., & Evans, S.F. (2004). Teenage antenatal clinics may reduce the rate of preterm birth: A prospective study. *BJOG, 111*(6), 571–578.

Raneri, L., & Wiemann, C. (2007). Social ecological predictors of repeat adolescent pregnancy. *Perspectives in Sexual & Reproductive Health, 39*(1), 39–47.

Rayburn, W.F. (2007). Maternal and fetal effects from substance use. *Clinical Perinatology, 34*(4), 559–571.

Rees, S., & Inder, T. (2005). Fetal and neonatal origins of altered brain development. *Early Human Development, 81*(9), 753–761.

Reid, V., & Meadows-Oliver, M. (2007). Postpartum depression in adolescent mothers: An integrative review of the literature. *Journal of Pediatric Health Care, 21*(5), 289–298.

Reidpath, D., & Allotey, P. (2003). Infant mortality rate as an indicator of population health. *Journal of Epidemiology & Community Health, 57*, 344–346.

Rentschler, D.D. (2003). Pregnant adolescents' perspectives of pregnancy. *MCN: Maternal Child Nursing, 28*(6), 377–383.

Reynolds, A., Temple, J., Suh-Ruu, O., et al. (2007). Effects of a school-based, early childhood intervention on adult health and wellbeing. *Archives of Pediatrics & Adolescent Medicine, 161*(8), 730–739.

Rideout, V., Vandewater, E., & Wartella, A. (2003). *Zero to six: Electronic media in the lives of infants, toddler and preschoolers.* Menlo Park, CA: Kaiser Family Foundation.

Rivkin, M., Davis, P., Lemaster, J., et al. (2008). Volumetric MRI study of brain in children with intrauterine exposure to cocaine, alcohol, tobacco, and marijuana. *Pediatrics, 121*(4), 741–750.

Roberto, A., Zimmerman, R., Carlyle, K., & Abner, E. (2007). A computer-based approach to preventing pregnancy, STD, and HIV in rural adolescents. *Journal of Health in the Community, 12*(1), 53–76.

Robertson, A. (2003). *Working with the young and pregnant.* Birth International: Specialist in Birth & Midwifery. Retrieved August 18, 2008 from http://www.acegraphics.com.au/articles/andrea17.html.

Roisman, G., & Fraley, R. (2008). A behavior-genetic study of parenting quality, infant attachment security, and their covariation in a nationally representative sample. *Developmental Psychology, 44*(3), 831–839.

Rosenthal, J., Rodewald, L., McCauley, M., et al. (2004). Immunization coverage levels among 19- to 35-month-old children in 4 diverse medically underserved areas of the United States. *Pediatrics, 113*(4), 296–302.

Roush, S., Murphy, T., & the Vaccine-Preventable Disease Table Working Group. (2007). Historical comparisons of morbidity and mortality for vaccine-preventable diseases in the United States. *The Journal of the American Medical Association, 298*(18), 2155–2163.

Rydz, D., Srour, M., Oskoui, M., et al. (2006). Screening for developmental delay in the setting of a community pediatric clinic: A prospective assessment of parent-report questionnaires. *Pediatrics, 118*(4), E1178–E1186.

Safe Kids Worldwide (SKW). (2007). *Burn and scalds safety.* Washington, DC: Author.

Salafia, C., Charles, A., & Maas, E. (2006). Placenta and fetal growth restriction. *Clinical Obstetrics & Gynecology, 49*(2), 236–256.

Save the Children. (2008). *State of the world's mothers, 2008.* Westport, CN: Author.

Save the Children. (2008). *State of the world's mothers: Closing the survival gap for children under 5.* Westport, CN: Author.

Schnitzer, P.G. (2006). Prevention of unintentional childhood injuries. *American Family Physician, 74*(11), 1864–1872.

Schatz, J., & Roberts, C. (2007). Neurobehavioral impact of sickle cell disease in early childhood. *Journal of the International Neuropsychological Society, 13*, 933–943.

Schroth, R., Brothwell, D., & Moffatt, M. (2007). Caregiver knowledge and attitudes of preschool oral health and early childhood caries (ECC). *International Journal of Circumpolar Health, 66*(2), 153–167.

Schuetze, P., Eiden, R., & Coles, C. (2007). Prenatal cocaine and other substance exposure: Effects on infant autonomic regulation at 7 months of age. *Developmental Psychobiology, 49*(3), 276–289.

Schwimmer, J., Burwinkle, T., & Varni, J. (2003). Health-related quality of life of severely obese children and adolescents. *JAMA, 289*, 1813–1819.

ScoutNews. (April 3, 2008). *More than 90,000 U.S. infants are victims of abuse or neglect.* HealthDay News. Retrieved August 18, 2008 from http://www.nlm.nih.gov/medlineplus/print/news/fullstory_63001.html.

Seipone, K., Ntumy, R., Smith, M., et al. (2004). Introduction of routine HIV testing in prenatal care: Botswana, 2004. *Morbidity and Mortality Weekly Report, 53*(46), 1083–1086.

Shearer, W.T. (2008). Breastfeeding and HIV infection. *Pediatrics, 121*(5), 1046–1047.

Sheiham, A. (2006). Dental caries affects body weight, growth and quality of life in preschool children. *British Dental Journal, 201*, 625–626.

Shirazian, N., Mahboubi, M., Emdadi, R., et al. (2008). Comparison of different diagnostic criteria for gestational diabetes mellitus based on the 75-g glucose tolerance test: A cohort study. *Endocrinology Practice, 14*(3), 312–317.

Sidebotham, P., & Heron, J. (2003). Child maltreatment in the "children of the nineties": The role of the child. *Child Abuse & Neglect, 27*, 337–352.

Silk, H., Douglass, A., Douglass, J., & Silk, L. (2008). Oral health during pregnancy. *American Family Physician, 77*(8), 1139–1144.

Sims, T., & Sims, M. (2005). Tobacco use among adolescents enrolled in Wisconsin Medicaid program. *Wisconsin Medical Journal, 104*(7), 41–46.

Singhal, A. (2007). Does breastfeeding protect from growth acceleration and later obesity? *Nestle Nutrition Workshop Series: Pediatric Program, 60*, 15–25 (discussion 25–29).

Singh, S., & Darroch, J. (2000). Adolecent pregnancy and childbearing: Levels and trends in developing countries. *Family Planning Perspectives, 32*, 14–23.

Smith, D., Johnson, A., Pears, K., Fisher, P., & DeGarmo, D. (2007). Child maltreatment and foster care: Unpacking the effects of prenatal and postnatal parental substance use. *Child Maltreatment, 12*(2), 150–160.

Smith, L., LaGasse, L., Derauf, C., et al. (2006). The infant development, environmental, and lifestyle study: Effects of prenatal methamphetamine exposure, polydrug exposure, and poverty on intrauterine growth. *Pediatrics, 118*(3), 1149–1156.

Smith, L.E., Greene, M.A., & Singh, H.A. (2002). Study of the effectiveness of the U.S. safety standard for child resistant cigarette lighters. *Injury Prevention, 8*, 192–196.

Smithbattle, L. (2007). Learning the baby: An interpretive study of teen mothers. *Journal of Pediatric Nursing, 22*(4), 261–271.

Smoots, E. (2008). *Beware of gum disease's full-body potential.* Everett, WA: The Daily Herald. Retrieved August 18, 2008 from http://www.heraldnet.com/apps/pbcs.dll/article?AID=/20080212/LIVING/220434718.

Snider, J. (2007). News: Reducing sugary beverage consumption in childhood may lessen chronic disease risk. *Journal of the American Dental Association, 138*(2), 160.

Spear, H.J. (2004). Personal narratives of adolescent mothers-to-be: Contraception, decision making, and future expectations. *Public Health Nursing, 21*(4), 338–346.

Spear, H.J. (2006). Breastfeeding behaviors and experiences of adolescent mothers. *MCN: American Journal of Maternal Child Nursing, 31*(2), 106–113.

Spector, J.M., & Daga, S. (2008). Preventing those so-called stillbirths. *Bulletin of the World Health Organization, 86*(4), DOI: 10.1590/S0042-96862008000400017.

Steele, R.W. (2005). *Prevention of communicable disease in childhood.* American Academy of Pediatrics National Conference & Exhibition, October 8–11, 2005. Washington, DC. Retrieved August 18, 2008 from http://www.medscape.com/viewarticle/520832.

Stein, A., Thompson, A., & Waters, A. (2005). Childhood growth and chronic disease: Evidence from countries undergoing the nutrition transition. *Maternal and Child Nutrition, 1*(3), 177–184.

Steinhausen, H., Blattmann, B., & Pfund, F. (2007). Developmental outcome in children with intrauterine exposure to substances. *European Addiction Research, 13*(2), 94–1000.

Stringer, M., Ratcliffe, S., & Gross, R. (2006). Acceptance of hepatitis B vaccination by pregnant adolescents. *MCN: American Journal of Maternal Child Nursing, 31*(1), 54–60.

Struck, J. (2003). Four-state FAS consortium: Model for program implementation and data collection. *Neurotoxicology & Teratology, 25*(6), 643–649.

Strunk, J.A. (2008). The effect of school-based health clinics on teenage pregnancy and parenting outcomes: An integrated literature review. *Journal of School Nursing, 24*(1), 13–20.

Substance Abuse & Mental Health Services Administration (SAMHSA). (September 3, 2004). *Pregnant women in substance abuse treatment: 2002.* The DASIS Report. Retrieved from http://www.drugabusestatistics.samhsa.gov/2k4/pregTX/pregTX.pdf.

Taylor, J., Geller, L., Risica, P., et al. (2008). Birth order and breastfeeding initiation: Results of a national survey. *Breastfeeding & Medicine, 3*(1), 20–27.

Tempfer, T. (2005). *Offering guidance to parents: Child temperament, managing colic, and youth sport participation.* Paper presented at the 26th Annual Conference of the National Association of Pediatric Nurse Practitioners (NAPAP), Phoenix, AZ.

Ten Hoope-Bender, P., Liljestrand, J., & MacDonagh, S. (2006). Human resources and access to maternal health care. *International Journal of Gynecology & Obstetrics, 94*, 226–233.

Thomas, D., Leicht, C., Hughes, C., et al. (2003). *Emerging practices in the prevention of child abuse and neglect.* Washington, DC: USDHHS.

Thomson Healthcare. (June 2007). *The healthcare costs of having a baby.* Santa Barbara, CA: Author.

Tinker, A., Paul, V., & Ruben, J. (2006). The right to a healthy newborn. *International Journal of Gynecology & Obstetrics, 94*, 269–276.

Tough, S., Siever, J., Leew, S., et al. (2008). Maternal mental health predicts risk of developmental problems at 3 years of age: Follow up of a community based trial. *BMC: Pregnancy and Childbirth, 8*(1), 16–20.

Tsai, J., Floyd, R., Green, P., & Boyle, C. (2007). Patterns and average volume of alcohol use among women of childbearing age. *Maternal and Child Health Journal, 11*, 437–445.

Tsujimoto, S. (2008). The prefrontal cortex: Functional neural development during early childhood. *Neuroscientist,* doi: 10.1177/1073858408316002.

Turck, D. (2007). Later effects of breastfeeding practice: The evidence. *Nestle Nutrition Workshop Series: Pediatric Program, 60*, 31–39 (discussion 39–42).

United States Department of Health and Human Services. (2000). *Healthy people 2010.* [Conference ed., Vols. 1 & 2]. Washington, DC: U.S. Government Printing Office.

United States Department of Health and Human Services. (USDHHS). (2006). *Healthy People 2010 Midcourse Review.* Washington, DC: U.S. Government Printing Office.

United States Department of Health and Human Services (USDHHS). (2007). *Women's Health USA 2007.* Health Resources & Services Administration. Rockville, MD: Author.

United States Department of Health and Human Services (USDHHS). (2008). *Child maltreatment 2006.* Administration on Children, Youth & Families. Washington, DC: U.S. Government Printing Office.

University of Chicago Medical Center. (2008). *Sickle cell disease.* Retrieved October 14, 2008 from http://www.uchospitals.edu/online-library/content=P00101.

Usta, I., Zoorob, D., Abu-Musa, A., Naassan, G., & Nassar, A. (2008). Obstetric outcome of teenage pregnancies compared with adult pregnancies. *Acta Obstetrics & Gynecology Scandanavia, 87*(2), 178–183.

Van Pampus, M., & Aarnoudse, J. (2005). Long-term outcomes after preeclampsia. *Clinical Obstetrics & Gynecology, 48*(1), 489–494.

Vance, J., Boyle, F., Najman, J., & Thearle, M. (2002). Couple distress after sudden infant or perinatal death: A 30-month follow up. *Journal of Paediatric Child Health, 38*(4), 368–372.

Wagner, J., Jenkins, B., & Smith, C. (2006). Nurses' utilization of parent questionnaires for developmental screening. *Pediatric Nursing, 32*(5), 409–412.

Wang, L., & Pinkerton, K. (2008). Detrimental effects of tobacco smoke exposure during development on postnatal lung function and asthma. *Birth Defects Research. Part C, Embryo Today: Reviews, 84*(1), 54–60.

Watkins, M.L., Rasmussen, S.A., Honein, M.A., et al. (2003). Maternal obesity and risk for birth defects. *Pediatrics, 111*, 1152–1158.

Weber, M.K., Floyd, R.L., Riley, E.P., & Snider, D.E. (2002). National task force on fetal alcohol syndrome and fetal alcohol effect: Defining the national agenda for fetal alcohol syndrome and other prenatal alcohol-related effects. *Morbidity and Mortality Weekly Report, 51*(RR14), 9–12.

Weck, R., Paulose, T., & Flaws, J. (2008). Impact of environmental factors and poverty on pregnancy outcomes. *Clinical Obstetrics & Gynecology, 51*(2), 349–359.

Wiggins, P.K. (2001). *Why should I nurse my baby?* Franklin, VA: L.A. Publishing.

Wigle, D., Arbuckle, T., Turner, M., et al. (2008). Epidemiologic evidence of relationships between reproductive and child health outcomes and environmental chemical contaminants. *Journal of Toxicology & Environmental Health. Part B, Critical Reviews, 11*(5–6), 373–517.

Williams, D. (2002). *Postpartum psychosis: A difficult defense.* Cable News Network (CNN). Retrieved August 18, 2008 from http://archives.cnn.com/2001/LAW/06/28/postpartum.defense/.

Wold, C., & Nicholas, W. (2007). Starting school healthy and ready to learn: Using social indicators to improve school readiness in Los Angeles. *Preventing Chronic Disease, 4*(4). Retrieved August 18, 2008 from http://www.cdec.gov/pcd/issues/2007.Oct/07_0073.htm.

World Bank. (2008). *Brain development.* Retrieved August 18, 2008 from http://web.worldbank.org/KQUAYBVT10.

World Health Organization. (2008a). *Maternal mortality remains high in much of the developing world.* Retrieved August 18, 2008 from http://www.who.int/reproductive-health/publications/.maternal_mortality_2005/index.html.

World Health Organization. (2008b). *New world health report spotlights mother and child health.* Retrieved August 18, 2008 from http://www.euro.who.int/mediacentre/PR/2005/20050406_1?PrinterFriendly=1&.

Worrall, G. (2008). Bronchiolitis. *Canadian Family Physician, 54*(5), 742–743.

Yiallourou, S., Walker, A., & Horne, R. (2008). Effects of sleeping position on development of infant cardiovascular control. *Archives of Disease in Childhood*, doi: 10.1136/adc.2007.132860.

Yorita, K., Holman, R., Sejvar, J., et al. (2008). Infectious disease hospitalizations among infants in the United States. *Pediatrics, 121*(2), 244–252.

Yost, J., & Li, Y. (2008). Promoting oral health from birth through childhood; Prevention of early childhood caries. *MCN: American Journal of Maternal Child Nursing, 33*(1), 17–23.

Zero to Three. (n.d.). *Frequently asked questions: Brain development.* Retrieved October 14, 2008 from http://www.zerotothree.org/site/PageServer?pagename=ter_key_brainFAQ.

Zhou, F., Shefer, A., Kong, Y., & Nuorti, J. (2008). Trends in acute otitis media-related health care utilization by privately insured young children in the United States, 1997–2004. *Pediatrics, 121*(2), 253–260.

Ziegler, P., Hanson, C., Ponza, M., et al. (2006). Feeding Infants and Toddlers Study: Meat and snack intakes of Hispanic and non-Hispanic infants and toddlers. *Journal of the American Dietetic Association, 106*[1 Suppl. 1], S107–S123.

Zwicker, J., & Harris, S. (2008). Quality of life of formerly preterm and very low birth weight infants from preschool age to adulthood: A systematic review. *Pediatrics, 121*(2), E366–E376.

Selected Readings

Akinbami, L.J., & Schoendorf, K.C. (2002). Trends in childhood asthma: Prevalence, health care utilization, and mortality. *Pediatrics, 110*(2), 315–322.

American Academy of Pediatrics. (2003). Oral health risk assessment and establishment of the dental home. *Pediatrics, 111*(5), 1113–1116.

Araojo, R., McCune, S., & Feibus, K. (2008). Substance abuse in pregnant women: Making improved detection a good clinical outcome. *Clinical Pharmacology & Therapeutics, 83*(4), 520–522.

Beckwith, J.B. (2003). Defining the sudden infant death syndrome. *Archives of Pediatrics and Adolescent Medicine, 157*, 286–290.

Campbell, S., Spieker, S., Burchinal, M., et al. (2006). Trajectories of aggression from toddlerhood to age 9 predict academic and social functioning through age 12. *Journal of Child Psychology & Psychiatry, 47*(8), 791–800.

Caplan, L., Erwin, K., Lense, E., & Hicks, J. (2008). The potential role of breast-feeding and other factors in helping to reduce early childhood caries. *Journal of Public Health Dentistry*, ePub ahead of print PubMed PMID: 18384535.

Centers for Disease Control & Prevention (CDC). (May 15, 2007c). *Learn the signs. Act early. Cerebral palsy fact sheet.* Retrieved August 18, 2008 from http://www.cdc.gov/ncbddd.autism/ActEarly/cerebral_palsy.html.

Centers for Disease Control & Prevention (CDC). (2008). *Poisoning in the United States: Fact sheet.* Retrieved August 18, 2008 from http://www.cdc.gov/ncipc/factsheets/poisoning.htm.

Currie, J. (2005). Health disparities and gaps in school readiness. *The Future of Children, 15*(1), 117–138.

Dalziel, S., Lim, V., Lambert, A., et al. (2007). Psychological functioning and health-related quality of life in adulthood after preterm birth. *Developmental Medicine & Child Neurology, 49*(80), 597–602.

Dehaene-Lambertz, G., Hertz-Pannier, L., & Dubois, J. (2006). Nature and nurture in language acquisition: Anatomical and functional brain-imaging studies in infants. *Trends in Neuroscience, 29*(7), 367–373.

Dennison, E., Sydall, S., Rodriguez, A., et al. (2004). Polymorphism in the growth hormone gene, weight in infancy, and adult bone mass. *Journal of Clinical Endocrinology & Metabolism, 889*(10), 4898–4903.

Dworkin, P. (2003). Enhancing developmental services in child health supervision: An idea whose time has truly arrived. *Pediatrics, 114*, 827–831.

Fegran, L., Helseth, S., & Fagermoen, M. (2008). A comparison of mothers' and fathers' experiences of the attachment process in a neonatal intensive care unit. *Journal of Clinical Nursing, 17*(6), 810–816.

Fukuda, S., Mizuno, K., Kawai, S., et al. (2008). Reduction in cerebral blood flow volume in infants complicated with hypoxic ischemic encephalopathy resulting in cerebral palsy. *Brain Development, 30*(4), 246–253.

Goodlin-Jones, B., Sitnick, S., Tank, K., et al. (2008). The children's sleep habits questionnaire in toddlers and preschool children. *Journal of Developmental & Behavioral Pediatrics, 29*(2), 82–88.

Hodges, E.A. (2003). A primer on early childhood obesity and parental influence. *Pediatric Nursing, 29*(1), 12–22.

Kimmel, S.R. (2002). Vaccine adverse events: Separating myth from reality. *American Family Physician, 66*(11), 2113–2120.

Kramer, M., Goulet, L., Lyndon, J., et al. (2001). Socioeconomic disparities in preterm birth: Causal pathways and mechanisms. *Paediatric & Perinatal Epidemiology, 15*[Suppl. 2], 104–123.

Kupferminc, M.J. (2005). Thrombophilia and preeclampsia: The evidence so far. *Clinical Obstetrics & Gynecology, 48*(2), 406–415.

Laudert, S., Liu, W., Blackington, S., et al. (2007). Implementing potentially better practices to support the neurodevelopment of infants in the NICU. *Journal of Perinatology, 27*[Suppl. 2], S75–S93.

Li, R., Ogden, C., Ballew, C., et al. (2002). Prevalence of exclusive breastfeeding among U.S. infants: The third national health and nutrition examination survey: Phase II: 1991–1994. *American Journal of Public Health, 92*(7), 1107–1110.

Lobato, M., Sun, S., Moonan, P., et al. (2008). Underuse of effective measures to prevent and manage pediatric tuberculosis in the United States. *Archives of Pediatric & Adolescent Medicine, 162*(5), 426–431.

Macdonald, H., Beeghly, M., Grant-Knight, W., et al. (2008). Longitudinal association between infant disorganized attachment and childhood posttraumatic stress symptoms. *Developmental Psychopathology, 20*(2), 493–508.

MacLean, L.M., Estable, A., Sims-Jones, N., & Edwards, N. (2002). Concurrent transitions in smoking status and maternal role. *Journal of Nursing Scholarship, 34*(1), 30–39.

McCarthy, M., Herbert, R., & Brimacombe, M. (2002). Empowering parents through asthma education. *Pediatric Nursing, 28*(5), 465–504.

Montgomery, D., Plate, C., Alder, S., et al. (2006). Testing for fetal exposure to illicit drugs using umbilical cord tissue vs meconium. *Journal of Perinatology, 26*(1), 11–14.

Olds, D.L., Robinson, J., O'Brien, R., et al. (2002). Home visiting by paraprofessionals and by nurses: A randomized, controlled trial. *Pediatrics, 110*(3), 486–496.

Papiernik, E., & Goffinet, F. (2004). Prevention of preterm births, the French experience. *Clinical Obstetrics & Gynecology, 47*(4), 755–767.

Ramasubbu, R., Masalovich, S., Peltier, S., et al. (2007). Neural representation of maternal face processing: A functional magnetic resonance imaging study. *Canadian Journal of Psychiatry, 52*(11), 726–734.

Rasinski, K.A., Kuby, A., Bzdusek, S.A., et al. (2003). Effect of a sudden infant death syndrome risk reduction education program on risk factor compliance and information sources in primarily black urban communities. *Pediatrics, 111*(4), E347–E354.

Reime, B., Schucking, B., & Wenzlaff, P. (2008). Reproductive outcomes in adolescents who had a previous birth or an induced abortion compared to adolescents' first pregnancies. *BMC: Pregnancy & Childbirth, 31*(8), 4–12.

Ryan, A.S., Wenjun, Z., & Acosta, A. (2002). Breastfeeding continues to increase into the new millennium. *Pediatrics, 110*(6), 1103–1109.

Sadler, L., Swartz, M., Ryan-Krause, P., et al. (2007). Promising outcomes in teen mothers enrolled in a school-based parent support program and childcare center. *Journal of School Health, 77*(3), 121–130.

Saewyc, E.M. (2003). Influential life contexts and environments for out-of-home pregnant adolescents. *Journal of Holistic Nursing, 21*(4), 343–367.

Salt, A., & Redshaw, M. (2006). Neurodevelopmental follow-up after preterm birth: Follow-up after two years. *Early Human Development, 82*(3), 185–197.

Schempf, A.H. (2007). Illicit drug use and neonatal outcomes: A critical review. *Obstetrics & Gynecology Surveys, 62*(11), 749–757.

Sidebottom, A., Birnbaum, A., & Stoddard-Nafstad, S. (2003). Decreasing barriers for teens: Evaluation of a new teenage pregnancy prevention strategy in school-based clinics. *American Journal of Public Health, 93*(11), 1890–1892.

Simard, V., Nielsen, T., Tremblay, R., et al. (2008). Longitudinal study of preschool sleep disturbance: The predictive role of maladaptive parental behaviors, early sleep problems, and child/mother psychological factors. *Archives of Pediatric & Adolescent Medicine, 162*(4), 360–367.

Stoelhorst, G., Rijken, M., Martens, S., et al. (2005). Changes in neonatology: Comparison of two cohorts of very preterm infants (gestational age <32 weeks): The Project on Preterm and Small for Gestational Age Infants 1983 and the Leiden Follow-Up Project on Prematurity 1996–1997. *Pediatrics, 115*(2), 396–405.

Underwood, K., Rubin, S., Deakers, T., & Newth, C. (2007). Infant botulism: A 30-year experience spanning the introduction of botulism immune globulin intravenous in the intensive care unit at Children's Hospital Los Angeles. *Pediatrics, 120*(6), E1380–E1385.

van Zeijl, J., Mesman, J., Stolk, M., et al. (2007). Differential susceptibility to discipline: The moderating effect of child temperament on the association between maternal discipline and early childhood externalizing problems. *Journal of Family Psychology, 21*(4), 626–636.

Walters, M., Boggs, K., Ludington-Hoe, S., et al. (2007). Kangaroo care at birth for full term infants: A pilot study. *MCN: American Journal of Maternal Child Nursing, 32*(6), 375–381.

Willinger, M., Ko, C.W., Hoffman, H.J., et al. (2003). Trends in infant bed sharing in the United States, 1993–2000: The National Infant Sleep Position Study. *Archives of Pediatrics and Adolescent Medicine, 157*, 43–49.

Zigler, E., Pfannenstiel, J., & Seitz, V. (2008). The Parents as Teachers program and school success: A replication and extension. *Journal of Primary Prevention, 29*(2), 103–120.

Internet Resources

Black Infant Health Program, California Department of Public Health: *http://www.cdph.ca.gov/PROGRAMS/BIH/Pages/default.aspx*

Centers for Disease Control & Prevention (CDC) (child development resources for families): *http://www.cdc.gov/ncbddd/child/links.htm*

Centers for Disease Control & Prevention (CDC) (fact sheets on developmental disorders and developmental milestones): *http://www.cdc.gov/ncbddd/autism/ActEarly/pdf/hcp_pdfs/Fact%20Sheets.pdf*

Child Welfare League of America: *http://www.cwla.org*

Kaiser Family Foundation (statistics by state, US): *http://www.statehealthfacts.org/*

March of Dimes (birth defects, prenatal care): *http://www.marchofdimes.com/*

Maternal Child Health Bureau (resources & information): *http://mchb.hrsa.gov/*

National Clearinghouse on Child Abuses & Neglect (state reporting laws and other resources): *http://www.calib.com/nccanch/statutes*

National Council on Alcoholism and Drug Dependence: *http://www.ncadd.org*

National Institute on Alcohol Abuse and Alcoholism: *http://www.niaaa.nih.gov*

National Institute of Child Health & Development—*Back to Sleep* Campaign to prevent SIDS: *http://www.nichd.nih.gov/sids*

National Network for Child Care: *http://cyfernet.ces.ncsu.edu/cyfdb/browse_2pageAnncc.php?subcat=Health+and+Safety&search=NNCC&search_type=browse*

National Organization on Fetal Alcohol Syndrome: *http://www.nofas.org*

Reading is Fundamental (choosing young children's books): *http://www.rif.org/parents/articles/Choosing_Books.mspx*

The National Healthy Mothers, Healthy Babies Coalition (HMHB): *http://www.hmhb.org*

Zero to Three (information and resources on infant and young child brain development): *http://www.zerotothree.org/site/PageServer?pagename=homepage*

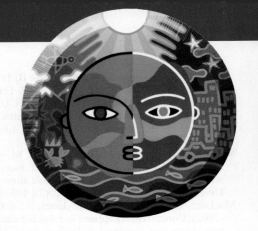

22

School-age Children and Adolescents

KEY TERMS

Anorexia nervosa
At risk of overweight
Attention deficit
  hyperactivity disorder
  (ADHD)
Binge eating
Bulimia
Learning disability
Overweight
Pediculosis

LEARNING OBJECTIVES

Upon mastery of this chapter, you should be able to:

◆ Identify major health problems and concerns for U.S. school-age children and adolescent populations.

◆ Explain how health status can influence academic achievement.

◆ State the recommended immunization schedule for school-age children and adolescents.

◆ Examine the trends in mortality and injury among school-age children and adolescents and identify the most important areas needing intervention.

◆ Discuss *Healthy People 2010* objectives affecting adolescents and the barriers that may be involved in attaining these objectives.

◆ Describe types of programs and services that promote health and prevent illness and injury of school-age children and adolescent populations.

"Youth isn't always all it's touted to be."
—Lawana Blackwell, *The Dowry of Miss Lydia Clark, 1999*

According to Erick Erickson's developmental framework, the school-age and adolescent years are a time of task mastery and development of competence and self-identity (Encyclopedia of Childhood & Adolescence, 1998). During these years, children grow physically, as well as emotionally and socially. They move from the total control of parents and families during infancy and toddler years to deriving more and more influence from outside the home—from school, teachers, peers, and other groups.

The challenges of childhood and adolescence include developmental issues, school concerns, behavioral and learning problems, emotional and mental health issues, and the risk behaviors characteristic of teenage years. This chapter explores the health needs of school-age children and adolescents and describes various services that address those needs, along with the community health nurse's role in assisting families with children.

SCHOOL—CHILD'S WORK

In the United States in 2005, about 55.8 million school-age children and adolescents (5 to 18 years old) attended more than 123,000 public and private schools (Federal Interagency Forum on Child and Family Statistics, 2004; National Center for Education Statistics [NCES], 2005). In 2008, the U.S. population ages 0 to 17 was composed of 57% White, 15% Black, 4% Asian, 21% Hispanic, and 5% other groups (Federal Interagency Forum on Child and Family Statistics [FIFCFS], 2004).

Children and adolescents spend most of their waking hours in school. Their academic success can predict future education, employment, and income. The quality of their educational experiences (e.g., teacher–child interactions) can influence learning (Pianta, Belsky, Vandergrift, Houts, & Morrison, 2008). These children are the parents, workers, leaders, and decision makers of tomorrow, and their future success depends in good measure on achievement of their educational goals today (Burgess, Gardiner, & Propper, 2006). Child health has been linked to school success—healthy children are found to be more motivated and prepared to learn (Centers for Disease Control & Prevention [CDC], 2008a; O'Connell, 2005), and coordinated school health programs are linked to academic achievement (Murray, Low, Hollis, Cross, & Davis, 2007). This is well known to school nurses and public health nurses (PHNs) working in schools.

HEALTH PROBLEMS OF SCHOOL-AGE CHILDREN

The well-being of children has been a subject of great concern in the United States since the days of Lillian Wald. For many years, international organizations, including the World Health Organization (WHO), the United Nations Children's Fund (formerly, United Nations International Children's Education Fund [UNICEF]), and U.S. governmental agencies, nonprofit groups, and charitable foundations have focused their resources on improving the health and well-being of children. Nonetheless, the needs of millions of children in the United States and worldwide remain unmet.

Even in the wealthiest nations, many children face complex and often chronic health problems that cause them to miss school days or participate only marginally in the classroom. Because childhood is a critical period during which certain behaviors or health conditions are known to lead to more serious adult illnesses, it is vital for community health nurses and school nurses to screen children and identify problems early (Forrest & Riley, 2004). The chronic health problems of children younger than age 18 are often characterized by severity (e.g., persistence of symptoms and impact on social functioning) and duration (usually longer than 3 to 12 months) and may include:

- Diabetes
- Asthma
- Autism
- Cystic fibrosis
- Spina bifida
- Neuromuscular disorders
- Juvenile rheumatoid arthritis
- Seizure disorders
- Hemophilia
- Congenital heart disease
- Attention deficit hyperactivity disorder (ADHD).

Other conditions may also be defined as chronic, such as allergies, ear infections, and sinusitis; hearing or speech disorders; or even childhood obesity. Some chronic conditions may affect a child socially and emotionally, as well as physically. School attendance and relationships with family and peers may be affected.

Chronic Diseases

Stomachaches, headaches, colds, and flu are frequent complaints of school-age children, but it is not uncommon for this same age group to be afflicted with some type of chronic disease: Between 6.5% and 18% of children are estimated to have a significant chronic condition (Schmidt, Petersen, & Bullinger, 2003). Common chronic problems include hay fever, sinusitis, dermatitis, tonsillitis, asthma, and hearing difficulties. Chronic health problems such as these can affect a child's ability to learn and/or his physical and social development. Other more serious conditions, such as diabetes, sickle cell anemia, or seizure disorders, have definite effects on academic achievement (Taras & Potts-Datema, 2005a).

The numbers of children with chronic conditions are increasing, and more children with significant health problems are present in schools (Perrin et al., 2007). In the school setting, some children require specialized physical health care procedures, such as catheterization or suctioning. The U.S. Supreme Court ruled that even complex nursing services (i.e., ventilator care) must be provided by schools, even though school nurses are not always present in each school building every day (American Academy of Pediatrics Committee on Children With Disabilities [AAPCCWD], 2000). (See Chapter 30 for more on school nursing.) The Individuals with Disabilities Education Act (IDEA) or Section 504 of the Rehabilitation Act of 1973 (AAPCCWD, 2000; National Dissemination Center for Children with Disabilities, n.d.) mandates that services must be provided for children identified as *disabled*. Many conditions may be characterized as disabling under these two laws, including autism, deafness or hearing impairment, blindness or vision impairment, emotional disturbances, mental retardation, specific learning disabilities, speech or language impairments, or other health impairments (e.g., ADHD, asthma). Once they have been characterized as disabled, children may qualify for special educational services. Children with chronic health conditions that can affect learning (e.g., diabetes, seizure disorders) may receive medications or other related services while in school, to maintain their health and promote their ability to learn (Merck, 2005).

Chronic diseases of childhood and adolescence affect the entire family and can lead to developmental and social issues for children, as well as missed school days and eventual school failure (Centers for Disease Control & Prevention [CDC], 2008a; Schmidt, Petersen, & Bullinger, 2003).

Asthma

Asthma is the most common chronic disease of childhood. In 2003, it was estimated that 13% of children younger than age 18 have at some time been diagnosed with asthma (Forum on Child & Family Statistics [FCFS], 2005). Non-Hispanic Black children exhibited the highest asthma attack rates at 13%, compared with 8% for White children and 7% for Hispanic children; overall, about 6% of children reported an episode within the past year (FCFS, 2005).

Although reasons for the increasing cases of asthma are somewhat unclear, experts speculate that better recognition and diagnosis of the disease; overcrowded conditions; and exposure to air pollution (indoor or outdoor), allergens, and irritants in the environment are probable culprits and may trigger asthma attacks. Many schools have high levels of allergens and irritants. Children and adolescents with asthma may have attacks triggered by infections, exposure to cigarette smoke, stress, strenuous exercise, or weather changes (e.g., cold, wind, rain) (Daisey, Angell, & Apte, 2003; FCFS, 2005).

Pediatric asthma led to a high rate of hospitalizations for preventable conditions in 2004—155 per 100,000, second only to pediatric gastroenteritis and substantially higher than the rate of 31.5 per 100,000 for short-term diabetes complications—and further contributed to rising health care costs (Russo, Jiang, & Barrett, 2007). Treatment for chronic asthma usually includes inhaled corticosteroids, but acute symptoms may involve inhaled beta$_2$ agonists and sometimes anticholinergics (Courtney, McCarter, & Pollart, 2005). Parent and child education, along with adequate primary medical care, can help decrease the number of emergency room visits (Boudreaux, Emond, Clark, & Carmargo, 2003; Courtney et al., 2005).

Teaching families to reduce allergens in their homes by controlling dust mites, vacuuming frequently, preventing animal dander and the entry of pollen into the home, and avoiding mold and mold spores may help minimize asthma symptoms for many children (Asthma & Allergy Foundation of America, 2007). School nurses and PHNs often work with students, families, and physicians to develop an asthma action plan to control, prevent, or minimize the untoward effects of acute asthma episodes. The goal is to control asthma symptoms and minimize school absences resulting from asthma (Courtney, et al., 2005). Asthma triggers are noted, and school staff are taught to assist the child in avoiding these triggers. Peak flow meters can be used to determine early signs of asthma problems and to facilitate early interventions. Approximately 27% of schools reported having these available for asthmatic students, and 68% allowed students to self-administer their inhalable asthma medications (CDC, 2004).

Monitoring asthma medications and teaching proper methods of inhaler use are also vital school nursing or PHN functions. Although the link between asthma and academic achievement is not definitive, some evidence exists that school nurse case management of asthmatic children can lead to fewer absences, fewer hospitalizations, and reduced emergency room visits (Taras & Potts-Datema, 2005b; Levy, Heffner, Stewart, & Beeman, 2006).

Autism

Autism is a complex developmental disorder that is usually first noticed within the first few years of life. A child's communication skills and interaction with others is most often affected, along with obsessive behavior and narrowed interests. Behaviors associated with autism include:

- Language problems (no language, delay in language, repetitive use of language)
- Motor mannerisms (rocking, hand flapping, object twirling)
- Fixation on objects (restricted interests)
- No spontaneous play or make-believe play; no interest in peers (problems making friends)
- Little or no eye contact (may also resist hugging)

The estimated lifetime expense for an autistic child averages $3.5 to $5 million (Autism Society of America [ASA], 2008). Autism is not a new disorder—descriptions of autistic behavior have been identified in 18th century writings. Currently, the Autism Information Center estimates the prevalence of autism at one in 150 children, with boys four times more likely than girls to have the disorder (2007). Because autism is a "spectrum disorder" that presents differently among individuals, behaviors and severity can vary widely (ASA, 2008).

The cause of autism is not clear—some genetic links have been found, but environment may also be a factor. There is a higher risk of subsequent children having autism in a family with one autistic child (National Institute of Neurological Disorders & Stroke [NINDS], 2008). It is often associated with other disorders (e.g., congenital rubella syndrome, phenylketonuria [PKU], fragile X syndrome, tuberous sclerosis), but with early intervention some children's symptoms improve, and they can lead near-normal adult lives (Autism Information Center, 2007; NINDS, 2008).

PHNs may come in contact with families dealing with autism through work in well-child or immunization clinics. It is important to educate parents that parenting practices are now known *not* to be a cause of autism and that multiple, large-scale research studies on childhood immunizations have shown no relationship between immunization and autism (Autism Information Center, 2007; NINDS, 2008).

Diabetes

Diabetes is another common chronic illness in children, with the National Institutes of Health's (NIH) National Diabetes Education Program (NDEP, 2006) reporting that nearly one in every 400 to 600 children has type 1 diabetes. Both type 1 and type 2 diabetes are found in school-age children. Type 2 diabetes is rising almost exponentially in this age group, leading some scientists to call this a major public health crisis. Newly diagnosed type 2 diabetes in children has increased from less than 5% before 1994 to 30% and 50% in more recent years (NDEP, 2006). This epidemic is thought to stem from increasing rates of childhood obesity, sedentary lifestyle, and the predisposition of certain ethnic groups (e.g., American Indian, Mexican American) to the disease. A family history of type 2 diabetes may also play a role.

Younger children with type 1 diabetes, especially those who use insulin pumps, may need careful monitoring, something that is not always possible for the school nurse, who is often assigned to several school sites and may not be present when problems arise. A multidisciplinary team approach to care is needed, coordinating family, school staff, and physician collaboration.

Children and adolescents with diabetes may be reluctant to comply with medical regimens, although strict adherence has proved to reduce later microvascular complications (NDEP, 2006). Testing blood sugar levels and taking insulin at school can be frustrating and cause children to feel singled out or different from their peers. One study found that adolescents with type 1 diabetes have significantly higher rates of depression than those without diabetes (Kanner, Hamrin, & Grey, 2003). It is important for school nurses and PHNs to understand each child's unique concerns and to alert teachers and school personnel to the signs and symptoms (as well as treatment) of hypoglycemia.

In addition to the obvious emergency health-related concerns for diabetic children, a classic study showed that diabetes-related severe hypoglycemia affects memory tasks (Hershey, Bhargava, Sadler, White, & Craft, 1999). Over time, memory deficits can affect learning and progress in school, and this has been substantiated by later research (Taras & Potts-Datema, 2005a). Moreover, obesity and overweight have been found to correlate with "poorer levels of academic achievement" (Taras & Potts-Datema, 2005c, p. 291).

It is imperative to teach children and families that nutrition, oral antidiabetes medications or insulin administration, physical activity, and blood glucose testing are vital strategies to keep blood glucose levels as close to normal as possible (NDEP, 2006). The prevention of type 2 diabetes through education and improvement in exercise, nutrition, and lifestyle can be one of the most important areas of focus for health professionals who work with the school-age population—including PHNs who may come into contact with them during immunization or child health clinics. Health education and health promotion to decrease childhood obesity and sedentary lifestyles may help stem the tide of type 2 diabetes in children and adolescents (see Levels of Prevention Pyramid).

Juvenile Rheumatoid Arthritis

Juvenile rheumatoid arthritis is a painful autoimmune disorder characterized by persistent joint swelling and stiffness with periods of remission and flare-up. It is treated with nonsteroidal anti-inflammatory drugs (NSAIDs), disease-modifying antirheumatic drugs (DMARDs) such as methotrexate, and sometimes corticosteroids or newer biologic response modifiers (National Institute of Arthritis and Musculoskeletal and Skin Diseases, 2004; Wilkinson, Jackson, & Gardner-Medwin, 2003). Exercise is often an important component of therapy, and an adapted physical education program may be developed for these children. Long-term sequelae may result,

and many adolescents with this disorder require additional support and counseling (Bowyer et al., 2003).

Seizure Disorders

Seizure disorders are not uncommon in the school-age population. Epilepsy is a disorder of the brain in which neurons sometimes transmit abnormal signals. Epilepsy is considered to be one of the most common disabling neurologic conditions, and it is most common in the very young and in elderly populations (CDC, 2007a). About 40% of children with epilepsy between the ages of 4 and 15 have "one or more additional neurological disorders" (Silver, 2004a). For almost 85% to 90% of those diagnosed, seizures can usually be controlled with medications (Freeman, Freeman, Kossoff, & Kelly, 2006). Vagus nerve stimulators are used in some cases after other treatments have failed (Buchhalter & Jarrar, 2003; NINDS, 2008). Rectal diazepam is commonly prescribed for younger children and those with developmental disabilities, yet nurses are not always available to make an appropriate nursing assessment of the child before the drug is given to stop a seizure (Fitzgerald, Okos, & Miller, 2003; Epilepsy Foundation, 2003). Often, school secretaries or health aides are trained to give the emergency medication—highlighting the conflict between education laws and nurse practice acts. Treatment of epilepsy has been greatly enhanced by the use of newer antiepilepsy drugs (AEDs) specific to the pediatric population and, in some cases, by a diet rich in proteins and fats and low in carbohydrates—a *ketogenic diet* (Freeman et al., 2006).

It is important to monitor medication compliance and teach school staff about first-aid measures for seizure victims. When teachers are anxious about having a child with epilepsy in the classroom, educational programs for them and other school staff members can be provided by community health nurses or school nurses to allay fear and promote appropriate and timely care (Price, Murphy, & Cureton, 2004).

Family dynamics are also a consideration, as behavior problems can arise from "deficient family mastery and parent confidence in managing their child's discipline" (Austin, Dunn, Johnson, & Perkins, 2004). Children and adolescents with seizure disorders may feel embarrassed or be the victims of teasing or bullying. They may exhibit signs of school avoidance, or they may have problems learning. The side effects of antiepileptic medications may lead to problems with memory and learning, as well as changes in behavior. Moreover, seizures can affect short-term memory or language functions, and almost 50% of children with learning disabilities have epilepsy (Silver, 2004a). It is important for school nurses to work with children with epilepsy and to teach all students about the disease process and the need for empathy and understanding.

Childhood Cancers

In 2007, cancer ranked as the leading cause of death from disease among U.S. children between the ages of 1 and 14. Given the generally good health of children in this age group, however, this alarming ranking is actually low, at one to two cases per 10,000 children (National Cancer Institute [NCI], 2008). Most childhood cancers are blood cell cancers (e.g., leukemias) or cancers of the central nervous system or brain.

LEVELS OF PREVENTION PYRAMID

SITUATION: The public health nurse and children with type 2 diabetes
GOAL: By using the three levels of prevention, negative health conditions are avoided, promptly diagnosed and treated, and/or the fullest possible potential is restored.

Tertiary Prevention

Rehabilitation	Primary Prevention
	Health Promotion & Education
• Monitor the child's health	• Continue to promote a healthy lifestyle that includes appropriate food choices and daily physical activity within the limitations of type 2 diabetes
• Work closely with the child, family, physician, and teacher to ensure proper follow-up	**Health Protection**
• Be alert to monitor for any possible complications (e.g., medication side effects)	• Educate the teachers on safety precautions for children in their classroom diagnosed with type 2 diabetes
	• Monitor children taking medications for type 2 diabetes (e.g., over- or under-dosage and adverse reactions)

Secondary Prevention

Early Diagnosis	Prompt Treatment
• Teach older children to calculate their BMI	• Initiate referrals for health care provider follow-up in collaboration with parents of students at risk for type 2 diabetes
• Monitor BMI scores	
• Yearly screenings for height and weight (calipers are useful)	• Initiate referrals to health care providers in collaboration with parents of students with signs and symptoms of type 2 diabetes
• Complete health histories on at-risk children	

Primary Prevention

Health Promotion & Education	Health Protection
• Educate to promote good nutrition and a physically active lifestyle	
• Provide classroom contact in the early primary grades to encourage children to make good food choices	
• Limit passive activities and increase sports and physical activity	
• Teach older children how to make better food choices at fast food restaurants	

Acute lymphoblastic leukemia is the most common childhood cancer. Childhood cancers, especially leukemias, now have better outcomes than ever before. Five-year survival rates for childhood cancers increased by almost 80% from 1996 to 2003, generally as a result of treatment advances (NCI, 2008). More than 70% of childhood cancers are now considered curable, with survivors more concerned about later complications of treatment than about cancer recurrence (Wallace et al., 2001). However, children who have been treated with chemotherapy and/or radiation may develop a second primary cancer, and the risk of leukemia may be increased (NCI, 2008).

Acquired immune deficiency syndrome (AIDS), high levels of ionizing radiation, Down syndrome, and other genetic syndromes (e.g., Gorlin syndrome) have been linked to a higher risk for some childhood cancers. Pesticide exposure may be a factor, but research findings have not been decisive. Parental smoking may be linked to an increased cancer risk, but evidence for this is also inconclusive (NCI, 2008).

Because many children return to school after initial hospitalization and treatment for cancer, school nurses or PHNs can help make this transition easier by educating classmates about cancer (e.g., it is not contagious), helping the children make necessary adjustments, and vigilantly protecting any immunocompromised students from communicable diseases (VanDenBurgh, 2003).

Behavioral and Learning Problems

Other childhood health problems, less easy to detect and measure but often just as debilitating, are those of emotional, behavioral, and intellectual development. Although these problems are not new, awareness and concern have increased as the rates of occurrence for other life-threatening childhood diseases have diminished. Emotional or behavior problems and learning disabilities are prevalent in childhood. In a national survey, 8% of girls and 16% of boys reported having been diagnosed with ADHD or learning disability—the most commonly reported problems. Three times more boys than girls reportedly have ADHD, and boys are more likely to have a comorbid learning disability (CDC, 2005).

Learning Disabilities

Children and adults who have average or above-average intelligence and who demonstrate significant difficulties in one or more areas of learning (e.g., reading, writing, mathematics) may have a **learning disability**. Thinking and organization skills can also be affected. Learning disabilities may occur in one area or be overlapping—they are often lifelong conditions (NINDS, 2007). Causes of learning disabilities and emotional behavioral problems appear to have genetic, environmental, and cultural influences. Approximately 5% to 10% of students have a learning disability, formally defined as a "neurologically based processing disorder" (Silver, 2006). A U.S. Department of Education survey in 2001 revealed that 68% of those with learning disabilities were male (Cortiella, 2008). The number of children with learning disabilities in the lowest economic group is twice that in the highest economic group (CDC, 2002a). Children characterized as being in fair or poor health were more than four times as likely to have a learning disability and three times as likely to have ADHD as children with excellent, very good, or good health status (CDC, 2002a).

Children with learning disabilities can be helped through special education services. Students must first be carefully diagnosed through psycho-educational testing; then, special education or resource teachers can build on the child or adolescent's strengths while working to compensate for weaknesses (NINDS, 2007). Some learning disabilities are apparent in early school years, whereas others do not present problems until later, in early adolescence. Battles over homework, poor grades, acting out in school, or frequent child complaints about school, teachers, or schoolwork, are often harbingers of learning disabilities. Common signs of learning disabilities are (Silver, 2006):

◆ Reading problems
◆ Writing problems (fine motor control and handwriting; problems with spelling, grammar, punctuation, capitalization; difficulty controlling flow of thoughts)
◆ Math problems (problems learning and understanding concepts, missing steps or sequencing of problems and placement of numbers in columns)
◆ Language problems (cannot quickly process what is heard, problems with multiple instructions, difficulty organizing thoughts and speaking in classroom situations)
◆ Motor problems (problems with fine-motor planning activities, such as tying, cutting, coloring, and gross-motor planning, such as jumping and running; trouble with visual–motor activities, such as hitting or catching a ball)

If learning disabilities are not dealt with in childhood and adolescence, they can lead to later, more serious problems related to employment and relationships. Approximately 19% of students diagnosed with learning disabilities reported being suspended or expelled from school, arrested, or fired by their employers (Cortiella, 2008).

Attention Deficit Hyperactivity Disorder

Attention deficit hyperactivity disorder (ADHD) is a cluster of problems related to hyperactivity, impulsivity, and inattention. Its estimated prevalence has ranged from 3% to 5%, representing about 2 million children (National Institute of Mental Health [NIMH], 2006). Others have reported much higher overall rates (7%), and around 10% of 3 to 17 year-old males in 2004 were diagnosed by a health professional as having ADHD (Child Trends, 2006), and the disorder continues to be diagnosed with increasing frequency (Damico, Tetnowski, & Nettleton, 2004). One study found the rate of ADHD diagnosis had more than tripled over 10 years, with the largest increase among low-income and poor children in the 12- to 18-year-old age group (Olfson, Garneroff, Marcus, & Jensen, 2003). Although there were fewer treatment visits, an increase was noted in stimulant prescriptions during this same period. Others have noted the trend of increasing pharmacologic treatment of ADHD (Damico et al., 2004). Another study found a positive association between stimulant treatment for ADHD and age, male gender, fewer child dependents, higher income, white communities, and living in the Midwest or South (Cox, Motheral, Henderson, & Mager, 2003). Girls, on the other hand, are at increased risk for not receiving appropriate services because they often do not exhibit the hyperactivity component and often are not appropriately diagnosed.

Although a number of parents believe that sugar, food coloring agents, or other food additives may worsen ADHD symptoms in their children, research shows no behavioral or learning differences in double-blind studies using sugar and sugar substitutes. Some research shows that prenatal exposure to nicotine and psychosocial adversity are associated with ADHD (Biederman & Faraone, 2002; NIMH, 2006). Symptoms of ADHD may be related to such diverse causes as lead poisoning and traumatic brain injuries, but new research focuses on the inherited tendencies for problems with dopamine receptors and transporter genes, along with evidence of decreased blood flow in the prefrontal regions of the brain and smaller brain volumes in the frontal lobe, caudate nucleus, cerebellum, and temporal gray matter (NIMH, 2006). These findings support a neurobiologic basis for the condition (Kelly, Margulies, & Castellanos, 2007). Some evidence indicates that children with ADHD who are medicated properly later show white matter volumes consistent with control subjects, indicating that medication can restore brain volume to a more normal level (NIMH, 2006). Some family and twin studies reveal a higher heritability factor (0.8) for ADHD than for other psychiatric disorders, and researchers consider ADHD a "familial and highly heritable disorder" (Thapar, Langley, O'Donovan, & Owen, 2006, p. 714; Weiss & Murray, 2003). In families that have children with ADHD, about 25% of close relatives also had ADHD—much higher than the general population estimate of 5% (NIMH, 2006).

Not all behaviors related to ADHD, such as hyperactivity, may truly be ADHD (Silver, 2004b). Health and psychological professionals must take a careful history and note if sudden family changes may have recently occurred (e.g., divorce, death, family crises) that may cause children to behave erratically. Untreated chronic middle ear infections, undetected temporal lobe seizures, and anxiety or depression can also be the source of some behavior problems that mimic ADHD, as can other brain disorders (NIMH, 2006). Although some health professionals believe that many of the symptoms found in people with ADHD are part of the normal spectrum of human behavior, others note that people with ADHD have functional impairment in academic, social, or occupational areas resulting from their problem behaviors. Noted differences have even been reported in the results of electroencephalograms (Swartwood et al., 2003). Nursing researchers have documented qualitative data from children and adolescents who described their difficulties (Kendall, Hatton, Beckett, & Leo, 2003).

At each stage of development, those with ADHD are presented with distinct challenges. For example, children in elementary school are often involved in conflicts with peers and have problems in organizing tasks. They may be more prone to accidents, and may have more school-related problems, such as grade retention and suspension or expulsion. They often have problems with grooming and handwriting, and they exhibit difficulty sleeping and making friends. As adolescents, 80% still exhibit symptoms of inattentiveness, hyperactivity, and impulsiveness. Compared with non-ADHD teens, they may have more conflict with their parents, poorer social skills, and ongoing problems at school. They may face more difficulty driving and are more prone to injury while driving, biking, or walking than are their peers. They are also more likely to use tobacco and alcohol, spend less time with their families, and more often experience negative moods (Child Trends, 2006). As young adults, they are less likely to be enrolled in college, more likely to have begun sexual activity at an earlier age and to have been treated for a sexually transmitted disease (STD), and more likely to experience lower job performance ratings than their peers (Child Trends, 2006). In adulthood, they tend to have more marital and occupational problems. They often have less formal education and lower levels of savings. Poor social skills continue to be an issue (Barkley, Fischer, Smallish, & Fletcher, 2002; Child Trends, 2006; Weiss & Murray, 2003).

ADHD is sometimes found with associated disorders, such as communication or language disorders and learning disabilities. About half of ADHD children and adolescents have learning or other mental disorders (Child Trends, 2006). Common comorbid conditions are bipolar, depressive, and anxiety disorders, as well as conduct disorders and oppositional defiant disorder (Biederman & Faraone, 2002; Child Trends, 2006). At an earlier age of onset, ADHD is associated with more parental reports of child aggressive behavior, whereas at a later age of onset, ADHD is associated with more anxious/depressive symptoms (Connor et al., 2003). For some children, ADHD might even be a precursor of a child-onset subtype of bipolar disorder (Masi et al., 2003). Differentiating between the two conditions can be difficult, as bipolar disorder in children can present as a chronic mood problem, with some symptoms related to depression, irritability, and elation (NIMH, 2006).

Collaboration among the child's family, school, and physician is needed to diagnose ADHD and to plan appropriate interventions and educational accommodations. Although parents have a wealth of knowledge about the child, teacher confirmation of ADHD-related behaviors is very important. School nurses and PHNs can assist parents in recognizing the symptoms of ADHD and in obtaining appropriate treatment and follow-up. A multimodal treatment approach is recognized as most effective. This includes medication, usually methylphenidate (Ritalin, Metadate, or Concerta), dextroamphetamine (Dexedrine or Dextrostat), or amphetamine (Adderall); school accommodations for learning problems; and social skills training for the child with ADHD (NIMH, 2006). Family and individual counseling, parent support groups, and training in behavior management techniques, as well as family education about the condition, are also essential features of this treatment method. Not all children and adolescents respond to medication—about 10% do not—and medication dosage must be carefully monitored and adjusted.

The main goal of medical treatment for school-age children is academic improvement. If this does not occur, medication may need to be changed or discontinued. Parental depressive symptoms and severity of ADHD symptoms in children have been found to decrease the rate of response to medication and combined treatments (Owens et al., 2003). School nurses and community health nurses can work closely with school staff, parents, and physicians in determining the efficacy of treatment regimens.

Parents often voice concern about giving their children a stimulant medication to treat ADHD, and some families pursue alternative treatments. One study revealed that 54% of parents used some type of complementary and alternative medicine (e.g., acupuncture, nutritional supplements, diet), and 11% did not discuss this fact with their child's physician (Chan, Rappaport, & Kemper, 2003). Some promising results with neurofeedback were found in a German study (Fuchs, Birbaumer, Lutzenberger, Gruzelier, & Kaiser, 2003). A new nonstimulant medication, atomoxetine (Strattera), has been used in children but has also been linked to increased suicidal thoughts or attempts.

Parental resistance to treatment may result from side effects (e.g., problems with sleep, appetite, greater anxiety) or stem from fears about later abuse of substances. As adolescents, those with ADHD may experiment with alcohol and other substances earlier than non-ADHD teens do—hyperactivity has been shown to predict low self-esteem, leading to social withdrawal and abuse of substances (Tarter, Kirisci, Feske, & Vanyukov, 2007). However, a good deal of research indicates that treatment with medication for ADHD in childhood does not lead to an increased risk for substance use or abuse in adulthood, and some studies found that adolescents who consistently took their ADHD medications were actually less likely to use or abuse substances (Barkley et al., 2003; NIMH, 2006).

Behavioral and Emotional Problems

It is estimated that 1 in 20 children and adolescents "have one or more significant behavioral problems in school." and that a very small percentage of them receive any consistent, specialized mental health care (Hennessy & Green-Hennessy, 2000, p. 591). Between 10% and 15% of children and adolescents have symptoms of depression. About 20% of school-age children display behaviors consistent with oppositional defiant disorder (e.g., hostile, stubborn, disobedient, belligerent), and about 10% of children between the ages of 9 and 17 have been diagnosed with conduct disorder. Symptoms of this disorder, sometimes thought to be a more severe form of antisocial behavior than oppositional defiant disorder, include behaviors that "violate the rights of others and age-appropriate social standards and rules" (American Academy of Child & Adolescent Psychiatry [AACAP], 2008). These behaviors can include destruction of property, fire setting, cruelty to animals or people, and/or bullying and threatening behavior (Kazdin, 2008). Schizophrenia in childhood affects one in 40,000 children under age 12, and adult schizophrenia, which affects one in 100 people, usually begins in young adulthood (age 18 for males, age 25 for females). Bipolar disorder, most often found in adults, is also found in children and adolescents. Early identification of children and adolescents at risk for developing bipolar disorder may be accomplished through the use of behavior checklists and other psychometric tools that reveal higher scores related to aggression, delinquent behavior, and attention problems, or withdrawal and anxiety/depression (Giles, DelBello, Stanford, & Strakowski, 2007). It is important to find referral sources for these children and their families, and this may be difficult in more rural or outlying areas (Kazdin, 2008).

School-age problem behaviors stem from many causes, some of them genetic and others environmental. Corporal punishment may be a risk factor for antisocial behavior (Kazdin, 2008), and a large-scale national study found that parental corporal punishment negatively contributed to behavioral problems in preschool and first-grade children. It was thought both to trigger and maintain child behavior problems, and decreasing this parental behavior could be associated with better child mental health and lower levels of behavior problems (Mulvaney & Mebert, 2007). Children are barometers of their environment. The current rate of divorce in the United States is double what it was in the 1950s; over the last 30 years, the percentage of children living in two-parent families decreased from 85% to 69%, and more than 26% of children today live with one parent, usually their mother (Schor, 2003).

Children of divorce are more likely to exhibit behavior problems, with children who are products of highly contentious divorces most at risk. School nurses can be alert to early symptoms and refer parents to marital counseling or suggest family therapists. Some schools also offer support groups for children of divorce.

School refusal is found in 1% to 5% of school-age children and differs from truancy. It is commonly a symptom of emotional distress—usually anxiety or depression—but may also be associated with oppositional-defiant disorder, ADHD, or other disruptive behavior disorders. School refusal is most commonly found in children ages 5, 6, 10, and 11, and rates are similar between boys and girls and for all socioeconomic levels (Fremont, 2003). Children usually present to the school nurse or PHN with headaches and/or abdominal pains. They may throw tantrums, cry, or exhibit panic and fear to their parents in an attempt to stay home from school. Sometimes, children are afraid of something in the school environment (e.g., bullies, teachers, test-taking), or they may have a type of separation anxiety. Family enmeshment or detachment, or high levels of family conflict, may contribute to school refusal problems. The best interventions include early return to school, with parental involvement in school, systematic desensitization (graded exposure to the classroom), relaxation training, and counseling being the most effective (Fremont, 2003). Occasionally, antidepressant medications are used as well. Community health nurses can serve as a liaison among the child, family, school, and health care/mental health care providers to promote a positive outcome.

Disabled Children

Children with disabilities account for more than 10% of the total school-age population. Between 2003 and 2004, over 6,500 students were classified as disabled, or 14% of school-age students. The most commonly-cited disabilities are specific learning disability, speech or language disability, mental retardation, emotional disability, and hearing impairments (National Center for Education Statistics, n.d.). The prevalence of disability in children has increased greatly over the past 30 years, more so for Blacks than for Whites (Newacheck, Stein, Bauman, & Hung, 2003). Many children with perceived disabilities or problems are referred for assessment and possible placement in special education programs each year. However, most children receive special services in a regular classroom because *full inclusion* or *mainstreaming* legislation mandates that fewer children be segregated into special classes or separate schools.

Problems Associated with Economic Status

After reaching a low point in 2000, in 2004, childhood poverty in the United States rose to 18% (Koball & Douglas-Hall, 2006). This increase in poverty did not vary by parents' place of birth, employment status, or educational level, leading many to speculate that this jump in the poverty rate reflects overall economic conditions. According to the Children's Defense Fund (CDF, 2008a), one in 13 children lives in extreme poverty, and one in six are poor. Every 35 seconds, a baby is born into poverty (CDF, 2008b). It is in society's best interest to care for its children, because they will become the taxpayers of tomorrow. In the past, single-parent families (usually without an adult man present), welfare reform, and economic trends that keep less well-educated populations from entering all but the most menial jobs combined to produce a powerful synergistic effect on children and adolescents (Shields & Behrman, 2002).

Poverty has profound and lasting effects on children. More than 20% of low-income children between the ages of 6 and 17 have some type of mental health problem (Chau & Douglas-Hall, 2007). Children living in poverty have poorer health and are more likely to suffer from a chronic health condition; they are more likely to be born prematurely or at a lower birth weight. They are also more likely to experience depression and mental health problems and engage in more health-risk behaviors (e.g., smoking, early sexual activity), and they account for more adolescent delinquent behaviors and pregnancy (Cauthen, 2005; Child Trends Databank, 2008).

As adults, these children will be more likely to have lower occupational status and lower wages. Poor children and adolescents are at higher risk for negative cognitive outcomes and learning problems, resulting in fewer school days, lower math and reading scores, more grade failures, and earlier high school dropout (Child Trends Databank, 2008; National Center for Children in Poverty, 2008). A recent study found family wealth as a significant partial predictor of test scores in school-age children. The disparity in this study was stunning—white families owned more than 10 times the assets of black families and white children's test scores were significantly higher than those of black children (Yeung & Conley, 2008).

The social, emotional, and behavioral problems of some poor children may be the end result of disproportionate exposure to environmental toxins, parental substance abuse, maternal depression, trauma and abuse, divorce, violent crime, low-quality child care, inadequate nutrition, and decreased cognitive stimulation and exposure to vocabulary in early childhood and infancy (Child Trends Databank, 2008).

The relationship between lower socioeconomic status and poor health persists throughout childhood and adolescence (Chen, Martin, & Matthews, 2006), and poor adolescent and adult health are associated with childhood poverty (Cauthen, 2005). A longitudinal study in New Zealand by Poulton and colleagues (2002) found that childhood poverty can lead to health problems in adulthood (e.g., poor cardiovascular health, periodontal disease), even if socioeconomic status later increases.

Welfare reforms enacted in 1996 (i.e., The Personal Responsibility and Work Opportunity Reconciliation Act [PRWORA]) have been successful in moving many families from welfare to work. By 2000, the number of families receiving cash assistance fell to half the number served in 1996 (Shields & Behrman, 2002). However, employment rates that increased during the mid-1990s have once again fallen in the face of a declining job market in the mid-2000s (Parrott & Sherman, 2006). More than 1 million single mothers are now in the "no work, no welfare" group—with no jobs and no government support. The decline in social worker caseloads has been linked to a drop in service to qualifying families, rather than a reduction in the numbers of poor families (Parrott & Sherman, 2006).

Funding cuts to the Food Stamp Program, decreased benefits to legal immigrants, and reductions in Medicaid eligibility have impacted many poor families. Reduced allotments of food stamps to households with mixed citizens/noncitizens have led to child citizens of noncitizen parents reporting persistent and higher levels of food insecurity (Van Hook & Stamper-Balistreri, 2003). An Illinois study found that those affected by welfare reform decreased their food stamp participation while turning more to the special supplemental food program for Women, Infants, and Children (WIC) as a source of essential food items for their children. Researchers posited that cash assistance and food stamps are more closely linked and identified as "welfare programs," whereas WIC has the connotation of a "public health program" (Lee, Mackey-Bilaver, & Goerge, 2003, p. 609).

Safety-net programs—specifically, WIC and the Food Stamp program—have been shown to reduce the risk of nutrition-related problems (e.g., anemia, nutritional deficiency, failure-to-thrive). They have also been associated with a reduction in the risk of child abuse and neglect (Lee, Mackey-Bilaver, & Chin, 2006). The negative impact of welfare reform has also been noted in lower rates of first-trimester prenatal care (Gavin, Adams, Manning, Raskind-Hood, & Urato, 2007). Forty percent of families remaining uninsured 1 year after leaving welfare rolls (Seecombe, Newsom, & Hoffman, 2006) and one-third of those timed-off of welfare reported housing problems, lack of access to medical care, and insufficient food (Lindhorst & Mancoske, 2006). In a comparison of Temporary Assistance for Needy Families (TANF) and Aid to Families with Dependent Children (AFDC) recipients, those leaving TANF had a decline in economic status whereas AFDC leavers reported increases (Ozawa & Yoon, 2005). Children in families in which welfare benefits were reduced or terminated due to sanctions (usually related to inability to find work or comply with program rules) had greater odds of hospitalizations and food insecurity (Cook et al., 2002). One longitudinal study found that, after 3 years, children in the child welfare or child protective system had stable insurance coverage, a finding partially attributable to the persistence of social workers finding available coverage for children in this vulnerable group or the movement of the children into the foster care system (Raghavan, Aarons, Rosch, & Leslie, 2008).

The Personal Responsibility and Work Opportunity Reconciliation Act did provide needed changes in child support enforcement—in 2005, over 50% of families in programs received child support, up from 20% in 1996 (Parrott & Sherman, 2006). And, despite problems with welfare reform, some studies show that school-age children in families that participate in these programs do better in school and exhibit fewer behavior problems than those from families that do not participate. More negative outcomes, however, were found for adolescents, even though employment and income levels increased (Morris, Huston, & Duncan et al., 2001). Some small but significant improvements in parenting practices of participating mothers were also noted (Chase-Lansdale & Pittman, 2002). There is a need for high-quality child care and after-school programs to support these families (Fuller, Kagan, Caspary, & Gauthier, 2002). Some studies indicate that about half the families who leave welfare for work actually have fewer economic resources than they had while on welfare. A good number return to the welfare rolls because of their inability to survive in the work world (Loprest, 2001).

Although almost 13 million U.S. children live in families with incomes below the federal poverty level ($20,650 for a family of 4 in 2006), economists note that families need about twice the income of the federal poverty level to survive (Fass & Cauthen, 2007). These families are characterized as low-income, and more than 28 million children live in these circumstances. Millions more children live in moderate-income families that have inadequate child care, limited health insurance, limited access to higher education, and poor housing. In fact, a classic study by Vissing and Diament (1997) surveyed more than 3,600 high school students in New Hampshire and Maine and found that between 5% and 10% had been homeless during the past year. Almost 20% lived in distressing situations and were at risk of being homeless. About 19% of poor children have no health insurance; overall, 11.7% of children are uninsured (Fass & Cauthen, 2007). In some states, this figure is 30%, even though more than 90% of uninsured children have one or more parents who work, and more than 66% have family incomes greater than the poverty level (see Chapters 6 and 25).

Some specific physical health problems are related to poverty (e.g., lead poisoning, iron deficiency anemia, increased susceptibility to illness). Children living in poorer neighborhoods are exposed to higher levels of community violence and may be more prone to seeing the world as a hostile and dangerous place; they are often also exposed to higher levels of family violence and are more at risk of subsequent mental health issues (Linares, 2008). A longitudinal study of childhood poverty and its relationship to health status found that "the greater the number of years spent living in poverty, the more elevated was overnight cortisol and the more dysregulated was the cardiovascular response" (Evans & Kim, 2007, p. 953). This study demonstrated the physiologic effects of poverty, mediated by increased social and physical risk factors (e.g., substandard housing, environmental toxins, crowding, noise, greater family conflict, harsher parenting styles). Earlier research showed an association between crowding and noisy conditions and hypertension (Evans & Kim, 2007). The results reported by Evans and Kim (2007) align with previous research demonstrating that exposure to early childhood poverty leads to later morbidity in adulthood: "an early history of poverty appears to set children on a life-course trajectory of ill health" (p. 956).

Many school-age children suffer from the effects of poverty-related hunger. It is difficult to concentrate and learn properly if meals are often skipped or if food consistently does not provide enough nourishment (Taras, 2005). Alaimo, Olson, and Frongillo (2001) found that younger school-age children were more likely to have had difficulty getting along with other children, to have seen a psychologist, and to have repeated a grade if they reported food insufficiency. Food-insufficient adolescents were more likely to have had problems getting along with other children, to have seen a psychologist, and to have been suspended from school. Food insufficiency is defined as a child reporting that "his or her family sometimes or often did not get enough food to eat" (p. 44). Weinreb and colleagues (2002) studied the effects of hunger on preschool and school-age children. They found that, even after controlling for variables, such as housing status, mother's distress, child life events, and low birth weight, severe hunger was a predictor for adverse outcomes of both physical health (i.e., chronic illness) and mental health (e.g.,

anxiety, depression, internalizing behavior problems). In a U.S. Department of Agriculture (USDA) survey (2006), only about half of food-insecure households reported use of any of the largest federal food assistance programs, such as food stamps, free or reduced school lunches, and WIC. Thus, children go hungry because many eligible families do not use these services. Only 60% of eligible people are enrolled in the Food Stamp program, and even lower numbers of eligible working poor participate—about 51%. In 2005, about 40% of food stamp beneficiaries lived in extreme poverty, and the average monthly income for all participants was $648. Those children who participate in school lunch and breakfast programs suffer fewer of the side effects of hunger that affect learning; however, not all schools participate in these programs (Food Research and Action Center, 2007).

Death from Injuries

The loss of children's lives that results from all injuries combined suggests a staggering loss to society in the number of years of productive life lost. For children between the ages of 1 and 19, unintentional injury is the leading cause of death, and motor vehicle injury was the leading cause of injury death between 1999 and 2002 (Bernard, Paulozzi, & Wallace, 2007). Approximately 16,000 deaths yearly are the result of childhood injuries, 70% of them unintentional (Schnitzer, 2006). For the 1- to 9-year-old age group, motor vehicle/traffic injury, drowning, and fire/burn injuries were the top three causes of injury death. The injury death rate for this age group is 10.4 per 100,000, with rates for American Indians and Alaska Natives two times higher and for Blacks 1.8 times higher than for Whites (Bernard et al., 2007). Leading causes of nonfatal injuries that result in hospitalization are falls, poisoning, scald burns, and traffic crashes (Schnitzer, 2006).

For the 10- to 19-year-old age group, the overall injury death rate was 30.9 per 100,000, but for those 15 to 19 years old, the rate rises to 52 per 100,000. Motor vehicle/traffic injuries, drowning, and poisoning are the three leading causes of injury death, and Hispanics had higher rates than Whites for drowning (Bernard et al., 2007). A large-scale study examining the risk factors for passenger deaths in fatal motor vehicle crashes found that in more than 21% of cases of child passenger fatalities, alcohol was a factor. When drivers were younger than age 18, the greatest risk factors for death were most often associated with drivers younger than age 16, failure to use seat belts or other restraints, and driving on high-speed roads (Winston, Kallan, Senserrick, & Elliott, 2008). Suicides in the 10- to 19-year-old group more commonly involved firearms for Whites and Blacks, but suffocation/hanging was more prevalent for Alaska Natives/American Indians, Asian/Pacific Islanders, and Hispanics.

For all racial and ethnic groups, death rates were higher for infants and late adolescents, and dropped during the middle years. Homicide rates were highest for Black children in all age groups (Bernard et al., 2007). Injuries not resulting in death often cause permanent disabilities, or emotional and physical consequences for children and their families (Safe Kids USA, 2008).

For children and adolescents ages 6 to 19, the "choking game" is an often-misreported cause of death (CDC, 2008b). This involves self-strangulation, or strangulation by a friend through the use of hands or a noose, causing a brief euphoric high due to cerebral hypoxia. Most of the victims are male (estimated at almost 87%), and the average age is estimated at 13.3 years. Most parents were unaware of this potentially fatal activity until a child's death occurred, but warning signs such as bloodshot eyes; disorientation after being alone; belts, scarves, and ropes tied to doorknobs or bedroom furniture; and marks on the neck should lead parents to suspect this dangerous activity (CDC, 2008b).

Childhood unintentional injury deaths in the United States have declined by more than 45% in the past 20 years (Safe Kids USA, 2008) but are still much higher than in other developed countries (Deal et al., 2000). It is estimated that the cost of childhood unintentional injuries in 2000 resulted in $58 billion in medical bills, lost wages to caregivers, and other services (Safe Kids USA, 2008).

Community health nurses can promote injury prevention and control through education, promotion of engineering and environmental protection strategies, and legislative advocacy (Schnitzer, 2006). PHNs can advance the prevention of unintentional injuries and deaths by working with families to initiate consistent use of seat belts and child safety seats in vehicles, and the use of helmets and other protective gear for children riding bikes and skateboarding. Where water is a natural hazard, wearing life jackets while boating and swimming can help decrease accidental drowning. Promotion of smoke and carbon monoxide detectors, poison prevention, and sudden infant death syndrome (SIDS) education can help to further decrease injury death rates (Safe Kids USA, 2008). Teaching parents about presetting hot water heaters to lower than 130°F, recognizing the hazards of infant walkers, storing matches and lighters safely, and using pool fencing can help prevent common unintentional injuries (Schnitzer, 2006). Advocacy for stricter seat belt and child safety seat enforcement, as well as programs to provide child safety seats and bicycle helmets, has been shown to affect injury rates (Bernard et al., 2007).

Community health nurses can work with their local health departments and community action groups to provide seats and helmets to families who cannot afford them, and can encourage local police offices to enforce seat belt and safety seat laws.

Communicable Diseases

The mortality rates of school-age children 5 to 14 years old are comparatively low and have decreased substantially over the last century (Arias & Smith, 2003), a reduction that can be attributed to the effective prevention and control of the acute infectious diseases of childhood. Although mortality rates are low, morbidity due to communicable diseases among school children is high. Worldwide, communicable diseases are the leading cause of death (The World Bank, 2008). Children between ages 5 and 14 are most often affected by respiratory illnesses, followed by infectious and parasitic diseases, injuries, and digestive conditions. Among school children, the incidence rates of measles, rubella (German measles), pertussis (whooping cough), infectious parotitis (mumps), and varicella (chickenpox) have dropped considerably because of widespread immunization efforts (see Figure 22.1 for Childhood Immunization Schedule).

Over the past several decades, the incidence of vaccine-preventable diseases has generally decreased, although in 2003–2004, reported cases of mumps, hepatitis A, pertussis, and measles increased in some areas of the United States (Maternal and Child Health Bureau, 2006). Some of these illnesses carry potentially serious complications, such as birth defects from rubella and nerve deafness from mumps. Ten percent of the reported pertussis cases in 2004 occurred in infants younger than 6 months of age who had not yet received the scheduled doses of the vaccine; however, cases occurred across age groups, and increases were posted for the 3 preceding years (Maternal and Child Health Bureau, 2006).

One Wisconsin study found 261 cases of rubella and mumps in one county, and 47% of the children with confirmed cases reported using the weight room in a particular high school. An important finding was that 84% of children with reported vaccine histories had received five or more doses of pertussis vaccine, indicating that booster vaccinations may be required for adolescents and adults (Sotir et al., 2008).

Vigorous campaigns have been undertaken by health departments to get children immunized. An immunization for mumps, measles, and rubella (MMR) has been available for more than 25 years, and newer vaccines for *Haemophilus influenzae* type b (Hib), hepatitis A and B, and varicella have been developed and are now included in the childhood immunization schedule. Meningococcal, pneumococcal, and rotavirus vaccines have also been added, along with yearly influenza vaccines for all children younger than age 5 and human papillomavirus for girls age 11 and above (Advisory Committee on Immunization Practices, 2008a,b).

As increasing numbers of school-age children must show proof of required vaccinations before they are allowed to enroll in school, the percentages of children in this age group who are immunized against specific diseases may continue to rise. However, some studies reveal that immunization compliance for adolescents is a continuing problem due to lack of sufficient insurance coverage and poor systems for tracking and recall (Schaffer, Humiston, Shone, Averhoff, & Szilagyi, et al., 2001). Also, more parents of young children are choosing not to immunize their children, invoking religious or personal belief exceptions. This practice has led to outbreaks of vaccine-preventable diseases: In the first 4 months of 2008, confirmed and reported measles cases numbered 64—the greatest number for any year since 2001 (Reinberg, 2008).

Other considerations regarding communicable diseases involve their seasonality (e.g., mumps and varicella peak in April, pertussis and typhoid fever peak in August) and how climate change may affect the incidence and distribution of communicable diseases, especially vector-borne and water- and food-borne diseases (Shah, Smolensky, Burau, Cech, & Lai, 2006; Greer, Ng, & Fisman, 2008).

In the adolescent population, sexually transmitted infections (STIs) are more common, and 15- to 19-year olds are at greater risk of contracting an STI than older adults (Maternal and Child Health Bureau, 2006). Chlamydia is the most common STI, with a rate of 1,579 per 100,000; genital human papillomavirus (HPV) is also commonly found in adolescents and a relatively new vaccine is now available (see Figure 22.2, Adolescent Immunization Schedule).

With the marked rise in community-acquired methicillin-resistant *Staphylococcus aureus* (CA-MRSA), PHNs and school nurses must be alert when skin infections or other conditions do not resolve quickly in children and adolescents (Pallin, Egan, Pelletier, Espinola, Hooper, & Camargo, 2008).

Recommended Immunization Schedule for Persons Aged 0–6 Years—UNITED STATES • 2008

For those who fall behind or start late, see the catch-up schedule

Vaccine ▼ Age ►	Birth	1 month	2 months	4 months	6 months	12 months	15 months	18 months	19–23 months	2–3 years	4–6 years
Hepatitis B[1]	HepB	HepB	see footnote 1			HepB					
Rotavirus[2]			Rota	Rota	Rota						
Diphtheria, Tetanus, Pertussis[3]			DTaP	DTaP	DTaP	see footnote 3	DTaP				DTaP
Haemophilus influenzae type b[4]			Hib	Hib	Hib[4]	Hib					
Pneumococcal[5]			PCV	PCV	PCV	PCV				PPV	
Inactivated Poliovirus			IPV	IPV		IPV					IPV
Influenza[6]						Influenza (Yearly)					
Measles, Mumps, Rubella[7]						MMR					MMR
Varicella[8]						Varicella					Varicella
Hepatitis A[9]						HepA (2 doses)				HepA Series	
Meningococcal[10]										MCV4	

Range of recommended ages

Certain high-risk groups

This schedule indicates the recommended ages for routine administration of currently licensed childhood vaccines, as of December 1, 2007, for children aged 0 through 6 years. Additional information is available at www.cdc.gov/vaccines/recs/schedules. Any dose not administered at the recommended age should be administered at any subsequent visit, when indicated and feasible. Additional vaccines may be licensed and recommended during the year. Licensed combination vaccines may be used whenever any components of the combination are indicated and other components of the vaccine are not contraindicated and if approved by the Food and Drug Administration for that dose of the series. Providers should consult the respective Advisory Committee on Immunization Practices statement for detailed recommendations, including for **high risk conditions**: http://www.cdc.gov/vaccines/pubs/ACIP-list.htm. Clinically significant adverse events that follow immunization should be reported to the Vaccine Adverse Event Reporting System (VAERS). Guidance about how to obtain and complete VAERS form is available at www.vaers.hhs.gov or by telephone, 800-822-7967.

1. Hepatitis B vaccine (HepB). *(Minimum age: birth)*
   At birth:
   • Administer monovalent HepB to all newborns prior to hospital discharge.
   • If mother is hepatitis B surface antigen (HBsAg)-positive, administer HepB and 0.5 mL of hepatitis B immune globulin (HBIG) within 12 hours of birth.
   • If mother's HBsAg status is unknown, administer HepB within 12 hours of birth. Determine the HBsAg status as soon as possible and if HBsAg-positive, administer HBIG (no later than age 1 week).
   • If mother is HBsAg-negative, the birth dose can be delayed, **in rare cases,** with a provider's order and a **copy of the mother's** negative HBsAg laboratory report in the infant's medical record.
   After the birth dose:
   • The HepB series should be completed with either monovalent HepB or a combination vaccine containing HepB. The second dose should be administered at age 1–2 months. The final dose should be administered no earlier than age 24 weeks. Infants born to HBsAg-positive mothers should be tested for HBsAg and antibody to HBsAg after completion of at least 3 doses of a licensed HepB series, at age 9–18 months (generally at the next well-child visit).
   4-month dose:
   • It is permissible to administer 4 doses of HepB when combination vaccines are administered after the birth dose. If monovalent HepB is used for doses after the birth dose, a dose at age 4 months is not needed.

2. Rotavirus vaccine (Rota). *(Minimum age: 6 weeks)*
   • Administer the first dose at age 6–12 weeks.
   • Do not start the series later than age 12 weeks.
   • Administer the final dose in the series by age 32 weeks. Do not administer any dose later than age 32 weeks.
   • Data on safety and efficacy outside of these age ranges are insufficient.

3. Diphtheria and tetanus toxoids and acellular pertussis vaccine (DTaP). *(Minimum age: 6 weeks)*
   • The fourth dose of DTaP may be administered as early as age 12 months, provided 6 months have elapsed since the third dose.
   • Administer the final dose in the series at age 4–6 years.

4. Haemophilus influenzae type b conjugate vaccine (Hib). *(Minimum age: 6 weeks)*
   • If PRP-OMP (PedvaxHIB® or ComVax® [Merck]) is administered at ages 2 and 4 months, a dose at age 6 months is not required.
   • TriHIBit® (DTaP/Hib) combination products should not be used for primary immunization but can be used as boosters following any Hib vaccine in children age 12 months or older.

5. Pneumococcal vaccine. *(Minimum age: 6 weeks for pneumococcal conjugate vaccine [PCV]; 2 years for pneumococcal polysaccharide vaccine [PPV])*
   • Administer one dose of PCV to all healthy children aged 24–59 months having any incomplete schedule.
   • Administer PPV to children aged 2 years and older with underlying medical conditions.

6. Influenza vaccine. *(Minimum age: 6 months for trivalent inactivated influenza vaccine [TIV]; 2 years for live, attenuated influenza vaccine [LAIV])*
   • Administer annually to children aged 6–59 months and to all close contacts of children aged 0–59 months.
   • Administer annually to children 5 years of age and older with certain risk factors, to other persons (including household members) in close contact with persons in groups at higher risk, and to any child whose parents request vaccination.
   • For healthy nonpregnant persons (those who do not have underlying medical conditions that predispose them to influenza complications) ages 2–49 years, either LAIV or TIV may be used.
   • Children receiving TIV should receive 0.25 mL if age 6-35 mos or 0.5 mL if age 3 years or older.
   • Administer 2 doses (separated by 4 weeks or longer) to children younger than 9 years who are receiving influenza vaccine for the first time or who were vaccinated for the first time last season, but only received one dose.

7. Measles, mumps, and rubella vaccine (MMR). *(Minimum age: 12 months)*
   • Administer the second dose of MMR at age 4–6 years. MMR may be administered before age 4–6 years, provided 4 weeks or more have elapsed since the first dose.

8. Varicella vaccine. *(Minimum age: 12 months)*
   • Administer second dose at age 4–6 years; may be administered 3 months or more after first dose.
   • Don't repeat second dose if administered 28 days or more after first dose.

9. Hepatitis A vaccine (HepA). *(Minimum age: 12 months)*
   • HepA is recommended for all children aged 1 yr (i.e., aged 12–23 months). The 2 doses in the series should be administered at least 6 months apart.
   • Children not fully vaccinated by age 2 years can be vaccinated at subsequent visits.
   • HepA is recommended for certain other groups of children, including in areas where vaccination programs target older children.

10. Meningococcal vaccine. *(Minimum age: 2 years for meningococcal conjugate vaccine (MCV4) and for meningococcal polysaccharide vaccine (MPSV4))*
   • MCV4 is recommended for children aged 2–10 years with terminal complement deficiencies or anatomic or functional asplenia and certain other high-risk groups. Use of MPSV4 is also acceptable.
   • Persons who received MPSV4 3 or more years prior and remain at increased risk for meningococcal disease should be vaccinated with MCV4.

The Recommended Immunization Schedules for Persons Aged 0–18 Years are approved by the Advisory Committee on Immunization Practices (www.cdc.gov/vaccines/recs/acip), the American Academy of Pediatrics (http://www.aap.org), and the American Academy of Family Physicians (http://www.aafp.org).

DEPARTMENT OF HEALTH AND HUMAN SERVICES • CENTERS FOR DISEASE CONTROL AND PREVENTION • SAFER • HEATHIER • PEOPLE™

CS103164

FIGURE 22.1 Childhood immunization schedule.

Recommended Immunization Schedule for Persons Aged 7–18 Years—UNITED STATES • 2008
For those who fall behind or start late, see the green bars and the catch-up schedule

Vaccine ▼ Age ▶	7-10 years	11-12 years	13-18 years
Diphtheria, Tetanus, Pertussis[1]	see footnote 1	Tdap	Tdap
Human Papillomavirus[2]	see footnote 2	HPV (3 doses)	HPV Series
Meningococcal[3]	MCV4	MCV4	MCV4
Pneumococcal[4]	PPV		
Influenza[5]	Influenza (Yearly)		
Hepatitis A[6]	HepA Series		
Hepatitis B[7]	HepB Series		
Inactivated Poliovirus[8]	IPV Series		
Measles, Mumps, Rubella[9]	MMR Series		
Varicella[10]	Varicella Series		

Legend:
- Range of recommended ages
- Catch-up immunization
- Certain high-risk groups

This schedule indicates the recommended ages for routine administration of currently licensed childhood vaccines, as of December 1, 2007, for children aged 7–18 years. Additional information is available at www.cdc.gov/vaccines/recs/schedules. Any dose not administered at the recommended age should be administered at any subsequent visit, when indicated and feasible. Additional vaccines may be licensed and recommended during the year. Licensed combination vaccines may be used whenever any components of the combination are indicated and other components of the vaccine are not contraindicated and if approved by the Food and Drug Administration for that dose of the series. Providers should consult the respective Advisory Committee on Immunization Practices statement for detailed recommendations, including for **high risk conditions**: http://www.cdc.gov/vaccines/pubs/ACIP-list.htm. Clinically significant adverse events that follow immunization should be reported to the Vaccine Adverse Event Reporting System (VAERS). Guidance about how to obtain and complete VAERS form is available at www.vaers.hhs.gov or by telephone, 800-822-7967.

1. Tetanus and diphtheria toxoids and acellular pertussis vaccine (Tdap). *(Minimum age: 10 years for BOOSTRIX® and 11 years for ADACEL™)*
- Administer at age 11–12 years for those who have completed the recommended childhood DTP/DTaP vaccination series and have not received a tetanus and diphtheria toxoids (Td) booster dose.
- 13–18 year olds who missed the 11–12 year Tdap or received Td only, are encouraged to receive one dose of Tdap 5 years after the last Td/DTaP dose.

2. Human papillomavirus vaccine (HPV). *(Minimum age: 9 years)*
- Administer the first dose of the HPV vaccine series to females at age 11–12 years.
- Administer the second dose 2 months after the first dose and the third dose 6 months after the first dose.
- Administer the HPV vaccine series to females at age 13–18 years if not previously vaccinated.

3. Meningococcal vaccine.
- Administer MCV4 at age 11–12 years and at age 13–18 years if not previously vaccinated. MPSV4 is an acceptable alternative.
- Administer MCV4 to previously unvaccinated college freshmen living in dormitories.
- MCV4 is recommended for children aged 2-10 years with terminal complement deficiencies or anatomic or functional asplenia and certain other high-risk groups.
- Persons who received MPSV4 3 or more years prior and remain at increased risk for meningococcal disease should be vaccinated with MCV4.

4. Pneumococcal polysaccharide vaccine (PPV).
- Administer PPV to certain high-risk groups.

5. Influenza vaccine.
- Administer annually to all close contacts of children aged 0–59 months.
- Administer annually to persons with certain risk factors, health-care workers, and other persons (including household members) in close contact with persons in groups at higher risk.

- Administer 2 doses (separated by 4 weeks or longer) to children younger than 9 years who are receiving influenza vaccine for the first time or who were vaccinated for the first time last season, but only received one dose.
- For healthy nonpregnant persons (those who do not have underlying medical conditions that predispose them to influenza complications) ages 2–49 years, either LAIV or TIV may be used.

6. Hepatitis A vaccine (HepA).
- The 2 doses in the series should be administered at least 6 months apart.
- HepA is recommended for certain other groups of children, including in areas where vaccination programs target older children.

7. Hepatitis B vaccine (HepB).
- Administer the 3-dose series to those who were not previously vaccinated.
- A 2-dose series of Recombivax HB® is licensed for children aged 11–15 years.

8. Inactivated poliovirus vaccine (IPV).
- For children who received an all-IPV or all-oral poliovirus (OPV) series, a fourth dose is not necessary if the third dose was administered at age 4 years or older.
- If both OPV and IPV were administered as part of a series, a total of 4 doses should be administered, regardless of the child's current age.

9. Measles, mumps, and rubella vaccine (MMR).
- If not previously vaccinated, administer 2 doses of MMR during any visit, with 4 or more weeks between the doses.

10. Varicella vaccine.
- Administer 2 doses of varicella vaccine to persons younger than 13 years of age at least 3 months apart. Do not repeat the second dose, if administered 28 or more days following the first dose.
- Administer 2 doses of varicella vaccine to persons aged 13 years or older at least 4 weeks apart.

The Recommended Immunization Schedules for Persons Aged 0–18 Years are approved by the Advisory Committee on Immunization Practices (www.cdc.gov/vaccines/recs/acip), the American Academy of Pediatrics (http://www.aap.org), and the American Academy of Family Physicians (http://www.aafp.org).

DEPARTMENT OF HEALTH AND HUMAN SERVICES • CENTERS FOR DISEASE CONTROL AND PREVENTION
SAFER • HEALTHIER • PEOPLE™

FIGURE 22.2 Adolescent immunization schedule.

CS103164

Referral to an infectious disease specialist may need to be considered.

Head Lice

Pediculosis (head lice) is a frustrating and common problem for many school-age children, and the incidence has been increasing over the past three decades (Guenther, 2007). It is estimated that 6 to 12 million children between the ages of 6 and 12 years become infested with head lice each year (Frankowski & Weiner, 2002). A study conducted by a school nurse in California found the highest incidence of head lice in her school district occurred among early elementary children, and that girls were three times more likely to have head lice than boys. Hispanic and White children had the highest rates of pediculosis, and Black children had the lowest rate (Estrada & Morris, 2000). Girls are thought to be at higher risk due to social behavior (closer contact, sharing of items), and close crowded conditions can also be a risk factor (Guenther, 2007). An infestation of *Pediculus humanus* var. *capitis,* the parasite that lives and feeds on the human scalp, can be an embarrassing nuisance to families of any socioeconomic level. These very tiny, wingless insects need blood to survive and can cause itching and skin irritation. They are most often found toward the nape of the neck, where hair is usually thickest, but their pearly white eggs (nits) are distributed all over the head. They are attached to the hair shaft with a glue-like substance and can be detected by careful examination of the scalp. Because nits hatch within 10 days, and the immature louse can reach reproductive maturity within 8 to 9 days, recurring cycles of infestation are common. If no treatment is given, the cycle repeats every 3 weeks (American Academy of Pediatrics, 2006; Hansen, 2004). Complete eradication generally requires that all nits be removed along with lice.

Head lice are most often transmitted by direct contact (head-to-head) or may be passed from infected to uninfected children through shared items such as combs and brushes, hats, scarves, sheets, and towels (items called *fomites*). Contrary to some popular myths, lice do not fly or jump, and they cannot be contracted from animals—they live only on humans (Aubrey, 2006). They do not survive long off the human head, only about 3 days (Guenther, 2007). Many schools have recurring outbreaks of head lice that can be traced back to particular families who have failed to completely eradicate an infestation (Hansen, 2004). Because of perceived social stigma, some families are defensive and unresponsive to attempts at education and intervention. Some schools resort to "no nit" policies and establish routine head lice examinations, with a goal of early detection and treatment. However, the American Academy of Pediatrics discourages such policies because they have not been effective in curbing head lice infestations and they often result in significant lost school days and negative social impact (Aubrey, 2006).

Treatment of head lice commonly includes over-the-counter insecticide shampoos, such as pyrethrin-based *RID*, *R&C*, *Pronto*, or *A200*. A permethrin cream rinse (*Nix*) has been a recommended choice for treatment (Frankowski & Weiner, 2002). Other treatments include lindane (Kwell), malathion (Ovide), oral antibiotic agents, such as Septra and Ivermectin, and occlusive agents such as petroleum jelly (Fawcett, 2003; Frankowski & Weiner, 2002; Jones & English, 2003). Solvents that aid in dissolving the "cement" that holds the nit in place have been shown to be helpful when using fine-tooth combs (e.g., Lice Meister)—these include white vinegar and formic acid (Guenther, 2007). The use of special combs and wet combing conditioners into affected hair has been shown in one study to be more effective than pediculicides (Dawes, 2005). In some cases, resistance to topical pediculicides has necessitated the use of other measures (Hansen, 2004).

School nurses and PHNs also need to educate families about reducing reinfestation by careful cleaning and treatment of any fomites (e.g., combs, hats, towels, sheets, clothing, upholstered furniture) and scrupulous nit removal. It is difficult, however, to prevent children—who are social creatures—from coming into close contact with one another and becoming reinfected. In some larger cities, entrepreneurs have started nit removal businesses (e.g., Nit Pickers, Hair Fairies) to assist parents with this tedious task.

Other Health Problems

Other health problems found in this age group are nutritional problems (primarily overeating and inappropriate food choices) and poor dental health. Obesity often begins in childhood and becomes a risk factor for cardiovascular disease and diabetes later in life (Institute of Medicine, 2006). The percentage of children who are overweight has risen over 15% between 1980 and 2004 (Fig. 22.3), despite the fact that food insecurity is found in over 11% of American households and affects over 13 million children (Cook, 2002).

Food allergies can also play a role in poor nutritional status, especially with school-age children and adolescents. Although 20% of children and adolescents may report a food allergy (Noimark & Cox, 2008), one study in England noted that only 2.3% of 11- and 15-year-old children actually demonstrated sensitivity upon skin testing and double-blind food challenges (Pereira, Venter, Grundy, Clayton, Arshad, & Dean, 2005). Food allergies can be especially problematic in the school setting (see Chapter 30), and new food labeling initiated in 2006 makes identification of the eight most common food allergens a much easier process (U.S. Food and Drug Administration, 2007).

Dental caries is another common problem among school-age children. Fourteen percent of U.S. school-age children have untreated cavities; over 21% of children living in poverty need treatment for dental caries (Forum on Child & Family Statistics [FCFS], n.d.).

Childhood Obesity

About one-third of U.S. children are classified as overweight or at risk of becoming overweight. The CDC uses the term **overweight**, rather than obese, in defining children who have a body mass index (BMI) at or above the 95th percentile. Children with a BMI between the 85th and 94th percentile are defined as **at risk of overweight** (CDC, 2007b). (See Display 22.1 for explanation and examples.) The obesity rate has tripled for preschool children and adolescents, but it has quadrupled for children 6 to 11 years of age (Institute of Medicine, 2006). Obese children are more likely to become obese adults. The Surgeon General reports that there is a 70% chance of adult overweight or obesity if an adolescent is overweight; if at least one parent is overweight, the risk jumps to

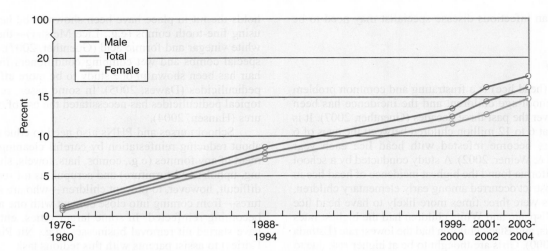

NOTE: Overweight is defined as body mass index (BMI) at or above the 95th percentile of the 2000 Centers for Disease Control and Prevention BMI-for-age growth charts. BMI is calculated as weight in kilograms divided by the square of height in meters.

SOURCE: Centers for Disease Control and Prevention, National Center for Health Statistics. *National Health and Nutrition Examination Survey.*

FIGURE 22.3 Percentage of children ages 6–17 who are overweight by gender, selected years 1976–2004. Retrieved July 31, 2008 from *http://www.childstats.gov/americaschildren06/hea4.asp#health4.*

80% (2007). Results of a recent Youth Risk Behavior Survey indicated that almost 80% of high school students surveyed ate fewer than five servings of fruits and vegetables the day before, and almost 84% drank fewer than three glasses of milk per day in the previous week (CDC, 2006a).

DISPLAY 22.1

EXPLANATION AND EXAMPLES OF OVERWEIGHT CLASSIFICATION FOR CHILDREN AND TEENS

Body mass index (BMI) is used as a screening tool to identify weight problems in children and teens. The criteria are different from those used for adults, as body fat differs between boys and girls, and the amount of body fat changes with age. BMI-for-age growth charts for boys and girls are available at: http://www.cdc.gov/growthcharts.

Weight Status Category	Percentile Range
Underweight	Less than the 5th percentile
Healthy weight	5th percentile to less than the 85th percentile
At risk of overweight	85th to less than the 95th percentile
Overweight	Equal to or greater than the 95th percentile

From Centers for Disease Control & Prevention. (2007b). *About BMI for Children & Teens.* Retrieved July 31, 2008 from http://www.cdc.gov/print.do?url=http%3A%2F%2Fwww.cdc.gov%2Fnccdphp%2Fdnpa%2Fbmi%2Fchildrens_BMI%2Fabout_childrens_BMI.htm.

The poor eating habits that develop during childhood are generally thought to persist into adulthood, contributing to the leading causes of death and disability—cardiovascular disease, cancer, and diabetes. Between 75% and 90% of cardiovascular disease is related to hypertension, tobacco use, diabetes, obesity, and inadequate physical activity (Gidding et al., 2005). Evidence of early atherosclerosis and fatty streaks has been found in autopsy studies of children as young as 6 years of age (Harrell, Pearce, & Hayman, 2003). Aside from its relationship with inactivity, television viewing has been associated with higher intake of fats, sweet and salty snacks, and carbonated drinks, and lower intakes of fruits and vegetables (Coon & Tucker, 2002). Watching television while eating meals has been shown to lead to increased frequency of poor food choices (Coon, Goldberg, Rogers, & Tucker, 2001; Boynton-Jarrett, Thomas, Peterson, Wiecha, Sobol, & Gortmaker, 2003). Food is the most heavily advertised product on children's television, and highly sweetened products (e.g., sweetened beverages and sugar-rich cereals), as well as fast food, are the most frequently advertised foods (Gidding et al., 2005). In a classic study of television commercials, researchers noted that children watch 21.3 commercials per hour and that almost half of the advertisements were for food (mostly those high in sugar, salt, and/or fat). Even with the change in child advertising rules, advertising for unhealthful foods has changed little (Taras & Gage, 1995).

As children move from elementary to middle school, their food choices change dramatically. Fad diets and peer pressure become more of an issue. Media fast food promotion, targeted to middle and high school students, is common. Diets most often include fast food French fries and hamburgers, pizza, and sweetened carbonated beverages. "Excess fat, trans fat, and added sugars . . . (and) insufficient consumption of micronutrients such as calcium, iron, zinc, and potassium, as well as vitamins A, D, and C and folic acid" are common in this age group (Gidding et al., 2005, p. 2,068). This is a time when school-based nutrition education programs can have an influence (Gidding et al., 2005; Perez-Rodrigo & Aranceta, 2001) (see Using the Nursing Process).

In longitudinal research, preschool children whose BMI was greater than the 85th percentile were five times more likely to continue to be overweight at age 12. Children younger than age 9 with a BMI between the 75th and 85th percentiles have been shown to have a 40% to 50% greater chance of being overweight by age 12 (Nader et al., 2006). Parents can help their younger children develop better habits by implementing suggestions recommended by the American Heart Association (Gidding et al., 2005), for example:

◆ Reduce added sugars (cereals, drinks, juices, etc.).
◆ Use unsaturated oils in cooking (no solid fats).

USING THE NURSING PROCESS

James Lopez is entering third grade. His teacher comes to you, the school nurse, because she is concerned about his poor performance in school. He frequently comes to school late and often puts his head on his desk and appears to be falling asleep. You notice that James has gained a significant amount of weight over the summer. His face is much fuller now than in his second grade picture.

Assessment (Initial Visits)

You call James' mother and make an appointment for a home visit.

You do a health history, noting family history of diabetes, current eating, and activity and sleeping patterns for James and the family, and determine whether he has a regular physician and insurance or Medicaid.

You assess his vital signs, height and weight, hearing, and vision.

You talk more with his teacher about his activity on the playground and any signs of excessive thirst, hunger, or general fatigue.

Nursing Diagnoses

After a home visit, a meeting with James' teacher, and two observations/interviews with James, you decide on the following nursing diagnoses:

1. Nutrition: more than body requirements related to James' eating as a way of coping and his sedentary lifestyle.
2. Altered family process related to mother's recent change from being a stay-at-home single mom to attending truck driving school (necessitating absences of several days at a time, with James cared for by a married teenage sister and her husband).

Findings, Plan, and Implementation

James has been eating large quantities of snack food and fast food meals for the last 3 months, since his mother started her training. He has also quit participating in soccer and baseball, because his mother can no longer provide transportation. His bicycle was recently stolen, and he spends a lot of time playing video and computer games. James misses his mother when she is away and says that he "stays up late watching television" and has "trouble getting up for school" when he is at his sister's house.

You plan to work with the family to refer James to his physician to rule out diabetes. A family meeting is scheduled so that you can provide some health education on childhood obesity and inactivity. You discuss some possible interventions that the family can put into place:

• Decrease reliance on fast food meals.
• Have a regular evening meal time and encourage less snacking.
• Provide fresh fruit and vegetable snacks and decrease purchases of high-calorie, high-fat snack foods.
• Decrease sedentary activity (e.g., video and computer games, television viewing) and increase physical activity (e.g., team sports, walking, bicycling, active outdoor games).
• Establish a reasonable bedtime and consistently enforce it.
• Offer referral for family counseling so that James can discuss his feelings in a safe environment.
• With the family's input, seek ways for James and his mother to keep in better contact and for his sister to gain a greater understanding of good parenting practices.
• Meet with the teacher, the family, and James to discuss ways to help with his school performance.
• Continue to monitor James' progress with monthly height and weight checks, personal interviews, home visits, and teacher conferences.

Evaluation

The physician reported that James does not have diabetes; however, if he continues to gain weight and remains inactive he is at a higher risk for type 2 diabetes. Evaluation of nursing diagnoses 1 and 2 includes the following goals:

• The family will report less reliance on fast food and more meals cooked at home.
• The family will report more purchases of fresh fruits and vegetables and fewer purchases of high-calorie, high-fat snacks.
• James will report more physical exercise (by the use of a calendar) and less hours spent in sedentary activity (corroborated by family).
• James will exhibit less tardiness and fewer signs of sleep deprivation at school, and his school performance will improve.
• James and his family will complete sessions with a family counselor.
• James' weight will remain stable or will decrease as his height increases over time.

◆ Adhere to recommended portion sizes on food labels.
◆ Serve fresh, frozen, or canned vegetables and fruits at every meal.
◆ Use lean cuts of meat and remove skin from poultry.
◆ Serve fish more often, and eat more beans and tofu.
◆ Limit high-calorie creamy sauces (e.g., cheese, Alfredo).
◆ Eat more whole grains (look for breads and cereals with whole grain as the first ingredient).
◆ Watch for high salt and/or sugar content in processed soups, prepared foods, cereals, and breads (read labels and select lower salt/sugar options).
◆ Use nonfat or skimmed milk/dairy products.
◆ Help your child to get 60 minutes of moderate to vigorous exercise daily.
◆ With increasing activity, allow more discretionary calories (e.g., low-nutrient dense snacks and beverages).

Inadequate Nutrition

Undernutrition can also have serious consequences, including effects on the cognitive development and academic performance of children (Cook, 2002; Hall et al., 2001). Research indicates that food insecurity in kindergarten is associated with poorer mathematics performance in children and in delayed reading performance and social skills for girls (Jyoti, Frongillo, & Jones, 2005). Irritability, lack of energy, and difficulty concentrating are only some of the problems that arise from skipped meals or consistently inadequate nutrition. Infection and illness that lead to loss of school days can affect academic progress and interfere with the acquisition of basic skills, such as reading and mathematics. One study in Brazil found a link between childhood undernutrition and later risk of adult chronic degenerative diseases (Sawaya, Martins, Hoffman, & Roberts, 2003).

In children, the rate of food insecurity between 2003 and 2005 was estimated to be 18% (Cook, 2002). A national study of food insecurity found that it was associated with overweight status in children between the ages of 12 and 17, especially girls and children living in poverty (Casey et al., 2006). Another large-scale study failed to find a link between food insecurity and overweight (Rose & Bodor, 2006).

Olson, Bove, and Miller (2007) conducted a qualitative and quantitative study to examine how childhood poverty–associated food deprivation may lead to adult obesity. They found that, in some cases, early deprivation influenced later food choices and that there was an active drive to avoid food insecurity. Women in their study also developed patterns of emotional eating, and they concluded that attitudes and behaviors toward food were formed in childhood as a response to deprivation. Food insecurity in childhood has been linked to both undernutrition and overnutrition, and is most harmful during critical periods of development; it is also linked to postponed medical care and medications, lack of routine well-child medical visits, and absence of a usual source of health care for children (Cook, 2002; Ma, Gee, & Kushel, 2008). Childhood hunger was reported at 50% (severe hunger 16%) in a study of low-income homeless mothers and school-age children in Massachusetts. Hunger was related to higher chronic illness and anxiety/depression (Weinreb et al., 2002).

Undernutrition is frequently associated with poverty and hunger, but social pressure to be thin can also spark purposeful undernutrition. Because prepubertal children often exhibit a period of adiposity before a growth spurt, they are at risk for developing eating disorders (Dietz & Gortmaker, 2001). A 5-year study of the frequency of reading magazine articles about dieting and weight loss found that girls who frequently read these magazines were two times more likely to engage in unhealthful weight-control measures (e.g., skipping meals, smoking more cigarettes, fasting) than those who did not read magazine articles about dieting and weight loss. Extreme weight-control measures (e.g., laxative use, vomiting) were found three times more often in high-frequency readers versus nonreaders (van den Berg, Neumark-Sztainer, Hannan, & Haines, 2007). A longitudinal study of adolescents found that dieting and unhealthful weight-control measures predicted eating disorders and obesity 5 years later, thus emphasizing the need to encourage healthy eating and physical activity in childhood (Neumark-Sztainer, Wall, Guo, Story, Haines, & Eisenberg, 2006). School nurses and PHNs can provide families with necessary information to promote healthy eating and exercise.

Inactivity

An association between poor eating habits and physical inactivity was found in studies of school-age children and adolescents (Chatrath, Shenoy, Serratto, & Thoele, 2002; Trost et al., 2001). Low levels of physical activity and more than 2 hours of watching television per day were found to be predictors of overweight status in a large longitudinal study of children (Rose & Bodor, 2006). More television watching, fewer family meals eaten together at home, and living in an unsafe neighborhood were also shown to be associated with overweight (Gable, Chang, & Krull, 2007). The Youth Risk Behavior Survey (YRBS) revealed that 67% of children surveyed who were enrolled in physical education classes did not attend class on a daily basis. In addition, fewer than 39% of respondents stated that they participated in either vigorous or moderate physical activity for at least 20 minutes on at least 3 of the past 7 days, and almost 45% watched 3 or more hours of television on school nights (CDC, 2006a). Increased physical activity was shown to decrease BMI in a large study of overweight girls and boys (Berkey, Rockett, Gillman, & Colditz, 2003). Children who watched television and were less physically active during after-school hours were more likely to become overweight by age 12 in one 12-year longitudinal study of almost 1,000 children (O'Brien et al., 2007).

School nurses and PHNs can work with families to increase their levels of physical activity and to encourage limited television viewing for school-age children. They can also advocate for increased physical education in the school setting, and for increased safe recreational opportunities in all neighborhoods.

Dental Health

Dental caries affects more than half of U.S. school-age children and is the most common chronic disease for that age group. School days are lost to dental problems and dental visits, and self-esteem, along with general growth and function, can be hindered (Sinclair & Edelstein, 2005). In a comparison of African refugee children with U.S. children, the rate of dental caries for refugee children was half that of U.S. children (Cote, Geltman, Nunn, Lituri, Henshaw, & Garcia, 2004). Poor children report twice the rate of untreated dental caries than do children from higher-income families (Division of Oral Health, 2008). One twin study found that traits for dental caries and sucrose sweetness preference exhibit an independent "genetic contribution" (Bretz et al., 2006, p. 1,156).

The cost for dental services in 2003 was estimated to be $68 billion (CDC, 2003). The peak incidence of dental caries is found among school-age children and adolescents, although the effects of decay are observed in adulthood as caries activity recurs or various restorations fracture or wear out and must be replaced. One study found that school-age dental decay could be predicted in toddlers by determining the frequency of brushing and other variables, thus emphasizing the importance of regular brushing for young children (Clarke, Fraser-Lee, & Shimono, 2001).

Fluoridated drinking water, the availability of school-provided fluoride rinse or gel, and dental sealant programs are cost-effective, proven methods of reducing dental caries in school-age children (Lam, 2008; Levy, 2003; Marinho, Higgins, Logan, & Sheiham, 2003). The CDC found that for every $1 spent on fluoridation, $38 is saved in dental treatment costs (Sinclair & Edelstein, 2005). Between 11% and 72% of poor children have been found to have early childhood caries, an infectious disease thought to be caused by *Streptococcus mutans* and exacerbated by poor dietary practices. Topical antimicrobial therapies show some promise in these cases (Berkowitz, 2003; Kroll & Nedley, 2007). Some research has also demonstrated an association between passive exposure to tobacco smoke and tooth decay (Aligne, Moss, Auinger, & Weitzman, 2003).

Access to necessary outpatient dental care is much less expensive (by a factor of 10) than inpatient treatment of symptoms (Sinclair & Edelstein, 2005). Yet, access to dental care is still problematic. Barriers to dental care are more prevalent among the poor and those who are institutionalized. When children have public or private dental coverage, their incidence of at least one preventive dental visit during the previous year was 30% higher than for uninsured children (Sinclair & Edelstein, 2005). In a national survey, more than 32% of children living in poverty had a need for dental care, and more than 36% of children living within 100% to 199% of the poverty level had untreated dental caries (FCFS, n.d.). Financial barriers and lack of education lead to poor dental health values and adversely affect the appropriate use of early dental services and conscientious personal oral health care. PHNs and other community health nurses working with school-age children and families can promote good dental health through education and advocacy, as well as through collaboration to provide adequate dental services to uninsured children.

ADOLESCENT HEALTH

Adolescence is a time of self-discovery, movement toward self-reliance, increasing opportunities, and pivotal choices that can affect the remainder of an individual's life. Adolescence generally begins with puberty and encompasses the ages between 10 and 24; it consists of early adolescence (ages 10 to 14), middle adolescence (15 to 17), and late adolescence

(18 to mid 20s). Adult society largely segregates adolescents and often has ambiguous expectations for them (Feldman & Elliott, 1990). Adolescents are part of a subculture, one with its own language, dress, social mores, and values. The tasks of adolescence remain fairly constant: Adolescents must become autonomous, come to grips with their emerging sexuality and the skills necessary to attract a mate, and acquire skills and education that can prepare them for adult roles, all while resolving identity issues and developing values and beliefs (Feldman & Elliott, 1990; Shaffer & Kipp, 2006). The search for and expression of developing identity, along with the strong drive for social acceptance, are evident in the personal home pages and blogs of adolescents on social networking Internet sites such as MySpace and Facebook (Schmitt, Dayanim, & Matthias, 2008).

Adolescents are generally healthy, but parents and teens may differ in their perceptions of the adolescent's health. Adolescents from lower income brackets frequently report poorer health than those from higher-income groups (Johnson & Wang, 2008). As with other population groups, socioeconomic level and health are inversely related for adolescents. Teens also exhibit inverse relationships between income level and health resilience, school achievement, and feeling that they are in good health (Starfield, Riley, Witt, & Robertson, 2002). Parental long-term unemployment is also negatively associated with adolescent self-reported health status and depressive symptoms and psychosomatic complaints. These, along with poor health behaviors related to lack of physical activity and drug use or smoking, contribute to self-perceived poor or fair health (Piko, 2007; Sleskova et al., 2006). Social stressors and strained relations with peers and parents are also related to health complaints, including psychosomatic complaints (Brolin-Laftman & Ostberg, 2006; Hjern, Alfven, & Ostberg, 2008). Common complaints of adolescents include fatigue, sleep deprivation, chronic insomnia, acne, and concerns about weight and body image (Chung & Cheung, 2008; Koch, Ryder, Dziura, Njike, & Antaya, 2008; Roberts, Roberts, & Duong, 2008; ter Bogt et al., 2006; ter Wolbeek, van Doornen, Kavelaars, & Heijnen, 2006). As children become adolescents, their sleep patterns change—they move from early risers/sleepers to staying up later and sleeping in later, or catching up on sleep over weekends. This transition becomes more apparent through high school (Gau & Soong, 2003). Sleep deprivation, along with television viewing time, has been related to increased BMI and blood pressure, and a poor body weight perception (being overweight or underweight) has predicted problem behaviors in both male and female adolescents (ter Bogt et al., 2006; Wells et al., 2008).

In the past, routine health care visits by adolescents were not commonplace. However, newer recommended vaccines and better awareness of the health needs of adolescents have resulted in better utilization of services. In 2003, about 73% of adolescents between the ages of 12 and 17 had one or more preventive medical visits. More than 51% had one or more visits due to illness or injury—the most common reasons being bronchitis or upper-respiratory infections and trauma-related problems (National Adolescent Health Information Center [NAHIC], 2008). In 2005, over 45% of adolescents ages 15 to 24 had emergency room visits, largely for contusions.

Hospitalization was most often related to childbirth, but trauma-related injuries (e.g., wounds, fractures) were also prominent. About 20% of 12- to 17-year olds with special health care needs do not get the health care services they need (NAHIC, 2008). About 87% of adolescents (ages 12 to 17) had insurance coverage in 2005; but the number drops to 55% for those ages 18 to 24. Hispanic adolescents have the least proportion of health insurance—public or private—and were the least likely to have had a health care visit in the past year (NAHIC, 2008).

Health literacy during adolescence is an important consideration. Teens are frequent users of mass media (Internet, television, radio, text messaging), and specific health-related educational interventions can be targeted to them by using these media (Manganello, 2007).

During the period that roughly encompasses the teen years, adolescents encounter many complex changes, physically, emotionally, cognitively, and socially (Steinberg, 2005). Rapid and major developmental adjustments create a variety of stresses with concomitant problems that have an impact on health. More recent advanced neuroimaging techniques have demonstrated marked changes in the adolescent brain, especially related to white and gray matter and the prefrontal cortex (Blakemore, den Ouden, Choudhury, & Frith, 2007; Casey, Jones, & Hare, 2008), along with other regions of the brain related to "attention, reward evaluation, affective discrimination, response inhibition, and goal-directed behavior," that help explain the cognitive and affective peculiarities of this developmental period (Yurgelun-Todd, 2007, p. 251).

The uneven changes in brain development may also help explain the risk-taking behaviors and higher incidence of unintentional injuries found in this population (Paus, 2005). Unintentional injuries were the leading cause of death in the 15- to 24-year-old age group. Most deaths in this adolescent/young adult age group are due to preventable causes (NAHIC, 2006b). The overall injury death rate for adolescents (10 to 19 years of age) was 30.9 per 100,000 between 1999 and 2002. A dramatic upward trend in these figures is apparent: the rate at age 10 is 6.9, but by age 19, it jumps to 72.1. Gender differences are also apparent: girls are much less likely than boys to engage in behaviors that put them at risk for injuries, resulting in more than twice the unintentional injury death rate for males than females between the ages of 15 and 19 (NAHIC, 2000).

The overall unintentional death rate for only motor vehicle–related injuries was 14.9 (Bernard et al., 2007). The death rate from motor vehicle–related injuries for this age group peaked during the 1970s and 1980s, then declined throughout the next 2 decades, although motor vehicle–related injuries remain the number one cause of injury mortality for this age group (Bernard et al., 2007; NAHIC, 2000). Considering that 99% of motor vehicle–related injuries are nonfatal, this death rate becomes even more alarming (NAHIC, 2000). Ethnic differences are noted, with Whites having higher death rates than other ethnic and racial groups (Fig. 22.4).

Health Objectives for Adolescents

Healthy People 2010 objectives are focused on improving the health of all Americans. Of the 476 objectives, 107 have been identified as relevant to the adolescent population (Park, Brindis, Chang, & Irwin, 2008). However, 21 specific objectives have been ranked as critical objectives related to adoles-

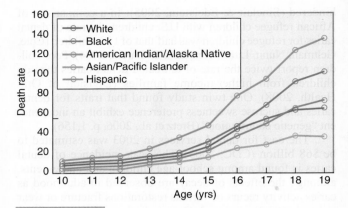

FIGURE 22.4 Rate of injury death among children aged 10–19 years, by race/ethnicity—United States, 1999–2002. Retrieved July 31, 2008 from www.cdc.gov/mmwr/preview/mmwrtml/ss5605al.htm?s_cid=ss5605a1_x.

cents and young adults (CDC, n.d.). Because much of the mortality and morbidity in this age group stems from risk-taking behaviors, many of these objectives address alcohol-related unintentional injuries, violent behaviors, and suicide and mental health issues, as well as more responsible reproductive health behaviors (Table 22.1). The 2007 midcourse review of these critical objectives found overall mortality trends at two times the 2010 target rate, although the 10- to 14-year-old rate is "on pace to reach the 2010 target" (p. 331). Unintentional injury results are mixed; motor vehicle–related crashes (with and without alcohol) increased slightly, but seat belt use also increased, and the number of adolescents reporting that they rode with a driver who had been drinking alcohol decreased. The objectives related to "homicide, physical fighting, and carrying a weapon have shown little or no improvement" (p. 331), and mental health objectives have shown mixed results. Suicide rates and reported attempted suicides are not significantly improved, and only modest increases are found in other objectives related to mood and treatment. Binge drinking and marijuana use demonstrate small decreases, and vigorous physical activity reports are basically unchanged. Tobacco use has gone down considerably, but obesity and overweight figures increased by more than 50%. The adolescent pregnancy rate decreased 34%—the best results of all 21 objectives—almost achieving the 2010 target rate, and related objectives are on pace to reach targets (e.g., never having sex, used a condom with last sexual contact). Chlamydia infection rates have increased, but may be an artifact of more sensitive testing and improved reporting (Park et al., 2008).

Because adolescents have less contact with the health care system than children, many conditions may go undetected. Also, a shift occurs from a childhood preponderance of physical conditions to more social behavioral problems in adolescence. Risk behaviors become much more evident, along with their attendant outcomes: unsafe sexual activity, substance use, violence, and motor vehicle–related issues (Michaud, 2008; Shaffer & Kipp, 2006).

Emotional Problems and Suicide

The adolescent years are a time of rapid growth and change. Hormonal influences may cause a teen to be emotional and

TABLE 22.1   *Healthy People 2010*: **21 Critical Health Objectives for Adolescents and Young Adults**

The 21 Critical Health Objectives represent the most serious health and safety issues facing adolescents and young adults (aged 10 to 24 years): mortality, unintentional injury, violence, substance abuse and mental health, reproductive health, and the prevention of chronic diseases during adulthood.

Obj. #	Objective	Baseline (year)	2010 Target
16-03. (a,b,c)	Reduce deaths of adolescents and young adults. 10–to 14–year-olds 15–to 19–year-olds 20–to 24–year-olds	21.5 per 100,000 (1998) 69.5 per 100,000 (1998) 92.7 per 100,000 (1998)	(per 100,000) 16.8 39.8 49.0
Unintentional Injury			
15-15. (a)	Reduce deaths caused by motor vehicle crashes. 15- to 24-year-olds	25.6 per 100,000 (1999)	[1]
26-01. (a)	Reduce deaths and injuries caused by alcohol- and drug-related motor vehicle crashes. 15- to 24-year-olds	13.5 per 100,000 (1998)	[1]
15-19.	Increase use of safety belts. 9th –12th grade students	84.0% (1999)	92.0%
26-06.	Reduce the proportion of adolescents who report that they rode, during the previous 30 days, with a driver who had been drinking alcohol. 9th –12th grade students	33.0% (1999)	30.0%
Violence			
15-32.	Reduce homicides. 10–to 14–year-olds 15–to 19–year-olds	1.2 per 100,000 (1999) 10.4 per 100,000 (1999)	[1] [1]
15-38.	Reduce physical fighting among adolescents. 9th –12th grade students	36.0% (1999)	32.0%
15-39.	Reduce weapon carrying by adolescents on school property. 9th –12th grade students	6.9% (1999)	4.9%
Substance Abuse and Mental Health			
26-11. (d)	Reduce the proportion of persons engaging in binge drinking of alcoholic beverages. 12- to 17-year-olds	7.7% (1998)	2.0%
26-10. (b)	Reduce past-month use of illicit substances (marijuana). 12- to 17-year-olds	8.3% (1998)	0.7%
18-01.	Reduce the suicide rate. 10–to 14–year-olds 15–to 19–year-olds	1.2 per 100,000 (1999) 8.0 per 100,000 (1999)	[1] [1]

U.S. Department of Health and Human Services
Centers for Disease Control and Prevention

Obj. #	Objective	Baseline (year)	2010 Target
18-02.	Reduce the rate of suicide attempts by adolescents that required medical attention. 9th –12th grade students	2.6% (1999)	1.0%
06-02.	Reduce the proportion of children and adolescents with disabilities who are reported to be sad, unhappy, or depressed. 4- to 17-year-olds	[2]	[2]
18-07.	Increase the proportion of children with mental health problems who receive treatment.	59.0% (2001)	66.0%
Reproductive Health			
09-07.	Reduce pregnancies among adolescent females. 15- to 17-year-olds	68.0 per 1,000 females (1996)	43.0 per 1,000
13-05.	(Developmental) Reduce the number of new cases of HIV/AIDS diagnosed among adolescents and adults. 13- to 24-year-olds	16,479 (1998) [4]	[3]
25-01. (a,b,c)	Reduce the proportion of adolescents and young adults with *Chlamydia trachomatis* infections. 15- to 24-year-olds		
	Females attending family planning clinics	5.0% (1997)	3.0%
	Females attending sexually transmitted disease clinics	12.2% (1997)	3.0%
	Males attending sexually transmitted disease clinics	15.7% (1997)	3.0%
25-11. (a,b,c)	Increase the proportion of adolescents (9th–12th grade students) who: Have never had sexual intercourse	50.0% (1999)	56.0%
	If sexually experienced, are not currently sexually active	27.0% (1999)	30.0%
	If currently sexually active, used a condom the last time they had sexual intercourse	58.0% (1999)	65.0%
Chronic Diseases			
27-02. (a)	Reduce tobacco use by adolescents. 9th–12th grade students	40.0% (1999)	21.0%
19-03. (b)	Reduce the proportion of children and adolescents who are overweight or obese. 12- to 19-year-olds	11.0% (1988-94)	5.0%
22-07.	Increase the proportion of adolescents who engage in vigorous physical activity that promotes cardiorespiratory fitness 3 or more days per week for 20 or more minutes per occasion. 9th –12th grade students	65.0% (1999)	85.0%

Note: Critical health outcomes are underlined, and behaviors that substantially contribute to important health outcomes are in normal font.

[1] 2010 target not provided for adolescent/young adult age group.
[2] Baseline and target inclusive of age groups outside of adolescent/young adult age parameters.
[3] Developmental objective – baseline and 2010 target coming soon.
[4] Proposed baseline is shown but has not yet been approved by the *Healthy People 2010* Steering Committee.

Source: U.S. Department of Health and Human Services. *Healthy People 2010*. Volumes 1 and 2. Washington, DC: U.S. Government Printing Office, November 2000. This information can also be accessed at *http://wonder.cdc.gov/data2010/*.

**U.S. Department of Health and Human Services
Centers for Disease Control and Prevention**

From Centers for Disease Control & Prevention (CDC). (n.d.). *21 Critical Health Objectives for Adolescents and Young Adults.* Retrieved July 31, 2008 from http://www.cdc.gov/HealthyYouth/adolescenthealth/NationalInitiative/pdf/21objectives.pdf.

unpredictable at times (SAMHSA, 2003). The influence of peers increases, and peer pressure may influence behavior. Teens test family rules and generally search for their own identity and individuality apart from the family. Most parents and teens ride out this period with love and understanding and no long-term negative effects. For some children, however, a real or perceived lack of emotional support can lead to temporary or permanent emotional problems. Longitudinal research through late childhood into adolescence reveals that harsh parenting practices in childhood and parental rejection in adolescence lead to shame and guilt that are associated with depression and delinquency (Stuewig & McCloskey, 2005). Also, gender differences in types and trajectories of emotional and behavioral problems have been noted, with more females developing adolescent-onset depression and males demonstrating more conduct problems at an earlier age of onset (Zahn-Waxler, Shirtcliff, & Marceau, 2008). Emotional problems can affect many, often subtle, aspects of an adolescent's life: for example, positive psychosocial adjustment has been linked to fewer traffic offenses in adolescents (Bingham, Shope, & Raghunathan, 2006).

Depression, schizophrenia, and eating disorders may first appear during adolescence. About 50% of mental health conditions begin before age 14, and 75% by age 21 (Knopf, Park, & Mulye, 2008). It is estimated through parent ratings that approximately 12% of 12- to 17-year-olds have a serious behavioral or mental health problem (12% of females and 12.3% of males; low-income youth were rated at almost 18%) (Knopf et al., 2008). Common adolescent mental health problems include depression, anxiety disorders, ADHD, and substance abuse problems. Mild depression affects over 25% of adolescents, but prevalence rates vary (Fig. 22.5). Depression is two times more likely among females (ages 15 to 20), and comorbidities (e.g., anxiety disorder, and addictive and conduct disorders) are not uncommon (Knopf et al., 2008). Researchers have concluded that between 20% and 25% of adolescents display symptoms of emotional distress, and about 10% have moderate to severe symptoms (Knopf et al., 2008). Adolescent brain maturation

may explain susceptibility to depression during this period of development (Andersen & Teicher, 2008).

Many adolescents are reluctant to seek help for emotional problems, or help may not be readily available to them. Most research shows that many adolescents with "significant emotional distress" fail to receive mental health treatment—estimates have ranged from 10% to less than 40% (Knopf et al., 2008, p. 9). Newer survey results have found that 21.3% of youth ages 12 to 17 have been given some type of mental health services, but the usual disparities apply (e.g., ethnicity, income level, rural versus urban locale). Treatment for serious mental health problems may include hospitalization or placement in a group home. However, primary care providers commonly evaluate children and adolescents for psychosocial problems in their everyday practice. Pediatricians report that almost 19% of patient visits concerned conduct or emotional problems or ADHD (Knopf et al., 2008).

Suicide is the third leading cause of death in adolescents and young adults (NAHIC, 2006a). A psychiatric diagnosis is found in 90% of suicide victims, with depression noted in over 50% of all cases (Shaffer, Gould, & Hicks, 2007). In 2003, the suicide rate in the 10- to 24-year age group was 6.8 per 100,000, down from the peak rate in the early 1990s. However, the rate increased by 8% between 2003 and 2004, reflecting the largest 1-year jump between 1990 and 2004 (Lubell, Kegler, Crosby, & Karch, 2007). It is interesting to note that, even though antidepressant medications have demonstrated effectiveness in reducing depressive symptoms in adolescents (the relationship between antidepressants and suicide has not been studied), the sudden rise in suicides in 2004 coincided with a large decline in antidepressant prescriptions. Also, selective serotonin reuptake inhibitors (SSRIs; among the more commonly prescribed antidepressant medications) are almost never found during autopsy of teen suicide victims (Shaffer et al., 2007; CDC, 2006c). In 2005, almost 17% of high school students reported that they seriously considered suicide in the previous 12 months (21.8% girls, 12% boys), and 8.4% made at least one suicide attempt—2.3% made an attempt that required medical attention (CDC 2007e; Lubell et al., 2007). Geographically, higher suicide rates occur in the West (i.e., Alaska, New Mexico, Montana), and the lowest rates are found in the northeastern United States (Shaffer et al., 2007). As teens age, they are more at risk for suicide: the rate increases from 1.2 per 100,000 for ages 10 to 14 to 12.1 for ages 20 to 24. Males are five times more likely to die from suicide than females, and male American Indian/Alaska Natives are two to four times more likely than other ethnic groups to die from suicide (NAHIC, 2006a).

Girls, especially Hispanic females, attempt suicide more frequently than boys (Lubell et al., 2007). An alarming finding is that suicide deaths by hanging or suffocation have dramatically increased for girls, whereas the use of firearms has decreased since 1997; poisoning has increased only slightly (National Youth Violence, 2007).

It is important to question a teen about her history of depression or feelings of hopelessness, as well as the quality and quantity of her social support systems and the availability of means to follow through on suicide threats (Bethell & Rhodes, 2008). School and discipline problems, family discord, and depression, as well as drug and alcohol abuse can increase the risk of suicide (NCIPC, 2007). Recent stressful events and preoccupation with suicide, as well as substance

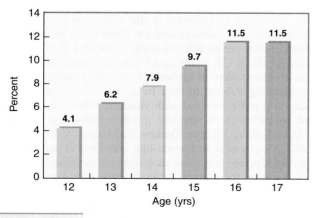

FIGURE 22.5 Prevalence of past-year major depressive episode among youth aged 12–17, by age: 2005. From Substance Abuse & Mental Health Services Administration (SAMHSA). (May 3, 2007). *The National Survey on Drug Use & Health Report.* Depression and the use of alcohol and other drug use among youths aged 12–17.

use, are also important to note. Gay, lesbian, and bisexual youth have high rates of suicidal ideation and suicide attempts, and for all youth, having a close family member who committed suicide doubles the risk (Shaffer et al., 2007). *Suicide contagion* refers to copycat suicides, especially among high school students, after a highly publicized suicide. This can lead to suicide clusters—deaths of three to seven adolescents over a 3- to 9-month period (Shaffer et al., 2007).

Suicide hotlines are often ineffective for adolescents, as they are infrequently used (Shaffer et al., 2007). Suicide prevention programs and direct intervention by counselors or school nurses to determine an adolescent's suicide intentions are the most effective school-based approaches (Eggert, Thompson, Randell, & Pike, 2002; May, Somal, Hurt, & DeBruyn, 2005). Hendin and colleagues (2001) noted that it is important for counselors to identify markers for attempted suicide, such as a precipitating event, intense affective state, suicide ideation or actions, deterioration in social or academic functioning, or increased substance abuse. Community health nurses and community mental health counselors may serve as consultants to schools in the development of sound prevention programs. Hallmarks of good prevention programs include school policies and inservice training on suicide prevention; collaboration among teachers, counselors, and nurses; student education on suicide prevention; peer assistance programs; school–family–community partnerships; activities that increase school connectedness; and crisis intervention teams. Suicide screening, education, and peer support have been found to significantly reduce the rates of self-reported suicide attempts (Aseltine & DeMartino, 2004). Some examples of programs used in high schools include *Suicide-Awareness Voices Education*, *Lifelines*, and *SOS: Signs of Suicide* (Shaffer et al., 2007).

A behavior that can sometimes accidentally result in suicide is *self-injury* or *cutting*. Adolescents with this abnormal behavior who overdose, cut, burn, or otherwise dangerously harm themselves are attempting to find relief from profound psychological pain. The physical injury distracts them from these painful emotions, possibly giving them a feeling of control or providing a means of feeling emotions when they are cut off from them. This behavior is found in 3% to 5% of the population, and most often begins in early adolescence or late childhood. It is more common in girls and in those with a family history of suicide or self-injury. Isolation, neglect, or abuse may predispose an adolescent to this behavior. Depression, borderline personality disorder, and eating disorders are commonly associated with self-injury. PHNs and school nurses can provide education to adolescents and families about this condition, and can work with schools to promote prevention strategies, such as early detection and referral to mental health providers (Mayo Clinic, 2006).

Violence

Arrests for violent youth crimes peaked in the decade between 1983 and 1993 (Surgeon General of the United States, 2002). The total costs of youth violence are more than $158 billion each year (CDC, 2007d). Nonfatal violent crimes (among youth ages 12 to 24) dropped by one-half between 1994 and 2004. Simple assault was 321 times more common than homicide (Dinkes et al., 2006). Homicide is the second leading cause of death for adolescents (ages 10 to 24), and is more common in males than females. Homicide rates for 10- to 24-year-olds peaked in the early 1990s, but decreased significantly by the end of that decade. Firearms are involved in most adolescent and young adult homicides (NAHIC, 2007).

Surveys show that between 15% and 40% of teens admit to having committed a serious violent offense by age 17, and serious youth violence is part of a constellation of risk-taking behaviors that also includes precocious sex, drugs, and guns (Surgeon General of the United States, 2002). Multiple longitudinal research studies show that delinquency peaks during middle adolescence—around age 16. Preadolescent delinquency, however, has been related to a pattern of persistent criminal behavior (Landsheer & van Dijkum, 2005). Children assault and kill other children at school and on the streets. More than 20,000 children and adolescents are killed or injured by firearms each year. Adolescents (between the ages of 15 to 19 years) account for almost 85% of all firearm injuries treated in emergency rooms or hospitals. Only 1% of all firearm-related deaths for school-age children occur on school grounds (Fingerhut & Kaufer-Christoffel, 2002).

Gangs are often associated with teen violence. However, the proportion of schools reporting gang activity has dropped (Surgeon General of the United States, 2002), and the overall number of gangs and gang members has decreased since 1996 (Egley & Ritz, 2006; National Youth Violence Prevention Center [NYVPRC], 2008). However, gangs have penetrated previously untouched areas; they are now found in every state and in smaller communities with populations of 25,000 or less (Egley & Ritz, 2006). In large cities, about one-quarter of homicides are considered gang-related; in Chicago and Los Angeles, more than half are gang-related (Egley & Ritz, 2006). In schools where gang activity is reported, higher drug availability and student victimization are found (NYVPRC, 2008). Incidents of high school shootings have raised concerns among parents and teachers. School violence has been linked to bullying (Nansel, Overpeck, Haynie, Ruan, & Scheidt, 2003) and school environments. Comprehensive school safety plans are advised; grants and technical assistance are available to local school districts through the federal government.

Cultural and environmental influences on youth include the violence to which children and adolescents are exposed. Increased aggressive behavior among children and teens has been attributed to violence in the environment, the home (spousal and child abuse), and the community, as well as to what children see on television and in movies. A large-scale study across 10 U.S. cities found that adolescents (even more than children) were at higher risk for being victimized and experiencing a threat to their lives. Adolescents were more likely also to be involved with violence outside their homes and to suffer from physical injuries related to violence (Harpaz-Rotem, Murphy, Berkowitz, Marans, & Rosenheck, 2007). A study of 9- to 15-year-olds who lived in public housing demonstrated that some adolescents who witness violence (not as victims themselves) suffer the same symptoms that victims of violence experience, for example, difficulty concentrating, vigilant/avoidant behavior, and intrusive thoughts and feelings (Howard, Feigelman, Li, Cross, & Rachuba, 2002). Violence is an increasing threat for teenagers. Middle school students are reported to fight more and experience bullying more than elementary school age children or high school students (Juvonen, Le, Kaganoff, Augustine, & Constant, 2004).

Bullying can result in depression, social anxiety, internalizing and psychosomatic symptoms, loneliness, and poor school performance (Arseneault et al., 2008; Wigfield, Lutz, & Wagner, 2005). Children or adolescents with anxiety or depression are also at increased risk of being the victims of bullying (Fekkes, Pijpers, Fredriks, Vogels, & Verloove-Vanhorick, 2006). The percentage of young adolescents who do not feel safe at school is increasing dramatically: In the most recent Youth Risk Behavior Survey, 18.5% of adolescents reported carrying a weapon to school during the past month, and more than 35.9% were involved in physical fights in the last year (CDC, 2006a).

Adolescents who are better connected to school are less likely to engage in violent behaviors. School climate is important in reducing the levels of violence in this age group (Brookmeyer, Fanti, & Henrich, 2006). High levels of parental support have been found to moderate the effects of witnessing violent acts, in that children with support are less likely to commit violent acts (Brookmeyer, Henrich, & Schwab-Stone, 2005).

Following the lead of the federal government with the implementation of the Safe and Drug-Free Schools and Communities Act, most schools have developed zero-tolerance policies to counteract and prevent violence (King, Wagner, & Hedrick, 2001). Many schools now have metal detectors and security guards, and some schools conduct random searches of students' lockers in an effort to prevent violence. However, a report from the American Psychological Association Zero Tolerance Task Force (2006) that examined 10 years of research studies, found that schools are no safer after the implementation of these widespread policies and that the policies can actually lead to increased violent and disruptive behavior and higher dropout rates. The task force found that a disproportionate number of Black and Hispanic students were expelled or suspended from school, and that zero-tolerance policies do not consider children's lapses in judgment as a normal aspect of development. They recommended adaptations to zero-tolerance policies to make them more flexible and individualized to students, school sites, and situations.

Substance Abuse

Substance abuse among young people was almost unknown before 1950, and rare before 1960. Now, adolescent drug experimentation and use pose serious physical and psychological threats. A national survey found that by the time they complete high school, 53% of teens report having tried an illicit drug, and 78% have consumed alcohol (Johnston, O'Malley, & Bachman, 2003). A more recent survey reported that 47% of high school seniors have tried an illicit drug, which reflects a slight improvement over earlier surveys (Johnston, O'Malley, Bachman, & Schulenberg, 2008). The most recent Youth Risk Behavior Survey found that 20.2% of high school students had used marijuana in the past month, and 54.8% of 12th-graders smoke marijuana regularly; 3.4% of high school students had used cocaine at some time. Over 43% reported that they currently drink alcohol (CDC, 2006a).

Why do adolescents turn to alcohol or illicit drugs? Acosta, Manubay, and Levin (2008) have described parallels between addictive behavior and obesity—especially personality, environmental risk factors, genetic predisposition, and

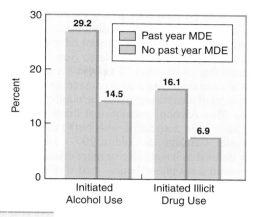

FIGURE 22.6 Percentages reporting past-year substance use initiation among persons aged 12–17 who were at risk for substance use initiation, by past year major depressive episode (MDE): 2005. From Substance Abuse & Mental Health Services Administration (SAMHSA). *The National Survey on Drug Use & Health Report.* (May 3, 2007). Depression and the use of alcohol and other drug use among youths aged 12–17.

common neurobiologic brain pathways. A large-scale, 25-year prospective longitudinal study in New Zealand found that gender, novelty-seeking behaviors, childhood conduct disorder, and parental illicit drug use predicted use of illicit drugs in 16- to 25-year-olds. Marijuana use, substance-using peers, and alcohol use were also factors (Fergusson, Boden, & Horwood, 2008; Fergusson, Horwood, & Ridder, 2007). Depression has also been linked to alcohol and substance use (Fig. 22.6). Can peers lure adolescents into alcohol and drug use? Most evidence reveals both genetic and environmental influences—in other words, those who were more prone by genetics to use substances "were more vulnerable to adverse influences of their best friends" (Harden, Hill, Turkheimer, & Emery, 2008).

Alcohol is the most frequently used substance for U.S. adolescents—it is their "drug of choice" (Faden, 2006, p. 1,011). Boys begin drinking at an earlier age than girls, usually around seventh and eighth grades. According to the 2005 Youth Risk Behavior Survey (CDC, 2006a), 43.3% of high school students reported drinking alcohol within the previous month. Early drinkers more often report academic problems, use of other substances, and delinquent behavior in middle and high school. A study found that, by the time they were young adults, people with a history of early alcohol use had problems related to abuse of other substances, employment problems, and criminal and violent behavior (Ellickson, Tucker, & Klein, 2003). Analysis of national survey data found that adolescents who begin first alcohol use before the age of 13 had significantly more involvement in violent behaviors and suicide attempts than those who delayed the initiation of alcohol (Swahn, Bossarte, & Sullivent, 2008). Early use of alcohol was found to be a marker for later alcohol and drug dependence in one longitudinal study (King & Chassin, 2007), and in a large-scale twin study, early regular drinking was significantly associated with later drug abuse and dependence, as well as with alcohol use and dependence that could not be fully explained by shared family factors or genetics (Grant et al., 2006). It is important to stress education and prevention in late childhood to delay the initiation of alcohol use.

A study on the effects of alcohol advertising on youth drinking rates (Snyder, Milici, Slater, Sun, & Strizhakova, 2006) found that youth (ages 15 to 26) who saw more advertising for alcohol drank more on average (each dollar spent per capita on alcohol advertising raised the number of drinks consumed by 3%). Alcohol promotional items (e.g., clothing, posters) have been associated with binge drinking (Fisher, Miles, Austin, Camargo, & Colditz, 2007). Binge drinking is generally defined as having five or more drinks at one time—usually within a couple of hours—and it often increases as adolescents get older (CDC, 2008c; Miller, Naimi, Brewer, & Jones, 2007). Binge drinking has been associated with poor academic achievement and other risk behaviors (e.g., sexual activity, smoking, using illicit drugs, riding with a driver who had been drinking, attempting suicide), and the more adolescents binge drink, the more they engage in risk behaviors (Miller et al., 2007).

Family drinking and perceived family norms related to drinking have been found to affect adolescents' perceptions of the benefits of drinking. This perception, in turn, predicts their drinking behavior (Epstein, Griffin, & Botvin, 2008). Parenting practices (e.g., monitoring, discipline, enforcing rules related to alcohol use) have also been found to have an influence on adolescent drinking behavior (Latendresse et al., 2008; Van der Vorst, Engels, Meeus, Dekovi, & Van Leeuwe, 2005).

Some research has suggested that adolescents who spend more meal times with their families are less likely to engage in alcohol and other substance use and are more likely to have better grades and fewer depressive symptoms (Eisenberg, Olson, Neumark-Sztainer, Story, & Bearinger, 2004). Family meal times have been shown to promote family cohesion and problem- and emotion-focused coping by encouraging parents to help their children feel part of the family and allowing them valuable time to coach them in effective methods for dealing with daily stresses and problems (Franko, Thompson, Affenito, Barton, & Striegel-Moore, 2008). To promote the health and welfare of adolescent children, it is vital to stress to families with young children the continued importance of family meals throughout adolescence.

Marijuana is the most commonly used drug among 14- to 17-year-olds—41.8% of high school seniors reported ever using marijuana (National Survey on Drug Use & Health [NSDUH], 2008). Use of marijuana by early adolescents fell, but middle to late adolescent use remained the same (Johnston et al., 2008). This is an important finding, because early marijuana use (before age 15) has been associated with a much greater likelihood of adult cocaine and heroin use and drug dependency (Office of National Drug Control Policy [ONDCP], 2008). Marijuana use has negative health effects, including anxiety, panic attacks, increased heart rate, frequent respiratory infections, impaired memory and learning, and tolerance. Regular marijuana smokers often have respiratory complications similar to those of tobacco smokers—cough, phlegm, respiratory infections, and airway obstruction (ONDCP, 2008).

Inhalant abuse is very common, and shows signs of resurgence (Johnston et al., 2008). Inhalant use begins in early adolescence—more 12- and 13-year-olds reported using inhalants than any other illicit drug. The most commonly reported inhalants used were shoe polish, glue or toluene, spray paints, and lighter fluid or gasoline (NSDUH, 2008). Other inhalants commonly used include amyl nitrite "poppers"; locker room deodorizers or "rush"; cleaning fluid, degreasers, or correction fluid; halothane, ether, or other anesthetics; lacquer thinner or other paint solvents; butane or propane gases; nitrous oxide or "whippets"; and other aerosol sprays (NSDUH, 2008). Inhalant abuse can result in severe nervous system damage or death. Control of legal products, such as spray paint, lighter fluid, household solvents, gasoline, and glue, is difficult, making this problem almost impossible to monitor adequately.

Other drugs that are used by adolescents and young adults include "club drugs" such as MDMA (Ecstasy), a synthetic drug with amphetamine and hallucinogenic properties; Rohypnol (the date rape drug that is often mixed with alcohol to produce sedative hypnotic effects); ketamine (a rapid-acting anesthetic); lysergic acid diethylamide (LSD), an hallucinogen originally popularized in the 1960s; and gamma hydroxybutyrate (GHB, a drug that is touted as a synthetic steroid in fitness clubs and that has been associated with sexual assaults). Rates of use for ketamine, Rohypnol, and GHB have declined over the past few years, but Psilocybin, or "magic mushrooms" are still widely used. Ecstasy use has generally declined but may become popular again among younger adolescents. Over-the-counter cold and cough medications containing the cough suppressant dextromethorphan are sometimes used to produce a "high," and between 4% and 7% of adolescents are reported to have used them (Johnston et al., 2008). Visits to the emergency department and deaths have occurred from the use of many of these drugs.

Cocaine use has remained steady in recent years, after peaking in the late 1990s. Heroin use fell below peak levels reached in 2001 but continues to remain steady. Smoking or snorting of heroin, which is popular among adolescents and young adults because they mistakenly believe it precludes the strong physical addictiveness of this drug, has been found to lead to injection drug abuse (Johnston, O'Malley, & Bachman, 2003). Methamphetamine (meth) use has demonstrated a consistent decline since 1999. It may also be smoked, along with marijuana, or injected. Meth labs are a public health hazard and can often be found in rural areas.

The illicit use of anabolic steroids is also difficult to monitor; however, 0.8% of 8th graders, 1.1% of 10th graders, and 1.4% of 12th graders report using steroids (Johnston et al., 2008). About one-third of high school students taking anabolic steroid are girls (Gober, Klein, Berger, Vindigni, & McCabe, 2006). Some coaches have, at times, turned a blind eye to steroid abuse, but educational campaigns to fight the rising level of abuse in adolescents have led to decreases in use since peak levels were reached in 2000. Sato, Schulz, Sisk, and Wood (2008, p. 647) report that animal models show "adolescent anabolic-androgenic steroid exposure increases aggression, and causes lasting changes in neurotransmitter systems." Other symptoms include irritability, increased risk-taking behavior, extreme mood swings, and euphoria, psychiatric conditions may be intensified or induced. Some have cautioned that withdrawal from steroids may be especially difficult for adolescents who are "vulnerable to hormonal swings" (Gober et al., 2006).

Adolescents are becoming more involved with prescription drugs, often found in their parents' medicine cabinets, purchased on the Internet, or bought from friends at school (McCabe et al., 2007). Teens may have "pharming parties," in which medication bottles are emptied onto tables and selected like candies (Hipp, 2006). Medications are often mixed with alcohol, and half of adolescents surveyed stated that they believed prescription medicines are safer than street drugs when used to produce a high (Partnership for a Drug-Free America, 2004). Ritalin, prescribed to students with ADHD, may be given or sold to others, but the most commonly used medications are OxyContin, Vicodin, tranquilizers, and sedatives. One in 20 high school seniors has tried OxyContin, and almost 10% of high school seniors have used Vicodin (Johnston et al., 2008). This trend is very disturbing because of society's nonchalant, casual attitude toward prescription medications and their easy access. Early onset (before age 13) of nonmedical use of prescription medications is a predictor of later prescription drug abuse and drug dependence (McCabe, West, Morales, Cranford, & Boyd, 2007).

Tobacco products are also easily acquired, often from parents. Almost 70% of high school students reported in 2001 that they had smoked a cigarette, and more than 23% reported that they purchased their own cigarettes from a store or gas station (CDC, 2002b). The most recent Youth Risk Behavior Survey found that fewer students reported trying cigarettes—46% of 12th graders and 22% of 8th graders. Only 23% of high school students had smoked cigarettes on one or more days within the last 30 days (CDC, 2006a). The use of smokeless tobacco, or "chew," has also declined. Social disapproval and heightened perception of health risks have most likely helped contribute to the downward trend of smoking and smokeless tobacco use, as have price increases and advertising bans (Johnston et al., 2008). Also, comprehensive merchant education programs have reduced illegal sales to minors (Tobacco Information & Prevention Source, 2001). In a study of adolescents who use tobacco, addictive symptoms have been shown to begin to appear within the first few weeks of initiating smoking, highlighting the need to continue to attack this problem even though rates have been in decline over the past few years (DiFranza, 2008). Smoking cessation programs for adolescents must take into account their levels of nicotine dependence and stress, as well as the effectiveness of cognitive coping methods (Siqueira, Rolnitzky, & Rickert, 2001). Adolescents with negative affect also have a more difficult time when trying to quit smoking (Stevens, Colwell, Smith, Robinson, & McMillan, 2005). An Internet-based virtual reality world, along with real-time motivational interviewing by experienced smoking-cessation counselors, is an innovative program showing promise with adolescent smokers (Woodruff, Conway, Edwards, Elliott, & Crittenden, 2007). In addition, parental influence and monitoring have been shown to have an effect on adolescent smoking behavior (Dick et al., 2007).

Primary health care providers do not always question adolescents about smoking, drinking, and use of other substances. PHNs and community health nurses can provide information to teens about smoking cessation programs and promote primary prevention by educating children and adolescents to choose not to smoke or engage in other health-risk behaviors. They can also encourage physicians and parents to question and monitor adolescents about smoking and the use of tobacco products.

Teen Sexuality and Pregnancy

Teenage pregnancies, sexually transmitted diseases (STDs), and HIV/AIDS are public health concerns associated with the sexual activity of adolescents. In the 2005 Youth Risk Behavior Survey, almost 47% of high school students reported ever having sexual intercourse, and almost 63% used a condom during their last sexual intercourse (CDC, 2006a). Early sexual debut has been associated with delinquency, as well as with other negative outcomes (Armour, 2007). The United States leads most developed nations in rates of teenage pregnancy, abortion, and childbearing. The United States has the second highest teen pregnancy and birth rates among 46 developed countries, largely because U.S. adolescents are less likely to use or consistently use contraception (Darroch, Singh, Frost, & the Study Team, 2001; Singh & Darroch, 2000). Hamilton, Martin, and Ventura (2007) report that, since 1991, pregnancy and birth rates for 15- to 19-year-old girls have declined by 34%; in 2006, however, rates increased for the first time (from 40.5 per 1,000 to 41.9). The rate for Hispanic adolescent girls is 83 per 1,000. For non-Hispanic whites, the rate is 26.6 per 1,000. For black teens it is 63.7 per 1,000 (CDC, 2008d). The downward trend for teen pregnancy rates has been attributed largely to better use of contraception (77%), rather than less sexual activity (23%) (Santelli, Lindberg, Finer, & Singh, 2007).

Young mothers are at high risk of bearing infants with low birth weight, and they are more likely to smoke tobacco. They are also less likely to receive adequate prenatal care or to gain the recommended weight during pregnancy. Adolescent mothers are at a greater risk than mothers over age 20 to experience a complication of pregnancy (e.g., anemia, hypertension, premature labor), and the risk increases for those under age 15 (Briggs, Hopman, & Jamieson, 2007; March of Dimes, 2007; Usta, Zoorob, Abu-Musa, Naassan, & Nassar, 2008). The babies of adolescent mothers are more likely to die before 1 year than are babies born to 20- to 30-year-old mothers, and low-birth-weight babies are more common among 15- to 19-year-old mothers than among older mothers (March of Dimes, 2007). Adolescent mothers are also at risk for a greater number of physical, psychological, and social problems, including dropping out of high school, reliance on public assistance, limited earning potential, social isolation, and mental disorders (Boden, Fergusson, & Horwood, 2008; East et al., 2007; Reid et al., 2007). A longitudinal study found that "teen mothers' life trajectories reflected legacies of unequal life chances that began in childhood and persisted into their 30s," but that those who were from higher socioeconomic groups "fared better over time" (Smithbattle, 2007, p. 409). Adolescent girls living with a single parent or not living with either parent have higher teen birth rates than those who live with both parents (Forum on Child & Family Statistics, 2006). Adolescents report positive outcomes, but also that teen parenting is "hard," and they recognize that their current and future lives are profoundly affected (Herrman, 2006; Herrman, 2008, p. 42). A retrospective cohort study of women in their 70s and 80s found that those who had been teenage mothers had a higher risk of death than women who bore children after age 20, and they also had a higher prevalence of heart and lung disease, and cancer (Henretta, 2007). Also, those who choose to end their pregnancies by abortion may encounter other physical and psychosocial complications.

By 18 years of age, 7 of 10 males and 6 of 10 females have had sexual intercourse. As such, it would behoove U.S. society to provide effective sexuality education. Two thirds of U.S. school districts report that they have policies in place to provide sexuality education to students, and 86% of those require abstinence education—35% require abstinence-only education. Ninety percent of teachers report that students should be given instruction on contraception; however, 25% are prohibited from including contraception in their lessons. No conclusive evidence suggests that abstinence-only sexuality education delays sexual activity in adolescents, but research shows that it may discourage the use of contraception among sexually active teens. More comprehensive sexuality education programs (e.g., teaching about both abstinence and contraception) have delayed sexual activity in adolescents, decreased the number of sexual partners, and—when adolescents are sexually active—increased the use of contraceptives (Alan Guttmacher Institute, 2002). Teaching about contraception did not increase the risk of adolescent sexual activity or STDs, but it did decrease the risk of pregnancy in a study of abstinence-only versus comprehensive sexual education programs in a national survey of adolescents (Kohler, Manhart, & Lafferty, 2008).

Pregnancy prevention programs can be effective in reducing teen pregnancy and birth rates, as well as in reducing the number of second births to teenage mothers. A South Carolina program, The Second Chance Club, revealed a lower repeat teen birth rate as a positive result (Key, O'Rourke, Judy, & McKinnon 2005). In Maryland, a home visiting program for adolescent mothers improved parenting scores and school continuation rates, although it did not reduce rates of depression or repeat pregnancies (Barnet, Liu, DeVoe, Alperovitz-Bichell, & Duggan, 2007). A small study of mostly African American 14- to 19-year-old abstinent girls found four themes: self-respect (I am worth it), potential negative consequences of sex (Hold on, there's a catch), impact of mothers (Mama says . . . think before you let it go), and influence of boys/other peers (Boys will be boys). Building on self-esteem and family influences, researchers cited the need to develop interventions to help adolescents maintain abstinence and delay of sexual activity (Morrison-Beedy, Carey, Cote-Arsenault, Seibold-Simpson, & Robinson, 2008).

Primary care providers often miss opportunities to provide counseling on prevention of pregnancy, HIV, and STDs (Burstein, Lowry, Klein, & Santelli, 2003; Ellen, Lane, & McCright, 2000). Nurses can provide information and counseling on emergency contraception and collaborate with schools to promote effective pregnancy prevention programs (Haynes, 2007; Key et al., 2005). It is important for community health nurses to provide education and health counseling on these subjects.

Sexually Transmitted Diseases

More than 20 diseases can be transmitted sexually; only the most common are reportable. Each year, about half of the STD cases occur among the 15- to 24-year-old age group, even though they represent only 25% of the population of sexually active individuals. The annual cost of STD cases in the United States averages $11 to $17 billion (Grassia, 2007). These diseases include syphilis, gonorrhea, chlamydia, human papillomavirus (HPV), and herpes simplex virus. Approximately 30 of the 100 known types of HPV strains are sexually transmitted; some of these are related to cervical cancer and others lead to genital warts. Gardasil, a vaccine effective against some forms of HPV-related disease, can be administered in three doses to 11- to 12-year-old girls (Grassia, 2007).

Chlamydia, gonorrhea, and syphilis are other STDs found in the adolescent population. It is estimated that the prevalence rate for chlamydia in Black women is 13.95%; the overall prevalence is estimated at just over 4% (Miller et al., 2004). The highest age-specific gonorrhea rate among women occurred in the 15- to 19-year-old age group (CDC, 2006b). The rates of syphilis have increased between 2004 and 2006, and gonorrhea rates for 15- to 19-year-old men increased over 8% between 2005 and 2006 (CDC, 2006b). Compared with adults, adolescents (10 to 19 years) and young adults (20 to 24 years) are at increased risk for acquiring STDs/STIs. Reasons for this may include a greater likelihood of multiple sex partners, unprotected intercourse, and selection of higher-risk partners. Barriers to improvement include lack of health insurance and transportation, concerns about confidentiality, and lack of quality STD prevention services or clinics targeted to younger age groups (CDC, 2006b). Adolescent girls also have a physiologically amplified susceptibility to chlamydia infection because of increased cervical ectopy (CDC, 2006b). Serious complications from STDs include pelvic inflammatory disease (PID), sterility, increased risk of cancers of the reproductive system, and, with syphilis, blindness, mental illness, and death. There are also complications for the unborn children of those infected with STDs (Illinois Department of Public Health [IDPH], 2003). Medication-resistant strains of gonorrhea are spreading, especially in parts of Europe, the Middle East, and Asia, as well as in California and Hawaii (Grassia, 2007).

Even though death rates from HIV/AIDS have dramatically fallen, new HIV infections reported annually do not reflect the same steep decline. New medications are thought to be the cause of the declining death rate, whereas new cases are increasing within adolescent and young adult populations. Adolescents who were perinatally infected during the 1980s and 1990s demonstrate generational HIV. "Most pediatric HIV cases occur in 15- to 14-year-olds, and there have been no reductions in the last four years" (Grassia, 2007). New HIV infections among adolescent girls are equal to or greater than the number of cases reported in adolescent males. Teenage girls more often acquire infection through heterosexual encounters, whereas male cases are more often attributed to homosexual activity (National Institutes of Health, 2006). Sixty percent of female adolescents living with HIV are Black (Child Health USA, 2004).

A study completed at Carnegie Mellon University noted that most sexually active adolescent girls know little about STDs, becoming familiar with them only after being diagnosed with one (2006). Researchers found that, except in the case of HIV/AIDS, adolescent girls surveyed were unable to list basic facts about eight common STDs. Because schools generally focus on HIV/AIDS education, the researchers posited that other STD education was lacking. An earlier study found that girls who watched an interactive CD on sexual education were more likely than those not viewing the CD to become abstinent (2006). Effective methods of preventing STDs and HIV/AIDS include reduction of sexual activity among adolescents. This can be done by promoting abstinence or delaying sexual initiation, as well as by fostering safer-sex messages that promote the use of condoms. As noted earlier, sex education is effective at both delaying the onset of sexual activity and increasing the use of contraception in adolescents who are already sexually active. It is also effective in increasing safer-sex practices, knowledge of birth control method efficacy, and overall sexual knowledge (Lindau, Tetteh, Kasza, & Gilliam, 2008). A comprehensive review of 73 studies of programs to reduce adolescent sexual risk taking, unintended pregnancy, and STDs revealed strong evidence that such programs can delay sex, increase condom or contraceptive use, and reduce teen pregnancies. The most effective programs included specific sex/HIV education curricula and certain intensive multi-modal youth development programs (Kirby, 2002).

Acne

Between 79% and 95% of adolescents in Western societies have acne, leading some researchers to suspect environmental influences (Cordain et al., 2002). Acne is generally recognized as a genetic disease; three of four children whose mother or father had acne as a teenager will also have it (National Institute of Arthritis and Musculoskeletal and Skin Diseases [NIAMSD], 2004). Acne begins during puberty (10 to 12 years of age) with the increase in circulating male hormones that stimulate sebaceous glands in the skin. The excess sebum (oil) causes irritation in the pores and results in a buildup of cells, leading to whiteheads. Open pores are known as blackheads. A red and inflamed pustule can develop or, in serious cases of acne, cysts or nodules can form. This can lead to pitting and scarring if not treated.

It is now known that greasy foods and chocolate do not cause acne but may be aggravating factors (along with stress, environmental irritants, and certain cosmetics) in susceptible adolescents. Common treatment regimens include skin cleansers, peelers, and medications to decrease sebaceous gland activity. Girls are often prescribed oral contraceptives, which have been shown to be effective in treating acne (Rosen, Breitkopf, & Nagamani, 2003). Benzoyl peroxide is used to kill bacteria on the skin and in the pores. It may be sold over-the-counter (OTC) or by prescription. Other OTC medications include salicylic acid and resorcinol. Retin A (a topical vitamin A ointment), glycolic acid, and alpha-hydroxy acids help to peel the impacted cells from the pores. Isotretinoin (Accutane) reduces the size and activity of sebaceous glands but can cause liver or kidney dysfunction. Because of an extremely high risk of birth defects, female adolescents taking Accutane are prescribed oral contraceptives (NIAMSD, 2004). Oral antibiotics may be prescribed, and corticosteroids may be injected directly into the comedones. New topical therapies include dapsone gel (Aczone) and clindamycin phosphate/tretinoin combination gel (Ziana) (Del Rosso, 2007).

The best preventive measures are keeping the skin clean, eating a balanced diet that includes fresh fruits and vegetables, drinking lots of water, and getting adequate sleep. It is important for male adolescents to shave carefully and for all teens with acne to avoid touching their faces or picking at their blemishes. Adolescents with severe acne may need to be referred to dermatologists who specialize in this skin disorder.

Poor Nutrition and Eating Disorders

Poor nutrition and obesity are not uncommon among adolescents, whose diets often consist of snacks with limited nutritional value interspersed among unhealthful meals. Increased fast food consumption has been tied to the increase in obesity in the United States (Brinkley, Eates, & Jekanowski, 2000). A national study found that adolescents and young adults got more of their energy intake from restaurants and fast food outlets than from home, with increased consumption of pizza, cheeseburgers, and salty snacks (Nielsen, Siega-Riz, & Popkin, 2002). The eating behavior of adolescents is influenced by many things, among them psychosocial factors, family and peers, availability of fast food, and mass media marketing (Story, Neumark-Sztainer, & French, 2002). Girls are more at risk for problems with nutrition for several reasons: they tend to diet inappropriately, to have more finicky eating habits, and to be less physically active than teenage boys. Boys typically eat large quantities of food, which increases the likelihood of obtaining adequate nutrients, and they also tend to be more physically active than girls. A large study of high school students found that "consumption of fruits and vegetables and a healthful breakfast and lunch related both to family and individual factors"; as family situations deteriorated, the percentage of adolescents who ate a healthful breakfast or lunch decreased (Young & Fors, 2001, p. 487).

Issues with body image and control are at the heart of anorexia nervosa and bulimia nervosa, common problems for adolescent girls. **Anorexia nervosa** is an eating disorder with an emotional etiology that is characterized by body image disturbance (i.e., girls see themselves as fat although they may be extremely thin), an intense fear of becoming fat or gaining weight, and refusal to maintain adequate body weight (i.e., BMI of 18 or greater). **Bulimia** is an eating disorder characterized by recurrent episodes of binge eating with repeated compensatory mechanisms to prevent weight gain, such as vomiting (purging type) and fasting or exercise (nonpurging type).

Binge eating, also a recognized eating disorder, involves recurrent episodes of binge eating without fasting, self-induced vomiting, or other compensatory measures (Bulik, Sullivan, & Kendler, 2000). Self-esteem, depressive symptoms, and emotional eating are very sensitive predictors of binge eating. Low levels of support from peers can also be linked to binge eating, and binge eating is associated with an increased risk of becoming overweight or obese (Stice, 2002).

A woman's lifetime risk of developing a bulimic syndrome is estimated to be 8%; the estimated risk of developing an anorexic syndrome is 3% (Patton , Selzer, Coffey, Carlin, & Wolfe, 2000). These diseases have emotional causes that pose complex challenges to treatment. Nutrition education, psychological counseling, and cognitive-behavioral techniques that teach clients how to control stimuli, substitute alternative behaviors, and use positive visualization are all part of treatment; development of a support network is also important. Self-concept is often distorted and self-esteem is low; therefore, activities are initiated to improve the adolescents' feelings about themselves and to bolster their coping mechanisms. Medications (e.g., antidepressants) have been helpful in treating some adolescents with eating disorders (Sharma, 2001). In a sample of adolescents enrolled in a treatment program for bulimia nervosa, 62% had a comorbid diagnosis—generally a major mood disorder. Over 65% had consumed alcohol and 30% had used an illicit drug (Fisher & le Grange, 2007).

The key to prevention may be tied to girls' perceptions of their appearance and education about the risks of dieting. One study indicated that adolescent girls who were severe dieters were 18 times more likely to develop an eating disorder than those who did not diet. Even moderate dieters were at risk; they were five times more likely to develop an eating disorder. Psychiatric morbidity was also a factor; it increased risk sevenfold. Exercise is seen as a more viable alternative than extreme dieting for adolescents who want to control their weight (Patton et al., 2000). Girls who engage in dieting and unhealthful methods of weight control in middle school and high school are three times more likely to become overweight 5 years later than girls who did not diet. They were also found to be at higher risk for using laxatives, diuretics, diet pills, and engaging in binge eating and self-induced vomiting (American Dietetic Association, 2006).

HEALTH SERVICES FOR SCHOOL-AGE CHILDREN AND ADOLESCENTS

A number of programs serve the health needs of school-age children and adolescents. Community health nurses play a major and vital role in delivering these services. Such programs fall into three categories that approximate the three practice priorities of community health nursing practice: illness prevention, health protection, and health promotion.

Preventive Health Programs

Among programs to prevent physical illness and other health problems are immunizations and tuberculosis (TB) testing, as well as school- and community-based education and support programs. Private and public counseling programs and other social services are also geared to promote health and prevent illness.

Immunizations and TB Testing

Low immunization levels for adolescents, particularly among the poor, and increased disease rates signal the need for constant surveillance, outreach programs, and better documentation and educational efforts (Vandermeulen et al., 2008). Community health nurses are deeply involved in each of these preventive activities. Health departments and schools often work collaboratively to provide immunization services. Compulsory immunization laws are helpful in carrying out these preventive services, but recent survey results reveal that the *Healthy People 2010* targets for adolescent vaccination coverage have yet to be met (Jain & Stokley, 2007).

In the recent past, adolescents were only given "catch up" vaccinations (those missed in childhood), except for a tetanus/diphtheria booster. Now, recommended immunizations include tetanus/diphtheria/acellular pertussis (Tdap), meningococcal vaccine (MCV4), pneumococcal polysaccharide vaccine (PPV), both hepatitis A and B, influenza vaccine, and HPV vaccine for girls—along with any missed vaccines (e.g., polio, varicella) (see Fig. 22.2). Often, school nurses and community health nurses work with nurse volunteers to provide immunization clinics at elementary and middle schools; these are convenient for adolescents and their parents (Mark, Conklin, & Wolfe, 2001).

Although immunization clinics may improve rates of compliance, it is recommended that 11- to 12-year-olds be scheduled for routine health care visits to their physicians, so that immunizations can be administered, checked, and updated (Jain & Stokley, 2007). Adolescents who have not had chickenpox and have not received prior vaccination should be given the varicella virus vaccine. In a recent national survey of adolescents, 69% reported a history of chickenpox, and over 65% of those without a disease history reported receiving the vaccine (Jain & Stokley, 2007). Only 60.1% of adolescents had Tdap coverage, and MCV4 vaccination was only complete in less than 12% of adolescents surveyed (Jain & Stokley, 2007).

In addition to immunizations required for school entry, many states or local school districts now require TB skin tests for school-age children and adolescents. Children have a much higher risk of disease progression than do adults. Annual testing is often recommended for children and adolescents from high-risk populations (Pediatric Tuberculosis Collaborative Group, 2004). Targeted TB skin testing identifies adolescents and children at risk for latent TB who could benefit from treatment to prevent progression of the disease. The following questions should be asked to determine risk:

- ◆ Was the child born outside the United States? If so, where? (Asian, African, Latin American, and Eastern European births require TB skin testing.)
- ◆ Has the child traveled outside the United States? If so, where and with whom? (If child stayed with friends/family in Latin America, Asia, Africa, or Eastern Europe for 1 week or more, TB skin testing should occur.)
- ◆ Has the child been exposed to anyone with TB? Who? Did contact person have active or latent TB? When was child exposed and what was the nature of contact? (Notify the local health department if the child had contact with person having TB.)
- ◆ Does the child have close contact with a person who had a positive TB skin test? (Other questions may relate to contact with persons who have HIV, have been in jail or shelters, or are injection drug users; or if the child ingested raw milk/products? Does the child live in a household with member(s) who were born or traveled outside the United States?)

Positive skin tests for children and adolescents have three cut-off points (Pediatric Tuberculosis Collaborative Group, 2004):

- ◆ Induration greater than or equal to 5 mm (if child has close contact with known or suspected TB, if child or adolescent is suspected of having TB disease, if child or adolescent's immune system is suppressed)
- ◆ Induration greater than or equal to 10 mm (if child or adolescent is at an increased risk of disseminated disease or if child or adolescent has been exposed to cases of TB disease)
- ◆ Induration greater than or equal to 15 mm (if child is 4 years old or older and has no known risk factors)

Education and Social Services

The health education of school-age children and adolescents includes a wide variety of approaches and can range from the basics of hand-washing for elementary school students (Guinan, McGuckin, & Ali, 2002; White et al., 2001) to hearing conservation for students who like to listen to loud music (Folmer, Griest, & Martin, 2002).

Parental support services are commonly available through many public and private agencies, including churches. These services can have long-range effects on the health of school-age children, because emotionally healthy parents and stable families offer a healthful environment and support system for children and can facilitate their progress in school. In most states, community health nurses provide teaching and counseling services to parents in their homes and in groups. School nurses, school mental health counselors, and school psychologists also organize parent support groups in local schools. This is particularly important during periods of transition (e.g., from elementary to middle school, from middle to high school). Discussing parenting concerns and increasing parents' understanding of normal child growth and development helps to allay fears and prevent problems. Through such efforts, family violence and abuse can be averted. Reduction in rates of divorce and the attendant consequences may also be a benefit of strengthening family resilience.

Family planning programs, often stationed strategically in inner cities, near schools, or in school-based clinics, provide birth control information and counseling to young people. In some communities, the school-based clinic dispenses condoms. In most states, adolescents have the right to consent for sexual and reproductive health care without parental permission (English, 2007). Community health nurses, in collaboration with an interdisciplinary team, are usually the primary care providers in these programs. Their major goals are to prevent teenage pregnancy, educate teens about reproduction and contraception, and encourage responsible sexual behavior. Teaching parents about adolescent sexuality is important, as parents can influence their child's sexual behavior (Morrison-Beedy et al., 2008; Rupp & Rosenthal, 2007).

Providing STD services and HIV/AIDS education can be a daunting task. Many young people with STDs are often afraid or embarrassed to seek help, and others who have been exposed to the HIV virus may not know that they are infected (Carnegie Mellon University, 2006; Ellen, Lane, & McCright, 2000; Grassia, 2007). Gay and bisexual young men are particularly at risk, as are youth who have been sexually abused (Godin et al., 2003; Saewyc et al., 2006). Furthermore, community health professionals receive very little training in these areas and may be uncomfortable and judgmental in their approaches. Quality services that are easily accessible, provide anonymity for clients, are age-appropriate or targeted to adolescents, and are staffed with health care providers who exhibit nonjudgmental attitudes are better able to attract young people who need help. Some argue that drastic changes in the provision of services to young people—achievable through working to ensure economic development, privatization of prevention activities, and employment of innovative models and strategies—are needed to effect change (Johnson, Carey, Marsh, Levin, & Scott-Sheldon, 2003; Rotheram-Borus, 2000).

Vulnerable groups, particularly minority youth, inner-city residents, incarcerated youth, and homosexuals, are reached through STD clinics, HIV testing sites in clinics and health departments, family planning clinics, private health care providers, schools, juvenile rehabilitation facilities, and employers (Godin et al., 2003). Community health nurses are available in most of these settings; they are usually the professionals who deal most directly with these clients. Improved public awareness and education, screening of high-risk groups, appropriate treatment of infected people, and identification and treatment of sexual partners can reduce the threat of STDs.

Physicians are also concerned about the health risks common to adolescents. Pediatricians, especially, have instituted better history taking, more consistent monitoring, and anticipatory guidance for risks from unintentional and intentional injury, substance abuse, and sexual activity (Boekeloo et al., 2003; Pbert et al., 2003). Community health nurses need to collaborate with local physicians and other community care providers to ensure that adequate education and social services are available to school-age children and adolescents.

Educational efforts to prevent risk-taking behaviors that can lead to adverse health conditions have been effective. An examination of 44 studies that used interventions to reduce HIV in adolescents over a 15-year period revealed that reductions in sexual risk were greater for subjects who received HIV risk-reduction intervention than for those in comparison groups. The increased use of condoms, condom use negotiation skills, and sexual partner communication, along with delaying the onset of sexual activity and decreasing the number of sexual partners, were the outcomes of intensive behavioral interventions (Johnson et al., 2003). Peer educators are also effective in promoting personal responsibility and safer sexual behaviors, as well as in enhancing leadership roles and positive self-image (Fongkaew, Fongkaew, & Suchaxaya, 2007; Merakou & Kourea-Kremastinou, 2006).

Peer education can also be used to influence other risk behaviors. School-based educational program have also been effective (Mahat, Scoloveno, Ruales, & Scoloveno, 2006). A drug prevention curriculum for eighth graders was found to decrease misuse of alcohol, marijuana, and tobacco in a randomized trial. At-risk ninth graders also participated in the curriculum and had five booster lessons; positive results were noted among ninth grade girls (Ellickson, McCaffrey, & St. Clair, 2007). The effectiveness of a universal drug abuse prevention program (e.g., drug refusal skills, self-management, general social skills) was studied in 29 inner-city middle schools. About one-fifth of the subjects were considered to be at high risk for substance abuse. Participating high-risk youth reported less drinking, smoking, inhalant use, and polydrug use at the 1-year posttest than did high-risk youth in the control group (Griffin et al., 2003). In addition to school-based education, peer leadership, and parental education and involvement, community-wide task forces have been developed to lobby for local legislation and to strengthen community–school ties.

Media campaigns for tobacco use prevention have been successful, as have some school-based education programs (Schar, Gutierrez, Murphy-Hoefer, & Nelson, 2006; Tingle, DeSimone, & Covington, 2003). Community health nurses often work in conjunction with law enforcement officials, school district administrators, and other community agencies to ensure compliance with local regulations and prevent or delay the use of tobacco products. Information on smoking cessation and resources to help prevent tobacco use by children and adolescents is available through the Foundation for a Smokefree America (for more information, see the Internet Resources section at the end of this chapter).

Health Protection Programs

Safety and Injury Prevention

Accident- and injury-control programs serve a critical role in protecting the lives of school-age children and adolescents. They are cost-effective: Seat belt laws, child safety seats, and helmet laws have saved millions of dollars in medical care (Child Safety Network, 2005). Efforts to prevent motor vehicle accidents, a major cause of death, include driver education programs, better highway construction, improved motor vehicle design and safety features, and continuing research into what causes various types of crashes. Injury prevention and reduction have been addressed through strategies such as state laws requiring the use of safety restraints, installation of driver and front passenger airbags, substitution of other modes of travel (air, rail, or bus), lower speed limits, stricter enforcement of drunk driving laws, graduated drivers licenses for teenagers, safer automobile design, and helmets for motorcyclists, bicycle riders, and skaters.

Students Against Drunk Driving (SADD) and Friday Night Live activities can promote more responsible driving habits among teens. Communities can also work with law enforcement officials to ensure compliance with mandatory seat belt laws and to promote safe speeds and appropriate driving behaviors near schools. In 1999, the public health efforts to improve motor-vehicle safety were noted as a "20th century public health achievement" by the CDC because of the 90% decline in death rates between 1925 and 1997 despite the tenfold increase in miles traveled.

Safety programs also seek to protect school-age children and adolescents from the hazards of poisonings, ingestion of prescription or OTC drugs, product-related accidents (unsafe toys, bicycles, skateboards, skates, play ground equipment, and furniture), and recreational accidents, including drowning and sports-related injuries. Safety services assume various forms. Poison control centers in many localities offer information and emergency assistance, and have been shown to save $290 per $43 of call cost (Child Safety Network, 2005). Whereas the Federal Consumer Product Safety Commission monitors the safety of products, education programs in schools or through local fire or police departments teach school-age children about bicycle and water safety, fire dangers, and hazards related to poisoning. Generally, the community health nurse can educate families to recognize potentially hazardous situations and encourage efforts to eliminate them. Working with school nurses and school district officials to reduce playground hazards can contribute to the reduction of school-related injuries.

Environmental hazards and other dangers await school-age children and adolescents in the workforce. Between 1992 and 2000, 67 adolescent workers (under age 18) died, and 77,000 teen workers were treated in emergency rooms for work-related injuries in 1998. Because generally only one-third of work injuries are treated in the emergency room, it is believed that the number of teens experiencing work-related injuries is closer to 230,000. Close to 40% of teens injured on the job felt that they were "permanently injured in some way" (National Institute of Occupational Safety & Health [NIOSH], 2003, p. 2). One report states that the highest number of work-related injuries to youths younger than age 18 occurred in eating establishments and food stores (Mardis & Pratt, 2003), although the federal government lists agricultural work and retail trades as the location of most adolescent worker deaths. About 30% of teen worker fatal injuries occur in family businesses (NIOSH, 2003). Deaths caused by exposure to toxic vapors, electrocution, and work-related motor vehicle accidents are not uncommon. Community health nurses can join with occupational health nurses and school nurses to teach parents and children about the dangers and

risks inherent in the workplace, and they can work with local employers to ensure safe working conditions and reasonable hours of employment that do not interfere with school. Adolescent workers, depending upon social class and income backgrounds, may accrue either benefits or harm to their future education and employment because of high school jobs (Staff & Mortimer, 2008).

Infectious Diseases

Programs that protect school-age children and adolescents against infectious diseases encompass such efforts as closing swimming pools that have unsafe bacteria counts, conducting immunization campaigns in conjunction with influenza or measles outbreaks, and working with hospital pediatric units to reduce the incidence and threat of iatrogenic disease. Prevention of community-acquired MRSA is a new challenge for public schools, and PHNs may work with school nurses or others to provide educational programs covering a variety of infectious diseases (Alex & Letizia, 2007). Epidemiologic investigations, especially with school sports teams, may be necessary to determine the cause of outbreaks (Nguyen, Mascola, & Bancroft, 2005).

Child Protective Services

In 1974, the National Center for Child Abuse and Neglect was established as a result of the Child Abuse Prevention and Treatment Act. The center collects and analyzes information on child abuse and neglect, serves as an information clearinghouse, publishes educational materials on the subject, offers technical assistance, and conducts research into the problem (Children's Bureau, 2006).

An estimated 1 million to 2.5 million cases of child abuse and neglect are reported annually in the U.S. (American Academy of Pediatrics [AAP], 2007; Administration for Children and Families [ACF], 2006). Most victims suffered from neglect (64.1%), but approximately 16% were physically abused, almost 9% were sexually abused, 6.6% were psychologically abused, and more than 2% were medically neglected (ACF, 2006). In 2005, almost 1,500 children died from injury or neglect—and it is estimated that 50% to 60% of child abuse/neglect deaths are unrecorded. Fathers or male caretakers are most often responsible for physical abuse fatalities; mothers are more often associated with deaths stemming from neglect (Child Welfare Information Gateway, 2008). The estimated actual cost related to child abuse in 2007 was $103.8 billion, but the untold suffering and loss are incalculable (Wang & Holton, 2007). Consequences for affected children include lower self-esteem, depression, suicide, self-abuse, substance abuse, eating disorders, less empathy for others, antisocial behavior, delinquency, aggression, violence, low academic achievement, and sexual maladjustment (Dake, Price, & Murnan, 2003; Stuewig & McCloskey, 2005). Long-term emotional, social, cognitive, and physical consequences often follow abused children into adolescence and adulthood—posttraumatic stress disorder, poor attachment and problems with trust, difficulties with language development and abstract reasoning, high-risk health behaviors, and abusive or violent behavior (Wang & Holton, 2007).

Neglectful families are generally profiled as having high levels of adult problems, reports of stressful life events, and a higher incidence of maternal depression, and these families often live at or below the poverty level. One study found that those mothers who were more highly educated, had fewer stressful life events, and had more positive encounters with social services generally were better able to provide physically for their children (Casady & Lee, 2002). Children and adolescents who are raised in blended homes (where one parent is not their biologic parent) are at greater risk of physical or sexual abuse (McRee, 2008). Adolescents who run away, act out at school, commit illegal acts, or engage in high-risk behaviors (e.g., drug abuse, sexual promiscuity) may be exhibiting externalizing behaviors in response to years of abuse and neglect. Young adults who have been arrested for general or violent offenses and those who use illicit drugs are more likely to have been abused or neglected in adolescence (Smith, Ireland, & Thornberry, 2005). Verbal abuse of a child by parents is a predictor of adolescent dating violence, and paternal physical abuse can predict sexual victimization as an adolescent (Rich, Gidycz, Warkentin, Lo, & Weiland, 2005).

Services to protect children from abuse are not as well developed or as effective as safety and injury-protection programs, for a variety of reasons. Most child abuse occurs in the home, so only the most blatant situations become evident to outsiders (Spivey et al., 2008). Child social workers are also often unable to assess recurrent risk of child maltreatment, even when families continue in their caseloads (Dorsey, Mustillo, Farmer, & Elbogen, 2008). A wish to avoid legal involvement keeps others from reporting suspected cases, although this attitude is changing among professionals who work with children and other community members. Teachers (16.5%), lawyers and police officers (15.8%), and social services staff (10%) were the three highest reporters of child abuse in 2006; other mandated reporters include medical staff, mental health workers, day care workers, and foster care providers (Children's Bureau, 2006).

In some areas, community health nurses are working together with social workers, mental health workers, and substance abuse counselors as part of a team that provides services to families. Improved training of mandated reporters, such as teachers and physicians, has led to better reporting of abuse; as professionals and the public become more aware of the problem, an increase in reporting has occurred. Child abuse prevention education programs can be found in many public health departments and through some school districts as a primary preventive intervention. Primary prevention of child maltreatment can also occur through home visiting programs utilizing public health nurses. These visits can also help to connect high-risk families to the community and promote better child outcomes (Russell, Britner, & Woolard, 2007).

Families often have many time constraints that can lead to difficulties in providing adequate social support and sufficient opportunities for teaching children socialization skills and appropriate methods of coping with stress. Family stressors can cause parental conflict and lead to disruptions in parent–child relationships. Outcomes for children are worse when these situations occur early in childhood and continue for longer periods of time (Schor & American Academy of Pediatrics Task Force on the Family, 2003). Programs that target at-risk families, especially adolescent mothers and young couples prone to partner violence or harsh parenting practices, may help to prevent later child

abuse (Moore & Florsheim, 2008). PHNs, school nurses, and other nurses working in the community setting must be vigilant for signs of family stress, harsh parenting practices, family violence, and other risk factors for child abuse and neglect and provide resources and respite as needed (Taylor, Baldwin, & Spencer, 2008).

Child death review teams are found at state and local levels and, through their work, improvements in interagency collaboration, procurement of more comprehensive data sets, and identification of gaps in child protective services have led to better services for families and prosecution of abusers, along with improvements in child protective and other community supportive services (Child Welfare Information Gateway, 2008).

Oral Hygiene and Dental Care

School-based programs that provide fluoride rinses and dental sealants and promote tooth brushing and nutrition education for dental health can be found in most areas of the country. Fluoridation of community water supplies is considered the most effective, safe, and low-cost means of protecting the dental health of children and adolescents. Fluoridation of drinking water, school-provided fluoride rinse or gel, and dental sealant programs are cost-effective and can reduce dental caries (Lam, 2008; Levy, 2003; Marinho et al., 2003; Sinclair & Edelstein, 2005).

Fluoride makes teeth less susceptible to decay by increasing the resistance of tooth enamel to the bacterially produced acid in the mouth. Since 1945, public water supplies have been fluoridated at relatively low cost to communities. Water fluoridation has been ranked as one of the 10 greatest public health achievements of the 20th century (Division of Oral Health, 2008).

Some individuals and groups oppose fluoridation because of possible adverse effects (including fluorosis, which can cause mottling of tooth enamel). Research results have been mixed, although most studies have supported the low risk of water fluoridation and the benefits of decreased caries. A longitudinal study found that adults (ages 18 to 45) who grew up with fluoridation and a greater emphasis on preventive dentistry had significantly reduced dental caries, compared with the previous cohort studied (Brown, Wall, & Lazar, 2002). In the United States, because of children's potential for multiple exposures to fluoride through drinking water, processed foods and beverages, toothpaste, gels, and rinses, physicians may prescribe lower doses of fluoride supplements or deem that they are not needed (American Dietetic Association, 2008). In addition to regular dental care, good nutrition, and proper oral hygiene, community health nurses can promote public water fluoridation as an important program for protecting children's dental health.

Health Promotion Programs: Nutrition and Exercise

Nutrition and weight-control programs form another important set of health promotion services. Children need to learn sound dietary habits early in life to establish healthy lifelong patterns. Being overweight during childhood or adolescence may persist into adulthood and may increase the risk for some chronic diseases later in life (Institute of Medicine,

2006). Some school programs teach and provide good nutrition and encourage eating patterns that prevent obesity (Baranowski et al., 2003; Food & Nutrition Service, 2008). A number of weight-control programs for overweight children and adolescents are available through schools, health departments, community health centers, health maintenance organizations, and private groups.

Children and adolescents are particularly vulnerable to media and peer pressures with regard to their food choices. Because of increased rates of childhood obesity and a greater awareness of the need for better nutrition in adolescence, legislative support to limit soft drink sales at public schools is growing (Fletcher, 2003). Parents and children are becoming more aware of the need to cut consumption of saturated fat, salt, sugar, and overprocessed foods in order to feel and look better. The community health nurse, through nutrition education and reinforcement of positive practices, plays a significant role in promoting the health of children.

Summary

Physical health and illness, developmental issues, schooling, behaviors, and emotional and mental problems are major concerns for all Americans and especially for U.S. school-age and adolescent populations. Children and adolescents are important population groups to community health nurses, because their physical and emotional health can affect not only their academic achievement but also the future of society. This population group particularly needs the guidance and direction that can be provided by community health nurses. Among the health problems that affect learning and achievement in school-age children are chronic diseases, such as asthma, autism, and diabetes; behavioral and learning problems, such as ADHD and learning and other disabilities; poverty; injuries; communicable diseases, such as measles and mumps; and dietary problems involving inadequate nutrition, obesity, inactivity, and poor dental health.

One nationwide measure to prevent communicable diseases is the federally and state-mandated immunization program for school-age children and adolescents. Among vaccines given on schedule throughout childhood are those that prevent polio, smallpox, diphtheria, tetanus, typhoid, and many other diseases, so that these diseases will not be passed from one person to another in epidemic proportion.

Mortality rates for children and adolescents have decreased dramatically since the early 1900s, but morbidity rates remain high. Children and adolescents are vulnerable to many illnesses, injuries, and emotional problems, often as a result of a complex and stressful environment. Violence against children and deaths due to homicide occur in the United States at alarming rates. Unintentional injuries, suicide, and homicide are the leading threats to life and health for adolescents. Other health problems include alcohol and drug abuse, unplanned pregnancies, STDs and HIV/AIDS, and poor nutrition. All of these problems create major challenges for the community health nurse who seeks to prevent illness and injury among children and adolescents and to promote their health.

Among the objectives for children and adolescents proposed by *Healthy People 2010*, some key goals are reduction of alcohol-related unintentional injuries; declines in violent behaviors, suicide, and mental health issues; and more responsible reproductive health behaviors. Barriers to achieving these goals vary. Some include economic inequities; lack of sufficient immunization, educational, and community-supported health programs; and the presence of risk behaviors typical among developing youth. Community health nurses play a large role in promoting the health of young people, their families, and communities through education programs and by developing strategies to support healthy growth and development and prevent risky behaviors that lead to injury, teen pregnancy, and sometimes death. Health services for children and adolescents span three categories: prevention, health protection, and health promotion. The community health nurse plays a vital role in each. Preventive services may include immunization programs, parental support services, family planning programs, services for those with STDs, and alcohol and drug abuse prevention programs. Health protection services often include accident and injury control, programs to reduce environmental hazards and control infectious diseases, and services to protect children and adolescents from child abuse and neglect. Health promotion services may include programs in nutrition and weight control, along with HIV/AIDS prevention, and smoking, alcohol, and drug abuse education. Community health nurses are integral to the health and well-being of children and adolescents, through their work with families, schools, and other community agencies. ■

ACTIVITIES TO PROMOTE CRITICAL THINKING

1. You are a community health nurse assigned to work at a school. You learn that more than 20% of the students in this school district are being treated with Ritalin, Concerta, Adderall, or some other medication for treating ADHD. What issues should you consider in determining whether these medications are being appropriately prescribed?

2. What is the major cause of death among school-age children? What community-wide interventions could be initiated to prevent these deaths? Select one intervention and describe how you and a group of community health professionals might develop this preventive measure.

3. A 14-year-old girl from a middle-class family and a 14-year-old girl from a poor family both come to the health department clinic where you work. The girls have similar symptoms that possibly indicate gonorrhea. Would your assessment and intervention be the same for the two girls? What are your values and attitudes toward people with diseases that are sexually transmitted? Does social class, race, age, or sex make any difference in how you feel about them? What is one action the community health nurse can take to prevent such diseases in this population group?

4. Discuss possible methods of doing nutritional assessments in school-age children and adolescents. What programs could be instituted to encourage healthier diets and increased exercise? What other factors might need to be considered? How could you, as a community health nurse, work with schools and

parents to increase physical activity and improve nutrition for school-age children and adolescents?

5. A new elementary school to which you have been assigned has repeated outbreaks of head lice and very limited access to health care. Using the Internet, research causes for recurrent head lice infestations and effective over-the-counter treatment products. Are head lice most often found seasonally? Discuss possible education programs you might implement or other innovative methods of treatment and control you might be able to institute.

References

Acosta, M., Manubay, J., & Levin, F. (2008). Pediatric obesity: Parallels with addiction and treatment recommendations. *Harvard Review of Psychiatry, 16*(2), 80–96.

Administration for Children & Families. (2006). *Questions & answers support: How many children are abused and neglected each year?* Retrieved August 1, 2008 from http://faq.acf.hhs.gov/cgi-bin/acfrightnow.cfg/php/enduser/std_adp...Y2hfdHlwZT1hbnN3ZXJzLnNYXJjaaF9ubCZwX3BhZ2U9MQ**&p_lli=&p_topview=1.

Advisory Committee on Immunization Practices. (2008a). *Recommended Immunization Schedule for Persons 0–6 years.* Retrieved August 1, 2008 from http://www.cdc.gov/vaccines/recs/schedules/downloads/child/2008/08_0-6yrs_schedule_pr.pdf.

Advisory Committee on Immunization Practices. (2008b). *Recommended Immunization Schedule for Persons 7–18 years.* Retrieved August 1, 2008 from http://www.cdc.gov/vaccines/recs/schedules/downloads/child/2008/08_7-18yrs_schedule_pr.pdf.

Alaimo, K., Olson, C., & Frongillo, E. (2001). Food insufficiency and American school-aged children's cognitive, academic, and psychosocial development. *Pediatrics, 108*(1), 44–53.

Alan Guttmacher Institute. (2002). *Facts in brief: Sexuality education.* Retrieved August 1, 2008 from http://guttmacher.org/pubs/fb_sex_ed02.pdf.

Alex, A., & Letizia, M. (2007). Community-acquired methicillin-resistant staphylococcus aureus: Considerations for school nurses. *Journal of School Nursing, 23*(4), 210–214.

Aligne, C.A., Moss, M.E., Auinger, P., & Weitzman, M. (2003). Association of pediatric dental caries with passive smoking. *Journal of the American Medical Association, 289*(10), 1258–1260.

American Academy of Child & Adolescent Psychiatry. (2008). *Child and adolescent mental illness and drug abuse statistics.* Retrieved August 1, 2008 from http://www.aacap.org/cs/root/resources_for_families/child_and_adolescent_mental_illness_statistics.

American Academy of Pediatrics. (2006). *Section 3: Summaries of infectious diseases: Pediculosis capitis (head lice).* Red Book Online. Retrieved August 1, 2008 from http://www.aapredbook.aappublications.org/cgi/content.extract/2006/1/3.92.

American Academy of Pediatrics. (2007). *Parenting corner Q&A: Child abuse.* Retrieved August 1, 2008 from http://www.aap.org/publiced/BKO_ChildAbuse.htm.

American Academy of Pediatrics Committee on Children With Disabilities. (2000). Provision of educationally-related services for children & adolescents with chronic diseases & disabling conditions. *Pediatrics, 105*(2), 448–451.

American Dietetic Association. (2006). *Predicting obesity and eating disorders among adolescents.* Retrieved May 17, 2006 from http://www.eatright.org/cps/rde/xchg/ada/hs.xsl/home_8741_ENU-HTML.htm.

American Dietetic Association. (2008). *Fluoride and fluoridation.* Retrieved August 1, 2008 from http://www.ada.org/public/topics/fluoride/fluoride_article01.asp.

American Psychological Association Zero Tolerance Task Force. (2006). *Are zero tolerance policies effective in the schools? An evidenciary review and recommendations.* Retrieved August 1, 2008 from http://www.apa.org/ed/cpse/zttreport.pdf.

Andersen, S., & Teicher, M. (2008). Stress, sensitive periods and maturational events in adolescent depression. *Trends in Neuroscience, 31*(4), 183–191.

Arias, E., & Smith, B. (2003). Deaths: Preliminary data for 2001. *National Vital Statistics Reports, 51*(5), 1–44.

Armour, S. (2007). *Delaying sex can have positive effects for adolescents.* Medical News. Retrieved February 27, 2007 from http://www.news-medical.net/?id=22218.

Arseneault, L., Milne, B., Taylor, A., et al. (2008). Being bullied as an environmentally mediated contributing factor to children's internalizing problems: A study of twins discordant for victimization. *Archives of Pediatric & Adolescent Medicine, 162*(2), 145–150.

Aseltine, R., & DeMartino, R. (2004). An outcome evaluation of the SOS suicide prevention program. *American Journal of Public Health, 94*(3), 446–451.

Asthma & Allergy Foundation of America. (2007, Fall). Reduce the allergens in your home. *Fresh AAIR, 2.*

Aubrey, A. (2006). *Moms and pros tackle lice.* Morning Edition, National Public Radio. Retrieved November 30, 2006 from http://www.npr.org/templates/story/story.pp?storyId=6556831.

Austin, J., Dunn, D., Johnson, C., & Perkins, S. (2004). Behavioral issues involving children and adolescents with epilepsy and the impact of their families: Recent research data. *Epilepsy & Behavior, 5*[Suppl. 3], 33–41.

Autism Information Center. (2007). *Autism spectrum disorders overview.* Retrieved August 1, 2008 from http://www.cdc.gov/ncbddd/autism/overview.htm.

Autism Society of America. (2008). *About autism.* Retrieved August 1, 2008 from http://www.autism-society/org/site/PageServer?pagename=about_home.

Baranowski, T., Baranowski, J., Cullen, K., et al. (2003). The fun, food, and fitness project (FFFP): The Baylor GEMS pilot study. *Ethnicity and Disease, 13*[Suppl. 1], S30–S39.

Barkley, R., Fischer, M., Smallish, L., & Fletcher, K. (2002). The persistence of attention-deficit/hyperactivity disorder into young adulthood as a function of reporting source and definition of disorder. *Journal of Abnormal Psychology, 111*(2), 279–289.

Barkley, R., Fischer, M., Smallish, L., & Fletcher, K. (2003). Does the treatment of attention-deficit/hyperactivity disorder with stimulants contribute to drug use/abuse? A 3-year prospective study. *Pediatrics, 111*(1), 97–109.

Barnet, B., Liu, J., DeVoe, M., et al. (2007). Home visiting for adolescent mothers: Effects on parenting, maternal life course, and primary care linkage. *Annals of Family Medicine, 5*(3), 224–232.

Berkey, C., Rockett, H., Gillman, M., & Colditz, G. (2003). One-year changes in activity and in inactivity among 10- to 15-year old boys and girls: Relationship to change in body mass index. *Pediatrics, 111*(4), 836–843.

Berkowitz, R.J. (2003). Causes, treatment, and prevention of early childhood caries: A microbiologic perspective. *Journal of the Canadian Dental Association, 69*(5), 304–307.

Bernard, S., Paulozzi, L., & Wallace, L.J.D. (2007, May 18). Fatal injuries among children by race and ethnicity: United States, 1999–2002. *Morbidity and Mortality Weekly Report.* Retrieved August 1, 2008 from http://www.cdc.gov/mmwr/preview/mmwrhtml./ss5605a1.htm?s_cid=ss5605a1_x.

Bethell, J., & Rhodes, A. (2008). Adolescent depression and emergency department uses: The roles of suicidality and deliberate self-harm. *Current Psychiatry Reports, 10*(1), 53–59.

Biederman, J., & Faraone, S. (2002). Current concepts on the neurobiology of attention-deficit/hyperactivity disorder. *Journal of Attention Disorders, 6*[Suppl. 1], S7–S16.

Bingham, C., Shope, J., & Raghunathan, T. (2006). Patterns of traffic offenses from adolescent licensure into early young adulthood. *Journal of Adolescent Health, 39*(1), 35–42.

Blakemore, S.J. (2008). The social brain in adolescence. *Nature Reviews: Neuroscience, 9*(4), 267–277.

Blakemore, S.J., den Ouden, H., Choudhury, S., & Frith, C. (2007). Adolescent development of the neural circuitry for thinking about intentions. *Social, Cognitive & Affective Neuroscience, 2*(2), 130–139.

Boden, J., Fergusson, D., & Horwood, J. (2008). Early motherhood and subsequent life outcomes. *Journal of Child Psychology & Psychiatry, 49*(2), 151–160.

Boekeloo, B., Bobbi, M., Lee, W., et al. (2003). Effect of patient priming and primary care provider prompting on adolescent-provider communication about alcohol. *Archives of Pediatrics and Adolescent Medicine, 157*(5), 433–439.

Boudreaux, E., Emond, S., Clark, S., & Camargo, C. (2003). Race/ethnicity and asthma among children presenting to the emergency department: Differences in disease severity and management. *Pediatrics, 111*(5), E615–E621.

Bowyer, S., Roettcher, P., Higgins, G., et al. (2003). Health status of patients with juvenile rheumatoid arthritis at 1 and 5 years after diagnosis. *Journal of Rheumatology, 30*(2), 394–400.

Boynton-Jarrett, R., Thomas, T., Peterson, K., Weicha, J., Sobol, A., & Gortmaker, S. (2003). Impact of television viewing patterns on fruit and vegetable consumption among adolescents. *Pediatrics, 112*(6), 1321–1326.

Bretz, W.A., Corby, P. M., Melo, M.R., et al. (2006). Heritability estimates for dental caries and sucrose sweetness preference. *Journal of Evidence Based Dental Practice, 51*(12), 1156–1160.

Briggs, M., Hopman, W., & Jamieson, M. (2007). Comparing pregnancy in adolescents and adults: Obstetric outcomes and prevalence of anemia. *Journal of Obstetrics & Gynecology, Canada, 29*(7), 546–555.

Brinkley, J., Eales, J., & Jekanowski, M. (2000). The relation between dietary changes and rising U.S. obesity. *International Journal of Obesity and Related Metabolic Disorders, 24*(8), 1032–1039.

Brolin-Laftman, S., & Ostberg, V. (2006). The pros and cons of social relations: An analysis of adolescents' health complaints. *Social Science & Medicine, 63*(3), 611–623.

Brookmeyer, K., Fanti, K., & Henrich, C. (2006). Schools, parents, and youth violence: A multilevel, ecological analysis. *Clinical Child & Adolescent Psychology, 35*(4), 504–514.

Brookmeyer, K., Henrich, C., & Schwab-Stone, M. (2005). Adolescents who witness community violence: Can parent support and prosocial cognitions protect them from committing violence? *Child Development, 76*(4), 917–929.

Brown, L., Wall, T., & Lazar, V. (2002). Trends in caries among adults 18 to 45 years old. *Journal of the American Dental Association, 133*(7), 827–834.

Buchhalter, R., & Jarrar, J. (2003). Therapeutics in pediatric epilepsy, Part 1: The new antiepileptic drugs and the ketogenic diet. *Mayo Clinic Proceedings, 78,* 359–370.

Bulik, C., Sullivan, P., & Kendler, K. (2000). An empirical study of the classification of eating disorders. *American Journal of Psychiatry, 157*(6), 886–895.

Burgess, S., Gardiner, K., & Propper, C. (2006). School, family, and county effects on adolescents' later life chances. *Journal of Family & Economic Issues, 27*(2), 155–184.

Burstein, G., Lowry, R., Klein, J., & Santelli, J. (2003). Missed opportunities for sexually transmitted diseases, human immunodeficiency virus, and pregnancy prevention services during adolescent health supervision visits. *Pediatrics, 111*(5), 996–1001.

Carnegie Mellon University. (2006). *Teens unaware of sexually transmitted diseases until they catch one, Carnegie Mellon study finds*. ScienceDaily. Retrieved January 4, 2006 from http://www.sciencedaily.com/releases/2006/01/060103182708.htm.

Casady, M.A., & Lee, R.E. (2002). Environments of physically neglected children. *Psychological Reports, 91*(1), 711–721.

Casey, B.J., Jones, R., & Hare, T. (2008). The adolescent brain. *Annals of the New York Academy of Science, 1124,* 111–126.

Casey, P.H., Pippa, M.S., Gossett, J.M., et al. (2006). The association of child and household food insecurity with childhood overweight status. *Pediatrics, 118*(5), E1406–E1413.

Cauthen, N. (2005). *Family economic (in)security: A view from the states*. National Center for Children in Poverty. Retrieved November 30, 2005 from http://www.nccp.org/publications/pub_647.html.

Centers for Disease Control and Prevention (CDC). (2002a). *Summary health statistics for U.S. children: National health interview survey*. Vital and Health Statistics, Series 10, No. 208. Washington, DC: Author.

Centers for Disease Control and Prevention (CDC). (2002b). Trends in cigarette smoking among high school students: United States, 1991–2001. *Morbidity and Mortality Weekly Report*. Retrieved August 1, 2008 from http://www.cdc.gov/mmwr/preview/mmwrhtml/mm5119a1.htm.

Centers for Disease Control and Prevention (CDC). (2003). *Improving oral health*. Retrieved August 1, 2008 from http://www.cdc.gov/nccdphp/bb_oralhealth/index.htm.

Centers for Disease Control and Prevention (CDC). (2004). *Addressing asthma in schools*. Retrieved July 30, 2004 from http://www.cdc.gov/HealthyYouth/Asthma.

Centers for Disease Control and Prevention (CDC). (2005). QuickStats: Percentage of children aged 5–17 years ever having diagnosis of ADHD or LD by sex and diagnosis: United States, 2003. *Morbidity and Mortality Weekly Report*. Retrieved November 4, 2005 from http://www.cdc.gov/mmwR/preview/mmwrhtml/mm5443a8.htm.

Centers for Disease Control and Prevention (CDC). (2006a, June 9). Youth Risk Behavior Surveillance, United States, 2005. *Morbidity and Mortality Weekly Report, 55,* No. SS-5.

Centers for Disease Control and Prevention (CDC). (2006b). *Sexually transmitted diseases surveillance 2006: Special focus profiles adolescents and young adults*. Retrieved August 1, 2008 from http://www.cdc.govSTD/STATS/adol.htm.

Centers for Disease Control and Prevention (CDC). (2006c). Suicide trends among youths and young adults aged 10–24 years: United States, 1990–2004. *Morbidity and Mortality Weekly Report*. Retrieved September 7, 2006 from http://www.cdc.gov/mmwr/preview/mmwrhtml/mm5635a2.htm.

Centers for Disease Control and Prevention (CDC). (2007a). *One of the nation's most common disabling neurological conditions*. Retrieved August 1, 2008 from http://www.cdc.gov/print.do?url=http%3A%2F%2Fwww.cdc.gov%2Fepilepsy%2F.

Centers for Disease Control and Prevention (CDC). (2007d). *Youth violence: Fact sheet*. Retrieved August 1, 2008 from http://www.cdc.gov/print.do?url=http%3A//www.cdc.gov/ncipc/factsheets/yvfacts.htm.

Centers for Disease Control and Prevention (CDC). (2007e). *Suicide*. Retrieved August 1, 2008 from http://www.cdc.gov/ncipc/dvp/Suicide/SuicideDataSheet.pdf.

Centers for Disease Control and Prevention (CDC). (2008a). *Student health and academic achievement*. Retrieved August 1, 2008 from http://www.cdc.gov/HealthyYouth/health_and_academics/index.htm.

Centers for Disease Control and Prevention (CDC). (2008b). Unintentional strangulation deaths from the "choking game" among youths aged 6–19 years: United States, 1995–2007. *Morbidity and Mortality Weekly Report, 57*(6), 141–144.

Centers for Disease Control and Prevention (CDC). (2008c). *Alcohol: Frequently answered questions*. Retrieved August 1, 2008 from http://www.cdc.gov/alcohol/faqs.htm#11.

Centers for Disease Control and Prevention (CDC). (2008e). *Adolescent reproductive health: Home*. Retrieved August 1, 2008 from http://www.cdc.gov/reproductivehealth/AdolescentReproHealth/.

Centers for Disease Control and Prevention (CDC). (n.d.). *Healthy People 2010: 21 critical objectives identified by the adolescent health work group*. Retrieved October 14, 2008 from http://www.healthypeople.gov/search/stat_21crobj.htm.

Chan, E., Rappaport, L., & Kemper, K. (2003). Complementary and alternative therapies in childhood attention and hyperactivity problems. *Journal of Developmental and Behavioral Pediatrics, 24*(1), 4–8.

Chase-Lansdale, P.L., & Pittman, L.D. (2002). Welfare reform and parenting: Reasonable expectations. *The Future of Children, 12*(1), 167–186.

Chatrath, R., Shenoy, R., Serratto, M., & Thoele, D. (2002). Physical fitness of urban American children. *Pediatric Cardiology, 23*(6), 608–612.

Chau, M., & Douglas-Hall, A. (2007). *Low-income children in the United States: National and state trend data, 1996–2006*. National Center for Children in Poverty. Retrieved August 1, 2008 from http://www.nccp.org/publications/pub_672.html.

Chen, E., Martin, A., & Matthews, K. (2006). Socioeconomic status and health: Do gradients differ within childhood and adolescence? *Social Science & Medicine, 62*(9), 2161–2171.

Child Health USA. (2004). *Adolescent HIV infection*. Maternal Child Health Branch. Retrieved August 1, 2008 from http://mchb.hrsa.gov/mchirc/chusa_04/pages/0465ahi.htm.

Child Safety Network. (2005, November 28). *Injury prevention: What works? A summary of cost-outcome analysis for injury prevention programs*. Pacific Institute for Research & Evaluation. Retrieved August 1, 2008 from http://notes.edc.org/HHD/CSN/csnpubs.nsf/cb5858598bf707d58525686d005ec222/a2126ad88e9d48408525722d007da14c?OpenDocument.

Child Trends Databank. (2006). *ADHD*. Retrieved August 1, 2008 from http://www.childtrendsdatabank.org/indicators/76ADHD.cfm.

Child Trends Databank. (2008). *Children in poverty*. Retrieved August 1, 2008 from http://www.childtrendsdtabank.org/indicators/4poverty.cfm.

Child Welfare Information Gateway. (2008, March). *Child abuse and neglect fatalities: Statistics and interventions*. Children's Bureau, Administration for Children & Families. Retrieved August 1, 2008 from http://www.childwelfare.gov/pubs/factsheets/fatality.cfm.

Children's Bureau. (2006). *Child Maltreatment 2006*. U.S. Department of Health & Human Services, Administration for Children & Families. Retrieved August 1, 2008 from http://www.acf.hhs.gov/programs/cb/pubs/cm06/cm06.pdf.

Children's Defense Fund. (2008a). *Trends in child poverty and extreme child poverty*. Retrieved August 1, 2008 from http://www.childrensdefense.org/site.PageServer?pagename=research_family_income_2006childpovertytrends.

Children's Defense Fund. (2008b). *Moments in America for children*. Retrieved August 1, 2008 from http://www.childrensdefense.org/site/PageServer?pagename=research_national_data_moments.

Chung, K., & Cheung, M. (2008). Sleep-wake patterns and sleep disturbance among Hong Kong Chinese adolescents. *Sleep, 31*(2), 185–194.

Clarke, P., Fraser-Lee, N.J., & Shimono, T. (2001). Identifying risk factors for predicting caries in school-aged children using dental health information collected at preschool age. *Journal of Dentistry in Children, 68*(5), 373–378.

Connor, D., Edwards, G., Fletcher, K., et al. (2003). Correlates of comorbid psychopathology in children with ADHD. *Journal of the American Academy of Child and Adolescent Psychiatry, 42*(2), 193–200.

Cook, J.T. (2002). Clinical implications of household food security: Definitions, monitoring, and policy. *Nutrition in Clinical Care, 5*(4), 152–167.

Cook, J.T., Frank, D.A., Berkowitz, C., et al. (2002). Welfare reform and the health of young children: A sentinel survey in 6 U.S. cities. *Archives of Pediatric & Adolescent Medicine, 156*(7), 678–684.

Coon, K., Goldberg, J., Rogers, B., & Tucker, K. (2001). Relationships between use of television during meals and children's food consumption patterns. *Pediatrics, 107*(1), e7.

Coon, K.A., & Tucker, K.L. (2002). Television and children's consumption patterns: A review of the literature. *Minerva Pediatrics, 54*(5), 423–436.

Cordain, L., Lindeberg, S., Hurtado, M., et al. (2002). Acne vulgaris: A disease of Western civilization. *Archives of Dermatology, 138*(12), 1584–1590.

Cortiella, C. (2008). *National study follows youth with learning disabilities from high school to adult life*. Great Schools. Retrieved August 1, 2008 from http://www.schwablearning.org/print_resources.asp?type=article&r=717%20&popref=http%3A//www.schwablearning.org/articles/aspx%3Fr%3D717.

Cote, S., Geltman, P., Nunn, M., et al. (2004). Dental caries of refugee children compared with U.S. children. *Pediatrics, 114*(6), E733–E740.

Courtney, A.U., McCarter, D.F., & Pollart, S.M. (2005). Childhood asthma: Treatment update. *American Family Physician, 71*, 1959–1969.

Cox, E., Motheral, B., Henderson, R., & Mager, D. (2003). Geographic variation in the prevalence of stimulant medication use among children 5 to 14 years old: Results from a commercially insured U.S. sample. *Pediatrics, 111*(2), 237–243.

Daisey, J., Angell, W., & Apte, M. (2003). Indoor air quality, ventilation, and health symptoms in schools: An analysis of existing information. *Indoor Air, 13*(1), 53–64.

Dake, J., Price, J., & Murnan, J. (2003). Evaluation of a child abuse prevention curriculum for third-grade students: Assessment of knowledge and efficacy expectations. *Journal of School Health, 73*(2), 76–82.

Damico, J., Tetnowski, J., & Nettleton, S. (2004). Emerging issues and trends in attention deficit hyperactivity disorder: An update for the speech-language pathologist. *Seminars in Speech & Language, 25*(3), 207–213.

Darroch, J., Singh, S., Frost, J., & The Study Team. (2001). Differences in teenage pregnancy rates among five developed countries: The roles of sexual activity and contraceptive use. *Family Planning Perspectives, 33*(6), 244–250, 281.

Dawes, M. (2005). Wet combing compared with pediculicides for head lice: Single blind randomized study. *Student British Medical Journal, 10*, 338–339.

Deal, L., Gomby, D., Zippiroli, L., & Behrman, R. (2000). Unintentional injuries in childhood: Analysis and recommendations. *The Future of Children, 10*(1). Retrieved October 14, 2008 from http://www.futureofchildren.org/pubs-info2825/pubs-info_show.htm?doc_id=69724.

Del Rosso, J. (2007). Newer topical therapies for the treatment of acne vulgaris. *Cutis: Cutaneous Medicine for the Practitioner, 80*(5), 400–410.

Dick, D., Viken, R., Purcell, S., et al. (2007). Parental monitoring moderates the importance of genetic and environmental influences on adolescent smoking. *Journal of Abnormal Psychology, 116*(1), 213–218.

Dietz, W.H., & Gortmaker, S.L. (2001). Preventing obesity in children and adolescents. *Annual Review of Public Health, 22*, 337–353.

DiFranza, J. (2008). Hooked from the first cigarette. *Scientific American, 298*(5), 82–87.

Division of Oral Health. (2007). *Children's oral health*. Retrieved August 1, 2008 from http://www.cdc.gov/print.do?lurl=http%3A%2F%2Fwww.cdc.gov%2ForalHealth%2Ftopics%2Fchild.htm.

Dinkes, R., Cataldi, E.F., Kena, G., & Baum, K. (2006). *Indicators of School Crime and Safety: 2006* (NCES 2007–003/NCJ 214262). U.S. Departments of Education and Justice. Washington, DC: U.S. Government Printing Office.

Division of Oral Health. (2008). *Community water fluoridation: Overview.* Retrieved August 1, 2008 from http://www.cdc.gov/Fluoridation/.

Dorsey, S., Mustillo, S., Farmer, E., & Elbogen, E. (2008). Caseworker assessments of risk for recurrent maltreatment: Association with case-specific risk factors and reports. *Child Abuse & Neglect, 32*(3), 377–391.

East, P., Reyes, B., & Horn, E. (2007). Association between adolescent pregnancy and a family history of teenage births. *Perspectives on Sexual & Reproductive Health, 39*(2), 108–115.

Eggert, L., Thompson, E., Randell, B., & Pike, K. (2002). Preliminary effects of brief school-based prevention approaches for reducing youth suicide risk behaviors, depression, and drug involvement. *Journal of Child and Adolescent Psychiatric Nursing, 15*(2), 48–64.

Egley, A., & Ritz, C. (2006, April #1). Highlights of the 2004 National Youth Gang Survey. *OJJDP Fact Sheet*, No. FS-200601. Office of Justice Programs, U.S. Department of Justice.

Eisenberg, M., Olson, R., Neumark-Sztainer, D., et al. (2004). Correlations between family meals and psychosocial well-being among adolescents. *Archives of Pediatric & Adolescent Medicine, 158*(8), 792–796.

Ellen, J., Lane, M., & McCright, J. (2000). Are adolescents being screened for sexually transmitted diseases? A study of low-income African American adolescents in San Francisco. *Sexually Transmitted Infections, 76,* 94–97.

Ellickson, P., McCaffrey, D., & St. Clair, P. (2007). *School-based drug prevention among at-risk adolescents: Effects of ALERT plus.* Santa Monica, CA: Rand Corporation.

Ellickson, P., Tucker, J., & Klein, D. (2003). Ten-year prospective study of public health problem associated with early drinking. *Pediatrics, 111*(5), 949–955.

Encyclopedia of Childhood and Adolescence. (1998). *Erikson's theory.* Retrieved October 14, 2008 from http://findarticles.com/p/articles/mi_g2602/is_0002/ai_2602000230.

English, A. (2007). Sexual and reproductive health care for adolescents: Legal rights and policy challenges. *Adolescent Medicine: State of the Art Reviews, 18*(3), 571–581, viii–ix.

Epilepsy Foundation. (2003). *Children often not given Diastat in school: Denied participation in school activities.* Retrieved August 1, 2008 from http://www.epilepsyfoundation.org/epilepsyusa/schooldiastat.cfm.

Epstein, J., Grifin, K., & Botvin, G. (2008). A social influence model of alcohol use for inner-city adolescents: Family drinking, perceived drinking norms, and perceived social benefits of drinking. *Journal of Studies on Alcohol & Drugs, 69*(3), 397–405.

Estrada, J., & Morris, R. (2000). Pediculosis in a school population. *Journal of School Nursing, 16*(3), 32–38.

Evans, G., & Kim, P. (2007). Childhood poverty and health: Cumulative risk exposure and stress dysregulation. *Childhood Poverty & Health, 18*(11), 953–957.

Faden, V. (2006). Trends in initiation of alcohol use in the United States: 1975 to 2003. *Alcoholism Clinical & Experimental Research, 30*(6), 1011–1022.

Fawcett, R.S. (2003, September 15). Ivermectin use in scabies. *American Family Physician.* Retrieved August 1, 2008 from http://www.aafp.org/afp/AFPprinter.20030915/1089.html?print=yes.

Federal Interagency Forum on Child and Family Statistics. (2004). *Pop3: Percentage of U.S. children ages 0–17 by race and Hispanic origin, 1980–2004.* Retrieved August 1, 2008 from http://www.childstats.gov/americaschildren06/tables/pop3.asp?popup=true.

Feldman, S.S., & Elliott, G.R. (Eds.). (1990). *At the threshold: The developing adolescent.* Cambridge, MA: Harvard University Press.

Fekkes, M., Pijpers, F., Fredriks, F., et al. (2006). Do bullied children get ill, or do ill children get bullied? A prospective cohort study on the relationship between bullying and health-related symptoms. *Pediatrics, 117*(5), 1568–1574.

Ferguson, D., Horwood, L., & Ridder, E. (2007). Conduct and attentional problems in childhood and adolescence and later substance use, abuse and dependence: Results of a 25-year longitudinal study. *Drug and Alcohol Dependence, 88*(Suppl. 1), S14–S26.

Fergusson, D., Boden, J., & Horwood, L. (2008). The development of antecedents of illicit drug use: Evidence from a 25-year longitudinal study. *Drug & Alcohol Dependence*, in press.

Fingerhut, L., & Kaufer-Christoffel, K. (2002). Firearm-related death and injury among children and adolescents. *The Future of Children, 12*(2), 25–38.

Fisher, L., Miles, I., Austin, S., Camargo, C., & Colditz, G. (2007). Predictors of initiation of alcohol use among US adolescents: Findings from a prospective cohort study. *Archives of Pediatric & Adolescent Medicine, 161*(10), 959–966.

Fisher, S., & le Grange, D. (2007). Comorbidity and high-risk behaviors in treatment-seeing adolescents with bulimia nervosa. *International Journal of Eating Disorders, 40*(8), 751–753.

Fitzgerald, B., Okos, A., & Miller, W. (2003). Treatment of out of hospital status epilepticus with diazepam rectal gel. *Seizure, 12,* 52–55.

Fletcher, E. (2003, May 30). *Senate votes to move the fizz off-campus.* The Sacramento Bee. Retrieved January 29, 2004, from http://nl.newsbank.com/nlsearch/we/Archives?p_product=SB&p_theme=sb&p_action=search&p_maxdocs=200&s_dispstring=allfields(Senate%20votes%20move%20fizz%20off-campus)%20AND%20date()&p_field_advanced-0=&p_text_advanced-0=("Senate%20votes%20move%20fizz%20off-campus")&p_perpage=10&p_sort=YMD_date:D&xcal_useweights=no.

Folmer, R., Griest, S., & Martin, W. (2002). Hearing conservation education programs for children: A review. *Journal of School Health, 72*(2), 51–57.

Fongkaew, W., Fongkaew, K., & Suchaxaya, P. (2007). Early adolescent peer leader development in HIV prevention using youth-adult partnership with schools approach. *Journal of the Association of Nurses in AIDS Care, 18*(2), 60–71.

Food Research & Action Center (FRAC). (2007, June). *State of the states: 2007. A profile of food & nutrition programs across the nation.* Washington, DC: Author.

Food & Nutrition Service. (2008). *About school meals: FAQs.* Retrieved October 15, 2008 from http://www.fns.usda.gov/cnd/About/faqs.htm

Forrest, C., & Riley, A. (2004). Childhood origins of adult health: A basis for life-course health policy. *Health Affairs, 23*(5), 155–164.

Forum on Child & Family Statistics (FCFS). (n.d.). *HC4.B Oral health: Percentage of children ages 2–17 with untreated dental caries (cavities) by age, poverty status & race & Hispanic origin, 1999–2002 and 2003–2004.* Retrieved August 1, 2008 from http://www.childstats.gov/americaschildren/tabls/hc4b.asp.

Forum on Child & Family Statistics (FCFS). (2005). *America's children in brief: Key national indicators of well-being. Asthma, 2005.* Retrieved August 1, 2008 from http://www.childstats.gov/americaschildren06/specfeatures_2005spe1.asp.

Forum on Child & Family Statistics (FCFS). (2006). *Family structure and adolescent well-being, 2005.* Retrieved August 1, 2008 from http://www.childstats.gov/americaschildren06/specfeatures_2005spe4cf.asp.

Franko, D., Thompson, D., Affenito, S., et al. (2008). What mediates the relationship between family meals and adolescent health issues. *Health Psychology, 27*[2 Suppl.], S109–S117.

Frankowski, B., & Weiner, L. (2002). Head lice. *Pediatrics, 110*(3), 638–643.

Freeman, J.M., Freeman, J., Kossoff, E., & Kelly, M. (2006). *The ketogenic diet: A treatment for children & others with epilepsy.* New York: Demos Medical Publishing LLC.

Fremont, W. (2003). School refusal in children and adolescents. *American Family Physician, 68,* 1555–1560, 1563–1564.

Fuchs, T., Birbaumer, N., Lutzenberger, W., et al. (2003). Neurofeedback treatment for attention-deficit/hyperactivity disorder in children: A comparison with methylphenidate. *Applications in Psychophysiological Biofeedback, 28*(1), 1–12.

Fuller, B., Kagan, S., Caspary, G., & Gauthier, C. (2002). Welfare reform and child care options for low-income families. *The Future of Children, 12*(1), 97–120.

Gable, S., Chang, Y., & Krull, J. (2007). Television watching and frequency of family meals are predictive of overweight onset and persistence in a national sample of school-aged children. *Journal of the American Dietetic Association, 107*(1), 53–61.

Gau, S., & Soong, W. (2003). The transition of sleep-wake patterns in early adolescence. *Sleep, 26*(4), 449–454.

Gavin, N., Adams, E., Manning, W., et al. (2007). The impact of welfare reform on insurance coverage before pregnancy and the timing of prenatal care initiation. *Health Services Research, 42*(4), 1564–1588.

Gidding, S.S., Dennison, B.A., Birch, L.L., et al. (2005). Dietary recommendations for children and adolescents: A guide for practitioners. *Circulation, 112,* 2061–2067.

Giles, L., DelBello, M., Stanford, K., & Strakowski, S. (2007). Child Behavior Checklist profiles of children and adolescents with and at high risk for developing bipolar disorder. *Child Psychiatry & Human Development, 38*(1), 47–55.

Gober, S., Klein, M., Berger, T., et al. (2006). Steroids in adolescence: The cost of achieving a physical idea. *NASP Communique, 34*(7). Retrieved August 1, 2008 from http://www.nasponline.org/publications/cq/cq347steroids.aspx.

Godin, G., Michaud, F., Alary, M., et al. (2003). Evaluation of an HIV and STD prevention program for adolescents in juvenile rehabilitation centers. *Health, Education & Behavior, 30*(5), 601–614.

Grant, J., Scherrer J. F., Lynskey, M. T., et al. (2006). Adolescent alcohol use is a risk factor for adult alcohol and drug dependence: Evidence from a twin design. *Psychological Medicine, 36*(1), 109–118.

Grassia, T. (2007). *HIV/AIDS & STDs: Know the regional epidemiology of STDs when treating adolescent patients.* Infectious Disease News. Retrieved March 30, 2007 from http://infectiousdiseasenews.com/200703/stds.asp.

Greer, A., Ng, V., & Fisman, D. (2008). Climate change and infectious diseases in North America: The road ahead. *Canadian Medical Association Journal, 178*(6), 715–722.

Griffin, K., Botvin, G., Nichols, T., & Doyle, M. (2003). Effectiveness of a universal drug abuse prevention approach for youth at high risk for substance use initiation. *Preventive Medicine, 36*(1), 1–7.

Guenther, L. (2007). *Pediculosis.* Retrieved November 1, 2007 from http://www.emedicine.com/med/topic1769.htm.

Guinan, M., McGuckin, M., & Ali, Y. (2002). The effect of a comprehensive handwashing program on absenteeism in elementary schools. *American Journal of Infection Control, 30*(4), 217–220.

Hall, A., Khanh, L., Son, T., et al. (2001). An association between chronic undernutrition and educational test scores in Vietnamese children. *European Journal of Clinical Nutrition, 55*(9), 801–804.

Hamilton, B.E., Martin, J.A., & Ventura, S.J. (2007). Births: Preliminary data for 2006. *National Vital Statistics Reports, 56*(7). Hyattsville, MD: National Center for Health Statistics.

Hansen, R.C. (2004). Overview: The state of head lice management and control. *The American Journal of Managed Care, 10*(9), [Suppl.], S260–S263.

Harden, K., Hill, J., Turkheimer, E., & Emery, R. (2008). Gene-environment correlation and interaction in peer effects on adolescent alcohol and tobacco use. *Behavior Genetics,* doi: 10.1007/s10519-008-9202-7.

Harpaz-Rotem, I., Murphy, R., Berkowitz, S., et al. (2007). Clinical epidemiology of urban violence: Responding to children exposed to violence in ten communities. *Journal of Interpersonal Violence, 22*(11), 1479–1490.

Harrell, J., Pearce, P., & Hayman, L. (2003). Fostering prevention in the pediatric population. *Journal of Cardiovascular Nursing, 18*(2), 144–149.

Haynes, K. (2007). An update on emergency contraception use in adolescents. *Journal of Pediatric Nursing, 22*(3), 186–195.

Hendin, H., Maltsberger, J., Lipschitz, A., et al. (2001). Recognizing and responding to a suicide crisis. *Suicide and Life Threatening Behaviors, 31*(2), 115–128.

Hennessy, K., & Green-Hennessy, S. (2000). Estimates of children and adolescents with school-related behavioral problems. *Psychiatric Services, 51*(5), 591.

Henretta, J. (2007). Early childbearing, marital status, and women's health and mortality after age 50. *Journal of Health & Social Behavior, 48*(3), 254–266.

Herrman, J. (2006). The voices of teen mothers: The experience of repeat pregnancy. *The American Journal of Maternal Child Nursing, 31*(4), 243–249.

Herrman, J. (2008). Adolescent perceptions of teen births. *Journal of Obstetrical, Gynecological & Neonatal Nursing, 37*(1), 42–50.

Hershey, T., Bhargava, N., Sadler, M., et al. (1999). Conventional versus intensive diabetes therapy in children with type 1 diabetes: Effects on memory and motor speed. *Diabetes Care, 22*(8), 1318–1324.

Hipp, D. (2006). Generation Rx: New category of substance abuse emerging in America. *Prevention Talk,* No. 22. SAMHSA.

Hjern, A., Alfven, G., & Ostberg, V. (2008). School stressors, psychological complaints and psychosomatic pain. *Acta Paediatrica, 97*(1), 112–117.

Howard, D., Feigelman, S., Li, X., et al. (2002). The relationship among violence victimization, witnessing violence, and youth distress. *Journal of Adolescent Health, 31*(6), 455–462.

Illinois Department of Public Health. (2003). *Adolescents at risk: Statistics on HIV/AIDS, STDs and unintended pregnancies.* Retrieved January 25, 2004, from http://www.idph.state.il.us/public/respect/hiv_fs.htm

Institute of Medicine. (2006, September). *Progress in preventing childhood obesity: How do we measure up?* Retrieved August 1, 2008 from http://www.iom.edu/Object.File/Master/36/984/11722_reportbrief.pdf.

Jain, N., & Stokley, S. (2007). National vaccination coverage among adolescents aged 13–17 years: United States, 2006. *Morbidity and Mortality Weekly Report, 56*(34), 885–888.

Johnson B., Carey M., Marsh K., et al. (2003). Interventions to reduce sexual risk for the human immunodeficiency virus in adolescents, 1985–2000: A research synthesis. *Archives of Pediatrics and Adolescent Medicine, 157*(4), 381–388.

Johnson, S., & Wang, C. (2008). Why do adolescents say they are less healthy than their parents think they are? The importance of mental health varies by social class in a nationally representative sample. *Pediatrics, 121*(2), 307–313.

Johnston, L., O'Malley, P., Bachman, J., & Schulenberg, J. (2008). *Monitoring the Future national results on adolescent drug use: Overview of key findings, 2007.* [NIH Publication No. 08-6418]. Bethesda, MD: National Institute on Drug Abuse.

Johnston, L. D., O'Malley, P. M., & Bachman, J. G. (2003). *National survey results on drug use from the Monitoring the Future study, 1975-2002. Volume II: Secondary school students.* (NIH Publication No. 03-5376). Bethesda, MD: National Institute on Drug Abuse.

Jones, K., & English, J. (2003). Review of common therapeutic options in the United States for the treatment of pediculosis capitis. *Clinical Infectious Diseases, 36*(11), 1355–1361.

Juvonen, J., Le, V., Kaganoff, T., et al. (2004). *Focus on the wonder years: Challenges facing the American middle school.* Santa Monica, CA: Rand Corporation.

Jyoti, D., Frongillo, E., & Jones, S. (2005). Food insecurity affects school children's academic performance, weight gain, and social skills. *Journal of Nutrition, 135,* 2831–2839.

Kanner, S., Hamrin, V., & Grey, M. (2003). Depression in adolescents with diabetes. *Journal of Child and Adolescent Psychiatric Nursing, 16*(1), 15–24.

Kazdin, A. (2008). Treatment of antisocial behavior in children and adolescents. *Eye on Psi Chi, 12*(3), Article 1. Retrieved April 15, 2008 from http://www.psichi.org/pubs/articles/article_683.asp.

Kelly, A., Margulies, D., & Castellanos, F. (2007). Recent advances in structural & functional brain imaging studies of attention-deficit/hyperactivity disorder. *Current Psychiatry Reports, 9*(5), 401–407.

Kendall, J., Hatton, D., Beckett, A., & Leo, M. (2003). Children's accounts of attention-deficit/hyperactivity disorder. *Advances in Nursing Science, 26*(2), 114–130.

Key, J., O'Rourke, K., Judy, N., & McKinnon, S. (2005). Efficacy of a secondary adolescent pregnancy prevention program: An ecological study before, during and after implementation of the Second Chance Club. *International Quarterly of Community Health Education, 24*(3), 231–240.

King, K.A., Wagner, D.I., & Hedrick, B. (2001). Safe and drug-free school coordinators' perceived needs to improve violence and drug prevention programs. *Journal of School Health, 71,* 236–241.

King, K., & Chassin, L. (2007). A prospective study of the effects of age of initiation of alcohol and drug use on young adult substance dependence. *Journal of Studies on Alcohol & Drugs, 68*(2), 256–265.

Kirby, D. (2002). Effective approaches to reducing adolescent unprotected sex, pregnancy and childbearing. *Journal of Sexuality Research, 39*(1), 51–57.

Knopf, D., Park, J., & C., Mulye, T. (2008). *The mental health of adolescents: A national profile, 2008.* National Adolescent Health Information Center. Retrieved October 14, 2008 from http://nahic.ucsf.edu/downloads/MentalHealthBrief.pdf

Koball, H., & Douglas-Hall, A. (2006). *The new poor: Regional trends in child poverty since 2000.* National Center for Children in Poverty. Retrieved August 30, 2006 from http://www.nccp.org/publications/pub_672.html.

Koch, P., Ryder, H. F., Dziura, I., et al. (2008). Educating adolescents about acne vulgaris: A comparison of written handouts with audiovisual computerized presentations. *Archives of Dermatology, 144*(2), 208–214.

Kohler, P., Manhart, L., & Lafferty, W. (2008). Abstinence-only and comprehensive sex education and the initiation of sexual activity and teen pregnancy. *Journal of Adolescent Health, 42*(4), 344–351.

Kroll, D., & Nedley, M. (2007). Dental caries: State of the science for the most common chronic disease of childhood. *Advances in Pediatrics, 54*(1), 215–239.

Lam, A. (2008). Increase in utilization of dental sealants. *Journal of Contemporary Dental Practice, 9*(3), 81–87.

Landsheer, J., & van Dijkum, C. (2005). Male and female delinquency trajectories from pre- through middle-adolescence and their continuation in late adolescence. *Adolescence, 40*(160), 729–748.

Latendresse, S., Rose, R., Viken, R., et al. (2008). Parenting mechanisms in links between parents' and adolescents' alcohol use behaviors. *Alcoholism, Clinical & Experimental Research, 32*(2), 322–330.

Lee, B.J., Mackey-Bilaver, L., & Chin, M. (2006). *Effects of WIC & food stamp program participation on child outcomes.*

Contractor & Cooperator Report No. 27. Economic Research Service: USDA.

Lee, B.J., Mackey-Bilaver, L., & Goerge, R.M. (2003). The patterns of food stamp and WIC participation under welfare reform. *Children & Youth Services, 25*(8), 589–610.

Levy, M., Heffner, B., Stewart, T., & Beeman, G. (2006). The efficacy of asthma case management in an urban school district in reducing school absences and hospitalizations for asthma. *Journal of School Health, 76*(6), 320–324.

Levy, S.M. (2003). An update on fluorides and fluorosis. *Journal of the Canadian Dental Association, 69*(5), 286–291.

Linares, L.O. (2008). *Community violence: The effects on children.* Retrieved August 1, 2008 from http://www.aboutourkids.org/articles/community_violence_effects_children?print=1.

Lindau, S., Tetteh, A., Kasza, K., & Gilliam, M. (2008). What schools teach our patients about sex: Content, quality and influences on sex education. *Obstetrics & Gynecology, 111*[2 Pt. 1], 256–266.

Lindhorst, T., & Mancoske, R. (2006). The social and economic impact of sanctions and time limits on recipients of Temporary Assistance to Needy Families. *Journal of Sociology & Social Welfare, 33*(1), 93–114.

Loprest, P. (2001). *How are families that left welfare doing? A comparison of early and recent welfare leavers.* Assessing the New Federalism Policy Brief No. B-36. Washington, DC.

Lubell, K., Kegler, S., Crosby, A., & Karch, D. (2007). Suicide trends among youths and young adults aged 10–24 years: United States, 1990–2004. *Morbidity and Mortality Weekly Report, 56*(35), 905–908.

Lubell, K., Kegler, S., Crosby, A., & Karch, D. (2007, September 7). Suicide trends among youths and young adults aged 104 years—United States, 1990-2004. *Morbidity & Mortality Weekly Report (MMWR), 56*(35), 905–908.

Ma, C., Gee, L., & Kushel, M. (2008). Associations between housing instability and food insecurity with health care access in low-income children. *Ambulatory Pediatrics, 8*(1), 50–57.

Mahat, G., Scoloveno, M., Ruales, N., & Scoloveno, R. (2006). Preparing peer educators for teen HIV/AIDS prevention. *Journal of Pediatric Nursing, 21*(5), 378–384.

Manganello, J.A. (2007). Health literacy and adolescents: A framework and agenda for future research. *Health Education Research,* doi: 10.1092/her/cym069.

March of Dimes. (2007). *Teenage pregnancy.* Retrieved August 1, 2008 from http://www.marchofdimes.com/printableArticles/14332_1159.asp.

Mardis, A., & Pratt, S. (2003). Nonfatal injuries to young workers in the retail trades and service industries in 1998. *Journal of Occupational and Environmental Medicine, 45*(3), 316–323.

Marinho, V., Higgins, J., Logan, S., & Sheiham, A. (2003). Systematic review of controlled trials on the effectiveness of fluoride gels for the prevention of dental caries in children. *Journal of Dental Education, 67*(4), 448–458.

Mark, H., Conklin, V., & Wolfe, M. (2001). Nurse volunteers in school-based hepatitis B immunization programs. *Journal of School Nursing, 17*(4), 185–188.

Masi, G., Toni, C., Perugi, G., et al. (2003). Externalizing disorders in consecutively referred children and adolescents with bipolar disorder. *Comparative Psychiatry, 44*(3), 184–189.

Maternal and Child Health Bureau. (2006). Vaccine-preventable diseases. *Child Health USA 2006.* Retrieved August 1, 2008 from http://www.mchb.hrsa.gov/chusa_06/healthstat/0300hs.htm.

May, P., Somal, P., Hurt, L., & DeBruyn, L. (2005). Outcome evaluation of a public health approach to suicide prevention in an American Indian tribal nation. *American Journal of Public Health, 95*(7), 1238–1244.

Mayo Clinic. (2006). *Self-injury/cutting.* Retrieved August 1, 2008 from http://www.maoclinic.com/print/self-injury/DS))775/DSESCTION=all&METHOD=print.

McCabe, S., Boyd, C., & Young, A. (2007). Medical and nonmedical uses of prescription drugs among secondary school students. *Journal of Adolescent Health, 40*(1), 76–83.

McCabe, S. E., West, B.T., Morales, M., Cranford, J.A., & Boyd, C.J. (2007). Does early onset of non-medical use predict prescription drug abuse and dependence? Results from a national study. *Addiction, 102,* 1920–1930.

McRee, N. (2008). Child abuse in blended households: Reports from runaway and homeless youth. *Child Abuse & Neglect, 32*(4), 449–453.

Merakou, K., & Kourea-Kremastinou, J. (2006). Peer education in HIV prevention: An evaluation in schools. *European Journal of Public Health, 16*(2), 128–132.

Merck. (2005). *Caring for sick children & their families: Children with chronic health conditions.* Merck professional manual. Retrieved August 1, 2008 from http://www.merck.com/mmpe/sec19/ch268/ch268c.html.

Michaud, P.A. (2008). Adolescent medicine: From clinical practice to public health. *Georgian Medical News, 156,* 61–65.

Miller, W.C., Carol, A., Ford, M.D., et al. (2004). Prevalence of chlamydial and gonococcal infections among young adults in the United States. *JAMA, 291*(18), 2229–2236.

Miller, J., Naimi, T., Brewer, R., & Jones, S. (2007). Binge drinking and associated health risk behaviors among high school students. *Pediatrics, 119*(1), 76–85.

Moore, D., & Florsheim, P. (2008). Interpartner conflict and child abuse risk among African American and Latino adolescent parenting couples. *Child Abuse & Neglect, 32*(4), 463–475.

Morris, P., Huston, G., Duncan, D., et al. (2001). *How welfare and work policies affect children: A synthesis of research.* New York: Manpower Demonstration Research Corporation.

Morrison-Beedy, D., Carey, M., Cote-Arsenault, D., et al. (2008). Understanding sexual abstinence in urban adolescent girls. *Journal of Obstetrical, Gynecological & Neonatal Nursing, 37*(2), 185–195.

Mulvaney, M., & Mebert, C. (2007). Parental corporal punishment predicts behavior problems in early childhood. *Journal of Family Psychology, 21*(3), 389–397.

Murray, N., Low, B., Hollis, C., et al. (2007). Coordinated school health programs and academic achievement: A systematic review of the literature. *Journal of School Health, 77*(9), 589–600.

Nader, P., O'Brien, M., Houts, R., et al. (2006). Identifying risk for obesity in early childhood. *Pediatrics, 118*(3), E594–E601.

Nansel, T., Overpeck, M., Haynie, D., et al. (2003). Relationship between bullying and violence among U.S. youth. *Archives of Pediatric and Adolescent Medicine, 157*(4), 348–358.

National Adolescent Health Information Center. (2000). *Fact sheet on unintentional injuries: Adolescents & young adults.* San Francisco, CA: Author, University of California San Francisco.

National Adolescent Health Information Center. (2006a). *Fact sheet on suicide: Adolescents & young adults.* San Francisco, CA: Author, University of California San Francisco.

National Adolescent Health Information Center. (2006b). *Fact sheet on mortality: Adolescents & young adults.* San Francisco, CA: Author, University of California San Francisco.

National Adolescent Health Information Center. (2007). *Fact sheet on violence: Adolescents & young adults.* San Francisco, CA: Author, University of California San Francisco.

National Adolescent Health Information Center. (2008). *Fact sheet on health care access & utilization: Adolescents & young adults.* San Francisco, CA: Author, University of California San Francisco.

National Cancer Institute. (2008). *Fact sheet: Childhood cancers, questions & answers.* Retrieved August 1, 2008 from http://www.cancer.gov/cancertopics.factsheet/Sites-Types/childhood/print?page=&keyword.

National Center for Children in Poverty. (2008, February). *How maternal, family & cumulative risk affect absenteeism in early schooling: Facts for policymakers.* Columbia University. Retrieved August 1, 2008 from http://www.nccp.org/publications/pdf/text_802.pdf.

National Center for Education Statistics. (2005). *Digest of education statistics. Table 84: Number of public school districts and public and private elementary and secondary schools: Selected years, 1969–70 through 2003–04.* Retrieved August 1, 2008 from http://www.nces.ed.gov/programs/digest/d05/tables/dt05_084.asp.

National Center for Education Statistics (NCES). (n.d.). *Fast facts: how many students with disabilities receive services?* U.S. Department of Education. Retrieved October 14, 2008 from http://nces.ed.gov/fastfacts/display.asp?id=64.

National Diabetes Education Program. (2006). *Overview of diabetes in children and adolescents.* Retrieved August 1, 2008 from http://ndep.nih.gov/diabetes/youth/youth_FS.htm#Statistics.

National Dissemination Center for Children With Disabilities. (n.d.). General information about disabilities: Disabilities that qualify infants, toddlers, children and youth for services under the IDEA. *NICHCY: Academy for Educational Development.* Retrieved August 1, 2008 from http://www.nichcy.org/pubs/genresc/gr3.pdf.

National Institute of Arthritis & Musculoskeletal & Skin Diseases. (2004). *Rheumatoid arthritis.* Retrieved August 1, 2008 from http://www.niams.nih.gov/Health_Info/Rheumatic_Disease/default.asp.

National Institutes of Health. (2006). *Adolescent HIV infection and disease.* National Institute of Child Health & Human Development. Retrieved August 1, 2008 from http://www.nichd.nih.gov/about/org/crmc/pama/prog_hivadol/index.cfm?renderforprint=1.

National Institute of Mental Health. (2006). *ADHD.* Retrieved August 1, 2008 from http://www.nimh.nih.gov/health/publications/adhd/summary.shtml.

National Institute of Neurological Disorders and Stroke (NINDS). (2007). *NINDS learning disabilities information page.* Retrieved August 1, 2008 from http://www.ninds.nih.gov/disorders/learningdisabilities/learningdisabilities.htm?css=print.

National Institute of Neurological Disorders and Stroke (NINDS). (2008). *Autism fact sheet.* Retrieved August 1, 2008 from http://www.ninds.nih.gov/disorders/autism/detail_autism.htm?css=print.

National Institute of Neurological Disorders & Stroke (NINDS). (2008). *NINDS epilepsy information page.* Retrieved October 14, 2008 from http://www.ninds.nih.gov/disorders/epilepsy/epilepsy.htm

National Institute of Occupational Safety and Health (NIOSH). (July 2003). *Preventing deaths, injuries, and illnesses of young workers.* Washington, DC: Author.

National Survey on Drug Use & Health. (2008, March 13). Inhalant use across the adolescent years. *The NSDUH Report.* Retrieved August 1, 2008 from http://oas.samhsa.gov/2k8/inhalants/inhalants.pdf.

National Youth Violence Prevention Resource Center. (2007). *Youth suicide fact sheet.* Retrieved October 15, 2008 from http://www.safeyouth.org/scripts/facts/suicide.asp#pop.

Neumark-Sztainer, D., Wall, M., Guo, J., et al. (2006). Obesity, disordered eating, and eating disorders in a longitudinal study of adolescents: How do dieters fare 5 years later? *Journal of the American Dietetic Association, 106*(4), 559–568.

Newacheck, P.W., Stein, R.E., Bauman, L., & Hung, Y.Y. (2003). Disparities in the prevalence of disability between black and white children. *Archives of Pediatric and Adolescent Medicine, 157*(3), 244–248.

Nguyen, D., Mascola, L., & Bancroft, E. (2005). Recurring methicillin-resistant staphylococcus aureus infections in a football team. *Emerging Infectious Diseases, 11*(4), 526–532.

Nielsen, S., Siega-Riz, A., & Popkin, B. (2002). Trends in food locations and sources among adolescents and young adults. *Preventive Medicine, 35*(2), 107–113.

Noimark, L., & Cox, H. (2008). Nutritional problems related to food allergy in childhood. *Pediatric Allergy & Immunology, 19*(2), 188–195.

O'Brien, M., Nader, P.R., Houts, R.M., et al. (2007). The ecology of childhood overweight: A 12-year longitudinal analysis. *International Journal of Obesity, 31*(9), 1469–1478.

O'Connell, J. (2005, January 24). Healthy children ready to learn: A white paper on health, nutrition, and physical education. *California Department of Education.* Retrieved August 1, 2008 from http://www.cde.ca.gov/eo/in/se/yr05healthychildrenwp.asp?print=yes.

Office of National Drug Control Policy (ONDCP). (2008). *Drug facts: Marijuana.* Retrieved August 1, 2008 from http://www.whitehousedrugpolicy.gov/drugfact/marijuana/index.html.

Olfson, M., Gameroff, M., Marcus, S., & Jensen, P.S. (2003). National trends in the treatment of attention deficit hyperactivity disorder. *American Journal of Psychiatry, 160*(6), 1071–1077.

Olson, C., Bove, C., & Miller, E. (2007). Growing up poor: Long-term implications for eating patterns and body weight. *Appetite, 49*(1), 198–207.

Owens, E., Hinshaw, S., Kraemer, H., et al. (2003). Which treatment for whom for ADHD? Moderators of treatment response in the MTA. *Journal of Consulting and Clinical Psychology, 71*(3), 540–552.

Ozawa, M., & Yoon, H. (2005). "Leavers" from TANF and AFDC: How do they fare economically? *Social Work, 50*(3), 239–249.

Pallin, D.J., Egan, D., Pelletier, A., et al. (2008). Increased U.S. emergency department visits for skin and soft tissue infections, and changes in antibiotic choices, during the emergence of community-associated methicillin-resistant *Staphylococcus aureus. Annals of Emergency Medicine, 51*(3), 291–298.

Park, M., Brindis, C., Chang, F., & Irwin, C. (2008). A midcourse review of the *Healthy People 2010* critical health objectives for adolescents and young adults. *Journal of Adolescent Health, 42*, 329–334.

Parrott, S., & Sherman, A. (August 17, 2006). *TANF at 10: Program results are more mixed than often understood.* Washington, DC: Center on Budget & Policy Priorities.

Partnership for a Drug-Free America. (2006, May 15). *Generation Rx: National study confirms abuse of prescription and over-the-counter drugs.* Retrieved October 15, 2008 from http://www.drugfree.org/Portal/DrugIssue/Research/Teens_2005/Generation_Rx_Study_Confirms_Abuse_of_Prescription.

Patton, G., Selzer, R., Coffey, C., et al. (2000). Onset of adolescent eating disorders: Population based cohort study over 3 years. *British Medical Journal, 318*(20), 765–768.

Paus, T. (2005). Mapping brain maturation and cognitive development during adolescence. *Trends in Cognitive Science, 9*(2), 60–68.

Pbert, L., Moolchan, E., Muramoto, M., Winickoff, J., Curry, S., Lando, H., et al. (2003). The state of office-based interventions for youth tobacco use. *Pediatrics, 111*(6), e650–e660.

Pediatric Tuberculosis Collaborative Group. (2004). Targeted tuberculin skin testing and treatment of latent tuberculosis infection in children and adolescents. *Pediatrics, 114*, 1175–1201.

Pereira, B., Venter, C., Grundy, J., et al. (2005). Prevalence of sensitization to food allergens, reported adverse reaction to foods, food avoidance, and food hypersensitivity among teenagers. *Journal of Allergy & Clinical Immunology, 116*(4), 884–892.

Perez-Rodrigo, C., & Aranceta, J. (2001). School-based nutrition education: Lessons learned and new perspectives. *Public Health Nutrition, 4*(1A), 131–139.

Perrin, J.M., Bloom, S.R., & Gortmaker, S.L. (2007). The increase of childhood chronic conditions in the United States. *JAMA, 297*(24), 2755–2759.

Pianta, R., Belsky, J., Vandergrift, N., et al. (2008). Classroom effects on children's achievement trajectories in elementary school. *American Educational Research Journal,* doi: 10.3102/0002831207308230.

Piko, B. (2007). Self-perceived health among adolescents: The role of gender and psychosocial factors. *European Journal of Pediatrics, 166*(7), 701–708.

Poulton, R., Caspi, A., Milne, B.J., et al. (2002). Association between children's experience of socioeconomic disadvantage and adult health: A life-course study. *Lancet, 360*(9346), 1640–1645.

Price, V., Murphy, S., & Cureton, V. (2004). Increasing self-efficacy and knowledge through a seizure education program for special education teachers. *Journal of School Nursing, 20*(1), 43–49.

Raghavan, R., Aarons, G., Rosch, S., & Leslie, L. (2008). Longitudinal patterns of health insurance coverage among a national sample of children in the child welfare system. *American Journal of Public Health, 98*(3), 478–484.

Reid, V., & Meadows-Oliver, M. (2007). Postpartum depression in adolescent mothers: An integrative review of the literature. *Journal of Pediatric Health Care, 21*(5), 289–298.

Reinberg, S. (2008). *Measles outbreak rises to 64 cases, most since 2001.* The Washington Post. Retrieved August 1, 2008 from http://www.washingtonpost.com/wp-dyn/content/article2008/05/01/AR2008050102633_pf.html.

Rich, C., Gidycz, C., Warkentin, J., et al. (2005). Child and adolescent abuse and subsequent victimization: A prospective study. *Child Abuse & Neglect, 29*(12), 1373–1394.

Roberts, R., Roberts, C., & Duong, H. (2008). Chronic insomnia and its negative consequences for health and functioning of adolescents: A 12-month prospective study. *Journal of Adolescent Health, 42*(3), 294–302.

Rose, D., & Bodor, J. (2006). Household food insecurity and overweight status in young school children: Results from the Early Childhood Longitudinal Study. *Pediatrics, 117*(2), 464–473.

Rosen, M., Breitkopf, D., & Nagamani, M. (2003). A randomized controlled trial of second- versus third-generation oral contraceptives in the treatment of acne vulgaris. *American Journal of Obstetrics and Gynecology, 188*(5), 1158–1160.

Rotheram-Borus, M. (2000). Expanding the range of interventions to reduce HIV among adolescents. *AIDS, 14*[Suppl. l], S33–S40.

Rupp, R., & Rosenthal, S. (2007). Parental influences on adolescent sexual behaviors. *Adolescent Medicine: State of the Art Reviews, 18*(3), 460–470, vi.

Russell, B., Britner, P., & Woolard, J. (2007). The promise of primary prevention home visiting programs: A review of potential outcomes. *Journal of Prevention & Intervention in the Community, 34*(1–2), 129–147.

Russo, A., Jiang, J., & Barrett, M. (August 2007). *Trends in potentially preventable hospitalizations among adults and children, 1997–2004.* Statistical brief 36: Healthcare Cost & Utilization Project. Agency for Healthcare Research & Quality.

Saewyc, E., Skay, C., Richens, K., et al. (2006). Sexual orientation, sexual abuse, and HIV-risk behaviors among adolescents in the Pacific Northwest. *American Journal of Public Health, 96*(6), 1104–1110.

Safe Kids USA. (April 29, 2008). *Accidental injury death rate of children 14 and under down by 45 percent since 1987, says Safe Kids USA 20th anniversary report.* [Press release]. Retrieved April 28, 2008 from http://www.usa.safekids.org/tier3_cd.cfm?content_item_id=25671&folder_id=300.

Santelli, J.S., Lindberg, L.D., Finer, L.B., & Singh, S. (2007). Explaining recent declines in adolescent pregnancy in the

United States: The contribution of abstinence and improved contraceptive use. *American Journal of Public Health, 97*(1), 150–156.

Sato, S., Schulz, K., Sisk, C., & Wood, R. (2008). Adolescents and androgens, receptors and rewards. *Hormones & Behavior, 53*(5), 647–658.

Sawaya, A., Martins, P., Hoffman, D., & Roberts, S. (2003). The link between childhood undernutrition and risk of chronic diseases in adulthood: A case study of Brazil. *Nutrition Review, 71*[5 Pt. 1], 168–175.

Schaffer, S., Humiston, S., Shone, L., et al. (2001). Adolescent immunization practices: A national survey of U.S. physicians. *Archives of Pediatric and Adolescent Medicine, 155*(5), 566–571.

Schar, E., Gutierrez, K., Murphy-Hoefer, R., & Nelson, D.E. (March 2006). *Tobacco Use Prevention Media Campaigns: Lessons Learned From Youth In Nine Countries.* Atlanta, Ga: U.S. Department of Health and Human Services, Centers for Disease Control and Prevention, National Center for Chronic Disease Prevention and Health Promotion, Office on Smoking and Health.

Schmidt, S., Peterson, C., & Bullinger, M. (2003). Coping with chronic disease from the perspective of children & adolescents: A conceptual framework and its implications for participation. *Child Care, Health & Development, 29*(1), 63–75.

Schmitt, K., Dayanim, S., & Matthias, S. (2008). Personal homepage construction as an expression of social development. *Developmental Psychology, 44*(2), 496–506.

Schnitzer, P.G. (2006). Prevention of unintentional childhood injuries. *American Family Physician, 74*(11), 1864–1869.

Schor, E.L., & American Academy of Pediatrics Task Force on the Family. (2003). Family pediatrics: Report of the task force on the family. *Pediatrics, 111*(6), 1541–1571.

Seecombe, K., Newsom, J., & Hoffman, K. (2006). Access to health care after welfare reform. *Inquiry, 43*(2), 167–178.

Shaffer, D. & Kipp, K. (2006). *Developmental psychology: Childhood and adolescence.* London: Thomson Learning.

Shaffer, D., Gould, M., & Hicks, R. (March 14, 2007). *Teen suicide fact sheet.* New York: Columbia University.

Shah, A., Smolensky, M., Burau, K., et al. (2006). Seasonality of primarily childhood and young adult infectious diseases in the United States. *Chronobiology International, 23*(5), 1065–1082.

Sharma, A. (2001). Anorexia nervosa and bulimia nervosa: An appraisal. *Drugs Today, 37*(4), 229–236.

Shields, M.K., & Behrman, R.E. (2002). Children and welfare reform: Analysis and recommendations. *The Future of Children, 12*(1), 5–26.

Silver, L. (2004a). Epilepsy and learning disabilities. *Learning Disabilities Association of America.* Retrieved August 1, 2008 from http://www.ldanatl.org/aboutId/professionals/print_ epilepsy_ld.asp.

Silver, L. (2004b). Doctor to doctor: Information on attention-deficit/hyperactivity disorder for pediatricians and other physicians. *Learning Disabilities Association of America.* Retrieved August 1, 2008 from http://www.ldanatl.org/aboutId/ professionals/doctor_to_doctor.asp.

Silver, L. (2006). Doctor to doctor: Information learning disabilities for pediatricians and other physicians. *Learning Disabilities Association of America.* Retrieved August 1, 2008 from http://www. ldanatl.org/aboutId/professionas/doctor_to_doctor.asp.

Sinclair, S., & Edelstein, B. (February 23, 2005). *CHDP policy brief: Cost effectiveness of preventive dental services.* Dental Health Project. Retrieved August 1, 2008 from http://www.cdc.gov/OralHealth/publications/library/burdenbook/ pdfs/CDHP_policy_brief.pdf.

Singh, S., & Darroch, J. (2000). Adolescent pregnancy and childbearing: Levels and trends in developing countries. *Family Planning Perspectives, 32,* 14–23.

Siqueira, L., Rolnitzkyi, L., & Rickert, V. (2001). Strategies promoting smoking cessation in adolescents: The role of nicotine dependence, stress, and coping mechanisms. *Archives of Pediatric & Adolescent Medicine, 155,* 489–495.

Sleskova, M., Salonna F., Geckova, A.M., et al. (2006). Does parental unemployment affect adolescents' health? *Journal of Adolescent Health, 38*(5), 527–535.

Smith, C., Ireland, T., & Thornberry, T. (2005). Adolescent maltreatment and its impact on young adult antisocial behavior. *Child Abuse & Neglect, 29*(10), 1099–1119.

Smithbattle, L. (2007). Legacies of advantage and disadvantage: The case of teen mothers. *Public Health Nursing, 34*(5), 409–420.

Snyder, L., Milici, F., Slater, M., Sun, H., & Strizhakova, Y. (2006). Effects of alcohol advertising exposure on drinking among youth. *Archives of Pediatrics & Adolescent Medicine, 160*(1), 18–24.

Sotir, M.J., Cappozzo D.L., Warshauer D.M., et al. (2008). A countywide outbreak of pertussis: Initial transmission in a high school weight room with subsequent substantial impact on adolescents and adults. *Archives of Pediatric & Adolescent Medicine, 162*(1), 79–85.

Spivey, M., Schnitzer, P., Kruse, R., et al. (2008). Association of injury visits in children and child maltreatment reports. *Journal of Emergency Medicine,* doi: 10.1016/j.jemermed. 2007.07.025.

Staff, J., & Mortimer, J. (2008). Social class background and the 'school to work' transition. *New Directions for Child and Adolescent Development, 119,* 55–69.

Starfield, B., Riley, A., Witt, W., & Robertson, J. (2002). Social class gradients in health during adolescence. *Journal of Epidemiology & Community Health, 56,* 354–361.

Steinberg, L. (2005). Cognitive and affective development in adolescence. *Trends in Cognitive Science, 9*(2), 69–74.

Stevens, S., Colwell, B., Smith, D., et al. (2005). An exploration of self-reported negative affect by adolescents as a reason for smoking: Implications for tobacco prevention and intervention programs. *Preventive Medicine, 41*(2), 589–596.

Stice, E. (2002). *Certain behaviors can predict binge-eating disorders in teenage girls.* Center for the Advancement of Health. Retrieved March 14, 2002 from http://hbns.org/newsrelease/ eatingdisorder3-14-02.cfm.

Story, M., Neumark-Sztainer, D., & French, S. (2002). Individual and environmental influences on adolescent eating behaviors. *Journal of the American Dietetic Association, 102*[Suppl. 3], S40–S51.

Stuewig, J., & McCloskey, L. (2005). The relation of child maltreatment to shame and guilt among adolescents: Psychological routes to depression and delinquency. *Child Maltreatment, 10*(4), 324–336.

Substance Abuse & Mental Health Services Administration (SAMHSA). (2003). *Mental, emotional & behavioral disorders of childhood & adolescence.* Retrieved August 1, 2008 from http://mentalhealth.samhsa.gov/publications/allpubs/ CA-006/default.asp#6.

Surgeon General of the United States. (2002). *Youth violence: A report of the surgeon general.* Retrieved August 1, 2008 from http://www.surgeongeneral.gov/library/youthviolence/ toc.html.

Surgeon General of the United States. (2007). The Surgeon General's call to action to prevent and decrease overweight and obesity: Overweight in children and adolescents. Retrieved August 1, 2008 from http://www.surgeongeneral.gov/topics/ obesity/calltoaction/fact_adolescents.htm.

Swahn, M., Bossarte, R., & Sullivent, E. (2008). Age of alcohol use initiation, suicidal behavior, and peer and dating violence victimization and perpetration among high-risk, seventh-grade adolescents. *Pediatrics, 121*(2), 297–305.

Swartwood, J., Swartwood, M., Lubar, J., & Timmermann, D. (2003). EEG differences in ADHD-combined type during baseline and cognitive tasks. *Pediatric Neurology, 3,* 199–204.

Taras, H. (2005). Nutrition and student performance at school. *Journal of School Health, 75*(6), 199–213.

Taras, H., & Gage, M. (1995). Advertised foods on children's television. *Archives of Pediatric & Adolescent Medicine, 149*(6), 649–652.

Taras, H., & Potts-Datema, W. (2005a). Chronic health conditions and student performance at school. *Journal of School Health, 75*(7), 255–266.

Taras, H., & Potts-Datema, W. (2005b). Childhood asthma and student performance at school. *Journal of School Health, 75*(8), 296–312.

Taras, H., & Potts-Datema, W. (2005c). Obesity and student performance at school. *Journal of School Health, 75*(8), 291–295.

Tarter, R., Kirisci, L., Feske, U., & Vanyukov, M. (2007). Modeling the pathways linking childhood hyperactivity and substance use disorder in young adulthood. *Psychology of Addictive Behaviors, 21*(2), 266–271.

Taylor, J., Baldwin, N., & Spencer, N. (2008). Predicting child abuse and neglect: Ethical, theoretical and methodological challenges. *Journal of Clinical Nursing, 17*(9), 1193–1200.

ter Bogt, T., van Dorsselaer, S., Monshouwer, K., et al. (2006). Body mass index and body weight perception as risk factors for internalizing and externalizing problem behavior among adolescents. *Journal of Adolescent Health, 39*(1), 27–34.

ter Wolbeek, M., van Doornen, L., Kavelaars, A., & Heijnen, C. (2006). Severe fatigue in adolescents: A common phenomenon? *Pediatrics, 117*(6), 1078–1086.

Thapar, A., Langley, K., O'Donovan, M., & Owen, M. (2006). Refining the attention deficit hyperactivity disorder phenotype for molecular genetic studies. *Molecular Psychiatry, 11*(8), 714–720.

Tingle, L., DeSimone, M., & Covington, B. (2003). A meta-evaluation of 11 school-based smoking prevention programs. *Journal of School Health, 73*(2), 64–67.

Tobacco Information and Prevention Source. (2001). *Fact sheet: Minors' access to tobacco*. National Center for Chronic Disease Prevention and Health Promotion. Retrieved August 1, 2008 from http://www.cdc.gov/tobacco/sgr/sgr_2000/factsheets/factsheet_minor.htm.

Trost, S., Kerr, L, Ward, D., & Pate, R. (2001). Physical activity and eterminants of physical activity in obese and non-obese children. *International Journal of Obesity Related to Metabolic Disorders, 25*, 822–829.

United States Department of Agriculture (USDA). (2006). *WIC program coverage: How many eligible individuals participated in the Special Supplemental Nutrition Program for Women, Infants, & Children (WIC): 1994 to 2003?* Retrieved August 1, 2008 from http://www.fns.usda.gov/aone/MENU/Published/WIC/FILES/WICEligibles.pdf.

United States Food & Drug Administration. (February 2007). Food allergies: What you need to know. *Food Facts*. Center for Food Safety & Applied Nutrition. Retrieved August 1, 2008 from http://www.ldanatl.org/aboutId/professionals/doctor_to_doctor.asp.

Usta, I., Zoorob, D., Abu-Musa, A., et al. (2008). Obstetric outcome of teenage pregnancies compared with adult pregnancies. *Acta Obstetricia et Gynecologica Scandinavica, 878*(2), 178–183.

van den Berg, P., Neumark-Sztainer, D., Hannan, P., & Haines, J. (2007). Is dieting advice from magazines helpful or harmful? Five-year associations with weight-control behaviors and psychological outcomes in adolescents. *Pediatrics, 119*(1), E30–E37.

VanDenBurgh, K. (2003). Childhood cancer in the classroom: Information for the school nurse. *School Nurse News, 20*(2), 28–33.

Vandermeulen, C., Roelants M., Theeten, H., et al. (2008). Vaccination coverage in 14-year-old adolescents: Documentation, timeliness, and sociodemographic determinants. *Pediatrics, 121*(3), 428–434.

Van der Vorst, H., Engels, R., Meeus, W., et al. (2005). The role of alcohol-specific socialization in adolescents' drinking behaviour. *Addiction, 100*(1), 1464–1476.

Van Hook, J., & Stamper-Balistreri, K. (2003). Ineligible parents, eligible children: Food stamps receipt, allotments, and food insecurity among children of immigrants. *Children & Youth Services Review, 25*(8), 589–610.

Vissing, Y.M., & Daiment, J. (1997). Housing distress among high school students. *Social Work, 42*(1), 31–41.

Wallace, H., Blacklay, A., Eiser, C., et al. (2001). Developing strategies for long-term follow up of survivors of childhood cancer. *British Medical Journal, 323*(7307), 271–274.

Wang, C., & Holton, J. (2007). *Total estimated cost of child abuse and neglect in the United States*. Prevent Child Abuse America. Retrieved August 1, 2008 from http://www.preventchildabuse.org/about_us/media_releases/pcaa_pew_economic_impact_study_final.pdf.

Weinreb, L., Wehler, C., Perloff, J., et al. (2002). Hunger: Its impact on children's health and mental health. *Pediatrics, 110*(4), E41.

Weiss, M., & Murray, C. (2003). Assessment and management of attention-deficit hyperactivity disorder in adults. *Canadian Medical Association Journal, 168*(6), 715–722.

Wells, J., Hallal, P.C., Reichert, F.F., et al. (2008). Sleep patterns and television viewing in relation to obesity and blood pressure: Evidence from an adolescent Brazilian birth cohort. *International Journal of Obesity*, doi: 10.1038/ijo.2008.37.

White, C., Shinder, F., Shinder, A., & Dyer, D. (2001). Reduction of illness absenteeism in elementary schools using an alcohol-free instant hand sanitizer. *Journal of School Nursing, 17*(5), 258–265.

Wigfield, A., Lutz, S., & Wagner, A.L. (2005). Early adolescents' development across the middle school years: Implications for school counselors. *Professional School Counseling, 9*(2), 112–119.

Wilkinson, N., Jackson, G., & Gardner-Medwin, J. (2003). Biologic therapies for juvenile arthritis. *Archives of Diseases in Childhood, 88*(3), 186–191.

Winston, F., Kallan, M., Senserrick, T., & Elliott, M. (2008). Risk factors for death among older child and teenaged motor vehicle passengers. *Archives of Pediatric & Adolescent Medicine, 162*(3), 253–260.

Woodruff, S., Conway, T., Edwards, C., et al. (2007). Evaluation of an internet virtual world chat room for adolescent smoking cessation. *Addictive Behavior, 32*(9), 1769–1786.

World Bank. (2008). *Communicable diseases: Summary*. Retrieved August 1, 2008 from http://web.worldback.org/WBSITE/EXTERNAL/NEWS/0,,contentMDK:20040888~menuPK:34480~pagePK:34370~theSitePK:4607,00.html.

Yeung, W., & Conley, D. (2008). Black-White achievement gap and family wealth. *Child Development, 79*(2), 303–324.

Young, E.M., & Fors, S.W. (2001). Factors related to the eating habits of students in grades 9–12. *Journal of School Health, 71*(10), 483–488.

Yurgelun-Todd, D. (2007). Emotional and cognitive changes during adolescence. *Current Opinions in Neurobiology, 17*(2), 251–257.

Zahn-Waxler, C., Shirtcliff, E., & Marceau, K. (2008). Disorders of childhood and adolescence: Gender and psychopathology. *Annual Review of Clinical Psychology, 27*(4), 275–303.

Selected Readings

American Youth Policy Forum. (n.d.). *Background fact sheet: How severe is America's juvenile crime problem?* Retrieved August 1, 2008 from http://www.aypf.org/publications/lesscost/pages/fact02.html.

Armour, S., & Haynie, D. (2007). Sexual debut and delinquency. *Journal of Youth & Adolescence, 36*, 141–152.

Ault, K., & Reisinger, K. (2007). Programmatic issues in the implementation of an HPV vaccination program to prevent cervical cancer. *International Journal of Infectious Diseases, 11*[Suppl. 2], S26–S28.

Bailey, M., Zauszniewski, J., Heinzer, M., & Hemstrom-Krainess, A. (2007). Patterns of depressive symptoms in children. *Journal of Child & Adolescent Psychiatric Nursing, 20*(2), 86–95.

Baker, L., & Cavender, A. (2003). Promoting culturally competent care for gay youth. *The Journal of School Nursing, 19*(2), 65–72.

Bartlett, R., Holditch-Davis, D., & Belyea, M. (2007). Problem behaviors in adolescents. *Pediatric Nursing, 33*(1), 13–18, 35–36.

Boardman, J.D. (2006). Self-rated health among US adolescents. *Journal of Adolescent Health, 38*(4), 401–408.

Brindis, C., Morreale, M., & English, A. (2003). The unique health care needs of adolescents. *Future of Children, 13*, 117–135.

Burton, D.L. (2008). An exploratory evaluation of the contribution of personality and childhood sexual victimization to the development of sexually abuse behavior. *Sex Abuse, 20*(1), 102–115.

Cavanagh, S., Riegel-Crumb, C., & Crosnoe, R. (2007). Early pubertal timing and the education of girls. *Social Psychology Quarterly, 70*, 186–198.

Chen, A., & Thompson, E. (2007). Preventing adolescent risky sexual behaviors: Parents matter! *Journal of Specialists in Pediatric Nursing, 12*(2), 119–122.

Connell, A., Dishion T., Yasui, M., & Kavanagh, K. (2007). An adaptive approach to family intervention: Linking engagement in family-centered intervention to reductions in adolescent problem behavior. *Journal of Consulting & Clinical Psychology, 75*(4), 568–579.

Cotton, S., & Bery, D. (2007). Religiosity, spirituality, and adolescent sexuality. *Adolescent Medicine State of the Art Reviews, 18*(3), 471–483.

Crosnoe, R. (2007). Gender, education, and the experience of obesity. *Sociology of Education, 80*, 241–260.

Fergusson, D., Horwood, L., & Ridder, E. (2005). Show me the child at seven: The consequences of conduct problems in childhood for psychosocial functioning in adulthood. *Journal of Child Psychology & Psychiatry, 46*(8), 837–949.

Flores, G., & Tomany-Korman, S. (2008). Racial and ethnic disparities in medical and dental health, access to care, and use of services in US children. *Pediatrics, 121*(2), 286–298.

Hatmaker, G. (2003). Development of a skin cancer prevention program. *The Journal of School Nursing, 19*(2), 89–92.

Kuperminc, G., & Allen, J. (2001). Social orientation: Problem behavior and motivations toward interpersonal problem solving among high risk adolescents. *Journal of Youth & Adolescence, 30*(5), 597–622.

Magee, T., & Roy, C. (2008). Predicting school-age behavior problems: The role of early childhood risk factors. *Pediatric Nursing, 34*(1), 37–44.

Martin, J.L. (2008). Peer sexual harassment: Finding voice, changing culture: An intervention strategy for adolescent females. *Violence Against Women, 14*(1), 100–124.

McCabe, M., & Ricciardelli, L. (2003). Body image and strategies to lose weight and increase muscle among boys and girls. *Health Psychology, 22*(1), 39–46.

Mears, C., & Knight, J. (2007). The role of schools in combating illicit substance abuse. *Pediatrics, 120*(6), 1379–1384.

Mejdell-Awbrey, L., & Juarez, S. (2003). Developing a nursing protocol for over-the-counter medications in high school. *The Journal of School Nursing, 19*(1), 12–16.

O'Donnell, L., Myint-U, A., O'Donnell, C., & Stueve, A. (2003). Long-term influence of sexual norms and attitudes on timing of sexual initiation among urban minority youth. *Journal of School Health, 73*(2), 68–75.

Plomin, R., & Walker, S. (2003). Genetics and educational psychology. *British Journal of Educational Psychology, 73*(1), 3–14.

Roberts, T., & Ryan, S. (2002). Tattooing and high-risk behavior in adolescents. *Pediatrics, 110*(6), 1058–1063.

Sen, B., & Swaminathan, S. (2007). Maternal prenatal substance use and behavior problems among children in the U.S. *Journal of Mental Health Policy & Economics, 19*(4), 189–206.

Smith, C., Ireland, T., & Thornberry, T. (2005). Adolescent maltreatment and its impact on young adult antisocial behavior. *Child Abuse & Neglect, 29*(10), 1099–1119.

Solomon, B., Bradshaw, C., Wright, J., & Cheng, T. (208). Youth and parental attitudes toward fighting. *Journal of Interpersonal Violence, 23*(4), 544–560.

Thornton, N., Hamiwka, L., Elisabeth, L., et al. (2008). Family function in cognitively normal children with epilepsy: Impact on competence and problem behaviors. *Epilepsy & Behavior, 12*(1), 90–95.

Timmermans, M., van Lier, P., & Koot, H. (2008). Which forms of child/adolescent externalizing behaviors account for late adolescent risky sexual behavior and substance use? *Journal of Child Psychology & Psychiatry, 49*(4), 386–394.

United States Department of Agriculture (USDA). (2008). *Team nutrition.* Food & Nutrition Service. Retrieved August 1, 2008 from http://www.fns.usda.gov/tn/.

Winiewska, B., Baranowska, W., & Wendorff, I. (2007). The assessment of comorbid disorders in ADHD children and adolescents. *Advances in Medical Science, 52*[Suppl. 1], 215–217.

Yan, A., Chiu, Y., Stoesen, C., & Wang, M. (2007). STD/HIV-related sexual risk behaviors and substance use among U.S. rural adolescents. *Journal of the National Medical Association, 99*(12), 1386–1394.

Ybarra, M., Diener-West, M., & Leaf, P. (2007). Examining the overlap in internet harassment & school bullying: Implications for school intervention. *Journal of Adolescent Health, 41*[6 Suppl. 1], S42–S50.

Internet Resources

Adolescent Health (Guide for State/Communities): *http://www.cdc.gov/HealthyYouth/AdolescentHealth/Guide/order.htm*

Alcohol & Advertising Podcast: *http://www2a.cdc.gov/podcasts/player.asp?f=4032*

Allergy/Asthma Toolkit: *http://www.aaaai.org/members/allied_health/tool_kit/*

Child Behavior & How Parents Can Change Behaviors: *http://familydoctor.org/online/famdocen/home/children/parents/behavior/201.printerview.html*

Drug Abuse Prevention Guide: *http://www.drugabuse.gov/pdf/prevention/RedBook.pdf*

Food Allergies: *http://www.cfsan.fda.gov/~dms/ffalrgn.html*

Foundation for a Smokefree America: *http://www.tobaccofree.org/*

Injury Prevention Program (children 12 and under): *http://www.aap.org/familoy/tippmain.htm*

Learning Disabilities: *http://www.ldonline.org/index.php*

Marijuana Myths & Facts: *http://www2a.cdc.gov/podcasts/player.asp?f=4032*

MyPyramid for Kids: *http://www.mypyramid.gov/kids/index.html*

School Action Plans for Food Allergies: *http://www.foodallergy.org/school/guidelines.html*

Sports Head Injuries: *http://www.cdc.gov/ncipc/tbi/Coaches_Tool_Kit.htm*

Youth Violence Prevention: *http://www.cdc.gov/ncipc/dvp/bestpractices.htm*

23

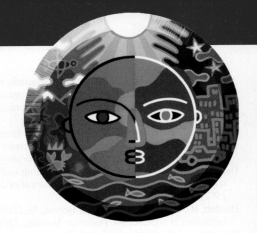

Adult Women and Men

LEARNING OBJECTIVES

Upon mastery of this chapter, you should be able to:

◆ Identify key demographic characteristics of women and men throughout the adult lifespan.

◆ Provide a health profile of adult women and men living in the United States.

◆ Discuss the major chronic illnesses found in adult women and men in the United States.

◆ Compare and contrast the manifestations of chronic illnesses in adult women and men.

◆ Identify desirable primary, secondary, and tertiary health promotion activities designed to improve the health of women and men.

◆ Describe the role of the community health nurse in promoting the health of adult women and men across the lifespan.

❝Male and female represent the two sides of the great radical dualism. But in fact they are perpetually passing into one another. Fluid hardens to solid, solid rushes to fluid. There is no wholly masculine man, no purely feminine woman. ❞
—Margaret Fuller (1810–1850), *Woman in the Nineteenth Century, 1845*

KEY TERMS

Adult
Anorexia nervosa
Binge eating
Bisexual
Bulimia nervosa
Cancer
Cardiovascular disease
Chronic fatigue and immune dysfunction syndrome (CFIDS)
Chronic lower respiratory disease
Diabetes mellitus
Erectile dysfunction
Gay
Health disparities
Health literacy
Life expectancy
Menopause
Obesity
Prostate
Substance use
Transgender
Unintentional injuries

The term *adult* has many different meanings in society. To children, an adult is anyone in authority, including a 14-year-old babysitter. As people age, they tend to redefine the term upward. It is not unusual, for example, to hear an elderly person describe a couple in their mid-30s as "kids." The United States Criminal Justice System distinguishes between adults and juveniles for purposes of delimiting types of crimes and possibilities for punishment, and labor legislation provides different protections for children than for adult workers. Even hospitals and health care systems vary somewhat as to the ages at which they distinguish pediatric and geriatric clients from middle-aged adults.

How would you characterize an adult? Does your definition rest solely on age, or is it influenced by other factors, such as marital status, employment status, financial independence, amount of responsibility for self and others, and so on? For the purposes of this chapter, an **adult** is defined as anyone 18 years of age or older. Obviously, there are tremendous differences in health profiles and health care needs as people age. As adults enter their middle years (35–65), they experience many normal physiologic changes. However, some changes are the result of disease, environment, or lifestyle and can be slowed through behavior change. A physical profile of middle-aged adults is organized by body systems and can be found in Display 23.1.

Throughout history, the health care needs of women and men have differed more often then they have been alike. Many health promotion and health protection programs are designed specifically for women or for men. Mammography screening programs and prenatal clinics are designed with a woman's health in mind. Teaching testicular self-examination and prostate cancer screening are health promotion programs for men. Programs in many areas, such as cardiac rehabilitation, stress management, and dating violence prevention, may have had one gender in mind at one time but are now established as programs for both genders. Nevertheless, morbidity and mortality statistics, historical development of research foci, and workforce changes required that the health care needs of women and men be examined separately. This chapter focuses on the health of women and men across the adult lifespan.

DEMOGRAPHICS OF ADULT WOMEN AND MEN

Mortality statistics are considered the most reliable indicator of the health status of a population. In 2004, a total of 2,397,615 people died in the United States. The crude death rate was 816.5 per 100,000 for all ages. Causes of death varied by age, sex, and ethnicity, but the 10 leading causes of death for all people in rank order included the following (National Center for Health Statistics [NCHS], 2007):

1. Diseases of the heart 652,486
2. Malignant neoplasms 553,888
3. Cerebrovascular diseases 150,074
4. Chronic lower respiratory diseases 121,987
5. Unintentional injuries 112,012
6. Diabetes mellitus 73,138
7. Alzheimer's 65,965

DISPLAY 23.1	PHYSICAL PROFILE OF MIDDLE-AGED ADULTS BY BODY SYSTEM
Body System	**Physical Characteristic**
Skeletal system	Intervertebral disks flatten over time
Integumentary system	Decreased secretions by sebaceous glands leads to drier skin
	Sweat glands diminish in size and number
	Skin loses elasticity and is more prone to wrinkles
	Hair bulbs lose melanin usually resulting in gray hair by age 50
Muscular system	Muscle fibers decrease by approximately 10%
	Lean body mass is replaced by adipose tissue
	Decreased grip strength occurs at this age
Endocrine and reproductive system	Menses stops
	Synthesis of estrogen decreases
	Tissues of the reproductive system (e.g., cervix and uterus) gradually atrophy
	Uterine changes make pregnancy less likely
	Intercourse may be more painful due to diminishing natural lubrications
Neurologic system	Nerve impulses are conducted 5% slower
	Cognition is unaffected, although there is a gradual loss of neurons
	Eyesight is poorer due to loss of elasticity in the lens
	Auditory discrimination of certain tones and consonants gradually decreases
Cardiovascular system	By age 50, the heart's efficiency may be only 80%
	Elasticity of heart and blood vessels decreases
	Cardiac output decreases
Respiratory system	Elasticity of lungs decreases
	Breathing capacity decreases to 75% due to diminished strength of chest wall muscles
Urinary system	Decreased glomerular filtration rate appears in women
	Loss of bladder tone and tissue atrophy may lead to incontinence or possibly prolapse
	In men, an enlarged prostate may result in nocturia or dribbling

8. Influenza and pneumonia 59,664
9. Nephritis, nephritic syndrome 42,480
and nephrosis
10. Septicemia 33,373

Diseases of the heart and malignant neoplasms accounted for more than 50% of deaths in 2004, and these diseases are the top two causes of death both for women and men. However, cerebrovascular diseases were the third leading cause of death for women and unintentional injuries were the third leading cause of death in men.

Since the beginning of the 21st century, the top 10 causes of death have remained the same. This was a major shift from the turn of the 20th century, when communicable diseases, such as tuberculosis and pneumonia, were leading causes of death. The shift from communicable to chronic illness can be attributed to the significant advances in public health, prevention, technology, and biomedical research.

LIFE EXPECTANCY

Life expectancy is the average number of years that an individual member of a specific cohort (usually a single birth year) is projected to live. It is another standard measurement that is used to compare the health status of various populations, typically calculated from age-specific death rates. Health statistics often report life expectancy figures for birth and 65 years of age (see Table 23.1).

In the United States, life expectancy has increased consistently over time. Between 1990 and 2004, life expectancy at birth increased 3.4 years for men and 1.6 years for women. The gap between men and women narrowed from 7.0 years in 1990 to 5.2 years in 2004. There are however, differences in the life expectancy between Whites and Blacks for both sexes. In 2004, life expectancy at birth for Whites was 5.0 years longer than for Blacks (NCHS, 2007).

Globally, the life expectancy in the United States trails that of more than 20 other countries (Table 23.2). Japan reports the highest life expectancy figures. In all countries, disparities exist between female and male life expectancy, some as much as 13 years. The smallest disparity can be found between women and men living in Canada.

HEALTH DISPARITIES

One of the goals of *Healthy People 2010* is to eliminate **health disparities**. A health disparity is defined as a difference in health status that occurs by gender, race or ethnicity, education or income, disability, geographic location, or sexual orientation (U.S. Department of Health and Human Services [USDHHS], 2000). Disparities in health occur when one segment of the population has a higher incidence of disease or mortality rate than another, or when survival rates are less for one group than another (Institute of Medicine, 2002). Often, persons with the greatest health burden have the least access to information, communication technologies, health care, and supporting social services. Interdisciplinary, collaborative, public, and private approaches, as well as public–private partnerships are needed to develop strategies to address this goal of *Healthy People 2010*.

HEALTH LITERACY

Health literacy is defined as the degree to which individuals have the capacity to obtain, process, and understand basic health information and services needed to make appropriate health decisions. The ability to read and understand health information is key to managing health problems. Low health literacy contributes to health disparities, and it has been documented as an increasing problem among certain racial and ethic groups, non-English speaking populations, and persons over 65 years of age in the United States (Kutner, Greenberg,

TABLE 23.1 Life Expectancy at Birth and 65 Years of Age According to Sex: United States, Selected Years, 1900–2004

Year	At Birth			At 65 Years		
	Both Sexes	Male	Female	Both Sexes	Male	Female
1900	47.3	46.3	48.3	11.9	11.5	12.2
1950	68.2	65.6	71.1	13.9	12.8	15.0
1960	69.7	66.6	73.1	14.3	12.8	15.8
1970	70.8	67.1	74.7	15.2	13.1	17.0
1980	73.7	70.7	77.4	16.4	14.1	18.3
1990	75.4	71.8	78.8	17.2	15.1	18.9
1995	75.8	72.5	78.9	17.4	15.6	18.9
2000	76.9	74.1	79.5	17.5	16.0	19.0
2004	77.8	75.2	80.4	18.7	17.1	20.0

Extracted from National Center for Health Statistics (2007). *Health, United States, 2006 with Chartbook on Trends in the Health of Americans.* (DHHS Pub. No. 1232.) Hyattsville, MD: Public Health Service.

TABLE 23.2 Life Expectancy at Birth for Selected Countries by Sex

	Female	Male	Disparity
Japan	85.2	78.3	6.9
France	83.0	75.8	7.2
Switzerland	83.0	77.8	5.2
Spain	83.5	75.8	7.7
Canada	82.1	77.2	4.9
Australia	82.6	77.4	5.2
Greece	80.7	75.4	5.3
Germany	81.2	75.4	5.8
United States	79.9	74.5	5.4
Russian Federation	72.0	58.9	13.1

Extracted from National Center for Health Statistics (2007). *Health, United States, 2006 with Chartbook on Trends in the Health of Americans.* (DHHS Pub. No. 1232.) Hyattsville, MD: Public Health Service.

Jin, & Paulsen, 2006). See Chapter 11 for additional information on health education.

MAJOR HEALTH PROBLEMS OF ADULTS

Morbidity and mortality among adults varies substantially by age, gender, race, and ethnicity. The six leading causes of death are presented in this section. Diseases of the heart (coronary heart disease) and cerebrovascular diseases (stroke) are the first and third causes of death in adults and are discussed together. Malignant neoplasms (cancer), chronic lower respiratory diseases, unintentional injuries, and diabetes mellitus are discussed separately. Other selected additional major causes of death are covered in detail in other chapters: suicide (Chapter 27), Alzheimer disease (Chapter 24), and homicide (Chapters 17 and 20).

Coronary Heart Disease and Stroke

An estimated one in three adults (79,400,000) have cardiovascular disease (CVD). More than 16% of all deaths among adults aged 25 to 64 years are due to CVD, primarily coronary heart disease (CHD), and stroke. Everyday, nearly 2,400 Americans die of CVD. In 2007, CVD was projected to cost more than $431.8 billion, which includes health services, medications, and lost productivity (Centers for Disease Control [CDC], 2007a; Rosamond et al., 2007) (Fig. 23.1).

Risk factors contributing to CHD can be separated into two categories: personal and hereditary. Personal risk factors include gender, age, race/ethnicity, cholesterol level (specifically the ratio of low-density to high-density lipoproteins), diabetes, obesity, physical inactivity, high blood pressure, and cigarette smoking. The most modifiable of these factors are cholesterol, high blood pressure, cigarette smoking, obesity, and physical inactivity. Heredity obviously cannot be changed. The likelihood of heart disease or stroke multiplies with the increasing number of risk factors present.

Disparities in heart disease have remained consistent. The incidence is higher in men than in women and higher in the Black population than the White. Death rates (per 100,000) in 2004 were 335.7 for White males and 448.9 for Black males. White females had a death rate of 239.3 compared to the rate for Black females, 331.6. Over the last 10 years, death rates from CHD have declined by 25%. The age-adjusted mortality from heart disease declined 16% between 2000 and 2004 (NCHS, 2006; Rosamond et al., 2007) (Table 23.3).

For persons who have a heart attack, disparities also exist in treatment outcomes. When compared to men, women in general have poorer outcomes; 44% of women who have a

TABLE 23.3 Primary Risk Factors for Coronary Heart Disease and Symptoms of Heart Attack in Adults

Risks	Symptoms
• Age	• Pain: Chest, neck, jaw, arm, stomach, or back
• Gender, male	
• Race, African American	• Chest: Pressure, squeezing, or fullness
• Family history	• Shortness of breath
• Sedentary lifestyle	• Cold sweat
• Excess body weight	
• Hypertension	• Nausea
• Diabetes mellitus	• Lightheadedness
• Hyperlipidemia	
• Cigarette smoking	

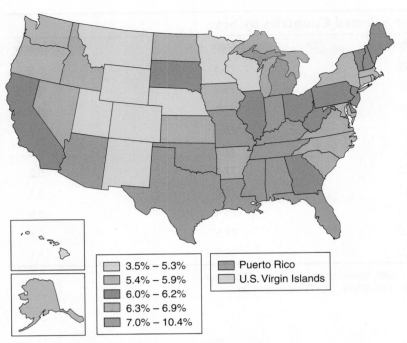

3.5% – 5.3%
5.4% – 5.9%
6.0% – 6.2%
6.3% – 6.9%
7.0% – 10.4%

Puerto Rico
U.S. Virgin Islands

*Age adjusted to the 2000 U.S. standard population of adults.

From Centers for Disease Control and Prevention. (2007). Prevalence of Heart Disease–United States, 2005, *Morbidity and Mortality Weekly Report, 56*(6), 113–118.

FIGURE 23.1 Prevalence of cardiovascular disease. Self-reported prevalence of history of myocardial infarction or angina/coronary heart disease among adults aged 18 years and older.

heart attack die within 1 year, compared with 27% of men. At older ages, women who have heart attacks are twice as likely to die within a few weeks (USDHHS, 2000).

Approximately 700,000 Americans suffer strokes each year, and strokes account for almost one in 16 deaths in the United States (Rosamond et al., 2007). Disparities also exist among people with strokes. In 2004, women accounted for 61% of all U.S. stroke deaths. Each year, approximately 46,000 more women than men have a stroke. Men are at a greater risk of having a stroke at a younger age than women; however this difference dissipates with age. Blacks are twice as likely to have their first stroke earlier than their White counterparts. In the southeastern United States (the "Stroke Belt"), stroke death rates for both Blacks and Whites are higher than in any other part of the country (Gorelick, 2004).

The hallmark Framingham Heart Study identified major risk factors associated with the development of CVD and the effects of related factors such as blood triglycerides, gender, and psychosocial issues. The study began in 1948 under the direction of National Heart Institute, now known as the National Heart, Lung, and Blood Institute (NHLBI). At that time, the death rates from CVD were rising, but little was known about the general causes of heart disease and stroke. The researchers recruited 2,336 men and 2,873 women between the ages of 30 and 62 in an effort to identify common factors or characteristics that contribute to CVD. Every 2 years, these individuals were scheduled for an extensive medical history, physical examination, and laboratory tests. In 1971, the study enrolled 5,124 of the original participants' adult children and their spouses, and currently, a third generation (the children of the Offspring Cohort) is being recruited and examined. Findings from the Framingham Heart Study continue to make important scientific contributions regarding the development

and treatment of CVD and related health issues (NHLBI, 2002).

Cancer

Cancer is a major chronic illness and the second leading cause of death in the United States. Currently the National Cancer Institute (NCI) estimates that 10.5 million Americans are living with cancer. Approximately 70% of all cancers are diagnosed in persons 55 years of age and older and, as individuals age, they are more likely to develop cancer. It is estimated in 2007 that 1,444,920 new cancer cases will be diagnosed. Blacks are more likely to develop and die of cancer. Over their lifetime, men living in the United States are more likely to develop cancer than women. The National Institutes of Health (NIH) 2006 estimates the overall costs for cancer are $206.3 billion (American Cancer Society [ACS], 2007).

Cancer is caused by internal and external factors. External factors include tobacco smoke, chemicals, radiation, and infectious organisms. Internal factors are inherited gene mutations, hormones, immune conditions, and gene mutations that occur from metabolism. These factors can occur in isolation or together to initiate illness. About 30% of all cancer deaths and 87% of lung cancer deaths are attributed to smoking. Smoking-related diseases remain the most preventable cause of death in the United States (ACS, 2007).

Lung and bronchial cancers are the number one cause of cancer deaths among adults. In 2007, it was estimated that 70,880 or 26% of the female cancer deaths and 89,310 or 31% of the male cancer deaths were related to lung and bronchus cancers (ACS, 2007). Cigarette smoking is the predominant risk factor for lung cancer. Quantity of cigarettes smoked and the number of years smoking increase an individual's risk of developing lung cancer. Other risk factors include occupational or environmental exposure to secondhand smoke, radon, asbestos, genetic susceptibility, and a history of tuberculosis. Current efforts to reduce mortality by early detection have been unsuccessful. The National Lung Screening Trial is currently assessing whether screening individuals at high risk with spiral computerized tomography (CT) or standard chest X-ray will reduce cancer deaths. Results are expected in 2010 (ACS, 2007).

Colon and rectal cancers are the third most common cancers in adults. Among adults, an estimated 153,760 cases of colon and rectal cancers are expected to occur in 2007, and 52,180 deaths. The risk of developing colorectal cancer increases with age and 90% of all cases are diagnosed in individuals 50 years of age or older. Other risk factors include certain inherited genetic mutations, personal or family history of polyps or colorectal cancer, and personal history of chronic inflammatory bowel disease. Screening for colon and rectal cancer should begin at age 50 for men and women who are at average risk (ACS, 2007) (see Display 23.2).

Chronic Lower Respiratory Diseases

Chronic Lower Respiratory Disease (CLRD) comprises three major conditions: chronic bronchitis, emphysema, and asthma. The term chronic obstructive pulmonary disease (COPD) includes emphysema and chronic bronchitis. Chronic lower respiratory disease is the fourth leading cause of death in the United States. Every year, approximately $43 billion is spent on direct and indirect health care costs related to chronic lower respiratory diseases (American Lung Association [ALA], 2006a).

Tobacco smoking is the major risk factor for developing COPD, accounting for about 80% of cases. The remaining 20% of COPD cases are attributable to environmental exposures and genetic factors. Over the past several years, the number of women dying of this disease surpassed the number of men. This increase is probably related to the increase in smoking by women, relative to men, since the 1940s. Chronic bronchitis sufferers are more likely to be between 18 and 44 years of age and female, whereas emphysema sufferers are mostly over age 65 and male. Both conditions are more commonly found among Whites than Blacks and among people living in the southern United States (ALA, 2006b, 2006c; NCHS, 2007).

Asthma appears to have a strong genetic basis, with 30% to 50% of all cases due to an inherited predisposition. Women are 6% more likely to be diagnosed with asthma than are men. In 2004, the prevalence of the disease in the Black population was 24% higher than in the White population. Over 4.5 million work days are lost each year due to asthma (ALA, 2006a, 2006b).

Unintentional Injuries

Unintentional injuries refers to any injury that results from unintended exposure to physical agents, including heat, mechanical energy, chemicals, or electricity. The top five causes of unintentional injuries include motor vehicle crashes, fire arms, poisoning, falls, and suffocation. Together, these causes account for approximately 80% of all injury deaths. In 2004, a total of 112,012 Americans died of injuries from a variety of causes. For persons under age 35, unintentional injuries are the leading cause of death. It is estimated that more than 20,000 adults ages 25 to 64 will die in motor vehicle crashes each year. The costs related to these deaths take into account wages and productivity losses, medical expenses, administrative expenses, motor vehicle damage, and employer's uninsured costs. In 2005, the average cost per fatal incident was $1,150,000. The cost of a nonfatal disabling injury was $52,900 in the same year (Finkelstein, Corso, & Miller, 2006; NCHS, 2006; National Center for Injury Prevention and Control [NCIPC], 2005; National Safety Council, 2006). In 2006, unintentional injuries in the United States included:

◆ Motor vehicle crashes: The leading cause of death among persons 25–44 years of age
◆ Suicide and homicide: The second and third leading causes of death for persons 25–34 years of age
◆ Falls: The leading cause of nonfatal injury related to emergency department visits by persons 25–64 years of age.

A disabling injury is one that results in restriction of normal activities of daily living (ADLs) beyond the day on which the injury occurred. Disabling injuries occur disproportionately among the young and the elderly. Seat belts, helmets, smoke detectors, and poison control centers save billions of dollars in direct and indirect medical costs. These primary and secondary prevention strategies save lives and money.

An *unsafe condition* is any environmental factor, either social or physical, that increases the likelihood of an unintentional injury. An icy walkway is an example of an unsafe condition; although it poses a hazard, it does not cause an injury, but only makes it more likely that an injury will occur. *Injury prevention* and *injury control* refer to any effort to prevent injuries or lessen their severity. These efforts often focus on assessment of the environment for unsafe conditions, such as loaded guns in the home or asbestos in school buildings and workplaces.

Diabetes Mellitus

Diabetes mellitus is the sixth leading cause of death in the United States. Current prevalence is based on national estimates for 2005, with 20.8 million people having diabetes (diagnosed 14.6 million, undiagnosed 6.2 million), representing 7% of the population. Of these diabetics, 20.6 million are women and men 20 years of age and older (50% are under the age of 60). Men are affected more than are women, with a prevalence of 10.9 for men and 9.7 for women. Differences also exist related to race and ethnicity, as American Indians and Alaska Natives are 2.2 times more likely and non-Hispanic Blacks are 1.8 times more likely to have diabetes than Whites. Overall, recent incidence was 1.5 million new cases in 2005 (American Diabetes Association [ADA], n.d.b; CDC, 2005b) (see Fig. 23.2).

Diabetes is a major chronic health condition that puts individuals at risk for other serious health conditions including heart disease and stroke, hypertension, blindness, kidney disease, and nervous system disease (i.e., neuropathy, which is a loss of sensation or pain in the feet or hands). Because diabetes can affect any part of the body, damage to other body systems can be minimized by good blood glucose control (assessed by hemoglobin A1C) (ADA, n.d.a; CDC, 2005b).

DISPLAY 23.2	SCREENINGS AND CHECK-UP SCHEDULE FOR ADULTS

	How Often	Ages 20–39	Ages 40–49	Age 50+
Physical Exam: Performed to review overall health status. Have a thorough physical examination and discuss health-related concerns and topics.	Every 3 years Every 2 years Every year	X	X	X
Blood Pressure: High blood pressure can have no symptoms, but can cause permanent damage to body organs and systems.	Every year	X	X	X
Blood Tests and Urinalysis: Screens for various illnesses and diseases, such as high cholesterol, kidney, or thyroid disorders, before problems or symptoms occur. Can be done at time of physical exam.	Every 3 years Every 2 years Every year	X	X	X
EKG: Electrocardiogram screens for heart abnormalities or problems.	Baseline–age 30 Every 4 years Every 3 years	X	X	X
Tetanus Booster	Every 10 years	X	X	X
Flu Vaccine	Every year	X	X	X
Rectal Exam: Screens for hemorrhoids, lower rectal problems, colon, and prostate cancer	Every year	X	X	X
PSA Blood Test (Men): Prostate specific antigen (PSA) is produced by the prostate. Levels increase when there is an infection, enlargement, or cancer. Screening for Black men and men with a family history should start at age 45.*	Every year		*	X
Clinical Breast Exam (Women): Breast exam by health care provider	Every year	X	X	X
Mammography (Women): Screening should begin at age 40 unless high-risk*	Every year		*	X
Pelvic Exam and Pap Smear (Women): A pelvic exam is performed to evaluate the size and position of the vagina, cervix, uterus, fallopian tubes, and ovaries. A Pap test is performed to look for changes in the cells of the cervix, such as dysplasia or cancer.	Every year Every 3 years after 3 consecutive negative pap smears	X	X	X
Self Exams: *Testicles* are examined to find lumps. *Skin* is checked to look for signs of changing moles, freckles, or early skin cancer. *Breasts* are examined to find abnormal lumps in their early stages.	Monthly	X	X	X
Hemoccult: Screens the stool for microscopic amounts of blood that can be the first indication of polyps or colon cancer	Every year		X	X
Colon–Rectal Health: A flexible endoscope is used to examine the rectum, sigmoid, and descending colon for cancer at its earliest stages. The exam also detects polyps that can progress to cancer if not found early.	Every 3–4 years			X
Chest X-ray: Should be considered in smokers over the age of 45.	Discuss with physician		X	X
Bone Health: Bone mineral density is measured.	Baseline As needed		X	X

Adapted from Brott, A., & The Blueprint for Men's Health Advisory Board. (2006). Blueprint for Men's Health: A Guide to Healthy Lifestyle, p. 64. Online: Men's Health Network.

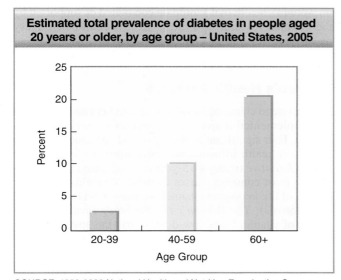

Estimated total prevalence of diabetes in people aged 20 years or older, by age group – United States, 2005

SOURCE: 1999-2002 National Health and Nutrition Examination Survey estimates of total prevalence (both diagnosed and undiagnosed) were projected to year 2005.

FIGURE **23.2** General diabetes chart.

Substance Use

According to the Centers for Disease Control and Prevention (CDC), **substance use** refers to the selected use of potentially dangerous substances including alcohol, tobacco products, drugs, inhalants, and other substances that can be consumed, inhaled, injected, or otherwise absorbed into the body with possible damaging effects. It is a serious and continuing problem among adult women and men living in the United States. In 2005, an estimated 22.2 million persons were classified with substance dependency or abuse in the past 12 months (Substance Abuse and Mental Health Services Administration [SAMHSA], 2006).

In the United States, approximately 75,000 deaths are attributed to alcohol use each year. In 2004, 48% of adults 18 years of age and older reported being a current regular drinker (at least 12 drinks in the past year). Among males, 57% reported being a current regular drinker as compared to females at 38%. Whites are also more likely to be current drinkers than other ethnic groups. Excessive alcohol use is the third leading lifestyle-related cause of death for people living in the United States. More than 39% of automobile fatalities were alcohol related in 2004. The social and economic cost of alcohol abuse exceeds $184 billion annually in the United States (Mokdad, Marks, Stroup, & Gerberding, 2004; Stahre, et. al, 2004; World Health Organization, 2004).

Smoking is associated with a significant increase in CVD and cancer. In 2005, approximately 21% of U.S. adults were current cigarette smokers, 2.2% cigar smokers, and 2.3% used smokeless tobacco. Among cigarette smokers, more men smoke (23.9%) than women (18.1%). American Indians and Alaska Natives (32%) smoke more cigarettes than Blacks (21.5%) and Whites (21.9%). Four of the *Healthy People 2010* objectives are related to tobacco use,

and there was no change between 2004 and 2005, which indicates a lack of progress in decreasing tobacco use. Smoking across the United States costs $97.2 billion yearly in health care costs and lost productivity, and smoking-related diseases claim an estimated 430,700 lives annually. At least 8.6 million people in the United States have at least one serious illness caused by smoking (ALA, 2006a; CDC, 2005a, 2006d).

Illicit drug use refers to use and misuse of illegal and controlled drugs. The primary illicit drugs used in the United States are cocaine, ecstasy, heroin, marijuana, and methamphetamine. Rates of illicit drug use are associated with age. In 2005, the highest rate was among persons between ages 18 and 20 (22.3%). The rate was 18.7% among those between ages 21 and 25, and drug use continued to decline with age (SAMHSA, 2006).

Abuse of prescription drugs is the misuse of prescription drugs for nonmedical reasons. The illegal use of prescription drugs is one of the fastest-growing forms of drug abuse and is becoming a major public health concern. In 2004, about 48 million persons aged 12 or older (20%) had misused prescription drugs in their lifetime. Young adults aged 18 to 25 had a higher prevalence of dependence or abuse for pain relievers, tranquilizers, and stimulants compared to persons in other age groups. Men generally had higher rates than women for misuse of pain relievers, stimulants, and methamphetamine (SAMHSA, 2006). This issue is covered in greater detail in Chapter 27.

Obesity

Obesity is defined as having a body mass index (BMI) of 30 or greater, and is becoming the nation's number one health problem. *Morbid obesity* is having a BMI of 40 or greater. One of the *Healthy People 2010* objectives is to reduce to 15% the prevalence of obesity among adults in the United States. In 2005, it was estimated that 23.9% of the U.S. population was obese and 3% morbidly obese. In the same year, obesity prevalence was 24.2% among men and 23.5% among women. Obesity was greatest among Blacks (33.9%). Between 1995 and 2005, a significant increase in obesity occurred, 15.3% to 23.9%, among adults 18 years of age or older. This continued increase underscores the need for additional measures to educate persons regarding healthier lifestyle choices, increasing physical activity, and decreasing caloric intake. The number of gastric bypass surgeries and other bariatric procedures performed on obese adults 18 to 44 years of age more than tripled between 1999 and 2004. These procedures were more common among women than men. Obesity-related medical expenses are estimated to range from $87 million in Wyoming to $7.7 billion in California (CDC, 2006c; NCHS, 2007)

WOMEN'S HEALTH

Women have not been the focus of medical attention throughout the centuries. Health benefits achieved by women were incidental compared to men. Advances in women's health are very recent and primarily an advantage for women living in Western countries, where the women's or feminist movement has made major inroads.

Overview of Factors Influencing Women's Health

Women's rights in the United States started in the second half of the 19th century and over time addressed issues directly or indirectly impacting the health of women: voting rights, labor laws, reproductive rights and violence against women (Imbornoni, 2006). This section of the chapter looks at women's health concerns over the adult lifespan and the major causes of acute and chronic illness and death; and the issues, trends, and policies that have affected women.

Women's health is still overlooked in much of the world. Only in the past few decades has the health of women been a formidable issue in the United States, coming not so coincidently with the modern women's feminist movement that began in the 1960s. The landmark publication *The Feminine Mystic* (Friedan, 1997) helped launch the modern women's movement by critically examining the role of women in American society (Fox, 2006). The Boston Women's Health Book Collective publication (2005), *Our Bodies, Ourselves*, represented the first book to explore women's health issues, exclusively written by and for women (Norsigian et al., 1999).

Feminists paved the way for women to have their voices heard on many health, social, and political issues. Women sought out higher education opportunities in greater numbers and entered workplaces once solely occupied by men, especially during and after World War II. These positive changes escalated women toward greater equality and, with equality, came the freedom—and pressure—for women to compete with men in their social and work settings. Issues in women's health were discovered as a result of research that now more regularly includes women. The importance of women's research was reaffirmed in the NIH Revitalization Act of 1993, Subtitle B—Clinical Research Equity Regarding Women and Minorities to "identify projects for research on women's health that should be conducted or supported by the national research institutes; identify multidisciplinary research relating to research on women that should be so conducted or supported . . . " (NIH, 1993, Sec. 486).

Women's Health Research

In response to changing priorities, researchers have designed and implemented major studies that focus exclusively on women. Four significant studies have and continue to provide important health information about women. *The Women's Health Initiative* (a major 15-year research program addressing the most common causes of death, disability, and poor quality of life in postmenopausal women—CVD, cancer, and osteoporosis); *The Women's Health Study* (evaluating the effects of vitamin E and low-dose aspirin therapy in primary prevention of CVD and cancer in apparently healthy women); *The Nurses' Health Study I* (investigating the potential long-term consequences of the use of oral contraceptives); and *The Nurses' Health Study II* (studying oral contraceptives, diet, and lifestyle risk factors in a population younger than the original Nurses' Health Study cohort).

The *Women's Health Initiative* (WHI) addressed CVD, cancer, and osteoporosis and was one of the largest U.S. prevention studies of its kind, spanning 15 years, starting in 1991. The three major components of the WHI were a randomized controlled clinical trial of promising but unproven approaches to prevention; an observational study to identify predictors of disease; and a study of community approaches to developing healthful behaviors. This study was sponsored by the NIH and the NHLBI, involving 161,808 women ages 50 to 79, and was considered to be one of the most far-reaching clinical trials for women's health ever undertaken. These studies have ended; however, the women are now participating in a follow-up phase, which will last until 2010.

The *Women's Health Study* is a randomized, double-blind, placebo-controlled clinical trial sponsored by both NHBLI and the NCI. It is the first large clinical trial to study the use of low-dose aspirin to prevent heart attack and stroke in women 45 years of age and older. This study began in 1991 and will continue through March 2009 for additional observation and follow-up of the original 28,345 participants. Current findings indicate that low-dose aspirin does not prevent first heart attacks or death from cardiovascular causes in women; however, stroke was found to be 17% lower in the aspirin group (Cook et al., 2005).

The *Nurses Health Study I*, a prospective study that began in 1976, enrolled 122,000 registered nurses ages 30 to 55 from 11 states, who responded to 170,000 mailed questionnaires. Every 2 years, participants received a follow-up questionnaire with questions about diseases and health-related topics including smoking, hormone use, and menopausal status. Later in the study, questions regarding diet and nutrition and quality of life were added. The study is still ongoing. Some findings to date indicate night-shift work can influence melatonin levels, which may increase risk for certain cancers (Schernhammer et al., 2004) and smoking can influence endometrial cancer at an early age (Viswanathan et al., 2005).

The *Nurses Health Study II* represented women who started using oral contraceptives in adolescence, hence a population with long-term exposure during early reproductive years. Participants were between 25 and 42 years of age, and

---

What Do You Think?

A woman's dressing style that included a tightly laced corset was popular from the late 1700s throughout the late 1800s in Germany, England, and the United States. It was brought into question by an anatomist, S. T. von Sommerring, in 1793. He identified compression of rib cages and internal organs as contributing to digestive problems, fainting, and shortness of breath. For the next century, dress reformers advocated looser lacing and clothes that allowed for a more natural movement. However, these reformers belonged to the "radical fringe" of the feminist movement and the tiniest waists, regardless of their impact on health, continued to be in vogue as the "hourglass" figure was sought by middle class and upper class women. More recently, hiatal hernias caused by overly tight girdles and corsets have been termed "Sommerring's syndrome" in tribute to the first physician to warn of the dangers, more than 200 years ago.

Adapted from Fee, E., Brown, T. M., Lazarus, J., & Theerman, P. (2002). The effects of the corset. *American Journal of Public Health*, 92, 1085.

116,686 women were enrolled and followed forward in time. Every 2 years, participants received a follow-up questionnaire and were surveyed about diseases and health-related topics including smoking, hormone use, pregnancy history, and menopausal status. These women also received nutrition assessment and quality-of-life assessment later in the study.

Women's Health Promotion Across the Lifespan

What health care needs do women have that are different from those of men? Is there a need to look at health promotion throughout the life cycle of adult women? How is the health of an 18-year-old different from that of a 50-year-old woman? Most of us would have no trouble agreeing that women have different health care needs that must be considered, and that these needs vary with age. Knowing what the needs are is essential to knowing how to help women promote their health.

Healthy People 2010 *Goals for Women*

As a nation, we have been focusing on improving the health of all citizens through the Healthy People initiatives. *Healthy People 2000* set a standard for change and improvement in objectives that were met or exceeded in some areas and were far from being reached in others. In that initiative, the objectives in 14 areas focused specifically on women's health issues. In *Healthy People 2010,* the focus is still on improving the nation's health, but the objectives have been reevaluated. Objectives have been eliminated, broadened, expanded, or tailored to meet the changing needs of society. However, many still focus on the health of women (Display 23.3). As the community health nurse works with women at various stages in the life cycle, the objectives in *Healthy People 2010* can give structure to program planning and services offered to women in the community at the primary, secondary, and tertiary levels of prevention.

Young Adult Women (18 to 35 Years)

Women in the earlier years of adulthood have different tasks to accomplish and issues to address than do women in later adulthood, and the transition from adolescence to adulthood can be stressful. According to Erickson (Stevens, 1983), the major developmental tasks that young women need to accomplish are forming an identity and the development of intimacy. Behaviors associated with young adulthood include attracting and choosing a significant other for the long-term and establishing a home. This task is phrased as such to include lesbian women—women who have sexual intercourse with other women. However, not all such women in this age group have "come out" or revealed to others that they are lesbian or **bisexual**—having sexual intercourse with people of both sexes. Young women during this stage also prepare and choose a life's work that is personally satisfying, plan for children by using a variety of parenting models (childbirth, adoption, foster parenting), and develop a personal philosophy that encompasses meaningful and comforting spiritual beliefs that are consistent with day-to-day living.

Women in this age group tend to be healthy. Unfortunately, during this period many women engage in health-risk behaviors such as physical inactivity, eating poorly, partici-

pating in unprotected sexual intercourse, and smoking. Some, if not all, of these behaviors may have been established in adolescence and represent modifiable behaviors. If not addressed, these behaviors can contribute significantly to the leading causes of morbidity and mortality: diseases of the heart and vascular systems, cancers, chronic respiratory diseases, and diabetes (McCracken, Jiles, & Blanck, 2007). The majority of health concerns for many of these women are related to eating disorders, reproductive health and sexually transmitted infections (STIs), physical activity, mental health and mood disorders, and substance use.

Eating Disorders

Eating disorders are complex, chronic illnesses primarily affecting young women. The cause of these disorders is not clear, however, the incidence is on the rise in the United States and other parts of the world. The three most common are anorexia nervosa, bulimia nervosa, and binge eating. **Anorexia nervosa** is an eating disorder that is marked by weight loss, emaciation, a disturbance in body image, and a fear of weight gain. Persons affected lose weight either by excessive dieting or by purging themselves of ingested calories. This illness is typically found in industrialized nations and usually begins in the teen years. Young women are 10 to 20 times more likely than young men to suffer from the disorder. The young woman claims to feel fat even when she is emaciated, and refusal to maintain body weight can be life-threatening due to electrolyte disturbances, anemia, and secondary cardiac arrhythmias. If anorexia nervosa is suspected, the client must be referred to a health care provider for follow-up as soon as possible (Office on Women's Health [OWH], 2000, 2006a).

A related disorder, **bulimia nervosa**, is marked by recurrent episodes of binge eating, self-induced vomiting and diarrhea, excessive exercise, strict dieting or fasting, and an exaggerated concern about body shape and weight. In many ways, the two disorders are similar, except that women with anorexia nervosa rarely binge eat. The community health nurse should refer a woman suspected of practicing bulimic behaviors to an appropriate health care provider (OWH, 2000, 2007). Females in careers in which low weight is required (e.g., modeling, entertainment), individuals who have been sexually abused or who come from families with a history of eating disorders, and individuals with low self-esteem and a history of not being "in control" or with communication and emotional difficulties are at greater risk for either disorder.

Binge eating is an eating disorder characterized by repeated episodes of uncontrolled eating. It is the newest clinically recognized disorder. The onset of this disorder is usually in late adolescence and the early 20s, and starts following significant weight loss from dieting. Typically, individuals with this disorder eat quickly, eat until they are uncomfortably full, eat when they are not hungry, eat large amounts of food alone, have difficulty expressing their feelings, have difficulty controlling impulses and stress, and feel depressed about overeating. Of note, many persons who binge are obese. Therefore, these individuals are at risk for type 2 diabetes, high cholesterol, gallbladder disease, depression, heart disease, and some cancers (OWH, 2000, 2005).

Overall, eating disorders are not gender specific, as some men are affected—one male to every 10 females. Currently,

---

DISPLAY 23.3 | *HEALTHY PEOPLE 2010* OBJECTIVES FOR WOMEN (INCLUDING EIGHT DEVELOPMENTAL OBJECTIVES)

1. Reduce the breast cancer death rate, from 27.9 deaths per 100,000 women to 22.3 deaths per 100,000.
2. Reduce the death rate from cancer of the uterine cervix, from 3.0 deaths per 100,000 to 2.0 deaths per 100,000 women.
3. Increase the proportion of women who receive a Pap test; from 92% to 97% for women older than 18 years of age who have ever received a Pap test, and from 79% to 90% for women who have received a Pap test within the preceding 3 years.
4. Increase the proportion of women aged 40 years and older who have received a mammogram within the preceding 2 years, from 67% to 70%.
5. (Developmental) Decrease the proportion of pregnant women with gestational diabetes.
6. Increase the proportion of pregnancies that are intended, from 51% to 70%.
7. Reduce the proportion of births occurring within 24 months after a previous birth, from 11% to 6%.
8. Increase the proportion of women at risk for unintended pregnancy (and their partners) who use contraception, from 93% to 100%.
9. Reduce the proportion of women experiencing pregnancy despite use of a reversible contraceptive method, from 13% to 7%.
10. Reduce pregnancies among female adolescents, from 68 pregnancies per 1000 girls aged 15-17 years to 43 pregnancies per 1000.
11. Reduce maternal deaths, from 7.1 maternal deaths per 100,000 live births in 1998 to 3.3 per 100,000 in 2010.
12. Reduce maternal illness and complications due to pregnancy, from 32.2 maternal complications per 100 deliveries during labor and delivery in 1998 to 20.0 in 2010.
13. (Developmental) Reduce ectopic pregnancies and postpartum complications, including postpartum depression.
14. Increase the proportion of pregnant women who receive early and adequate prenatal care, from 83% beginning in the first trimester of pregnancy to 90%, and increase early and adequate prenatal care, from 74% in 1997 to 90% in 2010.

15. (Developmental) Increase the proportion or pregnant women who attend a series of prepared childbirth classes.
16. Reduce cesarean deliveries among low-risk women (full-term, singleton, vertex presentation), from 18% to 15% among women with no prior cesarean delivery, and from 72% to 63% among women with prior cesarean delivery.
17. (Developmental) Increase the proportion of mothers who achieve a recommended weight gain during their pregnancies.
18. Increase abstinence from alcohol, cigarettes, and illicit drugs among pregnant women: alcohol, from 86% to 94%; binge drinking, from 99% to 100%; cigarette smoking, from 87% to 99%; and illicit drug use, from 98% to 100%.
19. Increase the proportion of mothers who breast feed their babies in the early postpartum period, from 64% to 75%; at 6 months, from 29% to 50%; at 1 year, from 16% to 25%.
20. Reduce anemia among low-income pregnant women in their third trimester, from 29% to 20%.
21. (Developmental) Reduce iron deficiency among pregnant females.
22. (Developmental) Reduce human immunodeficiency virus (HIV) infections associated with heterosexual contact in adolescent and young adult women aged 13 to 24 years.
23. (Developmental) Increase the proportion of sexually active women aged 25 years and younger who are screened annually for genital chlamydia infections.
24. (Developmental) Increase the proportion of pregnant women screened for STDs (including HIV infection and bacterial vaginosis) during prenatal health care visits, according to recognized standards.
25. Increase smoking cessation during pregnancy, from 14% smoking cessation during the first trimester of pregnancy to 30%.

Adapted from U.S. Department of Health and Human Services. (2000). *Healthy people 2010: Understanding and improving health* (2nd ed.). Washington, DC: U.S. Government Printing Office.

---

the perception is that White females are affected more than other ethnic groups; however, trends indicate that individuals from other ethnic groups also may suffer from eating disorders. The community health nurse can play a vital role in identifying persons affected and referring them to appropriate health care providers or self-help groups. A screening tool that may be helpful in this effort is the Malnutrition Universal Screening Tool (Duffin, 2006; Malnutrition Advisory Group, 2003; Murphy, 2007; OWH, 2000).

Reproductive Health

By age 25, at least 50% of childbearing women have given birth, at least once. Women need to be as healthy as possible

to have positive pregnancy outcomes. Based on published research and the input of experts, the CDC has put forth recommendations for preconception care. The main goal of preconception care is to "provide health promotion, screening, and interventions for women of reproductive age to reduce risk factors that might affect future pregnancies" (Johnson et al., 2006, p. 3). Recommendations for preconception care address consumer awareness, individual responsibility, minimizing health problems, access to care, disparities, and research. Although *Healthy People 2010* does not specifically address preconception care, at least 18 of the objectives for women are directly related (see Display 23.3). Community health nurses have been at the forefront of maternal and child heath for decades, and they must

DISPLAY 23.4	NURSING CARE PLAN MATRIX FOR HEALTH PROMOTION, YOUNG ADULTS—18 TO 35

Community health nurses can use this matrix to individualize teaching, services, and/or care to young adult clients. Use the questions to stimulate the development of an individualized approach that is client-focused and -driven with the community health nurse acting as the catalyst. In any or all of these areas, the community health nurse may (1) discuss issues and commend the client for positive attitudes and behaviors (example: when the client is making healthful decisions, such as condom use for his/her health and the health of significant others), (2) discuss the issues and guide the client to resources that will enhance more positive behaviors and decisions (example: flu shot clinic or healthy lifestyle program for adults), or (3) discuss the issues and inform the client that immediate changes must be made to protect the health of self or others and inform/utilize the appropriate resources as soon as possible (example: follow-up for symptoms related to suspected STI).

1. *Life partner*. Ascertain whether the client is looking for a life partner or is choosing to live a single life. Discuss how the single life is satisfying for the client and ways to make it richer.

   Discuss settings in which client can meet others (male or female, based on sexual preference) with similar interests, philosophy, and outlook, such as work settings, school settings, faith communities, recreational communities, and the like.

   Discuss what the client is looking for in a potential life partner; expectations for the relationship; what the client contributes; how the client compromises and resolves conflict, and other issues. If in a relationship, what is good; what needs improving; how to initiate change.

2. *Life's work*. How is the client preparing for his/her life's work (education, formal training, on the job training)? Will the life's work provide resources for client's life plans? Will the work choice provide long-term satisfaction? Is the work choice a "stepping stone" to another work role? How will/does he handle work and rearing children? What

needs changing or can be improved in the work/children arrangement?

3. *Planning for children*. What knowledge does he/she have about family planning? What methods fit best with his/her philosophy, religious beliefs, lifestyle? What are the long-term effects of the choices? How many children is the client planning to rear? Has he/she thought through the ramifications of this number? If choosing not to have (or unable to have) children how will he/she deal with this? Does he/she want alternative suggestions for raising a child (adoption, foster parenting) or information about interacting with children (volunteering)?

4. *Maintaining physical and mental health*. In this area, the community health nurse needs to explore all areas of health promotion and protection. This will include discussions regarding primary and secondary prevention. Primary prevention discussions could include:
   - Diet and nutrition
   - Physical and leisure activities
   - Safe sex practices
   - Periodic health examinations
   - Personal safety—seat belts, protective helmets, dating violence, etc.
   - Immunizations
   - Regular use of sun screen
   - Stress reduction activities
   Secondary prevention discussions could include:
   - Breast self-examination
   - Testicular self-examination
   - Smoking cessation
   - Pelvic exams and pap smears
   - Counseling and support at times of stress

5. *Developing a life's philosophy*. Discuss client's personal life satisfaction, which may include religiosity and spirituality, living in congruence with cultural/ethnic/family beliefs and expectations, and coming to a comfortable level of satisfaction with life choices, having few regrets.

---

continue to strive to incorporate components of preconception care into their practices. Nurses must advocate for their clients to influence public policy, which has the potential to improve access to care for many women and improve pregnancy outcomes (Johnson et al., 2006).

Sexual health and STIs are important health concerns for young women. Sexual activity typically commences in adolescence and continues throughout the lifespan. Sexually transmitted infections are epidemic in the United States, especially among young adults (see Chapter 8). Many of the common infections are asymptomatic, but not always. The two most common STIs affecting women are *Chlamydia* and gonorrhea. It is estimated that approximately 2.8 million cases of *Chlamydia* occur in the United States each year, and females 20 to 24 years of age have the second highest rate, preceded

by 15- to 19-year-old adolescents. Gonorrhea rates have reached a plateau in recent years, but the prevalence is still 115.6 per 100,000 persons. Both *Chlamydia* and gonorrhea are underdiagnosed, which can have deleterious consequences for women. If treatment is delayed, women can develop pelvic inflammatory disease, chronic pelvic pain, ectopic pregnancy, and infertility (CDC, 2006e).

Community health nurses working with females need to provide factual information to increase women's knowledge of STI risk. This information should be a part of frank discussions regarding condom use, sexual partners (male and female), type of sexual activity (oral, anal, vaginal), the life-threatening consequences of an undiagnosed STI, and undesirable pregnancy outcomes. Outside of abstinence, condom use is the first line of prevention against STIs.

EVIDENCE-BASED PRACTICE

Bridging Financial Gaps

A two-group pretest/posttest experiment was designed and implemented to examine the effect of an education program on knowledge and perceived risk of sexually transmitted infections (STIs). The Sexually Transmitted Infection Knowledge Survey and the Perceived Risk of Sexually Transmitted Infection Survey were used to measure knowledge and perceived risk among 104 women of childbearing age at two universities. The education program included a presentation on condoms, dental dams, and instructions on proper use. In addition, an informational brochure was provided. No education intervention or brochure was provided for the comparison group. Outcomes indicated that participants in the intervention group improved their STI knowledge and perceived risk from participating in a 30-minute educational intervention ($p = 0.0001$).

Sexually transmitted infections are a major burden on the already overtaxed public health system. More than 12 million new cases are diagnosed annually, and more than $8 billion is spent to diagnose and treat STIs and their complications in the United States. When interacting with clients who are sexually active, nurses need to consider incorporating brief educational interventions about STIs into client care; nurses cannot assume that persons are knowledgeable. The more informed individuals are about STI transmission and prevention, the more likely they are to protect themselves.

Reference:

Johnson-Mallard, V., Lengacher, C.A., Kromrey, J.D., Campbell, D.W., Jevitt, C.M., Daley, E., *et al.* (2007). Increasing knowledge of sexually transmitted infection risk. *The Nurse Practitioner*, *32*(2), 26–32.

Adult Women (35 to 65 Years)

Women in the adult age group of 35 to 65 years have established themselves into patterns of living that have served them well or ill. During this period, the results of years of choices may present themselves in the form of chronic illnesses. Nevertheless, many women in this age group have time to change their health habits to possibly reverse encroaching chronic illnesses. For other women, lifestyle choices and undetected diseases have shortened their lifespans, and large numbers of women in this age group are dying prematurely.

Menopause and Hormone Replacement Therapy

Women in this age group experience **menopause**, a time that marks the permanent cessation of menstrual activity, usually occurring between the ages of 45 and 55 years. However, it can occur as early as age 30. Natural menopause is defined as cessation of menstrual periods for 12 consecutive months, with no other apparent cause. Surgical removal of the ovaries produces menopause, and 600,000 total hysterectomies are performed each year in the United States. At least one in three women has had a hysterectomy by the age of 60. Symptoms of menopause vary among women and last from months to years. They range from hardly noticeable in some women to very severe in others. Symptoms include nervousness, hot flashes (flushes), chills, excitability, fatigue, mood disorders (apathy, mental depression, crying episodes), insomnia, palpitations, vertigo, headache, numbness, tingling, myalgia, urinary disturbances, and vaginal dryness (OWH, 2006b).

In 2002, researchers found an increased rate of breast cancer, ovarian cancer, heart disease, and stroke among healthy women in the Women's Health Initiative study who were taking combined estrogen and progestin hormone replacement therapy (HRT). The initial reaction to this information was a dramatic decline in prescribing by physicians, which included both combined HRT and estrogen alone. The debate over the risk versus benefit of long-term HRT is ongoing.

One benefit of HRT use is to support bone health. A long-term effect of low estrogen levels is osteoporosis. After menopause, lower estrogen levels affect the balance between bone removal and bone replacement. Overtime, the bone loses density, becomes fragile, and factures easily. Bone density is, however, influenced by other factors such as heredity, race, physical activity, and nutrition. Among healthy postmenopausal women, calcium with vitamin D supplementation resulted in a small improvement in hip bone density, but did not significantly reduce hip fracture. Medications such as biphosphates (Fosamax, Boniva, and Actonel) can improve bone density (OWH, 2006b).

Heart Disease

Diseases of the heart are the number one killer of women. In 2004, a total of 330,513 women in the United States died of heart disease. A racial disparity exists, with death rates related to CVD for Black women at 331.6 compared to 239.3 for White women in the same year. The most common heart problem, coronary heart disease, is underdiagnosed, undertreated, and under-researched in women. In addition, women have higher mortality after heart attack and poorer outcomes than do men, which may be related to delayed diagnosis and treatment. Risk factors for heart disease in women are age, family history, race and ethnicity (higher prevalence among Black women), physical inactivity, obesity, diabetes mellitus, high blood pressure, high cholesterol, and cigarette smoking (American Heart Association [AHA], n.d; NCHS, 2007).

Family history and advancing age cannot be changed, but women can make lifestyle changes to alter other risk factors. The remaining risk factors are issues that the community health nurse can discuss with female clients in this age group. Community health nurses can help raise awareness regarding heart disease when working with women at the individual, family, or aggregate levels. Some important facts that can be shared are that only 13% of women view heart disease as a health threat, even though it is number-one killer of women; 64% of women who die suddenly of coronary heart disease had no previous symptoms; one in 2.6 female deaths are from CVD, compared with one in 30 from breast cancer; women have atypical heart symptoms or less acute chest pain, which may delay them from seeking care; women are less likely to complete secondary prevention programs; and hormone therapy does not reduce coronary events. An excellent lay resource is "*Go Red for Women*" a public awareness program of the American Heart Association (AHA) to help improve knowledge (AHA, 2007; NCHS, 2007; Rosenfeld, 2006).

Cancer

Cancer is the second leading cause of death for women, killing 267,058 women in the United States in 2004. Genetic abnormality plays a role in cancer (possibly linked to environmental exposures), but only 5% of cancers are hereditary. Thus, the vast majority of cancers are random, and the majority occur in middle age. The lifetime risk of a woman getting cancer is one in three. Overall, Blacks are more likely to develop cancer and die. To help address this disparity, community health nurses can provide more opportunities for education and screening for this population (ACS, 2007; NCHS, 2007).

Breast cancer is the most common cancer among women; however, more women die of lung cancer. In 2007, it is estimated that 40,460 breast cancer–related deaths will occur. Overall, the death rates from breast cancer have declined since 1990, and the biggest decline was for women under 50 years of age. This can be attributed to early detection and improvements in treatment. The sooner breast cancer is discovered, the more successfully it is treated. By engaging in routine breast self-examinations (BSE), having regular mammograms, eating a diet low in fat and high in fruits and vegetables, breast-feeding (if possible), and avoiding prolonged use of estrogen replacement therapy, a woman is doing what she can to promote breast health. The community health nurse has many resources available to provide information and to teach BSE individually to women in their homes, small groups in clinics, or in various other community settings (see Chapter 12) (ACS, 2007). See Table 23.4.

Women should begin BSE at age 20 and continue monthly for the remainder of their lives. Clinical breast examination, conducted by a health care provider, should be done as a part of routine gynecologic or health examinations every 3 years for women 20 to 40 years of age and then annually. Mammography is not usually recommended for women younger than 40 years of age, but is recommended annually thereafter. Women who have a first-degree relative with breast cancer (mother, sister), a breast cancer gene (BRCA 1 or BACA 2), or have had previous breast cancer are at a higher risk for developing the disease than other women in the general population. Therefore, these individuals need to consult their physicians regarding timelines for screenings (ACS, 2007).

Papanicolaou (Pap) smears have improved early detection and prevention of cervical cancer dramatically. Both the incidence and the death rates for cervical cancer have declined dramatically in recent decades due to treatment of preinvasive cervical lesions. The major risk factors for this disease are infection with certain types of the human papillomavirus (HPV), unprotected intercourse at an early age, and multiple sex partners. In 2007, it was estimated that 11,150 new cases of cervical cancer would be diagnosed in the United States, contributing to 3,670 deaths among women from this disease. The 5-year survival rate for this cancer if prompt treatment is initiated is 92%, making it one of the most successfully treated cancers. Community health nurses can continue to improve screening and early diagnosis through education and advocating for low-cost screening, which will allow many at-risk elderly, low-income, and rural women access to regular Pap screenings. In addition, making women aware of the HPV vaccine Gardasil, approved by the U.S. Food and Drug Administration in 2006 for use in girls between the ages of 9 and 26, may reduce the incidence of cervical cancer in upcoming decades (ACS, 2007).

Ovarian cancer is the second most frequently diagnosed gynecologic cancer and contributes to more deaths than any other cancer of the reproductive system. In the past two decades, ovarian cancer has declined less than 1%, mostly because of a lack of ovarian cancer screening and early detection. For this reason, it is imperative that women have annual pelvic exams, especially those who are at risk (women have had breast cancer or a family history, BRCA 1 or BRCA 2 gene, previous ovarian cancer). The 5-year survival rate is 44% compared to cervical (77%) and breast (88.5%). Therefore, community health nurses need to continue to stress the importance of early detection for a disease that, in 2007, killed more than 15,000 women (ACS, 2007).

Chronic Fatigue and Immune Dysfunction Syndrome

Chronic fatigue and immune dysfunction syndrome (CFIDS) is characterized by persistent and debilitating fatigue and additional nonspecific symptoms such as sore throat, headache, painful muscles, joint pain, difficulty thinking, and loss of short-term memory. CFIDS affects as many as 500,000 persons in the United States, and 80% of those diagnosed with the syndrome are women between 25 and 45 years old. Rest does not relieve the fatigue. Symptoms may wax and wane, and are difficult to validate objectively, but they are subjectively debilitating. Symptoms can last for months or years. Because the cause is unknown, there is no specific treatment and no prevention suggestions. Treatment is focused on supportive care for the associated pain, depression, and insomnia. The community health

TABLE 23.4 Breast Cancer Death Rates Among All Women—2006	
(Age-Adjusted Rates per 100,000)	
Women	**Rate**
All Women	24.4
White	23.9
Black	32.2
Hispanic	15.6
American Indian/Alaska Native	14.8
Asian/Pacific Islander	12.7

Extracted from National Center for Health Statistics (2007). *Health, United States, 2006 with Chartbook on Trends in the Health of Americans*. (DHHS Pub. No. 1232.) Hyattsville, MD: Public Health Service.

nurse can assess activity level and degree of fatigue, emotional response to the illness, and coping ability. Emotionally supportive family members and health care providers are helpful. Referring women to mental health career counseling, or a local support group is helpful for many women and within the role of the community health nurse (CDC, 2006a; Edwards, Thompson, & Blair, 2007)

MEN'S HEALTH

Gender is among the numerous factors that influence health. More male neonates die at birth, and men are more likely to die earlier from a chronic illness than women. This is evidenced by the difference in life expectancy between men and women: in the United States, women survive an average of 6 years longer than men (Plumb & Brawer, 2006).

Overview of Factors Influencing Men's Health

The concept of masculinity is an influencing factor in men's health. Men are socialized to be independent and conceal their vulnerability. Therefore, even when they are aware of their personal physical or mental problems, they are less likely to access the health care system. How the male identity is maintained can include activities that are hazardous to their health, and the result is a high death rate from unintentional injuries among young men. Examples of these activities include working in dangerous jobs, engaging in behaviors that lead to increased risk of homicide or car crashes, excessive alcohol consumption, smoking, substance use, and unsafe sex practices (Galdas, Cheater, & Marshall, 2005; Gough, 2006; Lonczak, Neighbors, & Donovan, 2007).

Currently, there is no Office on Men's Health in the U.S. Department of Health and Human Services, but legislation to establish such an office has been introduced. This office would mirror the work of the existing Office on Women's Health and be responsible for coordinating the men's health awareness, prevention, and research efforts that are now being conducted by federal and state government.

Factors that contribute to the deteriorating state of men's health include a lack of quality health education programs for men, health care services that are only accessed half as much by men when compared to women, and a lack of male gender-specific research (Men's Health Network, 2003). Considering all of these factors, the community nurse must determine the health care needs of men at various stages, and how he can best meet these needs throughout the adult lifespan.

Men's Health Promotion Across the Adult Lifespan

In the early years of young adulthood (between 18 and 35 years), men continue to grow and mature. Adult men aged 35 to 65 years have reached maturity, the peak of their physical and intellectual development, and their greatest earning power. What specific needs do men in these age groups have? Are their needs being met through services provided?

Healthy People 2010 Goals for Men

Although *Healthy People 2010* has 25 health objectives specifically for women and just five specifically for men,

---

DISPLAY 23.5	*HEALTHY PEOPLE 2010* OBJECTIVES FOR MEN

3-7.   Reduce the prostate cancer death rate, from 32 prostate cancer deaths per 100,000 males to 28.8 deaths per 100,000.

9-6.   (Developmental) Increase male involvement in pregnancy prevention and family planning efforts.

13-2. Reduce the number of new AIDS cases among adolescent and adult men who have sex with men, from 17,847 new cases of AIDS in 1998 to 13,385 new cases in 2010.

13-4. Reduce the number of new AIDS cases among adolescent and adult men who have sex with men and inject drugs, from 2,122 new cases of AIDS in 1998 to 1,592 new cases in 2010.

13-6. Increase the proportion of sexually active persons who use condoms, from 23% to 50%.

Adapted from U.S. Department of Health and Human Services. (2000). *Healthy people 2010: Understanding and improving health* (2nd ed.). Washington, DC: U.S. Government Printing Office.

---

hundreds apply to both women and men of all ages. The five men's objectives focus on prostate health, reproductive health, and disease prevention among men, especially men who have sex with men (MSM) (see Display 23.5).

Young Adult Men (18 to 35 Years)

The young adult male has many tasks to accomplish. These tasks include the acquisition of training or education that will lead to a personally and financially rewarding career; selecting a compatible lifetime companion and establishing a life together; finding comfort with and meaning to existence through practicing and internalizing a belief and value system that works for him; actively planning for having (or not having) children; and participating in the betterment of the greater community, both actively (volunteering, committee work, leadership positions) and passively (voting, being a good citizen, obeying laws).

Depending on his attitudes and practices before a man enters this age group, he may or may not be enticed to experiment or continue with the use of tobacco, alcohol, or illicit drugs. Experimentation or usage of these substances can occur in college, the military, or working at a full-time job. Young men also engage in behaviors or take risks without thinking about the consequences. They respond to challenges such as drag racing, exceeding speed limits, and binge drinking. This is an important age group for the community health nurse to reach with health information, because the decisions made in the more formative years of this stage affect how these clients live the rest of their lives. The nurse can meet with young adult men in work settings, on college campuses, on military bases, at single-adult groups sponsored by religious communities and other organizations, and in health clubs and bars.

Another issue to address during the early years is the young man's attitudes and beliefs toward sex and sexual experimentation. Young men may question their sexuality as they mature, and during this stage some men come to the realization that they are homosexual. **Gay** is the commonly accepted term for a homosexual—a person who has sexual interest in, or has sexual intercourse exclusively with, members of his or her own sex. Some men choose to have sex with men as well as women; these men are bisexual. Some men who have sex with either men, women, or both often do not consider themselves to be gay or bisexual. These men are categorized as men who have sex with men (MSM). When taking a sexual history, community health nurses must ask men if they have sex with women, men, or both.

Transgender, another term associated with sexuality, is used to describe individuals who experience and/or express their gender differently from what people might expect. These individuals express characteristics that do not correspond with the person's apparent or presumed gender. An example is when a presumed male chooses to put on make-up and clothes that a female would traditionally wear. Some transgender individuals define themselves as *female-to-male* or *male-to-female* and may take hormones and/or undergo medical procedures to enhance or make permanent their gender selection, including sex reassignment surgery. Others prefer to simply be called *male* or *female*—the gender they present to others, whether or not they have undergone medical reassignment.

Sexual experimentation, whether heterosexual or homosexual, can place young men at risk for diseases that affect their long-term health or are life-threatening. Men who are sexually active can reduce the possibility of being infected with a STI by limiting the number of sexual partners and using condoms consistently and correctly. Condoms also serve as a form of birth control for men. *Monogamy*, having sex with only one partner, and abstinence can further reduce or eliminate the chance of contracting an STI. Community health nurses can serve as a resource for young men and can help them obtain free or low-cost condoms and treatment for STIs.

Human Immunodeficiency Virus and Men

Despite advances in the prevention and treatment of human immunodeficiency virus (HIV), the disease continues to disproportionately impact men in the United States. In 2005, an estimated 342,148 adult and adolescent males were living with HIV in the 33 states with confidential name-based reporting. This represents 73% of the total HIV/AIDS cases. Among those cases, 61% reported being exposed through male-to-male sexual contact, 18% through injection drug use, and 7% through male-to-male sexual contact and injection drug use; however, only 5% to 7% of male adults and adolescents in the United States self-identify as MSM. When examining trends in the disease based on race and/or ethnicity, the burden of the disease has shifted from White men to Black and Hispanic men. Approximately 64% of the men living with HIV are Black or Hispanic (CDC, 2006b, 2007b).

Alcohol and illicit drug use are known to decrease social inhibitions and increase the risk for HIV transmission through risky sexual behaviors (i.e., lack of condom use) and the sharing of needles or other injection equipment. Community health nurses must be able to talk openly and nonjudgmentally with men about their use of substances and their sexual relationships. These conversations can be challenging, but they have to occur if the number of HIV infections is to be reduced (Blake & Jones Taylor, 2006).

EVIDENCE-BASED PRACTICE

The Global Community

A study was implemented to examine the effects of a multifaceted HIV/AIDS educational intervention on the knowledge, attitudes, and willingness of 208 Chinese nurses to care for persons living with human immunodeficiency virus (HIV). A pretest, posttest, quasi-experimental design was employed. The intervention consisted of a 5-day workshop that included lectures interspersed with activities designed to elicit discussion of participants' values and personal feelings about HIV/acquired immune deficiency syndrome (AIDS). The content included HIV epidemiology, natural history, transmission route, and clinical care. In addition, human sexuality, addictive disease, and bereavement were addressed. The outcome variables included HIV/AIDS knowledge, attitude toward persons living with HIV/AIDS, and willingness to provide nursing care. At baseline, HIV/AIDS knowledge was low, and participants were neutral in their attitudes and willingness to care for infected individuals. Knowledge, attitudes toward persons with HIV/AIDS, and willingness to provide nursing care improved at the conclusion of the educational intervention ($p = 0.001$).

The HIV/AIDS epidemic challenges nurses to increase their knowledge about providing effective HIV/AIDS prevention and care. As the epidemic expands, nurses are being called upon to deliver competent and compassionate care to persons living with the disease and their families. Comprehensive and interactive HIV/AIDS educational programs can contribute to international efforts to increase knowledge and improve attitudes toward caring for persons living with HIV/AIDS.

Reference:

Williams, A.B., Wang, H., Burgess, J., Wu, C., Gong, Y., & Li, Y. (2006). Effectiveness of an HIV/AIDS educational programme for Chinese nurses. *Journal of Advanced Nursing, 53*(6), 710–720.

Testicular Cancer

The risk for testicular cancer is a health problem that young men should be aware of even before early adulthood. The disease occurs most often in men between 20 and 39 years of age. Men with a personal history of undescended testicles or a family history of testicular cancer have the highest risk of developing this cancer (ACS, 2007; National Cancer Institute, 2005). It is a rare form of cancer and is not on the list of objectives for men in *Healthy People 2010*. However, if detected early, this cancer is highly curable. It is beneficial to the overall health of a young man to know how to do a testicular self-examination (TSE), and teaching men how to perform this exam appropriately is an important role for the community health nurse (see Display 23.6).

The choices a man makes during these years establish healthy eating, work, rest, and exercise habits that will benefit him for a lifetime. Men should follow the diet recommended foods in the U.S. Department of Agriculture's Food

DISPLAY 23.6	PERFORMING TESTICULAR SELF-EXAMINATION (TSE)

- TSE should be performed monthly.
- TSE should be done right after a hot shower or bath. The scrotum is most relaxed then, which makes it easier to examine the testicles.
- Examine one testicle at a time. Use both hands to gently roll each testicle (with slight pressure) between your fingers. Place your thumbs over the top of your testicle, with the index and middle fingers of each hand behind the testicle, and then roll it between your fingers.
- The epididymis, which feels soft, rope-like, and slightly tender to pressure, is located at the top of the back part of each testicle. This is a normal lump.
- One testicle (usually the right one) is slightly larger than the other; this is normal.
- When examining each testicle, feel for any lumps or bumps along the front or sides. Lumps may be as small as a piece of rice or a pea.
- If there are any swellings, lumps, or changes in the size or color of a testicle, or if there is any pain or achy area in your groin, let your doctor know right away.
- Lumps or swelling may not be cancer, but a physician should be consulted.

Adapted from Testicular Cancer Resource Center. (2006). *How to do a testicular self-examination.* Retrieved May 14, 2007 from http://tcrc.acor.org/tcexam.html.

Guide Pyramid, considering his personal likes and dislikes (2005). He and his family will benefit if he is able to balance work and home, doing his best in both settings. Establishing a pattern of rest that allows his body to recover and refresh from a day full of meaningful activities will help him look forward to each day. He should establish an exercise routine that meets his personal needs, fits his skills and talents, and includes some physical activities that involve his family.

These choices provide him with the knowledge that he is doing everything he can to keep himself healthy and to prevent the two major killers of men—heart disease and cancer. However, there are additional considerations. Typically, young adult clients have few interactions with health care providers in any given year. It is often assumed that young adult males in this age range are not at risk for physical or psychological disease. This is a myth. It is important for people in this age group to have regular health checkups, to be assessed for early signs of disease and discuss health promotion activities.

Adult Men (35 to 65 Years)

Men in the developmental stage between 35 and 65 years of age are often faced with caring for both their own children and their aging parents and in-laws. The physical, economic, and emotional demands can be great: older adults may have extended care needs while, simultaneously, the family must bear the economic burdens of putting children through college. Meanwhile, men are adjusting to the reality that their career path is probably set and many of their life choices have been made.

The term "midlife" is applied to the first half of this age period. It is a time when many men focus on a reappraisal of values, priorities, and personal relationships. As the term "midlife crisis" implies, this can be one of the more difficult stages of life. It can be an emotional time of doubt and anxiety when a man becomes uncomfortable with the idea that his life is half over. He may believe that he has not accomplished enough, or he may struggle to find new meaning or purpose in his life. Men may experience boredom with their personal life, job, or partners, and desire to make changes in these areas may occur (Wilcox et al., 2006).

The later years in this stage, ages 50 to 64, involve preparation for retirement. In anticipation of retirement, these years are marked by expanded social relationships and pursuit of new hobbies to fill increased leisure time, along with anticipating finishing of a career and accumulation of the best retirement benefits. The decisions made during these years will play out over the rest of a man's life and could alter how a spouse or long-term partner lives out their years. Health problems that were left undiagnosed when the man was younger begin to emerge. Peers may be suffering and succumbing to diseases, and a man begins to adjust to the potential loss of loved ones, particularly a spouse or long-term companion (Miner-Rubino, Winter, & Stewart, 2004).

Successful navigation of this stage can be fulfilling but may require a man to enhance his self-care skills. This includes having a positive attitude toward aging, one that examines the benefits of maturity, finds a balance between work and home, and maintains a healthy lifestyle by eating balanced meals and obtaining regular exercise. The community health nurse can provide anticipatory guidance to men approaching this stage and help them with ways to manage life more effectively.

Reproductive Health

During this stage, especially when a man has decided that his family is complete, he may choose a permanent form of birth control. For men, permanent birth control can be obtained through a surgical procedure called a *vasectomy*. A vasectomy includes removal of all or a segment of the vas deferens, so that sperm cannot be released. The procedure is routinely conducted on an outpatient basis and is minimally invasive. The procedure takes about 30 minutes. Vasectomies are to be considered permanent, however with the advent of microsurgical techniques, vasectomy reversals are now possible. Vasectomies have grown in popularity since development in the 19th century, and about 500,000 men in the United States choose to undergo the procedure each year (Dassow & Bennett, 2006).

Erection problems are common among men of all ages, but especially in men as they age. **Erectile dysfunction** (ED), sometimes called "impotence," is the repeated inability to get or keep an erection firm enough for sexual intercourse. The word "impotence" may also be used to describe other problems that interfere with sexual intercourse, such as lack of sexual desire and problems with ejaculation or orgasm. Using the term *erectile dysfunction* makes it clear that those other problems are not involved (American Urological Association [AUA], 2006b; Wessell, Joyce, Wise, & Wilt, 2007).

Since an erection requires a specific sequence of events, ED can occur when any of the events are disrupted. The sequence includes nerve impulses in the brain, spinal column, and area around the penis, and response in muscles, fibrous tissues, veins, and arteries in and near the corpora cavernosa. Damage to nerves, arteries, smooth muscles, and fibrous tissues, often as a result of disease, is the most common cause of ED. Diseases such as diabetes, kidney disease, chronic alcoholism, multiple sclerosis, atherosclerosis, vascular disease, and neurologic disorders, account for about 70% of ED cases. Between 35% and 50% of men with diabetes experience ED (National Institute of Diabetes and Digestive and Kidney Diseases [NIDDKD], 2005; Sun et al., 2006).

Lifestyle choices that contribute to heart disease and vascular problems also increase the risk of ED. Smoking, being overweight, and lack of exercise are possible causes of ED. Surgery (especially radical prostate and bladder surgery for cancer) can injure nerves and arteries near the penis, causing ED. Injury to the penis, spinal cord, prostate, bladder, and pelvis can lead to ED by harming nerves, smooth muscles, arteries, and fibrous tissues of the corpora cavernosa. In addition, many common medicines—antihypertensives, antihistamines, antidepressants, tranquilizers, appetite suppressants, and cimetidine—can produce ED as a side effect (AUA, 2006b).

In diagnosing ED, the medical history should include whether or not erections occur at other times. If an erection can be achieved with masturbation or upon awakening, the problem is probably not physical and is related to stress or an emotional problem. Treatment for ED usually proceeds from least to most invasive. For some men, making a few healthy lifestyle changes may solve the problem. Smoking cessation, weight loss, and increased physical activity may help some men regain sexual function. Cutting back on any drugs with harmful side effects is considered next. For example, drugs for high blood pressure work in different ways. If a particular drug is causing problems with erection, a different class of blood pressure medicine might work just as well. Psychotherapy and behavior modifications in some men should be considered (AUA, 2006b; Laumann et al., 2007).

Drugs for treating ED can be taken orally, injected directly into the penis, or inserted into the urethra at the tip of the penis. In March 1998, the FDA approved sildenafil citrate (Viagra), the first pill to treat ED. Since that time, vardenafil hydrochloride (Levitra) and tadalafil (Cialis) have also been approved. Viagra, Levitra, and Cialis all belong to a class of drugs called phosphodiesterase (PDE) inhibitors. Taken an hour before sexual activity, these drugs work by relaxing smooth muscles in the penis during sexual stimulation and allow increased blood flow (Shabsigh et al., 2006).

Heart Disease and Men

Cardiovascular disease (CVD) is a term that refers to the broadest category of diseases that affect the heart and blood vessels. More than 37 million men (about one in three) have some form of CVD. The number of deaths among men from this disease exceeds 300,000 deaths annually. CVD accounts for more deaths in men than cancer, lung disease, accidents, and diabetes combined. Compared to White men, Black men are more likely to die of CVD and Hispanic men are less likely (NCHS, 2007; Rosamond et al., 2007).

In the 44-year follow-up of the Framingham Heart Study participants and the 21-year follow-up of their offspring, researchers found that the average annual rate of a major cardiovascular event among men 35 to 44 years of age was seven per 1,000.

It is estimated that between 70% and 89% of sudden cardiac events occur in men and that 50% of these men had no previous symptoms of disease. The average age of a first heart attack for men is 66 years. Men who have a heart attack before age 65 have an almost 50% chance of dying within 8 years (Rosamond et al., 2007).

Major risk factors for heart disease in men include hypertension, hyperlipidemia, tobacco use, diabetes, lack of physical activity, excessive alcohol consumption, and low daily fruit and vegetable consumption. When working with adult men, the community health nurse should educate men about the importance of modifying factors that increase their risk of developing CVD. Knowing the signs and symptoms of a heart attack and how to access emergency medical treatment are also important topics that the community health nurse should discuss with adult males.

Prostate Health

Prostate health is another concern that may occur later in this life stage. The **prostate** is a doughnut-shaped cluster of glands located at the bottom of the bladder, about halfway between the rectum and the base of the penis. The prostate encircles the urethra. The walnut-sized gland produces most of the fluid in semen. Men can experience infection (prostatitis), prostate enlargement (benign prostatic hypertrophy), and prostate cancer.

Benign prostatic hypertrophy (BPH) is very common, and affects about one-third of men over age 50. The primary risk factor for developing BPH is age. Symptoms of BPH are caused by an obstruction of the urethra and gradual loss of bladder function, which results in incomplete emptying of the bladder. The symptoms of BPH vary, but the most common ones involve changes or problems with urination, such as hesitant, interrupted, or weak urinary stream; urgency or leaking of urine; and more frequent urination, especially at night. Men often report the symptoms of BPH before the physician diagnoses it through a digital rectal examination (DRE). Treatment for BPH can include medication or surgery to reduce the size of the prostate (AUA, 2006a; Rados, 2006).

Prostate cancer is the most frequently diagnosed cancer in men. The ACS estimated that there were almost 219,000 new cases of the disease and about 27,050 deaths from prostate cancer in 2007. For unknown reasons, the incidence rates are significantly higher in Blacks than in Whites. Age, ethnicity, and family history of the disease are the only well-established risk factors. More than 65% of all prostate cancers are diagnosed in men age 65 years or older. If it is detected early, the cancer may be curable. The ACS recommends that screening of men who are at average risk should begin at age 50 years and should include a blood test to assess levels of prostate specific antigen (PSA) and a DRE.

Individuals at higher risk for developing the disease (Black men or men with a family history) should begin screening at age 45 (ACS, 2007; Constantinou & Feneley, 2006).

Treatment for prostate cancer depends on the man's age, overall health status, and stage of the disease. Treatment options include surgery to remove all or part of the prostate (prostatectomy), radiation, and hormone therapy. Surgery, radiation, and hormone therapy all have the potential to disrupt sexual desire and performance, temporarily or permanently. Urinary dysfunction and urinary incontinence are common side effects that can occur after surgery or radiation. Rather than immediate treatment, watchful waiting or careful observation is an option that may be appropriate for older men with limited life expectancy and/or less aggressive tumors. A community health nurse can reinforce or clarify information shared with the man by his health care provider, discuss his treatment options with him and his family, and provide the support they may need if prostate cancer is diagnosed.

ROLE OF THE COMMUNITY HEALTH NURSE

The community health nurse works with adults in all age groups using the three levels of prevention—primary, secondary, and tertiary—as a guide. Interventions are conducted at the individual, family, groups, and aggregate levels to make progress toward the *Healthy People 2010* objectives (see Levels of Prevention Pyramid; Display 23.2).

Client teaching by the community health nurse is a major factor in preventing and managing of chronic diseases. The challenge to the nurse is to be prepared to discuss issues, backed up with knowledge of and access to the appropriate community resources, to meet client needs. What the nurse can accomplish can be quite dramatic in terms of reducing days in the hospital because of chronic disease, improving quality of life for the chronically ill person, and preventing a combination of unhealthful habits from becoming causative factors in new cases of chronic disease. A nursing care plan matrix can guide the community health nurse in discussing areas of health promotion and protection with the client. An example of a Nursing Care Plan Matrix for Young Adults can be found in Display 23.4.

Primary Prevention

Primary prevention activities focus on education to promote a healthy lifestyle. Much of the community health nurse's time is spent in the educator role. When working with individuals, the community health nurse should encourage routine health examinations, healthy eating habits, adequate sleep, moderate drinking, and no smoking. Among aggregates, the community health nurse focuses on community needs for services and programs that will keep that population healthy, such as providing flu clinics, teaching sexual responsibility, and preventing STIs.

The community health nurse may collaborate with community leaders and other stakeholders in designing programs, work with committees to secure funding, or approach the state legislature to lobby for needed changes to state laws and policies governing the health of adults. At other times, the nurse works with small groups of adults who could benefit from making healthy choices in diet, relaxation, and physical activity. Likewise, it is not unusual for the community health nurse to work with an individual to promote healthy living.

Secondary Prevention

Secondary prevention focuses on screening for early detection and prompt treatment of diseases. Throughout the lifespan, screening tests can help adults to identify disease early (see Display 23.2). A significant amount of the community health nurse's time is spent in assessing the need for, planning, implementing, or evaluating programs that focus on the early detection of diseases. This is followed with teaching to prevent further damage from the disease in progress or to prevent the spread of the disease if it is communicable. Examples of secondary prevention programs include establishing mammography clinics, teaching breast and testicular self-examination, and conducting blood pressure, blood glucose, BMI, and cholesterol screenings. Wherever adults gather in groups, this is a good place to provide both primary and secondary health care and prevention services.

Tertiary Prevention

The tertiary level of prevention focuses on rehabilitation and preventing further damage to an already compromised system. Many adults that a community health nurse works with have chronic diseases, conditions resulting from another disease, or longstanding injuries with resulting disability. Ideally, negative health conditions can be prevented. If not, the next best thing is for them to be diagnosed early, without damage to an individual's health. But if negative health conditions have not been treated or brought under control, then the individual is at a tertiary level of prevention. At this level of prevention, the nurse focuses on maintaining quality of life.

Depending on the client's age, tertiary prevention can be simple or very complicated. A 19-year-old man who breaks his leg while skiing needs information about using crutches safely, a reminder to eat protein foods for bone healing, and a reminder to return to his health care provider to get the cast removed or if he experiences various symptoms. He needs no additional help from others. Tertiary prevention in this case is easy. On the other hand, a 62-year-old woman who is 70 pounds overweight with out-of-control blood glucose levels, symptoms of congestive heart failure, and difficulty walking more than 20 feet has much to accomplish in order to feel healthy. Can the nurse help the woman lose weight? Will weight loss bring her diabetes under control and alleviate congestive heart failure symptoms? With some weight reduction, will she be able to walk more easily? Or, will the woman feel better with physical therapy and a different medication regimen? Is there a quicker, safer, and better approach? On assessment, the nurse discovers that the woman has been as much as 80 pounds overweight for 40 years. Will this information alter the nurse's approach to helping this woman? What additional information does the nurse need?

Caring for people at the tertiary level of prevention can become quite complicated, because so many systems become involved. In addition, all people function within many social systems, which may include family expectations, roles people have within the family, expected behaviors, community

LEVELS OF PREVENTION PYRAMID

SITUATION: Breast Cancer
GOAL: Using the three levels of prevention, negative health conditions are avoided or promptly diagnosed
and treated, and the fullest potential is restored.

Tertiary Prevention

Rehabilitation	Primary Prevention	
	Health Promotion & Education	**Health Protection**
• Recovery at home with return to activities of daily living within 2 weeks	• Maintains periodic follow-up with health care provider, follow-up mammogram at 6 months and 12 months, and as recommended by health care provider • Education regarding risk for other cancers (ovarian, etc.)	• Continues to practice breast self-exam (BSE) and receive mammograms as required; receives screening for ovarian cancer—transvaginal ultrasonography and blood test for tumor marker CA125

Secondary Prevention

Early Diagnosis	Prompt Treatment
• Identification of lump in left breast; appointment made with health care provider for evaluation • Receives mammogram and sonogram	• Needle aspiration of lump followed by cytologic studies • Lumpectomy with removal of two suspicious lymph nodes • Low-dose radiation

Primary Prevention

Health Promotion & Education	Health Protection
• Education regarding how to perform the BSE • Education regarding timelines for BSE and mammograms • Education regarding environmental exposure and breast cancer (smoking, alcohol, chemicals) • Education regarding low-fat diet and maintaining a BMI less than 29	• Avoidance of environmental exposures that may contribute to cancer • Performs monthly BSE and obtains mammogram as appropriate

system knowledge and involvement, personal expectations, motivation, and support. Working at the tertiary level involves all of the nurse's skills in addition to community resources and a client who can be or wants to be motivated.

Summary

The 20th century saw a shift in the leading causes of death, from communicable to noncommunicable diseases. Currently, the five leading causes of death in adults are diseases of the heart, malignant neoplasms, cerebrovascular diseases, chronic lower respiratory diseases, and unintentional injuries—none of which are communicable. The health care needs of adults are of great concern. Many needs are the same for both women and men, but the important differences were addressed in this chapter.

Adults have health care needs that change as they age. Diet and exercise, obesity, substance use, safety, and healthy lifestyle choices are issues that adults must consider throughout their lives. Heart disease and cancers remain important concerns for both men and women, and health decisions made as a young adult can have a major impact on a person as he ages.

Chronic illness is an issue of increasing concern for both men and women as life expectancies increase. Community health nurses should use the three levels of prevention to promote health across the lifespan. Primary prevention activities focus on education to promote a healthy lifestyle. Secondary prevention focuses on screening for early detection and prompt treatment of diseases. The community health nurse's role at this stage is to assess the need for, plan, implement, or evaluate programs that focus on the early detection of diseases, and to educate clients to prevent further damage from, or spread of, the disease. The tertiary level of prevention focuses on rehabilitation and prevention of further damage to an already compromised system. At this level of prevention, the nurse focuses on maintaining quality of life. ■

ACTIVITIES TO PROMOTE CRITICAL THINKING

1. Using the local newspaper, select three articles that relate to a preventable chronic disease. For each article, summarize the content, identify the likely cause, and describe how the disease may have been prevented.

2. You are asked to offer a weight-control program for 12 young adults who are residents in an apartment complex that has monthly programs related to health and wellness. The ages of the intended participants range from 20 to 35. What steps would you take to develop a successful program?

3. Using the Internet and school library, research a chronic disease associated with men aged 35 to 65. Write a two-page paper in which you identify selected concerns and discuss both personal responsibility and societal responsibility regarding management of this health problem.

4. Using the Internet and school library, research a chronic disease associated with women aged 35 to 65. Write a two-page paper in which you identify selected concerns and discuss both personal responsibility and societal responsibility regarding management of this health problem.

References

American Cancer Society, Inc. (2007). *Cancer facts and figures 2007*. Retrieved May 1, 2007 from http://www.cancer.org/docroot/stt/stt_0.asp.

American Diabetes Association. (n.d.a). *All about diabetes*. Retrieved April 29, 2007 from http://www.diabetes.org/about-diabetes.jsp.

American Diabetes Association. (n.d.b). *Diabetes statistics*. Retrieved April 29, 2007 from http://www.diabetes.org/diabetes-statistics.jsp.

American Heart Association. (n.d.). *Cardiovascular disease statistics*. Retrieved May 1, 2007 from http://www.americanheart.org/presenter.jhtml?identifier=4478.

American Heart Association. (2007). *Go red for women*. Retrieved June 9, 2007 from http://www.goredforwomen.org/.

American Lung Association. (2006a). *Lung disease data: 2006*. Retrieved May 15, 2007 from http://www.lungusa.org.

American Lung Association. (2006b). *Trends in asthma morbidity and mortality*. Retrieved May 15, 2007 from http://www.lungusa.org/atf/cf/<7A8D42C2-FCCA-4604-8ADE-7F5D5E762256>/ASTHMA06FINAL.PDF.

American Lung Association. (2006c). *Trends in chronic bronchitis and emphysema*. Retrieved May 8, 2007 from http://www.lungusa.org/atf/cf/<7A8D42C2-FCCA-4604-8ADE-7F5D5E762256>/COPD06.PDF.

American Urological Association. Education and Research, Inc., Benign Prostatic Hyperplasia Guideline Update Panel. (2006a). *Guidelines on the management of benign prostatic hypertrophy*. Retrieved May 15, 2007 from http://www.auanet.org/guidelines/main_reports/bph_management/preface_toc.pdf.

American Urological Association. Education and Research, Inc., Erectile Dysfunction Guideline Update Panel. (2006b). *The management of erectile dysfunction: An update*. Retrieved May 15, 2007 from http://www.auanet.org/guidelines/main_reports/edmgmt/content.pdf.

Blake, B.J., & Jones Taylor, G.A. (2006). A portrait of HIV infection among men in the United States. *Journal of the Association of Nurses in AIDS Care, 17*(6), 3–13.

Boston Women's Health Book Collective. (2005). *Our bodies, ourselves: A new edition for a new era*. New York: Simon and Schuster.

Centers for Disease Control and Prevention (CDC). (2005a). Cigarette smoking among adults: United States, 2004. *Morbidity and Mortality Weekly Report, 54*(44), 1121–1124.

Centers for Disease Control and Prevention (CDC). (2005b). *National diabetes fact sheet: General information and national estimates on diabetes in the United States, 2005*. Atlanta, GA: U.S. Department of Health and Human Services. Retrieved May 15, 2007 from http://www.cdc.gov/diabetes/pubs/pdf/ndfs_2005.pdf.

Centers for Disease Control and Prevention (CDC). (2006a). *Chronic fatigue syndrome*. Retrieved May 15, 2007 from http://www.cdc.gov/cfs/cfsbasicfacts.htm.

Centers for Disease Control and Prevention (CDC). (2006b). *HIV/AIDS surveillance report 2005*, Vol. Atlanta: U.S. Department of Health and Human Services. Retrieved May 14, 2007 from http://www.cdc.gov.hiv/topics/surveillance/resources/reports/2005report/pdf/2005SurveillanceReport.pdf.

Centers for Disease Control and Prevention (CDC). (2006c). State-specific prevalence of obesity among adults: United States, 2005. *Morbidity and Mortality Weekly Report, 55*(36), 985–1010.

Centers for Disease Control and Prevention (CDC). (2006d). Tobacco use among adults: United States, 2005. *Morbidity and Mortality Weekly Report, 55*(42), 1145–1148.

Centers for Disease Control and Prevention (2006e) *Trends in reported sexually transmitted diseases in the United States, 2005*. Retrieved May 15, 2007 from http://www.cdc.gov/std/stats05/trends2005.htm.

Centers for Disease Control and Prevention (CDC). (2007a). *Heart disease facts and statistics*. Retrieved May 2, 2007 from http://www.cdc.gov/HeartDisease/facts/.htm#facts.

Centers for Disease Control and Prevention (CDC). (2007b). *HIV/AIDS and men who have sex with men (MSM)*. Retrieved May 14, 2007 from http://www.cdc.gov/hiv/topics/msm/index.htm.

Constantinou, J., & Feneley, M.R. (2006). PSA testing: An evolving relationship with prostate cancer screening. *Prostate Cancer and Prostatic Diseases, 9*, 6–13.

Cook, N.R., Lee, I., Gaziano, J.M., et al. (2005). Low-dose aspirin in the primary prevention of cancer. *Journal of the American Medical Association, 294,* 47–55.

Dassow, P., & Bennett, J.M. (2006). Vasectomy: An update. *American Family Physician, 74*(12), 2069–2074.

Duffin, C. (2006). Call for better identification of eating disorders in primary care. *Nursing Standard, 21*(14–16), 10.

Edwards, C.R., Thompson, A.R., & Blair, A. (2007). An "overwhelming illness": Women's experiences of learning to live with chronic fatigue syndrome/myalgic encephalomyelitis. *Journal of Health Psychology, 12*(2), 203–214.

Finkelstein, E.A., Corso, P.S., & Miller, T.R. (2006). *Incidence and economic burden of injuries in the United States.* Retrieved April 25, 2007 from http://www.us.oup.com/us/catalog/general/subject.Medicine/PublicHealth/?view=usa&ci.

Fox, M. (2006, February 5). *Betty Friedan, who ignited cause in 'feminine mystique,' dies at 85.* New York Times. Retrieved May 8, 2007 from http://www.nytimes.com/2006/02/05/national/05friedan.html.

Friedan, B. (1997). *The feminine mystique.* New York: W.W. Norton and Company.

Galdas, P.M., Cheater, F., & Marshall, P. (2005). Men and health help-seeking behavior: Literature review. *Journal of Advanced Nursing, 49,* 616–623.

Gorelick, P.B. (2004). TIA incidence and prevalence: The stroke belt perspective. *Neurology, 62*(8), S12–S14.

Gough, B. (2006). Try to be healthy, but don't forgo your masculinity: Deconstructing men's health discourse in the media. *Social Science & Medicine, 63,* 2476–2488.

Imbornoni, M. (2006). *Women's rights movement in the United States: Timeline of key events in the American Women's Rights Movement.* Retrieved March 19, 2008 from http://www.infoplease.com/spot/womenstimeline1.html.

Institute of Medicine (2002). *Unequal treatment: Understanding racial and ethnic disparities in health care.* Retrieved May 1, 2007 from http://www.iom.edu/Object.File/Master/4/175/.

Johnson, K., Posner, S.F., Biermann, J., et al. (2006). Recommendations to improve preconception health and health care: United States. *Morbidity and Mortality Weekly Report, 55*(RR06), 1–23. Retrieved May 15, 2007 from http://www.cdc.gov.mmwr/PDF/rr/rr5506.pdf.

Johnson-Mallard, V., Lengacher, C.A., Kromrey, J.D., et al. (2007). Increasing knowledge of sexually transmitted infection risk. *The Nurse Practitioner, 32*(2), 26–32.

Kutner, M., Greenberg, E., Jin, Y., & Paulsen, C. (2006). *The health literacy of America's adults: Assessment of adult literacy* (NCES 2006-483). U.S. Department of Education, Washington, D.C. Retrieved May 1, 2007 from http://nces.ed.gov/pubs2006/2006483.pdf.

Laumann, E.O., West, S., Glasser, D., et al. (2007). Prevalence and correlates of erectile dysfunction by race and ethnicity among men aged 40 or older in the United States: From the male attitudes regarding sexual health survey. *Journal of Sexual Medicine, 4*(1), 57–65.

Lonczak, H.S., Neighbors, C., & Donovan, D.M. (2007). Predicting risky and angry driving as a function of gender. *Accident Analysis and Prevention, 39,* 536–545.

Malnutrition Advisory Group. (2003). *Malnutrition universal screening tool.* Retrieved May 15, 2007 from http://www.bapen.org.uk/pdfs/must/must_full.pdf.

McCracken, M., Jiles, R., & Blanck, H.M. (2007). *Health behaviors of the young adult U.S. population: Behavioral Risk Factor Surveillance System, 2003.* Preventing Chronic Disease. Retrieved May 8, 2007 from http://www.cdc.gov/pcd/issues/2007/apr/06_0090.htm.

Men's Health Network. (2003). *The silent health crisis.* Retrieved May 14, 2007 from http://www.menshealthnetwork.org/library/silenthealthcrisis2003a.pdf.

Miner-Rubino, K., Winter, D.G., & Stewart, A. (2004). Gender, social class, and subjective experience of aging: Self-perceived personality change from early adulthood to late midlife. *Personality & Social Psychology Bulletin, 30*(12), 1599–1610.

Mokdad, A.H., Marks, J.S., Stroup, D.F., & Gerberding, J.L. (2004). Actual causes of death in the States, 2000. *The Journal of the American Medical Association, 291,* 1238–1245.

Murphy, K. (2007). The skinny on eating disorders. *Nursing Made Incredibly Easy!, 5*(3), 40–48.

National Cancer Institute (NIH). (2005). National Cancer Institute Fact Sheet. *Testicular cancer: Questions and answers.* Retrieved May 14, 2007 from http://www.cancer.gov/images/Documents/ffd243f5-320c-4eae-af09-77db37da14ce/fs6_34.pdf.

National Center for Health Statistics (NCHS). (2006). *The economic costs of injuries among adults.* Retrieved May 15, 2007 from http://www.cdc.gov/ncipc/factsheets/CostBook/Cost_of_Injury-Adults.htm.

National Center for Health Statistics (NCHS). (2007). *Health, United States 2006: Chartbook on trends in the health of Americans.* Retrieved May 1, 2007 from http://www.cdc.gov/nchs/data/hus/hus06.pdf#tocappii.

National Center for Injury Prevention and Control. (2005). *Unintentional injury activities: 2004.* Retrieved May 2, 2007 from http://www.cdc.gov.ncipc/pub-res/unintentional_activity/2004/activity04.htm.

National Heart, Lung, and Blood Institute (NHLBI). (2002). *Framingham Heart Study.* Retrieved May 14, 2007 from http://www.nhlbi.nih.gov/about/framingham/index.html.

National Institute of Diabetes and Digestive and Kidney Diseases (NIDDKD). (2005). *Erectile dysfunction,* NIH Publication No. 06-3923. Retrieved May 15, 2007 from http://kidney.niddk.nih.gov/kudiseases/pubs/pdf/ErectileDysfunction.pdf.

National Institutes of Health Revitalization Act. (1993). *Subtitle B-Clinical research equity regarding women and minorities.* Retrieved May 9, 2007 from http://orwh.od.nih.gov/inclusion/revitalization.pdf.

National Safety Council. (2006). *Estimating the costs of unintentional injuries, 2005.* Retrieved May 2, 2007 from http://www.nsc.org/lrs/satinfo/estcost.htm.

Norsigian, J., Diskin, V., Doress-Worters, P., et al. (1999). *The Boston Women's Health Book Collective and our bodies, ourselves: A brief history and reflection.* Retrieved May 8, 2007 from http://www.amwa-doc.org/index.cfm?objectid=E1FAA89F-D567-0B25-5CB8A9C1C826FDE8.

Office on Women's Health (USDHHS). (2000). *Eating disorders.* Retrieved May 15, 2007 from http://www.4women.gov/owh/pub/factsheets/eatingdis.htm.

Office on Women's Health (USDHHS). (2005). *Binge eating disorder.* Retrieved May 15, 2007 from http://www.4women.gov/faq/bingeeating.pdf.

Office on Women's Health (USDHHS). (2006a). *Anorexia nervosa.* Retrieved May 15, 2007 from http://www.4woman.gov/faq/easyread/anorexia-etr.pdf.

Office on Women's Health (USDHHS). (2006b). *Menopause and menopause treatments.* Retrieved May 15, 2007 from http://www.forwomen.gov/faq/Menopause.pdf.

Office on Women's Health (USDHHS). (2007). *Bulimia nervosa.* Retrieved May 8, 2007 from http://www.4woman.gov/faq/Easyread/bulnervosa-etr.htm#a.

Plumb, J.D., & Brawer, R. (2006). The social and behavioral foundation of men's health: A public health perspective. *Primary Care Clinics in Office Practice, 3,* 17–34.

Rados, C. (2006). *Prostate health: What every man needs to know.* Retrieved May 15, 2007 from http://www.fda.gov/fdac/features/2006/306_prostate.html.

Rosamond, W., Flegal, K., Friday, G., et al., (2007). Heart disease and stroke statistics—2007 update. *Circulation, 115,*

E69–E171. Retrieved May 2, 2007 from http://circ.ahajournals. org.cgi/reprint/115/5/e69.

Rosenfeld, A.G. (2006). State of the heart: Building science to improve women's cardiovascular health. *American Journal of Critical Care, 15*, 556–566.

Schernhammer, E.S., Hankinson, S.E., Rosner, B., et al. (2004). Job stress and breast cancer risk: The Nurses' Health Study. *American Journal of Epidemiology, 160*, 1079–1086.

Shabsigh, R., Seftel, A.D., Rosen, R.C., et al. (2006). Review of time of onset and duration of clinical efficacy of phosphodiesterase type 5 inhibitors in treatment of erectile dysfunction. *Journal of Urology, 68*, 689–696.

Stahre, M.A., Brewer, R.D., Naimi, T.S., et al. (2004). Alcohol-attributable deaths and potential life lost: United States, 2001. *Morbidity and Mortality Weekly Report, 53*(37), 866–870.

Stevens, R. (1983). *Erik Erikson: An introduction.* New York: St. Martin's Press, Inc.

Substance Abuse and Mental Health Services Administration. (2006). *Results from the 2005 National Survey on Drug Use and Health: National findings* (Office of Applied Studies, NSDUH Series H-30, DHHS Publication No. SMA 06-4194). Rockville, MD.

Sun, P., Cameron, A., Seftel, A., et al. (2006). Erectile dysfunction: An observable marker of diabetes mellitus? A large national epidemiological study. *Journal of Urology, 176*, 1081–1085.

Testicular Cancer Resource Center. (2006). *How to do a testicular self-examination.* Retrieved May 14, 2007 from http://tcrc. acor.org/tcexam.html.

U.S. Department of Agriculture. (2005). *MyPyramid.* Retrieved June 9, 2007 from http://www.mypyramid.gov/index.html.

U.S. Department of Health and Human Services. (2000). *Healthy People 2010: Understanding and improving health* (2nd ed.). Washington, DC: U.S. Government Printing Office.

Viswanathan, A.N., Feskanich, D., De Vivo, I., et al. (2005). Smoking and the risk of endometrial cancer: Results from the Nurses' Health Study. *International Journal of Cancer, 114*(6), 996–1001.

Wessell, H., Joyce, G.F., Wise, M., & Wilt, T.J. (2007). Erectile dysfunction. *Journal of Urology, 177*, 1675–1681.

Wilcox, B.J., He, O., Chen, R., et al. (2006). Midlife risk factors and healthy survival in men. *The Journal of the American Medical Association, 296*, 2343–2350.

Williams, A.B., Wang, H., Burgess, J., et al. (2006). Effectiveness of an HIV/AIDS educational programme for Chinese nurses. *Journal of Advanced Nursing, 53*, 710–720.

World Health Organization (2004). *Global status report on alcohol 2004.* Retrieved May 15, 2007 from http://www.who.int/ substance_abuse/publications/global_status_report_2004_ overview.pdf.

Selected Readings

Barrett, J.E., Plotnikoff, R.C., Courneya, K.S., & Raine, K.D. (2007). Physical activity and type 2 diabetes: Exploring the role of gender and income. *Diabetes Educator, 33*(1), 128–143.

Channing Laboratory. (2005). *The nurses' health study.* Retrieved May 9, 2007 from http://www.channing.harvard.edu/nhs/.

Daly, C., Clemens, F., Sendon, J.L.L., et al. (2006). Gender differences in the management and clinical outcome of stable angina. *Circulation, 113*, 490–498.

Doggrell, S. (2007). Do vardenafil and tadalafil have advantages over sildenafil in the treatment of erectile dysfunction? *International Journal of Impotence Research, 19*(3), 81–95.

Dorsey, R.R., Songer, T.J., Zgibor, J.C., & Orchard, T.J. (2006). Influences on screening for chronic diabetes: Complications in type 1 diabetes. *Disease Management, 9*(2), 93–101.

Erikson, E. (1990). Erikson's development stages. *Patient Teaching.* Loose Leaf Library, Springhouse Corporation. Retrieved May 8, 2007 from http://www.honolulu.hawaii.edu/intranet/ committees/FacDevCom/guidebk/teachtip/erikson.htm.

Fox, C.S., Coady, S., Sorlie, P.D., et al. (2007). Increasing cardiovascular disease burden due to diabetes mellitus: The Framingham Heart Study. *Circulation, 115*, 1544–1550.

Garavalia, L.S., Decker, R.N., Reid, K.J., et al. (2007). Does health status differ between men and women in early recovery after myocardial infarction. *Journal of Women's Health, 16*(1), 93–101.

Gay and Lesbian Medical Association and LGBT health experts. (2001). *Healthy People 2010 companion document for lesbian, gay, bisexual, and transgender (LGBT) health.* San Francisco: Gay and Lesbian Medical Association. Retrieved May 1, 2007 from http://www.lgbthealth.net.

Harper, S., & Lynch, J. (2005). Defining health disparities. In *Methods for measuring cancer disparities: Using data relevant to healthy people 2010 cancer-related objectives.* (pp. 17–18). NCI Cancer Surveillance Monograph Series, Number 6. Bethesda, MD: National Cancer Institute, NIH Publication No. 05-5777. Retrieved May 2, 2007 from http://seer.cancer.gov/publications/ disparities/md_defining.pdf.

Holmes-Rovner, M., Stableford, S., Fagerlin, A., et al. (2005). Evidence-based patient choice: A prostate cancer decision aid in plain language. Retrieved May 14, 2007 from http://scholar. google.com/scholar?hl=en&lr=&q=BMC+Medical_Informat ics+and+Decision+Making%2C+5%2816%29+prostate+ca ncer&btnG=Search.

Infoplease. (2007). *Women's rights movement in the U.S.: Timeline.* Pearson Education, publishing as Infoplease. Retrieved May 8, 2007 from http://www.infoplease.com/spot/womenstimeline1. html.

Jackson, R.D., LaCroix, A.Z., Gass, M., et al. (2006). Calcium plus vitamin D supplementation and the risk of fractures. *The New England Journal of Medicine, 354*, 669–683.

Kirby, R.S., & Kirby, M. (2005). The urologist as an advocate of men's health: 10 suggested steps toward helping patients achieve better overall health. *Journal of Urology, 66*(5A), 52–56.

McCullagh, J., Lewis, G., & Warlow, C. (2005). Promoting awareness and practice of testicular self-examination. *Nursing Standard, 19*(51), 41–49.

National Center for Health Statistics. (2006). *Accidents/ unintentional injuries.* Retrieved May 2, 2007 from http://www.cdc.gov/nchs/fastats/acc-inj.htm.

National Center for Injury Prevention and Control. (2007). *WISQARS fatal injuries: Leading causes of death reports.* Retrieved May 2, 2007 from http://webappa.cdc.gov/sasweb/ ncipc/leadcaus.html.

National Heart, Lung, and Blood Institute. (2005). *Women's Health Study NCT00000479.* Retrieved May 2, 2007 from http:// clinicaltrials.gov/ct/show/NCT00000479.

National Institutes of Health. (n.d.). *Women's Health Initiative.* U.S. Department of Health and Human Services. Retrieved May 1, 2007 from http://www.whi.org/.

National Safety Council. (2006). *Estimating the costs of unintentional injuries, 2005.* Retrieved May 2, 2007 from http://www. nsc.org/lrs/satinfo/estcost.htm.

Office on Women's Health. (2006). Importance of calcium for bone health throughout the life span. *Clinical Courier, 24*(5). Retrieved May 14, 2007 from http://www.4women.gov/ healthpro/edu/Clinical_Courier_17.pdf.

Parker, E.D., Schmitz, K.H., Jacobs, D.R., et al. (2007). Physical activity in young adults and incident hypertension over 15 years of follow-up: The CARDIA study. *American Journal of Public Health, 97*, 703–709.

Pleis, J.R., & Lethbridge-Cejku, M. (2006). Summary health statistics for U.S. adults: National Health Interview Survey, 2005. National Center for Health Statistics. *Vital and Health Statistics*

Series, 10(232). Retrieved May 2, 2007 from http://www.cdc.gov/nchs/data/series/sr_10/sr10_232.pdf.

Rossouw, J.E., Prentice, R.L., Manson, J.E., et al. (2007). Postmenopausal hormone therapy and risk of cardiovascular disease by age and years since menopause. *The Journal of the American Medical Association, 297*, 1465–1477.

Sadovszky, V.V., Kovar, C.K., Brown, C., & Armbruster, M. (2006). The need for sexual health information: Perceptions and desires of young adults. *The American Journal of Maternal/Child Nursing, 31*(6), 373–379.

Substance Abuse and Mental Health Services Administration. (2006). *Misuse of prescription drugs: Prevalence and recent trends in misuse of prescription drugs.* Retrieved May 2, 2007 from http://www.oas.samhsa.gov/prescription/Ch2.htm.

Travison, T.G., Shabsigh, R., Araujo, A.B., et al. (2007). The natural progression and remission of erectile dysfunction: Results from the Massachusetts male aging study. *The Journal of Urology, 177*, 241–246.

Vaillan, G.E., DiRago, A.C., & Mukamal, K. (2006). Natural history of male psychological health, XV: Retirement satisfaction. *American Journal of Psychiatry, 163*, 682–688.

Valenti, W.M. (2007). Health literacy, HIV, and outcomes. *AIDS Reader, 17*, 124–126.

Walter, L.C., Bertenthal, D., Lindquist, K., & Konety, B.R. (2006). PSA screening among elderly men with limited life expectancies. *The Journal of the American Medical Association, 296*, 2336–2342.

Weinmann, S., Richert-Boe, K., Glass, A.G., & Weiss, N.S. (2004). Prostate cancer screening and mortality: A case-control study (United States). *Cancer Causes and Control, 15*(2), 133–138.

Westermeyer, J.F. (2004). Predictors and characteristics of Erikson's life cycle among men: A 32 year longitudinal study. *International Journal of Aging and Human Development, 58*(1), 29–48.

Wright, D., & Sathe, N. (2005). *State estimates of substance use from the 2002–2003 national surveys on drug use and health (DHHS Publication No. SMA 05-3989, NSDUH Series H-26).* Rockville, MD: Substance Abuse and Mental Health Services Administration, Office of Applied Studies. Retrieved May 2, 2007 from http://www.oas.samhsa.gov/topics.cfm.

Internet Resources

American Cancer Society, Inc.: *http://www.cancer.org*
American Diabetes Association: *http://www.diabetes.org*
American Heart Association: Go Red for Women: *http://www.goredforwomen.org*
American Public Health Association (APHA): *http://www.apha.org*
American Red Cross: *http://www.redcross.org*
Centers for Disease Control and Prevention (CDC): *http://www.cdc.gov*
Centers for Disease Control and Prevention, National Center for Health Statistics: *http://www.cdc.gov/nchs*
Harvard Men's Health Watch: *http://www.health.harvard.edu/newsletters/*
Health Resources and Services Administration: *http://www.hrsa.gov/*
Institute of Medicine: *http://www.iom.edu/*
Men's Health Network: *http://www.menshealthnetwork.org*
National Cancer Institute: *http://www.cancer.gov*
National Heart, Lung, and Blood Institute: *http://www.nhlbi.nih.gov*
National Institute of Allergy and Infectious Diseases: *http://www.niaid.nih.gov*
National Institute of Environmental Health Sciences: *http://www.niehs.nih.gov*
National Institutes of Health: *http://www.nih.gov*
National Women's Health Center: *http://www.4women.gov*
Office of Research in Women's Health: *http://orwh.od.nih.gov*
U.S. Department of Health and Human Services: *http://dhhs.gov*
Wise Woman: *http://www.cdc.gov/wisewoman*
World Health Organization: *http://www.who.int/en/*

24

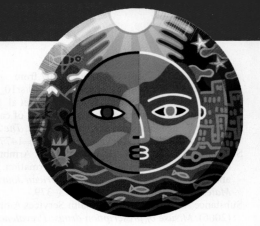

Older Adults: Aging in Place

LEARNING OBJECTIVES

Upon mastery of this chapter, you should be able to:

◆ Describe the global and national health status of older adults.

◆ Identify and refute at least four common misconceptions about older adults.

◆ Identify four types of elder abuse.

◆ Describe characteristics of healthy older adults.

◆ Provide an example of primary, secondary, and tertiary prevention practices in the elderly population.

◆ Identify four chronic conditions most commonly found in the elderly population.

◆ Discuss four primary criteria for effective programs for older adults.

◆ Describe various types of living arrangements and care options as older adults age in place.

◆ Describe the difference between hospice and palliative care.

◆ Describe the future of an aging America and the role of the community health nurse.

"We are encouraging Americans of all ages to live healthier lives. Healthy living can prevent diseases and certain disabilities, and it can ensure that today's older persons—as well as future generations—not only live longer, but also better."
—Josefina G. Carbonell, Assistant Secretary for Aging, U.S. Department of Health and Human Services (Administration on Aging, 2007a, p. 1).

KEY TERMS

Ageism
Alzheimer's disease (AD)
Assisted living
Board and care homes
Case management
Continuing care retirement
  communities (CCRCs)
Custodial care
Elder abuse
Elite-old
Frail elderly
Geriatrics
Gerontology
Hearty elderly
Hospice
Intermediate care
Long-term care
Osteoporosis
Palliative care
Personal care homes
Respite care
Senility
Skilled nursing facilities

Older Americans constitute a large and rapidly growing population group. If you aren't already part of it, you will be in the future. Perhaps your parents and grandparents are in that group now. Improved medical care, advances in public health standards, and focus on prevention have contributed to dramatic increases in life expectancy in the United States. Average life expectancy at birth rose from 47.3 in 1900 to 76.9 in 2000 (He, Sengupta, Velkoff, & DeBarros, 2005). According to U.S. Census Bureau projections, a substantial increase in the number of older people will occur during the 2010 to 2030 period, due to (1) increasing life spans and (2) aging baby boomers (people born between 1956 and 1964). By 2030, there will be 71 million American older adults, accounting for roughly 20% of the U.S. population (Centers for Disease Control [CDC] & Merck Co. Foundation, 2007).

The future older population is expected to be better educated than the current one. The increased levels of education will most likely accompany better health, higher incomes, more wealth, and consequently a higher standard of living in retirement. As people retire at younger ages and in better health, they will require programs and services that support preventive health measures, and thus provide opportunities for continued wellbeing and enhanced quality of life, and contribute to overall longevity (CDC & Merck Co. Foundation, 2007).

By 2030, the nation's health care spending is expected to increase by 25% due to projected numbers of aging adults that will require care (He et al., 2005). The cost of providing health care for an American 65 years and older is three to five times greater than the cost for someone younger (CDC, 2003a). The number of people over the age of 65 who will require health care services will create challenges, as well as opportunities, for our already overburdened, understaffed, and ever changing health care system. From 1990 to 2001, the U.S. expenditures for home health and nursing home care doubled, and are expected to continue to rise (CDC, 2003a). Although tremendous efforts have been made to develop and promote preventive health programs and services, the outcomes and benefits of these efforts may not be seen for many years (He et al., 2005; Schwappach, Boluarte, & Suhrcke, 2007).

For community health nursing, the growing aging population will present opportunities for nurses to work with communities to strengthen and build programs and services that focus on supporting the aging population's highest functional level. Like other nursing specialty areas, the community health nurse will be in the position to advocate for the needs of an aging population and work with other agencies and organizations involved with health care delivery to ensure that seniors have access to high quality health care and comprehensive services that address their unique and complex problems.

This group's potential for longevity will bring on myriad problems including poor retirement planning and dwindling finances, increased living costs and increasing chronic disease and disability, diminishing functional capacity, and ongoing losses. Despite preventive and supportive services, it is estimated that at least 40% of the population over the age of 75 will require extensive health care services late in their lives (CDC & Merck Co. Foundation, 2007; Lorenz et al., 2004). Those without adequate access to care will suffer more long-term consequences (Rahimi, Spertus, Reid, Bernheim, & Krumholz, 2007). Significant economic, environmental, and social changes create a demand for greater protective and preventive services for older adults in addition to requiring adjustments in health care provision patterns (He et al., 2005; Martini, Garrett, Lindquist, & Isham, 2007; Lorenz et al., 2004).

This chapter focuses on population-based nursing for the elderly. There are four fundamental requirements for effective nursing of any population:

1. Know the characteristics of the population.
2. Set aside stereotypes based on misconceptions about the population.
3. Know the health needs of the population as a basis for nursing intervention.
4. View the population from an aggregate, public health perspective that emphasizes health protection, health promotion, and disease prevention.

This chapter first examines the characteristics of the aging population in the United States and the global challenge of an aging society. Some myths and misconceptions about the elderly are described, and ageism is discussed. Four types of elder abuse are reviewed along with factors that contribute to the abuse of seniors. Next, the primary, secondary, and tertiary health needs of older adults are explored. Finally, population-based health services and nursing interventions applied to the health of the aging population are discussed in light of cost containment and comprehensive care at the beginning of the new millennium.

HEALTH STATUS OF OLDER ADULTS

The growth in the number and proportion of older adults living in the United States is unprecedented in our nation's history. The proportion of individuals aged 65 and older is projected to increase from 12.4% in 2000 to almost 20% by the year 2030 (CDC, 2003a). People are living longer as a result of improved health care, eradication and control of many communicable diseases, use of antibiotics and other medicines, healthier dietary practices, safer global water supplies, regular exercise, and accessibility to a better quality of life including education and social services. Increased life expectancy reflects, in part, the success of public health interventions, but public health programs must now respond to new challenges including the growing burden of chronic illness, injuries, disabilities, increasing concerns about future caregiving, and rapidly rising health care costs (CDC & Merck Co. Foundation, 2007; Lorenz et al., 2004; Martin & Sheaff, 2007).

As noted earlier, life expectancy at birth in the United States has increased from age 47.3 in 1900 to 76.9 in 2000 (He et al., 2005). Those born between 1946 and 1964, often referred to as "baby boomers," will begin to reach age 65 in 2011. By the year 2030, it is estimated that 20% of the entire U.S. population will be over age 65 (CDC & Merck Co. Foundation, 2007; U.S. Census Bureau, 2007). During that period, the U.S. population age 19 and under will drop—to 26.2% and 26%, respectively (U.S. Census Bureau, 2007).

The rising number of older adults increases demands on the public health system and on medical and social services and health care delivery. Chronic diseases, which affect older adults disproportionately, contribute to disability, diminish quality of life, and increase health care costs. As more and more Americans reach age 65, society is increasingly challenged to help them grow old with dignity and comfort (Kapo, Morrison, & Liao, 2007). Chronic diseases and conditions are also a part of aging, and 59% of those over 65 years of age in the United States report arthritis as a leading cause of disability (CDC, 2003b). Diabetes and Alzheimer disease affect one in five and one in 10 of those age 65 and older, respectively, and are expected to have even greater effects on the U.S. health care system in the next few decades (CDC, 2003a). Two key challenges that are new to the public health arena, although they have long been the target of health care and aging services professions, are preventing and treating cognitive decline and addressing end-of-life issues (Kettl, 2007; Richardson, Sullivan, Hill, & Yu, 2007; Mitchell, Teno, Intrator, Feng, & Mor, 2007). Meeting these challenges, along with the increasing number of individuals with chronic conditions, is critical to ensuring that the aging population can look forward to their later years.

Global Demographics

In 1950, there were 131 million people worldwide over the age of 65. By 1995, that number had increased to 371 million, and it should double again between 2000 and 2025. It is estimated that there could be 1.4 billion elderly worldwide by the year 2050 (International Institute for Applied Systems Analysis [IIASA], 2007). The elderly comprised 5.2% of the world population in 1950, growing only to 6.2% in 1995. But by 2050 one tenth of the population will be over the age of 65 (IIASA, 2007). In most of the world, the population of those over 80 years of age is growing faster than any other population age group (United Nations [UN], 2003a). The largest increases in absolute numbers of older persons will occur in developing countries, with China most likely to have an extraordinary rise in the proportion of elderly as their birth rates decline (IIASA, 2007). By 2050, Asia is predicted to be home to 63% of the world's elderly (UN, 2003a). Because of this demographic shift along with altered societal expectations, changes in attitudes and social policies worldwide are needed; many countries have few or no social programs, pensions, or health care services available for their elderly populations (UN, 2003b).

Life expectancy at birth around the world now ranges from 32.2 to 83.5 years (Central Intelligence Agency [CIA], 2007). Life expectancy has increased in developing countries since 1950, although the amount of increase varies. A higher life expectancy at birth for females compared with males is almost universal, with the average gender differential estimated for 2007 at approximately 4 years worldwide (67.8 years for females, 63.8 for males) (CIA, 2007). These high percentages are in part the result of extended lifespan, but they also reflect low birth rates in many countries. Presently, the world population is at roughly 6.6 billion people, but population projections continue to project increases (7.79 billion by 2025, 8.75 by 2050) despite lower birth rates in many countries (CIA, 2007; IIASA, 2007).

The median age of the world's population is 28 years, and this has been increasing due in part to declining fertility and a 20-year increase in the average life span during the second half of the 20th century (CIA, 2007; UN, 2003b). These factors, combined with elevated fertility in many countries during the 2 decades after World War II (i.e., the Baby Boom), will result in increased numbers of persons aged 65 and over as outlined above (IIASA, 2007). Worldwide, another 10 years will be added to the average lifespan by the year 2050 (CDC, 2003a).

National Demographics

As a result of demographic transitions including declining infant and childhood mortality, lower fertility rates, and improvements in adult health, the shape of the global age distribution is changing. By 2005, the age distribution in developed countries represented a larger proportion of older to younger populations. For developing countries, age distribution is projected to have similar proportions by 2025-2050 (UN, 2003a).

Estimates for 2007 reveal the average life expectancy at birth for Americans as 78 years (CIA, 2007). However, there are disparities in life expectancy among various subgroups in the population. Life expectancy is highest for White Americans and lowest for Black Americans, who have the highest death rates of any of America's racial and ethnic groups (Gist, 2007). Although life expectancies have been increasing for all Americans in general, a variety of factors have caused those figures to level off in recent years. These include unhealthy lifestyles; societal problems, such as deaths caused by firearms, substance abuse, and human immunodeficiency virus/acquired immunodeficiency syndrome (HIV/AIDS); and the rise of Alzheimer disease (AD) among the elderly (Gist, 2007).

The Hispanic, Black, and Asian populations have been expanding and are projected to grow substantially through 2025 (Campbell, 1996). The health status of racial and ethnic minorities of all ages lags far behind that of nonminority populations. For a variety of reasons, older adults may experience the effects of health disparities more dramatically than any other population group. In an effort to help address these health disparities, the Racial and Ethnic Approaches to Community Health (REACH 2010) Program supports community-based coalitions in the design, implementation, and evaluation of innovative strategies to reduce or eliminate health disparities among racial and ethnic minorities (CDC, 2006a). Methods utilized include "capacity building, targeted actions, community/system change, widespread risk/ protective behavior change, (and) health disparity reduction" (p. 2). An example of one of these programs is highlighted in Display 24.1. One of the two goals of *Healthy People 2010*, the comprehensive set of health objectives for the nation, is to eliminate health disparities among different segments of the population, and current research has shown that although many efforts—such as aspirin use for high-risk adults, tobacco-use screening and brief intervention, colorectal cancer screening for adults over age 50, and immunization for pneumococcal disease for those age 65 and older—can be very effective, they are not always implemented or consistently utilized (Maciosek, Coffield, Edwards, Flottemesch, Goodman, & Solberg, 2006).

Nevertheless, older people are healthier than ever before. Increasing numbers of capable elderly people are

DISPLAY 24.1   RACIAL AND ETHNIC APPROACHES TO COMMUNITY HEALTH (REACH)—DETROIT, MICHIGAN

High rates of diabetes-related hospital discharges and diabetes-related mortality were noted in both southwest and eastern areas of Detroit, Michigan. Public health nurses and other officials also checked statistical data and found that 43% of African Americans in Detroit were overweight, whereas 33% of Whites were overweight. Almost half of all residents reported that they had a sedentary lifestyle, and one-third stated that they engaged in no physical activities during their leisure time. Many of these people were older adults and elderly.

It was decided that this problem had to be addressed at multiple levels: with individuals and families (changing behaviors), social support systems, community agencies and services, and by making changes in policies and programs offered by Detroit Community Health & Social Services. They formed a partnership, based upon the principles of community-based participatory research (see Chapter 4). They began by collecting additional data on the prevalence of diabetes, the accessibility of quality health care services, and what community resources were available that promoted healthy lifestyles. They also looked for acceptable models of community-based interventions and gathered perspectives from members of the community by holding family focus groups.

They began educating their target population, and conducted diabetes education and self-management classes over a period of 5 to 6 weeks. They had good results with retention of REACH participants (80%), and significant improvements in both physical activity and dietary knowledge and behavior. Self-care behaviors and diabetes problem areas were also significantly improved ($p < .05$), as were levels of hemoglobin A1C. Hypertension was also decreased, from a baseline of 54.1% of REACH participants to 42.4% at the 6-month mark.

This multilevel, community-based intervention made marked improvements on several outcome measures for the targeted population. What type of disease or problem is most prevalent in your area? With whom could you collaborate to design interventions? Which levels would you want to address? How would you measure success (which outcomes would you select)?

Two Feathers, J., Kieffer, E., Palmisano, G., Anderson, M. et al. (2005). Racial and ethnic approaches to community health (REACH). Detroit partnership: Improving diabetes-related outcomes among African American and Latino adults. *American Journal of Public Health, 95*(9), 1552–1560.

---

living independently, and the **hearty elderly**—people older than 65 years of age who maintain a high level of wellness and activity, well above present expectations for that age—are increasing in number. Most people older than 65 years of age not only maintain independent living but also continue to contribute to society (Ostbye et al., 2006). Many continue to work and stay involved in community programs and activities. Some have become valuable volunteers, helping others in such community activities as hospice and literacy programs for adults, serving as foster grandparents, working in libraries and homeless shelters, or providing services such as Meals on Wheels. Research has shown a connection between positive health effect and community involvement/participation, volunteering, and other forms of social capital (Kim & Kawachi, 2006).

Not only are more people living into old age, but also, once they get there, they are living longer. Eliopoulos (2004) characterizes those between the ages of 65 and 75 as "young-old," whereas those between 75 and 85 years are labeled "old-old" (p. 5). The number of people living into "older" old age (75 years and older) is increasing. Forty percent of elderly people in the United States are among the "oldest old" (85–100 years)—0.2 million in the year 2000—and more than 200,000 are among the **elite-old**, or centenarians (Eliopoulos, 2004).

Some 72 million people will be entering old age, significantly affecting health care resources, housing options for older adults, and national longevity statistics. As the number of "old-old" people increases, so too will the need for assistance with activities of daily living (ADLs) and other services. Many people will be involved with the care and disposition of the **frail elderly**, those older than 85 years of age who need assistance in attending to ADLs such as dressing, eating, toileting, and bathing, and researchers are seeking effective methods of providing respite to caregivers and reducing costs (Mason et al., 2007).

In the United States, approximately 80% of all persons aged 65 years and older have at least one chronic condition, and 50% have at least two (CDC, 1999; National Center for Health Statistics, 2002). Death is only part of the picture of the burden of chronic disease among older Americans. These conditions can cause years of pain, disability, and loss of function and independence before resulting in death. In addition to chronic conditions that require ongoing monitoring and management, the community health nurse should anticipate the needs of many older adults who will face the loss of a spouse, helpmate, or companion and who may experience loneliness, social isolation, and depression.

In the total U.S. population, almost twice as many women as men (12.4% versus 7%) live below the poverty level, and this trend continues into old age (Gist, 2007). More than one in ten older Americans (10.1%) are poor, and many live in profound poverty. They are unable to afford clothing, recreation, transportation, or other items that most people consider necessary for mental health, social status, and continued personal growth. The differences among various ethnic groups experiencing poverty in old age are broad. Among White older adults, 8.9% were found to live below the poverty level, whereas 21.9% of African American elders and 21.8% of Hispanic elders live in poverty. Hispanic women who lived alone or with nonrelatives had the highest proportion of poverty at 50.5% (Administration on Aging, 2002a). Those elderly living barely above the poverty level ("near-poor") represent even greater numbers: 30% of Whites, 34% of Latinos, 28% of African Americans, 32% of Asian/Pacific Islanders, and 41% of American Indian/Alaska Natives live under 200% of the federal poverty level—proportions much higher than the nonelderly population (The Henry J. Kaiser Family Foundation, 2003).

The education level of the older population is increasing. The percentage of older adults who have completed high school increased between 1970 and 1998 (from 28% to 67%), and this trend is expected to continue to rise to 83% by 2030 (American Geriatric Society, 2007). These figures are predicted to change as the United States witnesses a trend toward a more educated senior population because of the significant numbers of baby boomers who completed high school and entered college during and since the 1960s. The number of seniors with bachelor's degrees is expected to increase from 15% to 24% (American Geriatric Society, 2007). With higher levels of education should come broader health consumerism and better quality of life.

DISPELLING AGEISM

Stereotyping older adults and perpetuating false information and negative images and characteristics regarding older adults is called **ageism**. These stereotypes often arise from negative personal experience, myths shared throughout the ages, and a general lack of current information. Ageism is a term that describes negative stereotyping of older adults and discrimination because of older age. Unfortunately health concerns and symptoms in the elderly are often overlooked or dismissed as part of the normal aging process (Moore, 2002). By becoming more aware of myths and realities of aging, community health nurses can improve the health and quality of life of the growing elderly population (Salzman, 2006). Ageism can interfere with effective practice and prevent the kind of comprehensive and interdisciplinary services and care that aging persons need and deserve (Ory, 2003). Ageism has an impact on both society and culture, even though most individuals are not aware of it. Ageism creates needless fear, waste, illness, and misery (Palmore, 2005).

Misconceptions About Older Adults

Most people know little about aging and may have negative stereotypes about old people. Community health nurses must guard against ageism in their practice by dispelling common misconceptions.

Misconception: Most Older Adults Cannot Live Independently

Although over 900,000 seniors live in assisted living residences and more than 1.1 million live in some type of senior housing community, most American seniors are below age 85 and live with their spouse (American Geriatric Society, 2007). In fact, 55% of older Americans were reported to be married and living with their spouse in 2000 (Administration on Aging, 2002a; American Association of Homes and Services for the Aging [AAHSA], 2007). Ninety-four percent of elderly individuals live in the community, outside formal facilities or institutions (Ebersole & Hess, 2004). About 30% live alone, and

others live with friends or in the homes of nonrelatives with room and board provided (Administration on Aging, 2002a). In some homes, assistance with ADLs is provided. Over 150,000 are provided services and care through adult day care (AAHSA, 2007). Alternative-housing arrangements are also available—group-living situations for older adults in which many types of housing and care possibilities are offered. This concept is not new, but these centers are being built now in greater numbers to meet the needs of a growing segment of the older adult population. These situations are well suited to those who desire such comprehensive living choices and have the financial means for the housing and care arrangements provided. About 745,000 seniors live in these continuing care retirement communities (AAHSA, 2007). The average waiting list time for an eligible older adult to be placed in an affordable senior housing unit is over 13 months (AAHSA, 2007).

Over 4% of those age 65 and older in 2000 lived in nursing homes, and the current percentage is still below 5%. By the age of 85 and above in 2000, that percentage increased to 18.2%. By 2020, it is estimated that 12 million seniors will need some form of long-term care (AAHSA, 2007). The average age of older adults in residential care is getting higher and is currently about 85 years. Such facilities typically are not chosen by the hearty elderly or by totally independent young-elders, who prefer to receive services that allow them to remain in their own homes—commonly referred to as Aging in Place (Hill, Thorn, Bowling, & Morrison, 2002; Administration on Aging, 2002b). Despite popular notions, only a small minority of older Americans move to warmer climates after retirement (National Association of Area Agencies on Aging, 2007).

Most elders who are vigorous and functioning independently live in their own homes. Only about 6% live in institutions such as skilled nursing facilities, extended care facilities, supervised living facilities, and AD centers, and not all of these are permanent residents. Many are recovering from illnesses or undergoing rehabilitation after an injury or surgery and will return to their living situation in the community within a matter of weeks (Hill et al., 2002).

Misconception: Chronologic Age Determines Oldness

The aging process is quite distinct among older people, and they age at widely disparate rates. Some people still play golf, drive a car, and participate in social and community activities at age 85; others are frail and cannot move about well, needing assistance with their ADLs. Some prefer to equate "real age" with biological age, not chronological age; this depends on how well an individual takes care of him- or herself physically and mentally (RealAge, 2007). Exercise, nutrition, vitamins, seat belt use, and other factors are thought to play a role in healthy aging. Physical, social, and mental health parameters, life experiences, and genetic traits all combine to make aging an individualized process (see Levels of Prevention Pyramid).

Misconception: Most Elderly Persons Have Diminished Intellectual Capacity or Are Senile

Recent research is proving several myths about cognition to be incorrect, notably the beliefs that aging is a time of irreversible mental decline and that dementia is universal and

LEVELS OF PREVENTION PYRAMID

SITUATION: Making a healthy transition into a satisfying retirement.

GOAL: Using the three levels of prevention, negative health conditions are avoided, promptly diagnosed, and treated, and/or the fullest possible potential is restored.

Tertiary Prevention

Rehabilitation

Primary Prevention

Rehabilitation	Health Promotion & Education	Health Protection
• Adapt to changed roles with spouse and significant others • Maintain health while assessing increasing dependency needs, including alternative housing, modifications in transportation, and changing health care needs	• Periodically review and update will, insurances, and other important documents as needed • Keep beneficiaries or executors aware of changes in and location of documents and personal wishes regarding end-of-life care, and funeral/burial arrangements	

Secondary Prevention

Early Diagnosis

Prompt Treatment

Early Diagnosis	Prompt Treatment
• Plan or participate in a celebration activity • Reflect on past successes and contributions to the workforce	• Allow time for adaptation to this life transition • Organize new free time into satisfying and enriching activities

Primary Prevention

Health Promotion & Education

Health Protection

Health Promotion & Education	Health Protection
• Early preparation—emotionally and financially • Avocation planning (preretirement workshops, support groups, financial planning)	

---

inevitable (Alzheimer's Association Medical and Scientific Advisory Council, 2005). As such, researchers and health professionals have begun to focus on opportunities to maintain or possibly improve cognitive health. Cognitive health is defined as a combination of mental processes we commonly think of as "knowing," including the ability to learn new things, intuition, judgment, language, and remembering. Studies show that intelligence, learning ability, and other intellectual and cognitive skills do not decline with age. Cognitive deficits are caused by certain risk factors. Nutritional status has been singled out as a physical health variable that influences cognitive functioning, particularly memory performance, regardless of a person's age. Mild cognitive impairment is viewed as "the transitional stage between normal aging and dementia" and can include deficiencies in language (slower with words), visual-spatial ability (difficulty with proportions when drawing a box, for instance), executive function (decision making), and memory (recent memory more difficult) (*Medical News Today,* 2006). Generally, older people are capable of making their own decisions; they want and need the freedom to make choices and to be as independent as their limitations will allow.

Senility, although not a legitimate medical diagnosis, is a term widely used by the lay public to denote deteriorating mental faculties associated with old age. A recent Mayo Clinic study of close to 4,000 people from a general population in Minnesota found that 12% of 70- to 89-year-olds had mild cognitive impairment—a condition often undiscovered except by close family members living with the elderly person. This increased with age, as only 9% of those 70 to

79 were found to be cognitively impaired whereas 18% of those from 80 to 89 had cognitive impairment. Education mediated those effects, as only 8.5% of those with greater than 16 years were found to have impairment, but 25% of those with up to 8 years of education were mildly cognitively impaired (*Medical News Today*, 2006).

Certainly, Alzheimer disease and arteriosclerosis cause memory loss and altered behavior in the elderly, but many older adults have similar symptoms as a result of anxiety, loss, depression, or grief, or simply from side effects of medications or changes in their routines. These reactions need to be diagnosed by health care providers and differentiated from disease processes, and new research indicates that intellectual stimulation, social engagement, and physical activity may help maintain cognitive functioning in older adults (Butler, 2004). Bernick and colleagues (2005) found a slight decrease in cognitive changes/impairment in a large sample of adults over the age of 65 taking cholesterol-lowering statin drugs, indicating that more research is needed to better understand how to prevent cognitive impairment in older adults.

Misconception: All Older People Are Content and Serene

The picture of Grandma sitting serenely in her rocker with her hands folded in her lap is misleading. It is true that many older people have learned to accept, rather than fight, the hardships and vicissitudes of life. Yet, for most people, advancing age brings increasing physical, social, and financial problems. However, it is important to remember that to attain the status of senior citizen, defined as individuals 65 years or older, one has often exhibited a great deal of strength, tenacity, and capacity for adaptation, as well as a sense of humor about many of the trials, tribulations, and absurdities in life. These people are survivors, and survivors do not always sit contentedly in a rocking chair on the sidelines of life.

Mental health problems continue into old age. Depression, which can affect close to one in five elderly people, is sometimes confused with dementia because of such common symptoms as disorientation, failing memory, and eccentric behavior (National Alliance on Mental Illness [NAMI], 2003). For some, depression has been a lifelong battle, but for others, the first onset of depressive symptoms may occur in old age. The losses and grief experienced by seniors may lead to clinical depression that can be treated with medications and other therapies. Because elderly often do not seek treatment or even recognize that they may be clinically depressed, it is important for public health nurses (PHNs) to monitor their older clients carefully and ask them about changes in appetite, sleep patterns, and behavior. Suicide is not uncommon among the elderly—in fact the highest rates are among older White men (NAMI, 2003).

Misconception: Older Adults Cannot Be Productive or Active

The average American retires at 57.8 years, although the average worker plans to retire at age 61 (Pew Research Center, 2006). Prior to the 1990s, the average age of retirement had been declining. Now, it is moving upward. A recent trend has been for retirees to return to work; 12% in one survey reported they are currently working, most on a part-time basis (Pew, 2006). A recent AARP survey found that 28% of workers and 12% of current retirees do not feel confident about having sufficient money to pay for medical expenses during retirement; 15% of workers and 9% of retirees are not sure they even have enough money for basic monthly expenses. The survey also noted that 40% of those still working are concerned that their employers will not pay them their full pensions or will abolish retirement health benefits (Holley, 2006).

Labor force participation rates of those over 60 (not retired) have been increasing over the past decade for men and women age 62 to 64 (4% increase for men and 12% increase for women). For those age 70 and above, 15.8% of men and 8.7% of women in 1994 worked full time versus 20.7% of men and 12.8% of women in 2005 (Population Reference Bureau, 2006). Millions of Americans older than 65 years of age work full- or part-time, and many others, who are not included in labor statistics, work but do not report their earnings. An example is the grandmother who chooses to give up full-time employment in an unsatisfying job to baby-sit for three pre-school grandchildren and is paid in cash by her two children. The grandmother gets to spend time with growing grandchildren and supplement her retirement income, the parents feel comfortable that their mother is caring for their children, and the grandchildren are experiencing the joy of being with their grandparent. In another situation, active retired older adults assist with their two children's businesses. The mother types legal documents for the son's law practice during busy times, and the father helps out on Saturdays at the daughter's pool supply store. Everyone wins in these situations.

Work remains important to seniors. Healthy older people usually do not disengage or withdraw and isolate themselves from society; rather, they are active and involved. Remaining active—through a daily routine, purposeful behavior, and a positive view of life—produces the best psychological climate.

Misconception: All Older Adults Are Resistant to Change

People at any age can learn new information and skills. Research indicates that older people can learn new skills and improve old ones, including how to use a computer and the Internet. Learning occurs best in a self-paced, supportive environment (American Association of Retired Persons [AARP], 2005). Studies have demonstrated that even those in very old age can still learn new skills. One study from Germany instructed and trained very old adults (mean age of 84 years) in a new skill, and found that they could improve their perceptual speed with training, demonstrating "memory plasticity" (Singer, Lindenberger, & Baltes, 2003). Those between the ages of 60 and 80 performed at a higher level; however, this study demonstrated that the very old were still able to learn and perform a new skill. The elderly have spent a lifetime adapting to change, with varying measures of success. People older than 65 years grew up in an age when having an automobile was a luxury and many did not have a microwave oven, video recorder, or DVDs until they were in middle adulthood. Elders learned to adapt to these changes, and they are becoming increasingly computer literate today. The ability to change does not depend on age, but rather on personality traits acquired throughout life or, sometimes, because of socioeconomic difficulties. For example, elders living on fixed incomes may be faced with inflationary costs. This may cause them to vote against a school levy that would increase taxes, although they otherwise would be very supportive of schools because they value education.

Misconception: Social Security Will Not Be There When I Retire

The Social Security fund is not yet bankrupt. Although the government has borrowed from it, the trust fund growth is sufficient to keep Social Security solvent and paying full benefits until 2042; after that time, if the current tax cuts are continued and no changes are made, retirees at age 60 in 2040 will have their benefits reduced by 26% and benefits could continue to drop every year (Center on Budget & Policy Priorities [CBPP], 2004; Social Security Administration [SSA], 2006). By 2018, benefit payments will exceed revenues; however, interest earnings on the Social Security Trust Fund will continue to keep it solvent. By 2028, Treasury Bonds will have to be redeemed in order for the government to continue to make full payments to beneficiaries (CBPP, 2007).

Although there are concerns about Social Security, Medicare is in far worse condition. It will stay financially healthy only until 2013 (CBPP, 2007). Money still pours into the Medicare Trust Fund from payroll taxes, and not until 2019 will the administrators have to start tapping the general fund to meet 45% of their obligations to Medicare Part A benefits (Center for Medicare Advocacy, 2007). The large shortfall in Medicare is mostly due to health care costs that continue to rise and the $10 billion per year overpayments to private insurers (CBPP, 2007). In 2006, a new prescription drug benefit was added to Medicare (Part D), and by 2007, over 39 million people had enrolled in this benefit (Centers for Medicare & Medicaid Services, 2007). Seniors can choose between adding a prescription drug plan to their traditional Medicare Part A and Part B (standard plan) or selecting a Medicare Advantage plan with prescription drug benefits (health maintenance organization [HMO] or preferred provider organization [PPO]), and over 88% have enrolled in these plans (U.S. Department of Health & Human Services, 2006; Centers for Medicare & Medicaid Services, 2007). Premiums average $22 a month,

and those choosing the standard plan are faced with a coverage gap, termed the "donut hole." There is a yearly deductible of $265, and then copayments of 25% up to a limit of $2,400. After that is reached, seniors pay out of pocket for drugs up to $3,850, when they reach what is termed the "catastrophic limit" and are only required to pay up to 5% (or a set fee) for medications (Center for Medicare Advocacy, 2007a).

Even though there are reported problems with Social Security and 7 of 10 Americans believe that it will go bankrupt, most do not believe there is a crisis (Morin & Russakoff, 2005; Center for Medicare Advocacy, 2007b). The system is for the most part secure, and most people who will reach retirement age in the next few decades have experienced a lifestyle well beyond what could be supported by the Social Security benefits they are scheduled to receive. "Social security was never meant to be the sole source of income in retirement" (SSA, 2006, p.16). This system was designed so that current workers pay benefits for current retirees, and investments of their overpayments earn interest. Even though more taxes are currently collected than the amounts paid out, this is changing. The worker-to-beneficiary ratio is now 3.3-to-1, whereas in 1950 it was 16.5-to-1; the ratio is expected to drop to 2-to-1 by 2046 (SSA, 2006). This means that people must plan early and contribute to a retirement fund at work (or establish their own retirement fund if self-employed), invest, and save regularly (Daaleman, 2006). These multiple sources of income at the time of retirement will provide the resources necessary so that decisions about when to start or how to spend one's retirement can be based on personal preference rather than a restricted and fixed Social Security check.

Characteristics of Healthy Older Adults

No one knows conclusively all of the variables that influence healthy aging, but it is known that a lifetime of healthy habits and circumstances, a strong social support system, and a positive emotional outlook all significantly influence the resources people bring to their later years. Most people recognize a healthy older person when they meet one. See From the Case Files I for an example of healthy aging.

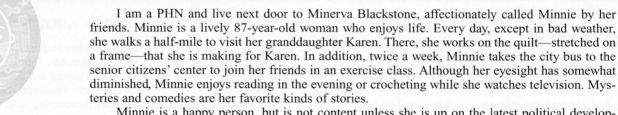

From the Case Files I

I am a PHN and live next door to Minerva Blackstone, affectionately called Minnie by her friends. Minnie is a lively 87-year-old woman who enjoys life. Every day, except in bad weather, she walks a half-mile to visit her granddaughter Karen. There, she works on the quilt—stretched on a frame—that she is making for Karen. In addition, twice a week, Minnie takes the city bus to the senior citizens' center to join her friends in an exercise class. Although her eyesight has somewhat diminished, Minnie enjoys reading in the evening or crocheting while she watches television. Mysteries and comedies are her favorite kinds of stories.

Minnie is a happy person, but is not content unless she is up on the latest political developments. She always has opinions on current events and expresses them with vigorous shakes of her curly white hair at her monthly group meeting on women and politics. She has a good appetite and generally sleeps well. Minor arthritis does not hamper her activities, nor does the hypertension that she controls by taking her medication with conscientious regularity. Minnie is enjoying a healthy, successful old age.

Carole Stokes, District PHN

What is healthy old age? As was mentioned earlier, the vast majority (94%) of our elderly, even those with chronic diseases or other disabilities, are living outside institutions and are relatively independent. Their ability to function is a key indicator of health and wellness and is an important factor in understanding healthy aging. Good health in the elderly means maintaining the maximum possible degree of physical, mental, and social vigor. It means being able to adapt, to continue to handle stress, and to be active and involved in life and living. In short, healthy aging means being able to function, even when disabled, with a minimum of help from others (CDC & Merck Co. Foundation, 2007).

Wellness among the older population varies considerably. It is influenced by many factors, including personality traits, life experiences, current physical health, and current societal supports and personal health behaviors including smoking, obesity, and excessive alcohol use. One way to measure healthy aging on a large scale is the degree to which states have met or exceeded targets on 11 of the *Healthy People 2010* older adult health indicators. For instance, we have already exceeded the goal of 70% of the population receiving mammograms within the past two years (75%). Colorectal screenings and checks for cholesterol have also been exceeded (63% versus 50% and 90% versus 80%, respectively). The number of people who currently smoke has also been reduced (CDC & Merck Co. Foundation, 2007). Other actions that can increase healthy aging include addressing health disparities among older adults, encouraging people to plan for end-of-life care and communicate their wishes through advance directives, improving oral health and increasing physical activity among seniors by promoting environmental changes, increasing adult immunization levels, and preventing falls (CDC & Merck Co. Foundation, 2007). Some elderly people demonstrate maximum adaptability, resourcefulness, optimism, and activity. Others, often those from whom we tend to draw our stereotypes, have disengaged and present a picture of dependence and resignation. Most of the elderly population fall somewhere in between these two extremes. Although the level of wellness varies among the elderly, that level can be raised. The goals in community health nursing are to maximize the wellness potential of elderly clients and to support their highest level of functional ability enabling them to remain independent. Nurses must analyze and build on an older person's strengths rather than focus on the difficulties or deficits. The goal for an aging population is to enable older people to thrive and have the highest quality of life for as long as possible, not merely to survive (Eliopoulos, 2004).

ELDER ABUSE

Elder abuse has reached epidemic proportions in the United States. Although estimates vary, it is believed that 4 to 6% of the elderly become victims of some form of abuse. One study estimated the frequency at between 2 to 10%. Recognition of elder abuse has been a relatively recent phenomenon (Dong, 2005; Lach & Pillemer, 2004). Some of the difficulty lies in the lack of national definitions of elder abuse or official statistics. There is also no uniform reporting law nationally (National Center on Elder Abuse, 2005). Elders are at increased risk for abuse due to social isolation, mental impairment, and dependency on others. **Elder abuse** is defined as the intentional or unintentional hurting, either physical or emotional, of a person who is age sixty or over. A recent large-scale survey of adult protective services (APS) revealed that there are 8.3 reports of abuse for every 1,000 American seniors (National Center on Elder Abuse, 2006). There are four general categories of elder abuse: (1) physical abuse, (2) psychological abuse, (3) neglect, and (4) financial abuse. It is important to note that financial abuse often accompanies one of the other forms of abuse. The financial abuse of seniors is a growing problem, often called the "Crime of the 21st Century." It is one of the most sinister forms of abuse. A senior can be financially stable and living independently one day, and become destitute and forced to live in a facility the next as a result of any one of the four types of abuse or a combination of abuses.

Sadly, most elder abuse occurs in the elder's home, and the abuser is usually a family member. Over 89% of alleged abuse occurs in a domestic setting, although abuse can occur in board and care or nursing home settings (National Center on Elder Abuse, 2005). In states reporting on the *2004 Survey of State Adult Protective Services*, almost half of all cases investigated were substantiated. Most victims of elder abuse are White (77.1%), and the majority of victims are reported to be over age 80 and female (National Center on Elder Abuse, 2006). The most common perpetrators of elder abuse are spouses or partners of elders. The next most frequent abuser is the adult child of the elder. An elder person in immediate danger should be removed from her environment (Gorbien & Eisenstein, 2005); however, elder abuse does not often come to the attention of PHNs or other providers of services to the elderly. It is estimated that five occurrences of neglect, abuse, exploitation, or self-neglect go unreported for every case that is reported. Financial exploitation is reported in only about 1 of 25 cases (National Center on Elder Abuse, 2005). Therefore, nurses working in the community with older adults must be vigilant for signs of elder abuse and knowledgeable about reporting laws.

Various state, local, and county agencies investigate and enforce elder abuse laws. The first agency to respond to a report of elder abuse in most states is APS. In some states, certain professionals are required or encouraged to report elder abuse. The people required to report elder abuse are generally doctors and nurses, psychologists, police officers, social workers, and employees of banks and other financial institutions. All elder abuse hotlines are free and anonymous (Gorbien & Eisenstein, 2005).

HEALTH NEEDS OF OLDER ADULTS

Effective nursing among any population requires familiarity with that group's health problems and needs. Aging, in and of itself, is not a health problem. Rather, aging is a normal, irreversible physiologic process. Its pace, however, can sometimes be slowed, as researchers are discovering, and many of the problems associated with aging can be prevented (Ebersole & Hess, 2004). The aging process is subtle, gradual, and lifelong. One can see remarkable differences among individuals in the rate of aging. Even in a single individual, various systems of the body age at different rates (Eliopoulos, 2004). Therefore, chronologic age cannot readily be a reliable indicator of health needs. However, the proportion of people with health problems increases with age, and as a group older adults are more likely than younger ones to suffer from multiple, chronic, and often disabling conditions requiring ongoing care and management.

The elderly, like any age group, have certain basic needs: physiologic and safety needs, as well as the needs for love and belonging, self-esteem, and self-actualization. Their physical, emotional, and social needs are complex and interrelated (Eliopoulos, 2004; Miller, 2003). The following sections discuss these needs according to primary, secondary, and tertiary prevention activities.

Primary Prevention

As discussed previously in this text, primary prevention activities involve those actions that keep one healthy. Such primary prevention activities as health education, follow-through of sound personal health practices (e.g., flossing, seat belt use, exercise), recommended routine screenings, and maintenance of an appropriate immunization schedule ensure that older adults are doing all that they can to maintain their health. The list in Display 24.2 includes strategies for successful aging. Taken from a variety of sources, it provides primary prevention activities the community health nurse can use when working with elders, either individually or in groups.

DISPLAY 24.2	STRATEGIES FOR SUCCESSFUL AGING

- Do at least 30 minutes of sustained, rhythmic, vigorous exercise four times a week.
- Eat "like a bushman" (a healthy diet of fruits, whole grains, vegetables, and lean meat).
- Get as much sleep and rest as needed.
- Maintain a sense of humor and deflect anger.
- Set goals and accept challenges that force you to be as alive and creative as possible.
- Don't depend on anyone else for your well-being.
- Be necessary and responsible; live outside yourself (give to others, become involved).
- Don't slow down. Stick with the mainstream. Avoid the shadows. Stay together. Maintain energy flow in a purposeful direction; aging need not be characterized by losses. Maintain contacts with family and friends, and stay active through work, recreation, and community.
- Get regular check-ups.
- Don't smoke—it's never too late to quit.
- Practice safety habits at home to prevent falls and fractures. Always wear seat belts when traveling by car.
- Avoid overexposure to the sun and the cold.
- If you drink, moderation is the key—when you drink, let someone else drive.
- Keep personal and financial records in order to simplify budgeting and investing—plan long-term housing and financial needs.
- Keep a positive attitude toward life—do things that make you happy.

Nutrition Needs

People who have maintained sound dietary habits throughout their life have little need to change in old age. Many have not established such habits, but may be required to do so because of disease processes such as diabetes or cardiovascular disease. It is generally believed that older people need to maintain their optimal weight by eating a diet that is low in fats, moderate in carbohydrates, and high in proteins with a daily calorie count of 1,200 to 1,600. Foods with "empty calories," such as salty snacks, candy, fatty foods, and alcohol, should be limited; they meet hunger needs by satisfying appetite only, while providing little nutrition. Cereals and whole grains, dried beans, and nuts can provide fiber needed by seniors, and eating colorful fruits and vegetables (rather than fruit juice) also contributes to fiber and may help to prevent macular degeneration (Center for the Advancement of Health, 2004). Another important thing to remind older adults to do is to drink adequate amounts of liquids, especially water. Eight glasses a day are recommended, and many older adults have a diminished feeling of thirst and can easily become dehydrated if they do not purposefully plan their fluid intake. Elders need less vitamin A, but more calcium and vitamin D (for healthy bones), more folic acid, and more vitamin B_6 and B_{12} (for cognitive health) than younger adults (Center for the Advancement of Health, 2004). Many communities offer meals to seniors, either at Senior Centers or by way of Meals on Wheels, through grants provided by the Elderly Nutrition Program (Administration on Aging, 2007b).

Major advances in the field of oral health including community water fluoridation, advanced dental technology, better oral hygiene, and more frequent use of dental services have had a substantial impact on the number of older adults who retain their natural teeth. Before the time of widespread fluoride use, it was common for people to lose most or all of their teeth by midlife (Ahluwalia, 2004). Most people can keep their natural teeth for a lifetime with preventive practices. Oral health is integral to general health and well being throughout one's life. A good deal of research has demonstrated the connection between oral health and general health due to chronic inflammation releasing cytokines and C-reactive protein causing endothelial damage and cholesterol plaque attachment in cardiovascular disease and stroke; poor oral health has also been associated with peripheral vascular disease, diabetes, and risk for death caused by pneumonia in nursing homes (Ahluwalia, 2004; Meurman, Sanz, & Janket, 2004; Rubinstein, 2005; Jurasek, 2002). Even those with dentures must be vigilant in maintaining oral health, as they are still at risk from inflammatory processes leading to diseases like pneumonia (Jurasek, 2002).

The oral health of older adults, however, is often neglected. Many older adults, especially those with limited or fixed incomes or cognitive limitations, are not able to maintain their oral health or visit a dentist on a regular basis. Medicare does not cover routine dental services. Maintaining oral health during the senior years is more difficult for many reasons: lack of dental insurance after retirement, economic disadvantages and limited incomes, decreased nutritional and fluid intake, changes in gums and increased periodontal disease, as well as a higher incidence of dry mouth (Gupta, Epstein, & Sroussi, 2006). "Over 400 commonly used medications can be the cause of a dry mouth," and certain disease processes produce dry mouth symptoms, but the elderly also have a natural decrease in saliva flow (Gupta et al., 2006; CDC, 2006b, p. 9). Saliva contains minerals for rebuilding of tooth enamel as well as "antimicrobial components" (CDC, 2006b, p. 9). Fluid intake and oral hygiene are appropriate topics for anticipatory guidance from PHNs for older adults.

We are very close to achieving the goal specified in Health People 2010 to reduce the number of adults with complete tooth loss to 20%. The percentage of U.S. adults aged 65 to 74 who experience complete tooth loss has declined from 55% (1957–1958) to 24% (1999–2002) (U.S. Department of Health & Human Services [USDHHS], 2000). Oral health and hygiene needs do not decrease with age. Eating, chewing, and swallowing should be an uncomplicated and natural process. Eating should remain a pleasurable social experience, preferably taking place in the company of others. Community health nurses can assist older adults with meal management by following the suggestions outlined in Display 24.3 and Figure 24.1.

In addition to maintaining a healthy diet, older adults are cautioned to limit the use of alcohol, avoid tobacco, drink fluoridated water or use fluoride toothpaste, and practice good oral hygiene and have regular dental checkups

---

DISPLAY 24.3 MEAL MANAGEMENT CONSIDERATIONS

- Complete a safety check with the older adult to assess the ability to operate stoves and microwave ovens. Include the elder's ability to reach, and put things on and off stove burners.
- Arrange cupboards so commonly used items can be reached from an easy standing level.
- Suggest use of turntables and long-handled "grabbers" while discouraging use of step stools or ladders.
- Assess the elder's typical meal for quality and availability—can be accomplished for all meals by doing a 24-hour dietary recall—begin with the most recent meal and work backwards.
- To ensure that elders eat an appropriate number of times a day, suggest that they "eat by the clock" or with a certain TV show.
- Help older adults build support system for sharing grocery shopping, cooking, and meals.
- Suggest they bake once a week for an activity or shop with another elder.
- Suggest buying convenience foods, making sure they have nutritional value, such as frozen vegetables or dinners.
- Consider community resources to assist with shopping, transportation, or meal preparation as needed. Keeping a continuous shopping list helps elders to remember needed grocery items, and provides a reference if someone offers to assist with shopping.
- Help elders consider increasing socialization by eating together with friends—rotating among three to four friends each week or eating out with friends, selecting restaurants that are physically and financially accessible.

(CDC, 2006b). They should also avoid the habitual use of laxatives, instead adding more fiber and bulk to their diet with fresh fruits and vegetables. Also inadequate fluid intake can contribute to bowel and bladder problems. Following a diet that includes eight or more 8-oz glasses of fluid (water, juices, tea) each day assists the gastrointestinal and genitourinary system in their functions. Increased physical activity and exercise helps keep an older adult's bowel patterns regular (Center for the Advancement of Health, 2004).

Exercise Needs

Older adults need to exercise; in fact, they thrive when exercise is incorporated into their daily routine (Burbank & Riebe, 2002). Research demonstrates that exercise and increased physical activity can slow the loss of bone density and increase the size and strength of muscles, including the heart, as well as increase the action of insulin and improve sleep and functional abilities of the elderly (Ballard, McFarland, Wallace, Holiday, & Roberson, 2004; Fahlman, Morgan, McNevin, Topp, & Boardley, 2007; Sato, Nagasaki, Kubota, Uno, & Nakai, 2007; USDHHS, 2000; Woo, Hong, Lau, & Lynn, 2007). Aging does not and should not involve passivity; instead, physical activity and movement contribute to the quality of intellectual and physical performance in old age. Exercise, such as a daily walk, can keep muscles in good tone, enhance circulation, and promote mental health and adequate sleep (Chen, Li, & Lin, 2007; Sato et al., 2007). Exercise may occur in connection with such activities as homemaking chores, gardening, hobbies, or recreation and sports. Often, such physical outlets are enjoyed in the company of other people, meeting social and emotional needs as well as physical ones. Even among the very old, an exercise routine that includes activities that improve strength, flexibility, and coordination may indirectly, but effectively, decrease the incidence of osteoporotic fractures by lessening the likelihood of falling (Ballard et al., 2004; Fahlman et al., 2007; Ettinger, 2003). Resistance training (with small dumbells or resistance bands), along with either Tai Chi or regular walking, has been shown to increase muscle strength, stability, and functional ability among seniors (Fahlman et al., 2007; Woo et al., 2007).

Public health nurses can encourage exercise among elderly clients and examine factors that prevent them from regularly exercising (Kressig & Echt, 2002). A recent study found that physical ailments were the most common barrier to exercise, whereas health concerns were the strongest motivators for older adults (Newsom & Kemps, 2007).

Economic Security Needs

Economic security is another major need for older adults. Worrying about finances is often one of the most debilitating factors of old age. Fearing the potential cost of major illness and not wanting to be a burden on family or friends, many older people conserve their limited finances by establishing frugal eating patterns, using health resources sparingly, not taking their medications or only taking medications in partial doses, reducing costs for home heating and cooling, and, in general, spending little on themselves (Eliopoulos, 2004). Elderly people sometimes have to choose between food, housing, and medications. Another factor that is driving up the cost of health care for the aging population is that many elderly clients wait

Modified MyPyramid for Older Adults

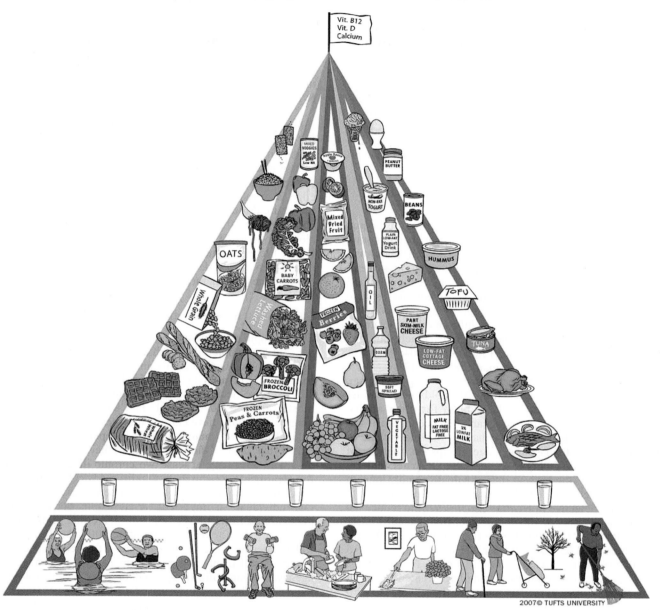

FIGURE 24.1 Modified MyPyramid for older adults. Copyright 2007 Tufts University. Reprinted with permission from Lichtenstein, A.H., Rasmussen, H., Yu, W.W., Epstein, S.R., Russell, R.M. Modified MyPyramid for Older Adults. *J Nutr.* 2008; 138:78–82.

until they are truly ill before seeking health care. In waiting for conditions to improve or go away, the elderly often miss out on important preventive health measures and community based programs that can maximize function and help the client maintain health at a higher level (Ezekowitz, Straus, Majumdar, & McAlister, 2003). Too often, the fear—let alone the reality—of financial difficulties prevents older adults from leading full and active lives (Stoller, 2003).

For older adults today who have lived many years past retirement and perhaps have not planned for sufficient financial security to maintain them throughout these additional, unexpected years, the fears are not unfounded. Putting older people in touch with appropriate community resources can do much to relieve the source of that stress and anxiety. The com-

munity health nurse can also provide information about potential consumer fraud (e.g., telemarketing schemes) targeted to the elderly. This is a form of financial abuse perpetrated by criminals who have no personal relationship with the victims, and seniors with retirement income, savings accounts, or property are disproportionately targeted (Cohen, 2006). Losses from this type of fraud can wipe out a lifetime of savings, and leave the older adult feeling foolish and helpless.

Psychosocial Needs

All human beings have psychosocial needs that must be met for their lives to be rich and fulfilling. Without healthy relationships with other people, life can be very lonely and lacking in quality. With advancing age, the psychosocial issues are many. A major issue that confronts the majority of our aging population is coping with multiple losses (Chong, 2007). In addition, maintaining independence, social interaction, companionship, and purpose is necessary for a healthy old age. Older adults who have maintained good health and have developed a supportive system of family and friends have more fulfilled lives (Owen, 2007). Programs such as Friendly Visitors, where volunteers regularly meet with isolated seniors either in their homes or long-term care facilities, can be an effective method of increasing social support for those who have no family members nearby (The Senior Source, 2007).

Coping with Multiple Losses

Elders experience multiple losses, including loss of income and prestige from a career once practiced or the economic stability of an enjoyable job; loss of space due to replacement of a larger residence by a much smaller home or apartment; and reductions in health and vitality that may result in limited movement or pain as a daily concern or may necessitate another move to a more dependent living environment. Repetitive losses occur as elders' significant others, relatives, friends, and acquaintances die; the "bereavement burden" may sometimes be hard to bear (Eliopoulos, 2004; Williams, Sawyer-Baker, Allman, & Roseman, 2007, p. 313).

Inadequate coping with the compounding losses can make an older person believe that life holds no meaning. Depression may be a difficult problem for older adults. Social and emotional withdrawal can often occur, as can suicide. Although older populations have a much lower rate of suicide attempts than younger age groups do, the rate of completed suicide is high. As mentioned earlier, elderly White men have the highest rate of suicide death. Concern for the increased suicide rates among older White men led to a key health objective in *Healthy People 2010*: to reduce the suicide rate to 38.9 per 100,000 people, from the 1987 baseline of 46.1 per 100,000 (USDHHS, 2000). By 1997, for White men aged 65 years or older, the suicide rate was 35.5 per 100,000, thus exceeding the 2010 goal. Because most elderly persons who commit suicide have visited their primary care provider in the last month of their lives, recognition and treatment of depression in health care settings is a promising way to prevent suicide in this age group.

Mortality after bereavement is high and can sometimes be prevented through nursing intervention. Loss and the mourning process among elders have been examined in many studies. It has been found that the ability to mourn prior states of one's self and the past is crucial to successful aging. Life review can be liberating and can provide energy for current living, including planning for the future; in one study higher levels of self-affirmation, confidence, self-esteem, and life satisfaction were noted (Chiang, Lu, Chu, Chang, & Chou, 2007). Although men and women experience similar levels of depression during early bereavement, it is often more difficult for men to seek and receive social support. One Israeli study found that more highly educated men had the greatest difficulty with bereavement (Manor & Eisenbach, 2003). Depression has been found to increase the risk of death for elderly who have lost a spouse, independent of age or bereavement.

The death of a spouse has effects upon the health of the surviving spouse, and depression can exacerbate these effects (Williams, 2005). In addition, grief over the loss of a spouse can continue for many years, as one study revealed. A large study of widows revealed that they "continued to talk, think, and feel emotions about their lost spouse decades later" — even as much as 20 years after their loss—indicating that the time course for grief is extensive (Carnelley, Wortman, Bolger, & Burke, 2006, p. 476).

In addition to preventing early deaths after the loss of a spouse, the greater goal for the nurse in promoting successful aging can be accomplished when the nurse recognizes the significance of accepting all the losses of aging. The loss of a spouse is much more frequent for women than for men (Eliopoulos, 2004; Carnelley et al., 2006). With this knowledge, a woman can age more successfully by planning for the future through anticipatory guidance, with the help of a community health nurse. Many women can expect to live alone for up to 20 years at the end of their life, because of a longer life expectancy and the fact that women in most cultures marry men older than themselves. The nurse can help to make these years meaningful and as healthy as possible.

Maintaining Independence

Older people need independence, and those who stay independent are happier. As much as possible, the elderly need to make their own decisions and manage their own lives. Even those with activity limitations because of disability can still exercise decision-making options about many, if not most, aspects of their daily living. Unfortunately, because many older adults have chronic diseases, it can be more difficult for them to maintain their independence. It is estimated that 75% of those over age 65 have one chronic illness, and 50% have at least two chronic illnesses (Agency for Healthcare Research & Quality [AHRQ], 2002). The need for autonomy—to be able to assert oneself as a separate individual—is important for all people. For the elderly person, with restrictions of life ever increasing, this need is even more pronounced (Eliopoulos, 2004; Miller, 2003). Independence helps to meet the need for self-respect and dignity. A self-management program, developed by a federal agency, is being utilized to prevent or delay disability among the elderly. The Chronic Disease Self-Management Program teaches patients to better manage their medications and symptoms, and to maintain greater functional ability. Those who have participated in this program have shown better communication with their physicians (and fewer MD visits and hospitalizations) and better coping and symptom management, along with more energy and increased exercise six months later. The reduced numbers of physician visits and emergency room visits, along with improvements in health status, energy, self-efficacy, and no further increases in disability, were noted at one year and two years postintervention (AHRQ, 2002). The good news is that the percentage of older adults becoming severely disabled has been gradually declining for over a decade, thought to be due to better awareness of the dangers of smoking, the need for better diet and exercise, new medications for cardiovascular and other diseases, and advances in eye surgery (Freudenheim, 2001).

The elderly need to have their ideas and suggestions heard and acted upon, and they ought to be addressed by their preferred names in a respectful tone of voice. Respect for the older adult is not a strong value in American society, but it is highly valued in Asian, Italian, Hispanic, and Native American cultures (Spector, 2004). Older people represent a rich resource of wisdom, experience, and patience that is often unacknowledged in the United States.

Social Interaction, Companionship, and Purpose

Older people need companionship and social interaction, particularly if they live alone. The company of other people and the companionship of a household pet offer avenues for expression and response and add meaning to life (Owen, 2007). Many studies of mortality patterns demonstrate that older adults living together have a greater survival rate and retain their independence longer than do those who live alone (Eliopoulos, 2004). As people age, their social networks weaken and community health nurses and others can help to improve their psychosocial health by working at individual, family, and community levels (Chong, 2007). The problem is of greatest significance for women, who outnumber men considerably in the later years and who live alone more frequently.

It is also important for older adults without companions to discover and develop a friendship with someone who can be considered a *confidante*, someone in whom the older adult can confide, share reflections on the past, and trust (Yang, 2006). It could be a close friend, a sibling, a son or daughter, or an acquaintance. This person is usually seen daily or talked with on the telephone each week. In particular, mothers and daughters form confidant bonds. Many women consider a sibling a confidant, especially if that person lives close by; this is especially true for childless and single women.

Meaningful activity is another need of the elderly that adds purpose to life. Some kind of active role in community life is essential for mental health, satisfaction, and self-esteem (Warburton, McLaughlin, & Pinsker, 2006). These activities can range from involvement in hobbies, such as gardening or crafts, to volunteer work or even full-time employment. Examples include the federally supported Foster Grandparents and Senior Companions programs, which engage the help of more than 20,000 seniors (Corporation for National & Community Service, 2007). These older adults work part-time offering companionship and guidance to handicapped children, the terminally ill, and other people in need.

Additional volunteering opportunities abound. Internationally, many older professionals join the Peace Corps, which was initiated in the early 1960s. In this program, people of all ages work for 2-year periods in global communities that are in need of services to improve personal health, education, environment, and the larger community (Peace Corps, 2007). On the national level, the newer AmeriCorps*VISTA (Volunteers in Service to America) programs are similar, but with a 1-year commitment; the volunteer lives among and at the economic level of the low-income people in the United States served by its projects. Retired people can volunteer to help others, donating their skills at a time in their lives when they are in transition from employment to retirement or to fill active retirement years (AmeriCorps, 2007). The Retired and Senior Volunteer Program (RSVP) engages seniors in a bevy of activities designed to improve people's lives and the environment (Senior Corps, 2007). Environmental Alliance for Senior Involvement (EASI) is a nonprofit coalition of aging, volunteer, and environmental organizations that began in 1991. It sponsors various environmentally focused programs, such as assisting the Hawk Mountain Sanctuary to protect birds of prey, or monitoring streams and other waterways for cleanliness (EASI, 2007).

Many older adults choose not to engage in long-term volunteering, and other programs are more appropriate for them. Elderhostel is a nonprofit organization with more than 25 years of experience providing high-quality, affordable, educational adventures for adults who are 55 years of age and older. It is the nation's first and the world's largest education and travel organization for older adults, offering "more than 8,000 learning adventures in all 50 states and more than 90 countries" (Elderhostel, 2007). Their theme-based, short-term (3 days to 3 weeks) educational programs are infused with a spirit of camaraderie and adventure. The success of this program is based on the fact that learning is a lifelong process that is rewarding at any age—and it is learning without any test or term papers! Elderhostel is inspired by the youth hostels and folk schools of Europe, but guided by the needs and interests of older citizens.

Safety Needs

People of all ages have safety needs, and safety issues are a major concern for older adults and the community health nurses who work with them. Several areas of focus are discussed here: personal health and safety, home safety, and community safety.

Personal health and safety includes three major areas: immunizations, prevention of falls, and drug safety. Immunizations are not just for children. Older adults are at risk not only of contracting influenza or pneumonia but of dying from them. During the last decade pneumococcal disease and influenza accounted for close to 40,000 annual deaths among those age 65 and above (CDC, 2003c). Other estimates put the annual death rate from influenza alone at over 41,000 (Dushoff, Plotkin, Viboud, Earn, & Simonsen, 2005). Although the overall influenza immunization rate among elders has steadily increased "from between 15% and 20% before 1980 to 65% in 2001," exceeding the *Healthy People 2000* target as early as 1997, some seniors still refuse to have yearly vaccinations (CDC, 2003c). Reasons most often cited by those 65 years and older for not getting flu shots are lack of knowledge that it is necessary, and concern that the flu shot might give them the flu or result in other side effects (CDC, 2004). Though steady increases have been shown overall, there remain racial and ethnic disparities in senior vaccination rates (Simonsen, Reichert, Viboud, Blackwelder, Taylor, & Miller, 2005, p. 265; CDC, 2003c). These racial and ethnic disparities were found even in groups who are usually most likely to avail themselves of health care services (e.g., those with higher education levels, those who have more frequent visits to health care providers). The reasons for the continuing disparity are not well understood, but are thought to be related to differences in care settings (lower vaccination rates with particular providers), lack of trust in providers, and communication problems, especially with those who do not speak English well. It appears that this problem can be solved with increased attention and consistency; the disparities are absent in Veterans Administration clinics where there are standing orders for influenza vaccination and systems that prompt providers to offer necessary vaccinations (Fiscella, 2005; CDC, 2004). When PHNs work with seniors, it is important to include outreach efforts, such as culturally targeting communication, reaching out to those providers serving this population, and offering vaccination clinics in underserved sections of the community (CDC, 2004).

Although pneumococcal vaccine coverage rates have also increased steadily from 38.4% in 1995 to 54.9% in 1999, improvement is still needed (Johnson, 2003). Only 16% of states met the *Healthy People 2000* goal of 60% vaccine coverage for a disease that is thought to result in over 175,000 hospitalizations annually (National Foundation for Infectious Diseases [NFID], 2002). Some question the validity of self-reported pneumococcal vaccination because this is, for most, a one time vaccination sometimes given many years before the survey is done, and it is often given with an influenza vaccine, causing confusion (Johnson, 2003). Despite the increases, coverage rates for certain racial and ethnic groups remain substantially below those of the general population (30% for Hispanics, 31% for African Americans) (NFID, 2002). Attempts to improve immunization coverage involve changing provider knowledge, attitudes, and behavior through reminders and standing orders, so that "missed opportunities" when seeing clients are prevented. One simple method is to ask clients about their beliefs and fears related to immunizations and then to address them directly and honestly (Fiscella, 2005). Additional opportunities for vaccinating people exist beyond the primary care setting, as community health nurses are well aware. People can be reached during emergency department visits, at neighborhood and senior centers, at religious facilities, and in other settings where elders may gather. Regardless of the site, a method for tracking and communicating vaccinations is needed so that vaccination information may be documented and shared with the elder's primary care provider. Some studies have reported that clinicians often fail to document immunizations for adult patients (Johnson, 2003). Immunizations protect more than the at-risk population; they protect society as a whole. People of any age with a chronic illness, such as heart disease, diabetes, or chronic respiratory disease, and people older than 65 years of age, should be encouraged to receive the flu vaccine each year and the pneumonia vaccine every 5 years.

Each year, approximately one-third of people older than 65 years of age who are independent and living on their own experience a fall, and falls occur for half of those over 80 years of age and for those individuals residing in long-term care settings (RAND Health, 2003; Hill-Westmoreland, Soeken, & Spellbring, 2002). Falls and the resulting injuries can have a dramatic impact on self-confidence and independence, often leading to decreased mobility, increased debility, and diminished quality of life as well as additional strain on health services. The injuries received from a fall can result in death, disability, nursing home admission, and direct medical costs. In 2003, a total of 1,700 persons aged 65 and older died from falls, and 1.8 million were treated in emergency departments for nonfatal injuries from falls. The average cost of health care due to a fall for a person 72 years and older has been estimated at close to $20,000. Falls cause the majority of hip fractures, which can often result in long-term functional impairments that may require admission to a nursing home for up to a year or more (CDC, 2007a; Stevens,

Corso, Finkelstein, & Miller, 2006). In 2000, medical costs were over $19 billion, and by 2020, the total cost of fall injuries could reach $43.8 billion (CDC, 2007a; Stevens et al., 2006). Causative factors involve both environmental hazards (e.g., lack of handrails and nonslip surfaces) and host issues (e.g., cognition, vision). Fall prevention, which involves education, strengthening and balance exercises, medication evaluation, and environmental improvements, is an important function of the community health nurse. Research has identified interventions that can reduce falls, but development and implementation of community-based programs remains limited (National Council on Aging, 2005; RAND Health, 2003; Rose, 2003). Use of a home safety checklist can give the nurse a baseline of information from which to begin teaching and providing interventions to ensure continued safety for many independent seniors who choose to remain in their homes (Display 24.4).

A significant safety issue for the older adult arises from adverse drug effects. Older people may need to take several medications to control the effects of chronic conditions, and their bodies can react differently than those of younger people (on whom most new drugs are tested). Absorption time is usually slower, distribution changes as drugs may stay in the body longer due to a higher percentage of fat stores, and reduced liver and kidney function affect clearance time for medications in elderly clients (Wooten & Galavis, 2005). Also, it is not unusual for older people to be taking four to six medications daily and filling 13 prescriptions or more each year. It is estimated that people over age 65 (13% of population) receive 30% of prescriptions and over half of all over the counter medications purchased (Wooten & Galavis, 2005; Bushardt & Jones, 2005). Elders often receive multiple prescriptions from multiple providers, and sometimes from multiple pharmacies, and are in danger of receiving double doses of the same or similar medications. This can happen, for instance, when one health care provider prescribes a name-brand medication and a second one writes a prescription for the same medication, but in generic form. Often, the elderly person has no idea that they are taking two doses of the same medication (Bushardt & Jones, 2005). Also, common medications like acetaminophen can be found in a variety of over the counter and prescription medications (e.g., cold remedies, arthritis topical ointments) and inadvertent overdosing can be a real problem (Bushardt & Jones, 2005). Most adverse drug events (ADEs) are due to drug interactions. The greater number of medications taken, the more likely there will be side effects (Wooten & Galavis, 2005). Multiple medications or complicated drug regimens for many older people can lead to unexpected and dangerous drug interactions or drug–disease interactions; sometimes medications are prescribed for symptoms that may actually be a side effect of an original medication, leading to a "prescribing cascade" (Wooten & Galavis, 2005). Medication side effects or drug interactions can lead to falls and further disability. Elderly clients need education about the drugs they take and their possible effects. They also need proper supervision of their overall medication intake, including complementary and alternative therapies (e.g., herbal treatments) and over the counter drugs. It is also important for all seniors to keep a list of their current medications and doses and to have this available in the event of an emergency. However, many hospitals and providers prefer the "brown bag method" of determining accurate medication information, in which they

DISPLAY 24.4 GUIDELINES FOR ASSESSING THE SAFETY OF THE ENVIRONMENT

Illumination and Color Contrast
- Is the lighting adequate but not glare producing?
- Are the light switches easy to reach and manipulate?
- Can lights be turned on before entering rooms?
- Are night lights used in appropriate places?
- Are there working flashlights close by (bedroom, kitchen, bath, living room)?
- Is color contrast adequate between objects such as a chair and floor?

Hazards
- Are there throw rugs, highly polished floors, or other hazardous floor coverings?
- If area rugs are used, do they have a nonslip backing and are the edges tacked to the floor?
- Are there cords, clutter, or other obstacles in pathways?
- Is there a pet that is likely to be running underfoot?

Furniture
- Are chairs the right height and depth for the person?
- Do the chairs have arm rests?
- Are tables stable and of the appropriate height?
- Is small furniture placed well away from pathways?

Stairways
- Is lighting adequate?
- Are there light switches at the top and bottom of the stairs?
- Are there securely fastened handrails on both sides of the stairway?
- Are all the steps even?
- Are the treads nonskid?
- Should colored tape be used to mark the edges of the steps, particularly the top and bottom steps?

Bathroom
- Are grab bars placed appropriately for the tub and toilet?
- Does the tub have skid proof strips or a rubber mat in the bottom?
- Has the person considered using a tub seat?
- Is the height of the toilet seat appropriate?
- Has the person considered using an elevated toilet seat?
- Does the color of the toilet seat contrast with surrounding colors?
- Is toilet paper within easy reach?

Temperature
- Is the temperature of the room(s) comfortable?
- Can the person read the markings on the thermostat and adjust it appropriately?
- During cold months, is the room temperature high enough to prevent hypothermia?
- During hot weather, is the room temperature cool enough to prevent hyperthermia?

Overall Safety
- How does the person obtain objects from hard-to-reach places?
- How does the person change overhead light bulbs?
- Are doorways wide enough to accommodate assistive devices?

- Do door thresholds create hazardous conditions?
- Are telephones easily accessible, especially for emergency calls?
- Would it be helpful to use a cordless portable phone or a cellular phone?
- Would it be helpful to have some emergency call system available?
- Does the person wear sturdy shoes with nonskid soles?
- Are smoke alarms present and operational?
- Is there a carbon monoxide detector (if the house has gas appliances)?
- Does the person keep a list of emergency numbers by the phone?
- Does the person have an emergency exit plan in the event of fire?

Bedroom
- Is the height of the bed appropriate?
- Is the mattress firm at the edges to provide enough support for sitting?
- If the bed has wheels, are they locked securely?
- Would side rails be a help or a hazard?
- When side rails are in the down position, are they completely out of the way?
- Is the pathway between the bedroom and bathroom clear of objects and adequately illuminated, particularly at night?
- Would a bedside commode be useful, especially at night?
- Does the person have sufficient physical and cognitive ability to turn on a light before getting out of bed?
- Is furniture positioned to allow safe use of assistive devices for ambulation?
- Is a telephone situated near the bed?

Kitchen
- Are storage areas used to the best advantage (e.g., are objects that are most frequently used in the most accessible places)?
- Are appliance cords kept out of the way?
- Are nonslip mats used in front of the sink?
- Are the markings on stoves and other appliances clearly visible?
- Does the person know how to use the microwave oven and other appliances safely?

Assistive Devices
- What assistive devices are used?
- Is a call light available, and does the person know how to use it?
- Would the person benefit from any assistive devices that are not being used?
- Are assistive devices being used safely and properly, or do they present additional hazards?

Adapted from Miller, C.A. (2003). *Nursing care of older adults: Theory and practice* (4th ed.). Philadelphia: Lippincott, Williams & Wilkins.

Environmental assessments and modifications are only part of an effective multifactorial fall prevention program. Medication assessment and medical evaluation (e.g., gait, balance, strength, vision, orthostatic blood pressure, and cognitive and functional status) need to be done, and an exercise program instituted (RAND, 2003).

are asked to bring everything they take with them (Wooten & Galavis, 2005). This is an area in which the community health nurse can intervene very effectively and with much success (see Display 24.5).

Safety in the community is an additional concern. Safety can involve many things, such as pedestrian and driving issues, crime and fear of crime against elders, and environmental factors such as sun exposure, pollution, heat, and cold.

Because of age-related changes in vision, hearing, mobility, and the effects of polypharmacy, elders are at risk in the community as pedestrians and as drivers. Automobile crashes and pedestrian injuries can be life-threatening events when elders are involved. As pedestrians, elders must be increasingly vigilant to traffic patterns, sidewalk irregularities, and the possibility of being a victim of street crime. Often out of necessity and pride, elders drive longer than their abilities permit. As people age, they are more prone to lapses in memory and attention, problems with depth perception and gauging distance of cars in traffic, reduced manual dexterity and reaction time, and impairment of other skills critical to driving safety (The Raw Story, 2007). Older adults age 65 and older have the second highest rate of death in car accidents, after those in the 15 to 24 age-range group. As the Baby Boomers age, this rate is expected to climb. The risk of death for a driver over the age of 85 is four times higher than for those 21 and younger (Agence France-Presse, 2007). Most accidents for people 65 years and older involve a seat-belted, sober driver, "pulling into the path of an oncoming vehicle during the day and dying several days after" the moderately severe collision (University of Virginia News, 2006, p.1). Because they generally have chronic diseases and are often frail, they are more susceptible to injury than younger drivers. Stopping driving is usually a difficult and painful decision for the elder to make. Some communities offer specialized driving classes for elders who want to continue to drive for as long as possible. At times, the car keys may have to be taken from the elder for her own safety and that of others. This may be necessary especially with elders who have dementia, AD, uncorrectable vision problems, or stroke-related physical or cognitive aftereffects. Only ten states require mandatory eye testing for drivers over 65 years of age, just five states require seniors to renew their drivers' licenses in person, and only two states require a mandatory road test (Agence France-Press, 2007). Public health nurses may need to consult with older adults and their families about determining when it is time for elders to stop driving.

Actual crime against elders in the community is lower than any other age group of the population: 2.8 per 1,000 cases for 65 and over versus 12 to 48.4 for those 50 to 64 years old and 20 to 24 years old, respectively (U.S. Department of Justice, 2006). However, the fear of crime among elders is often perceived as a major issue by the general public, and some research has shown both increased and decreased levels of fear in older adults (Acierno, Rheingold, Resnick, & Kilpatrick, 2004; Ziegler & Mitchell, 2003). Some researchers believe that the disposition to fear is more related to personality characteristics and other factors such as social isolation, depressive symptoms, and race (Acierno et al., 2004). Display 24.6 lists client-centered nursing interventions designed to reduce fear among older adults and empower them to feel safer in their communities.

Environmental factors can have an effect on the health and safety of elders when they are outside. Sun exposure, pollution, and exposure to heat and cold can have negative effects on older adults. They are vulnerable, as are infants and children, to climatic changes and should take a variety of preventive measures, including using sun block when gardening, reading, or walking outside for longer than 10 minutes, even on days with an overcast sky. Other measures include staying indoors on days when the air quality is poor or there is an air safety alert, drinking additional fluids, wearing protective covering, and limiting outdoor activities and exposure on days with elevated temperatures; and, conversely, limiting outdoor exposure and wearing appropriate

---

DISPLAY 24.5	**PROMOTING POLYPHARMACY SAFETY IN THE ELDERLY THROUGH MEDICATION REVIEW**

- Ask the client to bring all of her medications for you to examine.
- List all medications, along with dosage and time taken.
- Note the pharmacy or pharmacies where each prescription originates. Has more than one physician prescribed medications for the client?
- Ask about medical conditions and diseases for which she takes medications. Does the client have a clear understanding of each medication and its benefits and potential side effects?
- Ask the client for which condition or disease each medication is prescribed. Does the client understand the basic disease process and how the prescribed medication works?
- Are there duplicate medications (e.g., contain the same active ingredient, both a generic and a proprietary form)?
- What are the most common side effects of each medication?
- Is the dosage prescribed within the recommended range?
- Is the client experiencing any symptoms of potential drug interactions (e.g., nausea, headaches, dizziness)?
- Is one medication being used to treat possible side effects of another medication?
- Ask the client if she takes all medications as prescribed. Does she skip doses or medications?
- Does she use a daily/weekly pill box? Does she have some system of checking off when she has taken her medications each day?
- Is the client taking any medications that were prescribed for someone else?
- Is the client taking any over-the-counter or herbal remedies?

Adapted from: Wooten, J., & Galavis, J. (2005). *Polypharmacy: Keeping the elderly safe.* RNWeb. Retrieved August 18, 2008 from http://www.rnweb.com/rnweb/content/printContentPopup.jsp?id=172920; and Bushardt, R., & Jones, K. (2005). Nine key questions to address polypharmacy in the elderly. *Journal of the American Academy of Physician Assistants.* Retrieved August 18, 2008 from http://jaapa.com/issues/j20050501/articles/polypharm0505.htm.

DISPLAY 24.6 REDUCING THE FEAR OF CRIME

- Allow elder adults time to discuss their fears of crime.
- Facilitate a realistic self-assessment of their ability to avoid crime and to defend themselves.
- Teach basic safety and security techniques.
- Correct the elder's sensory losses if possible, such as by getting a hearing aid or glasses.
- Correct a physical disability if possible, such as by treating the pain of arthritis or obtaining physical therapy.
- Facilitate access to safe, reliable, and affordable transportation.
- Identify family members, friends, neighbors, or caregivers who can support efforts to leave the home on a more regular basis.
- Encourage an elder to make a daily telephone or e-mail contact with at least one supportive person.
- Encourage the elder to get to know his or her neighbors.
- Encourage elders to travel and conduct community activities and errands together.
- Encourage participation in local senior centers and other community-based programs.
- Refer to alternative housing options available for older adults.
- Provide information on local services that assist and support crime victims.

winter clothing, especially layers of clothes, on cold, snowy, or icy days (CDC, 2006c). Although sun exposure is beneficial in vitamin D production, older adults need to be careful about limiting their exposure. Teaching geographically and seasonally appropriate safety precautions is the responsibility of the community health nurse providing services to groups of elders in the community.

Spirituality, Advance Directives, Hospice, Palliative Care, and Preparing for Death

A final need of the elderly is preparing for a dignified death. In her classic work, Elisabeth Kübler-Ross (1975) described death as the final stage of growth and one that deserves the same measure of quality as other stages of life. Although death is a natural part of life, many older people fear death as an experience of pain, humiliation, discomfort, or financial concern for their loved ones. Sometimes, very aggressive and heroic medical treatments are offered to those near the end of their lives, often at the urging of family members (Richardson et al., 2007). Planning for a dignified death is an important issue for many older people, and PHNs can facilitate conversations among family members and provide necessary information and resources.

A commonly used option that takes a multidisciplinary approach to end of life care and needs is **hospice**. Hospice has been available in the United States since the mid-1970s. Hospice is more a concept of care than a specific place,

although some hospice organizations provide individuals with a place to die with dignity if they have no home or choose not to die at home. Hospice is an option for people with a "projected" life expectancy of six months or less and often involves palliative care (pain and symptom relief) as opposed to ongoing curative measures. Hospice enables many elderly clients to live their end days to the fullest, with purpose, dignity, grace, and support; in fact, one recent large scale study found that hospice patients survived 29 days longer than nonhospice patients (National Hospice & Palliative Care Organization, 2007). Hospice care focuses on all aspects of an individual's life and well being: physical, social, emotional, and spiritual (O'Brien, 2003). Individuals are permitted to go on and off hospice care as needed, or if they change their mind and decide to return to curative treatment. Some community health nursing agencies offer hospice programs staffed by their nurses. It is a service that has been well received by elders, meets important needs, and is growing in use. (See Chapter 32 for more.)

Palliative care consists of comfort and symptom management and does not provide a cure. For most chronic ongoing health conditions—such as diabetes, high blood pressure, congestive heart failure, arthritis, and chronic obstructive pulmonary disease—there are no cures, only symptom relief. Relative to the elderly population, which suffers from more chronic conditions than the rest of the population, palliative care should not be viewed as synonymous with hospice or end-of-life care. Rather, palliative care should be viewed as any care primarily intended to relieve the burden of physical and emotional suffering that often accompanies the illnesses associated with aging. Palliative care should be a major focus of care throughout the aging process, regardless of whether death is imminent within six months (Jerant, Azari, Nesbitt, Edwards-Goodbee, & Meyers, 2006).

Many seniors are now "pre-planning" their funerals. This option is gaining momentum in the senior population and allows individuals to make arrangements with a funeral home of their choice, selecting interment or cremation, a memorial service or a celebration of life gathering, music to be played, and other personal details. All options are chosen by the senior rather than leaving these choices and decisions solely to their family members. Other older adults may place less emphasis on the rituals, as was demonstrated by one elder who left these choices to her children by telling them, "Surprise me!"

Living wills and advance health care directives (AHCD), sometimes referred to as *advance directives*, are legal documents that instruct others about end-of-life choices should an individual be unable to make decisions on their own. An AHCD only becomes effective under the circumstances specified in the document. This document allows for appointment of a health care agent who will have the legal authority to make health care decisions on behalf of the patient, and for specific written instructions for future health care in the event of any situation in which the patient can no longer speak for herself. Having such documents prepared and making them known to significant others can ensure that wishes will be honored. These documents can provide clear directions for families and health care professionals and are gaining more recognition and importance as a result of increasing ethical dilemmas and challenges brought on by advances in technology (MedlinePlus, 2007a). Advance directives can be revoked or replaced at any time as long as the individual in question is capable of making her own decisions. It is recommended that these documents be reviewed every two years or so, or in the event of a change in health status, and revised to ensure that they continue to accurately reflect an individual's wishes (MedlinePlus, 2007a).

Secondary Prevention

Secondary prevention focuses on early detection of disease and prompt intervention (see Chapter 1). Much of the community health nurse's time is spent in educating the community on preventive measures and positive health behaviors. This includes encouraging individuals to obtain routine screening for diseases such as hypertension, diabetes, or cancer, which, if identified early, can be treated successfully (AHRQ, 2002). Many nurses, working in collaboration with community agencies, are in positions to establish screening programs based on the desires and demographics of the community and agency focus, making them accessible to the population being served.

Older adults need to be encouraged to follow the routine health-screening schedule prescribed by their clinic or health care provider. The health screening schedule described in Table 24.1 is based on the recommendations of Kaiser Permanente, Healthwise Handbook (2006), the largest Health Maintenance Organization in the world, that serves millions of clients, and is presented here as a guide. The United States Preventive Services Task Force (USPSTF) (AHRQ, 2007) proposed a more comprehensive view of interventions and recommendations for the periodic health examination of people older than 65 years of age. They identified age-specific, evidence-based preventive services guidelines that are outlined in Display 24.7.

Tertiary Prevention

Tertiary prevention involves follow-up and rehabilitation after a disease or condition has occurred or been diagnosed and initial treatment has begun. Chronic diseases that are common among older adults, such as heart failure, stroke, diabetes, cognitive impairment, or arthritis, cannot always be prevented, but can frequently be postponed into the later years of life through a lifetime of positive health behaviors (AHRQ, 2002). However, when they occur, the debilitating symptoms and damaging effects can be controlled through healthy choices encouraged by the community health nurse and recommended by the primary care practitioner (Hazard, 2003).

Although many older adults are considered generally healthy, 80% have at least one chronic condition and 50% have at least two (CDC, 2003b). A small proportion suffer more disabling forms of disease, such as chronic obstructive pulmonary disease (COPD), cerebral vascular accidents (CVAs), cancer, or diabetes mellitus (DM), the latter two requiring extensive care and ongoing medical management. The most common health problems of older people in the community are arthritis, reduced vision, hearing loss, heart disease, peripheral vascular disease, and hypertension. In 2002, the top three causes of death for U.S. adults aged 65 or older were heart disease (32% of all deaths), cancer (22%), and stroke (8%). These accounted for 61% of all deaths in this age group. The tragedy of these leading killers is that they are often preventable. Although the risk for disease and disability clearly increases with advancing age, poor health is not always an inevitable consequence of aging. Three behaviors—smoking, poor diet, and physical inactivity—were the root causes of almost 35% of U.S. deaths in 2000 (Mokdad, Marks, Stroup, & Gerberding,

TABLE 24.1　Recommended Health Screening/Immunizations—Older Adults

Test	Age 50–64	Age 65+	Comments
Men and Women			
Blood pressure	1–3 years	Yearly	More often if elevated
Total cholesterol	5 years	5 years	More often if elevated
Flexible sigmoidoscopy	10 years	10 years	—
Vision	4 years	2 years	—
Hearing	Not recommended	Once	Evaluate at regular health care practitioner visits
Pneumonia vaccine	Not recommended	Once	—
Influenza vaccine	Yearly	Yearly	—
Tetanus and diphtheria	10 years	10 years	After a closed/dirty wound if it has been >5 years
Women			
Breast self-examination	Monthly	Monthly	—
Pap test	2 years (after age 40)	2 years (after age 40)	After a hysterectomy by health care practitioner evaluation
Clinical breast examination	1–2 years	1–2 years	—
Mammogram	1–2 years	1–2 years	Frequency decided on an individual basis

(Adapted from Kaiser Permanente, 2006. Boise, ID: Author.)

nity health nurse working with these populations in the community.

Alzheimer's Disease

Alzheimer's disease (AD) was first described by Dr. Alois Alzheimer in a German medical journal in 1907. It is estimated that close to 5 million Americans suffer from Alzheimer's disease, and that the numbers of people developing this disease doubles every 5 years as people live beyond the age of 65 (National Institute on Aging, 2006a). With no cure in sight, this rate is expected to increase 27% by 2020, 70% by 2030, and it will more than triple by 2050 (Science Blog, 2003; National Institute on Aging, 2006a).

The occurrence of Alzheimer's disease is not a normal development in the aging process. It is characterized by a gradual loss of memory, decline in ability to perform routine tasks, disorientation, difficulty in learning, loss of language skills, impaired judgment and ability to plan, and personality changes. As the disease progresses these changes become so severe that they interfere with the individual's daily functioning, resulting in total dependence on others for care and eventually in death. Although the disease can last from 8 to 10 years, some people live 20 years after the onset of symptoms, and the current costs to Americans total $61 billion annually and Medicare costs for AD are expected to rise 54% by 2010 (Science Blog, 2003). Alzheimer disease is the fourth leading cause of death among the very old in the United States. Most people diagnosed with AD are older than 65 (called late-onset AD), and the incidence increases in the over-85 population. However, it is possible for the disease to occur in people between the ages of 30 and 60, but early-onset AD is usually considered an inherited form of the disease (National Institute on Aging, 2006a).

There is a simple way to describe the difference between the normal forgetfulness of aging and AD. From time to time, we all forget where we have put our keys, but people with early stage AD may notice that they tend to forget things more often—especially recent activities or events, or names of familiar things or people (National Institute on Aging, 2006a). Although these symptoms are bothersome, they are usually not serious enough to cause alarm. As the disease advances, the symptoms become serious enough to cause people with AD or their family members to recognize that things are not right and that help is needed. In the middle stages of AD, people eventually forget how to do simple tasks like brushing their teeth or combing their hair, and they begin to no longer be able to think clearly. They eventually have problems speaking, understanding, reading or writing, or recognizing people they have known for years. People who suffer from AD may become anxious or aggressive, and may wander away from home, thus requiring the need for total care (National Institute on Aging, 2006a).

There is no single test to identify AD. It is recommended that health care providers offer a comprehensive exam including a complete health history; physical exam; lab tests; neurologic, functional, and mental status assessments; and possible brain scans (National Institute on Aging, 2006a; Cherry, Vickrey, Schwankovsky, Heck, Plauche, & Yep, 2004). A comprehensive assessment is needed because many conditions, including some that are treatable or reversible (e.g., thyroid disease, depression brain tumors, drug reactions), may

---

DISPLAY 24.7 HEALTH MAINTENANCE PROGRAMS AND SERVICES FOR OLDER ADULTS

Resources for Community Health Nurses to Utilize With Clients

- Communication services (phones, emergency access to health care)
- Dental care services
- Dietary guidance and food services (such as Meals on Wheels, commodity programs, or group meal services)
- Escort and protective services
- Exercise and fitness programs
- Financial aid and counseling
- Friendly visiting and companions
- Health education
- Hearing tests and hearing-aid assistance
- Home health services (including skilled nursing and home health aide services)
- Home maintenance assistance (housekeeping, chores, and repairs)
- Legal aid and counseling
- Library services (including tapes and large-print books)
- Medical supplies or equipment
- Medication supervision
- Podiatry services
- Recreational and education programs (community centers, Elderhostel)
- Routine care from selected health care practitioners
- Safe, affordable, and ability-appropriate housing
- Senior citizens' discounts (food, drugs, transportation, banks, retail stores, and recreation)
- Social assistance services offered in conjunction with health maintenance
- Speech or physical therapy
- Spiritual ministries
- Transportation services
- Vision care (prescribing and providing eye glasses; diagnosis and treatment of glaucoma and cataracts)
- Volunteer and employment opportunities (Vista, RSVP)

Adapted from U.S. Preventive Services Task Force. (2000–2003). *Guide to clinical preventive services* (3rd ed.). Retrieved January 30, 2004 from *http://www.upstf.gov*

2004). The costs of chronic illness are high: one study found per capita Medicare expenditures increased from $211 (no chronic illness) to $13,973 with four or more chronic conditions and another study reported that someone age 65 and above with one serious chronic illness would spend between $1,000 and $2,000 more per year on health care (Wolff, Starfield, & Anderson, 2002; Joyce, Keeler, Shang, & Goldman, 2005). Although most elderly people experience relatively good health, almost all may expect to be chronically ill for an extended amount of time at the end of their lives (RAND Health, 2003). Chapter 26 expands on clients with disabilities and chronic illnesses and the role of the commu-

cause dementia-like symptoms. Physicians are now able to accurately diagnose 80% to 90% of people who show symptoms, but the only definitive diagnosis of AD is done at autopsy by the examination of brain tissue (National Institute on Aging, 2006a).

Probable causes of AD are many. Promising leads involve the role of neurotransmitters, proteins, metabolism, environmental toxins, and genes. Research has shown links between some genes and AD, with three gene variants identified for early-onset AD and one that boosts risk for late-onset. A recent study found that a new genetic link for late-onset AD, a variation in the gene SORL1, may be tied to levels of production of amyloid beta fragments that lead to plaques in the brains of AD patients (National Institute on Aging, 2007). Discovering the cause and a means of preventing AD, as well as better methods of earlier diagnosis, will be a significant achievement that may be realized in this century (National Institute on Aging, 2006b). Currently, 16 different agents are under study relative to AD, compared with 90 for cardiovascular disease; the medical community is not putting the same amount of effort into research for AD as it does for other diseases. This lack of research interest today affects what will be available for those in need tomorrow (Alzheimer's Association Medical and Scientific Advisory Council, 2005).

Medications may be prescribed, but many are largely experimental (National Institute on Aging, 2006a). At best, available medications "turn back the clock somewhat" with the disease worsening at a slower rate, or the drugs control some of the client's behaviors that jeopardize safety, thereby promoting caregiver management.

How does this disease affect the role of the community health nurse? Often, the person with AD is cared for at home until very late in the disease course. The intense care given these clients can be a constant drain on the emotional and physical reserves of their families and highlights the need for respite care (Mason et al., 2007). The client exhibits depression, agitation, sleeplessness, and anxiety, which can greatly upset the family's normal routine. In many situations, the main caregiver is an aged spouse. The stress of providing care puts the caregiver's health at risk, as well. The intensity of caregiving is aptly described in a book written for AD family members, *The 36-Hour Day* (Mace & Rabins, 2001). Another good book is *Staying Connected While Letting Go: The Paradox of Alzheimer's Caregiving* (Braff & Olenik, 2003). (See What Do You Think?)

Because so many elders afflicted with AD reside at home with their family members providing care, it is important for the community health nurse to monitor and assess the levels of stress on family members. The nurse can intervene as necessary and provide caregivers with methods to cope and adapt as needed, making applicable referrals. Most communities have resources for clients and their families. They may provide family and caregiver support groups, respite care, counseling, and legal or financial consultation. These services are available through local agencies, such as the Area Agency on Aging, but there are also government-sponsored national resources that offer information, referral services, and educational materials (e.g., Alzheimer's Association) all of which can be accessed by the community health nurse or the families in need. Some may find online support groups helpful. The nurse needs to know what resources are available in order to guide families to them (see Using the Nursing Process).

What Do You Think?

Have you heard of the *Best Friends* approach to Alzheimer's care? The approach has changed the caregiving approach to Alzheimer disease (AD) and is changing the live of caregivers, families, and clients. It improves the quality of life not only for clients with AD but also for those providing care. *Best Friends* is a groundbreaking and up-lifting method for the care of people with AD. It builds on the essential elements of friendship: respect, empathy, support, trust, and humor. These are the building blocks of a care model that is both effective and flexible enough to adapt to each person's remaining strengths and abilities. The *Best Friends* approach does not just prevent catastrophic episodes; it makes every day consistently reassuring, enjoyable, and secure.

From Bell, V., & Troxel, D. (2001). *The Best Friends staff: Building a culture of care in Alzheimer's programs.* Baltimore: Health Professions Press, and Bell, V., & Troxel, D. (1997). *The Best Friends approach to Alzheimer's care.* Baltimore: Health Professions Press. (*Best friends* is a trademark of Health Professions Press, Inc.)

Arthritis

Arthritis encompasses more than 100 diseases and conditions that affect joints, surrounding tissues, and other connective tissues, and is the leading cause of disability for adults in the United States (CDC, 2007b). Common forms include osteoarthritis, rheumatoid arthritis, gout, and fibromyalgia. Arthritis is a disease of both young and old, with two-thirds of sufferers younger than age 65. However, it is common among women and older adults, and over half of adults with heart disease or diabetes also have arthritis (CDC, 2007b). By 2030, it is estimated that 20% of Americans older than 65 will have osteoarthritis (OA) (National Institute of Arthritis & Musculoskeletal & Skin Diseases [NIAMS], 2006a).

Osteoarthritis is the most common form of arthritis. In this type of arthritis, the number of cartilage cells diminishes, cartilage becomes ulcerated and thinned, subchondral bone is exposed, and bony surfaces rub together resulting in joint destruction. This disease is no longer considered to be only a normal consequence of aging. Risk factors include obesity, repetitive mechanical overuse of a joint, and heredity. Classic symptoms include aching, stiffness, and limited motion of the involved joint. Discomfort increases with overuse and during damp weather. Acetaminophen is the first drug of choice; however, clients often find a combination of medications and daily routines that helps them the most. The nurse can best assist these clients by assessing the safety of a particular regimen and suggesting treatment changes as new research becomes available, including new medications, surgical options for joint replacement, and dietary changes (e.g., vitamins, foods high in essential fatty acids) (NIAMS, 2006a).

Rheumatoid arthritis (RA) is a progressive chronic condition that begins during young adulthood and becomes disabling as the disease continues, attacking tissues of the joints and causing systemic damage in the later years. It

USING THE NURSING PROCESS   WHEN WORKING WITH OLDER ADULTS

Assessment

Mr. and Mrs. Boxwell are in their late 70s and have lived modestly on a fixed income since Mr. Boxwell's retirement. However, their budget has been strained this year as they have had $300 to $400 a month in out-of-pocket expenses for prescription medications. Mrs. Boxwell confessed to you (the community health nurse visiting them after receiving a referral from the coordinator of the senior center they attend) that at times they will skip medication doses to make "ends meet" some months. They both take drugs for high blood pressure, and Mrs. Boxwell is diabetic and Mr. Boxwell has heart failure. They live in a small, older home, and their older model car is seldom driven as they report "the traffic is getting worse" and they have "come close to having a car crash two times" while they were driving in the past 3 months. They are receptive to your suggestions, and are trying to stay healthy and independent.

Nursing Diagnoses

1. The clients are at risk for an alteration in their health status due to insufficient finances to purchase needed medications for chronic diseases.
2. The clients are at risk for altered safety when driving related to chronic health problems, diminished driving skills, and a history of near automobile crashes.

Plan/Implementation

Diagnosis 1

The community health nurse will explore the clients' eligibility for Medicare Part D and Medicaid. It is possible these clients are eligible, yet unaware of these programs. The community health nurse will consult with the clients' primary health care provider and ask for a change in prescriptions from brand names to generic. Also, ordering some medications in larger doses that come in scored tablets may be less expensive, and the client can safely break the larger pills in half. Mrs. Boxwell will check with her present distributor of diabetic supplies about getting larger quantities, generic brands of syringes, alcohol pads, etc.

Diagnosis 2

Mr. Boxwell will look into selling their car, and exploring the bus schedule and other senior shuttle services that can be used to travel to the doctor and grocery store. Mr. and Mrs. Boxwell's daughter spends a day with them monthly and takes them wherever they want to go, as long as it is "a fun outing," and they will look into coordinating errands with her.

Evaluation

The couple is eligible for Medicare Part D, and this will help defray the out-of-pocket costs for medications. They have reduced medication costs as much as possible and report not missing any prescribed medications.

They sold their car and are negotiating the bus in good weather and using a taxi in the winter or when it is raining (they figured they save $1,000 a year in auto insurance, auto maintenance, and gasoline while the bus and taxi costs them about $22 a month).

Since the couple is receptive to the help you have provided, you initiate a discussion regarding their long-term plans for housing needs as they get older. They are not opposed to a senior housing option, and have been talking about it with their daughter. They are going to talk with a realtor about selling their house, explore some senior apartments with their daughter on her monthly visits, and review their budget.

---

affects diarthrodial (synovial-line) joints. This form of arthritis is an autoimmune disease that causes inflammation, deformity, and crippling. RA is treated with anti-inflammatory agents, corticosteroids, antimalarial agents, gold salts, and immunosuppressive drugs. Joint discomfort is often relieved by gentle massage, heat, and range-of-motion exercises (NIAMS, 2006b).

The community health nurse needs to be aware of the major differences between these two prevalent forms of arthritis. Recommended treatments, including physical therapy, diet, and medication, change as more evidence-based research is conducted on arthritis. It is important to keep up-to-date on treatments, as these conditions are treated in the community and affect a large portion of the midlife and older populations a PHN may serve.

Cancer

Cancers, which are characterized by the uncontrolled growth and spread of abnormal cells, steadily increase in incidence in aging adults. Leukemia and cancers of the digestive system, breast, prostate, and urinary tract increase with age (Ebersole & Hess, 2004). One popular theory is that as the body ages, the immune system declines, losing its ability to serve as a buffer against abnormal cancer cells that have been forming in the body throughout life. Other identified causes of cancer involve personal health behaviors such as tobacco and excessive alcohol use (American Cancer Society, 2002).

It is particularly important for the community health nurse to be aware of the increased incidence of cancer in older clients, because older people often under report symptoms that may be early signs of cancer. It is vital for PHNs, through assessments at clinics, on home visits, or during participation in screening programs, to encourage clients to report untoward symptoms in order to promote early detection, which gives clients their best chance of survival. Adherence to the health care practitioner's recommended schedule for health screening should be encouraged. In addition, being aware of and educating clients about the American Cancer Society's seven warning signals of cancer can possibly save their lives (Display 24.8).

DISPLAY 24.8 CAUTION

The seven warning signals of cancer can be remembered through the use of the mnemonic device, *CAUTION*, as follows:
1. **C**hange in bowel or bladder habits
2. **A** sore throat that does not heal
3. **U**nusual bleeding or discharge
4. **T**hickening or lump in breast or elsewhere
5. **I**ndigestion or difficulty in swallowing
6. **O**bvious change in wart or mole
7. **N**agging cough or hoarseness

(Source: The American Cancer Society)

Depression

Depression is one of the most common, and most treatable, of all the mental disorders in older adults. It is a major health concern in this population and can be life threatening if unrecognized and untreated. Biological, psychological, and social changes place older adults at high risk for the development and recurrence of depression. It is frequently related to multiple losses, such as retirement, a health change, or the death of a significant other. Depression is reported to be more common in women than in men (Ebersole & Hess, 2004). However, as mentioned earlier in this chapter, depression in men is more severe, resulting in suicide at a higher rate than among women. Higher levels of perceived social support are related to lower instances of depression among all people, especially the elderly, and women seem to make these supportive connections throughout life more effectively than men do. The nurturance, reassurance, and support women get from intimate relationships with other women are not often as highly developed in men, and for this reason, men display more symptoms of depression after a loss.

Community health nurses can help elders prevent the overwhelming signs and symptoms of depression related to losses by working with aggregates of elders in the community. Through senior centers, adult housing units, senior day care centers, or men's and women's groups at religious centers, the community health nurse can meet with seniors to offer support, teach strategies to improve the quality and quantity of support systems, invite mental health speakers to discuss the topic of depression prevention, and generally assess the holistic health status of the elders in that setting. The increased years added to life through the advances of the past few decades in medications and treatment should lead to healthy and happy later life for seniors, filled with activities that bring joy and contentment. Years lost to depression are a wasted resource that could be prevented through early intervention and medical management.

Diabetes

Diabetes mellitus (DM) affects the health of older people and limits their ability to perform activities. Among people 65 years and older in 1999-2000, 15.1% of men and 13.0% of women reported having diabetes. The prevalence of diabetes tends to be higher among Hispanics and non-Hispanic Blacks. The number of people with DM has increased six fold since 1958, and 95% of these have type 2 diabetes. Type 2 diabetes can often be prevented with adherence to proper diet and regular exercise with the addition of oral medications, when needed (Shashikiran, Vidyasagar, & Prabhu, 2004).

More Americans than ever suffer from various forms of DM, and the resulting rates of death and serious complications, such as adult blindness, kidney disease, and foot or leg amputations, are especially high for elders and racial and ethnic minority populations (Nwasuruba, Khan, & Egede, 2007). In the past, DM was not always managed effectively; fear and misinformation about the disease may hinder today's elders from getting an early diagnosis or from participating in effective teaching and instruction on how to manage DM.

Being diagnosed with DM can cause depression or anger, and the community health nurse must tailor educational programs to meet individual client needs. The plan should be comprehensive, with special emphasis placed on the areas in which each client needs information. For example, a spouse may be concerned about preparing meals that meet her husband's needs, whereas the husband may be more concerned with how the disease will affect his long days on the golf course or sexual functioning; in contrast, a single older woman may worry whether she can see well enough to draw up her insulin or can afford to pay for diabetic supplies and special foods. All newly diagnosed diabetics need a comprehensive overview of the disease process followed by an individualized approach for ongoing control and management of the disease.

Self-care behaviors (e.g., appropriate diet, glucose monitoring, medication management, foot care) are not often consistently practiced, yet they are necessary to promote good health and fewer complications (Nwasuruba et al., 2007). Community health nurses are ideally situated to meet group and individual needs. They have the resources and skills to plan and implement diabetic education classes for groups of elders, in addition to making home visits to address specific learning deficits that impact an individual's ability to manage their diabetes properly. The group setting allows elders to share their experiences, learn from each other, and benefit from the support of the group. Home visits permit the nurse to focus on an assessment of the client, home, family support, diabetic supplies and technique, and overall health management.

Cardiovascular Disease

Following arthritis and hearing impairment, hypertension is the third most frequent chronic condition for people older than 65 years. About 70% of those 65 and older have been diagnosed with hypertension, as have about 80% of those 75 years and older (CDC, 2006d). Hypertension increases with age and affects men more frequently than women. Hypertension is more prevalent and is less well controlled with medication in African Americans than in Whites (Kramer et al., 2004). Elders have difficulty managing ADLs if antihypertensive medications lower their blood pressure too dramatically. Hypotension leads to problems of safety, including a higher risk of falls, and blood pressure should be monitored by the PHN. Both hypertension and hypotension can have significant detrimental effects on the health of older adults.

Heart disease is the leading cause of death for both men and women in the United States (CDC, 2006e). Risk factors in the aging population associated with cardiovascular disease include tobacco use or exposure to tobacco smoke, inappropriate nutritional patterns, diabetes, high cholesterol, and lack of exercise. There are also regional differences in the pattern of deaths from heart disease: the southeastern coastal plains (Appalachia) and lower Mississippi River Valley (southern parts of Georgia and Alabama) have the highest death rates, and Blacks and Whites generally have higher rates of heart disease death than Hispanics or Asians and other races/ethnicities (CDC, 2006e).

Disease prevention is an important role for the community health nurse. Based on the knowledge of the prevalence of hypertension in older adults, the community health nurse can provide primary prevention by teaching community groups and individuals about this condition and ways to prevent its occurrence, and can provide secondary prevention by screening seniors on a regular basis.

Osteoporosis

Osteoporosis is a disease of bone in which the amount of bone is decreased and the strength is reduced. Osteoporosis is a generalized, persistent, and disabling disease that can overshadow every facet of an elder's overall functional level and independence. It causes acute and chronic pain, subsequent fractures, decreased physical activity, limited mobility, changes in body image, role changes, a reduction in ability to perform ADLs, and depression.

According to researchers, by 2025 osteoporosis related fractures and the associated costs are expected to increase by 48%, to more than 3 million fractures at a cost of $25.3 billion (Kuehn, 2005). In osteoporosis, calcium leaches from the bone mass and results in small holes forming in the bones. These empty spaces within the bone increase susceptibility to fractures of hip, wrist, or vertebra (McKeon, 2002). The risk of osteoporosis increases with age. As the disease progresses, other characteristics show up; e.g., compression of the vertebrae results in loss of height and the hunched back deformity known as dowager's hump.

Proper diet and exercise throughout life are now recognized as the most effective measure to maintain bone health. There is growing evidence that vitamin D supplementation can prevent fractures in the elderly (Bischoff-Ferrari et al., 2004); calcium supplementation is also critical. There are many FDA approved drugs to treat osteoporosis that can be prescribed by the primary care provider. Therefore, identification of risk factors and regular screenings is essential to prevent the progression of this debilitating disease.

Community health nurses can focus their teaching on primary prevention and ensure that people eat diets that are rich in vitamin D and calcium, and include calcium supplements as needed. Not smoking, maintaining a healthy weight, participating in weight bearing activities, and receiving ongoing bone density screenings are positive health behaviors that can contribute to strong bones throughout life. The value of hormone replacement therapy (HRT) in women—its benefits and possible long-term side effects—must be considered on the advice of the primary care provider, whose judgment should be based on the latest research findings along with the individual woman's needs.

APPROACHES TO OLDER ADULT CARE

In general, nursing service to seniors can be divided into two approaches: geriatrics and gerontology. In addition, healthy older adults can be effectively cared for in the community through case management approaches, which focus on all three types of services: primary, secondary and tertiary. The ultimate goal of community based case management for the aging population is to enhance the quality of care by decreasing fragmentation, maximizing resources, and providing the highest quality of care possible (Brickner, 2006; RAND Health, 2003b).

Geriatrics and Gerontology

Geriatrics is the medical specialty that deals with the health and social care of the elderly. A geriatrician is a medical doctor who has received specialized training in geriatrics. Geriatrics includes the physiology of aging, diagnosis and treatment of diseases affecting the aged and resulting from the aging process, and the complex psychosocial issues associated with the aging population. Geriatrics, like other medical specialties, with the exception of palliative care, focuses on abnormal conditions and the treatment and cure of those conditions (Eliopoulos, 2004). In the past, geriatric nursing focused primarily on the sick aged. As the profession of nursing has grown, the scope has broadened. Many nurses choose to be involved with community based nursing, focusing on prevention and improved health behaviors for the growing aging population.

Gerontology refers to the study of all aspects of the aging process, including economic, social, clinical, and psychological factors, and their effects on the older adult and on society. Gerontology is a broad, multidisciplinary practice, and gerontologic nursing concentrates on promoting the health and maximum functioning of older adults (Eliopoulos, 2004).

Community health nurses work with many types of older people. In one instance, the nurse may work to promote and maintain the health of a vigorous 80-year-old man who lives alone in his home. As another example, the nurse may give post surgical care at home to a 69-year-old woman, teaching her husband how to care for her, and helping them contact community resources for assistance with shopping, meals, housekeeping, and transportation services. Perhaps nursing intervention focuses on teaching nutrition and maintaining a healthful lifestyle for an extended family that includes a 73-year-old grandmother. The nurse may also lead a bereavement support group for senior citizens whose spouses have recently died. The possibilities are limitless and ever expanding.

A community health nurse works with older adults at the individual, family, and group levels. However, a community health perspective must also concern itself with the aggregate of older adults. There are many groups of seniors the PHN may choose to work with, such as those who attend an adult day care center, belong to a retirement community, live in a nursing home, or use Meals on Wheels. Others groups include residents of a senior citizens' apartment building, retired business and professional women, older post-cataract surgery patients at risk for glaucoma, the older poor, AD sufferers, and the homeless elderly. Work with elderly clients can also involve political advocacy.

Case Management and Needs Assessment

Case management involves assessing needs, planning and organizing services, and monitoring responses to care throughout the length of the care giving process, condition, or illness. This concept, which has been practiced by community health nurses for many years, focuses primarily on the health needs of clients. Social workers use case management to address their clients' social needs, including their financial problems. Some HMOs provide a coordinated system of services for their enrolled clients. However, many communities provide no such advocate for their older residents, and a more comprehensive, community-wide system needs to be developed to serve the entire older population. Such a system might be based in an agency specifically designed to serve as case manager or "agent" to assess clients' needs and assemble existing agencies and services to meet those needs (Mullin & Kelley, 2006; Barba et al., 2007).

Various techniques or tools are available to assess the needs of older adults:

◆ The Older Americans Resources and Services Information System (OARS), developed by Duke University Center for the Study of Aging and Human Development, utilizes two sections of one tool—OARS Multidimensional Functional Assessment Questionnaire (OMFAQ)—to determine levels of functioning in five areas (mental health, physical health, economic resources, social resources, and ability to perform ADLs), along with the extent and intensity of utilization, as well as perceived need, of services (Duke University, 2007). Administration time is about 45 minutes, and this tool is commonly used in research and to determine effectiveness of services, as well as assessment of functional status.

◆ The Barthel Index assesses functional independence and is often used to determine levels of disability or dependence of stroke victims with respect to ADLs. The Modified Rankin Scale (MRS) is another common tool used for this purpose (Sulter, Steen, & DeKeyser, 1999).

◆ The Katz Index of Activities of Daily Living is based on an evaluation of the functional independence or dependence of clients with respect to bathing, dressing, toileting, and related tasks. The Instrumental Activities of Daily Living Scale looks at an older adult's ability to perform such activities as using the telephone, shopping, doing laundry, and handling finances (Wallace, Shelkey, & The Hartford Institute for Geriatric Nursing, 2007; Ward, Jagger, & Harper, 1998).

◆ Other tools sometimes used with elderly clients include the Stanford 7-day Physical Activity Recall questionnaire (PAR), the Human Activity Profile (HAP), and the Physical Activity Scale for the Elderly (PASE). All of these tools measure physical activity and functioning (Johansen et al., 2001).

A frequently overlooked area of assessment is an elderly client's spiritual needs (Moberg, 2001; Hoffert, Henshaw, & Myududu, 2007). Religious dedication and spiritual concern often increase in later years. Limited ability or lack of transportation may prevent older people from attending religious services or engaging in spiritually enhancing activities. Self-health ratings, including clients' reports on their spiritual needs, provide another useful assessment technique.

HEALTH SERVICES FOR OLDER ADULT POPULATIONS

How well are the needs of older adults being met? To answer this question, other questions must be raised. Do health programs for the elderly encompass the full range of needed services? Are programs both physically and financially accessible? Do they encourage elderly clients to function independently? Do they treat senior citizens with respect and preserve their dignity? Do they recognize older adults' needs for companionship, economic security, and social status? If appropriate, do they promote meaningful activities instead of overworked games or activities such as bingo, shuffleboard, and ceramics? Are health care services and other social services provided based on evidence and research?

Criteria for Effective Service

Several criteria help to define the characteristics of an effective community health service delivery system for the elderly. Four, in particular, deserve attention.

For the delivery system of a community health service to be effective, it should be *comprehensive*. Many communities provide some programs, such as limited health screening or selected activities, but do not offer a full range of services to meet the needs of their senior citizens more adequately. Gaps and duplication in programs most often result from poor or nonexistent community-wide planning. Furthermore, such planning should be based on thorough assessment of the needs of the elderly population in that community. A comprehensive set of services should provide the following:

◆ Adequate financial support
◆ Adult day care programs
◆ Access to high quality health care services (prevention, early diagnosis and treatment, rehabilitation)
◆ Health education (including preparation for retirement)
◆ In-home services
◆ Recreation and activity programs that promote socialization
◆ Specialized transportation services

A second criterion for a community service delivery system is *coordination*. Often, older people go from one agency to the next. After visiting one place for food stamps, they go to another for answers to Medicare questions, another for congregate dining, and still another for health screenings. Such a patchwork of services reflects a system organized for the convenience of providers rather than consumers. It encourages misuse and discourages effective use. Instead, there should be coordinated, community-wide assessment and planning (Mollica, 2003). Communities must consider alternatives that can meet many needs in one location, such as multiservice agencies and interdisciplinary collaborative programs (AHRQ, 2002; RAND Health, 2003).

A coordinated information and referral system provides another link. Most communities need this type of information network, which contains a directory of all resources and services for the elderly and includes the name and telephone number of a contact person with each listing. Such a network is available in many communities and should be developed in those without one. A simplified information and referral system that includes one number, such as an 800 number, that can connect seniors with available resources and services is particularly helpful to older people. In an effort to better meet the needs of the elderly, a system of case-finding and referral services was instituted at four emergency departments in the Midwest, using screening assessments by the triage nurse and follow up, when needed, by a geriatric clinical nurse specialist (Mion, Palmer, Anetzberger, & Meldon, 2001).

In most communities, coordination is not present, or it is not done with any regularity or thoroughness. Many agencies in a given community do not coordinate services, but instead deliver their own services to the elderly in a patchwork and uncoordinated fashion (Mollica, 2003). Collaboration among those who provide services to seniors can provide vital information for planning and implementing needed programs. Even within the same health care system, collaboration and coordination of services are not always present. Kaiser-Bellflower, in Southern California, sought to improve end-of-life care by establishing improved connections between palliative and hospice care teams, along with staff members from disease management (RAND Health, 2003).

A third criterion is *accessibility*. Too often, services for the elderly are not conveniently located or are prohibitively expensive. Some communities are considering multiservice community centers to bring programs and services for the elderly closer to home (Artis, 2005). The Program of All-Inclusive Care of the Elderly (PACE) is one example of this. Comprehensive services are offered to eligible nursing home patients, including personal, health care, and housing services: e.g., adult day care, meals, social workers, nurses, primary care physicians, dentists, podiatrists, optometrists, prescriptions, medical specialists, and acute and nursing home care (RAND Health, 2003). More convenient and perhaps specialized transportation services and more in-home services, such as home health aides, homemakers, and Meals on Wheels, may further solve accessibility problems for many older adults. Federal, state, and private funding sources can be tapped to ease the burden on the economically pressured elderly population.

Finally, an effective community service system for older people should *promote quality programs*. This means that services should truly address the needs and concerns of a community's senior citizens and be based on scientific evidence (American Geriatric Society, 2006). Evaluation of the quality of a community's services for the elderly is closely tied to their assessed needs. What are the needs of this specific population group in terms of nutrition, exercise, economic security, independence, social interaction, meaningful activities, and preparation for death? Planning for quality community services depends on having adequate, accurate, and current data. Periodic needs assessment is a necessity to ensure updated information and initiate and promote quality services.

Services for Healthy Older Adults

Maintaining functional independence should be the primary goal of services for the older population. Assessment of needs and the ability to function and use of techniques such as OARS, the Instrumental Activities of Daily Living Scale, or other previously mentioned tools form the basis for determining appropriate services. Although many of the well elderly can assesses their own health status, some are reluctant to seek needed help (Nussbaum, 2006). Therefore, outreach programs serve an important function in many communities. They locate elderly people in need of health or social assistance and refer them to appropriate resources.

Health screening is another important program for early detection and treatment of health problems among older adults. Conditions to screen for include hypertension, glaucoma, hearing disorders, cancers, diabetes, anemias, depression, mild cognitive impairment, and nutritional deficiencies (Eliopoulos, 2004; Miller, 2003). At the same time, assessment of elderly clients' socialization, housing, and economic needs, along with proper referrals, can prevent further problems from developing that would compromise their health status (Mion et al., 2001).

Health maintenance programs may be offered through a single agency, such as an HMO, or they may be coordinated by a case management agency with referrals to other providers. These programs should cover a wide range of services needed by the elderly, such as those listed in Display 24.7.

Living Arrangements and Care Options

Three types of living arrangements and care options are available for elders. Some living arrangements are based on levels of care—from independent to skilled nursing care, and all levels of assistance in between. At times, seniors who remain in their own homes or apartments need home care services brought to them. Other seniors live with family members and go to an adult day care center during the day. The third category of living arrangements includes those that are short term. It may be a rehabilitation hospital for recovery and physical therapy related to a hip fracture, or respite care, which gives the usual caregiver a much-needed rest from 24-hour-a-day care giving and helps prevent "burnout." Families of terminally ill clients and those with severe dementia cared for at home often use respite services (Mason et al., 2007).

To meet the multiple housing and care giving needs of today's elders and in anticipation of the larger numbers to come, many options are becoming available. A range of housing types, from luxurious retirement communities with all amenities for the active and healthier senior to secure and more modestly priced or low-income apartments for independent senior living, are being built in most communities.

Day Care and Home Care Services

The majority of older adults want to remain in their own homes for the remainder of their lives and be as independent and in control of their lives as possible (AARP, 2007). Some struggle to appear to be doing well in maintaining their independence. Often, they fear that their children or others will make decisions for them that include leaving their homes. Home, whatever form it takes, is where these people believe they are the happiest (Eliopoulos, 2004; Miller, 2003).

There is increased emphasis on providing needed services for elders at home. This trend started several years ago when it became evident that people improved more quickly and at lower cost when they were cared for as outpatients in their own homes. Today's heightened emphasis on health care cost control gives added support for providing services at home. Given the increase in longevity, the potential for cost savings appears significant if dependent older people can be maintained at home. Doing so encourages functional independence as well as emotional wellbeing (AHRQ, 2002).

Home care provides services such as skilled nursing care, psychiatric nursing, physical and speech therapies, homemaker services, social work services, and dietetic counseling (see Chapter 32). Day care services offer a place where older adults can go during the day for social activities, nutrition, nursing care, and physical and speech therapies. Both services are useful for families who are caring for an elderly person, especially if the caregivers work and no one is at home or available during the day. One disadvantage to those remaining in their homes is that services for the dependent elderly in the community are often fragmented, inadequate, and inaccessible, and at times they operate with little or no maintenance of standards or quality control (Eliopoulos, 2004).

The dependent elderly need someone in the community to assess their particular needs; assemble, coordinate, and monitor the appropriate resources and services; and serve as their advocate. Some communities have Ombudsmen to serve this role. But, community health nurses can easily fill the role of case manager for elderly clients. This case management approach tailors services to the long-term needs of clients and enables them to function longer outside of institutions (Brickner, 2006).

Living Arrangements Based on Levels of Care

Although only 6% of the elderly population lives in **skilled nursing facilities**, such organizations remain the most visible type of health service for older adults (AAHSA, 2007). These facilities provide skilled nursing care along with personal care that is considered nonskilled or **custodial care**, such as bathing, dressing, feeding, and assisting with mobility and recreation. Currently, approximately 2 million elderly people are receiving nursing home care.

Long-term care services include those services that provide care for people at different stages of dependence for extended periods of time (Miller, 2003). New choices are now available and provide housing for larger numbers of elders than nursing homes do. There are currently roughly 7 million people with long-term care insurance policies, and the average premium for someone under age 65 is $1,337 a year (AAHSA, 2007). These policies will pay for skilled nursing care and long-term care facilities, as currently almost 40% of costs are paid by private funds and 40% by Medicaid (AAHSA, 2007).

Nursing home reform was promoted in 1987 with passage of the Omnibus Budget Reconciliation Act (OBRA), which put increased demands on facilities to provide competent resident assessment, timely care plans, quality improvement, and protection of resident rights starting in 1990 (Miller, 2003). This increased complexity of services has resulted in increased costs in these facilities. Staffing needs increase as care becomes more complex and the resident population grows. Licensed personnel must be knowledgeable decision-makers, managers of unskilled staff, staff educators, and role models, and efficient and effective administrators in an essen-

tially autonomous practice setting. And, as the elderly population grows, the need for greater numbers of both licensed and attendant staff becomes more evident. Because many of these jobs offer low pay and are without substantial benefits or a career ladder, it is projected that it will be difficult to find enough staff to meet the demands (RAND Health, 2003).

In the past, nursing homes had stigmas attached to them. Many people saw them as places that enforced dehumanizing and impersonal regulations, such as segregation of sexes, strict social policies, and sometimes overuse of chemical and physical restraints. Media attention to such conditions, together with current licensing regulations, should make these types of practices the rare exception. Gradually, the fear and despair associated with such facilities will begin to dissipate (National Citizen's Coalition for Nursing Home Reform, 2007). In addition, as competition comes from facilities offering lower levels of care (e.g., assisted living centers), residents in nursing homes who are receiving more minimal care may be attracted to move to other types of housing.

Even in institutions in which the quality of care is outstanding, costs are so high that family resources are soon depleted if not planned for long in advance of the need. Although Medicaid pays for skilled nursing costs if the client meets low income and asset requirements, and Medicare pays for a limited period of care, clients and families pay more than half of the total costs (Eliopoulos, 2004). Life savings that older parents had hoped to leave to their children may be quickly consumed, forcing them into indigence. It is estimated that average annual costs for nursing home care range from $75,000 for a private room and $65,000 for a semiprivate room (AAHSA, 2007).

Intermediate care facilities are less costly and still provide health care, but the amount and type of skilled care given are less than that provided in skilled nursing facilities. Frequently, older adults need **assisted living**, which generally means that they need assistance with everyday tasks such as bathing, eating, dressing, or using the bathroom (Medline Plus, 2007b). This is a less intense level of care than skilled nursing facilities provide. The average yearly cost of this type of care ranges from over $32,000 to $35,000 (AARP, 2007; AAHSA, 2007). Medicare and Medicaid generally pay only for care in skilled nursing facilities. Medicaid may pay for care in intermediate care facilities, but only after the client meets income and asset tests that leave them essentially indigent. Medicaid coverage of assisted living services is available in a few states that can grant Medicaid waivers. The average length of time a senior remains in an assisted living facility is 2 years (Bradford, 2001). Due to licensing restrictions, when someone becomes bedridden or needs additional assistance or skilled nursing care, they generally must move from assisted care into another facility.

Personal care homes (sometimes called board and care homes) offer 24-hour basic custodial care, such as bathing, grooming, and social support, but provide no skilled nursing services. Boarding homes, board and care homes, and residential care facilities often house a smaller number of elderly people in a residential home (often between five and eight) or a larger number in apartment type housing. These residents need only meals and housekeeping and can manage most of their own personal care, including medications (HelpGuide, 2007a). Costs can range from $350 to $3,500 per month, depending upon the amenities and services (HelpGuide, 2007a). Medicare only pays for medical care, not housing costs. Medicaid may help pay some assisted living costs and limited custodial home care, but not generally for housing costs related to personal care homes. Payment may come from private funds, Social Security, or Supplemental Security Income (aid to the aged, disabled, and blind) in some limited cases (HelpGuide, 2007b). Long-term care insurance usually covers only nursing home care, but some companies are expanding policy guidelines to include assisted living and personal care homes (HelpGuide, 2007b). Homes can serve special populations. Those focusing on the care of people with AD are physically designed with clients' safety and individual needs considered and are staffed with paraprofessionals trained to meet each person's needs.

The concept of **continuing care retirement communities (CCRCs)**, sometimes referred to as total life centers, allow seniors to "age in place," with flexible accommodations designated to meet their health and housing needs as these needs change over time. CCRCs are the most expensive long-term-care solution available to seniors; however, they provide all levels of living, from total independence to the most dependent, and are designed to meet the continuous living needs of older aging adults. Residents entering CCRCs sign a long-term contract that provides for housing, services, and nursing care, usually all in one location. Many seniors enter into CCRC contracts while they are healthy and active, knowing they will be able to stay in the same community and receive nursing care should this become necessary. Seniors who invest in a CCRC have adequately planned for housing and care for the remainder of their life, and have the financial means to support it; entrance fees can range from $20,000 to $400,000 and monthly fees from $200 to $2,500 (AARP, 2007b). Others may choose to remain in their own home because they do not desire consolidated living arrangements that include only older adults, or because they have not planned adequately for the expense. Nevertheless, demand is increasing for this type of housing option. Adults nearing retirement today are investigating this concept as a viable option as they actively plan for their retirement. Because of the demand, many of these centers have waiting lists, so older adults need to seek them out long before they intend to live there (AARP, 2007b).

Respite Care Services

Respite care is a service that is receiving increasing attention. It provides time off for caregivers, including family members, who care for someone who is ill, injured, or frail. An increasing number of older people are cared for in their home by a spouse or other family member on an unpaid basis. Almost 75% of persons receiving care at home rely exclusively on informal caregivers, usually women between the ages of 45 and 64 (AAHSA, 2007). The demands of such care can be exhausting unless the caregiver gets some relief (see Chapter 32). Respite care can take place in an adult day

---

PERSPECTIVES
VOICES FROM THE COMMUNITY

Continuing Care Centers— A Solution for Aging Adults

I am really sold on continuing care retirement communities! We have one in our area that is a big hit with our middle and upper income folks. The Otterbein-Lebanon Retirement Community is a model continuing care center and is one of five Otterbein Homes located in Ohio. With housing options for 1200 residents on a 1,500-acre campus in rural southeastern Ohio, older adults can choose housing options that include freestanding two- and three-bedroom homes, one-bedroom cottages, or apartment-style one- or two-bedroom or one-room studio units, where they live independently.

They are licensed for 296 beds, including assisted living options from one-room studio apartments (with limited facilities for meal preparation) to semiprivate rooms in which nurses oversee medication and staff is available to assist with personal care. If caregiving needs become greater, additional services are available. Both skilled nursing services and a freestanding 30-bed Alzheimer's living unit exist for the frailest older adults. This is a real advantage for my clients who want to remain in the same place, even as their physical condition may worsen.

Regardless of the living arrangement, the residents are free to come and go as they wish and all have access to congregate dining in their large and attractive restaurant-style dining room.

The retirement community is expanding. One hundred and ten patio homes were built in 1999–2000 with additional expansion planned.

The Otterbein-Lebanon Retirement Community also provides a health clinic, adult day care, and the other usual services found in a community: a bank, post office, ice cream parlor, a small convenience store, hairdresser, library, a church (with a 70-member choir, a bell choir, and men's and women's clubs), a thrift shop, and an arts and crafts shop open to the public. Because of the popularity of this Otterbein-Lebanon community, there is a waiting list for some independent living areas.

Many of the assisted living and skilled nursing beds are occupied by residents who moved into the independent living areas 10 to 15 years ago while they were in their 70s or 80s. Their ages now range from the late 80s to older than 100, and care needs have increased. This is wonderful because, in this type of setting, frail elderly people do not have to leave their community to get the care they need, and longtime friends are nearby to care for them or for companionship. It is not unusual to see many of the independent seniors volunteering to help feed frail elderly in the skilled nursing care units. In fact, residents volunteer more than 85,000 hours a year to the Otterbein-Lebanon Retirement Community. They know that when they need the care, a senior friend will be there for them.

Judy, 2008 PHN

center, in the home of the person being cared for, or even in a residential setting such as an assisted living facility or nursing home. Although there are different approaches to respite care, all have the same basic objective: to provide caregivers with *planned* temporary, intermittent, substitute care, allowing for relief from the daily responsibilities of caring for the care recipient (Eldercare, 2005). Respite care is sometimes available through agencies that provide volunteers to relieve caregivers; neighbors, churches, or volunteer organizations may be potential sources of assistance. Some skilled nursing facilities or **board and care homes** provide an extra room to give temporary institutional housing for the elderly while caregivers take a break over a weekend, for instance. Elderly clients may also need a change from the constant interaction with their caregivers. Long-term care insurance may cover some costs of respite care. The 2000 Older Americans Act Amendments provided funding for states to work through the National Family Caregiver Support Program (NFCSP) to address respite care specifically on the local level (Eldercare, 2005).

THE COMMUNITY HEALTH NURSE IN AN AGING AMERICA

Community health nurses can make a significant contribution to the health of older adults. Because these nurses are in the community and already have contact with many seniors, they are in a prime position to begin needs assessments and mutual planning for the health of this group. Case management is often a critical aspect of the nurse's role, because the community health nurse must know what resources are available and when and how to make referrals for these older clients (see From The Case Files II).

The availability and scope of health care services for the elderly are changing dramatically. The numbers and types of home care services, for example, are mushrooming. Many entrepreneurs, including nurses, who recognize the potential of this growing market, have begun offering goods and services targeted to older adults. Community health nurses must keep abreast of new developments, programs, regulations, and social and economic forces, along with their potential impacts on the provision of health services.

More importantly, community health nurses need to be proactive, designing interventions that maximize nursing's resources and provide the greatest benefit to elderly clients. For example, community health nurses might develop a case management program for older adults that comprises a community-wide assessment, information, and referral service. Such a program might contract with existing agencies to serve as a clearinghouse for the elderly and to channel clients to appropriate services. Financing of such a program might be based on tax dollars (if it is a public agency), grants, or some innovative fee-for-service reimbursement system.

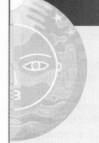

From the Case Files II

Johnny Jessup is 94 years old and lives with his wife, age 86, in a small mobile home on some acreage in a rural area of our county. He had mastoiditis as a child and lost a good deal of hearing. His vision is good, though, and he only wears glasses for reading. He was diagnosed with prostate cancer 20 years ago and still suffers from the radiation treatments he had at that time. He wears a protective "diaper" because he is often bowel incontinent. He is generally in good health, with no hypertension or evidence of heart disease. He spends most of his days outside, watering his berries, flowers, and fruit trees. He worked as a farmer and laborer—always outside—and he enjoys being in the sun and away from the television that his wife, Maude, likes to watch. He has difficulty hearing it, and when he turns up the volume, it "hurts her ears" and they argue over that. They have one son who lives in the same town, but who works long hours at his job. They speak by phone every other day, and he comes by to visit when he can. Their three grandsons are all away at college and they rarely see them.

As a young man, Johnny liked to dance, and he occasionally will go to the local senior center dances. Maude does not like to dance and will not accompany him there. This sometimes is a source of stress. Johnny likes to drink an "occasional cold beer," but he never drinks "hard liquor." He quit smoking 25 years ago, but he had been a heavy smoker from the age of 20. His appetite has usually been good, but he sometimes has difficulty eating fresh fruit or nuts because of his bowel problems. Maude has recently been having memory lapses and some difficulty remembering to turn off the stove and close the refrigerator door. She has trouble with a number of daily tasks. She likes to have someone bring them fast food as a treat every week, and they now require assistance with errands and most housekeeping tasks.

Recently, Johnny noticed that he was having more difficulty doing his outside chores. He seems more "weak" and "tired" and he has recently had quite a bit of "nausea and vomiting." Maude and Johnny's son took them for an appointment with his urologist and it was determined that his prostate-specific antigen (PSA) was slightly elevated.

You are a district PHN and have recently been assigned to the Jessup family to assess their functional limitations and provide them with information on resources they might need over the next few months. How would you begin your visit? How can you best determine their functional and physical limitations? What other assessments could be helpful (social, spiritual, mental/cognitive, etc.)? What resources and services might be helpful to them?

Many of the older population's health problems can be prevented and their health promoted. Changing to a healthier lifestyle is one of the most important preventive measures the nurse can emphasize. Education and support are key to the success of these changes.

The role of the community health nurse as a teacher is an important one. Educating the elderly about their health conditions, safety, and use of medications is another important way to prevent problems. Influenza and pneumonia can be prevented through regular health maintenance, which includes immunizations. Other problems associated with environmental conditions and the aging process, such as arthritis, diabetes, and some cancers, can be diagnosed and treated early, thereby minimizing their deleterious effect on functional independence.

Many types of accidents that frequently happen to older adults are preventable. Community health nurses can make a difference through their work with individuals, families, and aggregates in promoting and teaching safety measures to prevent such accidents. As discussed earlier, falls are a leading cause of injury and death for the elderly and result from a combination of internal factors (e.g., diseases, effects of medicines) and external factors (e.g., lighting, area rugs, lack of handrails) that are preventable or controllable (RAND, 2003; Australian Government Department of Health & Aging, 2004). Nurses can make a difference in the lives of older clients by using available materials and their own resources when teaching safety.

Community health nurses face a serious challenge in addressing the needs of the growing and aging elderly population. At the same time, nursing can be at the forefront of developing innovative health services for seniors, rising to meet the opportunity and the challenge.

Summary

The number of older adults (age 65 years and older) is increasing, and becoming a larger percentage of the overall population. Women commonly outlive men by a number of years, making women a larger part of this older population. With improved medicines and medical technology, many people are now living into their 80s and 90s in relatively good health. They are able to enjoy these later years and still make contributions to their families and society. This extended life expectancy is, of course, good news; however, it has also created a myriad of new health needs and concerns, not only for the older population, but also for health care facilities and professionals who deliver services to older adults.

Healthy longevity is the goal for the aging population and is a focus of *Healthy People 2010*. This means being able to function as independently as possible; maintaining as much physical, mental, and social vigor as possible; and adapting to life's changes while coping with the stresses and losses and still being able to engage in meaningful activity.

To promote and maintain health and prevent illness, older people need to be educated about their own health care needs. In particular, they should understand the potential hazards of drug interactions if they are taking multiple medications. They also need good nutrition and adequate exercise; they need to be as independent and self-reliant as possible; they need coping skills to face the possibility of financial insecurity and the loss of a spouse or other loved ones; they need social interaction, companionship, and meaningful activities; and they need to resolve anxieties regarding their own eventual death.

The most common health problems of older adults are chronic and often progressive conditions such as arthritis, vision and hearing loss, heart disease, hypertension, and diabetes, all of which can become disabling conditions. Other major causes of death or disability are cancer, cerebral vascular accidents, AD, and accidents and injuries resulting from falls, fires, or automobile crashes. Older adults also often suffer adverse side effects from taking multiple medications prescribed for various chronic conditions, and polypharmacy is a danger. Many of these health problems associated with old age are preventable to some extent, and early diagnosis and treatment of some conditions can minimize their adverse effects. Many accidents and injuries that render older adults unable to live independently are preventable.

Too frequently, older adults suffer from the emotional side effects of aging, such as feelings of distress and anxiety regarding their future; loneliness and social isolation when loved ones or friends die; and even depression, feeling that life is over and they have no purpose or meaningful function in life. However, older people can also enter this phase of life determined to keep physically and mentally healthy, interacting with others and making viable contributions to others and society.

Many programs are available to older adults, both for those who are healthy, hearty, and active, and for those who need some level of dependent or semi dependent care. Programs for hearty older people include health maintenance programs that cover a wide range of health services, wellness programs, health screening, outreach programs, social assistance programs, and information about volunteering and educational opportunities in the community. A variety of living arrangements and care options are available from which to choose, and can be tailored to the older person's desires and needs. These include the newest concepts of continuing care centers, which offer a full range of living arrangements—from totally independent living to skilled nursing services—all within one community. There are also facilities that provide skilled nursing and custodial care, assisted living, home care, day care, respite care, and hospice.

The community health perspective includes a case management approach that offers a centralized system for assessing the needs of older people and then matching those needs with the appropriate services. The community health nurse should also seek to serve the entire older population by assessing the needs of the population, examining the available services, and analyzing their effectiveness. The effectiveness of programs can be measured according to four important criteria (targeted to the specific needs of the population): comprehensiveness, effective coordination, accessibility, and quality.

The community health nurse can make significant contributions to the health of the older population as a whole by being aware of new developments and programs that become available, new regulations, and innovative social and economic forces and their impacts on the provision of health services. More importantly, the community health nurse can design interventions that maximize nursing resources and provide the greatest benefit to the older adult population. ∎

ACTIVITIES TO PROMOTE CRITICAL THINKING

1. Picture an elderly person who you know well or know a great deal about. Make a list of characteristics that describe this person. How many of these characteristics fit your picture of most senior citizens? What are your biases (ageisms) about the elderly?

2. If you were Minnie Blackstone's community health nurse (see From the Case Files I), what interventions would you consider using to maintain and promote her health? Why?

3. As part of your regular community health nursing workload, you visit a senior day care center one afternoon each week. You take the blood pressures of several people who are taking antihypertensive medications and do some nutrition counseling. The center accommodates 60 senior clients, and you would like to serve the health needs of the aggregate population. What are some potential health needs of this group? What actions might you consider taking at an aggregate level? With whom would you consult as you plan programs at the center?

4. Assume that you have been asked by your local health department to determine the needs of the elderly population in your community. How would you begin conducting a needs assessment? What data might you want to collect? How would you find out what services are already being offered and whether they are adequate?

5. Visit a continuing care center in your community. Assess the housing options, services, and health care provisions. Would you live here when you are older? How would you feel about a family member living here? What would you change if you could?

6. Using the Internet, locate innovative programs for elders in the community at the primary, secondary, and tertiary levels of care. Determine whether such programs could work in your community.

References

Acierno, R., Rheingold, A., Resnick, H., & Kilpatrick, D. (2004). Predictors of fear of crime in older adults. *Journal of Anxiety Disorders, 18*(3), 385–396.

Administration on Aging. (2002a). *A profile of older Americans: 2002. Poverty*. Retrieved August 1, 2008 from http://www.aoa.gov/prof/statistics/profile/8.asp.

Administration on Aging. (2002b). *A profile of older Americans: 2002. Living arrangements*. Retrieved August 1, 2008 from http://www.aoa.gov/prof/Statistics/profile/4_pf.asp.

Administration on Aging. (2007a). *Promoting healthy lifestyles*. Retrieved August 1, 2008 from http://www.aoa.gov/eldfam/Healthy_Lifestyles/Healthy_Lifestyles.asp.

Administration on Aging. (2007b). *Fact sheets: The Elderly Nutrition Program*. Retrieved August 1, 2008 from http://www.aoa.gov/press.fact/alpha/fact_elderly_nutrition_pf.asp.

Agency for Healthcare Research & Quality (AHRQ). (2002). Preventing disability in the elderly with chronic disease. *Research in Action, Issue 3*. Retrieved August 1, 2008 from http://www.ahrq.gov/research/elderdis.htm#fn1.

Agency for Healthcare Research & Quality (AHRQ). (2007). *Guide to clinical preventive services*. Retrieved August 1, 2008 from http://www.ahrq.gov/clinic/cps3dix.htm.

Ahluwalia, K. (2004). Oral health care for the elderly: More than just dentures. *American Journal of Public Health, 94*(5), 698.

Alzheimer's Association Medical and Scientific Advisory Council. (2005). Alzheimer's Association: 25 years of supporting science and shaping the Alzheimer's research agenda. *Alzheimer's & Dementia: The Journal of the Alzheimer's Association, 1*(1), 11–12.

American Association of Homes and Services for the Aging (AAHSA). (2007). *Aging services: The facts*. Retrieved August 1, 2008 from http://www.ashsa.or/aging_services/default.asp.

American Association of Retired Persons (AARP). (2002). Social security finances improve despite recession. *AARP Bulletin, 43*(5), 4.

American Association of Retired Persons (AARP). (2005). *Doing the math: Older adults online, 2005*. Retrieved August 1, 2008 from http://www.aarp.org/olderwierwired/owwresources/doing_the_math_older_adults_online.html.

American Association of Retired Persons (AARP). (2007a). *Long term care costs*. Retrieved August 1, 2008 from http://www.aarp.org/research/longtermcare/costs/ny_ltc_2007.html.

American Association of Retired Persons (AARP). (2007b). *Other options: Continuing Care Retirement Communities (CCRC)*. Retrieved August 1, 2008 from http://www.aarp.org/families/housing_choices/other_options/a2004-02-26-retirementcommunity.html.

American Cancer Society. (2002). *The history of cancer*. Retrieved August 1, 2008 from http://www.cancer.org/docroot/CRI/content/CRI_2_6x_the_history_of_cancer_72.asp?sitearea.

American Geriatric Society. (2006). *Highlights of the American Geriatrics Society 2006 Annual Scientific Meeting CME/CE*. Retrieved August 1, 2008 from http://www.medscape.com/viewprogram/5470_pnt.

American Geriatric Society. (2007). *Aging in the know: Trends in the elderly population*. Retrieved August 1, 2008 from http://www.healthinaging.org/agingintheknow/chapters_print_ch_trial.asp?ch=2.

AmeriCorps. (2007). *Frequently asked questions*. Retrieved August 1, 2008 from http://americorps.gov/assets/printable/printable.asp?tbl_cms_id=306.

Artis, B. (2005). Promoting health, building community. *Health Progress, 86*(2), 27–31.

Australian Government Department of Health & Aging. (2004). *An analysis of research on preventing falls and falls injury in older people: Community, residential care & hospital setting, 2004 update*. National Falls Prevention for Older People Initiative. Retrieved August 1, 2008 from http://www.health.gov.au/internet/wcms/Publishing.nsf/Content/health-pubhlth-publicat-document-falls_community-cnt.htm/$FILE/falls_community.pdf.

Ballard, J., McFarland, C., Wallace, L., et al. (2004). The effect of 15 weeks of exercise on balance, leg strength, and reduction in falls in 40 women aged 65 to 89 years. *Journal of the American Medical Women's Association, 59*(4), 255–261.

Barba, B.E., Tesh, A.S., & Kohlenberg, E. (2007). Recognizing the many facets of gerontological nursing. *Nursing Management, 38*(1), 36–41.

Bernick, C., Katz, R., Smith, N., et al. (2005). Statins and cognitive function in the elderly. *Neurology, 65*, 1388–1394.

Bischoff-Ferrari, H., Dawson-Hughes, B., Willett, W., et al. (2004). Effect of vitamin D on falls. *JAMA, 291*(16), 1999–2006.

Bradford, S.L. (2001). *Ten things your assisted-living facility won't tell you*. Retrieved August 1, 2008 from http://www.smartmoney.com/print/index.cfm?printcontent=/consumer/index.cfm?stoiry=200104192.

Braff, S., & Olenik, M.R. (2003). *Staying connected while letting go: The paradox of Alzheimer's caregiving*. New York: M. Evans & Co.

Brickner, E. (October/November 2006). Home care case management: A vital process for enhancing care and reducing costs. *Care Management, 17–20.*

Burbank, P.M., & Riebe, D. (2002). *Promoting exercise and behavior change in older adults: Interventions with the transtheoretical model.* New York: Springer.

Bushardt, R., & Jones, K. (2005). *Nine key questions to address polypharmacy in the elderly.* Retrieved August 1, 2008 from http://jaapa.com/issues/J20050501/articles/polypharm0505.htm.

Butler, R.N. (2004). Maintaining cognitive health in an ageing society. *The Journal of the Royal Society for the Promotion of Health, 124*(3), 119–121.

Campbell, P.R. (1996). *Population projections for states by age, sex, race, and Hispanic origin: 1995 to 2025.* U.S. Bureau of Census, Population Division, PPL-47. Retrieved August 1, 2008 from http://www.medicare.gov/medicarereform/drugbenefit.asp.

Carnelley, K., Wortman, C., Bolger, N., & Burke, C. (2006). The time course of grief reactions to spousal loss: Evidence from a national probability sample. *Journal of Personality & Social Psychology, 91*(3), 476–492.

Center for Medicare Advocacy. (2007b). *Medicare's solvency: Helped or harmed by the Medicare Act of 2003?* Retrieved August 1, 2008 from http://www.medicareadvocacy.org/Reform_MedSolvencyAndActof2003.htm.

Center for Medicare Advocacy. (2007a). *Medicare drug plan.* Retrieved August 1, 2008 from http://medicareadvocacy.org/CHOICES/ChoicesPartD.htm.

Center for the Advancement of Health. (2004). *Facts of Life, 9*(7), 1-2. Retrieved August 1, 2008 from http://www.cfah.org/pdfs/FOL_July%202004.pdf.

Center on Budget & Policy Priorities (CBPP). (April 23, 2007). *A brief analysis of the Social Security and Medicare Trustees' report.* Retrieved August 1, 2008 from http://www.cbpp.org/4-23-07health.htm.

Centers for Disease Control & Prevention. (1999). *Chronic disease notes and reports: Special focus healthy aging.* National Center for Chronic Disease Prevention and Health Promotion. Retrieved August 1, 2008 from http://www.cdc.gov/nccdphp/publications/cdnr/pdf/cdfall99.pdf.

Centers for Disease Control & Prevention. (2003a). Public health and aging: Trends in aging: United States and worldwide. *Morbidity and Mortality Weekly Report, 52*(06), 101–106.

Centers for Disease Control & Prevention (CDC). (2003b). *Trends in health and aging: Prevalence of selected chronic conditions by age, sex, and race.* Retrieved August 1, 2008 from http://209.217.72.34/aging/TableViewer/tableView.aspx?ReportId=380.

Centers for Disease Control & Prevention (CDC). (2003c). Racial/ethnic disparities in influenza and pneumococcal vaccination levels among persons aged ≥65 years: United States, 1989–2001. *Morbidity and Mortality Weekly Review, 23*(40), 958–962.

Centers for Disease Control & Prevention (CDC). (2004). Influenza vaccination and self-reported reasons for not receiving influenza vaccination among Medicare beneficiaries aged ≥65 years: United States, 1991–2002. *Morbidity and Mortality Weekly Review, 53*(43), 1012–1015.

Centers for Disease Control & Prevention. (2006a). *Racial and ethnic approaches to community health: Evaluation.* Retrieved August 1, 2008 from http://www.cdc.gov/reach.evaluation.htm.

Centers for Disease Control & Prevention. (2006b). *Fact sheet: Oral health for older Americans.* Retrieved August 1, 2008 from http://www.cdc.gov/OralHealth/factsheets/adult-older.htm.

Centers for Disease Control & Prevention. (2006c). *Extreme heat: A prevention guide to promote your personal health and safety.* Retrieved August 1, 2008 from http://www.bt.cdc.gov/disasters/extremeheat/heat_guide.asp.

Centers for Disease Control & Prevention. (2006d). *Prevalence of hypertension by age: United States, 1988–2002.* National Center for Health Statistics. Retrieved August 1, 2008 from http://www.cdc.gov/nchs/about/otheract/aging/quicktrends/qt-aging-02.png.

Centers for Disease Control & Prevention. (2006e). *Heart disease fact sheet.* Division for Heart Disease & Stoke Prevention. Retrieved August 1, 2008 from http://www.cdc.gov/dhdsp/library/fs_heart_disease.htm.

Centers for Disease Control & Prevention (CDC). (2007a). *Costs of falls among older adults.* Retrieved August 1, 2008 from http://www.cdc.gov/ncipc/factsheets/fallcost.htm.

Centers for Disease Control & Prevention (CDC). (2007b). *Chronic disease: Arthritis at a glance.* Retrieved August 1, 2008 from http://www.apps.nccd.cdc.gov/EmailForm/print_table.asp.

Centers for Disease Control & Prevention and the Merck Company Foundation. (2007). *The state of aging and health in America: 2007.* Whitehouse Station, NJ: The Merck Co. Foundation.

Centers for Medicare & Medicaid Services. (2007). *Medicare drug plans strong and growing.* Retrieved August 1, 2008 from http://www.cms.hhs.gov/PrescriptionDrugCovGenin/02_EnrollkmentData.asp.

Central Intelligence Agency (CIA). (2007). *The world factbook: Rank order: Life expectancy at birth.* Retrieved August 1, 2008 from http://www.cia.gov/library/publications/the-world-factbook/rankorder/2102rank.html.

Chen, K., Li, C., Lin, J., et al. (2007). A feasible method to enhance and maintain the health of elderly living in long-term care facilities through long-term, simplified tai chi exercises. *Journal of Nursing Research, 15*(2) 156–164.

Cherry, D., Vickery, B., Schwankovsky, L., et al. (2004). Interventions to improve quality of care: The Kaiser Permanente-Alzheimer's Association dementia care project. *American Journal of Managed Care, 10*(8), 553–560.

Chiang, K., Lu, R., Chu, H., et al. (2007). Evaluation of the effect of a life review group program on self-esteem and life satisfaction in the elderly. *International Journal of Geriatric Psychiatry,* (in press).

Chong, A.M. (2007). Promoting the psychosocial health of the elderly: The role of social workers. *Social Work in Health Care, 44*(1–2), 91–109.

Cohen, C.A. (2006). Consumer fraud and the elderly: A review of Canadian challenges and initiatives. *Journal of Gerontology in Social Work, 46*(3), 137–144.

Corporation for National & Community Service. (2007). *Foster grandparents: Make a difference in the life of a child.* Retrieved August 1, 2008 from http://www.nationalservice.gov/assets/printable/printable.asp?tbl_cms_id=32.

Daaleman, T.P. (2006). Reorganizing Medicare for older adults with chronic illness. *Journal of American Board of Family Medicine, 19*(2), 303–309.

Dong, X. (2005). Medical implications of elder abuse and neglect. *Clinical Geriatric Medicine, 21*(2), 293–313.

Duke University Center. (2007). *OARS: The method and its uses.* Center for the Study of Aging and Human Development. Retrieved August 1, 2008 from http://www.geri.duke.edu/sevice/oars.htm.

Dushoff, J., Plotkin, J., Viboud, C., et al. (2005). Mortality due to influenza in the United States: An annualized regression approach using multiple-cause mortality data. *American Journal of Epidemiology, 163*(2), 181–187.

Ebersole, P., & Hess, P. (2004). *Toward healthy aging,* 6th ed. St. Louis: Mosby.

Eldercare. (2005). *Respite care.* Retrieved August 1, 2008 from http://www.eldercare.gov/eldercare/Public/resources/fact_sheets/respite_care.asp.

Elderhostel. (2007). *Learn, travel & enjoy with not-for-profit Elderhostel.* Retrieved August 1, 2008 from http://www.elderhostel.org.

Eliopoulos, C. (2004). *Gerontological nursing,* 6th ed. Philadelphia: Lippincott Williams & Wilkins.

Environmental Alliance for Senior Involvement (EASI). (2007). *About EASI.* Retrieved August 1, 2008 from http://www.easi.org/modules.php?op=modload&name=PagEd&file=index&printerfriendly=1&page_id=15.

Ettinger, M.P. (2003). Aging bone and osteoporosis. *Archives of Internal Medicine, 163*(8), 2231–2235.

Ezekowitz, J., Straus, S., Majumdar, S., & McAlister, F. (2003). Stroke: Strategies for primary prevention. *American Family Physician, 68*(12), 2379–2386.

Fahlman, M., Morgan, A., McNevin, N., et al. (2007). Combination training and resistance training as effective interventions to improve functioning in elders. *Journal of Aging & Physical Activity, 15*(2), 195–205.

Fiscella, K. (2005). Commentary: Anatomy of racial disparity in influenza vaccination. *Health Services Research, 40*(2), 539–550.

Freudenheim, M. (May 8, 2001). Decrease in chronic illness bodes well for Medicare costs. *The New York Times.* Retrieved August 1, 2008 from http://query.nytimes.com/gst/fullpage.html?sec=health&res=9C05E5DF173BF93BA35756COA9679C8B63&fta=y.

Gist, J.R. (2007). *Population aging, entitlement growth, and the economy.* American Association of Retired Persons Public Policy Institute. Retrieved August 1, 2008 from http://www.aarp.org/ppi.

Gorbien, M.J., & Eisenstein, A.R. (2005). Elder abuse and neglect: An overview. *Clinical Geriatric Medicine, 21*(2), 279–292.

Gupta, A., Epstein, J., & Sroussi, H. (2006). Hyposalivation in elderly patients. *Journal of the Canadian Dentistry Association, 72*(9), 841–846.

Hazard, W.R. (2003). General internal medicine and geriatrics: Collaboration to address the aging imperative can't wait. *Annals of Internal Medicine, 139*(97), 597–598.

He, W., Sengupta, M., Velkoff, V., & DeBarros, K. (2005). *U.S. Census Bureau, Current Population Reports, P23–209, 65+ in the United States: 2005.* Washington, DC: U.S. Government Printing Office.

HelpGuide. (2007a). *Board and care homes for seniors.* Retrieved August 1, 2008 from http://www.helpguide.org/elder/board_care_homes_seniors_residential.htm.

HelpGuide. (2007b). *Payment options for senior housing and residential care.* Retrieved August 1, 2008 from http://www.helpguide.org/elder/paying_for_senior_housing_residential_care.htm.

Hill, R., Thorn, B., Bowling, J., & Morrison, A. (2002). *Geriatric residential care.* Mahwah, NJ: Lawrence Erlbaum Associates.

Hill-Westmoreland, E., Soeken, K., & Spellbring, A. (2002). A meta-analysis of fall prevention programs for the elderly. *How effective are they? Nursing Research, 51(1),* 1–8.

Hoffert, D., Henshaw, C., & Myududu, N. (2007). Enhancing the ability of nursing students to perform a spiritual assessment. *Nurse Educator, 32*(2), 66–72.

Holley, H. (May 2006). *Retirement planning survey among U.S. adults age 40 and older.* Retrieved August 1, 2008 from http://www.aarp.org/research/financial/retirementsaving/ret_planning.html.

International Institute for Applied Systems Analysis (IIASA). (2007). *Chapter 1: World population: Major trends.* Retrieved August 1, 2008 from http://www.iiasa.ac.at/Research/LUC/Papers/gkh1/chap1.htm.

Jerant, A.F., Azari, R., Nesbitt, R., et al. (2006). The Palliative Care in Assisted Living (PCAL) pilot study: Successes, shortfalls, and methodological implications. *Social Science in Medicine, 62*(1), 199–207.

Johansen, K., Painter, P., Kent-Braun, J., et al. (2001). Validation of questionnaires to estimate physical activity and functioning in end-stage renal disease. *Kidney International, 59,* 1121–1127.

Johnson, E.G. (2003). Pneumococcal vaccine rates in persons age 65 years and older: A U.S. Air Force medical facility record review. *Military Medicine, 168*(9), 706–709.

Joyce, G., Keeler, E., Shang, B., & Goldman, D. (2005). *The lifetime burden of chronic disease among the elderly.* Health Affairs. Retrieved August 1, 2008 from http://www.content.healthaffairs.org/cgi/content/abstract/hlthaff.w5.r18v1.

Jurasek, G. (2002). Oral health affect pneumonia risk in the elderly. *Pulmonary Reviews.Com, 7*(9). Retrieved August 1, 2008 from http://www.pulmonaryreviews.com/sep02/pr_sep02_oralhealth.html.

Kaiser Permanente Healthwise Handbook, 21st ed. (2006, revised). Boise, ID: Healthwise.

Kapo, J., Morrison, L., & Liao, S. (2007). Palliative care for the older adult. *Journal of Palliative Medicine, 10*(1), 185–209.

Kettl, P. (2007). Helping families with end-of-life care in Alzheimer's disease. *Journal of Clinical Psychiatry, 68*(3), 445–450.

Kim, D., & Kawachi, I. (2006). A multilevel analysis of key forms of community- and individual-level social capital as predictors of self-rated health in the United States. *Journal of Urban Health, 83*(5), 813–826.

Kramer, H., Han, C., Post, W., et al. (2004). Racial/ethnic differences in hypertension and hypertension treatment and control in the multi-ethnic study of atherosclerosis (MESA). *American Journal of Hypertension, 17*(10), 963–970.

Kressig, R.W., & Echt, K.V. (2002). Exercise prescribing: Computer application in older adults. *The Gerontologist, 42*(2), 273–277.

Kübler-Ross, E. (1975). *Death: The final stage of growth.* Englewood Cliffs, NJ: Prentice-Hall.

Kuehn, B. (2005). Better osteoporosis management a priority: Impact predicted to soar with aging population. *JAMA, 293*(20), 2453–2458.

Lach, M.S., & Pillemer, K. (2004). Elder abuse. *Lancet, 364,* 1263–1272.

Lorenz, K., Lynn J., Morton S.C., et al. (2004). *End-of-life care and outcomes: Summary.* Evidence Report/Technology Assessment: Number 110. AHRQ Publication Number 05-E004-1, December 2004. Agency for Healthcare Research and Quality, Rockville, MD. Retrieved August 1, 2008 from http://www.ahrq.gov/clinic/epcsums/eolsum.htm.

Mace, N.L., & Rabins, P.V. (2001). *The 36-hour day,* 3rd ed. [Large print.] Baltimore: Johns Hopkins University Press.

Maciosek, M., Coffield, A., Edwards, N., et al. (2006). Priorities among effective clinical preventive services: Results of a systematic review and analysis. *American Journal of Preventive Medicine, 31*(1), 52–61.

Manor, O., & Eisenbach, Z. (2003). Mortality after spousal loss: Are there socio-demographic differences? *Social Sciences & Medicine, 56*(2), 405–413.

Martin, J.E., & Sheaff, M.T. (2007). The pathology of ageing: Concepts and mechanisms. *Journal of Pathology, 211*(2), 111–113.

Martini, E.M., Garrett, N., Lindquist, T., & Isham, G.J. (2007). The boomers are coming: A total cost of care model of the impact of population again on health care costs in the United States by Major Practice Category (MPC). *Health Services Research, 42*[1 Pt. 1], 201–218.

Mason, A., Weatherly, H., Spilsbury, K., et al. (2007). A systematic review of the effectiveness and cost-effectiveness of different models of community-based respite care for frail older people and their caregivers. *Health Technology Assessment, 11*(15), 1–176.

McKeon, V.A. (2002, February/March). Exploring HRT. *AWHONN Lifelines,* 24–31.

Medical News Today. (2006). *Mild cognitive impairment prevalent in elderly population.* Retrieved August 1, 2008 from http://www.medicalnewstoday.com/printerfriendlynews.php?newsid=41039.

Medline Plus. (2007a). *Advance directives.* Retrieved August 1, 2008 from http://www.nim.nih.gov/medlineplus/advancedirectives.html.

Medline Plus. (2007b). *Assisted living.* Retrieved from http://www.nlm.nih.gov/medlineplus/assistedliving.html.

Meurman, J., Sanz, M., & Janket, S.J. (2004). Oral health, atherosclerosis, and cardiovascular disease. *Critical Reviews in Oral Biology & Medicine, 15*(6), 403–413.

Miller, C.A. (2003). *Nursing care of older adults: Theory and practice,* 4th ed. Philadelphia: Lippincott Williams & Wilkins.

Mion, L., Palmer, R., Anetzberger, G., & Meldon, S. (2001). Establishing a case-finding and referral system for at-risk older individuals in the emergency department setting: The SIGNET model. *Journal of the American Geriatric Society, 49*(10), 1379–1386.

Mitchell, S., Teno, J., Intrator, O., et al. (2007). Hospitalization of nursing home residents: The effects of states' Medicaid payments. *Journal of the American Geriatric Society, 55*(3), 432–438.

Moberg, D.O. (Ed.). (2001). *Aging and spirituality: Spiritual dimensions of aging theory, research, practice, and policy.* Binghamton, NY: Haworth Press.

Mokdad, A.H., Marks, J.S., Stroup, D.F., & Gerberding, J.L. (2004). Actual causes of death in the United States, 2000. *The Journal of the American Medical Association, 291*(10), 1238–1245.

Mollica, R. (2003). Coordinating services across the continuum of health, housing & supportive services. *Journal of Aging & Health, 15*(1), 165–188.

Moore, A.J., & Stratton, D.C. (2002). *Resilient widowers: Older men speak for themselves.* New York: Springer.

Morin, R., & Russakoff, D. (February 10, 2005). *Social Security problems not a crisis, most say.* Retrieved August 18, 2008 from http://www.washingtonpost.com/wp-dyn/articles/A12231-2005Feb9.html

Mullin, B., & Kelley, P. (2006). Diabetes nurse case management: An effective tool. *Journal of the American Academy of Nurse Practitioners, 18(1),* 22–30.

National Alliance on Mental Illness (NAMI). (2003). *Depression in older persons.* Retrieved August 18, 2008 from http://www.nami.org/PrinterTemplate.cfm?Section=By_Illness&template=/ContentManagement/ContentDisplay.cfm&ContentID=7515.

National Association of Area Agencies on Aging. (2007). *A blueprint for action: Developing a livable community for all ages.* Retried August 18, 2008 from http://www.n4a.org/pdf/07-116-n4a-blueprint4actionwcovers.pdf.

National Center for Health Statistics. (2002). *Health, United States, 2002, with chartbook on trends in the health of Americans.* Hyattsville, MD: Author.

National Center on Elder Abuse. (2006). *Abuse of adults aged 60+: 2004 Survey of Adult Protective Services.* Retrieved August 18, 2008 from http://www.elderabusecenter.org/pdf/2-14-06%2060FACT%20SHEET.pdf.

National Center on Elder Abuse. (2005). *Elder abuse prevalence and incidence.* Retrieved August 18, 2008 from http://www.elderabusecenter.org/pdf/publication/FinalStatistics050331.pdf.

National Citizen's Coalition for Nursing Home Reform. (2007). *Issue index.* Retrieved August 18, 2008 from http://www.ncc-nhr.org/public/245_2072_13432.cfm.

National Council on Aging. (2005). *Falls free: Promoting a national falls preventions action plan.* Retrieved August 18, 2008 from http://www.healthyagingprograms.org/resources/FallsFree_NationalActionPlan_Final.pdf.

National Foundation for Infectious Diseases. (2002). *Influenza and pneumococcal vaccines.* Retrieved August 18, 2008 from http://www.nfid.org/pressconf/flu02/release.html.

National Hospice & Palliative Care Organization. (2007). *New research finds patients do live longer under hospice care.* Retrieved August 18, 2008 from http://www.nhpco.org/i4a/pages/Index.cfm?pageID=54145.

National Institute of Arthritis & Musculoskeletal & Skin Diseases. (2006a). *Handout on health: Osteoarthritis.* Retrieved August 18, 2008 from http://www.niams.nih.gov/hi/topics/arthritis/oahandout.htm#1.

National Institute of Arthritis & Musculoskeletal & Skin Diseases. (2006b). *What people with rheumatoid arthritis need to know about osteoporosis.* Retrieved August 18, 2008 from http://www.niams.nih.gov/bone/hi/osteopososis_ra.htm.

National Institute on Aging. (2006a). *Alzheimer's disease fact sheet.* Retrieved August 18, 2008 from http://www.nia.nih.gov/Alzheimers/Publications/adfact.htm.

National Institute on Aging. (2003). Retrieved January 29, 2004 from http://www.nia.nih.gov.

National Institute on Aging. (2006b). *New brain imaging compound shows promise for earlier detection of Alzheimer's disease.* Retrieved August 18, 2008 from http://www.nia.nih.gov/Alzheimers/ResearchInformation/NewsReleases/20061220FDDNP.htm.

National Institute on Aging. (2007). *Scientists find new genetic clue to cause of Alzheimer's disease.* Retrieved August 18, 2008 from http://www.nia.nih.gov/Alzheimers/ResearchInformation/NewsReleases/PR20070114SORL1gene.htm.

Newsom, R.S., & Kemps, E.B. (2007). Factors that promote and prevent exercise engagement in older adults. *Journal of Aging & Health, 19*(3), 470–481.

Nussbaum, S.R. (2006). Prevention: The cornerstone of quality health care. *American Journal of Preventive Medicine, 31*(1), 107–108.

Nwasuruba, C., Khan, M., & Egede, L. (2007). Racial/ethnic differences in multiple self-care behaviors in adults with diabetes. *Journal of General Internal Medicine, 22*(1), 115–120.

O'Brien, M.E. (2003). *Spirituality in nursing: Standing on holy ground,* 2nd ed. Sudbury, MA: Jones & Bartlett.

Ory, M., Hoffman, M., Hawkins, M., et al. (2003). Challenging aging stereotypes: Strategies for creating a more active society. *American Journal of Preventive Medicine, 25*(3), [Suppl. 2], 164–171.

Ostbye, T., Krause, K., Norton, M., et al. (2006). Ten dimensions of health and their relationships with overall self-reported health and survival in a predominately religiously active elderly population: The Cache County study. *Journal of the American Geriatric Society, 54*(2), 199–209.

Owen, T. (2007). Working with socially isolated older people. *British Journal of Community Nursing, 12*(3), 115–116.

Palmore, E. (2005). Three decades of research on ageism. *The American Society on Aging: Generations, 29*(3), 87–90.

Peace Corps. (2007). *About the Peace Corps.* Retrieved August 18, 2008 from http://www.peacecorps.gov/index.cfm?shell=learn.whatispc.

Pew Research Center. (2006). *Working after retirement: The gap between expectations and reality.* Retrieved August 18, 2008 from http://www.pewresearch.org/pubs/320/working-after-retirement-the-gap-between-expectations-and-reality.

Population Reference Bureau. (2006). *Full-time work among elderly increases.* Retrieved August 18, 2008 from http://www.prb.org/Articles/2006/FullTimeWorkAmongElderlyIncreases.aspx.

Rahimi, A., Spertus, J., Reid, K., et al. (2007). Financial barriers to health care and outcomes after acute myocardial infarction. *The Journal of the American Medical Association, 297*(10), 1063–1072.

RAND. (2003a). *Evidence report and evidence-based recommendations: Falls prevention interventions in the Medicare population.* Retrieved August 18, 2008 from http://www.rand.org/pubs/reprints/2007/RAND_RP1230.sum.pdf.

RAND Health. (2003b). *Living well at the end of life: Adapting health care to serious chronic illness in old age.* Palliative Care Policy Center. Retrieved August 18, 2008 from http://www.medicaring.org/whitepaper/.

RealAge. (2007). *The science and philosophy behind RealAge.* Retrieved August 18, 2008 from http://www.realage.com/corporate/ra_faqs.aspx?pg=1#1.

Richardson, S., Sullivan, G., Hill, A., & Yu, W. (2007). Use of aggressive medical treatments near the end of life: Differences between patients with and without dementia. *Health Services Research, 42*(1), 183–200.

Rose, D.J. (2003). *Results of intervention research: Implications for practice.* Retrieved August 18, 2008 from http://www.generationsjournal.org/generations/gen26-4/article.cfm.

Rubinstein, H.G. (2005). Access to oral health care for elders: Mere words or action? *Journal of Dental Education, 69*(9), 1051–1057.

Salzman, B. (2006). Myths and realities of aging. *Care Management Journals, 7*(3), 141–150.

Sato, Y., Nagasaki, M., Kubota, M., et al. (2007). Clinical aspects of physical exercise for diabetes/metabolic syndrome. *Diabetes Research in Clinical Practice* (in press).

Schwappach, D., Boluarte, T., & Suhrcke, M. (2007). The economics of primary prevention of cardiovascular disease: A systematic review of economic evaluations. *Cost Effectiveness and Resource Allocation, 5.* Retrieved from http://www.pubmedcentral.nih.gov/articlerender.fcgi?tool=pubmed&pubmedid=17501999.

Science Blog. (2003). *New Alzheimer projections add urgency to search for prevention, cure.* Retrieved August 18, 2008 from http://www.scienceblog.com/community/older/2003/C/2003102.html.

Senior Corps. (2007). *RSVP.* Retrieved August 18, 2008 from http://www.seniorcorps.gov/about/programs/rsvp.asp.

Shashikiran, U., Vidyasagar, S., & Prabhu, M. (2004). Diabetes in the elderly. *The Internet Journal of Geriatrics & Gerontology, 1*(2). Retrieved August 18, 2008 from http://www.ispub.com/ostia/index.php?xmlFilePath=journals/ijgg/vol1n2/diabetes.xml.

Simonsen, L., Reichert, T., Viboud, C., et al. (2005). Impact of influenza vaccination on seasonal mortality in the US elderly population. *Archives of Internal Medicine, 165*(3), 265–272.

Singer, T., Lindenberger, U., & Baltes, P. (2003). Plasticity of memory for new learning in very old age a story of major loss? *Psychology & Aging, 18*(2), 306–317.

Social Security Administration. (2006). *Frequently asked questions about Social Security's future.* Retrieved August 18, 2008 from http://www.ssa.gov/qa.htm.

Spector, R.E. (2004). *Cultural diversity in health and illness,* 6th ed. Upper Saddle River, NJ: Prentice Hall.

Stevens, J.A., Corso, P.S., Fiinkelstein, E.A., & Miller, T.R. (2006). The costs of fatal and non-fatal falls among older adults. *Injury Prevention, 12*(5), 290–295.

Stoller, M.A. (2003). Perceived income adequacy among elderly retirees. *Journal of Applied Gerontology, 22*(2), 230–251.

Stone, C., & Greenstein, R. (2007, April 24). What the 2007 trustees' report shows about Social Security. Center on Budget & Policy Priorities. Retrieved October 18, 2008 from http://www.cbpp.org/4-24-07socsec.pdf.

Sulter, G., Steen, C., & DeKeyser, J. (1999). Use of the Bethel Index and Modified Rankin Scale in acute stroke trials. *Stroke, 30,* 1538–1541.

The Henry J. Kaiser Family Foundation. (2003). *Key facts: Race, ethnicity, and medical care (June 2003 update).* Menlo Park, CA: Author.

The Raw Story. (2007, May 16). US elderly brush up driving skills to stay behind the wheel. Retrieved October 18, 2008 from http://rawstory.com/news/afp/US elderly brush up driving skills 05162007.html.

The Senior Source. (2007). *Friendly Visitor program.* Retrieved August 18, 2008 from http://www.theseniorsource.org/pages/friendlyvisitor.html.

United Nations. (2003a). *The diversity of changing population age structures in the world.* Population Division, Department of Economic and Social Affairs. Retrieved August 18, 2008 from http://www.un.org/esa/population/meetings/Proceedings_EGM_Mex_2005/popdiv.pdf.

United Nations. (2003b). *United Nations Expert Group Meeting on social and economic implications of changing population age structures.* Department of Economic and Social Affairs, Population Division. Retrieved from http://www.un.org/esa/population/meetings/Proceedings_EGM_Mex_2005/index.htm.

University of Virginia News. (2006). *University of Virginia study: Car crashes are more deadly for seniors: Traffic fatalities expected to rise as baby boomers age.* Retrieved August 18, 2008 from http://www.virginia.edu/topnews/releases2006/20060613KentSeniorDrivers.html.

U.S. Census Bureau. (2000). *Projections of the total resident population by 5-year age groups, race, and Hispanic origin with special age categories: Middle series, 2006 to 2010.* Population Projections Program, Population Division. Retrieved August 18, 2008 from http://www.census.gov/population/projections/nation/summary/np-t4-c.txt.

U.S. Census Bureau. (2007). U.S. interim projections by age, sex, race, and Hispanic origin. Retrieved August 18, 2008 from http://www.census.gov/ipc/www.usinterimproj/.

U.S. Department of Health and Human Services. (2000). *Healthy people 2010.* [Conference ed., Vols. 1 & 2]. Washington, DC: U.S. Government Printing Office.

U.S. Department of Justice. (2006). *Criminal victimization in the United States, 2005: Statistical tables.* Retrieved August 18, 2008 from http://www.ojp.usdoj.gov/bjs/pub/pdf/cvus/current/cv0579.pdf.

U.S. Department of Health and Human Services (USDHHS). (2006). *Want to learn more about the new Medicare prescription drug coverage?* Retrieved October 18, 2008 from http://www.medicare.gov/MedicareReform/drugbenefit.asp.

Wallace, M., Shelkey, M., & The Hartford Institute for Geriatric Nursing. (2007). Katz Index of Independence in Activities of Daily Living (ADL). *Urology Nursing, 27*(1), 93–94.

Warburton, J., McLaughlin, D., & Pinsker, D. (2006). Generative acts: Family and community involvement of older Australians. *International Journal of Aging & Human Development, 63*(2), 115–137.

Ward, G., Jagger, C., & Harper, W. (1998). A review of instrumental ADL assessments for use with elderly people. *Reviews in Clinical Gerontology, 8,* 65–71.

Williams, B., Sawyer-Baker, P., Allman, R., & Roseman, J. (2007). Bereavement among African American and White older adults. *Journal of Aging & Health, 19*(2), 313–333.

Williams, J.R. (2005). Depression as a mediator between spousal bereavement and mortality from cardiovascular disease: Appreciating and managing the adverse health consequences of depression in an elderly surviving spouse. *Southern Medical Journal, 98*(1), 90–95.

Wolff, J., Starfield, B., & Anderson, G. (2002). Prevalence, expenditures, and complications of multiple chronic conditions in the elderly. *Archives of Internal Medicine, 162*(20), 2269–2276.

Woo, J., Hong, A., Lau, E., & Lynn, H. (2007). A randomized controlled trial of Tai Chi and resistance exercise on bone health, muscle strength and balance in community-living elderly people. *Age and Ageing, 36*(3), 262–268.

Wooten, J., & Galavis, J. (2005). *Polypharmacy: Keeping the elderly safe.* Retrieved August 18, 2008 from http://www.rnweb.com/rnweb/content/printContentPopup.jsp?id=172920.

Yang, Y. (2006). How does functional disability affect depressive symptoms in late life? The role of perceived social support and psychological resources. *Journal of Perceived Social Support & Psychological Resources, 47*(4), 355–372.

Ziegler, R., & Mitchell, D. (2003). Aging and fear of crime: An experimental approach to an apparent paradox. *Experimental Aging Research, 29*(2), 173–187.

Selected Readings

Akoyl, A.D. (2007). Falls in the elderly: What can be done? *International Nursing Review, 54*(2), 191–196.

Anderson, M.A. (Ed.). (2007). *Caring for older adults holistically,* 4th ed. Philadelphia, PA: F.A. Davis Co.

Bowling, A. (2007). Aspirations for older age in the 21st century: What is successful aging? *International Journal of Aging & Human Development, 64*(3), 263–297.

Centers for Disease Control & Prevention (CDC). (2006). *Growing stronger: Strength training for older adults.* Retrieved August 18, 2008 from http://www.cdc.gov/nccdphp/dnpa/physical/growing_stronger/index.htm.

Chernlack, P., & Chernlack, N. (Eds.). (2003). *Alternative medicine for the elderly.* New York, NY: Springer Publishing.

Clegg, A., Bradley, M., Smith, P., & Kirk, Z. (2006). Developing the nurse's role in the care of older people. *Nursing Older People, 18*(5), 26–30.

Fransen, M., Nairn, L., Winstanley, J., et al. (2007). Physical activity for osteoarthritis management: A randomized controlled clinical trial evaluating hydrotherapy or Tai Chi classes. *Arthritis and Rheumatism, 57*(3), 407–414.

Gray, S. (2003). Potentially inappropriate medication use in community residential care facilities. *The Annals of Pharmacotherapy, 37*(7), 988–993.

Hainer, T.A. (2007). Managing older adults with diabetes. *Journal of the American Academy of Nurse Practitioners, 18*(7), 309–317.

Hannah, J.M., & Friedman, J.H. (2006). *Taking charge: Good medical care for the elderly and how to get it.* Traverse City, MI: Old Mission Press.

Hash, K. (2006). Caregiving and post-caregiving experiences of midlife and older gay men and lesbians. *Journal of Gerontological Social Work, 47*(3–4), 121–138.

Hodge, W., Horsley, T., Albiani, D., et al. (2007). The consequences of waiting for cataract surgery: A systematic review. *Canadian Medical Association Journal, 176*(9), 1285–1290.

Irminger-Finger, I. (2007). Science of cancer and aging. *Journal of Clinical Oncology, 25*(14), 1844–1851.

Kean, R. (2006). Understanding the lives of older gay people. *Nursing Older People, 18*(8), 31–36.

Kennie, D.C. (2004). *Preventive care for elderly people.* New York, NY: Cambridge University Press.

Kohlenberg, E., Kennedy-Malone, L., Crane, P., & Letvak, S. (2007). Infusing gerontological nursing content into advanced practice nursing education. *Nursing Outlook, 55*(1), 38–43.

Landi, F., Onder, G., Carpenter, I., et al. (2007). Physical activity prevented functional decline among frail community-living elderly subjects in an international observational study. *Journal of Clinical Epidemiology, 60*(5), 518–524.

Lee, D., Gomz-Marin, O., Lam, B., et al. (2007). Severity of concurrent visual and hearing impairment and mortality: The 1986–1994 National Health Interview Survey. *Journal of Aging and Health, 19*(3), 382–396.

McCleane, G., & Smith, H. (Eds.). (2006). *Clinical management of the elderly patient in pain.* Binghamton, NY: Haworth Medical Press.

Milisen, K., Staelens, N., Schwendimann, R., et al. (2007). Fall prediction in inpatients by bedside nurses using the St. Thomas's Risk Assessment Tool in Falling elderly Inpatients (STRATIFY) instrument: A multicenter study. *Journal of the American Geriatric Society, 55*(5), 725–733.

Mollica, R. (2001). The evolution of assisted living. A view from the states. *Caring, 20*(8), 24–26.

Mosley, R., & Jett, K.F. (2007). Advance practice nursing and sexual functioning in late life. *Geriatric Nursing, 28*(1), 41–42.

National Institutes of Health. (2005). *Senior health: Exercise for older adults.* Retrieved August 18, 2008 from http://nihseniorhealth.gov/exercise/toc.html.

Petty, T.L., & Seebass, J.S. (Eds.). (2006). *Pulmonary disorders of the elderly: Diagnosis, prevention, and treatment.* Philadelphia: American College of Physicians.

Solomon, D., Polinski, J., Stedman, M., et al. (2007). Improving care of patients at-risk for osteoporosis: A randomized controlled trial. *Journal of General Internal Medicine, 22*(3), 362–367.

Tolson, D., Irene, S., Booth, J., et al. (2006). Constructing a new approach to developing evidence-based practice with nurses and older people. *Worldviews on Evidence-Based Nursing, 3*(2), 62–72.

U.S. Food & Drug Administration (FDA). (2007). *Medicines and older adults.* Retrieved August 18, 2008 from http://www.fda.gov/opacom/lowlit/medold.html.

Van Gool, C.H., Kempen, G.I., Pennix, B.W., et al. (2007). Chronic diseases and lifestyle transitions: Results from the Longitudinal Aging Study Amsterdam. *Journal of Aging and Health, 19*(3), 416–438.

Wagner, L., Capezuti, E., Brush, B., et al. (2007). Description of an advanced practice nursing consultative model to reduce restrictive siderail use in nursing homes. *Research in Nursing and Health, 30*(2), 131–140.

Wengreen, J., Munger, R., Corcoran, C., et al. (2007). Antioxidant intake and cognitive function of elderly men and women: The Cache County Study. *Journal of Nutrition, Health & Aging, 11*(3), 230–237.

Wolkove, N., Elkholy, O., Baltzan, M., & Palayew, M. (2007). Sleep and aging: 2. Management of sleep disorders in older people. *Canadian Medical Association Journal, 176*(10), 1449–1454.

Yaffe, K., Haan, M., Blackwell, T., et al. (2007). Metabolic syndrome and cognitive decline in elderly Latinos: Findings from the Sacramento Area Latino Study of Aging study. *Journal of the American Geriatric Society, 55*(5), 758–762.

Internet Resources

Administration on Aging: *http://www.aoa.gov*

Alzheimer's Disease Education and Referral Center (ADEAR): *http://www.nia.nih.gov/alzheimers*

AARP (formerly the American Association of Retired Persons): *http://www.aarp.org*

Association of Late Deafened Adults: *http://www.alda.org/*

Dementia: *http://www.dementia.com/home.jhtml?_requestid=847348*

Elderhostel: *http://www.elderhostel.org/*

Generations United: *http://www.gu.org/*

Gerontological Society of America: *http://www.geron.org/*

GriefNet: *http://www.griefnet.org/*

Healthy Aging (CDC): *http://www.cdc.gov/aging/*

Hearing Loss & Older Adults: *http://www.nidcd.nih.gov/health/hearing/older.asp*

Medications & Older People: *http://www.fda.gov/fdac/features/1997/697_old.html*

Modified Food Pyramid for Older Adults: *http://nutrition.tufts.edu/consumer/pyramid.html*

National Institute on Aging: *http://nihseniorhealth.gov/*

National Mental Health Information Center (Guide for Older Adults): *http://mentalhealth.samhsa.gov/publications/allpubs/KEN-01-0094/default.asp*

National Parkinson Foundation: *http://www.parkinson.org/NETCOMMUNITY/Page.aspx?&pid=201&srcid=-2*

Older Adults: Depression & Suicide Facts: *http://www.nimh.nih.gov/publicat/elderlydepsuicide.cfm*

Older Adult Drivers Fact Sheet (CDC): *http://www.cdc.gov/ncipc/factsheets/older.htm*

Older Adults and Sleep: *http://www.sleepfoundation.org/site/c.huIXKjM0IxF/b.2419289/k.290D/Aging_Gracefully_and_Sleeping_Well.htm*

Real Age: *http://www.realage.com/*

SPRY Foundation: *http://www.spry.org/sprys_work/education.html*

The Geezer Brigade: *http://www.thegeezerbrigade.com/*

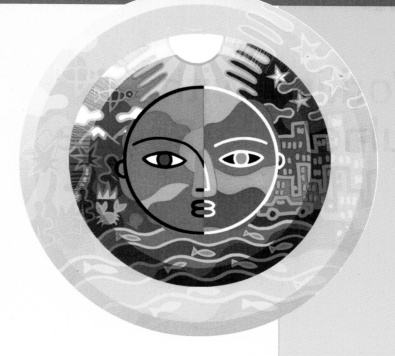

PROMOTING AND PROTECTING THE HEALTH OF VULNERABLE POPULATIONS

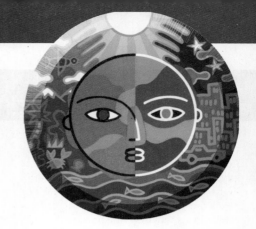

25

Working with Vulnerable People

LEARNING OBJECTIVES

Upon mastery of this chapter, you should be able to:

◆ Describe what the term "vulnerable populations" means.
◆ Describe and explain a conceptual model of vulnerability.
◆ Discuss the effects of vulnerability and relative risk.
◆ Differentiate between the concepts of social capital and human capital.
◆ Identify the key premise of the differential vulnerability hypothesis.
◆ List three of the most common factors related to vulnerability.
◆ Explain the socioeconomic gradient in health.
◆ Describe three types of health disparities.

❝*How far you go in life depends on your being tender with the young, compassionate with the aged, sympathetic with the striving, and tolerant of the weak and the strong—because someday you will have been all of these.*❞

—George Washington Carver

KEY TERMS

Differential vulnerability hypothesis
Environmental resources
Health disparity
Human capital
Participatory action research
Relative risk
Resilience
Social capital
Social determinants of health
Socioeconomic gradient
Socioeconomic resources
Vulnerability
Vulnerable populations

Vulnerability has been defined as being susceptible to neglect or harm, or being at risk of poor social, psychological, and/or physical health outcomes (Aday, 2001). The public health nurse (PHN) caseload is largely comprised of those who represent vulnerable populations. The term "vulnerable" comes from a Latin word that means *wound*, and **vulnerable populations** are groups who have a heightened risk of adverse health outcomes (Leight, 2003). They often have higher mortality rates, less access to health care (and disparities in the quality of care), are uninsured or underinsured, have lower life expectancy, and an overall diminished quality of life (Shi & Stevens, 2004; University of California Los Angeles [UCLA] Center for Vulnerable Populations Research, 2007). Some researchers feel that vulnerability stems from "developmental problems, personal incapacities, disadvantaged social status, inadequacy of interpersonal networks and supports, degraded neighborhoods and environments, and the complex interactions of these factors over the life course" (Mechanic & Tanner, 2007, p. 1220).

This section provides information on aggregates that are often considered vulnerable populations: the disabled and chronically ill, mentally ill and substance abusers, the homeless, and vulnerable groups living in rural and urban areas. Different researchers and authors characterize vulnerable populations in their own way. For the purposes of this introductory chapter, we will examine popular models and theories of vulnerability, as well as important concepts and contributing factors. We will also briefly discuss health disparities that often plague the more vulnerable members of our society, and the role of PHNs working with these groups. This chapter provides an overview of this subject and lays the foundation for further chapters within this section.

THE CONCEPT OF VULNERABLE POPULATIONS

Models and Theories of Vulnerability

A popular conceptual framework developed by a nursing professor and postdoctoral fellow at the University of California, Los Angeles examines three related concepts: resource availability, relative risk, and health status (Flaskerud & Winslow, 1998). They posit that a lack of resources (e.g., socioeconomic and environmental) increases a population's exposure to risk factors and reduces their ability to avoid illness. A community's health status can be observed by noting disease prevalence along with morbidity and mortality rates. Within this framework, the more risk a population faces, the greater the impact on their health status (e.g., higher morbidity and mortality rates). A feedback loop exists from health status to resource availability, as higher morbidity and mortality further deplete community resources (see Fig. 25.1).

To further define model components, Flaskerud and Winslow (1998) explain that **socioeconomic resources** can include such things as human capital (e.g., jobs, income, housing, education), social connectedness or integration (e.g., social networks or ties, social support or the lack of it, characterized by marginalization), and social status (e.g., position, power, role). **Environmental resources** deal mostly with access to health care and the quality of that care. The authors note the differential access to health care among

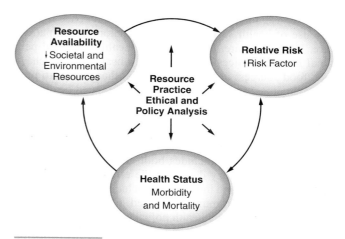

FIGURE 25.1 Vulnerable populations conceptual model. Adapted from Flaskerud, J. & Winslow, B. (1998). Conceptualizing vulnerable populations health-related research. *Nursing Research, 47*(2), 69–78.

the poor, different ethnic and racial groups, and other underserved populations. Decreased access to care can arise from many sources, including crime-ridden neighborhoods, insufficient transportation systems, lack of adequate numbers and types of providers, and limited choices of health care plans or no health insurance. **Relative risk** refers to exposure to risk factors identified by a substantial body of research as lifestyle, behaviors and choices (e.g., diet, exercise, use of tobacco, alcohol and other drugs, sexual behaviors), use of health screening services (e.g., immunizations, health promotion, use of seatbelts), and stressful events (e.g., crime, violence, abuse, firearm use). They note, for instance, that in populations of single-parent female-headed homes in poverty with little or no access to social programs, violence and homicide are more prevalent. They provide evidence of the link between poor health status and socioeconomic resource availability through the loss of income, jobs, and health insurance. In the case of environmental resources, high morbidity in an already underserved population will only exacerbate access problems.

Gelberg, Andersen, and Leake (2000) advanced The Behavioral Model for Vulnerable Populations that looked at population characteristics (predisposing and enabling factors and needs) as an explanation for health behaviors and eventual health outcomes. Predisposing factors included demographic variables (e.g., gender, age, marital status), social variables (e.g., education, employment, ethnicity, social networks), and health beliefs (e.g., values and attitudes toward health and health care services, knowledge of disease). Social structures (e.g., acculturation and immigration), sexual orientation, and childhood characteristics (e.g., mobility, living conditions, history of substance abuse, criminal behavior, victimization, or mental illness) were also considered as predisposing factors. Enabling factors included personal and family resources, as well as community resources (e.g., income, insurance, social support, region, health services resources, public benefits, transportation, telephone, crime rates, social services resources). Perceived health needs and population health conditions also were considered, as were health behaviors including diet, exercise, tobacco use, self-care, and adherence to care. The use of health services (e.g., ambulatory and inpatient care, long-term care, and alternative health care) and personal health practices (e.g., hygiene, unsafe sexual behaviors, food sources) combined with the other factors to produce outcomes, such as perceived and evaluated health and general satisfaction with health care services.

LuAnn Aday, a sociologist born and raised in rural Texas and a professor at the University of Texas School of Public Health, developed a Framework for Studying Vulnerable Populations that includes both macro and micro perspectives (2001). Aday describes the effects of policies on both communities and individuals, including social and economic policies, community-oriented health policies, and medical care and public health policies. She notes that community resources (e.g., strong neighborhoods, close ties between citizens) have a direct effect on individual resources (e.g., social status, social ties, human capital). For instance, a community with a high proportion of children, adolescents, and elderly, and a majority of single female-headed households will likely also be characterized by lower education levels, higher unemployment, and lower income levels, along with a subsequently higher relative risk of poor health status. When strong social networks are present and housing is adequate, the relative risk of poor psychological, social, or physical health decreases. Aday (2001) subscribes to a **differential vulnerability hypothesis** that "negative or stressful events (such as unemployment, divorce, or death of a loved one) hurt some people more than others" (p. 4). Even though we all are subjected to stressful events (nursing school, for instance), Aday cites research showing that low socioeconomic status (SES) groups, for example, are more adversely affected by stressful or negative events than those with higher SES. The "chronic psychosocial stresses" of lack of material resources and social marginalization experienced in childhood and early adolescence can make real physical changes by influencing "gene expression via neuroendocrine regulatory dysfunction" and are the basis of vulnerability to poor health in adulthood (Furumoto-Dawson, Gehlert, Sohmer, Olopade, & Sacks, 2007, p. 1238). The expression and interaction of these developmental genes with physical and social environments can produce long-term poor health outcomes. In other words, early chronic stressors can induce physiological changes that lead to later negative health outcomes.

Like Flaskerud and Winslow (1998), Aday notes that social status (e.g., age, gender, race, and ethnicity) affects social capital and human capital. **Social capital** consists of marital status, family structure, social ties and networks, and membership in voluntary organizations, such as church or clubs. Aday links **human capital** to investments in individuals' capabilities and skills (e.g., education, job training), and notes that it comprises jobs, income, housing, and education. Aday (2001) describes research showing that better health status is associated with higher education levels, and notes that the personal and political power of individuals and communities differentially affects their efforts to gain access to adequate schools, housing, and employment. "The social status and social capital resources of individuals and groups in a community influence the level of investments that are likely to be made in the schools, jobs, housing, and associated earning potential of the families and individuals living within it" (p. 8). Deficient social networks and social status

can lead to a cycle of poverty or vulnerability that can be difficult to break (Jones, 2003).

The importance of social capital is sometimes missed, as it can be subtle and less obvious than the lack of money or jobs. But the presence of friends and family, or someone to rely on in case of an emergency, can be invaluable in assisting individuals through many of life's difficulties. This can be very helpful to an individual while completing schooling or during employment. Social support, or a close confidant, can promote social and psychological health and help counteract the effects of stressful events. In our mobile society, many people live great distances from family members and have difficulty establishing new friendships. Those who live alone or who are socially isolated are at greatest risk, and PHNs should be aware of this and strive to provide additional support and resources (Aday, 2001).

Who Is Considered Vulnerable?

The most commonly cited causes of vulnerability or increased risk of poor health are income and education, along with race or ethnic background (Frist, 2005; Williams & Jackson, 2005). Aday (2001) includes the following factors and populations in her description of vulnerable populations:

- Income and education
- Age and gender
- Race and ethnicity
- Chronic illness and disability
- Human immunodeficiency virus (HIV)/acquired immune deficiency syndrome (AIDS)
- Mental illness and disability
- Alcohol and substance abuse
- Familial abuse
- Homelessness
- Suicide and homicide risk
- High-risk mothers and infants
- Immigrants and refugees

Other authors consider the uninsured and underinsured as vulnerable populations due to their difficulties with health care access and potential for poor health outcomes (Pauly & Pagan, 2007; Shi & Stevens, 2004). Single parents and those living in violent environments may also be recognized as vulnerable populations (Gitterman, 2001). Evans (2006) notes that those without liberty (e.g., prisoners, detainees) and rural populations, or those living in areas prone to natural disasters, are also vulnerable. As mentioned earlier, the higher SES groups generally have better access to health care and report that they are in better health. The very young and the very old have particular risk factors that increase their chances of poor health, as well as unique issues with access to health care. Some chronic illnesses and conditions are more prevalent in men than women, and vice versa. And, an extensive body of research substantiates the reality of health disparities and increased morbidity and mortality rates for racial and ethnic minorities (Aday, 2001; Byrd & Clayton, 2002; Institute of Medicine [IOM], 2003).

Prevalence of Vulnerable Populations and Causative Factors

Because many of the these conditions and categories have overlapping populations, it is difficult to access accurate data and statistics for each group or category. For example, someone with lower education and income may also be a member of a racial or ethnic minority and may have inadequate housing along with a chronic illness and high-risk births. Aday (2001) notes that rates of low birth weight and infant mortality, along with teenage pregnancy and inadequate prenatal care for mothers, are indicators of substantial problems in that particular area. Similar evidence for each of the listed areas reveals less than stellar progress toward *Healthy People 2010* objectives and further reiterates the gravity of the problem (Agency for Healthcare Research & Quality [AHRQ], 2006).

Root causes of vulnerability, such as SES, insurance coverage, and race or ethnicity, have been widely researched. Which factor is considered most important? The exact weight of the interaction of these variables has been difficult to ascertain. Haas and Adler (2001) have examined multiple, large-scale studies and determined that SES, race/ethnicity, and insurance coverage "each independently influence the utilization of health care and health status" (p. 28).

Poverty

If only one indicator is measured—poverty—it is evident that vulnerability touches a large segment of the American population, as well as the global one. Census data in 2005 indicated that about 37 million people in the United States live below the federal poverty level—$9,570 yearly for one person and $19,350 yearly for a family of four (Pugh, 2007; U.S. Department of Health & Human Services, 2007). Most disturbingly, over 43% of the poor live in deep or severe poverty—$5,080 per year for one person—and that level has been increasing dramatically. It grew 26% between 2000 and 2005 to reach the highest level in 32 years (Pugh, 2007). Almost one-third of those in deep poverty were under the age of 17, and about two-thirds were female and White. However, Blacks are 300% more likely to live in deep poverty than Whites (Pugh, 2007). In 2002, 12.1% of Americans were classified as living in poverty, with the rate for African Americans over two times higher than that of the total population (Semple, 2003).

How does poverty make one vulnerable to poor health outcomes? The obvious conclusion is that having less money also means being less able to afford adequate housing in a safe neighborhood. This may lead to fewer opportunities for exercise, especially if walking outside puts one at risk of becoming a victim of violence. Fewer community resources are usually available, such as gyms, grocery stores, and shopping areas. Lower income level is associated with less education and often results in a person having to work at jobs in which they are exposed to higher risks (e.g., mining), or the need to work at more than one job in order to make ends meet. Because of the lack of free time, one may be less likely to shop for fresh fruits and vegetables and to cook healthy meals, with a consequent reliance on fast foods. Inadequate childcare, lower social class, and stigmatization can cause ongoing psychological stress. There may be less control over transportation and work schedules, along with a greater degree of stress on the job and at home. Chronic stress takes a toll on one's body as it "can lead to health damage through neuroendocrine, sympathetic nervous system, vascular, and immune pathways" (Braveman, 2007, p. 2). The resulting consequences of chronic stress may lead to rapid aging and "induce health-damaging behaviors such as smoking" (Aday, 2005, p. 195) (see Perspectives: Student Voices).

Research has shown that poverty and lower education levels are associated with greater functional losses, certain diseases, more incidences of physical and cognitive impairment, and higher mortality rates (Crimmins, Hayward, & Seeman, 2004). Lower SES can affect health outcomes throughout life as different life trajectories encompass prenatal care, childhood learning activities, family experiences, educational and career opportunities, neighborhood environment, and opportunities for health care (Blackwell, Hayward, & Crimmins, 2001). As one example, poor prenatal nutrition can lead to type 2 diabetes and cardiovascular disease in later life (Aday, 2005).

Poverty and race/ethnicity are often intertwined, but SES is a better predictor of health outcomes in Whites than it is within other racial or ethnic groups (Crimmins, Hayward, & Seeman, 2004). Poor White populations suffer poor health outcomes, but in other racial or ethnic minorities, the association is much less straightforward.

If we examine just one aspect of poverty—access to healthy food—research has found that race and environment play a significant role. An audit of supermarkets and fast food restaurants in St. Louis, Missouri found that low-fat food options and fresh fruits and vegetables were more often found in higher-income, predominately White neighborhoods. African American and mixed-race areas, along with White high-poverty areas, were less likely to have access to these foods that are often crucial in making healthy dietary choices and adhering to federal dietary guidelines (Baker, Schootman, Barnidge, & Kelly, 2006).

Another risk factor for the poor is the finding that the highest amount of pollution is most often found in neighborhoods where there is more poverty, lower education levels, and higher rates of unemployment (Evans, 2006). Also, interventions like smoking cessation, have been shown to more often be accepted and successful among populations with higher levels of education, which are most often associated with higher income levels (Bulatao & Anderson, 2004).

At the population level, increases in total income and reductions in poverty levels are "strongly associated with subsequent improvements in population health" (Aday, 2005, p. 190). Income affects health, and poor health can affect the income of an individual as well as that of a nation (see Chapter 6). For a visual representation of the disparities found between the poor, near poor, and middle- to high-income groups, see *Healthy People 2010*—Health Disparities by Income, Figure 25.2.

Uninsured and Underinsured

If the number of uninsured are also classified as a vulnerable population, even more Americans join the ranks, because the majority of those without health insurance are working adults and are not eligible for Medicaid or Medicare. More than 45 million Americans in 2005 were without any form of health insurance coverage (Collins, Davis, Schoen, Doty, Kriss, & Holmgren, 2006). One year later, in 2006, that number jumped to 47 million (Hansen, 2007). The percentage of Whites who are uninsured is estimated at 12%, Blacks at 19%, and Latinos/ Hispanics at 34%, indicating racial and ethnic disparity in this area. In addition, about two-thirds of those who are uninsured are living in poverty, with many of them classed as the *working poor* (Collins, 2007; Haas & Adler, 2001). However, a good number of research studies

PERSPECTIVES
STUDENT VOICES

A Nursing Student's View of the Aftermath of Hurricane Katrina

I was beginning my last year of nursing school when Hurricanes Katrina and Rita hit the Gulf Coast of Louisiana and Mississippi. Like most people, I was fixated on the television coverage of this natural disaster. A lot of the round-the-clock coverage focused on New Orleans, and much of that city seemed to be under water. People in flooded areas were stranded on housetops, while families could be seen walking on highways to get to Red Cross shelters. A horrifying image that I recall clearly was one of yellow school buses, mostly underwater, that were part of the city's disaster plan and were supposed to be used to assist those without personal means of transportation to move to higher ground.

It was like watching a very bad dream. We have had disasters in this country, but I did not expect to witness the lack of organization and preparation that seemed to abound with Katrina. I couldn't understand why masses of people didn't leave the area before the storms hit, and why it took so long for the federal government to respond to the needs of American citizens. Those people who tried to leave found themselves delayed by the slowly moving parking lots that had once been interstate freeways. Even with personal transportation, evacuation was difficult!

What seemed very clear after Katrina was that there are large numbers of poor and vulnerable people in this country; I had not been previously aware of this. Did you know that most of those who died were poor and Black? This doesn't seem right; didn't we abolish segregation and advance civil rights? In our community health nursing class, we discussed vulnerable populations and read some articles about this disaster. We talked about health disparities. I had never really thought about that before, but it rings true to me now. Some groups of people have higher numbers of deaths and more problems with certain diseases than other groups. We do have different levels of health care for different groups, and some people can only access the health care system by coming to the ER.

I now have a better understanding of how things happened with Katrina. When you have little money, no reliable transportation, no extended support systems, and inadequate information about an impending disaster, you are vulnerable and at the mercy of government systems that often cannot respond quickly. I often wonder how I would fare if something happened suddenly, and I couldn't access cash from my bank account, or my car was low on gas, and I hadn't bought groceries in a couple of weeks. Would I be able to survive a natural disaster like an earthquake? I have family close by and many friends, some in nursing school, who could help me. That makes me less vulnerable, but I still should do a better job of being prepared.

Brooke, Nursing Student

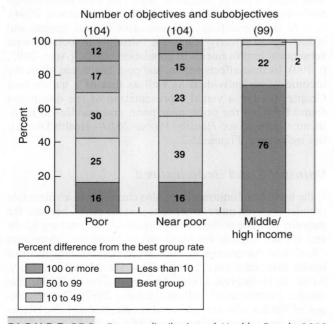

FIGURE 25.2 Percent distribution of *Healthy People 2010* objectives and subobjectives by size of disparity for income groups at the most recent data point. Adapted from http://www.healthy-people.gov/Data/midcourse/pdf/Executive Summary.pdf, Figure 13.

indicate that disparities in access to health care and sometimes health outcomes, independent of SES or race, are often found in uninsured populations (Haas & Adler, 2001).

A 2003 study found that at least 16 million Americans with health insurance could be classified as underinsured (Mahon, 2005). When that number is added to the uninsured population, at least 63 million of a total population of over 300 million people could be characterized as vulnerable (Hellander, 2006).

How does having inadequate or no health insurance lead to poor health outcomes? As explained in Chapter 6, those with few or no resources in this area do not utilize early screenings and preventive measures, and they delay getting treatment in an effort to save money. Because they don't often have regular health checks, they may lack a medical "home" or a consistent health care provider (Collins, 2007). Many utilize emergency rooms or urgent care facilities when their conditions worsen, and they have no real continuity of care (Davis, 2003). They only receive care for the problem at hand, and not always for underlying causes. They do not get regular physical examinations and may be inadequately immunized against common diseases. Thus, they are at risk for poorer general health as well (Himmelstein, Warren, Thorne, & Woolhandler, 2005). Also, when examination and subsequent treatment are delayed, diseases such as cancer or cardiovascular illness may result in earlier death.

Race and Ethnicity

The United States is a multiracial, multiethnic country. About one-third of the population belongs to a racial or ethnic minority group, and this proportion will continue to increase, as currently "45% of children under the age of 5 are minorities" (Population Reference Bureau, 2006, p. 1). Hispanics represent the largest minority group (about half of the 98 million total), and they are also the fastest-growing group, with a fertility rate of 2.80; the rate for non-Hispanic Whites is 1.85 (Haub, 2006). Blacks (13.3%), Asians (<5%), American Indians/Alaska Natives (1.5%), and Hawaiians/Pacific Islanders (<1%) also contribute to this minority population growth (Population Reference Bureau, 2006; U.S. Census Bureau, 2007).

Considering Hispanics alone, over 100 million Americans could potentially be part of a vulnerable group (U.S. Census Bureau, 2007). According to all major indicators of health, Hispanics, Blacks, and Native Americans are "more likely to be in poor health than are majority Whites" (Aday, 2001, p. 56). Although infant mortality, substance use and abuse, and HIV/AIDS prevalence, however, are lower for Asians overall, some Asians—most notably Southeast Asians—have poorer morbidity and mortality rates (Aday, 2001). Blacks and Hispanics report higher levels of metabolic and vascular diseases, as well as cognitive impairment (Crimmins, Hayward, & Seeman, 2004).

In 2005, Blacks represented 12.3% of the population, but they accounted for 40% of the total AIDS cases since the epidemic began in this country in 1981 (Andriote, 2005). Hispanics report higher incidences of diabetes, but are more often found to be obese—a condition that is linked closely with type 2 diabetes (Crimmins et al., 2004; Bulatao & Anderson, 2004). A recent study found an increased incidence of pulmonary embolism for Blacks, but no differences in hospital fatality rates (Schneider, Lilienfeld, & Im, 2006), whereas no racial or ethnic differences were noted in a study of interventions post myocardial infarction (Jacobi et al., 2007). Low birth weights and infant mortality are often more prevalent among Blacks (Nanyonjo, Montgomery, Modeste, & Fujimoto, 2007), and over a 15-year period, child mortality rates for Blacks and Hispanics have been consistently higher than those for Whites (Gitterman, 2001). Life expectancy for all minority races has been consistently lower than that of Whites since 1901. Life expectancy for Blacks was only 33.7 years in 1901, whereas for Whites it was 49.4 years—a difference of 15.7 years. The gap narrowed to 5.5 years by 2001, and to 4.7 years by 2004, but the racial/ethnic disparity still exists (Centers for Disease Control & Prevention [CDC], 2004, 2007).

Why does simply being a member of a racial/ethnic minority group make someone vulnerable? The reasons are complex and not well understood. Poorer health outcomes for Blacks have been attributed to cultural barriers, discrimination, and lack of access to appropriate health care (Evans, 2006). Some believe, as stated earlier, that race or ethnicity and poverty are related (Winkleby & Cubbin, 2004). But even when SES is controlled, racial disparities in health remain, especially among the Black population (Crimmins, Hayward, & Seeman, 2004; Chandra & Skinner, 2004). Some believe that the childhood experiences of the Black population may explain the disparity in mortality rates (Warner & Hayward, 2002) or that disparities may be related to differing cultural norms and values (Winkleby & Cubbin,

2004). Recent immigrants (i.e., foreign-born Mexican Americans) have healthier exercise and dietary patterns than those born inside the United States (Winkleby & Cubbin, 2004). Others note the generational link between minority group membership and low educational attainment (e.g., father's education level), and the tie between education and health (Crimmins, Hayward, & Seeman, 2004). A majority of Hispanics and Blacks have spent a lifetime at a lower level of educational attainment.

In examining racial and ethnic differences in the health of older people, Bulatao and Anderson (2004) note differential health and risk behaviors. For instance, Whites are less likely to get mammograms and Pap smears and more likely to smoke, whereas Blacks and Hispanics have more problems with obesity and report less physical activity or exercise. These differences in exercise were not explained by SES. Of note, health behaviors have been found to differ within racial and ethnic groups, especially by age, income, education, country of origin, and language spoken in the home. A high prevalence of unhealthy behaviors could be predicted for Hispanics born in the United States and/or those who spoke English when compared with Hispanics born in Mexico and/or speaking Spanish. They also differed by gender; women are more strongly affected than men, largely due to greater disparity in physical inactivity and obesity (Winkleby & Cubbin, 2004).

Some research has demonstrated racial differences in genetics that could offer an additional explanation for health disparities, whereas some subscribe to the mechanism of genetic risk and environmental risk exposure (Olden & White, 2005). Racial and ethnic genetic predisposition for disease development may be set in play by environmental triggers. Because multiple risk factors may react in a synergistic manner to cause disease, research is lacking to fully explain or predict this possible phenomenon. However, large, randomized trials have shown "race-specific drug response differences between Blacks and Whites" (p. 721).

Whatever the mechanism causing vulnerability among racial and ethnic groups, no one questions the difficulties they experience in accessing quality health care services (see *Healthy People 2010*—Health Disparities by Race/Ethnicity, Fig. 25.3).

VULNERABILITY AND INEQUALITY IN HEALTH CARE

Social Determinants of Health

Commonly acknowledged conditions (e.g., economic, social, environmental, genetic) are often associated with health outcomes, and are known as **social determinants of health**. The unequal distribution of these conditions among certain groups is thought to contribute to "persistent and pervasive health disparities" (Baker, Metzler, & Galea, 2005, p. 553). When we try to address health disparities, we must consider these social determinants and work on all levels—individual, aggregate, and population—to reduce them (Marmot & Wilkinson, 2006). For instance, most will acknowledge that a safe and nourishing diet is needed to be healthy. Safe and accessible drinking water is also required, as are adequate housing, a supportive environment, and appropriate levels of exercise. Political resources and social structures can also influence health, and "multiple

Characteristics: Race and Ethnicity

Population-based objectives	American Indian or Alaska Native	Asian	Native Hawaiian or other Pacific Islander	Two or more races	Hispanic or Latino	Black non-Hispanic	White non-Hispanic	Summary index
1-1. Health insurance: < 65 years (1997, 2003)*[1]							B	
1-3a. Counseled about physical activity: 18+ years (2001)*						B		
1-3b. Counseled about diet and nutrition: 18+ years (2001)*						B		
1-3c. Counseled about smoking cessation: 18+ years (2001)*	b						B	
1-3d. Counseled about reduced alcohol consumption: 18+ years (2001)*						B		
1-3f. Counseled about unintended pregnancy: females 15-44 years (1995)†						B		
1-3h. Counseled about management of menopause: females 45-57 years (2001)*					B			
1-4a. Source of ongoing care: all ages (1998, 2003)*[1]					↑		B	
1-4b. Source of ongoing care: < 18 years (1998, 2003)*[1]					↑↑		B	
1-4c. Source of ongoing care: 18+ years (1998, 2003)*[1]					↑		B	
1-5. Usual primary care provider (1996, 1999)*		2	2				B	
1-6. Delays or difficulties in obtaining needed health care (1996, 1999)*	b	2	2			b	B	
1-9a. Hospitalization for pediatric asthma: < 18 years (1996)†								
1-9b. Hospitalization for uncontrolled diabetes: 18-64 years (1996)†								
1-9c. Hospitalization for immunization-preventable pneumonia or influenza: 65+ years (1996)†								
1-10. Delay or difficulty in getting emergency care (2001)*							B	
1-15a. Access to home health care: 65+ years with long-term care needs (2001)*								
1-15b. Access to adult day care: 65+ years with long-term care needs (2001)*								
1-15c. Access to assisted living: 65+ years with long-term care needs (2001)*								
1-15d. Access to nursing home care: 65+ years with long-term care needs (2001)*								
1-16. Pressure ulcers: nursing home residents (1997, 1999)*								

Notes:

Data for objectives 1-3g, 1-7a through h, 1-8a through t, 1-11a through g, 1-12, 1-13a through i, and 1-14a and b are unavailable or not applicable. Objectives 1-2 and 1-3e were deleted at the midcourse.

Years in parentheses represent the baseline data year and the most recent data year (if available).

Disparity from the best group rate is defined as the percent difference between the best group rate and each of the other group rates for a characteristic (for example, race and ethnicity). The summary index is the average of these percent differences for a characteristic. Change in disparity is estimated by subtracting the disparity at baseline from the disparity at the most recent data point. Change in the summary index is estimated by subtracting the summary index at baseline from the summary index at the most recent data point. See Technical Appendix for more information.

The **best group rate** at the most recent data point.

B	The group with the best rate for specified characteristic.
b	Most favorable group rate for specified characteristic, but reliability criterion not met.
	Best group rate reliability criterion not met.

Percent difference from the best group rate

Disparity from the best group rate at the most recent data point.

- Less than 10 percent or not statistically significant
- 10-49 percent
- 50-99 percent
- 100 percent or more

Changes in disparity over time are shown when the change is greater than or equal to 10 percentage points and statistically significant, or when the change is greater than or equal to 10 percentage points and estimates of variability were not available.

Increase in disparity (percentage points)
- ↑ 10-49
- ↑↑ 50-99
- ↑↑ 100 or more

Decrease in disparity (percentage points)
- ↓ 10-49
- ↓↓ 50-99
- ↓↓ 100 or more

Availability of data.
- Data not available.
- Characteristic not selected for this objective.

* The variability of best group rates was assessed, and disparities of _ 10% are statistically significant at the 0.05 level. Changes in disparity over time, noted with arrows, are statistically significant at the 0.05 level. See Technical Appendix.

† Measures of variability were not available. Thus, the variability of best group rates was not assessed, and the statistical significance of disparities and changes in disparity over time could not be tested. See Technical Appendix.

[1] Baseline data by race and ethnicity are for 1999.

[2] Data are for Asians or Pacific Islanders.

[3] Baseline data only.

[4] Median ZIP code income levels: $25,000 or less, $25,001-$35,000, and more than $35,000.

FIGURE 25.3 Healthy People 2010: Health disparities by race/ethnicity. Adapted from http://www.healthypeople.gov/Data/midcourse/html/tables/dt/DT-01a.htm.

disadvantages and inequities are profoundly associated with poor health" (Baker, Metzler, & Galea, 2005, p. 554). Political and participatory action research are vital tools in reducing the effects of these conditions, as are methods of community empowerment (Metzler, 2007) (see Chapters 4 and 13).

In an effort to improve the health of disadvantaged groups, early public health efforts addressed social determinants of health, such as sanitation and poverty, along with living conditions and other environmental issues (Metzler, 2007). A quantitative tool, the Community Need Index, uses data on socioeconomic indicators than can lead to health disparity—income, education, housing, insurance coverage, and culture/language—and provides a score for each zip code in the United States (Roth & Barsi, 2005). This can be useful to researchers and policy makers, as well as PHNs. The present need to address underlying social conditions to improve health status is borne out by current research on race and socioeconomic class (Satcher, Fryer, McCann, Troutman, Woolf, & Rust, 2005; Isaacs & Schroeder, 2004). The federal government has acknowledged the need to improve social conditions that impact the health of our population:

> *Healthy People 2010* recognizes that communities, states, and national organizations will need to take a multidisciplinary approach to achieving health equity—an approach that involves improving health, education, housing, labor, justice, transportation, agriculture, and the environment, as well as data collection itself. (U.S. Department of Health & Human Services, 2000, p. 16)

Socioeconomic Gradient of Health

A series of large-scale, longitudinal studies in England, the now classic Whitehall studies, divided British civil servants into socioeconomic groups based upon their occupational status (e.g., executives to unskilled workers). What they discovered, over time, was an improvement in mortality and morbidity rates as the level of occupation and pay increased. Those at the lowest levels had the poorest health, but as they moved up the salary scale and occupational level, their health improved. What makes this so interesting is that all of the workers had basic health insurance coverage and free medical care—no real problems with access to health care existed. Even when the researchers adjusted for diet, exercise, and smoking, the gradient persisted, although it was less pronounced (Marmot, Ryff, Bumpass, Shipley, & Marks, 1997; Marmot et al., 1991). One of the studies found higher prevalence of heart disease for all participants at the lower end of the social stratus. It also found death rates for diabetic participants to be about 200% higher in the lowest social group when compared to the highest (Chaturvedi, 1998).

This inverse relationship between social class or income and health has been termed the **socioeconomic gradient**. It has been found in populations around the world, although not always unfailingly, and has been related to poor health outcomes regarding incidence of stroke in Swedish women (Kuper, Adami, Theorell, & Weiderpass, 2007); diabetes morbidity and mortality in a multinational population (Chaturvedi, 1998); cancer mortality in U.S. males (Singh, Miller, Hankey, Feuer, & Pickle, 2002); South Korean adolescent mortality rates, especially by suicide, circulatory disease, and "transport accident death" (Cho, Khang, Yang, Harper, & Lynch, 2007, p. 50); disability and functional limitation in the U.S. population (Minkler, Fuller-Thomson, & Guralnik, 2006); chronic illness, such as diabetes, hypertension, mental problems, and respiratory diseases in Australia (Glover, Hetzel, & Tennant, 2004); and mortality from acute myocardial infarction in industrialized countries (Alboni, Amadei, Scarfo, Bettiol, Ippolito, & Baggioni, 2003).

The socioeconomic gradient has also been noted in behaviors such as smoking—it is highest among those who are from the working class and who have low income and low educational levels (Barbeau, Krieger, & Soobader, 2004). The gradient is also apparent in studies of hospital deaths. Hospital mortality rates in England and Wales among low SES patients admitted for elective surgery demonstrated a statistically significant difference from those of higher SES patients (Hutchings, Raine, Brady, Wildman, & Rowan, 2004). Low birth weights and breast-feeding also demonstrate a socioeconomic gradient. Lower levels of education and income are associated with higher rates of low birth weight, while those at the higher levels of occupation and income are more likely to breast-feed their infants than those at the lower levels (Finch, 2003; Heck, Braveman, Cubbin, Chavez, & Kiely, 2006). The differences between high and low social and economic groups can be viewed as a disparity in health outcomes.

Health Disparities

One definition of **health disparity** is a "chain of events signified by a difference in: (1) environment, (2) access to, utilization of, and quality of care, (3) health status, or (4) a particular health outcome that deserves scrutiny" (Carter-Porras & Baquet, 2002, p. 427). Health disparities may be unavoidable, such as health-damaging behaviors that are chosen by an individual despite health education and counseling efforts, but most are thought to be due to inequities than can be corrected (Carter-Porras & Baquet, 2002). A long-held belief about health inequities adopted by the World Health Organization (WHO) is that health differences that are avoidable and unnecessary are patently unfair and unjust (Whitehead, 1991). Health disparities can be objectively viewed as a disproportionate burden of morbidity, disability, and mortality found in a specific portion of the population in contrast to another.

Healthy People 2010 goals include increasing the quality and years of healthy life of Americans, along with the elimination of health disparities among segments of our population (U.S. Department of Health and Human Services, 2000.) However, some overall progress has been made on the first goal; many feel it has been at the expense of the second, and encourage a more focused approach to eliminating health disparities (Keppel, Bilheimer, & Gurley, 2007). The 2006 *National Health Care Disparities Report* reveals that disparities "remain prevalent" and that, while some disparities are decreasing, others are increasing (AHRQ, 2006, p. 2). Reported disparities exist in the areas of quality of health care, access to care, levels and types of care, and care settings; they exist within subpopulations (e.g., elderly, women, children, rural residents, disabled) and across clinical conditions.

Poor access to quality care and overt discrimination are examples of disparities under investigation (Williams & Jackson, 2005). Discrimination can occur during service delivery if health care providers are biased against a specific group or hold stereotypical beliefs about that group. Providers may also not be confident about providing care for a racial or ethnic group with which they are unfamiliar. Language may be a problem, as can cultural values and norms that are unfamiliar to providers. Patients can also react to providers in a way that promotes disparities; they may not trust the information given to them and may not follow it as explained, leading to inadequate care (IOM, 2003). A survey conducted in 2006 found that in a large sample of over 4,000 U.S. adults from 14 racial and ethnic groups, many of the minority respondents viewed their health care as more negative than the care received by Whites. A good number of them reported discrimination in the health care setting, and did not think that they would be able to receive the best care if they became ill. These differences persisted despite controlling for socioeconomic variables, although a good deal of variation occurred across the racial and ethnic groups (Blendon, et al., 2007). Another study involving "severely disadvantaged people with HIV infection" found that almost 40% reported "experiencing discrimination in the health care system" (Sohler, Li, & Cunningham, 2007, p. 347). Higher perceived discrimination was associated with HIV infection, homelessness, drug use, and race/ethnicity, emphasizing the perceived poor quality of care and difficulties with access to care.

Access to Care

The Institute of Medicine's (IOM, 2003) *Unequal Treatment: Confronting Racial and Ethnic Disparities in Health Care* noted a large body of research highlighting the higher morbidity and mortality rates among all racial and ethnic minority groups when compared to Whites. Differences in health care access were also explained—be it in the form of inadequate or no health insurance, problems getting health care, the quality of that care, fewer choices in where to go for care, or the lack of a regular health care provider. For instance, there are fewer numbers of health care providers in minority neighborhoods and thus it is more difficult for those living in these areas to find a medical home. Often, sufficient transportation is not available or clinic hours may be unrealistic for individuals working long hours (IOM, 2003).

Residential segregation, although illegal, still exists and can play a role in health disparities; people of color often live in poorer areas where alcohol and tobacco are more heavily marketed (Williams & Jackson, 2005). Many vulnerable populations, especially racial and ethnic minority groups and low-income populations, find health care at safety net hospitals and community clinics, where they are at the mercy of balanced budgets and vast bureaucratic systems (IOM, 2003). Other geographic factors can affect access to health care services (Coberley et al., 2007). For example, only 25% of pharmacies in non-White neighborhoods, compared with 72% in predominately White neighborhoods, stocked sufficient opioid drugs to meet the needs of palliative care patients in different New York neighborhoods (IOM, 2003). This lack of access to proper medication represents a disparity in health care. In a Canadian study (Lemstra, Neudorf, & Opondo, 2006), significantly different patterns of health care utilization were found in neighborhoods characterized as low income, and differences

were noted for a wide variety of conditions (e.g., all-cause mortality, coronary heart disease, diabetes, poisonings, and injuries). In 2004, a survey of medical directors at all federally qualified community health clinics revealed that it was more difficult for uninsured patients to obtain access to specialty services outside the clinics (e.g., diagnostic tests, referrals to specialists) than for Medicare and Medicaid patients or those with private health insurance (Cook et al., 2007).

Health care access is also problematic for other vulnerable groups. For example, services and resources for the mentally ill and substance abusers are often fragmented and inadequate, as are those for abusing families and homeless persons. Refugees and immigrants may have difficulty finding affordable and easily accessible health care, largely due to their lack of health insurance and the need to find care at free clinics or emergency rooms (Aday, 2001). When vulnerable individuals cannot get appropriate health care or treatment for illness or disease, for whatever reason, they are more likely to have health deficits.

Quality of Care

Quality of care should result in an "increased likelihood of desired health outcomes" and should be "consistent with current professional knowledge" (IOM, 2003, p. 31). It can include such things as patient safety issues, timeliness and effectiveness of patient care, and patient centeredness (AHRQ, 2006). Research indicates that racial and ethnic minority clients feel more comfortable and satisfied with care from a health care provider who comes from the same racial and/or ethnic group (IOM, 2003). However, a shortage of ethnically diverse health care providers exists. Despite racial and ethnic minorities comprising 28% of the U.S. population, less than 10% of registered nurses (RNs) represent these same minorities (National Advisory Council on Nurse Education & Practice, 2000).

Lack of access to quality health care services is common among racial and ethnic minority groups. In examining racial disparities in diabetes care, researchers noted that the differences in receipt of eye examinations was most likely due to Blacks receiving care at "lower-performing facilities" (Heisler, Smith, Hayward, Krein, & Kerr, 2003, p. 1221). Other measures, like poor control of hypertension and cholesterol, were thought to be due to disparities in care within the same facilities as Whites and not an indication of the inadequacies of the health care agency.

Communication can be a widespread factor in poor quality of care (Yeo, 2004). A recent study reported between 24% and 36% of low-income parents of children felt that the communication they had with their child's health care provider in a Spanish interview was "poor" (Clemans-Cope & Kenney, 2007, p. 206). Marginalized vulnerable populations, such as substance abusers, at-risk mothers and infants, abusing families, suicide- and homicide-prone individuals, and the mentally ill or disabled may feel that they are treated as "second class citizens," and cultural barriers and misunderstandings can lead to a discontinuation of recommended regimens. Poor health outcomes may result, as effectiveness of health care for vulnerable populations is not often considered or even well defined (Aday, 2001; Nanyonjo, Montgomery, Modeste, & Fujimoto, 2007).

WORKING WITH VULNERABLE POPULATIONS

The Role of Public Health Nurses

Historically, community and public health nurses have focused their efforts on the most vulnerable populations. In Lillian Wald's time, PHNs worked and lived among the tenements (see Chapter 2). Today, most PHNs travel a good distance to reach the homes of vulnerable clients, knowing that they can leave and go back to their comfortable circumstances when they choose to do so. Coming from various different circumstances, some nursing students feel unsure and insecure when going into certain areas of the community, and not everyone is comfortable working with vulnerable populations (Martino-Maze, 2005, 2006). Research has demonstrated that clinical work with vulnerable populations helps nursing students become more aware of inequities and promotes critical engagement and a commitment to social change (Reimer-Kirkham, Van Hofwegen, & Hoe-Harwood, 2005). Recognizing that demeaning or dehumanizing behaviors or language directed toward clients or neighborhoods exemplifies disrespect and is often fear-based, helps us all to focus our efforts (see Fig. 25.4). One PHN succinctly described this fear:

> All of us, at some level, have a fear of the disenfranchised, whether it's because we could be in that place or because there may be potential harm to us. But I seek to break that fear and see someone as a human. The more I work with her, the more I see her as human (Zerwekh, 2000, p. 47).

Working with vulnerable clients is an important component of students' clinical experiences, and necessary to better understand client circumstances and needs, as well as to be competent as nurses. What then is the PHN's role, and how can we be most effective when working with vulnerable groups?

Effective Caring

Our goal for clients is to help them develop their capabilities to "take charge of their own lives and make their own choices" by helping them identify all possible choices, guiding them to think through all of the issues and possible consequences, providing honest feedback, and affirming their reality (Zerwekh, 2000, p. 48). This can be challenging when working with the most vulnerable clients, as they are often the most disenfranchised and fearful of others. One nurse described vulnerable individuals as being behind a locked door—"the door is shut and you can't get back in" (Zerwekh, 2000, p. 50). Opening that door is the first step to working effectively with these clients. Engagement and development of rapport are essential. Because vulnerability often equates with feelings of powerlessness, the actions of community health nurses can either promote engagement or destroy any chances for rapport. A Canadian study found three phases of PHN–client engagement: getting past the fear, working to build trust, and "seeking mutuality" (Jack, DiCenso, & Lohfeld, 2005, p. 182). The personal values, experiences, characteristics, and actions of both nurses and clients influenced the speed at which this process took place and the eventual level of connection. Helping clients identify their fears and clearly defining the PHN role with the client and family were also important. Earlier research described the process as "finding common ground" and "building trust" (Jack, DiCenso, & Lohfeld, 2002, p. 59).

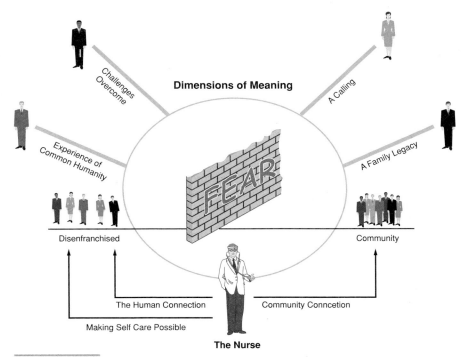

FIGURE 25.4   Breaking through the wall. Fearless caring with separated and often frightened clients has 10 themes that can be organized into three meta-themes: the Human Connection, the Community Connection, and Making Self-Care Possible. The nurse goes around the separating wall of fear. Adapted from Zerwekh, J. (2000). Caring on the ragged edge: Nursing persons who are disenfranchised. *Advances in Nursing Science, 22*(4), 47–61.

In a small qualitative study of expert PHNs with proven experience and a degree of success in working with disenfranchised populations, Zerwekh (2000) found three overarching themes—*human connection, community connection,* and *making self-care possible.* Those PHNs who can see the worth of clients as human beings and share their own humanity by expressing themselves and staying connected were part of the main theme of *human connection.* Another important component was becoming familiar with a client by learning about his past, his patterns, and the most effective means of communicating with him to draw him out. For the theme of *community connection,* subthemes of connecting clients to each other and to the community, as well as mediating bureaucratic red tape and occasionally making exceptions, were foremost, as was "haunting the case" or being a persistent advocate to get the client's needs met (p. 57). The meta-theme of *making self-care possible* was characterized by "getting them through emotionally" (p. 59), or being able to listen to and counsel clients who are often on the edge with their emotions (e.g., fear, anger). Additional components of this theme include teaching clients to have self-awareness and to better understand their bodies and their feelings, and coaching them to take control and foster their strengths. Confronting fear at the community level was another subtheme, as PHNs worked to break down barriers and work through longstanding prejudices and fears. Some authors believe that advocacy for vulnerable populations is an ethical responsibility for nurses who may need to help individuals and families find needed assistance (Erlen, 2006).

Working with disadvantaged populations can be challenging and exhausting, and the psychic distress should be "anticipated and addressed" (Beidler, 2005, p. 759; Beauchesne & Patsdaughter, 2005). Often, novice community health nurses feel overwhelmed and suffer "compassion fatigue" when confronted with the crushing realities that their vulnerable, disenfranchised clients face on a daily basis (p. 53). Feelings of guilt sometimes surface when nurses contrast their own life experiences with those of their clients. To be effective in working with vulnerable populations, it is often more helpful to donate money and items on a group level rather than an individual level, and to work for substantial changes in community attitudes. Also, it is vital to remain grounded in order to continue to have the necessary energy and compassion.

Empowerment

Chapter 13 discusses the concept of empowerment and applies it to the PHN role when working with communities. When dealing with individual clients, empowerment is defined as "an active, internal process of growth" that is reached by actualizing the full potential inherent within each client and occurring "within the context of a nurturing nurse–client relationship" (Falk-Raphael, 2001, p. 4). Public health nurses describe the process of empowerment as a two-way street, with clients gaining knowledge and skills and "acting on informed choices," but also further empowering the nurse to continue the work of empowerment (p. 6). In Paulo Freire's (1993) *Pedagogy of the Oppressed,* this reciprocity is explained as he notes that the oppressed (or vulnerable) liberate themselves as well as those who may oppress them (or the more advantaged members of society).

What community health nursing activities or actions are most effective in promoting empowerment among their vulnerable clients? In Falk-Raphael's (2001) qualitative study of PHNs and their clients, several themes were noted:

◆ *Having a client-centered approach,* denoted by flexibility in dealing with clients (e.g., "meeting them where they are"; "communicating at their level"; "backing off and following client's agenda," p. 6)

◆ *Developing a trusting relationship* based on mutual respect and dignity (e.g., clients as active partners with the PHN assuming more or less responsibility as needed; being empathetic, nonjudgmental, and "creating a safe environment," p. 7)

◆ *Employing advocacy,* both at an individual level as well as political advocacy (e.g., using their role and power as a professional to cut through bureaucratic red tape, connecting clients with available community resources, supporting clients in reaching their health goals, making their expertise available, and being a client resource as someone who is open and "available," p. 8)

◆ *Being a teacher and role model,* using a variety of strategies and providing opportunities for clients to safely practice new skills (e.g., teaching classes, providing individual coaching, providing positive reinforcement and support, demonstrating skills such as assertiveness and community action/ participation)

◆ *Capacity building* through encouraging and supporting of clients' work toward attainment of health goals (e.g., "reflective listening and an empathetic approach" focusing on strengths, not limitations; facilitating client "self-exploration" and providing encouragement for them to "act on their choices" while being "realistic about barriers to success;" or having expectations for client accountability regarding their decisions and actions (p. 9)

Outcomes of empowerment for clients included increased self-esteem and confidence, improved self-efficacy, and the ability to "reframe situations in a positive way" (p. 10). Clients also subsequently made better choices regarding their health and utilized resources more appropriately. They were better able to seek information and services, and became more politically active. Their focus became more proactive than reactive, and they felt that they could communicate more effectively to define boundaries or express feelings. Consequently, clients were also better able to collaborate with their health care providers, becoming more trusting partners in care by "taking ownership for their health" (p. 10). Some clients noted a newfound ability to see their communities in a more holistic way and looked for ways to change things for the better.

Making a Difference

Social scientists often frame the topic of vulnerability and risk by examining protective factors and resiliency at an individual level (McGee, 2006). **Resilience** is the ability to "bounce back" or recover from life's stressors without permanent injury. Some at-risk individuals fare better than others, but much of the research conducted on resiliency has dealt with life outcomes, not necessarily health (Gitterman, 2001). External support, along with temperament and other individual factors, has been associated with resiliency. This support can be from neighbors, friends, teachers, or others. Public health nurses can provide external support at both the individual and population levels (see Perspectives: Voices from the Community). For example, research has shown the effectiveness of social support, provided by nurses and health visitors, in promoting consistent program participation and positive social and health outcomes among low-income pregnant women (Shepard, Williams, & Richardson, 2004). Nurse visitation and support can also "successfully address informational needs and increase the likelihood that women will use existing community-based resources" (Tough, et al., 2006, p. 183).

Community health nurses can assist vulnerable individuals through "difficult life transitions" or stressful events (Gitterman, 2001, p. 23). They can also work as neighborhood nurses, becoming familiar with the community's resources and strengths. Through work with individual clients, PHNs can expand their empowerment strategies to serve the community. Being aware of the "pulse of the community" is vital, and can be accomplished not only through home visits but by attending community-level meetings and through the development of partnerships organized around specific health issues or community problems (SmithBattle, Diekemper, & Drake, 1999, p. 219). Community collaboratives can be formed, especially in areas with high-risk vulnerable populations, to address needs identified by the members of that community (Campbell-Grossman, Brage-Hudson, Keating-Lefler, & Ofe-Fleck, 2005). Early detection of problems at the community level can lead to the development of programs and services to provide early

intervention and avert costly tertiary care (Penprase, 2006; Salinsky & Gursky, 2006), or to proactively meet the needs of specific groups, such as low-income elderly (Artis, 2005).

To make a difference in the lives of vulnerable individuals, families, and communities, the community health nurse may need to reexamine the way in which public health nursing services are organized and delivered. To be effective in decreasing and eliminating health disparities, innovative and uncharted approaches may be necessary (Pritchard & de-Verteuil, 2007), and political advocacy to influence health policy should become a component of community health nursing practice (SmithBattle, Diekemper, & Drake, 1999; Salinsky &Gursky, 2006; Falk-Raphael, 2005). For example, because of the long-researched, strong connection between education and health outcomes noted in many classic studies (Marmot, Ryff, Bumpass, Shipley, & Marks, 1997), nurses and other public health professionals could become engaged with schools to reduce dropout rates and promote school completion by raising public awareness, organizing task forces, studying the reciprocity between health and school achievement, supporting school-based health education and quality teachers, and advocating for evidence-based practice (EBP) to improve dropout rates (Freudenberg & Ruglis, 2007).

Conducting Research with Vulnerable Populations

Until fairly recently, research studies were most often conducted utilizing middle-class, majority populations (IOM,

---

PERSPECTIVES
VOICES FROM THE COMMUNITY

A View of Katrina's Aftermath—Nurse Volunteer

I had never been a Red Cross volunteer before, but Katrina touched my heart and I signed up. Suddenly I was headed to New Orleans to help in a shelter. The sheer numbers of people streaming into the shelter astounded me—people who had lost everything. Some of these people had waited on housetops to be rescued. Others had walked for hours to reach the shelter. A common theme among them was their vulnerability. Many were members of vulnerable populations even before Katrina struck.

At first, most were relieved to be safe and dry. However, that changed as they realized what they had lost and how uncertain their futures were. Many of the older people and those with chronic illnesses had significant health problems that worsened while they were residents of the shelter. Although they were provided with food, it was sometimes difficult for them to get the exact food they needed for their special diets. Some of them did not have all of their medications, and it took some time to complete health histories and secure necessary prescriptions. The weather was very muggy and hot, and there was little privacy. Even though the governor had called out the National Guard, people had to protect their few belongings, as theft was rampant. Toilet and bathing facilities were inadequate,

space was limited, and fights often broke out between people who had been pushed to the limits of their composure.

People had to show identification in order to apply for emergency loans or to receive other assistance. Some of them had lost all documents in the flooding, or had lost things on the way to the shelter. Standing in line was physically difficult for many people, but lines were long and standing was necessary in order to get assistance.

Many people were displaced, and a good number of them were separated from their families and friends, with no idea whether they were dead or alive. It was difficult to reconnect people, as individuals were evacuated to diverse locations. Communication was often a problem until phone lines and cell towers were back up and running.

I was there to help and to listen and provide care, but sometimes I felt frustrated and ineffective. I wanted to advocate for people and improve on systems of care, but this was almost impossible in such an erratic and crisis-driven system. Better systems need to be in place before the next disaster strikes, especially for the most vulnerable. All in all, it was a rewarding experience, and I was able to make a difference for some people on an individual basis. But there were so many who needed significant and long-term assistance!

Helena, RN, PHN, Red Cross Volunteer

Adapted from Saunders, J. (2007). Vulnerable populations in an American Red Cross shelter after hurricane Katrina. *Perspectives in Psychiatric Care, 43*(1), 30–37.

2003). Vulnerable groups, such as racially and ethnically diverse populations or even women, were often excluded from mainstream research. The focus has changed, and now there is a recognized need for research into the mechanisms of health disparities among diverse populations. However, even when federal regulations called for inclusion of "special populations" in the 1990s, they required adherence to strict guidelines that sometimes discouraged researchers (Meaux & Bell, 2001, p. 241). This paternalistic stance denied many vulnerable groups access to the "benefits of research by 'protecting' them" (List, 2005, p. 54). To more equitably distribute information about effective treatments and EBP, it is important to investigate broadly and to include disadvantaged and disenfranchised individuals in current research studies and trials (Rogers, 2004).

Researchers interested in working with vulnerable populations perform a balancing act between accessing or recruiting vulnerable populations and protecting them (Meaux & Bell, 2001). Institutional Review Boards must always be utilized (see Chapter 4), and vulnerable populations (e.g., children, prisoners/other institutionalized individuals, mentally/ emotionally/physically disabled persons, pregnant women/ fetuses) require greater scrutiny and additional procedures (Polit & Beck, 2005). Ruof (2004) notes that special justifications are required when including vulnerable individuals or groups as research subjects in order to protect against potential human rights abuses. The *Annual Review of Nursing Research* (Fitzpatrick, Nyamathi, & Koniak-Griffin, 2007) highlights the state of nursing science with regard to research with vulnerable populations and the promotion of health disparities studies, as well as culturally appropriated interventions.

Because of the various restraints related to conducting research studies and the categorical nature of many research-oriented grants, research with vulnerable populations is often fragmented and isolated rather than interdisciplinary in nature, and thus it often fails to produce a clear picture (Aday, 2001). Ethical issues are often raised when research is conducted, especially with vulnerable populations (Beattie & VandenBosch, 2007). Questions concerning the ethical principles of autonomy, beneficence, and justice must be addressed. Research with vulnerable populations is carefully examined and generally requires a full review by all members of an institutional review board. The board examines the invasiveness of the study and the risk–benefit ratio. They also review the need for informed consents (Baren & Fish, 2005), the inducements that may be offered to participants (e.g., money), and any perception of coercion or undue influence over prospective participants (Singer & Bossarte, 2006). This is especially important with children and others who are not able to choose freely or may easily be coerced to participate (Lynn & Nelson, 2005; Locher, Bronstein, Robinson, Williams, & Ritchie, 2006).

Because public health agencies are continually collecting data in the capacity of evaluation and monitoring health status of populations, surveillance (e.g., reporting of certain diseases), and epidemiologic investigations (e.g., disease outbreaks, epidemics)—most often involving diverse vulnerable populations—it is especially necessary for them to delineate between these public health functions and research involving actual human subjects that should be evaluated by an institutional review board (Hodge, 2005). Most public health research deals with information applied to specific geographic populations, with the aim of benefiting that community, while human subjects research contributes to testing hypotheses that contribute to more "generalizable knowledge" (p. 127).

Participatory Action Research

Community-based participatory research or **participatory action research** (PAR) is often used among vulnerable populations around the world because it calls upon the expertise and perspectives of the community in identifying needs and developing appropriate interventions (Dickson & Green, 2001; Etowa, Thomas-Bernard, Oyinsan, & Clow, 2007; Schrader-McMillan, 2007). It is an iterative, cyclical process of problem identification and problem solving using reflection and analysis that empowers vulnerable disadvantaged people to effect change in their neighborhoods. It may begin with an investigator posing a research question to a group of individuals from a selected community. Feedback is given, and more information or data may be gathered and then collectively analyzed; this analysis becomes the basis for further actions. As interventions are suggested and community action moves forward, the community members are viewed as co-researchers and are invested in the outcomes and results. Corbett, Francis, and Chapman (2007) identify three main components of PAR:

◆ Problem inquiry
◆ Organization of participants
◆ Awareness and action

They also note the success of this research method with vulnerable groups such as immigrants/refugees, oppressed women, mentally ill or disabled individuals, and rural or inner-city poor, and in examining issues related to education, health, housing, and community development.

One example of the use of this research method was a study to engage at-risk adolescents in organizational change at two youth-serving government agencies (Schulman, 2006). Researchers and adolescent participants worked "as one" to "disrupt the status quo and spark social change" (p. 28). Discussion groups, journals, review of documents, and structured interviews were utilized to answer research questions about youth engagement and how well the two agencies incorporated that concept. Data were analyzed and key elements were identified and shared with the agencies, so that changes could be initiated. One outcome of the study was continued engagement of adolescent participants in social planning and agency programs.

Public health nurses are natural choices for involvement in PAR. Visibility and credibility in disadvantaged communities provide entrée for PHNs who may wish to partner with agency or university researchers wanting to engage vulnerable populations and address social justice facets of health disparities, but needing assistance in making the study operational (Malone, Yerger, McGruder, & Froelicher, 2006). The PHN's connections to vulnerable populations may provide ideas or suggest areas requiring further research and intervention.

Summary

Vulnerable populations are at a higher risk of poor health outcomes. Various models or theoretical frameworks examine personal and environmental resources and risks relative to vulnerability. Vulnerability is associated with increased risk for morbidity and mortality. Vulnerable groups can include chronically ill or disabled, high-risk mothers and infants, those with HIV/AIDS, and the mentally ill or disabled. Alcohol and substance abusers, the suicide and homicide prone, the homeless, abusing families, and immigrants or refugees can also be characterized as vulnerable. Poverty, age, gender, and race or ethnicity can also constitute vulnerability, as can being uninsured or underinsured, a single parent, and those with little or no education.

It is difficult to calculate the exact numbers of Americans who are members of vulnerable groups, largely because of the overlap in populations, but it involves a significant proportion of the total population. Low-income status is often associated with underinsurance or race and ethnicity, and may also be related to homelessness and high-risk births.

Social determinants of health are commonly associated with health outcomes. Such things as economic, social, environmental, and genetic factors are considered social determinants of health. The socioeconomic gradient—an inverse relationship between social class/income, and health—has been repeatedly demonstrated in research conducted around the world.

Health disparities are defined as differences in access to quality health care and health outcomes, and are usually characterized as avoidable and unfair. One of the two main goals of *Healthy People 2010* is to decrease health disparities; however, this outcome has not been as successful as increasing life expectancy. Many disparities occur along income/class or racial/ethnic lines. A good deal of research is under way to determine more specifically the causes and consequences of health disparities.

Community health nurses often work with vulnerable populations, and nurses must learn to break through barriers of fear—their own and that of their clients. To be effective, PHNs must establish a sense of trust and rapport with their clients by finding common ground. Connecting with clients and connecting clients to the community and its available resources are key factors in successful PHN–client relationships. Coaching and mentoring clients to solve their own problems and make necessary changes are also effective behaviors of community health nurses.

Empowerment strategies with individual clients can help them to meet their full potential, while also providing empowerment to the nurses working with them. Flexible, client-centered approaches, based on trust and mutual respect, have been found to be most effective. A nonjudgmental attitude and openness with clients lays the foundation for development of mentoring relationship. Public health nurses who work at empowering clients are advocates at the individual as well as political levels. They are a resource to clients without being paternalistic. They provide a safe place for clients to try to out skills and demonstrate new, healthier behaviors. They build capacity through active, reflective, empathetic listening, and serve as role models and teachers. Empowered clients have greater self-confidence and are better able to collaborate with health care providers. Often, they become more engaged with their communities and neighborhoods.

Resiliency, or the ability to recover from the stressors of life, can be accentuated by external support from friends, teachers, or nurses. Community health nurses can provide individual support as well as support and leadership in vulnerable communities. Political action can involve not only health policy issues, but political activism on the part of underserved populations to improve housing, education, and employment.

Vulnerable populations research may involve stricter guidelines and closer scrutiny from institutional review boards because of ethical considerations. Research with vulnerable populations may provide better treatments and health outcomes, and should be encouraged. Public health nurses may serve as a liaison between academic or agency investigators and vulnerable populations in the communities they serve. It is important to note the difference between public health functions (e.g., surveillance, epidemiologic studies) and human subjects research. Many public health agencies conduct studies of their programs and practices within a confined geographic area, to improve care for the populations they serve. These do not always require permission from institutional review boards.

Participatory action research (PAR) is often used with vulnerable populations, as it draws them into the research process. They join as partners with the investigators in assessing the needs of the community and designing interventions or marshalling resources for change.

This chapter covered some basic information about the role of the community health nurse when serving vulnerable populations. Other chapters in this section will deal with specific vulnerable groups. ▪

 ACTIVITIES TO PROMOTE CRITICAL THINKING

1. Identify at least four vulnerable groups within your community. Using the Flaskerud and Winslow (1998) model depicted in this chapter, determine the health status for each of these groups. Describe the relative risk for each group.

2. Find available community resources for each of the identified groups. Where are they located? How easily accessible are they? What outreach services do they provide for the vulnerable population they serve? Describe some socioeconomic resources—what areas are most deficient?

3. Pick a client from your community health nursing clinical assignment. In a respectful way, discuss your fears of working in the community and ask about any fears they may have experienced in permitting you access to their home. Outline ways in which you could build upon this mutual sharing to achieve mutual trust and rapport.

4. Talk to two expert PHNs and discuss with them the concept of empowerment. What strategies have they used with clients? Ask them to each share an example in which they felt that they made a real difference in the lives of their clients.

5. Locate a community collaborative that is addressing the needs of vulnerable groups in your community. Who are the members? Note the agencies represented. Are there any community members present? If possible, attend a meeting and determine the types of issues being discussed. Is there a sense of community involvement and participation?

References

Aday, L.A. (2001). *At risk in America: The health and health care needs of vulnerable populations in the United States,* 2nd ed. San Francisco, CA: Jossey-Bass.

Aday, L.A. (Ed.). (2005). *Reinventing public health: Policies and practices for a healthy nation.* San Francisco, CA: Jossey-Bass.

Agency for Healthcare Research & Quality (AHRQ). (2006). *National Healthcare Disparities Report.* Retrieved August 18, 2008 from http://www.ahrq.gov/qual/nhdr06/nhdr06high.pdf.

Alboni, P., Amadei, A., Scarfo, S., et al. (2003). In industrialized nations, a low socioeconomic status represents an independent predictor of mortality in patients with acute myocardial infarctions. *Italian Heart Journal, 4*(8), 551–555.

Andriote, J.M. (2005, May). *HIV/AIDS and African Americans: A state of emergency.* Population Reference Bureau. Retrieved October 15, 2008 from http://www.prb.org/Articles/2005/HIVAIDSandAfricanAmericansAStateofEmergency.aspx.

Artis, B. (2005). Promoting health, building community. *Health Progress, 86*(2), 27–31.

Baker, E.A., Metzler, M.M., & Galea, S. (2005). Addressing social determinants of health inequities: Learning from doing. *American Journal of Public Health, 95*(4), 553–555.

Baker, E.A., Schootman, M., Barnidge, E., & Kelly, C. (2006). *The role of race and poverty in access to foods that enable individuals to adhere to dietary guidelines.* Prevention of Chronic Disease. Retrieved August 18, 2008 from http://www.cdc.gov/pcd/issues/2006/jul/05_0217.htm.

Barbeau, E., Krieger, N., & Soobader, M. (2004). Working class matters: Socioeconomic disadvantage, race/ethnicity, gender, and smoking in NHIS 2000. *American Journal of Public Health, 94*(2), 269–278.

Baren, J., & Fish, S. (2005). Resuscitation research involving vulnerable populations: Are additional protections needed for emergency exception from informed consent? *Academic Emergency Medicine, 12*(11), 1071–1077.

Beattie, E.R., & VandenBosch, T.M. (2007). The concept of vulnerability and the protection of human subjects of research. *Research and Theory in Nursing Practice, 21*(3), 156–173.

Beauchesne, M., & Patsdaughter, C. (2005). Primary Care for the Underserved Conference: The evolution of an emerging professional culture. *Journal of Cultural Diversity, 12*(3), 77–88.

Beidler, S.M. (2005). Ethical considerations for nurse-managed health centers. *Nursing Clinics of North America, 40*(4), 759–770.

Blackwell, D., Hayward, O., & Crimmins, E. (2001). Does childhood health affect chronic morbidity in later life? *Social Science & Medicine, 52,*1269–1284.

Blendon, R., Buhr, T., Cassidy, E., et al. (2007). Disparities in health: Perspectives of a multi-ethnic, multi-racial America. *Health Affairs, 26*(5), 1437–1447.

Braveman, P. (2007). Do we have real poverty in the United States? *Preventing Chronic Disease, 4*(4). Retrieved August 18, 2008 from http://www.cdc.gov/pcd/issues/2007/.oct/07_0124.htm.

Bulatao, R., & Anderson, N. (Eds.). (2004). *Understanding racial and ethnic differences in health in late life: A research agenda.* Washington, DC: The National Academies Press.

Byrd, W.M., & Clayton, L.A. (2002). *An American health dilemma: Race, medicine, and health care in the United States 1900–2000,* Vol. II. New York: Routledge.

Campbell-Grossman, C., Brage-Hudson, D., Keating-Lefler, R., & Ofe-Fleck, M. (2005). Community leaders' perceptions of single, low-income mothers' needs and concerns for social support. *Journal of Community Health Nursing, 22*(4), 241–257.

Carter-Porras, O., & Baquet, C. (2002). What is a "health disparity"? *Public Health Reports, 117,* 426–434.

Centers for Disease Control & Prevention (CDC). (2004). *National Vital Statistics Reports,* Vol. 52, No. 14, February 18, 2004. Retrieved August 18, 2008 from www.cdc.gov/nchs/data/dvs/nvsr52_14t12.pdf.

Centers for Disease Control & Prevention (CDC). (2007). *Health, United States, 2006.* Retrieved August 18, 2008 from http//www.cdc.gov/nchs/data/hus/hus06/pdf#027.

Chandra, A., & Skinner, J. (2004). Geography and racial health disparities. In N. Anderson, R. Bulatao, & B. Cohen (Eds.). *Critical perspectives on racial and ethnic differences in health in late life.* (pp. 604–640). Washington, DC: The National Academies Press.

Chaturvedi, N. (1998). Socioeconomic gradient in morbidity and mortality in people with diabetes: Cohort study findings from the Whitehall study and the WHO multinational study of vascular disease in diabetes. *British Medical Journal, 316*(7125), 100–105.

Cho, H., Khang, Y., Yang, S., et al. (2007). Socioeconomic differentials in cause-specific mortality among South Korean adolescents. *International Journal of Epidemiology, 36*(1), 50–57.

Clemans-Cope, L., & Kenney, G. (2007). Low-income parents' reports of communication problems with health care providers: Effects of language and insurance. *Public Health Reports, 122*(2), 206–216.

Clementson, L. (September 26, 2003). *Number of people living in poverty in U.S. increases again.* The New York Times. Retrieved August 19, 2008 from http://www.nytimes.com/2003/09/26/ politics/26CND-CENS.html?ex=1224302400&en=d437a1843fd2&ei=5070.

Coberley, C., Puckrein, G., Dobbs, A., et al. (2007). Effectiveness of disease management programs on improving diabetes care for individuals in health-disparate areas. *Disease Management, 19*(3), 147–155.

Collins, S. (2007). *Congressional testimony: Universal health insurance: Why it is essential to a high performing health system and why design matters.* The Commonwealth Fund. Retrieved August 18, 2008 from http://www.commonwealthfund.org/publications/publications_show.htm?doc_id=506778#areaCitation.

Collins, S., Davis, K., Doty, M, Kriss, J., & Holmgren, L. (2006, April). *Gaps in Health Insurance: An All-American Problem.* The New York: Commonwealth Fund.

Cook, N., Hicks, L., O'Malley, J., Keegan, T., Guadagnoli, E., & Landon, B. (2007). Access to specialty care and medical services in community health centers. *Health Affairs, 26*(5), 1459–1468.

Corbett, A., Francis, K., & Chapman, Y. (2007). Feminist-informed participatory action research: A methodology of choice for examining critical nursing issues. *International Journal of Nursing Practice, 13,* 81–88.

Crimmins, E., Hayward, M., & Seeman, T. (2004). Race/ethnicity, socioeconomic status, and health. In N. Anderson, R. Bulatao, & B. Cohen (Eds.). *Critical perspectives on racial and ethnic differences in health in late life.* (pp. 310–352). Washington, DC: The National Academies Press.

Davis, K. (2003). The costs and consequences of being uninsured. *Medical Care Research and Review, 60*(2), S89–S99.

Dickson, G., & Green, K. (2001). Participatory action research: Lessons learned with aboriginal grandmothers. *Health Care for Women International 22*(5), 471–482.

Erlen, J.A. (2006). Who speaks for the vulnerable? *Orthopedic Nursing, 25*(2), 133–136.

Etowa, J., Thomas-Bernard, W., Oyinsan, B., & Clow, B. (2007). Participatory action research (PAR): An approach for improving Black women's health in rural and remote communities. *Journal of Transcultural Nursing, 18*(4), 349–357.

Evans, D.P. (2006). *The calm before the storm: Addressing race as a vulnerability before and after hurricane Katrina.* Retrieved August 18, 2008 from http://www.medscape.com/viewarticle523436.

Falk-Raphael, A.R. (2001). Empowerment as a process of evolving consciousness: A model of empowered caring. *Advances in Nursing Science, 24*(1), 1–16.

Falk-Raphael, A. (2005). Speaking truth to power: Nursing's legacy and moral imperative. *Advances in Nursing Science, 28*(3), 212–223.

Fitzpatrick, J., Nyamathi, A., & Koniak-Griffin, D. (2007). *Annual review of nursing research,* Vol. 25. New York: Springer.

Flaskerud, J.H., & Winslow, B.J. (1998). Conceptualizing vulnerable populations health-related research. *Nursing Research, 47*(2), 69–78.

Freudenberg, N., & Ruglis, J. (2007). Reframing school dropout as a public health issue. *Preventing Chronic Disease, 4*(4). Retrieved August 18, 2008 from http://www.cdc.gobv/pcd/issues/2007/oct/07_0063.htm.

Freire, P (1993). *Pedagogy of the oppressed.* New York: Continuum Publishing Co.

Frist, W.H. (2005). Perspective: Overcoming disparities in U.S. health care. *Health Affairs, 24*(2), 445–451.

Furumoto-Dawson, A., Gehlert, S., Sohmer, D., et al. (2007). Early-life conditions and mechanisms of population health vulnerabilities. *Health Affairs, 26*(5), 1238–1248.

Gelberg, L., Andersen, R., & Leake, B. (2000). The Behavioral Model for Vulnerable Populations: Application to medical care use and outcomes for homeless people. *Health Services Research, 34*(6), 1273–1302.

Gitterman, A. (Ed.). (2001). *Handbook of social work practice with vulnerable and resilient populations,* 2nd ed. New York: Columbia University Press.

Glover, J., Hetzel, D., & Tennant, S. (2004). The socioeconomic gradient and chronic illness and associated risk factors in Australia. *Australian & New Zealand Health Policy, 1*(1), 8.

Haas, J.S., & Adler, N.E. (2001). *The causes of vulnerability: Disentangling the effects of race, socioeconomic status, and insurance coverage on health.* Institute of Medicine. Retrieved August 18, 2008 from http://www.iom.edu/Object.File/Master/19/227/HaasAdlerPaper%2001%2016%2002.pdf.

Hansen, D. (2007). *Uninsured count jumps to 47 million.* American Medical News. Retrieved August 18, 2008 from http://www.ama-assn.org/amednews/2007/09/17/gvl10917.htm.

Haub, C. (2006, January). *Hispanics account for almost one-half of U.S. population growth.* Population Reference Bureau. Retrieved October 15,2008 from http://www.prb.org/ArticIes/2006/HispanicsAccountforAlmost OneHalfofUSPopulationGrowth.aspx.

Heck, K., Braveman, P., Cubbin, C., et al. (2006). Socioeconomic status and breastfeeding initiation among California mothers. *Public Health Reports, 121*(1), 51–59.

Heisler, M., Smith, D., Hayward, R., et al. (2003). Racial disparities in diabetes care processes, outcomes, and treatment intensity. *Medical Care, 41*(11), 1221–1232.

Hellander, I. (2006). A review of data on the U.S. health section: Spring 2006. *International Journal of Health Services, 36*(4), 787–802.

Himmelstein, D., Warren, E., Thorne, D., & Woolhandler, S. (February 2, 2005). Market Watch: illness and injury as contributors to bankruptcy. *Health Affairs,* DOI: 10.1377/hlthaff.w5.63.

Hodge, J.G. (2005). An enhanced approach to distinguishing public health practice and human subjects research. *The Journal of Law, Medicine and Ethics, 33*(1), 125–141.

Hutchings, A., Raine, R., Brady, A., et al. (2004). Socioeconomic status and outcome from intensive care in England and Wales. *Medical Care, 42*(10), 943–951.

Institute of Medicine. (2003). *Unequal treatment: Confronting racial and ethnic disparities in healthcare.* Washington, DC: The National Academies Press.

Isaacs, S., & Schroeder, S. (2004). Class: The ignored determinant of the nation's health. *New England Journal of Medicine, 351*(11), 1137–1142.

Jack, S., DiCenso, A., & Lohfeld, L. (2002). Opening doors: Factors influencing the establishment of a working relationship between paraprofessional home visitors and at-risk families. *Canadian Journal of Nursing Research, 34*(4), 59–69.

Jack, S.M., DiCenso, A., & Lohfeld, L. (2005). A theory of maternal engagement with public health nurses and family visitors. *Journal of Advanced Nursing, 49*(2), 182–190.

Jacobi, J., Parikh, S., McGuire, D., et al. (2007). Racial disparity in clinical outcomes following primary percutaneous coronary intervention for ST elevation myocardial infarction: Influence of process of care. *Journal of Interventional Cardiology, 20*(3), 182–187.

Jones, A. (2003). *Greatest health problem: The unending cycle of poverty.* National Catholic Reporter. Retrieved August 18, 2008 from http://natcath.org/NCR_Online/archives2/2003c/092603/092603e.php.

Keppel, K.G., Bilheimer, L., & Gurley, L. (2007). Improving population health and reducing health disparities. *Health Affairs, 26*(5), 1281–1292.

Kuper, H., Adami, H., Theorell, T., & Weiderpass, E. (2007). The socioeconomic gradient in the incidence of stroke: A prospective study in middle-aged women in Sweden. *Stroke, 38*(1), 4–5.

Leight, S.B. (2003). The application of a vulnerable populations conceptual model to rural health. *Public Health Nursing, 20*(6), 440–448.

Lemstra, M., Neudorf, C., & Opondo, J. (2006). Health disparity by neighbourhood income. *Canadian Journal of Public Health, 97*(6), 435–439.

List, J.M. (2005). Histories of mistrust and protectionism: Disadvantaged minority groups and human-subject research policies. *The American Journal of Bioethics, 5*(1), 53–56.

Locher, J., Bronstein, J., Robinson, C., et al. (2006). Ethical issues involving research conducted with homebound older adults. *Gerontologist, 46*(2), 160–164.

Lynn, M., & Nelson, D. (2005). Common (mis)perceptions about IRB review of human subjects research. *Nursing Science Quarterly, 16*(3), 264–270.

Mahon, M. (2005). *New study: At least 16 million adults lack adequate health insurance coverage.* The Commonwealth Fund. Retrieved August 18, 2008 from http://www.commonwealthfund.org/newsroom/newsroom_show.htm?doc_id=280619.

Malone, R., Yerger, V., McGruder, C., & Froelicher, E. (2006). "It's like Tuskegee in reverse": A case study of ethical tensions in institutional review board review of community-based participatory research. *American Journal of Public Health, 96*(11), 1914–1919.

Marmot, M., Ryff, C.D., Bumpass, L.L., et al. (1997). Social inequalities in health: Next questions and converging evidence. *Social Science and Medicine, 44*(6), 901–910.

Marmot, M., & Wilkinson, R. (Eds.). (2006). *Social determinants of health.* Oxford, UK: Oxford University Press.

Martino-Maze, C.D. (2005). Registered nurses' personal rights vs. professional responsibility in caring for members of underserved and disenfranchised populations. *Journal of Clinical Nursing, 14*, 546–554.

Martino-Maze, C.D. (2006). Registered nurses' willingness to serve populations on the periphery of society. *Journal of Nursing Scholarship, 38*(3), 301–306.

McGee, E.M. (2006). The healing circle: Resiliency in nurses. *Issues in Mental Health Nursing, 27*(1), 43–57.

Meaux, J., & Bell, P. (2001). Balancing recruitment and protection: Children as research subjects. *Issues in Comprehensive Pediatric Nursing, 24*, 241–251.

Mechanic, D., & Tanner, J. (2007). Vulnerable people, groups, and populations: Societal view. *Health Affairs, 26*(5), 1220–1230.

Metzler, M. (2007). Social determinants of health: What, how, why, and now. *Preventing Chronic Disease, 4*(4). Retrieved August 18, 2008 from http://www.cdc.gov/pcd/issues/2007/oct/07_0136.htm.

Minkler, M., Fuller-Thomson, E., & Guralnik, J. (2006). Gradient of disability across the socioeconomic spectrum in the United States. *New England Journal of Medicine, 355*(7), 695–703.

Nanyonjo, R., Montgomery, S., Modeste, N., & Fujimoto, E. (2007). A secondary analysis of race/ethnicity and other maternal factors affecting adverse birth outcomes in San Bernardino County. *Maternal and Child Health Journal,* DOI 10.1007/s10995-007-0260-x.

National Advisory Council on Nurse Education & Practice. (2000). *A national agenda for nursing workforce racial/ethnic diversity.* Washington, DC: U.S. Department of Health & Human Services, Bureau of Health Professions, Division of Nursing.

Olden, K., & White, S.L. (2005). Health-related disparities: Influence of environmental factors. *Medical Clinics of North America, 89*(4), 721–738.

Pauly, M.V., & Pagan, J.A. (2007). Spillovers and vulnerability: The case of community uninsurance. *Health Affairs, 26*(5), 1281–1292.

Penprase, B. (2006). Developing comprehensive health care for an underserved population. *Geriatric Nursing, 27*(1), 45–50.

Polit, D.F., & Beck, C.T. (2005). *Essentials of nursing research: Methods, appraisal & utilization,* 6th ed. Philadelphia:, Lippincott Williams & Wilkins.

Population Reference Bureau. (2006, May). *In the news: U.S. population is now one-third minority.* Retrieved October 15, 2008 from http://www.prb.org/Articles/2006/IntheNews-USPopulationIsNowOneThirdMinority.aspx?p=1.

Pritchard, C., & deVerteuil, B. (2007). Application of health equity audit to health visiting. *Community Practice, 80*(5), 38–41.

Pugh, T. (May 25, 2007). *U.S. economy leaving record numbers in severe poverty.* McClatchy Washington Bureau. Retrieved August 19, 2008 from http://www.commondreams.org/headlines07/0223-09.htm.

Reimer-Kirkham, S., Van Hofwegen, L., & Hoe-Harwood, C. (2005). Narratives of social justice: Learning in innovative clinical settings. *International Journal of Nursing Education & Scholarship, 2*(article 28).

Rogers, W.A. (2004). Evidence based medicine and justice: A framework for looking at the impact of EBM upon vulnerable or disadvantaged groups. *Journal of Medical Ethics, 30*(2), 141–145.

Roth, R., & Barsi, E. (2005). The community need index: A new tool pinpoints health care disparities in communities throughout the nation. *Health Progress, 86*(4), 32–38.

Ruof, M.C. (2004). Vulnerability, vulnerable populations, and policy. *Kennedy Institute of Ethics Journal, 14*(4), 411–425.

Salinsky, E., & Gursky, E. (2006). The case for transforming governmental public health. *Health Affairs, 25*(4),1017–1028.

Satcher, D., Fryer, G., McCann, J., et al. (2005). What if we were equal? A comparison of the black-white mortality gap in 1960 and 2000. *Health Affairs, 24*(2), 459–464.

Saunders, J.M. (2007). Vulnerable populations in an American Red Cross shelter after hurricane Katrina. *Perspectives in Psychiatric Care, 43*(1), 30–37.

Schneider, D., Lilienfeld, D., & Im, W. (2006). The epidemiology of pulmonary embolism: Racial contrasts in incidence and in-hospital case fatality. *Journal of the National Medical Association, 98*(12), 1967–1972.

Schrader-McMillan, A. (2007). Learning at the edges: Participatory action research and child maltreatment in post-war Guatemala. *Bulletin of Latin American Research, 26*(4), 516–532.

Schulman, S. (2006). Terms of engagement: Aligning youth, adults, and organizations toward social change. *Journal of Public Health Management & Practice, 12*(6), 26–32.

Shepard, V., Williams, K., & Richardson, J. (2004). Women's priorities for lay health home visitors: Implications for eliminating health disparities among underserved women. *Journal of Health & Social Policy, 18*(3), 19–35.

Shi, L., & Stevens, G. (2004). *Vulnerable populations in the United States.* San Francisco, CA: Jossey-Bass Publishers.

Singer, E., & Bossarte, R. (2006). Incentives for survey participation: When are they "coercive"? *American Journal of Preventive Medicine, 31*(5), 411–418.

Singh, G., Miller, B., Hankey, B., et al. (2002). Changing area socioeconomic patterns in U.S. cancer mortality, 1950–1998: Part I: All cancers among men. *Journal of the National Cancer Institute, 94*(12), 904–915.

SmithBattle, L., Diekemper, M., & Drake, M.A. (1999). Articulating the culture and tradition of community health nursing. *Public Health Nursing, 16*(3), 215–222.

Sohler, N., Li, X., & Cunningham, C. (2007). Perceived discrimination among severely disadvantaged people with HIV infection. *Public Health Reports, 122*(3), 347–355.

Tough, S., Johnston, D., Siever, J., et al. (2006). Does supplementary prenatal nursing and home visitation support improve resource use in a universal health care system? A randomized controlled trial in Canada. *Birth, 33*(3), 183–194.

University of California Los Angeles (UCLA) Center for Vulnerable Populations Research. (2007). *Who are vulnerable populations?* Retrieved August 19, 2008 from http://www.nursing.ucla.edu/orgs/cvpr/who-are-vunerable.html.

U.S. Census Bureau. (2007). *Minority population tops one million.* (Press Release). Retrieved October 15,2008 from http://www.certsus.gov/Press-Release/www/releases/archives/population/010048.html.

U.S. Department of Health & Human Services. (2000). *Healthy people 2010: Understanding and improving health,* 2nd ed. Washington, DC: U.S. Government Printing Office.

U.S. Department of Health & Human Services. (2007). *The 2005 HHS poverty guidelines.* Retrieved August 19, 2008 from http://aspe.hhs.gov/poverty/05poverty.shtml.

U.S. Department of Health and Human Services (USDHHS). (2000). *Healthy people 2010* (Conference ed., Vols. 1 & 2). Washington, DC: Author.

Whitehead, M. (1991). *The concepts and principles of equity and health.* Copenhagen, Denmark: WHO/EURO.

Williams, D.R., & Jackson, P.B. (2005). Social sources of racial disparities in health: Policies in societal domains, far removed from traditional health policy, can have decisive consequences for health. *Health Affairs, 24*(2), 325–334.

Winkleby, M., & Cubbin, C. (2004). Racial/ethnic disparities in health behaviors: A challenge to current assumptions. In N. Anderson, R. Bulatao, & B. Cohen (Eds.). *Critical perspectives on racial and ethnic differences in health in late life.* (pp. 450–483). Washington, DC: The National Academies Press.

Yeo, S. (2004). Language barriers and access to care. *Annual Review of Nursing Research, 22,* 59–73.

Warner, D.F., & Hayward, M.D. (2002). *Race disparities in men's mortality: The role of childhood social conditions in a process of cumulative disadvantage.* Paper presented at the annual meetings of the Population Association of America, Atlanta, May 9–11.

Zerwekh, J. (2000). Caring on the ragged edge: Nursing persons who are disenfranchised. *Advances in Nursing Science, 22*(4), 47–61.

Selected Readings

Aston, M., Meagher-Stewart, D., Sheppard-Lemoine, D., et al. (2006). Family health nursing and empowering relationships. *Pediatric Nursing, 32*(1), 61–67.

Braveman, P. (2006). Health disparities and health equity: Concepts and measurement. *Annual Review of Public Health, 27,* 167–194.

Clover, A., Browne, J., McErlain, P., & Vandenberg, B. (2004). Patient approaches to clinical conversations in the palliative care setting. *Journal of Advanced Nursing, 48*(4), 333–341.

Copeland, D.A. (2007). Conceptualizing family members of violent mentally ill individuals as a vulnerable population. *Issues in Mental Health Nursing, 28*(9), 943–975.

Deaton, A. (2002). Policy implications of the gradient of health land wealth. *Health Affairs, 21*(2), 13–30.

Ferrie, J., Martikainen, P., Shipley, M., & Marmot, M. (2005). Self-reported economic difficulties and coronary events in men: Evidence from the Whitehall II study. *International Journal of Epidemiology, 34*(3), 640–648.

Giger, J., Davidhizar, R., Purnell, L., et al. (2007). American Academy of Nursing Expert Panel report: Developing cultural competence to eliminate health disparities in ethnic minorities and other vulnerable populations. *Journal of Transcultural Nursing, 18*(2), 95–102.

Glass, T., & McAtee, M. (2006). Behavioral science at the crossroads in public health: Extending horizons, envisioning the future. *Social Science and Medicine, 62*(7), 1650–1671.

Grahan, H., Inskip, H., Francis, B., & Harmon, J. (2006). Pathways of disadvantage and smoking careers: Evidence and policy implications. *Journal of Epidemiology in Community Health, 60*[Suppl. III], ii7–ii12.

Gregson, S., Terceira, N., Mushati, P., et al. (2004). Community group participation: Can it help young women to avoid HIV? An exploratory study of social capital and school education in rural Zimbabwe. *Social Science & Medicine, 58*(11), 2119–2132.

Knudsen, E., Heckman, J., Cameron, J., & Shonkoff, J. (2006). Economic neurobiological and behavioral perspectives on building America's future workforce. *Proceedings of the National Academy of Science, 103*(27), 10155–10162.

Koch, T., & Kralik, D. (2006). *Participatory action research in health care.* Oxford, UK: Blackwell Publishing.

Kupperschmidt, B.R. (2006). Addressing multigenerational conflict: Mutual respect and "carefronting" as strategy. *Online Journal of Issues in Nursing, 11*(2). Retrieved August 19, 2008 from http://www.medscape.com/viewarticle/536481.

Lott, J. (2005). Module three: Vulnerable/special participant populations. *Developing World Bioethics, 5*(1), 30–54.

Mackenbach, J., & Howden-Chapman, P. (2003). New perspectives on socioeconomic inequalities in health. *Perspectives in Biology & Medicine, 46*(3), 428–444.

Office of Minority Health. (2007). *Eliminating racial & ethnic health disparities.* Retrieved August 19, 2008 from http://www.cdc.gov/omh/AboutUs/disparities.htm.

Ross, C., & Wu, C. (1995). The links between education and health. *American Sociological Review, 60,* 719–745.

Tembreull, C., & Schaffer, M. (2005). The intervention of outreach: Best practices. *Public Health Nursing, 22*(4), 347–353.

Thrane, C. (2006). Explaining educational-related inequalities in health: Mediation and moderator models. *Social Science and Medicine, 62*(2), 467–478.

Upvall, M.J., & Bost, M.L. (2007). Developing cultural competence in nursing students through their experiences with a refugee population. *Journal of Nursing Education, 46*(8), 380–383.

Vanderwerker, L., Chen, J., Charpentier, P., et al. (2007). Differences in risk factors for suicidality between African American and White patients vulnerable to suicide. *Suicide and Life Threatening Behavior, 37*(1), 1–9.

Wilcox, L.S. (2007). Onions and bubbles: Models of the social determinants of health. *Preventing Chronic Disease, 4*(4). Retrieved August 19, 2008 from http://www.cdc.gov/pcd/issues/2007oct/07_0126.htm.

Wilkinson, R., & Pickett, K. (2006). Income inequality and population health: A review and explanation of the evidence. *Social Science & Medicine, 62*(7), 1768–1784.

Woolf, S., Johnson, R., Phillips, R., & Philipsen, M. (2007). Giving everyone the health of the educated: An examination of whether social change would save more lives than medical advances. *American Journal of Public Health, 97*(4), 679–683.

Zahner, S., & Gredig, O. (2005). Public health nursing practice change and recommendations for improvement. *Public Health Nursing, 22*(5), 422–428.

Internet Resources

Center for Comparative Biology of Vulnerable Populations: *http://www.nicholas.duke.edu/ccbvp/about/about.html*

Centers for Population Health & Disparities: *http://www.niehs.nih.gov/research/supported/centers/disparities/index.cfm*

Duke University (information on research with vulnerable populations): *http://www.ors.duke.edu/irb/vulnerable/index.htm*

Economic Research Initiative on the Uninsured (links to abstracts of research articles on a variety of topics related to vulnerable populations): *http://eriu.sph.umich.edu/research/all_vulnerable.html*

Harvard/MGH Center on Genomics, Vulnerable Populations & Health Disparities: *http://www.cgvh.harvard.edu/*

Health Canada (environmental & workplace health): *http://www.hc-sc.gc.ca/ewh-semt/contaminants/vulnerable/index_e.html*

Healthy People 2010—Midcourse review: *http://www.healthypeople.gov/Data/midcourse/pdf/ExecutiveSummary.pdf*

International Society of Nurses in Genetics (counseling vulnerable populations): *http://www.isong.org/about/ps_vulnerable.cfm*

National Center on Minority Health & Health Disparities: *http://ncmhd.nih.gov/*

Office of Minority Health (USHHS/CDC): *http://www.omhrc.gov/*

PrepareNow.org (links to vulnerable population information): *http://www.preparenow.org/pop.html*

Prevention Institute (resources on health disparities): *http://www.preventioninstitute.org/healthdis.html*

UCLA Center for Vulnerable Populations Research: *http://www.nursing.ucla.edu/orgs/cvpr/*

University of Colorado at Boulder, Natural Hazards Center (gender & vulnerable populations): *http://www.colorado.edu/hazards/resources/web/gender_vulnerable.html*

University of Illinois at Chicago, Center for Reducing Risks in Vulnerable Populations: *http://www.uic.edu/nursing/crrvp/*

USDA Economic Research Service (information on food access and vulnerable populations): *http://www.ers.usda.gov/Briefing/VulnerablePopulations/*

U.S. Department of Health & Human Services (research with special classes of subjects): *http://www.hhs.gov/ohrp/irb/irb_chapter6ii.htm*

Vulnerable Populations & Health Care Conference Proceedings: *http://kaisernetwork.org/health_cast/hcast_index.cfm?display=detail&hc=2287*

World Health Organization (vulnerable populations/substance abuse programs): *http://www.who.int/substance_abuse/publications/vulnerable_pop/en/index.html*

Yale Center for Self & Family Management of Vulnerable Populations: *http://nursing.yale.edu/Centers/ECSMI/*

26

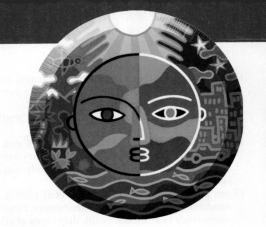

Clients with Disabilities and Chronic Illnesses

LEARNING OBJECTIVES

Upon mastery of this chapter, you should be able to:

◆ Discuss the national and global implications of disability and chronic illness.
◆ Describe the economic, social, and political factors affecting the well-being of individuals with disabilities and chronic illness.
◆ Provide an example of primary, secondary, and tertiary prevention practices for disabled individuals.
◆ Describe the Americans with Disabilities Act.
◆ Discuss the benefits of universal design for all persons.

❝*It was ability that mattered, not disability, which is a word I'm not crazy about using.*❞

—Marlee Matlin, Deaf Academy Award–Winning Actress

At some point in our lives, most of us will be diagnosed with a chronic illness or develop some type of disability. We may be lucky enough to get early diagnosis and treatment of our health conditions so that they can be easily managed. We might find ourselves temporarily incapacitated, unable to manage our daily lives, and needing assistance from others. We can hope our ability to resume more normal activities will return swiftly. An estimated 54 million Americans (almost 20% of the population) live with some ongoing level of disability (U.S. Department of Health and Human Services [USDHHS], 2005b). In 2006 alone, over 34 million persons reported limitations in their usual activities as the result of chronic conditions (USDHHS, 2008). The human costs associated with disabilities aside, the cost of direct medical care and indirect annual costs related to disability have reached almost $300 million in the United States alone.

In the *Final Review of Healthy People 2000* (USDHHS, 2001), the rates of some disabling conditions, such as significant hearing and vision impairments, decreased between 1991 and 2000. The rates of many other conditions however, either remained stable or increased during that same decade. In the ensuing years, disabilities and chronic health conditions continued to pose significant personal and public costs. The results of the *Midcourse Review: Healthy People 2010* (USDHHS, 2005a) demonstrate both positive and negative changes in the first half of the present decade. Many findings continue to cause concern for health professionals. For instance, arthritis remains the leading cause of disability in the United States. It affects approximately 43 million individuals and more than 20% of the adult population. Asthma remains a national health concern for all ages, most particularly for those under 18 years of age, and represents one of the four most common causes of chronic illness in children. Although asthma death rates for persons over 65 years have declined, racial and ethnic disparities persist. End-stage renal disease continues to increase, with over 45% of all new cases attributed to type 2 diabetes. Back pain will impact the lives of a staggering 80% of all people, with risk factors including age, fitness level, race, ethnicity, and occupation. Osteoporosis is estimated to be present in 10% of all persons over the age of 50 (USDHHS, 2005a), with the additional risk of serious injury or death following a fall. The need to address health issues of disability and chronic illness is vital to the well-being of affected individuals and families and crucial to the financial health of the country.

This chapter discusses important and necessary health promotion and preventive efforts at every level. Although treatment of chronic conditions has long been a mainstay of health care in the United States and globally, limited attention has been paid to the additional health promotion required to maintain and improve overall well-being of individuals with chronic conditions. Nor has enough attention been directed to those same needs for people with physical or psychological disabilities. This chapter begins with an overview of disabilities and chronic illnesses, then discusses the current national and global trends in addressing these issues. The various organizations that focus on improving the well-being of those affected, the impact on families, and the role of the community health nurse in addressing the chronic health care needs of individuals, families, and aggregates are discussed. The benefits of universal design and issues of easy access for all ages and abilities are also discussed.

PERSPECTIVES ON DISABILITY, CHRONIC ILLNESS, AND HEALTH

What does the word *disabled* mean to you? What thoughts come to mind when you think about the word as it applies to an individual? It is defined in one dictionary as "the incapacity to do something because of a handicap—physical, mental, etc." (Morehead & Morehead, 1995). Disability is linked with *inability*, which is defined as "the lack of ability to do something, whatever the reason, but usually through incompetence, weakness, lack of training, etc." (Morehead & Morehead, 1995). **Handicap** is explained in the same volume as "any encumbrance or disadvantage." **Chronic disease** is any illness that is prolonged, does not resolve spontaneously, and is rarely cured completely; these diseases are often preventable, and they pose a significant burden in terms of mortality, morbidity, and cost (Centers for Disease Control and Prevention [CDC], 2007). Each of these definitions provides a decidedly negative connotation, similar in nature to the typical societal view faced daily by people with disabilities.

Challenges differ from one individual to the next and require different degrees of accommodation. Fortunately, long-held negative views of disabled persons and their conditions are being replaced with new and more positive approaches that view individuals and their challenges from a more holistic standpoint.

International Classification of Functioning, Disability, and Health

One such change in thinking about disability and chronic illness was expressed in *International Classification of Functioning, Disability, and Health* (ICF), published by the World Health Organization (WHO) in 2001. This document, the result of 5 years of work, replaced *International Classification of Impairments, Disabilities, and Handicaps* (ICIDH) (World Health Organization [WHO], 1980). Even the change in terminology in the title showed the dramatic shift in thinking by the World Health Assembly; both *impairments* and *handicaps* were removed. In the revised document, **disability** serves as a broad term for impairments, activity limitations, or participation restrictions. It is linked with **functioning**, a term that encompasses all body functions, activities, and participation.

The ICF was an attempt to provide a universal classification system with standardized language and a way to view the domains of health from a holistic vantage point. It took into account body functions and structures, activities and participation, environmental factors, and personal factors. This allows a multidimensional evaluation of an individual's circumstances in terms of functioning, disability, and health. Melding the "medical model" of health and health care for disabled persons with the "social model," the ICF provided a biopsychosocial approach for assessing people with disabilities, emphasizing the observation that no two people with the same disease or disability have the same level of functioning.

The purpose of the ICF reaches far beyond simply categorizing the health status of people with disabilities. The specific aims of the document are (WHO, 2001, p. 5):

◆ Provide a scientific basis for understanding and studying health and health-related states, outcomes, and determinations
◆ Establish a common language for describing health and health-related states to improve communication between different users such as health care workers, researchers, policy makers, and the public, including people with disabilities
◆ Permit comparison of data across countries, health care disciplines, services, and time
◆ Provide a systematic coding scheme for health information systems

The document provides a roadmap for using the ICF, based on experience with the ICIDH for more than 20 years. Table 26.1 shows the current and potential uses of the document by various entities ranging from insurance companies and health care providers to policy makers and educators.

In addition to the just discussed definitions of disability and functioning, the following definitions serve to explain the ICF in terms of health (WHO, 2001, p. 10):

◆ **Body functions** are the physiologic functions of body systems and include psychological functions.
◆ **Body structures** are anatomic parts of the body such as organs, limbs, and their components.
◆ **Impairments** are problems in body function or structure, such as a significant deviation or loss.
◆ **Activity** is the execution of a task or action by an individual.

◆ **Participation** is involvement in a life situation, including personal and interpersonal roles and activities.
◆ **Activity limitations** are difficulties an individual may have in executing activities.
◆ **Participation restrictions** are problems an individual may experience when involved in life situations.
◆ **Environmental factors** make up the physical, social, and attitudinal environments in which people live and conduct their lives.
◆ **Personal factors** are the features of an individual's background, life, and living that are not part of a health condition or health status, such as gender, race, age, other health conditions, fitness, lifestyle habits, upbringing, coping styles, social background, education, profession, past and current experience, overall behavior pattern and character style, individual psychological assets, and other characteristics—all or any of which may play a role in disability at any level.

For the community health nurse, the ICF facilitates assessment of an individual client based on a wide range of factors. Disability or disease is just one factor to be considered in planning and implementing a care plan for clients in the community. Two individuals may have the same disability, such as a below-the-knee amputation, but their health and well-being can be quite different. One may have a more positive outlook, one may have more social support than the other, or one may suffer more than the other from additional health issues that impede rehabilitation. The community health nurse must always consider the totality of the situation, including the biologic, psychological, sociocultural, and environmental realms. Diseases and disabilities are conditions, yet a client may often be referred to as "the paraplegic" or "the amputee" and not by her name. This type of designation should be avoided: a disease or disability is something one has, not something one is. Figure 26.1 depicts the interactions among the various components addressed by the ICF in the evaluation and assessment of clients with disabilities. It can serve as a useful model for community health nursing practice in the overall assessment of people with disabilities.

TABLE 26.1	Applications of the International Classification of Functioning, Disability, and Health
Statistical Tool	Collection and recording of data: • Population studies & surveys • Management information systems
Research Tool	Measure: • Outcomes • Quality of life • Environmental factors
Clinical Tool	• Needs assessment • Matching treatments with specific conditions • Vocational assessment • Rehabilitation • Outcome evaluation
Social Policy Tool	• Social security planning • Compensation systems • Policy design and implementation
Educational Tool	• Curriculum design • Raising awareness • Undertaking social action

From World Health Organization. (2001). *International classification of functioning, disability and health.* Geneva, Switzerland: Author.

The World Health Report

The 2002 release of the annual report by the WHO (*The World Health Report 2002: Reducing Risks, Promoting Healthy Life*) set a new standard for addressing global health. It challenged the world community to focus more attention on unhealthy behaviors that lead ultimately to chronic disease, disability, and early mortality. The report stressed that, although infectious diseases and malnutrition require ongoing vigilance because they continue to plague many parts of the world, they are not the only threat. It is increasingly clear that lifestyle choices play a major role in morbidity and mortality levels in affluent and poor countries alike, and intervention at all levels (local, national, and international) is a high priority. With this new reality in mind, this document had a twofold purpose: to quantify the most important risks to health, and to assess the cost-effectiveness

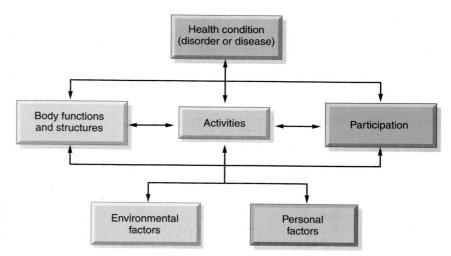

F I G U R E **26.1** Model of functioning and disability. From the World Health Organization (WHO). (2001). *ICF introduction.* Geneva, Switzerland: Author.

of interventions designed to reduce those risks. The overall goal was "to help governments of all countries lower these risks and raise the healthy life expectancy of their populations'" (WHO, 2002, p. 7).

No longer can health care providers across the globe continue to address acute illness by itself; lifestyle and behavior must be considered because of the impact they have on healthy years of life. The risks to health that the WHO report focused on include some that are the direct result of poverty, but many can be more aptly linked to excesses, notably in the more affluent countries. The 10 leading health risks are (1) underweight, (2) unsafe sex, (3) high blood pressure, (4) tobacco consumption, (5) alcohol consumption, (6) unsafe water, sanitation, and hygiene, (7) iron deficiency, (8) indoor smoke from solid fuels, (9) high cholesterol, and (10) obesity. Globally, these 10 health risks are responsible for more than 33% of all deaths and untold disability. Half of these risks—tobacco and alcohol consumption, high blood pressure, high cholesterol, and obesity—can be directly related to lifestyle and behavioral choices.

Nutrition is vital to health; nutritional imbalances can lead to severe chronic illness, disability, and premature death. Of the leading 10 health risks, five are directly related to consumption: underweight, hypertension, iron deficiency, high cholesterol, and obesity (WHO, 2002). The prevalence of obesity worldwide is estimated at more than 1 billion adults, with some 300 million who can be classified as clinically obese (WHO, 2008). In stark contrast, there are 170 million underweight children in poor countries, more than 3 million of whom will die each year from malnutrition. Being overweight increases the risk of coronary heart disease, stroke, diabetes, and some types of cancer. Malnutrition and the lack of important nutrients can lead to a wide array of preventable disabilities. For instance, the leading cause of acquired blindness in children is vitamin A deficiency, and the leading cause of mental retardation and brain damage is iodine deficiency (WHO, 2002).

The significance of the WHO report lies in its simplicity. If countries can make even minimal strides toward improving the health of their citizens, a dramatic improvement in health outlook can occur within those countries and worldwide. Governments must take a proactive role in addressing the preventive health care needs of their citizens

(Display 26.1). A shift in focus from the most high-risk individuals to the general population is essential. Primary and secondary prevention as the main focus is the approach that public health care professionals have stressed for decades. As difficult as it has been in the United States to implement a shift in emphasis to health promotion efforts, it will be interesting to see if this "call to action" by WHO will result in less emphasis on tertiary prevention. The old adage, "An ounce of prevention is worth a pound of cure," is most appropriate for the years ahead.

DISPLAY 26.1   **WORLD HEALTH ORGANIZATION RECOMMENDATIONS TO IMPROVE GLOBAL HEALTH**

- Government/health ministry support for scientific research, improved surveillance systems, and better access to global information
- Development of effective, committed policies for the prevention of health risks such as tobacco consumption, unsafe sex associated with HIV/AIDS, and unhealthy diet and obesity
- Implementation of cost-effectiveness analysis to identify the most cost-effective and affordable interventions to reduce priority health risks
- Collaborative efforts (intersectoral and international) to reduce major extraneous risk to health caused by unsafe water, poor sanitation, or lack of education
- Supportive and balanced approach in addressing these major health risks that includes government, community, and individual action
- Empowerment and encouragement of individuals to make positive, life-enhancing health decisions (such as eliminating tobacco use, excessive alcohol consumption, unhealthy diet, and unsafe sex)

Adapted from World Health Organization. (2002). *The world health report 2002: Reducing risks, promoting healthy life.* Geneva, Switzerland: Author.

Taken together, the ICF and the 2002 WHO report set a standard for health care in the 21st century. Chronic disease and disability prevention are vital to world health. The cost of health care treatment is high, but the cost in terms of lost productivity and decreased quality of life is even higher. Without control of preventable disability and chronic disease, these conditions could very well become the "new plagues" of the coming decades.

United Nations' Convention on the Rights of Persons with Disabilities

An estimated 650 million people live with disabilities worldwide (United Nations [UN], 2007a). Factoring in the nearly 2 billion family members affected by the disability, the WHO stressed that almost one-third of the world population is directly impacted by disabilities. The sheer magnitude of this issue, and the recognition that people with disabilities are a "significantly overlooked development challenge" across the world, led to the United Nations (U.N.) Convention on the Rights of Persons with Disabilities in 2006. The Convention was opened for signature in March 2007 and, as of May 2008, had been ratified by 129 countries. Specific principles of the convention include (United Nations [UN], 2007b):

◆ Respect for inherent dignity and individual autonomy, including the freedom to make one's own choices and independence of persons
◆ Nondiscrimination
◆ Full and effective participation and inclusion in society
◆ Respect for difference and acceptance of persons with disabilities as part of human diversity and humanity
◆ Equality of opportunity
◆ Accessibility
◆ Equality between men and women
◆ Respect for evolving capacities of children with disabilities and respect for the right of children with disabilities to preserve their identities

The convention, once entered into force, will be serviced by both the U.N. Department of Economic and Social Affairs (New York) and the Office of the High Commissioner for Human Rights (Geneva). The United States was not one of the signatories of the convention, joining countries such as Pakistan, the Russian Federation, Saudi Arabia, Switzerland, Ukraine, and Zimbabwe. Although the United States was an active participant in committee work on the convention and congratulated the convention's work, reasons cited for not signing the document appeared related to issues of sovereignty. In a December 2006 press release from Ambassador Richard Miller, U.S. Mission to the U.N. (2006), the following explanation was provided: "Our nation's commitment to the rights and dignities of persons with disabilities is embodied in our vast array of strong national laws, notably the historic Americans with Disabilities Act. . . . The United States believes that the most effective way for states to improve the real world situation of persons with disabilities from a legal perspective is to strengthen their domestic legal frameworks related to nondiscrimination and equality." The actual impact of the convention will only be realized in the coming years. Building on the Americans with Disabilities Act (ADA, discussed later in this chapter) the convention can only be viewed as a positive step in the progress toward equality. It should be noted that the National Council on Disability (NCD) has taken an approach to the convention that is profoundly different from the official U.S. government position. Noting the administration's concern that the convention would provide a baseline standard much lower than that provided for in the ADA, the NCD still urged the signing of the treaty. In a March 2007 letter to the President, they argued that signing the convention would provide "clear support for the principles of this landmark treaty and to continue our country's tradition as a world leader for people with disabilities" (National Council on Disability [NCD], 2008a, Preamble).

Healthy People 2010

The most influential document addressing health in the United States, *Healthy People 2010* (USDHHS, 2000) defines those areas of health and well-being that are most in need of attention. With its clearly delineated and measurable objectives, *Healthy People 2010* has far-reaching influence on national and state health initiatives, health care policy, research priorities, and funding. In terms of disability and chronic illness, *Healthy People 2010* has placed added emphasis on conditions expected to take a toll on the nation's health in the coming years. It also reflects a growing realization by health care providers, insurance companies, public health agencies, and health care facilities of the need to act proactively to avoid the economic toll that lack of attention can produce.

It is difficult to discuss *Healthy People 2010* (USDHHS, 2000) without some mention of *Healthy People 2000* (USDHHS, 1991). A comparison of the two documents reveals some striking differences regarding disabilities and chronic conditions. Increased attention has been given to the growing national need to reduce the incidence of disability and chronic disease and improve the health of people affected by them. In *Healthy People 2000,* only one priority area was devoted to disability and chronic illness. Priority Area 17, "Diabetes and Chronic Disabling Conditions," emphasized diabetes, with only limited attention to the broader range of other disabilities (asthma, chronic kidney disease, arthritis, deformities or orthopedic impairments, mental retardation, peptic ulcer disease, visual and hearing impairments, and overweight). In contrast, almost half of the *Healthy People 2010* focus areas directly address chronic illness and disability, and almost all of the focus areas can be related to these issues in some manner. Moreover, the section on "Disability and Secondary Conditions" is devoted exclusively to issues most relevant to people with disabilities.

The definition of disability in *Healthy People 2010* is somewhat different and more explicit than that used in the ICF (WHO, 2001); it is stated as "the general term used to represent the interactions between individuals with a health condition and barriers in their environment" (USDHHS, 2000, p. 25). Moreover, **people with disabilities** are "identified as having an activity limitation or who use assistance or who perceive themselves as having a disability" (USDHHS, 2000, p. 6–25).

This change in emphasis between the two documents was noted in *Healthy People 2010* (USDHHS, 2000), which cited lack of parity between disabled and nondisabled populations in terms of several selected objectives: leisure-time activity, use of community support programs, and receipt of clinical preventive services. One such example was the finding that the percentage of people with disabilities who reported some type of leisure-time activity was the lowest of any of the groups identified (including those older than 65 years of age and low-income persons). On the positive side, the percentage of people with disabilities who reported no leisure-time physical activity actually declined from the 1985 level of 35% to 29% in 1995, although it was still far short of the 2000 target of 20%. Additional disparities noted for people with disabilities included increased likelihood of being overweight, adverse effects from stress, and reduced rates of preventive services (e.g., tetanus boosters, Pap tests, breast examinations, and mammograms). Recognition that the health needs of disabled persons were not receiving needed attention resulted in increasing the priority of improving the health of people with disabilities.

Improving the health of the nation requires a multifaceted approach to improve parity among all individuals. *Healthy People 2010* states that "every person in every community across the nation deserves equal access to comprehensive, culturally competent, community-based health care systems that are committed to serving the needs of the individual and promoting community health" (USDHHS, 2000, p.16). The goal of *Healthy People 2010* specific to disabled persons is to "promote the health of people with disabilities, prevent secondary conditions, and eliminate disparities between people with and without disabilities in the U.S. population" (USDHHS, 2000, p. 6-8). Thirteen individual objectives have been selected to measure progress toward this goal (Table 26.2). The most significant changes in the *Healthy People 2010* objectives specific to disabled persons are the emphasis on healthy life-years and improved quality of life, similar to the recommendations by the WHO (2002). Although the issues of function stressed in the ICF (WHO, 2001) were not as explicit in *Healthy People 2010*, the 13 objectives indicate a growing emphasis on a holistic approach that recognizes that life satisfaction is just as important to health and well-being as preventive services. It also indicates a growing realization that healthy life-years for persons with disabilities equate to decreased health costs at local, state, and national levels, just as they do for persons without disabilities.

Building on the Healthy People initiative, in 2005, then current Surgeon General Richard Carmona released a *Call to Action to Improve the Health and Wellness of Persons with Disabilities* (USDHHS, 2005b). This document cited ongoing challenges faced by persons with disabilities and their families. Four major goals were proposed:

◆ People nationwide understand that persons with disabilities can lead long, healthy, productive lives.
◆ Health care providers have the knowledge and tools to screen, diagnose, and treat the whole person with a disability with dignity.
◆ Persons with disabilities can promote their own good health by developing and maintaining healthy lifestyles.
◆ Accessible health care and support services promote independence for persons with disabilities (p. 2).

The Surgeon General's attention to the need to "promote accessible, comprehensive health care that enables persons with disabilities to have a full life in the community with integration of services . . . ." (p. v) is in alignment with *Healthy People 2010* goals in this area. The emphasis placed on personal responsibility for maintaining a healthy lifestyle

---

TABLE 26.2 Healthy People 2010: Disability and Secondary Conditions— Objectives

- Include in the core of all relevant Healthy People 2010 surveillance instruments a standardized set of questions that identify "people with disabilities"
- Reduce the proportion of children and adolescents with disabilities who are reported to be sad, unhappy, or depressed
- Reduce the proportion of audults with disabilities who report feelings such as sadness, unhappiness, or depression that prevent them from being active
- Increase the proportion of adults with disabilities who participate in social activities
- Increase the proportion of adults with disabilities reporting sufficient emotional support
- Increase the proportion of adults with disabilities reporting satisfaction with life
- Reduce the number of people with disabilities in congregate care facilities, consistent with permanency planning principles
- Eliminate disparities in employment rates between working-age adults with and without disabilities
- Increase the proportion of children and youth with disabilities who spend at least 80% of their time in regular education programs
- Increase the proportion of health and wellness and treatment programs and facilities that provide full access for people with disabilities
- Reduce the proportion of people with disabilities who report not having the assistive devices and technology needed
- Reduce the proportion of people with disabilities reporting barriers to participation in home, school, work or community activities
- Increase the number of Tribes, States, and the District of Columbia that have public health surveillance and health promotion programs for people with disabilities and caregivers

From U.S. Department of Health and Human Services. (2000). *Healthy people 2010: Understanding and improving health.* Washington, DC: U.S. Government Printing Office.

---

is unique to this document; this approach is increasingly emphasized in health promotion education and will very likely be an important feature in efforts to reduce health care costs.

The development of *Healthy People 2020: The Road Ahead* is due for release in January 2010. This document will include the vision, mission, goals, focus areas, and objectives for the next decade. Utilizing an extensive review of current and evolving research and national surveys, as well as public and professional input, the document will provide a blueprint for the nation's health into the first quarter of the 21st century. This document will likely include insight gained from the earlier *Healthy People 2010* effort and the *Midcourse Review* released in 2005. One emerging issue noted in the *Midcourse Review* was the recognition of "insufficient inclusion of persons with disabilities in disaster management processes, training for first responders, county-level data to locate and evacuate persons with disabilities, and resources to meet disability needs during a disaster" (USDHHS, 2005a, p. 6-7). Of additional concern was the finding that two objectives moved away from their 2010 targets. A 7% increase occurred in the proportion of adults who expressed that negative feelings were impacting their lives; 32% in 2003 versus the 28% level reported in 1997. With respect to employment, the proportion of adults with disabilities who were employed dropped to between 1997 and 2003. As with the recession of 2001, the disproportionate impact of the economic instability of 2008 on persons with disabilities will likely reflect decreased progression toward the employment goals set for 2010. Although the national health priorities are not yet established, clearly, issues of depression, employment parity, and disaster preparedness will need to be addressed. In addition, as noted in the 2005 Surgeon General's *Call to Action*, personal responsibility for lifestyle choices will very likely have increasing emphasis.

CIVIL RIGHTS LEGISLATION

Policies such as *Healthy People 2010* are important features of an overall plan to address the health of people with disabilities and chronic diseases in the United States. Although it has a great deal of influence on the direction and type of programs initiated, policy alone cannot assure individuals with disabilities that the needed services and accommodations are or will be available. As has often been the case, an

act of legislation is vital to ensure that every individual's rights are protected and that legal recourse is available if such protection is denied. But, as is true for other issues of equality, legislation is only the first of many steps that must be taken. The struggle for civil rights for disabled persons in this country is still in its infancy, although it has begun to gain the level of attention that racial and gender equality receive.

The **Americans with Disabilities Act** (ADA) was signed into law in 1990 to protect the civil liberties of the many Americans living with disabilities. This legislation was the result of a long and difficult struggle. Individuals with disabilities and their advocates made their voices heard by repeatedly demanding an end to inferior treatment and lack of equal protection under the law, which impeded their daily lives. The ADA set the standard for a number of subsequent laws that, together with pre-ADA legislation, offer a broad spectrum of protections for disabled persons. These additional laws are listed in Table 26.3 and cover a variety of issues, including telecommunications, architectural barriers, and voter registration.

The ADA essentially "prohibits discrimination on the basis of disability in employment, state and local government, public accommodations, commercial facilities, transportation, and telecommunications [and] also applies to the United States Congress" (United States Department of Justice [USDOJ], 2005, p. 3). For an individual to be protected under the ADA, she must have a disability or some type of relationship or association with an individual who has a disability. The definition of a disabled person used in the application of the ADA is "a person who has a physical or

TABLE 26.3 Disability Rights Laws

Law	Summary	Contact
Telecommunications Act of 1996	Equipment and services are accessible	Federal Communications Commission (FCC)
Fair Housing Act (amended 1988)	Prohibits housing discrimination	U.S. Department of Housing and Urban Development (HUD)
Air Carrier Access Act	Prohibits discrimination in air transportation by domestic and foreign carriers	U.S. Department of Transportation
Voting Accessibility for the Elderly and Handicapped Act of 1984	Requires polling places to be physically accessible fo federal elections	U.S. Department of Justice—Civil Rights Division
National Voter Registration Act of 1993	"Motor Voter Act"—makes it easier to vote by increasing low registration rates by minorities and persons with disabilities	U.S. Department of Justice—Civil Rights Division
Individuals with Disabilities Education Act	Make available free public education in the least restrictive environment for all children with disabilities	U.S. Department of Education—Office of Special Education Programs
Rehabilitation Act	Prohibits discrimination in all federal programs or programs receiving federal financial assistance	Agency's Equal Employment Opportunity Office U.S. Department of Labor—Office of Federal Contract Compliance Programs U.S. Department of Justice
Architectural Barriers Act	Buildings constructed or altered with federal funds must meet federal accessibility standards	U.S. Architectural and Transportation Barriers Compliance Board

From the U.S. Department of Justice. (2005). *A guide to disability rights law*. Retrieved August 18, 2008 from: http://www.ada.gov./cguide.htm.

mental impairment that substantially limits one or more major life activities, a person who has a history or record of such an impairment, or a person who is perceived by others as having such an impairment" (USDOJ, 2005, p. 2). A listing of the specific impairments covered under the law is notably absent, leaving open a broad range of interpretations and legal challenges with respect to who is actually covered.

Although there is ongoing debate as to who is actually protected by the ADA, an equal amount of confusion exists as to who is actually required to comply with the provisions of the act and what specific actions are necessary. The following is a short summary of the ADA. All employers, including religious organizations with 15 or more employees, are subject to the act, as are all activities of state and local governments irrespective of size. Before 1994, the act applied only to employers with 25 or more employees. Public transportation, businesses that provide public accommodation, and telecommunications entities are all required to provide access for individuals with disabilities. It is important to note that the ADA does not override federal and state health and safety laws. However, successful legal challenges to those statutes have been made when they were clearly outdated or when it could be argued that the public safety was not actually at risk in a specific situation. Considerable gray areas exist within the ADA, leaving open the prospect of challenges by those who are subject to the law and those who are protected by it.

Individuals who believe that their legal rights under the ADA have been violated may seek remedy by filing a lawsuit or submitting a complaint to one of four federal offices, depending on the specific type of alleged violation: (1) the U.S. Department of Justice–Civil Rights Division, (2) any U.S. Equal Employment Opportunity Commission field office, (3) the Office of Civil Rights-Federal Transit Administration, or (4) the Federal Communications Commission. The process for filing a complaint is not a simple task, and many seek the assistance of attorneys, legal aid societies, or various private organizations, some of which are discussed later in this chapter (see Display 26.2).

DISPLAY 26.2	OFFICE OF CIVIL RIGHTS: COMPLIANCE WITH ADA

The responsibility of the U.S. Department of Justice, Office of Civil Rights (OCR), is to investigate complaints of alleged violations of the Americans with Disabilities Act (ADA). An example of one of those complaints involved a 22-year-old Connecticut woman with cerebral palsy. She had been placed in a nursing home because of changes in her living situation and health care status and wanted to move back into the community. The OCR intervened to ensure that the woman secured appropriate housing and that counseling and intensive case management services were in place when she moved back into the community. Without the protection afforded under the ADA, the outcome could have been much different.

Source: USDHHS (2006, September). *Delivering on the promise: OCR's compliance activities promote community integration.* Retrieved May 19, 2008 from Office for Civil Rights via: http://www.hhs.gov/ocr/complianceactiv.html.

In a report on the enforcement history of the ADA between its inception and 1999, the National Council on Disability (NCD) noted that many of the federal agencies charged with protecting the civil rights of disabled persons suffered from insufficient funding and lack of a coherent and unifying national strategy (NCD, 2000). The NCD recommendations included clarification of specific elements that provide a basis for evaluating agency performance and thereby serve to improve the full expression of the law as it was intended. These 11 elements or criteria are (1) proactive and reactive strategies, (2) communication with consumers and complainants, (3) policy and subregulatory guidance, (4) enforcement actions, (5) strategic litigation, (6) timely resolution of complaints, (7) competent and credible investigative processes, (8) technical assistance for protected persons and covered entities, (9) adequate agency resources, (10) interagency collaboration and coordination, and (11) outreach and consultation with the community. In a follow-up report in 2005, the NCD's ADA Impact Study, progress was noted in the following areas:

♦ Telephone relay services are being used at high levels, and changes in technology are making usage higher.
♦ Public transit systems in the United States have made dramatic progress in becoming more accessible, especially to wheelchair users.
♦ The percentage of Americans with disabilities voting in 2004 increased dramatically.
♦ The education gap between people with disabilities and people without disabilities is shrinking, and people with disabilities are attending postsecondary institutions in record numbers.
♦ People with disabilities are experiencing less discrimination in employment (NCD, 2005, p. 3).

It is important to those with disabilities and the professionals who serve them that a structure be in place to provide protection under the law, but this does not prevent discrimination, nor does the existence of such a structure suggest that immediate remedies will be available. Laws aside, the most difficult aspect of change comes when attempts are made to alter the perceptions and misunderstandings of others about people with disabilities. The perspective of one community member offers one such example (see Perspectives: Voices from the Community).

ORGANIZATIONS SERVING THE NEEDS OF THE DISABLED AND CHRONICALLY ILL

Although the impact of civil rights legislation cannot be underestimated, it did not come about without demands for change from the chorus of voices from all those who deal on a daily basis with the issue of disability (the individuals themselves, their families, coworkers, employers, and advocates). Without the hard work of those individuals and groups, it is unlikely that the efforts envisioned and accomplished by legislation would have occurred. Much of the credit for the legislative focus belongs to advocacy groups. The following section provides an overview of some of the groups that advocate for the disabled and chronically ill and their families. In serving those specific populations, they offer others an opportunity to learn more about the lives and struggles of disabled persons. Each of the organizations

PERSPECTIVES
VOICES FROM THE COMMUNITY

I was always such an active and healthy person, so when I was diagnosed with multiple sclerosis it hit me like a ton of bricks. Here I was with two small children and I was only 30 years old; it just wasn't fair. Some days are good and some days are just awful. I finally broke down and applied for one of those disabled parking stickers. The doctor had to approve it, and he said it was a good thing to help me save my energy for the important things, like taking care of my family. I hated to use it, but I was just getting so tired. What is so awful are the looks on people's faces when I park in the special areas near the door. I know I don't look like I'm sick. I just hate those looks—I can hear them saying under their breath, "She can't be sick . . . I'll bet that sticker is for a family member and she's just abusing it—how lazy!" If I wasn't so tired I'd park in the regular parking places.

Pat N., Tampa, Florida

listed offers a wide range of information, some of which can be accessed via the Internet. For community health nurses, these organizations provide a starting point for exploring specific topics pertinent to practice. They also can be a source of valuable information for clients and families to access on their own. Families who cannot afford Internet service or computers can use them at public libraries, most of which now offer this service. Many Internet sites are not reliable or accurate, so it is important for the nurse to prescreen any specific sites that are recommended to clients and their families.

Government

The NCD is an independent federal agency tasked with making recommendations to the President and to Congress about issues that face Americans with disabilities. The NCD has 15 Presidential appointees (all confirmed by the U.S. Senate) whose charge is to promote "policies, programs, practices, and procedures that guarantee equal opportunity for all individuals with disabilities, regardless of the nature or severity of the disability, and to empower individuals with disabilities to achieve economic self-sufficiency, independent living, and inclusion and integration into all aspects of society" (NCD, 2008b). In its 1986 report, *Toward Independence,* the NCD proposed that Congress should enact a civil rights law for people with disabilities; the result was the 1990 ADA.

Private

Many private organizations—local, national, and international—deal with a variety of disabilities and chronic diseases. Many of the better-known organizations such as the American Heart Association and the American Cancer Association are discussed in other chapters of this book and therefore are not covered here. Instead, examples of groups that deal most directly with disability and chronic illness are described. The reader is encouraged to search the Internet or

print resources for additional entities that deal with specific disabilities or chronic illnesses.

The National Association of the Deaf (NAD), headquartered in Washington, D.C., is a private, nonprofit organization that was established in 1880. As the oldest U.S. organization serving this population, it has the stated mission to "preserve, protect and promote the civil, human and linguistic rights of all deaf Americans" (National Association of the Deaf [NAD], 2008b, p. 1). Specific programs and activities that NAD is involved with include advocacy, captioned media, certification of **American Sign Language** (ASL) professionals and interpreters, legal assistance, and policy development and research (NAD, 2008a). ASL uses "handshapes" to communicate ideas and concepts; it is used primarily in America and Canada by the deaf community (Grayson, 2003). Display 26.3 offers a brief summary of sign languages.

The National Organization on Disability (NOD), headquartered in Washington, D.C., has as its mission statement "to expand the participation and contribution of America's 54 million men, women, and children with disabilities in all aspects of life" (National Organization on Disability [NOD], 2008, p. 1). An important contribution of NOD is the *2004 NOD/Harris Survey of Americans with Disabilities,* which sought to quantify the gaps between people with and without disabilities in terms of employment, income, education, health care, access to transportation, entertainment or going out, socializing, attending religious services, political participation/voter registration, life satisfaction, and trends (NOD, 2004). This was the fifth national survey sponsored by NOD since it was first initiated in 1986. Although improvements in all indicators have been demonstrated over this 18-year period, progress is described as both slow and modest in the final report. People with disabilities are more likely than nondisabled persons to have low incomes, are

---

DISPLAY 26.3　SIGN LANGUAGES IN BRIEF

- Sign languages are not universal
- Sign language is the use of "handshapes" and gestures to communicate ideas or concepts
- American Sign Language is a unique language with its own rules of grammar and syntax
- American Sign Language is primarily used in America and Canada and is the natural language of the deaf community
- International Sign Language (Gestuno) is composed of vocabulary signs from various sign languages for use at international events or meetings to aid communication
- Systems of Manually Coded English (i.e., Signed English, Signing Exact English) are not natural languages but systems designed to represent the translation of spoken language word for word

From Grayson G. (2003). *Talking with your hands, listening with your eyes. A complete photographic guide to American Sign Language.* Garden City Park, NY: Square One Publishers.

twice as likely to drop out of high school, are more likely to go without needed health care, and they report considerably lower satisfaction with life than persons without disabilities. The NOD Web site connects visitors to a rich variety of sources on community involvement, economic/employment topics, and access issues (*http://www.nod.org*).

The American Council of the Blind (ACB) was founded in 1961 and states as its purpose, "to improve the well-being of all blind and visually impaired people" (American Council of the Blind [ACB], 2008, p. 1). Services advertised by the organization include information and referral, scholarship assistance, public education, and industry consultation, as well as governmental monitoring, consultation, and advocacy. Some of the major issues currently being pursued by the organization include improved education and rehabilitation for the blind and increased production and use of reading materials for the blind and visually impaired.

Guide Dogs for the Blind is a nonprofit charitable organization established to train and make available guide dogs for the visually impaired (Guide Dogs for the Blind, 2008). The dogs and services are free, and the organization relies on donations. It currently has two training sites, one in California and one in Oregon, with puppy raisers located throughout the Western states. The organization can be reached through its Web site at *http://www.guidedogs.com*.

Another organization dealing with issues affecting the blind and visually impaired is the National Federation of the Blind (NFB). Founded in 1940, it seeks to help "blind persons achieve self-confidence and self-respect and to act as a vehicle for collective self-expression by the blind" (National Federation of the Blind [NFB], 2008, p. 1). Citing the need for assistance to the more than 1.1 million people in the United States who are blind, the organization fulfills its mission by providing public education, information and referral, and support for increased availability of materials in **Braille** (Display 26.4).

The oldest organization devoted to eliminating barriers for the blind and visually impaired is the American Foundation for the Blind (AFB), which was founded in 1921. The AFB advocates for the visually impaired through increased funding at the federal and state levels in areas such as rehabilitation research for older, visually impaired persons; improved literacy for the visually impaired, including use of Braille and

assistive technology; improved employment opportunities; and increased accessibility of technology. In addition, AFB houses the Helen Keller Archives, which contain her correspondence, photographs, and various personal items and documents (American Foundation for the Blind [AFB], 2008).

The Obesity Society has as its mission to promote "research, education and advocacy to better understand, prevent, and treat obesity and improve the lives of those affected" (Obesity Society, 2008). The organization addresses such issues as the need for attention to the impact of obesity on death and disability and for increased research, improved insurance coverage, and elimination of discrimination and mistreatment of people with obesity. The organization's Web site (*http://www.obesity.org*) offers informational literature covering topics that range from the global problem of obesity to treatment of obesity-related disability.

With growing awareness that, in many cases, human immunodeficiency virus (HIV)/acquired immune deficiency syndrome (AIDS) is a chronic condition, the long-term needs of those impacted by this disease are gaining attention. Hundreds of websites and organizations are available to provide information, assistance, and support. One website, *The Body: The Complete HIV/AIDS Resource* (2008) offers state-by-state links to a variety of resources. The site also includes resources in Canada and specific sites for American Indians and Alaskan Natives. The website can be accessed at *http://www.thebody.com/index/hotlines/other.html*.

Begun in the aftermath of World War I, the Disabled American Veterans organization has provided free services to military veterans seeking to obtain benefits for service-related injuries (Disabled American Veterans, 2008). The organization is not a government agency and receives no federal funds, instead providing services through membership dues and public contributions. The mission of the organization is to help disabled veterans build better lives for themselves and their families. With the growing number of military injuries resulting from the Iraq and Afghanistan conflicts, the organization finds its service delivery even more stretched. The volunteers provide transportation to Veterans Administration (VA) medical facilities and provide ongoing service at VA hospitals, clinics, and nursing homes. The organization's website can be accessed at *http://www.dav.org/*.

HEALTH PROMOTION AND PREVENTION NEEDS OF THE DISABLED AND CHRONICALLY ILL

Misconceptions Impede Improvement

Earlier, the influence of *Healthy People 2010* as it relates to people with disabilities was discussed. One of the most influential aspects of the document is its emphasis on a change in thinking within the health care community about the health promotion needs of people with disabilities. This shift is needed because the lack of health promotion and disease prevention activities for this population leads to an increase in the number and extent of **secondary conditions**, defined as "medical, social, emotional, mental, family, or community problems that a person with a disabling condition likely experiences" (USDHHS, 2000, p. 6-25). Approaching the health needs of disabled persons from the traditional standpoint of asking what medical, rehabilitative, or long-term care is needed has failed to reduce illness or improve the

---

DISPLAY 26.4	**WHAT IS BRAILLE?**

Braille takes its name from Louis Braille, an 18-year-old blind Frenchman who created a system of raised dots for reading and writing by modifying a system used on board sailing ships for night reading. Persons experienced in Braille can read at speeds of 200 to 400 words per minute, comparable to print readers. Braille consists of arrangements of dots to form symbols. The text can be written either by hand with a slate and stylus, with a Braille writing machine, or with the use of specialized computer software and a Braille embossing device attached to the printer.

Source: National Federation of the Blind. (2003). *What is Braille and what does it mean to the blind?* Retrieved May 19, 2008, from http://www.nfb.org/images/nfb/Publications/fr/fr15/Issue1/f150113.html.

overall well-being of the disabled or chronically ill. More-over, a number of misconceptions have resulted that impede progress in this area: (a) that all people with disabilities have poor health, (b) that public health activities need to focus only on preventing disability, (c) that there is no need for a clear definition of "disability" or "people with disabilities" in public health practice, and (d) that environment does not play a significant role in the disability process. Increased national attention to the needs of the disabled (those needs specific to disabled persons as well as needs that are universal to all) should greatly improve the outlook. This change of focus is clearly evident in the definition of **health promotion** used in *Healthy People 2010:* "efforts to create healthy lifestyles and a healthy environment to prevent medical and other second-ary conditions, such as teaching people how to address their health care needs and increasing opportunities to participate in usual life activities" (USDHHS, 2000, p. 6-25).

Missed Opportunities by Health Care Providers or Missed Opportunities to Affect Quality of Life

In this age of rapid growth in technology, it is easy to forget that clean water is a far more important commodity than hav-ing the latest prescription drug or surgical procedure. All of us, whether healthy, disabled, or chronically ill, require some

basic elements to maintain health. Those elements are the same all over the world and include clean air and water, a safe place to live, sunshine, exercise, nutritious food, socializa-tion, and the opportunity to be successful in life's pursuits. As self-evident as these health promoting elements may seem, for the millions of persons who deal with disability, chronic disease, or both, such basic needs seem too often to take sec-ond place to other issues. It is equally problematic that pre-ventive measures, most notably at the primary and secondary levels, are often nonexistent or lacking (see Evidence-Based Practice).

The issue of missed opportunities in health promotion and prevention is depicted in Figure 26.2. The focus of the health care delivery system is increasingly skewed toward secondary and tertiary prevention efforts, and limited emphasis is placed on the health promotion and primary pre-vention needs of the population. Although this is a concern for all persons, it is of particular importance for persons with disabilities and chronic illnesses, because they are more likely to have these needs ignored altogether. As Figure 26.2 shows, an entire area of issues may be addressed with a basically healthy person but not with a disabled or chronically ill individual. Some areas of secondary and ter-tiary prevention unique to persons with disabilities or chronic illnesses may be completely ignored. This nonre-ceipt of health promoting or preventive education or actions

EVIDENCE-BASED PRACTICE

Influenza Vaccine for Vulnerable Children

Influenza vaccination coverage was examined in an Italian study of children with chronic illnesses. The 274 children identified in the study were all at high risk of influenza complications as a result of their illness. The study sam-ple was obtained from the over 5,000 children (younger than 14 years of age) who presented at an emergency room in the first 4 months of 2003. High risk included conditions such as asthma, chronic pulmonary disease, hemodynamically significant cardiac disease, chronic metabolic disease, sickle cell anemia, and HIV infection. The study involved a parental questionnaire regarding medical history, influenza vaccination status for the past 3 years, and parental perceptions of the need for vaccina-tion. In addition, each of the children's pediatrician was contacted by phone to complete a separate survey regard-ing their opinions on the need for influenza vaccination in high risk children. The researchers found that children with asthma or cardiac disease showed the lowest rates of vaccination. Of particular interest was the finding that the "parents and primary care pediatricians had only a mar-ginal knowledge of influenza and the benefits of preven-tion" (p. 5253). The findings of this study support the need for improved vaccination rates for high risk children against influenza. Further, the lack of awareness by the pediatricians points to the need for increased professional educational efforts. Parents rely on their child's pediatri-cian for guidance on health promoting interventions such

as immunization, and that guidance should be clear, accu-rate, and up-to-date.

Nursing Implications
As this study emphasizes, children who are most at risk for severe sequel or even death from influenza may not be ade-quately immunized. The study findings are consistent with the results of the 2005 National Health Interview Survey showing that children with current asthma had a vaccina-tion rate of only 29%. Although this rate was higher than the reported rate for children without current asthma, it underscores the need to reduce barriers to vaccination in these children. One such method that can be utilized by the community health nurse is to vigorously promote the need for influenza vaccination with all parents, and especially with parents of children with chronic health conditions.

References:
Brim, S.N., Rudd, R.A., Funk, R.H., Callahan, D.B., & Euler, G.L. (2007). Influenza vaccination coverage among children with asthma—United States, 2004–05 influenza season. *Morbidity and Mortality Weekly Report, 56*(09), 193–196.
Esposito, S., Marchisio, P., Droghetti, R., Lambertini, L., Faelli, N., Bosis, S., et al. (2006). Influenza vaccination coverage among children with high-risk medical conditions. *Vaccine, 24,* 5251–5255.

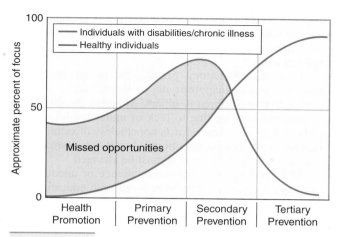

FIGURE 26.2   Difference in client focus between individuals with and without a chronic illness or disability.

vital to the health and well-being of those with disabilities or chronic illnesses is of grave concern. For example, issues such as sexuality are often not explored with the disabled or chronically ill. This skewed view of the lifestyles, behaviors, and needs of the disabled as "different" from those of the "able-bodied" is a clear example of lack of understanding by health professionals and the public alike.

It is likely that disability or chronic illness serves as the initial reason for an individual's encounter with the health care community, including the community health nurse. As a result, the disability or illness often drives the selection of prevention efforts, to the possible exclusion of other, equally important health issues. For example, for an individual with a primary diagnosis of type 2 diabetes, secondary prevention efforts often center on that disease (e.g., screening for diabetic retinopathy). The need to refer the client for a Pap test or a baseline mammogram may be overlooked. Likewise, the treatment plan may include a consultation with a dietitian but fail to address the basic needs for leisure-time activities, regular physical activity, a varied and interesting diet, fresh air and sunshine, and socialization—all of which may help prevent the development of depression, a common result of chronic illness. Display 26.5 offers several examples of missed opportunities in the areas of primary and secondary prevention. It is of particular concern to the practice of community health nursing that the broad range of health promotion and prevention needs of all clients be addressed.

A study by Wei, Findley, and Sambamoorthi (2006) demonstrated the risk for missed opportunities for clinical preventive services among women. Of the 3,183 individuals

---

DISPLAY 26.5   MISSED OPPORTUNITIES

Example 1
A 60-year-old woman, blind since birth, self-sufficient and active all of her life, has developed severe arthritis. She encounters a health care system that far too often focuses on her "disabilities" and not her "abilities." The focus is placed squarely on her tertiary health promotion needs, often at the expense of health-promoting or lifestyle-enhancing needs. The result is a failure to recognize that the "disability" of arthritis is likely no less and no more an issue for her than for a sighted person. She receives the same medication therapy as a sighted person but may not be offered a physical therapy program due to her disability. Her need for physical therapy is no less important, but locating an appropriate, safe, and easily accessible program requires some additional work on the part of her provider. At issue is that options potentially discussed with a sighted person are more apt to be omitted completely, which may negatively affect the client's overall health and well-being.

Example 2
A 20-year-old man with learning disabilities, who is employed at a local factory, receives a regularly scheduled physical examination with a new provider. He lives in a **congregate care facility**, which is an out-of-home facility that provides housing for people with disabilities in which rotating staff members provide care for 16 or more adults or any number of children/youth younger than 21 years of age. It excludes foster care, adoptive homes, residential schools, correctional facilities, and nursing facilities (USDHHS, 2000). The major finding of the examination is that he is due for a tetanus booster and should also begin the series for hep-

atitis A, because he lives in a high-risk area of the western United States. He takes the referral slip and leaves the office. One year later, at his regularly scheduled visit, it becomes clear that he never received his immunizations. Apparently, he didn't know what he was supposed to do with the paper, because he has difficulty reading, and he had no idea where to go to get his "shots." The primary prevention elements were provided, but clearly not in a manner appropriate for this individual. With additional explanation and follow-up, perhaps the outcome would have been quite different.

Example 3
A 34-year-old woman who has been severely obese since the birth of her last child (4 years ago) has not had a gynecologic examination since that birth. She is aware of the need to have regular examinations, yet she cannot bring herself to make an appointment. The reason is that she knows she will have to be weighed, and this terrifies her, especially because it is done in an open area where others can see. She finally gets the courage to call for an appointment and tells the clerk that she does not want to be weighed. The clerk's response is less than helpful and she is essentially told that it is "policy." She makes the appointment but does not keep it. This situation could have been handled in a compassionate manner, recognizing the painful experience that weighing is for many individuals and suggesting alternatives, one of which could have been simply to bypass the scales until after the interview and examination. At that point, the woman may have been more amenable to the measurement and a more discreet area could have been offered. In this case, the opportunities to provide primary, secondary, and tertiary prevention were lost.

sampled in this study, 23% were disabled. When compared to the other study participants, the disabled women were less likely to receive cancer screening (mammograms and Pap smears) within the recommended intervals. Interestingly, this group was more likely to receive influenza vaccination, cholesterol screening, and colorectal screenings as recommended. The researchers found that, overall, having a usual source of care and health insurance were predictive of preventive service receipt. They stressed the need for improving women's health care by identifying those who are most at risk and targeting efforts to reduce disparities.

Health Care Disparities and Discrimination

It is a growing concern to those who are disabled, and to their families and advocates, that the type and quality of the health-related services, referrals, and care that they receive may not be appropriate to their circumstances. This results in increased illness and disability and potentially decreased quality or length of life. One pointed example of this disparity involved a national sample of low-income female Medicaid recipients. Women with disabilities in this sample had lower rates of receipt of medical services, and were much less likely to receive cervical cancer screenings (Parish & Ellison-Martin, 2007). Although the women each had similar access to health care services, the disparities were of concern. Not surprisingly, those women with disabilities were less likely to report satisfaction with their care.

The issue of health care access was one of a number of elements explored in a study involving 932 independently living Massachusetts adults with a major disability (Wilber et al., 2002). The purpose of the study was to determine whether factors such as having a consistent primary care provider, access to health promotion or disease prevention programs, and accessible transportation were related to the number and severity of secondary conditions experienced. The findings suggested that the more independent the individual and the fewer obstacles faced, the fewer secondary conditions were reported. The study used the definition of secondary conditions in *Healthy People 2010*; the most notable findings were the high prevalence rates of fatigue, depression, spasms, and chronic pain.

Additional disparities may exist in services received by those with chronic illness and disabilities. Racial and ethnic differences in immunization rates were found in a study analyzing data from the National Health Interview Survey of almost 2,000 individuals with diabetes (Egede & Zheng, 2003). Even after controlling for access, health care coverage, and socioeconomic status, the rates of influenza and pneumococcal immunization were lower for certain racial/ethnic groups, primarily Blacks. What is not known from these results is whether the depressed immunization rates resulted from client acceptance issues, from differential provider recommendations, or from some combination of these factors.

A qualitative in-depth survey by Becker and Newsom (2003) that examined the issue of disparities found that economic status also appeared to affect dissatisfaction with health care among chronically ill African Americans. In this study, low-income individuals were less satisfied with both the quality and the quantity of their care than were middle-income respondents. The potential impact of low satisfaction for selected groups is of real concern in addressing the ongoing needs of those individuals. Although neither study was confirmatory, it is nevertheless an issue that needs to be explored further.

It is discriminatory practice when an individual receives unequal, inappropriate, or limited services compared with those offered to others. Although the difference in treatment is often due to lack of understanding of the needs of disabled persons, it is nonetheless discriminatory. Such bias may not be intentional, but it can dramatically affect the health of clients and must be changed.

The good news is that the incidence of unequal and inappropriate practices can be reduced with education and training of health care providers, agency staff, and insurance carriers. A crucial aspect of community health practice is to ensure that those individuals with disabilities or chronic illnesses are afforded the best possible care, treatment options, and opportunities to improve their health—the same options as are provided for nondisabled persons and those who do not suffer from chronic illness.

Health promotion and primary, secondary, and tertiary prevention activities are essential aspects of quality care for all persons. Those with disabilities require specialized attention to needs resulting from or related to their disabilities, yet they also require the same attention to health and well-being as the rest of the population. Community health nurses are in a prime position to advocate needed changes for those with disabilities and chronic illnesses. Such changes can include increased attention to health promotion and disease prevention needs, accessible and appropriate delivery of those services, and specialized treatment plans that incorporate the latest knowledge of a specific illness or disability (see Perspectives: Student Voices).

FAMILIES WITH A DISABLED OR CHRONICALLY ILL MEMBER

The Family's Role in Advocacy

Families that have a member with a chronic illness or disability face many challenges. They are required to navigate a health care system that they know little about and with which they often feel at odds. They serve as advocates for their member in need (whether child, spouse, or parent) and often feel tired and frustrated from their efforts, especially if they have been less than successful in meeting their goals. Many are forced to ask for or demand assistance from health care agencies, social services, or transportation sources to achieve the level of care needed by the family member. Many are required to open their home to others (e.g., community health nurses, social workers) to access the services. Families may have little understanding of what services they are entitled to because of language barriers, difficult agency policies, or disjointed service delivery.

The community health nurse is usually not the first health care professional that the family encounters. They may already have been through a lengthy struggle to receive assistance. In these circumstances, the nurse often is confronted by a frustrated family that distrusts yet another "professional." The nurse must gain the trust and confidence of the family by practicing consistency, following through with promised actions, and always being truthful.

PERSPECTIVES
STUDENT VOICES

For as long as I can remember, I have wanted to work with children. When I was finally accepted into the nursing program, I was so disappointed when I learned that we would only have 7 weeks in our pediatric rotation. Then, I found out about an opportunity to work with children at a school in my community health practicum—marvelous I thought. I just knew I'd be giving immunizations, physical assessments, and performing hearing checks. Then I found out that I would actually be working with school-aged children with disabilities and their parents in a special after-school health promotion program. The nurse I was assigned to asked me to come in before the program started, so that she could fill me in on the program and my role. It actually sounded great, and I was confident that I could handle this. Then she asked me something that made me worried; she asked if I had ever worked with a child who used a wheelchair, or had a continuous insulin pump, or had seizures. I told her that I had some experience in the hospital, and that I was sure that I would be prepared for any health care issues that might occur. "You misunderstand," she said, "that's not what I meant. Have you ever gotten to know a child with a disability?" I really hadn't, and it suddenly made me a bit worried. She explained to me that many people don't treat children with disabilities just like any other child. They also don't always know how to talk to the parents about their child. She suggested that one way to give me a bit of information was to go home and do some reading and look at some websites she recommended. One in particular, the National Organization on Disability (http://www.nod.org/), had a great feature called "Disability Etiquette Tips" that I have already found to be a big help with the kids and their parents. She also directed me to the Easter Seals Disability Services (http://www.easter-seals.com), which has a great deal of information on programs that are currently available for children and adults. I even learned that this organization used to be called the National Society for Crippled Children . . . I'm sure glad they changed the name.

Eileen S.

Not all problems that the family faces can be remedied, and even for problems that do have solutions, time and effort may be needed to obtain the desired result.

The Impact on Families

A literature review of the needs of parents with chronically ill children reported a number of common themes in the studies surveyed, among them the need for normalcy and certainty, the need for information, and the need for partnership (Fisher, 2001). Although these needs were associated with the presence of a chronically ill child in the family, the same needs are likely to occur in other families. These are certainly areas that can be addressed by the community health nurse in a practical way.

Wong and Heriot (2007), found somewhat similar results in their study of 35 parents of children with cystic fibrosis (CF). The parents who sought support from family and friends experienced less emotional distress than those who didn't, analogous to the need for partnership noted by Fisher (2001). Additional findings revealed that parents who used self-blame as a coping strategy were also more likely to report experiencing depression and were more likely to report lower levels of mental health in their children. Suggestions to assist the family include parental counseling to reduce self-blame, encouraging the children's important life goals, and providing information on available supportive social networks. With the current median life expectancy of patients with CF well above 30 years, the issue of long-term family support is vital.

One major obstacle for families with a disabled or chronically ill member may be obtaining needed **assistive devices and technology**. These are defined in *Healthy People 2010* as "any item, piece of equipment, or product system, whether acquired commercially, modified, or customized, that is used to increase, maintain, or improve the functional capabilities of individuals with disabilities" (USDHHS, 2000, p. 6-25). With constant changes in available equipment, financing, and technology, it is little wonder that families struggle to find the best alternatives. Just because the technology exists does not mean that it can be obtained. Often, the insurance carrier, whether private or governmental, sets limits on which products can be obtained or which brands are acceptable. The overriding issue of financing is no small hurdle. It is often left up to the family to learn about options and legal rights through a process of trial and error. Intervention by the community health nurse can greatly reduce the burden on the family. With so many product lines available on the Internet, the nurse can assist families in this area, especially those without access to or understanding of computer technology. It is equally helpful for the nurse to intervene with insurance providers if coverage of equipment is not easily obtained or to find sources of funding for the equipment from private agencies if possible. Referring families to community groups or organizations that provide specific assistance can be very helpful. Other families that share similar struggles can provide a vital link to needed services and can be contacted through self-help groups or other sources. Here, the community health nurse can provide expertise on available community resources.

Respite care is another area of great importance for families of the disabled and the chronically ill. It can be emotionally draining to meet the daily needs of a member who cannot perform self-care. This often leads to caregiver fatigue and increased stress. It is also important to recognize the effect of the situation on noncaregivers in the family, particularly nondisabled siblings of a disabled child. With focus placed on the needs of one member, children may feel that their own needs are not as important. This can lead to behavioral and health-related problems. Respite care offers some needed relief to the family and allows for uninterrupted attention to the nondisabled children. This service can occur within the home or at an outside facility. Respite care may be provided by a private organization at little or no cost to the family, or it may be quite expensive and require financing by the insurance company or by the family itself. Whatever the

USING THE NURSING PROCESS   WITH VULNERABLE POPULATIONS

Assessment

Anna Lopez is a mother of three children aged 2 to 9 years old. The eldest, Ernesto, was diagnosed with severe Down syndrome at birth. He is confined to a wheelchair, requires total care, and remains at home with his mother and younger siblings, who are not yet in school. Anna's husband works long hours as a computer repairman for a large company. The have health insurance, but it does not cover additional expenses, such as day care for Ernesto. The family has done very well in providing for Ernesto's needs, and they receive periodic visits from you, the community health nurse, to evaluate his condition and check on the feeding tube used for his nourishment. Physically, Ernesto is stable, but you notice that Anna has been increasingly withdrawn at the visits, rarely offering information, but responding to questions appropriately. She seems less engaged with her other children as well, only occasionally smiling at them.

Nursing Diagnoses

1. At risk for depression related to ongoing caregiver demands and lack of respite care
2. At risk for altered health status due to limited focus on self-care needs

Plan/Implementation

Diagnosis 1

The community health nurse will discuss with the client the need for a thorough physical assessment, including an evaluation for depression. The community health nurse will contact the insurance provider to discuss day care/respite options for Ernesto. If unavailable, local community organizations will be contacted for appropriate referrals. In addition, the need for more frequent visits to the family will be discussed with the insurance carrier to address the needs of the mother as caregiver.

Diagnosis 2

The community health nurse will discuss with the client her concerns about her overall physical and mental health and discuss some self-care options that may improve her well-being: improved nutrition, physical activity, leisure time options, and adjustment of family schedule to accommodate more free time for self-care.

Evaluation

The client was at first very reticent to make an appointment for an evaluation, but after thinking it over for a week and discussing it with her husband, she did so. Her husband was relieved that she had suggested the appointment, because he was growing increasingly concerned over her withdrawal but did not know how to bring up the subject. The family physician referred Anna to a psychologist for evaluation of the depression. The insurance carrier agreed to increase home visits on a short-term basis but did not have a respite care option available for Ernesto. Fortunately, a local faith-based community group was able to provide limited assistance to the family. They identified several members who had raised children with similar disabilities and were willing to stay with Ernesto and the other children once a week for 4 hours. This allowed Anna some free time to make appointments with her psychologist, shop, or visit friends. After several months, Anna has begun to smile more and seems much more relaxed at the home visits. The children are all doing fine, and the respite care is expected to continue for at least the next 6 months. The need for ongoing attention to her own self-care needs is emphasized with Anna by the community health nurse.

---

source, some type of respite care is often vital to the family's health and should be a priority in the overall treatment plan of the family (see Using the Nursing Process).

With the enactment of the 1996 welfare reform legislation (the Personal Responsibility and Work Opportunity Reconciliation Act), a number of significant changes were implemented that potentially affect families with a chronically ill child, especially those living in poverty. Changes included the stipulation of a 5-year lifetime limit on receipt of benefits, institution of work requirements, and elimination of entitlement to cash benefits. The impact of these changes is of growing concern within the public health community. Smith, Wise, and Wampler (2002) explored this issue in a study of knowledge of welfare reform among families with a chronically ill child. They found that respondents often had incomplete knowledge of work requirements, even if they were entitled to exemptions because their children received Supplemental Security Income. In those cases, 37% of the respondents were unaware that they qualified for work exemptions, and 70% had not applied for the exemptions. This indicates that eligible families might not be receiving the exemptions to which they are entitled, adding additional and unnecessary burdens to families already at risk.

Another study explored the relationship between welfare status, health insurance status, and the health and medical care received by children with asthma (Wood et al., 2002). The most significant findings were (a) children of parents who had been denied Temporary Assistance for Needy Families (TANF) experienced more severe asthma symptoms and had more acute care visits than children in families that did not access the welfare system, (b) children of recent TANF applicants were more likely to be uninsured or transiently insured than those who had not applied, and (c) recent TANF applicants had the poorest mental health scores. The significance of this study is that it demonstrated the high-risk status of those families with a chronically ill child and the need to provide access to health insurance and health services.

Even for families that are ineligible for public assistance, the issue of employment is generally of great significance. Employment options may be quite limited when a family has a member with special needs. The family may have to remain in a particular location to access needed health and social services, reducing the possibility of increased earning potential at a different location or in another field of employment. The working family members may choose less favorable employment options because the position is convenient or has more flexible hours. For instance, a person may take a part-time position at a local convenience store that does not pay particularly well in preference to a higher-paying, full-time factory position because the store is close to home and allows for frequent adjustments in schedule.

Having a chronically ill family member often means that working individuals must take time off from work. Although some legal protections are provided under the Family and Medical Leave Act of 1993, the Act does not apply in all situations. More importantly, it allows only for time off; it does not mandate payment during those periods. The choice becomes an issue of taking unpaid time off or continuing to work and deal with the needs of the family member as best one can. Some individuals choose to work part-time or not to work at all, so that they can care for family members. At a time when many families have two earners to help meet financial commitments, these families may have to rely on only one income. Limitations in income are particularly difficult when one considers the myriad needs of the disabled and chronically ill, many of which may not be covered by insurance.

Caregiver health needs and mental health status are yet another area of concern for families who must provide for a disabled or chronically ill member. One of the largest longitudinal studies in the United States, the Nurses' Health Study, provided the data for an investigation of the impact of informal caregiving on the mental health status of caregivers (Cannuscio et al., 2002). Using data collected over a 4-year period (1992–1996), the study found that women who provided 36 or more hours per week of care for a disabled spouse were six times more likely than noncaregivers to report depressive or anxious symptoms. The frequency of symptoms was elevated but less dramatic if the women cared for a disabled or ill parent as opposed to a spouse. The findings support the necessity of attention to the needs of caregivers, the majority of whom are women. A follow-up study by Cannuscio and colleagues (2004) found that higher weekly time commitment to informal care was associated with an increased risk of depression, regardless of level of social support. For those with few social ties and high spousal time commitment, the level of depressive symptoms was much higher. Interestingly, employment status didn't appear to have an impact on depressive symptoms of caregivers. Access to social ties was, however, strongly correlated with more positive health outcomes in the caregivers (Cannuscio et al., 2004). Poor health outcomes, both physical and mental, are of growing concern as the population ages and the need for family caregiving rises. Recognizing that caregivers within a family are at increased risk for poor health outcomes, the community health nurse must select appropriate interventions to address the health needs of the other family members.

Families of individuals with a disability or chronic illness are at increased risk for a number of negative consequences. Although families do not all have the same level of risk or disruption, the community health nurse should recognize the potential impact of the dependent member's needs on the entire family. Families may suffer from financial difficulties, poor physical or mental health, and a variety of other challenges. They are often ill prepared to deal with the complicated systems that must be accessed to obtain needed care. The community health nurse is in an optimal position to interpret those systems to the families and to advocate for the needed care, services, and equipment. The nurse must view the family holistically, recognizing additional needs that may develop as a result of the situation they currently face.

Universal Design

"**Universal design** is the design of products and environments to be usable by all people, to the greatest extent possible, without the need for adaptation or specialized design" (Mace, n.d.). The term "Universal Design" has been attributed to Ron Mace, founder of the Center for Universal Design (North Carolina State University). Mace, who had suffered from polio as a child, died suddenly in 1998, leaving behind a long legacy of advocacy on behalf of accessibility in design.

For those who live with a disability or chronic disease, and their family members, the issue of access is of utmost importance. As was noted earlier, the cost to a family to accommodate the needs of a disabled person can be enormous. Consider, that, as the U.S. population ages, more and more of us will have need of accessibility in housing, business, and recreation in order to remain active and healthy as long as possible. Accessibility was taken one step further in the concept of universal design, making tools, houses, and workplaces accessible to all. The cost of building our environments in a way that promotes access for all can be far less than the cost of remodeling those environments after the fact.

The issue of accessibility is not new. The ADA (discussed earlier) addresses issues of access in employment, governmental building, and public accommodations. The Fair Housing Accessibility Guidelines (HUD, 2008) published in 1990 provides for design and construction of multifamily dwellings (four or more units) in accordance with accessibility requirements. The specific provisions include:

◆ Public use and common use portions of the dwellings are readily accessible to and usable by persons with handicaps;
◆ All doors within such dwellings which are designed to allow passage into and within the premises are sufficiently wide to allow passage by persons in wheelchairs; and
◆ All premises within such dwellings contain the following features of adaptive design:
  1. An accessible route into and through the dwelling;
  2. Light switches, electrical outlets, thermostats, and other environmental controls in accessible locations;
  3. Reinforcements in bathroom walls to allow later installation of grab bars; and
  4. Usable kitchens and bathrooms such that an individual in a wheelchair can maneuver about the space.

Universal design incorporates access, but access does not necessarily imply universal design. The design of a community's built environment and its impact on individuals plays a role in the overall health and well-being of those living there. Universal design and access play a key role in this discussion, but the importance of accessible design is more far-reaching. According to the CDC, the built environment

> includes all of the physical parts of where we live and work (e.g., homes, buildings, streets, open spaces, and infrastructure). The built environment influences a person's level of physical activity. For example, inaccessible or nonexistent sidewalks and bicycle or walking paths contribute to sedentary habits. These habits lead to poor health outcomes such as obesity, cardiovascular disease, diabetes, and some types of cancer. (2006, p. 1)

For those with existing disabilities, assuring ease of access to all manner of recreation and exercise options is of paramount importance. For those who may develop disabilities or chronic illnesses, having the opportunities for healthy participation in physical activity may forestall or prevent the development of illness. For the community, having an environment that promotes rather than restricts a healthy lifestyle can be economically advantageous. Even schools have a role to play (CDC, 2008a). Building new schools away from residential areas decreases opportunities for exercise and after-school activities. As parents are increasingly forced to drive their children to school, the children remain sedentary, the pollution from cars is increased, and the risk of automobile accidents increases. Community design is a complicated and evolving issue, but the point remains: a healthier population may be achieved with attention to the environmental barriers that impede healthy lifestyles for all persons.

THE ROLE OF THE COMMUNITY HEALTH NURSE

This chapter has discussed a number of areas in which the community health nurse plays a key role. It is important to review those roles in the context of the individual, the family, and the community as prime areas for nursing intervention. Chapter 3 first examined the broad spectrum of roles that the professional nurse takes on within the community. It is helpful to review those roles and think about their application to disabled and chronically ill clients, their families, and the communities in which they live.

Table 26.4 provides a grid on which to record specific examples of the roles that community health nurses assume in relation to disabilities and chronic illnesses. Take note of each role that you participate in or observe while completing your clinical experience. If you cannot find examples of the various roles at each level, perhaps you can interview a community health nurse during your clinical experience and find examples of how she performs activities in each of those roles. You will probably find that, while addressing a single issue with a client, the community health nurse serves in a variety of roles and at different levels.

Consider as an example of the variety of roles and multilevel practice that the community health nurse assumes with respect to a 55-year-old female client who uses a wheelchair. The client has difficulty obtaining a gynecologic examination because of the lack of accessible examination tables at the local clinic; as a result, she has not had an examination for more than 20 years. Recognizing the need for a complete examination, the community health nurse arranges with the clinic to find appropriate alternatives that will aid the client in receiving the needed examination, possibly by ensuring that additional personnel are provided (Advocate Role–Individual Level).

Because this solution is temporary and less than optimal, the nurse contacts a number of clinics in neighboring communities and finds one that has appropriate equipment for people who have difficulty transferring to a standard examination table. Unfortunately, this clinic is 1 hour away. The nurse then contacts a number of other community health nurses and discovers that they also have a significant number of women clients with this problem who have not received a gynecologic examination in many years (Research Role–Community Level).

Through a coordinated effort with a local transportation company and the clinic, the nurse is able to arrange a twice-yearly gynecologic screening program for the women in the community who require special accommodations (Advocate and Coordinator Roles–Community Level). Information sheets that discuss the need for annual gynecologic examinations and advertise the program are distributed to area public health nurses, employers, and health clinics (Educator Role–Community Level). Data collection on examinations provided over the next few years shows a 65% increase in the number of women with special needs who have received a gynecologic examination within the past year (Research Role–Community Level).

TABLE 26.4	Roles of the Community Health Nurse		
Role	Individual	Family	Community
Clinician			
Educator			
Advocate			
Manager			
Collaborator			
Leaders			
Researcher			

This is not an uncommon scenario in the practice of community health nursing. Often, the needs of an individual open the door to areas of concern for many in a community and provide a basis for intervention that can benefit a larger population.

Like nursing practice in general, the role of the community health nurse with respect to disabilities and chronic illness requires broad and holistic practice. The complexity of issues surrounding these conditions requires creativity, tenacity, honesty, and, most of all, knowledge. Community health nurses who are informed about the issues that affect the disabled and chronically ill at local, state, and national levels are prepared to offer assistance to their clients and to their communities. Knowledge of civil rights for these individuals is crucial in serving as advocates.

The issues facing individuals and families with disabilities require strong and sustained efforts to achieve results. Although successes at the individual level are laudable, the extent to which the health and well-being of those affected is improved must be the ultimate goal. Community health nursing is in a prime position to initiate and support efforts to improve the health status of those populations. We can either leave the issues to other professionals or use our expertise and long history of caring for those less fortunate to make major and lasting changes. It is up to us.

Summary

The issue of disability and chronic illness is of growing importance in community health, both nationally and internationally. Through the efforts of the WHO, the international community has been challenged to provide increased attention to health promotion and disease prevention. Even in less developed countries, behavioral patterns linked to excesses in consumption (overweight and tobacco/alcohol use) have an impact on the quality and quantity of healthy years of life. The ICF provides a universal classification system that standardizes language and takes into account the biopsychosocial realms in health assessment and well-being of disabled persons. Along with the *World Health Report 2002*, this document now places the emphasis squarely on prevention of disease and disability. This means, of course, that the health promotion and disease prevention needs of the disabled and chronically ill must be given the same emphasis as the needs of those who are not disabled or ill.

The aging of the U.S. population and the rise in lifestyle-related illnesses such as diabetes and obesity are often linked with increasing rates of disability. Prevention of disability and disease is emphasized in *Healthy People 2010,* which serves as a wake-up call to Americans about the need to give serious attention to health promoting and disease prevention activities. In this current edition of *Healthy People,* unique emphasis is placed on health promotion and disease prevention needs of those with disabilities and chronic illness. It is no longer acceptable that these individuals be treated solely for tertiary health needs. Research has shown that when health promoting (lifestyle) issues are addressed with these clients, the rates of secondary conditions are reduced, including medical, social, emotional, mental, family, and community problems. Like the ICF, *Healthy People 2010* takes the position that disability and chronic conditions are not universally debilitating and that the overall well-being and health of these individuals must be a priority.

Legislation is but one step toward equality for those affected by disabilities and chronic illnesses. The ADA has provided for many improvements in accessibility and specific legal protections for the disabled, but it is only the beginning. Discrimination can occur at many levels; some is hurtful and intentional, but most results from misunderstanding of the needs and desires of disabled persons and their families. This may even occur in relation to the provision of health care because of lack of education. Improvement can be found only with increased community education programs for professionals and the public that target the myths and misunderstandings about those with disabilities and chronic illnesses.

Community health nurses are in a prime position to advocate for the health needs of the disabled and chronically ill. With a long history of serving those who are most vulnerable, community health nurses can help make needed changes at the individual, family, and community levels. Although it is often easier to focus on the needs of the individual, those needs are most often shared by many others. Nurses have long recognized the need to collaborate with other professionals in reaching the goal of improved health care for their clients; this continues to be an important aspect of successful efforts on behalf of the disabled and the chronically ill. It will take the concerted efforts of many to implement the changes necessary to improve the lives of those most affected, their families, and the communities in which they live.

The next time you have difficulty opening a door that is unusually heavy or struggle to open the lid of a jar or feel that you were treated differently than someone else in the receipt of services, take a moment to think. Think about the challenges, struggles, and pain that face so many citizens. Consider the impact of universal design at improving your life or the life of a family member or friend. Although many argue against improving accessibility of city streets and sidewalks because of the expense, those same people may one day find that they, too, are faced with trying to master a curb that is just a bit too high. ■

ACTIVITIES TO PROMOTE CRITICAL THINKING

1. Arrange to interview an individual with a disability (e.g., hearing, vision, mobility) about the challenges that he has faced in interactions with nondisabled persons.

2. Visit some of the nongovernmental sites listed under Internet Resources and read some of the personal stories that are included.

3. Take an inventory of your house or apartment and make a list of modifications you would need to make if you were suddenly confined to a wheelchair. Would you even be able to stay in your current residence?

4. As part of your regular clinical assignment in community health nursing, look at those clients and families who are dealing with either a disability or

chronic illness and assess how often you or other community health nurses have addressed health promotion activities (e.g., healthy eating, physical activity, leisure-time activities) with those clients.

5. Review your family history for chronic health conditions. Are you at risk? If so, what have you done to reduce your risk over the past 12 months?

References

American Council of the Blind. (2008). *Organizational profile.* Retrieved August 19, 2008 from http://www.acb.org/profile.html.

American Foundation for the Blind. (2008). *About AFB.* Retrieved August 19, 2008 from http://www.afb.org/.

Becker, G., & Newsom, E. (2003). Socioeconomic status and dissatisfaction with health care among chronically ill African Americans. *American Journal of Public Health, 93,* 742–748.

Cannuscio, C.C., Colditz, G.A., Rimm, E.B., Berkman, L.F., Jones, C.P., & Kawachi, I. (2004). Employment status, social ties, and caregivers mental health. *Social Science & Medicine, 58,* 1247–1256.

Cannuscio, C.C., Jones, C., Kawachi, I., Colditz, G.A., Berkman, L., & Rimm, E. (2002). Reverberations of family illness: A longitudinal assessment of informal caregiving and mental health status in the Nurses' Health Study. *American Journal of Public Health, 92,* 1305–1311.

Centers for Disease Control and Prevention. (2006). *Impact of the built environment on health.* Retrieved August 19, 2008 from http://www.cdc.gov/nceh/publications/factsheets/Impactof theBuiltEnvironmentonHealth.pdf.

Centers for Disease Control and Prevention. (2007). *Chronic disease prevention.* Retrieved August 19, 2008 from http://www.cdc.gov/nccdphp/.

Centers for Disease Control and Prevention. (2008a). *Children's health and the built environment.* Retrieved August 19, 2008 from http://www.cdc.gov/healthyplaces/healthtopics/children.htm.

Centers for Disease Control and Prevention. (2008b). *Summary health statistics for the U.S. population: National Health Interview Survey, 2006.* Washington, DC: Government Printing Office. Retrieved August 19, 2008 from http://www.cdc.gov/nchs/data/series/sr_10/sr10_236.pdf.

Disabled American Veterans. (2008). *Building better lives for disabled American veterans and their families.* Retrieved August 19, 2008 from http://www.dav.org/.

Egede, L.E., & Zheng, D. (2003). Racial/ethnic differences in adult vaccination among individuals with diabetes. *American Journal of Public Health, 93,* 324–329.

Esposito, S., Marchisio, P., Droghetti, R, Lambertini, L, Faelli, N., Bosis, S., et al. (2006). Influenza vaccination coverage among children with high-risk medical conditions. *Vaccine, 24,* 5251–5255.

Fisher, H.R. (2001). The needs of parents with chronically sick children: A literature review. *Journal of Advanced Nursing, 36,* 600–607.

Grayson, G. (2003). *Talking with your hands, listening with your eyes. A complete photographic guide to American Sign Language.* Garden City Park, NY: Square One.

Guide Dogs for the Blind. (2008). *About us.* Retrieved August 19, 2008 from http://www.guidedogs.com.

Mace, R. (n.d.). *About universal design: The Center for Universal Design.* Retrieved August 19, 2008 from http://design.ncsu.edu/cud/index.htm.

Morehead, P., & Morehead, A. (Eds.). (1995). *The new American Webster handy college dictionary.* New York: Penguin Books.

National Association of the Deaf. (2008a). *American Sign Language: Position statement National Association of the Deaf.*

Retrieved August 19, 2008 from http://www.nad.org/ASLposition.

National Association of the Deaf. (2008b). *Inside NAD: Mission statement.* Retrieved August 19, 2008 from http://www.nad.org/mission.

National Council on Disability. (1986). *Toward independence: An assessment of Federal laws and programs affecting persons with disabilities: With legislative recommendations.* Retrieved August 19, 2008 from http://www.ncd.gov/newsroom/publications/1986/publications.htm.

National Council on Disability. (2000). *Promises to keep: A decade of Federal enforcement of the Americans with Disabilities Act.* Retrieved August 19, 2008 from http://www.ncd.gov/newsroom/publications/2000/promises_1.htm.

National Council on Disability. (2005). *NCD and the Americans with Disabilities Act: 15 years of progress.* Retrieved August 19, 2008 from http://www.ncd.gov/newsroom/publications/2005/pdf/15yearprogress.pdf.

National Council on Disability. (2008a). *Finding the gaps: A comparative analysis of disability laws in the United States to the United Nations Convention on the Rights of Persons with Disabilities (CRPD).* Retrieved August 19, 2008 from http://www.ncd.gov/newsroom/publications/index.htm.

National Council on Disability. (2008b). *National Council on Disability: 30 Years of Disability Policy Leadership 1978–2008.* Retrieved August 19, 2008 from http://www.ncd.gov/.

National Federation of the Blind. (2003). *What is Braille and what does it mean to the blind?* Retrieved August 19, 2008 from http://www.nfb.org/images/nfb/Publications/fr/fr15/Issue1/f150113.html.

National Federation of the Blind. (2008). *About the NFB.* Retrieved August 19, 2008 from http://www.nfb.org/nfb/Default.asp.

National Organization on Disability. (2004). *Key findings: 2004 NOD/Harris Survey documents trends impacting 54 million Americans.* Retrieved August 19, 2008 from http://www.nod.org/index.cfm?fuseaction=Feature.showFeature&FeatureID=1422.

National Organization on Disability. (2008). *About us & quick links.* Retrieved August 19, 2008 from http://www.nod.org.

Obesity Society. (2008). *About the Obesity Society.* Retrieved October 14, 2008, from http://www.obesity.org/about/

Parish, S.L., & Ellison-Martin, M.J. (2007). Health-care access of women Medicaid recipients: Evidence of disability-based disparities. *Journal of Disability Policy Studies, 18,* 109–116.

Smith, L.A., Wise, P.H., & Wampler, N.S. (2002). Knowledge of welfare reform program provisions among families of children with chronic conditions. *American Journal of Public Health, 92,* 228–230.

The Body: The Complete HIV/AIDS Resource. (2008). *United States HIV/AIDS organizations.* Retrieved August 19, 2008 from http://www.thebody.com/index/hotlines/other.html.

United Nations. (2007a). *Relationship between development and human rights.* Retrieved August 19, 2008 from http://www.un.org/esa/socdev/enable/convinfodevhr.htm.

United Nations. (2007b). *Secretariat for the Convention on the Rights of Persons with Disabilities.* Retrieved August 19, 2008 from http://www.un.org/disabilities/default.asp?id=17.

U.S. Department of Health and Human Services. (1991). *Healthy People 2000: National health promotion and disease prevention objectives* (S/N 017-001-00474-0). Washington, DC: U.S. Government Printing Office.

U.S. Department of Health and Human Services. (2000). *Healthy People 2010: Understanding and improving health.* Washington, DC: Government Printing Office. Retrieved August 19, 2008 from http://www.health.gov/healthypeople/Document/.

U.S. Department of Health and Human Services. (2001). *Healthy People 2000 final review.* Retrieved August 19, 2008 from http://www.cdc.gov/nchs/data/hp2000/hp2k01.pdf.

U.S. Department of Health and Human Services. (2005a). *Midcourse review: Healthy People 2010*. Washington, DC: Government Printing Office. Retrieved August 19, 2008 from http://www.healthypeople.gov/data/midcourse/.

U.S. Department of Health and Human Services. (2005b). *The Surgeon General's call to action to improve the health and wellness of persons with disabilities*. Washington, DC: Government Printing Office. Retrieved August 19, 2008 from http://www.surgeongeneral.gov/library/disabilities/calltoaction/calltoaction.pdf.

U.S. Department of Health and Human Services. (2006). *Delivering on the promise: OCR's compliance activities promote community integration*. Retrieved August 19, 2008 from http://www.hhs.gov/ocr/complianceactiv.html.

U.S. Department of Housing and Urban Development (2008). *Fair housing accessibility guidelines*. Washington, DC: Government Printing Office. Retrieved August 19, 2008 from http://www.hud.gov/offices/fheo/disabilities/fhguidelines/fhefha1.cfm#background.

U.S. Department of Justice. (2005). *A guide to disability rights laws*. Retrieved August 19, 2008 from http://www.usdoj.gov/crt/ada/cguide.htm.

U.S. Mission to the United Nations. (2006). *Explanation of Position by Ambassador Richard T. Miller, U.S. Representative to the UN Economic and Social Council, on the Convention on the Rights of Persons with Disabilities, Agenda Item 67(b), in the General Assembly*. [USUN Press Release # 396(06)]. Retrieved August 19, 2008 from http://www.usunnewyork.usmission.gov/press_releases/20061213_396.html.

Wei, W., Findley, P.A., & Sambamoorthi, U. (2006). Disability and receipt of clinical preventive services among women. *Women's Health Issues, 16*, 286–296.

Wilber, N., Mitra, M., Walker, D.K., Allen, D., Meyers, A.R., & Tupper, P. (2002). Disabilities as a public health issue: Findings and reflections from the Massachusetts Survey of Secondary Conditions. *The Milbank Quarterly, 80*, 393–419.

Wong, M.G., & Heriot, S.A. (2007). Parents of children with cystic fibrosis: How they hope, cope and despair. *Child: Care, Health and Development, 34*, 344–354.

Wood, P.R., Smith, L.A., Romero, D., Bradshaw, P., Wise, P.H., & Chavkin, W. (2002). Relationships between welfare status, health insurance status, and health and medical care among children with asthma. *American Journal of Public Health, 92*, 1446–1452.

World Health Organization. (1980). International classification of impairments, disabilities, and handicaps. Geneva, Switzerland: Author.

World Health Organization. (2001). International classification of functioning, disability and health. Geneva, Switzerland: Author.

World Health Organization. (2002). *The World Health Report 2002. Reducing Risks, promoting healthy life*. Geneva, Switzerland: Author.

World Health Organization. (2008). *Obesity and overweight*. Retrieved August 19, 2008 from http://www.who.int/dietphysicalactivity/publications/facts/obesity/en/print.html.

Selected Readings

Bartlett, J.G., & Finkbeiner, A.K. (2006). *Guide to living with HIV infection: Developed at the Johns Hopkins AIDS Clinic*. Baltimore: Johns Hopkins University Press.

Becker, G., & Newsom, E. (2005). Resilience in the face of serious illness among chronically ill African Americans in later life. *Journal of Gerontology, 60B*(4), S214–S223.

Berke, E.M., Koepsell, T.D., Moudon, A.V., Hoskins, R.E., & Larson, E.B. (2007). Association of the built environment with physical activity and obesity in older adults. *American Journal of Public Health, 97*, 486–492.

Blomquist, K.B. (2007). Health and independence of young adults with disabilities: Two years later. *Orthopaedic Nursing, 26*, 296–309.

Brown, S. (2007). Universal design and me. *Inside MS, 25*(4), 43–44.

Chen, Y., Yi, Q., Wu, J., & Li, F. (2007). Chronic disease status, self-perceived health and hospital admissions are important predictors for having a flu shot in Canada. *Vaccine, 25*, 7436–7440.

Cohen, R.M. (2008). *Strong at the broken places: Five voices of illness, one chorus of hope*. New York: Harper Collins, Publishers.

Downing, M.J. (2008). The role of home in HIV/AIDS: A visual approach to understanding human-environment interactions in the context of long-term illness. *Home and Place, 14*, 313–322.

Dunlop, D.D., Song, J., Manheim, L.M., Daviglus, M.L., & Chang, R.W. (2007). Racial/ethnic differences in the development of disability among older adults. *American Journal of Public Health, 97*, 2209–2215.

Edwards, L. (2008). *A life disrupted: Getting real about chronic illness in your twenties and thirties*. New York: Walker & Company.

Fan, A.Z., Strine, T.W., Jiles, R., & Mokdad, A.H. (2008). Depression and anxiety associated with cardiovascular disease among persons aged 45 years and older in 38 states of the United States, 2006. *Preventive Medicine, 46*, 445–450.

Gee, G.C., Spencer, M.S., Chen, J., & Takeuchi, D. (2007). A nationwide study of discrimination and chronic health conditions among Asian Americans. *American Journal of Public Health, 97*, 1275–1282.

Grabar, S., Lanoy, E., Allavena, C., Mary-Krause, M., Bentata, M., Fisher, P., et al. (2008). Causes of the first AIDS – defining illness and subsequent survival before and after the advent of combined antiretroviral therapy. *HIV Medicine, 9*, 246–256.

Gruman, J. (2007). *Aftershock: What to do when the doctor gives you - or someone you love — a devastating diagnosis*. New York: Walker & Company.

Herwig, O. (Ed.). (2008). *Universal design: Solutions for a barrier-free living*. Basel, Switzerland: Birkhauser.

Jordon, W.A. (2008). *Universal design for the home: Great-looking, great-living design for all ages, abilities, and & circumstances*. Beverly, MA: Quarry Books, Inc.

Lehmann, I., & Crimando, W. (2008). Unintended consequences of state and federal antidiscrimination and family medical leave legislation on the employment rates of persons with disabilities. *Rehabilitation Counseling Bulletin, 51*(3), 159–169.

Lutz, B.J., & Bowers, B.J. (2003). Understanding how disability is defined and conceptualized in the literature. *Rehabilitation Nursing, 28*, 74–78.

Qui, Y., & Li, S. (2008). Stroke: Coping strategies and depression among Chinese caregivers of survivors during hospitalization. *Journal of Clinical Nursing, 17*, 1563–1573.

Richardson, L.C., Wingo, P.A., Zack, M.M., Zahran, H.S., & King, J.B. (2008). Health-related quality of life years in cancer survivors between ages 20 and 64 years. *Cancer, 112(6)*, 1380–1389.

Sun, H., Zhang, J., & Fu, X. (2007). Psychological status, coping, and social support of people living with HIV/AIDS in Central China. *Public Health Nursing, 24*, 132–140.

Thomsett, K., & Nickerson, E. (1993). *Missing words. The family handbook on adult hearing loss*. Washington, DC: Gallaudet University Press.

White, R.T., & Pope, C. (2008). *The globalization of AIDS*. Oxford, UK: Taylor & Francis, Inc.

Zhao, G., Ford, E.S., Li, C., & Mokdad, A.H. (2007). Compliance with physical activity recommendations in U.S. adults with diabetes. *Diabetic Medicine, 25*, 221–227.

Internet Resources

American Council of the Blind: *http://www.acb.org*
American Diabetes Association: *http://diabetes.org*
American Foundation for the Blind: *http://afb.org*

American Heart Association: *http://www.americanheart.org*
Center for Universal Design (NC State University): *http://www.design.ncsu.edu/cud/*
Disabled American Veterans: *http://www.dav.org/*
Easter Seals Disability Services: *http://www.easterseals.com/site/PageServer*
Family Health International: *http://www.fhi.org/en/index.htm*
Guide Dogs for the Blind: *http://www.guidedogs.com*
National Association to Advance Fat Acceptance: *http://naafa.org*
National Association of the Deaf: *http://www.nad.org*
National Center for Health Statistics: *http://www.cdc.gov/nchswww*
National Council on Disability: *http://www.ncd.gov*
National Federation of the Blind: *http://www.nfb.org*
National Institute of Diabetes & Digestive & Kidney Diseases: *http://www.niddk.nih.gov*

National Organization on Disability: *http://www.nod.org*
Obesity Society: *http://www.obesity.org*
Office of Minority Health Resource Center: *http://www.omhrc.gov*
Robert Wood Johnson Foundation: *http://www.rwjf.org*
The Body: The Complete HIV/AIDS Resource: *http://www.thebody.com/index/hotlines/other.html*
United States Access Board: *http://www.access-board.gov/*
U.S. Department of Health and Human Services, Office for Civil Rights: *http://www.hhs.gov/ocr*
U.S. Department of Justice (Americans with Disabilities Act Home Page): *http://www.usdoj.gov/crt/ada/adahom1.htm*
Universal Design Alliance: *http://www.universaldesign.org/*
Women with Disabilities (The National Health Information Center): *http://www.4woman.gov/wwd*

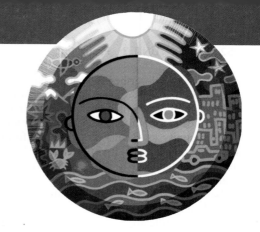

27

Behavioral Health in the Community

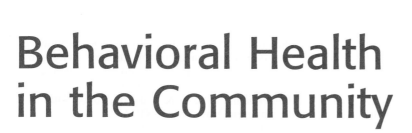

Upon mastery of this chapter, you should be able to:

◆ Discuss the incidence and prevalence of mental illness and substance use in the United States.

◆ Compare and contrast various theories on the etiology of substance use disorders.

◆ Discuss the treatment approaches at the community level related to behavioral health.

◆ Identify and describe community behavioral health resources.

◆ Identify the *Healthy People 2010* objectives for reducing substance use and addressing behavioral health needs in the United States.

◆ Discuss health-promoting interventions for community behavioral health.

◆ Describe the role of the community health nurse in the prevention of substance use and mental health disorders.

"Make your own recovery the first priority in your life."

—Robin Norwood

This chapter describes the role behavioral health plays in the overall health of a community and provides an overview of behavioral health prevention and treatment from the perspective of community health nursing practice with a focus on community level interventions. The following questions should be kept in mind while reading about the issues surrounding behavioral health: in what sense does behavioral health relate to the health of communities? What are the global implications related to an increase in mental health-related diagnoses and risky-to-dependent substance use? What is the role of a community health nurse in helping individuals, families, and communities to promote optimal mental health and responsible substance use and thereby decrease the prevalence and incidence of mental and substance use disorders (SUDs)?

BEHAVIORAL HEALTH TERMINOLOGY

Several terms that are useful for community health nurses working in the behavioral and mental health fields are defined below.

- ◆ **Community mental health nurse:** An individual whose practice is centered on the mental health needs of the populations served.
- ◆ **Community mental health:** A field of practice that seeks to promote the mental health of the community by preventing mental illness and addressing the needs of the mentally ill.
- ◆ **Community mental health centers (CMHCs):** Facilities that provide comprehensive, publicly funded services to the mentally ill population.
- ◆ **Mental health care system:** The collective programs designed for anyone with a mental illness. These programs may include treatments, services, or other types of supports, such as housing, employment, or disability benefits through government, private nonprofit, or private for-profit systems.
- ◆ **Mental health:** As defined in *Healthy People 2010*, mental health is "a state of successful mental functioning, resulting in productive activities, fulfilling relationships, and the ability to adapt to change and cope with adversity" (U.S. Department of Health and Human Services [USDHHS], 2000, p. 37).
- ◆ **Mental illness:** "Refers collectively to all diagnosable mental disorders [which] are health conditions that are characterized by alterations in thinking, mood, or behavior (or some combination thereof) associated with distress and/or impaired functioning" (USDHHS, 1999). The American Psychiatric Association (APA) (2000) further defines mental illness or mental disorder as "a clinically significant behavioral or psychological syndrome or pattern that occurs in a person and that is associated with present distress (e.g., a painful symptom) or disability (i.e., impairment in one or more important areas of functioning), or with a significantly increased risk of suffering, death, pain, disability, or an important loss of freedom . . . and is not merely an expectable and culturally sanctioned response to a particular event (e.g., the death of a loved one)" (p. xxxi).

- ◆ **Serious mental illness (SMI):** Mental illness that has compromised both the client's level of function and his or her quality of life is known as SMI. **Serious and persistent mental illness (SPMI)** is the preferred term for serious mental illness of a chronic nature. For example, schizophrenia is usually classified as an SPMI.
- ◆ **Addiction:** A complex neuro biobehavioral disorder characterized by impaired control, compulsive use, dependency, and craving for the activity, substance, or food. Relapses are possible even after long periods of abstinence (Armstrong, Feigenbaum, Savage, & Vourakis, 2006; National Institute on Drug Abuse [NIDA], 2004a).
- ◆ **Substance use disorders:** The spectrum of disorders that include substance abuse and dependence and are attributed to problematic consumption or illicit use of alcohol, tobacco, illicit, and legal drugs (Armstrong et al., 2006).
- ◆ **Levels of alcohol use** (National Institute on Alcohol Abuse and Alcoholism [NIAAA], 2007):

  Abstinence: Consumption of fewer than four standard drinks per year.
  Low-risk drinking: Low-level alcohol use that is not problematic (see below).
  Risky/hazardous use: Pattern of alcohol consumption that increases the risk of harmful consequences for the user or others.
  Harmful use: Alcohol consumption that results in consequences to physical and mental health.
  Alcoholism: Also known as "alcohol dependence," a disease that includes four symptoms: craving, loss of control, physical dependence, and tolerance.

- ◆ **Dependence:** An adaptive physiological state that includes craving, loss of control, physical dependence, and usually tolerance (NIAAA, 2007; NIDA, 2004a).
- ◆ **Screening:** A mechanism used to evaluate the presence of substance use problems and to estimate the probability of a specific disorder. This may include evaluation of a client's blood alcohol level or other tools, such as questionnaires (NIAAA, 2007).
- ◆ **Tolerance:** The need for significantly increased amounts of alcohol or drug to achieve intoxication or the desired effect or a markedly diminished effect with the continued use of the same amount of alcohol or drug (Armstrong et al., 2006).
- ◆ **Relapse:** Return to heavy alcohol, tobacco, or drug use after a period of abstinence or moderate use (NIAAA, 2007).

MENTAL HEALTH IN TRANSITION

The advances in research today and evolving best evidence-based practice models of mental health care are gaining ground across the world in various mental health centers of excellence. At the same time, numerous centers provide care with declining resources such that services are compromised. The science on brain structure functions and how learning occurs over time has impacted mental health services by expanding the possibilities of available therapies. Today, provision of care requires neurophysiologic, neurochemical, genetic, and endocrine considerations. This means that community health nurse approaches require holistic assessment that integrates physical, psychological, and sociocultural knowledge in the provision of care.

Several documents address the need for prevention and treatment for mental health disorders, such as *Healthy People 2010* (USDHHS, 2000), the National Health Promotion and Disease Prevention Objectives (2000), and the Report of the Surgeon General on Mental Health, submitted by David Satcher (USDHHS,1999). The health care goals addressed within *Healthy People 2010* (USDHHS, 2000) are relevant to community mental health nursing (see Table 27.1). Noted are improvements in mental health including reduction of suicide rates in the general population, reduction of suicide attempts by adolescents, reduction in the number of homeless persons with severe mental illness, and increase in employment of persons with serious mental illness. Several objectives focusing on treatment expansion for the mentally ill include the following:

1. Reduction of relapse rates for persons with eating disorders;
2. Increase in mental health screening and assessment in primary care settings;
3. Increase in the numbers of children and adults with mental illness who receive treatment;
4. Increase in treatment for persons with dual diagnosis (including substance abuse);

5. Increase in treatment for mentally ill persons in juvenile justice facilities and jails.

The Report of the Surgeon General on Mental Health (USDHHS, 1999) was the first Surgeon General's report ever published on the topic of mental health and mental illness. The report concluded that effective treatments are available for most adults with a serious mental illness who are age 18 and over and who currently or at any time during the past year have had a diagnosable mental, behavioral, or emotional disorder of sufficient duration to meet diagnostic criteria specified within DSM-IV, TR (Diagnostic and Statistical Manual for Mental Disorders, Text Revision; APA, 2000). The focus on the promotion of increased access to educational and employment opportunities for people with disabilities (both physical and psychiatric) was evident in President George W. Bush's New Freedom Initiative in 2001. The initiative also noted the need to increase access to assistive and universally designed technologies (2004). The Commission on Mental Health identified three impediments to the provision of quality mental health care on April 29, 2002 (Commission on Mental Health, 2003):

1. Stigma that surrounds mental illnesses
2. Unfair treatment limitations and financial requirements placed on mental health benefits in private health insurance
3. Fragmented mental health service delivery system

TABLE 27.1   *Healthy People 2010*—Summary of Objectives Focus Area 18

Goal: Improve mental health and ensure access to appropriate, quality mental health services.

Number	Objective
Mental Health Status Improvement	
18-1	Reduce the suicide rate
18-2	Reduce the suicide attempts by adolescents
18-3	Reduce the proportion of homeless adults who have serious mental illness (SMI)
18-4	Increase the proportion of persons with serious mental illness (SMI) who are employed
18-5	(Developmental) Reduce the relapse rates for persons with eating disorders including anorexia nervosa and bulimia nervosa
Treatment Expansion	
18-6	(Developmental) Increase the number of persons seen in primary health care who receive mental health screening and assessment
18-7	(Developmental) Increase the proportion of children with mental health problems who receive treatment
18-8	(Developmental) Increase the proportion of juvenile justice facilities that screen new admissions for mental health problems
18-9	(Developmental) Increase the proportion of adults with mental disorders who receive treatment
18-10	(Developmental) Increase the proportion of persons with co-occurring substance abuse and mental disorders who receive treatment for both disorders
18-11	(Developmental) Increase the proportion of local governments with community-based jail diversion programs for adults with serious mental illness (SMI)
State Activities	
18-12	State tracking of consumer satisfaction
18-13	State plans addressing cultural competence
18-14	State plans addressing elderly persons

Source: National Institutes of Health (NIH), Substance Abuse and Mental Health Services Association (SAMHSA). Retrieved August 20, 2008 from http://www.healthypeople.gov/document/HTML/Volume2/18Mental.htm.

Incidence and Prevalence of Mental Disorders

Mental illness is a global problem (World Health Organization [WHO], 2007). In its Global Burden of Disease Study, WHO showed that mental illness, including suicide, accounts for more than 15% of mortality worldwide. In the United States alone, more than 57.7 million people experience a diagnosable mental disorder (National Institute of Mental Health [NIMH], 2006a). Of this group, more than 6.5 million, including 4 million children and adolescents, are disabled by a SMI (USDHHS, 1999).

An estimated 7.6% of adults age 18 or older (approximately 16.4 million adults) reported at least one major depressive episode during the past year (Office of Applied Studies [OAS], 2007). More than 19 million Americans older than 18 years of age will suffer from a depressive illness at some time during their lives, and many of these individuals will be incapacitated for significant lengths of time by their illness. The age-adjusted suicide rate per 100,000 population for 2004 was 15.2% for men and 3.6% for women, with almost half of these with a diagnosed mental disorder (Centers for Disease Control and Prevention [CDC], 2006). Over two-thirds of suicides in the United States each year are caused by major depression. More than 2 million Americans 18 years of age and older, about 1% to 1.6% of the population, suffer from bipolar disorder, and an almost equal number of adults suffer from schizophrenia (NIMH, 2006a).

The poor, poorly educated, and the unemployed typically experience higher rates of mental illness than the general population. A large portion of the mentally ill population, many of whom are homeless, remain untreated in the community. The poor, disproportionately representative of racial and ethnic minorities, are even more vulnerable due to the lack of access to care and the questionable quality of the care that is received (Substance Abuse and Mental Health Services Administration [SAMSHA], 2003). The homeless are more likely to experience behavioral health issues, such as substance use disorders and mental illness. Alcohol use disorders (AUDs) are as high as 84% in homeless men and 58% of homeless women (D'Amore, Hung, Chiang, & Goldfrank, 2001; North, Eyrich, Pollio, & Spintznagel, 2004). The majority of hospital admissions among the homeless are for treatment of substance use or mental illness. In one study on the homeless, 33.2% of the population reported depression, and 9.6% had been professionally diagnosed with a mental illness other than depression (Greater Cincinnati Coalition for the Homeless, 2001).

Age influences the patterns of mental illness in the community. Each year about one of every five children and adolescents has the signs and symptoms of a mental health disorder described and defined by the APA in the fourth edition of DSM-IV, TR. The most commonly occurring conditions among American children ages 9 to 17 years are anxiety disorders, disruptive disorders, mood disorders, and substance use disorders. Attention-deficit/hyperactivity disorder (ADHD) affects approximately 3% to 5% of U.S. children, or about 2 million school-age children, with boys two to three times more likely to be affected than girls (NIMH, 2006a). Autism, a developmental disorder, affects 3.4 out of every 1,000 children ages 3 to 10 (NIMH, 2006a) and is four times more common in boys than in girls (NIMH, 2006b). For American adults, the most prevalent mental disorders are anxiety disorders, followed by mood disorders, especially major depression and bipolar disorder. Anxiety, depression, and schizophrenia present special problems for this age group—anxiety and depression because they contribute to such high rates of suicide, and schizophrenia because it is so persistently disabling. For the growing number of older adults, there is increased incidence of Alzheimer disease (8%–15% of adults age 65 and over); major depression (8%–20%); anxiety (11.4%), and other disabling mental disorders.

Gender differences also arise in the prevalence of certain mental disorders. Anxiety disorders and mood disorders, including major depression, occur twice as frequently in women as in men. Women of color, women on welfare, poor women, and uneducated women are more likely to experience depression than women in the general population. The three main types of eating disorders (anorexia, bulimia nervosa, and binge eating) also affect more women than men (Hudson, Hiripi, Pope, & Kessler, 2007).

Although suicide attempts are more common in women, men are more likely to be successful (National Center for Health Statistics [NCHS], 2004). Analysis of national suicide data from 1991 to 1996 suggested that White and African American widowed men younger than age 50 were at particular risk to commit suicide, compared with the general population of married men, and young African American men were most at risk (Luoma & Pearson, 2002). White men aged 85 and over, living alone, with a recent loss of a spouse or significant other account for 50% of suicides.

Cost of Mental Health Disorders

Adding to the heavy toll that mental illness exacts is the financial burden it creates. Costs associated with treatment of mental disorders—poor productivity, lost work time, and disability payments—are astronomical. The direct and indirect costs of mental illness and addictive disorders in the United States are greater than $273 billion annually. Furthermore, the cost to society when treatment is not provided for these illnesses is three times the cost of direct treatment (National Alliance on Mental Illness [NAMI], 2007). Certainly, these facts have policy implications and suggest the need for greater preventive and mental health-promoting efforts. The final report of the President's New Freedom Commission on Mental Health (2003) notes the governmental efforts to transform mental health care (see Display 27.1).

SUBSTANCE USE AND THE COMMUNITY HEALTH NURSE

Substances used in the United States that have the potential for dependence include alcohol, tobacco, and other drugs both legal and illegal. Substance use occurs across a continuum that includes abstinence, low-risk use, risky/hazardous use, harmful use, and dependence (Babor, Higgins-Biddle, Saunders, & Monteiro, 2001) (Fig. 27.1). From a community perspective, all substance use other than abstinence or low-risk use poses a threat to the overall health of the community as well as individuals and families. Reductions in substance use (including tobacco) are two of the 28 focus areas in *Healthy People 2010* (USDHHS, 2000). The community health nurse plays a vital role in developing successful prevention and treatment programs related to substance

DISPLAY 27.1	THE FINAL REPORT OF THE PRESIDENT'S NEW FREEDOM COMMISSION ON MENTAL HEALTH

Achieving the Promise: Transforming Mental Health Care in America

This *Final Report* conveys the Commission's bold vision for transforming the existing, often intimidating maze of mental health services into a coordinated, consumer-centered, recovery-oriented mental health system. Although barriers stand in the way, with national resolve and leadership, they will be overcome.

The Commission recognizes that historically Americans have assumed responsibility locally and regionally for working together to meet challenges and to support their neighbors and communities. A major step toward achieving the vision will require genuine collaborative efforts from all parties who deliver or use mental health services and supports. All must recognize the interwoven nature of the diverse programs that make up the mental health system and, in turn, must see where program flexibility and cooperation can be strengthened in the interest of consumers and families.

To transform the mental health care system, the Commission proposes a combination of goals and recommendations that together represent a strong plan for action. No single goal or recommendation alone can achieve the needed changes. No level or branch of government, no element of the private sector can accomplish needed change on its own. To transform mental health care as proposed, collaboration between the private and public sectors and among levels of government is crucial.

Mental illness is the only category of illness for which State and local governments operate distinct treatment systems, making comprehensive care unavailable in the larger health care system. Ultimately, this situation must change, but to do so requires health care reform beyond the Commission's scope.

> As has long been the case in America, local innovations under the mantle of national leadership can lead the way for successful transformation throughout the country.

Health care in America is at a pivotal point where reform must occur and mental health must share in that reform. The Nation has a vested interest and a tremendous stake in doing what is right to correct a system with problems that resulted from layering multiple, well-intentioned programs.

The integrated strategy outlined in this *Final Report* can achieve the transformation that will allow adults with serious mental illness and children with serious emotional disturbances to live, work, learn, and participate fully in their communities. Indeed, as has long been the case in America, local innovations under the mantle of national leadership can lead the way for successful transformation throughout the country.

As a Commission, we are grateful to the many strong and courageous individuals who gave their time, and in some cases traveled great distances to share their stories. It is for these individuals—as well as for the ones who continue to go unserved—that we must take swift, courageous action to transform the current maze of services, treatments, and supports into an efficient and cohesive mental health care delivery system. We owe them, their families, and future generations nothing less.

use in a community. These prevention programs are not limited to prevention of dependence but rather include the entire spectrum of use.

The community health nurse must begin with a basic understanding of the differences between substances of abuse since different substances pose different threats to the health of a community. This understanding can help the community health nurse match the community intervention to the substance in question, the desired outcome, and the particular needs of the target population. For example, the development of a tobacco smoking-prevention program in adolescents is quite different from a program to reduce drug-related intentional injuries.

Not only must the community health nurse understand the issues related to a specific substance of abuse (e.g.,

tobacco versus alcohol or versus cocaine), the nurse must also have a clear idea of the desired outcomes related to a treatment or prevention program. The key to successful community health interventions is to know initially what the over-arching goal of the intervention is. In other words, what aspect of substance use is the program addressing? To help in this process the nurse must also have a basic understanding of the different substances that have addictive potential (see Table 27.2), types of interventions available, the evidence to support their use, and the impact the substance use is having on the community. Examples of different over-arching goals include increasing access to treatment for SUDs, reducing alcohol-related motor vehicle crashes, reducing illicit drug related crime, or reducing secondary smoke exposure in public areas.

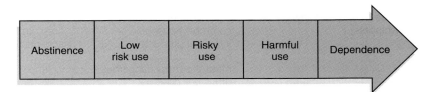

FIGURE 27.1 Continuum of substance use.

TABLE 27.2   Drugs Involved in Substance Abuse

Drug Type	Facts	Possible Signs of Use/Abuse	Possible Health Risks of Use/Abuse
Cannabis Hashish (hash, herb, kif) Hashish oil (hash oil, honey) Marijuana (grass, weed, dope, ganja, reefer, pot, Acapulco gold, Thai sticks)	Cannabis is made from the hemp plant, *Cannabis sativa*. When smoked or ingested produces mild euphoria, relaxation, and intense sensory perception. Users may develop tolerance and physical dependence. Sinsemilla is a highly potent form of marijuana.	Relaxation and euphoria Altered perceptions of time and space Hallucinations or anxiety attacks with sinsemilla use	Damage to heart and lungs Damage to brain nerve cells Memory disorders Temporary loss of fertility Psychological dependence
Depressants Alcohol (brew, juice, liquor) Barbiturates (downers, barbs) Benzodiazepines (Valium, Librium, tranquilizers) Chloral hydrate (knockout, Mickey Finn) Glutethimide (Doriden) Methaqualone (Quaalude, Ludes) Other Depressants (Equanil, Miltown, Noludar, Placidylm, Valmid)	Depressants depress or slow down the central nervous system by relaxing muscles, calming nerves, and producing sleep. Alcohol is a depressant. Depressants are composed of sedative-hypnotic and tranquilizer drugs. Depressants are addictive. Users of depressants develop a tolerance to the drugs, meaning larger doses must be taken each time to produce the same effect.	Relaxation and drowsiness; lack of concentration; disorientation; loss of inhibitions; lack of coordination; dilated pupils; slurred speech; weak and rapid pulse; distorted vision; low blood pressure; shallow breathing; staggering; clammy skin; fever, sweating; stomach cramps; hallucinations, tremors; and delirium	Liver damage; convulsions; addiction with severe withdrawal symptoms; coma; death due to overdose. For pregnant women: the newborn may be dependent and experience withdrawal or suffer from birth defects and behavioral problems
Hallucinogens Lysergic acid diethylamide (LSD) Phencyclidine (PCP, angel dust) Mescaline and peyote (Mesc, buttons, cactus) Psilocybin (mushrooms) Amphetamine variants (MDMA/Ecstasy, MDA/Love Drug, TMA, DOM, DOB, PMA, STP, 2.5-DMA) Phencyclidine analogues (PCE, PCPy, TCP) Other hallucinogens (Bufotenine, Ibogaine, DMT, DET)	Hallucinogens are psychedelic, mind-altering drugs that affect a person's perception, feelings, thinking, self-awareness, and emotions. A "bad trip" may result in the user's experiencing panic, confusion, paranoia, anxiety, unpleasant sensory images, feelings of helplessness, and loss of control. A "flash back" is a reoccurrence of the original drug experience without taking the drug again.	Dilated pupils, increased body temperature, heart rate, and blood pressure; sweating; loss of appetite; sleeplessness; dry mouth; tremors; hallucinations; disorientation; confusion; paranoia; violence; euphoria; anxiety; and panic	Agitation; extreme hyperactivity; psychosis; convulsions; mental or emotional problems; death
Inhalants Amyl nitrate (poppers, snappers) Butyl nitrate (rush, bolt, bullet) Chlorohydrocarbons (aerosol sprays, cleaning fluids) Hydrocarbons (solvents, airplane glue, gasoline, paint thinner) Nitrous oxide (laughing gas, whippets)	Inhalants are substances that are breathed or inhaled through the nose. Inhalants are depressants and depress or slow down the body's functions. Inhalants are normally not thought of as drugs because they are often common household or industrial products. However, inhalants are often the most dangerous drugs per dose.	Euphoria and lightheadedness; excitability; loss of appetite; forgetfulness; weight loss; sneezing; coughing; nausea and vomiting; lack of coordination; bad breath; red eyes; sores on nose and mouth; delayed reflexes; decreased blood pressure; flushing (skin appears to be reddish); headache; dizziness; and violence	Depression; damage to the nervous system and body tissues; damage to liver and brain; heart failure; respiratory arrest; suffocation; unconsciousness; seizures; heart failure; sudden death from sniffing

TABLE 27.2   Drugs Involved in Substance Abuse (*Continued*)

Drug Type	Facts	Possible Signs of Use/Abuse	Possible Health Risks of Use/Abuse
Narcotics Codeine (school boy) Heroin (H, harry, junk, brown sugar, smack) Meperidine (doctors) Methadone (dollies, methadose) Morphine (morpho, Miss Emma) Opium (Dover's powder) Other narcotics (Percodan, Talwin, Lomotil, Darvon, Numorphan, Percocet, Tylox, Tussionex, fentanyl)	Narcotics are composed of opiates and synthetic drugs. Opiates are derived from the seed pod of the Asian poppy. Synthetic drugs called opoids are chemically developed to produce the effects of opiates. Initially, narcotics stimulate the higher centers of the brain, but then slow down the activity of the central nervous system. Narcotics relieve pain and induce sleep. Narcotics, such as heroin, are often diluted with other substances (i.e., water, sugar) and injected. Other narcotics are taken orally or inhaled. Narcotics are extremely addictive. Users of narcotics develop a tolerance to the drugs, meaning larger doses must be taken each time to produce the same effect.	Euphoria; restlessness and lack of motivation; drowsiness; lethargy; decreased pulse rate; constricted pupils; flushing (skin appears to be reddish); constipation; nausea and vomiting; needle marks on extremities; skin abscess at injection sites; shallow breathing; watery eyes; and itching	Pulmonary edema; respiratory arrest; convulsions; addiction; coma; death due to overdose. For users who share or use unsterile needles to inject narcotics: tetanus, hepatitis, HIV/AIDS. For pregnant women: premature births; stillbirth, and acute infections among newborns
Steroids Anabolic-Androgenic (roids, juice, d-ball)	Steroids may contribute to increases in body weight and muscular strength. The acceleration of physical development is what makes steroids appealing to athletes and young adults. Anabolic-androgenic steroids are chemically related to the male sex hormone testosterone. Anabolic means to build up the muscles and other tissues of the body. Steroids are injected directly into the muscle or taken orally.	Sudden increase in muscle and weight; increase in aggression and combativeness; violence ("roid rage"); hallucinations; jaundice; purple or red spots on body, inside mouth, or nose; swelling of feet or lower legs (edema); tremors; and bad breath. For women: breast reduction, enlarged clitoris, facial hair and baldness, deepened voice. For men: enlarged nipples and breasts, testicle reduction, enlarged prostate, baldness.	Acne; high blood pressure; liver and kidney damage; heart disease; increased risk of injury to ligaments and tendons; bowel and urinary problems; gallstones and kidney stones; liver cancer. For men: impotence and sterility. For women; menstrual problems. For users who share or use unsterile needles to inject steroids: hepatitis, tetanus, AIDS
Stimulants Amphetamines (uppers, pep pills) Cocaine (coke, flake, snow) Crack (rock) Methamphetamines (ice, crank, crystal) Methylphenidate (Ritalin) Phenmetrazine (Preludin, Preludes) Other stimulants (Adipex, Cylert, Didrex, Ionamin, Melfiat, Plegine, Sanorex, Tenuate, Tepanil, Prelu-2)	Stimulants stimulate the central nervous system, increasing alertness and activity. Users of stimulants develop a tolerance, meaning larger doses must be taken to get the same effect. Stimulants are psychologically addictive.	Increased alertness; excessive activity; agitation; euphoria; excitability; increased pulse rate, blood pressure, and body temperature; insomnia; loss of appetite; sweating; dry mouth and lips; bad breath; disorientation; apathy; hallucinations; irritability; and nervousness	Headaches; depression; malnutrition; hypertension; psychosis; cardiac arrest; damage to the brain and lungs; convulsions; coma; death

From Spradley, B.W., & Allender, J.A. (1996). *Community health nursing* (4th ed.). Philadelphia: Lippincott-Raven.

Trends of Substance Use

How does the community health nurse start the process? First, it is important to know the trends related to substance use across different populations and communities. This information is useful to the community health nurse when developing a prevention program. If the target population is young adults, prevention of heavy episodic (binge) drinking may be a top concern because of the high prevalence of heavy episodic drinking in this population (Toumbourou, Stocwell, Neighbors, Marlatt, & Rehm, 2007). If the target population is the homeless adult then the community health nurse will need to know about chronic alcohol, cocaine, and heroin use in the local homeless community because of the high prevalence of SUDs in this population (Lynch & Greaves, 2000).

Difference Between Legal and Illegal Substance Use

The second step for the community health nurse is to appreciate the difference between legal and illegal substance use. Alcohol and tobacco are legal substances in the United States, but other drugs such as marijuana, heroin, and cocaine are illegal. Use of illegal drugs affects the community not only in relation to the morbidity associated with drug use in individuals but also in relation to problems of drug trafficking and other illegal activities engaged in by the user and the seller. Thus, cultural, environmental, and pharmacological differences related to a specific substance influence the type of community health interventions needed as well as the planned outcomes.

Consequences of Substance Use

The third step is to understand the consequences of substance use that affect a community as a whole. These consequences include violence, motor vehicle crashes, and injuries, especially related to alcohol and illicit drug use (Cherpitel, 2007). These risks are present in all age groups. For example, alcohol use increases the risk for injury in the elderly (Zautcke, Coker, Morris, & Stein-Spencer, 2002).

Another serious consequence to the community is the increased risk of morbidity and mortality related to substance use. This affects the community by decreasing the healthy work force and increasing the cost of providing health care. For example, although protective at low levels of use, alcohol in excess of recommended levels increases the risk of developing serious health consequences, such as cancer or heart disease (Bagnardi, Blangiardo, LaVecchia, & Corrao, 2001). There is no safe level of alcohol consumption during pregnancy; women who drink alcohol during pregnancy are at increased risk for having a baby with fetal alcohol spectrum disorder (FASD) or fetal alcohol syndrome (FAS) (NIAAA, 2006a). Members of the community with FASD and FAS require lifelong support, resulting in increased costs related to education, health care, and social services (Bloss, 1994).

Substance Use and the Environment

The last step is to view substance use from an environmental perspective. The impact of substance use varies based on the substance. Tobacco is an environmental pollutant. Exposure to secondary tobacco smoke increases the risk for health issues related to tobacco use including cancer and respiratory complications. Alcohol interacts with the environment in relation to point of sale. Sociologic studies have demonstrated an increase in motor vehicle crashes related to the location of bars and liquor stores, especially drive-through stores (Scribner, MacKinnon, & Dwyer, 1994, 1995).

The health care objectives addressed within *Healthy People 2010* (USDHHS, 2000) relevant to substance use are listed under Focus Area 26 (Table 27.3). The goal is to "reduce substance abuse to protect the health, safety, and quality of life for all, especially children." Among the 25 objectives listed are reducing the consequences of use, reducing actual use, reducing risk factors associated with harmful use, increasing access to treatment, and supporting policy initiatives.

TABLE 27.3	*Healthy People 2010*–Focus Area 26: Substance Abuse

Goal: Reduce substance abuse to protect the health, safety, and quality of life for all, especially children.

Number	Objective Short Title
Adverse Consequences of Substance Use and Abuse	
26-1	Motor vehicle crash deaths and injuries
26-2	Cirrhosis deaths
26-3	Drug-induced deaths
26-4	Drug-related hospital emergency department visits
26-5	Alcohol-related hospital emergency department visits
26-6	Adolescents riding with a driver who has been drinking
26-7	Alcohol- and drug-related violence
26-8	Lost productivity
Substance Use and Abuse	
26-9	Substance-free youth
26-10	Adolescent and adult use of illicit substances
26-11	Binge drinking
26-12	Average annual alcohol consumption
26-13	Low-risk drinking among adults
26-14	Steroid use among adolescents
26-15	Inhalant use among adolescents
Risk of Substance Use and Abuse	
26-16	Peer disapproval of substance abuse
26-17	Perception of risk associated with substance abuse
Treatment for Substance Abuse	
26-18	Treatment gap for illicit drugs
26-19	Treatment in correctional institutions
26-20	Treatment for injection drug use
26-21	Treatment gap for problem alcohol use
State and Local Efforts	
26-22	Hospital emergency department referrals
26-23	Community partnerships and coalitions
26-24	Administrative license revocation laws
26-25	Blood alcohol concentration (BAC) levels for motor vehicle drivers

Source: National Institutes of Health (NIH), Substance Abuse and Mental Health Services Association (SAMHSA). Retrieved August 20, 2008 from http://www.healthypeople.gov/document/HTML/Volume2/26Substance.htm#_Toc489757831.

EVIDENCE-BASED PRACTICE

Substance Use Prevention with Adolescents: What Works and What Does Not Work?

As nurses, when we move from an individual-based approach to a community-based approach we need to evaluate evidence from a population perspective. A major step in preventing SUDs is to focus on substance use in adolescents. A recent article by Toumbourou et al. (2007) provides us with a well-conducted systematic review of the literature related to the effectiveness of interventions aimed at reducing harm associated with adolescent substance use. A systematic review should be comprehensive and unbiased; it should use a strict scientific design to select and assess research articles. This article is a good example of a rigorous review and provides us with a broad overview of what works and what does not.

The authors examined evidence related to public health policies, harm reduction, prevention, screening, brief intervention, and treatment related to adolescents. They reported that public health policies related to substance use do work, such as taxation and ignition interlocks. They also reported that prevention interventions were more successful when the intervention was maintained over several years and used more than one strategy. They stated that screening and brief intervention holds promise as an effective means of reducing harmful alcohol or tobacco use and there is growing evidence that it may work with other drugs.

They concluded that harm reduction strategies were also effective in reducing harmful substance use. However, for treatment of SUDs with adolescents, the results were inconsistent. In addition, although there is evidence of the efficacy of many practices related to the prevention and treatment of SUDs in adolescents, more research is needed to demonstrate their effectiveness in real-world settings. Therefore, we can with confidence support a number of practices related to prevention of SUDs in adolescents but should also be aware of the need for more field research, especially in relation to treatment.

Prevalence of Substance Use and Substance Use Disorders

This section discusses the prevalence of substance use and SUDs. Different levels of use across populations are described based on the quantity, frequency, duration, and pattern of the use, as well as levels related to the prevalence of dependence. To obtain prevalence data related to substance use, surveys are conducted nationwide on a regular basis. The community health nurse can easily get updates on the results of surveys by accessing the websites of both the NIDA and NIAAA. Prevalence data are reported in different ways, and it is important to distinguish between the types of reports. Some reports focus on consumption rates based on gender, ethnic/racial group, or age group. Others focus on the prevalence of SUDs.

Alcohol

Over 50% of the adult population report current alcohol use. Alcohol is an integral part of the American culture, with 80% of adults reporting use of alcohol over their lifetime. In the United States and other countries, people use alcohol in religious ceremonies, celebrations, and sporting events, and as the beverage of choice at a meal. Unlike other drugs of abuse, alcohol can be consumed in moderation without resulting in alcohol dependence. To help distinguish risky and harmful use from responsible use of alcohol, NIAAA has published recommended drinking limits. For the general male adult population the recommended drinking limits are fewer than five standard drinks daily or 14 weekly. For the general female adult population the recommended drinking limits are fewer than four standard drinks daily or eight weekly, and for people age 65 and older, recommended drinking limits are no more that one standard drink daily or seven standard drinks weekly. The NIAAA recommends that pregnant women and women who may become pregnant abstain from alcohol (NIAAA, 2007).

A standard drink contains about 14 grams of alcohol (0.6 fluid ounces or 1.2 tablespoons) which is equivalent to one 12-ounce bottle of beer or wine cooler; 8 to 9 ounces of malt liquor; one 5-ounce glass of table wine; 3 to 4 ounces of fortified wine; 2 to 3 ounces of cordial, liqueur, or aperitif; 1.5 ounces of brandy; or 1.5 ounces of 80-proof distilled spirits (Fig. 27.2). Heavy use is defined as drinking more than the recommended limits per drinking day, at least five different days in a month. Episodic heavy drinking (binge drinking) is defined as drinking above the recommended limits per drinking occasion at least once in the past month (NIAAA, 2007).

Trends in alcohol use in the United States differ across subsets of the population. Young adults (age 18 to 25) have the highest incidence of problem drinking (Monti, Tevyaw, & Borsari, 2006). Based on recently published information, a little less than 5% of the total population met the criteria for alcohol dependence in 2001–2002. The highest percentage was in the 18 to 29 year age group (6.95%) and the lowest (1.2%) was in those over age 65 (Fig. 27.3) (Grant et al., 2004: NIAAA, 2004).

Although the reported prevalence of alcohol use disorders (AUDs) in the elderly is low, the prevalence of AUDs and alcohol-related consequences in the elderly may increase over the next few decades due to a cohort effect. Currently over 60% of baby boomers (age 45–64) consume alcohol (O'Connell et al., 2004). Another problem is underdetection of AUDs in this population. Thus, current estimates of AUDs in this population may not be a true picture.

One population with the highest prevalence of AUDs is the homeless; AUDs are as high as 84% in homeless men and 58% of homeless women (North et al., 2004). This high prevalence in a population most likely to experience problems with access to treatment can result in increased hospital admissions as well as increased alcohol-related morbidity (Salit, Kuhn, Hartz, Vu, & Mosso, 1998).

Tobacco

Tobacco use is the primary cause of one in every six deaths and is the most prevalent addictive disorder. Encouragingly there has been an overall decline in tobacco use over the

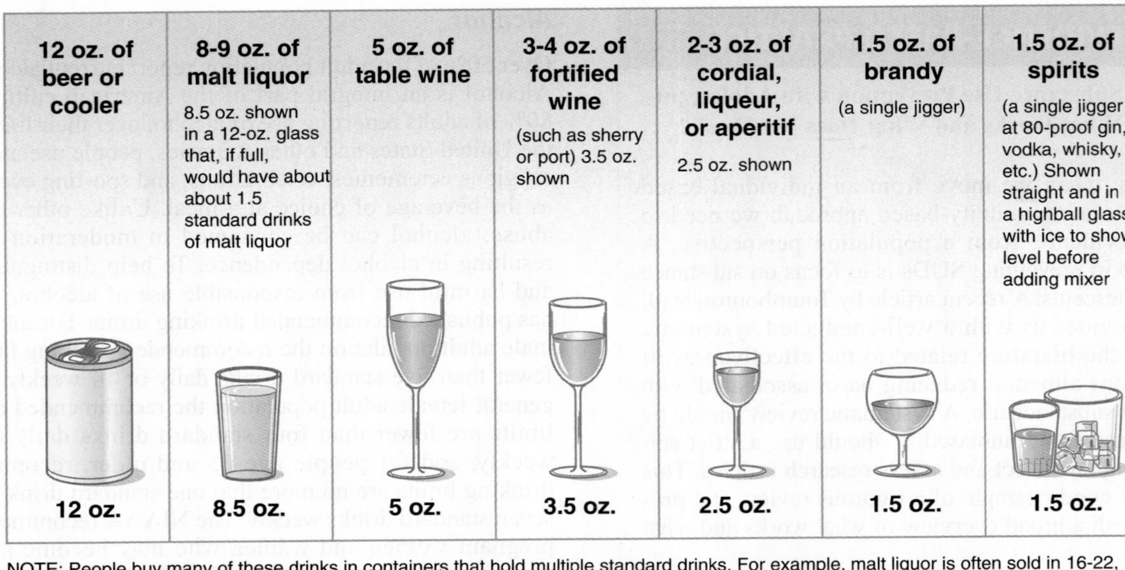

12 oz. of beer or cooler	8-9 oz. of malt liquor	5 oz. of table wine	3-4 oz. of fortified wine	2-3 oz. of cordial, liqueur, or aperitif	1.5 oz. of brandy	1.5 oz. of spirits
	8.5 oz. shown in a 12-oz. glass that, if full, would have about about 1.5 standard drinks of malt liquor		(such as sherry or port) 3.5 oz. shown	2.5 oz. shown	(a single jigger)	(a single jigger at 80-proof gin, vodka, whisky, etc.) Shown straight and in a highball glass with ice to show level before adding mixer
12 oz.	8.5 oz.	5 oz.	3.5 oz.	2.5 oz.	1.5 oz.	1.5 oz.

NOTE: People buy many of these drinks in containers that hold multiple standard drinks. For example, malt liquor is often sold in 16-22, or 40 oz. containers that contain between two and five standard drinks, and table wine is typically sold in 25 oz. (750 ml) bottles that hold five standard drinks.

FIGURE 27.2   Standard drink. Adapted from NIAAA (2007).

past decade, but this decline is not consistent across age groups and genders. An estimated 70.3 million Americans aged 12 or older consumed tobacco. Tobacco consumption includes cigarettes, pipes, cigars, and smokeless tobacco (chew). Between 2001 and 2006, daily tobacco use declined among eighth, tenth, and twelfth graders, but the decline in tobacco use is slowing. The high prevalence of tobacco use among youth is one of the top 10 statistical global public health highlights (WHO, 2007). Also, there is no decline in tobacco use among those with mental illness. Those with a mental illness other than schizophrenia have a prevalence of tobacco use two to four times higher. Ninety percent of those diagnosed with schizophrenia use tobacco (NIDA, 2006).

Other Drugs

The overall national statistics related to illicit drug use are encouraging. In a survey of students in the eighth, tenth, and twelfth grades, reported use of any illicit drug in the past month declined by almost 23% in a five-year period, from 19.4% in 2001 to 14.9% in 2006 (NIDA, 2006) (Fig. 27.4). However, illicit drug use continues in the United States especially among those aged 18 to 25.

Marijuana

Marijuana is the most frequently reported illicit drug. More than 94 million Americans age 12 and older have tried

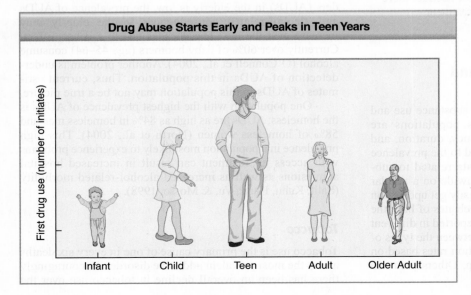

Drug Abuse Starts Early and Peaks in Teen Years

First drug use (number of initiates)

Infant   Child   Teen   Adult   Older Adult

FIGURE 27.3   Prevalence of drug abuse across the lifespan. Adapted from National Institute on Drug Abuse (2006). *Monitoring the Future Survey*. Retrieved August 19, 2008 from http://www.nida.nih.gov/DrugPages/MTF.html.

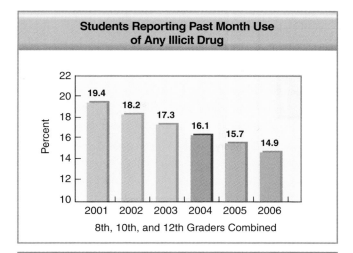

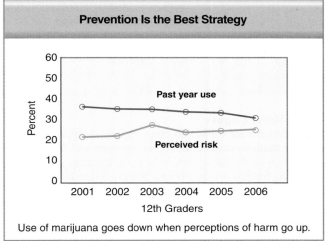

FIGURE 27.4 Trends in illicit drug use in youth. Adapted from National Institute on Drug Abuse. (2006). *Monitoring the Future Survey.* Retrieved August 19, 2008 from http://www.nida.nih.gov/DrugPages/MTF.html.

marijuana at least once, with most current users being adolescents and young adults. Lifetime use by 12th graders has declined slightly (NIAAA, 2006b). However, from 1992 to 2002 the prevalence of marijuana-related disorders increased particularly among older Americans, young Blacks, and Hispanic men (NIDA, 2004a; Zickler, 2005). Compton, Grant, Colliver, Glantz, and Stinson (2004) concluded that one explanation might be the increased potency of marijuana. Another explanation for the increase in use by older Americans may be a possible cohort effect among baby boomers.

Cocaine

Cocaine is a powerful addictive stimulant that directly affects the brain. In 2002, approximately 1.5 million Americans were dependent on or abusing cocaine, the majority of them males between the ages of 18 and 25. There are approximately 2 million current users of cocaine. In a study of 14 metropolitan areas, up to 49% of male offenders tested positive for cocaine. From 1992 to 2002, cocaine-related emergency department visits increased 33% (NIDA, 2004b).

Heroin

According to a 2003 survey, an estimated 3.7 million people had used heroin in their lifetime and more than 314,000 used it in the past year (NIDA, 2006). Most were over age 18 and male. Approximately 57.4% of past-year users were classified with a heroin use disorder. In 2002, approximately 93,000 emergency department visits were related to heroin use.

Meth, Ecstasy, and PCP

There are numerous other drugs of abuse. Examples include methamphetamine, MDMA (methylenedioxymethamphetamine or Ecstasy), phencyclidine (PCP), and inhalants. Methamphetamine use is spreading geographically especially into nontraditional drug use areas, such as the suburban and rural Midwest with an increase in "mom and pop" labs (NIDA, 2004a). MDMA has spread outside the club scene with an increase in emergency department visits related to MDMA. The use of PCP, a drug popularly in use during the late 1980s and early 1990s, has reemerged.

Prescription Drugs

Abuse of prescription drugs occurs across all age groups, and there has been a rise in prescription drug abuse among college students over the last few years (Whitten, 2006). Prescription drugs for managing pain, especially, can be misused. These drugs include oxycodone (OxyContin), a medication designed to alleviate pain related to cancer; hydrocodone (Vicodin); and meperidine (Demerol). Stimulant drugs such as methylphenidate (Ritalin) are also misused.

THEORETICAL FRAMEWORKS

Effective community and population-based interventions begin with the application of specific frameworks that help the planners identify why and how the intervention will work. Two theoretical frameworks used in community/public health science are *process theory* and *effect theory*. They are both part of the Logic Model of Program Theory and are used to plan the program, deliver the program, and evaluate the program (Issel, 2004). In relation to behavioral health, process theory helps the community health nurse identify the resources and structure needed to develop, implement, and evaluate the program. Effect theory provides the rationale for why the intervention will work (Fig. 27.5).

Effect Theory: Component of Program Theory

The challenge for the community health nurse in developing interventions related to behavioral health is the fact that both mental health and substance use have a strong behavioral component. Effect theory is a useful framework for behavioral health. There are four components to the theory: determinant theory, intervention theory, impact theory, and outcome theory (Issel, 2004). Determinant theory relates to what contributes to the health problem. This is an essential component since an intervention usually focuses on one or more determinants of the health problem, either by reducing risk or providing protection against the risk. Intervention theory relates to what is actually being done (see From the Case Files).

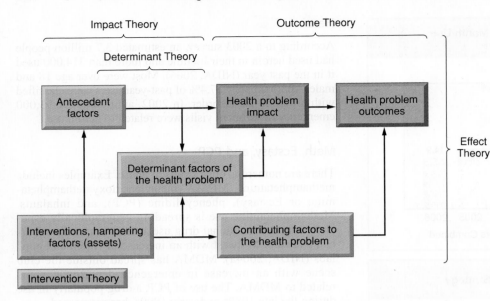

FIGURE 27.5 Elements of Effect Theory, incorporating need or problem statement components. From Issel, L.M. (2004). *Health planning and evaluation*. Boston: Jones and Bartlett Publishers, with permission.

From the Case Files

Smoking Cessation Program for Mothers in a Rural County

You have been working in the public health department well-child clinic in a rural Appalachian county and noticed that more than one-third of the mothers you are seeing are smokers and that their babies seem to be smaller than the babies of moms who do not smoke. When you mention smoking to individual mothers, they tell you they want to stop, but just are not able to. You are interested in putting together a smoking cessation program. You decide to use Issel's effect theory as a framework for building your intervention and convincing the county to fund the program. What data do you need before you begin to look at interventions (see strategy 1 below)? What data can you get using existing databases, and what data will you need to collect yourself? Once you have reviewed the data, you decide that you want to include smoking cessation as part of well-baby visits for all mothers who are current smokers. What do you need to do before you put together the program (see strategy 2 below)? After you have gathered all this information, what final piece is needed before you present your proposal to your public health department (see strategy 3 below)? If you are able to implement the program what immediate impact do you expect to have and what long-term outcomes are you hoping for?

Strategies
1. Preliminary data needed:
   a. Low-birth-weight rates compared to state and national rates. (Available vital statistics public health data)
   b. Low-birth-weight rates for smokers versus nonsmokers in your county, compared with the state and the nation. (Protected vital statistics public health data that will need approval from the state for you to access and analyze)
   c. Comparison of asthma rates in children in your county with smoke-free homes versus homes with a parent smoking. (Available survey data using prior studies, but may not be current. Will most likely need to conduct a survey at the county level. Check with state public health department for state level data.)
   d. County tobacco use rates based on gender and age, and trends among adolescent girls in your county schools compared to state and national rates. (Available public health survey data at state and national levels. May need to conduct a survey at the county level.)
2. A review of the evidence related to smoking-cessation interventions with women of childbearing age. Were any of the studies conducted with Appalachian women? Will you need to make some adjustments to interventions that work based on culture? Are there possible economic constraints for this population in relation to pharmacologic interventions? Are the time frames reasonable in your setting?
3. You need to do an analysis of the cost to implement the program, complete a cost–benefit projection, have clear program goals and objectives, and formulate a plan to evaluate the effectiveness of the program.

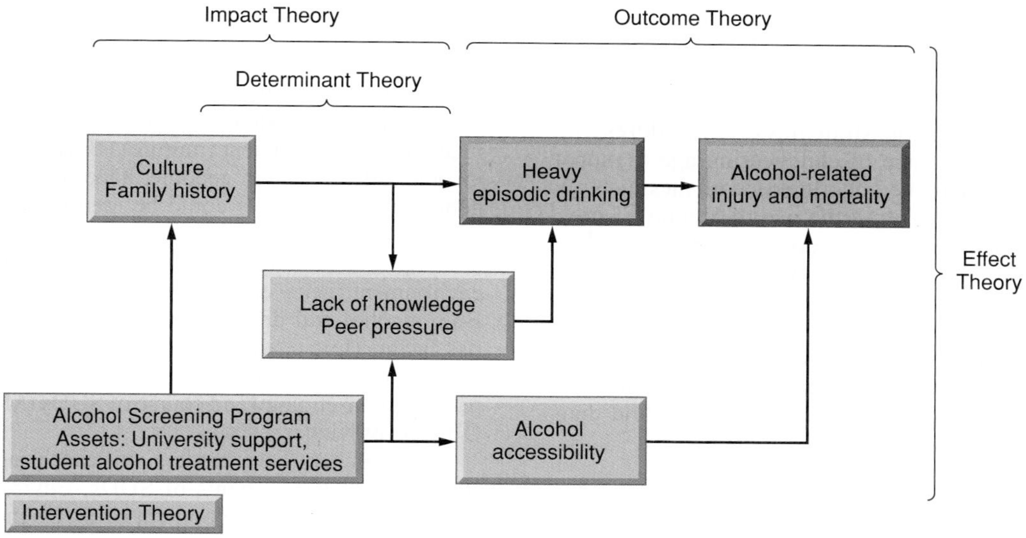

FIGURE 27.6 Elements of Effect Theory, example for reduction of alcohol-related injury and mortality in college students.

The desired health impact refers to the immediate impact expected from the program. For example, if the health problem is heavy episodic (binge) alcohol consumption among college students, a logical approach may be to institute an alcohol-screening program. For such a program the immediate *impact* for the program may be that 25% of students are screened and 75% of those who require a brief intervention and/or a referral for further assessment receive those interventions. However, the desired *outcome* of the program is an overall reduction in heavy episodic alcohol consumption on campus over the next 2 years. Remember that not all desired impact is related to change. The goal may be to stabilize, prevent, or maintain a health state or problem. Having a clear understanding of what a behavioral program can actually accomplish and what long-term goal it hopes to achieve prior to implementing the program will provide a clearer picture of how to proceed with the program.

When using effect theory to design a prevention program for behavioral health, a good place to start is to identify the specific health problem and then the desired health problem impact and health problem outcome (Fig. 27.6). As the program is developed, the community health nurse starts by identifying the antecedent factors that led to behavioral health problems. This provides a clear rationale for why the intervention should provide the desired impact.

Public Health Prevention Theory and Behavioral Health

Three public health models of prevention provide the nurse with a guide to decide what level of prevention is the focus of the program, the type of intervention to use, and the target population. The Centers for Disease Control and Prevention (CDC) (1992) presented two complementary prevention models: the primary, secondary, and tertiary prevention model based on the natural history of disease and the behavioral, clinical, and environmental model based on how the prevention technology is delivered (CDC, 1992; Savage, 2006).

Primary prevention is conducted when no disease is present in the target population, the primary goal being prevention of disease development. Secondary prevention is conducted when the disease is subclinical with no symptoms or early symptoms present, the goal being early identification and treatment. Tertiary prevention is conducted when disease is present with symptoms, the goal being to prevent consequences of the disease, such as disability or death.

Behavioral prevention includes a broad array of strategies aimed at changing lifestyles, (e.g., exercise, smoking cessation, balanced nutrition). It is a complex, sequential process targeted at individuals or groups. The goal of the intervention is to change behaviors that put the person at risk for developing the disease or to prevent consequences of the disease. Clinical prevention is based on the medical model for preventive services. It relies on one-to-one, provider-to-patient interaction and occurs within the traditional health care delivery system. Environmental prevention relies on a societal commitment for the implementation of the interventions and aims to alter the environment by reducing risk (e.g., community-wide decrease in availability of the substance, underage drinking law enforcement).

Another model used in the behavioral health field for developing prevention programs is the model used by the Institute of Medicine (IOM) based on Gordon's model: Classification of Disease Prevention. This model helps to frame the focus of the intervention, relying on three levels of prevention: universal, selected, and indicated. Universal prevention strategies address the entire population (national, local community, school, neighborhood), with messages and programs aimed, for example, at preventing or delaying the abuse of alcohol. Selective prevention strategies target subsets of the total population that are deemed to be at risk for alcohol abuse by virtue of their membership in a particular population segment. Indicated prevention strategies are designed to prevent the onset of abuse in individuals who do not meet DSM-IV, TR criteria for addiction, but who are showing early danger signs, such as falling grades and consumption of alcohol and other gateway drugs (Mrazek & Haggerty, 1994).

One example of the application of this model is a description of different interventions aimed at prevention of FAS. Universal prevention strategies would address the entire population of women of childbearing age (national, local community, school, neighborhood), with messages and programs aimed at preventing the use of alcohol if pregnancy is a possibility. Selective prevention strategies would target subsets of women of childbearing age who are deemed to be at risk for alcohol use by virtue of their membership in a particular population segment. Indicated prevention strategies would be designed to prevent the use of alcohol in pregnant women who had screened positive for alcohol use during pregnancy or already had a child diagnosed with FAS or FASD.

DETERMINANTS OF BEHAVIORAL HEALTH

What determines a person as mentally healthy or mentally ill, or as a casual substance user or a serious substance abuser, is complex. Genetics, environment, the societal frame of reference and context, and other factors play a role.

Determinants of Mental Health

Characterizing mental health versus mental illness is difficult because human beings evolve over the years with varied developmental tasks to achieve at each life stage while confronting day-to-day stressors associated with one's role functions. Complicating the issue is the frame of reference used in each society. Cultural beliefs differ regarding what one's behavior should or should not be and the level of tolerance for certain actions. There are expectations, standards, or legal parameters that put one's actions or behavior in a particular context that suggests health or illness. The APA (2003) defined mental health as *a state of being that is relative rather than absolute. The successful performance of mental functions shown by productive activities, fulfilling relationships with other people, and the ability to adapt to change and to cope with adversity.*

The process of adaptation can be a source of stress. Several factors influence each individual's perception of stress and subsequent response. Lazarus and Folkman (1984) define stress as the person's appraisal of the environment as "taxing" or endangering well-being. This implies that an event's significance is an individual personal experience. Certain elements are involved in this process: genetic factors, such as physical and psychological characteristics; learned patterns of coping or adaptation reinforced over time; and prevailing circumstances in each person's life. Correspondingly, the responses evoked may reflect adaptive or maladaptive functioning as evidenced by thoughts, feelings, and behaviors that are age-appropriate and congruent with sociocultural mores or standards. It is essential that individual coping mechanisms enable the person to function appropriately at home, work, and in various social settings. At times, the situation experienced may be perceived as overwhelming without adequate family or social support systems, thus creating a fertile ground for alcohol or drug dependency as a way of dysfunctional coping.

Determinants of Substance Use Disorders

Determining the etiology of SUDs has challenged researchers for decades. The debate has centered on *nature versus nurture*, that is, how much is related to genetics (nature) and how much to the environment (nurture) (Bozarth, 1990). With the mapping of the human genome, hope has increased that the genes related to SUDs could be identified. Genetics has a major role in the development of alcohol dependence, which is thought to be a multigenomic disorder influenced by the environment (gene–environment interaction) (Hardie, 2007). Both alcohol and drug dependence share common genetic risk factors (Luo et al., 2006). In addition to genetic heritability both personal and environmental factors are involved comparably in the etiology and course of SUDs (McLellan, Lewis, O'Brien, & Kleber, 2000).

Researchers have made significant progress in understanding the determinants of SUDs. Environmental influences connected to development of SUDs include influence of peers, lower socioeconomic status, partner use, and substance use by family members (Kendler et al., 2000; Kilpatrick et al., 2000). Individual factors associated with the development of AUDs include high antisocial behavior, high impulsivity, major depression, social anxiety problems, a history of childhood sexual abuse, hyperactivity, attention problems, and seminal events, such as loss of a spouse in the elderly (Knopik et al. 2004; Poikolainen, 2000; Reinherz et al., 2000).

SCREENING AND BRIEF INTERVENTION IN BEHAVIORAL HEALTH

This section discusses the use of screening in behavioral health as a means for preventing development of mental health and SUDs and for providing early intervention. As mentioned earlier, screening is the presumptive identification of an unrecognized disease or defect by the application of tests, examinations, or other procedures that can be applied rapidly. From an apparently well population, screening tests sort out persons who potentially have or are at increased risk for a disease from those who probably do not have the disease. Screening is the first step in a process that may or may not lead to a diagnosis of disease; it is not intended to be diagnostic. If a screening test result is positive, a diagnostic work-up should follow. Treatment should be initiated after a disease state is diagnosed.

Screening for Mental Health Disorders: BPRS, MADRS, CES-D10

The need for early detection has been highlighted in the New Freedom Commission on Mental Health report (2003). The reports calls for early mental health screening, assessment, and referral to mental health service programs. About 10% of children and adolescents in the United States have a mental illness that impairs functioning, yet only about 20% of this population receive treatment and services. It is critical that community health nurses focus on early detection and treatment of mental illness in this vulnerable population. Notably, suicide in the United States represents a major public health problem resulting in about 3,000 young lives lost every year. About 90% of those who commit suicide have a mental illness (USDHHS, 1999). Reducing suicide among youth requires mental health screening. Several mental health screening programs are available.

The National Depression and Anxiety Screening Day is an example of a community-level mental health awareness, disease-prevention program. The resources and materials, such as a comprehensive kit of materials, promotional information, media campaign, training, and technical assistance, are available by visiting the mental health screening website (see Internet Resources at the end of this chapter).

Every community health clinic can implement a routine screening program to capture mental illness problems early. Standardized screening tools for anxiety or depression are also available, such as the Brief Psychiatric Rating Scale (BPRS) (Fig. 27.7) (Overall & Gorham, 1988); the Beck Depression Scale, and the Montgomery Ashberg Depression Rating Scale (MADRS). The MADRS is known for its utility of administering the instrument from the practitioner standpoint given time constraints in the clinic.

A commonly used screening instrument for depression developed in the late 1970s is the Center for Epidemiologic Studies Depression Scale (CES-D) (Fig. 27.8) (Radloff, 1977). The CES-D and the shorter version, the CES-D 10, have established reliability and validity across populations and cultures and are widely used clinically to screen for depression (Andresen, Malmgren, Carter, & Patrick, 1994; Boey, 1999; Hann, Winter, & Jacobson, 1999; Radloff, 1991).

Screening for Substance Use and Substance Use Disorders

When screening for substance use there are three aspects of screening: screening for actual consumption, screening for at-risk drinking, and screening for SUDs. The use of substances represents a continuum of levels of consumption and associated risks for SUDs as well as health and social consequences related to substance use.

Brief Psychiatric Rating Scale

Indicate assigned patient age, psychiatric diagnoses, brief history of present illness and prior psychiatric history

0 = Not present   1 = Very mild   2 = Mild   3 = Moderate   4 = Moderate   5 = Severe
                                                                    severe

- SOMATIC CONCERN - preoccupation with physical health, fear of physical illness, hypochondriasis

- ANXIETY - worry, fear, over concern for present or future, uneasiness

- CONCEPTUAL DISORGANIZATION - though processes confused, disconnected, disorganized, disrupted

- GUILT FEELINGS - self-blame, shame, remorse for past behavior

- TENSION - physical and motor manifestation of nervousness, over-activation

- MANNERISMS & POSTURING - peculiar, bizarre unnatural motor behavior (except tic)

- GRANDIOSITY - exaggerated self-opinion, arrogance, conviction of unusual power or abilities

- DEPRESSIVE MOOD - sorrow, sadness, despondency, pessimism

- HOSTILITY - animosity, contempt, belligerence, disdain for others

- SUSPICIOUSNESS - mistrust, belief others harbor malicious or discriminatory intent

- HALLUCINATORY BEHAVIOR - perceptions w/o normal external stimulus

- MOTOR RETARDATION - slowed weakened movements or speech, reduced body tone

- UNCOOPERATIVENESS - resistance, guardedness, rejection of authority

- UNUSUAL THOUGHT CONTENT - odd, strange, bizarre thought content

- BLUNTED AFFECT - reduced emotional tone, reduction in formal intensity of feelings; flatness

- EXCITEMENT - heightened emotional tone, agitation, increased reactivity

- DISORIENTATION - confusion or lack of proper association for person, place or time

- NANDA: (Indicate appropriate nursing diagnoses based on observations noted)

FIGURE 27.7 Brief Psychiatric Rating Scale (BPRS). Modified: Andal, E.A. (2005). *Utilization of standardized psychiatric assessment tools in identifying NANDA and NIC-NOC*. N 352 Psychiatric Mental Health Nursing Course. California State University, Bakersfield. Overall, J.E., & Gorham, D.R. (1988). The Brief Psychiatric Rating Scale (BPRS): Recent developments in ascertainment and scaling. *Psychopharmacology Bulletin, 24*, 97–99.

During the past week:	Rarely or none of the time (less than 1 day)	Some or a little of the time (1-2 days)	Occasionally or a moderate amount of time (3-4 days)	Most or all of the time (5-7 days)
1. I was bothered by things that usually don't bother me.	0	1	2	3
2. I had trouble keeping my mind on what I was doing.	0	1	2	3
3. I felt depressed.	0	1	2	3
4. I felt that everything I did was an effort.	0	1	2	3
5. I felt hopeful about the future.	0	1	2	3
6. I felt fearful.	0	1	2	3
7. My sleep was restless.	0	1	2	3
8. I was happy.	0	1	2	3
9. I felt lonely.	0	1	2	3
10. I could not get going.	0	1	2	3

FIGURE 27.8 The Short Center for Epidemiologic Studies Depression Scale (CESD-10). From Radloff, L. (1977). The CES-D Scale: A self report depression scale for research in the general population. *Applied Psychological Measurement, 1,* 385–401. Stanford Patient Education Research Center. (n.d.). *Center for Epidemiologic Studies Short Depression Scale (CES-D 10).* Retrieved October 17, 2008 from http://patienteducation.stanford.edu/research/cesd10.pdf.

Level of Risk

Essentially, the continuum of use is based on the level of consumption (Fig. 27.1). This model is well developed in relation to alcohol consumption and serves as a model for understanding risk and how to interpret the screening results (Babor et al., 2001).

Screening Instruments: Self-reports

The recommendations for screening are well developed and validated in relation to alcohol use and tobacco use. There is less evidence to support the use of a specific screening approach related to other drug use, both illicit and licit. However, the evidence is growing and a growing body of literature supports screening for substance use as a standard of care for all health professionals (Hack & Adger, 2002). The difficulty is to choose a screening instrument that will allow the clinician to screen for consumption, pattern, duration of use, and SUDs, but not all screening instruments include all elements. The other difficulty is determining whether the screening instrument has known sensitivity and specificity in the target population. For most screening instruments the sensitivity and specificity information is based on a general population and may not be as reliable for populations such as pregnant women or the elderly (O'Connell et al., 2004; Savage et al., 2003).

Health researchers began developing and testing screening instruments aimed at identifying SUDs in the 1970s. Examples of these instruments include the Michigan Alcoholism Screening Test (MAST) (Selzer, 1971), the Drug Abuse Screening Test (Skinner, 1982), and the CAGE questionnaire (Ewing, 1984). These self-report instruments were developed for general adult populations with a focus on dependence. They were designed to distinguish persons who probably *are* dependent from those who apparently *are not.* If the clinician only uses a tool that screens for dependence and does not

screen for consumption or onset of consumption, then valuable clinical information may be missing since consumption in general puts a person at risk for negative consequences, such as injury and the potential of negative interactions with other medications. Thus levels and patterns of consumption are as important as early identification of an SUD.

For the community health nurse, screening programs are a valuable prevention tool. Prior to developing a screening program it is important to establish what the screening is for (consumption and/or SUDs) and the target population as well. Then an appropriate screening tool can be chosen.

Two main methods of screening for substance use are self-report and biologic markers. Self-report relies on the person to complete a screening instrument. Examples of screening instruments for alcohol use include the Alcohol Use Disorders Identification Test (AUDIT) (Fig. 27.9) (Babor et al., 2001) and the CAGE questionnaire (Ewing, 1984). Examples of screening instruments for drug use include the Drug Abuse Screening Test (DAST) (Skinner, 1982) and the Drug Use Screening Inventory (DUSI) (Tarter, 1990). These instruments vary based on length and whether or not they include questions related to quantity and frequency. For alcohol use, the screening instrument recommended by the NIAAA is the AUDIT (NIAAA, 2007). The WHO developed this instrument for use across populations, and it has established high reliability and validity across ethnic groups (Reinhart & Allen, 2007).

Biologic Screens

Biologic markers used to detect substance use include urine, blood, hair, saliva, breath, and meconium. In contrast to self-report, biologic markers provide either direct or indirect evidence of use (Helander, 2001). They are used with self-report as a means of providing corroborating evidence of use (Allen & Litten, 2001). Factors that influence sensitivity and specificity of biologic markers include other metabolic disorders or other diseases, medication use, and reliability of

During the past 6 months:

1. How often do you have a drink containing alcohol?
Never (0)
Monthly or less (1)
Two to four times a month (2)
Two to three times a week (3)
Four or more times a week (4)

2. How many drinks containing alcohol do you have on a typical day when you are drinking?
1 or 2 (0)
3 or 4 (1)
5 or 6 (2)
7 to 9 (3)

3. How often do you have six or more drinks on one occasion?
Never (0)
Less than monthly (1)
Monthly (2)
Weekly (3)

4. How often during the last year have you found that you were not able to stop drinking once you had started?
Never (0)
Less than monthly (1)
Monthly (2)
Weekly (3)

5. How often during the last year have you failed to do what was normally expected from you because of drinking?
Never (0)
Less than monthly (1)
Monthly (2)
Weekly (3)
Daily or almost daily (4)

6. How often during the last year have you needed a first drink in the morning to get yourself going after a heavy drinking session?
Never (0)
Less than monthly (1)
Monthly (2)
Weekly (3)
Daily or almost daily (4)

7. How often during the last year have you had a feeling of guilt or remorse after drinking?
Never (0)
Less than monthly (1)
Monthly (2)
Weekly (3)
Daily or almost daily (4)

8. How often during the last year have you been unable to remember what happened the night before because you had been drinking?
Never (0)
Less than monthly (1)
Monthly (2)
Weekly (3)
Daily or almost daily (4)

9. Have you or someone else been injured as a result of your drinking?
No (0)
Yes, but not in the last year (2)
Yes, during the last year (4)

10. Has a relative or friend, or a doctor or other health worker been concerned about your drinking, or suggested you cut down?
No (0)
Yes, but not in the last year (2)
Yes, during the last year (4)

AUDIT Score _____

FIGURE 27.9 Alcohol Use Disorders Identification Test (AUDIT). Adapted from Babor, T.F., Higgins-Biddle, J.C., Saunders, J.B., & Monteiro, M.G. (2001). *The Alcohol Use Disorders Identification Test: Guidelines for use in primary care* (2nd ed.). World Health Organization. Retrived February 8, 2007 from http://drugsandstuff.co.uk/drugs/resources/publication_pdfs_etc/auditbro.pdf.

the method (Musshuff & Daldrup, 1998; Sommers, Wray, Savage, & Dyehouse, 2003). They are rarely used in a community-based screening program due to the cost and the problems with obtaining biologic specimens. Various groups, such as legal authorities, employers, or sports programs, use biologic markers to verify alcohol or drug use.

When developing a screening program for substance use the community health nurse must take a number of things into account. First, a screening program has to be prepared to provide or be able to refer persons who have a positive screen to the appropriate level of services. Since substance use occurs across a continuum, a screening program may identify persons with risky use who may not have a substance use disorder. Therefore, a program should have links to clinically appropriate treatment services for nondependent substance users as well as for dependent substance users. This usually involves having linkages with community agencies that provide substance abuse treatment. Therefore, it is important to know communities' treatment capacity.

Brief Intervention for Positive Screens

When planning a screening program related to substance abuse, some of the participants in the program will screen positive for risky or hazardous use and are candidates for a Brief Intervention (BI). A BI for alcohol use can be done by any trained health care provider and can be completed in a short time. A BI generally lasts from 5 to 15 minutes, usually over one to three sessions. Strong research evidence exists for the use of BI for heavy or excess nondependent drinkers, especially those identified in primary care settings (NIAAA, 2007). As a whole, providing a BI is generally more effective in the year after delivery than if no intervention is given at all (Sommers, 2007). Less work has been done with other substances.

COMMUNITY-LEVEL INTERVENTIONS

As described in Chapter 15 the community health nurse begins with a community assessment in order to complete a community diagnosis. Once the nurse establishes a diagnosis, the next step is to decide on an intervention that can address the specific public health issue identified in the diagnosis. A good starting point in the development of community/public health intervention is to begin with the *Healthy People 2010* objectives (Tables 27.1 and 27.3). The nurse can review the objectives and locate the specific focus area that matches the community diagnosis. For example, if the community diagnosis relates to an increase in alcohol-related motor vehicle crashes in adolescents, there are two specific *Healthy People 2010* objectives related to that issue: reduction in motor vehicle crashes and deaths, and reduction in adolescents riding with a driver who has been drinking.

Level of Intervention from a Community Health Perspective

Once the nurse identifies the focus of the intervention, the next step is to determine the level of prevention (see Chapter 14 for more information on theoretical frameworks). First, the natural history of disease provides the framework for the traditional public health model of primary, secondary, and tertiary prevention. The next step is to decide on the type of intervention: clinical, environmental, or behavioral. The final model relates to the scope of the intervention: universal, selected, or indicated. Because a motor vehicle crash is an event rather than a disease, the desired outcome is to reduce the number of those events related to a behavior rather than a disease. Thus the prevention of SUDs is not the focus but rather the behavior of drinking while driving. Therefore, neither a screening program (secondary prevention) nor an alcohol treatment program (tertiary prevention) is needed. Considering also that almost all adolescents either drive or ride with other adolescents, a primary behavioral intervention using a universal approach would probably work best to address this problem.

Mental Health Community Interventions

"Integrative health assessment" has gained momentum in various health centers as a method for decreasing utilization of unwarranted procedures. The underlying premise here is that a person experiencing some personal trials and tribulations may manifest the stress through physical manifestations. There is greater recognition of the mind and body interaction. Accordingly, approaches to mental health promotion encompass physical, emotional, sociocultural, and intellectual considerations. Integrative health assessment is the process of identifying relevant factors, such as the following:

1. Treatment history relative to mental or emotions issues. This includes the visit to a psychologist or mental health professional for complaints of anxiety or periods of loneliness.
2. Personal life stressors. Each day, there are daily tasks relative to one's age and appropriate role function. This may be as a parent, provider, or

employee. Some subtle manifestations include irritability, impulsiveness, or frustration intolerance that the individual cannot cope with in a socially appropriate manner.
3. Disturbances in sleep, appetite, or energy level that are not attributable to a rational explanation given the person's daily lifestyle.
4. Complaints of chronic pain of somatic nature that is not attributable to a physical dysfunction.
5. History of abuse, trauma, substance use, and family history of mental illness.

One best practice of note is the Intermountain Healthcare program at Salt Lake City, Utah. Information about "mental health integration" can be accessed via the center's website (see Internet Resources).

Today, the community population is subjected to many uncertainties through instantaneous worldwide communication systems. Threats to personal or family safety are basic to mental health. Problems in global peace, the possibility of bioterrorism, or threats of natural disasters or calamities are unsettling. The exposure to fear and anxiety from disseminated information has untold psychological implications. For instance, the tragic news of the 2007 Virginia Tech student massacre immediately reached the global population via the Internet and was repeatedly aired via television and radio. Everyone felt shock and sorrow, although indirectly. It is clear that the psychological trauma imposed by events of this nature has implications for everyone's mental well-being.

Mental Health Promotion

As the field of mental health services has matured through advances in epidemiologic methods, research, and treatment, interest in illness prevention and health promotion has increased (USDHHS, 1999). Treatment and prevention of mental illness are important and ongoing priorities in community mental health, but promoting mental health, which is essential to healthier people for the future, needs greater emphasis.

Anticipated Outcomes of Mental Health Promotion

Mental health includes the successful performance of mental function that results in (1) productive activities, (2) fulfilling relationships, (3) the ability to adapt to change, and (4) the ability to cope with adversity. Targeting of these areas becomes a way of prioritizing in planning for health-promoting interventions. Designing programs in community mental health settings encourage productive activities (e.g., sports, hobbies), fulfilling relationships (e.g., foster grandparenting), adapting to change (e.g., volunteering), and coping with adversity (e.g., preparing for developmental crises) (USDHHS, 1999).

Interventions for Mental Health Promotion

Several different approaches can be used in designing interventions for mental health promotion. Two of them are discussed here: development of interventions to protect people who are potentially at risk for mental disorders, and promotion of healthy activities and lifestyles to the general public.

Risk-protective Activities

Epidemiologic data, along with the results of a growing body of other kinds of research, provide the community mental health nurse with increasing information about the factors that place people at risk for mental disorders. Targeting at-risk individuals with health promotion interventions gives them the resources needed to raise their own levels of health and protects them from mental disorders. It is known, for example, that consumption of alcohol, illegal drugs, and tobacco during pregnancy can damage the fetus. Consequently, extensive prenatal education and support programs can promote parental health and reduce this risk for the next generation. It also is known that abuse and neglect during childhood are risk factors for certain mental disorders. Promoting healthy parenting and stress-reducing activities through classes, group work, and other means can promote the health of parents and protect the health of their children.

Lifestyle and Behavior Activities

To promote the well-being of the public, health promotion interventions that are both life-sustaining and life-enhancing can be planned. Life-sustaining activities include proper nutrition and exercise, healthy sleep patterns and adequate rest, healthy coping with stress, and the ability to use family and community supports and resources. Health promotion programs in the community may address any or all of these. An example is educating schoolchildren about the food guide pyramid and encouraging healthy snacks and well-balanced meals in the home. Other examples include fitness programs for all ages, promotion of community playgrounds and walking or biking trails, and establishing networks of support in the community such as Meals on Wheels and other volunteer programs.

Life-enhancing activities include meaningful work, whether through or outside of employment, creative outlets, interpersonal relationships, recreational activities, and opportunities for spiritual and intellectual growth. Again, mental health promotion interventions can address any or all of these areas. For example, arts and crafts classes and fairs encourage creative expression, community sports events promote social outlets, participation in Elderhostel and other kinds of learning experiences promote spiritual and intellectual stimulation, volunteer programs encourage community participation, and classes to develop new skills promote meaningful vocation.

Role of the Community Mental Health Nurse

The nurse's role in community mental health is multifaceted; this has been evident throughout the chapter. First of all, the nurse must be able to *access and use epidemiologic data* to understand and serve the mentally ill population. This means identifying the incidence and prevalence of mental disorders, examining the causes and risk factors associated with mental illness, and identifying the needs of people with mental disorders. Nurses sometimes serve as part of the epidemiologic investigative team to conduct surveys and assist with data collection.

Advocacy

Next, an important part of the nurse's role with the mentally ill is *advocacy.* In this role, the nurse seeks to increase client access to mental health services, to reduce stigma and promote improved public understanding of this population, and to improve services in community mental health. The advocacy role requires being politically involved by serving on decision-making boards and committees, lobbying for legislative changes, and helping to influence mental health policy development that will better serve this population. Membership in state and national nursing organizations can be helpful in establishing collaborative partnerships to benefit the mentally ill. Membership in the National Alliance for the Mentally Ill (NAMI, 2001) or other advocacy groups can also effect positive change.

In any of these venues, the vision and expertise of the community mental health nurse can be used to advocate for enhancing existing services, developing new services, and increasing access for the mentally ill to all services.

Education

Another aspect of the nurse's role is *education.* The community mental health nurse teaches clients individually and in groups about their mental health conditions, their treatment protocols, ways to function more independently in the community, prevention and health-promoting strategies, and much more. The nurse also teaches the public through community education programs and has an educational role with caregivers, family and community members, and health care decision makers by providing information for service planning.

Case Management, Finding, and Referral

Case management for persons with SMIs is also part of the community mental health nurse's role. This includes screening, assessment, care planning, arranging for service delivery, monitoring, reassessment, evaluation, and discharge. It is often offered within the context of a community mental health center (CMHC). Case management helps the person with an SMI to access services and live as independently as possible.

The nurse's role also involves *case-finding and referral.* This means early identification of persons with mental disorders who are in need of treatment and referral of those persons to the appropriate resources for treatment. The purpose of this role is secondary prevention, because early identification and treatment help to ameliorate the severity of the mental disorder and promote a speedier recovery.

Collaboration

Finally, the nurse's role includes *collaboration.* Whether serving individual clients, groups, or populations, the nurse is part of the larger community mental health team and works in collaboration with many people to accomplish the goals of community mental health. The composition of the team—made up of clients, psychiatric nurses, physicians, social workers, nutritionists, epidemiologists, psychologists, health planners, and many more—is diverse and varies depending on the community health nurse's work setting. Collaboration allows for a pooling of professional expertise that enhances the quality and effectiveness of services for the mentally ill.

When working with the mentally ill, the nurse must be aware of issues of personal safety. Although most mentally ill clients are no more prone to violence than the population at large, conditions involving paranoia, hallucinations, or mania can increase clients' tendency toward physical violence. There are situations in which social workers, physicians, or nurses have been harmed by psychotic clients. Clients who are under the influence of drugs or alcohol pose a potentially serious threat to the nurse's safety. The nurse should be prepared for this eventuality with those clients suffering from addictions. Nurses working with this population must use caution in any situation that suggests danger and must take action immediately to protect themselves and their clients. This may require the nurse to take self-defense classes or assertiveness training or to carry protective gear. It may help to use an escort from a security service, collaborate with the police, or establish a "buddy system" in which two nurses work together in isolated or dangerous homes or areas. Additionally, the public health agency may consider hiring risk-management consultants to examine dangerous situations and recommend actions to preserve safety.

The nurse serving in community mental health plays many roles that are practiced in a variety of settings in collaboration with other members of the community mental health team. It is the challenge of this role and the opportunity to assist in raising the level of mental health for individuals and communities that make this field of practice so rewarding.

In this century (and beyond) community living is characterized by heightened stress and anxiety levels with daily life impacted by traffic congestion, rising fuel costs, threats of global warming and environmental pollution, increased divorce rates, deterioration of the basic family as a unit, continued reliance on the judicial system to resolve family and social conflicts, and incidence of crimes via the Internet. Indeed, individually and collectively, mental health and wellness must be a *national priority*. Healthy bodies necessitate a healthy mind.

Community organizations, religious groups, and educational institutions play critical roles in enhancing mental wellness by helping each person through the provision of family support as the basic unit of the community. The National Alliance on Mental Illness (NAMI) is a nationwide organization with chapters in each state and county. NAMI's website contains extensive information that can be utilized by both consumer and care provider. As a national organization, NAMI is committed to enhance the care of those with mental illness and improve the quality of life of those who are affected. NAMI has the "Families to Families" program designed to provide education to families and help them learn the requisite skills in caring for a mentally ill family member. Another NAMI program is called "Peer to Peer." This is a support group designed to help the consumers cope with the illness and live productive lives.

Nonprofit organizations focus on advocacy, education, service, and funding research endeavors. Mental Health America (formerly known as the National Mental Health Association [NMHA]) is a leading nonprofit organization that promotes mental health. In its position statement, the organization urged the federal government to address the need for comprehensive, community- and strengths-based, consumer- and family-driven mental health programs. The organization was established in 1909 as a reform movement by former psychiatric patient Clifford W. Beers who experienced abuse during his stay in public and private mental institutions.

Substance Use and Community-level Interventions

The National Alcohol Screening Day (NASD) is an example of a population-based nationwide screening program aimed at identifying persons with alcohol use disorders. The program is designed to be implemented on the community level in settings such as primary care, college campuses, the work place, or faith-based agencies. For a small registration fee, NASD supplies community organizations with a screening kit that provides all the necessary information needed to conduct the screening program. This model has the national organization providing the media support and the tools for conducting a community-screening program while the agency supplies the clinicians and facilities for conducting the screening program.

Another example of obtaining ready-made population-based screening programs is to use a company that specializes in conducting such programs. For example, an employer may need a more intensive screening program that includes biologic markers as well as self-report. These programs follow current legal requirements for screening and have higher costs. Another population-based approach to screening for substance use is online screening. A participant can complete a self-report screening tool. Such an approach helps protect the anonymity of the participant. To be effective the program should include a means to connect those who screen positive to health care providers.

Two government agencies provide a major resource for the community health nurse in the development, implementation, and evaluation of programs aimed at the prevention and treatment of SUDs: the Center for Substance Abuse Prevention (CSAP) and the Center for Substance Abuse Treatment (CSAT). They are both divisions of Substance Abuse and Mental Health Services Association (SAMHSA) and have user-friendly websites. Their published programs are evidenced-based and often include resources needed to implement the programs, such as brochures.

Community efforts are essential because only 10% of persons who are in need of treatment seek it. Using a broader community approach can result in reducing harm to the community, preventing the development of SUDs, and reducing the burden of disease on the population.

Policy-based Interventions

Not-for-profit, private for-profit, and governmental agencies play crucial roles in community health care. The provision of health care to the population requires multidisciplinary approaches that are driven by monetary reimbursements based on health care problems. Community mental health care policies may be instituted by local governments relative to administrative processes or procedural mechanisms. In contrast, however, at the national level the Tax Equity and Fiscal Responsibility Act (TEFRA), put in place in 1985, brought sweeping changes relative to capital outlay expenditures, hospital lengths of stay, and use of outpatient and home care services. This policy change directly and indirectly impacted the health care system.

Policies at the community or state levels aim to ensure the rights of individuals and public safety. Thus, cities or counties with appropriate jurisdiction over a geographic area develop policies and guidelines necessary to encourage mental health program development and implementations that address the needs of the community population. Depending on each county, certain rules or regulations apply. It is important to learn about the community agencies and interrelationships to other county service providers to ensure the coordination of care. At the local level are free-standing programs that focus on support for individuals, families, the indigent, or the homeless. Funding may come from charitable organizations or from local governments through grant moneys obtained from periodic requests for proposals (RFPs) or requests for applications (RFAs) issued by the local governing body. Other governmental agencies have roles in mental health by encouraging employee wellness in the workplace or through rules and regulations that encourage employers to provide benefits, such as mental health insurance, bereavement leave, or stress leave. The incidence of violence in the workplace has necessitated policy initiatives within the business community to respond by developing strategic plans and providing educational programs that address these issues.

Mental Health Policy

In June 2002, a 22-member commission was established by President George W. Bush to analyze the public and private mental health systems, visit innovative model programs throughout the United States, and hear testimony from the mental health systems' stakeholders and from the consumers of mental health care, their families, advocates, public and private providers, administrators and mental health researchers. Fifteen subcommittees were established to examine specific aspects of mental health services and delineate recommendations for improving delivery of care. The final report was submitted to the President in May 2003. The Commission's PowerPoint presentations are all available on-line (see the New Freedom Commission on Mental Health in the Internet Resources section at the end of this chapter). This provides guidance to health practitioners for the delivery and access to mental health services across the spectrum of care.

The WHO, at the international level, provides assistance to each country's policy makers and planners in developing a plan for the population's mental health by utilizing available resources including promoting human rights, enhancing health, and minimizing debility from mental disorders. Many projects involve technical assistance training on comprehensive strategic planning. The WHO Mental Health Policy Project is developing guidelines for use by countries. The guidelines will serve as a framework for the creation of policies and services that, when implemented, can lead to improved mental health care, treatment, and promotion. Specifically the project stresses that mental health outcomes can be optimized when:

◆ Mental health is an essential component of public health,
◆ Government policies and actions protect and promote the mental health and well-being of its peoples,
◆ Services are appropriate, accountable, accessible, and equitable, and
◆ People are treated in the least restrictive and intrusive manner. (WHO, n.d.)

Substance Use Policy

Policy related to substance use is defined broadly as any purposeful act on the part of a governmental or nongovernmental group to minimize or prevent adverse consequences related to use of potentially addictive substances. Specific strategies include implementing a law aimed at reducing use, such as taxation or a means to allocate resources related to prevention and/or treatment priorities (Babor et al., 2003).

One consistently used policy approach involves regulating the availability of the substance (AlcoholPolicyMD.com, 2005). In relation to illicit drugs, laws are in place that restrict availability through the classification of the drug. For alcohol and tobacco there are regulations on who may buy and who may sell the products. Other examples of governmental regulations related to alcohol and tobacco include drinking and driving laws, regulation of alcohol and tobacco promotion, regulations pertinent to bars, interlocks for individuals who drive drunk repeatedly, and limits on product outlet density (Toumbourou et al., 2007).

Policies in relation to alcohol and tobacco have a similar approach. Communities set policies that restrict both alcohol availability and consumption. This is done by controlling the number of alcohol outlets, regulating the current outlets, and setting laws that will allow the community to close problem outlets. These measures are implemented through policies related to zoning and the licensing of establishments that sell alcohol. Another measure has been to require responsible alcohol-service training for bartenders. Other examples include keg registration, stricter enforcement of underage sales of alcohol and tobacco, and controlling alcohol outlet density. Major efforts in relation to tobacco consumption in public areas have resulted in a drastic restriction of locations where tobacco users can smoke outside of their own home.

The focus of most policies related to illicit drugs has been to enact laws that criminalize the possession and sale of these substances. Other types of policies that have relevance, for example, are those enacted to prevent methamphetamine use. A number of states have restricted the sale of over-the-counter (OTC) medications that can be used to manufacture methamphetamine in home laboratories. The government enacted a major initiative when federal funding

---

DISPLAY 27.2 **HEALTHY PEOPLE 2010 LEADING HEALTH INDICATORS**

Top Ten Health Indicators
1. Physical Activity
2. Overweight and Obesity
3. Tobacco Use
4. Substance Abuse
5. Responsible Sexual Behavior
6. Mental Health
7. Injury and Violence
8. Environmental Quality
9. Immunization
10. Access to Health Care

was linked to a drug-free workplace. That is, any organization that receives federal funds, such as health care facilities that receive Medicare payments, must follow the SAMHSA guidelines (SAMHSA, n.d.).

Summary

Behavioral health is a key component in the health of a community. Six of the top ten health indicators from *Healthy People 2010* are closely linked to behavioral health issues: tobacco use, substance use, responsible sexual behavior, mental health, injury and violence, and access to health care (Display 27.2). In every community in the United States and the world, behavioral health directly or indirectly affects every other indicator of health. Harmful substance use overburdens the medical, social, economic, and criminal justice systems of communities and governments.

Researchers have devoted decades to determining the etiology of substance use disorders specifically with regard to *nature versus nurture*—in other words, whether SUDs occur as a result of genetics or environment. Both alcohol and drug dependence share common genetic risk factors, but are also influenced by environmental factors (influence of peers, lower socioeconomic status, partner use, and substance use by family members) and personal factors (high antisocial behavior, high impulsivity, major depression, social anxiety problems, a history of childhood sexual abuse, hyperactivity, attention problems, and seminal events).

Treatment related to behavioral health at the community level begins with a community assessment in order to establish a community diagnosis, followed by intervention that can address the specific public health issue identified in the diagnosis. The community health nurse can use *Healthy People 2010* objectives as a starting point in the development of an intervention.

The community health nurse must incorporate behavioral health in the assessment, planning, and developing of community health interventions and in the evaluation of outcomes. With this comes the need for administrative, managerial, or supervisory support with commitment not only from a philosophical perspective but from a resource perspective as well. Success comes with a unified approach to mental health and substance use, requiring application of research, utilization of best practice models at the clinical level, and education of all concerned. ■

ACTIVITIES TO PROMOTE CRITICAL THINKING

1. As a community health nurse, you have been asked to design and present a 2-hour program on suicide prevention to the entire student body of the local high school. This activity is representative of which level of prevention? What are some of the considerations involved in planning this program to promote optimal success? How might you measure the effectiveness of this intervention?

2. You are part of a multidisciplinary team whose goal is to identify families in your city who are at risk for crisis (e.g., single parent, divorce, teen pregnancy, loss of job) and develop a set of interventions. How would you determine who these families are? What interventions would be appropriate to meet their needs? What level of prevention would you be targeting?

3. You have met a few elderly men in your area who live alone and are widowed, and you have heard that there are others. Assuming your advocacy role in community mental health, you decide to take some action to ensure that their needs are being met. How would you determine the risks and needs for this group? What interventions would be appropriate to meet their needs?

4. Select a problem that places people at risk for mental disorders (e.g., child abuse and neglect, drug abuse) and do a search on the Internet to learn all you can about it. What is the incidence and prevalence of this problem? What interventions are most effective in addressing it? What can be done to prevent it?

References

AlcoholPolicyMD.com. (2005). *The relationship between alcohol availability and injury and crime.* Retrieved August 19, 2008 from http://www.alcoholpolicymd.com/press_room/brochures/bi_availability_crime.htm.

Allen, J.P., & Litten, R.Z. (2001). The role of laboratory tests in alcoholism treatment. *Journal of Substance Abuse Treatment, 20*(1), 81–85.

American Psychiatric Association. (2000). *Diagnostic and statistical manual of mental disorders.* [Text revision (DSM-IV-TR), (4th ed.)]. Washington, DC: Author.

American Psychiatric Association. (2003). *American psychiatric glossary,* 8th ed. Washington, DC: Author.

Andresen, E.M., Malmgren, J.A., Carter, W.B., & Patrick, D. L. (1994). Screening for depression in well older adults: Evaluation of the short form of the CES-D (Center for Epidemiologic Studies Depression Scale). *American Journal of Preventive Medicine, 10*(2), 77–84.

Armstrong, M., Feigenbaum, J., Savage, C.L., & Vourakis, C. (Eds.). (2006). *Addictions nursing, core curriculum,* 2nd ed. Raleigh, NC: International Nurses Society on Addiction.

Babor, T.F., Caetano, R., Casswell, S., et al. (2003). *Alcohol: No ordinary commodity: Research and public policy.* Oxford, England: Oxford University Press.

Babor, T.F., Higgins-Biddle, J.C., Saunders, J.B., & Monteiro, M.G. (2001). *The Alcohol Use Disorders Identification Test: Guidelines for use in primary care,* 2nd ed. World Health Organization. Retrieved February 8, 2007 from http://drugsandstuff.co.uk/drugs/resources/publications_pdfs_etc/auditbro.pdf.

Bagnardi, V., Blangiardo, M., LaVecchia, C., & Corrao, G. (2001) A meta-analysis of alcohol drinking and cancer risk. *British Journal of Cancer, 85,* 1700–1705.

Bloss, G. (1994). The economic cost of FAS. *Alcohol Health and Research World, 18*(1), 53–55.

Boey, K.W. (1999). Cross-validation of a short form of the CESD-D in Chinese elderly. *International Journal of Geriatric Psychiatry, 4*(8), 608–617.

Bozarth, M.A. (1990): Drug addiction as a psychobiologic process. In D.M. Warburton (Ed.). *Addiction controversies.* (pp. 112–134).

London: Harwood Academic Publishers. Retrieved August 19, 2008 from http://wings.buffalo.edu/aru/ARUreport04.html.

Centers for Disease Control and Prevention. (1992). A framework for assessing the effectiveness of disease and injury prevention. *Morbidity and Mortality Weekly Report, 41*(RR-3), (inclusive page numbers).

Centers for Disease Control and Prevention. (2006). Homicides and Suicides: National Violent Death Reporting System, United States, 2003–2004. *Mortality and Morbidity Weekly Report, 55*(26), 721–724.

Cherpitel, C.J. (2007). Alcohol and injuries: A review of international emergency room studies since 1995. *Drug and Alcohol Review, 26,* 201–214.

Commission on Mental Health. (2003). *Final Report for the President's New Freedom Commission on Mental Health.* Retrieved August 19, 2008 from http://www.mentalhealth commission.gov/background.html.

Compton, W.M., Grant, B.F., Colliver, J.D., Glantz, M.D., & Stinson, F.S. (2004). Prevalence of marijuana use disorders in the United States: 1991–1992 and 2001–2002. JAMA, 291(17): 2114–2121.

D'Amore, J., Hung, O., Chiang, W., & Goldfrank, L. (2001). The epidemiology of the homeless population and its impact on an urban emergency department. *Academic Emergency Medicine, 8,* 1051–1055.

Ewing, J.A. (1984). Detecting Alcoholism: The CAGE Questionnaire. *Journal of the American Medical Association, 252,* 1905–1907.

Grant, B.F., Dawson, D.A., Stinson, F.S., Chou, S.P., Dufour, M.C., & Pickering, R.P. (2004). The 12-month prevalence and trends in DSM-IV alcohol abuse and dependence: United States, 1991–1992 and 2001–2002. *Drug Alcohol Dependence,* 74(3), 223–234.

Greater Cincinnati Coalition for the Homeless. (2001). *Homeless in Cincinnati: A study of the causes and conditions of homelessness: Executive summary.* Cincinnati, OH: Author. Retrieved August 19, 2008 from http://www.airinc.org/Homelessness%20in% 20Cincinnat.htm.

Hack, M.R., & Adger, H. (2002). Strategic plan for interdisciplinary faculty development: Arming the nation's health professional workforce for a new approach to substance use disorders. *Substance Abuse, 23*(3), 1–12.

Hann, D., Winter, K., & Jacobson, P. (1999). Measurement of depressive symptoms in cancer patients: Evaluation of the Center for Epidemiological Studies Depression Scale (CES-D). *Journal of Psychosomatic Research, 46,* 437–443.

Hardie, T. (2007). Module 1: Alcohol and genetics. In C.L. Savage (Ed.). *A nursing education model for the prevention and treatment of alcohol use disorders.* Rockville MD: National Institute on Alcohol Abuse and Alcoholism.

Helander, A. (2001). Biologic markers of alcohol use and abuse in theory and practice. In D.P. Agarwal, & H.K. Seitz (Eds.). *Alcohol in health and disease.* (pp. 177–205). New York: Marcel Dekker.

Hudson, J.I., Hiripi, E., Pope, H.G., & Kessler, R.C. (2007). The prevalence and correlates of eating disorders in the National Comorbidity Survey Replication. *Biologic Psychiatry, 61,* 348–358.

Issel, L.M. (2004). *Health planning and evaluation.* Boston: Jones and Bartlett Publishers.

Kendler, K.S., Bulik, C.M., Silberg, J., Hettema, J.M., Myers, J., & Prescott, C.A. (2000). Childhood sexual abuse and adult psychiatric and substance use disorders in women: An epidemiological and co-twin control analysis. *Archives of General Psychiatry,* 57(10), 953–959.

Kilpatrick, D.G., Acierno, R., Saunders, B., Resnick, H.S., Best, C.L., & Schnurr, P.P. (2000). Risk factors for adolescent substance abuse and dependence: Data from a national survey. *Journal of Consulting and Clinical* Psychology, 68(1), 19–30.

Knopik, V.S., Heath, A.C., Madden, P.A., Bucholz, K.K., Slutske, W.S., Nelson, E.C., et al. (2004). Genetic effects on alcohol dependence risk: Re-evaluating the importance of psychiatric and other heritable risk factors. *Psychological Medicine,* 34,1519–1530.

Lazarus, R.S., & Folkman, S. (1984). *Stress, appraisal and coping.* New York: Springer Publishing.

Luo, X., Kranzler, H.R., Zuo, L., Wang, S., Schork, N.J., & Gelernter, J. (2006). Multiple *ADH* genes modulate risk for drug dependence in both African- and European-Americans. *Human Molecular Genetics,* 16(4), 380–390.

Luoma, J.B., & Pearson, J.L. (2002). Suicide and marital status in the United States, 1991–1996: Is widowhood a risk factor? *American Journal of Public Health, 92,* 1518–1522.

Lynch, R.M., & Greaves, I. (2000). Regular attendees to the accident and emergency department. *Journal of Accident and Emergency Medicine, 17,* 351–354.

McLellan, T.A., Lewis, D.C., O'Brien, C.P., & Kleber, H.D. (2000). Drug dependence, a chronic medical illness: Implications for treatment, insurance, and outcomes evaluation. *The Journal of the American Medical Association, 284,* 1689–1695.

Monti, P.M., Tevyaw, T.O., & Borsari, B. (2006). Drinking among young adults: Screening, brief intervention. *Alcohol Research and Health, 28*(4), 236–244.

Mrazek, P.J., & Haggerty, R.J. (Eds.). (1994) *Reducing risks for mental disorders: Frontiers for preventive intervention research.* Institute of Medicine. National Academy Press, Washington DC.

Musshoff, F., & Daldrup, T. (1998). Determination of biologic markers for alcohol abuse. *Journal of Chromatography B, 713,* 245–264.

National Alliance on Mental Illness. (2007). *State mental health parity laws 2007.* Retrieved July 5, 2007 from http://www. nami.org/Template.cfm?Section=Parity1&Template=/Content-Management/HTMLDisplay.cfm&ContentID=45368.

National Alliance for the Mentally Ill. (2001). *Families on the brink: The impact of ignoring children with serious mental illness.* Arlington, VA: Author.

National Center for Health Statistics. (2004). *Health, United States, 2004. With chartbook on trends in the health of Americans.* Hyattsville, MD: U.S. Department of Health and Human Services, Centers for Disease Control and Prevention.

National Institute on Alcohol Abuse and Alcoholism. (2004). *Twelve month prevalence of alcohol dependence.* Retrieved August 19, 2008 from http://www.niaaa.nih.gov/Resources/Database Resources/QuickFacts/AlcoholDependence/abusdep2.htm.

National Institute on Alcohol Abuse and Alcoholism. (2006a). *About Fetal Alcohol Syndrome and Fetal Alcohol Spectrum Disorders.* Retrieved August 19, 2008 from http://www.niaaa. nih.gov/AboutNIAAA/Interagency/AboutFAS.htm.

National Institute on Alcohol Abuse and Alcoholism. (2006b). *Frequently asked questions.* Retrieved August 19, 2008 from http://www.niaaa.nih.gov/FAQs/General-English/default.htm.

National Institute on Alcohol Abuse and Alcoholism. (2007). *Helping patients who drink too much: A clinician's guide.* Rockville MD: U.S. Department of Health and Human Services, National Institutes of Health.

National Institute on Drug Abuse. (2004a). *Info facts.* Retrieved February 20, 2007 from http://www.nida.nih.gov/pdf/infofacts/ NationTrends.pdf.

National Institute on Drug Abuse. (2004b). *Research report: Cocaine abuse and addiction.* Rockville MD: U.S. Department of Health and Human Services, National Institutes of Health.

National Institute on Drug Abuse (2006). *Monitoring the Future Survey.* Retrieved August 19, 2008 from http://www.nida.nih. gov/DrugPages/MTF.html.

National Institute of Mental Health. (2006a). *The numbers count. Mental disorders in America (revised).* [NIH Publication No.

06-4584]. Retrieved August 19, 2008 from http://www.nimh.nih.gov/publicat/numbers.cfm#Intro.

National Institute of Mental Health. (2006b). *Tiny, spontaneous gene mutations may boost autism risk.* Retrieved August 19, 2008 from http://www.nimh.nih.gov/press/gene-mutations-autism.cfm.

New Freedom Initiative. (2004). *The President's New Freedom Initiative for People with Disabilties: The 2004 Progress Report.* Retrieved August 19, 2008 from http://www.whitehouse.gov/infocus/newfreedom/toc-2004.html.

North, C., Eyrich, K.M., Pollio, D.E., & Spintznagel, E.L. (2004). Are rates of psychiatric disorders in the homeless population changing? *American Journal of Public Health, 94,* 103–109.

O'Connell, H., Chin, A., Hamilton, F., Cunningham, C., Walsh, J.B, Coakley, D., et al. (2004). A systematic review of the utility of self-report alcohol screening instruments in the elderly. *International Journal of Geriatric Psychiatry,* 19,1074–1086.

Office of Applied Studies, SAMSHA. (2007). *The NSDUH Report: Co-occurring Major Depressive Episode (MDE) and Alcohol Use Disorder among adults.* Retrieved August 19, 2008 from http://oas.samhsa.gov/highlights.htm#2k7Pubs.

Poikolainen, K. (2000). Risk factors for alcohol dependence: A case control study. *Alcohol and Alcoholism, 35*(2), 190–196.

Radloff, L. (1977). The CES-D Scale: A self report depression scale for research in the general population. *Applied Psychological Measurement, 1,* 385–401.

Radloff, L. (1991). The use of the Center for Epidemiological Studies Depression Scale in adolescents and young adults. *Journal of Youth and Adolescence, 20*(2), 149–166.

Reinhart, D.F., & Allen, J.P. (2007). The Alcohol Use Disorders Identification Test: An update of research findings. *Alcoholism Clinical and Experimental Research, 31*(2), 185–199.

Reinherz, H.Z., Giaconia, R.M., Hauf, A.M., Wasserman, M.S., & Paradis, A.D. (2000). General and specific childhood risk factors for depression and drug disorders by early adulthood. *Journal of the American Academy of Child & Adolescent Psychiatry, 39*(2), 223–231.

Salit, S.A., Kuhn, E.M., Hartz, A.J., et al. (1998). Hospitalization costs associated with homelessness in New York City. *The New England Journal of Medicine, 338,* 1734–1740.

Savage, C.L., Wray, J., Ritchey, P.N., Sommers, M., Dyehouse, J., & Fulmer, M. (2003). A critical review of current screening instruments related to alcohol consumption in pregnancy and a proposed alternative method. *Journal of Obstetrics, Gynecology and Neonatal Nursing, 32,* 437–446.

Savage, C.L. (Ed.). (2006). Chapter IV: Health promotion and risk reduction. In M. Armstrong, J. Feigenbaum, C. Savage, & C. Vourakis (Eds.). *Addictions nursing, core curriculum,* 2nd ed. Raleigh, NC: International Nurses Society on Addiction.

Scribner, R.A., MacKinnon, D.P., & Dwyer, J.H. (1994). Alcohol outlet density and motor vehicle crashes in Los Angeles County cities. *Journal of Studies on Alcohol, (44),* 447–453.

Scribner, R., MacKinnon, D., & Dwyer, J. (1995). The risk of assaultive violence and alcohol availability in Los Angeles County. *American Journal of Public Health, (85),* 335–340.

Selzer, M.L. (1971). The Michigan Alcoholism Screening Test: The quest for a new diagnostic instrument. *American Journal of Psychiatry, 127,* 1653–1658.

Skinner, H.A. (1982). The drug use screening test. *Addictive Behaviors, 7,* 363–371.

Sommers, M.S. (2007). Module IV: Treatment of hazardous (risky) or harmful alcohol use. In C.L. Savage (Ed.). *A nursing education model for the prevention and treatment of alcohol use disorders.* Rockville MD: National Institute on Alcohol Abuse and Alcoholism.

Sommers, M.S., Wray, J., Savage, C., & Dyehouse, J.M. (2003). Assessing acute and critically ill patients for problem drinking. *Dimensions of Critical Care Nursing, 22,* 76–89.

Substance Abuse and Mental Health Services Administration. (n.d.). *Drug Free workplace programs: Overview.* Retrieved August 19, 2008 from http://www.surgeongeneral.gov/library/mentalhealth/home.html.

Substance Abuse and Mental Health Services Administration. (2003). *National healthcare disparities report.* Retrieved August 19, 2008 from http://www.ahrq.gov/qual/nhdr03/nhdrsum03.htm#Inequality.

Tarter, R.E. (1990). Evaluation and treatment of adolescent substance abuse: A decision-tree method. *American Journal of Drug and Alcohol Abuse, 161,* 1–46.

Toumbourou, J.W., Stocwell, T., Neighbors, C., Marlatt, G.A., & Rehm, J. (2007). Interventions to reduce harm associated with adolescent substance use. *Lancet,* 369,1391–1401.

U.S. Department of Health and Human Services. (1999). *Mental health: A report of the Surgeon General.* Rockville, MD: Author. Retrieved August 19, 2008 from http://www.surgeongeneral.gov/library/mentalhealth/home.html.

U.S. Department of Health and Human Services. (2000). *Healthy People 2010: Understanding and improving health and objectives for improving health,* 2nd ed. 2 vols. Washington, DC: U.S. Government Printing Office.

Whitten, L. (2006). Studies identify factors surrounding rise in abuse of prescription drugs by college students. *NIDA Notes, 20*(4), 1, 6, 7.

World Health Organization. (2001). *Mental health: Strengthening mental health promotion.* Retrieved August 19, 2008 from http://www.who.int/mediacentre/factsheets/fs220/en/.

World Health Organization. (2007). *Ten statistical highlights in global public health.* Retrieved August 19, 2008 from http://www.who.int/whosis/whostat2006highlights/en/index1.html.

World Health Organization. (n.d.). *World Health Organization: Mental health policy.* Retrieved July 9, 2007 from http://www.who.int/mental_health/policy/MHPolicy_factsheet.pdf.

Zautcke, J.L., Coker, S.B., Morris, R.W., & Stein-Spencer, L. (2002). Geriatric trauma in the state of Illinois: Substance use and injury patterns. *American Journal of Emergency Medicine, 20,* 14–17.

Zickler, P. (2005). marijuana-related disorders, but not prevalence of use, rise over past decade. *NIDA Notes, 19*(6), 1–3.

Selected Readings

Amos, C., Peters, R.J., Williams, L., Johnson, R.J., Martin, Q., & Yacoubian, G.S. (2008), The link between recent sexual abuse and drug use among African American male college students: It's not just a female problem in and around campus. *Journal of Psychoactive Drugs, 40(2),* 161–166.

Chang, J.C., Dado, D., Frankel, R.M., Rodriguez, K.L., Zickmund, S., Ling, B.S. et al. (2008). When pregnant patients disclose substance use: Missed opportunities for behavioral change counseling. *Patient Education & Counseling, 72,* 394–401.

Dennison, C.R., & Hughes, S. (2008). New guideline for tobacco use and dependence provides arsenal of effective interventions. *Journal of Cardiovascular Nursing, 23,* 383–385.

Johnson, S., Needle, J., & Bindman, J.P. (Eds.). (2008). *Crisis resolution and home treatment in mental health.* New York: Cambridge University Press

Henderson, S. (Ed.). (2008). *Refugee mental health: An issue of child and adolescent psychiatric clinics.* St. Louis, MO: Elsevier.

Högberg, T., Magnusson, A., Ewertzon, M., & Lützén, K. (2008). Attitudes towards mental illness in Sweden: Adaptation and development of the Community Attitudes towards Mental Illness questionnaire. *International Journal of Mental Health Nursing,* 17, 302–310.

Huang, X., Ma, W., Shih, H., & Li, H. (2008). Roles and functions of community mental health nurses caring for people with schizophrenia in Taiwan. *Journal of Clinical Nursing, 17,* 3030–3040.

Hunter, A., Playle, J., Sanchez, P., Cahill, J., & McGowan, L. (2008). Introduction of a child and adolescent mental health link worker: Education and health staff focus group findings. *Journal of Psychiatric & Mental Health Nursing, 15,* 670–677.

Lewis, T. (2008). Assessing an older adult for alcohol use disorders. *Nursing, 38*(6), 60–61.

Mio, J.S., Barker, L.A., & Tumambing, J.S. (2008). *Multicultural psychology: Understanding our diverse communities.* Hightstown, NJ: McGraw-Hill.

Munro, I., & Edward, K. (2008). Mental illness and substance use: An Australian perspective. *International Journal of Mental Health Nursing, 17,* 255–260.

Salter, M. & Turner, T. (2008). *Community mental health care: A practical guide to outdoor psychiatry.* St. Louis, MO: Elsevier.

Stroul, B. A., & Blau, G. M. (Eds.). (2008). *The system of care handbook: Transforming mental health services for children, youth, and families.* Baltimore, MD: Paul H. Brookes Publishing Co., Inc.

White, J.H., & Kudless, M. (2008). Valuing autonomy, struggling for an identity and a collective voice, and seeking role recognition: Community mental health nurses' perceptions of their roles. *Issues in Mental Health Nursing, 29,* 1066–1087.

Internet Resources

Alcohol and health (current evidence): *http://www.alcoholandhealth.org*

Alcohol policies: *http://www.alcoholpolicymd.com/alcohol_policy/ama_policies.htm*

American Psychiatric Nurses Association: *http://www.apna.org/*

American Public Health Association (Alcohol, Tobacco, and Other Drugs [ATOD] Section): *http://www.apha.org/membergroups/sections/aphasections/atod/*

American Public Health Association (Mental Health Section): *http://www.apha.org/membergroups/sections/aphasections/mental/*

Drug Screening.org (online alcohol and drug screening tool): *http://www.drugscreening.org*

Intermountain Health Care: *http://intermountainhealthcare.org/xp/public/physician/clinicalprograms/primarycare/mentalhealth/*

International Nurses Society on Addictions: *http://www.intnsa.org*

International Society of Psychiatric-Mental Health Nurses: *http://www.ispn-psych.org/*

Mental Health America: *http://nmha.org*

National Alcohol Screening Day: *http://www.mentalhealthscreening.org/events/nasd/*

National Alliance on Mental Illness (NAMI): *http://www.nami.org/*

National Depression Screening Day (mental health screening tools): *http://www.mentalhealthscreening.org/events/ndsd/conduct.aspx*

National Institute of Mental Health: *http://www.nimh.nih.gov/*

New Freedom Commission on Mental Health: *http://www.mentalhealthcommission.gov/presentations/presentations.html*

SAMHSA [Substance Abuse and Mental Health Service Administration]—Substance use and mental health prevention: *http://ncadi.samhsa.gov/* (which includes the Center for Substance Abuse Treatment and the Center for Substance Abuse Prevention)

SAMHSA: Screening and Assessment for Family Engagement, Retention, and Recovery (SAFERR): *http://ncadistore.samhsa.gov/catalog/productDetails.aspx?ProductID=17633.*

SAMHSA: The NSDUH Report: Sexually Transmitted Diseases and Substance Use: *http://ncadistore.samhsa.gov/catalog/productDetails.aspx?ProductID=17622.*

SAMHSA: CSAT National Summit on Recovery: *http://partnersforrecovery.samhsa.gov/docs/Summit-Report.pdf*

Society of Behavioral Medicine: *http://www.sbm.org/*

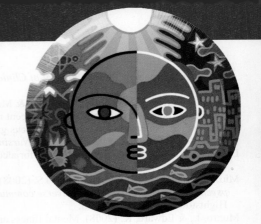

28

Working with the Homeless

LEARNING OBJECTIVES

Upon mastery of this chapter, you should be able to:

◆ Define the concept of homelessness.

◆ Describe the demographic characteristics of the homeless living in the United States.

◆ Discuss factors predisposing persons to homelessness.

◆ Compare and contrast the unique challenges confronting selected subpopulations within the homeless community.

◆ Examine the effects of homelessness on health.

◆ Analyze the extent and adequacy of public and private resources to combat the problem of homelessness.

◆ Assess your beliefs and values toward homelessness.

◆ Propose community-based nursing interventions to facilitate primary, secondary, and tertiary prevention in addressing the problem of homelessness.

"*Mid pleasures and palaces though we may roam,*
Be it ever so humble, there's no place like home."

—John Howard Payne (1791–1852)

KEY TERMS

Chronically homeless
Disenfranchised
Deinstitutionalization
Extremely low-income
Homelessness
Marginalized
Period prevalence counts
Point in time counts
Single-room occupancy
   (SRO) housing
Survival sex
Unaccompanied youth
Unsheltered (hidden)
   homeless

What was once considered unthinkable in a prosperous nation is now an expected occurrence in towns and cities across the United States. Drive through an inner-city or suburban community on any given day and you will see people on street corners holding signs reading "Hungry and homeless." Where is the public outcry in response to this scene? Has the American conscience been anesthetized to this form of human suffering? Or, is the need simply too overwhelming and the problems too far-reaching to mount an effective campaign to prevent such a tragedy?

The purpose of this chapter is to define the concept of **homelessness**, examine the factors contributing to homelessness, analyze the major issues confronting the homeless, and examine the role of the community health nurse in addressing the needs of the homeless.

Healthy People 2010 defines a person who lacks housing as being homeless. The definition also includes persons living in transitional housing or persons who spend the majority of nights in public or private facilities with temporary living quarters (Healthy People 2010, n.d.a). Table 28.1 outlines selected *Healthy People 2010* goals that relate to the homeless population.

The McKinney-Vento Homeless Assistance Act (Title 42 of the U.S. Code) defines a person as homeless who lacks a fixed, regular, adequate night time residence including supervised public or private shelters that provide temporary accommodations, institutional settings providing temporary shelter, or public or private places that are not designed for or used as a regular sleeping accommodation for human beings (e.g., cars, parks, camp grounds). Incarcerated individuals, however, are not considered homeless under this definition (National Coalition for the Homeless [NCH], 2006r).

The education subtitle of the McKinney-Vento Homeless Assistance Act expands on the definition of homelessness when addressing homeless children and youth. The Act includes as homeless those children who share housing with others due to economic hardship or loss of housing, are abandoned in hospitals, are awaiting placement in foster care, or are living in motels, trailer parks, or camping grounds (United States Department of Housing and Urban Development [USDHUD], n.d.c).

The Department of Housing and Urban Development interprets the McKinney-Vento definition of homeless to include only people living on the streets or in shelters or those facing imminent eviction (within 1 week). Although this definition may be appropriate for the urban homeless who are more likely to live on the street or in shelters, persons living in rural areas tend to cohabit with relatives or friends in overcrowded, substandard housing (NCH, 2006r).

SCOPE OF THE PROBLEM

It is difficult to estimate the number of people who are homeless, since homelessness is a temporary condition. Rather than trying to count the number of homeless people on a given day or week (**point in time counts**), it may be more prudent to measure the number of people who have been homeless over a longer time frame (**period prevalence count**s) (NCH, 2006m).

It is also difficult to locate and account for people who are homeless. Most estimates are based upon the number of people served in shelters or soup kitchens or the number of people who can easily be located on the streets. People who frequent places that are difficult to reach (e.g., cars, camp grounds, caves, box cars) are considered "**unsheltered**" or "**hidden**" **homeless**. Many people are unable to access shelters due to overcrowding and limited capacity. In rural areas, fewer housing options and resources are available for the homeless. As a result, people are forced to live temporarily with friends or family. Although still experiencing homelessness, these individuals may not be counted in homeless statistics or considered eligible for homeless services (NCH, 2006m).

The National Law Center on Homelessness and Poverty estimates that approximately 3.5 million people (of whom 1.35 million are children) experience homelessness in a given year. Approximately 1% of the U.S. population experiences homelessness each year. However, since this data is based on a survey of service providers, and since many homeless people are unable to access services, it is likely that the prevalence of homelessness is even higher. It is unlikely that researchers will ever be able to estimate the exact magnitude of homelessness in America (NCH, 2006m).

In 1996, the Interagency Council on Homelessness, in collaboration with 12 federal agencies, commissioned the United States Bureau of the Census to conduct a National Survey of Homeless Assistance Providers and Clients (NSHAPC). This was a landmark study based on a statistical sample of 76 metropolitan and nonmetropolitan areas, including cities and rural areas. The survey was initiated in response to the lack of national data on the homeless. The survey did not produce a national count of the number of homeless people, but it did provide information about the characteristics of homeless people who were able to access services (USDHUD, n.d.b). Although dated, this was the most recent survey of its kind until January 2007, when the Homelessness Research Institute of the National Alliance to End Homelessness published a report entitled "Homelessness Counts." This report used local point in time counts of communities across the United States

TABLE 28.1	Selected *Healthy People 2010* Goals Related to Homelessness
Overarching Goals	Increase quality and years of healthy life Eliminate health disparities
Related Focus Area Goals	Increase the proportion of persons who have a significant source of ongoing care Increase the proportion of persons with health insurance Reduce the proportion of families that experience difficulties or delays in obtaining health care or do not receive needed care for one or more family members

Source: Healthy People 2010. (n.d.b). Healthy People goals. Retrieved September 29, 2006 from http://www.healthypeople.gov/About/goals.htm. Healthy People 2010 (n.d.c). Retrieved August 22, 2008 from http://www.healthypeople.gov/hpscripts/KeywordResult.asp?n320=320&Submit=Submit.

to estimate the number of homeless people nationwide. The study reported that in January 2005 an estimated 744,313 people experienced homelessness. Of these, 56% were living in shelters and 44% were unsheltered (Homelessness Research Institute, 2007).

In 2005, The United States Conference of Mayors Task Force on Hunger and Homelessness conducted a survey of 24 cities across the nation. Seventy-one percent of the survey cities reported an increase in requests for emergency shelter during the past year. Requests for emergency shelter by homeless families with children increased in 63% of the survey cities. The number of emergency shelter beds for homeless people increased by 7%. People remained homeless for an average of 7 months. Eighty-seven percent of the cities reported an increase in the length of time people remained homeless. An average of 14% of shelter requests by homeless people and 32% of shelter requests by homeless families were reported to have gone unmet during the prior year. In 88% of the cities, emergency shelters may have turned away homeless families because of a lack of resources (U.S. Conference of Mayors, 2005).

DEMOGRAPHICS

Poverty is inextricably linked to homelessness. The increase in poverty and the growing shortage of affordable rental housing have led to a dramatic rise in homelessness over the past two decades (NCH, 2006r). Demographic groups more likely to be poor are also at greater risk of becoming homeless.

Age

In 2003, children under 18 accounted for 39% of the homeless population. Of these, 42% were under 5 years of age. Twenty-five percent of the homeless are between 25 and 34, and 6% are between 55 and 64 (NCH, 2006r).

Gender

Single homeless adults are more likely to be male than female. The U.S. Conference of Mayors (2005) survey found that single men comprised 43% and single women 17% of the homeless population. According to the NSHAPC survey, 77% of single homeless clients were male and 23% were female. The majority of homeless clients (85%) were single. Of parents in homeless families, 84% were female and 16% were male (USDHUD, n.d.b).

Ethnicity

The racial and ethnic makeup of the homeless population varies based upon geographic location. In urban areas, African American males constitute a large percentage of the homeless population while in rural areas the homeless are more likely to be White, Native American, or migrant workers (NCH, 2006r).

Families

Families with children comprise the fastest growing segment of the homeless population. Families with children represented 33% of the homeless population among the 24

American cities surveyed in the U.S. Conference of Mayors (2005) report. In rural areas, families, single mothers, and children represented the largest segment of homeless. According to the Homelessness Research Institute (2007), there were an estimated 98,452 homeless families in January 2005. Approximately 41% of the homeless population were members of families with children while 59% were individuals.

CONTRIBUTING FACTORS

A complex array of factors can result in individuals having to choose between necessities of daily living. Scarce resources limit choices. What would you do if you had to choose between eating and buying your child's medication? Housing consumes a substantial portion of one's income and is often the first asset to be lost. Many families find they are only a paycheck away from homelessness.

Poverty

In 2004, 12.7% of the U.S. population (37 million people) lived in poverty. Thirty-six percent of these were children. The increase in poverty rates over recent years may be attributed to declining wages, loss of jobs that offer security and carry benefits, an increase in temporary and part-time employment, erosion of the true value of the minimum wage, a decline in manufacturing jobs in favor of lower-paying service jobs, globalization and outsourcing, and a decline in public assistance. As wages drop, the potential to secure adequate housing wanes (NCH, 2006d,s). The U.S. Conference of Mayors (2005) found that a person must earn greater than minimum wage to afford a one- or two-bedroom apartment at 30% of income, the federal definition of affordable housing.

Many homeless shelters house people who are employed full time. The U.S. Conference on Mayors (2005) survey found that 15% of people in homeless situations in the cities surveyed were employed. The problem is compounded by a lack of affordable housing (particularly **single-room occupancy [SRO] housing** or housing units intended to be occupied by one person) and limited funding for housing assistance. As rental costs have increased and the number of available low-rent units has declined and federal support for housing assistance has dropped off, the housing gap has widened. People have been forced to pay high rents to obtain shelter. This situation leads to overcrowding and substandard housing (NCH, 2006e).

The average wait for Section 8 housing assistance is 35 months (U.S. Conference of Mayors, 2005). As a result, people remain in shelter situations for a longer period of time. With minimal turnover of shelter beds, shelters running at capacity are forced to turn people away. According to Burt (2006), the single most effective step to reduce the risk of homelessness is to increase housing for **extremely low-income** individuals (i.e., those earning 30% or less of the median income in an area) (National Low Income Housing Coalition (NLIHC), 2006 a,b).

Lack of Affordable Health Care

In the absence of affordable health care coverage, a serious illness or disability can lead to job loss, savings depletion, and even eviction. In 2004, approximately 45.8 million Americans (15.7% of the population) were without health care coverage. Approximately one-third of those in poverty have no health insurance. Those who are able to qualify for medical assistance may be reluctant to seek employment, fearing termination of benefits. Many others have limited coverage that requires higher co-pays or deductibles and does not cover major catastrophic illnesses (NCH, 2006f). An adverse health event can potentially plunge an individual into a homeless condition.

Employment

Many low-income wage earners hold jobs with nonstandard work arrangements. Temporary employees, day laborers, independent contractors, and part-time employees are examples of work arrangements that tend to pay lower wages, offer limited or no benefits, and have less job security. For persons with few or no job skills, it is virtually impossible to compete for jobs that offer a living wage. Barriers to employment among the homeless include lack of education and job skills; lack of transportation, day care, or other supportive services; and disabilities that make it difficult to pursue or retain employment (NCH, 2006d).

Domestic Violence

Victims of domestic violence often face a choice between living in an abusive situation or leaving and facing life on the streets. According to the U.S. Conference of Mayors (2005) report, 50% of the cities surveyed identified domestic violence as a primary reason for homelessness. Women who are victims of domestic violence may lack the resources necessary to escape an abusive environment and become independent. The lack of affordable housing, long waiting lists for housing and social services, and limited capacity of shelters to accommodate families in crisis only serve to exacerbate the problem (NCH, 2006b).

Mental Illness

Approximately 22% of the single adult homeless population suffers from severe mental illness (U.S. Conference of Mayors, 2005). **Deinstitutionalization** (being released from institutions into the community), coupled with limited access to services and inadequate discharge planning and referrals, may contribute to the number of severely mentally ill persons represented in the homeless population (NCH, 2006p).

Homeless persons with mental illness tend to remain homeless longer, be in poorer physical health, encounter more barriers to employment, have less support from significant others, and interface with the legal system more often than the homeless who do not have a mental disorder. Although the majority of the homeless mentally ill do not require institutionalization, the lack of community-based treatment and support services and affordable housing reinforce their homeless condition and trap them in a desperate cycle. Moreover, supplemental security income (SSI) benefit levels for persons with disabilities have not kept pace with inflation or the skyrocketing cost of rental housing.

Addictions Disorders

Rates of alcohol and drug abuse are disproportionately high among the homeless. Thirty percent of the homeless report problems with substance abuse (U.S. Conference of Mayors, 2005). For people already at risk for homelessness, the behaviors associated with an addictive disorder can create instability and jeopardize family and employment support nets. Once homeless, they may resort to drugs or alcohol to dull the pain of being homeless and ease the feelings of hopelessness that accompany such a desperate state. They may also turn to chemical substances in an attempt to self-medicate the disturbing symptoms of an untreated mental illness.

Although some homeless individuals may desire treatment to overcome their addictions, they often encounter obstacles that undermine their recovery and prevent them from obtaining the treatment they need. Limited access to care and lack of community resources make it difficult if not impossible to receive the services needed to achieve a successful recovery. There may be long waiting lists for addictions treatment, and homeless people who do not have phone access and are difficult to locate may be dropped from the waiting list. Lack of transportation and lack of the documentation needed to access programs (e.g., birth certificates, social security cards) further exacerbate the problem. Denial of SSI or Social Security Disability Insurance (SSDI) and Medicaid to persons with substance abuse related disabilities creates a huge barrier to achieving recovery support, proper medical care, and housing and income assistance. Moreover, the federal programs targeting homelessness, mental health, and addictions services (Treatment for Homeless Persons [THP] and Projects for Assistance in Transition from Homelessness [PATH]) lack the funding necessary to exert an impact that would effectively address this problem on a national level (NCH, 2006a).

Additional Variables

Additional variables impacting homelessness include personal or financial crisis, natural disasters, and personal choice. For example, Hurricanes Katrina and Rita, which devastated portions of the Gulf Coast in 2005, displaced many previously independent and self-sufficient individuals and families, rendering many homeless and in need of emergency shelter.

HOMELESS SUBPOPULATIONS

Although many of the struggles facing the homeless are universal, subpopulations within the homeless community are uniquely vulnerable. Often, these groups face additional burdens because of their special needs and challenges.

Homeless Men

According to the U.S. Conference of Mayors (2005) survey, men comprise approximately 48% of the homeless population. The majority of homeless men are single adults. Homeless men are more likely to be employed than their homeless female counterparts yet they usually hold temporary, low-wage jobs that offer little security. They are also more likely than homeless women to have uncontrolled substance abuse issues. This makes it more difficult for them to access shelters, which tend to require abstinence for admission (National Health Care for the Homeless Council [NHCHC], 2001).

Some men find themselves in a cycle of intermittent homelessness as they move back and forth between prisons, treatment centers, shelters, temporary housing, and the streets. Other men are at risk for becoming **chronically homeless**. These men may have significant health problems due to chronic substance abuse, lack of shelter, and poor access to health and social services (NHCHC, 2001). A chronically homeless adult is someone who has been homeless for long periods of time or has experienced repeated episodes of homelessness. In January 2005, approximately 23% of the homeless population was chronically homeless (Homelessness Research Institute, 2007).

Homeless men are more likely to be treated with disdain than other homeless subgroups (Perspectives: Voices from the Community). Some people perceive homeless men as largely to blame for their plight, believing that they are able

bodied and should be capable of working. Moreover, homeless men may suffer from disabilities that are not severe enough to warrant eligibility for health and social services. Often health and social programs give priority to women and children. Single, low-income men do not qualify for medical assistance unless they are disabled (NHCHC, 2001).

Homeless Women

The U.S. Conference of Mayors (2005) survey found that women comprised 17% of the homeless population. According to the NSHAPC survey, 23% of single homeless clients are female. Of parents in homeless families, 84% are female (USDHUD, n.d.b).

A high incidence of family violence occurs among homeless mothers, with 63% of homeless mothers reporting being violently abused by an intimate male partner. Ninety-two percent of homeless mothers report a history of physical or sexual assault either during their childhoods or in their adult years. This high rate of violence also correlates with a high rate of emotional disturbances among homeless mothers, including posttraumatic stress (three times the rate of other women), depression (twice the rate of other women), attempted suicide, and prior hospitalization for mental illness (NCFH, n.d.d; NCH, 2006h). Moreover, the potential for exposure to violence and sexual assault on the streets increases the risk for sexually transmitted infections (STIs) and traumatic injuries.

Homeless Children

In any given week, an estimated 200,000 children have nowhere to live. Approximately 1.4 million children experience homelessness over the course of a year. Forty-two percent of these children are under 5 years of age (U.S. Conference of Mayors, 2005).

Homeless families are the fastest growing segment of the homeless population. Most children living with homeless parents are young (42% are less than 6 years of age). Requests for emergency shelter for families have increased every year since 1985 (NCFH, n.d.c; National Resource and Training Center on Homelessness and Mental Illness [NRTCHMI], n.d.b). In 2005, 32% of requests for shelter by homeless families were denied due to lack of resources (U.S. Conference of Mayors, 2005) (see From the Case Files I).

The majority of homeless children and youth live in shelters, share housing with friends or relatives, or live in motels or camp grounds. More than 30% have been evicted from housing. Homelessness adversely affects children's mental health and can lead to emotional and behavioral problems. Common problems associated with child homelessness include anxiety, depression, and withdrawal (47% versus 18% of other children), as well as delinquent or aggressive behavior. Over 20% of homeless preschoolers have emotional problems severe enough to require professional intervention. Education is also compromised when one is homeless (NCH, 2006c). Although approximately 87% of homeless children are enrolled in school, only about 77% attend regularly. Some schools require a home address prior to enrollment. Other barriers include transportation to and from the shelter, lack of academic and medical records required for registration, unstable living arrangements necessitating multiple moves, and

---

PERSPECTIVES
VOICES FROM THE COMMUNITY

A Nurse's Viewpoint on Working with the Homeless

When I first decided to visit the homeless men's shelter, I was scared to death. Here I was, a veteran nurse with over 20 years experience in community health, and I was afraid. Afraid of what? I couldn't tell you. I suppose I harbored the stereotypes and negative images that most of us associate with homeless addicts. I remember passing this shelter years ago, looking out at the men hanging out on the street corner, and thinking to myself, "Please God, don't let my car break down!" I remember thinking "I would never set foot in a place like that."

Well, my views about homelessness were challenged to the core when I peered into the faces of those men, heard their stories, and began to feel their pain. Theirs were stories of broken lives and lost hope but also of courage in the face of suffering and the will to survive in the midst of great adversity. These men were as diverse as their stories. They were from all walks of life. They possessed incredible gifts and talents. They were musicians, artisans, businessmen, writers, and poets. They had families who loved them and families who left them. Left because they could not continue to watch them die a little each day and be destroyed themselves in the process.

So, here I am. Doing what I can to bring hope and healing. The irony is I came to bring hope and yet I am the one who is being healed. Healed in the broken areas of my life. Healed in my narrow view of life and my internal prejudices. It is a great privilege to serve these men.

Rita, Age 42

Reaching Out to Homeless Women and Children

Sheila Hendricks, a public health nurse for the Manchester City Health Department, and her colleagues were brainstorming ideas for how to reach the growing population of homeless women and children in their jurisdiction. They arranged a meeting with the director of a local rescue mission in the area. The mission provided emergency shelter to 100 homeless women and children each night. The women were allowed to remain at the shelter for 30 days provided they actively sought employment, social services, or educational opportunities. Families typically left during the day to seek jobs or other forms of assistance and returned in the evening for shelter. The community health nurses negotiated with the rescue mission to establish an on-site nursing clinic twice a week that would provide health education, screenings, and referrals on a drop-in basis. The hours of clinic operation were 4 p.m. to 8 p.m. to accommodate client schedules.

Assessment

After the clinic was in operation for 2 weeks, the following priority health issues began to emerge:

- Inadequate maternal and child nutrition
- Lack of primary health care services for women and children (e.g., immunizations, screenings, treatment for upper respiratory tract infections, dermatologic problems, asthma, hypertension)
- Depression
- High rate of reported sexually transmitted infections and HIV due to history of violence, survival sex, and injection drug use
- Untreated addiction disorders

Plan

The following diagnoses were developed (in order of priority):

- Impaired access to health and social services related to lack of insurance, scarce community-based resources, and lack of transportation
- Ineffective family coping related to untreated addictions, mental health issues, and history of intimate partner violence
- At risk for injury related to untreated addictions and mental health disorders, history of intimate partner violence, and hazards of street life
- Altered nutrition less than body requirements related to lack of resources to purchase nutritious foods, addictions disorders, and chronic health issues

After assessing priority needs and establishing relevant diagnoses, the nurses developed a plan of care for this population. The priority goal was to promote access to care by linking clients to essential health and social services. The rationale for establishing this goal as a top priority was that if clients were able to access needed services, the other diagnoses could potentially be addressed (e.g., need for counseling, health care, housing, education).

Implementation

A nurse practitioner was engaged from the health department to provide primary care services to the women and children at the shelter, including screening and treatment for sexually transmitted infections and treatment of common acute and chronic health conditions. Conditions requiring more extensive follow-up were referred to the local federally funded Health Care for the Homeless clinic. A social worker from the local social service agency was recruited to visit the mission on a monthly basis to assist clients in applying for housing and public assistance programs. Clients were referred to the local community mental health center for counseling related to addictions and violence issues. The nurses conducted health education programs and one-on-one counseling on topics such as parenting, coping, healthy eating, basic hygiene, and safety. They also offered health screenings for blood pressure, diabetes, HIV, and tuberculosis and provided referrals to the health department clinic for cancer screenings (e.g., mammograms, colorectal screening).

Evaluation

After the clinic had been in operation for 90 days, preliminary evaluation data revealed the following:

Sixty-five women and 28 children had frequented the clinic over the past 3 months. All 65 women received health promotion teaching and a resource packet for further reference. Eighty percent of clients who required referrals to outside agencies were successful in accessing care. Twenty-five women and 15 children were under the care of the nurse practitioner for acute or chronic health conditions. Ten cases of latent TB infection were identified through TB testing, and these clients were referred to the City Health Department TB clinic for follow-up treatment. Seven abnormal PAP smears were identified, and eight clients were diagnosed with sexually transmitted infections. Fifteen clients were found to be HIV positive. Clients with positive screenings were referred to the City Health Department or the local Health Care for the Homeless Clinic, where treatment was initiated. Forty women applied for social service benefits. Most of these clients are still awaiting the receipt of benefits.

urgent needs for food and shelter that take priority over education (NCFH, n.d.a; NRTCHMI, n.d.b).

Homeless children are more likely to repeat grades and to be diagnosed with learning disabilities and language impediments than other children. They are also more likely to go hungry and to experience physical or sexual abuse. Often, they have witnessed acts of violence (usually against their mother) or to have spent time apart from their immediate family (e.g., placed in foster care or with relatives) (NRTCHMI, n.d.b).

Homeless children are more likely to get sick than other children (NCFH, n.d.b). Common health complaints include ear infections, asthma, stomach problems, and speech difficulties. They are twice as likely to be hospitalized for illness. Homeless babies have higher rates of low birth weight than other infants and show significantly slower development. Ninety-seven percent of homeless children move each year, many up to three times a year. Twenty-eight percent of homeless children go to three or more schools in a given year (NRTCHMI, n.d.b).

Despite their many needs, homeless children do not have sufficient access to services. Most homeless preschool aged children are not in preschool programs. Approximately 20% of homeless children have no regular source of medical care. Less than one-third receive interventions for emotional disturbances. Only 50% to 60% of homeless families receive Medicaid and only 37% receive services to assist them in school (NCFH, n.d.a).

Homeless Youth

Homeless youth are persons under 18 who lack parental, foster, or institutional care. Homeless adolescents are sometimes referred to as "**unaccompanied youth**." They account for 3% of the urban homeless population (U.S. Conference of Mayors, 2005).

Factors contributing to youth homelessness include physical and sexual abuse, family addiction, parental neglect, strained relationships, or family financial crises that lead to family separation due to inadequate shelter, housing, or child welfare resources. A history of foster care placement is positively correlated with homelessness among youth. Moreover, some youth who are discharged from residential or foster care with inadequate housing or income support may find themselves homeless (NCH, 2006l). The majority of homeless adolescents believe they have no acceptable housing options (O'Sullivan & Lussier-Duynstee, 2006).

Homeless adolescents may have difficulty accessing emergency shelter because of shelter policies that prohibit older youth from the facility or because of a lack of bed space. Due to lack of education or job training skills, many resort to prostitution or **survival sex** (exchanging sex for food, shelter, or other basic necessities). As a result, homeless youth are at higher risk for human immunodeficiency virus (HIV), hepatitis, and sexually transmitted infections. Homeless youth also suffer disproportionately from anxiety, depression, malnutrition, conduct disorders, posttraumatic stress, and low self-esteem (NCH, 2006k) (see Evidence-based Practice).

Martijn & Sharpe (2006) found an increase in drug and alcohol diagnoses and criminal activity following home-

EVIDENCE-BASED PRACTICE

Treatment for Homeless Youth

How can we encourage homeless youth with mental health issues to remain in treatment? Darbyshire et al. (2006), in a qualitative study, investigated this question among 10 homeless youths in Australia. The youths were between 16 and 24 years of age and were suffering from mental health problems. The researchers sought to learn their perspectives on accessing and using health and social services. The study found that access to care was less of an issue than the actual quality of care delivered. Concerns were expressed regarding feeling labeled and stigmatized, receiving little time and attention, and being offered little explanation for the care being given. As a result, the youth felt a personal loss of control. Services were often fragmented, with one visit resulting in multiple referrals to other agencies. This magnified their sense of powerlessness, as it is often a challenge to access transportation or to negotiate the bureaucracies and nuances of each agency.

Trust and respect were foundational to facilitating engagement of the youth with health and social services. Acts of kindness, expressions of caring, active listening, and a nonjudgmental attitude facilitated trusting relationships and encouraged the youth to remain active in treatment or counseling. The findings suggest that a respectful, supportive climate is important in delivering health and social services to homeless youth with mental health issues.

Why might trust be hard to develop in this population? What can the CHN do to increase awareness among health and social service providers of the need to foster trusting, respectful encounters? What factors may have accounted for the young people's negative experiences with the health care system? How are perceptions influenced when persons seek care at times of personal crisis? Why would trust and respect, which are so basic to successful human encounters, be lacking? What are some of the unique stresses that health and social service professionals face when working with marginalized and disenfranchised groups?

lessness among youth. Homeless youth also experience a high rate of substance abuse, injuries, dermatological problems, and teen pregnancies. Barriers to accessing health care among homeless youth include fear of health care settings, long wait times, lack of insurance, concerns regarding confidentiality, confusion over need for parental consent, unclean facilities, lack of transportation, and fear of being judged by health care providers (Hagedorn, 2002). In a qualitative study of ten homeless youth aged 16 to 24 who had experienced mental health problems, Darbyshire and colleagues (2006) found that the most appreciated aspects of service delivery included receiving clear, specific information and advice; accessing multiple services in one location; and being treated with respect and dignity.

Homeless Families

The lack of affordable housing has contributed greatly to the rise in homeless families. In addition, an increase in the number of people uninsured has placed families at risk. A serious injury or illness can eradicate a family's savings and plunge a family into homelessness (NCFH, n.d.a).

More than 85% of homeless families are headed by single mothers. Although 70% of fathers of homeless children remain in contact with their children, most of these fathers do not live with the family. Families may be separated by shelter policies that prohibit admission of older boys or men. Sometimes, parents are forced to leave their children with family or friends or to place them in foster care to shelter them from becoming homeless (NCH, 2006h). According to the U.S. Conference of Mayors (2005), requests for emergency shelter by homeless families with children increased in 63% of the survey cities. In 57% of the cities, homeless families may have to separate in order to access emergency shelters.

A child is at greater risk for homelessness if his or her father becomes injured or ill, experiences a job loss, has a substance abuse issue, or becomes involved with the criminal justice system. Fifty percent of fathers of homeless children are unemployed. To assist homeless families, attention must be focused on promoting affordable housing; supporting education, job training, and child care; promoting access to school; expanding violence prevention and treatment services; and preventing unnecessary separation of families (NCH, 2006h; NRTCHMI, n.d.b).

Homeless Veterans

Approximately 40% of homeless men are veterans. On any given night, 200,000 veterans are homeless. Despite the number of homeless veterans, direct combat experience does not seem to be related to homelessness. Although homeless veterans are less likely to have been exposed to combat, they have an increased rate of mental illness and addiction disorders, suggesting that these factors have more to do with homelessness than whether someone has served in the military (NCH, 2006j).

Female homeless veterans represent about 1.6% of the homeless veteran population. They are more likely to be married and have serious psychiatric illnesses but less likely to be employed or have addictions disorders than their male counterparts. No difference exists in rates of mental illness or addictions between veteran and nonveteran homeless women (NCH, 2006j).

Although Black veterans are more likely to be homeless than their White veteran counterparts, the rate of homelessness among Black veterans is lower than among other nonveteran minorities. The reduced risk may be attributed to the educational opportunities and other benefits and entitlements afforded those with veteran status. The U.S. Department of Veteran Affairs (VA) administers the Domiciliary Care for Homeless Veterans (DCHV) and the Health Care for Homeless Veterans (HCHV) programs. These programs provide case management, residential treatment, and other services to homeless veterans and have been found to improve housing, employment, and access to care for the homeless veteran population (NCH, 2006j).

The Rural Homeless

Homeless people in rural areas are more likely to be White, female, married, working, homeless for the first time, and homeless for a shorter length of time. Because fewer shelters are available in rural areas, they are also less likely to live in shelters or in the streets. They are more likely to be found in cars or campers or living with relatives in substandard or overcrowded housing. As a result, they may not be considered "homeless" for reporting purposes. Moreover, the communities in which they live may not be able to access as much federal funding, because the statistics do not adequately reflect the magnitude of the problem. Families consisting of single mothers and children comprise the largest segment of the rural homeless population. Native Americans and migrant workers are likely to be among the rural homeless. Like urban homelessness, rural homelessness is largely a result of poverty and lack of affordable housing. Housing costs are lower in rural areas, but incomes are also lower (NCH, 2006q).

Homelessness in rural areas may be precipitated by structural or physical housing problems that force families to relocate to safer but more expensive housing. In addition, the lack of job opportunities, the distance between low-income housing and job sites, the lack of transportation, rising rents, geographic isolation, and lack of resources compound the problem. To address the needs of the rural homeless, the definition of homelessness needs to be expanded to include people living in temporary or substandard housing (NCH, 2006q).

The Older Homeless

As with other groups, the increase in homelessness among older Americans is due in part to poverty and the lack of affordable housing. Many older people live on a fixed income, rendering them more vulnerable to unexpected financial crisis and even homelessness. Isolation also contributes to homelessness. Many older people live alone and lack a support network. Some researchers define the "older homeless" as homeless persons 50 and older because of the decline in physical health that often accompanies street living. Approximately 9% of homeless persons are 55 or older (USDHUD, n.d.a). Since older persons tend to distrust crowds at shelters and clinics, they are more likely to stay on the streets. They are prone to criminal victimization and suffer from a variety of health conditions including chronic diseases and functional disabilities. The Social Security benefits to which many are entitled are inadequate to cover housing costs. They may also encounter difficulties applying for benefits (NCH, 2006l).

HEALTH CARE AND THE HOMELESS

Acute and chronic health problems prevail in the homeless population. Chronic health conditions such as tuberculosis (TB), HIV/acquired immune deficiency syndrome (AIDS), diabetes, hypertension, addictions, and mental disorders require ongoing monitoring and are often difficult to treat in a population that is transient and lacks stable housing (NCH, 2006f). It is difficult for the homeless to adhere to complex treatment regimens. For example, where would a homeless person find a refrigerator to store insulin? Where would someone keep supplies for dressings? How could someone with no access to transportation keep regular appointments with health care providers? How does a homeless person keep track of multiple appointment dates? How is a shelter resident, who receives the typical shelter diet high in carbohydrates, fats, and sodium, going to adhere to a low-salt or diabetic diet?

Many homeless people expend their time and energy trying to meet basic survival needs. Health care may take a backseat to finding food, clothing, or shelter. High costs and limited access to health care and negative experiences with the health care system can also result in avoidance or delays in seeking treatment (NHCHC, n.d.).

Frostbite, leg ulcers, and upper respiratory tract infections result from chronic exposure to adverse environmental conditions. The homeless are also at higher risk of trauma and criminal victimization, including muggings, beatings, and rape. When one is homeless, it is difficult to maintain adequate nutrition or personal hygiene or to have access to basic first aid (NCH, 2006f). Communicable diseases such as TB, HIV, hepatitis, and other infections threaten not only the homeless, but also the public in general.

Poverty, substance abuse, poor nutrition, and coexisting medical and psychiatric illnesses also predispose the homeless to severe oral health problems. Among adults aged 35 to 44, twice as many Blacks and African Americans as Whites have tooth decay. African Americans are more likely than Whites to have teeth extracted. Low education levels have been found to be strongly correlated with tooth loss. Oral and pharyngeal cancers tend to be diagnosed at later stages in African Americans than in Whites. Together, alcohol and tobacco account for 90% of all oral cancers (Healthy People 2010, n.d.d).

HIV infection rates among the homeless range from 3% to 20%. Persons with HIV/AIDS are at higher risk of homelessness, because HIV-related illness can impact job stability. Moreover, health care costs associated with treating the illness can place an enormous financial burden on a low-income family. Insufficient funds to adequately house the poor with HIV/AIDS may also contribute to homelessness among HIV-infected individuals. The prevalence of HIV among the homeless is three times greater than that of the general population. Homeless women and adolescents are at risk of acquiring HIV infection due to the high incidence of sexual abuse and exploitation in this population (NCH, 2006g).

"Health Care for the Homeless" was a model for homeless health care developed in 1985 through a 19-city demonstration project funded by the Robert Wood Johnson Foundation and the Pew Memorial Trust. In 1987, federal legislation (the McKinney Homeless Assistance Act) was passed that authorized federal funding for these programs (NHCHC, n.d.). Grants are awarded to community-based organizations that deliver high quality health care to homeless populations. Health Care for the Homeless projects can be found across the nation to address significant gaps in health care delivery for this vulnerable group in society.

RESOURCES TO COMBAT HOMELESSNESS

Both public and private sectors have promoted a variety of initiatives to address the problem of homelessness. These initiatives are intended to impact homelessness on the local, state, and national level and to ensure a coordinated, comprehensive, and systematic approach to addressing the problem of homelessness.

Public Sector

The McKinney-Vento Homeless Assistance Act (PL100-77) was the first and only major piece of federal legislation intended to address the problem of homelessness on a national level. This landmark legislation Act, passed by Congress in 1987, originally consisted of 15 programs to address the major, pressing needs of the homeless. These needs included emergency shelter, transitional housing, job training, primary health care, education, and housing. The current Act has been amended four times in an effort to expand its scope and strengthen its impact. In particular, the amendments made to the Act in 1990 represented significant milestones in advocating for the needs of the homeless. These amendments included the creation of the Shelter Care Plus program, which provides for housing assistance for persons with disabilities, mental illness, AIDS, and drug and alcohol addiction. Another amendment created a demonstration program within the Health Care for the Homeless program to provide primary care and outreach to at-risk and homeless children. In addition, the Community Mental Health Services Program was amended and retitled the Projects for Assistance in Transition from Homelessness (PATH). Finally, the amendments made in 1990 strengthened access to public education for homeless children and youth. For example, states were required to provide grant funding to local educational institutions to ensure access to free, appropriate education for homeless youth and children (NCH, 2006o).

Over the years, Congress has appropriated funding to enable implementation of this federal legislation. The extent of federal funding has fluctuated over the years. In recent years, some of the programs have been repealed or restructured in an effort to contain costs. Homeless advocates acknowledge that the Act was an important step in addressing homelessness, but the lack of adequate funding over recent years threatens its impact on a national level. Moreover, some homeless advocates believe that the legislation focuses more on emergency measures to address the crisis of homelessness rather than on promoting a proactive agenda to address the causes of homelessness (e.g., lack of good paying jobs with benefits, lack of access to affordable health care) (NCH, 2006o).

Another significant milestone in federal initiatives to reduce homelessness occurred in 2001, when the federal government adopted the goal of ending chronic homelessness in 10 years. To meet this goal, annual funding was appropriated to create new permanent supportive housing. These resources helped to stimulate the production of housing. Many communities followed the lead of the federal government and developed their own 10 year plans (Burt, 2006). Table 28.2 summarizes the nine titles of the McKinney-Vento Act. Table 28.3 presents selected federally sponsored programs for addressing the needs of the homeless.

Private Sector

The private sector has made a concerted effort to organize communities in the battle against homelessness by forming

TABLE 28.2   McKinney-Vento Homeless Assistance Act Titles I-IX

Title I	States findings by Congress and definition of homelessness
Title II	Establishes the Interagency Council on Homelessness, a Council comprised of 15 heads of federal agencies charged with providing leadership for activities that assist the homeless
Title III	Authorizes the Emergency Food and Shelter Program, administered by the Federal Emergency Management Agency (FEMA)
Title IV	Authorizes the emergency shelter and transitional housing programs administered by the Department of Housing and Urban Development (HUD) including the Emergency Shelter Grant Program, the Supportive Housing Demonstration Program, Supplemental Assistance for Facilities to Assist the Homeless, and Section 8 Single Room Occupancy Moderate Rehabilitation
Title V	Requires federal agencies to make available land and buildings for states, local governments, and agencies to use to assist the homeless
Title VI	Authorizes programs to provide health care services to the homeless, including Health Care for the Homeless program, Community Mental Health Services Block Grant Program, and two demonstration programs providing substance abuse and mental health treatment services to the homeless
Title VII	Authorizes the Adult Education for the Homeless Program, the Education of Homeless Children and Youth Program (administered by the Department of Education), the Job Training for the Homeless Demonstration Program (administered by the Department of Labor), and the Emergency Community Services Homeless Grant Program (administered by the Department of Health and Human Services)
Title VIII	Amends the Food Stamp Program to facilitate access by the homeless and expands the Temporary Emergency Food Assistance Program (administered by the Department of Agriculture)
Title IX	Extends the Veterans Job Training Act

Source: United States Department of Housing and Urban Development. (n.d.c). McKinney-Vento Homeless Assistance Act. Retrieved September 23, 2006 from http://www.hud.gov/offices/cpd/homeles/lawsandregs/mckv.cfm.

coalitions, alliances, and memberships that champion the causes of the homeless. These organized efforts are carried out at the national, state, and local level to positively impact the problem of homelessness in communities across the nation. Table 28.4 presents a list and description of selected resources in the private sector to combat homelessness.

ROLE OF THE COMMUNITY HEALTH NURSE

Community health nurses maintain a long tradition of providing care to the **marginalized** (persons excluded from mainstream society) and **disenfranchised** (persons deprived of rights) (Wilde et al., 2004). Community health nurses play a vital role in addressing the needs of the homeless. Settings for care include shelters, clinics, soup kitchens, churches, community centers, social service agencies, and even the streets (see Using the Nursing Process).

Trust is an essential ingredient in the development of a therapeutic relationship with the homeless. A caring, consistent relationship is more likely to engage people who are homeless into treatment (NRTCHMI, n.d.a). It is sometimes difficult to establish trust with clients who have experienced negative encounters with the health care system. Often these negative perceptions are intensified by limited resources, inadequate access to care, or prejudicial views. As with other vulnerable populations, the homeless struggle with feelings of powerlessness, loss of control, and low self-esteem. Victim blaming is common. Some members of society perceive the homeless as responsible for their own fate. It is not uncommon to hear people speak

about the homeless in derogatory terms or to suggest that the solution to the problem of homelessness is to simply "get a job."

Behaviors that would ordinarily be considered lawful in the privacy of one's home become criminal activity when they are exhibited in public. For example, the homeless can be arrested for loitering, sleeping, urinating, or drinking alcohol in public. These behaviors can trigger a criminal record, thereby jeopardizing future employment or housing opportunities. In some states, men can be incarcerated for failing to pay child support (NHCHC, 2001). Consider a man who is laid off from a low-wage job. He is unable to pay child support and is arrested. His violation generates a criminal record and compromises his ability to secure employment in the future. He becomes trapped in a cycle of poverty and homelessness that is difficult to escape.

Every nurse encounters new situations with prior assumptions and biases. When considering work with the homeless, it is important to clarify one's own beliefs and values about poverty, homelessness, addictions, and mental disorders. What has been your experience with the homeless? Have you ever observed a homeless individual asking for money or holding up signs at a busy intersection? What thoughts and feelings do encounters such as these provoke? Have you ever volunteered at a soup kitchen or food pantry, fed a group of homeless people, or donated food or clothing? Have you had the opportunity to get to know a homeless individual? Do you have a personal experience with homelessness or poverty? If so, how has it affected your understanding of what it means to be poor or homeless?

TABLE 28.3 Federally Sponsored Programs for the Homeless

The Interagency Council on Homelessness	The Interagency Council on Homelessness coordinates the federal response to homelessness and creates a national partnership with public and private sectors to reduce and end homelessness in the United States. The major activities of the Council include: (1) planning and coordinating federal programs to assist the homeless; (2) providing technical assistance and evidenced-based best practice information to the public and private sector; (3) monitoring and evaluating assistance provided to the homeless by public and private agencies; and (4) collaborating with communities and governmental bodies to end chronic homelessness (United States Interagency Council on Homelessness, 2006; 2003).
The Center for Mental Health Services	The Center for Mental Health Services, a center of the federal Substance Abuse and Mental Health Services Administration (SAMHSA), supports programs to assist the homeless mentally ill to access primary care, substance abuse, and mental health services, legal assistance, entitlements, and other supportive services. The Center develops models for delivering mental health services to the homeless that programs can then adopt and use. It also provides funding to states to deliver mental health services (SAMHSA, n.d.).
Projects for Assistance in Transition from Homelessness (PATH)	PATH is a grant program created under the McKinney Act to support the delivery of services to persons with severe mental illnesses, including those who are homeless or at risk of becoming homeless. SAMHSA provides technical support to states and local agencies, providing care through the PATH program (PATH, 2006).
The National Resource Center on Homelessness and Mental Illness	This Center operates under SAMHSA to develop workshops and training programs on service delivery to the homeless mentally ill. The Center maintains an extensive database of over 4000 articles (National Mental Health Information Center, n.d.; SAMHSA, n.d.).
Health Care for the Homeless (HCH)	The HCH program (a provision of the McKinney Act) awards grants to community-based organizations that seek to provide quality, accessible health care to the homeless. The HCH program is administered by the United States Department of Health and Human Services (USDHHS). Any local public or private nonprofit organization can apply for HCH funds. In 2004, 172 programs were awarded grants to serve over 600,000 homeless people per year (NCH, 2005).
The U.S. Department of Housing and Urban Development (HUD)	HUD provides funding for supportive housing for low-income families as well as low-income individuals with disabilities, and low-income elderly. Funds can be used for housing development or rental assistance (to cover the difference between what a resident can afford to pay and the cost to operate the project). Grants are also provided to public housing agencies to rehabilitate or replace dilapidated public housing structures. Persons applying for public housing face a long waiting period, sometimes up to as long as 10 years (NCH, 2006e).
The White House Office of Faith-based and Community Initiatives	This Office provides information on federal grants that are available to faith-based and community organizations to address the needs of the homeless (White House Office on Faith Based and Community Initiatives, n.d.). Grants catalog available at: (http://www.whitehouse.gov/government/fbci/grants-catalog-homelessness.html)

It may be helpful to interview people who work with the homeless or to visit clinics, shelters, or other settings where the homeless congregate or access services. How are homeless people treated? What is a typical day like for someone who is homeless? How often do homeless persons hear their names? How often are they looked in the eye when addressed by others? How often are they touched in a way that is therapeutic, respectful, and affirming? By reflecting on your personal values and by allowing yourself to get closer to the people and places that are a part of the experi-

ence of homelessness, you will gain a deeper understanding of the homeless condition and be better equipped to serve those suffering from homelessness.

To address the multifaceted problems associated with homelessness effectively, a comprehensive and holistic approach is needed. As such, the community health nurse is responsible for implementing primary, secondary, and tertiary preventive measures to prevent homelessness or to assist those who are homeless to obtain needed services (see Levels of Prevention Pyramid).

TABLE 28.4   Private Sector Initiatives to Combat Homelessness

National Coalition for the Homeless (NCH)	The National Coalition for the Homeless is a national network of persons committed to preventing and ending homelessness. This Coalition consists of homelessness activists, service providers, persons who have experienced homelessness or are presently homeless, and others who are concerned with the plight of the homeless. The Coalition works to address issues related to homelessness through activities that promote civil rights and economic, health care, and housing justice. Activities of the Coalition include organizing community events to raise awareness and promote the rights of the homeless, advocating for health policy that protects the homeless, educating the public on facts related to homelessness, and providing research and technical assistance. The NCH also supports local and statewide homeless and housing coalitions (NCH, 2006i). (http://www.nch.org)
The National Center on Family Homelessness	The National Center on Family Homelessness is a 501c3 nonprofit organization that seeks to end family homelessness in the United States through the development of innovative programs and services that provide long term solutions for family homelessness and through education of service providers, policy makers, and the public. (http://www.familyhomelessness.org)
National Coalition for Homeless Veterans	This Coalition seeks to end homelessness among veterans through public policy, collaboration, and building community capacity. (http://www.nchv.org)
National Alliance to End Homelessness	This national membership organization seeks to mobilize leaders in business, nonprofit agencies, service providers, political leaders, and citizens to end homelessness through research, education, and public policy reform. (http://www.endhomelessness.org)
National Center for Homeless Education	This national resource center provides research and information to help communities address the needs of homeless children, youth, and families. (http://www.serve.org/nche)
Commission on Homelessness and Poverty, American Bar Association	This Commission works with local and state bar associations and other organizations to develop pro bono programs to address the legal needs of the poor and homeless. (http://www.abanet.org/homeless)
Homes for the Homeless	This organization attempts to provide homeless families with education, employment training, and support services. (http://www.homesforthehomeless.com)
National Low-Income Housing Coalition	The National Low-Income Housing Coalition is a national membership organization dedicated to ending the housing crisis in America. A major priority of the Coalition is to promote legislation that provides funding for the production of rental housing for extremely low-income people (NLIHC, 2005). (http://www.nlihc.org)

Primary Prevention

Primary prevention includes advocating for affordable housing, employment opportunities, and better access to health care to prevent the downward spiral into homelessness. Strategies for preventing homelessness may include financial counseling to assist clients to better manage their money; assistance in locating sources of legal or financial aid to prevent eviction (e.g., loans or grants for emergency funds to help pay for rent, utilities, etc.); or assistance in accessing social services, temporary housing, or health care to avoid a housing, health, or family crisis (Anderson & McFarlane, 2004).

Health education that addresses primary prevention may focus on positive parenting skills, violence prevention, anger management, coping skills, healthy eating, or principles of basic hygiene. Immunization programs will help to prevent communicable disease in this high-risk population. Counseling victims of intimate partner violence and helping

them to locate safe shelters can also aid in the prevention of homelessness (Anderson &McFarlane, 2004). Addictions treatment is also important to prevent the likely consequences of untreated addiction: death, incarceration, institutionalization, or homelessness.

Secondary Prevention

The focus of secondary prevention measures is on the early detection and treatment of adverse health conditions. This requires a thorough assessment of client needs including the need for housing, health care, education, social services, and employment. Clients will also benefit from secondary prevention measures such as screening for communicable and chronic diseases (e.g., hepatitis, TB, STI, HIV, hypertension, diabetes, cancer).

Barriers to accessing services and the extent of community resources available to the homeless also need to be assessed (Anderson & McFarlane, 2004). Resources such

USING THE NURSING PROCESS

Conducting a Needs Assessment

As a faith community nurse working in a large church congregation, you are invited to develop an outreach program to minister to the needs of an inner-city mission that is receiving financial support from the church. You begin by visiting the Mission to conduct a needs assessment of its residents and to identify priority health issues. The shelter operates as a faith-based, nonprofit organization and is dedicated to serving the needs of homeless men with addictions. The shelter provides emergency overnight services and operates a 1-year residential faith-based addictions recovery program. Approximately 300 homeless male addicts visit the shelter daily. Staff and residents have expressed concerns regarding a recent outbreak of boils among residents.

Assessment data reveals the following issues:

- Approximately 80% of clients have a history of injection drug use.
- Clients sleep in dormitory-style accommodations and share bathroom facilities.

- An on-site barber shop operated by the residents provides haircuts for a nominal fee.
- Clients have access to a small recreational area with donated exercise equipment.
- Laundry services are available, and residents take their clothing to the laundry on alternate days to have it washed. Laundry is typically washed in cold water and at times the laundry runs out of detergent.

Questions:

1. What additional data would you wish to gather to address the outbreak of boils at the shelter? How would you collect this data?
2. What host, agent, and environmental factors may have contributed to the outbreak of boils?
3. Discuss appropriate nursing interventions to address the outbreak. Consider the following levels of prevention: Primary, Secondary, Tertiary.
4. What advocacy role might the CHN play in addressing this issue?

as shelters, soup kitchens, medical clinics, social service agencies, and supportive housing should be readily accessible to the homeless population. Consider hours of operation, wait times, acceptability of services, adequacy of services to meet needs, and transportation issues (Martin, 2003).

Lack of transportation can be a major barrier to accessing care. Some programs have responded to this need by adopting mobile health vans that provide care on street corners and in neighborhoods (Daiski, 2005). Clinics have also been established in shelters to facilitate client access. These clinics are often managed by nurses (Yousey & Carr, 2005). Nursing students also play an important role in promoting access to care for the homeless (Wilde et al., 2004).

The community health nurse should also consider the role of faith-based communities in providing physical and spiritual support to the homeless. Many places of worship have responded to the crisis of homelessness by offering food, shelter, counseling, medical care, and social services within the context of the faith community. Clinics have been built within faith communities to promote access to care.

Tertiary Prevention

Tertiary preventive measures attempt to limit disability and to restore maximum functioning. The goal is to provide rehabilitative care and support to clients who are already experiencing the consequences of homelessness. Often, homeless individuals suffer from chronic health conditions that have gone untreated for long periods of time. This neglect in attending to health needs results in significant disease morbidity. Treating complications of advanced disease, pro-

viding rehabilitative care, and offering counseling and support are important tertiary preventive strategies.

Case Management

At each level of prevention, the community health nurse functions as a case manager and coordinator of care to ensure seamless delivery of ser ces as people transition from one level of care to another. is often difficult for the homeless to keep track of multiple appointments, negotiate the bureaucracy of multiple agencies and services, or maintain communication with providers through follow-up phone calls, letters, or visits. With no permanent address or phone, homeless clients encounter obstacles to adhering to recommendations to follow-up on test results or to notify their provider if symptoms persist or worsen. The community health nurse can help to bridge these gaps in service delivery and promote more effective adherence to therapeutic regimens.

Advocacy

Advocacy is a vital dimension of the community health nurse's role in working with the homeless (Hatton et al., 2001). Advocacy entails working with different sectors of the community (including public officials, service providers, and persons living in the community) to develop innovative models for responding to the crisis of homelessness. Advocacy creates the broader systemic changes needed to end homelessness (NCH, 2006n). The community health nurse acts as an advocate at each level of prevention to effect positive change. For example, the nurse may advocate for mental health and substance abuse services to promote mental

LEVELS OF PREVENTION PYRAMID

SITUATION: Promoting health and preventing illness among homeless male addicts

GOAL: To apply the three levels of prevention to avoid adverse health conditions, diagnose and treat disorders promptly, and assist a homeless male addict population to maintain or regain optimal health.

Tertiary Prevention

Rehabilitation	Primary Prevention	
	Health Promotion & Education	*Health Protection*
• Provide case management of chronic health conditions • Advocate for supportive and transitional housing to enable homeless residents with addiction disorders to transition back into the community successfully	• Advocate for expansion of counseling, rehabilitative services, and addiction treatment programs for the homeless	

Secondary Prevention

Early Diagnosis	Prompt Treatment
• Conduct mass screenings for diseases commonly found in homeless male populations (TB, HIV, hepatitis, prostate cancer, colorectal cancer)	• Develop programs for health screening and early diagnosis and treatment in the community that are culturally sensitive and accessible to the homeless (e.g., mobile vans, faith community, or shelter-based clinics)

Primary Prevention

Health Promotion & Education	Health Protection
• Support employment and job training opportunities that assist clients to obtain jobs with livable wages and benefits • Advocate through housing coalitions and legislative efforts to promote affordable housing, employment opportunities, and better access to health care • Develop culturally sensitive health education programs that promote healthy coping, positive parenting, communication and relationship building, mental health, and injury and illness prevention • Promote programs that offer counseling and support to prevent continued high risk behaviors as a result of untreated addiction	• Advocate for legislation to protect citizens from environmental toxins and industrial wastes common to low-income areas • Provide immunization services to prevent communicable disease transmission • Counsel clients on proper nutrition, exercise, and basic hygiene to promote healthy lifestyles and prevent disease transmission • Advocate for funding for nutrition programs for the homeless and for homeless shelters that would allow for the purchase of nutritious foods

health and prevent homelessness (primary prevention). Alternatively, he or she may advocate for legislation to fund supportive housing, health care, or social services to benefit the homeless with chronically mental illness (NRTCHMI, n.d.a). The community health nurse (CHN) can also assume an advocacy role by becoming involved in local, state, or national coalitions or organizations devoted to protecting the rights of the homeless or by speaking out on legislation that impacts the homeless (NCH, 2006n).

Summary

Rising poverty and lack of affordable housing have led to a dramatic rise in homelessness over the past two decades. Poverty, lack of housing, domestic violence, mental illness, addictions, personal crises, and natural disasters are factors that may predispose persons to homelessness.

Homeless families represent the fastest growing segment of the homeless population. Acute and chronic health problems plague the homeless. Conditions such as HIV/ AIDS, diabetes, hypertension, addictions, and mental disorders are prevalent among the homeless and are difficult to treat because of the challenges associated with being homeless.

Both the public and private sectors have launched concerted efforts to combat the problem of homelessness through the passage of federal legislation (most notably the McKinney-Vento Homeless Assistance Act) and through the formation of national, state, and local coalitions and alliances to champion the cause of the homeless. Much remains to be done.

Community health nurses maintain a long and distinguished tradition of providing care to the marginalized. As such, they play a vital role in addressing the needs of the homeless in society. At the core of community nursing practice is the development of a trusting relationship. The community health nurse needs to examine his or her values and presuppositions regarding poverty and homelessness to be more effective in rendering care that is respectful, compassionate, and nonjudgmental. The community health nurse implements primary, secondary, and tertiary preventive measures to prevent homelessness or to assist those who are homeless to obtain needed services. Primary prevention includes advocating for affordable housing, employment opportunities, and improved access to health care to prevent the downward spiral into homelessness. Secondary prevention includes screening for communicable and chronic diseases and promoting access to affordable health care and social services. Tertiary prevention includes rehabilitative and supportive care and counseling.

The community health nurse also serves as a case manager to coordinate care and to assist clients to negotiate the bureaucracy of multiple agencies and services. Finally, the CHN acts as an advocate to promote the rights of the homeless and to speak out on legislation impacting homelessness. ■

⬡ ACTIVITIES TO PROMOTE CRITICAL THINKING

1. Reflect in writing on the meaning of "home." Share your reflections with someone experiencing homelessness.

2. Interview a homeless person regarding the most difficult choices he or she has had to make. What were the conditions surrounding these choices?

3. Volunteer to work at a soup kitchen or homeless shelter. Observe carefully the faces, sounds, attitudes, and activities. What is it like to share in the same spaces as those who are homeless? What would it be like to be receiving rather than giving service?

4. Consider joining a local coalition to support the cause of homelessness in your community.

5. Call or write your local legislator to advocate for legislation impacting the homeless and to share your thoughts and feelings about homelessness.

6. Attend a public meeting that addresses homelessness prevention or low-income housing. Listen to the debate and consider the divergent views. What are the political, economic, and social contexts underlying these views?

7. Perform a windshield survey in a low-income community. What resources are lacking? Where is the nearest bank, school, grocery store, or health clinic? What are the conditions of the roads, homes, and other buildings? How do you feel as you drive through the community? What do you think it would be like to live there?

References

Anderson, E., & McFarlane, J. (2004). *Community as partner: Theory and practice in nursing* (4th ed.). Philadelphia: Lippincott, Williams & Wilkins.

Burt, M. (2006). Testimony related to provisions of S. 1801, *The Community Partnership to End Homelessness Act of 2005*, 1–16. Retrieved August 21, 2008 from http://www.urban.org/ publications/900937.html.

Daiski, I. (2005). The health bus: Healthcare for marginalized populations. *Policy, Politics, and Nursing Practice, 6*(1), 30–38.

Darbyshire, P., Muir-Cochrane, E., Fereday, J., Jureidini, J., & Drummond, A. (2006). Engagement with health and social services: Perceptions of homeless young people with mental health problems. *Health and Social Care in the Community, 14*(6), 553–562.

Hagedorn, S. (2002). Caring for street youth: A nursing challenge. *Journal of School and Public Health Nursing, 7*, 34–37.

Hatton, D., Kleffel, D., Bennett, S., & Gaffrey, E. (2001). Homeless women and children's access to health care: A paradox. *Journal of Community Health Nursing, 18*(1), 25–34.

Healthy People 2010. (n.d.a). *Mental health and mental disorders.* Retrieved December 6, 2006 from http://www.healthypeople. gov/document/HTML/volume2/18mental.htm/.

Healthy People 2010. (n.d.b). *Healthy People goals.* Retrieved September 29, 2006 from http://www.healthypeople.gov/ Aboutgoals.htm/.

Healthy People 2010. (n.d.c). Search results. Retrieved August 21, 2008 from http://www.healthypeople.gov/hpscripts/ KeywordResult.asp?n320=320&Submit=Submit/.

Healthy People 2010. (n.d.d). *Oral health.* Retrieved December 6, 2006 from http://www.healthypeople.gov/document/html/ volume2/21oral.htm/.

Homelessness Research Institute. (2007). Homelessness Counts. *National Alliance to End Homelessness.* Retrieved January 10, 2007 from http://www.endhomelessness.org/content/general/ detail/1440/.

Martijn, C., & Sharpe, L. (2006). Pathways to youth homelessness. *Social Science and Medicine, 62*(1), 1–12.

Martin, B. (2003). Assisting homeless individuals to access health care. *Chart, 100*(2), 5.

National Center on Family Homelessness. (n.d.a). *America's homeless children.* Retrieved September 29, 2006 from http://www.familyhomelessness.org/pdf/fact_children.pdf/.

National Center on Family Homelessness. (n.d.b). *Homeless children: America's new outcasts.* Retrieved September 29, 2006 from http://www.familyhomelessness.org/pdf/fact_outcasts.pdf/.

National Center on Family Homelessness. (n.d.c). *Research on homeless and low-income housed families.* Retrieved September 29, 2006 from http://www.familyhomelessness.org/pdf/ fact_research.pdf/.

National Center on Family Homelessness. (n.d.d). *Violence in the lives of homeless women.* Retrieved December 4, 2006 from http://www.familyhomelessness.org/pdf/fact_violence.pdf/.

National Coalition for the Homeless. (2005, October). *Health Care for the Homeless program.* Retrieved September 29, 2006, from http://www.nationalhomeless.org/health/hchprogram.html/.

National Coalition for the Homeless. (2006a). *Addiction disorders and homelessness.* Retrieved September 29, 2006, from http://www.nationalhomeless.org/publications/facts.html/.

National Coalition for the Homeless. (2006b). *Domestic violence and homelessness.* Retrieved September 29, 2006, from http://www.nationalhomeless.org/publications/facts.html/.

National Coalition for the Homeless. (2006c). *Education of homeless children and youth.* Retrieved September 29, 2006 from http://www.nationalhomeless.org/publications/facts.html/.

National Coalition for the Homeless. (2006d). *Employment and homelessness.* Retrieved September 29, 2006, from http://www.nationalhomeless.org/publications/facts.html/.

National Coalition for the Homeless. (2006e). *Federal housing assistance programs.* Retrieved September 29, 2006, from http://www.nationalhomeless.org/publications/facts.html/.

National Coalition for the Homeless. (2006f). *Health care and homelessness.* Retrieved September 29, 2006, from http://www.nationalhomeless.org/publications/facts.html/.

National Coalition for the Homeless. (2006g). *HIV/AIDS and homelessness.* Retrieved September 29, 2006, from http://www.nationalhomeless.org/publications/facts.html/.

National Coalition for the Homeless. (2006h). *Homeless families with children.* Retrieved September 29, 2006, from http://www.nationalhomeless.org/publications/facts.html/.

National Coalition for the Homeless. (2006i). *Homeless self-help and empowerment projects.* Retrieved September 29, 2006, from http://www.nationalhomeless.org/publications/facts.html/.

National Coalition for the Homeless. (2006j). *Homeless veterans.* Retrieved September 29, 2006 from http://www.nationalhomeless.org/publications/facts.html/.

National Coalition for the Homeless. (2006k). *Homeless youth.* Retrieved September 29, 2006 from http://www.nationalhomeless.org/publications/facts.html/.

National Coalition for the Homeless. (2006l). *Homelessness among elderly persons.* Retrieved September 29, 2006 from http://www.nationalhomeless.org/publications/facts.html/.

National Coalition for the Homeless. (2006m). *How many people experience homelessness?* Retrieved September 29, 2006 from http://www.nationalhomeless.org/publications/facts.html/.

National Coalition for the Homeless. (2006n). *How you can end homelessness.* Retrieved September 29, 2006 from http://www.nationalhomeless.org/publications/facts.html/.

National Coalition for the Homeless. (2006o). *McKinney-Vento Act.* Retrieved September 29, 2006 from http://www.nationalhomeless.org/publications/facts.html/.

National Coalition for the Homeless. (2006p). *Mental illness and homelessness.* Retrieved September 29, 2006 from http://www.nationalhomeless.org/publications/facts.html/.

National Coalition for the Homeless. (2006q). *Rural homelessness.* Retrieved September 29, 2006 from http://www.nationalhomeless.org/publications/facts.html/.

National Coalition for the Homeless. (2006r). *Who is homeless?* Retrieved September 29, 2006 from http://www.nationalhomeless.org/publications/facts.html/.

National Coalition for the Homeless. (2006s). *Why are people homeless?* Retrieved September 29, 2006 from http://www.nationalhomeless.org/publications/facts.html/.

National Health Care for the Homeless Council. (n.d.). *The basics of homelessness.* Retrieved November 24, 2006 from http://www.nhchc.org/basics_of_homelessness.html/.

National Health Care for the Homeless Council. (2001, June). *Single males: The homeless majority.* *Healing Hands, 5*(3), 1–6. Retrieved December 4, 2006 from http://www.nhchc.org/healinghands.html.

National Low Income Housing Coalition. (2005). *About NLIHC.* Retrieved November 20, 2006 from http://www.nlihc.org/about/index.htm/.

National Low Income Housing Coalition. (2006a). *2006 Advocates guide to housing and community development policy.* Retrieved November 21, 2006 from http://www.nlihc.org/advocates/publichousing.htm/.

National Low Income Housing Coalition. (2006b). *Initial assessment of 2005 American Community Survey indicates growing housing cost burdens for lowest income households.* Retrieved December 4, 2006 from http://www.nlihc.org/research/06–04pdf/.

National Mental Health Information Center. (n.d.). *Homelessness.* Retrieved October 7, 2006 from http://mentalhealth.samhsa.gov/homelessness/links.asp/.

National Resource and Training Center on Homelessness and Mental Illness. (n.d.a). *Get the facts: Question #4—How can we end homelessness among people with serious mental illness?* Retrieved September 29, 2006 from http://www.nrchmi.samhsa.gov/facts/facts_question_4.asp.

National Resource and Training Center on Homelessness and Mental Illness. (n.d.b). *What about the needs of children that are homeless?* Retrieved September 29, 2006 from http://www.nrchmi.samhsa.gov/facts/facts_question_5.asp.

O'Sullivan, J., & Lussier-Duynstee, P. (2006) Adolescent homelessness, nursing, and public health policy. *Policy, Politics, and Nursing Practice, 7*(1), 73–77.

Projects for Assistance in Transition from Homelessness. (2006, September). *PATH.* Retrieved October 31, 2006 from http://pathprogram.samhsa.gov/.

Substance Abuse and Mental Health Services Administration. (n.d.). *Homelessness – Provision of mental health and substance abuse services.* Retrieved October 7, 2006 from http://mentalhealth.samsha.gov/scripts/pringpage.aspx?FromPage=http%3A/mentalhealth/.

United States Conference of Mayors-Sodexho, Inc. (2005). *Hunger and homelessness survey.* Retrieved September 29, 2006 from http://www.mayors.org/uscm/hungersurvey/2005/HH2005FINAL.pdf/.

United States Department of Housing and Urban Development. (n.d.a). *Facts about the homeless.* Retrieved October 31, 2006 from http://www.hud.gov/utilities/pring/print2cfm?page=80$^@http%3A%2Fwww%2Eh/.

United States Department of Housing and Urban Development. (n.d.b). *Homelessness: Programs and the people they serve – Highlights report.* Retrieved November 25, 2006 from http://www.huduser.org/publications/homeless/homelessness/highrpt.html/.

United States Department of Housing and Urban Development. (n.d.c). *McKinney-Vento Homeless Assistance Act.* Retrieved September 23, 2006 from http://www.hud.gov/offices/cpd/homeless/rulesandregs/law/.

United States Interagency Council on Homelessness. (2003). *Frequently asked questions.* Retrieved September 29, 2006 from http://www.ich.gov/faq/html/.

United States Interagency Council on Homelessness. (2006). *State and local initiatives.* Retrieved October 7, 2006 from http://www.ich.gov/slocal/index.html/.

White House Office on Faith Based and Community Initiatives. (n.d.). *The White House.* Retrieved December 4, 2006 from http://www.whitehouse.gov/government/fbci/grants-catalog-homelessness.html/.

Wilde, M., Albanese, E., Rennells, R., & Bullock, Q. (2004). *Public Health Nursing, 21,* 354–360.

Yousey, Y., & Carr, M. (2005). A health care program for home-less children using Healthy People 2010 objectives. *Nursing Clinics of North America, 40,* 791–801.

Selected Readings

Burke, J. (2005). Educating the staff at a homeless shelter about mental illness and anger management. *Journal of Community Health Nursing, 22*(2), 65–76.

Cohen, M.B. (2001). Homeless people. In A. Gitterman (Ed.) *Handbook of social work practice with vulnerable and resilient populations* (2nd ed., pp. 628–650). New York: Columbia University Press.

Hubber, A. (2005). An enthnonursing research study: Adults residing in a midwestern Christian philosophy urban homeless shelter. *Journal of Transcultural Nursing, 16*(3), 236–244.

Kushes, M. (2005). Revolving doors: Imprisonment among the homeless and marginally housed population. *American Journal of Public Health, 95,* 1747–1752.

Lashley, M. (2007). A targeted testing program for tuberculosis control and prevention among Baltimore City's homeless population. *Public Health Nursing, 24,* 34–39.

Nelson, G. (2005). A narrative approach to the evaluation of support-ive housing: Stories of homeless people who have experienced mental illness. *Psychiatric Rehabilitation Journal, 29*(2), 98–104.

Romeo, J. (2005). Down and out in New York City: A participant-observation study of the poor and marginalized. *Journal of Cultural Diversity, 12*(4), 152–160.

Savenstedt, S. (2005). Working with girls living on the streets in East Africa: Professionals' experiences. *Journal of Advanced Nursing, 50,* 489–497.

Sleath, B. (2006). Literacy and perceived barriers to medication taking among homeless mothers and their children. *American Journal of Health-System Pharmacy, 63*(4), 346–351.

Valios, N. (2005). You're not from round here. *Community Care,* Sept. 22–28(1591), 32–33.

Washington, O. (2005). Identification and characteristics of older homeless African American women. *Issues in Mental Health Nursing, 26*(2), 117–136.

Wilson, M. (2005). Health promoting behaviors of sheltered homeless women. *Family and Community Health, 28*(1), 51–63.

Internet Resources

Interagency Council on Homelessness: *http://www.ich.gov*

National Alliance to End Homelessness: *http://www.endhomelessness.org*

National Center on Family Homelessness: *http://www.familyhomelessness.org*

National Coalition for the Homeless: *http://www.nationalhomeless.org/*

National Health Care for the Homeless Council: *http://www.nhchc.org*

National Low Income Housing Coalition: *http://www.nlihc.org*

United States Department of Housing and Urban Development: *http://www.hud.gov*

United States Substance Abuse and Mental Health Services Administration: *http://www.samhsa.gov*

White House Office of Faith-Based and Community Initiatives: *http://www.whitehouse.gov/government/fbci/*

29

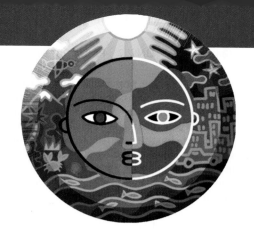

Issues with Rural, Migrant, and Urban Health Care

LEARNING OBJECTIVES

Upon mastery of this chapter, you should be able to:

◆ Define the terms *rural, migrant,* and *urban.*
◆ Discuss the population characteristics of rural residents.
◆ Describe five barriers to health care access for rural clients.
◆ Describe the migrant lifestyle.
◆ Identify at least three health problems common to migrant workers and their families.
◆ Discuss barriers and challenges to migrant health care.
◆ Identify common health disparities found among urban populations.
◆ Propose intervention strategies at the aggregate or community level to assure a healthier *built environment* in both rural and urban areas.
◆ Explain the concept of *social justice* and how it relates to public health nursing in urban areas.
◆ Compare and contrast the challenges and opportunities related to rural and urban community health nursing practice.

> *"No city should be too large for a man to walk out of in a morning."*
> —Cyril Connolly (1903–1974), British critic

KEY TERMS

Built environment
Critical access hospitals
Federally qualified health centers
Frontier area
Ghettos
Health professional shortage areas (HPSAs)
In-migration
Medically underserved areas (MUAs)
Metropolitan statistical area
Micropolitan statistical area
Migrant farmworkers
Migrant streams
Out-migration
Patterns of migration
Population density
Rural
Rural health clinics
Seasonal farmworkers
Social justice
Telehealth
Urban
Urban health
Urbanized area (UA)
Urban cluster (UC)
Urban health penalty
Urban planning

About half the population live in what is known as the suburbs, but the remainder live in one of two diametrically opposed areas: rural or urban. There is a good chance that many of you reading this book live in either very densely populated, bustling urban areas or in sparsely populated, somewhat isolated rural areas. Community health nursing in urban and rural areas requires not only general public health nursing knowledge and skills, but also a unique understanding of how these distinctive environments affect the health of the populations living there. Where you live can and does markedly affect your health outcomes, with rural and urban areas having distinctive problems and issues (van Dis, 2002). These differences are much more than just the ability to shop at "Wal-Mart versus Pottery Barn" (p. 108). Both rural and urban clients have health disparities and disadvantages, although they may be dissimilar in nature.

Rural nursing practice offers many opportunities. Nurses are respected community members—their judgment and opinions count. Rural nurses are key members of the health care team. They can make a difference in the lives of their neighbors, friends, and community. Rural public health nurses (PHNs) often struggle with helping clients gain access to quality health care and the inherent transportation problems found in isolated areas. The challenges are many, but the rewards are great.

Urban public health nurses often specialize in particular areas of interest. They deal with different types of problems, such as homelessness, overcrowding, bioterrorism threats, and violent crime. They are often called upon to advocate for their most vulnerable clients, and they develop collaborative relationships with other professionals. Urban community health nursing can also be very rewarding and satisfying.

This chapter addresses the special health needs and concerns of rural, migrant, and urban clients and the ways in which a community health nurse can address those needs. After reading the chapter, you may come to appreciate the many advantages that rural nurses enjoy and consider rural nursing as a practice choice, or you may find that being a PHN in an urban area offers you more opportunities for specialization and networking. Either way, your contributions can improve the health of populations living at both extremes.

DEFINITIONS AND DEMOGRAPHICS

Depending on one's geographic location, professional discipline, agency or institutional affiliation, or other frame of reference, the term *rural* has different and specialized meanings. Moreover, rural populations and characteristics have changed significantly over many years. These differences and their implications are described in this chapter.

Definitions of Rural

The term *rural* means different things to different people. The community health nurse needs to be aware of the precise meaning of the term as it is used in a particular agency, community, or piece of legislation, because differences in semantics can affect public policy regarding rural communities. For example, federal dollars are often distributed to communities based on rural or urban status.

The U.S. government provides several definitions of rural. These can seem confusing and complicated, but it is important to understand the terms and how they are used in federal programs and grant funding. The U.S. Census Bureau (2002) identifies **urban** as all "territory, population, and housing units located within an **urbanized area (UA)** or an **urban cluster (UC)**." A UA consists of densely settled territory with an area of population density of 1,000 people or more per square mile and with surrounding areas with population densities of at least 500 people per square mile. **Population density** refers to the number of persons per square mile—urban areas are much more densely populated than rural areas. The U.S. Census definition of *rural* is all territory, population, and housing units located outside UAs and UCs. Some counties, however, may include both rural and urban designations, as these designations do not follow municipal boundaries but rather denote population density (like the dense grouping of buildings that you might notice from an airplane).

For the 2000 Census, the U.S. Office of Management and Budget (OMB) reclassified the United States into metropolitan and micropolitan statistical areas. This newer nomenclature identifies a **metropolitan statistical area** as a core-based statistical area associated with at least one urbanized area that has a minimum population of 50,000. **Micropolitan statistical areas** are "core-based statistical areas" associated with at least one urban cluster of no less than 10,000 and no more than 50,000 people (U.S. Department of Agriculture [USDA], 2003a). Both metropolitan and micropolitan statistical areas comprise the central county or counties containing the core; also included are adjacent outlying counties that have a high degree of social and economic integration with the central county (based on the number of people who commute—generally considered 25% or more). With such a broad definition, micropolitan statistical areas can include both rural and urban areas. Before 2003, the OMB defined urban and rural in terms of metropolitan and nonmetropolitan counties. By making these changes, the numbers of people living in what used to be considered nonmetropolitan areas decreased from 55 to 49 million (USDA, 2003a).

The U.S. Department of Agriculture (USDA) rural–urban continuum examines metropolitan and nonmetropolitan areas on the basis of counties, and this provides different data apart from census reports. State and federal agencies recognize county-level jurisdictions and governments, and depend upon employment, income, and population data that are available on an annual basis (USDA, 2007a). Many states have offices of rural health or other agencies dealing with issues specific to rural populations.

For the purposes of this chapter, **rural** is defined as *communities with fewer than 10,000 residents and a county population density of less than 1,000 persons per square mile* (Table 29.1). This definition of rural is arbitrary because rural clients do not merely consider population density or community size when defining their *ruralness*. They have a multitude of reasons for defining their community as rural, such as distance from a large city, major occupations in the area (e.g., agriculture), or numbers of students in the local schools. If you have access to a small community, ask some of the residents the reasons why they consider their community to be urban or rural.

The term **frontier area** is used to designate sparsely populated rural places that are isolated from population centers

TABLE 29.1   Definitions of Rural

Source	Nomenclature	Definition
U. S. Bureau of the Census	Rural	All territory, population, and housing units located outside of urbanized areas (UAs) and urbanized clusters (UCs)
U. S. Office of Management and Budget	Micropolitan statistical area	A core-based statistical area associated with at least one urban cluster of at least 10,000 but <50,000 people.
U. S. Department of Agriculture Rural-Urban Continuum Codes	Completely rural	<2,500 urban population either adjacent to or not adjacent to metropolitan area.
U. S. Government	Frontier area	<6 people per square mile
Author	Rural	Communities with <10,000 residents and county population <1,000 people per square mile.

and services, but specific definitions vary (Rural Assistance Center [RAC], 2007a). A common definition of a frontier area is one with six or fewer persons per square mile, but others include not only population density but distance and travel time to market-service areas (RAC, 2007a; National Center for Frontier Communities, 2006). For instance, 60 miles or 60 minutes of driving on paved roads to the nearest 75-bed (or greater) hospital can constitute a frontier area. It is estimated that 3% of the U.S. population live in frontier areas that comprise 56% of the U.S. land areas; frontier areas are located in 38 states. States with either a high frontier population and/or high frontier land area include Alaska, Texas, Arizona, Montana, Wyoming, New Mexico, Colorado, North Dakota, and South Dakota (National Center for Frontier Communities, 2006). Rural–urban commuting area (Census data) is used to designate remote areas (RAC, 2007a).

Health issues of concern to rural areas may be of even greater concern to frontier areas. In rural health circles, the term **health professional shortage areas (HPSAs)**, defines urban or rural geographic areas, population groups, or facilities with chronic shortages of medical, dental, or mental health professionals. The federal government determines which areas are HPSAs. About 20% of the U.S. population live in areas that have been designated as HPSAs (Fig. 29.1). In **medically**

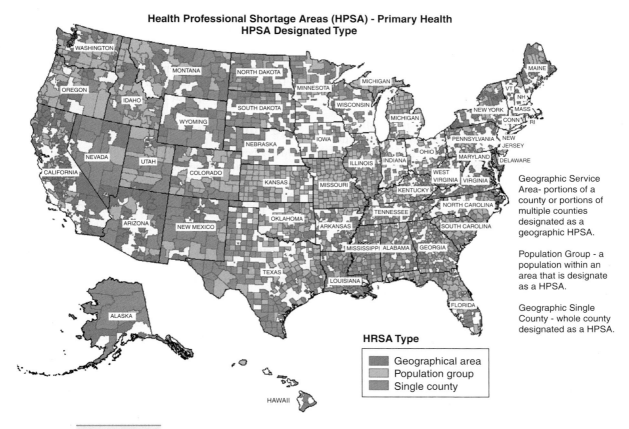

Health Professional Shortage Areas (HPSA) - Primary Health HPSA Designated Type

Geographic Service Area- portions of a county or portions of multiple counties designated as a geographic HPSA.

Population Group - a population within an area that is designate as a HPSA.

Geographic Single County - whole county designated as a HPSA.

HRSA Type

■ Geographical area
□ Population group
■ Single county

FIGURE 29.1   Health Professional Shortage Areas (HPSA) – Primary Health HPSA Designated Type. From: Modern-day slavery. (2005). *Palm Beach Post*. Retrieved October 23, 2008 from http://www.palmbeachpost.com/moderndayslavery/content/moderndayslavery/reports/gr. Used with permission.

underserved areas (MUAs), residents experience a shortage of health services; these areas are determined by the federal government using a score based on the shortage of primary care physicians, high infant mortality rates, high percentage of the population living below the poverty level, and a high proportion of residents over age 65 (Health Resources & Services Administration [HRSA], 2007a).

Population Statistics

The number of persons living in urban areas of the United States tripled since the mid-1800s, to 59,367,367 in 2000 (U.S. Census Bureau, 2000a). During the same period, the proportion of persons living in rural communities decreased from about 85% of the U.S. population to 21% (Ricketts, 1999; USDA, 2007a). By 2005, residents in nonmetropolitan counties dropped to just under 50 million (USDA, 2007a). The highest proportion of the rural population is located in the South (35%). The Midwest and West have approximately 23% of rural residents, and the Northeast has the smallest percentage (19%) (Eberhardt et al., 2001). About 11% of the population lives in what is now characterized as urban clusters (USDA, 2007b).

In 2003, of the 250 poorest counties in America, 244 are rural (Congressional Rural Caucus, 2004). Poverty and joblessness are common among rural Americans. Rural areas have a higher percentage of elderly, along with fewer physicians, nurses, hospitals, and other health care resources; almost one-third of rural adults report that they are in poor to fair health (Agency for Healthcare Research & Quality [AHRQ], 2007; Zigmond, 2007). A large-scale study found that rural workers were less likely than urban workers to be offered insurance. They also reported lower wages and were more often working in small businesses or were self-employed (Larson & Hill, 2005).

Rural areas have a slightly higher fertility rate than urban areas (Tarmann, 2003). However, this population growth related to births (termed *natural increase*) is offset by the loss of rural youth moving to more urban areas for education, jobs, and marriage (USDA, 2007c). The loss of 20- to 34-year-olds was greatest in the Northeast (29.1%) and Midwest (16.8%) for the period from 1990 to 2000 (Kirschner, Berry, & Glasgow, 2006).

Changing Patterns of Migration

Population changes in rural areas are usually related to natural increase through births or through **out-migration**, the process of residents moving out of rural communities and into urban places (USDA, 2007a). When American was a more rural country, there was more natural increase than out-migration, which caused continued growth in the rural population.

In the 1970s, the proportion of births decreased, but many people moved into rural communities, resulting in an increase in population. During the 1980s, the population trends shifted, as most rural areas lost population to out-migration as a result of economic recession and a serious farming crisis. During the first half of the 1990s, the population trend in rural communities changed to **in-migration**, an increase in residents moving into rural communities from urban places. White-collar workers were affected by changing technologies, and many young professionals with families elected to live in more rural settings (USDA, 2007a). Since 1995, however, the growth rate in many rural communities has decreased. Rural areas with textile jobs experienced out-migration, whereas immigrants moved to fill jobs in states with meat packing and other "food-and-fiber industries" (USDA, 2007a). Rural counties with "natural amenities," such as beautiful landscapes, desirable climates, or proximity to tourist areas (e.g., ski slopes, lakes, beaches, national parks), have experienced more growth (McGranahan & Sullivan, 2005). Some rural counties have noted increased employment opportunities, with Indian casinos and the proliferation of prisons, helping to stem some of the out-migration of young adults (Tarmann, 2003).

Natural amenity counties and other rural areas are also attractive to retired people, who are responsible for some of the in-migration to those areas. The older adults moving into rural areas are generally healthier, more financially secure, and better educated than the rural elderly population who are aging in place (Tarmann, 2003; USDA, 2007a). The rural West had an increase of 23% among those 75 years and older (Kirschner et al., 2006).

Population trends have many implications for the health services needed by rural people. The patterns of rural migration change shifting sand, adding to the challenge of planning resources for rural communities.

POPULATION CHARACTERISTICS

The following information is meant to describe, not stereotype, rural clients. Each rural community is unique, as are its residents. The community health nurse must determine whether the population characteristics discussed fit a specific rural community. The nursing student who plans to practice in the international arena will need to seek out relevant information about the specific rural population to be served.

Age and Gender

Elderly persons, those age 65 and older, are the fastest growing population in the United States in every location, including rural America. About 7% of the total U.S. population lives in rural counties, but 10% of the country's older population resides there (Tarmann, 2003). In 2000, close to two-thirds of those people 75 years and older living in rural areas were female (Kirschner et al., 2006). However, population projections through 2020 show that females will outnumber males in all but the oldest age groups, indicating a shift from a male-dominated to a female-dominated rural population (Maternal Child Health Branch, 2002). In 2002, 17.3% of rural women were between 65 and 90 years, compared with 13.8% of rural men and 13.4% of women in metropolitan areas—indicating a higher proportion of older rural women (Maternal Child Health Branch, 2005). Because of the preponderance of elderly in rural America, Medicare is a primary funding source for health care (HRSA, 2002).

The median age for nonmetropolitan areas in 2000 was over 35, approximately 4 years greater than for urban areas. The ratio of males per 100 females is slightly higher in nonmetropolitan areas when compared to suburban or metropolitan areas, but there are still more women than men (Kirschner et al., 2006). Population estimates of projected rural age distribution between 1996 and 2020 indicate (Maternal Child Health Branch, 2002) the following:

◆ 19% ages 0 to 14 years
◆ 12.2% between 15 and 24 years
◆ 11.9% ages 25 to 34
◆ 12.9% between 35 and 44 years
◆ 23.5% ages 45 to 64
◆ 20.2% over the age of 65

Population trends have a direct relationship to the kinds of health services that are needed in rural communities. Growing families with young children need maternity, pediatric, and family health medical services, along with dental care and mental health services. They also can benefit from health promotion and disease prevention activities. The elderly, on the other hand, need health care to manage increased numbers of chronic health conditions. Rural communities need to provide access to nursing homes and rehabilitative services, as well as to hospitals, clinics, and health promotion programs that serve the elderly and the entire community.

Race and Ethnicity

Rural areas have historically had less racial diversity than urban areas. In 1998, the U.S. Census Bureau estimated that 83.3% of nonmetropolitan (rural) residents were White, 9.1% were African American, 4.8% were Hispanic, 1.8% were American Indian or Alaskan Native, and 1% were Asian or Pacific Islander (Eberhardt et al., 2001). Racial and ethnic groups have historically been concentrated in certain

areas of the country—for example, Blacks in the rural South and American Indians in the rural Southwest and West, as well as Mexican Americans in the border states of the Southwest (Kirschner et al., 2006). However, these patterns are changing. Rapid Hispanic growth areas are found in the Midwest and Southeast (see Figs. 29.2 and 29.3).

Lower median age and higher birth rates signal faster growth of this population, and this can lead to a need for changing health policies and practices. For instance, in rural counties with a high elderly population and established caseloads of chronic disease patients, an influx of younger Hispanic populations may require a shift in policies and resources to include more pediatric and obstetric care (Kandel & Parrado, 2006). All of these changes influence geographic patterns of health status.

Education

Rural clients in the United States generally have lower educational attainment than those in urban areas. In 1998, some 15% of adults (25 years of age and older) in nonmetropolitan areas had college degrees, but this percentage increased to 15.5% in 2000. This compares with 26.6% of urban adults with college degrees in 2000. More than 23% of rural adults do not have a high school diploma—an all time low—compared with 18.7% of urban adults (USDA, 2003b).

Rural Hispanic people have the lowest percentage of educational attainment—more than half never finished high school and only 6.5% graduated from college. However, in counties with a rapid growth of Hispanic populations,

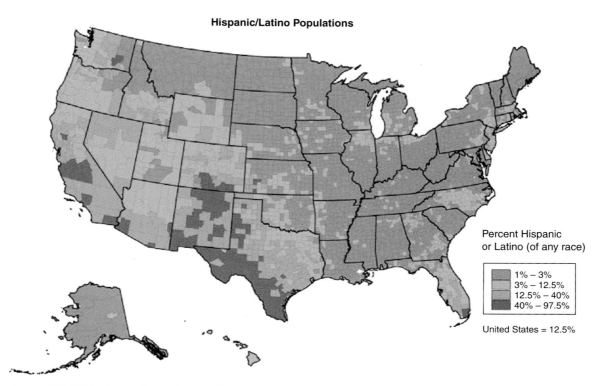

Hispanic/Latino Populations

Percent Hispanic or Latino (of any race)

◻ 1% – 3%
◻ 3% – 12.5%
◻ 12.5% – 40%
◼ 40% – 97.5%

United States = 12.5%

Source: United States Census Bureau, Census of Population and Housing, 2000
Note: Alaska and Hawaii are not to scale.

FIGURE 29.2 Hispanic/Latino populations.

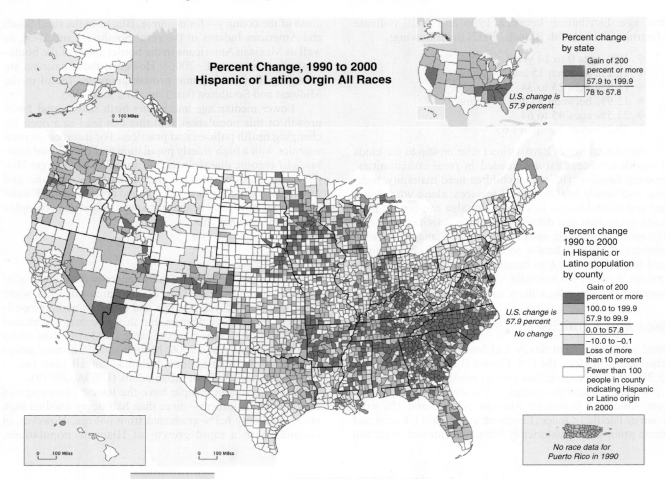

FIGURE 29.3 Percent change in Hispanic/Latino populations from 1990 to 2000.

enrollment in K–8 schools has grown by over 500% (Kandel & Parrado, 2006). For Blacks, urban residents were two times more likely to complete college than rural citizens, even though Black high school completion rates have jumped 12 points in the last decade (USDA, 2003b).

Lower levels of education are consistently and "highly correlated with persistent poverty," with 23.5% of adults over age 25 without a high school education living in poverty and only 7.1% for those with some college (USDA, 2003b, p. 4). Rural clients have little access to higher educational facilities, such as community colleges or universities close to home. Travel to urban areas for educational pursuits adds to the burden of obtaining additional education beyond high school.

Income, Housing, and Jobs

Some rural communities are home to some very wealthy residents, many of them landowners, business owners, farmers, or ranchers. On the average, however, the income of people in rural communities is lower than that of persons living in urban communities. This is reflected in higher unemployment and lower per capita income (Hummel, 2001). In 2004, some 4.5% of urban residents were unemployed, whereas unemployment was 5.7% for rural residents (Gibbs, 2004). Of the 386 counties noted for persistent poverty, 340 are rural. Over 14% of rural Americans live below the poverty level, and over 13% of

them report being hungry and having difficulty securing sufficient food for their families. In agricultural communities, over one-third of the residents have incomes below $15,000. In 2000, the median income for metropolitan households was $44,984, whereas the median rural income was $32,837. Poverty is deeply entrenched in rural America. In one-fourth of rural counties, 20% of people have lived below the poverty level for a minimum of four decades (Food Security Learning Center, 2007). The percentage of working poor in rural areas is higher than in urban areas (Merchant, Coussens, & Gilbert, 2006). In a number of low-income communities, up to 50% of income may derive from federal support through health and social services (HRSA, 2002).

Living in a rural area, however, has a number of economic advantages. The cost of land is lower than in urban areas; therefore, housing costs are also lower, with $79,000 as the median value, opposed to an urban median value of $121,000 in 1999 (Wills, 2002). Taxes are usually less, and restrictions on land use are not as stringent. Less expensive land is advantageous to businesses, such as manufacturing, which may need large parcels of land. However, transportation costs are higher and nonmetropolitan rural median housing values grew faster (57.9%) than any urban or suburban areas (around 35%) during the decade between 1989 and 1999 (Wills, 2002). This growth corresponded with rural in-migration, but posed several problems. For cash-strapped families whose house values rose, subprime mortgages allowed them to trade equity for cash, and foreclosure rates have now skyrocketed. In Minnesota, rural county foreclosures outpaced foreclosures in metropolitan counties (Oakes, 2008). Low-income families who are renters have found it difficult to find affordable housing (USDA, 2007d). Most low-income housing in rural areas consists of single-family homes, not large apartment complexes, and housing availability is problematic. A consistent problem in rural areas is housing quality; many units are substandard and in need of repair (Rural Assistance Center, 2007b; U.S. Department of Housing & Urban Development [USDHUD], 2007).

Some government assistance is available to help low-income renters. The USDA offers rent subsidies to low-income elderly or disabled residents of multifamily housing units through Section 521 (USDA, 2007d). Section 8, a rental voucher program administered by the U.S. Department of Housing and Urban Development (HUD), is targeted to very low-income families who can choose from privately owned rental housing (USDHUD, 2004). However, funds for this program are limited and applicants can wait years for approval. Both programs supplement participants' rental costs above 30% of their income.

Although many people equate farming with rural life, only 7.6% of rural employment is related to agriculture (HRSA, 2002). The United States is unique in that it feeds its population with a small proportion of workers committed to food production and still exports food products to the rest of the world. Rural workers are two times more likely than urban and suburban workers to earn only the minimum wage, and they are "more likely to be underemployed and are less likely to improve their employment circumstances over time" (HRSA, 2002).

When compared with urban areas, rural communities typically offer fewer job options. Types of rural work, such as crop agriculture, manufacturing, and forestry, vary by locale, and these employment opportunities have been diminishing along with concomitant decreases in population and the shift from a goods-based to a service-based economy (HRSA, 2002; Gibbs, Kusmin, & Cromartie, 2004). Examples of goods-producing industries in rural areas include yarn, thread, and fabric mills, and apparel industries, along with lumbering, mining, and agriculture. Construction and livestock agriculture are also included in this category. Service industries that have increased in rural areas include trucking, tourism (hotels/motels), department stores, banking, and insurance (Gibbs et al., 2004).

Even though rural salaries on the whole are less than urban, the evolution from goods- to a more service-based economy has spurred skills and earnings increases for rural residents, with Black women reporting the greatest gains (Gibbs et al., 2004). Rural areas have manufacturing, business, education, and service occupations just as urban communities do. In fact, in many rural communities, health care provides 15% to 20% of total jobs (HRSA, 2002). Education and government are also major employers.

Although the use of the telephone and Internet for commerce is now very common in urban and suburban areas, the "rural digital divide" still exists (HRSA, 2002). Smaller public health departments (those serving fewer than 25,000) are less likely to have access to the Web (Quiram, Meit, Carpender, Pennel, Castillo, & Duchicela, 2004). Many rural communities cannot provide access to Internet service, thus limiting the proliferation of information technology-based businesses and services (HRSA, 2002). The benefits of broadband services not only apply to wider employment opportunities, but also to job retraining, education, and medicine (Cooper, 2002). Where Internet services are readily available, higher-skilled "remote workers" can remain in rural areas while still providing high-tech services to clients across the country, thus reducing the out-migration of young adults (Berkes, 2005).

RURAL HEALTH ISSUES

Health concerns of populations in rural areas are related to the environment, occupations, injuries, and distance from health care providers. Environment issues particularly relate to agriculture and the health risks that accompany farming and other rural lifestyles.

Agriculture and Health

Although farming is not characteristic of all rural areas, where agricultural production occurs, both direct and indirect effects on health can exist (Merchant et al., 2006). The water, air, and soil can be affected by pesticides and fertilizers; air can be polluted by the dust created from plowing for crops. An "estimated 70% of antibiotics are used for nontherapeutic purposes in intensive livestock production," and this practice puts workers at risk for developing antibiotic-resistant infections (p. 4). Occupational exposures to wind-blown soil, organic dust, pesticides, mycotoxins, ammonia, animal dander, and hydrogen sulfite are only some of the air quality issues in rural areas. In Iowa, for instance, it is estimated that for every pound of corn harvested, two pounds of soil are "exported" (p. 7). Livestock growth-producing agents, along with radon, pesticides, and fertilizers, can contaminate ground water. Many rural residents depend on their own well water for drinking, and water quality is monitored only sporadically by well owners, and then usually only for "coliform bacteria and nitrates" (p. 19). About 30% of rural residents obtain drinking water from very small water systems, without the monitoring and regulations associated with large urban water suppliers.

Agricultural-related morbidity and mortality are relatively high. Agriculture ranks second, behind mining, in occupational death rate (Smith, 2007). The fatality rate for farming is 28 per 100,000, and almost 28,000 children and adolescents were injured in farming accidents in 2004 (National Institute for Occupational Safety & Health [NIOSH], 2007). Farming injuries can result from tractor rollovers, suffocations in grain bins, exposure to harmful substances, falls, fires or explosions, accidents with other farm equipment, and on- or off-road collisions. About 5% of injuries result in permanent disability, and worker-training programs to recognize hazards and prevent injuries are rare (Merchant et al., 2006). See Display 29.1 for two examples of agricultural accidents.

Almost 70% of farm families have a member working off the farm. This is sometimes due to required additional income, but most often attributed to a need for health insurance through outside employment (Merchant et al., 2006). This contributes to the time spent in travel and its attendant

DISPLAY 29.1	AGRICULTURAL ACCIDENTS

It was an average day for Sampson Parker, a part-time farmer in South Carolina who also worked in construction. He was trying to get a cornstalk out of the rusty old harvester when the glove he was wearing got stuck in the rollers of the machine and pulled his hand into it. He couldn't get it out and waited more than an hour-and-a-half for someone to come and rescue him. After his hand became numb, he pushed a metal rod into the machine to stop the rollers so that he could cut off his fingers with a penknife. But, the metal rod grinding against the rollers caused a spark and flames began to engulf the harvester. He described watching his skin melt like plastic and began cutting off his arm in order to free himself from the death-trap. He said he felt the nerves in his arm as he cut through them, but was determined not to die in the cornfield. As a tire blew from the heat, he fell and broke his bone, freeing himself from the harvester. He jumped into his van and drove to the front of his property, where a passing fire-fighter stopped to help him. Farmer Parker is now being fitted for a prosthetic arm and notes that this injury was due to his mistake, not the harvester's.

Source: *Sky News*, November 27, 2007. Retrieved August 20, 2008 from http://news.sky.com/skuynews/article/0,,30200-1294480,00.html.

Jason Silveira, a rambunctious 10-year-old living in the agriculturally rich San Joaquin Valley of California, was spending the day off from school with his younger sister and cousin at their grandparents' ranch in Plainview. He had just helped his grandfather load a bunch of leaves into a manure spreader attached to a tractor and asked his grandfather if he could ride along with him as he spread them onto a nearby field. His grandfather told Jason to return to the house, as he knew how dangerous farm equipment could be, but Jason decided to play a game of "cat and mouse"—running up to the spreader and falling back as it criss-crossed the field. His grandfather couldn't see him playing this dangerous game, as the tall, boxy implement obscured his view. The spreader has "three rows of tines that turn quickly when engaged," and as soon as his grandfather sensed something was wrong, he stood up from his seat—engaging a safety mechanism that stopped the spreader immediately (para 12). Jason's parents feel that this is what saved his life—as Jason had fallen and become entangled in the tines. Ambulance and fire crews used the Jaws of Life to cut the tines free from the spreader bars, although they were still embedded in Jason's head, neck, and torso. He was taken by helicopter to a regional trauma center where additional fire crews removed more of the bars before he was taken into the emergency room. He remained conscious throughout the ordeal—until he was taken to surgery where the tines were removed. One of the tines had entered the right side of his jaw, traveling diagonally through his head behind his sinus cavity, and another pierced his neck and fell out on the trip to the hospital. The third tine went through his ribs, but miraculously did not puncture his lungs. His parents reported that Jason came through surgery, but that they were still waiting for definitive news from his doctors.

Source: *Visalia Times-Delta*, November 24, 2007. Retrieved August 20, 2008 from http://www.visaliatimesdelta.com/apps/pbcs.dll/article?AID=/20071124/NEWS/711240324.

problems. Because of the lack of mass transit, rural commuting increases air pollution and the incidence of injury or death from traffic accidents.

The Built Environment in Rural Areas: Relationship to Health

Medicine will not be adequate to deal with the health challenges of the 21st century, not even with the help of the sequenced genome and advances in robotic surgery. Even though the United States spends one of every seven dollars on medical care, we will not significantly improve health and the quality of life unless we pay more attention to how we design our living environments. Healthy living environments include not just a clean and heated kitchen, bath, or bedroom, but also the landscape around us. Health for all, especially for the young, aging, poor and disabled, requires that we design healthfulness into our environments as well. (Richard Jackson [2001], National Center for Environmental Health, CDC)

The **built environment** consists of the development of housing, highways, shopping areas, and other manmade features added to the natural environment. As populated areas expand, stresses are placed on natural habitats, water supplies, and air quality (U.S. Environmental Protection Agency [EPA], 2007).

Urban sprawl is a concern in some rural areas, as people move from urban centers to more suburban environments. Urban encroachment into agricultural areas creates problems with air and water pollution, access to health care, and heat islands. *Heat islands* occur when green areas are exchanged for asphalt, resulting in temperature and ecosystem changes that can extend to more rural areas (Merchant et al., 2006). Ozone levels are often highest just outside the city, because "ozone is formed relatively slowly by the action of sunlight on oxides of nitrogen and hydrocarbons" (p. 72). Urban sprawl also causes problems with water pollution and the availability of water. Encroachment of housing areas into natural habitats or farmlands can lead to wider human exposure to pesticides, herbicides, and other hazards such as mosquito-borne illnesses. Mass transit is not often available in suburban areas, and almost never found in rural areas. Opportunities for health-promoting behaviors are often more limited in rural areas. Deteriorating (or no) sidewalks can be a barrier to walking in rural areas. Exercise or fitness facilities, bike paths, jogging trails, and other incentives for physical activity are also often lacking in rural communities. Obesity is prevalent in rural areas, and the physical environment, along with diet, plays a role in this epidemic (Merchant et al., 2006).

Rural roads are another concern because they are often narrow, without streetlights, and poorly maintained. Slow moving farm equipment traveling on these roads, along with speeding and failure to use safety restraints, has led to injury-related non–farm vehicle crashes in one Iowa study (Peek-Asa, Sprince, Whitten, Falb, Madsen, & Zwerling, 2007).

Self, Home, and Community Care

In one qualitative study of rural clients, health was described as "being able to function" at both work and play (Lee & Winters, 2004, p. 55). Historically, self-management of health care problems has been the most common way for rural people to cope with illness. This can be viewed as a strength, or it may be seen as a limitation. A rural mental health professional recently noted that the "culture of rural states" is often "one of self-sufficiency, traditional values, and patriarchal social structures" (Merchant et al., 2006, p. 41). Rural residents are often viewed as hardworking, traditional, hardy, self-reliant, and resistant to accepting help or services from outside agencies regarded by them as welfare-type programs (Lee & Winters, 2004; Phillips & McLeroy, 2004). Many rural clients are considered individualistic, independent, and resourceful. They often take care of illnesses or injuries on their own, or have a supportive network to help them get their health needs met (Lee & Winters, 2004). Small communities commonly have strong social networks, but this type of familiarity can lead to problems with privacy and confidentiality, as well as stigma regarding mental health or substance abuse treatment (HRSA, 2002).

Because cost, travel, weather, and distance are barriers to obtaining health services from formal health care providers, rural clients may employ a variety of folk treatments and home remedies before consulting a nurse or a physician; such clients tend to visit providers at a much later stage than do people in urban areas. Research reveals that rural residents have fewer visits to health care providers than their urban counterparts and are less likely to receive all recommended preventive screenings and services (Larson & Fleishman, 2003). They are also more likely to report poor or fair health (one in three adults), to have chronic diseases, such as diabetes, and to die from heart disease than are residents of urban areas (AHRQ, 2005). Rural residents receive care in a less timely manner than urban residents and utilize physicians who are more likely to provide care that is outside their specialty areas (AHRQ, 2002).

The low population density in rural areas makes service delivery more difficult, especially for those with special health needs such as the elderly, the disabled, and others (AHRQ, 2007). Suicide rates in rural areas, especially the rural West, can be as much as three times those in urban areas. Over twice the rate of anxiety and depression has been found in rural women, as opposed to urban women. And, less than half of rural community clinics or primary care settings accurately diagnosed depression in their patients. Designated mental health professional shortage areas are found in 60% of rural areas (Merchant et al., 2006).

Home health care (HHC) is particularly difficult in sparsely populated areas, both for patients and nurses.

| DISPLAY 29.2 | LOCATING A RURAL HOME HEALTH CLIENT |

The following written (verbatim) directions were given by a discharge planner to a case manager (home care nurse) when making a referral for Mary, a 67-year-old woman who lived 37 miles from the hospital:

> "Drive on the gravel road east of town until you get to the third set of mailboxes. Then, turn left; drive up the road until you see the old church; cross the broken bridge toward the river. Mary lives on the third farm. Her house has some trees and a fence around it" (p. 222).

It took the home health nurse over 2 hours to drive about 30 miles on the narrow country roads after the morning rain. The nurse had to stop four times to ask residents for additional directions and hints for finding Mary's house. It was finally located, hidden in a large group of trees. The total travel time for this visit was about 4 hours.

From Bushy, A. (2003). Considerations for working with diverse rural client systems. *Lippincott's Case Management, 8*(5), 214–223.

Locating addresses in very rural areas often takes additional skills. (See Display 29.2 for the story of a home health nurse trying to locate a client's home.) The benefits of HHC are worthwhile; it allows people to stay at home, supports their hardiness, and compensates for the long distance between home and formal health care. Adams and colleagues (2001) conducted a study to determine whether health status differed between rural and urban HHC clients and whether place of residence was a predictor of HHC direct care time. The study collected data from more than 2,500 episodes of patient care using items from the Outcome Assessment and Information Set (OASIS). Home health nurse time in the home was also measured. The study results showed significant differences in rural versus urban health status, with urban patients being healthier. Rural HHC clients were more ill and received more home health nurse time. This study demonstrated the need for higher Medicare reimbursement for rural patients and supported the importance of the availability of HHC for patients who need these services.

Access to Acute Care

Rural hospitals have a high risk for financial problems and closures, thus leaving rural patients stranded without services nearby and forcing them to drive long distances for inpatient care. The Balanced Budget Act of 1997 encouraged states to form rural health networks, improve emergency medical services, and improve the financial performance of rural hospitals by designating them critical access hospitals. **Critical access hospitals** (CAHs) are rural hospitals, located a minimum of 35 miles from the next hospital, or 15 miles if the terrain is mountainous or the only routes are on secondary roads (Rural Assistance Center, 2007c). One intention of this designation was to reduce the number of rural hospital closures by providing cost-based Medicare reimbursements, which differ from the prospective payments given to larger hospitals. Most CAHs are nonprofit, have limited lengths of stay and bed capacity, and are heavily dependent on Medicare and Medicaid funding (Pink et al., 2006).

Major Health Problems

Among major health problems affecting individuals in rural areas are cardiovascular disease, diabetes, and human immunodeficiency virus (HIV). Geography, economics, and rural lifestyle factors may account for the higher rate of these major health problems.

Cardiovascular Disease

When it comes to cardiovascular disease, "it is possible that geography is more powerful than any risk factor yet to be discovered" (Taylor, Hughes, & Garrison, 2002, p. 550). Geographic concentrations of cardiovascular disease and other diseases vary from one rural location to the next, possibly related to inadequate health care, distance from care, environmental exposures, infectious disease in the area, and other factors. These multidimensional elements interact in such a way to cause cardiovascular mortality statistics to vary among regions and ethnic groups.

Cardiovascular disease is a leading cause of death in the United States, with ischemic heart disease accounting for more than 60% of deaths (Eberhardt et al., 2001). Clear differences exist in the cardiovascular mortality rates between urban and rural residents. The rates of cardiovascular death from ischemic heart disease for men age 20 and older are highest in the most rural counties. In the South, both men and women are more likely to die of ischemic heart disease than in other parts of the country. In the West, rural adults have less heart disease than urban residents do.

There are many reasons for these data. Cardiovascular disease, like some other chronic diseases, is characterized by a long latency period. Residence of diagnosis is of less interest than residence 10 to 30 years prior to diagnosis (Dennis & Pallotta, 2001). Rural residents may ignore early cardiovascular symptoms and give little heed to preventive interventions such as exercise and low-fat diets. Other risk factors, such as smoking and poverty, affect cardiovascular health. Adults in rural counties are most likely to smoke (Doescher, Jackson, Jerant, & Hart, 2006). This may be related to "delayed access to medical and media resources that help change unhealthy behaviors, and lower educational attainment, which is strongly associated with smoking" (Eberhardt et al., 2001, p. 34). Rural residents are also more likely to be obese and to be more sedentary than urban counterparts (Hartley, Ziller, & MacDonald, 2002).

In addition, rural areas usually have less high-tech health care equipment available, which may affect outcomes for patients with cardiovascular emergencies. However, even low-tech differences can be found. One large-scale study, examining 135,759 Medicare patient records, found significant differences in receipt of recommended treatments for acute myocardial infarction (AMI) between patients in rural hospitals and urban hospitals. Rural patients were less likely to be given heparin, aspirin, and intravenous nitroglycerin than were urban patients, and they had a higher adjusted 30-day post-AMI death rate (Baldwin et al., 2004).

Diabetes

Rural populations are disproportionately affected by diabetes; the prevalence is generally greater in rural areas (5.54% versus 4.85%), and this is even more pronounced among Hispanics and Blacks (Hartley et al., 2002; HRSA, 2002; Mainous, Koopman, & Geesey, 2004). Causes for these differences are not always well understood, but one study reported less exercise, higher rates of smoking, and greater incidence of obesity in rural populations, all of which put them at a higher risk for type 2 diabetes (Hartley et al., 2002). Rural areas have been cited as promoting obesity "on a population level by encouraging physical inactivity and unhealthy food choices" (Boehmer, Lovegreen, Haire-Joshu, & Brownson, 2006, p. 411). Rural residents spend a great deal of time commuting to work or driving to essential services, and studies have demonstrated that for each additional hour spent driving per day, there is a "6% increase in the likelihood of obesity" (Frank, Andresen, & Schmidt, 2004, p. 87).

Rural populations also face greater barriers in diagnosis, treatment, and follow-up care. Some compliance issues with prescribed medication regimens may relate to the lack of health insurance and low-income levels in rural areas, but could also be due to lower health literacy and education levels. Other problems with accessing care may involve transportation and weather. The lack of appropriate services, such as certified diabetes educators or endocrinologists, is also common in rural America; expensive, up-to-date technologies requiring technical expertise are not readily available in most rural areas (Fraser, Skinner, & Mueller, 2006). Basic follow-up with podiatrists for diabetic foot care, ophthalmologists for retinal health, nutritionists, and health educators, as well as laboratory blood tests, can be extremely complicated for rural individuals who may have to travel great distances to access these services (Hartley et al., 2002). Programs targeted specifically to rural areas, usually provided by additional grant funding and personnel, have demonstrated success in reducing emergency department and outpatient visits for rural diabetics by providing group education on self-management and nutrition. Costs may be as low at $400 per person, but savings can be astronomical, as one study estimated 12% less coronary heart disease and 15% fewer microvascular disease events over 10 years (Balamurugan, Ohsfeldt, Hughes, & Phillips, 2006).

Human Immunodeficiency Virus Infection

Human immunodeficiency virus or HIV, the virus that causes acquired immunodeficiency syndrome (AIDS), was first identified among the urban U.S. population in the early 1980s. The Centers for Disease Control and Prevention (CDC) estimates that more than 1 million U.S. residents have HIV, and that more than one-quarter of them are unaware of their HIV infection and remain undiagnosed. In 2005, the estimated number of Americans with AIDS was 41,897, and the cumulative number had reached almost 1 million (CDC, 2007a). About 5% to 8% of all HIV cases in the United States are among rural populations, with the South being hardest hit and African Americans being the largest racial/ethnic group affected (University of California San Francisco [UCSF], 2006; Dean, Steele, Satcher, & Nakashima, 2005).

Among rural areas, 68% of new AIDS cases are from the South, and rates are increasing in this region while other regions of the country have rates that have either remained stable or posted only small increases from 2000 to 2003 (Reif, Geonnotti, & Whetten, 2006). Highest rural rates of HIV are found in the U.S.–Mexico border region, the Mississippi Delta, the Southeast, and Appalachia (Hall, Li, & McKenna, 2005). Also, 50% of rural AIDS cases are among African Americans (National Rural Health Association [NRHA], 2006; UCSF, 2006; Dean et al., 2005), although one study found that the number of heterosexually acquired HIV cases was significantly decreased for Black men (−2.9%) between 1999 and 2004. Researchers also noted significant increases among Hispanic men (6.1%) and women (4.5%) (Espinoza et al., 2007).

Early diagnosis and treatment of HIV/AIDS are issues that must be faced by all rural communities. Physicians, nurses, and other health practitioners need to be educated about the changing face of the disease. Because relatively few cases of HIV/AIDS may be present in any one rural community, specialized services are often not available, and it can be a challenge to stay up-to-date with the newest treatment protocols (NRHA, 2006). Each state health department has resource persons who can provide information to health professionals in rural communities about the HIV/AIDS epidemic and current treatment protocols.

It may be difficult for a person to seek diagnosis or treatment from a rural health practitioner. Confidentiality is an issue of concern, as is lack of anonymity. People with HIV/AIDS may fear the stigma of HIV/AIDS and the rejection that is often associated with it. They may have concern for their jobs or their position in the community if their diagnosis is divulged, and they frequently fear that health care workers will break confidentiality rules (NRHA, 2006). Instead, rural people may choose to seek out HIV/AIDS testing through an urban health care facility where they know no one. Returning to the community can be devastating because of the lack of needed support services and the fear of sharing their diagnosis with others.

Another issue that may arise is that of urban residents with rural roots who return to their home communities as their illness worsens. These people seek family support and can overwhelm their caregivers, especially if the caregivers do not seek support for themselves. Community health nurses are in a good position to assist families with any health issues and can offer to facilitate connections to other social, spiritual, financial, and health care providers. A recent study of HIV-positive women found that satisfaction with social support and coping that focused on managing HIV disease were the best predictors of adherence to medication regimens (Vyavaharkar et al., 2007).

Access to Health Care

Insurance, Managed Care, and Health Care Services

Health insurance in today's market is costly, especially for individual purchasers. Some people, therefore, forego health insurance for themselves and their families. As noted earlier, rural workers are less likely to be offered health insurance through their employers, often because they are either self-employed or due to the size or type of employers (Larson & Hill, 2005). Depending on their income, these people may or may not be eligible for Medicaid or State Children's Health Insurance Programs (S-CHIPs). Even people who are eligible for government health assistance may not apply because of their belief that it is a sign of weakness to accept a handout.

Historically, a traditional fee-for-service model delivered health care in rural and urban communities (see Chapter 6). However, it is challenging for rural providers to deliver the cost-effective, complex health care that rural persons need via solo or small group practices. Rural patients often utilize family practice clinics. The managed care model, which attempts to control costs and improve health care delivery, has slowly diffused into rural communities (AHRQ, 2002). One reason for the sluggishness is that rural practitioners are reluctant to become part of organizations whose "governance, values, and objectives rest in the hands of people who no longer live in the local community" (Rosenblatt, 2001, p. 9). Another reason is the low population density, making this type of health care insurance less profitable.

Building provider networks in rural communities is both time- and effort-intensive because rural providers are often inexperienced with managed care organizations (MCOs). The federal government provides support for **rural health clinics** in areas designated as underserved and nonurban (Finerfrock, 2006; Rural Assistance Center, 2007d). Specialized *migrant clinics* may also be located in rural areas with large migrant worker populations. Many of these are **federally qualified health centers** that provide care to underserved populations through Medicare, Medicaid, or a sliding fee scale (Rural Assistance Center, 2007e). Because only 9% of physicians work in rural areas (where 21% of the population resides), mid-level practitioners, such as physician assistants (PAs) and nurse practitioners (NPs), are often employed in these clinics (AHRQ, 2005; Evans et al, 2006). Also, specialists are most often found in metropolitan areas; rural areas are devoid of most of the smaller-specialty physicians, and residents have difficulty accessing these services (Rosenthal, Zaslavsky, & Newhouse, 2005).

Rural areas are characterized by a lack of "core health care services," defined as primary care, hospital care, emergency medical services, long-term care, mental health and substance abuse counseling services, dental care, and public health services, and it is noted that "the smaller, poorer, and more isolated a rural community is, the more difficult it is to ensure the availability of high-quality health services" (Committee on the Future of Rural Health Care, 2005, p. 1).

Many rural residents depend heavily on public health department services. Two-thirds of all health departments serve populations of fewer than 50,000 people (Rosenblatt, Casey, & Richardson, 2002). Many rural public health agencies are small and isolated, with a need for connections with other agencies in the region or state. Public health nurses "serve in various important capacities" in rural areas, and continuing education has been identified as the "most important training need" (Hajat, Stewart, & Hayes, 2003, p. 481). Rural public health departments generally have lower public funding for programs and services and a potential for "fragmentation of scarce resources" (Phillips & McLeroy, 2004, p. 1662). They also experience difficulty competing against urban agencies in access to grant funding and recruiting specialized staff. Transportation costs and adequate provision of a variety of services are other

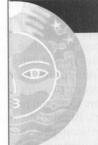

From the Case Files I

A Lesson in Rural Transportation

I live in a relatively large city of 450,000 people. When I started my community health nursing rotation, I was assigned to a rural county public health department in an adjoining county over 50 miles from my house. To make matters worse, when I got there for my first clinical day, my professor told me that I was assigned to see clients in an isolated community another hour away from the health department! There was nothing but farmland between the county seat and this small, forgotten oil town. This town didn't even have sidewalks, much less a fast-food restaurant! After I got over my frustration about traveling such long distances, I began to visit some of my families and started to actually enjoy my time with them. They were so appreciative and open to my suggestions. I really seemed to be making a difference. One older gentleman, Armando, was a diabetic who spoke very little English. He lived with his wife of 45 years, who spoke almost no English. Their children had moved away in order to go to school and get better jobs. His diabetes was not well controlled, and the rural health clinic FNP suggested that he see a specialist (actually an internist) in the county seat. I helped him make arrangements with the doctor for an early afternoon visit, and made sure that he could catch the county bus that ran between the smaller communities and the county seat. When I came back for a follow-up visit the next week, I was shocked to learn that Armando's appointment had been pushed back to 4:30 p.m. because of the doctor's involvement in hospital emergencies and, by the time Armando was finished with his appointment, the county bus service had ended. Armando, with no money and no one to call for a ride, began walking back to his home—over 52 miles away! About halfway home, the driver of a farm truck gave him a lift to a large cotton farm a few miles from his home. You can imagine my horror and embarrassment when I learned of this ordeal! I never realized how difficult it was for rural people to get to their medical appointments. I always had a car and could drive wherever my gas allowance could take me. I thought that the bus would not be a problem, but I learned my lesson. Now, I make sure that the physician's office understands the patient's circumstances and the importance of getting them back to the bus stop in time to make the last bus.

Andrea, Senior Nursing Student

issues faced by rural public health departments, and all of these issues affect the health of the populations served.

Barriers to Access

In rural areas, numerous access barriers to health care exist. The physical distance between place of residence and location of health care services can be considerable. Rural clients may be referred to a distant urban medical center for cancer therapy or other sophisticated care. Members of the population may be frustrated if they travel to a faraway site for care and do not have their problem resolved. Rural clients must be advised before they travel to make sure that the health care provider is not behind schedule or unable to see them; see From the Case Files I for a hard lesson learned by one PHN student.

Transportation can also be an issue, especially for people who do not drive or who lack dependable vehicles. Unpredictable weather adds to potential barriers for rural clients. Snow, ice, wind, and rain can make travel dangerous, even over short distances. Parents may decide not to risk driving on poorly maintained roads to get their children immunized or to have their own hypertension evaluated. Elderly people may choose to delay health care when long travel times, especially in isolated rural areas, are involved. As the seriousness of a condition increases, however, people often reverse their decisions (Basu & Mobley, 2006), and travel in emergency situations can be life-threatening, not only because of the emergency itself, but also because of the distance involved to get the ill or injured person to the nearest health care facility. According to a study by Branas and colleagues (2005), almost 47 million rural Americans do not have access to either Level I or Level II trauma centers within an hour's driving time, leaving them at higher risk for death from injuries. However, almost 43 million urban Americans can access 20 or more trauma centers (Level I or Level II) within an hour's time.

Limited choice of health care providers is a barrier for some rural residents. Fewer physicians, nurses, dentists, and other providers work in rural areas (AHRQ, 2007; HRSA, 2002). Those with special needs often must travel to urban medical centers to get required care. One study of disabled adults noted that they found their local rural physicians to be less familiar with their conditions, thus requiring these disabled patient to "teach" their health care provider. They also described rural public transportation as often unreliable and inaccessible (Iezzoni, Killeen, & O'Day, 2006). Another study involving children with special health care needs found that they were 17% more likely to have an unmet need for dental care than their urban counterparts, often because of difficulty accessing dental services, poverty, low levels of education, and lack of insurance (Skinner, Slifkin, & Mayer, 2006). As mentioned earlier, concerns about confidentiality or provider expertise sometimes cause clients to seek care from even more distant providers.

New Approaches to Improve Access

The *Healthy People 2010* objectives (USDHHS, 2000) mandate improvements in health education, health screening, immunizations, and disease morbidity for the United States. Creative ways of delivering these and other services to rural clients need to be explored. Access to care is a social justice issue: clients who live in rural areas should receive quality health care, regardless of where they choose to live.

One approach that has been successful in numerous rural areas is the use of *mobile clinics*. These clinics bring health care providers to remote places for health screenings, immunizations, dental care, mental health visits, and other services. Mobile health clinics are frequently staffed by NPs, and can improve access to health care for low-income residents. They often are available to residents on evenings and weekends and offer culturally sensitive and bilingual outreach, as well as care for uninsured clients (Santana, 2005).

School-based clinics are another approach that improves access, but may be less prominent in rural areas. These clinics provide available, community-based, affordable, and culturally acceptable care to well and sick children. Often grant-supported, school-based clinics facilitate the receipt of health education and primary care by children who are otherwise without easy access to health services (Gamm, Castillo, & Williams, 2004).

Telehealth, another approach to increasing access to care, provides electronically transmitted clinician consultation between the client and the health care provider. This option is especially useful for connecting home health nurses with their patients who need close monitoring at home. It is also useful for patient and professional health education, public health applications, and health administration. Specialty health care also may be accessed, with patients and providers connected via two-way audiovisual transmission over telephone lines or the Internet, thus obviating the need for patients to leave their residences. Streaming media, video conferencing, and store-and-forward imaging are just some of the applications commonly utilized (HRSA, 2007b). Clients can also be assessed quickly by interactive communication from physician offices, hospitals, and other sites. Telehealth technology may decrease visits to emergency departments and hospitalizations. Grants and other funding are available to promote the use of this technology (HRSA, 2007b; USDA, 2005).

Healthy People 2010 Goals

The two broad objectives of *Healthy People 2010* are (1) to increase quality and years of healthy life and (2) to eliminate health disparities. The report noted specific rural disparities: injury-related death rates are 40% higher in rural communities and 20% of the rural population is uninsured, compared with 16% of urban residents (USDHHS, 2000). Because of the unique health issues facing rural America, *Rural Healthy People 2010: A Companion Document to Healthy People 2010* was developed. Using surveys, literature reviews, and other methods of data collection and analysis, the 28 *Healthy People 2010* focus areas were examined for relevance to rural health. The following list represents a consensus of the top priorities addressed in *Rural Healthy People 2010* (Gamm, Hutchison, Dabney, & Dorsey, 2003):

- ◆ Access to health care:
  - Access to insurance
  - Access to primary care
  - Access to emergency medical services (EMS)
- ◆ Heart and stroke
  - Diabetes mellitus
  - Oral health
  - Tobacco use
  - Substance abuse
  - Maternal, infant, and child health
  - Nutrition and overweight
  - Cancer

Access issues ranked highest because of the disparity in insurance and availability of health care providers between urban and rural populations, as well as the unequal access to emergency medical services (Patterson, Probst, & Moore, 2006). Heart disease, stroke, and diabetes are significant problems among rural populations, leading to avoidable hospitalizations because of inadequate care and follow-up (Hartley et al., 2002; Okon et al., 2006; Gamm et al., 2003).

Oral health in rural areas is affected by the shortage of dentists (Gordon, 2007). Rural adults over age 65 more often report total tooth loss than do their urban counterparts, and dental visits for rural adults between the ages of 18 and 64 are fewer than for urban adults (Gamm et al., 2003; HRSA, 2002). Smoking prevalence in rural areas is higher than in urban areas, and the prevalence rate has changed little from the mid-1990s, despite tobacco education and cessation programs (Doescher et al., 2006). Alcoholism is more common in rural than suburban areas (Borders & Booth, 2007). Prevalence of illicit drug use is higher in rural America; rural eighth graders were found to be more likely to have used marijuana, alcohol, cocaine, and crack than urban eighth graders. They were twice as likely to use methamphetamines (National Center on Addiction & Substance Abuse, 2000; HRSA, 2002). Latino, American Indian, and Asian rural adolescents have more chronic illnesses than do adolescents in other racial/ethnic groups (Wickrama, Elder, & Abraham, 2007).

Children who have special health care needs and who live in rural areas are less likely to be have their health care provided by a pediatrician and more likely to have unmet health care needs due to unavailability of services or transportation problems (Skinner & Slifkin, 2007). Adolescent mortality is higher in rural areas, and early prenatal care among rural women, especially minorities and teens, continues to be low (Eberhardt et al., 2001; HRSA, 2002). Studies demonstrate that rural residence is a risk factor for obesity and overweight in children and women (Lutfiyya, Lipsky, Wisdom-Behounek, & Inpanbutr-Martinkus, 2007; Bove & Olson, 2006).

Cancer disparities are found in rural populations. For example, cervical cancer rates for rural women are statistically higher than for women living in urban areas (Bernard, Coughlin, Thompson, & Richardson, 2007). Both rural Blacks and Whites were found to be at increased risk for colon cancer when compared with urban populations (Kinney, Harrell, Slattery, Martin, & Sandler, 2006). One Iowa study found that less than half of rural residents were screened for colorectal cancer by their family physicians (Levy, Dawson,

Hartz, & James, 2006). Rural community health nurses need to consider the *Healthy People 2010* objectives and *Rural Healthy People 2010* priority areas as guides for improving the health status of rural communities throughout the decade.

MIGRANT HEALTH

You may never have seen migrant workers, yet you are a direct beneficiary of their labor. Have you ever thought about the people who harvest the fruits and vegetables that you eat? What would happen to the complex system of agricultural production and distribution if workers were not available to pick crops at peak harvest times? Have you ever thought about exactly who these people are, where they come from, where they live, or what their health is like? Migrant farmworkers are an integral part of the farming community in the United States and across the world (Cholewinski, 2005). The agricultural industry relies heavily on migrant workers to harvest the almost endless array of fresh produce that appears year-round in supermarkets across the United States as fresh, frozen, and canned fruits and vegetables. More than 3 million seasonal and migrant farmworkers provide labor for the $28 billion vegetable and fruit crops of the United States (National Center for Farmworker Health [NCFH], 2007a).

Despite their importance to American agriculture, migrant workers are rarely visible members of our society. They go unnoticed beyond the fringes of the camps and farms to which they travel to pursue their livelihood. Most come to the United States from other countries (93%), and of those, about 90% are from Mexico (Evans, Lantigua, Stapleton, Daughtery, & Piloto, 2005). They come with the hope of improving their impoverished lives. Some are legal residents, but most are undocumented aliens and live in fear of deportation. All endure backbreaking, menial labor for low wages and are often deprived of basic rights to safe working conditions, adequate sanitation, decent housing, quality education for their children, and health care.

MIGRANT FARMWORKERS: PROFILE OF A NOMADIC AGGREGATE

Maintaining a low public profile, migrant workers are, for the most part, marginalized from mainstream society. They remain unseen, unheard, poorly understood, and excluded from many programs that provide health care assistance for low-income people. The migrant worker is a kind of disenfranchised person, for whom no one wants to take responsibility. Yet the needs of these workers are great. They are plagued with different, more complex, and more frequent health problems than the general population (Formichelli, 2008). Common ailments include infectious diseases (e.g., tuberculosis [TB], parasites), gastrointestinal disorders, dermatitis due to pesticide exposure, emotional distress and depression, vision and eye problems, cancer, and chronic illnesses, such as asthma, bronchitis, diabetes, and hypertension. They are plagued by poverty, poor nutrition, substandard housing conditions, long hours and grueling, often unsafe, working conditions. Their demographics, socioeconomic conditions, and lifestyle resemble those of a Third World country despite the fact that they live and work in one of the most prosperous nations on Earth. Although migrant families are in dire need of health resources, various economic, cultural, and language barriers prevent this aggregate from accessing available health services. According to the Kaiser Commission (Rosenbaum & Shin, 2005), only 15% of migrant farmworkers have full health insurance—compared with 63% of all low-income adults—and only 20% of seasonal and migrant workers reported accessing any health care services between 1998 and 2000. Another study found that less than 10% of Mexican immigrants (documented and undocumented) who were in the United States less than 10 years reported ever going to an emergency department for care, compared with 20% of native-born Mexican Americans and Whites (King, 2007).

Migrant workers live and work in areas where health care practitioners are generally in short supply. In one study of California agricultural communities, 20% had no primary care physician available, while others had a ratio of one physician to 3,000 people (cited in Villarejo, 2003). These astounding facts makes it essential to understand the history, demographics, environment, culture, and health care needs of the migrant worker, so that PHNs can better assist them in protecting their health and the health of all citizens.

Historical Background

Both historically and internationally, farmers have rarely been able to permanently employ the large workforces needed to harvest their crops. Throughout the 19th century, however, the small, family-owned farms typical in the United States got through the harvest by using school children, neighbors, and local day laborers. As time went by, this became more and more difficult to accomplish. During the decade ending in 1929, over half a million Mexicans migrated to the United States, many drawn to work in seasonal agriculture. With the Great Depression, many of the small, independently run farms went bankrupt, and citizens were concerned about scarce employment opportunities. Because of this, state and federal governments were lobbied by civic groups to "round up Mexican Americans indiscriminately . . . and to 'repatriate' them to Mexico" (University of California, 2008a). Within a few years, the outbreak of World War II caused an increased need for food production and additional workers, as many U.S. workers joined the military. To keep abreast of the demand for produce, the larger surviving farms turned to migrant labor for help. The Emergency Labor Program—known as the Bracero Program—was enacted in 1942 to permit temporary Mexican immigration to provide needed workers for American agriculture and industry (University of California, 2008a). Between 1942 and 1964, more than 4 million Mexican workers participated in this program, leaving their families behind and coming to work in Californian fields. When this program ended, workers continued to cross the border to seek employment, often bringing along their families. Employers hired needed undocumented workers from Mexico, as well as Central and South America. Living apart from society, the plight of migrant farmworkers was largely ignored until exposure on a 1960 television documentary—Edward R. Murrow's *Harvest of Shame*—created a national outcry (Moyers, 2004). This led to the passage of the Migrant Health Act of 1962, which addressed the specific health needs of migrant workers for the first time in U.S. history.

The Migrant Health Act authorized delivery of primary and supplementary health services to migrant farmworkers

(HRSA, 2008). Federally funded migrant health clinics serve areas in the United States where significant numbers of migrant farmworkers gather. In 2004, these clinics served more than 675,000 seasonal and migrant farmworkers, a number far below the estimated 3+ million noted earlier (King, 2007). Services may be provided seasonally, on a temporary basis, or year-round. Staffing usually includes doctors, nurses, NPs, PAs, outreach workers, social workers, and dental and pharmacy workers, along with health educators. Transportation may also be a component in some areas. Primary and preventive health care services are provided to migrant workers and their families throughout more than 800 clinic sites (see Internet Resources at the end of this chapter for a map of your state). However, funding is often inadequate, and many clinics are not sufficiently staffed or operated to meet the health needs of migrant farmworkers and their dependents. Only a few centers are funded exclusively by migrant grant funding, and most are designated as "mixed grant" centers receiving funding from a variety of sources, including Medicaid in some instances (Rosenbaum & Shin, 2005, p. 16). Additionally, although these clinics exist throughout the United States, large geographic regions are not served well or at all. Other services, such as *promotora programs* that employ Hispanic lay health workers or nursing voucher programs providing NP services at participating clinics and nurse referrals to specialists, are available in some areas (King, 2007; Formichelli, 2008). Migrant workers in areas without migrant clinics or other targeted services must rely on local health departments and emergency rooms for health care, or they may simply go without needed care.

Demographics

Because migrant farmworkers constitute a mobile population with shifting composition, it is difficult to precisely determine their numbers or origins. Estimates of the number of migrant workers vary also because of the influx of illegal and undocumented workers. Approximately 70% of seasonal and migrant farmworkers permanently reside in the United States (Rosenbaum & Shin, 2005). Most of the estimated 3 to 5 million migrant farmworkers tend to be either newly arrived immigrants, with few connections, or established legal residents with limited opportunities and skills, who rely on farm labor for survival (NCFH, 2007a; 2007b). It is estimated that 1.3 million U.S. citizens are agricultural workers who move between states (Moyers, 2004). The majority of migrant and seasonal farmworkers (81%) were born outside the United States—mostly in Mexico (95%) and Latin America (2%)—although roughly 2% come from Asia and other countries (NCFH, 2007c). African Americans, Jamaicans, Haitians, and other ethnic groups are also represented (NCFH, 2007b). The pool of farmworkers is increasingly diverse in California, with people coming from Latin American and Asia, such as Hmong from Southeast Asia, Mixtec and Zapotec from Mexico, and Maya from Guatemala (Alderete, Vega, Kolody, & Aguilar-Gaxiola, 2000). Many of them speak little English (NCFH, 2007c). Most of the migrant workers are young, with an average age of 31, and half of them are under age 29. Roughly half of all farmworkers are married, and just under 50% of them are parents; about half of them have their families with them. Fifty percent of farmworkers are either citizens (22%), legal permanent residents of the United States (24%), or workers who possess temporary work permits (2%), according to the most recent government survey (U.S. Department of Labor, 2000). Eighty percent of them are male, and 84% report that they speak Spanish. Twelve percent speak English, and the reported median level of education was sixth grade (NCFH, 2007c). In addition, many mothers bring infants and young children to work with them, and the children spend their days strapped to their mother's back or playing among the pesticide-laden fields (Alderete et al., 2000; McCauley et al., 2006).

Farmworkers are defined as having income derived primarily from work in the agricultural industry (e.g., field and orchard crops, packing houses, food processing, horticulture, livestock). In a government survey, over 60% reported working in vegetable, fruit, or nut crops (U.S. Department of Labor, 2000).

Seasonal farmworkers generally live in one geographic location and are principally employed in agriculture (51% or more of their time), whereas **migrant farmworkers** meet that classification while moving to find agricultural work throughout the year, usually from state to state, and establishing temporary residences (Larson, 2000). Some live apart from their families, forming groups of single men; others travel with their entire families. The average migrant farmworker spends from June to September doing seasonal harvesting, with about 8 weeks on the road traveling from farm to farm for work, and is then unemployed unless other work, such as hauling or canning, is found (Sandhaus, 1998; Bacon, 2006). The main reason migrant workers immigrate is to find work, and most migrant farmworkers end up in areas where they already have social networks, such as family or acquaintances from their own areas of Mexico (Lindstrom & Lauster, 2001). Recent studies show that farmworkers reported being employed only 47% of the previous year in agriculture, and the number of weeks of farm work available to them dropped from 28 weeks to 25 weeks over a 6-year period for workers born outside the United States and from 24 to 23 weeks for native-born workers (Das, Steege, Baron, Beckman, & Harrison, 2001). Migrant workers with less than a year of experience in U.S. agriculture reported only 17 weeks of farm work (U.S. Department of Labor, 2000). Reports of annual income vary, from between $7,500 and $10,000 (Formichelli, 2008; U.S. Department of Labor, 2000), to a higher estimate of just under $15,000 in 2000 (Rosenbaum & Shin, 2005). Most farm workers have incomes below the federal poverty level—76% in 1993 and 60% in 2000 (Rosenbaum & Shin, 2005; NCFH, 2007c).

As an illustration of the working conditions and wages in the tomato fields of Florida, pickers work "10 to 12 hours a day picking tomatoes by hand, earning a piece-rate of about 45 cents for every 32-pound bucket" (Schlosser, 2007). An average work day consists of picking, carrying, and unloading about 2 tons of tomatoes. In Florida, abuses of migrant farm workers have included nonpayment of wages and forcing workers into debt, chaining workers in trailers at night, and charges of slavery. The U.S. Department of Justice has prosecuted roughly "a half a dozen cases of slavery" in the last decade (Schlosser, 2007). Families working in the cotton fields of Arizona report working long hours—from 3 a.m. to 2 p.m.; those working peak season in lettuce and broccoli fields have been known to work 14-hour days with only a half-hour lunch and two 15-minute breaks (Human Rights Watch, 2000).

States in Migrant Streams
Lines denote major migration patters

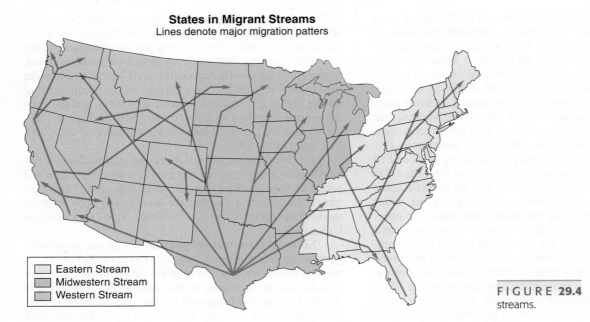

Eastern Stream
Midwestern Stream
Western Stream

FIGURE 29.4 States in migrant streams.

Migrant Streams and Patterns

Migrant farmworkers usually have their permanent residence, or *home base*, states with a traditionally high number of immigrants, like California, Texas, Florida, New York, or Illinois (King, 2007). From their home base, they mobilize as each new crop is ready for harvest. Following the harvest seasons of agricultural crops, migrant farmworkers move from place to place, usually along predetermined routes called **migrant streams** (Fig. 29.4). Some migrant farmworkers are multigenerational; that is, their families have been farmworkers for several generations, traveling the same streams for many years.

Three principal streams formulate the agricultural routes that migrant laborers follow. The *eastern stream* originates in Florida, where most of their time is spent, and extends up the East Coast through North Carolina, Tennessee, Kentucky, Virginia and other states east of the Mississippi, as far as north as Ohio, New Jersey, New York, Connecticut, Massachusetts, New Hampshire, Vermont, and Maine. The *midwestern stream* begins in southern Texas or northern Mexico and fans out across the United States, ending in the northwestern and midwestern states bordering Canada, both east and west of the Mississippi. The *western stream* originates in California and moves up the West Coast to all western states and from central California into North Dakota (Formichelli, 2008; Evans et al., 2005). Workers move from areas with cotton, tree fruits and nuts, and vegetable crops to other areas where they harvest watermelons, cantaloupes, and potatoes. About 17% of seasonal farmworkers "follow-the-crop" (Villarejo, 2003, p. 177).

Weather conditions and employment opportunities affect movement and patterns of migration. Because of the unpredictable nature of farm work, the three streams are not clearly delineated, pointing to more complex patterns of movement. In addition to the migrant streams, **patterns of migration** exist, with varying lengths of stay. In a *restricted circuit,* many people travel throughout a season within a small geographic area, following the crops. *Point-to-point*

migration entails leaving a home base for part of the year to travel to the same place or series of places along a route during the agricultural season, usually returning on a yearly basis. Almost 40% of seasonal farmworkers shuttle back and forth this way (Villarejo, 2003).

Nomadic migrant workers travel away from home for several years, working from farm to farm and crop to crop, relying on word of mouth about job opportunities. Nomadic workers are often younger males who send money home to their families (McLaurin & Morrison, 2006). Some of these workers eventually settle in the areas to which they have migrated, whereas others return to their home base. A given ethnic group usually follows its own particular stream and pattern of migration. New growth states, like Utah, Minnesota, Wisconsin, Nebraska, Kansas, Tennessee, and Arkansas, have seen immigrant populations double in the last 15 years (King, 2007). Some migrant workers find work in service-sector jobs and others labor in construction or landscaping, thus ending their need to constantly move with the crops.

Migrant Lifestyle

To understand the health needs of migrant farmworkers and their families, it is important to understand their lifestyle. Migrant workers and their families endure a transient and uncertain life, with long hours, stressful working conditions, low wages, and poor health care. Substandard housing, often unsafe working conditions, and language barriers make life even more difficult.

Migrant workers must confront the vagaries of an unpredictable world. Migrants typically remain in an area for only 6 to 8 weeks, working the fields 6 days a week from sunrise to sunset. Depending on weather and crop conditions, work may be plentiful one week and virtually gone the next. Because yearly income must be earned during the harvest season, all family members contribute to harvesting. Children are essential to the core group's economy and must help in the fields and at home (American Academy of Pediatrics,

2005). Migrant workers often drive night and day as they move from crop to crop. Typically, they travel with their children and only their most essential possessions, in aging cars, vans, and trucks. Occasionally, van loads of *solos*, or single men, migrate together. Their status is even more precarious, because they lack family support systems.

Depending on the economy and the crop, a migrant farmworker may earn as little as 40 cents per 5-gallon bushel of harvested crops. At that rate, a worker can earn up to $100 on a good day, but rain, poor harvest, injury, and disease make the average earnings only $30 to $60, causing annual income to fall below the poverty level (NCFH, 2007a). Men, women, and older children all work in the fields. Because inexpensive child care is seldom available, mothers often leave very young children alone playing in fields, where they are exposed to sun, chemicals, and dangerous machinery. Sometimes children are brought to the fields and left in cars or in cardboard boxes. Often a teenage girl or the mother of an infant may remain in the camp to baby-sit all the children; she is usually stranded there, because all available cars are used to take workers to the fields.

Migrant laborers learn about employment opportunities from recruiters, farm labor contractors, and crew leaders, as well as from other migrants. About one-third of California farm workers and 20% of those nationwide are usually employed through farm labor contractors (University of California, 2008b). Migrant laborers who travel in crews, or groups, are often employed by farm labor contractors, who act as the mediator between workers and the farmer (Bureau of Labor Statistics, 2007). They may also provide transportation, housing, and meals for the workers; they may also supervise their work in the fields (Farmworker Justice, 2007). The farmer usually pays the labor contractor, who, in turn, pays the workers. This can be viewed as a way for farmers to remove themselves from the responsibility of paying minimum wages to workers, providing worker's compensation, or meeting legal responsibilities (e.g., state and federal worker safety rules), and preventing union organizing because they employ the contractor, not the individual workers (Ruckelshaus & Goldstein, 2002). An unscrupulous crew leader can withhold payment and keep the migrant workers in constant debt.

Migrant Hero

César Chavez founded the National Farm Workers Association (NFWA; later changed to United Farm Workers [UFW]), the first union in agricultural labor history to successfully organize migrant farmworkers. As a child, he traveled with his family to harvest crops, but they rarely had enough food to eat and often lived in shacks. Work was frequently scarce, wages were low, and labor contractors cheated the family out of the money they earned. Moving to California during the Great Depression, the family became part of the migrant community. Chavez attended as many as 65 different schools, and after completing eighth grade, he dropped out of school to help support his family by working full-time in the fields.

Chavez organized many successful strikes and boycotts, the most famous one being the boycott of California grapes as a protest against the indiscriminate use of pesticides by growers. This boycott lasted for longer than 5 years,

and on two occasions he fasted as a protest against the use of agricultural pesticides. His efforts united people who, as individuals, had no significance in the power structure. His legacy is an example of how people build power together. He achieved great recognition, although he never owned a home or a car and never made more than $6,000 a year (United Farm Workers, 2006; Bruns, 2006). Throughout his life, he ignored personal hardships to continue the struggle with union victories and losses.

HEALTH RISKS OF MIGRANT WORKERS AND THEIR FAMILIES

A community with varied and profound health needs complicated by disease and social isolation, migrant farmworkers and their families are at risk. Migrant workers, often paid piece work, labor at a fast pace, largely without breaks, in order to take advantage of the short growing season (Connor, Rainer, Simcox, & Thomisee, 2007). Because seasonal earnings must last the entire year, the migrant farmworker generally avoids or delays seeking health care until illness becomes debilitating. When work is primary, health is eclipsed (King, 2007). Migrant farmworkers and their families suffer illnesses caused by poor nutrition, a lack of resources to seek care early in the disease process, and infectious diseases due to overcrowding and poor sanitation. National statistics on migrant seasonal workers are sparse, with much of the data regional and only sporadically collected. Some of the most shocking statistics include:

- The life expectancy of a migrant worker is much lower than the general population, with proportionally increased mortality from "injuries, tuberculosis, mental disorders, cerebrovascular disease, respiratory diseases, ulcers, hypertension, and cirrhosis" (Villarejo, 2003, p. 180).
- The migrant infant mortality rate is 25% to 30% higher than the national average (cited in Triantafillou, 2003).
- Migrant children are delayed for immunizations; one national study noted 75% of migrant children were behind on immunization or unimmunized (cited in Triantafillou, 2003).
- Parasites were reported in 20% to 80% of migrant farmworkers in North Carolina studies (cited in Triantafillou, 2003).
- Migrant workers have the highest rates of skin disorders; and chemicals, dust, and constant sun exposure are also a continual source of eye hazards (Connor et al., 2007).

Occupational Hazards

The hazards of agricultural employment, coupled with limited legal protection, jeopardize the health of the migrant farmworker. As mentioned earlier, agriculture ranks second, behind mining, in occupational death rate (Smith, 2007). Falls, cuts, muscle strains and sprains, and repetitive motion injuries (e.g., carpal tunnel syndrome) commonly afflict migrant laborers.

Migrant and seasonal farm work typically requires stooping, long hours working in wet clothes, working with sometimes contaminated soil and water, climbing, carrying heavy loads, and exposure to the sun and the elements. Failure to perform these activities on a rigid timetable dictated by seasons and weather can result in crop loss. This urgency compels farmworkers to work in all weather conditions, including extreme heat or cold, rain, bright sun, and humidity (Cooper et al., 2005).

In a small study of migrant workers, 41% of those reporting an injury were not provided medical care within 24 hours, and 24% got no care at all (NCFH, 2007d). Eye injuries (from tree branches, tools, or irritants) can cause serious problems. Some research suggests that farmworkers may be six times more likely than the general public to become infected with TB. Parasitic infections have been found to be 28% higher in migrant workers, and higher cancer rates have also been noted (NCFH, 2007d). Extreme cold can lead to frostbite, and overexposure to the sun may result in heat stroke; farm laborers are more often at risk for these conditions. Some plants, like tobacco and strawberries, release chemicals that are toxic to farmworkers who come in close contact with them (NCFH, 2007b).

Pesticide Exposure

Migrant farmworkers are at greater risk for pesticide poisoning when fields are sprayed or during initial reentry into the field. Many migrant camps are located within large open fields or on the periphery of crop land. Overhead pesticide sprayings then endanger not only those at work in the fields, but also those in the camp. If fields are not posted with warning signs, mass poisoning of farm workers can occur: one example in the central San Joaquin Valley of California involved lengthy exposure for 34 workers and necessitated subsequent hospital treatment (Villarejo, 2003). Two nurses, who as children worked alongside their families in the fields, noted "as the planes sprayed the fields, you could feel the drifts" and when the spray mixed with the early morning dew "the pesticide residue would be on your clothes and your skin—it looked like a white film" (Formichelli, 2008).

Contaminated water sources in the field enhance the absorption and spread of pesticides and organic compounds. Environmental Protection Agency (EPA) standards that bar entry to sprayed fields for at least 24 hours are often ignored. Pesticides can drift from the fields to contaminate food, yards, or children playing nearby. Children are at greater risk for pesticide-induced illnesses because of their higher metabolic rate, greater surface absorption, still developing organs, and possibility for chronic long-term exposure. It is estimated that 300,000 farmworkers suffer pesticide poisoning each year (NCFH, 2007b). Surveillance systems are only in place in eight states; only 30 states require that pesticide-related illnesses be reported. Reporting of pesticide-induced morbidity and mortality are not often required. California has the oldest pesticide surveillance system in the United States (McCauley, Anger, Keifer, Langley, Robson, & Rohlman, 2006), but, even with reporting laws, many cases are never recognized because workers do not seek medical care. Pesticide burns and rashes often go untreated because of lack of education about the dangers of pesticides and lack of available services. Migrant workers are often unaware of the hazards of pesticides. A study among adolescent Latino farmworkers found that 64.7% were traveling and working in the United States independent of their parents, and few reported having received

pesticide training; however, 21.6% of the sample reported that their current work involved mixing or applying agricultural chemicals (McCauley et al., 2006).

A Florida study indicated that farmworkers had a rather extensive lay knowledge of pesticide exposure, and that this could be combined with more required ethnical training to reduce poor health effects (Flocks, Monaghan, Albrecht, & Bahena, 2007). Even though it may be required of health care providers to report pesticide poisoning, it is often misdiagnosed because the symptoms can mimic those of viral infections or heat-related illness (Das et al., 2001; Triantafillou, 2003).

Symptoms of pesticide exposure include sore throat, runny nose, headache, watery eyes, drowsiness, itchy skin, abdominal pain, and nausea or vomiting. More severe symptoms may include sweating, salivation, blurred vision or pinpoint pupils, muscle twitching, or weakness and incontinence (especially with organophosphate or carbamate exposures). Finally, with the most severe exposures, seizures, respiratory depression, and unconsciousness or coma can occur (Migrant Clinician's Network, n.d.a; McCauley et al., 2006). Only a few categories of pesticides account for more than half of the cases of acute illness; these include inorganic compounds, carbamates, pyrethroids, and organophosphates (Das et al., 2001). Although the impact of acute pesticide poisoning is widely recognized, little is understood about the long-term effects of the repeated low-level exposures to which migrant farmworkers are constantly subjected. Some studies have noted memory problems, depression, neurologic deficits, miscarriages, and birth defects, along with respiratory problems, as being linked to chronic pesticide exposure (McCauley et al., 2006). A study of California agricultural counties found "an increased risk of death among developing babies, ranging from 40% to 120% among those whose mothers lived near crops where certain pesticides were sprayed" ("Living near where pesticides used may boost fetal deaths due to birth defects," 2001). Numerous studies have examined the link between exposure to pesticides and various neurologic problems and cancer—most often with organophosphate-based pesticides. Some pesticides have been suspected of leading to depression (Stallones & Beseler, 2002). Non-Hodgkin lymphoma, leukemia, prostate cancer, sarcomas and multiple myelomas have been associated with organophosphates, herbicides, and insecticides (Alavanja, Hoppin, & Kamel, 2004; Mahajan, Bonner, Hoppin, & Akavanja, 2006).

A large body of supportive research has indicated a link between Parkinson's disease, other neurologic disorders and pesticide exposure, but specific mechanisms have been difficult to pinpoint (Alavanja et al., 2004). One study revealed a 70% chance of development of Parkinson's disease for farm workers exposed to pesticides ("Study links pesticide exposure to Parkinson's disease," 2006). Display 29.3, Environmental Exposure History, is a helpful assessment tool for community health nurses working with migrant and seasonal workers to use to determine pesticide exposure. When a client presents with symptoms that may be suggestive of pesticide exposure, mnemonic prompts may help to clarify common symptoms (see Display 29.4).

Pesticide exposure can be a single event, may occur multiple times, or even be continuous. Health effects are thought to be a function of the frequency of exposure and the dose (Hiott, Quandt, Early, Jackson, & Arcury, 2006). Most

DISPLAY 29.3 — ENVIRONMENTAL EXPOSURE HISTORY

Do an exposure history to:
* Identify current or past exposures
* Reduce or eliminate current exposures
* Reduce adverse health effects.

Taking an Exposure History: Questions to Consider

Use the **I PREPARE** mnemonic:

I–Investigate potential exposures
* Have you ever felt sick after coming in contact with a chemical, pesticide, or other substance?
* Do you have any symptoms that improve when you are away from your home or workplace?

P–Present work:
* Are you exposed to solvents, dusts, fumes, radiation, loud noise, pesticides, or other chemicals?
* Do you know where to find Material Data Safety Sheets on chemicals that you work with?
* Do you wear personal protective equipment?
* Are work clothes worn home?
* Do co-workers have similar health problems?

R–Residence:
* When was your residence built?
* What type of heating system do you have?
* Have you recently remodeled your home?
* What chemicals are stored on your property?
* Where does your drinking water come from?

E–Environmental concerns
* Are there environmental concerns in your neighborhood (e.g., air, water, soil)?
* What types of industries or farms are near your home?
* Do you live near a hazardous waste site or landfill?

P–Past work
* What are your past work experiences?

* What is the longest job held?
* Have you ever been in the military, worked on a farm, or done volunteer or seasonal work?

A–Activities
* What activities and hobbies do you and your family engage in?
* Do you burn, solder, or melt any products?
* Do you garden, fish, or hunt?
* Do you eat what you catch or grow?
* Do you use pesticides?
* Do you engage in any alternative healing or cultural practices?

R–Referrals and resources (use these key referrals and resources)
* Agency for Toxic Substances & Disease Registry: *www.atsdr.cdc.gov*
* Association of Occupational & Environmental Clinics: *www.aoec.org*
* Environmental Protection Agency: *www.epa.gov*
* Material Safety Data Sheets: *www.hazard.com/msds*
* Occupational Safety & Health Administration: *www.osha.gov*
* Local health department, environmental agency, poison control center

E–Educate (a checklist)
* Are materials available to educate the patient?
* Are alternatives available to minimize the risk of exposure?
* Have prevention strategies been discussed?
* What is the plan for follow-up?

Source: http://www.cdc.gov/healthyplaces/. Adapted from http://www.migrantclinician.org/_resources/Iprepare_2page.pdf.

DISPLAY 29.4 — MNEMONIC PROMPTS TO DETERMINE ACUTE SYMPTOMS OF ORGANOPHOSPHATE EXPOSURE

SLUD	MUDDLES
Salivation	Miosis
Lacrimation	Urination
Urination	Diarrhea
Defecation	Diaphoresis
	Lacrimation
	Excitation of central nervous system
	Salivation

Source: Sanborn, M., Cole, D., Abelsohn, A., & Weir, E. (2002). Identifying and managing adverse environmental health effects: 4. Pesticides. *Canadian Medical Association Journal (CMJ), 166*(1), 1431–1436.

migrant workers come into contact with pesticides through their work. However, exposure to pesticides does not affect only those working in the fields. A Washington state study revealed that workers who thinned trees and plants were more likely to have higher levels of pesticide residues in their house and dust in their vehicles than were those working in other areas (e.g., picking or harvesting, planting or transplanting, pruning, loading plants, or even mixing or applying pesticides). These higher levels were not only present in the homes and vehicles of farmworkers, but pesticide metabolites were also found in their children's urine as well (Coronado, Thompson, Strong, Griffith, & Iuslas, 2004). A study of Virginia- and North Carolina-based farmworkers and their families found higher levels of organophosphate pesticide metabolites in the urine of these children and adults compared to national reference samples (Arcury, 2005). Organophosphates decrease the levels of acetylcholinesterase, found in nerve endings, and can be absorbed through the skin, inhaled, or ingested. All study participants had metabolites present, and farm work and housing close to agricultural fields were the common factors associated with exposure. Drifts from sprayed fields, residues on farmworker clothing, shoes, tools and skin, as well as food brought from the fields, are all potential sources of exposure. Vehicles can also become contaminated, as can carpeting and furniture. Contaminated clothing should be kept in separate hampers and laundered separately; workers need to be encouraged to leave boots and shoes outside their homes and to change clothing and shower before eating and playing with their children. In homes where more male workers were present, higher levels of pesticide metabolites were found (Arcury, 2005). Substandard housing was also a factor.

Substandard Housing and Poor Sanitation

In a classic article by Cole and Crawford (1991), a vivid example of one migrant camp in Alabama highlighted workers living in a converted chicken house. An upper portion of the wall had been removed for ventilation, creating easy access for insects and birds. A dirt floor, a single light bulb, and two portable toilets located a distance away were some of the other features. Two sinks in a common living area provided the only water for the almost 60 people who lived in the chicken house. Many did not have mattresses, and because the workers were harvesting potatoes, potato baskets conveniently served as the only furniture. Such living situations still exist today. A nurse who was the child of a migrant farmworker family noted that they "lived in houses that had been condemned," and that she once "fell into a well that was covered up by grass and dirt" (Formichelli, 2008).

Migrant farmworkers move frequently and often have great difficulty securing adequate housing. In the past, many growers or owners provided housing to migrant workers and their families. This practice has now become much less common, and only limited numbers of government-sponsored housing units are available for migrant workers. When private housing is available, it is often only offered at prices that outpace worker's wages (Ziebarth, 2006). Data are scant, but a large survey of migrant workers in the eastern, midwestern, and western migrant streams conducted by the Housing Assistance Council (HAC, 2001) revealed that only a quarter of the housing units were owned by employers. However, for those lucky enough to find employer-owned housing, over half of those units were offered without charge. Single-family homes (46%) and apartments (21%) are most common, but workers and their families also are housed in barracks or dormitories and in mobile homes (HAC, 2001; Ziebarth, 2006). The most serious housing problems were found in the Northwest region and in Florida. Over one-quarter of housing units were located adjacent to agricultural fields; in the eastern stream, this figure was much higher at 65% (HAC, 2001).

Families with children occupied 65% of both severely substandard and moderately substandard units (HAC, 2001). Eastern stream units were more often found to be severely or moderately substandard. Many of these included mobile homes. Substandard housing is far more common in the migrant population, as national surveys of U.S. households find only 5% to 2% of the total population, respectively, live in moderately or severely substandard housing (HAC, 2001). Dilapidated conditions were common, with 22% of units having at least one of four appliances or fixtures broken (e.g., bathtub, toilet, stove, refrigerator). Over half had

no working washing machine, compared to national estimates of fewer than one-quarter of households without washing machines (HAC, 2001). Structural problems, such as holes in the roof (15%), sagging frames or roofs (22%), or damage to foundations (15%), were common. Broken glass or window screens were noted in 36% of units, and peeling external paint was found in over 40% of units (HAC, 2001). Evidence of water damage was found in 29% of units, and 19% of them had rodent or insect infestations or other unsanitary conditions.

Crowding is also a problem, as many farmworkers, unable to find sufficient numbers of rental units, share housing—sometimes paying per-person costs. One Minnesota study found that construction trailer barracks, housing 15 to 20 single migrant workers, rented for $90 per month per person. Cinder-block duplexes cost $40 per month per worker, and some residential hotels, lacking hot water, rented rooms for almost $600 per month. Over 75% of respondents earned less than $7.50 per hour (Ziebarth, 2006). In the HAC study, almost one-third of migrant workers paid rental costs that were in excess of 30% of their gross incomes—the median income was $860 and the median housing cost was $380—defined as a "housing cost burden" (p. 10). The costs led to further crowding, as families doubled up to save expenses; 52% of all units were considered crowded. In those crowded units, 74% were occupied by adults and children. Nationally, only 2% to 3% of U.S. households live in housing that is characterized as crowded (HAC, 2001).

In the Minnesota study, 21% of workers experienced "discrimination when trying to find housing," and noted that landlords "don't rent to Hispanics" or families with large numbers of children (Ziebarth, 2006, p. 349). When housing cannot be found, workers and families may have to resort to paying rent to live in garages, barns, sheds, or chicken coops, or they may be forced to stay in their cars.

Agricultural fields are usually located in isolated areas on the outskirts of rural communities. While in these isolated fields, migrant workers often are not provided with sanitation facilities or fresh drinking water. The Occupational Safety and Health Administration (OSHA) mandates field sanitation (one toilet) and fresh drinking water for farms with 11 workers or more working together within a quarter-mile stretch of field (OSHA, 2008). Large corporate farms can, however, simply space workers out and legally avoid this regulation. Furthermore, one in six migrant or seasonal workers are employed on farms hiring 10 or fewer workers, where toilets and drinking water do not have to be provided.

Migrant Family Health

Because of frequent moves, migrant children are often educationally, socially, and physically disadvantaged. Their academic performance may be 10% to 30% below that of other students, as they are often called upon by their families to stay home from school to work, care for younger children, or attend to other household chores (Cooper et al., 2005). They are often socially estranged, constantly moving, and have difficulty finding health-promoting recreational activities. Some research has shown that children of Latino and Black migrant farmworkers exhibit a high degree of psychiatric problems—mostly anxiety-related—including separation anxiety and phobias (Triantafillou, 2003).

The children of migrant farmworkers receive only fragmented health care. Health problems of migrant children include general poor nutrition, anemia, vitamin A deficiency, increased risk for respiratory and ear infections, dental problems, lead and pesticide poisoning, intestinal parasites, skin infections, TB, and delayed development (American Academy of Pediatrics, 2005). Lack of awareness that minor symptoms, such as diarrhea or fever, may indicate a more serious underlying problem can cause delays in seeking medical attention, as can poverty and a lack of health insurance. An earache is minor, but it can lead to a major problem, such as deafness, if left untreated. Deafness is a frequently mentioned major health problem in the migrant population (Kerr, Lusk, & Ronis, 2002).

Migrant adolescents may be more likely to abuse substances, as they are more often "in contact with adult cultural environments" and under a good deal of stress related to poverty and frequent moves (Cooper et al., 2005, p. 7). They are less likely to graduate from high school, because their education is often interrupted. Stress from acculturation, poor working conditions, deficient social support, and poor family functioning have been associated with greater anxiety and depressive symptoms among farmworkers in the Midwest (Hiott, Grzywacz, Davis, Quandt, & Arcury, 2008).

A North Carolina study of farmworker stress found that 38% had "significant levels of stress"; the most stressful factors were identified as "difficulty finding a place to live," "not enough water to drink when I am working," "my partner is no longer with me," and being bothered "that other people use drugs" (Hiott et al., 2008, p. 36). Display 29.5 lists some stressors from the Hispanic Stress Inventory evaluation tool. Social isolation factors ranked slightly lower, but being away from friends and family were often mentioned. In this study of farmworkers immigrating mostly from Mexico, almost 42% met the classification as depressed, and over 18% had anxiety levels consistent with impaired functioning. The researchers concluded that social isolation had a stronger potential effect on anxiety, whereas poor working conditions were associated more with depression. The need for migrant workers to congregate in neighborhoods with others from their cultural background is an attempt to counter this social isolation. When they are surrounded by others who share their culture and speak their language, and when they can find familiar music, television, entertainment, and food, it helps to allay feelings of anxiety and depression. It is easy to understand why many migrant workers in specific migrant streams originate from the same states or communities in Mexico or other countries; it is an attempt to hold onto some semblance of their social networks as they migrate to the United States (Lindstrom & Lauster, 2001).

In the earlier cited study by Hiott and colleagues (2008), over one-third of respondents met the criteria for alcohol dependence. Alcohol use has been noted to be common among male migrant workers, and the stressors migrant farmworkers face related to their employment and acculturation put them at a higher risk for drug and alcohol abuse (Alderete et al., 2000; Finch, Catalano, Novaco, & Vega, 2003). Drugs and alcohol may be used as a means of coping with separation from family and social isolation (Florida International University, 2005).

Problems with substance abuse may also be associated with violence. Some studies report that 46% of children

DISPLAY 29.5	HISPANIC STRESS INVENTORY—BRIEF VERSION

Item	Yes	No
My spouse and I disagree about who controls the money.	❏	❏
My spouse expects me to be more traditional in relationships.	❏	❏
My spouse and I disagree on how to bring up our children.	❏	❏
I've questioned the idea that "marriage is forever."	❏	❏
There have been cultural conflicts in my marriage.	❏	❏
I've felt my spouse and I haven't communicated.	❏	❏
My spouse and I disagree on the language spoken at home.	❏	❏
Both my spouse and I have had to work.	❏	❏
My spouse hasn't adapted to American life.	❏	❏
I watch my work quality so others don't think I'm lazy.	❏	❏
My income is insufficient to support my family or myself.	❏	❏
Since I'm Latino I'm expected to work harder.	❏	❏
Since I'm Latino it's hard to get promotions/raises.	❏	❏
I've been criticized about my work.	❏	❏
I think my children used illegal drugs.	❏	❏
My children have been drinking alcohol.	❏	❏
My children received bad school reports/grades.	❏	❏
My children haven't respected my authority as they should.	❏	❏
My children's ideas about sexuality are too liberal.	❏	❏
My children have talked about leaving home.	❏	❏
There's been physical violence among my family members.	❏	❏
My personal goals conflict with family goals.	❏	❏
I've had serious arguments with family members.	❏	❏
Since I'm Latino it is difficult to find the work I want.	❏	❏
I thought I could be deported if I went to a social/government agency.	❏	❏
Due to poor English, people treat me bad.	❏	❏
Due to poor English, it's hard dealing with daily situations.	❏	❏

From Garcia, D. (1997). Assessing stress among migrant and seasonal farmworkers. *Streamline: The Migrant Health News Source, 3*(5), 1–5.

have witnessed some form of violence; 20% had witnessed a shooting and 11% had witnessed a murder (Triantafillou, 2003). Domestic violence affects migrant worker families, and childhood exposure to family violence has been found to be associated with behavioral and emotional problems, as well as carrying weapons (Villarejo, 2003). Also, recent surveys show that half of men who are frequent wife abusers also abuse their children (Family Violence Prevention Fund, 2008). Research on domestic violence in this vulnerable population is scant, but more than 1,000 battered farmworker women in a multicenter study were interviewed and researchers identified the typical profile as:

◆ Childbearing age (15–40)
◆ Hispanic
◆ Afraid of their partner
◆ Married or living with partner
◆ Drug or alcohol use by partner

The overall incidence was 20.6%. Fifty percent of abused women were pregnant at the time of the abuse (Migrant Clinician's Network, n.d.b). Nationally, just over 30% of women report sexual or physical abuse by a boyfriend or husband during their lifetime (Family Violence Prevention Fund, 2008). (See Chapter 20 for a more complete discussion of domestic violence.) What makes farmworker domestic violence so significant is the fact that these women often experience language barriers, do not have adequate access to health care, live isolated lives with little social support, and fear deportation if they report the abuse—all factors that lead them to endure their violent situation in silence. An example is related by one migrant women who shared one room with her husband, infant, and five single men. Her husband became increasingly violent and unpredictable. He began to beat her and the baby, and she was unable to predict what would initiate a violent attack. She finally fled when one of the men living with them also began beating her. She attributed the aggressive behavior to the powerlessness felt by the men. The Violence Against Women Act of 1994 affords protection for undocumented battered women and children by allowing them to seek legal immigration status without the help of their abusers (Migrant Clinician's Network, n.d.b). Public health nurses must be aware of these issues and what resources are available in the community (see Levels of Prevention Pyramid).

Infectious Diseases

As noted earlier, TB is a common infectious disease among farmworkers. Some studies find that between 37% and 44% of farmworkers tested positive for TB in mass screenings throughout the United States (NCFH, 2007d). Discussing the concern for TB, one epidemiologist said, "A Mexican farmworker with TB who begins treatment in New Mexico might travel during the summer all the way to Canada after the harvests, and, even if successfully treated, may well go home to Mexico in the winter, only to be reinfected by an untreated family member" (McCarthy, 2000, p. 1021). Because of frequent moves, poor access to health care, and social isolation, it is often difficult for migrant farmworkers to be accurately diagnosed and treated. Many factors may prevent them from successfully completing a treatment regimen, and language barriers, along with cultural differences, may preclude them from fully understanding the impact of their disease on themselves and others.

Migrant workers are at greater risk of HIV infection for many of the same reasons. HIV-positive status may be misunderstood and, because of stigmatization and fears of deportation, may be purposely hidden from health officials. Estimated HIV rates are reported to be between 2% and 13%, depending on geographic area and personal risk factors like drug abuse (McCoy, 2005). Others have noted that the rate of HIV infection in migrant farmworkers was 10 times greater than the national average, and that knowledge of HIV transmission in this population was deficient (Fitzgerald, Chakraborty, Shah, Khuder, & Duggan, 2003).

Economic Barriers and Limited Health Resources

Most migrant workers are unable to qualify for basic health and disability benefits such as Workers' Compensation, Social Security, occupational rehabilitation, and disability compensation because of undocumented status (NCFH, 2003). Only 7% to 11% of migrant workers have been granted Medicaid coverage (Villarejo, 2003), and federal legislation passed in 2006 requires proof of U.S. citizenship (e.g., passport, birth certificate) when applying for or renewing Medicaid coverage (King, 2007). As a group, migrant farmworkers have more difficulty accessing Medicaid than any other population.

Medicaid benefits have little value in the face of constant mobility, because they are not transferable from state to state. On one hand, although the low income of migrant workers meets the guidelines for state medical assistance, few families remain in one state long enough for the 30-day residency requirement. On the other hand, farmworker families may not qualify for Medicaid because, during certain months of the year, they earn more than the state's poverty limits. Ironically, migrant workers suffer from preventable and treatable diseases covered under Medicaid, but they are unable to obtain treatment. Some undocumented workers may be eligible for emergency Medicaid—a very limited benefit.

Although many are eligible for public programs such as Medicaid, food stamps, and the Women Infants, and Children (WIC) program, migrant farmworkers as a whole generally do not participate. They may fear immigration penalties or be totally unaware of the available benefits. Some are eligible for Social Security benefits but do not possess the ability to process their claim (NCFH, 2003). Workers who do not have valid Social Security numbers, but still have taxes withheld from their wages, are estimated to contribute $7 billion in Social Security taxes and about $1.5 billion in Medicare taxes—and most of them will never qualify for either Medicare or Social Security benefits (King, 2007).

Some think that undocumented workers are a drain on the U.S. economy, and illegal immigration is a hot-button topic. However, a substantial amount of research demonstrates that immigrants generally pay more money into the system than they extract from it. In 2005, approximately 7% of the Texas population were undocumented immigrants, and Texas spent $58 million that year for health care for undocumented immigrants. However, state revenues from undocumented immigrants exceeded what was spent on health care and education costs by almost $425 million (King, 2007).

LEVELS OF PREVENTION PYRAMID

SITUATION: Domestic Violence in the Migrant Population. Research is scant, however informal discussions occur among women and health care providers. Outreach workers sometimes possess lists of men who are abusive and their victims. Although the migrant lifestyle and experience is difficult for the entire family, women and children suffer most from family violence that the migrant way of life promotes. Isolation and subjugation to a patriarchal system usually prohibit migrant women from seeking help if they are abused. Fear of consequences and difficulty expressing negative views about husbands prevent women from speaking out. (Migrant Clinician's Network. *Domestic violence in the farmworker population.* Monograph Series, n.d.)

GOAL: Using the three levels of prevention, negative health conditions are avoided, promptly diagnosed and treated, and/or the fullest possible potential is restored.

Tertiary Prevention

Rehabilitation	Primary Prevention	
	Health Promotion & Education	**Health Protection**
• Promote family rehabilitation, with or without abuser in the home • Encourage ways to eliminate or reduce social and geographic isolation among vulnerable women	• Alleviate stressors of the migrant lifestyle, such as overcrowding and substandard living conditions • Provide emotional support and educate on what constitutes abuse • Promote self-esteem to the point where a woman can take control of her situation	• Encourage women to contact health care providers as they migrate • Encourage women to find appropriate lay community outreach workers for support • Encourage migrant women to unite and create and environment that allows them to speak up and out while supporting one another against abuse

Secondary Prevention

Early Diagnosis	Prompt Treatment
• Promptly identify an abused woman—through self-identification or by other family members or professionals—and remove her from the dangerous situation* • Keep communication lines open, be culturally sensitive, examine for injuries	• Secure the victim in a safe battered women's shelter • Assist victim to regain self-esteem

Primary Prevention

Health Promotion & Education	Health Protection
• Create awareness of the harsh living conditions that migrant families endure • Advocate for improved and safe living conditions on state and national levels • Provide adequate housing that eliminates overcrowding and offers privacy	• Train bilingual and bicultural lay migrant women on the issues of spousal abuse and help them form support groups • Provide opportunities for women and men to improve self-esteem which will change attitudes toward each other

*Secondary prevention is difficult because of limited financial resources, lack of transportation, no nearby friends or relatives for support, language barriers (e.g., non-English speaking), and limited safe shelters for battered women in rural areas.

Whatever your viewpoint on this issue, it is important to the public's health that basic health care services be available to vulnerable populations. Continued efforts must be made to conduct research assessing risks and hazards, especially those of pesticide exposure. Many government publications document the despair and isolation of migrant workers, yet very little has been done to address the living and working environments that contribute to diminished health. Although migrant workers are difficult to study as a mobile population, they are important as an integral part of our economy and because infectious disease in their sector increases health risks for all (Hirsch et al., 2002; Glasgow, Johnson, & Morton, 2004).

Unique Methods of Health Care Delivery and Primary Prevention

Because migrant health centers do not adequately meet the health needs of the entire migrant community, several innovative methods of health care delivery have been developed and implemented by community health nurses. Although changes are often minor and slow to occur in the migrant population, even minute changes are a milestone, because the migrant lifestyle does not support any type of health stability. Any progress made must be welcomed with recognition and support.

Mobile health vans staffed with bilingual community health nurses and lay workers can travel directly to migrant camps and are an effective strategy for outreach health screening and education. By going to migrant camps and delivering care where the clients live and work, especially during nonwork hours such as evenings and weekends, community health nurses increase health access and overcome barriers of culture and lack of child care. Although migrant families receive only fragmented acute care, a nurses' outreach team can succeed in encouraging migrant farmworkers to prevent illness with immunizations, good nutrition, and healthy lifestyles. A viable alternative to traditional medical clinics, the mobile nursing clinic provides primary care to an underserved population through health promotion, disease prevention, and early treatment. Mobile dental vans also provide services to migrant worker's children, often with arrangements made through school nurses, and dental care provided by dental schools or through partnerships (State of California, 2006). Migrant workers suffer from dental problems at a rate higher than the national average; dental caries and periodontal disease are twice the rate of the total population (Lukes & Miller, 2002).

The use of *promotoras*, lay community outreach workers, or *doulas*, usually trained childbirth assistants, have promoted health in migrant communities (Migrant Health, 2006). Some programs use *doulas* to provide classes on childbirth and other perinatal subjects in an interactive manner; these provide extensive case management services along with the traditional duties of childbirth coach. Because *doulas* and *promotoras* are generally members of the migrant community, they are readily accepted. Some *promotoras* teach parenting classes to avert child abuse and neglect, others may work with special populations to deter domestic violence or substance abuse. Some deal with prevention and early diagnosis of infectious diseases, and others facilitate early screening and treatment for cancer (Coughlin & Wilson, 2002). One program in South Texas, *Nuestra Salud*, specifically served women in the *colonias*—or unincorporated border areas between the United States and Mexico—to promote early detection and treatment of breast and cervical cancer (Migrant Health, 2006). Some *promotoras* migrate with workers and families to provide year-round support and resources.

Information Tracking Systems

Mobility impedes continuity of care, and the inadequate system of medical record keeping for the migrant population is particularly frustrating and challenging. Data information systems are vital components for monitoring the health status of individual farmworkers as they migrate. Furthermore, these data are essential for generating research and follow-up care as well as long-range health planning. They also help justify appropriation of monies to migrant health agencies. The Migrant Clinician's Network has instituted several tracking systems (2008). *TBNet* promotes the completion of TB treatment among migrant populations, and *Diabetes Track II* is geared toward those with diabetes and helps with monitoring and control. *CAN-Track* is a system for coordination of cancer care, and the newest tracking system, *Prenatal Health Network Project*, offers greater continuity for pregnant migrant women. *Heart Fax* is another system of tracking for those with cardiovascular disease.

Migrant children are susceptible to medical "feast or famine" and may be either overtreated or undertreated simply because their medical histories are unknown to current providers. One method for tracking the health status of migrant school-age children is through the Migrant Student Record Transfer System (MSRTS), a computerized system that collects and maintains health and academic records for migrant children (Branz-Spall, Rosenthal, & Wright, 2003). Records of migrant children collected by school nurses include data on personal and family history; immunization status; visual, auditory, and dental problems; nutritional status; and general physical condition. Although this tracking system does serve to enhance the health of migrant children, many do not attend school or do so only on a sporadic basis. The ability to track these children in the migratory lifestyle from work location to work location is often inadequate. Early intervention for migrating children is not always feasible, although it has been proven to greatly improve outcomes. The creation of a national database for information on the health status of adult migrant workers, paralleling the information included in the MSRTS, has also been suggested.

One such system, MiVIA ("my way" in Spanish), is putting health records online and making them available to migrant workers and their health care providers. Workers get a photo identification card, and their records can be accessed only by the use of a personal password. They can access their medical files, medications, a medical reference guide (bilingual), and other resources, such as local clinics and doctors, public transportation, and housing online, no matter their location (Barbassa, 2006). The program began in California's wine country, but is spreading to more distant locations.

THE ROLE OF COMMUNITY HEALTH NURSES IN CARING FOR A MOBILE WORKFORCE

Beyond barriers to health care, such as lack of health services, language, and cultural impediments; inadequate to non-existent transportation; financial strains; underinsurance;

and questionable residency status, which are by themselves formidable obstacles, the migrant lifestyle is fraught with challenges. Because of the insecurity and instability inherent in a mobile lifestyle, long-term health goals are difficult to establish and long-term follow-up of any chronic illness is doubtful. Nonetheless, community health nurses provide much-needed services using community resources, innovative thinking, tenacity, and sensitivity.

Strategies for improving the health status and resource use of migrant workers and their families include:

◆ Improving existing services
◆ Advocating and networking
◆ Practicing cultural sensitivity
◆ Using lay personnel for community outreach
◆ Utilizing unique methods of health care delivery
◆ Employing information tracking systems

Community health nurses are the major providers of migrant health services and have a crucial role in the development and management of interventions. In response to the growing need for available, accessible, and affordable health care for farmworker families, nurses are called on not only to understand the migrant lifestyle but also to help migrant families overcome the barriers to health care (see Perspectives: Voices from the Community).

An aggregate at risk, migrant workers suffer higher frequency of illness, more complications, and more long-term debilitating effects. Exacerbated by a magnitude of environmental and work stressors, the health of migrant families is also compromised by limited access to health care, mobility, language and cultural barriers, low educational levels, and few economic and political resources. Because migrant health needs are largely manageable within community settings, community health nurses are ideal health providers. Implementing health education at migrant camps, training lay health workers, and providing clinic hours to accommodate late workdays are successful interventions. Learning the language of the migrant workers and their unique cultures is also helpful in reaching this population. Community health nurses must advocate for the health of migrant workers, who have very little economic or political power, and also guide them through the complexities of a changing health care system.

In the past, male migrant workers traveled primarily in organized crews; now they are most often traveling in family units with women and children. Added attention must be given to family members exposed to the hazards of the migrant lifestyle. Even as many migrant workers settle into communities, the cycle of poverty continues as other workers arrive from impoverished countries. With a paucity of health

---

PERSPECTIVES: VOICES FROM THE COMMUNITY

"First of all, a nurse should expect the unexpected. Because of the migratory way of life . . . they do not always know where they will be next week or next month. Therefore we must understand that they do not always have their medical records, immunization records, or income records. Hours are very irregular, depending on what time the workers get in from the fields and what time the shifts are. Because of the distances we travel, we work anywhere from 8 to 12 hours a day. The most rewarding part of the job is bringing health services to the underserved and uninsured. The people are so gracious and appreciative of whatever services we provide."

J. S., RN, Michigan

"Since farmworkers come to our area for only 4 months of the year, it is rare that I care for a migrant woman through her entire pregnancy. I may diagnose her pregnancy, I may see her for three or four prenatal visits, or I may meet her only once before she goes into labor and delivers her baby. I struggle with the desire to make a difference in a short period of time and with the disappointment of not being able to follow-through."

C. K., CNM, RN, Pennsylvania

"Encourage clinicians to trust old diagnostic skills of palpation, auscultation, and careful listening. Exhaustive laboratory work or radiology studies are not likely to be welcomed by farm workers who seek relief of symptoms so

that they may return to work. Be warm and interested in the whole family. If you do not speak Spanish or Creole, work with translators who understand how you work. Use translators as . . . vehicles to get the information out and in. Eye contact and touch are crucial. Learning to be clinically relevant as well as competently utilizing a translator is an art, and takes time and experience to hone. Learning some phrases or some of the most frequently asked questions in the language of the farm worker should be encouraged. Even the attempt to speak the patients' language will build trust and confidence. These harvesters of the nation's food are very bright and resourceful people who travel great distances and undergo severe deprivation in order to work. The nobility of this pursuit is getting short shrift in the press and legislative bodies today, but the sheer enormity of the service [that] this group of oppressed people do for the rest of us needs to be acknowledged and honored by the clinicians who will provide primary health care to them and theirs."

W. H., RN, Michigan

"I'm dealing right now with Hispanic women, migrant workers, who do not have any access to prenatal care, none whatsoever. What I'm doing is creative financing, a lot of begging, a lot of pleading, a lot of being nice to people I don't even want to be nice to because it means that much to me for them to get help. So I find myself in situations that are sometimes uncomfortable, but nonetheless I do it because I feel that as a nurse that's my job. Having been a farmworker myself, I would want someone to do that for my mother, and they did."

Unidentified female nurse, Idaho Falls, Idaho

USING THE NURSING PROCESS   WHEN WORKING WITH MIGRANT FAMILIES

Background Data and Assessment

Elena Vasquez is a community health nurse in rural Central California. She had two migrant camps in her service area and realized that during her normal working hours she was missing the adults in the camps. She met with several farmworker families one evening and brainstormed with them. They discussed their health needs and what type of services they needed most. A similar meeting was held at the other camp. At both camps, the families were willing to work with the nurse to enhance needed health care services. The information gathered helped Elena formulate nursing diagnoses which led to innovative planning and implementation.

Nursing Diagnoses

1. Alteration in family health status related to hazardous working conditions, poverty, and mobility.
2. At risk for occupational and situational injury, illness, and stress due to poverty-level working and living conditions.
3. Inadequate and inaccessible health care services related to poverty, work hours, and mobility.

Plan and Implementation

Elena enthusiastically approached the health department administration with the innovative ideas she was formulating. The administrator agreed to try the plan Elena proposed for 3 months if Elena could find the personnel she needed and the results were positive.

She enlisted four other community health nurses, two social workers and several bilingual students from the local university's community health nursing class, which used the agency as a clinical site. Each team of nurses, a social worker, and three students drove to a camp once a week on a Tuesday or Thursday evening from 5 to 9 PM

(the professionals started their day at 1 PM on that day). They completed a family assessment for each family; established a health record for each person; conducted health appraisals; administered immunizations; enrolled families in the Women, Infants, and Children Supplemental Food Program (WIC); made early-evening dentist and doctor appointments and arranged transportation if needed; and held brief teaching sessions on safety, infant and child care, family planning, and any topic the people requested or Elena and her colleagues felt the families needed.

The students became as innovative as Elena. They gathered used clothing and household items from their fellow nursing students for distribution and got valuable practice teaching and delivering health care services. The volunteers' enthusiasm overflowed to the farmworkers. Some of the women planned an informal "day care" program after receiving child care classes from the nursing students. Some of the men organized a baseball team to play against the other camp on Sunday afternoons. Additional donations were solicited—toys and books for the day care program and bats and gloves for the ball teams.

Evaluation

The interventions were so successful that the program became a permanent service of the health department. In the following months, a nurse practitioner was added, along with a preschool teacher and students from the early elementary education program at the university. The two camps became popular with migrant workers, who stayed healthier and were more productive. In addition, the camp managers found the grounds being kept cleaner and had fewer complaints and less abuse of the cabins and shower areas. With improved health and productivity, several families were motivated to establish a permanent home in the community and not continue the migrant lifestyle.

---

resources, the community health nurse is sometimes the only health provider who can and will care for this population.

Providing care for migrant workers presents a challenge, requiring nurses to be innovative and to go beyond the boundaries of traditional health services (see Using the Nursing Process). Although many resources and programs exist to help migrant families, the needs are still overwhelming. By aligning with the goals of *Healthy People 2010* to improve the health of one of the most underserved populations, the community health nurse will also be improving the health of the nation as a whole.

URBAN HEALTH

Urban health considers those characteristics of the environment as they relate to the health of the population living within large cities. According to Galea and Vlahov (2005), the factors responsible for the health of urban residents reflect three broad themes: the physical environment, the

social environment, and access to health and social services. As opposed to rural areas, there is a noted "lack of connectedness in urban life," and lower overall levels of trust, along with weaker family and community ties (Leviton, Snell, & McGinnis, 2000, p. 864). Connectedness has been shown to be a protective factor, especially for adolescent risk behaviors. Inner-city neighborhoods are often observed to have "both conventional culture and street culture" (p. 865). Community involvement and social networks, often deficient in densely populated areas, are components of social capital (discussed in Chapter 25) and have been associated with positive health outcomes, such as mental and physical health and a longer lifespan (Leyden, 2003). Urban communities may be marked by negative social support, such as that found associated with drugs and gangs. Moreover, the "high concentration of poverty (in central cities) leads to social exclusion" and high stress levels from violence and social isolation (Vlahov et al., 2007). Urban communities are made up of multiethnic and diverse racial communities, and these groups are often socially and economically separate from what one might believe to be mainstream urban communities.

In 2000, The Johns Hopkins University founded the Urban Health Institute as a means to bolster support among an inner-city population. This "interface between the university and the Baltimore community" was created to improve the health and well-being of the residents of East Baltimore (Urban Health Institute, 2007). Its mission is to promote evidenced-based interventions to solve local, as well as national, health problems encountered in urban America. The New York Academy of Medicine has organized the Center for Urban Epidemiologic Studies to promote research that improves the health and well-being of urban populations by studying the social, biologic, and environmental influences on health (2007). The Academy sponsors the *Journal of Urban Health,* a "collaborative, multi-disciplinary, population-based research, with a special focus on low-income, disadvantaged populations" (2007). But how did the health of these urban communities evolve to such a state that targeted efforts are now required? It began in the 1800s.

HISTORY OF URBAN HEALTH CARE ISSUES

Urban living has a long and checkered history in the United States. Arriving immigrants increased population density, especially in the large eastern and midwestern cities. Millions of immigrants arrived in the United States between the mid-1800s and the early 1900s. Because most had some family or distant relatives who had arrived here earlier, they made their ways to where these people lived, hoping to receive temporary shelter while they sought work (Garb, 2003). Many came with large families and roomed with other large European and Eastern European families in tenements. Others came alone or as a nuclear family without close ties to others already living here. Nonetheless, they gathered in **ghettos**, thickly populated sections of cities inhabited predominantly by members of the same minority group. This enabled them to be with people from their homeland—people who knew the same language and the same ways.

As time went on, many families left ghetto communities and found housing in smaller towns or in the beginnings of suburbs. As described in the classic work by Cutler, Glaeser, and Vigdor (1997), the Irish left New York City in the early 20th century; then Blacks, coming from the South, moved in. Many Black families later left for outlying suburban areas, and Puerto Rican families moved in. Today, Haitian and Middle Eastern families inhabit some of the same neighborhoods. After 100 years, many of the same buildings continue to provide less than optimal shelter for a new group of immigrants. Although ghetto living provides a sense of belonging, for many it is temporary because it engenders more negatives than positives. Children and grandchildren of the original immigrants seek out a different life for themselves, away from the urban areas that are often riddled with crime, unsafe housing, and disease. Others, because of poverty, drugs, or being near-homeless, remain in urban slum areas (Cutler et al., 1997; Waltzer, 2000).

In a classic position paper, the American College of Physicians used the term **urban health penalty** to describe the "concentration of economic decline, job loss, and major health problems" afflicting inner-city populations experiencing health problems when healthier and wealthier residents moved to the suburbs, leaving poverty zones of economic and physical deterioration that act as determinants of health (1997, p. 485). Freudenberg, Galea, and Vlahov (2005) find urban health penalty associated with large cities that "concentrate poor people, and expose residents to unhealthy environments, leading to a disproportionate burden of poor health," and feel that it inaccurately likens "urbaness with class and race" (p. 2–3).

Who has been responsible for addressing the needs of these communities over the last hundred or more years? Who has been, or should have been, addressing the needs evolving among the urban communities? Two connected disciplines, urban planning and public health, have addressed these issues from the 19th century to the present. **Urban planning** worked to improve the welfare of individuals and communities by creating more healthful, efficient, attractive, and equitable places (Kochtitzky et al., 2006). The activities of urban planners usually include addressing the community's needs related to transportation, housing, commercial areas, natural resources, environmental protection, and health care infrastructure (Johansson, Svedung, & Andersson, 2006; Corburn, 2004).

Public health, of course, is directed at improving human well-being through assessing and ensuring the delivery of services at the community level. Together, these disciplines both addressed the needs of the identified vulnerable populations. Initially, during the late 19th and early 20th centuries, these two systems were linked in promoting health by facilitating physical activity through the creation of green space. They joined together in preventing infectious diseases by ensuring healthful drinking water and sewage systems. They also protected the community from exposure to hazardous substances related to industry by monitoring land uses and instituting zoning ordinances (Corburn, 2004; Kochtitzky et al., 2006). During the middle of the 20th century, the focus of planning and public health agencies drifted apart, partly because of their successes in limiting injury and health risk caused by inappropriate mixing of land use. The target of public health agencies shifted from investigating ways to improve the infrastructure to a focus on germ theories and immunizations (Corburn, 2004), challenges that were easier for physicians to address than changing environments. On the other hand, Corburn describes urban planning as switching its energy to "promoting economic development through large infrastructure and transportation projects. Planning shifted from attempting to restrain harmful spillovers from private market activities in urban areas to promoting suburban economic development" (p. 542). At about the same time, Rachel Carson's book *Silent Spring,* published in 1962, described the effects of pesticides on wildlife and the eventual effects on human health, thus initiating the *environmental justice movement,* and focusing environmental health professionals largely on toxic chemical exposures (Frumkin, 2005).

According to Kochtitzky and colleagues (2006), the disciplines of urban planning and public health have begun to collaborate once again, working together to improve transportation and air quality, and addressing national health issues such as injury prevention, physical activity, access to health care, energy use, and greenhouse gas emissions, along with disaster preparedness and response. This team effort is a natural partnership when addressing such concerns as physical activity and the provision of safe and accessible spaces (Geller, 2003). A study by Leyden (2003), for instance, found that "residents living in walkable, mixed-use neighborhoods are more likely to know their neighbors, to participate politically, to trust others, and to be involved socially," all components of social capital that have been shown to improve both mental and physical health (p. 1550). These joint ventures are significant in reaching those *Healthy People 2010* objectives directed at the prevention of chronic disease, injury prevention, and health promotion. Leaders at the CDC are concerned with factors that affect people and their environments, and support efforts that address the improvement of both physical and social environments as related to places to live, work, and play. The CDC's *Healthy Places* describes the components involved: interaction between environment and health, poorly planned growth leading to sprawl and increased used of vehicles, and healthy community design that promotes health and well-being (2007b). See Display 29.6 for a list of community design issues.

URBAN POPULATIONS AND HEALTH DISPARITIES

The majority of the world's populace now lives in cities, which is a change from long-held rural dominance (Vlahov et al., 2007; Vlahov, Gibble, Freudenberg, & Galea, 2004).

The greatest growth of large cities around the world is among less-wealthy nations, where urban slums are developing at a rapid rate (Vlahov & Gaklea, 2002). Depending upon the classification used, more than 30% of the U.S. populace still lives in central cities. Central cities with a population under 50,000 in 1990 grew more rapidly than those with more than 1 million people (U.S. Bureau of Census, 2000b). However, metropolitan areas outside central cities have had faster growth in recent years (U.S. Census Bureau, 2000b). More than 220 million people (almost 80% of the U.S. population) live in what are characterized as urban or metropolitan areas (U.S. Census Bureau, 2000c; Fleischman & Barondess, 2004). Roughly half of the populace lives in *suburban areas* (Collins-Perdue, Stone, & Gostin, 2003). About 80% of all North Americans live in towns and cities, and they spend 90% of their time indoors (Hancock, 2002).

Although some metropolitan areas have recorded substantial population losses in central-city areas (e.g., Milwaukee, Racine, and Waukesha, WI losses of 95.3%; Detroit, Warren, and Flint, MI, 91.7%; Rochester, Batavia, and Seneca Falls, NY, 543.7%; and the New Orleans area, 838.8%), others have logged substantial gains (e.g., San

---

| DISPLAY 29.6 | CENTERS FOR DISEASE CONTROL AND PREVENTION–SIGNIFICANT HEALTH ISSUES RELATED TO LAND USE (2007) |

Accessibility
Absence of ramps for wheelchairs; lack of depressed curbs (periodic breaks in curbs that act as ramps); narrow doorways that cannot accommodate various assistive devices, such as wheelchairs and walkers; lack of access to mass transit routes or other public services

Children's Health and the Built Environment
School design, increased obesity and diabetes, asthma, attention deficit hyperactivity disorder, parks and green spaces

Elders' Health and the Built Environment
Safe housing, appropriate public transportation, green spaces and recreational facilities, chronic diseases that limit mobility

Gentrification
Transformation of neighborhoods from low- to high-value, causing displacement of long-time residents due to higher taxes and rents

Health Impact Assessment
Effects of a policy, program, or projects on the health of a population and the distribution of those effects judged by tools, procedures, or methods. *The major steps in conducting a health issue assessment (HIA) include*
* screening (identify projects or policies for which an HIA would be useful)
* scoping (identify which health effects to consider)
* assessing risks and benefits (identify which people may be affected and how they may be affected)
* reporting (present the results to decision-makers)
* evaluating (determine the affect of HIA on the decision process)

Injury
Transportation planning and safety, bicycle- and motor vehicle-related unintentional injuries

Mental Health
Effect of community design and the built environment on stress levels and cognitive functioning

Physical Activity
Aspects of the home, workplace, and community environments influence a person's level of physical activity—the availability and accessibility of attractive stairwells, bicycle paths, walking paths, exercise facilities, and swimming pools, as well as the overall aesthetics of an environment, may play a role in determining the type and amount of physical activity people engage in

Respiratory Health and Air Pollution
Air quality and air pollutants' effects on asthma and other health conditions

Social Capital
Individual and communal time and energy available for such things as community improvement, social networking, civic engagement, personal recreation, and other activities that create social bonds between individuals and groups

Water Quality
Pollution of surface and groundwater; increased runoff from paved surfaces (streets, parking lots) causes increased erosion and silt and may affect water treatment plants

Source: CDC, 2007. *Designing and building healthy places.* Retrieved August 20, 2008 from http://www.cdc.gov/healthyplaces/.

Antonio, TX, a gain of 59%; Oklahoma City and Shawnee, OK, 39.3%; Jacksonville, FL, 37.4%; and Raleigh-Durham and Cary, NC, 29.1%) (Demographia, 2006). One example of how changes in population can adversely affect large cities is Cleveland, Ohio. Between 1950 and 2000, the population dropped from 915,000 to fewer than 500,000 people. This led to a smaller tax base and a greater proportion of poor residents, yet the city had the same maintenance expenses for sewers, water lines, and streets. Detroit, Michigan, lost roughly one-third of its population between 1975 and 1995, but the poverty rate doubled (Galea, Freudenberg, & Vlahov, 2005).

After the automobile became the mainstay of transportation, and with the housing boom and highway expansion occurring after WWII, the suburbs became "the place to be." People moved from large cities to more suburban areas, and shopping malls and schools followed. Cars became even more essential, because public transportation did not always extend into suburban areas thereby leading to long commute times, traffic congestion, and increased motor vehicle and pedestrian injuries and deaths (Frumkin, 2005; Srinivasan, O'Fallon, & Dearry, 2003). Although not all suburban areas have remained attractive and vital, an income gap persists between city and suburban residents. Poverty is two times greater in cities than in suburban areas (18.2% versus 8.6%); unemployment is also higher (8% versus 5%). In the 2000 Census, per capita income was $1,000 more for suburban residents than for city dwellers, despite the almost equal percentage of college-educated and professionally employed residents (Logan, 2002).

Today, the declining urban situation is not confined to a few large cities. To achieve the vision of "healthy people in healthy communities," as discussed throughout the *Healthy People 2010* document, more must be done to promote health and prevent disease in urban areas. Although some significant improvements have been made in the last decade, no more than 15% of the goals identified in *Healthy People 2000* have been achieved (Freudenberg, 2000; Duchon, Andrulis, & Reid, 2004). The primary reason for health disparity, as mentioned in Chapter 25, is the disproportionate burden of certain health and social problems among different populations—in this instance, urban areas. This is believed by some authors to be due to stress, economic inequity, perceptions of deprivation, racism, and lack of access to quality health care among some residents (Fleischman & Barondess, 2004).

Overcrowding and poor-quality housing have been found to have a direct relationship with poor mental health, developmental delay, and even to shorter stature (Bashir, 2002; Vlahov et al., 2007). In a large-scale study, Galea, Ahern, Rudenstine, Wallace, and Vlahov (2005) found that people living in neighborhoods "characterized by poorer features of the built environment" were between 29% and 58% more likely to report depression in the past 6 months, and 36% to 64% more likely to report lifetime depression when compared with people living in better built environments (p. 825). Certain characteristics of the built environment and socioeconomic status have been associated with the prevalence of sexually transmitted diseases/infections and cardiovascular disease mortality rates (Cohen et al., 2000; Diez-Roux et al., 2001). Hazardous waste landfill sites are often located in or near urban areas (Vlahov et al., 2007, p. 119). Air pollution and noise exposure, often associated with large inner cities, have been linked to asthma, cardiovascular death, hypertension, ischemic heart disease, and hearing impairment (Vlahov et al., 2007). A study of 95 urban communities, comprising about 40% of the U.S. population, revealed a statistically significant relationship between short-term changes in ozone and mortality; the relationship was even higher for respiratory and cardiovascular mortality (Bell, McDermott, Zeger, Samet, & Dominici, 2004). Lead poisoning has been more often reported in older, larger cities, as have poor nutrition and violent crime (Leviton et al., 2000).

Violence is often associated with large metropolitan cities. Urban youth are more likely to engage in violence than those from rural areas, although this varies among cities and neighborhoods (Leviton et al., 2000). U.S. Department of Justice (2007) crime statistics reveal that urban residents had the highest violent victimization rates in 2005 (six per 1,000 compared to four per 1,000 for both suburban and rural residents), and urban households continue to be the most vulnerable to property crime, motor vehicle theft, burglary, and other theft. Some researchers have associated higher crime rates in central cities with unemployment and urban economic change related to a shift from manufacturing to service-sector jobs along with high poverty rates (Oh, 2005).

Inner cities are often thought to be places with "above average . . . unemployment, full-time workers living on low pay, single parents and the sick and . . . disabled . . . living in poor quality and deteriorating housing conditions" (Wasylenki, 2001, p. 214). Dilapidated housing exposes residents to leaking pipes, cracks in walls and ceilings, peeling paint, broken windows, and pests such as cockroaches and rats (Rauh, Chew, & Garfinkel, 2002; Bashir, 2002; Leaderer et al., 2002). There is often limited access to adequate rental properties, and rent is often higher in large cities, making it difficult for low-income residents to find adequate housing. They are often forced to live in neighborhoods that do not facilitate outdoor activity or have markets that provide healthy foods, such as fresh fruits and vegetables (Dannenberg et al., 2003). Low-income housing, when available, is often plagued with construction and maintenance problems and is characterized by crowding, poor quality, high population density, and attendant health problems. Homelessness is more prevalent in urban areas than in rural areas (see Chapter 28). Deteriorated neighborhoods are associated with high crime levels and greater social isolation (Srinivasan et al., 2003). Sociologists Wilson and Kelling first proposed the "broken window theory" in 1982, noting that if a broken window goes unrepaired, soon all the windows are broken, and this sends a powerful message to residents that no one cares. Public health research has validated that a high "broken window index" (graffiti, litter, blighted housing, and abandoned cars) can independently predict neighborhood gonorrhea rates (Frumkin, 2005, p. A291; Cohen et al., 2000).

Population density, complexity, and racial/ethnic diversity are associated with urban areas. Central cities are often home to a large proportion of poor people and those from different racial and ethnic groups (Srinivasan, O'Fallon, & Dearry, 2003). Almost half of all Hispanics live in central cities (46.4%), most often Puerto Ricans and other Hispanics. Cubans live outside central cities within metropolitan areas (76%); only 21.2% of Whites live in central cities (Therrien & Ramirez, 2001). Problems such as HIV infection, asthma, cirrhosis, diabetes, violence (including homicide), unintentional injury, heroin abuse, preterm delivery, infant mortality, heart disease, cancer, and stroke affect the poor and people of color more than other groups, and these groups are increasingly concentrated in cities. As an illustration, in 1998, the age-adjusted death rate for heart disease among non-Hispanic Black people was 40% higher than the rate for non-Hispanic Whites (Phillips & Grady, 2002). A classic study by McCord and Freeman (1990) found that the mortality rates of Harlem residents between the ages of 5 and 65 years were higher than those in Bangladesh, which was then noted to have one of the lowest income levels in the world—a shocking finding. As noted in Chapter 25, poverty makes a significant difference in health status. A Canadian study found that those living in wealthier neighborhoods of Ontario had 45% shorter waiting times for angiograms and were 23% more likely to have an angiogram than residents in poorer areas. A larger percentage of patients with myocardial infarctions were from the lowest income level (Wasylenki, 2001).

Over the past 25 years, cities and their suburbs have become more alike, and the demographic and health profiles that were previously uniquely urban are now shared by "edge cities" and suburbs populated by poor and minority families. Political power has shifted to more affluent suburban areas, where the tax base and spending practices are greater, at the expense of these cities. Monies that once came to cities to support new resources have also declined. The U.S. Conference of Mayors (2005) estimates that additional expenses to cities due to unfunded federal mandates, such as the Americans with Disabilities Act (ADA) for example, run in the billions of dollars. While these changes were occurring, power shifted to the states and multinational corporations, which invested tax dollars and incentives in the growing suburbs. In the 20 years between 1970 and 1990, the number of people living in poor inner-city neighborhoods doubled (Freudenberg, 2000). These people live a marginal existence—substance abusers, poor elderly, undocumented immigrants, the very ill, and the disabled. They are economically trapped, as the inner city declines around them.

Urban health disparities present a challenge that can be addressed only by the joint effort of public health and urban planning bodies. Coalitions of public health professionals, planners, builders, and architects, along with transportation engineers and government officials are needed to promote healthy, sustainable communities (Srinivasan et al., 2003). President Clinton's 1999 Council on Sustainable Development defined *sustainable communities* as healthy places where both natural and historic resources are protected, employment is available, urban sprawl is contained, neighborhoods are safe, lifelong learning is promoted, health care and transportation are easily accessible, and all citizens have the opportunity to improve their quality of life.

As with all good plans, the sustainable development plan requires that the recipient of the planning be involved. Corburn calls this "democratizing the practice" (2004, p. 543). Communities that have been victimized through ineffective planning must be included in the decision-making process. This process will require the inclusion of the practical experience that residents bring to the table, alongside expert input. However, to ensure equitable participation and to level the discussions, the community must have access to all the necessary resources, such as technical, legal, and financial assistance.

The health of communities must be addressed from all levels of environmental impact (individual, community, and systems). Data must be included from the various environments, such as homes, workplaces, schools, and community spaces. These approaches then bring such action in line with what is often referred to as *environmental justice*, or the marriage of environmental health and civil rights (Frumkin, 2005, p. 290). A framework to ensure such justice requires that all individuals and communities have the right to work, play, and live in environments that are safe and healthy. It also requires that polluters are punished and required to provide compensation for damages and/or renovation.

SOCIAL JUSTICE AND THE COMMUNITY HEALTH NURSE

Justice is concerned with treating people fairly. *Distributive justice* refers to the justified distribution of burdens and benefits throughout society (see Chapter 4 for a discussion of distributive justice). In the United States, the distribution of goods and services is largely determined by the marketplace. Although equality is claimed as a social ideal, dramatic inequities are accepted as being determined by the law of the marketplace. In contrast, community health nursing is grounded in commitment to a just distribution of primary goods for all members of society (Drevdahl, Kneipp, Canales, & Shannon-Dorcy, 2001). The founder of American public health nursing, Lillian Wald, was in the forefront of social reform movements emphasizing just allocation of resources for the immigrant and poor laborer (Wald, 1971). At the start of the 21st century, PHNs have inherited her legacy, but are we living up to it?

The hardships faced by people in decaying urban areas is an example of social injustice. **Social justice** occurs when a society provides for the health needs and health care issues of all people by treating people fairly, regardless of where they live or who they are. It involves an "equitable bearing of burdens and reaping of benefits in society" (Drevdahl, Kneipp, Canales, & Shannon-Dorcy, 2001, p. 23). It is a widely held view that social justice is the foundation of public health nursing, and that premature death and disease or health and illness derive from the political, socioeconomic, and structural workings of society (Drevdahl, 2002; Fahrenwald, Taylor, Kniepp, & Canales, 2007). Community health nurses who practice social justice have broad and holistic views of health; they have strong convictions that health care is a basic human right, and that improving the health of communities is an example of social justice (Couto, 2000). Social justice deals with concepts of inclusion, participation, empowerment, and the recognition that diversity is a strength—not a limitation (Racher, 2007). Social justice "ensures distribution of life resources in a way that benefits the marginalized and constrains the self-interest of the privileged"; at its best, it implies complete impartiality (Schim, Benkert, Bell, Walker, & Danford, 2006, p. 73–74).

Public health nurses must have a heightened sense of the value of cultural, racial, and socioeconomic differences and an awareness that these differences are often turned into discrimination in health care services and policies. They must be determined to "extend the bonds of community to give everyone a firm place to stand as equally entitled to services from a health care system with a single high standard" (Couto, 2000. p. 4). Two programs represent this commitment to social justice on both national and international levels.

The Community Environmental Health Resource Center (CEHRC) in Washington, D.C., works with grassroots organizations engaged in the fight for social justice for low-income communities (Bashir, 2002; CEHRC, 2007). The primary focus is empowering residents and increasing economic opportunities to address the environmental health hazards posed by substandard housing. Children and other vulnerable persons in low-income urban communities are at greatest risk. The CEHRC addresses the major negative health outcomes of childhood asthma and lead poisoning, along with increased risk for depression and poor mental health, among people living in substandard housing in urban areas.

For more than 20 years, the goal of an international movement, *Healthy Cities*, has been to improve the conditions in urban areas, developing cities in which the focus is on "affordable housing, accessible transportation systems, employment for all who want to work, a healthy and safe environment with a sustainable ecosystem, and accessible health care services that focus on [illness] prevention and staying healthy" (Schim et al., 2006, p. 74). The World Health Organization (WHO) sponsors this program and works with local governments to develop healthy populations through capacity building and projects. It is now in its fourth phase, which focuses on healthy aging, health impact assessment, and healthy urban planning (WHO, 2007).

Where is nursing's role within the concept of social justice? Schim and colleagues (2006) propose a new meta-paradigm for urban health nursing. They propose a model that not only includes social justice along with the traditional concepts of *person, environment, health,* and *nursing,* but also places social justice at the center of this new approach. Their view is to interconnect social justice with the four basic constructs and promote its centrality in order to guide both "philosophical orientation (theory) and dynamic implementation process (practice) in nursing" (Schim et al., 2006, p. 74). They view social justice as a population-based concept, and note that having an individual patient focus can lead to "paternalism and racism" (p. 76). In their model, urban health nursing directs its practice to the systems and community- or population-based level, at which both political and economic solutions must be considered. Although most nurses in urban settings continue to provide service on the individual level, nurses should step back and analyze their practice and synthesize recommendations for a plan of action at the community planning table to better address the needs of the city or neighborhood.

For nurses, a key factor in the process is to emphasize the social justice perspective of *impartiality,* as defined originally by Barry (cited in Schim et al., 2006). This impartiality drives planning and action in a more *just* manner (i.e., as if neither side knew which position they were in: the advantageous [stronger bargaining] position or the disadvantageous [weaker bargaining] position). Thus, instead of an intervention or action being deemed *just* simply because it gives an advantage to one side or the other, it is done because its *outcome* is considered just or fair when viewed by a dispassionate outsider. The point of negotiations, then, is to get an equal share and no more. Self-interest is rationally put aside in favor of the greater good.

Therefore, although day-to-day practice usually includes individual services, the overall planning for change and improvement must occur from the perspective of the population level. From this level of practice, the construct of *person* incorporates the population level of aggregates, institutions, communities, states, and nations—not solely the individual. The concept of the *environment* at the individual level is often associated with physical and psychosocial influences. With a population focus, it incorporates economic and political structures that can influence health or illness and addresses community and global systems that must be utilized to initiate change and solutions.

Like the other constructs, *health* is expanded to include a population focus that recognizes sociopolitical influences. By acknowledging the health issues encountered at the individual, as well as the population level, the urban nurse can incorporate interventions that address the "dynamic institutional and societal environment" described by Schim and colleagues. In reflecting on the practice of urban nursing, the profession must believe that it requires more of a "population consciousness," something that is missing throughout most of undergraduate nursing education (Schim et al., 2006, p. 76).

At the same time, urban nursing practice requires cultural and racial competence in order to advocate for the communities served by nursing. Once nursing again accepts and embraces social justice as a focal concept within the practice, especially in urban and public health practices, it can challenge itself to develop more dynamic forms of advocacy and social responsibility that will not only affect its clients, but shape the education and training of future nursing professionals (Fahrenwald et al., 2007). This, in turn, should lead to an enhancement of the practice and research needed to contribute solutions for addressing health disparities in all settings.

The urban nursing profession must focus, much like public health nursing, on including both primary and secondary prevention—not only at the local or community level, but also include the state, national, and international levels, to enact change for the common good. The role of advocate in these practice settings must include not only the individual level, but also the community or population and systems levels. An example of such actions would include advocating for adequate funding of government health systems, such as Medicare and Medicaid, and helping to ensure that all communities are safe and healthy environments in which to live and work. To connect all populations to fair and just systems "requires available, accessible, affordable, and sustainable health care that is equitably and impartially distributed without regard to personal advantage and disadvantage" (Schim et al., 2006, p. 77). Drevdahl and colleagues (2001) remind us that "health is not something belonging only to those who have the means to pay for education, safe working environments, and health care services," but should be a benefit for all of us living together on this planet.

COMMUNITY HEALTH NURSING IN RURAL AND URBAN SETTINGS

The proportion of registered nurses (RNs) living in urban and rural areas mirrors the general population (79% versus 21%). The mean age for urban RNs is 43.4 years, whereas rural nurses average 43.1 years. The proportion of male RNs is similar in urban and large rural areas, but fewer male nurses work in small, isolated rural areas. Like the general population, the education level for nurses is higher in urban areas (46.6% with a baccalaureate or higher degree) than in rural areas (35.3% for large rural, 30.7% for small rural, 30.6% for isolated rural areas).

Working in a Rural Community

Rural nurses are more likely to work outside hospital settings than are urban RNs, and are more likely to commute outside their residential areas to work. For instance, while there are 719 RNs per 100,000 residents living in small rural areas, only 411 per 100,000 work there. Many rural RNs commute to larger rural areas or urban centers to earn higher wages (Skillman, Palazzo, Keepnews, & Hart, 2005). Rural community health nurses most often grew up in rural areas or lived for a time in small communities. They frequently have extended family there (Bushy, 2000). Rural PHNs are active members of their community and are highly respected professionals (Bushy, 2003).

The rural community health nurse plays many roles:

1. *Advocate*: Assists rural clients and families in obtaining the best possible care
2. *Coordinator/case manager*: Connects rural clients with needed health and social services, often assisting with information on transportation
3. *Health teacher*: Provides education to individuals, families, or groups on health promotion or other health-related topics (e.g., prepared childbirth, parenting, diabetes maintenance, home safety)
4. *Referral agent*: Makes appropriate connections between rural clients and urban service providers
5. *Mentor*: Guides new community health nurses, nursing students, and other nurses new to the rural community
6. *Change agent/researcher*: Suggests new approaches to solving patient care or community health problems based on research, professional literature, and community assessment
7. *Collaborator*: Seeks ways to work with other health and social service professionals to maximize outcomes for individual clients and the community at large
8. *Activist*: With a deep understanding of the community and its population, takes appropriate risks to improve the community's health

See From the Case Files II for a day in the life of a rural public health nurse.

Rural community health nurses have the opportunity to use autonomy in daily practice. Nurses must rapidly assume independent and interdependent decision-making roles because of the small workforce and large workload. Rural nurses are often generalists out of necessity—serving as a "jack-of-all-trades" and feeling that "you're it" (Rosenthal, 2005, pp. 42–44). Rural community health nurses learn to prioritize tasks quickly and work efficiently with others to get the job done. Referrals to other rural providers are facilitated because providers frequently know one another. The rural community health nurse has an advantage over urban nurses in that the rural health care system is smaller and easier to influence and change, but specialization is seldom possible and long-distance travel is generally a necessity (Bushy, 2003).

Anonymity is not easy for the rural community health nurse, who is always on duty. A trip to the grocery store on a Saturday morning may include interactions with rural clients

From the Case Files II

A Day in the Life of a Rural Public Health Nurse

Carol M. arrives at the Stevens County Public Health Department in rural America. She reviews her caseload for the day and begins her work. First, she telephones the principal of the local high school to let him know that she is able to speak next week to the Parent-Teacher Association about raising healthy adolescents (*health teacher*). Then, she calls the family of a hospitalized patient (*coordinator/case manager*) to plan the discharge of their family member. At 10:00 a.m., Carol makes a home visit to the Wesley family. The family members explain that they have been unable to enroll for needed food stamps because they do not understand the process. Carol gives the family an informational handout with phone numbers and addresses, so that they can contact the appropriate agency (*referral agent*) and even calls her neighbor who works at the office to inform her of the need for special attention for the family (*advocate*). At lunch, Carol runs into a social worker colleague and they discuss their concerns about the hospitalized individual with whom Carol spoke earlier in the day (*collaborator*). Both question whether the family will be able to manage the care needed for the patient without much outside support. After lunch, Carol returns to her office for a staff meeting and discusses a new charting system that she is recommending (*change agent/researcher*) for implementation by the department. At the same meeting, she agrees to work with a visiting community health nursing student during his rural practicum (*mentor*). That evening, Carol, as a concerned citizen, participates in a meeting at the town hall about issues related to local water quality. She addresses the group, giving them data and expresses concern (*activist*), then volunteers to lead others who are concerned about the issue. It is obvious that community health nurses like Carol M. often play many roles during the day. As a nursing student working in a rural community, you may have the opportunity to "try on" many of these roles.

and their families about their pressing health concerns. Rural nurses may experience role conflict, as neighbors often view them in all of their various roles—as nurse, "parent, spouse, and church member" (Rosenthal, 2005, p. 43). Rural community health nurses may have confidentiality and personal/professional boundary issues that have to be addressed. However, rural community health nurses are often respected, known, and trusted by the populations they serve (Bushy, 2000). Also, an "insider/outsider" mentality often exists in rural areas, as rural residents may tend to exclude nurses who have only lived in their communities for a short time or who want to remain less involved (Rosenthal, 2005, p. 43).

Rural community health nurses may experience the challenge of physical isolation from personal and professional opportunities associated with urban areas. Travel to cities for basic and continuing education can be a barrier. Rural nurses may also feel isolated in their clinical practices because of the scarcity of professional colleagues. Many rural community health nurses overcome these barriers and learn to appreciate the benefits of clinical practice in a rural setting by discussing their concerns with peers through professional organizations and seeking ways to combat isolation through online education or discussion groups (Bushy, 2003; Rosenthal, 2005).

The rural community health nurse often receives a salary that is lower than that of urban nurses in comparable positions (Skillman et al., 2005). However, there are benefits to rural nursing. Housing costs are usually lower than in larger cities, and long commutes to and from work on congested highways are often avoided, although rural driving can be hazardous. As a place to live and raise a family, rural communities offer a slower pace of life, open spaces, clean air, and friendly atmosphere. The smaller system of health care in a rural community can be advantageous to the community health nurse. It may be easier to understand the system and initiate planned change. There are many possibilities to enhance rural nursing practice, including continuing education by satellite or Internet, partnerships with larger medical centers, and invitations to clinical experts to provide on-site workshops. Grants can be written to facilitate these endeavors.

Working in an Urban Setting

Urban public health nursing can be very rewarding, and many nurses are drawn to urban areas where salaries are higher, and opportunities for advancement or additional education greater. In urban areas, there are a larger number of nurses, more schools of nursing, and more intensive recruitment efforts than in rural areas, although, inner-city areas, much like rural settings, have a more difficult time filling nursing vacancies (LaSala, 2000).

A study of three Western states, comparing rural and urban health departments, found similar per capita ratios of PHNs. However, urban heath departments had more PHN vacancies (70% versus 21%), and both reported difficulties recruiting NPs. More of the rural health agencies permitted part-time work, and this may have somewhat skewed results. Urban health departments employ a variety of personnel, including epidemiologists and nutritionists, who are not always found in rural health agencies, thus allowing for broader collaboration and in-depth services (Rosenblatt, Casey, & Richardson, 2002). Advanced PHNs are more

prevalent in larger urban areas, and they may assume a more population-focused practice—working at a systems level—in place of, or in addition to, the individual care they can provide (Mondy, Cardenas, & Avila, 2003).

The description of PHN duties in one large Midwestern city includes combinations of "home visiting, school assignments, clinic services, and other programs," with caseloads averaging between 90 and 140 families (Schulte, 2000, p. 5). Specialized positions are also common, with PHNs staffing TB and sexually transmitted diseases/infection clinics, serving assigned schools, providing staff development, or being assigned special projects such as screenings and disaster preparedness. The urban nurses in this study worked mainly with clients at or below the poverty level, and one nurse described the situation this way:

> The problems have gotten to be more. The economic situation—everything's gotten worse. The medical care is a mess—not as accessible. People are more mobile now, even more so than they were years ago . . . they think they left [home] . . . for a better place (p. 6).

Schulte (2000, p. 6) also noted that PHNs worked largely with "three interacting communities": the local physical communities to which they were assigned, the communities created by individual clients and families, and resource communities (those organized to provide services and goods to clients in need). The processes used by the urban community health nurses included:

- Forging working relationships
- Acting as a resource
- Detecting/asking the next question
- Making informed judgments
- Managing a sense of time
- Teaching
- Intervening with conditions influencing health
- Using physical dexterity.

In *forging a relationship*, PHNs began with creating a "perception of presence" by identifying themselves as a PHN and passing out their card with the instruction to the client to call upon them when needed. *Acting as a resource* involves dealing with "sensitive subjects" and requires "honesty, asking direct questions, and ignoring rude behavior." *Detecting and asking the next question* "means listening to more than what is said" (Schulte, 2000, p. 7). When a client is truly heard and all information is on the table, *making an informed judgment* is then possible. *Sense of time* includes the awareness of the long-term commitment of the community health nurse to the client and the belief that results can occur, despite the lack of progress or even regression on the part of some clients. An illustration of this concept was reported by one of the PHNs in the study:

> I had this one lady where I just sensed that something else was going on. She was . . . separated from her husband, but he would come over and demand his "right"—sex—and then he'd give her money. And I kept seeing this pattern in her life. So I started getting her to talk about what kind of childhood she had . . . and it came out that she had an abusive father who did the same thing—he'd rape her and then give her money. So I talked with her and then got her into counseling. I didn't see her (for awhile) and then she showed up at one of

my schools . . . and said, "You're the nurse who saw this and sent me for counseling." She told me that she went back to school, for her GED, and is now enrolled in college. It really helped change her (Schulte, 2000, pp. 7–8).

Teaching is described as an ongoing, interactive process that not only provides information about disease prevention and health promotion, but also helps clients navigate the health care system. *Intervening with conditions* that affect health draws on nursing knowledge and experience and involves interceding to reduce the affect of social, political, and economic determinants of health; it involves a "mix of knowledge, experience, intuition, and sensitivity" (p. 8). *Physical dexterity* is used when completing a health assessment of a client's physical condition.

Schulte (2000) found that urban PHNs create connections through caring processes and an underlying sense of regard for their clients as human beings. Community health nurses collaborate with their clients to develop their facility for long-term health promotion and improvement of their quality of life. Their ultimate goal is to empower clients to be self-sufficient. The centrality of caring is noted in the following PHN comment:

> Public health nursing is more than a job. . . . When I'm out there, I care about the people, about what happens to them. I don't think I'd make a really good public health nurse if I didn't care. You get results if they know you care—they're willing to make some change. If they don't think you care at all about them, why should they take a risk for you? I think public health nursing is all about caring about people (Schulte 2000, p. 8).

There are many points at which the community health nurse can make a difference in people's lives. Nurses provide services in deteriorating urban areas, with those living in poverty in all settings, and among all vulnerable populations. Nurses first need to assess themselves for their attitudes and preconceptions. Although access to care can be improved for many low-income people in urban areas, many clients simply need an advocate. The urban communities, and the poor or vulnerable people living in them, need strengthening and interventions that can be initiated by community health nurses using the nursing process as a guide.

Self-assessment

Confronting poverty and caring for vulnerable people from diverse backgrounds, whether in rural or urban areas, necessitates reflective assessment of one's own assumptions and beliefs. Because poverty may be prevalent over a lifetime, a good number of nursing students have personal or family experience of living in poverty. However, because the stigma is so great and fault finding is so pervasive in U.S. society, acknowledging and reflecting on this experience may well be painful. In contrast, because poverty is so hidden and frequently denied, some nursing students have lived apart from any knowledge of the human experience of poverty. They may have come to believe many of the negative stereotypes about poor people. Nursing students and practicing nurses need to ask such questions as "How have my judgments been shaped? How can I open myself to caring for those from whom most of society turns away?"

We learn from one another's stories. First, learn from your classmates, friends, and neighbors who are courageous enough to tell you their own experiences of living in poverty. Ask them and listen intently. Then, let your clients teach you. One honor that nurses have is the opportunity to work with people from all walks of life. You are particularly likely in clinical experiences in community health to meet impoverished, vulnerable individuals and families living outside the mainstream. See From the Case Files III about experiences of students, like yourself, through the eyes of their professors.

Improving Access

Even when government-sponsored health insurance and services are available, extensive barriers prevent many people from accessing services. The community health nurse serves as an advocate and bridge for families who need to gain access. Barriers to access associated with the clients themselves include reluctance to seek coverage because of feelings of pride, independence, or mistrust; feeling powerless; being unaware that such services exist or are worthwhile; lacking resources such as a telephone, transportation, or fare for children who need to go along because no babysitter is available; being illiterate; and preoccupation with meeting survival needs and competing life priorities instead of health needs (Bamberger et al., 2000).

Barriers associated with applying for health insurance include a system that is unfriendly and complicated. Paperwork is overwhelming and may be returned for correction; presentation of paid utility bills or other statements that are not often saved may be required. Informative materials may be too difficult to understand; programs may seek to restrict enrollments by restricting information. The process may require a car, a telephone, and appointments at inconvenient times. The nurse can intervene as a coach and guide, interpreting the system to the client and the client to the system. Likewise, the nurse can act as change agent to improve the system whenever possible.

Strengthening Communities

We are all connected. All of us as citizens have a stake in preventing the adverse hardships of poverty and ill health. All of society pays to support community members who do not contribute, to house those who are incarcerated, and to ignore the vulnerable. This weakens us. We fear crime in our homes, schools, businesses, and communities in general. Society is impaired by adults who are incapable of providing nurturing environments for their children. And the alienation of many groups in society erodes our sense of community as a nation.

The common good is enhanced by strengthening community resources, including investing in people of historically low status, developing and strengthening ties within families and among people involved in neighborhood mutual support, and redeveloping neighborhood resources (see Chapter 13). Whenever possible, the PHN voices support of economic redevelopment of neighborhoods to enhance schools, housing, and employment. The community health nurse can also work to promote subsidized carpools, school-to-work transition programs, universal health insurance, and inner-city economic-development programs.

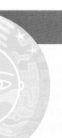

From the Case Files III

Examples from Community Health Nursing Instructors

Ann, a nursing faculty member at a small Roman Catholic college, had a one-to-one post clinical conference with a student and relays this conversation. The student had made many visits to an African American teen mother of two thriving children. The young mother lived in a dangerous housing project, and, although she locked him out of her second-floor apartment, her abusive boyfriend had been known to climb up the drainage pipe and over the porch roof. Sometimes, he forced open a window and beat her. The mother worked every day at a fast food establishment; her grandmother took care of the children. After a couple of months of weekly visits, the student exclaimed, "When I read her chart, I saw her as an immoral girl—a slut—and I expected her to be a loser. Now I can't believe what I've learned about how strong she is. She just keeps fighting for herself and for her kids to survive! She's a great mom and I told her so!"

Another faculty member, Sharon, who taught community health nursing in a Midwestern school of nursing was having an informal discussion with a student who related her experience of trying to get comfortable making home visits with low-income young women. She was making brave attempts at home visits to a pregnant woman, about her age, living in the deteriorating outskirts of a major city. She thought she had established rapport and was making headway developing trust with the client. One day the client asked the student, with concern in her voice, if she had "broken off her engagement." The flustered student then had difficulty explaining the absence of her engagement ring, which she had never mentioned but the client had obviously noticed. During the previous week, she had suddenly realized she was wearing this special ring in marginal neighborhoods and thought it best to leave it at home. Of course, she thought that she had to fabricate another reason to tell the client, but felt badly for being so judgmental when the client was identifying with the student and noted they had something in common.

Lynn, a new public health nursing faculty member from a large state university in the West was shocked and repulsed by the comment of one of her students during lecture one day. When discussing vulnerable populations in urban centers and rural areas, the point was made that poverty can be a generational phenomenon and that many of our clients may find it difficult to dig out of this circumstance. Social justice was discussed, along with the need for PHNs to become social activists in order to change political and socioeconomic factors that keep the status quo. One student, a Hispanic female from a middle class family, spoke up stating "they should all get jobs at McDonalds." This spurred further discussion about population-focused versus individual-focused interventions and approaches, and the need for all of us to be aware of our prejudices and stereotypical viewpoints.

Many caution well-intentioned professionals to beware when seeking solutions to vulnerability through the use of service programs alone. First, a whole population of people can become defined in terms of their problems instead of their strengths. In addition, citizens acting to help themselves within their community can be weakened when they are seen as clients requiring professional services. Finally, being dependent on multiple human services often has a disabling effect, reducing self-worth and leads to feelings of powerlessness.

Because human service interventions can have negative as well as positive effects, it is important to consider whether more community agencies are the answer to resolving community hardship. Community health planning should seriously consider an organizing process that builds community and that focuses on developing neighborhood competence to solve problems and create solutions for itself (see the discussion of community development in Chapter 15).

Summary

Rural clients are a unique aggregate. Community health nurses are key to ensuring the delivery of appropriate health services to this population. There are numerous definitions of the term *rural*. In this chapter, rural is defined as communities with fewer than 10,000 residents and a county population density of fewer than 1,000 people per square mile. The total number of people living in rural communities has increased over the last century. Since 1995, however, the growth rate in many rural communities has decreased. The elderly are a rapidly growing population in rural communities. Rural areas often have less diversity than urban cities, but that is changing in many areas. Rural clients generally have lower educational levels than urban clients, due in part to less access to higher education and lower-paying jobs. Income levels and housing costs are frequently lower than in larger cities.

Rural Healthy People 2010 identifies national goals applicable to rural communities. Many at-risk populations live in these communities, where there are often fewer employment opportunities, a lack of adequate housing, and limited access to health and social services. Rural elders may have more limited alternatives for housing if they can no longer live alone. Mental health services are limited, even though the need may be great. Numerous risks are associated with agriculture. The community health nurse must help this population identify hazards and practice injury prevention.

A community health nurse needs to engage in community assessment of the rural area as a part of orientation. It is helpful to identify the strengths of the community. Rural clients are frequently resourceful and often have a supportive network of people to meet their needs.

Access to health care is an important issue in rural communities. Health insurance may not be easily available, and is often not offered to self-employed and those working for smaller companies. Managed care organizations are diffusing into rural communities, and their long-term impact is uncertain. Barriers to access include distance, weather, transportation, and limited choice of providers. Some ways to improve access in these communities are school-based clinics, mobile health vans, and use of the latest technology. University-sponsored nursing centers that could serve rural populations should be explored.

Migrant farmworkers are an integral part of the farming community in the United States and across the world, however they are rarely visible members of our society. As members of a community with varied and profound health needs complicated by disease, social isolation, exposure to occupational hazards such as pesticide and dangerous farm equipment, substandard housing, and poor sanitation, migrant farmworkers and their families are at risk. Migrant children are often educationally, socially, and physically disadvantaged. Because migrant health centers do not adequately meet the health needs of the entire migrant community, several innovative methods of health care delivery have been developed and implemented by community health nurses, including mobile health vans and information tracking systems.

Rural community health nurses are key members of the professional community. Their roles include advocate, coordinator/case manager, health teacher, referral agent, mentor, change agent/researcher, collaborator, and activist. Community health nurses have challenges and opportunities related to their clinical practices. Confidentiality and personal/professional boundary issues may exist. Salaries for rural nurses may be lower than for nurses in urban areas. Rural community health nurses are highly respected individuals who make a difference in the communities they serve.

Urban health issues have existed for hundreds of years in the United States, and they continue today. Many disenfranchised and minority groups call inner cities home. In some downtown areas, upper-middle-class people are renovating old buildings and returning to the city, in the process moving out the poor literally to the streets. Although nursing services may often be delivered at the individual level, the true impact on health must address the community or population level. Key to recognizing the potential impact for improvement in the health disparities that exist is the acceptance of a social justice orientation that will empower nurses to address the required changes needed within the existing social, political, and economic systems. ▪

ACTIVITIES TO PROMOTE CRITICAL THINKING

1. Look on the Internet for six recent articles in both rural and urban newspapers relating to access to health care. After summarizing the content, identify barriers to access that are common to both and those that are different. What are the main themes relating to health and access to care?

2. Discuss with a classmate the common characteristics of rural, migrant, and urban clients. How can the PHN be better prepared to meet their unique needs? What are some specific challenges facing the PHN working in a rural area? In an urban area?

3. Describe some of the benefits of rural public health nursing.

4. Compare and contrast health, living, and working concerns between migrant workers and recent immigrants. Discuss how many recent immigrants from places such as Asia, Russia, or Iraq experience the same hardships as migrant workers do. How does nomadic lifestyle affect and differentiate the needs of migrant workers and recent immigrants?

5. If you are from a rural area, interview a peer who was raised in an urban setting (or vice versa). Compare your experiences with family, school, friends, entertainment, etc.

6. Look on the Internet for examples of community needs assessment from both rural and urban areas. What are the main findings of each? How do planned interventions differ? How are they similar?

7. Debate with a classmate the need for ready access to specialist medical care and sophisticated diagnostic equipment in all communities. Is this feasible? If not, how can services best be made available to urban and rural clients?

References

Adams, C.E., Michel, Y., DeFrates, D., & Corbett, C.F. (2001). Effect of locale on health status and direct care time of rural versus urban home health patients. *Journal of Nursing Administration, 31,* 244–251.

Agency for Healthcare Research & Quality (AHRQ). (2002). *Rural health care: AHRQ focus on research.* Retrieved August 21, 2008 from http://www.ahrq.gov/news/focus/focrural.htm.

Agency for Healthcare Research & Quality (AHRQ). (2005). *Health care disparities in rural areas.* Retrieved August 21, 2008 from http://www.ahrq.gov/research.ruraldisp/ruraldispar.htm.

Agency for Healthcare Research & Quality (AHRQ). (2007). *Improving health care for rural populations: Research in action.* Retrieved August 21, 2008 from http://www.ahrq.gov/research.rural.htm.

Alavanja, M., Hoppin, J., & Kamel, F. (2004). Health effects of chronic pesticide exposure: Cancer and neurotoxicity. *Annual Review of Public Health, 25,*155–197.

Alderete, E., Vega, W.A., Kolody, B., & Aguilar-Gaxiola, D. (2000). Lifetime prevalence of and risk factors for psychiatric disorders among Mexican migrant farmworkers in California. *American Journal of Public Health, 90*(4), 608–614.

American Academy of Pediatrics. Committee on Community Health. (2005). Providing care for immigrant, homeless, and migrant children. *Pediatrics, 115*(4), 1095–1100.

American College of Physicians. (1997). Inner-city health care. *Annals of Internal Medicine, 126*(6), 485–490.

Arcury, T.A. (2005). Organophosphate pesticide exposure in farmworker family members in Western North Carolina and Virginia: Case comparisons. *Human Organization, 64*(1).

Bacon, D. (October 11, 2006). Farmworkers' plight: No fruits for their labors. *San Francisco Chronicle.*

Balamurugan, A., Ohsfeldt, R., Hughes, T., & Phillips, M. (2006). Diabetes self-management education program for Medicaid recipients: A continuous quality improvement process. *Diabetes Educator, 32*(6), 893–900.

Baldwin, L., MacLehose, R., Hart, L., et al. (2004). Quality and care for acute myocardial infarction in rural and urban U.S. hospitals. *Journal of Rural Health, 20*(2), 99–108.

Bamberger, J.D., Unick, J., Klein, P., et al. (2000). Helping the urban poor stay with antiretroviral HIV drug therapy. *American Journal of Public Health, 90*(5), 699–701.

Barbassa, J. (March 8, 2006). Program puts migrant workers' health records online. *San Diego Union Tribune.*

Bashir, S.A. (2002). Home is where the harm is: Inadequate housing as a public health crisis. *American Journal of Public Health, 92*(5), 733–738.

Basu, J., & Mobley, L. (2006). *Illness severity and propensity to travel along the urban-rural continuum.* AHRQ Publication No. 06-R077. Washington DC: Agency for Healthcare Research & Quality.

Bell, M., McDermott, A., Zeger, S., et al. (2004). Ozone and short-term mortality in 95 U.S. urban communities, 1987–2000. *Journal of the American Medical Association, 292*(19), 2372–2378.

Berkes, H. (2005). *Outsourcing high-tech jobs to rural America.* National Public Radio: People & Places. Retrieved August 21, 2008 from http://www.npr.org/templates/story/story.php?storyid=4496502.

Bernard, V., Coughlin, S., Thompson, T., & Richardson, L. (2007). Cervical cancer incidence in the United States by area of residence, 1998–2001. *American Journal of Obstetrics and Gynecology, 110*(3), 681–686.

Boehmer, T., Lovegreen, S., Haire-Joshu, D., & Brownson, R. (2006). What constitutes an obesogenic environment in rural communities? *American Journal of Health Promotion, 20*(6), 411–422.

Borders, T., & Booth, B. (2007). Rural, suburban, and urban variations in alcohol consumption in the United States: Findings from the National Epidemiologic Survey on Alcohol & Related Conditions. *Journal of Rural Health, 23*(4), 314–321.

Bove, C., & Olson, C. (2006). Obesity in low-income rural women: Qualitative insights about physical activity and eating patterns. *Women's Health, 44*(1), 57–78.

Branas, C., McKenzie, E., & Williams, J. (2005). Access to trauma centers in the United States. *Journal of the American Medical Association, 293*, 2626–2633.

Branz-Spall, A., Rosenthal, R., & Wright, A. (2003). Children of the road: Migrant students, our national most mobile population. *The Journal of Negro Education, 72*(1), 55–62.

Bruns, R. (2006). *Cesar Chavez: A biography.* Westport, CN: Greenwood Publishing Group.

Bureau of Labor Statistics. U.S. Department of Labor. (2007). *Occupational employment & wages, May 2006.* Retrieved August 21, 2008 from http://www.bls.gov/oes/current/oes451012.htm.

Bushy, A. (2000). *Orientation to nursing in the rural community.* Thousand Oaks, CA: Sage.

Bushy, A. (2003). Considerations for working with diverse rural client systems. *Lippincott's Case Management, 8*(5), 214–223.

Centers for Disease Control & Prevention (CDC). (2007a). *HIV/AIDS statistics and surveillance.* Retrieved August 21, 2008 from http://www.cdc.gov/hiv/topics/surveillance/basic.htm#Main.

Centers for Disease Control & Prevention (CDC). (2007b). *About Healthy Places.* Retrieved August 21, 2008 from http://www.cdc.gov/healthyplaces/about.htm.

Cholewinski, R. (2005). Protecting migrant workers in a globalized world. *Migration Information Source.* Retrieved August 21, 2008 from http://www.migrationinformation.org/Feature/print.cfm?ID=293.

Cohen, D., Spear, S., Scribner, R., et al. (2000). Broken windows and the risk of gonorrhea. *American Journal of Public Health, 90*(2), 230–236.

Cole, A., & Crawford, L. (1991). Implementation and evaluation of the health resource program for migrant women in the Americus, Georgia area. In A. Bushy (Ed.). *Rural nursing,* Vol. 1. (pp. 364–374). Newbury Park: Sage Publications.

Collins-Perdue, W., Stone, L., & Gostin, L. (2003). The built environment and its relationship to the public's health: The legal framework. *American Journal of Public Health, 93*(9), 1390–1394.

Committee on the Future of Rural Health Care. (2005). *Quality through collaboration: The future of rural health.* Washington, DC: National Academic Press.

Community Environmental Health Resource Center. (2007). *About CEHRC.* Retrieved August 21, 2008 from http://www.cehrc.org/.

Congressional Rural Caucus, United States House of Representatives. (March 22, 2004). *Rural Caucus to host forum on job losses, economic decline in rural America.* [Press release].

Connor, A., Rainer, L., Simcox, J., & Thomisee, K. (2007). Increasing the delivery of health care services to migrant farm worker families through a community partnership model. *Public Health Nursing, 24*(4), 355–360.

Cooper, D. (November 15, 2002). DSL spells j-o-b-s for rural areas. *Telecommunications Americas.* Retrieved August 21, 2008 from http://findarticles.com/p/articles/mi_mONUH/is_13_36/ai_95791454/print.

Cooper, S., Cooper, S.P., Felknor, S., et al. (2005). Nontraditional work factors in farmworker adolescent populations: Implications for health research and interventions. *Public Health Reports, 120*(6), 622–629.

Corburn, J. (2004). Confronting the challenges in reconnecting urban planning and public health. *American Journal of Public Health, 94*(4), 541–546.

Coronado, G., Thompson, B., Strong, L., et al. (2004). Agricultural task and exposure to organophosphate pesticides among farmworkers. *Environmental Health Perspectives, 112*(2), 142–147.

Coughlin, S.S., & Wilson, K.M. (2002). Breast and cervical cancer screening among migrant and seasonal farmworkers: A review. *Cancer Detection and Prevention, 26*(3), 203–206.

Couto, R. (2000). Community health as social justice: Lessons on leadership. *Family and Community Health, 23*(1), 1–17.

Cutler, D., Glaeser, E., & Vigdor, J. (1997). *The rise and decline of the American ghetto.* [NBER Working Paper No. W5881]. Retrieved August 21, 2008 from: http://ssrn.com/abstract=225663.

Dannenberg, A., Jackson, R., Frumkin, H., et al. (2003). Public health matters. The impact of community design and land-use choices on public health: A scientific research agenda. *American Journal of Public Health, 93*(9), 1500–1508.

Das, R., Steege, A., Baron, S., et al. (2001). *International Journal of Occupational & Environmental Health, 7*(4), 303–305.

Dean, H., Steele, C., Satcher, A., & Nakashima, A. (2005). HIV/AIDS among minority races and ethnicities in the United States, 1999–2003. *Journal of the National Medical Association, 97*[7 Suppl.], 5S–12S.

Demographia. (2006). *Metropolitan & central city population: 2000–2005.* Retrieved August 21, 2008 from http://www.demographia.com/db-metrocore2005.htm.

Dennis, L., & Pallotta, S. (2001). Chronic disease in rural health. In S. Loue, & B. Quill (Eds.). *Handbook of rural health.* New York: Springer Publishing.

Diez-Roux, A., Merkin, S., Arnett, D., et al. (2001). Neighborhood of residence and incidence of coronary heart disease. *New England Journal of Medicine, 345*(2), 99–106.

Doescher, M., Jackson, J., Jerant, A., & Hart, L.G. (2006). Prevalence and trends in smoking: A national rural study. *Journal of Rural Health, 22*(2), 112–118.

Drevdahl, D., Kneipp, S., Canales, M., & Dorcy, K. (2001). Reinvesting in social justice: A capital idea for public health nursing? *Advances in Nursing Science, 24*(2), 19–31.

Drevdahl, D. (2002). Social justice or market justice? The paradoxes of public health partnerships with managed care. *Public Health Nursing, 19*(3), 161–169.

Duchon, L., Andrulis, D., & Reid, H. (2004). Measuring progress in meeting Healthy People goals for low birth weight and infant mortality among the 100 largest cities and their suburbs. *Journal of Urban Health, 81*(3), 323–339.

Eberhardt, M.S., Ingram, D.D., Makuc, D.M., et al. (2001). *Urban and rural health chartbook: Health, United States, 2001.* Hyattsville, MD: National Center for Health Statistics.

Espinoza, L., Hall, H., Hardnett, F., et al. (2007). Characteristics of persons with heterosexually acquired HIV infection, United States, 1999–2004. *American Journal of Public Health, 97*(1), 144–149.

Evans, C., Lantigua, J., Stapleton, C., et al. (2005). *Modern-day slavery: A Palm Beach Post special report.* Palm Beach Post. Retrieved August 21, 2008 from http://www.palmbeachpost.com/hp/content/moderndayslavery/reports/graphic1207.html.

Evans, T., Wick, K., Brock, D., et al. (2006). Academic degrees and clinical practice characteristics: The University of Washington Physician Assistant Program: 1969–2000. *Journal of Rural Health, 22*(3), 212–219.

Fahrenwald, N., Taylor, J., Kneipp, S., & Canales, M. (2007). Academic freedom and academic duty to teach social justice: A perspective and pedagogy for public health nursing faculty. *Public Health Nursing, 24*(2), 190–197.

Family Violence Prevention Fund. (2008). *The facts on domestic violence.* San Francisco, CA: Author.

Farmworker Justice. (2007). *Contingent workers.* Retrieved August 21, 2008 from http://www.fwjustice.org/Iummigration_Labor/ContingentWrks.htm.

Finch, B., Catalano, R., Novaco, R., & Vega, W. (2003). Employment frustration and alcohol abuse/dependence among labor migrants in California. *Journal of Immigrant and Minority Health, 5*(4), 1096–4045.

Finerfrock, B. (2006, May 10). *Rural health clinics technical assistance conference call presentation.* HRSA Rural Health Policy. [PowerPoint presentation]. Retrieved August 21, 2008 from http://ruralhealth.hrsa.gov/RHC/Basics01text.htm.

Fitzgerald, K., Chakraborty, J., Shah, T., et al. (2003). HIV/AIDS knowledge among female migrant farm workers in the Midwest. *Journal of Immigrant Health, 5*(1), 1573–3629 (online).

Fleischman, A., & Barondess, J. (2004). Urban health: A look out our windows. *Academic Medicine, 79*(12), 1130–1132.

Flocks, J., Monaghan, P., Albrecht, S., & Bahena, A. (2007). Florida farmworkers' perceptions and lay knowledge of occupational pesticides. *Journal of Community Health, 32*(3), 181–194.

Florida International University. (Fall 2005). *Migrant farm workers are vulnerable to HIV/AIDS.* Diversity Exchange. Retrieved August 21, 2008 from http://news.flu.edu/diversity/fall2005/classroom2.html.

Food Security Learning Center. (2007). *Rural poverty FAQs.* Retrieved August 21, 2008 from http://www.worldhungeryear.org/fslc/faqs/ria_070b.asp?section=14&click=8#1.

Formichelli, L. (2008). A harvest of hope. *Minority Nurse.* Retrieved August 21, 2008 from http://www.minortynurse.com/features/nurse_emp/07-09-01b.html.

Frank, L., Andresen, M., & Schmid, T. (2004). Obesity relationships with community design, physician activity, and time spent in cars. *American Journal of Preventive Medicine, 27*(2), 87–96.

Fraser, R., Skinner, A., & Mueller, K. (2006). *Elements of successful rural diabetes management programs.* Rural Policy Research Institute Center for Rural Health Policy Analysis. [Publication No. P2006-2].

Freudenberg, N. (2000). Time for a national agenda to improve the health of urban populations. *American Journal of Public Health, 90*(6), 837–840.

Freudenberg, N., Galea, S., & Vlahov, D. (2005). Beyond urban penalty and urban sprawl: Back to living conditions as the focus of urban health. *Journal of Community Health, 30*(1), 1–11.

Frumkin, H. (2005). Health, equity & the built environment. *Environmental Health Perspectives, 113*(51), A290–A291.

Galea, S., & Vlahov, D. (2005). Urban health: Evidence, challenges, and directions. *Annual Review of Public Health, 26,* 341–365.

Galea, S., Ahern, J., Rudenstine, S., et al. (2005). Urban built environment and depression: A multilevel study. *Journal of Epidemiology in Community Health, 59,* 822–827.

Galea, S., Freudenberg, N., & Vlahov, D. (2005). Cities and population health. *Social Science & Medicine, 60*(5), 1017–1033.

Gamm, L., Castillo, G., & Williams, L. (2004). Education and community-based programs in rural areas. In L. Gamm, & L. Hutchison (Eds.). *Rural Healthy People 2010: A companion document to Healthy People 2010,* Vol. 3. (pp. 1–9).

Gamm, L., Hutchison, L., Dabney, B., & Dorsey, A. (Eds.). (2003). *Rural Healthy People 2010: A companion document to Healthy People 2010,* Vol. 1. College Station, TX: Texas A&M University System Health Science Center. School of Rural Public Health, Southwest Rural Health Research Center.

Garb, M. (2003). Health, mortality, and housing: The "tenement problem" in Chicago. *American Journal of Public Health, 93*(9), 1420–1430.

Geller, A.L. (2003). Smart growth: A prescription for livable cities. *American Journal of Public Health, 93*(9), 1410–1415.

Gibbs, R. (September 12, 2004). *Rural dimensions of welfare reform.* [PowerPoint slide presentation]. Retrieved August 21, 2008 from http://www.ruralcommittee.hrsa.gov/Sept2004/Gibbstext.htm.

Gibbs, R., Kusmin, L., & Cromartie, J. (November 2004). *Low-skill jobs: A shrinking share of the rural economy.* Amber Waves. Retrieved August 21, 2008 from http://www.ers.esda.gov/AmberWaves/Scripts/print.asp?page=/November04/Features/lowskilljobs.htm.

Glasgow, N., Johnson, N., & Morton, J.W. (2004). *Critical issues in rural health.* Oxford, UK: Blackwell Publishing.

Gordon, D. (2007). *Rural health brief: Where have all the dentists gone?* National Conference of State Legislatures. Retrieved August 21, 2008 from http://www.ncsl.org/programs/health/ruraldent.htm.

Hajat, A., Stewart, K., & Hayes, K. (2003). The local public health workforce in rural communities. *Journal of Public Health Management & Practice, 9*(6), 481–488.

Hall, H., Li, J., & McKenna, M. (2005). HIV in predominately rural areas of the United States. *Journal of Rural Health, 21*(3), 245–253.

Hancock, T. (2002). From public health to the healthy city. In E. Fowler, & D. Siegel (Eds.), *Urban policy issues: Canadian perspectives* (2nd ed.) (pp. 277–297). Toronto, ON: Oxford University Press.

Hartley, D., Ziller, E., & MacDonald, C. (January 2002). *Diabetes and the rural safety net.* Maine Rural Health Research Center, Working Paper # 28.

Health Resources & Services Administration (HRSA). (2002). *One department serving rural America.* HHS Rural Task Force Report to the Secretary. HRSA Rural Health Policy. Retrieved August 21, 2008 from http://ruralhealth.hrsa.gov/PublicReport.htm#summary.

Health Resources & Services Administration (HRSA). (2007a). *Shortage designation.* Bureau of Health Professions. Retrieved August 21, 2008 from http://www.bhpr.hrsa.gov/shortage/.

Health Resources & Services Administration (HRSA). (2007b). *Telehealth.* Retrieved August 21, 2008 from http://www.hrsa.gov/telehealth/default.htm.

Health Resources & Services Administration (HRSA). (2008). *Migrant health center program.* Retrieved August 21, 2008 from http://bhpr.hrsa.gov/kidscareers/migrant_program.htm.

Hiott, A., Grzywacz, J., Davis, S., et al. (2008). Migrant farmworker stress: Mental health implications. *The Journal of Rural Health, 24*(1), 32–39.

Hiott, A., Quandt, S., Early, J., et al. (2006). Review of pesticide education materials for health care providers providing care to agricultural workers. *The Journal of Rural Health Care, 22*(1), 17–35.

Hirsch, J.S., Higgins, J., Bentley, M.E., & Nathanson, C.A. (2002). The social constructions of sexuality: Marital infidelity and sexually transmitted disease—HIV Risk in a Mexican migrant community. *American Journal of Public Health, 92*(8), 1227–1237.

Housing Assistance Council. (2001). *No refuge from the fields: Findings from a survey of farmworker housing conditions in the United States.* Washington, DC: Author.

Human Rights Watch. (2000). *Fingers to the bone: United States failure to protect child farmworkers.* Retrieved August 21, 2008 from http://www.hrw.org/report/2000/frmwrkr/.

Hummel, J. (2001). Population-based medicine: Links to public health. In J.P. Geyman, T.E. Norris, & L.G. Hart (Eds.). *Textbook of rural medicine.* (pp. 55–72). New York: McGraw-Hill.

Iezzoni, L., Killeen, M., & O'Day, B. (2006). Rural residents with disabilities confront substantial barriers to obtaining care. *HSR: Health Services Research, 41*(4), 1258–1275.

Jackson, R.J. (2001). *What Olmstead knew.* Western City Magazine. Retrieved August 21, 2008 from http://www.checnet.org/healthehouse/education/articles-detail-print.asp?Main_ID=565.

Johansson, A., Svedung, I., & Andersson, R. (2006). Management of risks in societal planning: An analysis of scope and variety of health, safety and security issues in municipality plan documents. *Safety Science, 44*(8), 675–688.

Kandel, W., & Parrado, E. (2006). Public policy impacts of rural Hispanic population growth. In W. Kandel, & D. Brown (Eds.). *Population change and rural society.* (pp. 155–176). New York: Springer Publishing.

Kerr, M., Lusk, S., & Ronis, D. (2002). Explaining Mexican American workers' hearing protection use with the health promotion model. *Nursing Research, 31*(2), 100–109.

King, M. (June 7, 2007). *Immigrants in the U.S. health care system: Five myths that misinform the American public.* Washington, DC: Center for American Progress.

Kinney, A., Harrell, J., Slattery, M., et al. (2006). Rural-urban differences in colon cancer risk in Blacks and Whites: The North Carolina Colon Cancer study. *Journal of Rural Health, 22*(2), 124–130.

Kirschner, A., Berry, E.H., & Glasgow, N. (2006). The changing demographic profile of rural America. In W. Kandel, & D. Brown (Eds.). *The changing faces of rural America.* (pp. 53–74). New York: Springer Publishing.

Kochtitzky, C., Frumkin, H., Rodriguez, R., et al. (2006). Urban planning and public health at CDC. *Morbidity & Mortality Weekly, 55*[Suppl. 02], 34–38.

LaSala, K.B. (2000). Nursing workforce issues in rural and urban settings: Looking at the difference in recruitment, retention and distribution. *Online Journal of Rural Nursing and Health Care, 1*(1), 8–17.

Larson, A.C. (2000). *Migrant and seasonal farmworker enumeration profiles study: Washington.* Vashon Island, WA: Larson Assistance Services.

Larson, S., & Fleishman, J. (2003). Rural/urban differences in usual source of care and ambulatory service use: Analyses of national data using Urban Influence Codes. *Medical Care. 41*(7 Suppl. 1). 65–74.

Larson, S., & Hill, S. (2005). Rural-urban differences in employment-related health insurance. *Journal of Rural Health, 21*(1), 21–30.

Lee, H., & Winters, C. (2004). Testing rural nursing theory: Perceptions and needs of service providers. *Online Journal of Rural Nursing and Health Care, 4*(1), 51–63.

Leviton, L., Snell, E., & McGinnis, M. (2000). Urban issues in health promotion strategies. *American Journal of Public Health, 90*(6), 863–866.

Levy, B., Dawson, J., Hartz, A., & James, P. (2006). Colorectal cancer testing among patients cared for by Iowa family physicians. *American Journal of Preventive Medicine, 31*(3), 193–201.

Leyden, K.M. (2003). Social capital and the built environment: The importance of walkable neighborhoods. *American Journal of Public Health, 93*(9), 1546–1551.

Lindstrom, D., & Lauster, N. (2001). Local economic opportunity and the competing risks of internal and U.S. migration in Zacatecas, Mexico. *International Migration Review, 35*(4), 1232–1256.

Living near where pesticides used may boost fetal deaths due to birth defects. (February 15, 2001). Science Daily. Retrieved August 21, 2008 from http://www.sciencedaily.com/releases/2001/02/01021475018.htm.

Logan, J.R. (2002). *The suburban advantage.* University of Albany: Lewis Mumford Center for Comparative Urban & Regional Research. Retrieved August 21, 2008 from http://www.s4.brown.edu/cen2000/CityProfiles/SuburbanReport/page1.html.

Lukes, S., & Miller, F. (2002). Oral health issues among migrant farmworkers. *Journal of Dental Hygiene, 76,* 134–140.

Lutfiyya, M., Lipsky, M., Wisdom-Behounek, J., & Inpanbutr-Martinkus, M. (2007). Is rural residency a risk factor for overweight and obesity for U.S. children? *Obesity, 15*(9), 2348–2356.

Mahajan, R., Bonner, M., Hoppin, J., & Akavanja, M. (2006). Phorate exposure and incidence of cancer in the Agricultural Health Study. *Environmental Health Perspectives, 114*(8), 1205–1209.

Mainous, A., Koopman, R., & Geesey, M. (August 2004). *Diabetes & hypertension among rural Hispanics: Disparities in diagnostics and disease management.* South Carolina Rural Health Research Center. Retrieved August 21, 2008 from http://rhr.sph.sc.edu/report/SCRHRC_Hispanics_Exec_Summary.pdf.

Maternal Child Health Branch. (2002). *Population characteristics: Women in rural areas.* Women's Health USA 2002. Retrieved August 21, 2008 from http://mchb.hrsa.gov/whusa02/Page_16.htm.

Maternal Child Health Branch. (2005). *Rural and urban health.* Women's Health USA 2002. Retrieved August 21, 2008 from http://mchb.hrsa.gov/whusa_05/pages/0433ruh.htm.

McCarthy, M. (2000). Fighting for public health along the USA-Mexico border. *The Lancet, 356,* 1020–1022.

McCauley, L., Anger, W.K., Keifer, M., et al. (2006). Studying health outcomes in farmworker populations exposed to pesticides. *Environmental Health Perspectives, 114*(6), 953–960.

McCord, C., & Freeman, H. (1990). Excess mortality in Harlem. *New England Journal of Medicine, 322,* 173–177.

McCoy, V. (2005, Fall). Migrant farm workers are vulnerable to HIV/AIDS. *Diversity Exchange.* Retrieved October 20, 2008 from http://www.osha.gov/SLTC/agriculturaloperabons/standards.html.

McGranahan, D., & Sullivan, P. (2005). *Farm programs, natural amenities, and rural development.* Amber Waves. Retrieved August 21, 2008 from http://www.ers.usda.gov/AmberWaves/February05/Features/FarmPrograms.htm.

McLaurin, J., & Morrision, S. (2006, September). *Reaching the underserved: A joint newsletter of the Migrant Clinicans' Network and the HCH Clinicians' Network.* Retrieved October 20, 2008 from http://www.nhchc.org/ReachingTheUnderserved0906.pdf.

Merchant, J., Coussens, C., & Gilbert, D. (2006). *Rebuilding the unity of health and the environment in rural America.* Washington, DC: National Academies Press.

Migrant Clinician's Network. (2008). *Women's health.* Retrieved August 21, 2008 from http://www.migrantclinician.org/excellence.women.

Migrant Clinician's Network. (September 2006). *Reaching the underserved: Connecting mobile and homeless people to the health disparities collaborative.* Retrieved August 21, 2008 from http://www.migrtantclinician.org/-resources/MC-HCH_September2006newsletter.doc.

Migrant Clinician's Network. (n.d.a). *Pesticides and lead: Hazards for migrant farm workers.* Retrieved August 21, 2008 from http://www.migrtantclinician.org/_resource/Pesticides_and_Lead.pdf.

Migrant Clinician's Network. (n.d.b). *Monograph series: Domestic violence in the farmworker population: Resources for clinicians.* Retrieved August 21, 2008 from http://www.migrantclinician.org/_resources/DVMonograph.pdf.

Migrant Health. (2006). *Migrant health promotion: Biennial report 2005–2006.* Retrieved August 21, 2008 from http://www.migranthealth.org/material_docs/Annual_Report2005-2006.pdf.

Mondy, C., Cardenas, D., & Avila, M. (2003). The role of an advanced practice public health nurse in bioterrorism preparedness. *Public Health Nursing, 20*(6), 422–431.

Moyers, B. (2004, May 28). *Migrant labor in the United States.* NOW. Retrieved August 21, 2008 from http://www.pbs.org/now/politics/migrants.html.

National Center for Farmworker Health (NCFH). (2007a). *Facts about farmworkers.* Retrieved August 21, 2008 from http://ncfh.org.

National Center for Farmworker Health (NCFH). (2007b). *Overview of America's farmworkers.* Retrieved August 21, 2008 from http://www.ncfh.org/aaf_01.php.

National Center for Farmworker Health (NCFH). (2007c). *Migrant and seasonal demographics fact sheet.* Retrieved August 21, 2008 from http://www.ncfh.org.

National Center for Farmworker Health (NCFH). (2007d). *Tuberculosis.* Retrieved August 21, 2008 from http://www.ncfh.org.

National Center for Farmworker Health. (2003). *Quick facts.* Retrieved August 21, 2008 from http://www.ncfh.org/factsheets.shtml.

National Center for Farmworker Health. (2007d). *Occupational safety.* Retrieved August 21, 2008 from http://www.ncfh.org.

National Institute for Occupational Safety & Health (NIOSH). (2007). *Agricultural safety.* Retrieved August 21, 2008 from http://www.cdc.gov/niosh/topics/aginjury/.

National Center for Frontier Communities. (2006). *2000 update: Frontier counties in the United States.* Retrieved August 21, 2008 from http://www.frontierus.org/2000update.htm.

National Center on Addiction & Substance Abuse. (2000). *No place to hide: Substance abuse in mid-size cities and rural America.* New York: Columbia University.

National Rural Health Association. (2006). *About rural HIV/AIDS.* Retrieved August 21, 2008 from http://wwwnrharural.org/opporty/sub/rural_HIV.html.

New York Academy of Medicine. (2007). *The Center for Urban Epidemiologic Studies.* Retrieved August 21, 2008 from http://www.nyam.org/initiatives/cues.shtml.

Oakes, L. (2008, January 23). *Mortgage foreclosures ripple into rural Minnesota.* Star Tribune. Retrieved August 21, 2008 from http://www.startribune.com/templates/Print_This_Story?sid=12337191.

Occupational Safety & Health Administration. (2008). *Agricultural operations standards.* Retrieved October 20, 2008 from http://www.osha.gov/SLTC/agriculturaloperations/standards.html.

Oh, J-H. (2005). Social disorganizations and crime rates in U.S. central cities: Toward an explanation of urban economic change. *The Social Science Journal, 42*(4), 569–582.

Okon, N., Rodriguez, D., Dietrich, D., Oser, C., Blades, L., Burnett, A., Russell, J., Allen, M., Chasson, L., & Helperson, S. (2006). Availability of diagnosis and treatment services for acute stroke in frontier counties in Montana and northern Wyoming. *Journal of Rural Health, 22*(3), 237–241.

Patterson, P., Probst, J., & Moore, C. (2006). Expected annual emergency miles per ambulance: An indicator for measuring availability of emergency medical services resources. *Journal of Rural Health, 22*(2), 102–111.

Peek-Asa, C., Sprince, N., Whitten, P., et al. (2007). Characteristics of crashes with farm equipment that increase potential for injury. *The Journal of Rural Health, 23*(4), 339–347.

Phillips, C.D., & McLeroy, K.R. (2004). Health in rural America: Remembering the importance of place. *American Journal of Public Health, 94*(10), 1661–1663.

Phillips, J., & Grady, P.A. (2002). Reducing health disparities in the twenty-first century: Opportunities for nursing research. *Nursing Outlook, 50*(3), 117–120.

Pink, G. H., Holmes, G. M., D'Alpe, C., Strunk, L. A., McGee, P., & Slifkin, R. T. (2006). Financial indicators for critical access hospitals. *Journal of Rural Health, 22,* 229–236.

Quiram, B., Meit, M., Carpender, K., Pennel, C., Castillo, G., & Duchicela, D. Rural Public Health Infrastructure. In L. Gamm. & L. Hutchison (Eds.) *Rural Healthy People 2010: A companion document to Healthy People 2010. Volume 3.* College Station, TX: The Texas A&M University System Health Science Center, School of Rural Public Health, Southwest Rural Health Research Center.

Racher, F. (2007). The evolution of ethics for community practice. *Journal of Community Health Nursing, 24*(1), 65–76.

Rauh, V., Chew, G., & Garfinkel, R. (2002). Deteriorated housing contributes to high cockroach allergen levels in inner-city households. *Environmental Health Perspectives, 110*(Suppl. 2), 323–327.

Reif, S., Geonnotti, K., & Whetten, K. (2006). HIV infection and AIDS in the Deep South. *American Journal of Public Health, 96*(6), 970–973.

Ricketts, T.C. (2001). The rural patient. In J.P. Geyman, T.E. Norris, & L.G. Hart (Eds.). *Textbook of rural medicine.* (pp. 15–26). New York: McGraw-Hill.

Rosenbaum, S., & Shin, P. (April 2005). *Migrant and seasonal farmworkers: Health insurance coverage and access to care.* The Kaiser Commission on Medicaid and the Uninsured. Menlo Park, CA: The Henry J. Kaiser Family Foundation.

Rosenblatt, R.A. (2001). The health of rural people and the communities and environments in which they live. In J.P. Geyman, T.E. Norris, & L.G. Hart (Eds.). *Textbook of rural medicine.* (pp. 3–14). New York: McGraw-Hill.

Rosenblatt, R.A., Casey, S., & Richardson, M. (2002). Rural-urban differences in the public health workforce: Local health departments in 3 rural Western states. *American Journal of Public Health, 92*(7), 1102–1105.

Rosenthal, K. (2005). What rural nursing stories are you living? *Online Journal of Rural Nursing and Health Care, 5*(1), 37–47.

Rosenthal, M., Zaslavsky, A., & Newhouse, J. (2005). The geographic distribution of physicians revisited. *HSR: Health Services Research, 40*(6), 1931–1952.

Ruckelshaus, C., & Goldstein, B. (2002). *From orchards to the internet: Confronting contingent work abuse.* Oakland, CA: National Employment Law Project.

Rural Assistance Center. (2007a). *Frontier frequently asked questions.* Retrieved August 21, 2008 from http://www.raconline. org/info_guides/frontier/frontierfaq.php.

Rural Assistance Center. (2007b). *Housing and homelessness frequently asked questions.* Retrieved August 21, 2008 from http://www.raconline.org/info_guides/housing/housingfaq.php.

Rural Assistance Center. (2007c). *CAH frequently asked questions.* Retrieved August 21, 2008 from http://www.raconline.org/ info_guides/hospitals/cahfaq.php#whatis.

Rural Assistance Center. (2007d). *Rural health clinics frequently asked questions.* Retrieved August 21, 2008 from http://www. raconline.org/info_guides/clinics/rhcfaq.php#whatis.

Rural Assistance Center. (2007e). *FQHC frequently asked questions.* Retrieved August 21, 2008 from http://www.raconline. org/info_guides/clinics/fqhcfaq.php@whatis.

Sanborn, M., Cole, D., Abelsohn, A., & Weir, E. (2002). Identifying and managing adverse environmental health effects: 4. Pesticides. *Canadian Medical Association Journal, 166*(1), 1431–1436.

Sandhaus, S. (1998). Migrant health: A harvest of poverty. *American Journal of Nursing, 98*(9), 52–54.

Santana, J. (2005, July). *Going out to the community: Mobile clinics bring health care to families of migrant farmworkers.* Mobile Health Clinics Network. Retrieved August 21, 2008 from http://www.mobilehealthclinicsnetwork.org/featured.html.

Schim, S., Benkert, R., Bell, S., et al. (2006). Social justice: Added metaparadigm concept for urban health nursing. *Public Health Nursing, 24*(1), 73–80.

Schlosser, E. (November 29, 2007). *Penny foolish.* The New York Times. Retrieved August 21, 2008 from http://www.nytimes. com/2007/11/29/opinion/29schlosser.html.

Schulte, J. (2000). Finding ways to create connections among communities: Partial results of an ethnography of urban public health nurses. *Public Health Nursing, 17*(1), 3–10.

Skillman, S., Palazzo, L., Keepnews, D., & Hart, D. (2005, January). *Characteristics of registered nurses in rural vs. urban areas: Implications for strategies to alleviate nursing shortages in the United States.* [Working paper No. 91.] WWAMI Center for Health Workforce Studies. Seattle: University of Washington.

Skinner, A., & Slifkin, R. (2007). Rural/urban differences in barriers to and burden of care for children with special health care needs. *Journal of Rural Health, 23*(2), 150–157.

Skinner, A., Slifkin, R., & Mayer, M. (2006). The effect of rural residence on dental unmet need for children with special health care needs. *Journal of Rural Health, 22*(1), 36–42.

Smith, D. (2007). *U.S. agriculture fatality statistics.* Texas Cooperative Extension. The Texas A&M University System. Retrieved August 21, 2008 from http://agsafety.tamu.edu/ US%AGRICULTURE%20FATALITY%20STATISTICS.pdf.

Srinivasan, S., O'Fallon, L., & Dearry, A. (2003). Creating healthy communities, healthy homes, healthy people: Initiating a research agenda on the built environment and public health. *American Journal of Public Health, 93*(9), 1446–1450.

Stallones, L., & Beseler, C. (2002). Pesticide illness, farm practices, and neurological symptoms among farm residents in Colorado. *Environmental Research, 90,* 89–97.

State of California, Managed Risk Medical Insurance Board. (August 2006). Mobile dentals. *Rural Health Demonstration Projects, 1*(11).

Study links pesticide exposure to Parkinson's disease. (2006). *Safety & Health, 174*(3), 18.

Tarmann, A. (2003a). *Revival of U.S. rural areas signals heartland no longer a hinterland.* Population Reference Bureau. Retrieved August 21, 2008 from http://www.prb.org/Articles/2003/ RevivalofUSRuralAreasSignalsHeartlandNoLongeraHinterland. aspx.

Taylor, H.A., Hughes, G.D., & Garrison, R.J. (2002). Cardiovascular disease among women residing in rural America: Epidemiology, explanations, and challenges. *American Journal of Public Health, 92,* 548–551.

Therrien, M., & Ramirez, R. (2001). *Population characteristics released March 2001 for March 2000 counts.* Las Culturas. Retrieved August 21, 2008 from http://www.lasculturas. com/aa/spec/blcensus2000a.htm.

Triantafillou, S.A. (2003). North Carolina's migrant and seasonal farmworkers. *North Carolina Medical Journal, 64*(3), 129–131.

United Farm Workers. (2006). *The story of Cesar Chavez.* Retrieved October 20,2008 from http://www.ufw.org/ page.php?inc=history/07.html&menu=rese arch.

University of California San Francisco (UCSF). (May 2006). *What are rural HJIV prevention needs?* Center for AIDS Prevention Studies. AIDS Research Institute. Retrieved August 21, 2008 from http://www.caps.ucsf.edu/pubs/FS/revrural.php.

University of California. (2008a). *Hispanic Americans: Migrant workers and Braceros (1930s–1964).* Calisphere: California Cultures. Retrieved August 21, 2008 from http://www. callisphere.universityofcalifornia.edu/calcultures/ethnic_groups/ subtopic3b.html.

University of California. (2008b). *Farm labor contracting.* Agricultural Personnel Management Program. Retrieved August 21, 2008 from http://are.berkeley.edu/APMP/pubs/flc/farmlabor.html.

Urban Health Institute. (2007). *About us: Creation of the Urban Health Institute.* Johns Hopkins University. Retrieved August 21, 2008 from http://www.jhsph.edu/urbanhealth/about_us/.

U.S. Census Bureau. (2000a). *Detailed tables: Urban and rural-universe total population.* Retrieved August 21, 2008 from: http://factfinder.census.gov.

U.S. Census Bureau. (2000b). *Population trends in metropolitan areas and central cities.* Retrieved August 21, 2008 from http://www.census.gov/prod/2000pubs/p25-1133.pdf.

U.S. Census Bureau. (2000c). *United States: Urban/rural and inside/outside metropolitan area.* Retrieved August 21, 2008 from http://factfinder.census.gov/servlet/GCTTable? _bm=y&-geo_id=&-ds_name=DEC_2000_SF1_U&- _lang=en&-mt_name=DEC_2000_SF1_U_GCTP8_US1 &-format=US-1&-CONTEXT=gct.

U.S. Census Bureau. (2002). *Census 2000 urban and rural classification.* Retrieved August 21, 2008 from http://www.census. gov/geo/www.ua/ua_2k.html.

U.S. Conference of Mayors. (June 2005). *Impact of unfunded federal mandates and cost shifts on U.S. cities.* Retrieved August 21, 2008 from http://www.usmayors.org/73rdAnnualMeeting/ mandates2005.pdf.

U.S. Department of Agriculture (USDA). (2003a). *Measuring rurality: New definitions in 2003.* Economic Research Service. Retrieved August 21, 2008 from: http://www.ers.usda.gov/ briefing/rurality/NewDefinitions/.

U.S. Department of Agriculture (USDA). (2003b). *Rural education at a glance.* Economic Research Service. Retrieved August 21, 2008 from http://www.ers.usda.gov/publlications/ rdrr98/rdrr98_lowres.pdf.

U.S. Department of Agriculture (USDA). (2007a). *Rural population & migration: Trend 2: Nonmetro population growth slows.* Economic Research Service. Retrieved August 21, 2008 from http://www.ers.esda.gov/BriefingPopulation/ NonMetro.htm.

U.S. Department of Agriculture (USDA). (2007b). *Measuring rurality: What is rural?* Economic Research Service. Retrieved August 21, 2008 from http://www.ers.usda.gov/Briefing/Rurality/ WhatIsRural.

U.S. Department of Agriculture (USDA). (2007c). *Rural population and migration: Trend 6: Challenges from an aging population.* Economic Research Service. Retrieved August 21, 2008 from http://www.ers.usda.gov/Briefing/Population/Challenges.htm.

U.S. Department of Agriculture (USDA). (2007d). *Multi-family housing: Rental assistance program (Section 521).* Rural Development Housing & Community Facilities Programs. Retrieved August 21, 2008 from http://www.rurdev.usda.gov/rhs/mfh/indiv_mfh.htm#Multi-Family.

U.S. Department of Agriculture (USDA). (December 5, 2005). *USDA awards over $29 million in distance learning and telemedicine grants.* [News Release No. 0526.05].

U.S. Department of Health and Human Services, Office of Rural Health Policy. (1998). *Definitions of rural: A handbook for health policy makers and researchers.* [Technical Issues Paper]. Bethesda, MD: Equal Three Communications.

U.S. Department of Health and Human Services. (January 2000). *Healthy people 2010,* Conference ed., Vols. 1 & 2. Washington, DC: U.S. Government Printing Office.

U.S. Department of Housing & Urban Development (USDHUD). (2004). *Section 8 rental voucher program.* Retrieved August 21, 2008 from http://www.hud.gov/progdesc/voucher.cfm.

U.S. Department of Housing & Urban Development (USDHUD). (2007). *Homes and communities.* Retrieved August 21, 2008 from: http://www.hud/gov/offices/cpd/economicdevelopment/programs/rhed/gateway/housing.htm.

U.S. Department of Justice. (2007). *Crime characteristics: Urban, suburban and rural.* Bureau of Justice Statistics. Retrieved August 21, 2008 from http://www.ojp.usdoj.gov/bjs.cvict_c.htm.

U.S. Department of Labor. (March 2000). *Findings from the National Agricultural Workers Survey (NAWS) 1997–1998.* [Research Report No. 8]. Washington, DC: Author.

U.S. Environmental Protection Agency (EPA). (2007). *Built environment.* Retrieved August 21, 2008 from http://www.epa.gov/sustainability/builtenvironment.htm.

U.S. Office of Management & Budget. (December 27, 2000). Standards for defining metropolitan and micropolitan statistical areas: Notice. *Federal Register, 65*(249), 82228–82238.

Villarejo, D. (2003). The health of U.S. hired farm workers. *Annual Review of Public Health, 24,* 175–193.

van Dis, J. (2002). Where we live: Health care in rural vs. urban America. *Journal of the American Medical Association, 87*(1), 108.

Vlahov, D., & Gaklea, S. (2002). Urbanization, urbanicity, and health. *Journal of Urban Health, 79*[4 Suppl. 1], S1–S12.

Vlahov, D., Freudenberg, N., Proietti, F., et al. (2007). Urban as a determinant of health. *Journal of Urban Health, 84*[3 Suppl.], i16–i26.

Vlahov, D., Gibble, E., Freudenberg, N., & Galea, S. (2004). Cities and health: History, approaches, and key questions. *Academic Medicine, 79*(12), 1133–1138.

Vyavaharkar, M., Moneyham, L., Tavakoli, A., et al. (2007). Social support, coping, and medication adherence among HIV-positive women with depression living in rural areas of the southeastern United States. *AIDS Patient Care STDS, 21*(9), 667–680.

Wald, L. (1971/1915). *The house on Henry Street.* New York: Dovr Publications. (Originally published by Henry Hold & Co., New York.)

Waltzer, K. (2000). *East European Jewish Detroit in the early twentieth century.* Judaism. Retrieved August 21, 2008 from http://findarticles.com/p/articles/mi_m0411/is_3_49/ai_6635396 6/print.

Wasylenki, D.A. (2001). Inner city health. *Canadian Medical Association Journal, 164*(2), 214–215.

Wickrama, K., Elder, G., & Abraham, W. (2007). Rurality and ethnicity in adolescent physical illness: Are children of the growing rural Latino population at excess health risk? *Journal of Rural Health, 23*(3), 228–237.

Wills, D.S. (2002). Rural housing prices grew rapidly in the 1990s. *Rural America, 17*(3), 47–56.

World Health Organization (WHO). (2007). *Healthy Cities and urban governance.* Retrieved August 21, 2008 from http://www.euro.who.int/healthy-cities/.

Ziebarth, A. (2006). Housing seasonal workers for the Minnesota processed vegetable industry. *Rural Sociology, 71*(2), 335–357.

Zigmond, J. (2007). Remote possibilities: Rural communities seek creative solutions as they grapple with a nurse shortage that's particularly acute outside metro areas. *Modern Healthcare, 37*(15), 26–28.

Selected Readings

Arcury, T., Preisser, J., Gesler, W., & Powers, J. (2005). Access to transportation and health care utilization in a rural region. *Journal of Rural Health, 21*(1), 31–38.

Avery, B., & Bashir, S. (2003). Public health advocacy forum. The road to advocacy: Searching for the rainbow. *American Journal of Public Health, 93*(8), 1207–1210.

Bayne, T., Higgs, Z., Gruber, E., & Bendel, B. (July 2002). *Eastern Washington access to health care consumer study.* Spokane, WA: Tina Bayne (Intercollegiate College of Nursing, 2917 W Fort George Wright Dr., Spokane, WA 99223).

Bazargan, M., Bazargan, S., CalderÂn, J., et al. (2003). Mammography screening and breast self-examination among minority women in public housing projects: The impact of physician recommendation. *Cellular And Molecular Biology (Noisy-Le-Grand, France), 49*(8), 1213–1218.

Brody, J., Moysich, K., Humblet, O., et al. (2007). Environmental pollutants and breast cancer: Epidemiologic studies. *Cancer, 109*[12 Suppl.], 2667–2711.

Calico, F., & Myers, W. (2007). *What makes rural health care work?* Alexandria, VA: National Rural Health Association.

Coburn, A.F., & Bolda, E.J. (1999). Rural elderly and long-term care. In T.C. Ricketts (Ed.). *Rural health in the United States.* (pp.179–189). New York: Oxford University Press.

Cox, H., Cash, P., Hanna, B., et al. (2001). Risky business: Stories from the field of rural community nurses' work in domestic violence. *Australian Journal of Rural Health, 9,* 280–285.

Craft-Rosenberg, M., Powell, S.R., & Culp, K. (2000). Health status and resources of rural homeless women and children. *Western Journal of Nursing Research, 22,* 863–878.

Dennis, L.K., & Pallotta, S.L. (2001). Chronic disease in rural health. In S. Loue & B.E. Quill (Eds.). *Handbook of rural health.* (pp. 189–207). New York: Kluwer Academic/Plenum.

D'Lugoff, M., Jones, W., Kub, J., et al. (2002). Tuberculosis screening in an at-risk immigrant Hispanic population in Baltimore city: An academic health center/local health department partnership. *Journal of Cultural Diversity, 9*(3), 79–85.

Estill, C.F., Baron, S., & Steege, A.L. (2002). Research and dissemination needs for ergonomics in agriculture. *Public Health Reports, 117*(5), 440–445.

Frates, J., Diringer, J., & Hoganm L. (2003). Models and momentum for insuring low-income, undocumented immigrant children in California. *Health Affairs, 22*(1), 259–263.

Gerberich, S. (2000). Care of homeless men in the community. *Holistic Nursing Practice, 14*(2), 21–28.

Hart, L., Larson, E., & Lishner, M. (2005). Rural definitions for health policy and research. *American Journal of Public Health, 95*(7), 1149–1155.

Hartley, D., Bird, D., & Dempsey, P. (1999). Rural mental health and substance abuse. In T.C. Ricketts (Ed.). *Rural health in the United States.* (pp. 38–51). New York: Oxford University Press.

Hayes, L., Quine, S., & Taylor, R. (2005). New South Wales trends in mortality differentials between small rural and urban communities over a 25-year period, 1970–1994. *The Australian Journal Of Rural Health, 13*(2), 71–76.

Hilton, B., Thompson, R., Moore-Dempsey, L., & Hutchinson, K. (2001). Urban outpost nursing: The nature of the nurses' work in the AIDS Prevention Street Nurse Program. *Public Health Nursing, 18*(4), 273–280.

Jackson, J., Doescher, M., Jerant, A., & Hart, L. (2005). A national study of obesity prevalence and trends by type of rural county. *Journal of Rural Health, 21*(2), 140–148.

Kaiser, K., Hays, B., Cho, W., & Agrawal, S. (2002). Examining health problems and intensity of need for care in family-focused community and public health nursing. *Journal of Community Health Nursing, 19*(1), 17–32.

Kalb, K., Cherry, N., Kauzloric, J., et al. (2006). A competency-based approach to public health nursing performance appraisal. *Public Health Nursing, 23*(2), 115–138.

Klinedinst, N. (2005). Effects of a nutrition education program for urban, low-income, older adults: A collaborative program among nurses and nursing students. *Journal of Community Health Nursing, 22*(2), 93–104.

Laditka, S., Laditka, J., Bennett, K., & Probst. J. (2005). Delivery complications associated with prenatal care access for Medicaid-insured mothers in rural and urban hospitals. *Journal of Rural Health, 21*(2), 158–166.

Lawsin, C., Borrayo, E., Edwards, R., & Belloso, C. (2007). Community readiness to promote Latinas' participation in breast cancer prevention clinical trials. *Health and Social Care in the Community, 15*(4), 369–378.

Loue, S., & Quill, B. (Eds.). (2001). *Handbook of rural medicine.* New York: Kluwer Academic/Plenum Publishers.

Maantay, J. (2002). Zoning law, health, and environmental justice: What's the connection? *The Journal Of Law, Medicine and Ethics: A Journal of The American Society Of Law, Medicine and Ethics, 30*(4), 572–593.

Magilvy, J.K., & Congdon, J.G. (2002). The crisis nature of healthcare transitions for rural older adults. *Public Health Nursing, 17,* 336–345.

Manthorpe, J. (2003). City challenges. *Nursing Older People, 15*(4), 10–13.

Mayer, M., Slifkin, R., & Skinner, A. (2005). The effects of rural residence and other social vulnerabilities on subjective measures of unmet need. *Medical Care Research and Review, 62*(5), 617–628.

McMurray, A. (2006). Peace, love and equality: Nurses, interpersonal violence and social justice. In: *Advances in Contemporary Nursing and Interpersonal Violence,* Vol. 4. vii–x.

Myhrvold, T. (2006). The different other—Towards an including ethics of care. *Nursing Philosophy, 7*(3), 125–136.

Nandi, A., Galea, S., Ahern, J., & Vlahov, D. (2005). Probable cigarette dependence, PTSD, and depression after an urban disaster: Results from a population survey of New York City residents 4 months after September 11, 2001. *Psychiatry, 68,* 99–310.

National Advisory Committee on Rural Health. (2002). *A targeted look at the rural health care safety net: A report to the Secretary.* U.S. Department of Health and Human Services.

Nettle, C., & Jones, S. (2001). Undergraduate community health nursing education in a neighborhood settlement house. *Journal of Community Health Nursing, 18*(2), 85–91.

Office of the U.N. High Commissioner for Human Rights. (n.d.). *Committee on migrant workers: Frequently asked questions (FAQs).* Retrieved August 21, 2008 from http://www.ohchr.org/english/bodies/cmw/faws.htm.

Pathman, D., Fryer, G., Green, L., & Phillips, R. (2005). Changes in age-adjusted mortality rates and disparities for rural physician shortage areas staffed by the National Health Service Corps: 1984–1998. *Journal of Rural Health, 21*(3), 214–220.

Poltavski, D., & Muus, K. (2005). Factors associated with incidence of inappropriate ambulance transport in rural areas in cases of moderate to severe head injury in children. *Journal of Rural Health, 21*(3), 272–277.

Probst, J., Moore, C., & Baxley, E. (2005). Update: Health insurance and utilization of care among rural adolescents. *Journal of Rural Health, 21*(4), 279–287.

Probst, J., Moore, C., & Baxley, E. (2005). Effects of race and poverty on perceived stress among rural women. In R.T. Coward, L.A. Davis, et al. (Eds.). *Rural women's health: Mental, behavioral and physical issues.* New York, NY: Springer Publishing Company.

Reimer-Kirkham, S., Van Hofwegen, L., & Hoe Harwood, C. (2005). Narratives of social justice: Learning in innovative clinical settings. *International Journal of Nursing Education Scholarship, 2*(1), [Article 28]. Retrieved August 21, 2008 from http://www.bepress.com/ijnes/vol2/iss1/art28.

Robbins, J., Hopkins, S., Mosley, B., et al. (2006). Awareness and use of folic acid among women in the lower Mississippi Delta. *Journal of Rural Health, 22*(3), 196–203.

Ritter, J. (May 3, 2007). Agricultural uncertainties worry pickers and growers: Low unemployment, change in migrant patterns among causes of labor shortage. *USA Today.*

Schoneman, D. (2002). Surveillance as a nursing intervention: Use in community nursing centers. *Journal of Community Health Nursing, 19*(1), 33–47.

Sistrom, M.G., Hale, P.J. (2006). Integrative review of population health, income, social capital and structural inequality. *Journal of Multicultural Nursing & Health, 12*(2), 21–27.

Steinbeck, J. (2002/1939). *The grapes of wrath.* (John Steinbeck Centennial Edition, 1902–2002). New York: Penguin USA.

Urban Health Initiative. (2003). *Using data in the decision making process.* Retrieved August 21, 2008 from http://www.urbanhealth.org/docs/Using%20Data%20for%20web.pdf.

Vlahov, D., Galea, S., & Freudenberg, N. (2005). Toward an urban health advantage. *Journal of Public Health Management & Practice, 11*(3), 256–258.

Ward-Griffin, C., & McKeever, P. (2000). Relationships between nurses and family caregivers: Partners in care? *Advances in Nursing Science, 22*(3), 89–103.

Weatherill, S., Buxton, J., & Daly, P. (2004). Immunization programs in non-traditional settings. *Canadian Journal Of Public Health. Revue Canadienne De Santé Publique, 95*(2), 133–137.

Williams, A., & Wold, J. (2000). Nurses, cholesterol, and small worksites: Innovative community intervention comparisons. *Family & Community Health, 23*(3), 59–75.

Internet Resources

American Community Survey (see how your community is changing): *http://www.census.gov/acs/www/*

Children's Health Fund (Medical Home Initiative—addresses needs of poor, medically-underserved children & families in isolated, rural areas): *http://www.childrenshealthfund.org/whatwedo/medical_home.php*

Children's Health Fund (Urban Health Initiative—addresses needs of children & families in urban areas): *http://www.childrenshealthfund.org/whatwedo/urbanhealthinitiative.php*

Community Environmental Health Resource Center (promotes social justice for low-income communities): *http://www.cehrc.org/*

Environmental Exposure History: *http://www.migrantclinician.org/_resources/Iprepare_2page.pdf*

Environmental & Occupational History (pesticide exposure): *http://www.epa.gov/pesticides/safety/healthcare/handbook/Chap03.pdf*

International Healthy Cities Foundation:
http://www.healthycities.org/
Johns Hopkins Urban Health Institute:
http://www.jhsph.edu/urbanhealth/
Map of Migrant Health Centers by State:
http://www.migrantclinician.org/healthcenters/
healthcenterdirectory.php
Migrant Clinician's Network (resources on migrant health,
pesticide exposure, directory of migrant health clinics):
http://www.migrantclinician.org
National Alliance for Hispanic Health:
http://www.hispanichealth.org
National Center for Farmworker Health, Inc.:
http://www.ncfh.org
National Center for Frontier Communities:
http://www.frontierus.org

National Rural Health Association:
http://www.nrharural.org/
N.Y. Academy of Medicine's Center for Urban
Epidemiologic Studies:
http://www.nyam.org/initiatives/cues-journal.shtml
Office of Rural Health Policy (HRSA):
http://ruralhealth.hrsa.gov/
Rural Assistance Center: *http://www.raconline.org*
Sinai Urban Health Institute: *http://www.suhichicago.org/*
Urban Health Initiative: *http://www.urbanhealth.org/*
USDA Rural Housing Resources:
http://www.nal.usda.gov/ric/ricpubs/housing.html
USDHUD (rental assistance information):
http://www.hud.gov/renting/index.cfm
WHO Health Cities and Urban Governance:
http://www.euro.who.int/healthy-cities

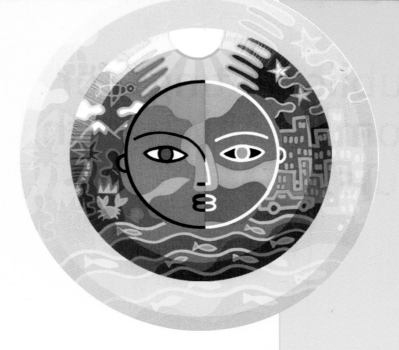

SETTINGS FOR COMMUNITY HEALTH NURSING

Public Settings for Community Health Nursing

LEARNING OBJECTIVES

Upon mastery of this chapter, you should be able to:

◆ Explain the focus of the nursing process and how public health nurses (PHNs) and other nurses working in the public sector use it to provide care in their communities.

◆ Describe how federal, state, and local public health infrastructures influence the population's health.

◆ Evaluate the potential benefits of school-based health centers, and discuss possible parental or community objections.

◆ Compare and contrast common roles and functions of PHNs, school nurses, and corrections nurses.

"A [community nurse] must first nurse. She must be of yet higher class and yet of fuller training than that of a hospital nurse because she has no hospital appliances at hand at all and because she has to take notes on the case for the doctor who has no one but her to report to him."

—Florence Nightingale, 1876 (as cited in Edgecomb, 2001)

Many nursing students are not aware of the vast employment opportunities available outside the hospital in public settings. This chapter will discuss several of these public health settings and the opportunities nurses can garner, particularly in services such as public health nursing, school nursing, or corrections nursing. This chapter is a practical explanation of the work of nurses in the public sector.

Although each of these nursing opportunities differs greatly, they have several characteristics in common. First, community nurses who work in a public setting still use the nursing process, but their client is a population or group of people, rather than an individual. Second, emphasis is placed on prevention of disease or disability. Third, community nurses employed in public settings work with a variety of people. They must be able to network and collaborate with other agencies and disciplines. For example, a nurse working in a correctional facility often collaborates with mental health workers and correctional officers. A nurse working in the public setting has many opportunities to be an advocate for individuals and the community, and may serve on regional task forces or advisory boards. In addition, public health nurses (PHNs) focus on population-based care. Nurses may perform individual care, especially correctional nurses; however, most of the focus is placed on the population as client. Finally, nurses who work in the public setting must be autonomous, flexible, creative thinkers who are self-directed and able to prioritize and use the nursing process to make educated decisions and plan care for their respective populations. Nurses who work in public settings must have the highest level of nursing, communication, problem-solving, and intellectual skills.

⊕ PUBLIC HEALTH NURSING

A **public health nurse** is a nurse who works to promote and protect the health of an entire population (American Nurses Association [ANA], 2007a). The most recent data specify that 448, 254 workers comprise the U.S. public health workforce (Gebbie, 2000). This workforce consists of epidemiologists, nurses, environmentalists, laboratory professionals, nutritionists, dental workers, social workers, and other health care providers. Of this group, PHNs are the largest, making up 10% of the workforce (or approximately 49,323 nurses). Most PHNs work for governmental bodies, with the majority (36,921) working for local, state, or territorial agencies. Another 4,300 PHNs work for the federal government, and approximately 8,000 are associated with volunteer agencies, such as the American Red Cross (Gebbie, 2000).

Looking at public health from a nursing perspective, approximately 14.9% of all registered nurses (RNs) work in public/community health settings (Health Resources & Services Administration [HRSA], 2006). Public or community agencies are the second largest employer of RNs, after hospitals (employing 56% of nurses). However, with the struggle to find adequate access to health care, along with its increased costs, more nursing care is being performed in a public or community setting. Unfortunately, you may not know of these wonderful employment opportunities available in the public sector. This section will describe the role and opportunities for RNs at the local, state, and federal levels of government. The focus will be on governmental agencies, because these agencies employ the majority of PHNs.

EDUCATION

The American Nurses Association (ANA) (2007a) recommends that an entry-level PHN should have a bachelor's degree in nursing. This is important because baccalaureate programs provide additional training in public health and leadership. Some states, such as California, require nurses to take additional classes and obtain certification beyond a bachelor's degree if the BSN program does not offer specific content (e.g., child abuse, public health didactic and practicum). Public health nurses working with specific populations, or in administration, should hold a master's degree. A PHN with a master's degree in community/public health nursing may take a national certification examination offered by the American Nurses Credentialing Center (ANCC) (2008). Many master's programs offer dual nursing and public health degrees, but not all. The emphasis on national certification is due to an ever-increasing need to keep the population protected from health threats, such as bioterrorism (especially after September 11, 2001), emerging diseases (e.g., pandemic flu), or natural disasters (e.g., hurricane Katrina).

KEY FUNCTIONS OF THE PHN IN THE PUBLIC SETTING

Public health nursing practice consists of many areas of expertise; it

- Focuses on the health of populations
- Reflects the needs and priorities of the community
- Requires caring relationships with individuals, families, communities, and systems
- Is grounded in cultural sensitivity, compassion, social justice, and a belief in the worth of all people (e.g., vulnerable populations)
- Encompasses all aspects of health (e.g., physical, emotional, mental, social, spiritual, and environmental)
- Uses strategies to promote health that are motivated by epidemiologic evidence
- Involves individual, as well as collaborative, strategies to achieve results
                    (Minnesota Department of Health, 2007)

In brief, the role of the PHN is to focus on the health of the public. Public health nurses combine their nursing and clinical knowledge of disease and the human response to it, along with public health skills, to accomplish their goals (Quad Council, 2007; ANA, 2007a). They apply the nursing process, not only with individuals but also with populations. Public health nurses are the critical link between data tracking (e.g., epidemiology) and clinical understanding of a disease or condition (Missouri Department of Health & Social Services [DHSS], 2006). Public health nurses use the data to prioritize their interventions to stop the spread of diseases, such as measles, and also to intercede with other concerns (e.g., childhood obesity). For example, PHNs may develop a campaign for children to wear bike helmets after an increase of fatal head injuries is noted in their area. A key emphasis of the PHN is prevention, and a key focus is educating and empowering the community. Several other differences exist between PHNs and nursing in general (see Table 30.1 for a comparison).

TABLE 30.1	Comparing Public Health and General Nursing	
Public Health Nursing	**General Nursing**
Population-based	Individual-based
Grounded in social justice	Grounded in a relationship of caring
Focuses on the greater good	Focuses on individual good (patient)
Health promotion & disease prevention	Restoration of health & function
Utilize & organize community resources	Manage resources at hand
Seek out clients in need	Take care of clients who come to them
Commitment to the community as a whole	Commitment to individual patient

Adapted from *Cornerstones of Public Health Nursing*, Minnesota Department of Health, 2007.

The population that PHNs focus on can be a geographic community (e.g., a state or municipality) or a focus group (e.g., adolescents or the elderly) spanning all socioeconomic levels. To accomplish this, PHNs often work with individuals or families at highest risk, and their motive is to improve, protect, and promote the health of the entire population. One of the goals that characterize PHNs, and differentiate their goals from those of other specialty disciplines, is achieving the greatest good for the majority of people (ANA, 2007a). (See Chapter 13 for an in-depth discussion of social justice.) This requires priority planning and a basic knowledge of the community.

For example, many issues exist in a community. In one community, a single child may have been hit by a car while riding his bike without a helmet. At the same time, in the same community, there may be 10 births to teen moms, 20 instances of drug overdose, and an outbreak of pertussis. The PHNs in that community must prioritize which issue to address first by deciding which issue impacts the most people and what interventions will help the population thrive (ANA, 2007a). Because each community is different, the priorities will vary among communities, once all factors are taken into account. Hence, *assessment* is a critical component of public health and a key tool for the nurses who work in the public sector (Institute of Medicine, 1988) (see Display 30.1).

Another way public health nursing differs from other areas in nursing is that PHNs must actively seek out and identify potential problems and situations (ANA, 2007a). Nurses who work in a hospital setting address the issues that come to them. If a nurse works in the intensive care unit (ICU) of a hospital, she will work with her assigned patient load. Public health nurses, on the other hand, are out in the community identifying the problems, not waiting for problems to come to them. For example, PHNs may participate in visits to childcare centers to note any safety hazards, ensure that rules and regulations are being followed, and that children are properly immunized. These visits are part of the priority of *assurance* identified by the Institute of Medicine (1988), noted in Display 30.1.

Public health nurses cannot perform all these activities alone. They need to collaborate with other partners and optimally use often limited resources. Public health nurses are in a unique situation because they work with their populations (i.e., clients) and with others to find the best solutions for a situation or problem.

For instance, PHNs may notice an increase in the number of measles cases in their community. They may then work with families to identify where and how the children were exposed to the disease, and with local health care providers to provide treatment and vaccinations for those at highest risk of exposure to and damage from measles. Public health nurses also work with school nurses and other school personnel to exclude from school attendance those children who are not adequately immunized against measles. This helps decrease the spread and potential harm due to measles. Public health nurses educate a variety of groups, such as parent–teacher associations (PTAs) and city or school officials, as to how measles spreads, what can be done to treat the disease, and the importance of herd immunity in protecting the public. Education thus empowers each group to be part of the solution. Finally, PHNs can work with public health officials to develop a policy for all new school entrants to receive a second booster of measles vaccine. *Policy development* is the third critical component of public health identified by the Institute of Medicine (1988) (see Display 30.1).

PUBLIC HEALTH FUNDING AND GOVERNMENTAL STRUCTURES

Public health nurses can work at any and all levels of government. Hence, it is important to understand the organizational structure, communication, and funding streams between the federal, state, and local levels of government (see Chapter 6 for more on the structure of the public health system). At each level, all three branches of the government are involved in public health, although often the legislative and executive branches play the most important roles, and this discussion will focus on these areas.

The legislative branch (meaning Congress, state legislatures, or local councils) mandates laws or policies and decides how much of the funding in its jurisdiction will be appropriated to public health. Much of the work for public

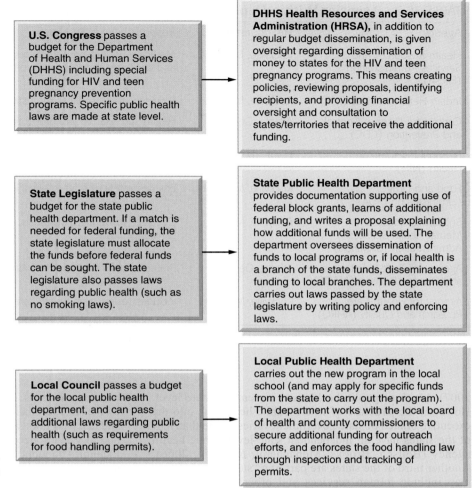

U.S. Congress passes a budget for the Department of Health and Human Services (DHHS) including special funding for HIV and teen pregnancy prevention programs. Specific public health laws are made at state level.

DHHS Health Resources and Services Administration (HRSA), in addition to regular budget dissemination, is given oversight regarding dissemination of money to states for the HIV and teen pregnancy programs. This means creating policies, reviewing proposals, identifying recipients, and providing financial oversight and consultation to states/territories that receive the additional funding.

State Legislature passes a budget for the state public health department. If a match is needed for federal funding, the state legislature must allocate the funds before federal funds can be sought. The state legislature also passes laws regarding public health (such as no smoking laws).

State Public Health Department provides documentation supporting use of federal block grants, learns of additional funding, and writes a proposal explaining how additional funds will be used. The department oversees dissemination of funds to local programs or, if local health is a branch of the state funds, disseminates funding to local branches. The department carries out laws passed by the state legislature by writing policy and enforcing laws.

Local Council passes a budget for the local public health department, and can pass additional laws regarding public health (such as requirements for food handling permits).

Local Public Health Department carries out the new program in the local school (and may apply for specific funds from the state to carry out the program). The department works with the local board of health and county commissioners to secure additional funding for outreach efforts, and enforces the food handling law through inspection and tracking of permits.

FIGURE 30.1 Examples of government organization in relation to public health.

health is carried out in the executive branch of government (Fig. 30.1). Because state and local organizations can be set up in a variety of ways, nurses must check with their local health department for specifics.

Federal Agencies

The federal government oversees national policy and funding, provides expertise, and sets a national agenda (Novick, Morrow, & Mays, 2008). Several federal organizations are part of the executive branch that oversees the health of the nation. The main organization involved with public health is the Department of Health and Human Services (DHHS), which is overseen by the Secretary of Health and Human Services. The Secretary of DHHS is appointed by the President, and is a member of the President's cabinet. Within DHHS are many agencies, including eight that specifically impact public health (Turnock, 2006). Table 30.2 provides additional detail regarding these eight agencies. Other federal agencies that also impact public health include the Environmental Protection Agency (EPA), the Department of Homeland Security, the Department of Agriculture, the Department of Education and the Department of Veterans Affairs.

These various organizations receive funding and directives from the U.S. Congress (i.e., the legislative branch of the federal government) as part of the DHHS budget process. In 2006, the overall budget of DHHS was $642 million (USD-HHS, 2006). It is the prime responsibility of DHHS and other agencies to ensure that legislative mandates are followed, policies carried out, and funds appropriately disseminated. State health entities receive a large portion of funds as part of *block grant funding.* These funds are lumped together to pay for some general use that states have identified (see Chapter 6 for more detailed information). *Healthy People 2010* and state needs assessments help set priorities for state funding. For example, the maternal and child health (MCH) block grants received by states are then used for reproductive health, child health, and immunizations. States with local health departments also disseminate a portion of these funds to the local level. In addition, state and local tax dollars are used to supplement various programs. Thus, the political leanings of state and local officials can strongly influence local health initiatives.

State Governments

The U.S. Constitution bestows states with the responsibility to safeguard the health of their citizens (Turnock,

TABLE 30.2   Agencies Within Department of Health and Human Services

Agency	Headquarters	Responsibility & Bureaus
Health Resources and Services Administration (HRSA)	Rockville, Maryland	Medically underserved—includes Medicare/Medicaid, HIV/AIDS, maternal and child, health professions, primary health care
Indian Health Services (IHS)	Rockville, Maryland	Provides health services for Native Americans (including Alaskan Natives)
Centers for Disease Control and Prevention (CDC)	Atlanta, Georgia	Health surveillance and prevention of disease and bioterrorism
National Institutes of Health (NIH)	Bethesda, Maryland	Medical research
Food and Drug Administration (FDA)	Rockville, Maryland	Ensures safety of food, medication, medical procedures, and equipment
Substance Abuse and Mental Health Services Administration (SAMHSA)	Rockville, Maryland	Oversees prevention, diagnosis, and treatment for mental health and substance abuse
Agency for Toxic Substances and Disease Registry (ATSDR)	Atlanta, Georgia	Protects public from environmental exposures
Agency for Health Care Research and Quality (AHRQ)	Rockville, Maryland	Includes research on health care quality and effectiveness

Source: http://www.dhhs.gov; Turnock, B.J. (2007). *Essentials of public health.* Sudbury, MA: Jones and Bartlett Publishers.

2007). Much of public health is overseen at a state level. However, the structure of where public health fits into the executive branch of state government varies. More than half of the states have an independent state-level public health agency (Beitsch, Brooks, Menachemi, & Grigg, 2006). Another third of the states are part of a "super agency" that may include human services and other state programs (Novick, Morrow, & Mays, 2008). The governor appoints a commissioner, or leading health official, to oversee public health and serve as a member of the governor's cabinet. These cabinet members are usually medical doctors, appointed by the governor. In recent years, state directors have also included social workers (e.g., Michigan) and public health professionals (e.g., Arkansas). In 2007, Governor Phil Bredesen appointed Susan Cooper, RN, MSN, as the first nurse to serve as public health commissioner for the state of Tennessee. The first nurses appointed to director of state offices of public health were Barbara Sabol and Gloria Smith in Kansas and Michigan (Feldman, 2008).

The purpose of state agencies is to carry forth regulations and policies determined by the federal government. Examples of these programs are the Medicaid, Medicare, and State Children's Health Insurance Programs (SCHIPs). Many of these programs may have specific federal requirements, but they also allow states the ability to personalize the programs to fit the state's individual needs. An example of such a program is the MCH block grant, which provides funding and guidelines for the states. However states determine which programs (e.g., reproductive health or children's health) will be funded and how they will be implemented.

Another example of federal leadership is the *Healthy People 2010* document that provides goals for a variety of health outcomes. States can use these outcomes, or develop additional performance measures, according to state charac-

teristics and needs. In addition, the state agency is influenced by the state legislative body, which oversees the state budget and can pass laws specific to the state. Each state is different due to varying needs, cultures, and political environments. Examples of public health laws at a state level include immunization requirements for school entrance, seat belt safety laws, and regulations regarding parental rights concerning birth control and abortion services for teens.

Local Public Health

Local health departments (LHDs) carry out state laws and policies (Turnock, 2007). They provide the most direct, immediate care of the population (Novick, Morrow, & Mays, 2008). For example, they may provide immunization clinics, track and treat cases of tuberculosis (TB) and other communicable diseases, and provide education on a variety of subjects (e.g., human immunodeficiency virus [HIV]/ acquired immune deficiency syndrome [AIDS] prevention, smoking cessation). They often carry out programs with funding from federal and state agencies. For instance, federal funding to address asthma may be obtained through the state agency, and local agencies may organize an educational program on asthma triggers in a local business where many community members work. State and local agencies do not work alone in such endeavors, however. Collaboration is very important in addressing the public health needs of a community. Public health agencies work with private organizations, hospitals, nonprofit groups, universities, and government agencies that oversee food and housing to meet citizens' needs.

Local health departments work with state health departments, some independently and some as dependent branches of the state agency. The size and services offered by a local agency also differ depending on state laws, structure, and wealth (Turnock, 2007). Half of LHDs in the United States have fewer than 20 employees (NACCHO, 2007). Thus, the number of LHDs per state can vary dramatically. For example, California has only 62 LHDs, whereas Massachusetts has the most with 324 (NACCHO, 2007). Nearly all LHDs (95%) employ nurses, who make up 24% of the total public health workforce at the local level (NACCHO, 2007).

NURSING ROLES IN LOCAL, STATE, AND FEDERAL PUBLIC HEALTH POSITIONS

Nurses can work in a variety of capacities at the various levels of government, which may cover most aspects of public health (Novick, Morrow, & May, 2008). Generally speaking, nurses who work at the local level of public health tend to provide direct service care. For example, they often administer immunizations, monitor patients with TB, provide education to school groups, provide cancer screenings, and track communicable disease rates. Local PHNs are the eyes and ears of their communities. Many PHNs working at the local level, especially in rural or small public health departments, may have a variety of responsibilities. For instance, a PHN may be a full-time employee whose time could be split into 50% cancer screening, 25% with the Women, Infant, and Children (WIC) program, and 25% on Medicaid outreach (see Display 30.2 for an example of a PHN's day). Public health nurses also serve in administrative roles within agencies, as well, where they may oversee an entire bureau or program, for example, or serve as supervisors for a group of PHNs.

Within each of the governmental agencies, programs may be arranged according to a particular subject area. For example, a PHN may work in the cardiovascular disease program, overseeing cholesterol screenings and promoting physical health and nutrition. A PHN could also work in the immunization program, promoting and tracking the immunization requirements of school-age children. The nurse may also be in charge of day care licensure requirements, traveling throughout the state and conducting inspections or writing policies. Or, the nurse could oversee a program to decrease sudden infant death syndrome (SIDS) in the state and track SIDS-related deaths. Thus, the variety of locations and programs are limitless for PHNs. The following is a brief overview of some of the main roles of nurses working at state and local health departments. Specific options and means by which PHNs serve as advocates and change agents to protect and promote the health of all are discussed, using the nursing process as an outline. Figure 30.2 provides a practical model of how PHNs use the nursing model and public health principles in their everyday functions.

Assess

An assessment of the situation is key to any nursing care. Public health nurses assess the situation in a variety of ways. They observe a great deal when they are in the community and when they conduct home visits. They also assess data to identify trends. Often nurses work with other public health personnel when assessing and tracking data, although nurses

---

DISPLAY 30.2	A TYPICAL DAY IN THE LIFE OF A PHN

8:00 a.m. Staff reproductive health clinic. Provide counseling regarding family planning services, as well as breast and other cancer screenings.

10:30 a.m. Make a home visit to a mother and baby who is not thriving. Conduct an examination of the baby and assess the living situation. Assist the mother regarding breastfeeding, nutrition, newborn care, and parenting.

12:30 p.m. Attend a lunch meeting of a newly formed coalition that is concerned about the increased rate of teen pregnancy in the city. Provide statistics from community, as well as firsthand knowledge of teens participating in the Women, Infants, and Children (WIC) program and the home visiting program. Offer expertise regarding how to approach the problem.

2:00 p.m. Investigate the case of a kindergartner who has TB. With the help of the school nurse, check immunization records of other students and staff. Contact the family to learn who else is exposed and at risk. Provide proper testing and education regarding the signs and symptoms of TB, the need for regular testing, and following the treatment regimen.

3:30 p.m. Staff cancer screening clinic performing Pap smears and providing counseling to women regarding risks of breast and cervical cancer. Follow-up with patients from last week's clinic whose results were questionable.

5:00 p.m. Finish paperwork and go home knowing the community's health was positively impacted today.

Adapted from *Public Health Nursing: Promoting and Protecting Health in Colorado.* Retrieved Sept 21, 2007 from http://www.cdphe.state.co.us/oll/phn/PHNBrochure.pdf.

---

may serve as specialists in epidemiology. For example, PHNs can use morbidity and mortality statistics to determine the leading causes of death nationally and locally. They can assess communicable disease rates to identify an outbreak before it becomes too widespread. They track how many people in the community are in compliance with immunizations to keep the herd immunity high and decrease the chance of outbreaks.

Public health nurses use census data to determine population growth. As an example, the census indicates that the number of individuals 65 years or older will double by 2030 (Bergman, 2006). Estimates indicate that in 2030, approximately 72 million, or one in five persons, will be over 65 years of age. This is important in planning for future activities and resources. Public health nurses also use prevalence data to determine which ethnic groups are at higher risk than others. For example, the PHNs at the Utah County Health department noticed an increase in STDs. Upon further investigation, they learned that the greatest increases were within the Hispanic population. Through this assessment they were able to successfully target interventions for this population (Page, 2006).

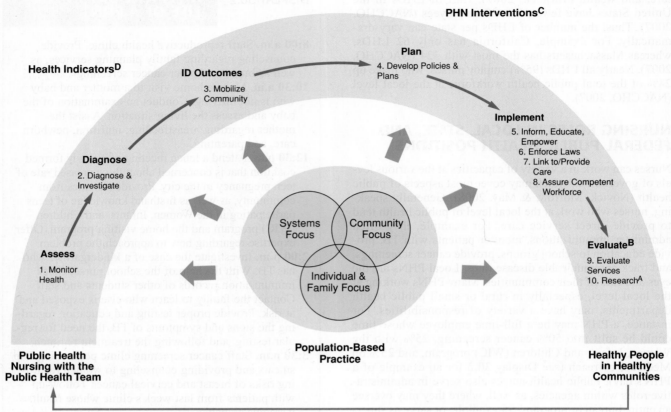

Public Health Nursing Practice Model*

PHN Interventions[C]

Health Indicators[D]

ID Outcomes
3. Mobilize Community

Plan
4. Develop Policies & Plans

Diagnose
2. Diagnose & Investigate

Implement
5. Inform, Educate, Empower
6. Enforce Laws
7. Link to/Provide Care
8. Assure Competent Workforce

Assess
1. Monitor Health

Systems Focus

Community Focus

Individual & Family Focus

Evaluate[B]
9. Evaluate Services
10. Research[A]

Public Health Nursing with the Public Health Team

Population-Based Practice

Healthy People in Healthy Communities

References:
(A) Public Health Functions Steering Committee. (1994, Fall). *Public Health in America*. Retrieved May 7, 2001, from the World Wide Web: http://health.gov/phfunctions/public.htm
(B) Quad Council of Public Health Nursing Organizations. (2007). *Public Health Nursing: Scope & Standards of Practice*. Washington D.C.: American Nurses Association.
(C) Minnesota Department of Health, Public Health Nursing Section. (2000). *Public Health Nursing Practice for the 21st Century: National Satellite Learning Conference; Competency Development in Population-based Practice October 5, November 2, December 7, 2000*. St. Paul, MN: Minnesota Department of Health Nursing Section. Retrieved May 7, 2001, from the World Wide Web: http://www.health.state.mn.us/divs/chs/phr/material.htm.
(D) U.S. Department of Health and Human Services. (2000). *Healhy People 2010*. (Vol. 1). McLean, VA: International Medical Publishing, Inc.

*Created by Los Angeles County DPH, Public Health Nursing with input from CCLHDND-Southern Region. This model serves as the basis for the CCLHDND California PHN Practice Model (05-2002).
© 2007 Los Angeles County DPH Public Health Nursing

FIGURE 30.2 Public health nursing model from Los Angeles Country.

Environmental risks are important to the public's health and are often assessed by nurses. For example, a PHN conducting blood tests noticed that students living in a mining community had elevated blood lead levels. This assessment information forms the basis for the nurse's intervention. Each nurse must assess his or her own community, because each has specific characteristics and needs. A community positioned next to a factory that emits fumes will have different issues than a rural community 90 miles away from any industry. At the same time, an outbreak of *Escherichia coli* in one town may identify a risk to the PHN in the neighboring town.

Diagnose

Assessment is key to diagnosing a situation or problem. For a PHN, diagnosis also includes identifying priorities for the many concurrent issues. Nurses who work in public settings

may perform skin tests or simple blood work in public clinics to determine TB exposure, or risk of diabetes, or other conditions (Southern Nevada Health District, 2005) (see From the Case Files I). Other nurses utilize microscopes to identify cases of vaginitis and cervicitis (George, 2007). This could all occur on the same day.

As nurses diagnose individual needs, they apply this information and watch for increased or decreased rates (e.g., of disease or injury) among the population. For instance, a nurse working in a public health clinic may notice an increase in the number of people diagnosed with diabetes. The nurse further assesses the situation to determine if it is a population need, and also the degree of the problem. Another PHN may assist with newborn genetic testing. Nurses are in the perfect position to identify issues and trends early on. As more is known regarding genetic trends, the PHN can use this information to advocate policies and laws that will impact a particular population.

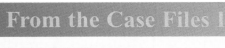

From the Case Files I

Tuberculosis Exposure

As a PHN you are alerted to a person who has an active TB case. He came into the health department for a chest x-ray after he failed his tuberculin skin test. The person has recently arrived by plane from another state. He stayed for a few weeks with family members in a small house, but now lives with friends in a small apartment. When talking to the patient, you note that he coughs often and does not cover his mouth.

- As a PHN what steps would you take to determine exposure?
- How will you determine who was exposed and will need to be tested?
- What questions can you ask to help determine when and how the patient was exposed to TB?
- What type of education will you provide to him?
- How can you ensure that the patient is compliant with medication treatment?
- Imagine that you are the school nurse of the patient's 8-year-old daughter who has also tested positive. What steps would you take?
- What would you do differently if you were a corrections nurse and the patient was an inmate?

Constant assessment and diagnosis are tools by which PHNs identify critical situations and prioritize issues that must be addressed first. Several documents have helped PHNs prioritize issues. *Healthy People 2010* identifies many of the nation's top priorities (USDHHS, 2000) (see Display 30.3). Public health performance standards also assist nurses in prioritizing needs (CDC, 2001; Quad Council, 2007). The Institute of Medicine (2003) has also identified a need for a greater focus on informatics and genomics.

Improved medical technology has supplied immunizations that have decreased the rates of many communicable diseases. This led to the emergence of new issues and priorities for PHNs, specifically, injury prevention and the management of chronic diseases (Beitsch, Brooks, Menachemi, & Grigg, 2006). World events have also placed additional emphasis on public health roles, including the global spread of TB, bioterrorism, pandemic influenza, and natural disasters (Beitsch, et al., 2006). Because of their nursing and epidemiologic skill, PHNs serve as critical members of emergency response teams, specifically regarding bioterrorism surveillance and preparedness (Atkins, Williams, Silenas, & Edwards, 2005). The nursing and epidemiologic skills they use when tracking outbreaks of communicable diseases, such as TB, are easily transferable to the communicable agents of bioterrorism (e.g., smallpox, anthrax).

Plan and Implement

Once PHNs have diagnosed and prioritized the needs of their community, they develop and carryout plans to address those needs. Development of care plans is an important function for nurses (Georgia, 2007). Many interventions require collaborating and working with other agencies. Education is also a key to many public health nursing interventions. However, education alone will not change behavior; thus, it is important to address the issue from many different angles, as well as at different levels. Public health nurses cannot solve all issues, but they can serve as advocates to influence those who can make the changes. The interventions are endless, but here are a few examples:

- Nurses conduct home visits to mothers at risk. They conduct family assessments to determine the level of psychological issues and education needed by the family regarding specific needs, such as responses to medication. They also help mothers receive needed psychological counseling by linking them to a local mental health agency.
- A nurse working in risk management develops and teaches an education program about workplace safety and ergonomics. She develops policies regarding shift hours and heavy lifting.
- A nurse serves as an advocate for a program that will assist children with special health care needs attend a clinic closer to home.
- A nurse develops a campaign for television, newspaper, and radio regarding the need to receive a flu shot. The nurse also includes incentives that target the elderly community who are at additional risk for developing complications from this illness.
- The nurse organizes a health clinic at local shelters providing foot care and screenings for blood pressure, diabetes, TB, and cholesterol, as appropriate.
- The nurse works with schools to educate teens regarding birth control and the impact of teen pregnancy. She includes counseling regarding STDs. She works with the community to ensure that a variety of teen-focused activities are available for this population.
- The nurse conducts home visits to new mothers who need assistance with breast-feeding and newborn care. The nurse also contacts the housing authority to report hazardous conditions in the housing project she has visited.
- The nurse helps identify resources for families without insurance to ensure that well-child and adult screenings are performed regularly in order to reduce health care costs associated with illness.

DISPLAY 30.3	HEALTHY PEOPLE 2010–PUBLIC HEALTH PRIORITIES

Healthy People 2010: Public Health

Healthy People 2010 provides the direction and goals for all public health nurse (PHNs). *Healthy People 2010* is used to guide prioritizing activities for PHNs. Specifically, PHNs focus on the ten leading indicators, which include:

- Physical activity
- Overweight and obesity
- Tobacco use
- Substance abuse
- Responsible sexual behavior
- Mental health
- Injury and violence
- Environmental quality
- Immunization
- Access to health care

Healthy People 2010: School Nursing

One objective directly relates directly to school nurse staffing:

7-4   Increase the proportion of the nation's elementary, middle, junior high, and senior high schools that have a nurse-to-student ratio of at least 1:750.

Other objectives that school nurses can use to help prioritize activities include:

6-9   Increase the proportion of children and youth with disabilities who spend at least 80% of their time in regular education programs.

8-20   (Developmental) Increase the proportion of the nation's primary and secondary schools that have official school policies ensuring the safety of students and staff from environmental hazards, such as chemicals in special classrooms, poor indoor air quality, asbestos, and exposure to pesticides.

14-23   Maintain vaccination coverage levels for children in licensed day care facilities and children in kindergarten through the first grade.

15-31   (Developmental) Increase the proportion of public and private schools that require use of appropriate head, face, eye, and mouth protection for students participating in school-sponsored physical activities.

19-15   (Developmental) Increase the proportion of children and adolescents aged 6 to 19 years whose intake of meals and snacks at schools contributes to good overall dietary quality.

22-8   Increase the proportion of the nation's public and private schools that require daily physical education for all students.

22-12   (Developmental) Increase the proportion of the nation's public and private schools that provide access to their physical activity spaces and facilities for all persons outside of normal school hours (that is, before and after the school day, on weekends, and during summer and other vacations).

24-5   (Developmental) Reduce the number of school or work days missed by persons with asthma due to asthma-related illness.

26-11   Reduce the proportion of persons engaging in binge drinking of alcoholic beverages.

Healthy People 2010: Corrections Nursing

13-8   Increase the proportion of substance abuse treatment facilities that offer HIV/AIDS education, counseling, and support.

13-9   (Developmental) Increase the number of state prison systems that provide comprehensive HIV/AIDS, sexually transmitted diseases, and tuberculosis (TB) education.

13-10   (Developmental) Increase the proportion of inmates in state prison systems who receive voluntary HIV counseling and testing during incarceration.

18-8   (Developmental) Increase the proportion of juvenile justice facilities that screen new admissions for mental health problems.

25-14   (Developmental) Increase the proportion of youth detention facilities and adult city or county jails that screen for common bacterial sexually transmitted diseases (STDs) within 24 hours of admission and treat STDs (when necessary) before persons are released.

26-19   (Developmental) Increase the proportion of inmates receiving substance abuse treatment in correctional institutions.

◆ The nurse organizes an immunization clinic at the local school after an outbreak of measles. The nurse also conducts classes at the school regarding communicable disease prevention and tobacco cessation.

◆ The nurse organizes a bicycle fair to educate the community regarding the need for bicycle helmets, in hopes of decreasing head injuries. She also works to develop public policy related to car seat usage and collaborates with local businesses in providing vouchers for discounts on car seats for low-income parents.

◆ The nurse, who is a paid lobbyist, works to change laws regarding smoking.

◆ A nurse, who is an elected member of the state legislature, sponsors a bill to increase funding for school nurses.

◆ After a hepatitis outbreak at a local business, the nurse conducts an assessment of the business and provides education classes and suggests policy changes to help guard against future outbreaks.

These interventions are based on evidence-based practice (EBP) (see Chapter 4). Below are some examples of EBP in public health nursing:

◆ Media campaigns targeting specific populations have been successfully used to educate and

EVIDENCE-BASED PRACTICE

Public Health Nursing

This study investigated the various health sources used by Vietnamese men in the Seattle area (Woodall, Taylor, Yasui, Ngo-Metzger, Burke, Thai, & Jackson, 2006). The sample was determined using the 2001 metropolitan telephone book and 23 last names that investigators at the University of California determined to be shared by 95% of Vietnamese families. From this population, 900 households were randomly selected to participate (509 chose to participate, 79% response rate). Before households were contacted, advertisements about the upcoming survey were publicized on posters in the community Vietnamese grocery stores. The survey was conducted in person by male bilingual and bicultural survey workers (participants had the option to participate in English or Vietnamese). Participants were asked where they received information regarding health and health care. The most common mediums used included Vietnamese newspapers/magazines (73%); English television (67%); Vietnamese television (64%); family members (63%); doctors/nurses and friends (58%); and Vietnamese radio (51%).

Nursing Implications

Results of past studies indicate Blacks, Hispanics, and Whites rely more on print media and doctors, whereas Korean Americans preferred newspapers. Family and radio were used much less. Thus, when PHNs and others want to target the Vietnamese population, they should include the message in Vietnamese newspapers/magazine. In addition, potentially effective messages can ask "Have you talked to your friends about. . . .?" These would be effective because family and friends are often the source of health information for Vietnamese American men.

It is critical for a PHN to understand her population and the best mediums to reach it, as each population or community may be different. Cultural sensitivity is key to successful community outreach. Constant assessment of a community helps PHNs stay up to date with issues and influential media.

Reference:

Woodall, E.D., Taylor, V.M., Yasui, Y., Ngo-Metzger, Q., Burke, N., Thai, H., & Jackson, J. C. (2006). Sources of health information among Vietnamese American men. *Journal of Immigrant and Minority Health, 8*(3), 263–271.

♦ Bike helmets have been proven to be effective in decreasing head injuries (Berg & Westerling, 2007).
♦ Hofler (2006) has described how nurses can effectively impact health policy.
♦ The American School Health Association has developed a toolkit to help nurses organize successful immunization programs (Boyer-Chu & Wooley, 2006).

Evaluate

The world in which PHNs work is always changing. It is crucial to constantly evaluate programs and interventions to determine if goals are reached. For example, a nurse may visit childcare facilities or senior centers to ensure that laws regarding licensure are being followed. Evaluating is often equated with assessing. Public health nurses also can evaluate data to determine whether various rates (e.g., infant mortality, or other health indicators) increase or decrease as a result of their interventions.

Another way that PHNs can determine if their interventions are effective is by becoming involved in research. Numerous researchers have studied the impact that PHNs have on improving population health and societal outcomes (Quad Council, 2007). Corrarino and Little (2006) found that case management and education provided by nurses to families decreased the number of hospital visits for children with asthma. Public health nurses who conducted home visits to these high-risk mothers have also improved the lives of mothers and their babies. Children in the intervention group were found to have increased achievement and intellectual functioning, along with decreased aggression and behavior problems (Olds, et al., 2004; Izzo, et al., 2005).

PUBLIC HEALTH NURSING CAREERS

Nurses who work at the state and federal levels tend to have consultant, or oversight-type, roles, and some nurses head programs that are specifically funded at the state and/or federal levels (e.g., HIV/AIDS, immunization programs). Some state-employed nurses may work in clinics for children with special health care needs. Some federally employed nurses may provide direct care in Indian Health Service clinics. Public health nurses at all levels may also be called upon to help during a disaster or communicable disease outbreak.

Among distinct opportunities at the federal level are those associated with the Department of Veteran's Affairs and DHHS. Agencies headed by DHHS include the National Institutes of Health (NIH), the Indian Health Service, the Health Resources and Services Administration Services (HRSA), the U.S. Food and Drug Administration (FDA), the Substance Abuse and Mental Health Services Administration (SAMSHA), and the Centers for Disease Control and Prevention (CDC).

Public health nurses in these agencies oversee and carryout the initiatives of *Healthy People 2010*, along with other program initiatives. Many of their functions are similar to those mentioned earlier. For example, they may oversee and develop programs, such as national surveys, that collect data used to determine priorities. Examples of these

promote healthy behavior (Beaudoin, Fernandez, Wall, & Farley, 2007).
♦ Health screenings have been shown to be a successful outreach effort for the homeless population (Krisberg, 2004).
♦ Soloman and Card (2004) have identified several school-based programs that successfully impact sexual activity and teen pregnancy.

PERSPECTIVES
VOICES FROM THE COMMUNITY

As an instructor of undergraduate nursing students, I want students to realize *public health nursing* is a wonderful and rewarding employment opportunity. Many students often enter the nursing program not knowing much about public health nursing. They may only get minimal exposure to public health and thus not understand who or what is involved in public health nursing. In so doing, they miss out on a wonderful opportunity to work with a variety of people. It may be helping new moms, or working with children and adolescents or the elderly. They may help give vaccinations or prepare for community disasters. They might teach about breastfeeding or conduct cancer screening clinics. They are out with the people ensuring the public's health.

Public health nurses are able to use the science of nursing because they need to understand the pathophysiology, anatomy, human development, and disease transmission. They may not do as many hands-on procedures as hospital nurses, but they still must keep up to date in knowledge, as they are often teaching. In addition, they must be quick and receptive thinkers who can work independently and creatively. Public health nurses also are the essence of the "art" of nursing. They must understand and relate to people, and understand social systems and human behavior. They are the voice for the most vulnerable and the champion of all.

Although PHNs may not see an immediate reward for their actions, as a nurse who works in the hospital does, PHNs make a long and lasting impact not just to an individual but to an entire society. They also have the opportunity to really be a patient advocate. They do this by helping well people stay well and by preventing illness. They also help those who are sick obtain medical access. Public health nurses can also be involved in public policy change that can help an entire community. Public health nursing encompasses the entire art and science of nursing.

Erin M.

surveys include the Behavioral Risk Factor Survey (BRFS), the Youth Risk Behavior Survey (YRBS), and the National Health Interview Survey (NHIS). Federally employed PHNs may also review state funding proposals for projects and ensure that guidelines are met. They are a resource for state and local health departments, and often are called upon as consultants. Nurses working at the NIH may assist in conducting research. For example, a nurse may study the effects of applying chemotherapy directly to a tumor, instead of through intravenous or central lines (U.S. Public Health Service Commissioned Corps, 2007). In addition to these opportunities, PHNs may work as clinicians for the Indian Health Services.

Indian Health Services

Indian Health Services (IHS) is responsible for providing healthcare to Native Americans (American Indians and Alaska Natives) (Turnock, 2007). The IHS provides services for approximately 1.5 million American Indians in 35 states (Turnock, 2007). Employment with the IHS allows a nurse to live in a variety of rural and urban settings and to work specifically with Native Americans, a vulnerable population. These nurses work and oversee health care services in clinics run by IHS. The clinics are usually focused on primary care and focus on general practice. They may work with patients who have diabetes, providing nutritional counseling and education; they may also provide immunizations, perform well-child examinations, or conduct HIV/AIDS screenings. Unique aspects of these jobs are that most clinics are located in remote areas of the country and face unique challenges. Some houses on Native American reservations may not have a telephone or consistent electricity, and these clients may have numerous special needs. This type of nursing is very challenging but can also be extremely rewarding.

Uniformed Public Health Nursing

Nurses can serve in each of the seven uniformed services of the U.S. Department of Defense (Army, Navy, Marine, Air Force); U.S. Department of Homeland Security (Coast Guard); U.S. Department of Commerce (National Oceanic and Atmospheric Administration [NOAA] Commissioned Corps); and the U. S. Public Health Services Commissioned Corps (USPHSCC) (NOAA, 2007; USPHSCC, 2007).

The **U.S. Public Health Service Commissioned Corps** (USPHSCC) is a group of 6,000 specially trained public health members who serve their country with the goal of protecting and promoting the health of the nation. The Corps was established in 1798, as part of an act to treat sick seaman in Marine hospitals. Over the years, the Corps expanded to oversee the health of immigrants entering the country and to assist in preventing/treating communicable disease outbreaks. The U.S. Surgeon General oversees the Commissioned Corps, and many of its officers are stationed at other federal agencies, such as the CDC and the FDA (USPHSCC, 2007).

Nurses are an integral part of the Corps. They provide nursing care and health care leadership around the world. Their focus is on improving health for the entire community by providing care, conducting research, or reviewing new medications. These nurses work in a variety of federal agencies, many of them listed earlier. On a daily basis, they may perform tasks similar to civilian nurses. However, as commissioned officers they can also be deployed to protect the nation's health. For example, USPHSCC nurses were some of the first on the scene to assist in the aftermath of hurricane Katrina (see Display 30.4). They may also be deployed in the case of a widespread communicable disease outbreak. Their activities can be international as well, in providing expertise and support on global issues such as the Asian tsunami or the worldwide spread of HIV/AIDS.

As commissioned officers, USPHSCC nurses are compensated in addition to their regular salaries and receive veteran's benefits, health insurance, access to military base lodging and recreational facilities, and other benefits. Officers are supported with tuition and other training opportunities to fur-

| DISPLAY 30.4 | UNITED STATES PUBLIC HEALTH SERVICE COMMISSIONED CORPS AND HURRICANE KATRINA |

Here is an example from an account in the *Journal of Professional Nursing* of how nurses from the United States Public Health Service Commissioned Corps (USPHSCC) are called upon to help during a national crisis. The authors of the article have "regular" positions with the federal government. At the time the article was written, two authors (Debisette and Brown) worked for the Bureau of Health Professions, part of the Health Resources and Services Administration (HRSA) in the U.S. Department of Health and Human Services. The third author (Chamberlain) worked as a nurse medical evaluations officer in the Office of Commissioned Corps Support Services.

As the threat of hurricane Katrina was imminent the USPHSCC nurses were deployed to Louisiana; they arrived the day before the storm hit land, and were some of the first to respond. In fact, nearly half of the 37 member team ($n = 15$) were nurses. The team was deployed to Baton Rouge to assist local personnel in setting up an 800-bed field hospital (including an intensive care unit) at the Pete Maravich Assembly Center at Louisiana State University. The USPHSCC nurses helped provide nursing care that included triage, treatment, stabilization, and transport to permanent facilities. They addressed the psychological, as well as physiologic, needs of the people as evacuees.

Having lost everything, the evacuees streamed into the center. Many of these evacuees, in addition to the trauma and shock associated with their losses, had special medical needs. Some needed dialysis, some were physically disabled, and some had diabetes.

USPHSCC nurses also ensured the safety and security of the people. For example, it was a USPHSCC nurse who realized that the electrical outage would create a failure of the water pump system, and alerted the command-ing officer. Knowing they would soon lose water, the nurses then filled bathtubs with water that was later needed for flushing toilets. The USPHSCC nurses covered gaps in care and worked long hours to ensure that the needs of everyone were met.

After working 3 weeks in the Baton Rouge area, the USPHSCC nurses traveled for 3 days with the American Red Cross and the Louisiana Department of Health and Hospitals to other parts of Louisiana to assess needs. They visited 270 shelters. They worked in teams of four (an environmental officer, a health provider trained in epidemiology, a local American Red Cross representative, and an RN). Each member had specific responsibilities. The nurses assessed the ability of the shelters to address the acute and chronic health care needs of the residents, either within the shelter or by accessing local health resources. They accomplished this assignment by interviewing various shelter staff using a standardized survey tool, as well as by direct observation.

The authors concluded from their experience with Katrina:

> Nurses are often caregivers, nurturers, and advocates. In addition, they are frequently called upon to take on the roles of educators, counselors, and as evidenced here, researchers. As representatives of the USPHS, they stood with strength and courage in the face of devastation. Most of all, they [were] leaders of compassion who appreciate[d] the love, sense of community, and love for their country that emanated from the people of Louisiana in the aftermath of Hurricane Katrina. (p. 272)

From Debisette, A.T., Brown, C.R., & Chamberlain, N. (2006). A nursing perspective from United States Public Health Service Nurses. *Journal of Professional Nursing, 22*(5), 270–272.

ther their education and advance their careers. Student tuition reimbursement and loan payment options are also available.

To qualify as a nurse in the Commissioned Corps, one must be a U.S. citizen, less than 44 years old, able to pass a physical examination, possess a bachelor's or higher degree from an accredited nursing program, pass the National Council Licensure Examination (NCLEX), and hold a valid nursing license from one of the 50 states, the District of Columbia, Puerto Rico, Guam, or the U.S. Virgin Islands. For more information on the USPHSCC, see the Internet Resources at the end of this chapter.

⊙ SCHOOL NURSING

School nurses save lives and assist in helping children so that they are able to learn and reach their greatest potential.

> School nursing is a specialized practice of professional nursing that advances the well-being, academic success, and life-long achievement of students. To that end, school

nurses facilitate positive student responses to normal development; promote health and safety; intervene with actual and potential health problems; provide case management services; and actively collaborate with others to build student and family capacity for adaptation, self-management, self-advocacy, and learning. (National Association of School Nurses [NASN], 2007a)

A **school nurse** works primarily with the students who attend the nurse's assigned schools, as well as with the families of those schoolchildren, members of the school staff and administration, health care providers, and other helping professionals within the school and community. In 2005, approximately 14.8 million school-age children attended over 95,000 public schools (U.S. Department of Education, 2006). These children are the parents, workers, leaders, and decision-makers of tomorrow, and their future success depends in good measure on achieving their educational goals today. Their school success is intertwined, to some degree, with the state of their health (Mitchell, 2000).

Think back to your own elementary and secondary schooling. Did you have access to a school nurse? If so, how did that person influence your health and the health of your peers? If you did not have a school nurse, how do you think a school nurse might have improved your school environment or educational experience? The school nurse is a key provider of a variety of services.

HISTORY OF SCHOOL NURSING

Beginning in the mid-1800s and continuing through the early years of the 20th century, mandatory education was instituted in the United States. The early years included health services often conducted by "medical inspectors," usually physicians. In New York City, where communicable disease was rampant, inspectors sent notes home with children with the message "you are sick—go home" and citing the reason for their exclusion from school (Vessey & McGowan, 2006, p. 255). The reasons for exclusion were largely the contagious illnesses commonly found among the tenements and crowded slums of the growing city. However, parents often did not receive these notes, or couldn't read them, and because families lacked resources, most children were left untreated and simply remained out of school as truants. No efforts were made by medical inspectors to follow up on excluded children. Because these excluded children played with healthy children after school hours, the levels of contagious illness actually worsened (Vesey & McGowan, 2006; Wolfe & Selekman, 2002). The absentee children promoted the spread of various communicable diseases (Woodfill & Beyrer, 1991). In 1902, the New York Board of Education contracted with Lillian Wald's Henry Street Settlement to provide a PHN to work with the families and schools to facilitate the return of healthy children to school. The nurse was Lina Rogers (she later married and added the name Struthers). She made home visits to follow-up on excluded children and was assisted by other Henry Street nurses in providing care, educating families about diseases and the need for hygiene, and working with other organizations to provide needed food, shoes, and clothing (Vessey & McGowan, 2006). In the first month of the school nurse experiment, 98% of children previously excluded from school for medical reasons were treated and readmitted (Woodfill & Beyrer, 1991). The board hired 12 more school nurses, and over the next few years, other cities and states began hiring nurses to work in the schools. School nurses have historically advocated for hot lunches, breakfast programs, and the need for increased health education in schools and for families (Abrams, 2005).

School nurses continue as a specialty branch of professional nursing that serves the school-age population. More than 50,000 school nurses are estimated to be working in schools today (Zaslow, 2006). However, according to the 2006 School Health Policies and Programs Study (SHPPS), many school nurses oversee multiple schools, and less than half of the schools had the nationally recommended ratio of one school nurse for every 750 students (Brener, Wheeler, Wolfe, Vernon-Smiley, & Caldart-Olson, 2007). Most schools (86.3%) had at least a part-time nurse, although some schools still report not having any school nursing services.

School nurses deliver services to students from birth through age 21 years. They also work with students' families and the school community in regular and special education schools, as well as other educational settings (e.g., preschools, court, and other community schools). Studies show that having a school nurse present increases health and social services and improves absentee rates (Guttu, Engelke, & Swanson, 2004; Telljohann, Price, Dake, & Durgin, 2004; Telljohann, Dake, & Price, 2004).

The role of the school nurse has expanded over the years, along with the increase in chronic conditions and challenges in accessing health care (Lear, 2007; Broussard, 2004). Federal law requires school systems to provide care for children with disabilities. The Individuals with Disabilities Education Act (IDEA), the Rehabilitation Act of 1973, and Title II of the Americans with Disabilities Act all mandate equal educational opportunities for all students, including children with complex medical conditions.

Legislative mandates and technology that has allowed low-birth-weight babies to survive, have led to a steady increase in the number of children with special health care needs attending school (U.S. Department of Education, 2006; Lakdawalla, Bhattacharya, & Goldman, 2004). It is now commonplace for children to attend school accompanied by feeding tubes, catheters, insulin pumps, and glucose monitors, as well as ventilators (Wolfe & Selekman, 2002). More children with life-threatening conditions have required schools to consider "do not resuscitate" orders and provide emergency care plans (Wolfe et al., p. 404).

In addition, the lack of access to health care has added extra burdens on schools as children come to school sick or miss additional days of school resulting from complications of illnesses that could have been easily treated in earlier stages. In 2006, approximately 6.9 million children (10%) did not have health insurance (Bloom & Cohen, 2006). Many children can access health care services only at school (Vessey & McGowan, 2006). Results from the most recent National Health Survey indicate that 5% of children missed 11 days of school or more in the past year because of illness. Children from families of lower socioeconomic status were twice as likely to miss 11 days of school or more than were children from families with higher income levels (9% versus 4%).

KEY ROLES OF THE SCHOOL NURSE

To understand the role of the school nurse, one must first realize that school health, like all health programs in the community, requires a great degree of collaboration (Brener et al., 2007). School nursing services are part of a coordinated school health program that provides school health services, health education, and health promotion programs for faculty and staff.

Liaison with the Interdisciplinary School Health Team

The nurse collaborates with counseling and psychological services, as well as physical education and nutrition services, working to provide a healthy school environment with family and community involvement (CDC, 2007a). Although the school nurse plays a central role, collaboration with many other individuals is important. The coordinated school health program includes eight components and involves a variety of professionals and other people ranging from teachers, administrators, and school staff to families. The components are:

- School health services (preventive services, referral)
- Health education (kindergarten through 12th grade curricula)
- Health promotion for faculty and staff (employee health)
- Counseling, psychological, and social services
- School nutrition services
- Physical education programs
- Healthy school environment
- Family and community involvement (partnership among school, families, community groups)

Positive Working Relationship with Administrators and Teachers

The school principal influences all phases of the school health program by promoting good school health through active support of the school's health services, participation in setting health-related policies, and tapping into community resources. The principal can reinforce positive efforts within the school, ranging from the health teaching in the classroom to the cleaning activities of the custodian. Because of the principal's influential position, it is absolutely essential for the nurse and principal to maintain a positive and cooperative working relationship.

Teachers, whether they are involved in regular instruction, physical education, or special education, play a major role in school health. Because they spend the most time with students, their observations, health teaching, and personal health habits have a profound effect on student health and the quality of school health services. The school nurse and teachers must collaborate constantly, as the school nurse provides information and guidance to teachers regarding students in their classrooms with specific health conditions and concerns and teachers report on students' health concerns and behaviors.

Other health team members, such as health educators, health coordinators, psychologists, audiologists, speech therapists, occupational therapists, physical therapists, counselors, health care providers, dentists, dental hygienists, social workers, security and juvenile justice personnel, health aides, and volunteers, may also be involved, depending on the size and financial resources of the school. All team members, including students, parents, bus drivers, and custodians, have a specialized role complementary to that of the school nurse. Consultation and referral among team members are crucial to the successful implementation of the school health program (Guttu, Engelke, & Swanson, 2004).

If the school system desires such services, a physician may work on a part-time consultative basis; however, fewer than 16% of school systems reported having a school physician (Brener et al., 2007). This role focuses largely on advising and consulting related to policy and medical-legal matters. A community physician may serve on a school advisory panel, acting as a liaison between the community, other health agencies, and the school. The physician or a nurse practitioner (NP) may become involved in student health appraisals, rescreenings, health problem interventions, sports physical examinations, or first aid support at sporting events.

Funding for school nursing comes from a variety of sources. School districts use support services funding for school nurses. Public health departments may also contribute funding, along with hospitals and other organizations. Federal Medicaid funding has been used to support some of the administrative and nursing services provided to children with special health care needs. Over the last 10 to 15 years, school districts have billed Medicaid for specific services provided in the school setting (e.g., case management of children with chronic illnesses such as diabetes and asthma). However, a recent ruling found that Medicaid funds were being misused and such reimbursement was stopped (USDHHS, Centers for Medicare and Medicaid, 2007). Many schools relied heavily on this funding, and school nurse positions will undoubtedly be eliminated if other funding is not forthcoming (NASN, 2007b).

RESPONSIBILITIES OF THE SCHOOL NURSE

The primary responsibilities of the school nurse are to prevent illness and to promote and maintain the health of the school community. The school nurse serves not only individuals, families, and groups within the context of school health, but also the school as an organization and its membership (students and staff) as aggregates. The school nurse identifies health-related barriers to learning, serves as a health advocate for children and families, and promotes health while preventing illness and disability (NASN, 2007a).

School nursing activities include care of children with special health needs, including nasogastric tube feedings, catheterization, insulin pumps, and suctioning; general and emergency first aid; vision, hearing, scoliosis, and TB screenings; height, weight, and blood pressure monitoring; oral health and dental education; immunization assessment and monitoring; medication administration; assessment of acute health problems; health examinations (especially for athletic participation or school entry); and referrals.

Other duties that a school nurse may have include training school staff in cardiopulmonary resuscitation (CPR), universal precautions, and first aid, and overseeing the health and wellness of school staff members. Many of these activities may be performed concurrently. See Display 30.5 for a typical day in the life of a school nurse. Each school nurse must assess and prioritize how to address the specific needs in each individual school and determine the order. This largely autonomous practice requires specific skills and training.

EDUCATION: SPECIAL TRAINING AND SKILLS OF THE SCHOOL NURSE

School nurses operate from one of two administrative bases: the school system or the public health department. In most localities, public or private school systems or districts hire school nurses, and they maintain a specialized, school-based practice. In this specialized role, the nurse can concentrate

DISPLAY 30.5	A DAY IN THE LIFE OF A SCHOOL NURSE

8:00 a.m. The nurse begins work at her assigned middle school. A parent brings in a controlled medication (narcotic) for her son who fractured his arm the day before. The school nurse works with the parent regarding the medication protocol of the school. The nurse advises that narcotics will affect the student's concentration and ability to learn.

8:15 a.m. Two students come into the office to take medications (dextroamphetamine [Dexedrine] and an antidepressant for concentration and focusing).

8:20 a.m. First acute illness of the day! A girl has vomited and is very nervous about being in middle school. The nurse calls home to learn that the student has been to her health care provider twice this week because of anxiety. The nurse helps to calm her and talk about the situation and then walks her back to class. The nurse talks to the teacher about the student's situation.

8:45 a.m. Three pupils come to the nurse's office complaining of sickness. The nurse assesses them and calls the parents to explain the situation and tells them of the current illness in the school.

9:00 a.m. A student arrives in the office holding her nose. She was playing volleyball when she collided with another student. She is afraid her nose is broken. The nurse assesses the situation, and determines that there is a possible fracture. The student's parents are contacted, and arrangements are made for the student to visit the doctor, where the diagnosis (fracture) is confirmed and the student is treated.

9:15 a.m. Nurse leaves the middle school and heads for her assigned elementary school (three blocks away). She has a meeting for an individualized education program (IEP). One student has attention deficit disorder and bipolar disorder, and so the student's parents and the educational team (which includes the school nurse) meet to determine how to best serve the student's needs while in school and set goals and objectives. The nurse's role includes educating teachers and staff about how to handle mood swings and outbursts. The nurse works with the student's health care provider regarding

medications and monitors the impact of the medications. The nurse also works with the parents regarding strategies and coping skills to use at home.

10:30 a.m. The nurse returns to the middle school and finds six students in her office. One has a bloody nose (and is applying pressure to stop the bleeding); two collided while in physical education class (and have ice on their heads); and three have fevers and upset stomachs and are waiting for parents to arrive. The students who have head injuries are assessed for concussions and neurologic concerns. Parents are contacted regarding signs to watch for when the students return home. One of the student's parents cannot be reached, so a note will be sent home with the same information.

11:00 a.m.–1:00 p.m. Lunch time! Ten students come in for their medications. Students arrive with playground injuries to assess and monitor, and parents return calls and arrive to sign out their children.

1:00 p.m. The nurse receives a call from the assistant principal requesting the nurse to come to the main office. A student has been found with cigarettes and lighters. The student is given information regarding smoking and drugs. The student lives with surrogate parents who need assistance in setting limits at home and at school.

1:30 p.m. All immunizations have been documented and entered for the year. The nurse prints the immunization report and identifies 177 students who are not up-to-date with state requirements. The nurse will need to contact and work with the parents of these students to help them achieve compliance. Students will not be allowed to return to school until the situation is resolved.

2:30 p.m. The nurse attends a meeting to create a behavior modification plan for a student who is having difficulty completing assignments.

3:00 p.m. The school day ends.

Adapted from Weirick, K. (2003). A typical day in the life of a school nurse. *New Mexico Nurse.*

time and effort solely on the school health program and develop specialized skills in school health assessment and intervention. Today, with the emphasis on delivery of health care at community sites where clients spend most of their time (e.g., schools for children, the workplace for adults), the nurse whose specialty is school health care seems better prepared to meet the complex needs of the school-age population.

In contrast, the school nurse who operates under the board of health's jurisdiction provides services to schools as one part of generalized public health nursing services to the community. The community health nurse working through the health department usually devotes only a portion of the workday to the school; she may have additional responsibilities, such as clinic nursing and home visits. This broader base

allows contact with preschoolers and their families, provides a stronger knowledge of the community and its resources, and promotes integration of in-school and out-of-school care.

Depending on the state of residence, a school nurse is usually an RN—frequently with additional education beyond the bachelor's degree in nursing, sometimes including a master's degree—who has primary responsibility for the health care of school-age children and school personnel in an educational setting. In some areas of the country, licensed practical nurses (LPNs) or licensed vocational nurses (LVNs) may be hired by school districts, but they must generally work under the supervision of an RN. *The Scope and Standards of School Nursing Practice* (2005) indicate that school nurses should, at minimum, possess a bachelor's degree. A school nurse functions as a promoter of health, an educator, counselor, advocate, manager, and deliverer of care (Brener et al., 2007). And these functions require a knowledge base derived from a baccalaureate nursing program. Many states (39.6%) require state school nurse certification and 29.2% of states have a policy indicating that school nurses must perform continuing education (Brener et al., 2007).

As the needs of school-aged populations become increasingly complex, some states require even more specialized training for school nurses. In California, for instance, school nurses are expected to hold a school health services credential. This credential is obtained through a post-baccalaureate program that includes a minimum of 24 semester units of course work in audiology, guidance and counseling, exceptional children, school health principles and practice, a practicum in school nursing, child psychology, and health curriculum development, in addition to other courses. However, most school nurse credential programs are now available only as part of a master's degree program. A national certification is available as well (*Careers in Focus,* 2006).

School nurse practitioners (SNPs) are RNs with advanced academic and clinical preparation (generally certification and a master's degree in nursing) along with a guided experience in physical assessment, diagnosis, and treatment, so that the SNP may provide primary care to school-age children. Many school districts see the advantage of having an SNP on staff, rather than using the limited services of a physician. Assessment, diagnosis, treatment, and referral of injuries, communicable diseases, or other health problems can be managed more efficiently by a NP who is educationally prepared to work holistically with the school-age population and is part of the educational setting. If this arrangement is impractical, an SNP who is available to school nurses for consultation or who is employed on a part-time basis can become the impetus for comprehensive school-based health services. Some school districts utilize SNPs to provide services to teachers and staff to promote wellness or to handle job-related injuries. Some research findings cite cost savings related to SNP services, as students and staff served by them experience fewer days of absenteeism (Perrin, Goad, & Williams, 2002).

As the population continues to become more diverse and the problems of children and their families grow in complexity, the school nurse with specialized training in school health, the education system, case management, and advanced practice nursing (e.g., NPs, clinical nurse specialists) becomes even more essential.

FUNCTIONS OF SCHOOL NURSING PRACTICE

The three main functions of school nursing practice are health services, health education, and promotion of a healthy school environment.

Health services include caring for individual students who have chronic conditions or acute situations, while at the same time thinking of the entire population and tracking trends. For example, the school nurse observes an increase in the number of students diagnosed with asthma and investigates ways to help all students with asthma. One way of doing this may be to organize an *Open Airways* course (developed by the American Lung Association) to assist students in identifying triggers and managing their own care. The goal of this course would be to decrease student asthma attacks.

Health Services for Chronic Conditions

The number of children afflicted with chronic diseases is rising, and 45% of those students are reported to have fallen behind in their schoolwork, whereas 58% are routinely reported absent from school (Guttu, Engelke, & Swanson, 2004). Commonly seen chronic problems include hay fever, sinusitis, dermatitis, tonsillitis, asthma, diabetes, seizure disorders, and hearing difficulties. In addition, acute illnesses such as stomachaches, headaches, colds, and flu are frequent complaints of school-age children. School nurses develop **individualized health plans (IHPs)** to ensure that students with special needs (e.g., chronic conditions) have these needs met. If these students attend the regular classroom, the plans may be known as **Section 504 plans**, named after the section of the Individuals with Disability Education Act that specifically allows for school accommodations with this population. For students in special education programs, nurses can coordinate IHPs with **individualized education programs (IEPs)** to develop health management goals for students. Medically fragile or technology-dependent students, who may require procedures such as suctioning or tube feeding, would have plans developed for *specialized physical health care procedures*. The four chronic conditions most often seen in school-age children are asthma, diabetes, seizures, and severe food allergies (Wolfe & Selekman, 2002).

Asthma

Asthma is the most common chronic disease of childhood. Although reports indicate morbidity and mortality from asthma has stabilized in the past few years, in 2006, an estimated 14% of children younger than age 18 were diagnosed with asthma (Bloom & Cohen, 2006). Non-Hispanic Blacks exhibit the highest asthma attack rates, and boys more often than girls reported an episode within the past year (Bloom & Cohen). Over half (54%) the children, ages 4 to 18, with asthma experienced school absences—missed "some school"—due to their asthma (Schulman, Ronca, & Bucuvalas, Inc. [SRBI], 2004). Children with asthma also tend to show comorbidities, such as depression and behavioral disorders (Blackman & Gurka, 2007). In such situations, school nurses work with students, their families, and their doctors to develop an *asthma action plan* to control, prevent, or minimize untoward effects of acute asthma episodes. Peak flowmeters can be used regularly to determine early signs of asthma problems. The activities of nurses acting as case managers have been found to decrease the number of emergency room visits and hospitalizations of school-age children with asthma (Levy, Heffner, Stewart, & Beeman, 2006).

Monitoring asthma medications and teaching proper methods of inhaler use are also vital school nursing functions. Many states (88%) allow students to carry quick-acting inhalers on their person (Brener et al., 2007). It often falls to school nurses to ensure that proper protocols and training are accomplished. A study of 19 school districts in North Carolina found a significant difference in outcomes for students with asthma in districts with a nurse-to-student ratio of more than one to 1,000 when compared to districts with a ratio of less than one to 1,000 (Guttu, Engelke, & Swanson, 2004).

Diabetes

Diabetes is another common chronic illness in young people: approximately 176,500 under age 20 have diabetes. This translates into one in every 400 to 600 children having type I diabetes (National Diabetes Education Program, 2006), and experts now conclude that both type 1 and type 2 diabetes mellitus are found in school-age children. One report estimates a 45% increase in adolescents with type 2 diabetes over the past 15 years (Pinhas-Hamiel & Zeitler, 2005). Type 2 diabetes is rising almost exponentially in adolescents, leading some scientists to frame it as a major public health crisis caused largely by obesity, sedentary lifestyle, and the predisposition to diabetes of certain ethnic groups.

Working with families and health care providers, school nurses assess and develop a care plan for diabetic students (Clark, Clasen, Stolfi, & Jaballas, 2002). School nurses work closely with the family to maintain confidentiality and at the same time ensure that the school is a safe environment for the child. A multidisciplinary team approach is needed, with family, school, and physician collaboration. Training for teachers and fellow classmates is also important. Teachers are often called upon to assist students with their insulin pumps or food management. Younger children with type 1 diabetes, especially those who use insulin pumps, may need careful monitoring—something that is not always possible for the school nurse, who may not be present where and when problems arise. If the child has an insulin reaction, fellow students should be taught to quickly get the teacher. A current initiative of the American Diabetes Association is to ensure that glucagon can to be administered by nonlicensed personnel, such as teachers (NASN, 2006b). However, many school nurses do not feel comfortable delegating this task or others like it. Delegation has become a safety issue that has reached many state boards of nursing and legislatures (Heschel, Crowley, & Cohen, 2005).

Testing blood sugar and taking insulin at school can be frustrating and can cause children to feel singled out or different from their peers. One study found that adolescents with type 1 diabetes have significantly higher rates of depression than those without diabetes (Guzman, 2004). Also, some schools do not permit blood sugar testing and insulin administration in classrooms, so that school health offices are often a place of refuge for diabetic students (Wolfe & Selekman, 2002). It is important for school nurses to understand each child's concerns and to alert teachers and school personnel to the signs and symptoms (as well as the treatment) of hypoglycemia. In addition to the obvious emergency health-related concerns for diabetic children, a classic study showed that diabetes-related severe hypoglycemia does affect memory tasks (Hershey, Bhargava, Sadler, White, & Craft, 1999). Over time, memory deficits can affect learning and progress in school.

Seizure Disorders

Seizure disorders are not uncommon in the school-age population. Epilepsy is a disorder of the brain in which neurons sometimes give abnormal signals. A person who suffers from epilepsy may have comorbidities including autism, depression, and anxiety (National Institute of Neurological Disorders and Stroke [NINDS], 2007). For almost 80% of those diagnosed, seizures can usually be controlled with medication (e.g., antiepileptic drugs specific to the pediatric population), surgical treatment, or a diet rich in proteins and fats and low in carbohydrates (a *ketogenic diet*) (NINDS, 2007).

It is important for school nurses to develop care plans to address seizure concerns during school hours. Care plans include monitoring medication compliance and teaching school staff about first-aid measures for seizure victims. Children and adolescents with seizure disorders may feel embarrassed or be the victims of teasing or bullying. They may exhibit signs of school avoidance. Nurses need to work with these children and to teach all students about the disease process and the need for empathy and understanding.

Food Allergies

The fourth leading chronic condition found in school settings is severe food allergies that can lead to anaphylactic shock. Such severe allergies result in approximately 30,000 emergency room visit each year (Food Allergy and Anaphylaxis Network, 2006). Eight common foods account for 90% of severe food allergies. They are fish, shellfish, soy, milk, egg, wheat, peanuts, and tree nuts (e.g., cashews, walnuts). Many common foods and school supplies (e.g., play dough) can contain hidden allergens, and care must be taken to prevent exposure. School nurses coordinate and work with students and their families, along with school personnel, to raise awareness and enlist caution. They also work with families and health care providers to ensure that epinephrine via an auto-injector (EpiPen) is available for the child in case of emergencies. Epinephrine reverses the body's allergic reaction to the allergen (Dey, 2008). Many states (66%) allow students to carry an EpiPen on their person because reactions can occur very quickly (Brener et al., 2007). School nurses coordinate and ensure that proper protocol is followed. School nurses also work with teachers and lunch room personnel to alert them of the allergy, explain what can happen in a case of anaphylaxis, and provide training on how to use the EpiPen or other needed medication.

Behavioral Problems and Learning Disabilities

Other often chronic childhood health problems are those of emotional, behavioral, and intellectual development. These are not always easy to detect and measure, and they can be debilitating. Although these problems are not new, awareness and concern have increased as the rates of occurrence for other life-threatening childhood diseases have diminished. Emotional or behavior problems and learning disabilities are prevalent during childhood, with approximately 22% of adolescents ages 14 to 17 years having a special health care need (Okumura, Pheeters, & Davis, 2007).

The causes of learning disabilities and emotional behavioral problems appear to have genetic, environmental, and cultural influences. The number of children with learning disabilities in the lowest economic group is twice that in the highest group (Bloom & Cohen, 2006). Children who were characterized as being in fair or poor health were more than five times as likely to have a learning disability and three times as likely to have attention deficit–hyperactivity disorder (ADHD) as children with excellent, very good, or good health status (Bloom & Cohen, 2006). High-risk children often come from families with a high incidence of child abuse (physical and sexual) and neglect. The number of children affected by parental drug use has surpassed that of children with disabilities caused by lead poisoning, another major contributor to developmental problems in children.

ADHD is a cluster of problems related to hyperactivity, impulsivity, and inattention (Dang, Warrington, Tung, Baker, & Pan, 2007). The CDC estimates 4.4 million school-age children between the ages of 4 and 17 have been diagnosed with ADHD (CDC, 2004). School nurses must be aware of the signs and symptoms and serve as an advocate for these children and their families. At each stage of development, those with ADHD are presented with distinct challenges. For example, children in elementary school may often have difficulty and conflict with peers, as well as problems organizing tasks. They may be more accident prone and may have more school-related problems, such as grade retention and suspension or expulsion.

They often have problems with grooming and with handwriting, and they exhibit difficulty sleeping. ADHD is sometimes found with associated disorders, such as communication or language disorders and learning disabilities. Common comorbid conditions are depression, anxiety disorders, and conduct disorders (Dang et al., 2007).

Behavioral and emotional problems of school-age children stem from many causes. School nurses can be alert to early symptoms and refer families for counseling. Some schools are also now offering support groups for children of divorce.

Collaboration is needed between the child's family, the school, and the child's health care provider to diagnose ADHD and effectively plan appropriate interventions and educational accommodations. Teacher confirmation of ADHD-related behaviors is very important. Numerous checklists and assessment tools are available, and school psychologists typically serve as a source for additional information and resources. School nurses can assist parents in recognizing the symptoms of ADHD and obtaining appropriate treatment and follow-up (Dang et al., 2007). A multimodal treatment approach may include stimulant medication, usually methylphenidate (Ritalin or Concerta), dextroamphetamine (Dexedrine) and amphetamine (Adderall), or antidepressants (such as Wellbutrin). Other treatment includes school accommodations for learning problems and social skills training for the child with ADHD (Dang et al., 2007). Family and individual counseling, parent support groups, and training in behavior management techniques, as well as family education about the condition, are also essential features of this method of treatment.

Not all children and adolescents respond to medication, and medication dosage must be carefully monitored and titrated. School nurses can assist parents in this task. The main goal of medication for school-age children is academic improvement. If this does not occur, medication may need to be changed or discontinued. School nurses and community health nurses can work closely with school staff, parents, and physicians in determining the efficacy of treatment regimens.

Medication Administration

Medication administration for a variety of conditions is an important responsibility for school nurses. In schools where a nurse is present every day, the nurse can personally oversee medication administration. Unfortunately, many nurses cover more than one school and so other school personnel (e.g., secretaries, health aides) oversee medication administration. Over half the states have laws allowing teachers or health aides to administer medication (Brener et al., 2007). In these situations, it is ideal for school nurses to provide training and audit records to ensure that proper guidelines are followed. Multiple studies show that medication errors increase when school nurses cover multiple schools and unlicensed personnel assist in medication administration (McCarthy, Kelly, & Reed, 2000; Ficca & Welk, 2005). Problems commonly occur with omission of doses because students fail to come to the office for medication administration. This is especially problematic with students taking insulin or antidiabetic drugs, antibiotics, and medication for ADHD.

Health Services to Prevent Illness and Injury

School nurses emphasize prevention, and focus many of their efforts on prevention of communicable disease (via immunizations) and of injuries.

Immunizations

Among schoolchildren, the incidence rates of measles (rubeola), rubella (German measles), pertussis (whooping cough), infectious parotitis (mumps), and varicella (chickenpox) have dropped considerably because of widespread immunization efforts, although these communicable diseases do still occur, and sometimes with serious complications such as birth defects from rubella and nerve deafness from mumps. Although the number of cases of *Haemophilus influenzae* infection and hepatitis B decreased between 2003 and 2004, there was an increase in the number of cases of pertussis, measles, mumps, and hepatitis A. In fact, during this time period (2003–2004), the number of pertussis cases was at its highest point since 1959 (Maternal and Child Health Bureau, 2006).

Low immunization levels in many areas, particularly among poor populations, and increased disease rates signal the need for constant surveillance, outreach programs, and educational efforts. School nurses are deeply involved in each of these preventive activities. Health departments and schools often work collaboratively to provide immunization services. Compulsory immunization laws for school entrance, which vary among states, have enabled public health personnel to carry out these preventive services. Nearly all states (94%) have a policy of excluding students from school if they are not adequately immunized (Brener et al., 2007). Only about 17% of states require TB skin testing before entering school.

School nurses often oversee and ensure that children are in compliance with school entrance laws regarding

EVIDENCE-BASED PRACTICE

School Nursing

A study was conducted to determine if the rates of absenteeism were lower at schools where students who received FluMist than at schools where students were not offered the treatment. FluMist was offered free of charge to students at the two experimental schools (64% compliance in school 1 and 46% compliance in school 2). Two other schools with school populations and attendance rates similar to the experimental schools were used as controls. Attendance rates were reviewed from all four schools once FluMist was offered. Those schools where students were offered FluMist statistically ($p < .001$) increased their attendance rates (95.3% to 96.1% and 93.9% to 95.8%) compared to the control schools' rates (94.6% to 94.4% and 94.6% to 94.7%). No significant differences were found in the number of absenteeism due to influenza. However this was self-reported and difficult to track. Wiggs-Stayner, Purdy, Go, McLaughlin, Tryzynka, Sines, and Hlaing (2006) concluded that on-site school immunization programs can be a positive primary prevention.

Nursing Implications

Although school nurses often work with individual children, they also look at the school community as a whole and should conduct interventions that will benefit the whole. School nurses must also collect data and determine the effectiveness of their treatments. Finally school nurses must also remember the goals of the institution in which they work (education) and strive to meet these goals (i.e., increased attendance) while at the same time protecting the public's health.

Reference:

Wiggs-Stayner, K. S., Purdy, T. R., Go, G. N., McLaughlin, N. C., Tryzynka, P. S., Sines, J. R., & Hlaing, T. (2006). The impact of mass school immunization on school attendance. *Journal of School Nursing, 22*(4), 219–222.

immunizations. They may call parents directly when they note that the student is out of compliance. They may also arrange to help the student get immunized by facilitating appointments or, in some school districts, providing the immunizations directly. The American School Health Association has developed a toolkit for school nurses and others to follow when developing successful immunization outreach programs in secondary schools where compliance is always difficult (Boyer-Chu & Wooley, 2006).

Safety

School nurses are also involved in ensuring that injury prevention efforts are encouraged. Emphasis on a healthful physical environment includes proper selection, design, organization, operation, and maintenance of the school building and playground equipment. Although no national

database collects information about school injuries, one study in Indiana found school injury rates of 2.5 per 100 students (Kaldahl & Blair, 2005).

Custodial personnel assist in the maintenance of school grounds, but school nurses must be aware of conditions and make recommendations to remedy unsafe situations. As school nurses provide first aid treatment for playground injuries they may observe trends (e.g., a high number of injuries where faulty playground equipment or other factors influence higher injury rates) and request action. When injury trends are noted, school nurses work with maintenance departments and administration to advocate change and prevent future injury. In addition, nearly half of the states have adopted a policy directing schools to complete a report when serious injury occurs on school properties (Brener et al., 2007). School nurses also assist with physical adaptations for students with special needs (e.g., ramps, electric doors); they work to ensure safety in and around schools; and they are mindful of visual, thermal, and acoustic factors in school buildings, as well as aesthetic values. Additionally, they promote sanitation and the safety of the school bus system as well as food services (Food-Safe Schools, 2004).

Health Education and Health Promotion

Another main function of school nursing practice involves education and health promotion. This includes planned and incidental teaching of health concepts and health curriculum development. In some states, school nurses even teach the regular health classes. Education may be one-on-one to help a child obtain better control over asthma or to explain to a newly diagnosed diabetic student what is occurring in his body. As an educator, the school nurse may also teach an entire class regarding a student's severe food allergy or the need for proper hand hygiene. The school nurse explains in simple terms what allergies are and helps students understand that allergies are not contagious, what to do in the case of an allergic reaction, and the importance of not sharing foods that may contain potential allergens (Wolfe & Selekman, 2002).

Because school nurses are trusted by students, students listen to them. Educational subjects are limitless, but should always apply to the specific needs of the children in the school. The nurse must use creativity and autonomy to identify and prioritize needs. A school nurse may also teach about basic first aid, nutrition, physical exercise, and seat belt safety, or provide information about careers in the health care professions.

In addition to lecture or verbal teaching, education may also be in the form of bulletin board notices, newsletters, or in-service presentations for educators and parents. These activities integrate health information with students' daily living experiences to build positive attitudes toward health and to establish sound health practices that will carry forward into adulthood.

Screenings: Opportunities for Teaching

Most local school districts provide some type of health screening services, usually through the school nurse or local health care providers. Although the goal of all screening is to promote early intervention, screening also provides the school nurse many opportunities to teach students and staff. Referral information resulting from screening results is usually given to parents, and school nurses may contact parents to encourage follow-through. Children who are not present for school screenings may not receive the benefits of these screenings (e.g., home schooled and private school students). School nurses often help to coordinate screening resources and benefits, and they often carry out additional screenings for students who were absent when mass screenings were held.

Vision

The 2006 School Health Policies and Programs Study (SHPPS) noted that 93.4% of reporting school districts offered vision screening (Brener et al., 2007). School nurses often oversee routine vision screenings at periodic intervals, so that vision problems that can interfere with learning may be detected and treated early (e.g., nearsightedness, farsightedness, strabismus, amblyopia). School nurses also are involved in follow-up to ensure that corrective eyewear is obtained. Local Lion's Clubs may be involved in paying for area optometrists to assist with or direct screenings or to provide follow-up care.

Hearing

Hearing screenings were reported by 92% of districts (Brener et al., 2007). These mass screenings are done to detect any serious hearing deficits that may be related to recurrent ear infections or some type of sensorineural hearing loss. (*Sensorineural hearing loss* involves the inner ear or the nerves leading from the inner ear. It is permanent and cannot be surgically or medically corrected [American Speech-Language Hearing Association, 2007]).

Miscellaneous Health Screenings

Height, weight, and sometimes blood pressure and cholesterol screenings are done on a regular basis to monitor normal growth and development and allow for early intervention with populations who are especially susceptible to hypertension and heart disease.

In some areas, scoliosis screening is also done, frequently during middle school years or in fifth grade, to permit early detection and referral for medical intervention (e.g,. bracing, surgery). Scoliosis may be congenital, but is often idiopathic (Lewis & Bear, 2002). Some 66% of districts reported performing scoliosis screenings (Brener et al., 2007). In Texas and some other areas of the country, acanthosis nigricans (hyperpigmentation from various causes, but sometimes a symptom of diabetes) screenings are being done to look for early markers of type 2 diabetes, especially in high-risk populations (Texas Department of Health Services, 2005).

Oral and Dental Health: Teaching and Referral

Dental caries affect more than half of school-age children and are the most common chronic disease for that age group. In 2006, about 7% of children ages 2 to 17 had unmet dental needs because their families could not afford dental care (Bloom & Cohen, 2006). An estimated 16.3 million children do not have any dental insurance, a rate 2.6 times greater than those who do not have medical insurance (Lewis,

Mouradian, Slayton, & Williams, 2007). Minority groups tend to have worst rates of dental caries. School days are lost to dental problems and dental visits, with poor children reporting almost 12 times more restricted-activity days from dental-related illness than children from families with higher incomes (CDC, 2005). The cost for dental services in 2006 was estimated to be $94 billion (CDC, 2007b).

School nurses can address dental health issues in a variety of ways. At a community level, they can educate the public about the benefits of dental fluoride treatments. They can advocate for fluoridation of drinking water, school-provided fluoride rinses or gels, and dental sealant programs. These are all cost-effective, proven methods of reducing dental caries in school-age children. At the classroom level, school nurses can provide dental education and provide toothbrushes, toothpaste, and floss to ensure that students are able to practice good dental hygiene habits. (Local organizations and businesses often will donate such supplies.) Many programs from the American Dental Association, the CDC, and other organizations provide resource materials. At an individual level, school nurses can assist in finding resources for those with no dental health insurance. Finally, school nurses can successfully educate parents, especially those who are immigrants or have different cultural beliefs, regarding the importance of oral and dental health (Brown, Canham, & Cureton, 2005).

Dental screenings or clinics may be conducted to determine the incidence of dental caries, especially in elementary school children, and to encourage follow-up with local dentists for necessary restorations. Only 29% of districts reported performing some type of oral health screening (Brener et al., 2007).

Promotion of a Healthful School Environment

A third function of school nursing practice includes maintaining and promoting a healthful school environment. Promotion of healthful school living emphasizes planning a daily schedule for monitoring healthful classroom experiences, extracurricular activities, school breakfasts and lunches, emotional climate, discipline programs, and teaching methods. It also includes screening, observing, and assessing to identify needs early and to report illegal drug use, suspected child abuse, and violations of environmental health standards. Health promotion involves the nurse in supporting the physical, mental, and emotional health of school personnel by being an accessible resource to teachers and staff regarding their own health and safety.

Proper Nutrition and Exercise

Many factors can affect the school environment—heating, cooling, lighting, safe playgrounds, and policies and practices to limit bullying and social aggression or other forms of school violence. The school cafeteria and physical education activities can promote health or contribute to obesity and sedentary lifestyles.

Obesity

Obesity rates have increased for all children. They have doubled for children between ages 2 and 5 and adoles-

LEVELS OF PREVENTION PYRAMID

HEALTH ISSUE: Obesity in a school setting

Tertiary Prevention

Rehabilitation

- Work closely with the child, family, physician, and teacher to decrease body mass index (BMI)

Primary Prevention

Health Promotion & Education

- Continue to promote healthy lifestyle choices and daily physical activity

Health Protection

Secondary Prevention

Early Diagnosis

- Conduct yearly screening of students' heights and weights to calculate BMI
- Complete health histories on at-risk children

Prompt Treatment

- Initiate referrals for health care provider follow-up in collaboration with parents of students at risk for obesity

Primary Prevention

Health Promotion & Education

- Limit passive activities and increase sports and physical activity
- Teach children how to make better food choices at fast food restaurants
- Educate children and teachers to promote good nutrition and a physically active lifestyle
- Promote a change of policy to take junk food out of vending machines

Health Protection

---

cents (ages 12–19) and tripled for those between ages 6 and 11 years. Approximately 9 million children over the age of 6 are considered obese (Institute of Medicine, 2005). Obesity-related hospital costs for children have tripled over the past two decades and have reached $129 million a year (Institute of Medicine, 2005). Obesity often begins in childhood and becomes a risk factor for cardiovascular disease and diabetes later in life. With the increase in child obesity rates, the number of children diagnosed with type 2 diabetes continues to rise. One report estimates a 45% increase in adolescents with type 2 diabetes over the past 15 years (Pinhas-Hamiel & Zeitler, 2005).

As children become older, families have less impact on food choices, and peers begin to have more influence. Results of the 2005 Youth Risk Behavior Survey (YRBS) indicate that 80% of those surveyed ate fewer than five servings of fruits and vegetables the day before the survey, and 84% drank fewer than three glasses of milk per day in the previous week (CDC, 2006).

School nurses can do many things to assist with the obesity epidemic. They can advocate for health and physical activity classes. Speroni, Earley, and Atherton (2007) found that a nurse-implemented program in the school decreased obesity among students. The 2005 YRBS revealed that 46% of children surveyed were not enrolled in physical education classes (CDC, 2006). Parents are supportive of increasing physical exercise and emphasizing nutritional foods in the school setting (Murphy & Polivka, 2007). A number of weight control programs for overweight children and adolescents are available through schools, health departments, community health centers, HMOs, and private groups.

Undernutrition

Poor nutrition and obesity are not uncommon among adolescents, whose diets often consist of snacks with limited nutritional value interspersed among unhealthful meals. *Undernutrition* can also have serious consequences, one being an impact on the academic performance of children. Irritability, lack of energy, and difficulty concentrating are only some of the problems that arise from skipped meals or consistently inadequate nutrition (Sweeney & Horishita, 2005). Infection and illness that lead to loss of school days can affect academic progress and interfere with the acquisition of basic skills, such as reading and mathematics. Undernutrition is frequently associated with poverty and hunger, but social pressure to be thin can also spark purposeful undernutrition.

School nurses can advocate for better nutritional choices in the lunch room and vending machines. This may include approaching the legislature to limit soft drink sales in public schools. They can also teach all grade levels regarding proper nutrition, and they can educate students and parents alike about nutritious snacks in contrast to snacks with little food value. School nurses may also work with staff to provide nutrition and exercise programs.

Eating Disorders

Eating disorders are another area of concern. Issues with body image and control are at the heart of *anorexia nervosa* and *bulimia nervosa*, common problems for adolescent girls. These diseases have emotional causes that pose complex challenges to treatment. School nurses must be aware of the signs and symptoms of eating disorders and be proactive in identifying students at risk. Scoliosis screenings are an optimal time to also observe for eating disorders, as examination of the spine allows for visualization of the body core. School nurses can work with students to develop a healthier self-concept and identify outside treatment resources (NASN, 2002).

Adolescent High-risk Behaviors

Mortality and morbidity rates for adolescents are low overall and demonstrate considerable improvement since the early 1900s. Many of the health issues that modern adolescents face are a result of their own choices and high-risk activity; for example, sexual activity, substance abuse, injury, and violence are all high-risk behaviors in which adolescents can choose to participate or not. The effects of such choices may not be discovered for many years. From 2003 to 2006, a good number of states developed policies to address alcohol and drug use (22% to 42%), sexually transmitted disease (STD) prevention (17.6% to 32%), suicide prevention (16% to 28%), and tobacco-use (19.6% to 40%) (Brener et al., 2007).

Sexual Activity: Teen Pregnancy and Sexually Transmitted Diseases

Sexual activity is a sensitive issue. However, the YRBS indicates that close to half of the 12th graders and one-third of all students who participated in the study were sexually active (CDC, 2006). Each year, about half of new STD cases in the United States occur among those between the ages of 15 and 24 (CDC, 2007c). The overall rates of syphilis, gonorrhea, chlamydia, human papillomavirus (HPV), and herpes simplex virus are climbing.

Providing STD services and HIV/AIDS education can be a daunting task. Young people with STDs are often afraid or embarrassed to seek help. Those who have been exposed to the HIV virus may not know that they are infected.

Although in some communities, the school-based clinic dispenses condoms, in other areas school nurses may be restricted in what safe-sex products they can provide. However, nurses *can* provide teens with education and with information about resources that are available outside of school property. School nurses can promote, at the local and state level, the HPV vaccine that guards against cervical cancer. They can also promote abstinence or delaying sexual initiation, as well as fostering safer-sex messages that promote the use of condoms. Sex education is effective at both delaying the onset of sexual activity and decreasing sexual activity in adolescents who are already sexually active. It is also effective in increasing safer-sex practices, knowledge of the efficacy of birth control methods, and overall sexual knowledge (Soloman & Card, 2004).

School nurses are sometimes restricted by state and/or district policies from addressing the issues of sex education and STD (including HIV) prevention. However, they can inform students and others in the community about the existence of multimodal youth development programs and family planning programs, which are often stationed strategically in inner cities, near schools, or in school-based clinics. These agencies are empowered to provide birth control information and counseling to young people.

Substance Abuse

Substance abuse among young people was almost unknown before 1950, and rare before 1960. Now, adolescent drug experimentation and use poses serious physical and psychological threats. By the time they complete high school, 20% of teens report having tried marijuana, 54% have used tobacco, and 74% have consumed alcohol (CDC, 2006). Over half (54%) of those who smoke have tried to quit, and 25% of those who have consumed alcohol tried it before they were 13 years old.

School nurses can assist in programs targeting all substance abuse. Successful programs focus on protective factors, instead of just high-risk behaviors. The programs focus more on the root causes, or why youth choose high-risk activities. When school nurses focus on developing and advocating for protective factors that assist youth to feel part of their community (Graves, Fernandez, Shelton, Frabutt, & Williford, 2005), they can help teens avoid the onset of substance abuse.

School nurses can also provide resources for smoking cessation and substance abuse programs. Hamilton, O'Connell, and Cross (2004) found that school nurses can be successful members of school smoking-cessation programs. In addition to school-based education, programs of peer leadership and parental education/involvement, and community-wide task forces have been developed to lobby for local legislation and strengthen community–school ties. School nurses can be advocates at a community level by lobbying the city council for tougher ordinances controlling advertising content and zoning (especially

LEVELS OF PREVENTION PYRAMID

HEALTH ISSUE: Cervical cancer

Tertiary Prevention

Rehabilitation

- Provide nursing support groups after hysterectomy and other treatment

Primary Prevention

Health Promotion & Education

Health Protection

Secondary Prevention

Early Diagnosis

- Promote regular Pap smears
- Provide Pap smear and high-risk screening counseling at local health fairs

Prompt Treatment

- Provide resources of medical services available for women diagnosed with cervical cancer

Primary Prevention

Health Promotion & Education

- Promote healthy lifestyle choices that will decrease risk of HPV (use of condoms, decrease tobacco use, food containing vitamin C and beta carotene)
- Provide HPV vaccine at appropriate age
- Educate public on risks related to cervical cancer (HPV vaccine, multiple sex partners)
- Educate women to get regular Pap smears

Health Protection

---

near schools). School nurses often work in conjunction with law enforcement officials, school district administrators, and other community agencies to ensure compliance with local regulations and prevent or delay tobacco use. Other groups, such as 4-H clubs, religious congregations, the Catholic Youth Organization, and Boy Scouts, use peer counseling to influence young people to assume responsibility for healthy lifestyles, with the goal of developing decision-making skills that lead to healthy lifestyle choices in adolescence and through adulthood. The school nurse participates in and supports existing programs in addition to counseling and referring young people who need help.

Mental Health Issues and Suicide

Depression, schizophrenia, and eating disorders may first appear during adolescence. It is estimated that one of 10 children suffers from a mental illness severe enough to impair them in some way (National Institute of Mental Health, 2008). Many adolescents are reluctant to seek help for emotional problems, or help may not be readily available to them. It is estimated that only one of five of those who need treatment actually receives it. Common mental health disorders in adolescence include anxiety, depression, ADHD, eating disorders, bipolar disorder, and schizophrenia (NIMH, 2008). Suicide is the third leading cause of death for young people between ages 15 and 24; it is the sixth leading cause of death in children between ages 5 and 14 (American Academy of Child & Adolescent Psychiatry [AACAP], 2004). In 2005, 20% of all high-school students reported that they had either seriously considered or attempted suicide in the past year (CDC, 2006). Girls attempt suicide more frequently than boys, but the actual suicide rate (those who successfully kill themselves) is higher among boys (AACAP, 2004). School nurses must be aware of the signs and symptoms of mental illness and suicidal intentions. They can work with school psychologists, social workers, and other mental health workers to address the needs of the students. They can also provide grief counseling to peers after a student commits suicide.

Abuse

In 2005, a total of 12 children in every 1,000 had substantiated reports of maltreatment, with younger children (0 to 13 years of age) at the greatest risk (Federal Interagency Forum on Child and Family Statistics, 2007). Girls tended to be maltreated more often than boys. Black, non-Hispanic youth were also at greater risk. Most victims suffered from neglect (USDHHS, 2008). Child abuse prevention education programs can be found in many school districts as a primary preventive intervention. School nurses are required by law to report suspected or confirmed cases of abuse. In addition, school nurses can educate teachers and other school personnel regarding the signs and symptoms of abuse. Abuse can also include issues related to bullying and school violence. For more information on health problems and issues concerning children and adolescents, see Chapter 22.

School-based Health Clinics

Because of the complex and intertwined emotional, physical, and educational needs of school-age children and adolescents, a more comprehensive interdisciplinary approach to services is needed than the piecemeal approaches attempted previously. School nurses are able to do much to influence school children's health. However, often they need to refer the children to a health care provider. Yet, more parents are working and less available to take care of their children's health care needs during the day. **School-based health centers (SBHC)** provide ready access to health care for large numbers of children and adolescents during school hours, reducing absences from school due to health care appointments. School-based health centers provide a variety of services in a user-friendly manner at a convenient location.

In 2005, there were more than 1,700 SBHCs in the United States, up from only 200 in 1990 (National Assembly on School-Based Health Care [NASBHC], 2007). These clinics are generally established inside the schools. They are distributed in high schools (39%), middle schools (18%), and elementary schools (23%). Some clinics provide services only to school children, whereas others extend services to their families and to other families with preschool-age children in the neighborhood. Most centers are open full time. Those located in middle or high schools may provide pregnancy testing and STD diagnosis and treatment, as well as birth control. However, many SBHCs do not provide contraceptive services on the school site because of school district policy or state law (NASBHC, 2007).

School-based health centers are staffed by interdisciplinary teams of helping professionals, paraprofessionals, and other staff and can include nurses, nurse practitioners, and social workers. Many hospitals, HMOs, and health departments are sponsors of these school clinics, because it is a cost-effective way to decrease visits to the emergency department and promote health, especially to underserved groups such as adolescents. Third-party billing, especially to access Medicaid funding, is increasingly more common among SBHCs, and private foundations have also been instrumental in providing financial and technical support.

School nurses support the clinics by referring students who need additional attention. In some areas, school-linked health centers are utilized. These clinics are not on school property, but may be nearby or easily accessible through mass transit. Schools refer students to these centers and have established collaborative, working relationships that promote information sharing and support.

Evaluation research has demonstrated that SBHCs are effective in increasing student access to health care. The majority (60%) of clients surveyed in Oregon indicated they would have not been able to receive care that day had it not been for the SBHC, and 68% said their health was improved due to the SBHC (Oregon State Government, 2007). School-based health centers also have been found to decrease absenteeism and school dropout rates of teenage mothers who attended the clinic (Barnet, Arroyo, Devoe, & Duggan, 2004).

SCHOOL NURSING CAREERS

School nurses must be able to work autonomously. They need excellent communication skills and the ability to prioritize and collaborate with many others. The pay for school nurses depends on location and employer (health department or school district). In some places, the wage may be lower than acute care nurses, but the health insurance and benefits package is usually quite extensive. School nurses are sometimes frustrated working in an educational setting, in which health may be a secondary priority, but their expertise is usually highly valued. In addition, school nurses may become involved with other issues in the school, such as violence prevention, that extend beyond the traditional role of the nurse.

There are many positive reasons to work as a school nurse: School nurses generally do not work on weekends, many have contracts that give them the summer off, and the daily work schedule and holidays often coincide with those of the nurse's own school-age children, thus allowing a parent to be home with children during off-school hours. Finally, for most of those employed as school nurses, it is a wonderful and rewarding experience to work with children whose eagerness and innocence can often refresh the soul. It is an opportunity to protect and heal our future leaders, who may become the ones who will protect and heal the world.

CORRECTIONS NURSING

Nurses who work within the criminal justice system—correctional facilities, prisons, jails, detention centers, substance abuse treatment programs—work with clients in a range of ages from juvenile to elderly, both male and female (ANA, 2007b). The facilities in which they work can hold just a few inmates or may house over 30,000 at one time (Office of Justice Programs [OJP], 2007). In 2006, there were 181,622 federal prisoners; 1,290,200 state prisoners; and 766,010 inmates in local jails, and the number of inmates is steadily rising (OJP, 2007). Tracking the number of nurses who work in correctional facilities is difficult. The last attempt, made in 2000, estimated the number to be 18,033 RNs (Spratley, Johnson, Sochalski, Fritz, & Spencer, 2002).

A great aspect of being a *school nurse* is being able to work with many different people. I like being able to work with people who aren't necessarily sick, but can benefit from my help. Additionally, school nurses must become familiar with resources and people in the community and surrounding areas. By making friends and connections in multiple facilities, occupations, and the like, school nurses can involve local resources as well as specific individuals in improving the population. That is an essential aspect to recognize: nurses shouldn't be alone in working with the community, they should involve as many people as possible, because community members should be active in improving their own area.

Unfortunately, working as a school nurse takes a lot of effort and is time-consuming. Even with the work that has been done at the school, it makes me wonder just how long our interventions will last. Unlike working in a hospital, where results come in just a few days, school nurses must work tirelessly for long periods of time to see the fruits of their labors. Resources aren't as readily available as they are for other types of nursing. Being a school nurse requires learning how to get funding for projects. School nurses often don't have models to work from, as each situation may be unique. They must be innovative, resourceful, and dedicated in order to stick with a project long enough for it to be beneficial to the population.

My overall opinion in working as a community nurse the past few weeks has changed. Being a school nurse has been hard, but rewarding. I know several students in my semester who don't really consider community nursing to be truly nursing practice. I would beg to differ; school nursing is probably the epitome of what nursing was meant to be. It is focused on service and improving the health and well-being of the populace. While nursing in the early days mainly dealt with fixing problems and injuries after they happened, everyone knows that an ounce of prevention is worth a pound of cure. Therefore, school nurses are doing the work that should benefit people the most. However, because their focus is on prevention, they seem to get little recognition for their work, since they are saving lives before they are endangered, they are saving teeth before they fall out, they are saving families before they are lost. I believe their work is pivotal to the improvement of society.

Neil P., School Nurse

HISTORY OF CORRECTIONS NURSING

Although the correctional system of prisons and jails has been around for a very long time, it historically provided minimal, if any, health care to inmates. Prison was a punishment, and the inmates were viewed as not deserving of care that was being paid for from public dollars. The situation did not change until 1976, when the U.S. Supreme Court issued its decision regarding *Estelle v. Gamble*. The Supreme Court ruled that not providing medical services inflicted pain and denied inmates their Eighth Amendment rights. This decision led to major reforms in the corrections health system. Medical providers were hired and inmates' rights were established. These rights included (ANA, 2007b, p 2):

- ◆ The right to access care
- ◆ The right to professional judgment
- ◆ The right to care that is ordered
- ◆ The right to informed consent
- ◆ The right to refuse treatment
- ◆ The right to medical confidentiality

Although the correctional health system is relatively new, it is under intense pressure from the courts to ensure that adequate and humane care is provided (ANA, 2007b). Several lawsuits have occurred, and unsolved issues in the correctional health care setting continue to be highlighted. Some main issues regard the provision of appropriate and timely patient care for inmates. Ensuring that inmates' health needs are met—along with the growing number of inmates and the increasing intensity of their health concerns—has imposed a huge financial burden on systems that are already overtaxed. Funding for correctional health care derives from public tax dollars. Keeping equipment up-to-date and avoiding shortcuts can be challenging. In an attempt to decrease costs and save money, most states utilize managed care organizations to provide some services for inmates. Correctional Medical Services (CMA) is the largest provider of prison health care in the nation. Some states may also utilize local HMOs (Restum, 2005).

Many institutions have a house clinic, medical unit, or infirmary. However, these clinics do not have the capability to provide all the services inmates may need. For example, if imaging procedures, such as magnetic resonance (MRI) or computed tomography (CT) scans are needed, or specialty consultations required, inmates must go to other sources outside of the prison or jail. In these instances, most corrections' facilities use managed health care systems.

Corrections nurses work in onsite medical units housed in criminal justice facilities. These facilities can be local jails, or may be at state and federal prison. The staff members in these units focus on the individual, immediate, and ambulatory care needs of the patients. They also attend to emergency needs and may help manage chronic conditions. They often provide screenings and preventive services. Corrections nurses have the potential to assist inmates to obtain optimal health and thus save taxpayer dollars.

The challenge of corrections nursing is to maintain the fundamental nature of nursing in a challenging environment that is not primarily focused on health care, and to remain nonjudgmental toward clients (ANA, 2007b). Today, corrections nurses work with a variety of clients.

Demographically, inmates differ from the general population. First, inmates have all committed some type of crime, with nearly half (52%) being violent crimes (OJP, 2007). National statistics indicate a larger portion of Black (3,042 per 100,000) and Hispanic (1,261 per 100,000) male inmates than White male inmates (487 per 100,000). Although males are still the majority population (88.6%), trends show an increase in the number of women in state or federal prisons (OJP, 2007). In addition, the inmate population is drawn disproportionately from lower socioeconomic backgrounds when compared with the general public. This increases their chances of having a long trajectory of poorer access to health care and treatment. Statistics show a greater disproportion of inmates who are chronically ill and have infectious diseases than the nonincarcerated population (ANA, 2007b).

EDUCATION

The preferred educational level for corrections nurses is a bachelor's degree. The level of skill, judgment, and autonomy needed by nurses who work in corrections is supported and developed within baccalaureate education. Some institutions may require additional coursework in criminal justice, decision-making, assessment, and administrative skills. Master's level nurses (specifically NPs) also are working in corrections, providing primary health care to inmates. National certification, through the National Commission on Correctional Health Care (NCCHC) as a certified correctional health professional (CCHP) or the American Correctional Association (ACA) as a certified corrections nurse (CCN), is available (ANA, 2007b).

FUNCTIONS OF CORRECTIONS NURSE

The prime responsibility of the corrections nurse is to restore and maintain the health of inmates by providing nursing care within correctional settings (ANA, 2007b). The work location does set corrections nurses apart as being the only nurses who enter their workplaces through metal detectors and grill gates and into a locked-down unit (FitzGerald, 2007). Yet, the knowledge and skill set of corrections nurses overlaps the knowledge and skill sets of many other nursing specialties.

Corrections nurses use public, community, and school health nursing skills, along with skills acquired from the emergency room, occupational health, mental health, orthopedics, and ambulatory care specialties. Like public, community, and school health nurses, corrections nurses are autonomous and must make decisions on their own. They track and screen for communicable diseases. They assist in setting up resources so that inmates who are released can continue getting medical treatment. They also educate inmates and promote healthful lifestyles among them.

Corrections nurses often work in clinic settings, assisting the health care provider in assessing medical situations. They review sick call requests to determine what and if any action needs to be taken, and by whom (nurse or physician). They may also oversee the medical unit beds that house patients who suffer from a variety of conditions, such as neurotrauma requiring critical care or kidney disease requiring dialysis. They provide nursing care for inmates with uncontrolled diabetes, those with pneumonia needing IV antibiotics, inmates with mental health issues, or those undergoing withdrawal ("detox") from years of substance abuse (Laffan, 2005). They participate in administering medications, as many inmates receive a variety of medications. In addition, by law, inmates must have a physical assessment within 14 days of admittance. Corrections nurses often perform these assessments. Corrections nurses also provide assessment and assistance in occupational safety issues.

Finally, corrections nurses are called upon to assist in medical emergencies, anywhere in the facility, such as helping with an accident in a woodshop or evaluating an inmate too sick to leave his cell. If inmates need to go to a hospital or appointment outside the correctional facility, a correctional officer generally accompanies them, not the nurse. With so many responsibilities and the uncertainty of new issues, it is imperative for corrections nurses to prioritize their day (see Display 30.6).

Several common health concerns face corrections nurses. These concerns are mental health, drug abuse, and communicable diseases. As the inmate population grows, an increase in elderly and female inmates creates additional health concerns for correctional nurses. The following sections briefly describe some of these concerns, along with examples of what corrections nurses may do to address the issue.

Mental Health Issues

The increasing number of inmates over the years may be attributed to the deinstitutionalization of individuals with mental illness in the 1970s. For example, in 1970, 368,000

PERSPECTIVES
VOICES FROM THE COMMUNITY

The prison is, in my opinion, a very good place to work. I believe that every student should experience nursing within corrections. I have worked floor nursing before, and working at the prison is much better. Although it can get crazy and chaotic from time to time, the atmosphere is much more laid back. Nurses at the prison seem to have a lot more autonomy than do nurses at other facilities or companies. The prison offers nurses a chance to experience many different skills. . . . You might not gain absolute proficiency in any one skill, but you will gain many skills, and you will become very good at many of them. The nice thing is that nurses come from many different backgrounds, and so they can and will certainly help you and teach you what they know to help with your own skill base. I guarantee that if you work at the prison, you will get to see and experience things that people in normal society will never get the opportunity to see. Come to the prison, and you will get to be a medical nurse, a psych nurse, a triage nurse, an orthopedic nurse, and you can get to do the medical/psychiatric intake screenings for all the new or parole violation inmates who come to the prison on a daily basis. There is probably more, but certainly keep your minds and options open for a great and secure career.

Travis H., correctional nurse

DISPLAY 30.6   A DAY IN THE LIFE OF A CORRECTIONAL NURSE

A day in my life depends on whether or not I am working at the infirmary or on the forensic unit. I will begin with the prison's infirmary.

I work 12-hour day shifts, so my day begins at 0600 and ends at 1830. As on any nursing unit or floor, I take report from the night shift charge RN. Within our infirmary, we have both a medical side and a psychiatric side where report is given. Following report, I decide with the other nurses whether or not I am going to be responsible for the medical or psychiatric patients, or the walk-ins (acute/emergency care patients). If I, for instance, take the medical side for the day, I will set up the medications and then wait for the other nurse to set up his or her medications for the psychiatric in-patients. We usually do what we call "pill line" together. Following pill line, I return to the nursing station and do my charting. Currently, we have a quadriplegic and paraplegic on our medical side who require a lot of personal care. We also have recently had several patients with MRSA (methicillin-resistant *Staphylococcus aureus*) requiring fairly extensive dressing/packing changes along with IV antibiotics. So with this in mind, following my charting, I will have officers escort the MRSA patients out to a trauma bed in order for me to perform the dressing change and/or administration of IV antibiotics (usually Vancomycin) that take 1 to 2 hours to complete. Following care, these inmates return to their medical cells, and I do my usual charting. The quadriplegic and paraplegic inmates have call lights, so I have to attend to their needs when called. This may consist of feedings, diaper changes, and repositioning. Depending on the day, I will administer showers or bed baths for them. We also currently have an inmate with Parkinson's disease and comorbid psychiatric disorder and neuropathy, who also requires a great deal of care. These are the types of inmates for whom we try to get compassionate releases, so that they can be sent out to nursing homes. Unfortunately, that has not happened yet. I say that because we are not staffed for this kind of care. With this kind of patient care, I tend to remain quite busy. Fortunately for me, the other nurses are very kind and help me along the way. Usually the nurse who does the psychiatric side does not have quite the "hands-on" patient care, and is usually very happy to help. In fact, we all help each other with our respective areas. Even though I am responsible for the medical in-patients, I still might take a walk-in or two and do some of the "q30-minute checks" on the psychiatric side. At the end of the day, I make sure that all my charting is done and then go on my way. There is quite a bit more actually involved, but it is difficult to explain all the situations that may develop.

On the forensic unit, I show up once again at 0600 and take report from the night RN. On this unit I, along with our one LPN, am responsible for passing all the medications and performing all the blood sugars and insulin administrations for the diabetics in the morning, noon, and afternoon. I have to perform an extensive mental health note on all the inmates in the maximum-security unit of this building, which consists of 10 to 12 inmates on average. I then have to do a less extensive mental health nursing note on all the inmates in our B-section bottom tier, which consists of approximately 20 to 24 inmates. Following all my charting, I enter in all the diabetic care and scan all the medications passed on our electronic MAR (medication administration record). Following all of these duties, I usually make sure that all the medications are current and check for any expired critical medications that might need reordering. I may have to do some blood draws and give some shots for those inmates on forced medications. I consider this unit more of a nursing management unit rather than a hands-on patient care unit.

I decided to work at the prison for a number of reasons. First, I began my nursing career at the state hospital and once I got sucked into the state system, I felt like working for the state throughout my career would be a very beneficial decision for me and for my family. The state offers great benefits, security, and a very good retirement. In the process of receiving my RN degree, I worked with a preceptor at the prison and enjoyed the opportunities that it offered. I really enjoyed the staff and the experience that they brought to the environment. Second, the environment was one in which I found a great deal of interest. During my clinical rotations at the prison, I was exposed to a world that many other people don't have the opportunity to experience. The prison environment certainly is not for everyone, but I felt it was for me. Once I received my RN license, I transferred from the state hospital to the prison, along with all my same benefits. Third, I love mental health nursing and that is what I am currently specializing in at the university. I am in my second year in the psych APRN program. It may sound strange that I just didn't stay at the state hospital, but I really wanted to gain the variety of medical experience the prison had to offer—on top of the mental health experience I already had. Once I graduate with my psych APRN, I plan to stay and retire after 20 years—which will only be about 12 more years—then teach perhaps until I fully retire and golf!

Travis H, Corrections Nurse

---

beds were available for mental health services, but by 1992 only 84,000 remained (ANA, 2007b). Many people suffering from mental illness were left without assistance or support. As a result, they became homeless and, in many cases, committed crimes.

Mental health is a major concern in correctional facilities. Mental health problems affect inmates three to five times more than they do people in the general population (Heines, 2005). At least half of all inmates have some type of mental health problem (James & Glaze, 2006). Those who suffer from mental illness are three times as likely to have been physically or sexually abused in their lifetime, and 4.5% of state and federal inmates experience at least one incident of sexual victimization by staff or other inmates while in prison (Beck & Harrison, 2007). At a state level, more than 70% of females and 55% of males in state prisons had some type of mental illness, and those with mental illness tended to have longer sentences (James & Glaze, 2006). That 74% of state inmates and 76% of local inmates with mental health concerns also suffer from substance abuse complicates the matter. Mental illness also impacts suicide rates. In 2002, the suicide rate in local jails (47 per 100,000) was three times higher than the rate in state prisons (Mumola, 2005). Inmates who committed violent crimes were twice as likely to commit suicide as those convicted of nonviolent crimes.

Corrections nurses provide a good deal of mental health nursing care and assist in identifying undiagnosed conditions. James and Glaze (2006) found that one in every three state inmates and one in every six local jail inmates indicated that he had received mental health treatment upon admission. A post-arrest diversion program, in which detainees can visit a psychiatrist within 24 hours of entering jail, has reduced recidivism from 70% to 19%, saving $2.5 million per year (Heines, 2005). A pre-arrest diversion program that trains police officers to identify persons with mental illness has also been successful in assisting with treatment and avoiding arrest.

Correctional nurses assist in multiple medication administrations per day to ensure that inmates receive the medications needed for their mental illnesses. They can also provide counseling regarding medication usage and assist inmates in understanding the side effects of their medication, which for some are many. Corrections nurses advocate for medication changes when they note severe side effects or a change in the mental status of inmates. Nurses can facilitate setting up medication support groups to allow inmates an opportunity to discuss concerns regarding their medications. They also can assist inmates in understanding the importance of taking their medication.

As inmates prepare to leave the institution, corrections nurses assist in finding outpatient mental health clinics and other resources that will provide support and further treatment for the inmate. Finally, corrections nurses can provide education and training to other corrections workers regarding signs and symptoms of mental illness and the impact mental health has on decision-making and the general health of a person.

Drug Abuse

Drug abuse by inmates is very high. Mumola and Karberg (2007) estimate that half of all federal prison inmates used drugs, which is a 5% increase from 1997. Female drug use increased by 11% during this same period. All types of drug use increased, except crack cocaine, which declined from 25% in 1997 to 21% in 2004. Drug treatment programs are essential in correctional facilities. Corrections nurses can assist in identifying those in need of the treatment and assessing their willingness to participate. Of the drug users in prison, 40% of state and 49% of federal inmates had participated in treatment programs (Mumola & Karberg, 2007). Corrections nurses also provide nursing care as patients withdraw from substances while in prison. Withdrawal can cause life-threatening symptoms that need immediate medical attention.

EVIDENCE-BASED PRACTICE

Corrections Nursing

Smith, Gates, and Foxcroft (2006) conducted a literature review to determine if therapeutic communities (TCs) effectively change behavior better than other substance abuse programs. TCs are commonly used in the prison setting as treatment for drug users. The authors searched numerous databases including MEDLINE, Psychinfo, CINAHL, SIGLE, EMBASE, and the Cochrane Central Register of Controlled Trials. Selection criteria for the review included randomly controlled studies (considered the gold standard of research) that compared TCs with other treatment, no treatments, or other types of TC. Seven studies were found to meet the criteria. The studies were difficult to compare due to the diverse populations being compared (TC versus community residence programs; residential versus day TC programs; standard TC versus abbreviated TC; TCs versus no treatment; TC versus mental health treatment). Of these seven studies only two were conducted in a prison setting. The results of both studies indicate that those who participated in TCs had fewer reincarcerations when compared with the comparison group (no treatment in one study and mental health treatment in the other study). However, Smith and colleagues concluded that minimal evidence exists to support TCs over other types of residential treatment programs. However, methodology and minimal numbers of studies contributed to the lack of comparable evidence.

Nursing Implications

It is important for nurses in any setting to know if the treatment they provide is based on evidence and is effective. It is inappropriate and unprofessional for nurses to perform activities and treatment just because it traditionally has always been done. It is also important for nurses to evaluate current treatment programs to ensure they are the most effective treatment available.

Reference:

Smith, L.A, Gates, S., & Foxcroft, D. (2006). Therapeutic communities for substance related disorder. *Cochrane Database Systems Review, 1,* CD005338.

In addition, corrections nurses can organize and provide support groups to assist inmates in staying sober and drug-free. They can advocate for the inclusion of Alcoholics Anonymous, Narcotic Anonymous, and Al-Anon services in the correctional facility. Counseling can be offered to assist inmates as they leave the facility, so that they do not return to prior bad habits if and when they return to areas where drug and alcohol use is rampant (Restum, 2005). Returning to this environment increases their chances of returning to substance abuse, and inmates leaving prisons or jails need to be connected to outside resources.

LEVELS OF PREVENTION PYRAMID

HEALTH ISSUE: Sexually transmitted disease (STD) in correctional facilities

Tertiary Prevention

Rehabilitation

- Work closely with inmates and physician to decrease side effects of STD (i.e., cervical cancer)

Primary Prevention

Health Promotion & Education
- Continue to promote responsible sexual behavior

Health Protection

Secondary Prevention

Early Diagnosis

- Provide STD screening upon entering facility
- Provide regular, routine STD screenings

Prompt Treatment

- Provide treatment for inmates diagnosed with STDs
- Promote facility policies that allow for STD screenings and early treatment

Primary Prevention

Health Promotion & Education

- Teach inmates how STDs are transmitted and what can be done to stop transmission (condoms, other preventive measures)
- Teach signs and symptoms of commonly occurring STDs
- Teach that gonorrhea and chlamydia are often asymptomatic, and so routine screening is important for individuals at risk

Health Protection

Communicable Disease

Several communicable diseases are of great concern in the correctional community. These include STDs including HIV/AIDS, TB, and hepatitis C. The concern of communicable disease is not only for the health of the inmate with the disease, but the susceptibility of all inmates, and ultimately the general public (if the inmate is released while still infected). Increased rates of these diseases are due to high-risk behaviors and increased rates of abusive behaviors, including rape (Restum, 2005).

A hallmark study, conducted by the RAND Corporation, indicated that inmates were four times as likely to have active TB, nine to ten times as likely to have hepatitis C, and five times as likely to be infected with HIV as the general population (Davis & Pacchiana, 2003). Data from the end of 2005 indicated that 18,953 male and 1,935 female inmates in state prisons have HIV/AIDS, and 176 state inmates died from AIDS (Maruschak, 2007). On a positive note, the rates of HIV infection have been steadily declining among inmates since 1999. The number of inmates suffering from

hepatitis C varies, but is estimated to be between 20% and 40% (Marcalino, Dhawan, & Rich, 2005). Inmates are at risk for hepatitis C because of the heavy drug use among prisoners.

Tuberculosis is widespread among prisoners and rates are much higher than in the general population. In 2003, TB rates of federal prison inmates were 6.9 times greater than the rates in the general public for a variety of reasons (MacNeil, Lobato, & Moore, 2005). Because many inmates are homeless and abuse alcohol and/or drugs, they are more susceptible to TB; to compound the problem, the closeness of living conditions in jails and prisons facilitates the quick spread of TB (Restum, 2005).

Correctional nurses must track rates of communicable diseases and provide education regarding the spread and treatment of those diseases. They must provide data on the number of cases of reportable diseases to the state health department. Corrections nurses can provide preventative care by offering immunizations to inmates. In addition, they can provide the necessary treatment for TB, STDs, and other diseases, and can assist in advocating for measures to decrease the spread of disease within correctional facilities.

Corrections nurses can assist institutions by providing initial screenings upon arrival of inmates and periodic screening for certain diseases. Beck and Maruschak (2004) found that 66% of state facilities had policies for regular hepatitis C screenings. However, these screening should not necessarily be for only those high at risk, such as drug abusers. Marcalino, Dhawan, and Rich (2005) found 66% of those who tested positive for hepatitis C did not report drug use. Screening based on risk may miss many of these inmates. Although female inmates are traditionally screened for *Chlamydia*, Tebb and colleagues (2005) found that a successful screening program tests for *Chlamydia* among adolescent males as well.

Corrections nurses can also evaluate inmates for complications, such as retinal hemorrhage and liver problems, especially in those suffering from hepatitis C (Heines, 2005). For chronic communicable diseases, such as HIV/AIDS, corrections nurses can facilitate and organize peer educator groups. These have been found to be successful in educating inmates on HIV/AIDS, substance abuse, and low self-esteem (Heines, 2005).

Successful programs also exist to assist inmates as they prepare for release. Corrections nurses can facilitate programs that empower inmates not to return to behaviors that increase their chance of contracting HIV (Myers, Zack, Kramer, Gerdner, Rucobo, & Costa-Taylor, 2005). Corrections nurses can also identify resources for inmates suffering from TB, so that they can continue their medication and treatment upon their release.

Future Trends

Due to advances in health care, longer prison terms, and more restrictive policies, inmates are older, sicker, and remain in prison longer than they did even 20 years ago. And historically, inmates have not taken good care of themselves. Hence, a 50-year-old inmate may have the health of a typical 65-year-old in the general public (ANA, 2007b). This surge in the inmate population is creating a lack of resources and beds for the aging inmate population.

Corrections nurses can increase efforts to empower inmates to take control of their health and can provide them with resources for health care access outside the prison, so that inmates will continue their care upon release. Corrections nurses can also be advocates and lobby state and federal legislatures to allocate funding for the additional resources needed within the prison system.

The female inmate population is also increasing. In addition to women's reproductive health issues, females tend to have higher rates of diabetes, HIV, STDs, mental illness, drug abuse, and emotional issues (ANA, 2007b). One study indicated that female inmates were also more likely to develop cervical cancer due to a lack of cancer screenings when in prison (Magee, Hult, Turalba, & McMillan, 2005). Corrections nurses can begin providing routine cervical and breast cancer screenings for female inmates. They can also provide counseling and emotional support.

Chronic disease, such as diabetes, heart disease, and asthma, are also increasing in the incarcerated population. Corrections nurses can facilitate chronic disease clinics to educate and empower inmates to better control their chronic conditions. To this end, corrections nurses need to conduct thorough family health histories, as many health conditions tend to have a genetic component, and employ screenings to identify conditions as soon as possible, so that early intervention can decrease complications and stop disease progression. They can follow-up by promoting better nutrition and exercise habits, and medication management.

CORRECTIONS NURSING CAREERS

Corrections nurses must have good mental health and assessment skills. They must be able to communicate well and be strong nursing advocates and strong advocates for their clients. They work in an intense environment where their safety could be threatened, and they must deal with clients who may be noncompliant, combative, and manipulative. Corrections nurses must also be very flexible and knowledgeable about a variety of nursing specialties.

Salaries depend upon the state, although they tend to be higher salaries than in other nursing fields. Moreover, corrections nurses usually receive extensive employee benefits and insurance packages as government employees. Despite this, nursing shortages still occur (California Department of Personnel Administration, 2005). Corrections nurses have the ability to see amazing and awe-inspiring recoveries from illnesses and injuries because they work with the same patients for a longer time than hospital-based nurses. Correctional nursing provides an opportunity to work with a vulnerable population and practice the true art and science of nursing. You use every nursing skill you have learned and advocate for a population that is in need. It is a challenging, rewarding career.

Summary

Nurses who work in public settings are critical to the health and well-being of their communities. Public health nursing interventions are essential in keeping our nation healthy. They may not be as visible as hospital nurses, who interact with each patient in the hospital, because PHNs often work from behind the scenes. Those who come in contact with them directly know of their worth, but much of the general population remains unaware of the role and the need for PHNs. Public health nurses deal with a number of issues including communicable diseases, chronic diseases, injuries, STDs, and substance abuse. They work with all ages, ethnicities, socioeconomic groups, and populations. Their emphasis is on health prevention and promotion.

School nurses work with school populations including students, their families and the school staff. They provide individual care and are the bridge between medical providers and schools. School nurses provide health care services, such as direct nursing care, first aid, and specialized health care for children with special needs. They also provide health protection measures such as immunizations and environmental assessments. Finally, school nurses provide health promotion activities including education, health screenings, immunizations, and staff wellness programs. School-based clinics are another means of providing care for the school population. Children and adolescents are important population groups for community health nurses because their physical and emotional health is vital to the future of society and because they require guidance and direction.

Corrections nurses work with inmates in federal, state, or local facilities, including drug treatment and juvenile detention centers. They provide individual care in facility clinics and infirmaries, while also identifying and developing programs to address major health concerns of inmates, including mental illness, drug and alcohol abuse, and communicable diseases. The inmate population is growing older, staying longer, and suffering more from chronic disease. This, along with an increase in female inmates, brings additional challenges for corrections nurses.

All three specialty areas impact the health of our communities. Due to the high level of nursing knowledge, communication skills, autonomy, and leadership needed for these nursing specialties, entry level should be at least a baccalaureate degree. Community nurses who work in public settings provide a valuable service needed to keep our nation healthy. ■

ACTIVITIES TO PROMOTE CRITICAL THINKING

1. As a government employee, a PHN must be careful not to lobby as part of her work duties. However, knowing the greatest health concerns of the population, how can PHNs serve as advocates for their clients (i.e., population) while remaining politically neutral?

2. What is the major cause of death among adolescents and children? What community-wide interventions could be initiated to prevent these deaths? Select one intervention and describe how you and a group of community health professionals might develop this preventive measure in your community. (Think outside the school setting.)

3. As a correctional nurse, you deal with people from a variety of backgrounds, social classes, and past crimes. How can your values and attitudes toward criminal activity impact your treatment of inmates? Does social class, race, age, or gender make any difference in how you feel about them?

4. One of the concerns expressed by correctional facility nurses is the antisocial behavior and manipulativeness of inmates, along with potential violence. How can a nurse working in a state prison effectively determine the health care needs of inmates?

5. Discuss possible methods of doing nutritional assessments in school-age children. What programs could be instituted to encourage healthier diets and increased exercise? What other factors might need to be considered? How could you, as a school nurse, work with schools and parents to increase physical activity and improve nutrition for school-age children and adolescents?

6. Describe possible benefits of school-based health centers (SBHCs). What are the most common mis-perceptions? What are frequent barriers to starting SBHCs? What steps can community health nurses take to promote community awareness and facilitate development of SBHCs in local schools?

7. Many of the chronic diseases plaguing society are attributable to people's behavior (such as eating habits, lack of exercise, tobacco use, etc.). Within your clinical group, debate the pros and cons of passing laws that restrict a person's right to behave as they wish, even if it impacts the overall population (increasing health care costs for all).

8. Most schools require that children entering school show proof of being fully immunized for a variety of communicable diseases. With a partner, discuss what would happen if schools no longer had this requirement. How else can immunizations be reinforced in the public?

9. Do you think that schools should require children with behavioral problems to be evaluated and required to take medication? Should taking that medication be a condition of their continuing enrollment? Who should pay for that evaluation and medication?

10. Many prisoners suffer from mental illness. List types of programs and/or support groups that the nurse could provide for these inmates. What about inmates not formally diagnosed with a mental illness?

11. Should inmates be required to pay for their health care (via work programs or other options) while in prison? Would it make them more accountable?

References

Abrams, S.E. (2005). Changing times, changing needs, changing programs. *Public Health Nursing, 22*(3), 267–268.

American Academy of Child & Adolescent Psychiatry. (2004). *Fact sheet: Teen suicide.* Retrieved August 11, 2008 from http://www.aacap.org/page.ww?name=Teen+Suicide&section=Facts+for+Families.

American Nurses Association (ANA). (2007a). *Public health nursing: Scope and standards of practice.* Silver Spring, MD: Nursesbook.org.

American Nurses Association (ANA). (2007b). *Corrections nursing: Scope and standards of practice.* Silver Spring, MD: Nursesbook.org.

American Nurses Credentialing Center. (2008). *Clinical nurse specialist in community/public health.* Retrieved August 11, 2008 from http://www.nursecredentialing.org/cert/PDFs/CNS_PublicCommunity.pdf.

American Speech-Language Hearing Association. (2007). *Type, degree, and configuration of hearing loss.* Retrieved August 11, 2008 from http://www.asha.org/public/hearing/disorders/types.htm.

Atkins, R.B., Williams, J.R., Silenas, R., & Edwards, J.C. (2005). The role of public health nurses in bioterrorism preparedness. *Disaster Management Response, 3*(4), 98–105.

Barnet, B., Arroyo, C., Devoe, M., & Duggan, A.K. (2004). Reduced school dropout rates among adolescent mothers receiving school-based prenatal care. *Archives of Pediatric and Adolescent Medicine, 158*(3), 262–268.

Beaudoin, C.E., Fernandez, C., Wall, J.L., & Farley, T.A. (2007). Promoting healthy eating and physical activity: Short-term effects of a mass media campaign. *American Journal of Preventive Medicine, 32*(3), 217–223.

Beck, A.J., & Harrison, L.M. (2007). *Sexual victimization in state and federal prisons reported by inmates, 2007* [NCJ 219414]. Bureau of Justice Statistics Special Report. Retrieved January 8, 2008 from http://www.ojp.usdoj.gov/bjs/pub/pdf/svsfpri07.pdf.

Beck, A.J., & Maruschak, L.M. (2004). *Hepatitis testing and treatment in state prisons* [NCJ 199173C]. Bureau of Justice Statistics Special Report. Retrieved January 8, 2008 from http://www.ojp.usdoj.gov/bjs/pub/pdf/httsp.pdf.

Beitsch, L.M., Brooks, R.G., Menachemi, N., & Grigg, M. (2006). Structure and functions of state public health agencies. *American Journal of Public Health, 96*(1), 167–172.

Berg, P., & Westerling, R. (2007). Decrease in both mild and severe bicycle-related head injuries in helmet wearing ages–trend analyses in Sweden. *Health Promotion International, 22*(3), 191–197.

Bergman, M. (2006, March 9). *Dramatic changes in U.S. aging highlighted in new census, NIH report.* U.S. Census Bureau News. Retrieved August 11, 2008 from http://www.census.gov/PressRelease/www/releases/archives/aging_population/006544.html.

Blackman, J.A., & Gurka, M.J. (2007). Developmental and behavioral comorbidities of asthma in children. *Journal of Developmental and Behavioral Pediatrics, 28*(2), 92–99.

Bloom, B., & Cohen, R.A. (2006). Summary health statistics for U.S. children: National health interview survey. National Center for Health Statistics. *Vital Health Statistics, 10*(234), 111–179. Retrieved August 11, 2008 from http://www.cdc.gov/nchs/data/series/sr_10/sr10_234.pdf.

Boyer-Chu, L., & Wooley, S.F. (2006). *Give it a shot!* American School Health Association. Retrieved January 7, 2008 from http://www.izta.org/PromisingPractices/Give%20it%20a%20Shot%20Toolkit.pdf.

Brener, N.D., Wheeler, L., Wolfe, L.C., et al. (2007). Health services: Results from the School Health Policies and Programs Study. *Journal of School Health, 77*(8), 464–486.

Broussard, L. (2004). School nursing: Not just Band-aids any more! *Journal of Specialists Pediatric Nursing, 9*(3), 77–83.

Brown, R.M., Canham, D., & Cureton, V.Y. (2005). An oral health education program for Latino immigrant parents. *Journal of School Nursing, 21*(5), 266–271.

California Department of Personnel Administration. (2005). *A comparison of total compensation of Registered Nurses in California public sector jurisdictions.* Retrieved August 11, 2008 from http://www.dpa.ca.gov/collbarg/news/Registered%20Nurses.htm.

Careers in Focus: Nursing, 3rd ed. (2006). New York: Ferguson (Infobase) Publishing.

Centers for Disease Control and Prevention (CDC). (2001). *National public health performance standards.* Retrieved August 11, 2008 from http://www.cdc.gov/od/ocphp/nphpsp/.

Centers for Disease Control and Prevention (CDC). (2004). *Attention-deficit/hyperactivity disorder: A new public health program.* Retrieved August 11, 2008 from http://www.cdc.gov/ncbddd/adhd/.

Centers for Disease Control and Prevention (CDC). (2005). *Preventing dental caries.* Retrieved August 11, 2008 from http://www.cdc.gov/nccdphp/publications/factsheets/Prevention/oh.htm.

Centers for Disease Control and Prevention (CDC). (2006). Youth Risk Behavior Surveillance 2005. *Morbidity and Mortality Weekly Report, 55*(SS–5).

Centers for Disease Control and Prevention (CDC). (2007a). *Healthy Youth! Coordinated School Health Program.* Retrieved August 11, 2008 from http://cdc.gov/healthyyouth/CSHP/.

Centers for Disease Control and Prevention. (2007b). *Fact sheet. Oral health problems: Painful, costly and preventable.* National Center for Chronic Disease Prevention and Health Promotion. Retrieved January 8, 2008 from http://www.cdc.gov/nccdphp/publications/aag/oh.htm.

Centers for Disease Control and Prevention (CDC). (2007c). *Sexually transmitted diseases: Surveillance 2006.* Retrieved August 11, 2008 from http://www.cdc.gov/std/stats/trends2006.htm.

Clark, D., Clasen, C., Stolfi, A., & Jaballas, E. (2002). Parent knowledge and opinions of school health services in an urban public school system. *Journal of School Health, 72*(1), 18–22.

Corrarino, J.E., & Little, A. (November 2006). *Breathing easy: A public health nursing/community coalition success story.* Paper presented at the meeting of the American Public Health Association, Boston, MA.

Dang, M.T., Warrington, D., Tung, T., et al. (2007). A school-based approach to early identification and management of students with ADHD. *Journal of School Nursing, 23*(1), 2–12.

Davis, L., & Pacchiana, S. (2003). *Prisoner reentry: What are the public health challenges?* Retrieved January 9, 2008 from http://www.rand.org/pubs/research-briefs/RB6013.

Dey, L.P. (2008). *About EpiPen®.* Retrieved August 11, 2008 from http://www.epipen.com/epipen_main.aspx.

Edgecombe, G. (2001). *Public health nursing past and future: A review of the literature.* Retrieved October 16, 2007 from http://www.rcm.org.uk/info/docs/060105163054-331-1.pdf.

Estelle v. Gamble. No. 75-929 (U.S. Supreme Court, 1976).

Federal Interagency Forum on Child and Family Statistics. (2007). *America's children: Key national indicators of well-being, 2007.* Retrieved August 11, 2008 from http://childstats.gov/americaschildren/famsoc7.asp.

Feldman, H. (2008). *Nursing leadership: A concise encyclopedia.* New York: Springer Publishing.

Ficca, M., & Welk, D. (2005). Medication administration practices in Pennsylvania schools. *Journal of School Nursing, 22*(3), 148–155.

FitzGerald, E. (2007). Inside job. *California Nurse, 103*(4), 10–19.

Food Allergy and Anaphylaxis Network. (2006). *Anaphylaxis and common food allergens [websites].* Retrieved August 11, 2008 from http://www.foodallergy.org/allergens/index.html.

Food-Safe Schools. (2004). *The food-safe schools action guide: Food safety for school nurses.* Retrieved August 11, 2008 from http://www.foodsafeschools.org/schoolnurse.php.

Gebbie, K. (2000). *The public health workforce enumeration.* Center for Health Policy, Columbia University: New York, NY. HRSA/ATPM Cooperative agreement #U76 AH 00001-03.

Georgia, State of. (2007). *State of Georgia job description.* Retrieved August 11, 2008 from http://www.gms.state.ga.us/jobdescriptions/jobsalarydetail.asp?jobcode=71122.

Graves, K.N., Fernandez, M.E., Shelton, T.L., et al. (2005). Risk and protective factors associated with alcohol, cigarette, and marijuana use during adolescence. *Journal of Youth and Adolescence, 34*(4), 379–387.

Guttu, M., Engelke, M.K., & Swanson, M. (2004). Does the school nurse-to-student ratio make a difference? *Journal of School Health, 74*(1), 6–9.

Guzman, S. (October 2004). Depression, a different kind of low. *Diabetes Forecast, 57*(10), 52–57. Retrieved January 7, 2008 from Proquest database.

Hamilton, G., O'Connell, M., & Cross, D. (2004). Adolescent smoking cessation: Development of a school nurse intervention. *Journal of School Nursing, 20*(3), 169–175.

Health Resources and Services Administration (HRSA). (2006). *The registered nurse population: Findings from the 2004 National Sample of Registered Nurses Survey: The registered nurse population 1980–2004.* Retrieved August 11, 2008 from http://bhpr.hrsa.gov/healthworkforce/rnsurvey04/.

Heines, V. (2005). Speaking out to improve the health of inmates. *American Journal of Public Health, 95*(10), 1685–1688.

Hershey, T., Bhargava, N., Sadler, M., et al. (1999). Conventional versus intensive diabetes therapy in children with type 1 diabetes: Effects on memory and motor speed. *Diabetes Care, 22*(8), 1318–1324.

Heschel, R., Crowley, A., & Cohen, S. (2005). State policies regarding nursing delegation and medication administration in child care settings: A case study. *Policy, Politics & Nursing Practice, 6*(2), 86–98.

Hofler, L.D. (2006). Learning from the best: The benefits of a structured health policy fellowship in developing nursing health policy leaders. *Policy, Politics and Nursing Practice, 7*(2), 110–113.

Individuals with Disabilities Education Act. (1975). 20 U.S.C. §§ 1400 et. seq., as amended and incorporating the Education of All Handicapped Children Act (EHA), 1975, P.L. 94-142, and subsequent amendments; Regulations at 34 C.F.R. §§ 300-303 [Special education and related services for students, preschool children, and infants and toddlers].

Institute of Medicine (IOM). (1988). *The future of public health.* Washington, DC: National Academies Press.

Institute of Medicine (IOM). (2003). *Who will keep the public healthy?* Washington, DC: National Academies Press. Retrieved January 7, 2007 from http://www.iom.edu/ Object.File/Master/24/562/EducatingPHFINAL.pdf.

Institute of Medicine (IOM). (2005). *Preventing childhood obesity: Health in the balance.* Washington, DC: National Academies Press.

Izzo, C.V., Eckenrode, J.J., Smith, E.G., et al. (2005). Reducing the impact of uncontrollable stressful life events through a program of nurse home visitation for new parents. *Prevention Science, 6*(4), 269–274.

James, D.J., & Glaze, L.E. (2006). *Mental health problems of prison and jail inmates* [NCJ213600]. Bureau of Justice Statistics Special Report. Retrieved January 8, 2008 from http://www.ojp.usdoj.gov/bjs/pub/pdf/mhppji.pdf.

Kaldahl, M.A., & Blair, E.H. (2005). Student injury rates in public schools. *Journal of School Health, 75*(1), 38–40.

Krisberg, K. (2004). UCLA students meeting needs of underserved. *Nation's Health, 34*(2), 13.

Laffan, S. (2005). "Inside look" on correctional nursing: A unique nursing specialty. *New Jersey Nurse.* Retrieved August 11, 2008 from http://findarticles.com/p/articles/ mi_qa4080/is_200501.ai_n11826429/print.

Lakdawalla, D.N., Bhattacharya, J., & Goldman, D.P. (2004). Are the young becoming more disabled? *Health Affairs, 23*(1), 168–176.

Lear, J.G. (2007). Health at school: A hidden health care system emerges from the shadows. *Health Affairs, 26*(2), 409–419.

Levy, M., Heffner, B., Stewart, T., & Beeman, G. (2006). The efficacy of asthma case management in urban school district in reducing school absences and hospitalizations for asthma. *Journal of School Health, 76*(6), 320–324.

Lewis, C., Mouradian, W., Slayton, R., & Williams, A. (2007). Dental insurance and its impact on preventive dental care visits for U.S. children. *Journal of the American Dental Association, 138*(3), 369–380.

Lewis, K.D., & Bear, B.J. (2002). *Manual of school health,* 2nd ed. St. Louis, MO: Saunders.

MacNeil, J.R., Lobato, M.N., & Moore, M. (2005). An unanswered health disparity: Tuberculosis among correctional inmates, 1993–2003. *American Journal of Public Health, 95*(10), 1800–1805.

Magee, C.G., Hult, J.R., Turalba, R., & McMillan, S. (2005). Preventive care for women in prison: A qualitative community assessment of the Papanicolaou test and follow-up treatment at a California state women's prison. *American Journal of Public Health, 95*(10), 1712–1717.

Marcalino, G.E., Dhawan, D., & Rich, J.D. (2005). A missed opportunity: Hepatitis C screening of prisoners. *American Journal of Public Health, 95*(10), 1739–1740.

Maruschak, L.M. (2007). *HIV in prisons, 2005* [NCJ 218915]. Bureau of Justice Statistics Bulletin. Retrieved January 8, 2008 from http://www.ojp.usdoj.gov/bjs/pub/pdf/hivp05.pdf.

Maternal and Child Health Bureau. (2006). Vaccine-preventable diseases. In *Child Health USA 2004.* U.S. Department of Health and Human Services, Health Resources and Services Administration. Retrieved January 7, 2008 from http:// www.mchb.hrsa.gov/chusa_06/healthstat/children/0311vpd.htm.

McCarthy, A.M., Kelly, M., & Reed, D. (2000). Medication administration in schools. *Journal of School Health, 709,* 371–376.

McGregor, A., Wheless, J., Baumgartner, J., & Bettis, D. (2005). Right-sided vagus nerve stimulation as a treatment for refractory epilepsy in humans. *Epilepsia, 46*(1), 91–96.

Miller, S.K. (2006). Jail health assessment practices: An analysis of national trends as compared to National Commission on Correctional Health Care recommendations. *Journal of Correctional Health Care, 12*(2), 104–117.

Minnesota Department of Health. (2007). *Cornerstones of public health nursing.* Retrieved August 11, 2008 from http://www.health.state.mn.us/divs/cfh/ophp/resources/docs/cor nerstones_definition_revised2007.pdf.

Missouri Department of Health and Senior Services (DHSS). (2006). *Role of the PHN.* Retrieved August 11, 2008 from http://www.dhss.mo.gov/LPHA/PHNursing?Role_PublicHealth Nurses.htm.

Mitchell, M. (2000). Schools as catalysts for healthy communities. *Public Health Reports, 115,* 222–227.

Mumola, C. (2005). *Suicide and homicide in state prisons and local jails* [NCJ 210036]. Bureau of Justice Statistics special report. Retrieved January 8, 2008 from http://www.ojp. usdoj.gov/bjs/pub/pdf/shsplj.pdf.

Mumola, C.J., & Karberg, J.C. (2007). *Drug use and dependence, state and federal prisoners, 2004.* [NCJ 213530]. Bureau of Justice Statistics special report. Retrieved August 11, 2008 from http://www.ojp.usdoj.gov/bjs/pub/pdf/dudsfp04.pdf.

Murphy, M., & Polivka, B. (2007). Parental perceptions of the schools' role in addressing childhood obesity. *Journal of School Nursing, 23*(1), 40–46.

Myers, J., Zack, B., Kramer, K., et al. (2005). Get connected: An HIV prevention case management program for men and women leaving California prisons. *American Journal of Public Health, 95*(10), 1682–1684.

National Assembly on School-Based Health Care (NASBHC). (2007). *School-based health center census: National census school year 2004–2005.* Retrieved December 21, 2007 from http://www.nasbhc.org/atf/cf/%7BCD9949F2-2761-42FB-BC7A-CEE165C701D9%7D/Census2005.pdf.

National Association of County and City Health Officers (NAC-CHO). (2007). *2005 National profile of local health departments study.* Retrieved July 21, 2007 from http://www.naccho.org/pubs/product1.cfm?Product_ID=15.

National Association of School Nurses (NASN). (2002). *Issue brief: School health nursing services role in health care: Eating disorders.* Retrieved August 11, 2008 from http://www.nasn.org/Default.aspx?tabid=269.

National Association of School Nurses and American Nurses Association. (2005). *School nursing: Scope and standards of practice.* Washington, DC: Author.

National Association of School Nurses (NASN). (2006b). *Diabetes in the school setting.* Retrieved August 11, 2008 from http://www.nasn.org/Default.aspx?tabid=216.

National Association of School Nurses (NASN). (2007a). *About us.* Retrieved August 11, 2008 from http:// www.nasn.org/Default.aspx?tabid=57.

National Association of School Nurses (NASN). (2007b). *Statement of Denise Herrmann, MS, RN, LSN, CPNP on behalf of the National Association of School Nurses before* the Committee on Oversight & Government Reform, U.S. House of Representatives concerning the administration's regulatory actions of Medicaid: The effects on patients, doctors, hospitals, and states. Retrieved August 11, 2008 from http://oversight.house.gov/documents/20071101111516.pdf.

National Diabetes Education Program. (2006). *Overview of diabetes in children and adolescents.* Retrieved August 11, 2008 from http://ndep.nih.gov/diabetes/youth/youth_FS.htm.

National Institute of Mental Health (NIMH). (2008). *Child and adolescent mental health.* Retrieved January 8, 2008 from http://www.nimh.nih.gov/health/topics/child-and-adolescent-mental-health/index.shtml.

National Institute of Neurological Disorders and Stroke (NINDS). (2007). *Curing epilepsy: The promise of research.* [NIH Publication No. 07-6120]. Retrieved August 11, 2008 from http://www.ninds.nih.gov/disorders/epilepsy/epilepsy_research.htm#Section1_2.

National Oceanic & Atmospheric Administration (NOAA). (2007). *About NOAA Corps.* Retrieved August 11, 2008 from http://www.noaacorps.noaa.gov/about/about.html.

Novick, L.F., Morrow, C.B., & Mays, G.P. (2008). *Public health administration: Principles for population-based management,* 2nd ed. Sudbury, MA: Jones and Bartlett Publishers: Sudbury Massachusetts.

Office of Justice Programs (OJP). (2007). *Prisoners in the United States, 1990–2006.* Retrieved July 27, 2007 from http://ojp.usdoj.gov/bjs/pub/pdf/pjim06.pdf.

Okumura, M.J., Pheeters, M.L., & Davis, M.M. (2007). State and national estimates of insurance coverage and health care utilization for adolescents with chronic conditions from the National Survey of Children's Health, 2003. *Journal of Adolescent Health, 41*(4), 343–349.

Olds, D.L., Kitzman, H., Cole, R., et al. (2004). Effects of nurse home-visiting on maternal life course and child development: Age 6 follow-up results of a randomized trial. *Pediatrics, 114*(6), 1550–1559.

Oregon State Government. (2007). *School-based heath centers: Quality health care for kids, 2007 status report.* Retrieved January 8, 2008 from http://oregon.gov/DHS/ph/ah/docs/2007_SBHC_Status_Report.pdf.

Page, J. (2006, August 17). *Sex-disease cases soar in Utah County.* Deseret News. Retrieved January 7, 2008 from http://findarticles.com/p/articles/mi_qn4188/is_20060817/ai_n16641786.

Perrin, K., Goad, S., & Williams, C. (2002). Can school nurses save money by treating school employees as well as students? *Journal of School Health, 72*(7), 305–307.

Pinhas-Hamiel, O., & Zeitler, P. (2005). The global spread of type 2 diabetes in children and adolescents. *Journal of Pediatrics, 146*(5), 693–700.

Quad Council. (2007). *The public health nursing shortage: A threat to the public's health.* Quad Council of Public Health Nursing.

Rehabilitation Act of 1973, Section 504. (1973). 29 U.S.C. §794 et seq., Regulations at 34 C.F.R. §104.

Restum, Z.G. (2005). Public health implications of substandard correctional health care. *American Journal of Public Health, 95*(10), 1689–1691.

Romano, C.A. (2007). *Profession: Nurse.* U.S. Public Health Service Commissioned Corps. USDHHS. Retrieved August 11, 2008 from http://commcorps.shs.net/profession/nurse/default.aspx.

Schulman, Ronca & Bucuvalas, Inc. (SRBI). (2004). *Children and asthma in America,* on behalf of GlaxoSmithKline. Retrieved August 11, 2008 from http://www.asthmainamerica.com/.

Selekman, J., & Gamel-McCormik, M. (2006). Children with chronic conditions. In J. Selekman, (Ed.). *School nursing: A comprehensive test.* (pp. 615–646). Philadelphia: F.A. Davis.

Soloman, J., & Card, J.J. (2004). *Understanding, selecting and replicating effective teen pregnancy prevention programs.*

Retrieved November 14, 2007 from http://www.teenpregnancy.org/works/pdf/MakingTheList.pdf.

Southern Nevada Health District. (2005). *PHN I & II.* Retrieved July 21, 2007 from http://www.southernnevadahealthdistrict.org/employment/public_health_nurse_I-II.htm.

Speroni, K.G., Earley, C., & Atherton, M. (2007). Evaluating the effectiveness of the Kids Living Fit trademark program (LKF): A comparative study. *Journal of School Nursing, 23*(6), 329–336.

Spratley, E., Johnson, A., Sochalski, J., et al. (2002). *The registered nurse population, March 2000: Findings from the national sample survey of registered nurses.* Washington, DC: USDHHS. Retrieved August 11, 2008 from http://bhpr.hrsa.gov/healthworkforce/reports/rnsurvey/rnss1.htm.

Sweeney, N.M., & Horishita, N. (2005). The breakfast-eating habits of inner city high school students. *Journal of School Nursing, 21*(2), 100–105.

Tebb, K.P., Pantell, R.H., Wibbelsman, C.J., et al. (2005). Screening sexually active adolescents for *Chlamydia trachomatis*: What about the boys? *American Journal of Public Health, 95*(10), 1806–1810.

Telljohann, S.K., Dake, J.A., & Price, J.H. (2004). Effect of full-time versus part-time school nurses on attendance of elementary students with asthma. *Journal of School Nursing, 20*(6), 331–334.

Telljohann, S.K., Price, J.H., Dake, J.A., & Durgin, J. (2004). Access to school health services: Differences between full-time and part-time school nurses. *Journal of School Nursing, 20*(3), 176–181.

Texas Department of Health Services. (2005). *Frequently asked questions: Implementation of laws on screening for Acanthosis Nigricans.* Retrieved August 11, 2008 from http://www.dshs.state.tx.us/schoolhealth/organscreen.shtm.

Turnock, B.J. (2006). *Public health: Career choices that make a difference.* Sudbury, MA: Jones and Bartlett Publishers.

Turnock, B.J. (2007). *Essentials of public health.* Sudbury, MA: Jones and Bartlett Publishers.

U.S. Department of Education, National Center for Education Statistics. (2006). *Digest of education statistics, 2005* (NCES 2006-030). Retrieved August 11, 2008 from http://nces.ed.gov/programs/digest/d06/.

U.S. Department of Health and Human Services. (2000). *Healthy People 2010: Understanding and improving health,* 2nd ed. Washington, DC: U.S. Government Printing Office.

U.S. Department of Health and Human Services (DHHS). (2006). *Department of Health and Human Services budget in brief.* Retrieved Sept. 21, 2007 from http://www.hhs.gov/budget/06budget/FY2006BudgetinBrief.pdf.

U.S. Department of Health and Human Services. Centers for Medicare and Medicaid. (2007). *Medicaid program: Elimination of reimbursement under Medicaid for school administration expenditures and costs related to transportation of school-age children between home and school.* [CMS–2287–F]. Retrieved December 27, 2007 from http://www.cms.hhs.gov/MedicaidGenInfo/Downloads/CMS2287F.pdf.

U.S. Department of Health and Human Services, Administration on Children, Youth and Families. (2008). *Child Maltreatment 2006.* Washington, DC: U.S. Government Printing Office.

U.S. Public Health Service Commissioned Corps. (2007). *U.S. Public Health Service Commissioned Corp.* Retrieved August 11, 2008 from http://commcorps.shs.net/default.aspx.

Utah County Job Description. (March 8, 2007). *Public Health Nurse.* Retrieved from July 21, 2007 from http://www.co.utah.ut.us/Dept/Pers/JobAnnounceDetails.asp.

Vessey, J., & McGowan, K. (2006). A successful public health experiment: School nursing. *Pediatric Nursing, 32*(3), 255–257.

Wolfe, L., & Selekman, J. (2002). School nurses: What it was and what it is. *Pediatric Nursing, 28*(4), 403–407.

Woodfill, M.M., & Beyrer, M.K. (1991). *The role of the nurse in the school setting: A historical perspective.* Kent, OH: American School Health Association.

Zaslow, J. (2006). *Is there a nurse in the house? A shortage of school needs rise.* Wall Street Journal Online: Career Journal.com. Retrieved August 11, 2008 from http://www.careerjournal.com/salaryhiring/industries/health/20061103-zaslow.html.

Selected Readings

Adams, S., & McCarthy, A. (2007). Evidence-based practice guidelines and school nursing. *Journal of School Nursing, 23*(3), 128–136.

Allen, K., Taylor, J., & Kuiper, R. (2007). Effectiveness of nutrition education on fast food choices in adolescents. *Journal of School Nursing, 23*(6), 337–341.

Bierschbach, J., Cooper, L., & Liedl, J. (2004). Insulin pumps: What every school nurse needs to know. *Journal of School Nursing, 20*(2), 117–123.

Browring-Lossock, E. (2006). The forensic mental health nurse: A literature review. *Journal of Psychiatric & Mental Health Nursing, 13*(6), 780–785.

Campbell, S., Fowles, E., & Weber, B. (2004). Organizational structure and job satisfaction in public health nursing. *Public Health Nursing, 21*(6), 564–571.

Canham, D., Bauer, L., Concepcion, M., et al. (2007). An audit of medication administration: A glimpse into school health offices. *Journal of School Nursing, 24*(31), 21–27.

Collins, S.E. (2007). Forensic nursing. *Pennsylvania Nurse, 62*(3), 5, 28.

Dang, M., Warrington, M., Tung, T., et al. (2007). A school-based approach to early identification and management of students with ADHD. *Journal of School Nursing, 23*(1), 2–12.

Donaghy, G. (2006). Men's health in prison. *Mental Health Nursing, 26*(3), 6.

DuPont, R., Bucher, R., Wilford, B., & Coleman, J. (2007). School-based administration of ADHD drugs decline, along with diversion, theft, and misuse. *Journal of School Nursing, 23*(6), 349–352.

Flanagan, N. (2006). Testing the relationship between job stress and satisfaction in correctional nurses. *Nursing Research, 55*(5), 316–327.

Fothegill, A., Palumbo, M., Rambur, B., et al. (2005). The volunteer potential of inactive nurses for disaster preparedness. *Public Health Nursing, 22*(5), 414–421.

Gagne, M. (2005). You work here? *Registered Nurse Journal, 17*(5), 22.

Holmes, D. (2005). Governing the captives: Forensic psychiatric nursing in corrections. *Perspectives in Psychiatric Care, 41*(1), 3–13.

Holmes, D., Perron, A., & Michaud, G. (2007). Nursing in corrections: Lessons from France. *Journal of Forensic Nursing, 3*(3–4), 126–131.

Hufft, A., & Kite, M. (2003). Vulnerable and cultural perspectives for nursing care in correctional systems. *Journal of Multicultural Nursing & Health, 9*(1), 18–26.

Litarowsky, J., Murphy, S., & Canham, D. (2004). Evaluation of an anaphylaxis training program for unlicensed assistive personnel. *Journal of School Nursing, 20*(5), 279–284.

Mavromichalis, C. (2003). Corrections nurse provides care behind bars. *Registered Nurse Journal, 15*(3), 17.

Moss, B. (2006). A captive audience: Inmates at Massachusetts' only women's prison have the opportunity of a lifetime to learn better self-care. *Nursing Spectrum—New England Edition, 10*(25), 8–9

Murphy, D. (2003). Public health in corrections. *Chart, 100*(2), 10–12.

O'Dell, C., O'Hara, K., Kiel, S., & McCullough, K. (2007). Emergency management of seizures in the school setting. *Journal of School Nursing, 23*(3), 158–165.

Pulcini, J., DeSisto, M., & McIntyre, L. (2007). An intervention to increase the use of asthma action plans in schools: A MASNRN study. *Journal of School Nursing, 23*(3), 170–176.

Robertson, J. (2004). Does advanced community/public health nursing practice have a future? *Public Health Nursing, 21*(5), 495–500.

Sakamoto, S., & Avila, M. (2004). The Public Health Nursing Practice Model: A tool for public health nurses. *Public Health Nursing, 21*(2), 179–182.

Sciscione, P., & Krause-Parello, C. (2007). No-nit policies in schools: Time for change. *Journal of School Nursing, 23*(1), 13–20.

Smith, K., & Bazini-Barakat, N. (2003). A public health nursing practice model: Melding public health principles with the nursing process. *Public Health Nursing, 20*(1), 42–48.

Stoddard, S., Kubik, M., & Skay, C. (2007). Is school-based height and weight screening of elementary students private and reliable? *Journal of School Nursing, 24*(1), 43–48.

Tousman, S., et al. (2007). Evaluation of a hand washing program for 2nd graders. *Journal of School Nursing, 23*(6), 342–348.

Weiskopf, C. (2005). Nurses' experience of caring for inmate patients. *Journal of Advanced Nursing, 49*(4), 336–343.

Weiss, C., Munoz-Furlong, A., Furlong, T., & Arbit, J. (2004). Impact of food allergies on school nursing practice. *Journal of School Nursing, 20*(5), 268–278.

Wold, J., Gains, S., & Leary, J. (2006). Use of public health nurse competencies to develop a childcare health consultant workforce. *Public Health Nursing, 23*(2), 139–145.

Zahner, S., & Gredig, O. (2005). Public health nursing practice change and recommendations for improvement. *Public Health Nursing, 22*(5), 422–428.

Zalumas, J., & Rose, C. (2003). Hepatitis C and HIV in incarcerated populations: Fights, bites, searches, and syringes! *Journal of the Association of Nurses in AIDS Care, 14*(5), [Suppl.]:S108–S115.

Internet Resources

Public Health Nursing

American Public Health Association: *http://www.apha.org*
Bureau of Health Professionals (in Health Resources & Services Administration): *http://bhpr.hrsa.gov*
Centers for Disease Control and Prevention: *http://www.cdc.org*
Civilian nursing opportunities: *http://www.usajobs.gov.*
Department of Health and Human Services: *http://www.dhhs.gov*
Department of Veteran's Affairs: *http://www.va.gov*
Federal government jobs: *http://www.usa.jobs*
Indian Health Services: *http://www.ihs.gov*
National Institutes of Health: *http://www.nih.gov*

Uniformed Nursing Services

Department of Commerce (National Oceanic & Atmospheric Administration Commissioned Corps):
http://www.noaacorps.noaa.gov
Department of Defense: *http://www.defenselink.mil*
Department of Homeland Security (Coast Guard):
http://www.uscg.mil
Public Health Services/Commissioned Corps:
http://commcorps.shs.net/default.aspx

School Nursing

American School Health Association (ASHA):
http://www.ashweb.org
Centers for Disease Control and Prevention-Division of Adolescent and School Health (DASH): *http://www.cdc.gov/HealthyYouth*

National Assembly on School-Based Healthcare. Information on School-Based Clinics: *http://www.nasbch.org*

National Association of School Nurses (NASN): *http://www.nasn.org* "School Nurse": *http://www.schoolnurse.com/*

Correctional Nursing

Academy of Correctional Health Professionals: *http://www.correctionalhealth.org*

American Correctional Association (ACA): *http://www.aca.org*

American Correctional Health Services Association (ACHSA): *http://www.achsa.org*

American Nurses Association: Corrections Nursing/Scope & Standards of Practice: *http://nursingworld.org/books/ pdescr.cfm?cnum=15*

Federal Bureau of Prisons: *http://www.bop.gov*

National Commission on Correctional Health Care (NCCHC): *http://www.ncchc.org*

United States Department of Justice: *http://www.usdoj.gov*

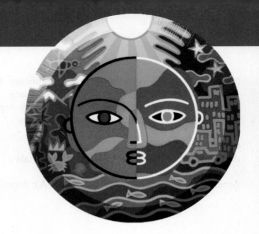

31

Private Settings for Community Health Nursing

LEARNING OBJECTIVES

Upon mastery of this chapter, you should be able to:

◆ State the historical roots of nurse-managed health centers.
◆ Identify the distinctiveness of various nurse-managed health center models.
◆ Describe funding sources for nurse-managed health centers.
◆ Articulate the importance of sustainability for nurse-managed health centers.
◆ State at least two roles of nurses in nurse-managed health centers.
◆ Describe the evolution of faith community nursing.
◆ Describe and differentiate among the roles of the faith community nurse.
◆ Identify the steps for establishing a practice as a faith community nurse.
◆ Describe the role of the occupational health nurse and other members of the occupational health team in protecting and promoting workers' health and safety.

"To insure good health: eat lightly, breathe deeply, live moderately, cultivate cheerfulness, and maintain an interest in life."

—William Londen

KEY TERMS

Best practices
Comprehensive primary care center
Congregational nurse
Contracts
Faith community
Faith community nurse
Federally qualified health center (FQHC)
Grant
Health ministry nurse
National Nursing Centers Consortium (NNCC)
Nurse-managed health center (NMHC)
Occupational and environmental health nurse
Outcomes
Parish nurses
Request for proposal (RFP)
Safety-net provider
Sustainability
Wellness center

Healthy People 2010: Understanding and Improving Health (U.S. Department of Health and Human Services [USDHHS], 2000) provided clear objectives for promoting health and preventing disease for the past decade. The next 10 years will see unprecedented changes and challenges in the nation's health. As we ponder what those changes will be, the preparation of *Healthy People: The Road Ahead* is in the beginning stages of development. This initiative will "reflect assessments of major risks to health and wellness, changing public health priorities, and emerging issues related to our nation's health preparedness and prevention" (USDHHS, 2008). With this new initiative, there will be ever increasing opportunities for community health nurses to make a difference in their communities. This chapter examines three distinct areas of practice in the community as potential options for your own professional road ahead.

Chapter 30 discussed a wide variety of practice opportunities in the public sector. This chapter will examine three unique private sector roles and practice environments available in the United States and in many other countries: nurse-managed health centers, faith community nursing, and occupational and environmental health nursing. Nurse-managed centers offer the opportunity for more autonomous practice and present excellent learning venues for nursing students. Many such centers are connected to academic nursing programs. Faith community nursing, begun in the mid-1980s, has gained increasing attention in many religious communities. Although the positions are frequently held by volunteers, there are increasing opportunities for paid employment. Occupational and environmental health is a specialty health practice that focuses on the health and well-being of the working population, including both paid and unpaid laborers, and therefore covers most of the country's able adults. This role provides the vital link between nursing and sound business practices. Each of these areas of practice offers community health nurses an avenue to address health disparities in their communities, increase years of healthy life, and provide holistic, client-centered care to meet the current and emerging health needs in their communities, as indicated in *Healthy People 2010*.

NURSE-MANAGED HEALTH CENTERS

Nursing centers, more recently termed **nurse-managed health centers (NMHC)**, are organizations that give clients access to professional nursing services, and are administered by nurses in partnership with the community in which they serve. In the mid-1980s, The American Nurses Association (ANA) Nursing Centers Task Force developed a definition of nursing centers that is still applicable today (Aydelotte, et al., 1987). Display 31.1 shows a modified version of that original definition. Although all NMHCs share the core elements of the ANA definition, they vary in their practice models. Services offered at NMHCs range from health promotion and wellness to conventional primary care (Torrisi & Hansen-Turton, 2005) (see Fig. 31.1).

Nurse-managed health centers have emerged as vital "safety net" health care providers in America's health care delivery system (Hansen-Turton & Miller, 2006). A "**safety-net provider**" is defined as one that, by mandate or mission, organizes and delivers a significant level of health care and other health-related services to the uninsured, Medicaid

---

DISPLAY 31.1	DEFINITION OF NURSING CENTER

Nursing centers—sometimes referred to as community nursing organizations, nurse-managed centers, nursing clinics, and community-nurse-managed health centers—are organizations that give clients and communities direct access to professional nursing services. Professional nurses in these centers diagnose and treat human responses to actual and potential health problems, and promote health and optimal functioning among target populations and communities. The services provided in these centers are holistic, client-centered, and affordable. Overall accountability and responsibility remain with the nurse executive/director. Nurse-managed health centers are not limited to any particular organizational configuration. Nurse-managed health centers can be free-standing businesses or may be affiliated with universities or other service institutions, such as home health agencies and hospitals. The primary characteristic of the organization is responsiveness to the health needs of populations. The nurse is responsible for all patient care and business operations.

Source: Aydelotte, M.K., Barger, S.E., Branstetter, E., et al. (1987). *The nursing center: Concept and design.* Kansas City, MO: American Nurses Association; and National Nursing Center Consortium. (2008). Modified version of the ANA 1987 *Nursing Centers Task Force* definition.

---

recipients, and other vulnerable populations (Health Resources and Services Administration, 2005).

Located in or near health professional shortage areas and medically underserved areas in both urban and rural communities, NMHCs are found in convenient sites where people live, work, learn, and worship. Oversight is provided by a nurse executive with an advanced degree. Traditionally, targets of service have been those who are least likely to be engaged in ongoing health care services for themselves and their family members. Currently, NMHCs serve both uninsured and underinsured population groups of all age.

NMHCs differ from other public health agencies and tertiary medical care facilities. Although some services overlap, the distinctiveness of NMHCs is found in the community orientation of the nurse-managed centers. This model is depicted by Lundeen's comprehensive community based primary health care model (Lundeen, 2005), in which NMHCs are referred to as *community nursing centers* and are the central figure in the model of health care utilized at the University of Wisconsin, Milwaukee (see Fig. 31.2).

Healthy People 2010

The publication of *Healthy People: The Surgeon General's Report on Health Promotion and Disease Prevention* (U.S. Department of Health, Education & Welfare, 1979) focused attention on the nation's health promotion and disease prevention activities. The current publication, *Healthy People 2010*, has two main goals: to increase quality of life and to eliminate health disparities (USDHHS, 2000). "Achieving

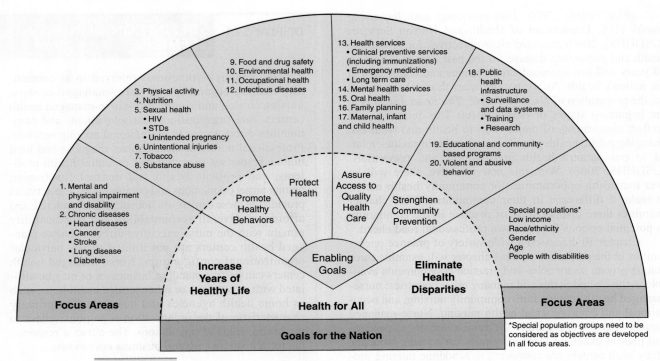

FIGURE 31.1 Vision of 2010: Healthy people in healthy communities. From U.S. Department of Health and Human Services, Office of Disease Prevention and Health Promotion. (1997). *Developing objectives for Healthy People 2010*. Washington, DC: U.S. Printing Office, p. 14.

Healthy People 2010 goals requires a long-term commitment to community collaboration and powerful, productive partnerships among many diverse people and groups" (Kinsey & Buchanan, 2008, p. 414). Nurse-managed health centers are an excellent venue to meet the goals of *Healthy People 2010*.

History of the Nurse-managed Model

Although today's NMHCs trace their roots to changes in national health care laws begun in the mid-1960s, the nursing model of holistic care that focuses on vulnerable populations

and integrates primary care and public health dates back to the 19th century. Florence Nightingale's passion for at-risk populations, as well as her success related to health reform, provides a model for NMHCs today. Lillian Wald, who founded the Henry Street Settlement, and Margaret Sanger, who initiated the first family planning clinic, are two examples of nurses providing holistic care to vulnerable populations (see Chapter 2). These nurse activists sought to resolve the 20th-century problems caused by immigration, urbanization, and industrialization in the United States (Beidler, 2005) (see From the Case Files I).

From the Case Files I

Caring for Vulnerable Populations at an NMHC

Ms. Jones is a 22-year-old mother of three small children who recently moved to Philadelphia. She brings her oldest child, age 6, to a local comprehensive primary care NMHC for school immunizations. During the course of the history and physical examination, the nurse-practitioner becomes aware that this mother also has two younger children, aged 2 and 3, at home. The family rents a small apartment in housing that was built in the mid-1950s. Ms. Jones reports that her mother (the children's grandmother) also resides with them. The grandmother is the child care provider while Ms. Jones works at a local hair salon. The grandmother smokes 1.5 to 2 packages of cigarettes daily; Ms. Jones reports that she is a nonsmoker. Upon further questioning, the nurse practitioner learns that the 3-year-old child has a chronic cough and occasional wheezing. Ms. Jones also confides to the nurse-practitioner that she recently missed two menstrual periods and is sexually active.

1. What are some possible health care needs of Ms. Jones? Her mother?
2. What screenings should be performed on Ms. Jones' children?
3. What other interdisciplinary team members should be involved in this family's health care?
4. What are some possible referrals that would benefit this family?

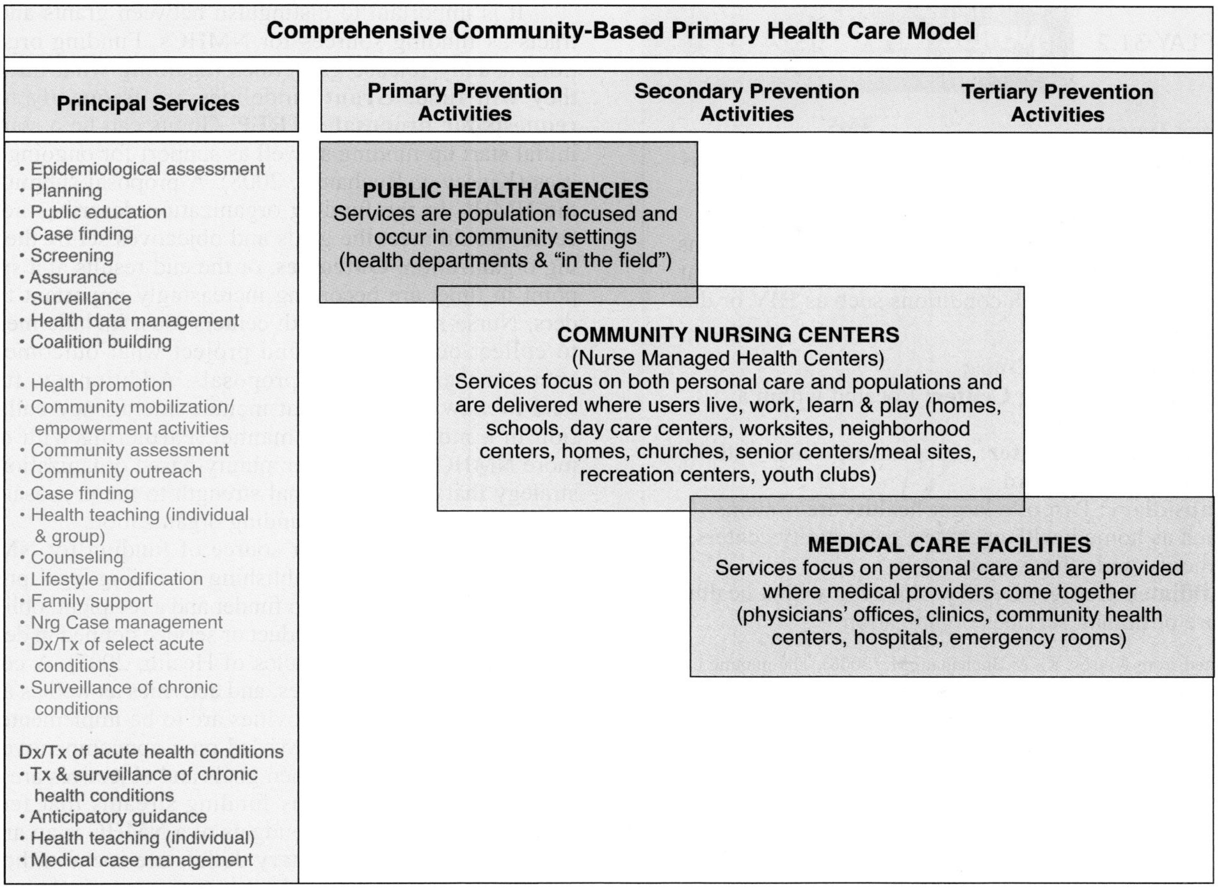

Comprehensive Community-Based Primary Health Care Model

Principal Services	Primary Prevention Activities	Secondary Prevention Activities	Tertiary Prevention Activities

- Epidemiological assessment
- Planning
- Public education
- Case finding
- Screening
- Assurance
- Surveillance
- Health data management
- Coalition building

- Health promotion
- Community mobilization/ empowerment activities
- Community assessment
- Community outreach
- Case finding
- Health teaching (individual & group)
- Counseling
- Lifestyle modification
- Family support
- Nrg Case management
- Dx/Tx of select acute conditions
- Surveillance of chronic conditions

Dx/Tx of acute health conditions
- Tx & surveillance of chronic health conditions
- Anticipatory guidance
- Health teaching (individual)
- Medical case management

PUBLIC HEALTH AGENCIES
Services are population focused and occur in community settings
(health departments & "in the field")

COMMUNITY NURSING CENTERS
(Nurse Managed Health Centers)
Services focus on both personal care and populations and are delivered where users live, work, learn & play (homes, schools, day care centers, worksites, neighborhood centers, homes, churches, senior centers/meal sites, recreation centers, youth clubs)

MEDICAL CARE FACILITIES
Services focus on personal care and are provided where medical providers come together (physicians' offices, clinics, community health centers, hospitals, emergency rooms)

FIGURE 31.2   Comprehensive Community-Based Primary Health Care Model. From Lundeen, S. (2005). *Lundeen's comprehensive community-based primary health care model.* Milwaukee, WI: UW, Milwaukee College of Nursing, with permission.

Since the late 1970s, in conjunction with the development of educational programs for nurse practitioners (NPs), faculties in schools of nursing have established nurse-managed health centers. Linkages have provided clinical sites for educating nurses at all levels and settings, as well as for faculty practice opportunities (Hansen-Turton & Miller, 2006). For example, one urban academic nursing center, La Salle Neighborhood Nursing Center in Philadelphia, Pennsylvania, involves students and faculty in primary and secondary prevention services to the community. Health fairs, immunization outreach and administration, after-school programs, home visiting, health literacy programs, case management for migrant workers, outreach to the homeless, and cable TV health videos are some of the initiatives that undergraduate and graduate students have been engaged in for almost two decades (Miller, 2007).

Today, NMHCs embody the traditional role of nurses, who have historically provided compassionate health care focusing on the special needs of society's most vulnerable: the poor, the aged, those experiencing social injustice, and those living in geographic areas with limited or no access to adequate health care facilities (National Nursing Centers Consortium, 2007). Unlike traditional health care venues that provide primary care and public health services, NMHCs include community participation in program development, implementation, and evaluation (Anderko, Bartz, & Lundeen, 2005).

Nursing Center Models

Several types of nursing centers exist; each reflects the community in which it is located and the particular services it offers (Gerrity & Kinsey, 1999). Academic-based nursing centers, which are located within schools of nursing, are common. In addition, hospital-based and free standing community-based NMHCs offer a mixture of primary care, health promotion, and disease prevention services (Hanson-Turton & Miller, 2006).

Hansen-Turton (2003, p. 150) states that NMHCs meet all of the requirements for **federally qualified health centers (FQHC)**, as defined in Section 330 of the Public Health Service Act. This is an especially important designation, as it enables centers to qualify for many funding sources vital to service provision that would not be available otherwise. To qualify, the centers must:

- Be located in a medically underserved area or serve a medically underserved population
- Have a nonprofit, tax-exempt, or public status
- Have a board of directors, a majority of whom must be consumers of the center's health services

---

DISPLAY 31.2 **NURSE-MANAGED HEALTH CENTER MODELS**

Center Types:

- **Wellness Center:** Provides public health as well as health promotion and disease prevention programs
- **Comprehensive Primary Care Center:** Provides traditional primary care and public health programs
- **Specialty Nursing Centers:** Provide programs that target specific health conditions such as HIV or diabetes

Organizational Structure:

- **Academic Nursing Center:** Located within a school of nursing
- **Free-standing Center:** Independent center with its own governing board
- **Subsidiary:** Part of a larger health care system, such as home health agencies, community centers, schools, and other venues
- **Affiliated Center:** Legal partnership with a health care or human services organization

Adapted from Kinsey, K., & Buchanan, M. (2008). The nursing center: A model for nursing practice in the community. In M. Stanhope & J. Lancaster, *Public health nursing: Population-centered health care in the community* (7th ed., p. 412). St. Louis, MO: Mosby, with permission.

◆ Provide culturally competent, comprehensive primary care services to all age groups
◆ Offer a sliding scale fee, and provide services regardless of ability to pay

The variety of nursing center models currently being used and their organizational structures demonstrate the diversity of contemporary NMHCs. Display 31.2 describes the three major types of centers (wellness, comprehensive primary care, and specialty nursing centers), along with the various organizational structures that influence their delivery models.

Funding for Nurse-managed Health Centers

As NMHCs vary in their models, so too do their methods of cost reimbursement, encompassing fee for service, sliding fees, grant support, third-party payments, and the cost-based reimbursement available to FQHCs (Torrisi & Hansen-Turton, 2005). Most nursing centers' operational and salary budgets entail a combination of these funding sources.

In the **comprehensive primary care centers**, advanced practice nurses (APNs) provide primary care services. Such services are usually reimbursable under Medicaid and managed care medical insurance plans. In the **wellness centers**, public health nurses and other interdisciplinary team members provide a range of primary and secondary prevention strategies. These services are usually not reimbursed by insurance plans, but are often covered by grants and contracts (Hansen-Turton & Miller, 2006). In addition, foundation support and private donations from community organizations and members provide fiscal support for NMHC initiatives.

It is important to distinguish between grants and contracts as funding sources for NMHCs. Funding organizations usually release guidelines regarding what initiatives they will fund. **Grant** guidelines are frequently termed **requests for proposal**, or **RFP**. Grants can be a source of initial start up funding as well as support for ongoing activities (Kinsey & Buchanan, 2008). A proposal submitted by the NMHC to the funding organization describes how the center would meet the goals and objectives set by the funding organization. **Outcomes**, or the end results at a specific point in time, are becoming increasingly important to funders. Nurse-managed health centers must include measures to collect outcome data and project what outcomes will occur in their submitted proposals. Additionally, funders tend to view initiatives that include interagency collaboration in a more favorable manner. Partnering with one or more NMHCs or other community-based organizations is a strategy that gives additional strength to the proposal when it is under review by the funding organization.

Contracts are another source of funding for NMHCs. **Contracts** are awards establishing a binding legal procurement relationship between a funder and a recipient, obligating the receiver to furnish a product or service defined in detail by the funder (National Institutes of Health, 2007). A contract has specific goals, objectives, and activities as well as a timeframe within which the activities are to be implemented and evaluated. Contracts are awarded on a noncompetitive basis and often are renewable when goals and objectives are met.

Managing the various funding streams that feed the personnel and operations budgets of a NMHC is an arduous task. To ensure that budgetary dollars are spent in the manner specified by the funding organization, meticulous record keeping and itemization of spending is another undertaking that the nurse executive or an operations coordinator of the NMHC must carry out. It is imperative that key personnel from NMHCs maintain precise records and submit accurate quarterly, semi-annual, or annual reports as specified in the grant or contract award.

Sustainability of Nurse-managed Health Centers

Sustainability, or the ability to carry on services and health promotion activities when funding is no longer available, is one of the main challenges of NMHCs. The challenge of sustainability is a common dilemma that funders and grantees both face at the end of an initiative's funding period (Cutler, 2002).

Nurse-managed health centers have much to offer toward resolving the national health care crisis facing vulnerable populations who are uninsured or underinsured. However, without the ability to maintain fiscal sustainability, NMHCs may fail to reach their full potential for positively influencing the future of health care (McBryde-Foster, 2005).

In the past, funders were often confronted either with the task of helping organizations find and secure other resources, or extending their own financial support to ensure the continuity of services. More recently, both public and private funders are stipulating that organizations describe detailed plans for sustainability after the award period ceases in their funding application. Cutler (2002) proposes "Critical Sustainability Questions" that can be used as a preliminary avenue of

DISPLAY 31.3	**CRITICAL SUSTAINABILITY QUESTIONS**

When applying to a funding organization, applicants should consider the following questions:

1. Assuming acceptable results, and assuming that the task will not be fully completed at the end of the grant period, is it expected that this initiative will continue beyond the period for which funding is available?
2. If so, what level of financial and other resources will be needed to continue?
3. What capacity-building measures are needed to make the initiative sustainable? How will these measures be implemented?
4. What is it about this initiative that is likely to attract interest and elicit support?
5. Who are the most likely future funders? (Be specific. If government, what level of government, what agency, what funding stream? If private, which foundation or other source?)
6. Is there a history of this entity supporting efforts (a) of this sort? and (b) of this size?
7. Would success in this effort obviate the need to spend resources on something else, and could that money be diverted to this effort? How?
8. Who within the anticipated funding organization would have to decide to fund, through what processes?

Source: Cutler, I. (2002). *End games: The challenge of sustainability.* Baltimore: Annie E. Casey Foundation Publisher, pp. 23–24.

DISPLAY 31.4	**NATIONAL NURSING CENTERS CONSORTIUM**

Vision
Keep the nation healthy through nurse-managed health care.

Mission
To strengthen the capacity, growth, and development of nurse-managed health centers to provide access to quality care for vulnerable populations and to eliminate health disparities.

Goals
1. Provide national leadership in identifying, tracking, and advising health care policy development.
2. Position nurse-managed health centers as a recognized mainstream health care model.
3. Foster partnerships with people and groups who share common goals.

Source: National Nursing Centers Consortium. (2008). Retrieved August 20, 2008 from http://www.nncc.us.

consideration for organizations such as NMHCs when completing a grant application for funding (see Display 31.3).

National Organization: The National Nursing Centers Consortium

In 1996, due to interest from several nursing center directors, staff, and community members to address all aspects of operations and to provide ongoing collaboration and continuing education, the Regional Nursing Centers Consortium (RNCC) of Pennsylvania, New Jersey, and Delaware was established. In the short span of 5 years, nursing centers nationwide were contacting the RNCC with inquiries related to all aspects of operations, funding, and sustainability. It soon became evident that the RNCC needed to expand its service area to meet the needs of NMHCs nationwide. In 2001, The **National Nursing Centers Consortium (NNCC)** was formed to represent NMHCs nationwide. Headquartered in Philadelphia, Pennsylvania, the NNCC expanded internationally in 2005 with the addition of a NMHC in Auckland, New Zealand. The vision, mission, and goals of the NNCC are found in Display 31.4.

Best Practices of Nurse-managed Health Centers

In contemporary health care, evidence-based practice (EBP) is the process of making clinical decisions based upon the best available research evidence, clinical expertise, and client preferences in the context of available resources (Melnyk & Fineout-Overholt, 2005). Nurse-managed health centers implement EBP via **best practices**, or the application of the best available evidence to improve practice (Youngblut & Brooten, 2001). Chapter 4 provides an extensive overview of EBP.

Annually, the NNCC conducts a *Best Practice Conference* at varied locations throughout the nation. This professional conference brings together nurses, staff members, funders, and political leaders to share best practices and participate in networking opportunities. Continuing education credits are awarded for attendance at scientific sessions. This is one example of how NMHCs set standards for quality improvement and promote professional growth among members.

Role of Students in Nurse-managed Health Centers

Undergraduate and graduate students from several disciplines play a vital part in the activities of NMHCs. These disciplines include, but are not limited to, nursing, social work, mental health, dental, nutrition, and speech-language-hearing science students. When students are assigned to a NMHC for their clinical experience, they become aware of the distinctiveness of nursing centers from other health care delivery systems and of the variety of models and organizational structures that exist, and they are active participants in the vital activities of the particular nursing center to which they are assigned. Most often, students are engaged in primary and secondary prevention strategies via health education, immunization, and screening programs. Students' roles are similar to those of their staff mentors, including advocate, case manager, educator, and referral agent. Faculty roles in NMHC academic models involve clinical supervision of undergraduate and graduate students assigned to the nursing center for their clinical experience (see From the Case Files II).

EVIDENCE-BASED PRACTICE

The Role of Community-based Practice Research

The importance of practice-based research networks (PBRNs) in primary health care research and the need for community based primary health research for addressing health disparities experienced by large populations in the United States, is addressed in this article. The unique community-based care delivered by nurses in NMHCs provides a distinct opportunity to combine the strengths of community-based practice research (CBPR) methods, found within a PBRN, to develop and test EBP that benefits health outcomes and decreases health disparities.

The Midwest Nursing Centers Consortium Research Network (MCCRN) was funded by a grant from the Agency for Healthcare Research and Quality in 2002 to begin to develop a collaborative program of PBPR with vulnerable populations across multiple NMHC sites. The research network began with 20 NMHCs, in operation from 3 to 17 years and representing thirteen Midwestern universities. By 2005, the MCCRN had 19 academic NMHCs based in 15 universities.

The original purposes of the MCCRN were to establish a practice-based research network for APNs who practice in NMHCs, establish a web-based system for data collection, and develop a collaborative program of CBPR with vulnerable populations that will inform primary care practitioners about health professional education and health care policy. Additional aims include linkages with other nursing PBRNs, to create a national network to generate knowledge about users of NMHCs, advanced practice nursing in community-based settings, and health outcomes among vulnerable and minority populations served by NMHCs.

The Robert Wood Johnson's Foundation Prescription for Health initiative provided funding for the first MNC-CRN's research study. This study, "Wellness for a Lifetime," took place in eight NMHCs at seven universities in five states. The primary purpose of this study was to evaluate outcomes of an accessible, culturally, and educationally appropriate physical activity and nutritional intervention for high-risk, low-income, ethnically diverse clients of NMHCs.

Findings included self-reported behavior changes (increase movement and physical activity) as well as intake of a more balanced diet (less junk food and increased fruits and vegetables). The major findings were:

- Twenty-one APNs participated; chart audits before and after the study revealed that APN assessment of physical activity levels (32.9% versus 47.5%) and nutritional status (30.5% versus 56.8%) improved significantly ($p < .01$).
- Clients were predominately women (84%), with an age range between 25 and 83 years and a diverse ethnic distribution of African American (44.4%), White (44.4%), Hispanic (9.9%), and Native American (1.1%).
- Of the 121 clients who signed consent forms, 82 started the program; of those, 20 clients withdrew during the study, for an overall retention rate of 50%.

Nursing Implications

Evidence from the first MNCCRN study suggests that a shift in the level of wellness in a large percentage of the population of the nation may depend upon the ability to create new models of health care and promotion that merge the traditional model of primary care with a public health approach to primary prevention and health promotion. Nurse researchers can work with community representatives to identify questions significant to populations served, plan and execute studies that include adequate numbers of participants from underrepresented populations, and generate evidence that can be translated back into best practices at NMHCs.

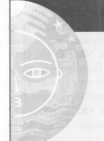

From the Case Files II

Health Screening at an NMHC

Public Health Nurses from an academic wellness NMHC and undergraduate student nurses are conducting blood pressure and glucose screenings at a church-sponsored health fair. For optimum participation, the event is conducted on Sunday from 10 a.m. to 2 p.m., before, during, and after church services. Approximately 50% of adults screened have hypertension and/or hyperglycemia. One African American male participant, who was asymptomatic, had severe hypertension (220/154) and was transported to the nearest hospital for evaluation.

1. What are the possible sequela of untreated hypertension and hyperglycemia?
2. What are some feasible referrals that the PHNs may have made for this aggregate?
3. What types of primary prevention strategies may benefit those attendees who had normal screening results?
4. In what ways do student nurses benefit from participating in this type of screening activity, such as participation at a health fair?

FAITH COMMUNITY NURSING

Faith community nursing is one of the newest nursing specialties, and one of the oldest means of health care delivery. For hundreds of years, deaconesses, sisters, and lay members of religious communities have been involved in ministering to the sick. This tradition was revitalized through the efforts of Reverend Dr. Granger Westberg, a hospital chaplain and Lutheran minister, in the 1960s. Westberg observed a great need for preventive and holistic health services, especially among the underserved. He estimated that one-third of the illnesses his patients experienced could have been prevented, or the severity reduced, by education and health promotion (Westberg, 1990). To address these needs, he launched several church-based holistic health clinics that were each staffed by a physician, nurse, and chaplain. These clinics provided health services to the underserved in the community for several years. The clinics eventually closed, but the experience led Reverend Westberg to recognize the unique ability of nurses to bridge the disciplines of medicine and religion, and assist the client in understanding the physical and spiritual influences on health. In 1985, Westberg initiated a pilot project in which nurses provided holistic, preventive health care for six Christian congregations in the Chicago area. These nurses were called *parish nurses*.

The surrounding community quickly recognized the positive impact of the parish nurses on the six congregations. More and more churches sought to incorporate a parish nurse into their staff. The parish nursing movement soon spread beyond Christian religious institutions and beyond the borders of the United States to Canada, Australia, and New Zealand. The International Parish Nurse Resource Center, formed in the 1980s, has provided educational programs and resources for nurses seeking to practice as a parish nurse for over two decades. The Health Ministries Association (HMA, 2008) provides additional resources and support for faith community nursing practice and was instrumental in developing the first *Scope and Standards of Parish Nursing Practice* (American Nurses Association/Health Ministries Association [ANA/HMA], 1998).

The original *Scope and Standards of Parish Nursing Practice* defined **parish nurse** as "a registered professional nurse who serves as a member of the ministry staff of a faith community to promote health and wholeness of the faith community . . ." (ANA/HMA, 1998, p.1). The term **faith community** was defined broadly as "an organization of families and individuals who share common values, beliefs, religious doctrine and faith practices . . . such as a church synagogue or mosque . . ." (ANA/HMA, 1998, p. 6). These definitions were carried over to the revised scope and standards published in 2005. In the *Faith Community Nursing: Scope and Standards of Practice* (ANA/HMA, 2005), the title of parish nurse was changed to faith community nurse (FCN) and the name of the specialty was changed to "faith community nursing" (ANA/HMA, 2005). Today, nurses who practice in a faith community may be referred to as a **faith community nurse** (FCN), parish nurse, **health ministry nurse**, or **congregational nurse** depending upon preference and the traditions of the faith community. No matter what title is used, a nurse who practices in a faith community is governed by the *Faith Community Nursing: Scope and Standards of Practice* (ANA/HMA, 2005).

What Do Faith Community Nurses Do?

Activities and interventions used by FCNs are as diverse as their faith communities. Authors have described key aspects of this specialty, which include meeting the emotional and spiritual support needs of the dying (O'Brien, 2006; Redmond, 2006; Weis, Schank, & Matheus, 2006) and serving as an advocate for individuals who are hospitalized, living at home, or in long-term care facilities (Patterson, 2007). Faith community nurses also provide health education by developing ongoing programs that provide essential health information. For example, Redmond (2006) developed a monthly health presentation she coined the "Health Spot," which was provided in conjunction with a women's church luncheon. Topics presented were related directly to health concerns common to older women who attended the luncheon. Redmond also developed a competitive walking program framed in a spiritual context to appeal to members of her faith community. Others have described the development of holistic exercise and wellness programs (White, Drechsel, & Johnson, 2006) and health education programs (DeHaven, et al., 2004).

Researchers have also explored what FCNs do. In a review of research, King (2004) concluded that caring, listening, being there, and providing health promotion and health screenings were common and effective interventions provided by the FCN. Anderson's (2004) study of parish nurses supports King's conclusions. Anderson found that providing holistic support was a major theme in FCN practice. Holistic support included actions that addressed physical, social, emotional, mental, and spiritual needs such as health education, counseling, referral to community agencies, advocacy on the client's behalf to meet needs and reduce complications, and mobilizing other members of the faith community to provide support such as visitation, meals, and transportation.

Although some of these interventions may seem different from traditional nursing, which emphasizes physical care, medication administration, and other prescribed treatments, all registered professional nurses including the FCN share the use of the nursing process (ANA, 2004). For the FCN, implementation of a plan of care incorporates actions that fall within one or more of the seven roles of the FCN (see Display 31.5).

Roles of the Faith Community Nurse

The goal of the FCN is the "protection, promotion and optimization of health and abilities; prevention of illness and injury; and responding to suffering within the context of the values, beliefs, and practices of the faith community. . . ." (ANA/HMA, 2005, p. 1). Health promotion outcomes may be primary, directed at prevention of disease, illness, or injury; secondary, focused on early detection and appropriate intervention; or tertiary, concerned with promoting a sense of well-being when preventing or curing a condition may not occur. To achieve the goal of faith community nursing, seven diverse nursing roles are central for the FCN to incorporate into practice.

Health Educator

A primary role of the FCN is as a health educator. Increasing awareness of health issues through health education is

DISPLAY 31.5	ASSURING CONGREGATIONAL HEALTH AND WHOLENESS

Roles of the Faith Community Nurse
1. Health educator
2. Health counselor
3. Advocate
4. Referral agent
5. Developer of support groups
6. Coordinator of volunteers
7. Integrator of faith and health

Accountability
1. ANA Scope and Standards of Nursing Practice
2. ANA Scope and Standards of Faith Community Nursing
3. Congregational standards
4. Institutional standards
5. ANA Social Policy Statement
6. ANA Code of Ethics for Nurses with Interpretive Statements
7. State nurse practice act
8. Patients rights

the foundation for health promotion and lifestyle changes. The FCN uses assessment skills to determine the health issues that may be present in the faith community and assesses the educational needs related to these issues. In the role of health educator, the FCN may provide individual and group education strategies such as providing health education materials, leading health education classes, or providing health screenings. The FCN may also develop educational displays or flyers, or write educational articles for the faith community newsletter or website (Patterson, 2006).

Health Counselor

When education alone is not sufficient for empowering the individual to initiate a change or seek assistance, health counseling may be indicated. In the health counseling role, the nurse seeks to understand the individual's perceptions, fears, and barriers that prevent the person from taking action. The FCN may use a five-step health counseling process described as the 5 A's: Ask, Advise, Assess, Assist, and Arrange (Fiore, et al., 2000). Using this process, the FCN asks about the person's perceptions related to a specific health concern, advises the person about the health concern and the benefits of taking health promoting actions, assesses the person's readiness to take action, offers assistance and guidance in planning ways to address the health concern, and arranges follow-up support.

Advocate

The third role of a FCN is that of an advocate, helping individuals obtain needed services or care whether in the hos-

pital, a long-term care facility, or at home. In the advocate role, the FCN uses knowledge of the health care system and awareness of safe and effective care practices to facilitate appropriate, timely intervention. Advocacy is indicated when dealing with vulnerable populations, such as older adults, children, or the homeless, who may not have the ability to speak for themselves or may lack the knowledge or awareness of what constitutes safe, effective care (Patterson, 2007).

Referral Agent

The FCN also functions as a referral agent by assisting and guiding the client through the health care system and connecting the client with needed community resources. Through networking with community agencies, the FCN is often aware of and able to access a variety of community resources that support the client's physical, social, financial, emotional, or spiritual needs.

Developer of Support Groups

Receiving emotional support from persons who share similar experiences can provide strength, comfort, knowledge, and a sense of empowerment. When the FCN discovers a need for a support group that is not currently available in the community at large, the FCN may fulfill the role of developer of support groups. The FCN develops groups tailored to the faith community needs such as coping with loss and grief, cancer, caregiver stress, chronic illness, single parenting, addiction recovery, and more. The FCN may lead or facilitate the support groups or may train others to fulfill those positions.

Coordinator of Volunteers

The health ministry mission of a faith community typically includes a variety of services and activities to provide holistic support of the physical, social, emotional, mental, and spiritual needs of its members. Such a diverse array of services cannot be provided by the FCN alone. In the role of coordinator of volunteers, the FCN recruits, trains, and coordinates other members of the faith community. Volunteers provide or assist with a variety of services such as home, hospital, or long-term care visitations; respite care; assisting with transportation needs of home-bound individuals; calling or sending cards to ill or injured members; and assisting with health screenings. Health ministry volunteers may include nurses, counselors, physical therapists, pharmacists, and other health care providers, as well as those with no health care background.

Integrator of Faith and Health

A distinctly unique role of the FCN is as integrator of faith and health. This role emphasizes the holistic relationship between physical, social, emotional, mental, and spiritual dimensions of the person. The FCN helps the person to improve health or enhance wellness by appreciating how the dimensions of the person are interconnected and by helping the person strengthen or support the weaker aspects, as needed.

Models of Faith Community Nursing Practice

Models of faith community nursing practice are diverse and may be categorized according to volunteer versus salaried positions with institutional versus faith-based sponsorship. The type of practice model adopted depends upon variables such as the number of faith community members served, the existing health ministry services in place, the faith community's governance structure and financial resources, and existing health care systems in the community at large.

Early in the development of faith community nursing, a large number of FCNs were part-time volunteers who were members of the faith community they were serving. Gradually, as communities experienced the positive effect of FCNs within their organizations and researchers validated the effectiveness of FCNs (Brown, 2006; Rethemeyer & Wehling, 2004; Rydholm, 2006), more and more faith communities began creating salaried positions for FCNs. Salaried FCNs may be employed full- or part-time by the faith community, by a group of faith communities, or by a health care system as part of their pastoral care community outreach.

Regardless of the model of practice utilized, integrating the FCN position into the faith community's organizational structure is recommended (Solari-Twadell & McDermott, 2005; Westberg, 1990; Westberg-McNamara, 2006). One way this integration can be provided is with the formation of a *health cabinet* or health and wellness committee within the faith community. The health cabinet was originally described as a way to provide health ministry for a faith community that is interested in adding a FCN to its staff (Westberg, 1990). The health cabinet includes members from the faith community who are interested in promoting and sponsoring health-related activities and programs for the faith community. Members may be nurses, other health care professionals, or persons with no health care background. The FCN functions as a member of the health cabinet and receives guidance and support from the cabinet in developing, promoting, and delivering programs and services to members of the faith community.

Becoming a Faith Community Nurse

The FCN practices community nursing with a high degree of independence and autonomy. Often, the FCN deals with clients experiencing complex health care situations who may have limited resources and extensive health-related needs. Recommended educational preparation for a FCN includes a bachelor's degree in nursing with community nursing experience as part of the program (ANA/HMA, 2005), and completion of additional education such as a *basic preparation course*. The basic preparation course addresses the roles of the FCN, and provides information on establishing, promoting, and maintaining a FCN practice. Participants gain experience in resolving complex client situations using scenarios and case studies.

Establishing a Faith Community Nursing Practice

Several steps are involved in creating a FCN position within a faith community. One of the first things to do is assess the community the nurse plans to serve, identifying the health needs of the faith community and the roles of the FCN that meet those needs. For example, a nurse might assess the demographics of the community and determine the most common health concerns and what education or health counseling needs the faith community may have. A needs assessment survey of the membership about health concerns, or topics of interest may be used. Questions to explore include: Does the faith community need support groups for members who are experiencing the stress of illness, injury, or loss and grief? Do the members of the faith community need more information or assistance to access existing community resources? Is there a need for health screening, respite care, or visitation for the sick or injured in their home, hospital, or long-term care facility?

Once the nurse has assessed the needs of the faith community, he can then identify how a FCN could help to meet those needs. He uses this information to seek the support of the faith community members and staff, usually through visits with key members of the faith community, including longstanding members and past and present board members. The nurse describes to these key members the roles of a FCN and how specific health needs of the faith community could be addressed by the services of a FCN, then solicits input from the staff and spiritual leaders of the faith community.

After key members and leaders of the faith community have verbalized support for adding a FCN to the organization's health ministry, the nurse must seek formal approval from the organization's governing body. The scope of services to be offered, time commitment expected, process of referral to the FCN, means of contacting the FCN, and other administrative aspects of the position should be negotiated before approval is finalized. The organization's bylaws, committee structure, and spiritual leader will determine the process for obtaining formal approval and will determine where the FCN will fit in the organizational structure. The approval process may require a formal presentation of the nurse's proposal to the board members or to the faith community as a whole.

Launching a FCN practice should begin after formal approval and after the nurse has prepared himself and the community for his role as a FCN. As a community health nurse practicing as a FCN, additional educational preparation such as a basic preparation course (mentioned earlier) is recommended. This course provides foundational knowledge for providing care encompassing the seven roles of the FCN, as well as guidance in establishing and maintaining a practice as a FCN.

Another aspect of preparation involves establishing community contacts and compiling information about community resources. The FCN should visit local health-related agencies, clinics, and hospitals and discuss services they provide and how the services can be accessed by members of his faith community. He may seek out community organizations such as the March of Dimes, American Cancer Society, and American Heart Association, which provide health information and online resources for health promotion activities.

If the faith community is not familiar with FCNs, the nurse will want to educate them about the roles of the FCN by describing specific activities that will be actively pursued, such as visitations, support groups, health classes, health screening, health counseling, and referral to community resources. The nurse should consider making presentations about faith community nursing to groups within the faith community, such as prayer circles, adult Sunday school, teen groups, and existing support groups. These presentations will provide multiple benefits for the FCN and the faith community: the nurse will become familiar with members of the faith community, and they will become familiar with the nurse and the services he will be offering.

In addition to providing presentations about faith community nursing to groups within the faith community, the nurse should consider other ways to inform members of his presence. If the faith community publishes a newsletter or has a website, including a brief introduction to faith community nursing and providing some personal background and professional experience information will help. The nurse may wish to develop flyers and/or brochures that describe what a FCN does and the services he will offer, distributing these from the faith community's office, bulletin board, or foyer. Business cards that provide name, contact information, and outline FCN services may be made available. Once these steps are completed and the foundation for practice has been laid, the nurse is ready to begin a new career path as a FCN.

OCCUPATIONAL HEALTH NURSING

Business and industry provide another group of settings for community health nursing practice. Employee health has long been recognized as making a vital contribution to individual lives, productivity of business, and the well-being of the entire nation. Organizations are expected to provide a safe and healthy work environment in addition to offering insurance for health care. More companies, recognizing the value of healthy employees, are going beyond offering traditional health benefits to supporting health promotional efforts. Some businesses, for example, offer healthy snacks such as fruit at breaks and promote jogging during the noon hour. A few larger corporations have built exercise facilities for their employees, provide health education programs, and offer financial incentives for losing weight or staying well. An increasing number of both large and small companies have recognized the benefits of occupational and environmental health nurses as part of their overall health promotion and wellness efforts.

ROLE OF THE OCCUPATIONAL AND ENVIRONMENTAL HEALTH NURSE

Community health nurses have a long history of involvement in occupational health. In 1895, the Vermont Marble Company hired the first industrial nurse in the United States to care for its employees and their families. At the time, it was an unusual demonstration of interest in employee welfare. The nursing service, which consisted mostly of home visiting and care of the sick, was free to employees and their families. Gradually, that role changed. World War II showed a marked increase in employment of industrial public health nurses, who practiced illness prevention and health education among employees at work.

In addition to emergency care and nursing of ill employees, the activities of many industrial nurses involved

safety education, hygiene, nutrition, and improvement of working conditions. Yet, a significantly high number of industrial injuries and sick employees kept many nurses too busy to do anything but care for the ill. They might see more than 75 patients a day in the plant dispensary, where they provided first aid and medications. Employee health programs have improved as socioeconomic and political pressures have created improved safety and health standards for the work environment. Similarly, these developments have changed and expanded the nurse's role. The role of an **occupational and environmental health nurse** is to ensure that the workforce is healthy and productive, as evidenced by the nursing practice standards developed by the Association of Occupational Health Nurses, Inc. (2008).

Special Skills and Demands

The nurse's role in occupational health, as previously mentioned, has traditionally focused on illness and injury care. This directly resulted from the knowledge and skills obtained in basic nursing education. During the last decade, a number of nursing education programs (primarily on the graduate level) have developed a specialty focus in occupational and environmental health. In addition, many continuing education programs provide occupational and environmental health nurses with updated information and skill training for identifying and assisting in the management of the physical, chemical, biologic, ergonomic, and psychosocial factors in the work environment that can affect worker health and safety. As a result, the occupational health nurse's role is not universal; it depends on the type and philosophy of the company, type and number of workers, health professionals involved, exposures and potential hazards in the work environment, and knowledge and skills of the nurse.

Internationally, occupational health nursing education is garnering attention. The World Health Organization (WHO), as expressed in the 2007 document *Workers' Health: Global Plan of Action,* takes the position that:

> Development of human resources for workers' health should be further strengthened by: further postgraduate training in relevant disciplines; building capacity for basic occupational health services; incorporating workers' health in the training of primary health care practitioners and other professionals needed for occupational health services; creating incentives for attracting and retaining human resources for workers' health, and encouraging the establishment of networks of services and professional associations. Attention should be given not only to postgraduate but also to basic training for health professionals in various fields such as promotion of workers' health and the prevention and treatment of workers' health problems. This should be a particular priority in primary health care. (World Health Organization [WHO], p. 6)

This WHO document was based on the earlier policy statement regarding occupational health disparities and the release in 2003 of a standardized occupational health nursing curriculum. These WHO efforts were the basis of a 2004–2005 study of undergraduate nursing programs in Turkey. Esin, Emiroglu, Aksayan, and Beser (2008) sought to determine the length of time devoted to occupational health nursing and the qualifications of the instructors.

Overall, the research indicated limited time spent in both theory and practical experiences, and faculty, although well qualified in public health nursing, had limited practical experience in the corporate sector, pointing to the need for a standardized curriculum in Turkey and other developing countries, as provided in the WHO documents.

Consistent with the WHO (2003) recommendations that occupational health nursing requires additional training and expertise beyond the basic level, U.S. nurses in this specialty are encouraged to seek certification through the American Board for Occupational Health Nurses, Inc. (ABOHN). Established in 1972, this independent nursing specialty board has the stated purposes of establishing standards and examinations for professional nurses in occupational health, elevating and maintaining the quality of occupational health nursing services, stimulating the development of improved educational standards and programs in the field of occupational health nursing, and encouraging occupational health nurses to continue their professional education (ABOHN, 2008).

Nurses who select the field of occupational health and safety encounter experiences that differ significantly from those found in an acute care setting. To make the adjustment, the nurse should be aware of the factors that make occupational health unique.

Unlike hospitals or ambulatory care centers, the workplace is a non–health care institution in which production or service (not health care) is the primary goal. The occupational and environmental health nurse participates in the organization's goals through activities that contribute to the productivity of the workforce.

An occupational and environmental health nurse in the organization is in a staff position, taking on the role of a consultant, educator, or role model in the workplace, but has no supervisory responsibilities or power to hire or fire workers. The nurse is generally responsible for management of the occupational health unit, serving the needs of employees and management personnel.

The occupational and environmental health nurse, especially in smaller organizations, may be the only nurse in the company. As a result, he has none of the on-site consultation and direction that are needed for comfortable, competent, and independent decision-making. Nurses who use critical thinking skills to develop a framework for independent problem-solving enhance their efficiency. A nurse who works alone may feel isolated and need to collaborate with the occupational health and safety team members.

There are various causes of job stress for the occupational and environmental health nurse, and there may be related personal, professional, and employer factors. The nurse may experience role ambiguity due to a lack of professional preparation or inadequate orientation and continuing education. The corporate culture and leadership may foster work overload, be nonsupportive, and have limited career opportunities for the nurse. Occupational and environmental health nurses need to apply strategies to reduce job stress and potential job strain by modeling health-affirming choices, networking with other nurses and professional organizations in the community, and setting appropriate occupational health standards.

The client base served in occupational health is a well-adult population with whom long-term contact is possible.

Occupational and environmental health nurses, therefore, have the chance to know their clients well and have opportunities to work with them through various stages of personal as well as health service–related incidents. Such continuity of health care can challenge occupational health nurses to use all of the community health nursing model interventions—education, engineering, and enforcement.

Finally, the practice focus is oriented to the aggregate; the nurse serves a worker population. Environmental factors significantly influence the health and safety of workers. Therefore, occupational health nurses need to constantly monitor the work environment and assess the health needs of the entire worker population to identify those at risk, particularly workers in hazardous lines of work, and to develop prevention, promotion, and protection programs (see Display 31.6).

Community-based Occupational Health Nursing

Agencies external to business and industry also provide occupational and environmental health nursing services. Historically, public health nurses from visiting nurse associations made home visits to sick employees and their families. In subsequent years, public health agencies provided part-time nursing services to small companies. These services included supervising the work environment, conducting health examinations, keeping records, teaching about and counseling on health issues, providing first aid, giving immunizations, and referring workers to community resources. More recently, community health nursing services have offered health screening and health promotion programs. Furthermore, occupational and environmental health nurse consultants based in state departments of health provide consultation and continuing education programs to nurses employed in occupational health settings.

Hospital-based occupational health programs, large medical–industrial health clinics, and insurance companies also provide occupational and environmental health nursing services. These services may be in the form of direct care (rehabilitation of an injured worker) or indirect care (consultation on implementing regulations regarding record keeping or compiling health statistics).

A continuing unmet need is attending to the health of workers in smaller companies. These companies have more hazards because equipment and controls are often inadequate. They seldom, if ever, have a health professional on site. Attempts have been made by some communities to provide needed health protection services, but no sustained efforts exist. Community health nurses are in a position to accept this challenge and develop a system that will ensure ongoing service to this high-risk population.

Members of the Occupational Health Team

Today, the two professionals who generally provide on-site occupational health services are the occupational and environmental health nurse and the safety engineer. Other members of the interprofessional team may include an industrial hygienist, epidemiologist, toxicologist, and occupational physician. However, these specialists usually are employed only by large corporations, or they provide only selected part-time services on a contractual basis. Therefore, the

DISPLAY 31.6	OCCUPATIONAL AND ENVIRONMENTAL HEALTH NURSING CARE PLAN

Evelyn Robbins has been the Occupational and Environmental Health Nurse at ABC Metals for 4 years. She works with management, the company physician (who works at ABC Metals 2 days a week), union representatives, unit foremen, individual employees, and representatives from the community businesses and neighborhoods surrounding the plant. The company employs 400 workers—380 in manufacturing, primarily an assembly line making telephone electrical boxes, and 20 management and administrative staff.

Recently, 12 employees came to the worksite clinic complaining of hand injuries that had not occurred before. Ms. Robbins treated the wounds, reported the occurrences to the foremen involved, and reported the incidents to management. In addition, she wanted to explore the cause of these injuries so that they could be interrupted. She used the nursing process in her exploration.

Assessment
- Tour the areas where the incidents occurred
- Inquire among the foremen to determine whether there was a change in routine, equipment, employee assignment, or product being manufactured
- Ask injured employees what they were doing when the injury occurred
- Reassess wounds for likenesses and differences; for example, was it the right or left hand and was it on the same part of the hand in each case?

Diagnoses
- Wounds occurred in factory areas where a new piece of equipment had been installed
- Injured employees did not receive orientation to the equipment

Plan
- Plan to work with foremen to provide an orientation for all employees who work with the new equipment
- Plan an orientation program (with foremen, union representative, and one employee from each unit in the factory) for all employees before working with new equipment in the future, to prevent further injuries

Implementation
- Implement the orientation for employees who work with the new equipment
- Initiate the orientation program as new equipment is introduced into the factory

Evaluation
- Have there been any new equipment-related injuries in the factory?
- Has there been any change in general safety in the factory related to the increased focus on safety with new equipment.

position of occupational and environmental health nurse in a large company or of the community health nurse who serves smaller companies is the cornerstone of occupational health.

Collaboration may take time, but it is worth the investment. The occupational health nurse must gain the respect and trust of management and establish open communication to influence company policies regarding the nature and scope of health programs.

Depending on the size of the company and its products or services, the occupational health nurse may also collaborate with any or all of the following people: insurance carriers, union representatives, employee assistance counselors, industrial hygienists, safety engineers, company or outside lawyers, toxicologists, human resources personnel, and the community. Any comprehensive assessment of employee health and safety problems, as well as any health promotion program, requires cooperation and assistance from many people working in various departments within the organization.

Finally, the occupational health team is not complete without the workers themselves. Employees can help identify problems and needs while contributing to decision-making about health programs. Their cooperation in implementing and evaluating programs is essential for an effective health protection and promotion effort.

Future Trends

A broad goal for occupational health is to promote and maintain the highest level of physical, social, and emotional health for all workers. In practice, this goal is only beginning to be realized in selected instances. Nevertheless, it is a worthy and, more importantly, an essential objective in the realization of an energized and productive working community.

However, the rapid and fundamental changes in U.S. businesses and the economy in the 1990s and 2000s have added four critical issues that affect the practice of occupational and environmental health nursing. First, the downturn in the global economy, and in the economy of the United States specifically, has skeletonized many worksites, shut down companies, eliminated night or evening shifts, or moved companies to less expensive communities. In addition, several major scandals have eliminated jobs within hours, such as in the Enron and Worldcom corporations, and in those major banks involved in risky home loans that resulted in unprecedented housing foreclosures across the country. Second, increasing worldwide competition requires businesses to remain competitive by reducing or controlling operating costs at the lowest level possible. Third, an increase in technologic hazards requires a sophisticated approach as well as knowledge of toxicology, epidemiology, ergonomics, and public health principles. Fourth, health care costs continue to escalate at faster rates than most company profits do.

Current occupational and environmental health nurse practices will continue to evolve to meet future needs. The focus will shift from one-on-one health services to a new role involving broader environmental, business, and research skills. One such example of this changing role was an Australian study of nurses' perceptions of their current and future roles in occupational health practice (Mellor & St. John, 2007). The researchers found that wellness, management, and research were the more important activities identified. Their findings suggest that educational efforts should focus on wellness-based models of practice, research, and negotiating skills for the workplace.

Current occupational health nurse activities include the following:

- Supervising care for emergencies and minor illnesses
- Counseling employees about health risks
- Following up with employees' workers' compensation claims
- Performing periodic health assessments
- Evaluating the health status of employees returning to work

Future occupational health nurse activities will involve the following:

- Analyzing trends (health promotion, risk reduction, and health expenditures)
- Developing programs suited to corporate needs
- Recommending more efficient and cost-effective in-house health services
- Determining cost-effective alternatives to health programs and services
- Collaborating with others to identify problems and propose solutions

As we move further into the 21st century, occupational and environmental health nurses and management will share the goal of developing a healthy, productive, and profitable company. A healthy company consists of healthy and productive employees, and healthy employees mean lower health care costs. Lower costs result in an increased competitive edge and higher profits. Higher profits can make more resources available to support more programs and to improve employee health.

The occupational and environmental health nurse will particularly need skills in effective communication, leadership, change management, research, business acumen, and assertiveness. These tools will be crucial for effectively interpreting the occupational health nurse's role and promoting ideas. The success of programs developed by the occupational health nurse depends on establishing positive working relationships with the other team members. Nurses involved in occupational health have a unique opportunity to help shape the health profile of the working population. An example of this type of effort was the study by Hyeonkyeong, Wilbur, Kim, and Miller (2007) linking high job insecurity with increased risk for lower-back work-related musculoskeletal disorders among long-haul flight attendants. Their findings point to the need for occupational health nurses in the airline industry to be aware of the potential relationship between job tasks and work-related psychosocial factors.

The degree of the occupational nurse's influence depends on how the nurse defines the occupational and environmental health nurse role. Also, the nurse must be able to overcome the many obstacles found in the occupational setting, including restrictive company policies, misunderstanding of the nurse's role, and lack of time for innovative program development. The nurse's role in occupational health, therefore, varies considerably. It ranges from providing only emergency care for on-the-job injuries or illness to establishing comprehensive policies and programs covering health promotion, accident and disease prevention, and innovative care for disease and disability.

Occupational and environmental health nursing demands a great deal from the nurse. Individual needs in the workplace always compete for the nurse's time and take attention away from aggregate needs, often to the detriment of the latter. To maintain a proper focus on aggregate needs requires discipline and commitment—commitment based on a different mindset and the realization that the health and productivity of workers are interrelated with the health of the community.

Summary

Healthy People 2020 will guide both public and private sector nursing practice well into the next decade. Community health nurses have a number of options available to them as they seek to address the myriad health issues facing our communities. For many, the opportunities may present to assume roles in a variety of nontraditional settings, including nurse-managed health centers, faith community nursing, and occupational and environmental health nursing. All three settings offer the community health nurse the opportunity to address health disparities in their communities, promote healthy lifestyles, and improve the overall health and well-being of their respective populations.

Nurse-managed health centers have emerged as critical safety net providers in America's health care delivery system. Various nursing center models exist and are located in health professional shortage areas or medically underserved areas in urban and rural communities. Interdisciplinary teams of APNs, social workers, substance abuse counselors, community health outreach workers, and students from varied disciplines, provide services that generally focus on primary and secondary prevention strategies. Lundeen's comprehensive community based primary health care model demonstrates how NMHCs are distinct from public health agencies and medical care facilities. Funding sources for NMHCs include reimbursement from various organizations, sliding scale fees, grants, contracts, foundation support, and private support via gifts. Sustainability is an ongoing challenge in all NMHC models. An international organization to strengthen the capacity, growth, and development of NMHCs is The National Nursing Center Consortium. Nurse-managed health centers identify, develop, and share best practices. Nurse leaders and staff from NMHCs engage in sociopolitical activities to raise awareness of the outcomes generated by the nursing center model. These activities are implemented to raise awareness of the role of NMHCs in the health care system and to promote sustainability of the centers. Undergraduate and graduate students from various disciplines engage in all aspects of NMHC activities and augment the interdisciplinary team.

Faith community nurses practice community nursing within a unique setting—a faith community. A FCN may provide services to a single faith community or may coordinate services for multiple communities. The FCN addresses the physical, social, emotional, mental, and spiritual needs of the faith community through the roles of health educator, health counselor, referral agent, advocate, developer of support groups, coordinator of volunteers, and integrator of faith and health.

Occupational and environmental health nursing applies the philosophy and skills of nursing, community, and environmental health to protect and promote the health of people in their workplaces. The occupational and environmental health nurse's role is evolving as business becomes more competitive and health care costs escalate at a frightening rate. That expanded role will include analyzing current trends, recommending more cost-effective and innovative in-house health services, and collaborating with other members of the multidisciplinary occupational health team, including management, to develop appropriate programs.

Each of these three professional practice areas provides a unique opportunity for community health nursing practice. Escalating health care costs, increasing numbers of uninsured and underinsured, and the many gaps in services experienced by so many in our communities present an unprecedented opportunity for community health nurses. The many unmet needs in our communities can be addressed, but only if nurses are willing to take the "road less traveled," as did Lillian Wald and the other pioneers of nursing. As you ponder your options for practice, consider the challenges and the many benefits of these and the many other practice areas in your community. Perhaps you cannot envision yourself in this type of service at this point in your career. A time may come, however, when you are afforded the chance to participate in your own faith community health education efforts, refer a client to a nurse-managed health center, or possibly collaborate with an occupational and environmental health nurse to address an emerging health issue in your community. ■

ACTIVITIES TO PROMOTE CRITICAL THINKING

1. You are practicing as a newly hired nurse in a NMHC. What assessments would you conduct to determine the needs for the local community that surrounds the NMHC? What sources of data (qualitative and quantitative) would be useful to you during your assessment?

2. Based upon your findings in the previous question, what public policy issues are apparent in this community? How could you, as a nurse working in this NMHC, impact public policy in the future? What key legislators would you contact? How would you accomplish this?

3. Locate a NMHC in your community. Interview a nurse practitioner or public health nurse employed there. Ask the nurse to describe the type of NMHC model he works in. Ask the nurse about *Best Practices* performed in his role. If you cannot locate a NMHC in your local community, search online via the National Nursing Center Consortium's website at www.nncc.us for a NMHC. E-mail the nurse listed as the contact person and ask him the questions in activity 2.

4. This chapter covers the role of the faith community nurse. Search for information about this area of community health nursing in your community. Do you know a faith community nurse? If so, plan to observe his practice for a few hours and explore what the role entails in this faith community.

5. Figure 31.1 depicts the major focus areas identified to meet the nation's goals of increasing years of healthy life and eliminating health disparities. Which of these focus areas is addressed by each of the three areas of practice discussed in this chapter? Which of these focus areas do you see as most critical to each area of practice?

6. This chapter covers the role of the occupational and environmental health nurse. Search for information about this specialty area of nursing in your community. Do you know an occupational health nurse? If so, plan to observe his practice for a few hours and explore what the role entails in this organization.

References

American Association of Occupational Health Nurses, Inc. (2008). *Standards of Occupational and Environmental Health Nursing.* Retrieved October 24, 2008 from http://www.aaohn.org/practice/standards.cfm

American Board for Occupational Health Nurses, Inc. (2008). *Are you an occupational or employee health nurse?* Retrieved August 12, 2008 from http://www.abohn.org/.

American Nurses Association. (2004). *Nursing: Scope and standards of practice.* Silver Spring, MD: Nursesbooks.org.

American Nurses Association/Health Ministries Association. (1998). *The scope and standards of parish nursing practice.* Washington, DC: American Nurses Publishing.

American Nurses Association/Health Ministries Association. (2005). *Faith community nursing: Scope and standards of practice.* Silver Spring, MD: Nursesbooks.org.

Anderko, L., Bartz, C., & Lundeen, S. (2005). Practice-based research networks: Nursing centers and communities working collaboratively to reduce health disparities. *Nursing Clinics of North America, 40*(4), 747–758.

Anderson, C.M. (2004). The delivery of health care in faith-based organizations: Parish nurses as promoters of health. *Health Communication, 16*(1), 117–128.

Aydelotte, M.K., Barger, S.E., Branstetter, E., Fehring, R.J., Lindgren, K., et al. (1987). *The nursing center: Concept and design.* Kansas City, MO: American Nurses Association.

Beidler, S. (2005). Ethical considerations for nurse-managed health centers. *Nursing Clinics of North America, 40*(4), 759–770.

Brown, A. (2006). Documenting the value of faith community nursing: Faith nursing online. *Creative Nursing, 2,* 13.

Cutler, I. (2002). *End games: The challenge of sustainability.* Baltimore: Annie E. Casey Foundation.

DeHaven, M.J., Hunter, I.B., Wilder, L., Walton, J.W., & Berry, J. (2004). Health programs in faith-based organizations: Are they effective? *American Journal of Public Health, 94,* 1030–1036.

Esin, M.N., Emiroglu, O.N., Aksayan, S., & Beser, A. (2008). Undergraduate occupational health nursing education in Turkey: A national survey. *International Nursing Review, 55,* 156–163.

Fiore, M.C., Bailey, W.C., Cohen, S.J., Dorfman, S.F., Goldstein, M.G., Gritz, E.R., et al. (2000, October). *Treating tobacco use and dependence—Quick Reference Guide for Clinicians.* Rockville, MD: U.S. Department of Health and Human Services, Public Health Service. Retrieved June 1, 2008 from http://www.surgeongeneral.gov/tobacco/tobaqrg.htm.

Gerrity, P., & Kinsey, K. (1999). An urban nurse managed primary health care center: Health promotion in action. *Family Community Health, 21*(4), 29–40.

Hansen-Turton, T. (2003). The quest for sustainability gets closer: CMS funds nurse-managed health center congressional demonstration. *Policy, Politics, and Nursing Practice, 4,* 147–152.

Hansen-Turton, T., & Miller, M.E. (June 2006). Nurses and nurse-managed health centers fill healthcare gaps. *The Pennsylvania Nurse, 18.*

Health Ministries Association. (2008). *About HMA.* Retrieved August 12, 2008 from http://www.hmassoc.org/about_us.php.

Health Resources and Services Administration. (2005). *Medicare Part D and safety net providers.* Retrieved August 12, 2008 from: http://www.hrsa.gov/medicare/modelcontract.htm.

Hyeonkyeong, L., Wilbur, J., Kim, M.J., & Miller, A.M. (2007). Psychosocial risk factors for work-related musculoskeletal disorders of the lower-back among long-haul international female flight attendants. *Journal of Advanced Nursing, 61,* 492–502.

King, M.A. (2004). Review of research about parish nursing practice. *Online Brazilian Journal of Nursing, 3*(1). Retrieved June 1, 2008 from http://www.uff.br/nepae/objn301king.htm.

Kinsey, K., & Buchanan, M. (2008). The nursing center: A model for nursing practice in the community. In M. Stanhope, & J. Lancaster (Eds.). *Public Health Nursing: Population-centered health care in the community,* 7th ed. (pp. 409–428). St. Louis, MO: Mosby.

Lundeen, S. (2005). *Lundeen's comprehensive community-based primary health care model.* Milwaukee, WI: UW, Milwaukee College of Nursing.

McBryde-Foster, M. (2005). Break-even analysis in a nurse-managed center. *Nursing Economics, 23*(1), 31–34.

Mellor, G., & St. John, W. (2007). Occupational health nurses' perceptions of their current and future roles. *Journal of Advanced Nursing, 58,* 585–593.

Melnyk, B.M., & Fineout-Overholt, E. (2005). *Evidence-based practice in nursing and healthcare: A guide to best practice.* Philadelphia: Lippincott Williams & Wilkins.

Miller, M.E. (2007). *Annual report: La Salle Neighborhood Nursing Center.* Philadelphia: La Salle University.

National Institutes of Health, Office of Extramural Research. (2007). *Glossary and acronym list.* Retrieved August 12, 2008 from http://grants.nih.gov/Grants/glossary.htm.

National Nursing Centers Consortium. (2007). *Mission, vision, goals.* Retrieved August 12, 2008 from http://www.nncc.us/about/vision.html.

O'Brien, M. (2006). Parish nursing: Meeting spiritual needs of elders near the end of life. *Journal of Christian Nursing, 23*(1), 28–33.

Patterson, D.L. (March 2006). The head is connected to the heart bone: Parish nurses as teachers. *The Clergy Journal,* 29–30.

Patterson, D.L. (2007). Eight advocacy roles for parish nurses. *Journal of Christian Nursing, 24*(1), 33–35.

Redmond, G. (2006). Developing programs for older adults in a faith community. *Journal of Psychosocial Nursing, 44*(11), 15–18.

Rethemeyer, A., & Wehling, B.A. (2004). How are we doing? Measuring the effectiveness of parish nursing. *Journal of Christian Nursing, 21*(2), 10–12.

Rydholm, L. (2006). Documenting the value of faith community nursing: Saving hundreds, making cents: A study of current realities. *Creative Nursing, 2,* 10–13.

Solari-Twadell, P.A., & McDermott, M.A. (2005). *Parish nursing: Development, education, and administration.* St. Louis, MO: Elsevier.

Stanhope, M., & Lancaster, J. (2008). *Public health nursing: Population-centered health care in the community,* 7th ed. St. Louis, MO: Mosby.

Torrisi, D., & Hansen-Turton, T. (2005). *Community and nurse-managed health centers: Getting them started and keeping them going.* Philadelphia: Springer.

U.S. Department of Health Education and Welfare (1979). *Healthy People: The Surgeon General's report on health promotion and disease prevention.* Washington, DC: U.S. Government Printing Office.

U.S. Department of Health and Human Services. (2000). *Healthy People 2010: Understanding and improving health,* 2nd ed. Washington, DC: U.S. Government Printing Office. Retrieved August 12, 2008 from http://www.healthypeople.gov.

U.S. Department of Health and Human Services. (2008). *Healthy People 2020: The road ahead.* Retrieved August 12, 2008 from http://www.healthypeople.gov/hp2020/.

Weis, D., Schank, M.J., & Matheus, R. (2006). The process of empowerment: A parish nurse perspective. *Journal of Holistic Nursing, 24*(1), 17–24.

Westberg, G.E. (1990). *The parish nurse: Providing a minister of health for your congregation.* Minneapolis, MN: Augsburg.

Westberg-McNamara, J. (2006). *The health cabinet: How to start a wellness committee in your church.* Cleveland. OH: Pilgrim Press.

White, J.A., Drechsel, J., & Johnson, J. (2006). Faithfully fit forever: A holistic exercise and wellness program for faith communities. *Journal of Holistic Nursing, 24*(2), 127–131.

World Health Organization. (2003). *WHO Europe occupational health nursing curriculum: WHO European strategy for continuing education for nurses and midwives.* Retrieved June 1, 2008 from http://www.euro.who.int/document/e81556.pdf.

World Health Organization. (2007). *Workers' health: Global plan of action.* Retrieved June 1, 2008 from http://www.who.int/gb/ebwha/pdf_files/WHA60/A60_R26-en.pdf.

Youngblut, J., & Brooten, D. (2001). Evidenced-based nursing practice: Why is it important. *AACN Clinical Issues, 12,* 468–476.

Selected Readings

American Association of Occupational Health Nurses. (2008). *The occupational and environmental health nursing profession.* Retrieved August 12, 2008 from http://www.aaohn.org/press_room/fact_sheets/profession.cfm.

Krothe, J.S., & Clendon, J.M. (2006). Perceptions of effectiveness of nurse-managed clinics: A cross-cultural study. *Public Health Nursing, 23,* 242–249.

Mosack, V., Medvene, L.J., & Wescott, J. (2006). Differences between parish nurses and parish nurse associates: Results of a statewide survey of an ecumenical network. *Public Health Nursing, 23,* 347–353.

Naumanen, P. (2007). The expertise of Finnish occupational health nurses. *Nursing and Health Sciences, 9,* 96–102.

Occupational Safety and Health Administration. (2002). *OSHA fact sheet.* Retrieved June 1, 2008 from http://www.osha.gov/OshDoc/data_General_Facts/jobsafetyandhealth-factsheet.pdf.

Patterson, D.L. (2003). *The essential parish nurse: ABCs for congregational health ministry.* Cleveland, OH: Pilgrim Press.

Ramos, E.I. (2006). Occupational health nurses and case management. *Nursing Economics, 24*(1), 30–40.

Solari-Twadell, P.A., & McDermott, M.A. (1999). *Parish nursing: Promoting whole person health within faith communities.* Thousand Oaks, CA: Sage.

Strasser, P.B., Maher, H.K., Knuth, G., & Fabrey, L.J. (2006). Occupational health nursing: 2004 practice analysis report. *American Association of Occupational Health Nurses Journal, 54*(1), 14–23.

Westberg-McNamara, J. (2006). *Health and wellness: What your faith community can do.* Cleveland, OH: Pilgrim Press.

Internet Resources

Nurse Managed Health Centers

Agency for Health Care Research and Quality: *http://www.ahrq.gov*

Department of Health Resources and Services Administration: *http://www.hrsa.gov*

Healthy People 2010: *http://www.healthypeople.gov*

Institute for Nursing Centers: *http://www.nursingcenters. org/index.html*

National Nursing Centers Consortium: *http://www.nncc.us/*

Nurse Family Partnership: *http://www.nursefamilypartnership. org/index.cfm?fuseaction=home*

Faith Community Nursing

Faith Community Nurse Network of the Greater Twin Cities: *http://www.fcnntc.org/*

Health Ministries Association, Inc.: *http://www.hmassoc.org/*

Interfaith Health and Wellness Association: *http://www.ihwassoc. org/nursing.html*

International Parish Nurse Resource Center: *http://www. parishnurses.org/*

Marquette University College of Nursing—Parish Nurse: *http://www.marquette.edu/nursing/Continuing/Parish.shtml*

New Jersey State Nurses Association—Forum of Faith Community Nurses: *http://www.njsna.org/displaycommon.cfm? an=1&subarticlenbr=41*

New Zealand Faith Community Nurses Association: *http://www. faithnursing.co.nz/*

Parish Nurse Center, Carroll College: *http://www.carroll.edu/ ~parishnurse/linkpage.htm*

Parish Nurse Institute: *http://parishnursing. communityhealthministry.net/*

University of Maryland, Baltimore—Parish Nursing Health Information Resources: *http://www.parishnursing.umaryland.edu/ whatis.asp*

Occupational Health Nursing

American Association of Occupational Health Nurses: *http:// www.aaohn.org/*

American Board for Occupational Health Nurses, Inc.: *http:// www.abohn.org/*

Centers for Disease Control and Prevention—Workplace Safety and Health: *http://www.cdc.gov/Workplace/*

Haz-Map (U.S. National Library of Medicine): *http://hazmap. nlm.nih.gov/*

Healthy Arkansas—Worksite Wellness: *http://www.arkansas.gov/ ha/worksite_wellness/index.html*

Healthy South Dakota—New Worksite Wellness Tools: *http://www. healthysd.gov/Workplace.html*

Medline Plus—Occupational Health: *http://www.nlm.nih.gov/ medlineplus/occupationalhealth.html*

National Institute of Environmental Health Sciences—Occupational Health: *http://www.niehs.nih.gov/health/topics/population/ occupational/*

National Institute for Occupational Safety and Health—Browse Occupational Safety and Health Topics: *http://www.cdc.gov/ niosh/topics/safety.html*

U.S. Department of Labor, Occupational Safety & Health Administration–Nursing in Occupational Health: *http://www. osha.gov/dts/oohn/ohn.html*

Wellness Councils of America: *http://www.welcoa.org/*

Wisconsin Department of Health & Family Services—Worksite Wellness Resource Kit: *http://www.dhfs.state.wi.us/Health/ physicalactivity/Sites/Worksitekit.htm*

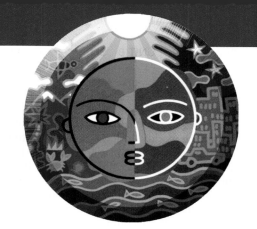

32

Clients Receiving Home Health and Hospice Care

KEY TERMS

CMS (Centers for Medicare and Medicaid Services)
Community-based long-term care
Home-bound
Hospice
Medicare Home Health Benefit
Medicare Hospice Benefit
Medicare Prospective Payment System
OASIS (Outcome and Assessment Information Set)
Palliative interventions
Responsive use of self
Visiting nurse associations

LEARNING OBJECTIVES

Upon mastery of this chapter, you should be able to:

◆ Summarize the history and contemporary circumstances of home health and hospice care.

◆ Describe Medicare standards for home health and hospice programs.

◆ Explain family caregiver burdens of providing home care.

◆ Explain how Medicare reimburses home health and hospice care.

◆ Describe essential characteristics of home health and hospice nursing practice.

◆ Identify unique challenges of infection control, medication management, fall prevention, use of technology, and nurse safety during home visits.

◆ Contrast the goals of home health care and hospice.

◆ Explain the gaps in home health care and hospice and the need for a coherent community-based long-term care program in the United States.

"People from all walks of life agree that someone who is sick deserves, in principle, compassion and care."

—Paul Farmer, American anthropologist and physician

891

A home health nurse sits in an upscale condominium with a frail, elderly gentleman tethered to his home oxygen unit and suffering air hunger as he struggles to speak of the "good old days" when he was young, full of vigor, and taking on the world. During her next visit to a trailer park, she inspects an infected pressure sore that has become smaller and cleaner with each home visit as the client's wife carefully follows through with wound care teaching. Next, she monitors the pulmonary and cardiac status of a patient newly discharged to his aging bungalow, detecting early signs of cardiac decompensation, and treating them at home in close collaboration with his physician. At that same time, her hospice nurse colleague walks into family chaos with a mother in pain and vomiting at the end of her life, and then leaves with everyone calm and the patient comfortable. These are the kinds of experiences that make up the daily lives of nurses who work with home care and hospice clients. Indeed, home health and hospice programs allow nurses to practice what some see as the very heart of compassionate and highly skilled nursing care. Home health care and hospice programs are expanding and are the work settings for more and more nurses.

Home health care is discussed in the first section of this chapter, followed by an overview of hospice care. The reader is also referred to the discussions in Chapter 19 on working with families, Chapter 20 on violence in families, Chapter 24 on care of the older adult, and Chapter 26 on chronic illness.

⊙ OVERVIEW OF HOME HEALTH CARE

The need for health care at home continues to accelerate. Drastic changes in financing and more people living with complex illness have contributed to this trend. For example, early hospital discharges resulting from third-party payers' efforts toward cost containment have forced clients to return home quickly to recuperate from surgeries and severe illnesses. Likewise, a growing population survives and yet suffers from complex chronic and life-threatening illness that they struggle to manage at home. Advanced technologies such as telehealth monitoring, intravenous (IV) antibiotics, total parenteral nutrition (TPN), dialysis, and mechanical ventilation are routinely provided and maintained in the client's home. As the population ages, and particularly now that the baby boomer generation is entering their elder years, home health nursing is challenged to respond. Professional home health care agencies seek to maximize the client's level of independence and to minimize the effects of existing disabilities through noninstitutional services. Professional home health services aim to decrease rehospitalization and prevent or delay institutionalization (Martinson, Widmer, & Portillo, 2002; Rice, 2006). The National Association for Home Care and Hospice (NAHC at http://www.nahc.org) provides a variety of direct services to members, including the publication *Caring* and monthly newsletters.

This section explores the evolution of home health care in the United States; describes home health agencies, clients, and personnel; and examines Medicare criteria and documentation. Finally, the unique characteristics of home health nursing are explored.

HISTORY AND POLITICS OF HOME HEALTH

Throughout human history, health care has been provided at home by family members. In the United States, the Ladies Benovelent Society in Charleston, South Carolina, made the earliest known (1813) organized effort to care for the sick poor at home (Buhler-Wilkerson, 2007). Later in the 19th century, it became possible for women to become nurses trained in the manner of Florence Nightingale, and wealthy women began to hire them as visiting nurses and to sponsor visiting nurse services. In 1893, Lillian Wald began home visiting in New York City and is famed for professionalizing visiting nursing. One of her most famous innovations was the establishment of insurance coverage for home care. Between 1909 and 1952, 100 million home visits were made to the policy holders of Metropolitan Life Insurance Company. Then, as now, the needs for cost containment and therefore quick discharge were in diametric opposition to nursing goals of providing needed care at the patient's side as long as needed.

In the latter half of the 20th century, as hospitals became increasingly effective in providing acute care, more people survived to live with debilitating chronic illness and disability, and referral to home care was used to discharge those nonacute patients from the hospital (Buhler-Wilkerson, 2007). The **visiting nurse associations** (VNAs) struggled with patched-together community support until 1965, which began the era of the **Medicare Home Health Benefit**, designed to respond to the medical needs of those convalescing from acute illness.

The Medicare Home Health Benefit was established with certain goals in mind. It was designed to provide intermittent home visits, in which nurses and therapists would instruct clients and families in self care. Home health nursing was clearly differentiated from longer nursing shifts in which nurses stayed in the home for several hours at a time. The period of visiting was to be brief and provide direct personal care just temporarily until patients and families could care for themselves. Neither health promotion nor long-term care was valued or reimbursed. Families were expected to manage long-term care alone. Whereas nurses had previously controlled their own practice, services under the new benefit were viewed as extensions of medical care, with physicians certifying needed services for short-term treatment of sickness.

The number of Medicare-certified home care agencies grew rapidly until enactment of the Balanced Budget Act (BBA) of 1997, which sought explicitly to reduce federal payments for home health care by changing payment from reimbursement for each visit to the **Medicare Prospective Payment System** that determined Medicare payment rates based on patient characteristics and need for services (Kulesher, 2006). The BBA resulted in a closure of 36% of the nation's Medicare-certified home health agencies and a dramatic decline in the number of patients served, with particular impact on the most vulnerable patients over 85 years old who need intensive services. As a result, some agencies currently deny care to those whose complex nursing needs exceed expected reimbursement. Both cost and number of visits have declined while rates of wound healing failures, incontinence, and psychosocial problems have worsened

(Schlenker, Powell, & Goodrich, 2005). The long-term effect on emergency care and hospitalization is being monitored. The diminished patient contact and increased documentation associated with these restrictive Medicare policies is distressing for home health nurses, who are most satsified when they have control over their practice and are able to provide quality patient care (Ellenbecker, Boylan, & Samia, 2006).

It is important to be aware that a distinct difference exists between professional and nonprofessional home care services provided to clients. Professional home care is provided by professionals with licenses, certification, or specific qualifications. These professionals typically work for home care agencies with internal and external standards that guide the provision of their services. Nurses, social workers, physical therapists, occupational therapists, and home health aides are examples of professional home care practitioners. In contrast, there are home care organizations that provide nonprofessional home care and those who sell equipment for home care.

HOME HEALTH AGENCIES

The mix of Medicare-certified home health care agencies includes voluntary nonprofits, hospital-based agencies, proprietary for-profit agencies, governmental agencies, or agencies not federally certified to provide care.

Voluntary nonprofit agencies traditionally have a charitable mission and are exempt from paying taxes. They are financed with nontax funds such as donations, endowments, United Way contributions, and third-party provider payments. If nonprofit agencies make any money, they reinvest it back into the agency. Voluntary agencies are usually governed by a voluntary board of directors; they are considered community-based because they provide services within a well-defined geographic location. Whereas in the past VNAs were assured of receiving almost all of the home care referrals in their community, the proliferation of other agencies has eroded their traditional base and put them in a competitive mode. The number of nonprofit home health agencies is diminishing across the country.

Hospital-based agencies comprise about one-quarter of Medicare-certified agencies (NAHC, 2004). A hospital may operate a separate department as a home health agency. It may be nonprofit or generate revenue for the hospital. Hospital-based agencies are governed by the sponsoring hospital's board of directors or trustees. The referrals to such hospital-based agencies usually come from the hospital staff itself, and the missions of the agency and the sponsoring hospital are similar. The same is true for rehabilitation and skilled-nursing facilities with home health departments.

For-profit proprietary agencies can be governed by individual owners, but many are part of large, regional or national chains that are administered through corporate headquarters. Proprietary agencies are expected to turn a profit on the services they provide, either for the individual owners or for their stockholders. They are required to pay taxes on profits generated. Although some participate in the Medicare program, others rely solely on "private-pay" clients. For-profit home care agencies now comprise over half the number of Medicare-certified agencies (NAHC, 2004).

Some city and county government agencies also provide home care services. They are created and empowered through statutes enacted by legislation. Services are frequently provided by the nursing divisions of state or local health departments and may or may not combine care of the sick with traditional public health nursing services, including health promotion, illness prevention, communicable disease investigation, environmental health services, and maternal–child care. Funding comes from taxes and is usually distributed on the basis of a per capita allocation.

Many agencies providing services in the home remain outside the federal Medicare system that reimburses skilled nursing. These *noncertified* agencies are usually private and derive their funding from direct payment by the client or from private insurers. They may be governed by individual owners or by corporations. For instance, some agencies offer "private duty" shifts of registered nurses, licensed practical nurses, various therapists, or home health aides who are usually paid for "out of pocket" rather than reimbursed by insurance or Medicare. Other services include unskilled assistance in the home with homemaking or housekeeping. Some of these agencies provide live-in personal care. Some organizations provide *durable medical equipment* (DME), such as wheelchairs, commodes, beds, or oxygen. Other services provide high-technology pharmacy services.

CLIENTS AND THEIR FAMILIES

The client in home health care is not only the individual patient but also the family and any significant others. The nurse must consider how the environmental, political, economic, cultural, and religious dimensions impact the client's illness and ability to meet the goals outlined in the plan of care.

Home care recipients are predominantly white women. More than two-thirds are over age 65 (NAHC, 2004). The most common diagnoses managed at home are cardiovascular, with the five top conditions identified as essential hypertension, heart failure, diabetes, chronic skin ulcers, and osteoarthritis. Most home health clients are admitted after hospitalization.

Individuals recovering from severe illness or living with debililtating chronic illness rely on family members or other sources of unpaid assistance. One in five American households contains a person who provides informal caregiving for an adult family member or friend (Schumacher, Beck, & Marren, 2006). Almost two-thirds are women with an average age of 46, although people can become caregivers at any age. Frail elderly caregivers are especially vulnerable to deterioration of their own health due to their caregiving burden. Family caregiving tasks range from personal care such as bathing and feeding to sophisticated skilled care, including managing tracheostomies or IV lines. Primary caregivers are those who assume the daily tasks of care, while secondary caregivers assume intermittent responsibilities such as shopping or transportation.

These informal caregivers assume a considerable physical, psychological, and economic burden in the care of their loved one at home. When layered on top of existing responsibilities, caregiver tasks compete for time, energy, and attention. As a result, caregivers often describe themselves as emotionally and physically drained and may very much need information about resources to assist them: Likewise, the economic cost of providing home care places a significant burden on informal caregivers. Out-of-pocket expenditures include medications, transportation, home medical equipment, supplies, and respite services. These costs may be nonreimbursable and are often invisible, but they are very real to families struggling to provide care on a fixed income. While family members compassionately assume their responsibilities, their collective burden in our society as a whole is mounting. Home health nurses must continually assess the strain on caregivers as they seek to develop realistic plans of care.

HOME HEALTH CARE PERSONNEL

The largest number of home care employees are nurses and home care aides (NAHC, 2004). Registered nurses and licensed practical nurses represent just under half of full time equivalent (FTE) positions in Medicare-certified agencies. Home care aides, physical therapy staff, occupational therapists, social workers, and administrative personnel comprise the rest of the home health team. The business and office personnel of a home health agency are critical to the agency's ability to deliver services to clients. Home health nurses must acquire an understanding of the financial aspects of their clients' care and provide this information to the agency staff, so that appropriate and full reimbursement can be obtained for the services provided.

REIMBURSEMENT FOR HOME HEALTH CARE

Home health services are reimbursed by both corporate and governmental third-party payers as well as by individual clients and their families. Corporate payers include insurance companies, health maintenance organizations (HMOs), preferred provider organizations (PPOs), and case-management programs. Government payers include Medicare, Medicaid, the military health system (TRICARE), and the Veterans Administration system. These governmental programs have specific conditions for coverage of services, which are often less flexible than those of corporate payers. For a general description of these reimbursement systems, see Chapter 6. The Medicare policies for home health programs set the precedent for all other reimbursement sources and are discussed below.

Medicare Criteria and Reimbursement

Medicare is the largest single payer for home care services in the United States and has set the standard in establishing reimbursement criteria for other payers. Therefore, it is essential that home care nurses seek to understand the complex Medicare home health requirements and rules for determining eligibility for home care services. It is important to acknowledge that a person may be in dire need of care at home, yet not meet eligibility standards for home health care under Medicare. Five criteria must all be met to be eligible for reimbursement by Medicare (Display 32.1). Consider the implications of these requirements. Documentation must justify that the plan of care is medically "reasonable and necessary." The person must be under the care

---

DISPLAY 32.1 | **MEDICARE HOME HEALTH ELIGIBILITY**

1. The type of services and frequency provided must be reasonable and necessary. To determine whether this criterion is met, the client's current health status, medical record, and plan of care are evaluated. If a care plan has been ineffective with a client over a long period of time, continuation of that care plan would not be considered reasonable. Therefore, comprehensive documentation is essential to validate that the provided care was both reasonable and necessary.
2. The client must be **home-bound**. This means that the client leaves the home with difficulty and only for medical appointments or adult day care related to the client's medical care.
3. The plan of care must be entered onto specific Medicare forms. The forms require very specific information regarding the client's diagnosis, prognosis, functional limitations, medications, and types of services needed. The home health nurse often has the primary responsibility for ensuring that the forms are completed appropriately.
4. The client must be in need of a skilled service. In the home, skilled services are provided only by a nurse, physical therapist, or speech therapist. *Skilled nursing services* include skilled observation and assessment, teaching, and performing selected procedures requiring nursing judgment.
5. Services must be intermittent and part-time.

---

of a physician. He or she must be "homebound" and in need of services that Medicare narrowly defines as "skilled." A person who is "homebound" must be confined to home except for visits to the physician, outpatient dialysis, adult day center, or outpatient chemotherapy and radiation therapy. "Skilled" services are restrictively defined and include selected aspects of nursing, physical therapy, or speech therapy. Home visits must be "intermittent" and time limited. Extensive documentation is required according to Medicare specifications. All of these requirements are subject to contradictory interpretations, which can put an agency's reimbursement at risk.

The Medicare Prospective Payment System (PPS) pays an agency for a 60-day "episode of care." All services and many medical supplies must be provided under the payment amount adjusted to geographic location and determined by the patient's clinical and functional status at the start of care, as well as the projected need for services over the anticipated 60-day period. When the patient is admitted, the patient is comprehensively assessed using a lengthy tool called the **Outcome and Assessment Information Set (OASIS)**. Clinical, functional, and service scores are calculated from selected OASIS items.

In the ongoing campaign to hold down the federal budget by diminishing health costs, home health care faces the ongoing threat of freezes or cuts in payment. For example, in Spring of 2007, the **Centers for Medicare and**

PERSPECTIVES
VOICES FROM THE COMMUNITY

It is vital to develop an expanded vision about the health care needs of frail elders and the kinds of services that are needed in the community. Sometimes, after nurses have been working in Medicare home health for a while, they may begin to identify with the Medicare guidelines. Too often, I have heard experienced home health nurses say about a patient living with severe chronic illness, "She doesn't deserve services. She doesn't have skilled needs." In contrast, I would hope knowledgeable nurses would say to families and decision makers, "She needs and deserves services, but the Medicare home health benefit will not pay for them. Our agency cannot continue to provide care because of the limits imposed on us. We'll do everything possible to find help for her, but resources are limited." This kind of insight leads to patient advocacy, development of community networks, and becoming outspoken about needed changes in health policy. Visiting nurses witness the struggles of chronically ill people living at home; we must not abandon them.

Beth L., Nursing Instructor

Medicaid Services (CMS) proposed reduction in reimbursement, justified by their claim that patients' needs have been exaggerated in documentation submitted to them (CMS, 2007). They also require payment adjustment based on agency submission of data on selected quality measures. In 2007, the Medicare Payment Advisory Commission (MedPAC) recommended to Congress that payments be frozen and that patients co-pay for each illness visit (Markey, 2007). These proposals overlook the reality that home health care is a cost-effective alternative to hospital and nursing home care. As home health care is restricted to save money and reduce fraud, greater amounts will need to be spent for inpatient care when people cannot cope in the absence of health care assistance at home (see Perspecives: Voices from the Community).

Medicare Documentation

Initially, every patient must be assessed using the OASIS tool, which determines reimbursement, is integral to agency surveys and certification, and collects information used to measure quality. OASIS assessment requires combining observation and interview to determine functional status, since clients often report what they wish to be true, rather than actual ability (Godfrey, 2005). Selected quality outcomes are measured and data released on the CMS website, which is accessed as "Home Health Compare" (http://www.medicare.gov/ HHCompare). Display 32.2 identifies selected quality measures. Note that the expectation is that of improving function, not simply stabilizing function, and consider the implications of this standard for very disabled patients.

   The Medicare Plan of Care is also completed by the nurse at admission; it must be signed by the physician. It is

---

DISPLAY 32.2   SELECTED HOME HEALTH QUALITY MEASURES

Higher Percentages Are Better
- Percentage of patients who get better at walking or moving around
- Percentage of patients who get better at getting in and out of bed
- Percentage of patients who have less pain when moving around
- Percentage of patients whose bladder control improves
- Percentage of patients who get better at bathing
- Percentage of patients who get better at taking their medicines correctly (by mouth)
- Percentage of patients who are short of breath less often
- Percentage of patients who stay at home after an episode of home health care ends
- Percentage of patients with improvement in status of surgical wound

Lower Percentages Are Better
- Percentage of patients who had to be admitted to the hospital
- Percentage of patients who need urgent, unplanned medical care
- Percentage of patients with deteriorating wound status

Source: http://www.medicare.gov/HHCompare.

---

then used to assess agency complicance with Medicare and state requirements. Obviously, great pains must be taken to assure accuracy. All follow-up services must match the plan of care. Likewise, OASIS answers and Plan of Care answers must match.

HOME HEALTH NURSING PRACTICE

The practice of home health nursing has roots in community health nursing (American Nurses Association, 1999). The nurse provides home health nursing care to acute, chronic, and terminally ill clients of all ages in their homes while integrating community health nursing principles that focus on the environmental, psychosocial, economic, cultural, and personal health factors affecting a client's and family's health status and well-being. Home health is a unique field of nursing practice that requires a synthesis of community health nursing principles with the theory and practice of medical/surgical, geriatric, mental health, and other nursing specialties. The official journal of the Home Healthcare Nurses Association (HHNA), *Home Healthcare Nurse*, is the primary source of up-to-date nursing knowledge in this rapidly changing field of practice. The stories of home health nurses emphasize shared humanity and promotion of client autonomy (Stulginsky, 1993a, 1993b). The effective home health nurse must

- ◆ Deliberately build trust.
- ◆ Sense "where people are" and suspend judgment.
- ◆ Develop a connection at the first visit.

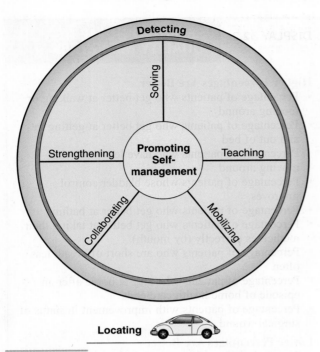

FIGURE 32.1 Home Health Nursing Caregiving Wheel.

♦ Develop "giant antennae" to detect cues in the home.
♦ Face persistent distractions during home visits.
♦ Help people solve their own problems.
♦ Keep priorities fluid.
♦ Determine how to keep the unstable client safe until the next visit.
♦ Thoughtfully maintain boundaries between personal and professional life.
♦ "Make do" with limited supplies.
♦ Face immense challenges with time management and paperwork demands.
♦ Constantly think of personal safety in neighborhoods and homes.

Nursing Practice During the Home Visit

The practice competencies of home health nurses can be illustrated with the Home Health Nursing Caregiving Wheel (Fig. 32.1).

Locating the Client and Getting Through the Door

The first step in making a home visit is finding where the person lives, which might involve telephone instructions, a map, or a global positioning system (GPS) unit. For most home health nurses, locating clients involves driving their own cars to the home. Sometimes nurses drive agency cars, and occasionally transportation may involve a bus, subway, boat, or airplane. Directions and household identification can be unclear. In rural areas, tracking down clients can involve vague instructions involving barns, bridges, trees, and other colorful local landmarks (see From the Case Files for an example). When families are unstable, clients may not be staying in households designated on the nurse's paper-

work. They may have moved in with relatives or friends or back home alone, despite major care needs. Locating is especially challenging when neighbors or even family members live in fear, for whatever reason.

Even when the wheels stop at the correct household, there is the challenge of getting through the closed door and making the connection. *Always remember that you are a guest in the home.* Respect and attentive listening are the foundation. Agendas must be laid aside initially as the nurse focuses on the concerns and realities of both client and family. SmithBattle, Drake, and Diekemper (1997) describe **responsive use of self** as the process expert nurses use to come to understand the lives of vulnerable clients in the community. Assumptions and stereotypes are overturned in the process of discovering how clients live, what they believe, and who comprises their family and community.

Other nursing approaches that build the initial therapeutic nurse–client connection include helping with immediate problems that the family identifies. Start where they want in ways that make sense to them. Emphasize positives to the extent possible, rather than telling people what they are doing wrong and need to change. Autonomy should be respected, and the family should be empowered by actions recognizing that they are in charge of their lives. At the same time, the nurse must be up front and truthful regarding the medical and nursing problems that need resolution. For example, a nurse might say, "You might lose your foot if we cannot work together to figure out a plan of care that works. Let's think together about what we can do to prevent it." Since these well-tested relational strategies for developing caring connections run contradictory to the current Medicare requirements for immediate completion of the lengthy OASIS survey tool on admission, the wise nurse needs to focus on sensitively developing initial connections as well as completion of the OASIS.

Hub of the Family Caregiving Wheel: Promoting Self-management

Home health nursing involves home visits to promote independence rather than dependence on the home health team. Lasting health improvement is only possible when the home health nurse works with the client/family to make decisions that are truly their own. Although financial incentives push home health nurses to minimize the number of visits and duration of service, pressuring a client or family to adopt the agency agenda denies any sense of partnership and can backfire, resulting in nonadherence to the therapeutic regimen. This can place a nurse in a no-win situation.

Every effort is made to develop capacity for self-care, so that the home team can safely withdraw. Obviously, this is quite appropriate for those recoving from an episode of acute illness, but it can be quite difficult when clients are living with severe chronic illness and do not have adequate caregivers to provide needed care without outside nursing assistance. Pressures to discharge are resulting in some patients discharged from home health care agencies while unable to manage care at home; indeed, a proportion of elderly clients are currently discharged from home health agencies with unresolved wound and incontinence issues (Flynn, 2007). Currently, no governmental program assures long-term care for those people unable to care for themselves. The home

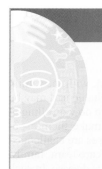

From the Case Files

Locating the Client's Home

"You can't miss our place," Diane had reassured me on the phone. I slowed in front of the decrepit Sunrise Motel, its roof partially collapsed, and reviewed my notes. I was supposed to turn right on the unmarked gravel road just after the abandoned motel and continue until the road ended. I proceeded slowly through an evergreen tunnel past an old green truck body resting belly up. A little girl perhaps 5 years old, came from around the truck and joined two grade-school-aged boys playing Frisbee in a clearing. I asked them where Diane Quimby lived, and they pointed around a curve in the road. In a moment, I came to a stop near a large wood and metal shed with smoke coming out of a crooked metal pipe in the roof. I knocked. No answer. I heard dialogue from "General Hospital" coming from inside. I knocked again and shouted, "Hello! It's the nurse." "Come on in!" a loud voice responded.

I pushed open the door. There was no knob. Illuminated by one weak lamp, I could just make out a round face with wire rim glasses and a long gray-blond braid. Here was Diane, sitting on a sagging sofa facing a TV tray and watching a flickering black-and-white television. I could see a wooden table in a corner, three mismatched dinette chairs, and a couple of cots against the wall. The air was hazy with the smell of wood smoke.

Diane invited me to pull up a chair. "We're worried about your infections," I began. Diane had unstable, insulin-dependent diabetes and high blood pressure. In June, surgeons had removed her gangrenous left foot with an amputation that ended just below the left knee. Now there was an infection in the wound that had not healed despite extended use of antibiotics.

During the course of the visit, I learned that Diane had no tub or shower for bathing. She also had no money for dressings and no supplies. Since Diane's vision was impaired, her 9-year-old grandson was doing the dressing changes. Until the latest surgery, Diane worked as a cook in a local "boarding home" for frail elders. She was 66 years old and had Medicare coverage. I learned that Diane was the legal guardian for two grandchildren, ages 5 and 9.

Apply the nursing process to comprehensively identify and prioritize nursing diagnoses and propose interventions. Use the Home Health Nursing Caregiving Wheel to guide your care planning.

health nurse must work closely with agency social workers to mobilize resources to care after the agency leaves.

Rim of the Home Health Caregiving Wheel: Detecting

Nurses in the home are challenged by an extraordinarily complex environment with much to investigate and frequently many distractions to ignore. Detecting is an all-encompassing, never-ending assessment process as the nurse seeks to understand the client's health in the context of home (Zerwekh, 1991). The nurse keeps her ears and eyes "wide open." The home environment surrounds the nurse with sounds, sights, and scents that need to be comprehended in light of the client's needs. Who lives in the home? How do they interact? Who are the caregivers, and how do they care? What is the relevance of culture and religion in the life of the household? How does the physical environment impact patient safety and security? Is there drug paraphernalia in the living room? Can the bathroom tub be used? The questions are endless. Sometimes the underlying etiologies of illness can be discovered by scrutinizing the "big picture" in the home. The OASIS format provides the baselines for the first visit, and then the nursing assessment broadens with each visit as the nurse continually widens her lens to take it all in. Home visits reveal discoveries that can never be imagined in clinic or hospital settings. Take for example the client whose refrigerator no longer chills and whose impaired vision prevents awareness of the expanding family of roaches in the kitchen.

Spokes of the Home Health Caregiving Wheel: Collaborating, Mobilizing, Strengthening, Teaching, Solving Problems

Home health nursing competencies that radiate from the hub and contribute to promotion of self-care and family care include *collaborating* with multiple team members and *mobilizing resources* in the community that can sustain the client after discharge. The home health care nurse usually is the coordinator of all other home health team members. Working with the social worker, she proposes needed connections with community services. Likewise, *strengthening* involves development of self-management or family caregiving ability. People learn that they can give injections, manage IV lines, safely take complex drug regimens, provide rehabilitation for loved ones after stroke, and perform countless other skills that they do not believe possible until a nurse shows them and they discover that they can do it themselves.

The home health nurse is constantly *teaching* clients and/or family caregivers through concrete explanation, discussion, and modeling behavior. Teaching facts is no assurance of behavior change and improved management of a health problem. Underlying factors influencing health behavior must be diagnosed and addressed. Health coaching, also called *motivational interviewing*, has demonstrated effectiveness in improving chronic disease management by getting patient and family to be actively involved (Huffman, 2007). Instead of telling people what to do, this involves asking people how they would like to change, "What worries you the most?" Those concerns and relevant feelings must be validated, and the nurse leads the person to consider options for change. The solution develops through a mutual, participatory process. Ultimately, people are responsible for their own health decisions.

Finally, home health nursing competency requires flexibility and creativity in *solving* health care problems and the challenges of everyday living. All outcomes of care can be achieved only by adapting to the skills and resources available in the home. Although people of all socioeconomic backgrounds present with severe health problems requiring home health nursing, many families live on the margins. Inderwies (in Cohen, 2007) vividly describes her 32 years of visiting the "have-nots, can-nots, and will-nots" (p. 15). By this, she refers to people living on the margins of society who have few resources, little capability, and frequent resistance to being told what to do. Their housekeeping may be terrible. Their interactions may be abusive. Witnessing lives in some homes requires an awareness of self and every effort to reach beyond preconception and judgment. Caring in the homes of those living "on the ragged edge" of society necessitates a strong commitment to discovering and honoring shared humanity (Zerwekh, 2000). Sometimes awareness of our own limitations should lead to referral to another home health nurse rather than imposing our own fear and/or anger on vulnerable clients.

Home Health Nursing Case Management

The home health nurse is the case manager for each client and responsible for coordination of the other professionals and paraprofessionals involved in the client's care.

She plans visit frequency and duration. Will home visits be made twice weekly, once weekly, or every day? For how long will visits continue? As the care is provided and the client's condition improves, the home health nurse determines whether the frequency of visits should be reduced or whether the client can be discharged.

She is the primary contact with the client's physician, collaborating on the initial plan of care, reporting changes in the client's condition, and securing changes in the plan of care.

The nurse conducts case conferences among team members to share information, discuss problems, and plan actions to effect the best possible outcomes for the client. Medicare mandates such case conferences every 60 days in home care. The nurse case manager supervises the paraprofessionals, such as home health aides, who also serve the home-bound client. This may entail visiting the client at a time when the home health aide is present to observe the care provided.

The home health nurse must know who is going to pay for services from the first visit to the time of discharge from the agency. If the client does not have a source of payment for the care that is needed, the agency must determine whether the client will receive the care free of charge or at a reduced rate. Many agencies have a sliding fee scale, which means that the charge for the services is based on the client's ability to pay.

Selected Nursing Challenges in the Home

Working in the home immerses the nurse in challenges unlike anything encountered in controlled institutional environments.

Some of these include infection control, medication safety, risk for falls, technology at home, and nurse safety.

Infection Control

Home health nurses frequently need to work with the family to prevent infection in clients who are debilitated and may be immunocompromised; in addition, many are now dwelling at home with invasive medical devices that make them especially vulnerable to infection. Likewise, nurses are challenged to consider how to protect the home health care team, family, and community from a client with contagious disease. In such cases, all people living in the home will need instruction. Some households have inadequate facilities to control disease transmission. There may be no access to running water, no heating unit to boil equipment, or inadequate facilities to dispose of contaminated equipment. These conditions necessitate the development of creative solutions to control infection. Complexities of the home environment require the nurse to carefully consider exactly how microorganisms are likely to exit the body, how might they be transmitted, and how are they likely to enter the body of another individual. Households cannot be organized like hospital units with isolation rooms. The nurse must decide when gloves are absolutely essential, when protecting clothing with a gown is needed, when a mask should be worn, and what environmental surfaces are likely to be contaminated and must be scrupulously cleaned. How should soiled tissues or dressings, dishes, and laundry be handled? What is realistic and can actually be carried out by client and family? As in the hospital environment, hands are the main vehicle for transmission of contagion, and hand hygeine is the main intervention that must be emphasized. To guide the nurse, home health agencies have adapted infection control policies and procedures based on the Centers for Disease Control and Prevention's isolation precautions (Siegel, Rhinehart, Jackson, Chiarello, et al., 2007).

Medication Safety

Home health nurses assume major responsibility for medication safety. The home health client taking multiple medications is at particular risk of multiple errors in self-administration, including incorrect medication, dose, time, interval, or route. Often doses are missed or doubled. Clients may discontinue a drug or not complete the full course. Sometimes, the drug or drugs ordered are inappropriate considering the patient's condition at home.

The home presents risks of medication errors that are different from those found in hospital or nursing home (Mager, 2007). Every visiting nurse has stories of finding drawers and cupboards filled with multiple prescriptions from multiple physicians, some current and some many years old. Polypharmacy becomes very obvious at home. Even if the client is well organized and taking every drug prescribed, those prescriptions may have originated from several providers over time and may have contradictory side effects. Sometimes medication errors at home include failure to clearly reconcile hospital or nursing home orders with home discharge orders. Although medication boxes can helpfully organize medications, they can also confuse new or impaired users. Distraction, visual impairment, forgetfulness, depression, and cognitive impairment are common causes of unintentional medication noncompliance. The home health nurse investigates how the medication is taken by reviewing and reconciling the current list of medications and having the patient explain and demonstrate the process he goes through. Intervention requires clear and repeated instruction, updating the medication list, charting or diagramming the schedule for medication taking, and assuring that the client or caregiver knows how to use the medication box.

Some of the reasons for intentional noncompliance are knowledge deficit, unacceptable side effects, no immediately obvious consequence when the drug is stopped, resistance to authority, perception of personal weakness if needing medication, and prohibitive cost. As the cost of prescriptions is shifted onto people living with chronic illness, drug spending goes down, with partial adherence or total discontinuation of therapy by clients who cannot afford their medication. It is not surprising to note that health then deteriorates and clients with diseases such as congestive heart failure and diabetes come to need intensive medical intervention (Goldman, Joyce, & Zheng, 2007). The home health nurse seeks to nonjudgmentally elicit reasons and mutually figure out solutions that manage medications at home and prevent intensive medical interventions.

Risk for Falls

Elders living at home have a 35% to 40% chance of falling; fear of falling is a serious problem in the aging, especially in those with debilitating illness (Stanley, Blair, & Beare, 2005). Physiological risk factors include orthostatic hypotension and cardiac dysrhythmias, dizziness, neurologic and musculoskeletal effects on gait and balance, urinary urgency, impaired hearing or vision, alcohol or drug abuse, and medication effects impairing alertness, balance, urinary frequency, and blood pressure. Clients should be observed as they move through their home and carry out activities of daily living. It is important to investigate factors that obstruct movement or threaten balance. The nurse in the home should inspect sidewalks, stairs, and surfaces outside the home; floor, rugs, electrical cords, stairs, lighting, and clutter inside the home; kitchen safety; and bathroom features including grab bars and a raised seat for the toilet and safety modifications for the bathtub. Common home modifications, such as eliminating throw rugs and loose mats and the use of nonslip bath mats have a significant protective effect. Display 32.3 lists teaching guidelines to prevent falls.

Technology at Home

Home health nurses teach patients and family to manage a wide array of complex technologies. Home regimens often require mini-intensive care units. In the past, the average home had a limited capacity for technology; medication was swallowed and food and fluid were consumed with the aid of fork and spoon. Now, the IV needle has evolved into venous access devices and plastic IV fluid bags can be stacked in the refrigerator and hung from the arm of a lamp. The household becomes home to dialysis, ventilators, enteric and IV nutrition, vasopressors—the list goes on. Nurses teach clients and families to manage it all; we become the guardians and advocates of complex regimens

| DISPLAY 32.3 | TEACHING TO PREVENT FALLS |

- Discuss fear of falling as normal and then urge preventive approaches.
- Identify environmental hazards and explain need for change.
- Encourage highest possible level of physical activity considering ability.
- Explain importance of reporting health status changes that increase risk of falls.
- Explain importance of recognizing sensory changes and correcting immediately.
- Teach regular blood pressure monitoring.
- Emphasize slowing down when moving and changing positions.
- Emphasize safe footware and foot care.
- Explore strategy for responding to a fall, including calling for help and getting up.
- Demonstrate safe body mechanics to lift heavy objects and to move immobilized family members.

Modified from Stanley, M., Blair, K.A., & Beare, P.G. (2005). *Gerontological nursing: Promoting successful aging with older adults,* 3rd ed. Philadelphia: F.A. Davis, with permission.

that require multiple nursing visits. Paradoxically, our primary mission is to be guardians and advocates for the well-being of client and family. Consider the human impact when the machines and the sickbed become the center of household activities. "We can slip so easily into the struggle to keep the technological regime functioning. However, nurses and other professionals in the home are in the pivotal position to witness the impact, to document the impact, and to assist clients to construct their lives in a meaningful way, so that neither illness nor medical regimes are the only reason for being" (Zerwekh, 1995, p. 12). Sometimes, we can foster dialogue with clients and families to consider the benefits and burdens of continuing technologies. Consider four reasons why technology may be inappropriate: (1) the technology is not achieving a therapeutic purpose, (2) the therapeutic purpose can be met more simply, (3) complications of the intervention outweigh benefits, and (4) the resulting quality of life does not justify the technology.

Recent information technologies being adopted by home health care agencies significantly improve quality of client care. These include medical records available instantly on the nurse's laptop and daily telemedicine monitoring of electrocardiogram, blood pressure, oxygen saturation, and other vital measures.

Nurse Safety

Every home health care agency should have a carefully developed program to assure the safety of personnel traveling to homes. Many work closely with local police departments to identify the wisest process for visiting dangerous neighborhoods and isolated rural areas. Display 32.4 lists practices for safe home visiting.

DISPLAY 32.4	SAFE HOME VISITS

- Carry a cellular phone.
- Be sure the agency knows your itinerary.
- Clarify directions before travel. Carry a map.
- Make joint visits or request security escort if safety is threatened. Refuse to visit when there is strong evidence of personal danger. Consult the police.
- Call to schedule the visit and do not go into the home without invitation.
- Dress simply without expensive jewelry. Do not carry large amounts of cash. Keep wallet or purse locked in the car.
- Wear an agency badge.
- Follow family directions about how to get by in their neighborhood and when to come in or leave their home. Patients and families usually will protect their nurse.

THE FUTURE OF CARE IN THE HOME

In conclusion, it can be seen that present-day Medicare home health care intervenes during brief episodes of acute medical trouble, relies on family at home as caregivers, and is expected to get in and out of the home as inexpensively as possible. Consider instead that the true needs of the frail elderly or severely disabled require prolonged psychosocial support, personal care, housekeeping, promotion of health, prevention of deterioration, and early detection of medical problems. In other words, they need case managment that extends over months and years. For this to happen, the United States must develop a **community-based long-term care** system. Home health care leaders look to a future of reinventing themselves by moving into new lines of business to meet these needs (Cohen, 2007). Some baby boomers will be able to afford these services by paying out of their own pockets for a network of elder management services. Most baby boomers will need the development of a national community-based long-term care benefit. Refer to Display 32.5 for a list of *Healthy People 2010* objectives related to home health and hospice care (U.S. Department of Health & Human Services [USDHHS], 2000).

⊛ OVERVIEW OF THE HOSPICE MOVEMENT

The contemporary circumstances of death in America are often dehumanizing; most people die in hospitals and long-term care institutions, surrounded by strangers. Uncertainty and denial often prevail during the final stage of life because prognoses are uncertain and many serious illnesses are now treated aggressively until the last breath. The battle against the "evil" of death seems to be the primary emphasis, with patient, family, and professionals wanting to believe that it is possible to win the final struggle. In the 21st century, fatal conditions have been turned into expensive chronic illnesses. Too often, discomfort is not relieved and treatment causes further suffering. And as the period of disability extends and the body deteriorates, social isolation develops. The modern preoccupation with action, productivity, and beauty has little interest in the process of dying. In dramatic

DISPLAY 32.5	HEALTHY PEOPLE 2010 HOME HEALTH AND HOSPICE CARE OBJECTIVES

Remember that *Healthy People 2010* has two broad goals: to eliminate health disparities and to increase quality and years of healthy living. A vital concept for elders is that of "compressing morbidity." This means that we seek to promote healthy lives and to diminish (compress) the time they are suffering with disabling illness. Any health care system developed to provide long-term care for the elderly and those with chronic illness should maximize function and independence. How might such a system work?

Specific *HP 2010* objectives related to home health and hospice care include:

1-4. Increase the proportion of persons who have a specific source of ongoing care.

1-5. Increase the proportion of persons with a usual primary care provider.

1-6. Reduce the proportion of families that experience difficulties or delays in obtaining health care or do not receive needed care for one or more family members.

1-15. Reduce the proportion of adults with long-term care needs who do not have access to the continuum of long-term care services. (Midcourse revision)

Sources: U.S. Department of Health and Human Services. (2000). *Healthy People 2010: Understanding and improving health* (2nd ed.). Washington, DC: U.S. Government Printing Office.

U.S. Department of Health and Human Services. (2006). *Healthy People 2010: Midcourse review.* Washington, DC: U.S. Government Printing Office.

contrast to the dehumanization of death, the **hospice** movement has developed to humanize the end-of-life experience and provide palliative care. **Palliative interventions** relieve suffering without curing underlying disease. The hospice movement has emphasized four major changes in end-of-life care: (1) care should attend to body, mind, and spirit; (2) death must not be a taboo topic; (3) medical technology should be used with discretion; and (4) clients have a right to truthful discussion and involvement in treatment decisions (McIntosh & Zerwekh, 2006). Table 32.1 contrasts mainstream medical focus with hospice. This section explores the evolution of hospice care in the United States, describes hospice agencies, and examines Medicare criteria for hospice reimbursement. It concludes with an exploration of the unique characteristics of hospice nursing practice.

EVOLUTION OF HOSPICE CARE

In medieval Europe, hospices were refuges for the sick and dying. The contemporary hospice movement originated in England, where Dame Cicely Saunders founded St. Christopher's Hospice in 1967 (McIntosh & Zerwekh, 2006). Dr. Saunders was credentialed as a nurse, social worker, and

TABLE 32.1   Contrasts Between Home Health and Hospice

Hospice	Home Health
Emphasis is on quality of life and comfort.	Emphasis is on rehabilitation and physiological stabilization.
Focus is on health of whole family.	Focus is on health of client.
Plan of care is guided by client choice.	Plan of care is determined by medical need.
Nurse is case manager until death.	Nurse is case manager until home health discharge.
Client chooses how to live last days.	Priority is given to correcting physiologic imbalances.
Intermittent visits increase in frequency as death become imminent.	Intermittent visits decrease in frequency as client stabilizes.
Nurses are expert in symptom control.	Symptom control is domain of physician with some nurses having expertise.
Sedatives and opioids are expertly adjusted to eliminate suffering.	Sedatives and opioids are used hesitantly to reduce suffering.
End-of-life disease course is managed to avoid crises.	End-of-life problems tend to be seen as medical crises.
Goal is for symptoms at end of life to be managed at home if possible.	Client is brought to hospital for unmanaged symptoms.
Spiritual care is focus of whole team.	Spiritual needs are met by own clergy.
Survivors have bereavement support.	No bereavement support is provided.

Adapted from Zerwekh, J. (2002). Home care of the dying. In I. Martinson, A. Widmer, & C. Portillo. *Home health care nursing*. Philadelphia: W.B. Saunders, with permission.

physician. She developed a unique program based both on compassion and skillful relief of physical discomfort through around-the-clock analgesics administered by mouth. It had been previously assumed that only injections, administered sparingly, could be used for terminal pain control. The first hospice in the United States was established in 1974 in Branford, Connecticut, by Florence Wald, Dean of the Yale School of Nursing. Because even in the 1970s, there was concern about saving money by shortening hospital stays and keeping people out of the hospital, hospices in the United States came to focus on providing care in the home. To that end, Congress established the Medicare hospice benefit in 1982, with the intention of keeping people at home, yet receiving comprehensive services that are less expensive than hospitalization.

Hospice characteristics have changed over time. Initially, nearly all clients suffered from terminal cancer; presently, people with a variety of end-stage diseases are admitted. Diseases that were once rapid death sentences have now turned into chronic life-limiting diseases. With prognoses difficult to predict and denial of death a continuing issue, hospice referrals are now made very late in the disease process. Brief hospice stays make it difficult to significantly help families and clients before death occurs. Another transition in hospice is the move from charity to business (McIntosh & Zerwekh, 2006). With highly reliable Medicare payment, for-profit hospices have expanded and are competing in many communities for the hospice "market share."

HOSPICE SERVICES AND REIMBURSEMENT

As in home health care, Medicare has determined the way services are provided. The **Medicare Hospice Benefit** requires that a client who has a prognosis of 6 months or less must sign up for the comfort-focused hospice benefit and waive the regular hospice benefit. This mandates that the client acknowledges a terminal prognosis and chooses comforting care instead of life-extending care. When this choice is made, the hospice coordinates care in all settings, functioning both as clinical and financial case manager (McIntosh & Zerwekh, 2006). The government pays a flat rate to the hospice for each day the patient receives care. There are four payment levels: (1) routine home care with intermittent visits, (2) continuous home care when the patient's condition is acute and death is near, (3) inpatient hospital care for symptom relief, and (4) respite care in a nursing home to relieve family members. Eighty percent of care has to be provided at home or in a nursing home that has become the person's permanent residence.

Hospices coordinate home care and direct inpatient care if needed. The emphasis is on palliation, with a focus on physical, psychosocial, and spiritual comfort. A strong emphasis is placed on caring for the entire family. The hospice team includes nurse, physician, home health aides, physical and occupational therapists, social workers, volunteers, palliative medication and medical equipment specialists, and bereavement counselors. Staff meet regularly to explore together the challenges of assuring comfort at the end of life.

Volunteers fill an important need in hospice care. They act as companions to the client when the family must be somewhere else or is away for short respite. They run errands for family members, shop, organize hot meals prepared by friends and neighbors, baby-sit children in the family, and perform other services as needed.

HOSPICE NURSING PRACTICE

The nurse's role is central in the hospice interdisciplinary team. She functions as case manager and visits the client more frequently than other members of the team. Nurses work in close collaboration with physicians to assure management of symptoms often change rapidly as the end of life nears. In addition to home visits focusing on palliation and interdisciplinary planning, hospice nurses rotate through 24-hour call 7 days a week to assure continuous availability by telephone and visits for emergent problems reported by client or family. Hospice nursing competencies and challenges are similar to those described for home health nurses, with the added expertise needed to relieve physical and emotional suffering of terminally ill people and their families. The American Nurses Association (ANA), in collaboration with other groups, has published standards of practice for hospice and palliative nursing (2007), as well as pain management nursing (2005). These practice standards provide guidance in this specialized field of nursing.

Hospice caregiving can be illustrated as a tree, strongly rooted in the process of nurses deliberately practicing self-care for themselves (Fig. 32.2). This tree has been drawn to explain the expert competencies of hospice nurses who were interviewed to capture the essence of their practice (Zerwekh, 1995, 2006). Each of the hospice nursing practices visualized by the tree diagram is briefly summarized below.

Roots of Hospice Nursing: Sustaining Oneself

Effective hospice nurses understand that to care for others, they must care for themselves. Without strong healthy roots, the tree will not thrive. *Sustaining oneself* requires deliberate effort to maintain one's own physical, emotional, and spiritual well-being. Knowing oneself, identifying sources of stress, and learning how to care for oneself are important. Expert hospice nurses keep themselves healthy by maintaining a balance between giving and receiving, letting go of predetermined agendas and idealistic hopes to achieve more than is humanly possible, being emotionally open and clear, and deliberately replenishing themselves to restore their energy (Zerwekh, 2006). "Rooted in self care, we are able to reach out with courage to the broken and terrified at the end of their lives" (p. 60). Examine the Evidence-based Practice feature about the risk of compassion fatigue. Of note: The contemporary work environment of most nurses actually causes more stress than everyday witnessing of suffering and death (Vachon, 2001); emphasis on productivity and finances, with limits placed on nurse empowerment and resources, can be quite disheartening. Leaders must seek to develop a caring culture that respects nurse autonomy in the face of these challenges.

The Trunk Reaching Upward: Connecting, Speaking Truth, and Encouraging Choice

Rooted in self-care, hospice nurses practice *connecting*, which refers to the centrality of relationships in providing hospice care. The hospice nurse seeks to understand the emotional and spiritual distress common to the end of life, particularly the progressive experience of loss after loss. Guided by that understanding, hospice nurses emphasize attentive

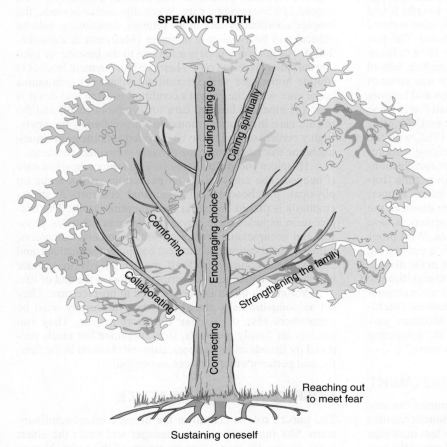

SPEAKING TRUTH

Guiding letting go

Caring spiritually

Encouraging choice

Comforting

Collaborating

Strengthening the family

Connecting

Reaching out to meet fear

Sustaining oneself

FIGURE 32.2 The Hospice Caregiving Tree.

EVIDENCE-BASED PRACTICE

Compassion Fatigue

Do you wonder how hospice nurses sustain compassionate practice as they work day in and day out with suffering patients who always die? Abendroth and Flannery (2006) investigated "compassion fatigue" among 216 nurses in 22 Florida hospices. They defined compassion fatigue as a traumatic stress reaction resulting from helping a person suffering from traumatic events. Symptoms in hospice nurses included being preoccupied with the patient, feeling overwhelmed with work, feeling "on edge" due to helping, losing sleep over patient's trauma, feeling "bogged down" by the system, depression, memory loss, headaches, and having "frightening" thoughts. The central theme was intense identification with patients that resulted in vicarious experiences of anxiety and pain.

Staying healthy as a hospice nurse requires a high level of self-awareness to "purposefully enter into the world of a suffering person to understand his or her experience, while maintaining enough detachment to be of practical usefulness and to retain our own emotional health" (Zerwekh, 2006, p. 50). Abendroth and Flannery note the value of being able to debrief after experiencing a patient's death. Nurses working in this area must be supported emotionally by their agency and must also recognize their own need to share stories and speak openly about sorrow, anger, and fear.

References:

Abendroth, M., & Flananery, J. (2006). Predicting the risk of compassion fatigue. *Journal of Hospice and Palliative Nursing, 8*(6), 346–356.

interdisciplinary team members share information and work interdependently. The hospice nurse coordinates the plan of care and day-to-day efforts to provide physical and psychosocial comfort. She supervises practical nurses and nursing assistants. The physician is responsible for medical care and serves as liaison with the client's primary care physicians. Social workers, spiritual counselors, and volunteers are integral members of the hospice team. The hospice interdisciplinary team is constantly challenged to work creatively together to find solutions for complex end-of-life suffering with emotional, spiritual, and physical components.

Strengthening the Family

The death of a family member causes great disruption for all involved. When family members are in a caregiving role in the home, they experience significant personal suffering. They are vulnerable to physical and emotional illness themselves. The process of taking care involves managing the illness and all practical assistance, seeking information and resources, and preparing for death itself (Stetz & Brown, 1997). Family members often are caught up with family issues and struggles with the health-care system. An extremely important hospice nursing role involves strengthening family members' abilities as caregivers. Teaching caregiving requires creative teaching methods and flexibility. Often the hospice nurse is able to help family members communicate with each other, gather them together, and act as an intermediary if necessary.

Comforting

Hospice nurses develop extensive expertise in pain and symptom management. Contemporary medical/surgical nursing textbooks discuss the essentials in this field, and advanced knowledge is developed through experience, continued education, and reading. Display 32.6 lists fundamental palliative

listening to understand each individual's unique story. This requires quieting your own thoughts to truly hear what is being expressed. Sometimes listening involves simply being present in the moment, paying attention. Having heard the client's story, it is important for hospice nurses to speak honestly when other professionals and family feel obliged to keep being cheerful and positive. Hospice nurses openly seek to speak truthfully about many issues that can be painful to discuss. *Speaking truth* is visualized as encircling the entire top of the caregiving tree. Hospice nurses bring up difficult subjects, so that the client is freed to speak about his greatest fears and concerns. Sometimes it leads to joint problem solving and *encouraging choice* through informed decision making. After truth has been discussed and the client has made a decision, the hospice nurse often advocates for client wishes against the resistance of various authorities. Remember that these are the final decisions in a dying person's life.

Collaborating

Interdisciplinary teamwork is an essential branch on the tree. Hospice team members communicate around the table and are constantly consulting each other. The hospice

DISPLAY 32.6 — FUNDAMENTALS OF PALLIATIVE CARE

- Make no assumptions about what is wrong.
- Believe the patient's report of symptoms.
- Relieve discomfort to the extent that the patient chooses and finds acceptable.
- Investigate the biologic, psychosocial, and spiritual dimensions of discomfort.
- Anticipate symptoms and relieve them before they occur again.
- Use nursing and complementary (integrative) interventions.
- Become an expert in the use of palliative medication.
- Continually evaluate the effectiveness of interventions.
- Choose the least complex and most manageable interventions that patients and families can manage themselves at home.
- Never give up. Persist in trying different palliative strategies.

principles and Display 32.7 identifies four important components of pain relief.

Spiritual Practice and Letting Go

As death draws near, spiritual needs intensify, with the final search for meaning, reconciliation, hope, and transcendence beyond the limits of human lived experience (Touhy & Zerwekh, 2006). Hospice nurses recognize spiritual distress and practice spiritual caring interventions that include respect for beliefs and spiritual practices and fostering reconciliation if there is a problem with estrangement from family, friends, and faith tradition. They deliberately try to keep their minds uncluttered by distracting preoccupations, so that they can listen attentively and promote life review. Cassidy (1998) states that spiritual care at the end of life involves being a companion on the dying person's journey, even when we would rather escape walking with them along the frightening path through darkness.

Guiding letting go is a truly unique nursing practice that involves helping the client to let go of former activities and hopes, including life itself. This involves listening to intense emotions and helping the person and family find resolution. Sometimes it involves participating in a vigil at the bedside of the dying person and encouraging loved ones to say their final words of farewell.

ETHICAL CHALLENGES IN HOSPICE NURSING

The hospice nurse confronts striking ethical challenges at the end of life. "To nurse at the end of life, you need to become conscious of how value-laden the choice of medical and nursing interventions can be. We practice in the middle of an ethical minefield. . . . Naming and clarifying ethical issues is a prominent nursing role. . . . We must strengthen our voice and ask, 'Is what we are doing good for this person and family?'" (Zerwekh, 2006, pp. 180–181). Wide-ranging issues

include respect or disregard for client autonomy, relief or disregard for client suffering, and avoidance of killing at the very end of life. The hospice nurse needs to develop her own knowledge of nursing and medical ethics in order to question the ethical implications of interventions and to advocate for client and family.

THE FUTURE OF HOME HEALTH AND HOSPICE

Given a rapidly expanding population of elders living longer with challenging chronic illnesses, home health and hospice care in the home will soon need to transform into a community-based long-term care system that doesn't discharge after an acute episode or admit only at the very end of life. In response to out-of-control medical inflation, federal and state governments have sought to hold down expenses in all areas, including restrictions on home health and hospice care. However, costs keep rising in step with technologic and pharmacologic innovation and marketing. Containing costs will eventually force a shift in services from expensive institutional and high-technology interventions to community-based home services.

The entire model for service provision in the home must change to a health care delivery system that continuously serves those living with disabling and terminal illness to maximize well-being at home, anticipate and prevent crises, and minimize emergent and inpatient interventions. The Medicare definitions of home-bound, medical necessity, and skilled nursing must become extinct. Likewise, the current hospice admission requirement that a person must discontinue treatment in order to receive hospice services is outdated. Reception of hospice services should be based on client choice and the reality of a terminal diagnosis. A sustainable, affordable (Callahan, 1999) approach to care in the home will require ongoing case management to coordinate and manage resources with incentives that control cost while assuring quality of life and comfort. Community resources will need to be mobilized to develop interdisciplinary and volunteer teams. Clients and family caregivers will need education and supportive networks. Homemaking and personal care will be the bedrock to keep people at home as long as possible. Nurses, nurse practitioners, and home visiting physicians will need to have the diagnostic and therapeutic resources to monitor physiologic status and intervene in the home. Telehealth and home monitoring will be essential. The focus must change from doing everything possible to prolong physiologic survival to promoting meaningful and comfortable lives. Nurses will have an active role in this process.

Summary

Community health nurses have an important role in working with elders who receive home care or hospice services. As the population continues to age, the need for nurses to work with older adults where they live, as they are discharged from acute care settings earlier and earlier and, if they are terminally ill, during their final months and days, will only increase.

There are many types of home care agencies: voluntary, proprietary, hospital-based, official, homemaker, and hospice. Care is provided by formal and informal caregivers.

Professional staff members, such as nurses, social workers, therapists, and certified nursing assistants, work in collaboration with family members, and, in some situations, with friends and neighbors.

Hospice is a fairly new concept in the United States, but has a longer history in England. Medicare covers hospice care without the restrictions experienced by nonhospice home care clients. Hospice programs provide holistic care to clients during the last months of life. Many programs are home-based, and they often are a service offered by a home health agency. In addition to in-home hospices, inpatient hospices exist; these can be located in a free-standing building, in part of a skilled nursing facility, or in a section of an acute care facility. The focus of hospice care is not aimed at cure, and it employs holistic caregiving practices that involve family members, professionals, and volunteers.

The nurse provides direct physical nursing care both in home health care and with hospice clients. In additon, the nurse teaches clients, family members, and volunteers; supervises; and case manages. Assessing clients to determine health status and eligibility for additional services and acting as a client advocate occurs with both groups of clients. Determining the frequency and duration of services occurs in home care. With both home care and hospice clients, the nurse must become familiar with the requirements of documentation to promote continuity of care and ensure reimbursement. ■

ACTIVITIES TO PROMOTE CRITICAL THINKING

1. Go to the *Healthy People 2010* website at http://www.healthypeople.gov/. Look up Objective 1.15: *Long-term care and rehabilitative services.* What specific services are included in this objective? Now access the *Healthy People 2010 Midcourse Review* (USDHHS, 2006). Again look up Objective 1.15: Are there changes/revisions to the original objective? How are home health and hospice care addressed in each document? In planning for *Healthy People 2020*, what changes would you propose to this objective to improve access to quality health services?

2. Search the Internet for home health and hospice agencies in your city or town. Select two agencies and compare the employment opportunities of each. How do these job descriptions and the published pay ranges compare to hospitals in your area? What are the benefits of working in home health and hospice? Will the agency hire new graduates, or do they require prior acute care experience?

3. John S., age 58 years, was recently diagnosed with liver cancer following years of heavy alcohol consumption. At the urging of his physician, his wife contacted the local hospice agency for assistance. You have been assigned this case. When you arrive at John's house, his wife tells you that he refuses to see you and is continuing to drink alcohol. She is very distressed and begins to cry. How would you

handle this situation? What are some of the issues inherent in this case?

4. Review your personal health insurance policy or that of a family member. What coverage, if any, is provided for home health or hospice care? What restrictions are stated in the coverage—total reimbursement, source of care, length of service? Do you think this will be adequate to meet your or your family member's needs? What other options might be available to help defray the cost of this type of care?

References

American Nurses Association. (1999). *Scope and standards of home health nursing practice.* Washington, DC: American Nurses Foundation.

American Nurses Association/American Society for Pain Management Nursing. (2005). *Pain management nursing: Scope and standards of practice.* Washington, DC: American Nurses Foundation.

American Nurses Association/Hospice and Palliative Nurses Association. (2007). *Hospice and palliative nursing: Scope and standards of practice.* Washington, DC: American Nurses Foundation.

Buhler-Wilkerson, K. (2007). No place like home: A history of nursing and home care in the U.S. *Home Healthcare Nurse, 25*(4), 253–259.

Callahan, D. (1999). *False hopes: Overcoming the obstacles to a sustainable, affordable medicine.* New Brunswick, NJ: Rutgers University Press.

Cassidy, S. (1988). *Sharing the darkness: The spirituality of caring.* London: Darron, Longman and Todd.

Centers for Medicare and Medicaid Services. (2007). *CMS proposes payment changes for Medicare home health services.* Retrieved August 12, 2008 from http://www.cms.hhs.gov.

Cohen, B. (January 2007). Best of care: Most difficult of circumstances. *Caring, 26*(1), 13–23.

Ellenbecker, C.H., Boylan, L.N., & Samia, L. (2006). What are home healthcare nurses are saying about their jobs. *Home Healthcare Nurse, 24*(5), 315–324.

Flynn, L. (2007). Managing the care of patients discharged from home health: A quiet threat to patient safety? *Home Healthcare Nurse, 25*(3), 184–190.

Godfrey, S. (2005). Conquering the dilemma of improving function. *Home Healthcare Nurse, 23*(11), 703–706.

Goldman, D.P., Joyce, G.F., & Zheng, Y. (2007). Prescription drug cost sharing: Associations with medication and medical utilization and spending and health. *Journal of the American Medical Association, 298*, 61–69.

Huffman, M. (2007). Health coaching: A new and exciting technique to enhance patient self-management and improve outcomes. *Home Healthcare Nurse, 25*(4), 271–276.

Kulesher, R.R. (2006). Impact of Medicare's prospective payment system on hospitals, skilled nursing facilities and home health agencies: How the balanced budget act of 1997 may have altered service patterns for Medicare providers. *The Health Care Manager, 25*(3), 198–205.

Mager, D.R. (2007). Medication errors and the home care patient. Safety in practice. *Home Healthcare Nurse, 25*(3), 151–155.

Markey, C. (2007). What might the 110th Congress have in store for home health and hospice care in 2007–2008? *Home Healthcare Nurse, 25*(5), 343–344.

Martinson, I. M., Widmer, A.G., & Portillo, C.J. (2002). *Home health care nursing,* 2nd ed. Philadelphia: W.B. Saunders.

McIntosh, E., & Zerwekh, J. (2006). Hospice and palliative care. In J. Zerwekh (Ed.). *Nursing care at the end of life.* Philadelphia: F.A. Davis.

National Association for Home Care and Hospice. (2004). *Basic statistics about home care.* Retrieved August 12, 2008 from http://www.nahc.org/facts/.

Rice, R. (2006). *Home care nursing practice: Concepts and applications,* 4th ed. St. Louis, MO: Mosby.

Schlenker, R.E., Powell, M.C., & Goodrich, G.K. (2005). Initial home health outcomes under prospective payment. *Health Services Research, 40*(1), 177–193.

Schumacher, K.L., Beck, C.A., & Marren, J. (2006). Family caregivers. *American Journal of Nursing, 106*(8), 40–48.

Siegel, J.D., Rhinehart, E., Jackson, M., Chiarello, L., & Healthcare Infection Control Practices Advisory Committee. (2007). *Guideline for isolation precautions: Preventing transmission of infectious agents in healthcare settings* 2007. Atlanta, GA: Centers for Disease Control and Prevention. Retrieved August 23, 2007 from http://www.cdc.gov/ncidod/dhqp/pdf/isolation2007.pdf.

SmithBattle, L., Drake, M.A., & Diekemper, M. (1997). The responsive use of self in community health nursing practice. *Advances in Nursing Science, 20,* 75–89.

Stanley, M., Blair, K.A., & Beare, P.G. (2005). *Gerontological nursing: Promoting successful aging with older adults,* 3rd ed. Philadelphia: F.A. Davis.

Stetz, K.M., & Brown, M.A. (1997). Taking care: Caregiving to persons with cancer and AIDS. *Cancer Nursing, 20*(1), 12–22.

Stulginsky, M.N. (1993a). Nurses' home health experience: Part I: the practice setting. *Nursing and Health Care, 14*(8), 402–407.

Stulginsky, M.N. (1993b). Nurses' home health experience: Part II: the unique demands of home visits. *Nursing and Health Care, 14*(9), 476–485.

Touhy, T., & Zerwekh, J. (2006). Spiritual caring. In J. Zerwekh (Ed.). *Nursing care at the end of life.* Philadelphia: F.A. Davis.

U.S. Department of Health and Human Services. (2000). *Healthy People 2010: Understanding and improving health,* 2nd ed. Washington, DC: U.S. Government Printing Office.

U.S. Department of Health and Human Services. (2006). *Healthy People 2010: Midcourse review.* Washington, DC: U.S. Government Printing Office.

Vachon, M. (2001). The nurse's role: The world of palliative care nursing. In B.R. Ferrell, & N. Coyle (Eds.). *Textbook of palliative nursing.* New York: Oxford University Press.

World Health Organization. (2007). *WHO's pain relief ladder.* Retrieved August 12, 2008 from http://www.who.int/cancer/palliative/painladder/en/index.html.

Zerwekh, J. (1991). Tales from public health nursing true detectives. *American Journal of Nursing, 91*(10), 30–36.

Zerwekh, J. (1995). High-tech home care for nurses. *Home Healthcare Nurse, 13*(1), 9–14.

Zerwekh, J. (2000). Caring on the ragged edge: Nursing persons who are disenfranchised. *Advances in Nursing Science, 22,* 47–61.

Zerwekh, J. (2006). *Nursing care at the end of life.* Philadelphia: F.A. Davis.

Selected Readings

Abbey, J., Froggatt, K. A., Parker, D., & Abbey, B. (2007). Palliative care in long-term care: A system in change. *International Journal of Older People Nursing, 1*(1), 56–63.

Arber, A. (2007). "Pain talk" in hospice and palliative care team meetings: An ethnography. *International Journal of Nursing Studies, 44,* 916–926.

Carlson, M. D., Morrison, R. S., Holford, T. R., & Bradley, E. H. (2007). Hospice care: What services do patients and their families receive? *Health Services Research, 42,* 1672–1690.

Crist, J. D., Michaels, C., Gelfand, D. E., & Phillips, L. R. (2007). Defining and measuring service awareness among elders and caregivers of Mexican descent. *Research & Theory for Nursing Practice, 21*(2), 119–134.

Gazelle, G. (2007). Understanding hospice — An underutilized option for life's final chapter. *New England Journal of Medicine, 357,* 321–324.

Gray, J. (2007). Protecting hospice patients: A new look at falls prevention. *American Journal of Hospice & Palliative Medicine, 24,* 242–247.

Hartman, L., Jarosek, S. L., Virnig, B. A., & Durham, S. (2007). Medicare-certified home health care: Urban-rural differences in utilization. *Journal of Rural Health, 23,* 254–257.

Hawranik, P. G., & Strain, L. A. (2007). Giving voice to informal caregivers of older adults. *Canadian Journal of Nursing Research, 39*(1), 156–172.

Kraft, L., & Scott, P. (2007). Computerized client assessments: A change in practice. *Canadian Nurse, 103*(5), 28–31.

Kubler-Ross, E., & Kessler, D. (2005). *On grief and grieving: Finding the meaning of grief through the five stages of loss.* New York: Scribner.

Polzien, G. (2007). Where we have been and where we are going: Implications for home health. *Home Healthcare Nurse, 25,* 408–411.

Roberts, D., Tayler, C., MacCormack, D., & Barwich, D. (2007). Telenursing in hospice palliative care. *Canadian Nurse, 103*(5), 24–27.

Shaw, S., Meek, F., & Bucknall, R. (2007). A framework for providing evidence-based palliative care. *Nursing Standard, 21*(40), 35–38.

Siegler, E.L., Murtaugh, C.M., Rosati, R.J., Schwartz, T., Razzano, R., Sobolewski, S., et al. (2007). Improving communication at the transition to home health care: Use of an electronic referral system. *Home Health Care Management & Practice, 19*(4), 267–271.

Siskowski, C., Diaz, M., Connors, L., & Mize, N. (2007). Hospice & palliative care. Recognition and assessment of caregiving youth in hospice and home health care. *Home Healthcare Nurse, 25,* 433–438.

Spitz, B., Fraker, C., Meyer, C.P., & Peterson, T. (2007). Evolution of evidence-based guidelines for home care: Wisconsin's experience. *Home Healthcare Nurse, 25,* 327–334.

Internet Resources

Center to Advance Palliative Care: *http://www.capc.org*

Centers for Medicare and Medicaid Services: *http://www.cms.hhs.gov/oasis*

Family Caregiver Alliance: *http://www.caregiver.org*

Home Health care Nurses Association: *http://www.hhna.org*

Hospice and Palliative Nurses Association: *http://www.hpna.org*

Medicare: telephone 1-800-633-4227, *http://www.medicare.gov*

National Association for Home Care and Hospice: *http://www.nahc.org*

National Hospice and Palliative Care Organization: *http://www.nhpco.org*

Index

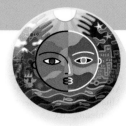